Anesthesiologist's Manual of Surgical Procedures

Third Edition

Anesthesiologist's Manual of Surgical Procedures

THIRD EDITION

Editors

Richard A. Jaffe, M.D., Ph.D.
Professor of Anesthesia and Neurosurgery

and

Stanley I. Samuels, M.B., B.Ch., F.F.A.R.C.S.
Professor of Anesthesia, Emeritus

With 159 Contributors

Stanford University School of Medicine
Stanford, California

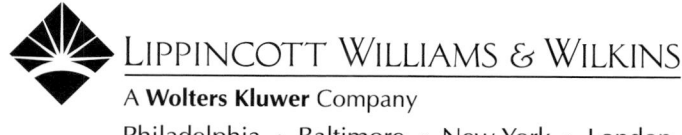

LIPPINCOTT WILLIAMS & WILKINS
A **Wolters Kluwer** Company
Philadelphia · Baltimore · New York · London
Buenos Aires · Hong Kong · Sydney · Tokyo

Acquisitions Editor: R. Craig Percy
Developmental Editor: Dee Mosteller
Developmental Assistants: Timothy Reiley, Eileen Wolfberg
Production Editor: Robert Pancotti
Manufacturing Manager: Benjamin Rivera
Cover Designer: Christine Jenny
Indexer: Dee Mosteller
Compositor: QualiType, Inc.
Printer: Quebecor World Taunton

Illustrations new to this edition were rendered by Jennifer Smith.

Library of Congress Cataloging-in-Publication Data
Anesthesiologist's manual of surgical procedures / editors, Richard A. Jaffe, Stanley I. Samuels.
—3rd ed.
        p. ; cm.
    Includes bibliographical references and index.
    ISBN-13: 978-0-7817-4332-7
    ISBN-10: 0-7817-4332-X
    1. Anesthesiology—Handbooks, manuals, etc. 2. Surgery, Operative—Handbooks, manuals, etc. 3. Operations, Surgical—Handbooks, manuals, etc. I. Jaffe, Richard A.
        II. Samuels, Stanley I.
    [DNLM: 1. Anesthesia—methods. 2. Surgical Procedures, Operative. WO 235 A5795 2004]
RD82.2.A54 2004
617.9'6—dc22
                                                                    2003059514

Care has been taken to confirm the accuracy of the information presented and to describe generally accepted practices. However, the authors, editors, and publisher are not responsible for errors or omissions or for any consequences from application of the information in this book and make no warranty, expressed or implied, with respect to the currency, completeness, or accuracy of the contents of the publication. Application of this information in a particular situation remains the professional responsibility of the practitioner.

The authors, editors, and publisher have exerted every effort to ensure that drug selection and dosage set forth in this text are in accordance with current recommendations and practice at the time of publication. However, in view of ongoing research, changes in government regulations, and the constant flow of information relating to drug therapy and drug reactions, the reader is urged to check the package insert for each drug for any change in indications and dosage and for added warnings and precautions. This is particularly important when the recommended agent is a new or infrequently employed drug.

Some drugs and medical devices presented in this publication have Food and Drug Administration (FDA) clearance for limited use in restricted research settings. It is the responsibility of the health care provider to ascertain the FDA status of each drug or device planned for use in their clinical practice.

10 9 8 7 6

This book is respectfully dedicated to
our friend, mentor, teacher, and colleague,

C. Philip Larson, Jr, MD, MS

TABLE OF CONTENTS

Contributors xxi

Foreword xxxi

Acknowledgments xxxii

Preface xxxiii

1.0   Neurosurgery 1

  1.1   Intracranial Neurosurgery 3

  *Surgeons: Gary K. Steinberg, Robert L. Dodd, Gordon T. Sakamoto, Lawrence M. Shuer,
  Steven D. Chang, John R. Adler* **Anesthesiologists:** *Richard A. Jaffe, Stanley I. Samuels,
  C. Philip Larson, Jr.*

    Craniotomy for intracranial aneurysms   **4**
    Craniotomy for cerebral embolectomy   **13**
    Craniotomy for intracranial vascular malformations   **15**
    Craniotomy for extracranial-intracranial revascularization (EC-IC bypass)   **21**
    Craniotomy for tumor   **26**
    Craniotomy for skull tumor   **31**
    Craniotomy for trauma   **32**
    Microvascular decompression of cranial nerve   **37**
    Bifrontal craniotomy for CSF leak   **40**
    Transoral approach to the cervicomedullary junction and odontoid   **42**
    Transsphenoidal resection of pituitary tumor   **44**
    Ventricular shunt procedures   **47**
    Craniocervical decompression (Chiari malformation)   **51**
    Stereotactic neurosurgery   **52**

  1.2   Functional Neurosurgery 57

  Surgeons: Gary Heit, Lawrence M. Shuer **Anesthesiologists:** *Richard A. Jaffe, Stanley I. Samuels*

    Functional neurosurgery: the surgical treatment of pain, movement disorders,
       and epilepsy—Introduction   **58**
    Stereotactic procedures: deep brain stimulation, pallidotomy, thalamotomy   **59**
    Surgical analgesia: spinal cord stimulation, intrathecal pumps, and cortical stimulation   **61**
    Vagal nerve stimulation   **64**
    Epilepsy surgery   **66**
    Surgery for spasticity   **69**

  1.3   Spinal Neurosurgery 71

  Surgeons: Raju S. V. Balabhadra, Daniel H. Kim, Lawrence M. Shuer
  Anesthesiologist: *C. Philip Larson, Jr.*

    Anterior fusion/fixation of the upper cervical (C1-C2) spine   **73**
    Posterior fusion/fixation of the upper cervical spine   **75**
    Anterior fusion/fixation of the mid and lower cervical spine   **77**
    Posterior fusion/fixation of the mid and lower cervical spine   **80**
    Anterior cervicothoracic spine surgery   **82**

Anterior thoracic spine surgery **87**
Posterior thoracic spine surgery **89**
Anterior lumbar/lumbosacral spine surgery **91**
Posterior lumbar spine surgery **93**
Posterior lumbar fusion and instrumentation **94**
Combined anterior and posterior instrumentation of the thoracic and lumbar spine **96**

1.4   Extracranial Neurosurgery 101

Surgeons: Gary K. Steinberg, Robert L. Dodd, Lawrence M. Shuer
Anesthesiologists: Richard A. Jaffe, Stanley I. Samuels, C. Philip Larson, Jr.

Carotid endarterectomy **102**
Percutaneous procedures for trigeminal neuralgia **108**

2.0   Ophthalmic Surgery 113

Surgeons: Christopher J. Engelman, Peter R. Egbert, Weldon W. Haw, Michael W. Gaynon
Anesthesiologists: Stanley I. Samuels, Richard A. Jaffe

Cataract extraction with intraocular lens insertion **114**
Corneal transplant **115**
Trabeculectomy **116**
Ectropion repair **118**
Entropion repair **119**
Ptosis repair **120**
Eyelid reconstruction **122**
Pterygium excision **123**
Anesthetic considerations for ophthalmic surgical procedures under MAC **124**
Repair of ruptured or lacerated globe **126**
Dacryocystorhinostomy (DCR) **129**
Enucleation **131**
Orbitotomy—anterior and lateral **132**
Retinal surgery **134**

3.0   Otolaryngology—Head and Neck Surgery 139

Surgeons: Willard E. Fee, Jr., Winston C. Vaughan, Joseph B. Roberson, Jerome Hester,
Robert J. Troell, Robert W. Riley, Nelson B. Powell, Kasey K. Li
Anesthesiologists: Vladimir Nekhendzy, Edward R. Baer, Michael W. Champeau

Introduction—Surgeon's perspective **140**
Introduction—Anesthesiologist's perspective **141**
Tonsillectomy and/or adenoidectomy **143**
Laryngoscopy/bronchoscopy/esophagoscopy **146**
Nasal surgery **153**
External sinus surgery **155**
Endoscopic sinus surgery **157**
Ear surgery **160**
Parotidectomy: superficial, total, radical **163**
Submandibular gland excision **166**
Neck dissection: functional, modified radical, radical **168**
Laryngectomy: total, supraglottic, hemi **173**
Glossectomy **177**
Maxillectomy **178**
Tracheostomy **182**
Intubation for epiglottitis **186**
Skull base surgery **187**
Reconstructive surgery for sleep-disordered breathing **193**

4.0   **Dental Surgery**   **199**

Surgeons: Sabine C. Girod, Stephen A. Schendel   *Anesthesiologists: Richard A. Jaffe,*
Stanley I. Samuels

Temporomandibular joint arthroscopy/arthrotomy   **200**
Oral surgery   **201**
Restorative dentistry   **202**

5.0   **Thoracic Surgery**   **205**

Surgeons: Richard I. Whyte, Walter B. Cannon, Jessica S. Donington
Anesthesiologists: John L. Chow, Jay B. Brodsky

Introduction—surgeon's perspective   **206**
Lobectomy, pneumonectomy   **208**
Wedge resection of lung lesion   **215**
Chest-wall resection   **218**
Repair of pectus excavatum or carinatum   **219**
Thoracoplasty   **222**
Drainage of empyema   **223**
Tracheal resection   **226**
Excision of mediastinal tumor   **229**
Mediastinoscopy   **231**
Bronchoscopy—flexible and rigid   **235**
Anesthetic considerations for laser resection   **238**
Video-assisted thoracoscopy surgery (VATS)   **240**
Thymectomy   **243**
Excision of blebs or bullae   **246**
Lung-volume reduction surgery   **249**
Bronchopulmonary lavage   **252**
Lung transplant   **255**

6.0   **Cardiovascular Surgery**   **257**

6.1   **Cardiac Surgery**   **259**

Surgeons: R. Scott Mitchell, Norman E. Shumway   *Anesthesiologists: J. Kent Garman,*
Lawrence C. Siegel

Cardiopulmonary bypass   **260**
Coronary artery bypass graft surgery   **266**
Left ventricular aneurysmectomy   **271**
Aortic valve replacement   **272**
Mitral valve repair or replacement   **275**
Tricuspid valve repair   **279**
Septal myectomy/myotomy   **282**
Pacemaker insertion   **284**
Pericardiectomy   **287**

6.2   **Minimally Invasive Cardiac Surgery**   **291**

Surgeon: James I. Fann   *Anesthesiologist: Lawrence C. Siegel*

Port-access coronary revascularization   **293**
Off-pump and minimally invasive coronary artery bypass grafting   **295**
Limited thoracotomy and port-access approach to mitral valve surgery   **300**

6.3   **Vascular Surgery**   **307**

Surgeons: James I. Fann, R. Scott Mitchell, Stephen T. Kee, Michael D. Dake
Anesthesiologist: Pieter Van der Starre

Carotid endarterectomy (vascular)   **308**
Repair of thoracic aortic aneurysms   **310**
Endovascular stent-grafting of aortic aneurysms   **313**
Repair of acute aortic dissections and dissecting aneurysms   **317**
Repair of aneurysms of the thoracoabdominal aorta   **322**
Surgery of the abdominal aorta   **327**
Infrainguinal arterial bypass   **331**
Arterial embolectomy   **335**
Lumbar sympathectomy   **336**
Upper extremity sympathectomy   **339**
Venous surgery—thrombectomy or vein excision   **341**
Surgery for portal hypertension—shunt and nonshunt procedures   **343**
Arteriovenous access for hemodialysis   **349**
Permanent vascular access   **351**
Venous surgery—vein stripping and perforator ligation   **354**
Varicose vein stripping   **355**

6.4   **Heart/Lung Transplantation**   **359**

Surgeons: James I. Fann, Bruce A. Reitz   *Anesthesiologists: J. Kent Garman, Lawrence C. Siegel*

Surgery for heart transplantation   **360**
Surgery for lung and heart/lung transplantation   **365**

7.0   **General Surgery**   **375**

7.1   **Esophageal Surgery**   **377**

Surgeon: Richard I. Whyte   *Anesthesiologist: John L. Chow*

Esophagostomy   **378**
Esophageal diverticulectomy   **379**
Management of esophageal perforation   **381**
Esophagomyotomy   **382**
Esophagogastric fundoplasty   **384**
Esophagectomy   **385**

7.2   **Stomach Surgery**   **391**

Surgeons: H. Ward Trueblood, Myriam J. Curet   *Anesthesiologists: Kevin A. Malott, Jay B. Brodsky*

Gastric resections   **392**
Oversew gastric or duodenal perforation   **394**
Operations for peptic ulcer disease   **396**
Open operations for morbid obesity   **399**
Gastrostomy placement   **403**

7.3   **Intestinal Surgery**   **405**

Surgeon: Harry A. Oberhelman   *Anesthesiologist: Kevin A. Malott*

Duodenotomy   **406**
Open appendectomy   **407**
Excision of Meckel's diverticulum   **408**
Enterostomy   **410**

Continent ileostomy pouch (Kock) **412**
Small-bowel resection with anastomosis **413**
Enterolysis **415**
Closure of enteric fistulae **416**

7.4 **Colorectal Surgery** **419**

Surgeons: Andrew A. Shelton, Mark Lane Welton   *Anesthesiologist: Afshin Abdollahi*

Laparoscopic colorectal surgery **420**
Total proctocolectomy **420**
Segmental (partial) colectomy **423**
Stoma closure or peristomal hernia repair **426**
Operations for rectal prolapse **429**
Rectal surgery **431**
Anal fistulotomy/fistulectomy **433**
Hemorrhoidectomy **434**
Operations for fecal incontinence **435**

7.5 **Hepatic Surgery** **439**

Surgeons: Samuel K. S. So, Harry A. Oberhelman   *Anesthesiologist: Hendrikus J. M. Lemmens*

Hepatic resection **440**
Hepatorrhaphy **441**

7.6 **Biliary Tract Surgery** **445**

Surgeon: Mark A. Vierra   *Anesthesiologist: Hendrikus J. M. Lemmens*

Open cholecystectomy **446**
Biliary drainage procedures **448**
Excision of bile duct tumor **450**
Choledochal cyst excision or anastomosis **451**

7.7 **Laparoscopic General Surgery** **455**

Surgeon: Myriam J. Curet   *Anesthesiologists: Sunita G. Sastry, Brendan Carvalho, Sheila E. Cohen*

Laparoscopic esophageal fundoplication **456**
Laparoscopic Heller's myotomy—antireflux procedure **458**
Laparoscopic cholecystectomy—common duct exploration **459**
Laparoscopic splenectomy **463**
Laparoscopic adrenalectomy **466**
Laparoscopic bowel resection **469**
Laparoscopic appendectomy **472**
Laparoscopic inguinal hernia repair **475**
Laparoscopic bariatric surgery **477**
Anesthesia for laparoscopy in pregnancy **480**

7.8 **Pancreatic Surgery** **483**

Surgeon: J. Augusto Bastidas   *Anesthesiologist: Martin Angst*

Operative drainage for pancreatitis **484**
Drainage of pancreatic pseudocyst **485**
Pancreaticojejunostomy **486**
Pancreatectomy **488**
Whipple resection **490**

7.9   Peritoneal Surgery   495

Surgeon: Harry A. Oberhelman   Anesthesiologist: Martin Angst

Exploratory or staging laparotomy   **496**
Splenectomy   **499**
Excision of intraabdominal, retroperitoneal tumors   **501**
Drainage of subphrenic abscess   **502**
Inguinal herniorrhaphy   **504**
Femoral herniorrhaphy   **505**
Repair of incisional hernia **506**
Repair of abdominal dehiscence   **507**

7.10   Breast Surgery   511

Surgeons: Irene L. Wapnir, Stefanie S. Jeffrey   Anesthesiologist: Lindsey Vokach-Brodsky

Breast biopsy   **512**
Sentinel lymph node biopsy   **513**
Breast-conserving surgery and mastectomy ± reconstruction   **516**

7.11   Endocrine Surgery   519

Surgeons: Mark Koransky, Ralph Greco   Anesthesiologist: Frederick G. Mihm

Excision of thyroglossal duct cyst   **520**
Thyroidectomy   **521**
Parathyroidectomy   **526**
Adrenalectomy   **530**

7.12   Liver/Kidney Transplantation   537

Surgeons: Stéphen Busque, Maria T. Millan, Dev M. Desai, Carlos O. Esquivel
Anesthesiologists: Timothy Angelotti, Hendrikus J. M. Lemmens

Kidney transplantation—cadaveric and live-donor   **538**
Cadaveric kidney/pancreas transplantation   **539**
Live-donor nephrectomy—laparoscopic and open   **543**
Kidney transplant nephrectomy   **545**
Liver transplantation   **547**
Living-donor liver transplantation   **559**
Multiorgan procurement   **560**

7.13   Trauma Surgery   567

Surgeons: David A. Spain, J. Augusto Bastidas   Anesthesiologist: Linda E. Foppiano

Initial assessment and airway management for trauma surgery   **568**
Emergency tube thoracostomy   **569**
Emergency department thoracotomy   **571**
Exploratory surgery for neck trauma   **572**
Chest trauma: pericardial window, release of tamponade, repair of cardiac laceration   **576**
Chest trauma: repair of great vessels   **577**
Chest trauma: pneumonectomy, lobectomy, repair of tracheobronchial injury   **579**
Abdominal trauma: damage control   **582**
Abdominal trauma: hepatic and splenic injuries   **583**
Abdominal trauma: vascular injuries   **585**
Pediatric trauma: airway and vascular access   **589**

8.0   **Obstetric/Gynecologic Surgery   591**

    8.1   **Gynecologic Oncology   593**

        Surgeons: O. W. Stephanie Yap, Amreen Husain, Daniel S. Kapp, Nelson N. Teng
        Anesthesiologists: Ian Carroll, Meyer H. Rosenthal

        Staging laparotomy for ovarian, fallopian tube, and primary peritoneal cancer   **594**
        Second-look/reassessment laparotomy for ovarian cancer   **597**
        Radical vulvectomy   **601**
        Conization of the cervix   **605**
        Anesthetic considerations for laser therapy to vulva, vagina, cervix   **608**
        Suction curettage for gestational trophoblastic disease   **610**
        Pelvic exenteration   **613**
        Exploratory laparotomy, hysterectomy/BSO for uterine cancer   **618**
        Radical hysterectomy   **621**
        Interstitial perineal implants   **624**
        Laparoscopic surgery in gynecologic oncology   **627**

    8.2   **Gynecology/Infertility Surgery   631**

        Surgeons: Bertha Chen, Eva D. Littman, Amin A. Milki, Lynn M. Westphal
        Anesthesiologist: Karen A. Giarrusso

        Dilatation and curettage (D&C)   **632**
        Therapeutic abortion, dilatation and evacuation (D&E)   **633**
        Hysteroscopy   **636**
        Pelvic laparotomy   **639**
        Transvaginal oocyte retrieval (TVOR)   **641**
        Infertility operations/in vitro fertilization   **643**
        Hysterectomy—vaginal or total abdominal   **647**
        Anterior and posterior colporrhaphy, enterocele repair, vaginal sacrospinous suspension   **652**
        Operations for stress urinary incontinence   **654**

    8.3   **Obstetric Surgery   659**

        Surgeons: M. Mark Taslimi, Yasser El-Sayed   *Anesthesiologists: Brendan Carvalho, Sheila E. Cohen*

        Cesarean section—lower segment and classic   **660**
        Medical and surgical management of postpartum hemorrhage   **666**
        Repair of uterine rupture   **668**
        Postpartum tubal ligation   **669**
        Repair of vaginal/cervical lacerations   **672**
        Cervical cerclage—elective and emergent   **674**
        Removal of retained placenta   **677**
        Management of uterine inversion   **679**

    8.4   **Laparoscopic Procedures for Gynecologic Surgery   683**

        Surgeon: Camran R. Nezhat   *Anesthesiologist: Lindsey Vokach-Brodsky*

        Laparoscopic surgery for endometriosis   **684**
        Laparoscopic surgery for ectopic pregnancy   **687**
        Laparoscopic myomectomy   **688**
        Laparoscopic hysterectomy   **690**

9.0   **Urology**   **695**

Surgeons: Harcharan S. Gill, Fuad S. Freiha   *Anesthesiologists: Steven A. Deem, Ronald G. Pearl*

Diagnostic transurethral (endoscopic) procedures   **696**
Therapeutic transurethral procedures (except TURP)   **697**
Transurethral resection of the prostate (TURP)   **699**
Open prostate operations   **703**
Nephrectomy   **706**
Operations on the renal pelvis and upper ureter   **709**
Cystectomy   **712**
Open bladder operations (other than cystectomy)   **715**
Inguinal operations   **718**
Penile operations   **721**
Scrotal operations   **723**
Perineal operations   **726**
Vaginal operations   **728**

10.0   **Orthopedic Surgery**   **731**

    10.1   **Hand Surgery**   **733**

    Surgeons: Vincent R. Hentz, Gordon A. Brody   *Anesthesiologist: Eric Rey Amador*

    Darrach procedure   **734**
    Dorsal stabilization and extensor synovectomy of the rheumatoid wrist   **735**
    Metacarpophalangeal and interphalangeal joint arthroplasty   **736**
    Arthrodesis of the wrist   **737**
    Total wrist replacement   **738**
    Thumb carpometacarpal joint fusion/arthroplasty/stabilization   **739**
    Excision of ganglion of the wrist   **743**
    Palmar and digital fasciectomy   **744**
    Repair of flexor tendon laceration   **745**
    Tendolysis of flexor or extensor tendon (with capsulotomy of joints)   **748**
    Wrist arthroscopy   **749**
    Carpal tunnel release   **750**
    Repair of fractures and dislocations of the distal radius, carpus, and metacarpals   **753**
    Digit and hand replantation   **755**

    10.2   **Shoulder/Arm Surgery**   **759**

    Surgeons: Amy L. Ladd, Andrew C. Karich   *Anesthesiologist: Eric Rey Amador*

    Arthroscopic shoulder surgery   **760**
    Surgery for subacromial impingement, rotator cuff tears, and acromioclavicular joint arthritis   **762**
    Surgery for shoulder dislocations or instability   **765**
    Glenohumeral shoulder arthroplasty   **769**
    Shoulder girdle procedures   **773**
    Brachial plexus surgery   **775**
    Arm surgery   **778**

    10.3   **Spine Surgery**   **781**

    Surgeon: Eugene J. Carragee   *Anesthesiologists: C. Philip Larson, Jr., Stanley I. Samuels, Richard A. Jaffe*

    Minimally invasive posterior lumbar discectomy (microdiscectomy)   **782**
    Anterior spinal reconstruction and fusion—thoracic and thoracolumbar spine   **784**
    Anterior spinal reconstruction and fusion—lumbosacral spine   **787**

10.4   Hip, Pelvis, Upper Leg Surgery   795

Surgeons: Michael J. Bellino, Stuart B. Goodman   Anesthesiologist: Frederick G. Mihm

Open reduction and internal fixation (ORIF) of pelvis or acetabulum   **796**
Closed reduction and external fixation of the pelvis   **798**
Open reduction and internal fixation (ORIF) of acetabulum fractures   **799**
Osteotomy and bone graft augmentation of the pelvis   **802**
Arthrodesis of the sacroiliac joint   **804**
Amputations about the hip and pelvis: disarticulation of the hip and hindquarter amputation   **805**
Arthroplasty of the hip   **808**
Arthrodesis of the hip   **811**
Synovectomy of the hip   **812**
Open reduction and internal fixation (ORIF) of proximal femoral fractures   **815**
Open reduction and internal fixation (ORIF) of distal femoral fractures   **818**
Open reduction and internal fixation (ORIF) of the femoral shaft with plate   **819**
Intramedullary nailing of femoral shaft   **820**
Repair of nonunion/malunion of proximal third of femur, proximal femoral osteotomy
    for osteoarthritis   **822**
Closed reduction and external fixation of femur   **823**

10.5   Knee Surgery   825

Surgeons: John J. Csongradi, Stuart B. Goodman   Anesthesiologist: Frederick G. Mihm

Arthroplasty of the knee   **826**
Arthrodesis of the knee   **827**
Open reduction and internal fixation (ORIF) of patellar fractures   **829**
Repair or reconstruction of knee ligaments   **830**
Patellar realignment   **831**
Arthroscopy of the knee   **833**
Knee arthrotomy   **834**
Repair of tendons—knee and leg   **835**

10.6   Lower Leg, Ankle, Foot, and Other Lower-Extremity Procedures   839

Surgeon: John J. Csongradi   Anesthesiologist: Frederick G. Mihm

Open reduction and internal fixation (ORIF) of the tibial plateau fracture   **840**
Intramedullary nailing, tibia   **841**
External fixation, tibia   **842**
Open reduction and internal fixation (ORIF) of distal tibia, ankle, and foot fractures   **843**
Repair nonunion/malunion, tibia   **844**
Arthroscopy of the ankle   **845**
Ankle arthrotomy   **846**
Ankle arthrodesis   **847**
Repair/reconstruction of ankle ligaments   **848**
Amputation through ankle (Syme)   **849**
Amputation, transmetatarsal   **850**
Lengthening or transfer of tendons, ankle, and foot   **851**
Amputation above the knee   **852**
Amputation below the knee   **854**
Fasciotomy of the thigh   **857**
Fasciotomy of the leg   **858**
Biopsy, leg and foot   **861**
Biopsy or drainage of abscess/excision of tumor   **862**

11.0   Plastic and Reconstructive Surgery   865

    11.1   Facial Cosmetic Surgery   867

        Surgeons: *Lonny L. Ross, David M. Kahn*   ***Anesthesiologist:*** *Tara Cornaby*

        Introduction to cosmetic facial surgery   **868**
        Facelift and necklift   **869**
        Browlift and blepharoplasty   **872**
        Rhinoplasty   **878**
        Facial laser resurfacing   **881**

    11.2   Nonfacial Aesthetic Surgery   883

        Surgeons: *David M. Kahn, Jeffrey D. Pardun, George W. Commons*
        Anesthesiologists: *Lindsey Vokach-Brodsky, Bruce D. Halperin*

        Augmentation mammoplasty   **884**
        Reduction mammoplasty   **885**
        Mastopexy/breast lift   **887**
        Abdominoplasty   **889**
        Liposuction   **892**

    11.3   Craniofacial Surgery   895

        Surgeons: *Lonny L. Ross, Stephen A. Schendel*   ***Anesthesiologists:*** *Tara Cornaby,*
        Stanley I. Samuels, Richard A. Jaffe

        Repair of facial fractures   **897**
        LeFort osteotomies   **902**
        Mandibular osteotomies/genioplasty   **905**

    11.4   Functional Restoration   909

        Surgeons: *Yvonne L. Karanas, James Chang, David M. Kahn, Jeffrey D. Pardun,*
        William C. Lineaweaver, Kenneth C. W. Hui   ***Anesthesiologist:*** *Tara Cornaby*

        Microsurgery—free flap procedures   **910**
        Microsurgery—replantation   **913**
        Breast surgery—introduction   **914**
        Breast reconstruction   **915**
        Chest-wall reconstruction   **920**
        Pressure-sore reconstruction   **923**

    11.5   Burn Surgery   927

        Surgeon: *Kenneth K. Yim*   ***Anesthesiologist:*** *Melissa T. Berhow*

        Free skin graft for burn wound   **928**

12.0   Pediatric Surgery   933

    12.1   Pediatric Neurosurgery   935

        Surgeon: *Stephen L. Huhn*   ***Anesthesiologists:*** *William W. Feaster, C. Philip Larson, Jr.*

        Craniofacial surgery   **936**
        Closure of myelomeningocele   **938**
        Surgical correction of spinal dysraphism   **941**
        Craniotomy for vein of Galen malformation   **943**
        Ventriculoscopy and third ventriculostomy   **945**

12.2   Pediatric Ophthalmic Surgery   949

Surgeon: D. M. Alcorn   *Anesthesiologist:* Alice A. Edler

Strabismus surgery   950

12.3   Pediatric Otolaryngology   953

Surgeons: Anna H. Messner, Kay W. Chang   *Anesthesiologists:* Cathy R. Lammers, Gregory B. Hammer

Introduction—Surgeon's perspective   954
Myringotomy and tympanostomy tube placement   954
Tonsillectomy and adenoidectomy   956
Bronchoscopy/esophagoscopy   959
Laryngoscopy, supraglottoplasty, excision of laryngeal lesions   960
Removal of branchial cleft cyst or thyroglossal duct cyst   963
Incision/drainage of deep neck abscess   964
Cricoid split, laryngotracheoplasty   966
Choanal atresia repair   968
Pediatric tracheostomy   970

12.4   Pediatric Cardiovascular Surgery   971

Surgeons: V. Mohan Reddy, Frank L. Hanley   *Anesthesiologists:* M. Gail Boltz, Chandra Ramamoorthy

Surgery for atrial septal defect (ostium secundum)   972
Surgery for atrioventricular canal defect   975
Surgery for ventricular septal defect   979
Surgery for patent ductus arteriosus   981
Surgery for coarctation of the aorta   984
Surgery for tetralogy of Fallot   988
Surgery for total anomalous pulmonary venous connection   993
Surgery for complete transposition of the great arteries   996
Surgery for truncus arteriosus   1000
Surgery for tricuspid atresia   1003
Surgery for double-outlet right ventricle   1006
Surgery for hypoplastic left heart syndrome   1008

12.5   Pediatric General Surgery   1013

Surgeons: Baird M. Smith, Christine Matthes-Kofidis, MD   *Anesthesiologists:* Brenda Golianu, Gregory B. Hammer

Resection of cystic hygroma, branchial cleft cyst, thyroglossal duct cyst, or other cervical mass   1014
Esophagus—foreign body removal and dilation   1016
Repair of tracheoesophageal fistula and esophageal atresia   1018
Mediastinal mass—biopsy or resection   1021
Neonatal lung resection   1024
Drainage of empyema   1027
Repair of pectus excavatum/carinatum   1029
Esophageal replacement, colon interposition, Waterston procedure, gastric tube placement   1031
Repair of congenital diaphragmatic hernia   1034
Pyloromyotomy for pyloric stenosis   1038
Abdominal tumor: resection of neuroblastoma, Wilms' tumor, hepatoblastoma   1040
Laparotomy for intestinal perforation, necrotizing enterocolitis   1043
Repair of biliary atresia and choledocal cysts   1046
Repair of abdominal wall defects: omphalocele/gastroschisis   1049
Pullthrough for Hirschsprung's disease   1053

Pullthrough for imperforate anus, cloaca   **1056**
Repair of inguinal and umbilical hernias, hydrocele   **1058**
Surgery for the undescended testicle   **1061**
Resection of sacrococcygeal teratoma   **1062**
Anesthesia for minimally invasive surgery in pediatric patients   **1064**

12. 6   Pediatric Urology   1067

Surgeons: Jeffrey B. Marotte, Linda M. Dairiki Shortliffe   Anesthesiologists: Cathy R. Lammers, Gregory B. Hammer

Kidney and upper urinary tract operations   **1068**
Transurethral procedures   **1071**
Open bladder operations   **1073**
Penile surgery   **1075**
Genital procedures (clitoroplasty, vaginoplasty, urethroplasty)   **1076**
Inguinoscrotal procedures   **1079**
Laparoscopic procedures   **1081**

12.7   Pediatric Orthopedic Surgery   1083

Surgeons: Lawrence A. Rinsky, Todd Lincoln, James Chang, Amy L. Ladd
Anesthesiologists: Komal Kamra, Alice A. Edler

Percutaneous pinning of displaced supracondylar humerus fracture   **1084**
Closed or open reduction of displaced lateral condyle humerus fracture   **1085**
Aspiration and injection of unicameral bone cyst   **1086**
Release for torticollis   **1088**
Pollicization of a finger   **1089**
Syndactyly repair   **1090**
Posterior spinal instrumentation and fusion   **1093**
Anterior spinal fusion for scoliosis ± instrumentation   **1095**
Pelvic osteotomy   **1097**
Acetabular augmentation (shelf) & Chiari osteotomy   **1099**
Ober fasciotomy, Yount-Ober release   **1101**
Hip, open reduction ± femoral shortening   **1102**
Adductor release or transfer, psoas release   **1103**
Pinning of slipped capital femoral epiphysis (SCFE)   **1105**
Flexible intramedullary nailing of long-bone fractures   **1106**
Proximal femoral osteotomy   **1108**
Epiphysiodesis   **1110**
Sofield procedure   **1111**
Limb lengthening   **1113**
Patellar realignment   **1115**
Tendon transfer, lengthening (posterior tibial)   **1117**
Triple arthrodesis and Grice procedure (extraarticular subtalar arthrodesis)   **1118**
Surgical correction of clubfoot   **1119**
Surgery for epidermolysis bullosa   **1125**

12.8   Surgery for Craniofacial Malformations   1129

Surgeons: Lonny L. Ross, Stephen A. Schendel, Laurence M. Shuer
Anesthesiologists: Louise Fukurawa, Gregory B. Hammer

Surgical correction of craniosynostosis   **1130**
Major secondary craniofacial surgical procedures   **1134**
Cleft lip repair—unilateral/bilateral   **1137**

Palatoplasty   **1140**
Pharyngoplasty   **1142**
Alveolar cleft repair with bone graft   **1144**
Secondary cleft lip/nasal surgery   **1145**
Otoplasty   **1149**

13.0   Out-of-Operating Room Procedures   1151

13.1   Adult Procedures   1153

Surgeons: Charles DeBattista, Joan K. Frisoli, Stephen T. Kee, L. Bing Liem, Michael P. Marks, Erik J. Sirulnick, Daniel Y. Sze   Anesthesiologists: Jay B. Brodsky, John L. Chow, J. Kent Garman, Leland H. Hanowell, Richard A. Jaffe, Stanley I. Samuels, Richard C. Shinaman

Anesthesia for out-of-operating room procedures   **1154**
Electroconvulsive therapy (ECT)   **1154**
Interventional neuroradiology   **1158**
Direct current (DC) cardioversion   **1162**
Implantation of cardioverter-defibrillator (ICD)   **1165**
Transjugular intrahepatic portosystemic shunt (TIPS)   **1169**
Imaging and image-guided procedures   **1173**
Tracheobronchial stenting   **1178**
Radiofrequency ablation   **1182**

13.2   Pediatric Procedures   1187

Authors: Sarah S. Donaldson, Anne M. Dubin, Jeffrey A. Feinstein, Gary E. Hartman, Stanton B. Perry, Michael V. Sattah, Kalyani R. Trivedi   Anesthesiologists: M. Gail Boltz, Gregory B. Hammer, Cathy R. Lammers, Chandra Ramamoorthy, Glyn D. Williams

Pediatric radiation therapy   **1188**
Pediatric cardiac catheterization and electrophysiology   **1192**
Pediatric oncologic procedures   **1198**
Upper/lower GI endoscopy   **1199**
Cross-sectional imaging (CT, MRI)   **1201**
Extracorporeal membrane oxygenation (ECMO)   **1203**

14.0   Office-Based Anesthesia   1205

Surgeons: David A. Berman, Vernon J. Adams, Jr., Azeem K. Lakha
Anesthesiologist: Terri D. Homer

Introduction—Anesthesiologist's Perspective   **1206**
Laser skin resurfacing   **1207**
Office dental rehabilitation under deep iv sedation   **1209**
Dental implants and bone grafting   **1211**

15.0   Emergency Procedures for the Anesthesiologist   1213

Anesthesiologists: Frederick G. Mihm, Myer H. Rosenthal

Emergency cricothyrotomy   **1214**
Periocardiocentesis   **1216**
Arterial cutdown   **1217**
Emergency needle/catheter thoracostomy   **1218**

Appendices

Authors: *Sandra Leigh Bardas, Stephen P. Fischer, Raymond R. Gaeta, Brenda Golianu, Julie Good, Alvin Hackel, Gregory B. Hammer, Richard A. Jaffe, Cathy R. Lammers, C. Philip Larson, Jr., Sean Mackey, Stanley I. Samuels, Clifford A. Schmiesing*

A. **Preoperative considerations   A1**
B. **Standard adult anesthetic protocols   B1**
C. **Standard perioperative pain management   C1**
D. **Standard pediatric anesthetic protocols   D1**
E. **Standard pediatric postoperative pain management   E1**
F. **Table of drug interactions   F1**
G. **Special considerations for latex allergy   G1**
H. **Acronyms and abbreviations   H1**

Subject Index   I-1

CONTRIBUTORS

Afshin Abdollahi, MD
Clinical Instructor of Anesthesia
Stanford University Medical Center
(*Colorectal Surgery*)

Vernon J. Adams, Jr., DMD
Assistant Clinical Professor of Pediatrics, Plastic and
Dental Surgery
Stanford University School of Medicine
Acting Chief, Pediatric Dental Services
Lucile Salter Packard Children's Hospital at Stanford
(*Office-Based Dental Procedures*)

John R. Adler, MD
Professor of Neurosurgery
Stanford University School of Medicine
(*Stereotactic Neurosurgery*)

D. M. Alcorn, MD
Associate Professor of Ophthalmology and Pediatrics
Director, Pediatric Ophthalmology and Strabismus
Services
Stanford University School of Medicine
(*Pediatric Ophthalmic Su*rgery)

Eric Rey Amador, MD
Clinical Instructor of Anesthesia
Stanford University Medical Center
(*Hand, Shoulder/Arm Surgery*)

Timothy Angelotti, MD, PhD
Assistant Professor of Anesthesia
Stanford University School of Medicine
(*Kidney, Pancreas Transplantation; Multiorgan
Procurement*)

Martin S. Angst, MD
Assistant Professor of Anesthesia
Stanford University School of Medicine
(*Pancreatic, Peritoneal Surgery*)

Edward R. Baer, MD
Adjunct Clinical Assistant Professor of Anesthesia
Associated Anesthesiologists
Stanford University Medical Center
(*Otolaryngology–Skull Base Surgery*)

Raju S. V. Balabhadra, MD
Clinical Fellow
Department of Neurosurgery
Stanford University Medical Center
(*Spinal Neurosurgery*)

Sandra Leigh Bardas, RPh, BS
Clinical Pharmacist
Stanford University Medical Center
(*Drug Interactions*)

J. Augusto Bastidas, MD
Assistant Professor of Surgery
Stanford University Medical Center
(*Pancreatic, Trauma Surgery*)

Michael J. Bellino, MD
Staff Physician
Department of Orthopedic Surgery
Stanford University Medical Center
(*Orthopedic Surgery–Hip, Pelvis, Upper Leg*)

Melissa T. Berhow, MD, PhD
Department of Anesthesia
Santa Clara Valley Medical Center
San Jose, CA
(*Burn Surgery*)

David A. Berman, MD
Medical Director, Berman Skin Institute
Palo Alto, CA
Medical Staff, Stanford University Hospital
(*Office-Based Dermatologic/Laser Surgery*)

M. Gail Boltz, MD
Assistant Professor of Anesthesia
Division of Pediatric Anesthesia
Stanford University Medical Center
Lucile Salter Packard Children's Hospital at Stanford
(*Pediatric Cardiovascular Surgery*; *Pediatric Cardiac
Catheterization*)

Jay B. Brodsky, MD
Professor of Anesthesia
Stanford University School of Medicine
(*Thoracic, Stomach, Laparoscopic Surgery; Adult Out-
of-OR Procedures*)

Gordon A. Brody, MD
Sports, Orthopedics, and Rehabilitation
Medicine Associates
Menlo Park, CA
(*Hand Surgery*)

Stéphan Busque, MD, MSc, FRCSC
Director
Adult Kidney and Pancreas Program
Stanford University School of Medicine
(*Kidney, Pancreas Transplantation*)

Walter B. Cannon, MD
Clinical Professor of Cardiothoracic and Thoracic
Surgery
Stanford University School of Medicine
(*Thoracic Surgery*)

Eugene J. Carragee, MD
Professor of Orthopedic Surgery
Director, Orthopedic Spine Center
Stanford University Medical Center
(*Orthopedic Spine Surgery*)

Ian Carroll, MD
Fellow, Pain Management
Department of Anesthesia
Stanford University Medical Center
(*Gynecologic Oncology*)

Brendan Carvalho, MBBCh, FRCA
Clinical Instructor of Anesthesia
Stanford University Medical Center
(*Laparoscopic, Gynecologic, Obstetric Surgery*)

Michael W. Champeau, MD
Clinical Associate Professor of Anesthesia
Associated Anesthesiologists
Stanford University School of Medicine
(*Surgery for Sleep Disorders*)

James Chang, MD
Associate Professor of Plastic and Reconstructive Surgery
Stanford University School of Medicine
Program Director for Plastic Surgery
Stanford University Medical Center
(*Functional Restoration; Pediatric Hand Surgery*)

Kay W. Chang, MD
Assistant Professor of Pediatric Otolaryngology
Stanford University School of Medicine
Staff Surgeon, Lucile Salter Packard Children's Hospital
(*Pediatric Otolaryngology*)

Steven D. Chang, MD
Assistant Professor of Neurosurgery
Stanford University School of Medicine
(*Intracranial, Stereotactic Neurosurgery*)

Bertha Chen, MD
Assistant Professor of Gynecology and Obstetrics
Stanford University School of Medicine
(*Gynecologic Surgery*)

John L. Chow, MD, MS
Assistant Professor of Anesthesia
Stanford University School of Medicine
(*Thoracic, Esophageal Surgery; Adult Out-of-OR Procedures*)

Sheila E. Cohen, MB, ChB, FRCA
Professor of Anesthesia
Director, Obstetrical Anesthesia
Stanford University School of Medicine
(*Laparoscopic, Gynecologic, Obstetric Surgery*)

George W. Commons, MD
Clinical Assistant Professor of Functional Restoration
Stanford University School of Medicine
(*Liposuction*)

Tara Cornaby, MD
Clinical Instructor of Anesthesia
Stanford University Medical Center
(*Cosmetic Facial Surgery; Craniofacial Surgery; Functional Restoration*)

John J. Csongradi, MD
Director, Department of Pediatric Orthopedic Surgery
Santa Clara Valley Medical Center
San Jose, CA
Clinical Associate Professor of Orthopedic Surgery
Stanford University School of Medicine
(*Orthopedic Surgery–Knee, Lower Leg, Ankle, Foot*)

Myriam J. Curet, MD, FACS
Associate Professor of Surgery
Stanford University Medical Center
(*Bariatric Surgery; Laparoscopic General Surgery*)

Michael D. Dake, MD
Associate Professor of Radiology
Division of Cardiovascular and Interventional Radiology
Stanford University School of Medicine
(*Endovascular Stent-Grafting*)

Charles DeBattista, MD
Associate Professor of Psychiatry
Stanford University School of Medicine
(*Electroconvulsive Therapy*)

Steven A. Deem, MD
Associate Professor of Anesthesia
University of Washington
Seattle, WA
(*Urology*)

Dev M. Desai, MD
Clinical Instructor of Surgery
Division of Multiorgan Transplant
Stanford University Medical Center
(*Liver Transplantation; Multiorgan Procurement*)

Robert L. Dodd, MD, PhD
Resident in Neurosurgery
Stanford University School of Medicine
(*Intracranial, Extracranial Neurosurgery*)

Sarah S. Donaldson, MD, FACR
Professor of Radiation Oncology
Stanford University School of Medicine
Chief of Pediatric Radiation Oncology
Lucile Salter Packard Children's Hospital at Stanford
(*Pediatric Radiation Therapy*)

Jessica S. Donington, MD
Assistant Professor of Thoracic Surgery
Stanford University School of Medicine
(*Thoracic Surgery*)

Anne M. Dubin, MD
Associate Professor, Department of Pediatrics
Stanford University School of Medicine
Pediatric Services, Lucile Salter Packard Children's
Hospital at Stanford
(*Pediatric Cardiac Catheterization*)

Alice A. Edler, MD
Assistant Professor of Anesthesia
Stanford University School of Medicine
(*Pediatric Ophthalmic, Orthopedic Surgery*)

Peter R. Egbert, MD
Professor of Ophthalmology
Stanford University School of Medicine
(*Ophthalmic Surgery*)

Yasser El-Sayed, MD
Clinical Assistant Professor of Maternal-Fetal Medicine
Department of Gynecology and Obstetrics
Stanford University School of Medicine
(*Obstetric Surgery*)

Christopher J. Engelman, MD
Glaucoma Fellow
Devers Eye Institute
Ophthalmology Clinical Fellow,
Good Samaritan Hospital, Portland, OR
(*Ophthalmic Surgery*)

Carlos O. Esquivel, MD, PhD
The Arnold and Barbara Silverman Professor of
Pediatric Transplantation
Professor of Surgery and Chief
Division of Transplantation
Stanford University Medical Center
(*Liver Transplantation; Multiorgan Procurement*)

James I. Fann, MD
Assistant Professor of Cardiothoracic Surgery
Stanford University Medical Center
Surgeon, Department of Cardiovascular Surgery
Veterans Administration–Palo Alto Health Care System
Palo Alto, CA
(*Minimally Invasive Cardiac Surgery; Vascular Surgery;
Heart/Lung Transplantation*)

William W. Feaster, MD
Clinical Professor of Anesthesia
Stanford University School of Medicine
(*Pediatric Neurosurgery*)

Willard E. Fee, Jr, MD
Sewell Professor of Otolaryngology
Department of Surgery
Stanford University School of Medicine
(*Otolaryngology*)

Jeffrey A. Feinstein, MD, MPH
Assistant Professor of Pediatrics
Associate Director
Pediatric and Congenital Cardiac Catheterization
Lucile Salter Packard Children's Hospital at Stanford
Stanford University Medical Center
(*Pediatric Cardiac Catheterization*)

Stephen P. Fischer, MD
Associate Professor of Anesthesia
Stanford University School of Medicine
Medical Director
Anesthesia Preoperative Evaluation Clinic at Stanford
(*Preoperative Laboratory Testing/Diagnostics*)

Linda E. Foppiano, MD
Assistant Professor of Anesthesia
Stanford University School of Medicine
(*Trauma Surgery*)

Fuad S. Freiha, MD, FACS
Chief of Urologic Oncology
Professor of Urology
Stanford University School of Medicine
(*Urology*)

Joan K. Frisoli, MD, PhD
Assistant Professor of Radiology
Stanford University Medical Center
(*TIPS*)

Louise Furukawa, MD
Clinical Instructor of Anesthesia
Stanford University School of Medicine
(*Repair of Craniofacial Malformations*)

Raymond R. Gaeta, MD
Associate Professor of Anesthesia
Director of Pain Management Services
Stanford University School of Medicine
(*Adult Perioperative Pain Management*)

J. Kent Garman, MD, MS, FACC
Associate Professor of Anesthesia
Stanford University School of Medicine
(*Cardiac Surgery; Heart/Lung Transplantation;
Adult Out-of-OR Procedures*)

Michael W. Gaynon, MD
Clinical Associate Professor of Ophthalmology
Stanford University School of Medicine
(*Retinal Surgery*)

Karen A. Giarrusso, MD
Clinical Instructor of Anesthesia
Stanford University School of Medicine
(*Gynecology/Infertility Surgery*)

Harcharan S. Gill, MD
Associate Professor of Urology
Stanford University School of Medicine
(*Urology*)

Sabine C. Girod, MD, DDS, PhD
Assistant Professor of Oral and Maxillofacial Surgery
Division of Plastic and Reconstructive Surgery
Stanford University Medical Center
(*Dental Surgery*)

Brenda Golianu, MD
Assistant Professor of Anesthesia and Pain Management
Stanford University School of Medicine
(*Pediatric General Surgery; Standard Pediatric Pain
Management*)

Julie Good, MD
Clinical Instructor of Pediatric Pain Management
Department of Anesthesia
Stanford University Medical Center
Lucile Salter Packard Children's Hospital at Stanford
(*Standard Pediatric Pain Management*)

Stuart B. Goodman, MD, PhD, FRCSC, FACS
Professor of Orthopedic Surgery
Stanford University School of Medicine
(*Orthopedic Surgery–Hip, Pelvis, Upper Leg, Knee*)

Ralph Greco, MD
Johnson and Johnson Distinguished Professor of
Surgery
Chief, Division of General Surgery
Director, General Surgery Residency Program
Stanford University School of Medicine
(*Endocrine Surgery*)

Alvin Hackel, MD
Professor of Anesthesia and Pediatrics, Emeritus
Stanford University School of Medicine
Lucile Salter Packard Children's Hospital at Stanford
(*Latex Allergy Considerations*)

Bruce D. Halperin, MD
Adjunct Clinical Associate Professor of Anesthesia
Associated Anesthesiologists
Stanford University Medical Center
(*Liposuction*)

Gregory B. Hammer, MD
Associate Professor of Pediatrics in Anesthesia
Stanford University School of Medicine
Associate Director, Pediatric Intensive Care Unit
Lucile Salter Packard Children's Hospital at Stanford
(*Pediatric Otolaryngology, General, Urology, Surgery
for Craniofacial Malformations; Pediatric Out-of-OR
Procedures; Pediatric Anesthetic Protocols and
Postoperative Pain Management*)

Frank L. Hanley, MD
Professor of Cardiothoracic Surgery
Division of Pediatric Cardiovascular Surgery
Stanford University School of Medicine
(*Pediatric Cardiovascular Surgery*)

Leland H. Hanowell, MD
Clinical Associate Professor of Cardiovascular
Anesthesia
Stanford University Medical Center
Professor Emeritus of Anesthesia
University of California–Davis
(*Adult Out-of-OR Procedures*)

Gary E. Hartman, MD
Professor of Pediatric Surgery
George Washington University School of Medicine
Chief of Pediatric Surgery
Children's National Medical Center
Washington, DC
(*ECMO*)

Weldon W. Haw, MD
Assistant Professor of Ophthalmology
Clinical Chief, Ophthalmology
Stanford University Medical Center
(*Ophthalmic Surgery*)

Gary Heit, MD, PhD
Assistant Professor of Neurosurgery
Stanford University School of Medicine
(*Functional Neurosurgery*)

Vincent R. Hentz, MD
Professor of Surgery
Chief, Division of Plastic and Reconstructive Surgery
Stanford University School of Medicine
(*Hand Surgery*)

Jerome E. Hester, MD
Attending Surgeon, Department of Surgery
Stanford University Medical Center
Facial Reconstructive Surgical and Medical Center
Palo Alto, CA
(*Surgery for Sleep Disorders*)

Terri D. Homer, MD
Clinical Educator, Department of Anesthesia
Associated Anesthesiologists
Stanford University Medical Center
(*Office-Based Anesthesia*)

Stephen L. Huhn, MD
Assistant Professor of Neurosurgery
Stanford University School of Medicine
Chief of Pediatric Neurosurgery Services
Lucile Salter Packard Children's Hospital at Stanford
(*Pediatric Neurosurgery*)

Kenneth C. W. Hui, MD, FACS
Plastic Surgeon
Hong Kong, Republic of China
(*Scalp Replantation*)

Amreen Husain, MD
Assistant Professor of Gynecology and Obstetrics
Stanford University School of Medicine
(*Gynecologic Oncology*)

Richard A. Jaffe, MD, PhD
Professor of Anesthesia and Neurosurgery
Stanford University School of Medicine
(*Intracranial, Functional, Extracranial Neurosurgery;
Ophthalmic Surgery; Dental Surgery; Orthopedic
Spine Surgery; Craniofacial Surgery; Adult Out-of-OR
Procedures; Adult Anesthetic Protocols*)

Stefanie S. Jeffrey, MD, FACS
John and Marva Warnook Faculty Scholar in Cancer
Research
Associate Professor of Surgery
Division of Surgical Oncology
Stanford University School of Medicine
(*Breast Surgery*)

David M. Kahn, MD
Assistant Professor of Surgery
Division of Plastic and Reconstructive Surgery
Stanford University School of Medicine
(*Facial Cosmetic Surgery; Nonfacial Aesthetic Surgery;
Functional Restoration*)

Komal Kamra, MD
Clinical Instructor of Anesthesia
Stanford University School of Medicine
(*Pediatric Orthopedic Surgery*)

Daniel S. Kapp, MD
Professor of Radiation Oncology
Stanford University School of Medicine
(*Gynecologic Oncology*)

Yvonne L. Karanas, MD
Assistant Professor of Surgery
Division of Plastic and Reconstructive Surgery
Stanford University School of Medicine
(*Functional Restoration*)

Andrew C. Karich, MD
Sports Medicine Fellow
Southern California Orthopedic Institute
Van Nuys, CA
(*Shoulder/Arm Surgery*)

Stephen T. Kee, MD
Associate Professor of Radiology
Division of Cardiovascular and Interventional
Radiology
Stanford University School of Medicine
(*Endovascular and Tracheobronchial Stent-Grafting; RF
Ablation*)

Daniel H. Kim, MD, FACS
Associate Professor of Neurosurgery
Director
Spinal Neurosurgery and Reconstructive Peripheral
Nerve Surgery
Stanford University School of Medicine
(*Spinal Neurosurgery*)

Mark Koransky, MD
Chief Resident, General Surgery
Stanford University Medical Center
(*Endocrine Surgery*)

Amy L. Ladd, MD
Associate Professor of Hand and Upper Limb Surgery
Stanford University School of Medicine
Chief of Pediatric and Upper Extremity Clinic
Lucile Salter Packard Children's Hospital at Stanford
(*Shoulder/Arm Surgery; Pediatric Hand Surgery*)

Azeem K. Lakha, DMD
Clinical Instructor of Plastic and Reconstructive Surgery
Stanford University Medical Center
Oral and Maxillofacial Surgeon
Palo Alto, CA
(*Office-Based Dental Procedures*)

Cathy R. Lammers, MD, FAAP
Assistant Professor of Anesthesia and Pain Management
University of California–Davis Medical Center
Director of Pediatric Anesthesia
University of California–Davis Children's Hospital
Sacramento, CA
(*Pediatric Otolaryngology, Urology; Pediatric
Out-of-OR Procedures; Latex Allergy Considerations*)

C. Philip Larson, Jr, MD, CM
Professor of Anesthesia and Neurosurgery, Emeritus
Stanford University School of Medicine
Professor of Clinical Anesthesia
David Geffen School of Medicine at University of
California–Los Angeles
(*Intracranial, Spinal, Extracranial Neurosurgery;
Orthopedic Spine Surgery; Pediatric Neurosurgery;
Adult Anesthetic Protocols*)

Hendrikus J. M. Lemmens, MD, PhD
Associate Professor of Anesthesia
Stanford University Medical Center
(*Hepatic, Biliary Surgery; Liver Transplantation*)

Kasey K. Li, DDS, MD
Clinical Instructor
Sleep Disorders Clinic and Research Center
Stanford University School of Medicine
(*Surgery for Sleep Disorders*)

L. Bing Liem, DO
Clinical Associate Professor of Cardiovascular Medicine
Stanford University Medical Center
Electrophysiologist, Department of Cardiology
Palo Alto Medical Foundation, Palo Alto, CA
(*DC Cardioversion; ICD Placement*)

Todd Lincoln, MD
Assistant Professor of Orthopedic Surgery
Stanford University School of Medicine
Lucile Salter Packard Children's Hospital at Stanford
(*Pediatric Orthopedic Surgery*)

William C. Lineaweaver, MD, FACS
Professor of Surgery
Division of Plastic Surgery
University of Mississippi Medical Center
(*Scalp Replantation*)

Eva D. Littman, MD
Clinical REI Fellow in Obstetrics and Gynecology
Stanford University Medical Center
(*Infertility Surgery*)

Sean Mackey, MD, PhD
Assistant Professor of Anesthesia and Pain Medicine
Stanford University School of Medicine
(*Adult Perioperative Pain Management*)

Kevin A. Malott, MD
Clinical Instructor of Anesthesia
Stanford University School of Medicine
(*Stomach, Intestinal Surgery*)

Michael P. Marks, MD
Chief of Interventional Neuroradiology
Director of Neuroradiology Stanford Stroke Center
Associate Professor of Radiology and Neurosurgery
Stanford University Medical Center
(*Interventional Neuroradiology*)

Jeffrey B. Marotte, MD
Resident, Department of Urology
Stanford University Medical Center
(*Pediatric Urology*)

Christine Matthes-Kofidis, MD
Research Assistant
Department of Pediatric Surgery
Stanford University School of Medicine
(*Pediatric General Surgery*)

Anna H. Messner, MD
Assistant Professor of Surgery/Otolaryngology Surgery
Stanford University Medical Center
Chief of Pediatric Otolaryngology
Lucile Salter Packard Children's Hospital at Stanford
(*Pediatric Otolaryngology*)

Frederick G. Mihm, MD
Professor of Anesthesia
Associate Medical Director, Intensive Care Units
Stanford University Medical Center
(*Endocrine Surgery; Orthopedic Surgery of
Lower Extremities; Emergency Procedures for
Anesthesiologists*)

Amin A. Milki, MD
Associate Professor of Obstetrics and Gynecology
Stanford University Medical Center
(*Infertility Surgery*)

Maria T. Millan, MD
Assistant Professor of Surgery
Division of Multiorgan Transplantation
Stanford University School of Medicine
(*Kidney, Pancreas Transplantation*)

R. Scott Mitchell, MD
Professor of Cardiothoracic Surgery
Stanford University School of Medicine
(*Cardiac, Vascular Surgery*)

Vladimir Nekhendzy, MD
Assistant Professor of Anesthesia
Chief of ENT Anesthesia
Stanford University Medical Center
(*Otolaryngology Surgery*)

Camran R. Nezhat, MD
Director of Endoscopy Training Center
Clinical Professor of Gynecology and Obstetrics and
Surgery
Stanford University School of Medicine
(*Laparoscopic Procedures for Gynecologic Surgery*)

Harry A. Oberhelman, MD, FACS
Professor Emeritus, Division of Gastrointestinal Surgery
Stanford University School of Medicine
(*Intestinal, Hepatic, Peritoneal Surgery*)

Jeffrey D. Pardun, MD
Resident in Plastic and Reconstructive Surgery
Stanford University Medical Center
(*Nonfacial Aesthetic Surgery; Functional
Reconstruction*)

Ronald G. Pearl, MD, PhD
Chairman, Staff Physician, VCF Affairs Administrator
Department of Anesthesia
Stanford University School of Medicine
(*Urology*)

Stanton B. Perry, MD
Associate Professor of Pediatric Surgery
Stanford University School of Medicine
Director of Pediatric and Congenital Catheterization and
Interventional Cardiology Services
Lucile Salter Packard Children's Hospital at Stanford
(*Pediatric Cardiac Catheterization*)

Nelson B. Powell, MD
Associate Clinical Professor
Co-Director, Sleep Disorders Clinic and Research
Center
Stanford University Medical Center
(*Surgery for Sleep Disorders*)

Chandra Ramamoorthy, MD
Associate Professor of Anesthesia
Director of Pediatric Cardiac Anesthesia
Stanford University Medical Center
(*Pediatric Cardiovascular Surgery; Pediatric Cardiac
Catheterization*)

V. Mohan Reddy, MD
Associate Professor of Cardiothoracic Surgery
Chief of Pediatric Surgery
Stanford University School of Medicine
(*Pediatric Cardiovascular Surgery*)

Bruce A. Reitz, MD
Professor and Chairman
Department of Cardiothoracic Surgery
Stanford University School of Medicine
Chief, Pediatric Cardiac Surgical Service
Lucile Salter Packard Children's Hospital at Stanford
(*Heart/Lung Transplantation*)

Robert W. Riley, DDS, MD
Associate Clinical Professor
Sleep Disorders Clinic and Research Center
Stanford University Medical Center
(*Surgery for Sleep Disorders*)

Lawrence A. Rinsky, MD
Professor of Orthopedic Surgery
Stanford University School of Medicine
Chief of Pediatric Orthopedics
Lucile Salter Packard Children's Hospital at Stanford
(*Pediatric Orthopedic Surgery*)

Joseph B. Roberson, MD
CEO/Managing Partner
California Ear Institute at Stanford
(*Otolaryngology–Skull Base Surgery*)

Myer H. Rosenthal, MD, FACCP
Professor of Anesthesia, Medicine, and Surgery
Stanford University School of Medicine
(*Gynecologic Oncology, Emergency Procedures for
Anesthesiologists*)

Lonny L. Ross, MD, FRCSC
Assistant Professor of Plastic Surgery
University of Manitoba
Director, Craniofacial Anomalies Clinic of Manitoba,
Children's Hospital at University of Manitoba
Winnipeg, Manitoba, Canada
(*Facial Cosmetic Surgery; Craniofacial Surgery;
Surgery for Craniofacial Malformations*)

Gordon T. Sakamoto, MD
Resident, Department of Neurosurgery
Stanford University Medical Center
(*Intracranial Neurosurgery*)

Stanley I. Samuels, MB, BCh, FFARCS
Professor of Anesthesia, Emeritus
Stanford University School of Medicine
(*Intracranial, Functional, Extracranial Neurosurgery;
Ophthalmic Surgery; Dental Surgery; Orthopedic
Spine Surgery; Craniofacial Surgery; Adult Out-of-OR
Procedures; Adult Anesthetic Protocols*)

Sunita G. Sastry, MBBS, FRCPSC
Assistant Professor of Anesthesia
Stanford University Medical Center
(*Laparoscopic General Surgery*)

Michael V. Sattah, MD
Chief Resident, Department of Radiation Oncology
Stanford University Medical Center
(*Pediatric Radiation Therapy*)

Stephen A. Schendel, MD, DDS, FACS
Professor of Plastic Surgery/General Surgery
Stanford University School of Medicine
Director, Craniofacial Anomalies Center
Lucile Salter Packard Children's Hospital at Stanford
(*Dental Surgery; Craniofacial Surgery; Surgery for Craniofacial Malformations*)

Clifford A. Schmiesing, MD
Assistant Professor of Anesthesia
Stanford University School of Medicine
(*Preoperative Anesthesia Considerations*)

Steven Shafer, MD
Professor of Anesthesia
Veterans Administration–Palo Alto Health Care System
Palo Alto, CA
(*TIVA*)

Andrew A. Shelton, MD
Assistant Professor of Surgery
Stanford University school of Medicine
(*Colorectal Surgery*)

Richard C. Shinaman, MD
Department of Anesthesia
Stanford University Medical Center
(*Adult Out-of-OR Procedures*)

Linda M. Dairiki Shortliffe, MD
Professor and Chair
Department of Urology
Stanford University School of Medicine and
Lucile Salter Packard Children's Hospital at Stanford
(*Pediatric Urology*)

Lawrence M. Shuer, MD
Professor of Neurosurgery
Stanford University School of Medicine
Chief of Staff
Stanford University Hospital and Clinics
(*Intracranial, Functional, Spinal, Extracranial Neurosurgery; Surgery for Craniofacial Malformations*)

Norman E. Shumway, MD, PhD
Professor of Cardiovascular and Cardiothoracic Surgery, Emeritus
Stanford University School of Medicine
(*Cardiac Surgery*)

Lawrence C. Siegel, MD
Attending Anesthesiologist
Veterans Administration-Palo Alto Health Care System
Palo Alto, CA
(*Cardiac Surgery; Minimally Invasive Cardiac Surgery; Heart/Lung Transplantation*)

Erik J. Sirulnick, MD
Clinical Fellow of Cardiovascular Medicine
Stanford University Medical Center
(*DC Cardioversion, ICD Placement*)

Baird M. Smith, MD
Assistant Professor of Pediatric Surgery
Stanford University School of Medicine
(*Pediatric General Surgery*)

Samuel K. S. So, MD, FACS
Professor of Surgery
Director of Liver Cancer Program and Asian Liver Program
Stanford University Medical Center
(*Hepatic Surgery*)

David A. Spain, MD
Professor of Surgery
Chief of Trauma/Surgical Critical Care
Stanford University Medical Center
(*Trauma Surgery*)

Gary K. Steinberg, MD, PhD
Lacroute-Hearst Professor and Chairman
Department of Neurosurgery
Stanford University School of Medicine
Chief of Neurosurgery
Stanford University Medical Center
(*Intracranial, Extracranial Neurosurgery*)

Daniel Y. Sze, MD, PhD
Associate Professor of Cardiovascular and Interventional Radiology
Stanford University Medical Center
(*Imaging, Image-Guided Procedures*)

M. Mark Taslimi, MD
Clinical Professor of Maternal and Fetal Medicine
Department of Obstetrics and Gynecology
Stanford University School of Medicine
(*Obstetric Surgery*)

Nelson N. Teng, MD, PhD
Associate Professor of Gynecology and Obstetrics
Chief, Division of Gynecologic Oncology
Stanford University School of Medicine
(*Gynecologic Oncology*)

Kalyani R. Trivedi, MD
Senior Clinical Fellow, Department of Pediatric Cardiology
Stanford University Medical Center
Lucile Salter Packard Children's Hospital at Stanford
(*Pediatric Cardiac Catheterization*)

Robert J. Troell, MD
Clinical Instructor of Surgery and Sleep Disorders
Clinic and Research Center
Stanford University Medical Center
(*Surgery for Sleep Disorders*)

H. Ward Trueblood, MD
Clinical Professor of Surgery
Division of General Surgery
Stanford University School of Medicine
(*Stomach Surgery*)

Pieter Van der Starre, MD, PhD
Associate Professor of Anesthesia
Stanford University School of Medicine
(*Vascular Surgery*)

Winston C. Vaughan, MD
Department of Otolaryngology
Stanford University Medical Center
Stanford Sinus Center
(*Endoscopic Sinus Surgery*)

Mark A. Vierra, MD
Staff Surgeon
The Community Hospital of Monterey
Monterey, CA
(*Biliary Tract Surgery*)

Lindsey Vokach-Brodsky, MBChB, FFARCS
Assistant Professor of Anesthesia
Stanford University School of Medicine
(*Breast Surgery; Laparoscopic Procedures for
Gynecologic Surgery; Nonfacial Aesthetic Surgery*)

Irene L. Wapnir, MD
Associate Professor of Surgery
Stanford University Medical Center
(*Breast Surgery*)

Mark Lane Welton, MD
Associate Professor of Surgery
Chief of Colorectal Surgery Service
Stanford University School of Medicine
(*Colorectal Surgery*)

Lynn M. Westphal, MD
Assistant Professor of Obstetrics and Gynecology
Stanford University School of Medicine
(*Infertility Surgery*)

Richard I. Whyte, MD
Associate Professor and Head of Thoracic Surgery
Stanford University School of Medicine
(*Thoracic, Esophageal Surgery*)

Glen D. Williams, MBChB, FFA
Associate Professor of Anesthesia
Stanford University School of Medicine
Lucille Salter Packard Children's Hospital of Stanford
(*Pediatric Radiation Therapy*)

O. W. Stephanie Yap, MD
Fellow, Gynecologic Oncology
Department of Gynecology and Obstetrics
Stanford University Medical Center
(*Gynecologic Oncology*)

Kenneth K. Yim, MD, FACS
Chief, Division of Plastic Surgery
Director, Burn Unit
Santa Clara Valley Medical Center
San Jose, CA
(*Burn Surgery*)

FOREWORD

One of the rewarding aspects of being an anesthesiologist is the opportunity to participate in a diversity of surgical procedures. We provide anesthesia for general surgery, thoracic surgery, neurosurgery, orthopedic surgery, plastic surgery, pediatric surgery, cardiovascular surgery, and obstetric and gynecologic surgery. Within each of these subspecialties, there are a bewildering array of procedures, each having its own specific anesthetic implications. Although some anesthesiologists do specialize in one specific area, most of us must always be prepared to handle cases from multiple surgical subspecialties. The *Anesthesiologist's Manual of Surgical Procedures* is designed for these anesthesiologists, who, in the course of a week, may have a list that includes such diverse cases as craniocervical decompression of a Chiari malformation, skull base surgery, ventricular septal myectomy/myotomy, laparoscopic splenectomy, TIPS procedure, and a Darrach procedure.

Finding relevant information on an unfamiliar and/or uncommon surgical procedure and its anesthetic implications can be a difficult, frustrating, and time-consuming task. The anesthesiologist can seek information from surgical or anesthesia colleagues, from books and publications in a personal or institutional library, or from electronic searches and sources. It is, however, often difficult to identify a colleague with the appropriate knowledge, and our print and electronic sources often discuss the disease process and the surgery, without directly addressing the important anesthetic implications. The first edition of the *Anesthesiologist's Manual of Surgical Procedures*, published in 1994, provided a fast, efficient way to find the information that is most relevant to the anesthesiologist. Each chapter was written jointly by surgeons and anesthesiologists with broad knowledge and experience in that particular surgical area. For each procedure, the surgical considerations, a summary of procedural issues, and the preoperative, intraoperative, and postoperative anesthetic considerations were reviewed in a concise, easy-to-follow manner. The consistent format throughout the book allowed the reader to develop a rapid approach to finding the information that is most relevant to a specific procedure.

The third edition continues this basic approach, while adding chapters and significantly expanding coverage in multiple areas, including functional neurosurgery, minimally invasive cardiac surgery, reconstructive/plastic surgery, and office-based anesthesiology. The expanding role of laparoscopy is well represented in the revisions of many chapters. In addition, several chapters have had major revisions and/or additional procedures added. These include neurosurgery, otolaryngology, thoracic surgery, stomach surgery, craniofacial surgery, functional restoration, and pediatric surgery. The number of illustrations has been increased significantly, making it easier for the reader to understand the specifics of the surgical procedures. The chapters and procedures are supplemented by eight appendices, which cover preoperative considerations, standard adult anesthetic protocols, perioperative pain management, pediatric anesthetic protocols, pediatric postoperative pain management, drug interactions, and latex allergy. The combination of the specific procedures discussed in the body of the book with the general approaches described in the appendices allows complete planning of an anesthetic for a typical patient in most surgical procedures.

This third edition documents the rapid growth that has occurred in surgery and anesthesia over the past five years. The editors have significantly improved both the quality and quantity of chapters, while maintaining those unique factors that have made the book an invaluable reference for all anesthesiologists over the past decade.

Ronald G. Pearl, M.D., Ph.D.
Professor and Chair of Anesthesia
Stanford University School of Medicine
July, 2003

ACKNOWLEDGMENTS

We gratefully acknowledge the indispensable organizational, copy editing, and production skills of our Developmental Editor, Dee Mosteller. Once again, the challenges of dealing with more than 700 procedures, 159 contributors and two very heavy-handed editors almost defy description, and definitely exceed the bounds of normal human endurance.

We would also like to thank our Contributors; the editorial staff at Lippincott Williams & Wilkins—most particularly our Executive Editor, Craig Percy, and his assistant, Timothy Reiley, for their patient and enthusiastic support of this project—our typesetters at QualiType, Inc., for service above and beyond; Jennifer Smith and QualiType, Inc., for greatly enhancing our artwork; Eileen Wolfberg, our perfect word processor; and a special thanks to our special proofreader, Donna J. Allison, Ph.D.

This edition is built upon the foundation of its predecessors and, thus, includes material from prior editions. We remain grateful to the following former contributors, some of whose words continue to live on in the present edition: Edward J. Alfrey, John G. Brock-Utne, Sally R. Byrd, Carter Cherry, Annette C. Cholon, Donald C. Dafoe, Jayshree B. Desai, John A. Duncan III, Babak Edraki, Talmage D. Egan, Brett G. Fitzmaurice, Edward C. Gabalski, Ronald N. Gibson, Rona G. Giffard, Alexandra J. Golby, Gordon R. Haddow, W. LeRoy Heinrichs, R. Harold Holbrook, Jr., Steven K. Howard, Amar Kaur, Alexsander R. Komar, Peter S. Kosek, Steven P. LaPointe, George Lederhaas, Yuan-Chi Lin, Padma Malipedi, M. Thomas Margolis, James B. D. Mark, Steven R. Miller, Robert J. Moynihan, Alexander M. Norbash, B. Hannah Ortiz, Kristi L. Peterson, Paul T. Pitlick, Barry H.J. Press, Jon W. Propst, Emily F. Ratner, Edward T. Riley, Cathy M. Russo, Jan T. Rydfors, Velerig Selivanov, Charles P. Semba, Carol A. Shostak, Gerald D. Silverberg, Robert J. Singer, Lynn D. Solem, James M. Stone, E. Price Stover, Jeffrey D. Swenson, David J. Terris, Andrew E. Turk, George F. Van Hare, Lars M. Vistnes, Robert J. Weigel, and David D. Yuh.

PREFACE

We naively assumed that the preparation of a third edition of the *Anesthesiologist's Manual of Surgical Procedures* would proceed easily, given our experience and the insights gained from the previous editions – we were wrong.

✳ ✳ ✳

The goals of the third edition are unchanged from those of the first—that is, to provide an easily accessible source of clinically relevant information about a wide variety of both common and not-so-common surgical procedures. As with the first edition, this one does not pretend to be either a textbook of anesthesia or a textbook of surgery. Indeed, in the formulation of an anesthetic plan, there is no substitute for experience and sound clinical judgment.

Those familiar with the preceding editions will notice that the format and organization of this edition remain unchanged. White-space throughout the book has been reduced to help disguise the significantly increased content, the result of adding eight new chapters and dozens of new procedures. Every existing procedure was reviewed and revised as necessary to reflect current practices.

Once again, we have made extensive use of abbreviations, medical symbols, and telegraphic sentence structure to present a large quantity of information in a condensed format. While we realize that it may be aesthetically more pleasing to read, "Hypoxia or hypercapnia can lead to the development of tachycardia and hypertension," it takes up a lot less space to write, "$\uparrow PaCO_2$ or $\downarrow PaO_2 \rightarrow \uparrow HR + \uparrow BP$."

Finally, we have again attempted to incorporate the many constructive comments we received from our readers and reviewers of the previous editions. In the final analysis, it must be left up to you, the reader, to decide if we have created an improved and more balanced edition the third time around.

Richard A. Jaffe and Stanley I. Samuels
Stanford University School of Medicine
July, 2003

1.0 NEUROSURGERY

Surgeons

Gary K. Steinberg, MD, PhD (*Neurovascular surgery*)
Robert L. Dodd, MD, PhD (*Neurovascular surgery*)
Gordon T. Sakamoto, MD (*General neurosurgery*)
Lawrence M. Shuer, MD (*General neurosurgery*)
Steven D. Chang, MD (*General neurosurgery, Stereotactic neurosurgery*)
John R. Adler, MD (*Stereotactic neurosurgery*)

1.1 INTRACRANIAL NEUROSURGERY

Anesthesiologists

Richard A. Jaffe, MD, PhD
Stanley I. Samuels, MB, BCh, FFARCS
C. Philip Larson, Jr, MD, MS

CRANIOTOMY FOR INTRACRANIAL ANEURYSMS

SURGICAL CONSIDERATIONS

Gary K. Steinberg and Robert L. Dodd

Description: Intracranial aneurysms are focal protrusions arising from vessel wall weaknesses at major bifurcations on the arteries at the base of the brain (some frequent sites of aneurysms are shown in Fig. 1.1-1), and are most commonly treated by microsurgical clip ligation. The high rate of mortality and morbidity from aneurysmal rupture necessitates treatment for symptomatic lesions. Treatment for asymptomatic lesions generally is recommended when the lifetime risk of rupture exceeds the risk of treatment. The most important surgical considerations include: clinical presentation, aneurysm size and location, patient age and neurologic status, and medical comorbidities. Aneurysm rupture into the subarachnoid spaces is the most common clinical presentation; however, symptoms from mass effect of enlarging aneurysms or ischemic symptoms from emboli also may occur. Aneurysm morphology, size, and location are important in determining the surgical approach, and these aneurysm characteristics, as well as patient age, condition, and comorbidities, affect the overall outcome. The **Hess and Hunt clinical grading system** (Table 1.1-1) has been proven useful in describing patients with ruptured intracranial aneurysms, since it has been shown to have prognostic value, in terms of ultimate clinical outcome. Grading is based on the neurologic examination and ranges from Grade I (minimal headache, no neurologic deficit) to Grade V (moribund).

Through a **craniotomy** or **craniectomy**, using microscopic techniques, the parent vessel giving rise to the aneurysm is identified. The aneurysm neck is isolated, and a small, nonferromagnetic alloy spring clip is placed across the aneurysm neck, excluding it from the circulation. A **frontotemporal (pterional) craniotomy** normally is used to approach anterior circulation aneurysms. This requires extensive drilling of the medial sphenoid wing (pterion) and allows access to most aneurysms on the anterior and lateral Circle of Willis vessels: internal carotid-paraclinoid/superior hypophyseal artery; internal carotid-ophthalmic artery; posterior communicating artery; anterior choroidal artery; internal carotid artery bifurcation; middle cerebral artery; and anterior communicating artery. Posterior circulation aneurysms are approached via a pterional or subtemporal exposure (upper basilar artery, posterior cerebral artery, superior cerebellar artery), a suboccipital exposure (vertebral artery, posterior inferior cerebellar artery), or a combined subtemporal and suboccipital exposure (basilar trunk, vertebrobasilar junction). Circulatory arrest under CPB with deep hypothermia (16-20°C) is used for repairing some giant (> 2.5 cm) aneurysms.

Usual preop diagnosis: Cerebral aneurysm; subarachnoid hemorrhage (SAH); intracerebral hemorrhage; progressive neuro-logical deficits (mass effect on cranial nerves or CNS structures); TIAs; cerebral infarct

SUMMARY OF PROCEDURES

	Anterior Circulation Aneurysms	Posterior Circulation Aneurysms	Circulatory Arrest (CPB) W/Deep Hypothermia
Position	Supine, head in Mayfield head-rest, turned 30-45° to side away from aneurysm, vertex dropped (Fig 1.1-5)	⇐ Or lateral decubitus, head lateral in Mayfield headrest	⇐ + Both groins must be accessible for arterial + venous cannulation; access to chest for defibrillation.
Incision	Frontotemporal	⇐ Or temporal, temporosuboccipital or suboccipital	⇐
Special instrumentation	Operating microscope; aneurysm clips; radiolucent table and headrest for intraop angiography	⇐ + Aperture clips to accommodate cranial nerves and critical vessels.	⇐ + CPB pump; femoral cannulae; defibrillator; CUSA for partially thrombosed aneurysms
Unique considerations	Temporary arterial clipping; mild hypothermia (33°C); intraop angiography with access to femoral artery; electrophysiological monitoring (SEPs, BAERs); brain relaxation; ± lumbar subarachnoid CSF drainage; dexamethasone 8-12 mg iv	⇐	⇐ + No manipulation of brain retractors after systemic heparinization; meticulous attention to hemostasis
Antibiotics	Nafcillin (1-2 g iv q 6 h) + cefotaxime (1 g iv q 6 h)	⇐	⇐

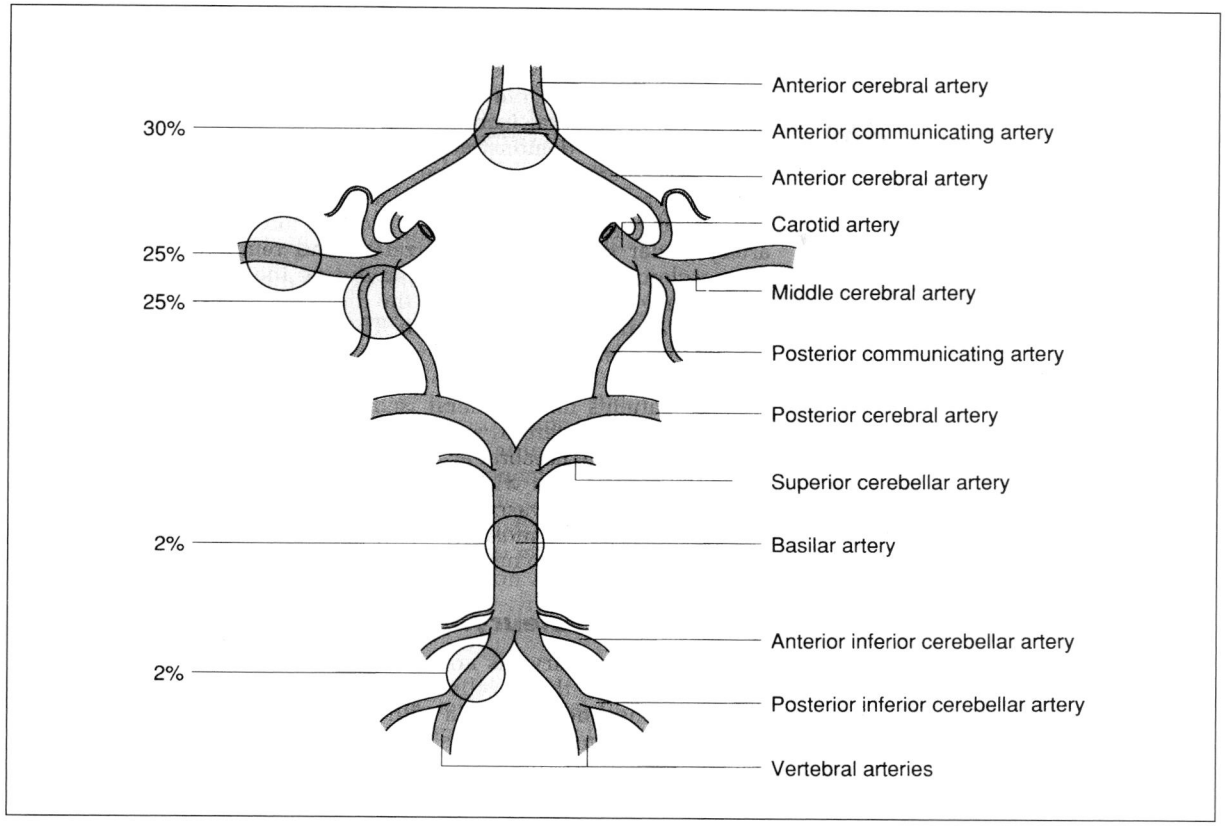

Figure 1.1-1. Locations of aneurysms of the circle of Willis, and their relative occurrence. (Reproduced with permission from Greenfield LJ, et al: *Surgery: Scientific Principles and Practice*, 3rd edition. Lippincott Williams & Wilkins, 2001.)

	Anterior Circulation Aneurysms	Posterior Circulation Aneurysms	Circulatory Arrest (CPB) W/Deep Hypothermia
Surgical time	3-5 h	3-6 h	6-8 h
Closing considerations	Rewarming	⇐	⇐
EBL	250-1000 ml	⇐	2000-4000 ml
Postop care	ICU × 1-7 d; postop CBF monitoring. Transcranial Doppler (TDC) monitor	⇐	⇐ + ICP monitoring
Mortality	Unruptured: 0.5% Ruptured:	1.5%	5-10% (giant aneurysms)
	Hunt and Hess grades I-III: < 10% (See Table 1.1-1.)	< 15%	5-15%
	Hunt and Hess grades IV-V: 20-40% (See Table 1.1-1.)	20-50%	15-50%
Morbidity	Neurological: 5-20%	10-30%	10-50%
	Cranial nerve injury	⇐	⇐
	Stroke	⇐	⇐
	Hydrocephalus	⇐	⇐
	Hyponatremia	⇐	⇐
	Respiratory failure: Rare	⇐	⇐
	Thromboembolism: Rare	⇐	⇐
	CSF leak: Rare	⇐	⇐
	Infection: Rare	⇐	⇐
	Massive blood loss: Rare	⇐	⇐
Pain score	3-4	3-4	4-5

PATIENT POPULATION CHARACTERISTICS

Age range	30-70 yr
Male:Female	44:56
Incidence	12/100,000/yr for ruptured aneurysms with SAH
Etiology	Idiopathic (probably acquired and related to hemodynamic stress at arterial branch points, although may have congenital predisposition to loss of internal elastic lamina); traumatic; infectious; familial
Associated conditions	Polycystic kidney disease; coarctation of the aorta; Marfan syndrome; Ehlers-Danlos syndrome; intracranial AVMs; aortic aneurysm; fibromuscular dysplasia; pseudoxanthoma elastica; Rendu-Osler-Weber syndrome

---

Table 1.1-1. Hunt-Hess Grading System for Aneurysmal SAH*

Grade	Description
I	Asymptomatic, or minimal headache and slight neck stiffness
II	Moderate-to-severe headache, neck stiffness, no neurological deficit (except cranial nerve palsy)
III	Drowsiness, confusion, or mild focal deficit
IV	Stupor, moderate-to-severe hemiparesis, possible early decerebrate rigidity, and vegetative disturbances
V	Deep coma, decerebrate rigidity, moribund

*The presence of serious systemic disease—such as hypertension, diabetes, severe arteriosclerosis, chronic pulmonary disease, and angiographic vasospasm—results in placement in the next less-favorable category.

ANESTHETIC CONSIDERATIONS

(Procedures covered: craniotomy for intracranial aneurysms; craniotomy for cerebral embolectomy)

PREOPERATIVE

Aneurysms may occur in any age group, although they generally become symptomatic and are diagnosed in young or middle-aged adults who are usually in otherwise good health. Most patients have warning Sx before the first major bleed, but these tend to be mild and nonspecific (e.g., headache, dizziness, orbital pain, slight motor or sensory disturbances). The symptoms are generally disregarded by both patients and physicians.

Respiratory	Respiratory complications (e.g., pulmonary edema, pneumonia, ARDS, PE) are the most common nonneurologic causes of death following SAH. Pulmonary aspiration may have occurred as the result of a neurological deficit from an intracranial hemorrhage. **Tests:** As indicated from H&P.
Cardiovascular	Generally, these patients do not have other cardiovascular diseases, although intracerebral aneurysms occur more commonly in patients with certain congenital disorders, such as polycystic disease of the kidneys, coarctation of the aorta, fibromuscular hyperplasia, and Marfan and Ehlers-Danlos syndromes. Patients who have had a recent intracranial hemorrhage from leaking or rupture of a cerebral aneurysm are prone to develop systemic HTN, hypovolemia,[1] and ECG abnormalities. The HTN is thought to be due to autonomic hyperactivity, and is generally treated with antihypertensive medication, which should be continued up to the time of anesthesia and surgery. Why hypovolemia occurs following SAH is not clear, but may be due in part to cerebral vasospasm and to sustained bed rest. ECG abnormalities occur in most patients following an intracranial hemorrhage and may represent subendocardial injury 2° catecholamine release. Dysrhythmias (most commonly PVCs) occur in 30-80% of patients, and ischemic changes (typically T-wave inversion and S-T-segment depression) are seen in > 50%. Appropriate preop preparation includes ECG characterization of the abnormality. If patient has Hx of ischemic heart disease, ECHO and cardiac enzyme studies may be helpful in determining whether ECG changes are due to heart disease or 2° intracranial hemorrhage. **Tests:** ECG; others as indicated from H&P.
Neurological	Seldom do aneurysms produce neurological Sx by enlarging to the point that they compress adjacent neural tissue or cause ↑ICP. If an intracranial hemorrhage occurs, the neurological dysfunction will

Neurological, cont. vary, depending on the site and extent of the hemorrhage. These patients may complain of severe HA, be confused and disoriented, have a motor deficit of one or more extremities, or be comatose. A major complication of an intracerebral hemorrhage is the development of cerebral vasospasm, which, if severe, will cause worsening of the neurological deficits. Vasospasm is usually mild in the first 4 d after the bleed, peaks at ~7-8 d, and usually is resolved within 2-3 wk. The exact mechanism for the vasospasm is not known, but it is believed that the precipitating agent is free Hb, which causes release of vasospastic substances from brain tissue. Treatment of vasospasm usually involves support of BP (occasionally, induced HTN), hydration to normovolemia, and systemic Ca^{++} antagonists (e.g., nimodipine, nicardipine). Although control of BP is important in all patients with aneurysms, it is particularly critical in this subset of patients. Any substantial increase in BP may cause a serious rebleed, permanent neurological deficits or death; any substantial decrease in BP may cause cerebral ischemia and infarction in the area of the original bleed. Arterial catheterization and continuous beat-to-beat monitoring of BP prior to induction of anesthesia is essential in these patients.
Tests: CT; MRI; cerebral angiogram, which the anesthesiologist should examine preop to identify the nature and site of the aneurysm.

Hematologic Thrombocytopenia may develop following SAH.
Tests: Hct; PT; PTT

Laboratory CT or MRI scan; cerebral angiogram; others as indicated from H&P.

Hepatic Hepatic dysfunction following SAH is not uncommon (24% in one series).
Tests: LFTs, as indicated from H&P.

Premedication If medication is desirable, small doses of midazolam 1-3 mg iv are preferable to opiates. Detailed discussion with the patient about the anesthetic plan, with appropriate reassurance, is essential. Should an intracranial aneurysm leak or rupture in the immediate preop period, its signs may be difficult to distinguish from those associated with excessive responses to premedication.

INTRAOPERATIVE

Anesthetic technique: GETA. The goals of anesthesia for this operation are to: (1) maintain optimum CPP (cerebral MAP minus cerebral venous or intracranial pressure, whichever is greater), but be prepared to decrease CPP rapidly and profoundly if intracranial hemorrhage occurs during surgical clipping; (2) decrease intracranial volume (blood and tissue) to optimize working space for surgeons within the cranial compartment, thereby minimizing the need for surgical retraction of brain tissue; and (3) minimize metabolic rate and $CMRO_2$, with the expectation that the brain will tolerate severe hypotension and ischemia if sudden decreases in MAP and, hence, CPP become necessary.

Induction STP 2-5 mg/kg (or propofol 1-2 mg/kg iv) to provide amnesia and ↓ cerebral blood volume by inducing cerebral vasoconstriction. Fentanyl 7-10 μg/kg iv to blunt response to intubation and provide analgesia for the first hs of surgery. Pancuronium 0.1 mg/kg, vecuronium 0.15 mg/kg, or rocuronium 0.7-1 mg/kg to provide muscle relaxation for tracheal intubation and positioning patient.

Maintenance Isoflurane ≤ 1% (≤ 0.6% if EP monitoring is used), inspired with O_2. N_2O > 50% is not used because of its potential for reversing the protective effects of STP.[7,20] Propofol (75-100 μg/kg/min) may be used to further ↓ cerebral blood volume, ↓ cerebral metabolism, and ↓ $CMRO_2$. Generally, if pancuronium is used, no additional NMBs are needed; however, if movement is of concern, rocuronium 10 μg/kg/min will provide adequate neuromuscular blockade. A remifentanil infusion (0.05-0.1 μg/kg/min) can be used to supplement the anesthetic without interfering with EP monitoring.

Emergence With the start of dural closure, consider changing the anesthetic to low-dose sevoflurane (e.g., 0.5%) or low-dose desflurane (e.g., 2%) in 50% N_2O, supplemented with a low-dose remifentanil infusion (e.g., 0.05 μg/kg/min). As recovery from anesthesia occurs, the patient's BP generally will increase in response to the emergence stimuli. Titration of β-adrenergic blocking drugs (e.g., labetalol or esmolol) and/or vasodilators (e.g., SNP) may be needed; if so, the dose should be stabilized before transport to ICU. (See Control of BP, below.) The inhalation agent can be D/C'd at the time of dressing application. Most patients will breathe spontaneously and can be extubated uneventfully while on the remifentanil infusion. If the brain has not been injured by the surgical procedure, the patient should awaken within 10 min after cessation of remifentanil administration. As the patient is awakening, it is important to assure full reversal from neuromuscular blockade and close regulation of BP. If the patient begins to cough on ETT, either it should be removed or cough reflex suppressed

Emergence, cont.	with iv lidocaine (0.5-1 mg/kg). Patient is placed in bed in a 30° head-up position and transported to ICU for monitoring overnight. Supplemental O_2 should be administered and close regulation of BP maintained. Prophylactic antiemetics (e.g., droperidol 0.625 mg or metoclopramide 10 mg, ondansetron 4 mg or dolasetron 12.5 mg) should be given 30 min before extubation.	
Blood and fluid requirements	IV: 16-18 ga × 2 NS/LR @ < 10 ml/kg + UO Expand blood volume with albumin 5% if Hct > 30%. Albumin + PRBC if Hct < 30%	What fluid and how much to give depends on patient's condition. If blood volume is normal, crystalloid fluid should not exceed 10 ml/kg beyond that required to replace UO. If blood volume is low because of vasospasm or prolonged bed rest, albumin 5% is given if Hct > 30%; combinations of albumin and blood, if Hct is < 30%.
	Hetastarch may → coagulopathy.[3]	Hetastarch 6% may be used in place of albumin, but do not exceed 20 ml/kg because of its potential for inducing a coagulopathy.
Control of brain volume (ICP)	Hyperventilate to $PaCO_2$ = 25-30 mmHg ($PetCO_2$ = 20-25 mmHg). PaO_2 >100 mmHg ↓ fluids < 10 ml/kg + UO STP or propofol infusion ↓ isoflurane < 1% Mannitol 0.5-1 g/kg ± Furosemide 0.3 mg/kg Control BP & CVP: low normal. ± Steroids ± Lumbar CSF drain Head up 20-30°	↓$PaCO_2$ → ↓cerebral vascular volume (better surgical access) + ↑CBF to ischemic areas ('Robin Hood' effect) + ↓anesthetic requirements + ↑lactic acid buffering. Mannitol/furosemide → ↓K^+; monitor level and replace as necessary. If mannitol is administered too rapidly, ↓BP may occur, probably from peripheral vasodilation. CSF drain often placed after induction of anesthesia, and may be opened as required.
Monitoring	Standard monitors (see p. B-1). Arterial line ± Bladder temperature CVP line UO (Foley catheter) ± Evoked potentials[6]	Direct monitoring of arterial pressure is essential because of the marked fluctuations in BP that may occur, necessitating hypertensive or hypotensive drug therapy, as well as need for ABGs. Recording transducer should always be at the level of the head rather than the heart. Monitoring CVP is desirable in virtually all patients to assess adequacy of fluid therapy intraop and postop. The catheter also is essential for infusion of vasoactive drugs commonly used during and/or after this operation. Localization of the catheter can be determined by CXR, ECG tracing (noting P-wave changes), or pressure-wave contour and value as the catheter is withdrawn from the right atrium.
Hypothermia	Thermal blanket Cool-air blower (Polar Air) Cold OR	Mild hypothermia (33-34°C) is used in some centers to ↓$CMRO_2$ and to ↓susceptability to ischemic injury. $CMRO_2$ decreases about 7% for every degree C decrease in brain temperature (30% ↓ @ 33°C). This level of hypothermia does not interfere appreciably with coagulation, nor is it generally associated with cardiac dysrhythmias. Warming is begun several h before the conclusion of the operation by using a thermal blanket and Bair Hugger, warming inspired gases, and increasing the ambient temperature in the OR. Usually, by the time the operation is completed, patient temperature is near normal.
Control of BP	During application of head fixation device (Mayfield): remifentanil 100-200 μg Prior to clipping: ↓MAP to ~80% of baseline.	Control of BP is critical to the successful outcome of the case. ↑↑BP → ↑↑transmural pressure across the aneurysmal wall → rupture of the aneurysm. Many neurosurgeons apply a temporary clip on the major feeding vessel(s) in advance of clipping the aneurysm. This technique collapses

Control of BP, cont.	Temporary clipping of major feeding vessel: ↑MAP to 110-120% of baseline. In event of aneurysmal rupture: ↓MAP to 40-50 mmHg, if necessary. Postclipping: MAP usually kept @ 80-100 mmHg. If HR > 80 bpm, esmolol 50-200 μg/kg/min to ↓HR to 50-60 bpm. If HR already slow, or if esmolol alone does not satisfactorily control BP, administer SNP 0.1-2 μg/kg/min to desired effect.	the aneurysm and makes the clipping easier and less likely to cause inadvertent rupture. If this technique is used, it is essential for the anesthesiologist to ↑BP 20-30% above baseline pressure to maximize collateral flow while the feeding vessel(s) is occluded. Phenylephrine is preferred because it has minimal dysrhythmogenic potential. If it becomes necessary to ↓BP, use esmolol and/or SNP. Responses to vasoactive drugs are much easier to regulate if a normal blood volume has been established and maintained throughout the anesthetic period.
Positioning	For most aneurysms: Supine, head turned Three-point fixation (beware of marked ↑BP with use of pins). Use shoulder roll. ✓ and pad pressure points. ✓ eyes.	Anesthetic gas hoses and all monitoring and vascular catheter lines are directed to patient's side or feet, where the anesthesiologist is positioned during surgery. Antiembolism stockings and SCDs used to minimize DVT. Shoulder roll to ↓brachial plexus stretch. Remifentanil (2-4 μg/kg) to minimize ↑BP during skull pinning.
Complications	Hypothermia (mild)	Many patients can be extubated safely at core T > 35°C with active rewarming.

POSTOPERATIVE

Complications	Intracranial hemorrhage Stroke Cerebral vasospasm	If any of these complications occur, it is likely that the patient's trachea will have to be reintubated and the patient transported to CT scanner for further neurological evaluation or possible reoperation.
Pain management	Meperidine (10-20 mg iv prn) Codeine (30-60 mg im q 4 h prn)	Meperidine will ↓ postop shivering.
Tests	CT scan, if any change in neurological status	

References

1. Brazenor GA, Chamberlain MJ, Gelb AW: Systemic hypovolemia after subarachnoid hemorrhage. *J Neurosurg Anesthesiol* 1990; 2:42-9.
2. Chang SD, Steinberg GK: Management of intracranial aneurysm. *Vascular Medicine* 1998; 3:315-26.
3. Cully MD, Larson CP Jr, Silverberg GD: Hetastarch coagulopathy in a neurosurgical patient. *Anesthesiology* 1987; 66(5): 706-7.
4. Dangor AA, Lam AM: Anesthesia for cerebral aneurysm surgery. *Neurosurg Clin North Am* 1998; 9:647-59.
5. Dodd RL, Steinberg GK: Aneurysms. *Encyclopedia of the Neurological Sciences*. Academic Press, San Diego: 2003 (in press).
6. Drake CG, Peerless SJ, Ferguson GG: Hunterian proximal arterial occlusion for giant aneurysms of the carotid circulation. *J Neurosurg* 1994; 81:656-65.
7. Hartung J, Cottrell JE: Nitrous oxide reduces STP-induced prolongation of survival in hypoxic and anoxic mice. *Anesth Analg* 1987; 66(1):47-52.
8. Lopez JR, Chang SD, Steinberg GK: The use of electrophysiological monitoring in the intraoperative management of intracranial aneurysms. *J Neurol Neurosurg Psychiatry* 1999; 66:189-96.
9. Maier CM, Steinberg GK, eds: *Hypothermia and Cerebral Ischemia: Mechanisms and Clinical Applications*. Humana Press. Totowa NJ: 2003 (in press).
10. Mayer SA, LiMandri G, Sherman D, Lennihan L, Fink ME, Solomon RA, DiTullio M, Klebanoff LM, Beckford AR, Homma S: Electrocardiographic markers of abnormal left ventricular wall motion in acute subarachnoid hemorrhage. *J Neurosurg* 1995; 83:889-96.
11. Mayer SA, Lin J, Homma S, Soloman RA, Lennihan L, Sherman D, Fink ME, Beckford A, Klebanoff LM: Myocardial injury and left ventricular performance after subarachnoid hemorrhage. *Stroke* 1999; 30:780-6.
12. Molyneux A, et al: International Subarachnoid Aneurysm Trial (ISAT) of neurosurgical clipping versus endovascular coiling in 2143 patients with ruptured intracranial aneurysms: a randomized trial. *Lancet* 2002; 360(9342):1267-74.

13. Ojemann RG, Ogilvy CS, Heros RC, Crowell RM: *Surgical Management of Cerebrovascular Disease*. Williams & Wilkins, Baltimore: 1995.
14. Samson DS, Batjer HH: *Intracranial Aneurysm Surgery: Techniques*. Futura Publishing Co, Mount Kisco: 1990.
15. Schmidek HH, Sweet WH, eds: *Operative Neurosurgical Techniques: Indications, Methods, and Results*, Vols I-II. WB Saunders, Philadelphia: 2000.
16. Steinberg GK, Drake CG, Peerless SJ: Deliberate basilar or vertebral artery occlusion in the treatment of intracranial aneurysms. Immediate results and long-term outcome in 201 patients. *J Neurosurg* 1993; 79:161-73.
17. Sundt TM Jr: *Surgical Techniques for Saccular and Giant Intracranial Aneurysms*. Williams & Wilkins, Baltimore: 1990.
18. Weir B: *Aneurysms Affecting the Nervous System*. Williams & Wilkins, Baltimore: 1987.
19. Warner DS, Zhou JG, Ramani R, Todd MM, McAllister A: Nitrous oxide does not alter infarct volume in rats undergoing reversible middle cerebral artery occlusion. *Anesthesiology* 1990; 73(4):686-93.
20. Wilkins RH, Rengachary SS, eds: *Neurosurgery*, Vols 1-3. McGraw-Hill, New York: 1996.
21. Youmans JR, ed: *Neurological Surgery*, Vols 1-6. WB Saunders, Philadelphia: 1996.

ANESTHETIC CONSIDERATIONS FOR CRANIOTOMY FOR GIANT INTRACRANIAL ANEURYSMS

(Requiring deep hypothermic circulatory arrest)

PREOPERATIVE

Aneurysms are classified as 'giant' when they are > 2.5 cm in diameter. These giant aneurysms represent ~5% of all aneurysms. They occur twice as often in women, usually become symptomatic in the 4th or 5th decade of life, and present particularly difficult surgical challenges:[5] (1) their large size makes direct visualization of the vascular anatomy difficult; (2) vascular branches essential to maintaining flow to normal brain may be an integral part of the giant aneurysm and cannot be included in the clipping without causing permanent neurological injury; (3) standard aneurysm clips may not occlude a large, turgid aneurysm, or may slip or move, once applied; and (4) giant aneurysms may rupture during dissection or clip application, resulting in severe neurological morbidity or mortality. Many of these aneurysms are amenable to coiling or other interventional radiologic techniques. For those requiring craniotomy, a special anesthetic and surgical management, using deep hypothermia to 18°C, achieved with fem-fem CPB and temporary circulatory arrest, is employed.[4] These techniques decompress the aneurysm, making it easier to clip, and protect the brain during circulatory arrest. The duration of cardiac arrest may be as long as 45 min.

Respiratory	None unless patient has Hx of smoking or has sustained pulmonary aspiration as a result of a neurological deficit from an intracranial hemorrhage. **Tests:** As indicated from H&P.
Cardiovascular	Generally, these patients do not have other cardiovascular diseases. (See Anesthetic Considerations for Intracranial Aneurysms, p. 6.) **Tests:** ECG; others as indicated from H&P.
Neurological	These patients usually present with complaints of intermittent or persistent headaches or visual disturbances that are probably due to aneurysmal compression of adjacent neural tissue or ↑ICP. If an intracranial hemorrhage occurs, neurological dysfunction varies, depending on site and extent of the hemorrhage. Cerebral vasospasm is a major complication of intracranial hemorrhage (see discussion in Anesthetic Considerations for Intracranial Aneurysms, p. 6). **Tests:** CT; MRI; angiogram. The anesthesiologist should examine the cerebral angiogram preop to visualize the size and site of aneurysm.
Hematologic	T&C for 6 U PRBCs. **Tests:** Hct; PT; PTT; hemogram; others as indicated from H&P.
Laboratory	Other tests as indicated from H&P.
Premedication	If premedication is desirable, small doses of midazolam (e.g., 1-5 mg) are preferable to opiates. Detailed discussion with patient about the anesthetic plan, with appropriate reassurance, is effective in reducing premedication requirements. Should an intracranial aneurysm leak or rupture in the immediate preop period, it may be difficult to distinguish this event from changes associated with excessive responses to premedication.

INTRAOPERATIVE

Anesthetic technique: GETA. The goals of anesthesia for this procedure are to: (1) provide adequate surgical anesthesia; (2) ↓ intracranial volume (blood and tissue) and optimize working space within the cranial compartment, thereby minimizing the need for surgical retraction of brain tissue; and (3) ↑ tolerance of the brain to ischemia by decreasing $CMRO_2$, which occurs with the use of deep hypothermia, barbiturate therapy, and isovolemic hemodilution.

Induction	STP 10-20 mg/kg or propofol 2-3 mg/kg iv to provide amnesia and ↓ CBV by inducing cerebral vasoconstriction. Fentanyl 7-10 μg/kg iv to provide analgesia for the first hours. Vecuronium 0.15 mg/kg or rocuronium 0.7-1 mg/kg to provide relaxation for intubation and positioning.	
Maintenance	STP 20 mg/kg by continuous infusion, to be completed within 2 h of induction, for a total dose of 30-40 mg/kg, or propofol 100-200 μg/kg/min administered by constant-infusion pump. These doses provide additional amnesia and ↓ CBV and $CMRO_2$. Isoflurane ≤ 1%. N_2O not used because of its potential for reversing the protective effects of STP.[1,4] An additional dose of NMB is administered just prior to the start of CPB.	
Emergence	Because of the length and nature of the operation, and the potential for temporary neurological injury, it is advisable to leave the ETT in place immediately postop, and send patient to the ICU on controlled ventilation. If patient begins to cough, the reflex should be suppressed with opiates, NMBs, and/or LTA sprayed down the ETT. The patient is placed in bed in a 30° head-up position and transported to ICU for overnight monitoring. Supplemental O_2 should be administered and close regulation of BP maintained. Prophylactic antiemetic (e.g., droperidol 0.625 mg or metoclopramide 10 mg, ondansetron 4 mg, or dolasetron 12.5 mg) should be given 30 min before extubation.	
Blood and fluid requirements	IV: 16 ga × 2 NS/LR @ 1-2 ml/kg/h PRBC 4-6 U	Cold NS up to 10 ml/kg, + a volume equal to UO, is administered during surgery.
Isovolemic hemodilution	5% albumin 8 × 250 ml NS 4 × 1000 ml CPD bags	Albumin and NS are placed in a refrigerator at 4°C the night before surgery to be used for cooling during isovolemic hemodilution. After induction of anesthesia, a 2nd arterial or large-vein cannula is placed for removal of blood into CPD bags. Generally, about 1000 ml of blood are removed and replaced with 1 L of cold albumin 5%. This usually → ↓Hct to 22-26%. Frequent intraop Hct checks are appropriate. The withdrawn blood is held at room temperature for reinfusion at the conclusion of operation. In addition, the perfusate from the CPB unit is spun down and packed cells returned to patient.
Control of brain volume (ICP)	Hyperventilate to $PaCO_2$ = 25-30 mmHg. Limit crystalloid < 10 ml/kg + UO. Limit isoflurane ≤ 1%. High-dose STP Mannitol 1 g/kg ± Furosemide 0.3 mg/kg ± Lumbar CSF drainage Dexamethasone 8-12 mg	Ventilation is controlled and TV and RR adjusted such that $PaCO_2$ ranges from 25-30 mmHg. There are several advantages to hypocarbia, including: ↓CBV to provide more surgical working space, thereby lessening need for vigorous retraction of brain tissue; improving regional distribution of CBF by preferentially diverting blood to potentially ischemic areas of the brain; better buffering of brain lactic acid that may form as a result of focal ischemia; and decreasing anesthetic requirement.
Monitoring	Standard monitors (see p. B-1). Temperature = esophageal, bladder and brain surface Arterial line × 1-2 CVP (triple-lumen) line UO	 CVP line is used for infusions of esmolol, SNP, and phenylephrine. Frequent checks are made of Hct, electrolytes, ACT values, before, during, and after CPB. Keep UO > 0.5 ml/kg/hr.
Control of BP	Maintain BP normal-to-20% below normal with esmolol infusion, SNP or propofol.	BP control is critical to successful surgery. ↑BP during induction or prior to CPB will ↑ transmural pressure across the aneurysmal wall and ↑ likelihood of rupture. Prior to

Control of BP, cont.	Phenylephrine	CPB, BP is generally kept to normal-to-20% below normal for patient, using anesthetic agents alone or with an esmolol infusion to ↓HR to a range of 50-60 bpm. If desired level of BP is not achieved with this combination, SNP or propofol infusion may be added. SNP also facilitates both cooling and rewarming because of its vasodilatory effect. If a vasoconstrictor is needed, particularly during CPB while patient is still cold, a pure α-adrenergic stimulant, such as phenylephrine, is preferred because of its minimal dysrhythmogenic potential.
Positioning	Shoulder roll 180° table rotation ✓ and pad pressure points. ✓ eyes. Circuit extension tubes Antiembolism stockings and SCD	Anesthetic gas hoses and all monitoring and vascular catheter lines are directed to patient's feet. Make sure that all will reach the foot of operating table. Antiembolism stockings and SCDs used to minimize DVT.

Deep hypothermia and CPB	Surface cooling:
	  Thermal blanket
	  Ice packs
	  SNP infusion
	
	Heparinization
	
	Rewarming
		Surface cooling is begun as soon as induction is complete, using thermal blankets above and below patient, ice packs and infusion of cold fluids during establishment of isovolemic hemodilution, and infusion of SNP, as tolerated, to induce cutaneous vasodilatation.
		Once the neurosurgeons have exposed the giant aneurysm and determined that it cannot be clipped without resorting to CPB, systemic **heparinization** (load: 300 U/kg; maintenance: 100 U/kg/h) is established, and patient is put on CPB using fem-fem bypass and cooled to ~18°C. During CPB cooling, the heart will usually fibrillate between 22-26°C. Once 18°C is reached, the CPB unit is shut off to deflate the aneurysm; it may be activated and shut off several times during clipping to evaluate adequacy of the surgical occlusion of the aneurysm and to apply additional clips. **Total circulatory arrest time should not exceed 45 min.**
		When clipping is complete, CPB is resumed and **warming** instituted. Partial CPB is continued until normal cardiac rhythm is established, and body temperature reaches ~36°C. Once partial CPB is D/C, patient will tend to cool unless vigorous efforts at warming are continued. Warming the OR and iv fluids, and use of warming lights and Bair-Hugger will facilitate the warming process. ACT analysis is performed to establish that heparin reversal is complete 5-10 min after protamine (1 mg/100 U heparin activity). Blood is sent for clotting studies, and Plts, FFP, and calcium gluconate are administered as needed. Hetastarch 6% is not used in these patients because of its potential for inducing a coagulopathy.[1]

Complications	↓↓BP 2° failure to maintain circulating volume Dysrhythmias 2° ↓K+ from diuresis and cold	

POSTOPERATIVE

Complications	HTN Vasospasm Intracranial hemorrhage, stroke	HTN Rx: esmolol + SNP titrated to effect Vasospasm Rx: fluid-loading

Complications, cont	Hypothermia	Patient should be rewarmed to 36-37°C before terminating CPB.
	Hypervolemia	
	Coagulopathy	✓ coag status.
	DVT	
	Seizures	Sz Rx: Phenytoin (1 g iv slowly to avoid ↓BP)
	PE	★ **NB:** PE incompatible with dextrose-containing solutions.
Pain management	Meperidine (10-20 mg iv prn)	Meperidine minimizes postop shivering.
	Codeine (30-60 mg im q 4 h prn)	
Tests	CT scan	If any question about neurological status arises, a CT scan is performed postop.
	Coag panel	Coagulation studies are needed early postop to assure normal coagulation.

References

1. Cully MD, Larson CP Jr, Silverberg GD: Hetastarch coagulopathy in a neurosurgical patient. *Anesthesiology* 1987; 66(5): 706-7.
2. Hindman BJ, Todd MM, Gelb AW, Loftus CM, Craen RA, Schubert A, Mahla ME, Torner JC: Mild hypothermia as a protective therapy during intracranial aneurysm surgery: a randomized prospective pilot trial. *Neurosurgery* 1999; 44:23-32.
3. Lawton MT, Raudzens PA, Zabramski JM, Spetzler RF: Hypothermic circulation arrest in neurovascular surgery: evolving indications and predictors of patient outcome. *Neurosurgery* 1998; 43:10-20.
4. Silverberg GD: Giant aneurysms: surgical treatment. *Neurol Res* 1984; 6(1-2):57-63.
5. Steinberg GK, Chung M: Giant cerebral aneurysms: Morphology and structural pathology. In *Giant Cerebral Aneurysms*. Olwad IA, Barrow DL, eds. American Association of Neurological Surgeons, Park Ridge: 1995, 1-11.
6. Steinberg GK, Drake CG, Peerless SJ: Deliberate basilar or vertebral artery occlusion in the treatment of intracranial aneurysms: Immediate results and long-term outcome in 201 patients. *J Neurosurg* 1993; 79:161-73.
7. Whittle IR, Dorsch NW, Besser M: Giant intracranial aneurysms: diagnosis, management, and outcome. *Surg Neurol* 1984; 21(3):218-30.
8. Young WL, Lawton MT, Gupta DK, Hashimoto T: Anesthetic management of deep hypothermic circulatory arrest for cerebral aneurysm clipping. *Anesthesiology* 2002; 96:497-503.

CRANIOTOMY FOR CEREBRAL EMBOLECTOMY

SURGICAL CONSIDERATIONS

Gary K. Steinberg and Robert L. Dodd

Description: While intravenous or endovascular intra-arterial thrombolysis is the current standard therapy for intracranial intravascular clots, embolic occlusion of a major intracranial vessel occasionally requires microsurgical embolectomy. In particular, when the embolus is a large atherosclerotic plaque or foreign body (such as a balloon or microcoil from endovascular treatment), surgery may be the treatment of choice. Since cerebral ischemia often proceeds to irreversible infarction before the surgeon can restore blood flow, early diagnosis is of the utmost importance, and several studies have demonstrated that the best results from embolectomy occur when the procedure is performed within 6 h following the onset of a neurologic deficit.

A standard craniotomy is fashioned as previously described for other lesions involving the vasculature at the skull base (see p. 4), and the occluded intracranial artery is exposed using microsurgical techniques. The involved arterial segment is isolated, temporarily occluded with miniature clips, and an arteriotomy is performed to remove the thrombus or embolus (Fig 1.1-2). The arteriotomy is then closed and blood flow reestablished.

Usual preop diagnosis: Stroke; TIA; intracranial arterial occlusion; catheter embolization to intracranial artery

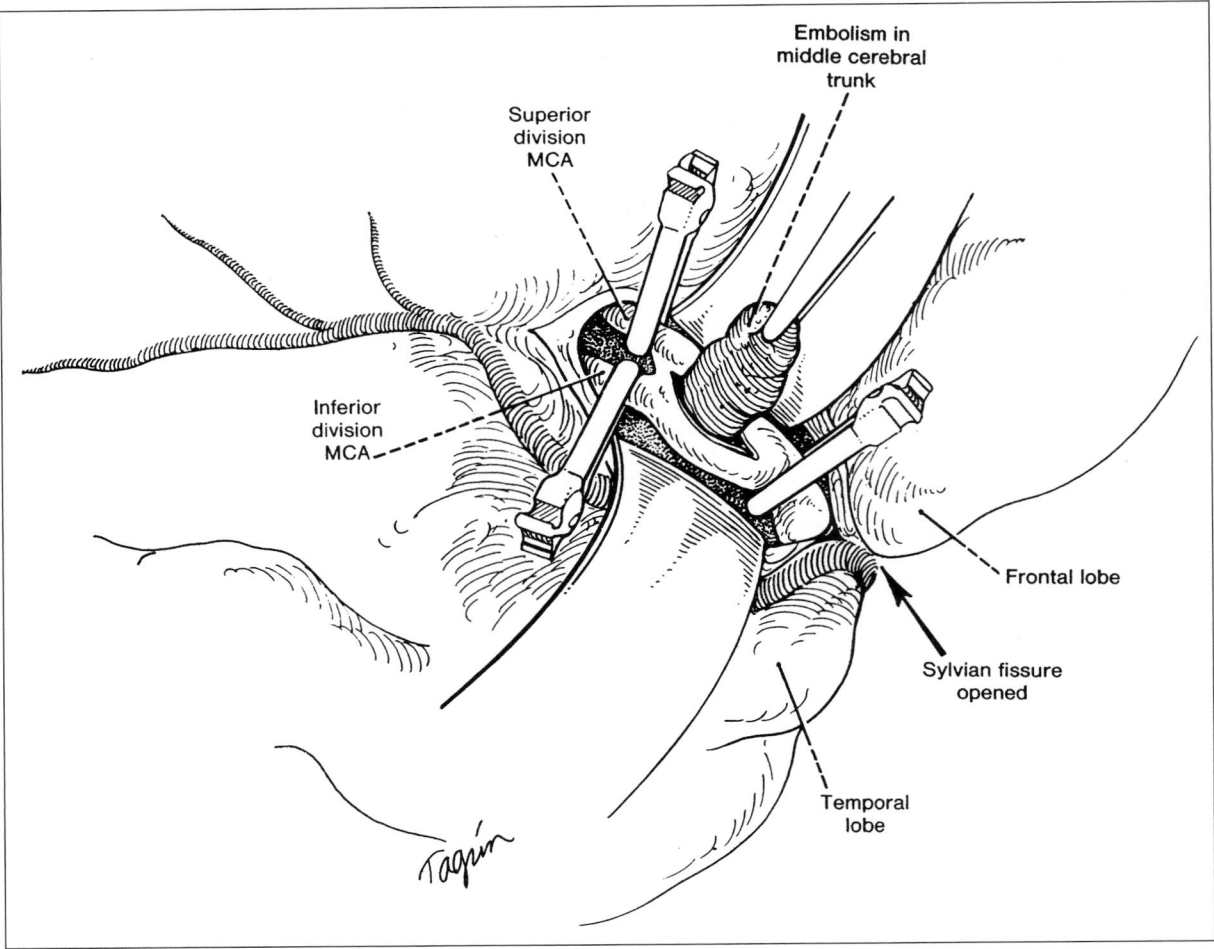

Figure 1.1-2. Middle cerebral artery (MCA) embolectomy. Exposure of right MCA in the sylvian fissure and removal of an embolus from the MI segment. (Reproduced with permission from Ojemann RG, Ogilvy CS, Crowell RM, Heros RC: *Surgical Management of Neurovascular Disease*, 3rd edition. Williams & Wilkins, 1995.)

SUMMARY OF PROCEDURE

Position	Supine or lateral decubitus
Incision	Frontal, temporal, or occipital
Special instrumentation	Microscopic instruments (fine forceps, miniature vascular clips, operating microscope)
Unique considerations	Neuroprotective agents during arterial segment occlusion (barbiturates, mannitol), mild hypothermia (33°C)
Antibiotics	Nafcillin (1-2 g iv q 6 h) + cefotaxime (1 g iv q 6 h)
Surgical time	3-4 h
Closing considerations	Avoid ↓BP (MAP 80-100 mmHg). Induced mild HTN (MAP 90-110) during temporary arterial occlusion.
EBL	100-250 ml
Postop care	Control BP (MAP 80-100 mmHg); start aspirin postop d 1; ICU: 1-2 d.
Mortality	5-10%
Morbidity	Intracerebral hemorrhage
	Stroke
	MI: Rare
	Thromboembolism: Rare
	Respiratory failure: Rare
	Infection: Rare
Pain score	3-4

PATIENT POPULATION CHARACTERISTICS

Age range	50-80 yr
Male:Female	1:1
Incidence	Rare
Etiology	Atherosclerosis; carotid artery disease; atrial fibrillation; iatrogenic endovascular catheter complication
Associated conditions	HTN; CAD; PVD; carotid artery disease; hyperlipidemia; smoking; alcohol abuse; obesity; atrial fibrillation

ANESTHETIC CONSIDERATIONS

See Anesthetic Considerations for Craniotomy for Intracranial Aneurysms, p. 6.

References

1. Gomez CR, Orr SC, Soto RD: Neuroendovascular rescue: interventional treatment of acute ischemic stroke. *Curr Treat Options Cardiovasc Med* 2002; 4:405-19.
2. Kakinuma K, Ezuka I, Takai N, Yamamoto K, and Sasaki O. The simple indicator for revascularization of acute middle cerebral artery occlusion using angiogram and ultra-early embolectomy. *Surg Neurol* 1999; 51:332-41.
3. Ojemann RG, Ogilvy CS, Heros RC, Crowell RM: *Surgical Management of Cerebrovascular Disease*. Williams & Wilkins, Baltimore: 1995.
4. Pikus HJ, Heros RC: Stroke: indications for emergent surgical intervention. *Clin Neurosurg* 1999; 45:113-27.
5. Schmidek HH, Sweet WH, eds: *Operative Neurosurgical Techniques: Indications, Methods, and Results*, Vols I-II. WB Saunders, Philadelphia: 2000.
6. Sundt TM Jr: *Surgical Techniques for Saccular and Giant Intracranial Aneurysms*. Williams & Wilkins, Baltimore: 1990, 467-76.
7. Touho H, Morisako T, Hashimoto Y, Karasawa J: Embolectomy for acute embolic occlusion of the internal carotid artery bifurcation. *Surg Neurol* 1999; 51:313-20.
8. Wilkins RH, Rengachary SS, eds: *Neurosurgery*, Vols 1-3. McGraw-Hill, New York: 1996.
9. Youmans JR, ed: *Neurological Surgery*, Vols 1-6. WB Saunders, Philadelphia: 1996.

CRANIOTOMY FOR INTRACRANIAL VASCULAR MALFORMATIONS

SURGICAL CONSIDERATIONS

Gary K. Steinberg

Description: Intracranial vascular malformations are congenital abnormalities that cause intracranial hemorrhage, seizures, headaches, progressive neurological deficits, or audible bruits. Intracranial vascular malformations comprise high-flow, arteriovenous malformations (AVMs); low-flow, angiographically occult vascular malformations (AOVMs), including cavernous malformations, 'cryptic' AVMs, capillary telangiectasias and transitional malformations; and low-flow, venous angiomas (developmental venous anomalies). **Microsurgical resection** is the optimal treatment for these lesions, although preop endovascular embolization, and preop or postop focused **stereotactic radiosurgery** (heavy particle or photon) may be useful adjuncts.

Most moderate-sized and large **AVMs** (> 3 cm diameter) are resected using a standard **scalp flap** and with **craniotomy** centered over the area of the AVM. The patient is positioned appropriately to place the craniotomy site uppermost in the field and parallel to the floor. For instance, a patient with a left frontal AVM would be positioned supine, head turned to the right, a left frontal or bicranial scalp flap raised and a left frontal craniotomy bone flap removed. A patient with a right medial occipital AVM would be positioned in the left lateral decubitus position with head turned semiprone and a right occipital scalp flap and craniotomy performed. Smaller AVMs (< 3 cm diameter), many low-flow AOVMs, and many deep-seated vascular malformations (AVMs and AOVMs) require a small, **stereotactic craniotomy**. This is performed by attaching a stereotactic base frame to the patient's skull (using local anesthetic and sedation). Next, a CT or MRI scan is obtained, using a radiopaque localizer fixed to the base frame. The location of the AVM in relation to the frame is calculated, using a computer and stereotactic geometric principles. The patient is taken to the OR, intubated fiber optically (because of the frame position), and positioned for surgery. A three-dimensional arc frame is fixed to the base frame, and coordinates are set to localize the vascular malformation within the brain.

In many centers, this traditional approach has been replaced with a **frameless OR surgical navigation system**. With this frameless system, small radiopaque localizers are glued to the scalp, an MRI or CT scan is obtained, and the patient is taken to the OR, anesthetized, and positioned for surgery. The surgical navigation system reference is attached to the headrest and microscope and calibrated. The location of the AVM is calculated, using a computer and stereotactic geometric principles. A small scalp flap and a small craniotomy (a few cm in diameter) can be fashioned precisely for microscopic exposure of the malformation. Microsurgical resection of brain stem and thalamic vascular malformations often necessitate special positioning.

Usual preop diagnosis: Cerebral AVM; dural AVM; cavernous malformation; angiographically occult vascular malformation; intracerebral hemorrhage; subarachnoid hemorrhage; seizures; epilepsy; progressive neurological deficit; migraine or vascular headaches

SUMMARY OF PROCEDURES

	Standard Craniotomy (High-Flow AVM)	Stereotactic Craniotomy (Low-Flow AOVM)	Brain Stem/Thalamic Vascular Malformations
Position	Supine, lateral, Concorde (modified prone) (Fig 1.1-3)	⇐	Lateral, Concorde, or semisitting (Fig 1.1-4)
Incision	Frontal, temporal, parietal, occipital, suboccipital, or combination	⇐	Suboccipital (midline), paramedian or occipital
Special instrumentation	Operating microscope; irrigating bipolar coagulation; radiolucent table and headrest. Sundt mini aneurysm and micro AVM clips. Access to femoral artery for intraop angiography.	⇐ + Surgical navigation system	⇐
Unique considerations	Induced hypotension (MAP 60-65 mmHg) during resection, use of neuroprotective agents (see Craniotomy for Aneurysms, pp. 6-7). Relaxed brain. Mild hypothermia (33°C); ± lumbar CSF drain.	Use of neuroprotective agents and relaxed brain (see Craniotomy for Aneurysms, pp. 6-7).	⇐
Antibiotics	Nafcillin (1-2 g iv q 6 h) + cefotaxime (1 g iv q 6 h)	⇐	⇐
Surgical time	4-10 h	2-5 h	3-6 h
Closing considerations	Maintain MAP 65-75 mmHg. Avoid ↑venous pressure. For supratentorial vascular malformations, administer additional anticonvulsants; give loading dose of phenytoin (1 g iv for adults) if not previously on anticonvulsants.	Keep MAP 70-90 mmHg. ⇐ ⇐	⇐ ⇐ No anticonvulsants necessary
EBL	500-3000 ml	< 250 ml	⇐
Postop care	ICU × 1-2 d. Maintain MAP 65-75 mmHg for 1 d. ICP monitoring, ventricular drain; normovolemic in ICU.	ICU × 1 d; normovolemic in ICU	⇐
Mortality	1-10%, depending on AVM size, location, and venous drainage pattern	< 0.5%	< 2%

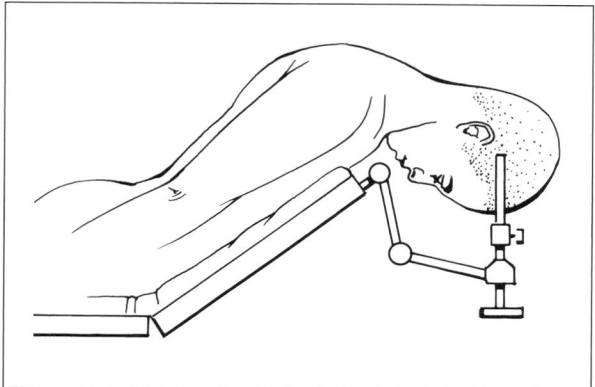

Figure 1.1-3. Concorde (modified prone) position for resection of posterior fossa vascular malformations.

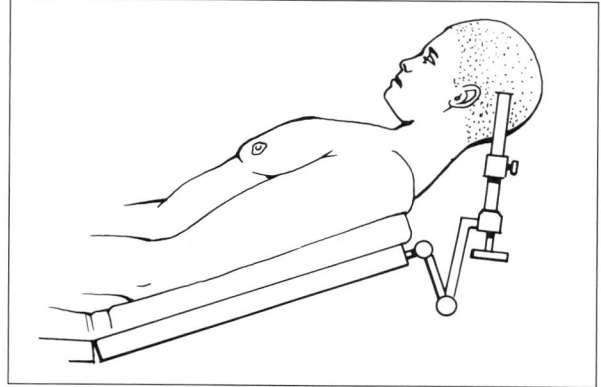

Figure 1.1-4. Semisitting position for resection of deep posterior corpus callosum or thalamic vascular malformations.

	Standard Craniotomy (High-Flow AVM)	Stereotactic Craniotomy (Low-Flow AOVM)	Brain Stem/Thalamic Vascular Malformations
Morbidity	Overall: 5-30%	< 5%	10-50% (transient)
	Neurological	⇐	⇐
	Intracranial hemorrhage	⇐	⇐
	Cerebral edema	⇐	⇐
	Stroke	⇐	⇐
	Hydrocephalus	⇐	⇐
	Massive blood loss: Occasional	⇐	⇐
	Thromboembolism: Rare	⇐	⇐
	Infection: Rare	⇐	⇐
Pain score	3-4	3-4	3-4

PATIENT POPULATION CHARACTERISTICS

Age range	15-40 yr (most common), 41-60 yr (less frequent)
Male:Female	1:1
Incidence	0.5-1% of U.S. population
Etiology	Congenital; traumatic for dural AVM
Associated conditions	Von Hippel-Lindau disease; Rendu-Osler-Weber syndrome; familial cavernous malformation syndrome

ANESTHETIC CONSIDERATIONS

PREOPERATIVE

AVMs are direct arterial-to-venous communications without intervening capillary circulation. With the gross and radiologic appearance of 'a bag of worms,' they can occur anywhere in the brain or spinal cord, varying in size from small lesions called 'cryptic malformations' to very large lesions occupying a major portion of a cerebral hemisphere. Thought to be congenital, AVMs usually do not manifest themselves clinically until patients are in their late teens or 20's. Typically, these patients are otherwise healthy. On histological exam, the vessel walls are thin and lack a muscular layer; consequently, the vessels exhibit loss of normal vasomotor control or responsiveness to changes in $PaCO_2$. Treatment consists of surgical excision, radiologic embolization, or stereotactic radiosurgery, alone or in combination.[14,15] **Stereotactic localization** is essential for safe excision of deep-seated AVMs (e.g. , those located in the corona radiata, basal ganglia, visual center, cerebellar white matter, or corpus callosum).

Respiratory	Not usually significant unless patient has Hx of smoking, or has pulmonary aspiration as a result of a neurological deficit from an intracranial hemorrhage. **Tests:** As indicated from H&P.
Cardiovascular	Generally, these patients do not have other cardiovascular diseases. Occasionally, ECG changes are noted following intracranial hemorrhage and may represent subendocardial injury 2° catecholamine release. **Tests:** ECG; others as indicated from H&P.

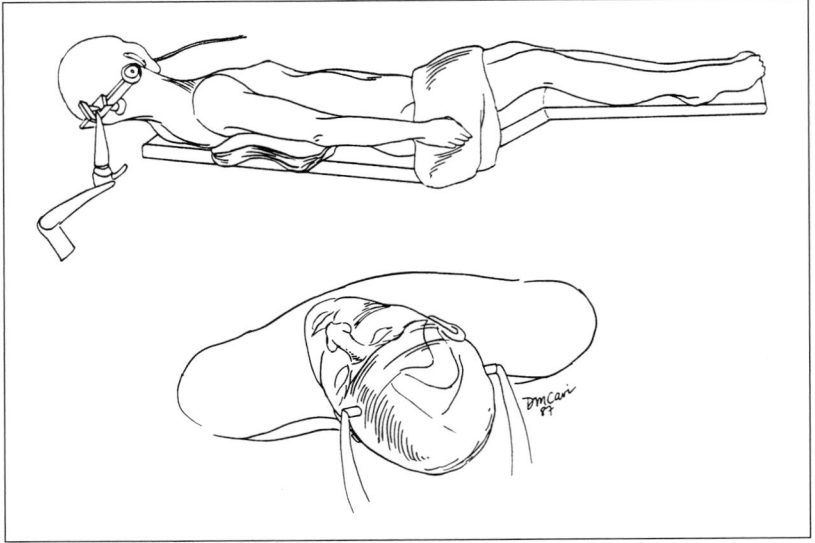

Figure 1.1-5. Supine position, head elevated above heart, turned 30-45° to side, vertex dropped for approach to anterior circulation aneurysms and frontal vascular malformations. (Reproduced with permission from Long DM: *Atlas of Operative Neurosurgical Technique*, Vol 1. Williams & Wilkins: 1989.)

Neurological	Presenting Sx depend on location and size of AVM, and whether it is a low- or high-flow lesion. Hemorrhage with resultant neurological deficit is the most common Sx, although patients also may present with intractable seizure disorder, recurrent HAs, or Sx of cerebral ischemia, including seizures 2° high-flow AV shunts, causing an intracerebral steal. Surgical treatment is essential to prevent future hemorrhage (incidence of 3-4%/yr) and substantial mortality (6-30%) or severe morbidity (15-80%).[17] Unlike hemorrhages from an intracerebral aneurysm (generally intraventricular), hemorrhages from an AVM are usually intraparenchymal; hence, they are seldom associated with cerebral vasospasm. **Tests:** CT; MRI; cerebral angiogram. Preop cerebral angiogram indicates size and location of the AVM, and whether it is likely to be a low- or high-flow lesion.
Hematologic	After surgery for AVM, it is fairly common for surrounding brain tissue to swell and vascular surgery sites to bleed. The cause of this is unknown, but it may be related to diversion of former AVM blood flow into the surrounding vasculature, producing a fragile hyperemic state. Thus, it is advisable to obtain coag studies preop and stage excision over more than one sitting when the AVM is large. **Tests:** Hct; PT; PTT; Plt count
Laboratory	CBC; other tests as indicated from H&P.
Premedication	If medication is desirable, small doses of midazolam (e.g., 1-3 mg iv) are useful. Detailed discussion with patient about the anesthetic plan, with appropriate reassurance, is essential.

INTRAOPERATIVE

Anesthetic technique: GETA. The goals of anesthesia for this operation are to: (1) maintain a somewhat decreased (10-20% below normal) CPP to lessen blood loss during excision of the AVM (CPP = cerebral arterial pressure minus cerebral venous pressure or ICP, whichever is greater); (2) decrease intracranial volume (blood and tissue) to optimize surgical working space within the cranial compartment and minimize the need for surgical retraction of brain tissue; (3) ↓ $CMRO_2$ to lessen the dependence, at least acutely, of normal brain on vessels feeding the AVM. For stereotactic surgery, scalp localizing markers are attached. The patient is then sent to MR or CT, where the exact coordinates defining the AVM and critical adjacent structures are established. The patient is brought to OR and anesthesia is induced.

Induction	STP 2-5 mg/kg or propofol 2-3 mg/kg iv provides amnesia and ↓CBV by inducing cerebral vasoconstriction. Fentanyl 9-10 μg/kg iv provides analgesia for the first hours. High-dose opiates used as a primary anesthetic technique do not alter CBF or $CMRO_2$ enough to provide any special benefits beyond their GA effects. Vecuronium (0.15 mg/kg), rocuronium (0.7-1 mg/kg), or pancuronium (0.1-1 mg/kg), provide muscle relaxation for intubation and patient positioning. If patient is in a stereotactic frame, ET intubation must be accomplished before anesthesia is induced, because the frame partially occludes the mouth, making conventional laryngoscopy impossible. Oral fiber optic intubation of the trachea is the easiest method for accomplishing this.

Maintenance	Isoflurane 1% or less (0.6% maximum if EP monitoring is used) with 1:1 O_2/N_2O. Propofol 75-150 μg/kg/min by continuous infusion may be administered to provide $\downarrow$CBV and $\downarrow$CMRO$_2$. Mild hypothermia (33°C) provides additional cerebral protection (see below). Additional neuromuscular blocking drugs are usually not necessary, but can be administered if patient movement is of concern. A remifentanil infusion (0.05-0.1 μg/kg/min) can be used to supplement the anesthetic without affecting EP monitoring.	
Emergence	With the start of dural closure, consider changing the anesthetic to low-dose sevoflurane (e.g., 0.5%) or low-dose desflurane (e.g., 2%) in 50% N_2O, supplemented with a low-dose remifentanil infusion (e.g., 0.05 μg/kg/min). As recovery from anesthesia occurs, the patient's BP generally will increase in response to the emergence stimuli. Titration of β-adrenergic blocking drugs (e.g., labetalol or esmolol) and/or vasodilators (e.g., SNP) may be needed; if so, the dose should be stabilized before transport to ICU. (See Control of BP, below.) The inhalation agent can be D/C'd at the time of dressing application. Most patients will breathe spontaneously and can be extubated uneventfully while on the remifentanil infusion. If the brain has not been injured by the surgical procedure, the patient should awaken within 10 min after cessation of remifentanil administration. As the patient is awakening, it is important to assure full reversal from neuromuscular blockade and close regulation of BP. If the patient begins to cough on ETT, either it should be removed or cough reflex suppressed with iv lidocaine (0.5-1 mg/kg). Patient is placed in bed in a 30° head-up position and transported to ICU for monitoring overnight. Supplemental O_2 should be administered and close regulation of BP maintained. Prophylactic antiemetics (e.g., droperidol 0.625 mg or metoclopramide 10 mg, ondansetron 4 mg or dolasetron 12.5 mg) should be given 30 min before extubation.	
Blood and fluid requirements	IV: 16 ga × 2 NS/LR @ < 10 ml/kg + UO	If blood volume is normal, NS/LR—not to exceed 10 ml/kg beyond that required to replace UO—is given. If hypovolemic, albumin 5% is given if Hct > 30%; combinations of albumin and blood, if Hct < 30%.
Hypothermia	Thermal blanket Cool air blower (or Polar Air) Cold OR	Mild hypothermia (33°-34°C) is used in some centers for cerebral protection and to $\downarrow$ brain size.[16] CMRO$_2$ decreases ~7% for every degree C decrease in brain T; so at 33°C, cerebral metabolism is decreased about 30% below normal. This level of hypothermia does not interfere appreciably with coagulation, nor is it generally associated with cardiac dysrhythmias. Warming is begun several h before the conclusion of surgery by using a thermal blanket and/or Bair-Hugger, warming inspired gases, and increasing the ambient temperature in OR. Usually by the time the operation is completed, patient T is near normal.
Control of brain volume (ICP)	Hyperventilate to PaCO$_2$ = 25-30 mmHg or PetCO$_2$ = 20-25 mmHg. Limit isoflurane ≤ 1%. Limit fluids.	$\downarrow$PaCO$_2$ has several advantages, including $\downarrow$cerebral vascular volume, which provides surgeons more working space and lessens need for vigorous retraction of brain tissue. $\downarrow$PaCO$_2$ also improves the regional distribution of CBF by: preferentially diverting blood to potentially ischemic areas of the brain; better buffering of the brain lactic acid that may form as a result of focal ischemia; and decreasing anesthetic requirement.
	High-dose STP Mannitol 0.5-1 g/kg Furosemide 0.3 mg/kg Lumbar CSF drainage	If AVM is superficial, decreasing brain volume is less important, and the first 4 techniques listed (at left) are usually sufficient. If AVM is deep, the additional listed therapies may be needed.
Monitoring	Standard monitors (see p. B-1). + Bladder temperature Arterial line CVP line UO	Direct monitoring of arterial pressure before induction is essential for rapid control of BP. Transducer should always be placed at the level of the head rather than the heart, since CPP is arterial pressure at the brain level minus CVP or ICP, whichever is higher. Monitoring CVP via a right atrial catheter is desirable in virtually all patients to assess adequacy of fluid therapy and for infusion of vasoactive drugs. Localization of the catheter can be determined

Monitoring, cont.		by CXR, ECG tracing, noting P-wave changes, or pressure-wave contour and value as the catheter is withdrawn from the right atrium. If patient has a high-flow AVM causing a large AV shunt, venous blood may appear arterialized (or bright red) during central venous catheterization, suggesting that the operator has punctured an artery rather than a central vein.
Control of BP	Isoflurane/sevoflurane Esmolol infusion SNP infusion Maintain normovolemia.	Close regulation of BP during induction and prior to excision of AVMs may be less critical than for aneurysmal surgery.[16] Once surgical excision is under way, however, modest decreases in MAP ($\leq$ 20% below normal) using isoflurane, alone or in combination with esmolol and/or SNP, should be used to prevent excessive bleeding. Responses to vasoactive drugs are much easier to regulate if normal blood volume has been established and maintained throughout the anesthetic period.
Positioning	Shoulder roll 3-point fixation ✓ and pad pressure points. ✓ eyes. 180° rotation Antiembolism stockings, SCDs	For most AVMs, patient is supine, head turned laterally in 3-point fixation, a roll under shoulder on the side of operation (Fig 1.1-5). Anesthetic hoses and all monitoring/vascular catheter lines are directed toward patient's feet or side. Make sure that all will reach the foot of operating table. Antiembolism stockings and SCDs used to minimize DVT. Remifentanil (4-5 μg/kg) to minimize ↑BP during skull pinning.

POSTOPERATIVE

Complications	Neurological deficits Cerebral edema and ↑ICP Intracerebral hemorrhage	If these complications occur, the patient likely will have to be reintubated and transported to the CT scanner for further neurological evaluation or possible reoperation. Careful regulation of BP is essential to avoid postop hemorrhage.
	Seizures	★ Sz Rx: Phenytoin (1 g loading dose). **NB:** Incompatible with dextrose-containing solutions.
Pain management	Meperidine 10-20 mg iv Codeine (30-60 mg im q 4 h prn)	Meperidine minimizes postop shivering.
Tests	CT scan	If neurological status changes.

References

1. Al-Rodhan NR, Sundt TJ, Piepgras DG, Nichols DA, Rufenacht D, Stevens LN: Occlusive hyperemia: a theory for the hemodynamic complications following resection of intracerebral arteriovenous malformations. *J Neurosurg* 1993; 78:167.
2. Berntman L, Welsh FA, Harp JR: Cerebral protective effect of low-grade hypothermia. *Anesthesiology* 1981; 55(5): 495-8.
3. Chang SD, Lopez JR, Steinberg GK: The usefulness of electrophysiologic monitoring during resection of central nervous system vascular malformations. *J Stroke Cerebrovasc Dis* 1999; 8:412-22.
4. Cully MD, Larson CP Jr, Silverberg GD: Hetastarch coagulopathy in a neurosurgical patient. [Letter] *Anesthesiology* 1987; 66(5):706-7.
5. Fleetwood IG, Steinberg GK: Arteriovenous malformations. *Lancet* 2002; 359:863-73.
6. Mohr JP: Arteriovenous malformations of the brain in adults. *N Engl J Med* 1999; 340:1812-18.
7. Ojemann RG, Ogilvy CS, Heros RC, Crowell RM: *Surgical Management of Cerebrovascular Disease.* Williams & Wilkins, Baltimore: 1995.
8. Sano T, Drummond JC, Patel PM, Grafe MR, Watson JC, Cole DJ: A comparison of the cerebral protective effects of isoflurane and mild hypothermia in a model of incomplete forebrain ischemia in the rat. *Anesthesiology* 1992; 76(2):221-8.
9. Schmidek HH, Sweet WH, eds: *Operative Neurosurgical Techniques: Indications, Methods, and Results,* Vols I-II. WB Saunders, Philadelphia: 2000.
10. Smith RM, Stetson JB: Therapeutic hypothermia. *N Engl J Med* 1961; 265:1097-1103, 1147-51.
11. Stein B, Soloman R: Arteriovenous malformations of the brain. In: *Neurological Surgery.* Youmans JR, ed. WB Saunders, Philadelphia: 1990, 1831-63.

12. Steinberg GK, Chang SD: Surgical management of angiographically occult vascular malformations of the brain stem, thalamus and basal ganglia. In: *Neurosurgical Atlas.* Rengachary SS, ed. American Association of Neurological Surgeons, Park Ridge: 1999, 129-33.

13. Steinberg GK, Chang SD, Gerwitz RJ, Lofly JR: Microsurgical resection of brain stem, thalmic and basal ganglia angiographically occult vascular malformation. *Neurosurgery* 2000; 46:260-71.

14. Steinberg GK, Chang SD, Levy RP, Marks MP, Frankel K, Marcellus M: Surgical resection of intracranial arteriovenous malformations following stereotactic radiosurgery. *J Neurosurg* 1966; 84:920-8.

15. Steinberg GK, Marks MP: Intracranial arteriovenous malformations: Therapeutic options. In: *Cerebrovascular Disease,* Batjer HH, ed. Lippincott-Raven Publishers, Philadelphia: 1997; 727-42.

16. Steinberg GK, Stoodley MA: Surgical management of intracranial arteriovenous malformations. In *Operative Neurosurgical Techniques,* 4th edition. Schmidek HH, ed. WB Saunders, Philadelphia: 2000, 1363-91.

17. Steinberg GK, Vanefsky MA: Management of the patient with an angiographically occult vascular malformation. In: *Perspectives in Neurological Surgery,* Hadley MN, ed. Quality Medical Publishing, St. Louis: 1994; 5:18-39.

18. Szabo MD, Crosby G, Sundaram P, Dodson BA, Kjellberg RN: Hypertension does not cause spontaneous hemorrhage of intracranial arteriovenous malformations. *Anesthesiology* 1989; 70(5):761-3.

19. Wilkins RH: Natural history of intracranial vascular malformations: a review. *Neurosurgery* 1985; 16(3):421-30.

20. Wilkins RH, Rengachary SS, eds: *Neurosurgery,* Vols 1-3. McGraw-Hill, New York: 1996.

21. Youmans JR, ed: *Neurological Surgery,* Vols 1-6. WB Saunders, Philadelphia: 1996.

22. Young WL, Kader A, Ornstein E, Baker KZ, Ostapkovich N, Pile-Spellman J, Fogarty-Mack P, Stein BM: Cerebral hyperemia after arteriovenous malformation resection is related to "breakthrough" complications but not to feeding artery pressure. The Columbia University Arteriovenous Malformation Study Project. *Neurosurgery* 1996; 38:1085-95.

CRANIOTOMY FOR EXTRACRANIAL-INTRACRANIAL REVASCULARIZATION (EC-IC BYPASS)

SURGICAL CONSIDERATIONS

Gary K. Steinberg and Robert L. Dodd

Description: Extracranial-intracranial (EC-IC) revascularization procedures are performed when: (1) deliberate occlusion of a major cervical artery (carotid or vertebral) is necessary and inadequate collateral CBF is available; or (2) stenosis or occlusion of major cervical or intracranial arteries causes TIA or stroke, despite the use of maximum medical therapy (aspirin, heparin, or Coumadin). The chief causes of stenosis or occlusion are atherosclerotic disease, radiation injury, and moyamoya disease. The subset of patients who benefit from revascularization are those whose radiographic and metabolism studies demonstrate that they have ↓CBF and poor or absent vascular reserve. The most important surgical considerations include site of stenosis, adequacy of donor graft, and patient age.

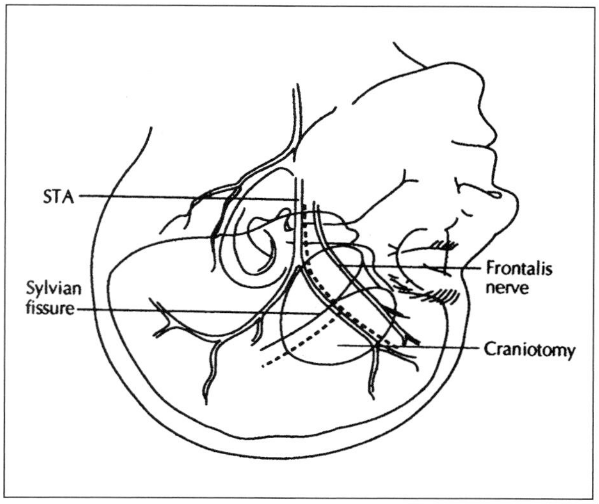

A standard craniotomy is fashioned as previously described for other lesions involving the vasculature around the skull base, and the intracranial site of anastomosis is exposed using microscopic techniques. Typically, a donor extracranial scalp artery is anastomosed to an intracranial artery distal to the site of stenosis. When scalp vessels are inadequate, an interposition vein segment can be sutured

Figure 1.1-6. Typical skin incision for EC-IC bypass. The main incision is planned over the superficial temporal artery (STA) with a Textension to allow exposure of the bone. (Reproduced from Chang SD, Steinberg GK: Superficial temporal artery to middle cerebral artery anastomosis. *Tech Neurosurg* 2000; 6(2):86-100.)

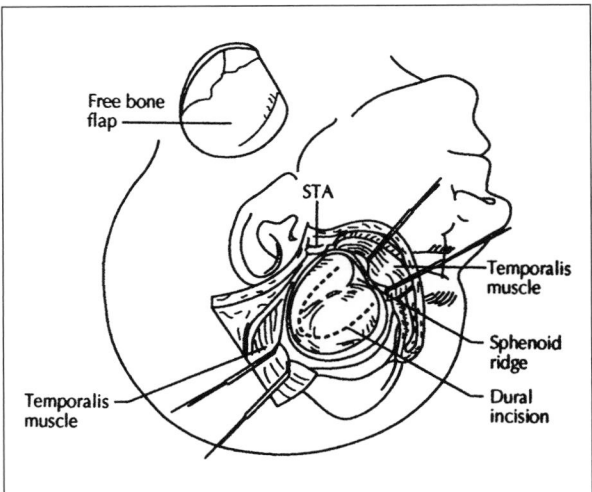

Figure 1.1-7. After the STA is dissected out, the temporalis muscle is divided and the bone flap is made to allow exposure of the brain over the anterior sylvian fissure. (Reproduced from Chang SD, Steinberg GK: Superficial temporal artery to middle cerebral artery anastomosis. *Tech Neurosurg* 2000; 6(2):86-100.)

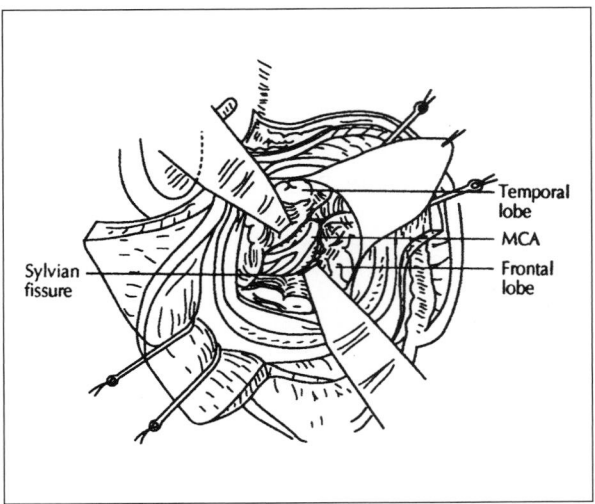

Figure 1.1-8. A middle cerebral artery (MCA) recipient vessel is identified. The sylvian fissure can be split to allow identification of a larger, more proximal branch of the MCA, preferably an M3 branch. (Reproduced from Chang SD, Steinberg GK: Superficial temporal artery to middle cerebral artery anastomosis. *Tech Neurosurg* 2000; 6(2):86-100.)

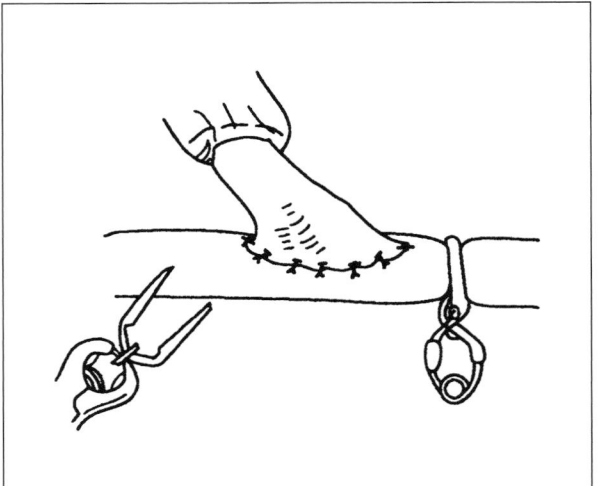

Figure 1.1-9. When the anastomosis is complete, the vascular clips are removed. (Reproduced from Chang SD, Steinberg GK: Superficial temporal artery to middle cerebral artery anastomosis. *Tech Neurosurg* 2000; 6(2):86-100.)

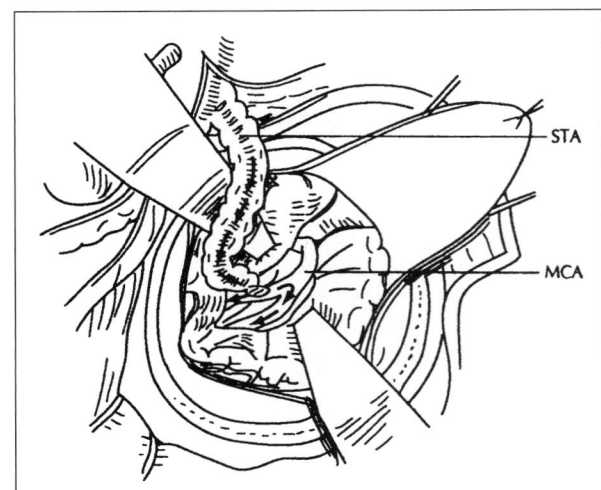

Figure 1.1-10. The completed anastomosis shows the STA positioned such that flow is directed toward the proximal portions of the MCA. (Reproduced from Chang SD, Steinberg GK: Superficial temporal artery to middle cerebral artery anastomosis. *Tech Neurosurg* 2000; 6(2):86-100.)

to a cervical artery and then anastomosed to the designated intracranial artery. The most common EC-IC procedure is a **superficial temporal artery (STA)-to-middle cerebral artery (MCA) branch anastomosis** (See Figs 1.1-6-1.1-10). Other grafts include STA-to-posterior cerebral artery, STA-to-superior cerebellar artery, occipital artery-to-posterior inferior cerebral artery or interposition saphenous vein segment graft from the cervical external carotid artery to the middle cerebral artery, posterior cerebral artery or superior cerebellar artery.

Variant procedure or approaches: Encephalo-duro-arterio-synangiosis (EDAS) is a variant procedure wherein the STA is dissected circumferentially with its adventitia in the scalp, left in continuity and laid on the surface of the brain after opening the dura. **Omentum-to-brain transposition** is another variant, wherein the omentum, with its luxuriant blood supply, is lengthened, left attached to the right gastroepiploic artery, tunneled subcutaneously in the chest and neck, and laid over a large area of poorly vascularized cerebral cortex after opening the dura. Sometimes a free omental graft is transposed to the brain by anastomosing the omental gastroepiploic artery and vein to the superficial temporal artery and vein. Revascularization is induced by angiogenesis factors and growth substances secreted by the omentum.

Usual preop diagnosis: Stroke; TIA; carotid artery stenosis (inaccessible to carotid endarterectomy); carotid artery occlusion; middle cerebral artery stenosis or occlusion; vertebral artery stenosis or occlusion; basilar artery stenosis or occlusion; moyamoya disease (cerebral ischemia due to occlusion of vessels at base of the brain)

SUMMARY OF PROCEDURES

	EC-IC Bypass	EC-IC Bypass With Vein Graft	Omentum-to-Brain Transposition
Position	Supine or lateral decubitus	⇐	⇐
Incision	Frontal, parietal, temporal, occipital, or a combination of these, depending on area to be vascularized.	⇐ + Medial aspect of leg and thigh for harvesting greater saphenous vein	⇐ + Vertical abdominal incision for harvesting omentum; chest/neck incision for tunneling
Special instrumentation	Microscopic instruments; microvascular Doppler to identify scalp donor artery course and confirm graft patency.	⇐ + Tunneling instruments	⇐
Unique considerations	Neuroprotective agents (barbiturates, mannitol) and induced mild HTN (MAP 90-110 mmHg) during cross-clamp of recipient intracranial artery. Avoid excessive brain relaxation. Mild hypothermia (33°C). Dexamethasone 8-12 mg iv.	⇐ + Attention to proper alignment of vein when tunneled, to avoid kinking; heparinization if major cervical artery (carotid, vertebral) is temporarily occluded.	⇐ + Avoid devascularizing omentum during dissection and compromise to omental blood supply during tunneling and skin closure.
Antibiotics	Nafcillin (1-2 g iv q 6 h) + cefotaxime (1 g iv q 6 h)	⇐	⇐
Surgical time	3-5 h	⇐	⇐
Closing considerations	Careful attention to hemostasis. Avoid compromise of graft with dural closure, bone replacement or scalp closure.	⇐	⇐
EBL	< 100 ml	⇐	100-500 ml
Postop care	Start aspirin on POD 1; monitor for subdural hygroma (CSF fluid collection in subdural space); ICU × 1 d.	⇐	⇐
Mortality	< 0.5%	⇐	⇐
Morbidity	Subdural hygroma: Rare	⇐	–
	Wound infection: Rare	⇐	⇐
	Stroke: Rare	⇐	⇐
			Abdominal hernia: Rare
Pain score	3	3	3

PATIENT POPULATION CHARACTERISTICS

Age range	40-80 yr; 2-20 yr for moyamoya disease
Male:Female	1:1 for atherosclerotic disease; 1:1.4 for moyamoya disease
Incidence	Thromboembolic stroke common, but indications for EC-IC bypass rare; 1/million/yr for moyamoya disease
Etiology	Atherosclerosis; embolism from heart or carotid artery
Associated conditions	HTN; CAD; PVD; hyperlipidemia; smoking; alcohol abuse; obesity; moyamoya disease

ANESTHETIC CONSIDERATIONS

PREOPERATIVE

EC-IC bypass is used to make an anastomosis between external (usually superficial temporal artery) and internal carotid circulations. Patients with symptomatic moyamoya disease or bilateral carotid stenosis or occlusion also seem to be good candidates for EC-IC bypass, especially since there are no other forms of therapy which have proven to be effective.

Respiratory	None unless patient has Hx of smoking or has sustained pulmonary aspiration 2° neurological deficit. **Tests:** As indicated from H&P.
Cardiovascular	These patients may have generalized vascular disease, including CAD, so a careful cardiac Hx, physical exam, and ECG analysis should be done. If findings are positive, consider a more complete evaluation, including ECHO and coronary angiography. Be aware that cardiac insufficiency is the cause of about half of the deaths in patients with cerebrovascular disease. **Tests:** Consider ECG, others as indicated from H&P.
Neurological	Patients present with Sx of focal ischemic lesions. Cerebral angiography to r/o other causes of TIAs and characterize collateral circulation. Regional CBF studies generally not helpful because measurement does not distinguish between low flow due to cerebrovascular obstruction from low flow due to low metabolic demands 2° prolonged cerebral ischemia. **Tests:** CT; MRI; angiogram
Hematologic	Anticoagulants or platelet-suppressive drugs (e.g., aspirin) should be D/C'd at least 1 wk before surgery to avoid excessive bleeding. **Tests:** Hct; PT; PTT; hemogram
Laboratory	Tests as indicated from H&P.
Premedication	If medication is desirable, small doses of midazolam (e.g., 1-3 mg iv) are useful. Detailed discussion with patient about the anesthetic plan, with appropriate reassurance, is essential.

INTRAOPERATIVE

Anesthetic technique: GETA. The goals of anesthesia for this procedure are to: (1) provide adequate surgical anesthesia; (2) ↓ intracranial volume (blood and tissue) to optimize working space within the cranial compartment, thereby minimizing the need for surgical retraction of brain tissue; and (3) ↑ tolerance of the brain to ischemia by decreasing $CMRO_2$ with the use of mild hypothermia (33°-34°C) and barbiturate or propofol therapy, and maximizing flow to the ischemic area through collateral channels by maintaining BP at normal or somewhat elevated values.

Induction	STP 2-5 mg/kg (or propofol 1-2 mg/kg iv) to provide amnesia and ↓ cerebral blood volume by inducing cerebral vasoconstriction. Fentanyl 7-10 μg/kg iv to blunt response to intubation and provide analgesia for the first hs of surgery. Pancuronium (0.1 mg/kg), vecuronium 0.15 mg/kg, or rocuronium 0.7-1 mg/kg to provide muscle relaxation for tracheal intubation and positioning patient.
Maintenance	Isoflurane ≤ 1% inspired with O_2/N_2O (≤ 50% N_2O because of its potential for reversing the protective effects of STP for focal ischemia). STP (2-5 mg/kg) or propofol (2-3 mg/kg) is given just before surgical occlusion of the cerebral vessel in preparation for anastomosis. This dose is given over 5-10 min to avoid sudden ↓BP. The concentration of isoflurane is decreased during STP or propofol administration.
Emergence	Generally, ETT can be removed at the conclusion of anesthetic, unless the operation has been particularly long or complex. Prophylactic antiemetic (e.g., metoclopramide 10 mg and ondansetron 4 mg) should be given 30 min before extubation.
Blood and fluid requirements	IV: 18 ga × 2 NS/LR @ < 10 ml/kg + UO CVP (triple-lumen)	CVP with multiple stopcocks for connection of esmolol, SNP, phenylephrine infusions. One lumen is used for monitoring CVP.
Control of brain volume (ICP)	↓fluids < 10 ml/kg + UO STP or propofol infusion ↓isoflurane < 1%, or sevoflurane < 2% Mannitol 0.5-1 g/kg	Generally, vigorous control of brain volume is not necessary since surgeon is working with cerebral vessels on the surface of the brain. If necessary, ventilation is controlled and TV and RR are adjusted such that $PaCO_2$ = ~30 mmHg. Hypocarbia may cause unwanted cerebral vasoconstriction in these patients.

Monitoring	Standard monitors (see p. B-1). ± Bladder temperature Arterial line CVP (triple-lumen catheter) UO	
Control of BP	Maintain normal BP.	Maintenance of normal BP is important because of the dependence of flow on collateral circulation, particularly during temporary occlusion of the surgical vessel being anastomosed. If a vasoconstrictor is needed, a pure α-adrenergic stimulant, such as phenylephrine, is preferred because it has minimal dysrhythmogenic potential. Responses to vasoactive drugs are much easier to regulate if a normal blood volume has been maintained throughout the anesthetic period.
Positioning	✓ and pad pressure points. ✓ eyes. Shoulder roll Antiembolism stockings, SCDs	Anesthetic hoses and monitoring and vascular lines directed to patient's feet where anesthesiologist is positioned during surgery. Used to minimize DVT.
Deliberate hypothermia	Cold-water circulating blanket and cold-air blanket Maintain body temperature of ~33-34°C. Warm OR and iv fluids.	Surface cooling is begun as soon as induction of anesthesia is complete, using a cold-water circulating blanket underneath patient and a cold-air blanket (e.g., Polar Air) above the patient. When anastomosis is nearly complete, vigorous efforts at warming, including warming OR and iv fluids, are initiated.
Complications	Seizures Stroke Hemorrhage at anastomosis	★ Sz Rx: Phenytoin (1 g loading dose). **NB:** Incompatible with dextrose-containing solutions.

POSTOPERATIVE

Complications	Localized scalp necrosis	Major complications uncommon; localized scalp necrosis unique to this procedure.
Pain management	Meperidine (10-20 mg iv prn) Codeine (30-60 mg im q 4 h prn)	
Tests	Cerebral angiogram	Cerebral angiography documents patency of graft and collateral flow.
	Regional blood flow studies	Some centers have the capability of performing regional blood flow studies.
	CT scan	If any question about neurological status, a CT scan is performed.

References

1. Adams HP, Powers WJ, Grubb RL, Clarke WR, Woolson RF (for the Carotid Occlusion Surgery Study): Preview of a new trial of extracranial-to-intracranial arterial anastomosis. *Neurosurg Clin North Am* 2000; 36:613-24.
2. Chang SD, Steinberg GK: Other surgical options for stroke prevention. In: *Cerebrovascular Disease: Pathophysiology, Diagnosis and Management.* Ginsberg M, Bougosslavsky J, eds. Blackwell Science, Cambridge: 1998, 1945–63.
3. Chang SD, Steinberg GK: Superficial temporal artery to middle cerebral artery anastomosis. *Techniques in Neurosurgery* 2000; 6:86-100.
4. Cockcroft KM, Steinberg GK: Cerebral revascularization. In *Principles of Neurosurgery,* 2nd edition. Grossman RG, Loftus CM, eds. Lippincott-Raven, Philadelphia: 1999, 367-84.
5. Firlick AD, Newell DW, Steinberg GK, eds: Cerebral revascularization. *Neurosurg Clin North Am* 2001; 12(3).
6. Ojemann RG, Ogilvy CS, Heros RC, Crowell RM: *Surgical Management of Cerebrovascular Disease.* Williams & Wilkins, Baltimore: 1995.
7. Schmidek HH, Sweet WH, eds: *Operative Neurosurgical Techniques: Indications, Methods, and Results,* Vols I-II. WB Saunders, Philadelphia: 2000.
8. Schmiedek P, Piepgras A, Leinsinger G, Kirsch CM, Einhupl K: Improvement of cerebrovascular reserve capacity by EC-IC arterial bypass surgery in patients with ICA occlusion and hemodynamic cerebral ischemia. *J Neurosurg* 1994; 81:236-44.

9. Steinberg GK, ed: Cerebral revascularization techniques. *Techniques in Neurosurgery* 2000; 6(2).

10. Wilkins RH, Rengachary SS, eds: *Neurosurgery*, Vols 1-3. McGraw-Hill, New York: 1996.

11. Yonekawa Y, Gots Y, Ogata N: Moyamoya disease: diagnosis, treatment and recent achievement. In *Stroke: Pathophysiology, Diagnosis and Management*, 2nd edition. Barnett HJM, Mohr JP, Stein BM, Yabu F, eds. Churchill Livingstone, New York: 1992, 721-47.

12. Youmans JR, ed: *Neurological Surgery*, Vols 1-6. WB Saunders, Philadelphia: 1996.

CRANIOTOMY FOR TUMOR

SURGICAL CONSIDERATIONS

Steven D. Chang and Lawrence M. Shuer

Description: Tumors of the brain fall into various categories, including supratentorial or infratentorial (Table 1.1-2), and intraaxial or extraaxial (Table 1.1-3). The surgical approach depends on the location of the lesion, the need for brain relaxation, and whether exposure will require brain resection. Patient positioning generally depends on the location and surgical approach to the tumor (Table 1.1-4). Once positioned, the patient's head typically is placed in a Mayfield pin fixation system to prevent head movement during surgery.

Several types of incisions are used for these procedures. **Linear incisions** can be used to resect small tumors over the convexity or when using a midline approach to the posterior fossa, and often have the advantage of a more rapid wound closure. **Curvilinear** or **horseshoe-shaped incisions** are commonly used for larger tumors. Once the skull is exposed, burr holes are made with a craniotome and the bone is cut with a cranial saw. Some surgeons routinely use a **free-bone flap**, in which the bone is completely removed and stored for the duration of the case. Other surgeons turn an **osteoplastic flap**, where the bone is left attached to muscle and/or pericranium to keep it partially vascularized. When performing certain posterior fossa resections (e.g., a retromastoid craniotomy or low suboccipital craniotomy), the surgeon may choose to remove the bone without replacement, performing a **craniectomy** instead of a craniotomy. Once the bone is removed, the dura is opened either in a stellate or curvilinear fashion. The method of dural opening generally is based on size of the bone opening and proximity to venous sinuses. The surgeon then proceeds with tumor removal if it is on the surface, or with brain retraction/resection if the tumor is deep to the surface. At this point, the surgeon may request anesthetic interventions for brain relaxation (osmotic diuresis, hyperventilation) and specific BP control (↓BP if bleeding occurs). Once the tumor is removed, hemostasis is achieved and the dura is closed. The bone flap is replaced, and the skin is closed with suture. Patients typically are extubated after cranial surgery, as it is paramount to obtain a neurologic exam as soon after surgery as possible. Patients undergoing a craniotomy almost always require a postop ICU course.

Electrophysiologic monitoring detects changes in SSEP, brain stem auditory evoked potentials (BAEP), and motor cranial nerve EMGs. Such monitoring is commonly used for tumors of the brain stem and skull base, or when resecting tumors in critical locations. Early changes in electrophysiologic monitoring potentials alert the surgeon and anesthesiologist to manipulate BP, and enhance extent of retraction and surgical approach to the tumor to minimize the likelihood of a postop deficit.

Image-guided navigation involves the use of a computerized workstation that can track position of specific instruments before and during the operation. This allows the surgeon to: 1) plan appropriate skin and bone openings, 2) choose an optimal trajectory to the tumor, and 3) achieve a volumetric resection of the tumor. Image-guided navigation involves obtaining a CT or MRI scan prior to the start of the surgical procedure; the time required to obtain this study is usually offset by a shorter operative time.

Mild hypothermia is often utilized when resecting tumors in eloquent areas of the brain, since hypothermia has been shown to provide neuroprotection. **CSF drainage** usually is accomplished by use of a lumbar drain. Lumbar drainage typically is used in common tumors, including cerebellopontine angle tumors, pineal region tumors, or tumors associated with significant edema.

Awake craniotomies typically are reserved for tumors adjacent to or within the receptive or expressive speech areas of the dominant cortex. Patients are sedated during cranial opening, and are awakened once the dura is open. Direct cortical

Table 1.1-2: Common Tumor Location (Supratentorial vs Infratentorial)

Supratentorial	Infratentorial
Metastatic tumors	Metastatic tumors
Astrocytoma/glioblastoma	Acoustic neuromas
Oligodendroglioma	Meningiomas
Ependymoma	Hemangioblastoma
Meningioma	Medulloblastoma
Choroid plexus papilloma	
Craniopharyngioma	
Primitive neuroectodermal tumor	

Table 1.1-3: Intraaxial (Within-the-Brain Parenchyma) vs Extraaxial (Outside-the-Brain Parenchyma)

Intraaxial Tumors	Extraaxial Tumors
Astrocytoma/glioblastoma	Meningioma
Metastatic tumors	Acoustic neuroma
Oligodendroglioma	Choroid plexus papilloma
Ependymoma	
Hemangioblastoma	Craniopharyngioma
Medulloblastoma	
Primitive neuroectodermal tumor	

Table 1.1-4: Common Patient Positions Based on Tumor Location

Supine: Most supratentorial tumors in the frontal, temporal, or anterior parietal lobe. Tumors of the lateral ventricles and third ventricle. Tumors of the anterior two thirds of the interhemispheric fissure.

Lateral: Tumors of the posterior or lateral parietal lobe, posterior temporal lobe, cerebellopontine angle, or lateral cerebellum. Tumors of the posterior ventricular horn.

Prone: Tumors of the occipital lobe, most midline cerebellar tumors, and tumors of the fourth ventricle. Tumors of the posterior one-third interhemispheric fissure and the tentorium.

Sitting: Tumors of the pineal region. Tumors of the fourth ventricle or midline cerebellum.

stimulation is performed to determine the relationship between the tumor and the speech centers. The patient continues to converse during the tumor resection to ensure that surgical resection does not affect language function.

Variant procedure or approaches: Patient position varies depending on tumor location and surgeon preference (Table 1.1-4). Tumors on the convexity, or surface, of the brain may require minimal brain relaxation or exposure. Deep tumors or tumors around the brain stem or skull base, however, may require substantial brain relaxation and retraction for optimal exposure. For deep tumors or tumors within or adjacent to critical structures, the operating microscope is commonly used.

Usual preoperative diagnosis: Glioma; glioblastoma; astrocytoma; oligodendroglioma; ependymoma; primitive neuroectodermal tumor; meningioma; craniopharyngioma; choroid plexus papilloma; hemangioblastomas; medulloblastoma; acoustic neuroma; brain metastasis

SUMMARY OF PROCEDURE

Position	Supine, lateral, prone, or sitting
Incision	Linear or curvilinear, based on location of tumor
Special instrumentation	Operating microscope, laser, CUSA, electrophysiologic monitoring, image-guided navigation, mild hypothermia, CSF drainage, awake craniotomy
Unique considerations	ETT must be taped securely in a location satisfactory to the surgeon; anode or RAE tube is helpful in certain situations. Brain relaxation techniques may be required. The patient with ↑ICP may require special consideration for induction of anesthesia. Awake craniotomy requires special iv anesthesia without ETT tube.
Antibiotics	Nafcillin 2 g iv; cefotaxime 1 g
Surgical time	1-12 hr
Closing considerations	Possible requirement for dural graft. Drain often left in the epidural or subgaleal space. Good BP control during closing and extubation to prevent hemorrhage into tumor resection bed.
EBL	25-500 ml
Postoperative care	ICU or close observation unit × 1-3 d. Fluid and electrolytes require frequent monitoring. BP may need to be controlled with antihypertensives.
Mortality	0-5% (mortality higher for tumors in critical locations)

Morbidity	Infection: 1%
	Neurological: neurologic disability, nerve injury: 0-10%
	Endocrine disorder
	CSF leak: 1-3%
	Venous sinus injury, air embolus
	Massive blood loss
Pain score	2-7

PATIENT POPULATION CHARACTERISTICS

Age range	Infant–85 yr (usually 20-60 yr)
Male:Female	~1:1
Incidence	Common neurosurgical procedure
Etiology	Neoplastic

ANESTHETIC CONSIDERATIONS
(Procedures covered: craniotomy for tumor; craniotomy for skull tumor)

PREOPERATIVE

Typically this is a healthy patient population, apart from Sx attributable to intracranial pathology ($\uparrow$ICP, Sz, HA, N/V, visual disturbances, etc.).

Respiratory	No special considerations, unless indicated from H&P.
Cardiovascular	Benign or malignant brain tumors cause edema formation in adjacent normal brain tissue, which may → $\uparrow$ICP. If ICP increases sufficiently to cause herniation of the brain stem, patients develop the 'Cushing triad' of HTN, bradycardia, and respiratory irregularity. These changes will resolve when ICP is reduced, so vigorous attempts to regulate BP and HR prior to craniotomy are not warranted. Once the diagnosis of brain tumor is made, most patients are placed on high-dose steroid therapy to lessen edema in surrounding normal brain. Steroids are extremely effective in this setting, and Sx of $\uparrow$ICP will often abate.
	Tests: Consider ECG; others as indicated from H&P.
Neurological	Patients may present with complaints of HA, N/V, recent onset of Sz, visual changes, neurological deficits from compression of motor area, or as a result of hemorrhage from the tumor or edema in surrounding normal brain. Document preop physical findings.
	Tests: A CT scan or MRI will delineate the site and size of the tumor, especially if iv contrast material, such as gadolinium, is administered to enhance the margins of the tumor.
Laboratory	Other tests as indicated from H&P.
Premedication	Standard premedication (except for patients with the possibility of $\uparrow$ICP → no sedation).

INTRAOPERATIVE

Anesthetic technique: Small tumors, particularly those located in deeper brain structures, may be localized and resected using stereotactic or image-guidance techniques. Generally, scalp markers or a stereotactic frame are placed on patient's head; then patient is taken to CT/MR for determination of the exact tumor site. GETA is almost invariably used for tumor removal, although MAC is used on rare occasions when the surgeon needs to assess motor or sensory function during resection of tumor adjacent to critical motor or speech areas.

Induction	If patient is in a stereotactic frame, or a difficult intubation is anticipated, orotracheal intubation will need to be accomplished before induction of GA. Awake fiber optic intubation (see p. B-6) is the best choice, since fitting a mask on the face with the stereotactic frame in place is impossible. Once the airway is secured, anesthesia usually is induced with STP (3-5 mg/kg) or propofol (2-3 mg/kg) and fentanyl (3-5 μg/kg), in combination with a NMR (e.g., vecuronium 0.1 mg/kg or pancuronium 0.1 mg/kg). To minimize $\uparrow\uparrow$BP and $\uparrow\uparrow$ICP with ET intubation, it is important that the patient be well anesthetized (and paralyzed) before undertaking laryngoscopy. Induction doses of STP, propofol, or midazolam may not be sufficient to abolish increases in MAP, CPP and, hence, $\uparrow$ICP associated with laryngoscopy and tracheal intubation. Consider using remifentanil (2-3 μg/kg) as part of the induction technique.

Maintenance	Isoflurane $\leq$ 1% ($\leq$ 0.6% if EP monitoring is used), inspired with O_2. N_2O > 50% is not used because of its potential for reversing the protective effects of STP.[5,15] Propofol (75-100 μg/kg/min) may be used to further $\downarrow$ cerebral blood volume, $\downarrow$ cerebral metabolism, and $\downarrow$ CMRO$_2$. Generally if pancuronium is used, no additional NMBs are needed; however, if movement is of concern, rocuronium 10 μg/kg/min will provide adequate neuromuscular blockade. A remifentanil infusion (0.05-0.1 μg/kg/min) can be used to supplement the anesthetic without interfering with EP monitoring.	
Emergence	With the start of dural closure, consider changing the anesthetic to low-dose sevoflurane (e.g., 0.5%) or low-dose desflurane (e.g., 2%) in 50% N_2O, supplemented with a low-dose remifentanil infusion (e.g., 0.05 μg/kg/min). As recovery from anesthesia occurs, the patient's BP generally will increase in response to the emergence stimuli. Titration of β-adrenergic blocking drugs (e.g., labetalol or esmolol) and/or vasodilators (e.g., SNP) may be needed; if so, the dose should be stabilized before transport to ICU. (See Control of BP, below.) The inhalation agent can be D/C'd at the time of dressing application. Most patients will breathe spontaneously and can be extubated uneventfully while on the remifentanil infusion. If the brain has not been injured by the surgical procedure, the patient should awaken within 10 min after cessation of remifentanil administration. As the patient is awakening, it is important to assure full reversal from neuromuscular blockade and close regulation of BP. If the patient begins to cough on ETT, either it should be removed or cough reflex suppressed with iv lidocaine (0.5-1 mg/kg). Patient is placed in bed in a 30° head-up position and transported to ICU for monitoring overnight. Supplemental O_2 should be administered and close regulation of BP maintained. Prophylactic antiemetics (e.g., metoclopramide 10 mg and ondansetron 4 mg) should be given 30 min before extubation.	
Blood and fluid requirements	IV: 16-18 ga × 2 NS/LR @ 2-3 ml/kg/h	Brain tumors (e.g., meningioma) can be highly vascular. To minimize postop cerebral edema, limit NS/LR to $\leq$ 10 ml/kg + replacement of UO. If volume is needed, administer albumin 5% as required.
Monitoring	Standard monitors (see p. B-1). Arterial line CVP line UO ± Doppler ± BAER, SSEP	If the tumor is in the posterior fossa and patient is in the seated position, a Doppler precordial monitor is necessary.
Positioning	✓ and pad pressure points. ✓ eyes.	For brain tumors in the frontal, parietal, or temporal lobes, patient will be supine with head in Mayfield-Kees skeletal fixation, turned to the side and a roll under the shoulder on the operative side (Fig 1.1-5). For occipital or posterior fossa tumors, patient may be prone or, occasionally, sitting (see Anesthetic Considerations for Cervical Neurosurgical Procedures, Positioning, p. 85). Acoustic neuromas are generally most easily removed with patient in the lateral ('park-bench') position with a roll under the axilla. Patient generally lies on a bean bag which, when aspirated, holds her/him firmly in the lateral position.
Control of ICP	Control BP & CVP = low normal. PaO_2 > 100 mmHg $\downarrow$ fluids < 10 ml/kg + UO $\downarrow$ isoflurane < 1%, or sevoflurane < 2% Steroids Hyperventilate to $PaCO_2$ = 25-30 mm Hg ($PetCO_2$ = 20-25 mmHg). Mannitol 0.5-1 g/kg ± Furosemide 0.3 mg/kg	Patients with intracranial tumors may be on the steep portion of the intracranial compliance curve such that any increase in intracranial volume may → ↑↑ICP. Transient increases in ICP—even up to 50-60 mmHg—are tolerated, provided they are promptly terminated. Sustained increases in ICP > 25-30 mmHg are associated with severe neurologic injury and poor outcome. $\downarrow PaCO_2$ → $\downarrow$ CBV (providing better surgical access) + ↑CBF to ischemic areas ('Robin Hood' effect) + $\downarrow$ anesthetic requirements + ↑lactic acid buffering. Mannitol/furosemide → $\downarrow K^+$; monitor level and replace as necessary. If mannitol is administered too rapidly, profound

Control of ICP, cont.	± Lumbar CSF drain Head up 20-30°	↓BP will occur, probably from peripheral vasodilation. CSF drain often placed after induction of anesthesia, and may be opened as required to ↓CSF volume and pressure.

POSTOPERATIVE

Complications	Seizures Neurologic deficits Tension pneumocephalus Hemorrhage requiring reexploration Edema and ↑ICP	★ Sz Rx: Phenytoin (1 g loading dose). **NB:** Incompatible with dextrose-containing solutions. In seated position, additional rare, but possible complications include quadriplegia from excessive flexion of head or tension pneumocephalus from air in cerebral cavities. Severe tension pneumocephalus may delay emergence from anesthesia or cause postop neurologic deficits.
Pain management	Meperidine (10-20 mg iv prn) Codeine (30-60 mg im q 4 h)	Meperidine minimizes postop shivering.
Tests	CT scan	If patient exhibits any delay in emergence from anesthesia and surgery, or any new neurologic deficits emerge postop, a CT scan is invariably obtained.

References

1. Apuzzo MLJ: *Brain Surgery: Complication, Avoidance and Management.* Churchill Livingstone, New York: 1993, 175-688.
2. Black PM: Brain tumors. *N Engl J Med* 1991; 324(21):1471-6, 1555-64.
3. Chang SD, Lopez JR, Steinberg GK: Intraoperative electrical stimulation for identification of cranial nerve nuclei. *Muscle Nerve* 1999; 22:1538-43.
4. Djuric S, Milenkovic Z, Klopcic-Spevak M, Spasic M: Somatosensory evoked potential monitoring during intracranial surgery. *Acta Neurochir* (Wein) 1992; 119:85-90.
5. Domaingue CM, Nye DH: Hypotensive effect of mannitol administered rapidly. *Anaesth Intensive Care* 1985; 13(2):134-6.
6. Domino KB, Hemstad JR, Lam AM, Laohaprasit V, Hamberg TA, Harrison SD, Grady MS, Winn HR: Effect of nitrous oxide on intracranial pressure after cranial-dural closure in patients undergoing craniotomy. *Anesthesiology* 1992; 77(3):421-5.
7. Eng C, Lam AM, Mayberg TS, Lee C, Mathisen T: The influence of propofol with and without nitrous oxide on cerebral blood flow velocity and CO_2 reactivity in humans. *Anesthesiology* 1992; 77(5):872-9.
8. Grady RE, Horlocker TT, Brown RD, Maxson PM, Schroeder DR: Neurologic complications after placement of cerebrospinal fluid drainage catheters and needles in anesthetized patients: implications for regional anesthesia. Mayo Perioperative Outcomes Group. *Anesth Analg* 1999; 88:388-92.
9. Grosslight KR, Foster R, Colohan AR, Bedford RF: Isoflurane for neuroanesthesia: risk factors for increases in intracranial pressure. *Anesthesiology* 1985; 63(5):533-6.
10. Guthrie BL, Adler JR, Jr: Computer-assisted preoperative planning, interactive surgery, and frameless stereotaxy. *Clin Neurosurg* 1992; 38:112-31.
11. Hoffman WE, Edelman G, Kochs E, Werner C, Segil L, Albrecht RF: Cerebral autoregulation in awake versus isoflurane-anesthetized rats. *Anesth Analg* 1991; 73(6):753-7.
12. Kochs E, Hoffman WE, Werner C, Thomas C, Albrecht RF, Schulte am Esch J: The effects of propofol on brain electrical activity, neurologic outcome, and neuronal damage following incomplete ischemia in rats. *Anesthesiology* 1992; 76(2): 245-52.
13. Kondziolka D, Lunsford LD: Intraoperative navigation during resection of brain metastases. *Neurosurg Clin North Am* 1996; 77:267-77.
14. Manninen PH, Raman SK, Boyle K, el-Beheiry H: Early postoperative complications following neurosurgical procedures. *Can J Anaesth* 1999; 46:7-14.
15. Milde LN, Milde JH, Lanier WL, Michenfelder JD: Comparison of the effects of isoflurane and STP on neurologic outcome and neuropathology after temporary focal cerebral ischemia in primates. *Anesthesiology* 1988; 69(6):905-13.
16. Minton MD, Grosslight KR, Stirt JA, Bedford RF: Increases in intracranial pressure from succinylcholine: prevention by prior nondepolarizing blockade. *Anesthesiology* 1986; 65(2):165-9.
17. Pinaud M, Lelausque JN, Chetanneau A, Fauchoux N, Menegalli D, Souron R: Effects of propofol on cerebral hemodynamics and metabolism in patients with brain trauma. *Anesthesiology* 1990; 73(3):404-9.
18. Pollock BE: Management of patients with multiple brain metastases. *Contemp Neurosurg* 1999; 21:1-6.
19. Steinberg GK, Grant G, Yoon EJ: Deliberate hypothermia. In *Intraoperative Neuroprotection*, Andrews RJ, ed, Williams and Wilkins: Baltimore: 1996, 65-84.
20. Van Hemelrijck J, Fitch W, Mattheussen M, Van Aken H, Plets C, Lauwers T: Effect of propofol on cerebral circulation and autoregulation in the baboon. *Anesth Analg* 1990; 71(1):49-54.
21. Zakhary R, Keles GE, Berger MS: Intraoperative imaging techniques in the treatment of brain tumors. *Curr Opin Oncol* 1999; 11:152-6.

CRANIOTOMY FOR SKULL TUMOR

SURGICAL CONSIDERATIONS

Gordon T. Sakamoto, Lawrence M. Shuer, and Steven D. Chang

Description: Tumors of the skull fall into the classification of other bony tumors. Examples of types of skull tumors often requiring surgery include eosinophilic granuloma, histiocytosis, hemangioma, osteoma, epidermoid, dermoid tumor, metastatic tumors, osteosarcoma, fibrous dysplasia, and meningioma. They may occur anywhere on the skull. The exact positioning of the patient depends on the location of tumor. For example, the sitting position often is used for tumors in the occipital or suboccipital regions and the supine position is used for frontal, temporal, or parietal tumors. Some surgeons prefer the lateral position for temporal or parietal bone lesions and the prone position for occipital and some suboccipital bone lesions. The patient's head is placed in a head holder (either pins, suction cup, horseshoe, or Shea headrest). The bone usually is removed by creating burr hole(s) and then cutting a flap with the neuro bone saw. In the suboccipital or posterior fossa craniotomy, the bone often is removed piecemeal with either a drill or a series of rongeurs. The dura usually is not opened unless it is involved with the tumor. The surgeon may elect to perform a **cranioplasty** to cover the defect, depending on size and location of the bone defect. The defect can be repaired using methylmethacrylate at the time of surgery, or bone may be harvested from either another location on the skull or another site (hip or rib) for reconstruction. Once the reconstruction is completed, the skin incision is closed. Occasionally, the tumor of the skull will be approached intracranially, if its location favors that approach. Examples include tumors of the petrous portion of the temporal bone or fibrous dysplasia involving the optic canal.

Usual preop diagnosis: Eosinophilic granuloma; histiocytosis; hemangioma; osteoma; epidermoid; dermoid tumor; metastatic tumors; osteosarcoma; fibrous dysplasia; meningioma

SUMMARY OF PROCEDURE

Position	Supine, lateral, prone, or sitting
Incision	Dependent on location of tumor
Special instrumentation	Neuro drill
Unique considerations	ETT must be taped securely in a location satisfactory to the surgeon. Anode or RAE tube may be helpful in certain situations.
Antibiotics	Cefazolin 1 g iv
Surgical time	1-4 h
Closing considerations	Drain often left in epidural space. Surgeon often requests control of BP to avoid hemorrhage into the bed of tumor.
EBL	25-500 ml
Postop care	ICU or close observation unit
Mortality	0-2% (higher for tumors in critical locations)
Morbidity	Usually < 5%:
	Infection
	Neurological disability
	CSF leak
	Massive blood loss—venous sinus injury
Pain score	2-5

PATIENT POPULATION CHARACTERISTICS

Age range	Infant–85 yr (usually 20-60 yr)
Male:Female	~1:1
Incidence	Unknown
Etiology	Neoplastic

ANESTHETIC CONSIDERATIONS

See Anesthetic Considerations following Craniotomy for Tumor, p. 28. Note, however, that patients with skull tumors rarely have problems with ICP.

Reference

1. Sawaya RE, Kroll S, Wecht DA, Ligon BL: Tumors of the scalp and skull. In *The Practice of Neurosurgery*. Tindall GT, Cooper PR, Barrow DL, eds. Williams & Wilkins, Baltimore: 1996, 1371-84.

CRANIOTOMY FOR TRAUMA

SURGICAL CONSIDERATIONS

Gordon T. Sakamoto, Lawrence M. Shuer, and Steven D. Chang

Description: Head injuries occasionally require emergent surgical procedures to evacuate mass lesions or debride contused or contaminated brain. The majority of these injuries are supratentorial. The surgical procedure depends on the exact type and location of the injury (e.g., epidural, subdural, intracerebral hematomas, or depressed skull fracture); however, most traumatic injuries can be addressed through a wide frontotemporiparietal craniotomy. Often the entire head is shaved and placed in a headrest (pins, suction cups, or horseshoe). If the C-spine has not been cleared, the patient may be placed in a lateral position to minimize neck involvement. For a standard trauma craniotomy, the scalp incision starts anterior to the tragus and continues superiorly in a question-mark type path, ending in the frontal area (Fig 1.1-11). This incision can be modified according to the location and extent of the injury. The skin is reflected and the skull is perforated with a cranial drill. If the patient's condition deteriorates rapidly, the temporal burr hole can be enlarged quickly to a craniectomy for decompression before continuing with the craniotomy. A chronic, subdural hematoma may be drained through burr holes. If there is a clot, depressed fracture, or penetrating wound, a formal bone flap is elevated. Wide exposure is used to visualize and control sources of bleeding. Mass lesions and associated contused brain parenchyma are identified and removed (Fig 1.1-12). For penetrating head injuries or depressed skull fractures, the wound is debrided, foreign bodies are removed, bleeding is controlled, and the dura is repaired if lacerated. Depending on the injury and the presence of brain swelling, it may be necessary to close the dura with pericranium, fascia lata, or bovine pericardium. Additionally, the bone flap may be left out to compensate for brain swelling and replaced later. A subgaleal drain may be inserted and brought out through a separate incision. An ICP monitor may be placed at the end of the procedure.

Usual preop diagnosis: Epidural hematoma; subdural hematoma; intracerebral hematoma; depressed skull fracture; cerebral contusions; gunshot wound of the brain

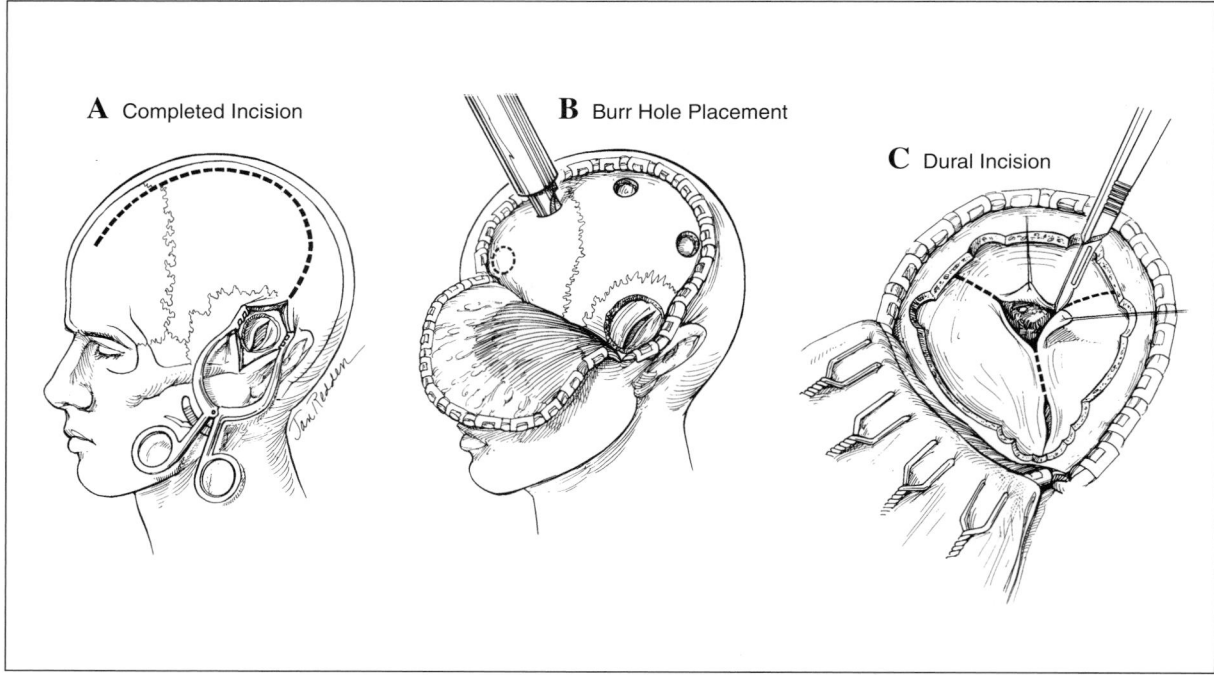

Figure 1.1-11. In an acute subdural hematoma: (A) A burr hole is made, followed by craniectomy, and the incision is extended upward to form a large question mark, the medial extent of which follows the midline. (B) Additional burr holes are made, with the medial ones 1.5 cm off the midline to avoid injury to the major venous structures and granulations. The anterior burr hole is placed above the frontal sinus (the size of which can be estimated from preop radiographs). (C) The dura can be opened with a Y- or X-shaped incision, with a flap being based on the superior sagittal sinus. (Reproduced with permission from Grossman RG, Loftus CM: *Principles of Neurosurgery*, 2nd edition. Lippincott-Raven, 1999.)

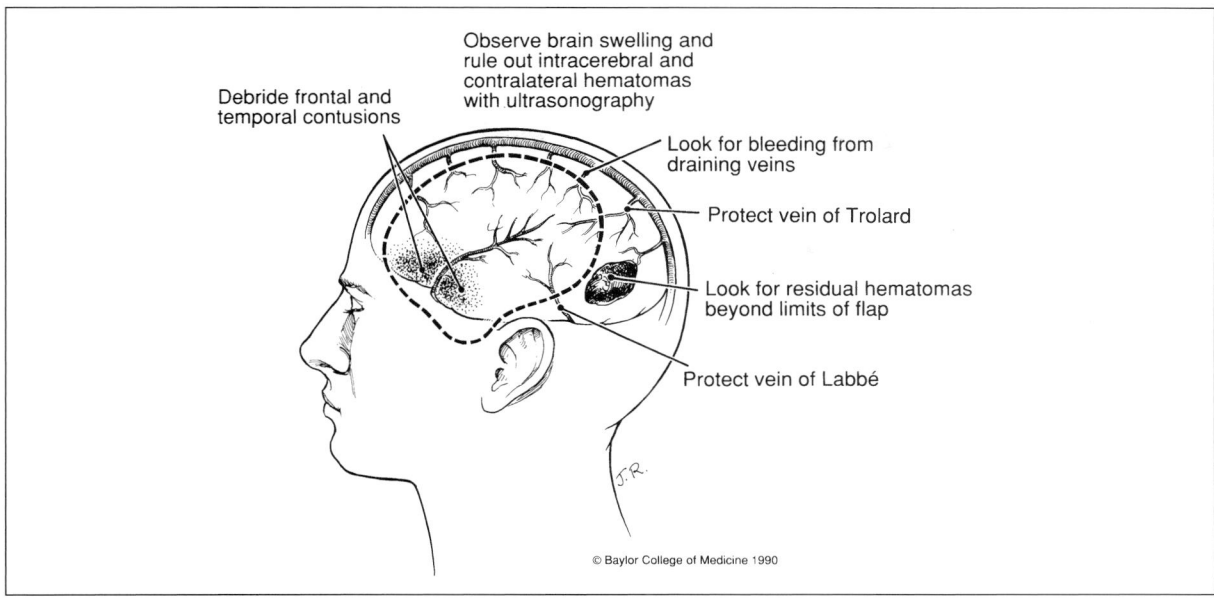

Figure 1.1-12. Precautions to be taken during a craniotomy for subdural hematoma. (Reproduced with permission from Grossman RG, Loftus CM: *Principles of Neurosurgery*, 2nd edition. Lippincott-Raven, 1999.)

SUMMARY OF PROCEDURE

Position	Supine, lateral, prone, or sitting, depending on site of injury
Incision	Varies with location of injury (typical incision shown in Fig 1.1-11)
Unique considerations	The patient may have ↑↑ICP. Because incipient herniation and/or associated injuries may be a concern, timing is critical. C-spine precautions may be necessary.
Antibiotics	Nafcillin 1-2 g iv + cefotaxime 1 g iv
Surgical time	1.5-6 h
Closing considerations	Application of head dressing may jostle ETT at end of case → ↑BP. Patient may stay intubated postop. ICP monitor may be placed. Phenytoin may be given for seizure prophylaxis.
EBL	25-500 ml
Postop care	ICU or close observation unit until stable. Fluid and electrolytes require frequent monitoring, as the patient may develop SIADH. BP may need to be controlled with vasodilator and β-blocker infusions.
Mortality	10-50%, depending on lesion; higher for acute subdural hematomas, lower for epidural hematomas.
Morbidity	Morbidity depends on lesion; morbidity from craniotomy itself is low.
	Infection
	Neurologic disability
	Nerve injury
	CSF leak
	Endocrine disorders:
	SIADH
	Panhypopituitarism
	Diabetes insipidus (DI)
	Massive blood loss: venous sinus injury
Pain score	2-4

PATIENT POPULATION CHARACTERISTICS

Age range	Infant–85 yr (usually 15-40 yr)
Male:Female	2:1
Incidence	Relatively common
Etiology	Trauma
Associated conditions	Abdominal injuries; C-spine fractures

ANESTHETIC CONSIDERATIONS

PREOPERATIVE

Head injury is the leading cause of death of persons < 24 yr old.[3] A penetrating injury of the skull usually will cause major damage to the brain as a result of diffuse neuronal injury and hemorrhage into brain tissue. Surgery is necessary to control intracranial bleeding, to debride the wound, and to remove bone fragments, foreign material, and damaged brain so that the cranial vault can better accommodate the brain swelling that inevitably occurs. Head injury also can be focal in nature, most commonly in the form of an epidural, subdural, or intracranial hematoma. Epidural hematomas form between the skull and dura, and are usually due to bleeding from an artery (e.g., anterior cerebral or middle meningeal). Hence, time is of the essence and rapid evacuation and control of the bleeding is essential if permanent neurological injury is to be avoided. Subdural bleeding occurs between the dura and the leptomeninges lining the brain surface. This bleeding is usually venous in origin, and usually occurs more gradually. Focal intracranial hemorrhages may be either arterial or venous, and, as with subdural hematomas, must be evacuated if they are enlarging.

Respiratory

Localized injuries to the frontal or parietal lobes may not cause any respiratory changes. If ↑ICP, respirations may become slow (< 10/min) and deep, and result in substantial hypocapnia. Many patients with head injuries demonstrate partial airway obstruction from the tongue falling back into the posterior pharyngeal space. If this occurs, or if the patient is comatose and unable to protect the airway and prevent aspiration of gastric contents, immediate tracheal intubation should be performed. Head injuries in the region of the occipital lobes may → apnea.
Tests: As indicated from H&P and as time allows.

Cardiovascular

Most patients with head injuries evidence ↑BP and ↑HR. If ICP increases sufficiently to cause herniation of brain stem, patients develop the 'Cushing triad' of ↑BP, ↓HR and irregular respiration. These changes resolve when ↑ICP is relieved, so vigorous attempts to regulate BP prior to craniotomy are not warranted. Patient, however, should be taken to OR as quickly as possible.
Tests: As indicated from H&P, and as time allows.

Neurological

Neurological evaluation of the head-injured patient is based on the Glasgow Coma Scale (Table 1.1-5). The scale involves evaluation of three functions: eye opening, verbal response, and motor response. Using this scoring system, the severity of brain injury may be classified as mild (13-15 points), moderate (9-12 points), or severe (8 points or less). By definition, any patient having 8 points or less is in coma. Additional useful neurological examinations include assessment of pupillary size and reactivity to the light, reflex responses, and evidence of asymmetry or flaccidity of the extremities or decerebrate or decorticate posturing. Head-injured patients whose neurological function is deteriorating rapidly, and in whom an epidural or subdural hemorrhage is suspected, should be taken to OR immediately.
Tests: CT scan

Hematologic

Severe head injury may be associated with a progressively worsening coagulopathy, resulting in a clinical picture similar to that of DIC. The reason for this is not known, but the brain is rich in thromboplastin and other coagulation factors.
Tests: Hct; PT; PTT; others as indicated from H&P.

Laboratory

Other tests as indicated from H&P, and as time permits.

Premedication

Usually none

INTRAOPERATIVE

Anesthetic technique: GETA

Induction

↑ICP is likely in most patients with head injury requiring operation, and induction of anesthesia is best accomplished with drugs that ↓ICP. If patient is hemodynamically stable and not hypovolemic, induction with STP (2-5 mg/kg), propofol (1.5-3 mg/kg), ± fentanyl (2-5 μg/kg) is satisfactory. If hemodynamically unstable, etomidate (0.1-0.4 mg/kg) is suitable for induction. Ketamine is not used because of its ability to ↑ICP. If patient is comatose, anesthetic requirement is less, needing only O_2 and muscle relaxant, or N_2O 60% or low-dose isoflurane (≤ 0.5%) or sevoflurane (< 1%). A nondepolarizing muscle relaxant (vecuronium [0.1 mg/kg] or rocuronium [1 mg/kg]) is administered for ET intubation.[17] Succinylcholine can be used if a 'defasciculating' dose of a nondepolarizing NMB is administered first.[14] Nasotracheal intubation is not recommended for patients with maxillary and/or basilar skull fractures because of the potential for inserting the tube through the fracture site into the brain.

Table 1.1-5. Glasgow Coma Scale (GCS)			
Category	**Score**	**Category**	**Score**
I. Eyes open:		III. Best motor response:	
Never	1	None	1
To pain	2	Extension (decerebrate rigidity)	2
To verbal stimuli	3	Flexion abnormal (decorticate rigidity)	3
Spontaneously	4	Flexion withdrawal	4
		Patient localizes pain	5
II. Best verbal response:		Patient obeys	6
None	1		
Incomprehensible sounds	2		
Inappropriate words	3	I + II + III Total = 3-15	
Patient disoriented and converses	4		
Patient oriented and converses	5		

Induction, cont.	To minimize ↑↑BP and ↑↑ICP with ET intubation, consider remifentanil (2-5 μg/kg iv) 1-2 min before laryngoscopy. In hypovolemic patients, hydration with a mixture of crystalloid and colloid should be initiated prior to induction.
Maintenance	The ideal drug for maintenance of anesthesia decreases ICP and $CMRO_2$, maintains cerebral autoregulation, redistributes flow to potentially ischemic areas, and provides protection for the brain from focal ischemia. STP or propofol meet these criteria and are excellent anesthetics for the head-trauma patient, provided the circulation tolerates these drugs.
	Isoflurane is regarded as the best volatile agent for patients undergoing neurosurgical procedures. Although isoflurane causes dose-dependent increases in CBF and volume and, hence, ↑ICP, these effects tend to be mitigated by the prior administration of STP, hyperventilation, and by limiting the inspired isoflurane concentration to ≤ 1%. At < 1% isoflurane, CBF responses to changes in $PaCO_2$ are maintained, and cerebral autoregulation remains intact.[7] Finally, isoflurane appears to provide protection from incomplete focal ischemia. Sevoflurane (≤ 2%) is also a good choice for maintenance because of its low solubility and, hence, rapid emergence. Its CNS properties appear to be similar to those of isoflurane.
	N_2O may be administered, recognizing that it is a modest cerebrovascular dilator, thereby increasing ICP, an effect that would not be desirable in patients with a space-occupying lesion. Also, N_2O does not appear to provide any cerebral protection in the presence of incomplete focal ischemia,[12] and, in fact, may attenuate the protective effects of STP or isoflurane.[13]
	Generally, no further NMBs are administered beyond that used for tracheal intubation. With adequate anesthesia, and head in Mayfield-Kees skeletal fixation, patient movement of any consequence is highly unlikely. Furthermore, it is useful to see movement of an extremity as an indicator of inadequate depth of anesthesia.
Emergence	Because recovery from head injury is so unpredictable, it is generally advisable to leave the ETT in place and maintain controlled hyperventilation until there is sufficient clinical evidence that normal neurological recovery is occurring. Prophylactic antiemetic (e.g., metoclopramide 10 mg and ondansetron 4 mg) should be given 30-60 min before extubation.
Blood and fluid requirements	Possible marked blood loss IV: 16-18 ga × 1 NS @ 2-4 ml/kg/h ± Albumin	Blood transfusion is often necessary. To minimize postop cerebral edema, total crystalloid volume should be limited to < 10 ml/kg + replacement of UO. Glucose-containing solutions should be avoided; blood glucose levels should be maintained between 80-200 mg%. If volume is needed, albumin 5% should be administered.
Control of blood loss	Low normal BP HR = 50-70	Blood loss is best minimized by maintaining MAP at low normal for that patient. Controlled ↓BP generally is not used unless bleeding becomes profuse and difficult to con-

Control of blood loss, cont.		trol. HR is easily controlled with an esmolol infusion, and if additional ↓MAP is needed, SNP is begun. ↓BP is better treated with volume replacement than vasopressors.
Monitoring	Standard monitors (see p. B-1). ± Arterial line ± CVP line ± UO	For minor head injuries, no special monitoring is needed. If the injury is extensive or unknown, or if the patient is unstable, invasive monitoring is mandatory.
Positioning	✓ and pad pressure points. ✓ eyes.	For occipital or posterior fossa injuries, patient may be prone or sitting (see Anesthetic Considerations for Cervical Neurosurgical Procedures, Positioning, p. 85). Otherwise, patient will be supine with head in Mayfield-Kees skeletal fixation and turned to the side, and a roll placed under the shoulder on the operative side.
Control of ICP	Adequate anesthesia Head up 20-30° STP or propofol infusion	Patients with skull fractures or intracranial bleeding may be on the steep portion of intracranial compliance curve such that any increase in intracranial volume may cause ↑↑ICP. Transient increases in ICP—even up to 50-60 mmHg—are tolerated, provided they are promptly terminated. Sustained increases in ICP > 25-30 mmHg are associated with severe neurologic injury and poor outcome.
	Hyperventilation to $PaCO_2$ = 25-30 mmHg PaO_2 >100 mmHg	Hypocarbia is a potent cerebral vasoconstrictor, thereby decreasing cerebral blood volume and ICP. It should be recognized that some patients with diffuse brain injury will have lost cerebrovascular sensitivity to $PaCO_2$, such that hyperventilation will have little or no effect on vascular volume (or brain size). Maintaining PaO_2 will prevent cerebral vasodilatation from hypoxemia. Despite maintaining adequate ventilation, oxygenation, and BP, patients with diffuse head injury often exhibit arterial and CSF lactic acidosis, a further indication of the metabolic derangement that exists in the brain from the injury.[12]
	Keep MAP low normal.	Control MAP and cerebral venous pressure so that CPP is maintained in the normal range for that patient. Because most patients with head injury of any consequence lose cerebral autoregulation, ↑CPP → ↑cerebral blood volume and ↑ICP. Also, with loss of autoregulation, ↓BP should be avoided to avoid cerebral ischemia. In severe, diffuse head injury with loss of autoregulation, some parts of the brain may exhibit 'luxury perfusion,' while other areas exhibit severe ischemia.[5]
	Mannitol 1 g/kg	With mannitol at a dose of 1 g/kg, vigorous diuresis will commence in about 30 min (if blood volume is adequate), and brain shrinkage will follow. It is often necessary to provide supplemental potassium (20-30 mEq iv slowly).
	Furosemide 10-20 mg	Simultaneous administration of furosemide (10-20 mg) is recommended to avoid the transient increases in cerebral blood volume and ICP that accompany mannitol administration. If mannitol is administered too rapidly, profound hypotension will occur, probably from peripheral vasodilatation.

POSTOPERATIVE

Complications	Seizures	★ Sz Rx: phenytoin (1 g loading dose). **NB:** Incompatible with dextrose-containing solutions.
	Neurologic deficits Hemorrhage	Some patients with severe head injury remain unconscious for weeks or months, without evidencing any substantial

Complications, cont.	Edema ↑ICP	neurological recovery. A late complication of head injury is hydrocephalus requiring a shunt procedure.
Pain management	Codeine (30-60 mg im q 4 h)	
Tests	CT scan ICP monitor	Unless neurological recovery is rapid, periodic CT scans are obtained postop to follow the intracranial changes. In addition, in many institutions, a device for monitoring ICP postop is placed at the time of operation.

References

1. Bouma GJ, Muizelaar JP, Choi SC, Newlon PG, Young HF: Cerebral circulation and metabolism after severe traumatic brain injury: the elusive role of ischemia. *J Neurosurg* 1991; 75:685-93.
2. Bullock RM, Chesnut RM, Clifton GL, et al: Management and prognosis of severe traumatic brain injury. Part I: Guidelines for the management of severe traumatic brain injury. *J Neurotrauma* 2000; 17:451-553.
3. Cooper PR: Traumatic intracranial hematomas. In *Neurosurgery*. Wilkins RH, Rengachary SS, eds. McGraw-Hill, New York: 1985, 1657-69.
4. Domaingue CM, Nye DH: Hypotensive effect of mannitol administered rapidly. *Anaesth Intensive Care* 1985; 13(2):134-6.
5. Kelly DF, McBride DQ, Becker DP: Surgical Management of Severe Closed Head Injury in Adults. In *Operative Neurosurgical Techniques: Indications, Methods, and Results*. Schmidek HA, Sweet WH, eds. WB Saunders, Philadelphia: 2000, 61-90.
6. King LR, McLaurin RL, Knowles HC Jr: Acid-base balance and arterial and CSF lactate levels following human head injury. *J Neurosurg* 1974; 40(5):617-25.
7. Kochs E, Hoffman WE, Werner C, Thomas C, Albrecht RF, Schulte am Esch J: The effects of propofol on brain electrical activity, neurologic outcome, and neuronal damage following incomplete ischemia in rats. *Anesthesiology* 1992; 76(2): 245-52.
8. Marion DW, Penrod LE, Kelsey SE, Obrist WD, Kochanek PM, Palmer AM, Wisniewski SR, DeKosky ST: Treatment of traumatic brain injury with moderate hypothermia. *N Engl J Med* 1997; 336:540-6.
9. Minassian AT, Dube L, Guilleux AN, et al: Changes in intracranial pressure and cerebral autoregulation in patients with severe traumatic brain injury. *Crit Care Med* 2002; 30:1616-22.
10. Piek J: Medical complications in severe head injury. *New Horiz* 1995; 3:534-9.
11. Reinert MM, Bullock R: Clinical trials in head injury. *Neurol Res* 1999; 21:330-8.
12. Stirt JA, Grosslight KR, Bedford RF, Vollmer D: "Defasciculation" with metocurine prevents succinylcholine-induced increases in intracranial pressure. *Anesthesiology* 1987; 67(1):50-3.
13. Van Hemelrijck J, Fitch W, Mattheussen M, Van Aken H, Plets C, Lauwers T: Effect of propofol on cerebral circulation and autoregulation in the baboon. *Anesth Analg* 1990; 71(1):49-54.
14. White RJ, Likavec MG: The diagnosis and initial management of head injury. *N Engl J Med* 1992; 327(21):1507-11.

MICROVASCULAR DECOMPRESSION OF CRANIAL NERVE

SURGICAL CONSIDERATIONS

Gordon T. Sakamoto, Lawrence M. Shuer, and Steven D. Chang

Description: Microvascular decompression is used to treat various disorders of the cranial nerves, including trigeminal neuralgia, hemifacial spasm and, more rarely, glossopharyngeal neuralgia. Trigeminal neuralgia is characterized by brief episodes of intense, stabbing facial pain along the distribution of the trigeminal nerve. This pain usually can be elicited by gentle stimulation of the affected area. Hemifacial spasm is characterized by paroxysmal repetitive twitching of the facial muscles. The twitching usually starts with the muscles around the eye and can progress to involve the rest of the facial muscles. Glossopharyngeal neuralgia is characterized by paroxysmal pain that involves the ear and throat. Typically, the pain is described as 'stabbing' and radiates from one site to the other. Swallowing, cold beverages, talking, or coughing can elicit the pain. All of these conditions are usually unilateral and are thought to be caused by cross-compression of a cranial nerve by a vascular structure (usually a superior cerebellar artery). To perform microvascular decompression, a linear incision is made behind the ear on the affected side (Fig 1.1-13A). Dissection is taken down to

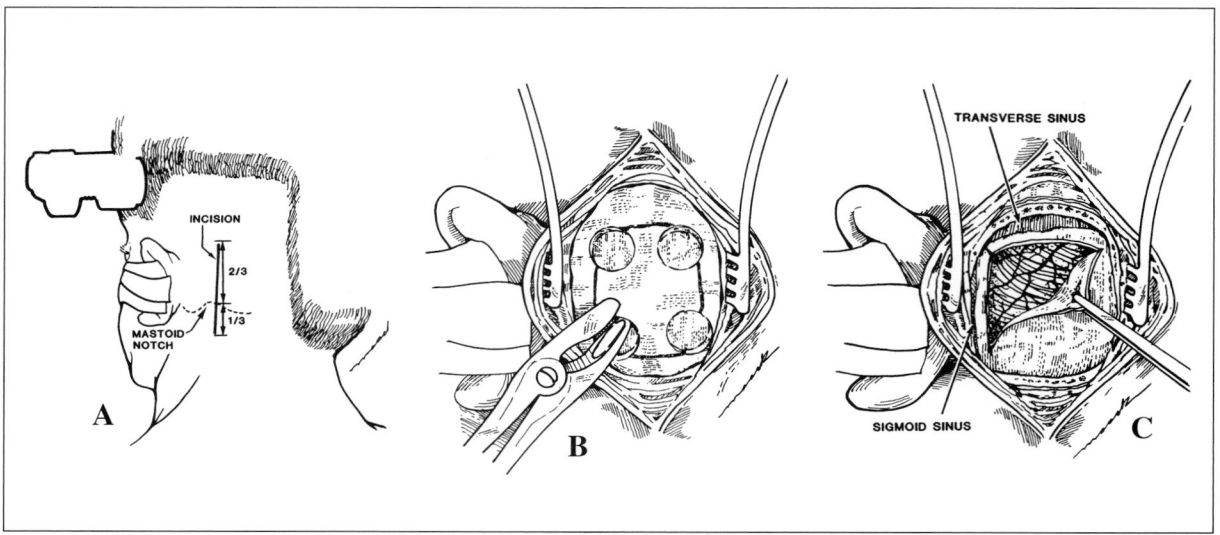

Figure 1.1-13 Microvascular decompression: (A) Location of incision. (B) Enlargement of burr holes into craniectomy with a rongeur. (C) Dural opening on the left side. Note position of venous sinuses. (Reproduced with permission from Wilson CB: *Neurosurgical Procedures: Personal Approaches to Classic Operations*. Williams & Wilkins, 1992.)

the skull, and several burr holes are made. The burr holes can be enlarged into a **craniectomy** (Fig 1.1-13B) or used for elevation of a bone flap. The craniectomy is placed below the transverse sinus and medial to the sigmoid sinus to allow access to the cerebellopontine angle. Any venous sinus bleeding is controlled and the dura is opened (Fig 1.1-13C). With brain relaxation, the cerebellum is retracted. The operating microscope allows the surgeon to explore the involved cranial nerve. If an offending vessel is identified, it is carefully dissected off the nerve and shredded Teflon felt or a small, plastic sponge is placed to keep the vessel from returning to its original position. In the case of trigeminal or glossopharyngeal neuralgia, occasionally a **partial section of the nerve** is performed, if no offending vessel is identified. Partial section of the 9th or 10th cranial nerve may cause some vasomotor instability. BAERs, facial nerve monitoring, and EMGs can be measured intraop to protect the cranial nerves. Once the cranial nerve has been decompressed, the dura is closed, and the wound is closed in layers. The main variations in this procedure are in patient positioning and surgeon's preference of monitoring modalities. Patient positioning may be lateral, prone, supine, or sitting. Intraop, mannitol (1 g/kg) and a lumbar drain (for CSF removal) may be needed for brain relaxation. Success rate is typically 75-95%, with a recurrence rate as high as 3.5% per year.

Usual preop diagnosis: Trigeminal neuralgia; tic douloureux; hemifacial spasm; tinnitus; glossopharyngeal neuralgia

SUMMARY OF PROCEDURE

Position	Normally, lateral ('park-bench'), head elevated 30°; upper shoulder retracted caudally
Incision	Retroauricular (mastoid) (See Fig. 1.1-13A.)
Special instrumentation	Operating microscope; cranial perforator; ± facial nerve monitoring; ± EMG; ± BAER
Unique considerations	Risk of air embolus in head-elevated positions
Antibiotics	Cefotaxime 1 g + nafcillin 1-2 g iv
Surgical time	2-3 h
EBL	25-250 ml
Postop care	ICU or close observation unit. Observe for change in neurologic status (e.g., level of alertness, response to commands), usually for 12-24 h.
Mortality	0.2-2%
Morbidity	Facial sensory deficit: 25%
	Aseptic meningitis: ≤ 20%, usually occurring 3-7 d postop
	Facial weakness: 2%
	Deafness: 1%; hearing loss: 3%
	Infection
	CSF leak
	Massive blood loss 2° vertebral artery injury or sinus laceration
Pain score	4-6

PATIENT POPULATION CHARACTERISTICS

Age range	40-85 yr (usually 60-70 yr)
Male:Female	~2:3
Incidence	4/1,000,000 (trigeminal neuralgia); 0.06/100,000 (glossopharyngeal neuralgia)
Etiology	Vascular compression of cranial nerve; multiple sclerosis plaque
Associated conditions	HTN; multiple sclerosis

ANESTHETIC CONSIDERATIONS

PREOPERATIVE

Microvascular decompression involves a full craniotomy for decompression of a nerve that is causing facial pain and/or spasm of facial muscles. Generally, these patients have trigeminal neuralgia or tic douloureux that has not been responsive to medical management (carbamazepine [Tegretol] therapy) and percutaneous rhizotomy or glycerol injection has failed.

Respiratory None unless the patient has a long-standing Hx of smoking and has COPD.

Cardiovascular Many patients will have Hx of idiopathic HTN and take any one of a variety of antihypertensive medications. Good control of BP preop is important because it will make intraop and postop management of BP easier.

Neurological The presenting symptom is pain ± muscle spasm in the maxillary and/or mandibular division of the trigeminal nerve, unaccompanied by any motor or sensory deficits.

Laboratory None, except for routine preop studies.

Premedication Generally, patients for these procedures are elderly and do not require any special premedication. Midazolam 2-4 mg im will provide amnesia for the preop events, if that is desired by patient or surgeons.

INTRAOPERATIVE

Anesthetic technique: GA is necessary because a full craniotomy is performed. ICP is not increased in these patients, so special precautions in that regard are not necessary. Brain shrinkage, however, is important to provide the surgeon with sufficient space to identify and relieve the pressure on the offending nerve without requiring excessive brain retraction in the process.

Induction Induction is best accomplished with drugs that cause brain shrinkage, including STP (2-5 mg/kg) or propofol (1-2 mg/kg), followed by neuromuscular blockade and ET intubation.

Maintenance Standard maintenance (p. B-3) is usually satisfactory. BP is maintained in the normal range during the operation. Hyperventilation to achieve a $PaCO_2$ of 25-30 mmHg is helpful in decreasing brain size and providing adequate space for the surgeon to work. Once the nerve has been isolated, hyperventilation can be terminated and brain size can be allowed to return to normal. Sometimes the surgeon also will insert a spinal drain to remove CSF during the operation and improve exposure. The drain usually is opened at the time of dural opening and closed as soon as surgery on the nerve is complete.

Emergence The ETT is removed at the conclusion of operation. Postop HTN may need to be controlled with esmolol and/or SNP by continuous pump infusion. Prophylactic antiemetic (e.g., metoclopramide 10 mg and ondansetron 4 mg) should be given 30 min before extubation.

Blood and fluid requirements Minimal blood loss
IV: 18 ga × 1
NS @ 2-4 ml/kg/h

Mannitol 0.5-1 mg/kg is sometimes necessary to provide sufficient brain shrinkage to permit adequate surgical exposure.

Monitoring Standard monitors (see p. B-1).
Arterial line
CVP line
± EMG and/or SSEP

Sometimes EMG and/or SSEP monitoring of the facial nerve is performed.

Positioning ✓ and pad pressure points.
✓ eyes.
Pillow between legs

Patients usually will be positioned laterally in the 'park-bench' position. Padding of the axillae and elbows and placing a pillow between the legs are necessary. A bean bag is often used to hold patient stable in the lateral position.

POSTOPERATIVE

Complications	Bleeding Brain edema	Major complications from this operation are uncommon, and postop recovery is usually uneventful. On rare occasion, significant brain edema or bleeding may be experienced.
Pain management	Codeine (30-60 mg im q 4 h)	
Tests	CT scan, if neurological recovery is delayed.	

References

1. Elias WJ, Burchiel KJ: Microvascular decompression. *Clin J Pain* 2002; 18(1):35-41.
2. Jannetta PJ: Supralateral exposure of the trigeminal nerve in the cerebellopontine angle for microvascular decompression. In *Brain Surgery: Complication, Avoidance and Management.* Apuzzo MLJ, ed. Churchill Livingstone, New York: 1993, 2085-96.
3. Lonser RR, Arthur AS, Apfelbaum RI: Neurovascular decompression in surgical disorders of cranial nerves V, VII, IX. In *Operative Neurosurgical Techniques: Indications, Methods, and Results.* Schmidek HA, Sweet WH, eds. WB Saunders, Philadelphia: 2000, 1576-88.

BIFRONTAL CRANIOTOMY FOR CSF LEAK

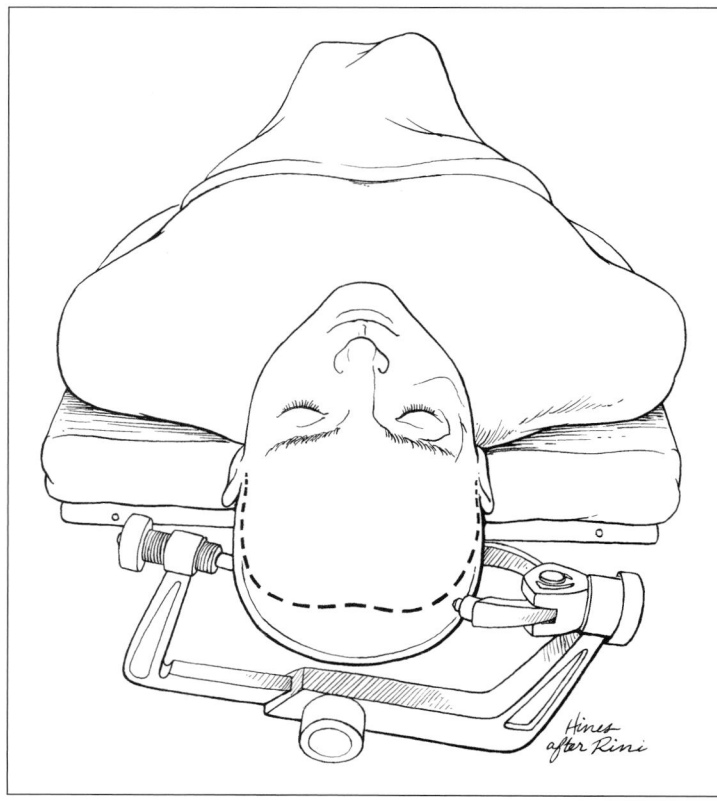

SURGICAL CONSIDERATIONS

**Gordon T. Sakamoto,
Lawrence M. Shuer, and
Steven D. Chang**

Description: CSF leaks may develop 2° trauma and, occasionally, to tumors or congenital malformations. Most of these leaks involve the floor of the anterior cranial fossa, with drainage through the auditory canal, nasopharynx, sinus air cells, or other less common routes. The surgical repair for this type of problem is typically through a **bifrontal craniotomy**. The patient is placed in a supine position and his/her head is stabilized with pins (Mayfield headrest). A bicoronal skin

Figure 1.1-14. Patient positioning for bifrontal craniotomy with bicoronal skin incision outlined. This position allows the frontal lobes to separate from the anterior cranial fossa with minimal retraction on the frontal lobes. (Reproduced with permission from Tindall GT, Cooper PR, Barrow DL: *The Practice of Neurosurgery.* Williams & Wilkins, 1996.)

incision (Fig 1.1-14) permits placement of burr holes and elevation of a bifrontal free-bone flap. If the frontal sinuses are entered, the mucosa is stripped and the sinus is packed with antibiotic-soaked Gelfoam. The dura is opened over the inferiomedial frontal lobes and the sagittal sinus is ligated. An intradural exploration is undertaken to determine the site of the leak. Brain relaxation is usually necessary to reduce the need for mechanical retraction, and may require intraop mannitol, hyperventilation, or the placement of a lumbar drain. The frontal lobes are elevated, and the olfactory tracts are often sacrificed. If the site of the leak can be determined, the dural repair can be performed using fascia lata, pericranium, or bovine pericardium. It usually is necessary to strip the dura off the anterior cranial fossa to complete the repair. Defects in the bone can be plugged with a variety of materials (e.g., pericranial flap, fat, muscle, bone, or wax). Once the repair is complete, the dura can be closed and the bone flap replaced, often with a drain left in the epidural space. At this point, brain relaxation is no longer required. The wound is closed with glial stitches and skin closure.

A combined approach may be used for CSF leaks 2° tumor that invades dura and the cribriform plate. In these cases, the procedure often is performed with an otorhinolaryngologist. The intracranial part of this procedure is identical to the bifrontal craniotomy, except that bone and tumor are removed at the floor of the anterior cranial fossa. The extracranial part of this procedure is performed by the otorhinolaryngologist, who approaches the sinonasal region endoscopically or through a lateral rhinotomy or degloving gingival incision. The extracranial approach is chosen to complement the cranial exposure and a common space is created between the two operative fields. Closure involves isolating the two operative fields once again. The dural repair is as above. The mucosa of the nasal cavity is replaced with the use of a skin graft.

Usual preop diagnosis: CSF leak or rhinorrhea; fracture of the anterior cranial fossa; intracranial encephalocele; cribriform plate tumor; olfactory neuroblastoma (tumor of the olfactory epithelium)

SUMMARY OF PROCEDURE

Position	Supine
Incision	Bicoronal (Fig 1.1-14)
Special instrumentation	Operating microscope (optional)
Unique considerations	Brain relaxation desired; lumbar subarachnoid catheter; fascia lata graft
Antibiotics	Nafcillin 1-2 g + cefotaxime 1 g iv
Surgical time	2-3.5 h, depending on extent of leak or lesion
Closing considerations	Drain often left in epidural space. Application of head dressing will jostle patient and ETT → ↑BP.
EBL	75-500 ml
Postop care	ICU or close observation unit
Mortality	≤ 5%
Morbidity	Usually < 5% for all complications
	Infection
	CSF leak
	Neurologic disability
	Nerve injury
	Massive blood loss: venous sinus injury
Pain score	3-5

PATIENT POPULATION CHARACTERISTICS

Age range	15-65 yr
Male:Female	~3:2
Incidence	Relatively rare neurosurgical procedure
Etiology	Traumatic; congenital; neoplastic

ANESTHETIC CONSIDERATIONS

See Anesthetic Considerations following Transsphenoidal Resection of Pituitary Tumor, p. 45.

References

1. Couldwell WT, Weiss MH: Cerebrospinal fluid fistulas. In *Brain Surgery: Complication, Avoidance and Management.* Apuzzo MLJ, ed. Churchill Livingstone, New York: 1993, 2329-42.
2. Osguthorpe J, Patel S: Craniofacial approaches to tumors of the anterior skull base. *Otolaryngol Clin North Am* 2001; 34(6): 1123-42.

TRANSORAL APPROACH TO THE
CERVICOMEDULLARY JUNCTION AND ODONTOID

SURGICAL CONSIDERATIONS

Gordon T. Sakamoto, Lawrence M. Shuer, and Steven D. Chang

Description: The transoral approach provides excellent access to the odontoid process of the C2 vertebral body, as well as the skull base just anterior to the brain stem (Fig 1.1-15). This is important for conditions where there is pressure on the ventral brain stem or spinal cord →Sx: HA, impaired ambulation, hyperreflexia, paresthesias, neurogenic bladder, etc. Common indications for this approach include basilar impression (upward translocation of the odontoid process) (Fig 1.1-16A); degeneration of the odontoid due to rheumatoid disease (Fig 1.1-17A); fracture of the odontoid, and resection of extradural tumors, such as chordomas and metastases. In these cases, the operation is performed through the oral cavity with an incision in the posterior wall of the pharynx. Special retractors hold the mouth open and keep the tongue out of the way. Fluoroscopic guidance helps the surgeon maintain proper trajectory. Intraop monitoring of evoked potentials (i.e., SSEP or BAER) and use of the operative microscope help avoid injury to the brain stem and spinal cord. The dissection is carried down to expose the anterior arch of C1 and body of C2. To decompress the region, the anterior arch of C1 and the odontoid process are removed. For basilar impression, a portion of the clivus may need to be removed to gain access to the dens (Fig 1.1-16B). For rheumatoid arthritis, the pannus (thickened fibrous tissue) surrounding the dens is also removed (Fig 1.1-17B). If an extradural tumor is found, it is resected in a piecemeal fashion. If a CSF leak occurs, the dura can be closed with fascia, muscle, fibrin glue, or thrombin-soaked Gelfoam. Upon completion of the decompression, the mucosa is closed. It may be necessary to fuse the occiput to the upper C-spine to correct any cervical instability. This may take place at the same time, or at a later date. C-spine precautions normally are used during and after the case. The patient may be in traction with tongs or a halter.

Variations in procedure: A fiber optic nasal intubation or tracheostomy may be necessary to gain adequate exposure and maintain ventilation. It also may be necessary to split the soft palate, hard palate, tongue, and/or mandible to obtain adequate exposure.

Usual preop diagnosis: Basilar impression (platybasia); odontoid fracture; rheumatoid arthritis with atlantoaxial instability and anterior impingement of the cord; chordoma; metastatic tumor

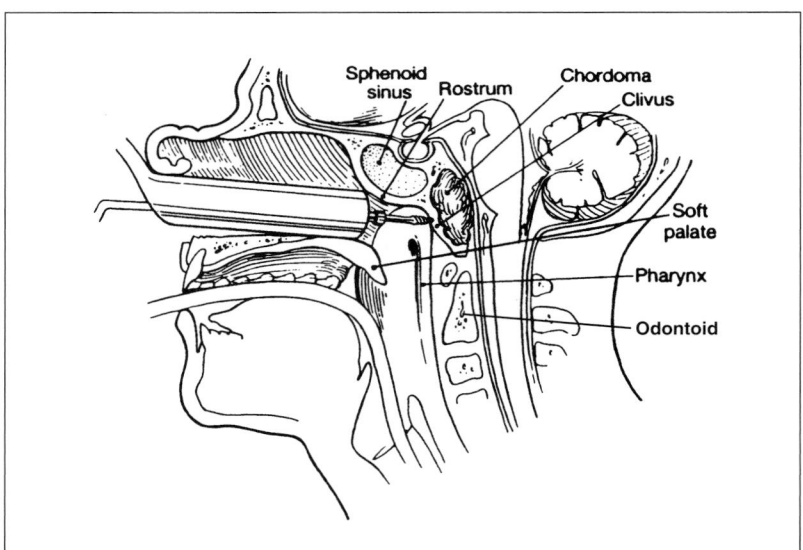

Figure 1.1-15. Inferior exposure of the clivus and chordoma. (Reproduced with permission from Grossman RG, Loftus CM: *Principles of Neurosurgery*, 2nd edition. Lippincott-Raven, 1999.)

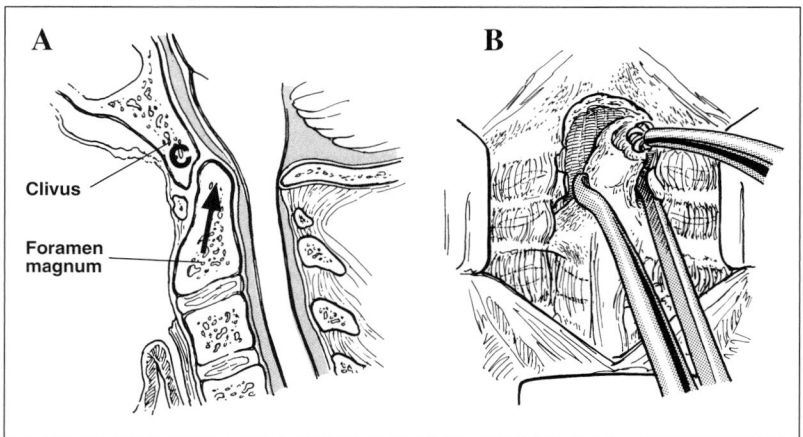

Figure 1.1-16. (A) Basilar impression. The dens has moved superiorly into the foramen magnum (arrow). (B) Removal of the dens with a drill. The arch of C1 and a portion of the clivus has been removed. (Reproduced with permission from Donald PJ: *Surgery of the Skull Base*. Lippincott-Raven, 1998.)

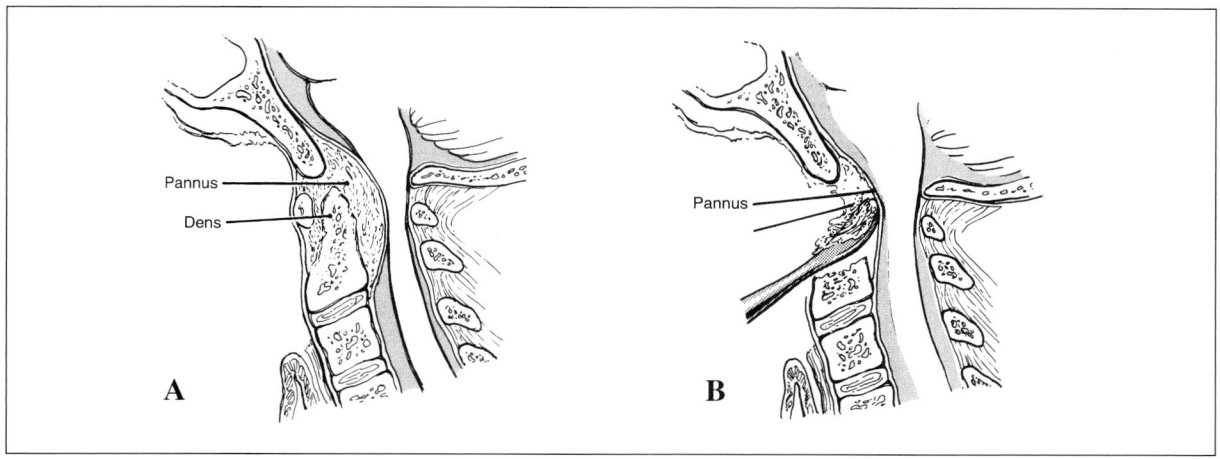

Figure 1.1-17. (A) Pannus formation in a patient with rheumatoid arthritis. (B) Removal of pannus. (Reproduced with permission from Donald PJ: *Surgery of the Skull Base*. Lippincott-Raven, 1998.)

SUMMARY OF PROCEDURE

Position	Supine; head in traction or pins
Incision	Back of oropharynx
Special instrumentation	Operating microscope; I.I.; intraop monitoring = SSEP or BAER; micro drill; intraoral retractors for exposure
Unique considerations	FOL may be necessary. ETT must be taped securely in a location satisfactory to surgeon. Anode or RAE tube may be helpful. Occasionally, a **tracheostomy** is performed in advance.
Antibiotics	Ampicillin (or vancomycin) 1 g iv + cefotaxime 1 g
Surgical time	2.5-3 h
Closing considerations	Patient may remain intubated postop. C-spine precautions may be necessary.
EBL	25-250 ml
Postop care	ICU or close observation unit; monitor airway for swelling (✓ for stridor).
Mortality	0-3%
Morbidity	All < 5%:
	Infection
	CSF leak
	Neurological
	Massive blood loss
Pain score	2-4

PATIENT POPULATION CHARACTERISTICS

Age range	18-85 yr (usually 20-60 yr)
Male:Female	~1:2
Incidence	Rare (See Associated conditions.)
Etiology	Neoplastic; traumatic; congenital; degenerative
Associated conditions	Rheumatoid arthritis (atlantoaxial subluxation in 25%; basilar compression in 8%); traumatic injury

ANESTHETIC CONSIDERATIONS

See Anesthetic Considerations following Transsphenoidal Resection of Pituitary Tumor, p. 45.

References

1. Hadley MN, Spetzler RF, Sonntag VKH: The transoral approach to the superior cervical spine. *J Neurosurg* 1989;71(1): 16-23.
2. Vangilder JC, Menezes AH: Craniovertebral abnormalities and their neurosurgical management. In *Operative Neurosurgical Techniques: Indications, Methods, and Results*. Schmidek HA, Sweet WH, eds. WB Saunders, Philadelphia: 2000, 1934-45.

TRANSSPHENOIDAL RESECTION OF PITUITARY TUMOR

SURGICAL CONSIDERATIONS

Gordon T. Sakamoto, Lawrence M. Shuer, Steven D. Chang

Description: The transsphenoidal approach to the sella turcica is a direct procedure used to gain access to the pituitary gland and sella region and is associated with relatively fewer complications than a craniotomy. The procedure usually is performed through a sublabial incision in the maxillary gingiva or via an incision in or alongside the nose. An otorhinolaryngologist may participate in obtaining the exposure, which involves creating a tunnel to the sphenoid sinus through a plane between the septum of the nose and nasal mucosa. Once the sphenoid sinus is reached, it is entered by removing a portion of the vomer. The mucosa of the sphenoid sinus is stripped and the sella is entered by removing a portion of the sella floor (Fig 1.1-18A). Under fluoroscopic guidance and with the aid of the operating microscope, the surgeon can operate safely within the region of the pituitary gland. Alternatively, a variety of other imaging techniques may be employed. Frameless stereotaxy, three-dimensional computer-assisted neuronavigation, intraop MRI, intraop ultrasound, and/or an endoscope can be used to assist with planning and performance of the surgery. Once the sella floor is removed, the dura is opened and the tumor is removed with a series of microdissectors and suctioned out with curettage. Following tumor removal, the surgeon may harvest fat, muscle, or fascia from the thigh or abdomen to pack into the sella to reduce free intrasellar space and serve as a graft to seal the dura if CSF is found (Fig 1.1-18B). Resorbable materials, such as Gelfoam and fibrin glue, also may be used to pack and seal the sella. The floor of the sella can be reconstructed with bone salvaged from the exposure. In order to obtain closure, the sphenoid sinus also may be packed and sealed with the same materials used to close the sella.

Usual preop diagnosis: Pituitary tumor; prolactin-secreting tumor; growth hormone-secreting tumor (acromegaly); ACTH-secreting tumor (Cushing's disease); visual compromise 2° intrasellar tumor; craniopharyngioma; meningioma; Forbes-Albright syndrome (galactorrhea-amenorrhea syndrome)

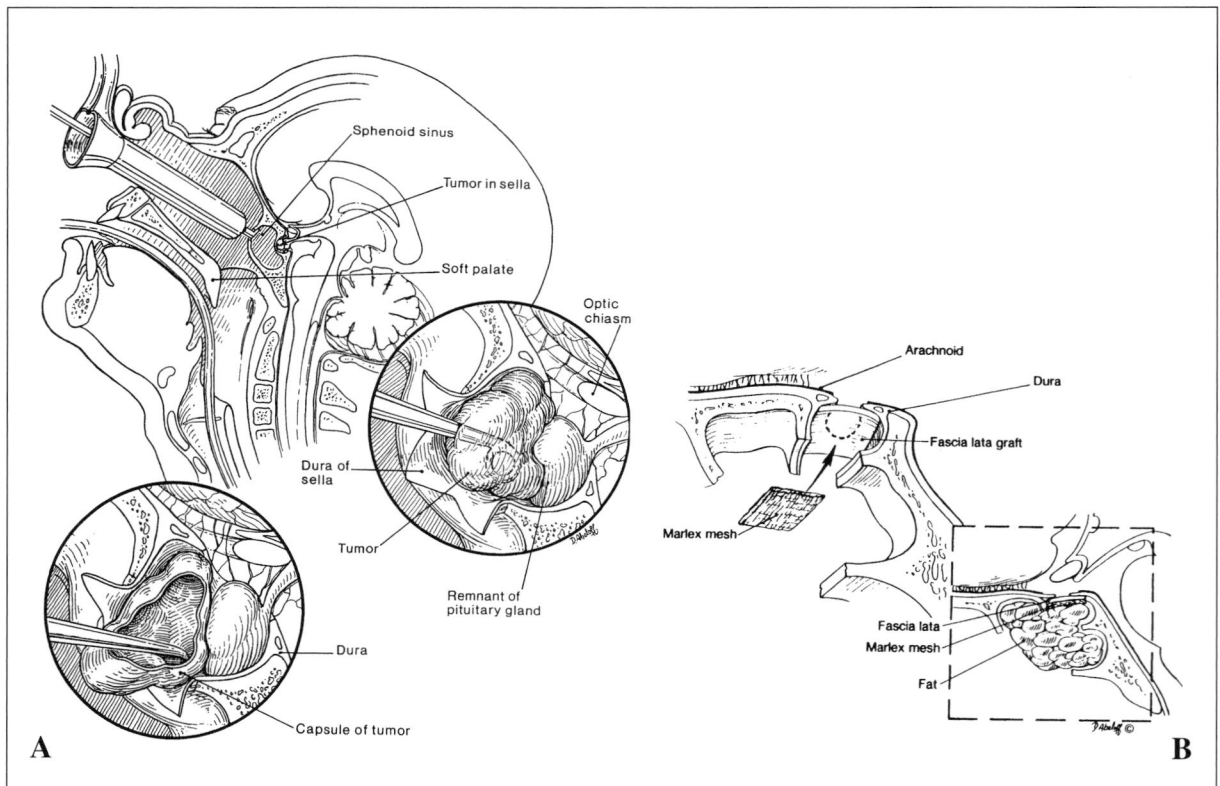

Figure 1.1-18. The transnasal/transsphenoidal removal of a pituitary tumor. (A, upper) The rostrum of the sphenoid is removed and mucosa of the sinus exenterated. (A, middle and lower) The floor of the sella is removed, the dura opened, and the tumor removed using microcurettes. (B) Fat taken from the subcutaneous tissue at the time of the fascial resection is utilized to fill the sphenoid and hold the graft material in position. (Reproduced with permission from Grossman RG, Loftus CM: *Principles of Neurosurgery*, 2nd edition. Lippincott-Raven, 1999.)

SUMMARY OF PROCEDURE

Position	Supine, head elevated 30°
Incision	Sublabial, maxillary gingiva; abdomen or thigh for fat graft
Special instrumentation	Operating microscope; I.I.; micro drill; laser (occasionally); neuronavigation
Unique considerations	ETT must be taped securely in a location satisfactory to surgeon. Anode or RAE tube may be helpful. Dissection in the nasal cavity can be noxious stimulus, thus elevating BP and ICP and risking air embolus.
Antibiotics	Ampicillin (or vancomycin) 1 g iv + cefotaxime 1 g iv
Surgical time	2.5-3 h
Closing considerations	Possible abdominal or thigh-fat graft. Closure quite fast, requiring only gingival suture and nasal packs.
EBL	25-250 ml
Postop care	ICU or close observation unit; fluid and electrolytes require frequent monitoring as the patient may develop diabetes insipidus (DI) transiently following this procedure.
Mortality	1%
Morbidity	Anterior pituitary insufficiency: 19.4%
	DI: 17.8%
	Sinusitis: 8.5%
	Septum perforation: 6.7%
	CSF leak: 3.9%
	Epistaxis: 3.4%
	Loss of vision: 1.8%
	Meningitis: 1.5%
	Carotid artery injury: 1.1%
Pain score	2-4

PATIENT POPULATION CHARACTERISTICS

Age range	18-85 yr (usually 30-50 yr)
Male:Female	~1:2
Incidence	3/1000 (autopsy studies)
Etiology	Neoplastic; traumatic
Associated conditions	Cushing's disease; acromegaly; amenorrhea/galactorrhea

ANESTHETIC CONSIDERATIONS

(Procedures covered: bifrontal craniotomy for CSF leak; transoral approach to cervicomedullary junction, odontoid; transsphenoidal resection of pituitary tumor)

C. Philip Larson, Jr.

PREOPERATIVE

Endocrine   Tumors of the pituitary gland are either nonfunctional or secretory. If nonfunctional, they will produce Sx either by their mass effect on adjacent pituitary tissue, or because of extension outside of the sella turcica. Rarely, the mass effect may cause the clinical picture of panhypopituitarism requiring preop treatment with thyroxine, glucocorticoid, and vasopressin. Functional tumors secrete varying quantities of prolactin (→ lactation), growth hormone (→ acromegaly) and ACTH (→ adrenal hyperplasia).
Tests: Preop endocrine studies, including serum and urinary levels of pituitary, thyroid, and adrenal hormones; appropriate replacement therapy established before proceeding with surgery.

Respiratory   No special requirements, unless patient has acromegaly,[2] in which case large facial features, long neck, large tongue, and redundant soft tissue in the oropharynx may make mask fit and ET intubation difficult. If these patients evidence hoarseness or inspiratory stridor, they should have a full clinical and radiological evaluation of the upper airway.
Tests: As indicated from H&P.

Cardiovascular	No special requirements unless patient has acromegaly, in which case they may have HTN, ischemic heart disease, or diabetes. **Tests:** As indicated from H&P.
Neurological	Secretory tumors of the pituitary are usually small, confined to the sella, rarely cause ↑ICP, and produce Sx of endocrine dysfunction early in their growth. In contrast, nonfunctional pituitary tumors may not produce Sx until they extend beyond the boundaries of the sella, causing HAs or pressure effects on the optic chiasm, producing visual field defects. **Tests:** A CT or MRI will delineate the site and size of the tumor, especially if iv contrast material, such as gadolinium, is administered to enhance the margins of the tumor.
Musculoskeletal	If growth hormone is the primary secretant, patient will exhibit Sx of acromegaly, including large hands, feet, head, and tongue. **Tests:** As indicated from H&P.
Laboratory	Hct and others as indicated from H&P.

INTRAOPERATIVE

Anesthetic technique: GETA is required for this operation, since the surgical approach is through either the nose or the mouth above the maxillary gum line and behind the nose.

Induction	If a difficult intubation is anticipated, orotracheal intubation will need to be accomplished before induction of GA. Awake FOL is the best choice (see p. B-6). Since these tumors generally are confined to the sella turcica and, hence, ICP usually is not increased, a standard induction technique is appropriate (see p. B-2). If ↑ICP is of concern, induction should be similar to that used for patients with other kinds of brain tumors (see Anesthetic Considerations for Craniotomy for Tumor, p. 28). Since the surgeon will be working from the patient's right side, the ETT must be positioned at the far left side of the mouth. Consider using a wire-reinforced tube to prevent kinking while surgeon is working in mouth. An oral airway should not be used.
Maintenance	Standard maintenance (see p. B-3). Generally, no further NMBs are administered beyond ET intubation. With adequate anesthesia, and the head in Mayfield-Kees skeletal fixation, patient movement of any consequence is highly unlikely. Also, it is useful to see movement of an extremity as an indicator of inadequate depth of anesthesia. Ventilation is controlled with PaCO$_2$ maintained in the normal range. Hyperventilation is not desirable because it makes it more difficult for the neurosurgeon to locate the tumor in the sella and establish that it has been removed in its entirety.
Emergence	At the conclusion of surgery, a decision must be made regarding extubation of the trachea. If the patient evidences normal emergence from anesthesia, the ETT should be removed before vigorous coughing ensues. Before removing the ETT, however, the anesthesiologist must make certain that all blood accumulated in the back of the throat is suctioned out, and that oropharyngeal packs placed in the back of the throat by the surgeon have been removed. The surgeon will have packed the nose at the end of operation, forcing the patient to be an obligatory mouth breather until the nasal packs are removed. If there is any question about airway patency because of a large tongue, small mouth, or soft-tissue redundancy in the oropharynx, the ETT should be left in place until patient is fully awake from anesthesia. Prophylactic antiemetic (e.g., metoclopramide 10 mg and ondansetron 4 mg) should be given 30 min before extubation.

Blood and fluid requirements	Minimal blood loss usual Potential large blood loss IV: 16-18 ga × 1 NS/LR @ 4-8 ml/kg/h	Blood loss is minimal, unless the surgeon inadvertently enters the internal carotid artery or cavernous sinus during the course of dissection and drilling into the sella.
Control of blood loss	Deliberate hypotension	Controlled ↓BP not used in this operation unless bleeding becomes profuse, diffuse, or hard to control.
Monitoring	Standard monitors (see p. B-1). Arterial line CVP line UO ± Doppler	Monitor for VAE in semisitting position.

Positioning	✓ and pad pressure points. ✓ eyes. Shoulder roll Table turned 180°		The surgeon will use an operating microscope, which means that the anesthesiologist will be positioned near patient's feet. Anesthetic hoses and intravascular lines must be long enough to be accessible.

POSTOPERATIVE

Complications	Hypopituitarism Diabetes insipidus (DI)	Replacement therapy with steroids is necessary until normal pituitary function returns. Occasionally, patients will develop DI postop, as evidenced by polyuria and ↓urine-specific gravity. Rarely, this may occur near the conclusion of anesthetic, necessitating vigorous fluid replacement and vasopressin therapy (5-10 U sc or im bid).
Pain management	Codeine (30-60 mg im q 4 h)	
Tests	CT scan	If a patient exhibits any delay in emergence from anesthesia and surgery, or any new neurologic deficits emerge postop, a CT scan is invariably obtained.

References

1. Chan VWS, Tindal S: Anesthesia for transsphenoidal surgery in a patient with extreme giantism. *Br J Anaesth* 1998; 60: 464-8.
2. Ciric I, et al: Complications of transsphenoidal surgery: Results of a national survey, review of the literature, and personal experience. *Neurosurgery* 1997; 40(2):225-36.
3. Elias JW, Laws ER Jr: Transsphenoidal approaches to lesions of the sella. In *Operative Neurosurgical Techniques: Indications, Methods, and Results*. Schmidek HA, Sweet WH, eds. WB Saunders, Philadelphia: 2000, 373-84.
4. Fahlbusch R, Honegger KR, Paulus W, Huk W, Buchfelder M: Surgical treatment of craniopharyngiomas: experience with 168 patients. *J Neurosurg* 1999; 90:237-50.
5. Matjasko J: Perioperative management of patients with pituitary tumors. *Semin Anesth* 1984; 111:155-67.
6. Semple PL, Laws ER: Complications in a contemporary series of patients who underwent transphenoidal surgery for Cushing's Disease. *J Neurosurg* 1999; 91:175-9.

VENTRICULAR SHUNT PROCEDURES

SURGICAL CONSIDERATIONS

Gordon T. Sakamoto, Lawrence M. Shuer, and Steven D. Chang

Description: Many conditions exist whereby it is necessary to shunt CSF from the ventricles to another body cavity where it can be absorbed readily. The most common condition is hydrocephalus, where there is dilation of the ventricular system due to an obstruction in the flow of CSF or decreased absorption of CSF by the arachnoid villi. Hydrocephalus is commonly treated by diverting CSF to the peritoneal cavity via a ventriculoperitoneal shunt (**VP shunt**). Most shunt systems have one-way, pressure-dependent valves to regulate the flow of CSF. These valves usually have a preset pressure setting (e.g., low, medium, high). Newer valves have externally adjustable opening pressures, flow-regulating devices, and/or antisiphon systems to prevent overshunting.

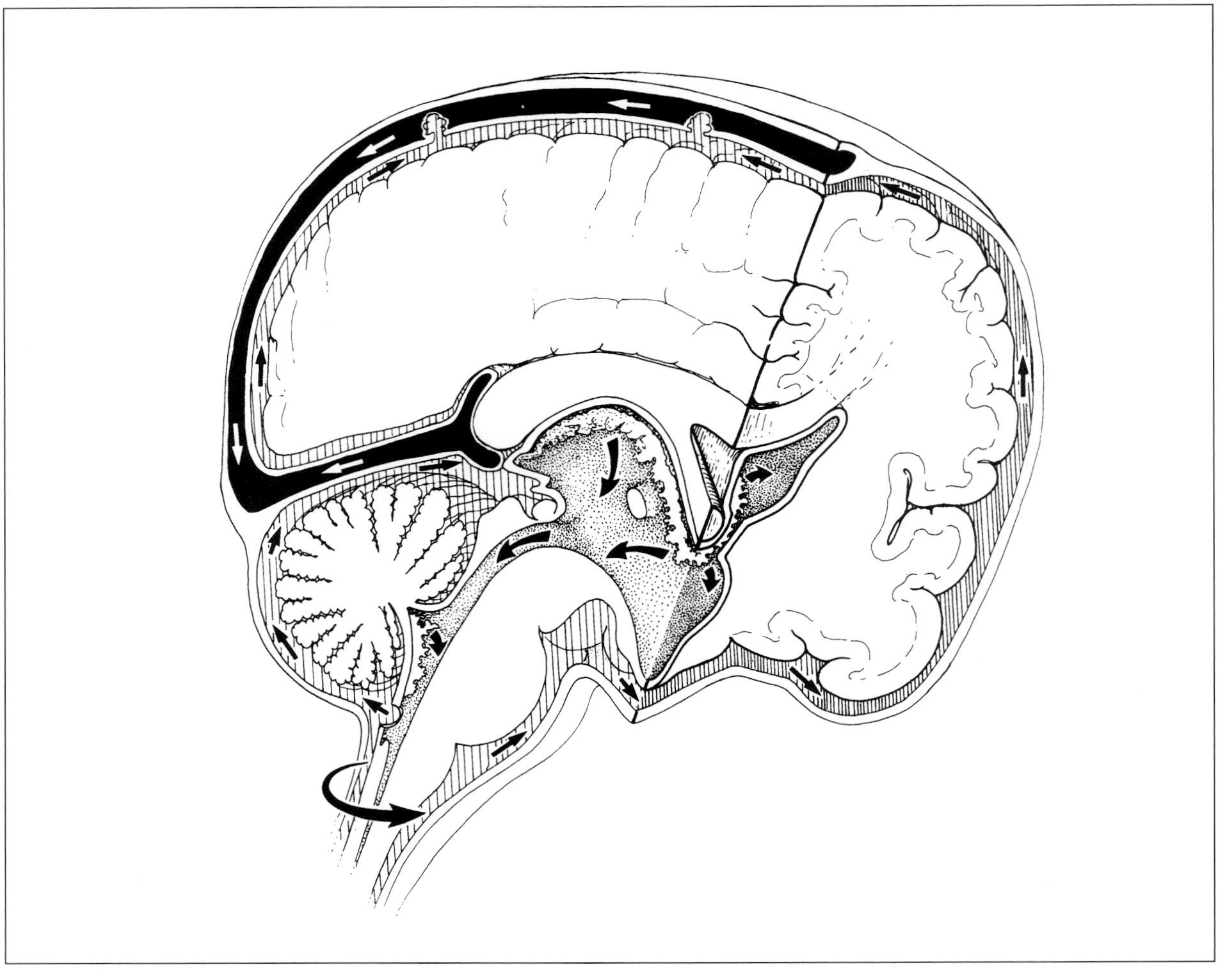

Figure 1.1-19. Pathways of CSF flow and potential sites of obstruction. (Reproduced with permission from Tindall GT, Cooper PR, Barrow DL: *The Practice of Neurosurgery*, Vol III. Williams & Wilkins, 1996. Orig. from Scott RM: *Hydrocephalus. Concepts in Neurosurgery*, Vol III. Williams & Wilkins, 1990.)

To insert a VP shunt, the patient is positioned so that the cranial incision and abdominal incision are aligned in the same plane. The scalp is shaved (usually over the frontal or parietal region) and a continuous surgical field is created from head to abdomen. The cranial incision is made over the intended region of cannulation of the ventricle, and a burr hole is made in the cranium. A subgaleal pocket is created for the valve, usually behind the ear. A separate incision is made in the abdomen and dissection is carried down to the level of the peritoneum. A catheter is then passed subcutaneously from the abdominal incision to the cranial incision with a special tunneling instrument (Fig 1.1-20A). It may be necessary to use one or more incisions between the head and the abdomen to thread the catheter. The valve is connected to the peritoneal catheter and placed in the subgaleal pocket. A ventricular catheter is then inserted into the ventricle (Fig 1.1-20B) and a small amount of CSF is drained to check placement and patency of the catheter. The catheter is then connected to the valve, and CSF flow through the entire shunt system is checked by draining some CSF from the distal end of the peritoneal catheter. The distal end is placed into the peritoneal cavity and all wounds are closed. Any component of the shunt may malfunction; thus, it may be necessary to test each component at the time of revision to identify the problem. To test the patency of the ventricular catheter, it is disconnected form the valve and CSF should flow freely through it. A saline-filled manometer can be attached to the valve to measure the opening pressure of the valve. The manometer should drain spontaneously until the opening pressure of the valve is reached. An elevated opening pressure may indicate a valve malfunction or a distal occlusion. If a distal occlusion is suspected, gentle irrigation may clear it, but externalization may be necessary.

Variant procedure or approaches: Endoscopy, fluoroscopy, ultrasound, or intraop MRI may be used to help place the catheter into the ventricle. The ventricular catheter can be placed in either lateral ventricle; occasionally, both lateral ventricles are cannulated. This procedure also is used to shunt the fourth ventricle and, sometimes, subarachnoid cysts and subdural hygromas. The distal end alternatively may be placed in the pleural cavity or the right atrium (ventriculoatrial

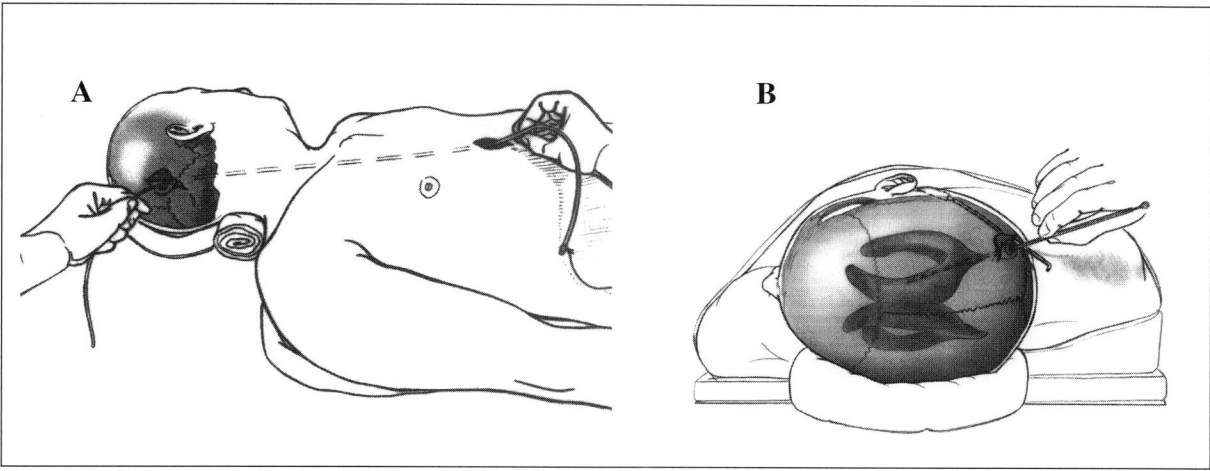

Figure 1.1.-20. (A) The catheter is threaded from the abdominal incision to the cranial incision. (B) Insertion of the ventricular catheter. (Reproduced with permission from Meyer FB: *Atlas of Neurosurgery: Basic Approaches to Cranial and Vascular Procedures.* Churchill Livingstone, 1999).

or **VA shunt**). If the distal end of the catheter is placed into the pleural cavity, a Valsalva maneuver is performed upon closure to reinflate the lung. To place the distal end into the atrium, a vein is cannulated in the neck (usually IJ or EJ), and the catheter is fed into the atrium under fluoroscopic guidance. It may be necessary to inject radiopaque contrast to verify proper placement.

Usual preop diagnosis: Hydrocephalus; obstructive or communicating hydrocephalus; aqueductal stenosis; Dandy-Walker malformation (cystic dilation of the fourth ventricle and incomplete formation of the cerebellar vermis); occult hydrocephalus; normal-pressure hydrocephalus; subarachnoid cyst; subdural hygroma

SUMMARY OF PROCEDURES

	VP Shunt	VA Shunt
Position	Supine, with head turned to contralateral side	⇐
Incision	Scalp, either coronal and retroauricular, or parietal; + neck and abdomen	Scalp, either coronal and retroauricular or parietal; + neck
Special instrumentation	Ventricular endoscope (optional)	⇐ + I.I.
Unique considerations	Patient to be treated as if there is ↑ICP.	⇐
Antibiotics	Cefotaxime 1 g iv and nafcillin 1-2 g iv	⇐
Surgical time	1 h	⇐
EBL	5-25 ml	⇐
Postop care	PACU → room; usually kept flat for 24 h.	⇐
Mortality	< 1%	⇐
Morbidity	Infection: < 15% Neurological: Intracranial bleed: < 1% Subdural hematoma: < 1% Hardware failure: < 1%	⇐
Pain score	4-6	2-4

PATIENT POPULATION CHARACTERISTICS

Age range	Newborn-elderly
Male:Female	1:1
Incidence	Common
Etiology	Congenital (3-4/1000 live births); acquired; neoplastic; infectious; posthemorrhagic
Associated conditions	Myelodysplasia; spina bifida (95% incidence); intraventricular hemorrhage; intraventricular tumor

ANESTHETIC CONSIDERATIONS

PREOPERATIVE

Ventricular shunts (VP and VA) are inserted to ameliorate hydrocephalus or cyst formations, which may be either congenital or acquired.

Cardiovascular	↑ICP → ↑BP & ↓↓HR (Cushing's response) **Tests:** As indicated from H&P.
Neurological	The most common presenting Sx is HA. If hydrocephalus is severe, Sx of ↑ICP (>15 mmHg) (e.g., N/V, drowsiness, papilledema, Sz, and focal neurological defects) develop.
Laboratory	Tests as indicated by H&P.
Premedication	Usually not required; should be avoided in patients with ↑ICP.

INTRAOPERATIVE

Anesthetic technique: GETA

Induction	If ↑ICP, iv induction with STP (2-5 mg/kg) or propofol (1-2 mg/kg) is preferred, because of their ability to decrease cerebral blood volume and, hence, to decrease ICP. ET intubation is accomplished with the use of a NMB (e.g., vecuronium [0.1 mg/kg] or rocuronium [0.7-1 mg/kg]).
Maintenance	Isoflurane ≤ 1% or sevoflurane < 2%, inspired with N_2O/O_2 mixture, to maintain O_2 sat ~99%. Depending on duration of operation, additional doses of vecuronium (0.1 mg/kg) or rocuronium (0.2 mg/kg) may be needed. Maintain normal temperature in children by keeping OR warm (78°F) and using a forced-air warming blanket. Ventilation should be controlled. TV and frequency should be adjusted such that the $PetCO_2$ = 35-40 mmHg. Hyperventilation and hypocarbia are undesirable because they make cannulation of the ventricle(s) more difficult for the surgeon. Maintain normotension.
Emergence	ETT is removed at the conclusion of the anesthetic. Prophylactic antiemetic (e.g., metoclopramide 10 mg and ondansetron 4 mg) should be given 30 min before extubation.
Blood and fluid requirements	IV: 18-20 ga × 1 NS/LR @ 4-6 ml/kg/h	Administer crystalloid, usually NS. Blood is rarely, if ever, necessary.
Monitoring	Standard monitors (see p. B-1).	
Positioning	Table turned 180° ✓ and pad pressure points. ✓ eyes.	Supine with a bolster under the shoulder on the operative side. The head, chest, and abdomen are prepped, so all anesthesia equipment and lines must be at the sides of the patient.
Complications	Valve malfunction	Major intraop complications from this operation are rare.

POSTOPERATIVE

Pain management	Children < 2 yr: Tylenol suppositories (10-15 mg/kg q 4 h) Adults: meperidine 10-20 mg iv prn

References

1. Drake JM, Iantosca MR: Current systems for cerebrospinal fluid shunting and management of pediatric hydrocephalus: Endoscopic and image-guided surgery in hydrocephalus. In *Operative Neurosurgical Techniques: Indications, Methods, and Results*, Schmidek HA, Sweet WH, eds. WB Saunders, Philadelphia: 2000, 573-94.
2. Drake JM, Kestle JRW, Tuli S: CSF shunts 50 years on—past, present and future. *Childs Nerv Syst* 2000;16:800-4.
3. Drake JM, Sainte-Rose C: *The Shunt Book*. Blackwell Scientific, New York 1995.

CRANIOCERVICAL DECOMPRESSION (CHIARI MALFORMATION)

SURGICAL CONSIDERATIONS

Gordon T. Sakamoto, Lawrence M. Shuer, Steven D. Chang

Historically, congenital hindbrain abnormalities characterized by cerebellar descent were known collectively as **Arnold-Chiari malformations**; now they are known as **Chiari malformations**. In these abnormalities, portions of the cerebellum protrude through the foramen magnum and may compress the brain stem and upper cervical spinal cord at this level. Frequently, the malformation is accompanied by a **syringomyelia**, a condition in which CSF is located abnormally within the spinal cord. In **Chiari I** malformation, the cerebellar tonsils are herniated through the foramen magnum. In the more severe **Chiari II** malformation, the tonsils, vermis, fourth ventricle, pons, and medulla are displaced caudally through the foramen magnum. Chiari II malformations are usually found in infants and are associated with myelomeningoceles. **Type III** malformations are the most severe, and have a poor prognosis. In order to make room for structures at the craniocervical level, decompression is necessary. This procedure may be performed in either the prone, 3/4 prone, or seated position. A midline incision is made, and a suboccipital craniectomy decompresses the foramen magnum. The posterior arch of C1 is removed and as many upper cervical lamina as are needed to fully decompress the malformation are removed. Next, the dura is opened and the tonsils are dissected apart under microscopic guidance to gain an opening to the fourth ventricle (Figure 1.1-21A & B). The cerebellar tonsils can be reduced to facilitate the outflow of CSF from the fourth ventricle. A stent or a shunt may be placed in the fourth ventricle and brought out to the subarachnoid space to ensure adequate drainage of the fourth ventricle. The dura is closed loosely with autologous pericranium, fascia lata, or bovine pericardium (Fig 1.1-21C). This creates a widely patent cisterna magna and prevents constriction of the corticomedullary junction.

Usual preop diagnosis: Chiari Malformation I or II, Arnold-Chiari malformation; syringomyelia

SUMMARY OF PROCEDURE

Position	Prone or sitting
Incision	Midline posterior, posterolateral thigh for fascia lata graft (optional)
Special instrumentation	Operating microscope
Unique considerations	Risk of air embolus; brain stem manipulation can cause BP and pulse instability.
Antibiotics	Cefotaxime 1 g and nafcillin 1 g iv
Surgical time	2.5-3.5 h
Closing considerations	Application of head dressing with consequent head movement → ↑BP and need for BP control.
EBL	25-250 ml
Postop care	ICU or constant observation unit; neurological function monitored.
Mortality	0-3% (usually respiratory arrest)
Morbidity	Respiratory depression: 14% up to 5 d postop
	All others < 5%:
	Infection
	Neurological: dysphagia and ↓gag reflex
	Aseptic meningitis
	CSF leak
	Massive blood loss; vertebral artery or transverse sinus injury
Pain score	5-7

PATIENT POPULATION CHARACTERISTICS

Age range	Infant-70 yr; Chiari I: average age = 41 yr
Male:Female	~1:1
Incidence	Relatively rare neurosurgical procedure
Etiology	Congenital; acquired, S/P lumboperitoneal shunting
Associated conditions	Hydrocephalus; syringomyelia; scoliosis; myelodysplasia

ANESTHETIC CONSIDERATIONS

See Anesthetic Considerations for Cervical Neurosurgical Procedures, p. 83.

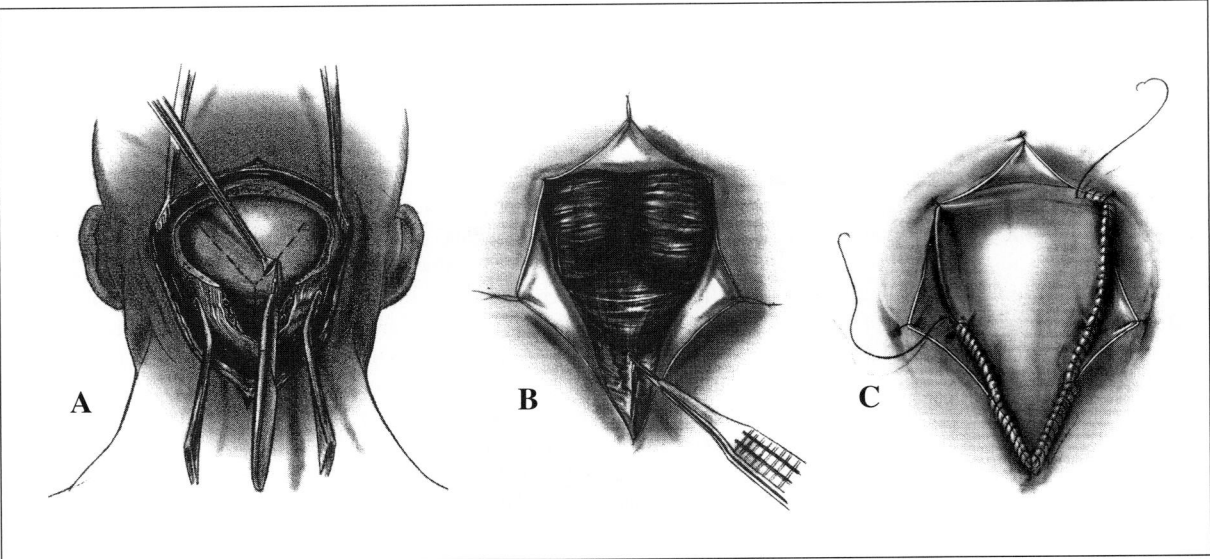

Figure 1.1-21. (A) A Y-shaped dural incision is made through the occipital craniectomy and laminectomy. (B) Opening the arachnoid mater to gain access to the cerebellar tonsils and fourth ventricle. (C) Loose closure of dura with graft. (Reproduced with permission from Meyer F: *Atlas of Neurosurgery: Basic Approaches to Cranial and Vascular Procedures.* Churchill Livingstone: 1999.)

References

1. Klekamp J, Batzdorf U, Samii M, Bothe HW: The surgical treatment of Chiari I malformation. *Acta Neurochir* 1996; 138: 788-801.
2. Rhoton AL: Microsurgery of syringomyelia and the syringomyelia-Chiari complex. In *Operative Neurosurgical Techniques: Indications, Methods, and Results.* Schmidek HA and Sweet WH, eds. WB Saunders, Philadelphia: 2000, 1955-69.

STEREOTACTIC NEUROSURGERY

SURGICAL CONSIDERATIONS

Steven D. Chang and John R. Adler

Description: Stereotaxis applies simple rules of geometry to radiologic images to allow precise localization within the brain. Such techniques can be applied to a variety of neurosurgical procedures, providing up to 1-mm accuracy. This precision makes it possible to perform certain intracranial procedures less invasively. Methods include both frame-based and frameless systems, as well as specific stereotactic applications for functional neurosurgery and radiosurgery.

Frame-based stereotaxy: Stereotactic localization was developed using frames and, despite the widespread use of image-guided, 'frameless' stereotactic systems for craniotomies, frame-based stereotaxy continues to be used commonly for biopsies and cyst drainage. These procedures begin with the attachment of a frame to the patient's head using four pins or screws that anchor it to the skull. This is typically done outside the OR, using local anesthetic and sometimes light sedation. In the cooperative adult, frame application takes only 5-10 min; however, GA typically is used for children. Once the frame is in place, access to the patient's airway is restricted. A key for emergency removal of the frame is kept with the patient at all times. With the stereotactic frame in place, CT, MRI, and/or cerebral angiography are used for target identification and localization. During imaging, a set of fiducials (radiographically visible markers) is attached to the frame. These markers provide the geometric reference points needed for localization. Data from imaging studies are

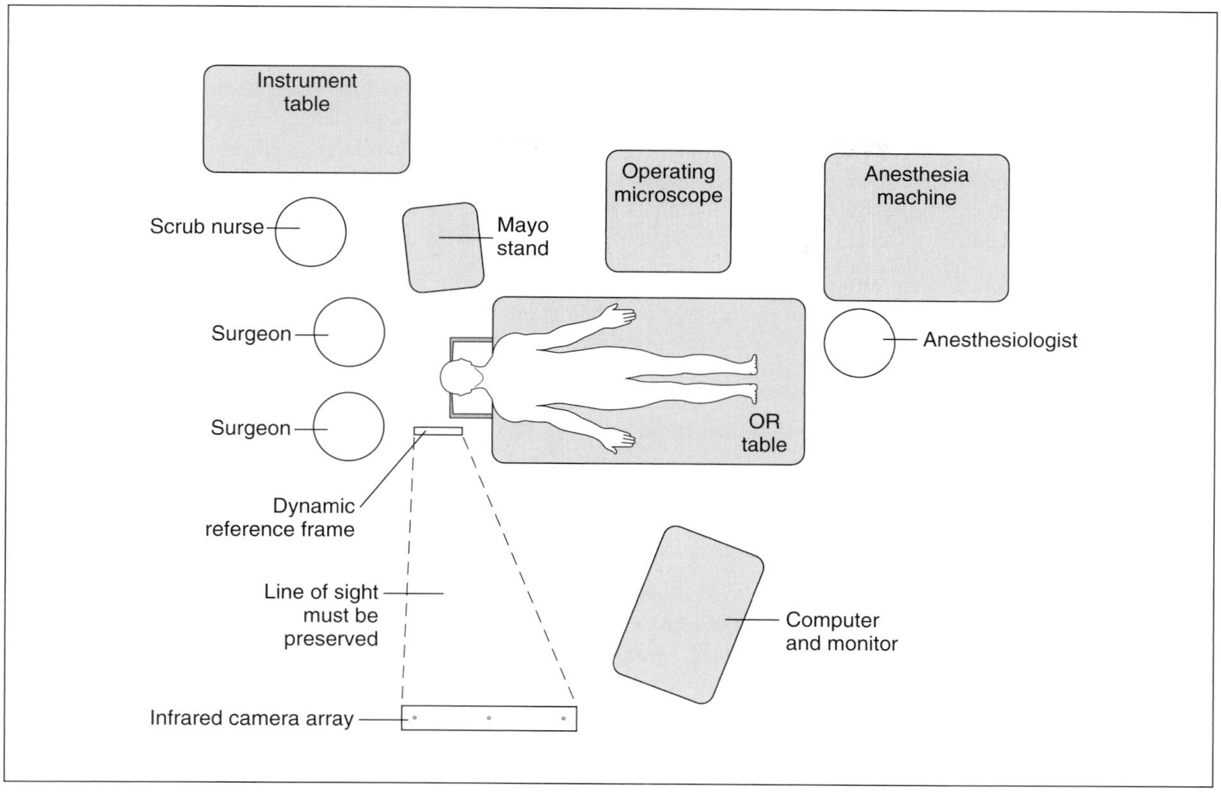

Figure 1.1-22. OR layout for frameless stereotactic surgery.

used to calculate, by hand or computer, the spatial coordinates of the target(s). In nearly all cooperative patients, there is no need for sedation or analgesia during this stage of the procedure.

Frame-based stereotaxy is used most frequently for biopsy of intracranial lesions; however, drainage of cystic lesions or placement of a catheter or depth electrodes also can be performed. These common procedures involve relatively minor surgery, usually requiring only light sedation and local anesthesia. After prepping and draping, specialized operating tools are attached to the stereotactic frame. These instruments provide spatial guidance throughout the surgical procedure. A burr or twist drill hole is the usual form of intracranial access. Maximal sedation is needed during drilling and dural opening. Anesthetic considerations include ensuring adequate oxygenation and ventilation, which may be compromised by the sterile drapes. Additionally, sedation should be light enough at times to allow the neurosurgeon to test gross neurologic function, such as extremity movement, both during and immediately after biopsy. At the completion of the case, the frame is removed and the patient is brought to the recovery room.

Image-guided 'frameless' stereotaxy: Over the last several years, techniques have been developed to provide neurosurgeons with a real-time computer display of position and trajectory. Spatial information is displayed on high-speed computer work stations as two-dimensional images and 3-D renderings obtained from CT and/or MRI. These devices have the added advantage of being frameless; instead of a frame providing a system of reference, small markers (fiducials) are affixed to the scalp and forehead with adhesive. Advances in image-guided navigation also allow the incorporation of ultrasound and endoscopy to provide intraop updating of the preop radiographic images.

Image-guided surgery begins with an imaging study performed with fiducials in place. The remainder of the case is performed in the OR, usually under GA. Once the patient's head is appropriately positioned, the locations of the fiducials are entered into a computer, using any one of several different commercially available digitizing techniques. The most common system uses triangulation of infrared light from LEDs to determine the position of a pointer in space. The computer calculates the position of the pointer with respect to the patient and displays on the monitor the images from the scan with a representation of the pointer superimposed. Since the process of localization assumes a constant frame of reference, it is important that fiducials do not move between the time of imaging and registration in the OR. A further refinement—the dynamic reference frame—may be affixed to the craniotomy headrest to allow intraop repositioning of the patient. The OR must be set up to accommodate the computer and monitor as well as to allow a direct line-of-sight between the operative site and an array of infrared sensors. (See Fig 1.1-22.) Care must be taken to avoid patient movement during the initial registration of the fiducials, as this induces a component of error with respect to the accuracy of the navigation system. Furthermore, during the actual procedure, the position of the camera array system must be preserved to maintain system accuracy.

The spatial information provided to neurosurgeons by image guidance can be used to access deep or critically located lesions through the most direct trajectory and a smaller craniotomy. These techniques have been used primarily during craniotomy for tumor or vascular malformation; however, image guidance also can be used for biopsy or other smaller procedures. As with most craniotomies, GA is used. Maneuvers that alter the spatial relationship of the intracranial contents, such as hyperventilation or diuresis, will result in brain shift relative to the presurgical images and should be avoided if possible, particularly during the early stages of surgery.

Radiosurgery: This technique allows the ablation of small tumors and vascular malformations through the closed cranium with focused doses of radiation. In contrast to other stereotactic operations, radiosurgery is performed outside the OR, using a linear accelerator or other specialized irradiation device. Cooperative adults need little or no sedation during the procedure. Children, however, almost always require GA from the beginning of frame placement through the actual treatment, which may last from 5-8 h. Consequently, anesthesia must be administered at several locations in the hospital, as well as during transport between these sites. Ideally, GA is initiated in the imaging suite just prior to frame placement. After transport to the recovery unit, the child is maintained under anesthesia while radiosurgical treatment is being planned, which takes from 1-3 h. The patient is then transported to the radiosurgery suite, still anesthetized, and treatment is performed. Depending on complexity, radiosurgery itself may last from 1-2 h. At the completion of treatment, the stereotaxic frame is removed and the child is awakened.

Functional Neurosurgery (see p. 58+ for full discussion of these procedures): Surgery using precisely placed lesions (e.g., **pallidotomy, thalamotomy**) or stimulators for the treatment of movement disorders, pain, and certain psychiatric syndromes is encompassed by the term 'functional stereotaxy.' These techniques depend on absolutely precise localization and are usually frame-based. Concurrent neuroanatomic localization using electrophysiologic techniques is often used. In order to preserve neural potentials and allow the patient to cooperate with neurologic testing, no GA is used. These procedures begin, as do other frame-based cases, with placement of the frame and imaging. In the OR, a burr hole is made with the patient under local anesthesia. The patient must remain awake and cooperative with his or her head immobilized throughout a several-hour procedure, which may require patient participation in various neurologic tests. Production of the lesion itself is brief and painless. After closure, the frame is removed and the patient is monitored in a postop observation unit.

Usual preop diagnosis: Brain disease requiring biopsy; brain tumor; vascular malformation; Parkinson's disease; pain syndromes; psychiatric syndromes; cyst drainage

SUMMARY OF PROCEDURES

	Frame-Based Biopsy	**Frameless Craniotomy**	**Pediatric Radiosurgery**	**Functional Neurosurgery**
Position	Supine or prone	Sitting, supine, prone, or lateral	Supine or prone	Supine, head fixed to floor stand
Incision	0.5-2 cm, scalp	1-12 cm, scalp	None	1-3 cm, scalp
Special instrumentation	Stereotactic treatment arc	Sensor array, pointer, computer, monitor, dynamic reference frame	Linear accelerator (LINAC)	Electrophysiologic monitoring equipment, lesion generator, stimulator
Unique considerations	Key for emergency: removal of frame	1. Minimize brain shift. 2. No patient movement during registration. 3. Clear line-of-sight between camera and dynamic reference frame.	Extended anesthesia in several different locations	Patient must be awake, able to cooperate with testing.
Antibiotics	Cefazolin 1 g	Nafcillin 1-2 g + cefotaxime 1 g	None	Cefazolin 1 g
Surgical time	0.5-1.5 h	2-6 h	5-8 h	2-6 h
EBL	< 10 ml	20-1000 ml	None	< 100 ml
Postop care	PACU	ICU	PACU	Neuroobservation unit
Mortality	< 0.5%	1%	None	< 1%

	Frame-Based Biopsy	**Frameless Craniotomy**	**Pediatric Radiosurgery**	**Functional Neurosurgery**
Morbidity	Overall: < 1% Symptomatic intracerebral hemorrhage	Infection Air emboli Hemorrhage Stroke Sz Worsening edema	N/V: 2-3%	N/V: 1-10% Intracerebral hemorrhage New neurologic deficits
Pain score	2	4	2	2

PATIENT POPULATION CHARACTERISTICS

Age range	All ages	⇐	0-12 yr	18-90 yr
Male:Female	1:1	⇐	⇐	⇐
Incidence	Uncommon	Unusual	⇐	Rare
Etiology	Tumor; infection; AIDS; demylinating syndromes	Tumor; vascular malformations; epilepsy	⇐	Parkinson's disease; pain syndromes; psychiatric syndromes

ANESTHETIC CONSIDERATIONS

PREOPERATIVE

Neurosurgical procedures are performed using stereotactic control when the lesion is small and/or is located deep within brain tissue, or as a means of obtaining a biopsy of a lesion for diagnosis. For example, focal, deep-seated AVMs may be resected under stereotactic control. These patients are often otherwise healthy.

Neurological   Neurological Sx vary (depending on site and size of the lesion) and they should be carefully documented. In addition to the usual tests, a CT or MRI scan is obtained preop with the frame in place to determine stereotactic coordinates. Once the coordinates are established, the frame or fiducial markers must not be moved until the operation is complete.

Laboratory   Tests as indicated from H&P.

INTRAOPERATIVE

Anesthetic technique: GETA or MAC. In adults, fiducial markers or a stereotactic frame are placed before surgery and the patient is taken to the radiologic suite for CT/MRI scan to determine stereotactic coordinates. The patient is then brought to OR with the frame or fiducial markers in place. The key for removing the stereotactic frame must be readily available in the event of an airway emergency. Biopsies generally are done under local anesthesia with MAC. If a complete resection is planned (e.g., AVM resection), GETA is used. In children, it is usually necessary to induce GA before placing the frame, thus necessitating the maintenance of GA during the CT/MRI scan. The child is then moved to the OR, still anesthetized, and the operation is completed.

Induction   If MAC is planned, O_2 by nasal prongs is administered, and the patient is lightly sedated with combinations of propofol 25-50 μg/kg/min ± midazolam 1-4 mg/kg in divided doses to provide amnesia ± remifentanil 0.02-0.05 μg/kg/min to provide analgesia. It is important that the patient be able to communicate with the surgeon as needed throughout the operation. For functional neurosurgery (e.g., pallidotomy), sedation should be minimized to preserve normal electrophysiological activity. If GETA is needed in a framed stereotactic procedure, FOL is necessary before inducing anesthesia because the frame precludes intubation by direct laryngoscopy (see p. B-6). Once ET intubation is established, anesthesia may be induced with STP 2-5 mg/kg or propofol 1-2 mg/kg, followed by a nondepolarizing NMB to facilitate positioning of patient.

Maintenance   If GA is used, maintenance is the same as for a tumor (see Anesthetic Considerations for Craniotomy for Tumor, p. 28) or AVM (see Anesthetic Considerations for Craniotomy for Intracranial Vascular Malformations, p. 17). If children are to be transported from the site of placement of the stereotactic frame to the radiologic suite and then to the OR, it is best to use a propofol infusion (e.g., 75-150 μg/kg/min) with spontaneous or controlled ventilation to assure adequate ventilation and oxygenation during transport and study. Opiates and nondepolarizing NMBs should not be administered until the child is in the operating suite.

Emergence	ETT generally is removed at the conclusion of the operation. Prophylactic antiemetic (e.g., metoclopramide 10 mg and ondansetron 4 mg) in adults should be given 30 min before extubation.	
Blood and fluid requirements	IV: 16-18 ga × 2 (adults); 20-22 ga (children) NS/LR @ 4-6 ml/kg/h	Blood loss is minimal since the volume of tissue removed is small.

Monitoring	If local anesthesia: standard monitors (see p. B-1).
	If GA:
	  Arterial line
	  CVP line
	  UO	

Positioning	✓ and pad pressure points. ✓ eyes.	

POSTOPERATIVE

Complications	Bleeding	Focal bleeding may occur postop, causing onset of a neurological deficit.
Pain management	Vicodin (1-2 mg po q 4 h prn)	
Tests	CT or MRI scan, if a new neurological deficit occurs.	

References

1. Baker KC, Isert PR: Anaesthetic considerations for children undergoing stereotactic radiosurgery. *Anaesth Intensive Care* 1997; 25(6):691-5.
2. Burchiel KJ: Image-based functional neurosurgery. *Clin Neurosurg* 1992; 39:314-30.
3. Chang SD, Adler JR, Hancock SL: Clinical uses of radiosurgery. *Oncology* 1998; 12(8):1181-91.
4. Glidenberg PL: Stereotactic surgery—the past and the future. *Stereotact Funct Neurosurg* 1998; 70(2-4):57-70.
5. Glidenberg PL, Tasker RR, eds: *Textbook of Sterotactic and Functional Neurosurgery*. McGraw-Hill, New York: 1997.
6. Glidenberg PL, Woo SY: Multimodality program involving stereotactic surgery in brain tumor management. *Stereotact Funct Neurosurg* 2000; 75(2-3):147-52.
7. Heilbrun MP, ed: *Stereotactic Neurosurgery*. Williams & Wilkins, Baltimore: 1988.
8. Kondziolka D: Functional neurosurgery. *Neurosurgery* 1999; 44(1):12-20.
9. Maciunas, RJ: Stereotactic radiosurgery. *Nat Med* 1996; 2(6):712-13.
10. Ohye C: The idea of stereotaxy toward minimally invasive neurosurgery. *Stereotact Funct Neuorsurg* 2000; 74(3-4):185-93.
11. Ross DA: Minimalism through stereotactic technique. *Clin Neurosurg* 1996; 43:317-23.
12. Vannier MW, Marsh JL: Three-dimensional imaging, surgical planning, and image-guided therapy. *Radiol Clin North Am* 1996; 34(3):545-63.

Surgeons

Gary Heit, MD, PhD
Lawrence M. Shuer, MD (*Epilepsy surgery*)

1.2 FUNCTIONAL NEUROSURGERY

Anesthesiologists

Richard A. Jaffe, MD, PhD
Stanley I. Samuels, MB, Bch, FFARCS

FUNCTIONAL NEUROSURGERY:
THE SURGICAL TREATMENT OF PAIN,
MOVEMENT DISORDERS, AND EPILEPSY

INTRODUCTION

Gary Heit

Functional neurosurgery consists of the treatment of chronic pain, epilepsy, and movement disorders. Each of these disease states has a distinctive anesthetic requirement dictated by the specific pathophysiology and subsequent intraop objectives. Procedures may be performed under local anesthesia, conscious sedation, or GA, and can be divided into ablative or augmentative techniques. With the exception of the treatment of epilepsy, ablative techniques are not recommended because of their unpredictable duration of effect and irreversible nature of the lesion. Neuroaugmentation (electrical stimulation or continuous local drug administration) tends to produce more lasting benefits and, more importantly, can be changed to meet fluctuations in the patient's symptoms.

The key to successful functional neurosurgical therapies is target identification. Many targets can be identified anatomically on appropriate radiographic studies. Within those targets (and in some that are not resolvable with imaging studies), however, there is a functional subdivision that often needs physiological identification. For pain management, this involves the identification of a target nucleus, as well as the appropriate somatotopic location matching the patient's complaints. In the case of movement disorders, target location is often the region that is involved in the tremor generation, or motor activity. This region can be closely associated with an area involved in higher cognitive behavior. Thus, the need for physiological identification often dictates a specific anesthetic technique.

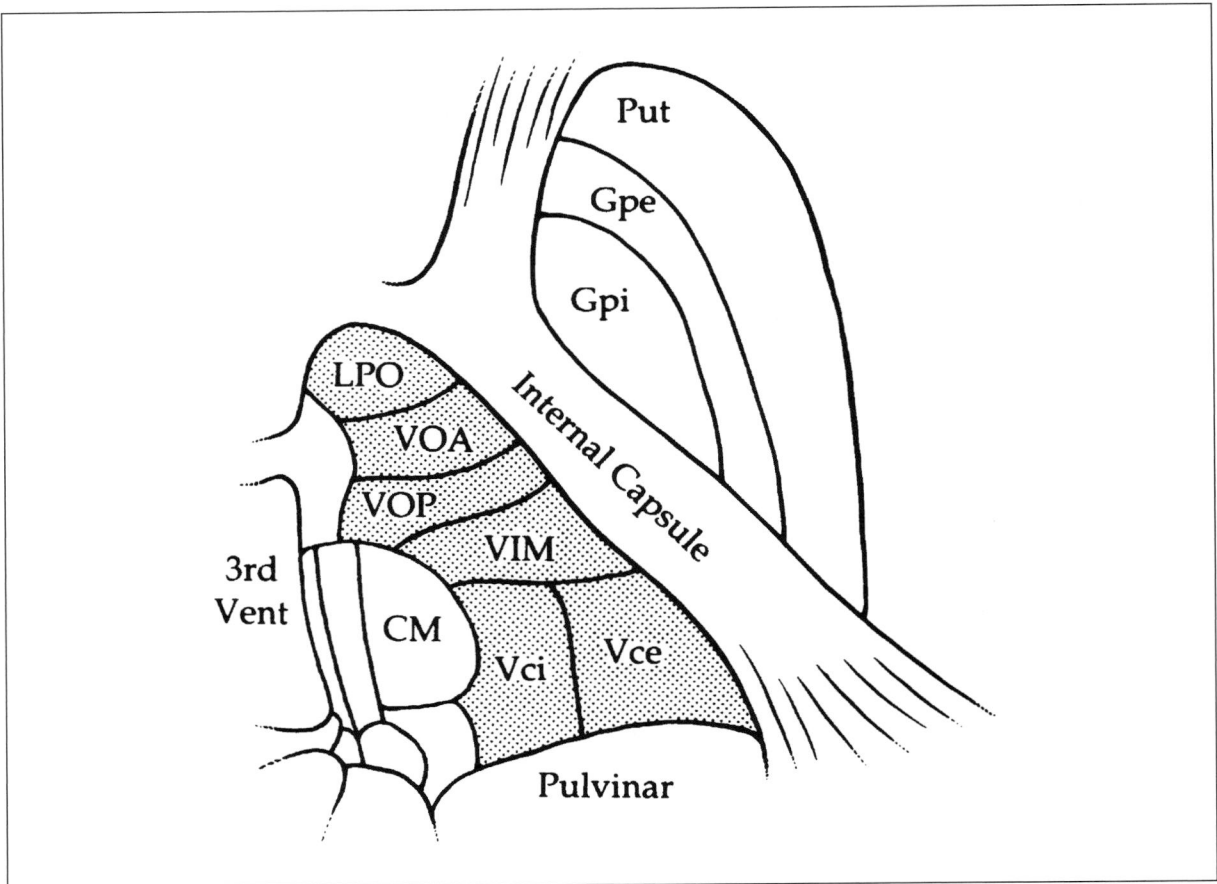

Figure 1.2-1. Topographical anatomy of the ventrolateral thalamus. CM = centrum medianum; GPe = external segment of globus pallidus; GPi = internal segment of globus pallidus; Put = putamen; LPO = lateropolaris; VOA = ventrooralis anterior; VOP = ventrooralis posterior; VIM = ventrali intermedius; Vce and Vci = ventralis caudalis externus and internus. (Reproduced with permission from Grossman RG, Loftus CM: *Principles of Neurosurgery*, 2nd edition. Lippincott-Raven, 1999.)

STEREOTACTIC PROCEDURES: DEEP BRAIN STIMULATION, PALLIDOTOMY, AND THALAMOTOMY

SURGICAL CONSIDERATIONS

Description: Most procedures are currently performed with **frame-based stereotactic techniques**, with intracranial access achieved via a burr hole or twist drill. There is a trend to use 'frameless' stereotactics based on optical systems, although they are less accurate. Two approaches to identification of the functional target are used following initial stereotactic CT or MRI radiographic localization; both require patient cooperation. In one approach, the target is confirmed by assessing symptomatic resolution during high-frequency macrostimulation and by identifying surrounding structures using their characteristic stimulation-evoked responses. In the other approach, before stimulation testing, single-neuron recordings are performed to localize the appropriate target through somatotopic kinesthetic and/or somatosensory responses. In an awake patient, appropriate stimulation is delivered to the skin, or by passive and active movement of the joints. This technique

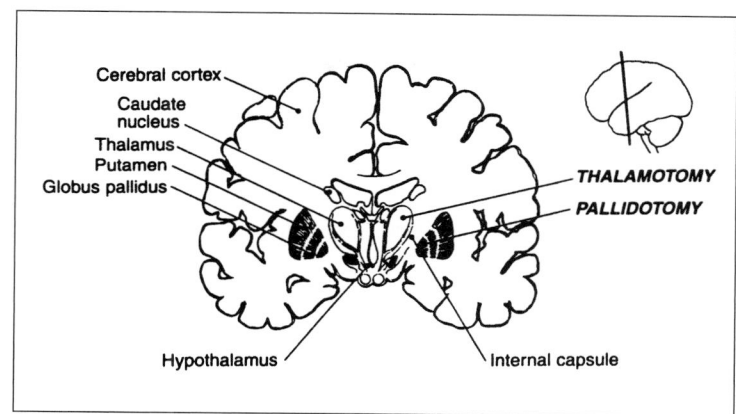

Figure 1.2-2. Anatomical locations for therapeutic lesions (thalamotomy and pallidotomy) for the surgical treatment of Parkinson's disease. Inset shows the plane of the coronal section through the diencephalon, identifying the lesions. (Reproduced with permission from Mason LJ, Cojocaru TT, Cole DJ: Surgical intervention and anesthetic management of the patient with Parkinson's disease. In *International Anesthesiology Clinics: Topics in Neuroanesthesia.* Jaffe RA, Giffard RG, eds. Little, Brown, Boston: 1996 4(34):141.)

utilizes specialized high-impedance microelectrodes and amplifiers susceptible to interference from monitoring equipment, which may necessitate manual measurements of BP and clinical assessment of oxygenation. Anesthesia or sedation can modify neuronal activity significantly and, thus, interfere with functional mapping. For example, propofol has been shown to inhibit globus pallidus neurons for several minutes beyond its behavioral effects. Additionally, many of these agents have been shown to change evoked potential (EP) responses, raising the possibility that they could alter stimulation thresholds for either the internal capsule or optic tract. Thermal ablation typically is performed with a radiofrequency (RF) lesion generator operating at 500 kHz, which may interfere with some types of monitoring equipment; however, the ablation process only lasts approximately 12-30 sec.

A variety of movement disorders are amenable to surgical treatment. They can be divided into akinetic (e.g., Parkinson's) and hyperkinetic (e.g., dystonias, tremor, spasticity) syndromes. Idiopathic **Parkinson's disease** is best treated with **deep brain stimulation (DBS)** targeted to a functional subcomponent of either the subthalamic nucleus or globus pallidus interna (posteroventral **pallidotomy**, or PVP, Fig 1.2-2). Tremor syndromes are treated by DBS, targeting of the ventral intermedius thalamic nucleus (**thalamotomy** or stimulation), while dystonias are treated by stimulation of the globus pallidus interna. **Spasticity** (p. 69) is not treated stereotactically, but through the administration of intrathecal baclofen (GABA-like synaptic inhibition) in the lumbar cistern via an internalized pump system. Abrupt loss of intrathecal infusion of baclofen, however, can quickly lead to a serious withdrawal syndrome with dysautonomia, circulatory collapse, and death within hours. Spasticity refractory to intrathecal baclofen may be amenable to selective dorsal root rhizotomy performed through an open laminectomy.

For **DBS**, implantation of the intracranial electrode is performed under local anesthesia to permit monitoring of behavioral and physiologic responses. A 2- to 3-cm linear incision (burr-hole access) or stab wound (twist-drill access), generally is placed in front of the coronal suture and 10-50 mm from the midline; generally placed in the frontal bone. Minimal or no sedation is used, as patient cooperation is necessary during the functional mapping component of the case. If single-neuron recordings are used, avoid propofol, since it can produce prolonged suppression of target neuronal activity. If sedation is needed, use a low-dose (0.01-0.05 µg/kg/min) remifentanil infusion. Local anesthetics should not contain epinephrine. Avoid central-acting β-blockers (e.g., propranolol), which suppress tremor activity in target neurons. Sedation with meperidine in patients taking selegiline is contraindicated. No dopaminergic antagonist (e.g., metoclopramide, droperidol) should be given to Parkinsonian patients or patients with dopamine-responsive dystonia. To enhance single-cell responses, withhold medications prescribed for target symptoms for 8-24 h. In some cases (e.g., Parkinson's disease), this may result in a rebound HTN requiring active treatment; however, patients will resume their medications postop (often in the post-anesthesia recovery area) and the HTN will resolve. The **implantable pulse generator (IPG)** may be placed in an infraclavicular subcutaneous pocket at the time of the intracranial electrode implantation. Implantation of the IPG and subcutaneous tunneling of the electrode lead can be done under MAC, but is best tolerated under GETA. To facilitate intubation, the calverial wound is closed temporally and the stereotactic frame is removed. Closure consists of a single, interrupted suture for stab wounds or two-layer suture/staple closure for a burr hole. IPG pockets are closed in two layers. The subcutaneous layer is closed with absorbable sutures and the skin is closed with staples or suture.

Usual preop diagnosis: Medically intractable idiopathic Parkinson's disease with disabling L-Dopa-induced dyskinesia, bradykinesia, or rigidity; severe fluctuations in medication responses; dystonia musculorum deformans; post-CVA dystonia; occasionally, torticollis; tremor; movement disorders

SUMMARY OF PROCEDURE

Position	Supine
Incision	Linear (burr holes); stab-wound (twist drill)
Unique considerations	Minimal/no sedation. BP ↑ in patients who have their antihypertensive medications withheld. Manual vital sign monitoring as electronic monitors may interfere with single-cell recordings.
Antibiotics + other meds	Cefazolin 1 g; dexamethasone 6-8 mg
Surgical time	3-9 h
EBL	25-150 ml
Postop care	Continue antibiotics, Parkinson's medications. BP may ↓. Maintain MAP 90 mmHg to prevent postop bleeding. ICU
Mortality	< 0.5%
Morbidity	Overall: 8-27%
	Infection
	Hardware failure: Rare
	Intracranial hemorrhage
	Cognitive disturbances
Pain score	2-3

PATIENT POPULATION CHARACTERISTICS

Age range	12-80 yr
Male:Female	1:1
Incidence	Becoming common
Etiology	Idiopathic; genetic
Associated conditions	Dystonia

ANESTHETIC CONSIDERATIONS

See Anesthetic Considerations following Surgical Analgesics, p. 62.

References:

1. Benabid A, Pollak P, Gao D, Hoffman D, Limousin P, Gay E, Payen I, Benazzouz A: Chronic electrical stimulation of the ventralis intermedius nucleus of the thalamus as a treatment of movement disorders. *J Neurosurg* 1996; 84:203-14.
2. Guridi J, Lozana A: A brief history of pallidotomy. Neurosurgery 1997; 41(5):1169-83.
3. Heit G. Murphy G, Jaffe R, Golby A, Silverberg GS: The effects of propofol on human globus pallidus neurons. *Stereotact Funct Neurosurg* 1997; 67(1-2):74.
4. Joint C, Nandi D, Parkin S, Gregory R, Aziz T: Hardware-related problems of deep brain stimulation. *Move Disord* 2002; 17(Suppl 3):S175-80.

SURGICAL ANALGESICS: SPINAL CORD STIMULATION, INTRATHECAL PUMPS, AND CORTICAL STIMULATION

SURGICAL CONSIDERATIONS

Description: Chronic pain arises from a variety of etiologies. It can involve both neuropathic and nociceptive processes and occur in a variety of anatomical distributions (e.g., radicular versus a hemibody pattern). Therapeutic interventions are dictated by the pathophysiology of the pain, its qualitative nature, etiology, and the patients' prognosis. Common procedures for chronic pain are directed at the spinal cord, and may consist of epidural or intrathecal medications or electrical stimulation.

For **chronic spinal cord stimulation** (e.g., postlaminectomy syndrome) an epidural electrode is implanted either percutaneously or via an open laminectomy. **Percutaneous electrodes** are easier to implant and have less associated surgical pain. The surgical electrode (implanted via laminectomy) confers greater mechanical stability in the epidural space. Additionally, given its larger contact size, it can generate higher current densities with less drain on the implanted system. For percutaneous electrodes, a small skin incision is made 2-3 vertebral levels caudal to the target region of the spinal cord. For 'surgical paddle' electrodes, the skin incision is made 1-2 levels caudal to the target zone of the spinal cord, and a laminectomy is performed to provide access to the epidural space. Incisions are closed in the standard fashion.

In either technique, patient cooperation is required during intraop test stimulation. The procedures are done in the prone or lateral position with consequent implications for airway management in the sedated patient. Localization of the electrodes is accomplished initially based on radiographic criteria; however, these localizations are only approximate, and it is recommended that the electrode placement be confirmed by intraop stimulation. The patient needs to be sufficiently alert to communicate the quality, distribution, and intensity of the stimulation-induced paresthesias. To assess efficacy, the electrode may be externalized and percutaneous stimulation used for assessment. If there is > 50% reduction in pain, the patient may return to the OR for internalization of the implantable pulse generator (IPG). Postop, these patients can have an exacerbation of pain, particularly if neuropathic in nature. They may require iv lidocaine or ketamine infusions to return them to their preop baseline, even with a functioning and appropriately located stimulating electrode.

For **pain of central origin** (e.g., poststroke, multiple sclerosis, and trigeminal nerve pathology), surgical procedures are directed at the thalamus and cortex. Thalamic interventions include stereotactic insertion of stimulating electrodes into sensory thalamus. **Thalamic DBS** requires awake mapping of the somatotopic representation of the affected body part through either microelectrode mapping or stimulation-induced paresthesias. For medically intractable neuropathic pain syndromes, **epidural motor cortex stimulation** has shown great promise. Functional mapping of the motor cortex for epidural stimulation can be done with anatomical and physiological mapping under GA via a craniotomy; and the anesthetic should be tailored to minimize interference with EP recording. The incision consists of a 5- to 10-cm linear or 5 × 10 cm trapezoidal incision placed over and paralleling the motor cortex.

Identification of the appropriate location on the motor strip can be done initially with epidural mapping using SSEPs elicited from the part of the body where the pain originates. In cases of denervation syndromes, SSEP may not be present and the minimum intensity point for epidural stimulation-induced movements is used. In rare cases, the surgeon may elect to perform the surgery awake to facilitate mapping. To assess efficacy, the electrode may be externalized and percutaneous stimulation assessed for overall therapeutic efficacy. If there is > 50% reduction in pain, the patient will return to the OR for internalization of the IPG. Closure consists of calverial reconstruction with externalization of leads. The craniotomy incision is closed in the standard fashion. If a percutaneous trial is done, the IPG implant requires a second GETA with reopening of wounds.

The current surgical 'gold standard' for the treatment of trigeminal neuralgia is **microvascular decompression of the trigeminal nerve** in the prepontine cistern (see p. 37). In patients who are poor surgical candidates, treatment is accomplished with ablative procedures aimed at the gasserian ganglia, using hemolytic, mechanical, or radiofrequency (RF) techniques. Patients who fail gasserian ganglion interventions or have atypical facial pain are candidates for **thalamic DBS** or **motor cortex stimulation**. Surgical treatments for trigeminal neuralgia, however, may become obsolete, given the advent of **stereotactic radiosurgical ablative techniques**. These systems utilize multiple beams of radiation focused on the nerve to achieve pain relief equivalent to microvascular decompression without the attendant complications of an invasive neurosurgical procedure.

For pain unresponsive to spinal cord stimulation or because of unacceptable side effects of parental medications, continuous intrathecal administration of analgesics can be accomplished with an **indwelling system**. An incision is made over the L3-4, L4-5 or L5-S1 spinous process and a second incision is placed in the RLQ of the abdomen. A tunnel tool is used to bring the catheter from the lumbar spinal region to the abdomen. This tunnel is rarely tolerated without GETA or deep sedation. Intrathecal narcotics (typically morphine), can achieve satisfactory results, since therapeutic drug concentrations can be achieved at the level of spinal opiate μ-receptors without influencing higher CNS opiate systems. This therapeutic intervention can be assessed through a percutaneous catheter trial. Patients who experience ≥ 50% reduction in pain are candidates for a **totally implanted pump system**. These are low-morbidity procedures (5-10%) with infections and hardware failures constituting the greatest problems. Abrupt cessation of medications—through either patient noncompliance with refill schedules (10-12 wk) or hardware failure—however, can lead to a serious withdrawal syndrome.

Usual preop diagnosis: Chronic pain

SUMMARY OF PROCEDURE

Position	Prone/lateral
Incision	2-3 levels ↑ target area (spinal and stimulation) + laminectomy; L3, 4, 5 (intrathecal pump) + 2nd incision RLQ of abdomen.
Unique considerations	Patient communication important; therefore, avoid oversedation. Copious use of local anesthetics (avoid overdosing).
Antibiotics	Cefazolin 1 g
Surgical time	1.5-3 h
EBL	< 25 ml
Postop care	May have ↑ pain
Mortality	< 0.5%
Morbidity	Overall: 5-10% Infection Hardware failure Withdrawal Sx
Pain score	3-8

PATIENT POPULATION CHARACTERISTICS

Age range	20-75 yr
Male:Female	1:1
Incidence	Common
Etiology	Iatrogenic; neuropathic; traumatic
Associated conditions	Opiate dependency

ANESTHETIC CONSIDERATIONS

(Procedures covered: DBS, pallidotomy, thalamotomy; spinal cord stimulation, intrathecal pumps, cortical stimulation)

PREOPERATIVE

Parkinson's disease is the most common movement disorder, affecting ~1% of the population > 60 yr. It is caused by the loss of dopaminergic neurons in the substantia nigra → ↓dopamine (dopamine/acetylcholine imbalance) in basal ganglia → movement disorder. Medical treatment is directed primarily to restoring dopamine levels by increasing the availability of the dopamine precursor (L-dopa), inhibiting liver dopa decarboxylase (carbidopa, usually given in combination with L-dopa as Sinemet), by releasing endogenous dopamine (amantadine [Symmetrel]) and by blocking MAO-B (selegiline [Eldepryl]). Medical treatment also may include dopamine agonists (pergolide [Permax]; bromocriptine [Parlodel]), and acetylcholine antagonists (amantadine [Symmetrel], benztropine [Cogentin]) to correct the dopamine/acetylcholine imbalance. Patients presenting for surgery have failed medical therapy, and will have been taken off their antiparkinsonian medications 8-24 h before surgery. This will maximize their symptoms to help assess treatment effects intraop; thus, preop assessment on the day of surgery will be difficult.

Respiratory	Autonomic dysfunction → esophageal dysfunction → ↑risk of aspiration. Patients typically have ↓vital capacity 2° rigidity, dyskinesia → ↓respiratory function and ↓cough. Laryngospasm and respiratory failure may occur following withdrawal of antiparkinsonian medications. **Tests:** CXR; consider ABG; PFTs may be difficult to obtain.
Cardiovascular	Autonomic dysfunction → orthostatic hypotension. Dopamine replacement therapy → cardiac dysrhythmias, ↓BP, and hypovolemia. In patients taking selegiline (MAOI): meperidine → ↑↑BP, rigidity, agitation; sympathomimetics → exaggerated ↑BP.

Neurological	The primary Sx of Parkinson's disease include rigidity, tremor, bradykinesia, muscle weakness. Secondary symptoms include dementia, depression, and speech difficulty. Patients may alternate between a state of immobility and one of exaggerated tremor (which may interfere with intraop monitoring).	
Renal	Urinary retention is common.	
Gastrointestinal	Autonomic dysfunction → gastroparesis, ↑incidence of reflux. Poor nutrition. Pharyngeal muscle dysfunction → dysphagia.	
Laboratory	As indicated from H&P.	
Premedication	None. These patients often will have received small doses of fentanyl and/or midazolam to facilitate placement of the stereotactic frame.	

INTRAOPERATIVE

Anesthetic technique: MAC, with minimal or no sedation, as patient cooperation is essential for the success of the procedure.

Induction	Low-dose remifentanil (0.01-0.05 μg/kg/min) may be used for sedation.	
Maintenance	BP control is important to minimize the risk of intracranial hemorrhage. MAP should be kept at or, preferably, somewhat below normal for that patient. This usually can be accomplished without an arterial line by using small doses of atenolol (0.5-1 mg increments iv) and/or an infusion of NTG titrated to effect. Atenolol is prefered over other parenteral β-blockers because its CNS penetration is limited → minimal effect on central tremor. Postop BP control can be continued by using NTG paste applied 30-60 min before the end of the procedure. In the event of an airway emergency, a means of releasing the patient from the stereotactic frame must be readily available.	
Emergence	Antiparkinsonian medication should be given when the procedure is complete. The patient is usually transported to the PACU, then to the neurology ward for postop monitoring.	
Blood and fluid requirements	Minimal blood loss IV: 18-20 ga × 1 NS/LR @ 1-2 ml/kg/h	IV should be placed in the ipsilateral arm (relative to side of surgery).
Monitoring	Standard monitors (see p. B-1).	Exaggerated tremors in these patients may interfere with monitoring. It may be helpful to place the BP cuff on a leg (less tremor). No monitor should be placed on contralateral arm, which must be kept free for testing. Monitors (oximeter, BP, gas analyzer) may interfere with intraop electrophysiology and may need to be replaced with manual techniques during this period.
Positioning	✓ and pad pressure points. ✓ stereotactic frame clearance.	Patient comfort may be improved by placing pillows under the knees to relieve lower back strain.
Complications	Intracerebral hemorrhage	Dx: ↓mental status and hemiparesis. CT scan usually required to confirm Dx. Emergency craniotomy may be necessary.
	Loss of airway	Rx: remove stereotactic frame and secure airway.

POSTOPERATIVE

Complications	Intracranial hemorrhage Motor deficit Visual field deficit Aphasia	Intracranial hemorrhage may require emergency craniotomy.
Tests	None	
Pain management	Usually not necessary	

References:

1. North RB: Spinal cord stimulation patient selection. In *Surgical Management of Pain.* Burchiel KJ, ed. Thieme Medical Pub, NY: 2002, 527-34.

2. Pagura JR, Rabello JR, Cerueira de Lima W: Microvascular decompression for trigeminal neuralgia. In *Textbook of Stereotactic and Functional Neurosurgery.* Gildenberg PL, Tasker RK, eds. McGraw Hill, NY: 1998, 1715-21.

3. Tsubokawa T: Motor cortex stimulation for the relief of central deafferented pain. In *Surgical Management of Pain.* Burchiel KJ, ed. Thieme Medical Pub, NY; 2002, 555-64.

VAGAL NERVE STIMULATION

SURGICAL CONSIDERATIONS

Description: The surgical treatment of medically intractable epilepsy consists of either **surgical resection** of the epileptic site (see p. 66) or **vagal nerve stimulation (VNS)**. For patients who are not candidates for resective surgery, VNS can be a viable surgical strategy. Although it is a low-morbidity procedure, its efficacy also is low. VNS tends to produce a 50% or greater reduction of Sz in ~48% of patients after 18 mo of stimulation.[1] By contrast, **temporal lobectomy** for patients with medial temporal lobe epilepsy has an 80-85% chance of making the patient seizure-free, while using only one anticonvulsant medication, or none at all. Surgery for **extratemporal epilepsy** originating in neocortex has a 50% chance of making the patient seizure-free, in the absence of a structural lesion. (If an anatomical abnormality is present, then that figure increases to ~75%.) In general, the complication rate is ~7%, dependent on the exact location of the Sz foci and its relationship to eloquent cortex.

Two incisions are used for VNS: one left anterior cervical, placed ~at the C6-7 level, with a second incision in the left infraclavicular region for placement of the implantable pulse generator (IPG). Some surgeons perform the procedure through a carotid-type incision and place the IPG caudally through blunt dissection. During surgery, the interface between the vagal nerve and the electrode is tested with electrical stimulation. Fortunately, this is associated with a very low incidence of bradycardia and extremely rare reports of asystole. All resolve with cessation of stimulation and administration of atropine. The surgeon should inform the anesthesiologist when vagal stimulation is about to begin. The incisions are closed using the standard technique; however, since many patients are developmentally delayed, the final skin layer is often closed with a subcutaneous technique that does not require subsequent removal.

Usual preop diagnosis: Epilepsy

SUMMARY OF PROCEDURE

Position	Supine
Incision	Anterior cervical (C6-7) + infraclavicular (for IPG)
Unique considerations	Bradycardia → asystole during stimulation phase
Antibiotics	Cefazolin 1 g
Surgical time	1.5 h
EBL	< 50 ml
Postop care	Observe for ↑Sz activity postop × 8 h
Mortality	< 0.5%
Morbidity	Overall, low
	Infection: 2%
	Hardware failure: Rare
	Nerve/vascular injury (similar to carotid surgery)
Pain score	1-2

PATIENT POPULATION CHARACTERISTICS

Age range	6-80 yr
Male:Female	1:1
Incidence	Uncommon
Etiology	Idiopathic, typically
Associated conditions	Developmental delay

ANESTHETIC CONSIDERATIONS

PREOPERATIVE

Antiepileptic medication, such as phenytoin, will abolish seizure disorders in most patients, but some develop intolerable side effects; others are refractory to medical therapy. Surgical ablation of the Sz focus may be the only effective therapy for some patients. For patients who are not candidates for ablative procedures, the placement of a vagal nerve stimulator may be a viable alternative.

Neurologic	The only common neurological finding is a Hx of uncontrollable Sz, either focal or generalized. Obtain a description of Sz and prodromal Sx.
Gastrointestinal	Abnormal liver function may be associated with use of valproate and carbamazepine. **Tests:** LFT and others as indicated from H&P.
Hematologic	Phenytoin/phenobarbital → ↓Hct; carbamazepine/valproate/ethosuximide/primidone → ↓Plt; carbamazepine/primidone → ↓WBC. **Tests:** CBC and others as indicated from H&P.
Laboratory	Tests as indicated from H&P.
Premedication	Standard premedication (see p. B-2) is usually appropriate.

INTRAOPERATIVE

Anesthetic technique: GETA

Induction	Standard induction (see p. B-2). Once anesthesia is induced, a nondepolarizing NMR is administered.
Maintenance	Standard maintenance (see p. B-3). Generally, no further NMBs are administered beyond that used for tracheal intubation.
Emergence	No special considerations. Prophylactic antiemetic (e.g., metoclopramide 10 mg or ondansetron 4 mg) should be given 30-60 min before extubation.
Blood and fluid requirements	Minimal blood loss IV: 18 ga NS/LR @ 4-6 ml/kg/h
Monitoring	Standard monitors (see p. B-1).	O_2 sat and $ETCO_2$ monitoring will indicate the adequacy of ventilation and oxygenation.
Positioning	✓ and pad pressure points. ✓ eyes.
Complications	Asystole Sz	Rarely (< 1%), the SA node is innervated by the left vagus nerve. In those patients, vagal stimulation may result in severe bradycardia or asystole. Rx: Stop stimulation; atropine 0.5 mg iv ± CPR.

POSTOPERATIVE

Complications	Seizure	Sz precautions may be necessary. Monitor carefully for altered mental status.
Pain management	Usually mild discomfort	Rx: See p. C-2.
Tests	No routine tests	

References:

1. Augustinsson LE, Ben-Menachem E: Vagal nerve stimulation for the treatment of refractory seizures. In *Textbook of Stereotactic and Functional Neurosurgery*. Gildenberg PL, Tasker RK, eds. McGraw Hill, NY: 1998, 1715-21.
2. Mason LJ, Cojocaru TT, Cole DJ: Surgical intervention and anesthetic management of the patient with Parkinson's disease. In *Topics in Neuroanesthesia*. Jaffe RA, Giffard RG, eds. Little, Brown, Boston: 1996; 34(4):133-50.

EPILEPSY SURGERY

SURGICAL CONSIDERATIONS

Lawrence M. Shuer and Gary Heit

Description: In the U.S., the prevalence of epilepsy is approximately 5-20/1,000 (0.5-2%), meaning that at least 1.5 million people have epilepsy.[2] In childhood, the incidence and prevalence is higher, with 90% of all new cases occurring before the age of 20. Intractable epilepsy is defined as persistent seizure activity of such frequency or severity that prevents normal function and/or development. This diagnosis is made only after an adequate trial of anticonvulsant medication(s), with therapeutic levels, has been documented. Of all those with epilepsy, 10-20% prove to be intractable; it is estimated that ~20-30% of patients with intractable epilepsy may benefit from a surgical procedure.[5]

The causes of epilepsy are varied, ranging from idiopathic to neoplastic. Epilepsy surgery is most beneficial in patients with partial epilepsy 2° a structural lesion. Most commonly, this lesion is located in the temporal lobe, and the most common operation is a **temporal lobectomy**, in both children and adults. Cerebral dominance and, hence, the location of speech, must be determined using a preop Wada test (intracarotid amobarbital injection to localize language function).[1] Studies to define the epileptogenic focus include simultaneous recordings of video/EEG and high-resolution MRI and PET scans. Temporal lobe surgery may involve removal of only the structural lesion and associated epileptogenic cortex, cortical resection alone, excision of the amygdala and hippocampus, or removal of the entire anterior temporal lobe, with the extent of posterior resection dependent on dominance. Depending on the involved center, intraop electrocorticography may be used, requiring neuroleptic anesthesia. In addition, the speech center may need to be identified intraop, necessitating an awake procedure. These differing options will significantly alter the choice of anesthesia and must be established before surgery.

A standard **temporal lobectomy** is detailed as follows: The patient is placed supine on the operating table with the head turned 90° and held with pin fixation. A 'question mark' temporal incision is often used, and hemostasis is achieved with skin clips. A flap—either a free temporal bone flap or an osteoplastic flap, based on the temporalis muscle—is elevated with a high-speed craniotome. A **subtemporal craniectomy** allows visualization of the entire anterior temporal lobe. The dura is opened, widely exposing the anterior 6-6.5 cm of the temporal lobe. Labbe's vein must be preserved. At this point, surface and/or depth electrocorticography may be employed and **inhalation anesthetics must not be used**. After mapping the lesion, amygdala and hippocampus or anterior temporal lobe is removed. Temporal lobectomy involves resection of both the lateral and medial temporal structures, and is commonly performed in two steps. Often an operating microscope will be used to completely resect medial structures, including the uncus and hippocampal formation. Injury to the brain stem, 3rd and 4th cranial nerves, and either the middle cerebral or posterior cerebral arteries, can occur; these are known complications of this surgery. Closure of the dura, bone flap, and scalp is routine.

Variant procedure or approaches: There are four common variant procedures. The first is sectioning of the corpus callosum, known as a **corpus callosotomy**. This is commonly used for patients with atonic seizures or partial seizures with secondary generalization. Either the anterior two-thirds or the entire corpus callosum is divided in the midline. The approach is the same as any transcallosal, intraventricular procedure, and uses a bifrontal, paramedian scalp incision and elevation of free-bone flap adjacent to the midline in the region of the coronal suture. Injury to the sagittal sinus is possible and must be avoided. In addition, numerous bridging veins across the interhemispheric fissure must be preserved to avoid venous congestion and possible infarction. The right cerebral hemisphere is gently retracted from the falx, exposing the paired anterior cerebral arteries and underlying corpus callosum. If an anterior two-thirds transection is performed, an intraop x-ray is required to determine the posterior border.

The second variant is either a **frontal**, **temporal**, or **occipital craniotomy** for resection of a structural, epileptogenic focus, such as a tumor or AVM. This procedure may use **stereotaxic localization** and the resultant craniotomy may be performed in the stereotaxic head frame, which alters the method of intubation. The subsequent craniotomy is similar to the excision of any structural lesion, with the exception of intraop electrocorticography of surrounding cortex, if used. Such monitoring alters the choice of anesthetic.

The third variant is a diagnostic procedure involving placement of **surface and/or depth electrodes**. This may be performed with or without stereotaxic localization. Often only burr holes, outlining the future craniotomy flap, are used. After placement, the electrodes are externalized, and postop the patients's naturally occurring Sz are recorded, in conjunction with video monitoring, to register the clinical presentation with the onset of ictal activity. This recording/observation period may last for several d. The patient is then returned to the OR and the epileptogenic focus resected.

The fourth alternative is **selective amygdalohippocampectomy**, a variation of the standard anterior temporal lobectomy. In this procedure, the surgeon makes a cortical incision in the anterior temporal lobe and exposes and resects the amygdala and hippocampus, sparing the remaining portions of the temporal lobe. This procedure is sometimes used on the dominant side of the brain in an effort to lower the risk of postop speech and language dysfunction.

Usual preop diagnosis: Temporal lobe epilepsy; partial epilepsy; intractable epilepsy

SUMMARY OF PROCEDURE

Position	Supine, rarely prone for occipital lesions; table turned 180°
Incision	Temporal question mark, reverse question mark, paramedian, frontal, or occipital
Special instrumentation	Operating microscope; Cavitron; bipolar cautery; surface electrode grids and strips; depth electrode
Unique considerations	Electrocorticography requiring neuroleptic anesthesia; awake procedures for mapping of temporal and/or frontal speech areas; stereotaxic craniotomy and lesionectomy
Antibiotics	Nafcillin 1-2 g + cefotaxime 1 g iv
Surgical time	3 h
EBL	Minimal for diagnostic procedures; 250-500 ml with craniotomy (adults)
Postop care	After craniotomy, ICU for 12-24 h
Mortality	< 1%
Morbidity	Hemiplegia
	Dysphasia
	Ophthalmoplegia
	Brain stem surgery
Pain score	1-3

PATIENT POPULATION CHARACTERISTICS

Age range	2-50 yr
Male:Female	1:1
Incidence	150,000/yr (new cases of epilepsy): ~10% eventually present for surgery/yr (1500)
Etiology	Idiopathic (mesial temporal sclerosis); infectious (brain abscess, encephalitis); traumatic (glial scar); vascular (AVM, infarct); neoplastic (glioma, hamartoma, ganglioglioma); congenital (cortical dysplasia)
Associated conditions	Tuberous sclerosis; Sturge-Weber syndrome; infantile hemiplegia; encephalitis; hemimegalencephaly

ANESTHETIC CONSIDERATIONS

PREOPERATIVE

Epilepsy is a common disorder among young adults. Antiepileptic medication, such as phenytoin, will abolish seizure disorders in most patients, but some develop intolerable side effects to such medications; others are refractory to medical therapy. Surgical ablation of the seizure focus may be the only effective therapy for some patients if they are to become self-sufficient. Several operations may be done, the most common being placement of surface or depth electrodes to determine the focus of the Sz, with subsequent temporal lobectomy for removal of the focus. In some cases, the lesion may be very focal and amenable to stereotactic localization and removal.

Neurological	Usually the only neurological finding is a Hx of uncontrollable seizures, either focal or generalized. Obtain a description of Sz and prodromal Sx.
	Tests: A Wada test (intracarotid injection of a barbiturate) usually is performed to determine whether the area of proposed surgery has any cerebral dominance or speech function.
Gastrointestinal	Abnormal liver function may be associated with valproate and carbamazepine use.
	Tests: LFT and others as indicated from H&P.
Hematologic	Phenytoin/phenobarbital → ↓Hct; carbamazepine/valproate/ethosuximide/primidone → ↓Plt; Carbamazepine/primidone → ↓WBC
	Tests: CBC and others as indicated from H&P.
Laboratory	Tests as indicated from H&P.
Premedication	Standard premedication (see p. B-2) is usually appropriate.

INTRAOPERATIVE

Anesthetic technique: Local anesthesia and GETA. The placement of surface or depth electrodes is done under GETA, as is a temporal lobectomy in the nondominant hemisphere. If the seizure focus is in the dominant hemisphere and/or if there is any question about possible neurological injury by temporal lobectomy, the procedure is performed under local anesthesia, with intraop localization of the seizure focus. In this case, the patient should be told that the operation will be performed under local anesthesia, that every effort will be made to control discomfort, and that he/she will be expected to respond to some pictures and questions once the head is opened and the seizure area is identified. The patient should also be told that he/she probably will be amnesic for the operative events.

Induction	Standard induction (see p. B-2). If a difficult intubation is anticipated (e.g., stereotactic frame), orotracheal intubation is best accomplished before induction of GA. An awake fiber optic intubation is the best technique (see p. B-6). Once anesthesia is induced, a nondepolarizing neuromuscular relaxant is administered.
Maintenance	Standard maintenance (see p. B-3). Generally, no further NMBs are administered beyond that used for tracheal intubation. With adequate anesthesia, and the head fixed in the Mayfield-Kees skeletal fixation, patient movement of any consequence is highly unlikely. Furthermore, it is useful to see movement of an extremity as an indicator of inadequate depth of anesthesia.
Emergence	No special considerations. Prophylactic antiemetic (e.g., metoclopramide 10 mg and ondansetron 4 mg) should be given 30 min before extubation.

Wake-up testing: At some institutions, an asleep-awake-asleep technique is used in which the patient is placed under GETA for positioning and craniotomy. After surgical exposure of the seizure area, the patient is allowed to awaken to assess neurologic function while areas of the brain are stimulated. When the seizure focus has been adequately delineated, GA is reinstituted for the remainder of the operation. An excellent anesthetic technique under these circumstances includes the use of N_2O and sevoflurane for amnesia, and remifentanil (0.05-2 μg/kg/min) by continuous infusion for analgesia. The advantage of these drugs is that they are quickly eliminated, allowing for rapid emergence for the awake component of the procedure, followed by rapid reinduction of anesthesia when the testing period is over. To allow the patient to talk during the awake portion of the procedure, the ETT must be removed. This is best accomplished by inserting a small or medium-sized tube changer through the ETT before it is removed. The tube changer can then be used as a guide for reinsertion of the ETT, and it will not prevent normal vocalization by the patient during the awake phase.

Local anesthesia: Initial sedation may be achieved with a combination of midazolam (0.07 mg/kg) and fentanyl (2-3 μg/kg). Nasal prongs should be placed on the patient and supplemental O_2 administered. If local anesthesia is used, continuous pump infusions of propofol (50-150 μg/kg/min) and an opiate (e.g., remifentanil 0.05-2 μg/kg/min) are extremely effective in providing amnesia and analgesia, while allowing the anesthesiologist to awaken the patient for about 30-60 min of testing, once the temporal lobe has been exposed surgically.

Blood and fluid requirements	Moderate blood loss IV: 18 ga × 2 NS/LR @ 4-6 ml/kg/h	If local anesthesia used, two iv cannulae are useful–one for fluid administration, another for infusion of anesthetic and other drugs. Alternatively, one peripheral iv and a CVP cannula are inserted. Blood transfusions seldom are needed for this operation since blood loss is usually < 500 ml.
Monitoring	Standard monitors (see p. B-1). Arterial line ± CVP line UO	O_2 sat and $ETCO_2$ monitoring will indicate the adequacy of ventilation and oxygenation.
Positioning	Table rotated 180° ✓ and pad pressure points. ✓ eyes.	Semisitting position with head held in Mayfield-Kees skeletal fixation and rotated laterally with a roll under the shoulder on the operative side. Anesthetic hoses and intravascular lines must be long enough to be accessible.
Complications	Anxiety Agitation Sz	Local anesthetic toxicity may produce agitation and seizures. Iced NS or LR should be immediately available for Sz control to flood cortical surface.

POSTOPERATIVE

Complications	Seizure	Monitor carefully for altered mental status.

Complications, cont.	Bleeding Cerebral edema	
Pain management	Codeine 30-60 mg im q 4 h	Avoid oversedation.
Tests	CT scan	If a patient exhibits any delay in emergence from anesthesia and surgery, or any new neurologic deficits appear, a CT scan is invariably obtained.

References

1. Blume WT, Grabow JD, Darley FL, Aronson AE: Intracarotid amobarbital test of language and memory before temporal lobectomy for seizure control. *Neurology* 1973, 23(8):812-19.
2. Hauser WA: *Epilepsy: Frequency, Causes, and Consequences.* Demos, New York: 1990, 21-48.
3. Kofke WA, Tempelhoff R, Dasheiff RM: Anesthetic implications of epilepsy, status epilepticus, and epilepsy surgery. *J Neurosurg Anesthesiol* 1997; 9:349-72.
4. Manninen PH, Burke SJ, Wennberg R, Lozano AM, El Beheiry H: Intraoperative localization of an epileptogenic focus with alfentanil and fentanyl. *Anesth Analg* 1999; 88:1101-6.
5. NIH Consensus Development Conference. *Consensus Statement: Surgery for Epilepsy.* 1990, Mar 19-21; 8(2):2, and *JAMA* 1990; 264:729-33.
6. Zimmerman RS, Sirven JI: An overview of surgery for chronic seizures. *Mayo Clinic Proceedings* 2003; 78(1):109-17.

SURGERY FOR SPASTICITY

SURGICAL CONSIDERATIONS

Description: Neurologic conditions associated with spasticity of the extremities include spinal cord injury, multiple sclerosis, stroke, etc. The spasticity is often managed with oral medications. An alternative approach is to infuse baclofen (GABA-agonist that decreases frequency and amplitude of tonic impulses to the muscle spindles) into the subarachnoid space via an implanted pump. When these therapeutic modalities fail, it may be necessary to perform surgery. Some of the procedures are destructive in that a lesion is placed in certain nerves or the spinal cord to destroy the reflex arc that is contributing to the spasticity. There are both percutaneous and open techniques for placing the lesion. In the **open procedures**, a **laminectomy** is performed (see Posterior Lumbar Spine Surgery, p. 93). In a case where a **myelotomy** is to be performed, the lower spinal cord is exposed and incised at the appropriate location to interrupt the reflex arc. In certain cases, selective electrical stimulation can be performed on isolated dorsal rootlets from the involved extremity. Abnormal responses in the extremities are monitored via EMG and direct observation. When abnormal responses are detected, that particular rootlet is divided (**dorsal rhizotomy**). This procedure is somewhat tedious and requires that stable anesthetic conditions be maintained so that appropriate monitoring can be carried out during the procedure. The surgeon usually must sacrifice 40-60% of the dorsal rootlets in cases of spastic diplegia found in cerebral palsy.

Variant procedure or approaches: Percutaneous **radiofrequency (RF) rhizotomy** is another procedure used for spasticity. A thermal lesion is placed in the appropriate dorsal roots with a RF generator. Needles are passed into the neural foramen via a posterolateral trajectory for levels L1-L5, and then from a midline approach to the S1 root. The needle position is determined by A-P and lateral fluoroscopy and by stimulus mapping. Stimulating current is delivered via an electrode passed through the needle. A low-level stimulating current causes muscle twitching in the appropriate leg if the needle is in the proper location. Once placed and verified, the RF generator is used to produce the lesion. At the termination of this procedure, the patient's legs should be flaccid. Patients with spinal cord injury producing anesthesia below T10 may not require additional anesthetic for the procedure.

Usual preop diagnosis: Spasticity; multiple sclerosis; spinal cord injury

SUMMARY OF PROCEDURES

	Open Rhizotomy or Myelotomy	RF Rhizotomy
Position	Prone	⇐
Incision	Midline	Needles placed in lumbar region
Special instrumentation	EMG monitor; nerve stimulator	RF generator; fluoroscope
Unique considerations	Anesthetic that allows EMG recordings	May not require anesthesia if anesthetic below waist (spinal cord surgery).
Antibiotics	Nafcillin 1 g iv + cefotaxime 1 g iv	None
Surgical time	4 h	2 h
Closing considerations	Surgeon may wish to test dural closure with Valsalva maneuver.	
EBL	50-250 ml	Negligible
Postop care	Head flat; PACU → room	⇐
Mortality	< 1%	⇐

Morbidity	All < 5%:
	    CSF leak
	    Infection
	    Hemorrhage
	    Neurological impairment
		⇐

Pain score	4	2

PATIENT POPULATION CHARACTERISTICS

Age range	3-55 yr
Male:Female	~3:2
Incidence	Relatively uncommon neurosurgical procedure
Etiology	Hyperactivity of gamma stretch reflex
Associated conditions	Multiple sclerosis; cerebral palsy; spinal cord injury

ANESTHETIC CONSIDERATIONS

See Anesthetic Considerations for Surgical Correction of Spinal Dysraphism, Pediatric Neurosurgery, p. 942.

References

1. Kennemore DE: Percutaneous electrocoagulation of spinal nerves for the relief of pain and spasticity. In *Radionics Procedure Technique Series*. Radionics, Burlington MA: 1978.
2. Peacock WJ, Staudt LA, Nuwer MR: A neurosurgical approach to spasticity: selective posterior rhizotomy. In *Neurosurgery Update*, Vol II. Wilkins RH, Rengachary SS, eds. McGraw-Hill, New York: 1991, 403-7.

Surgeons

Raju S.V. Balabhadra, MD
Daniel H. Kim, MD, FACS
Lawrence M. Shuer, MD

1.3   SPINAL NEUROSURGERY

Anesthesiologist

C. Philip Larson, Jr., MD, MS

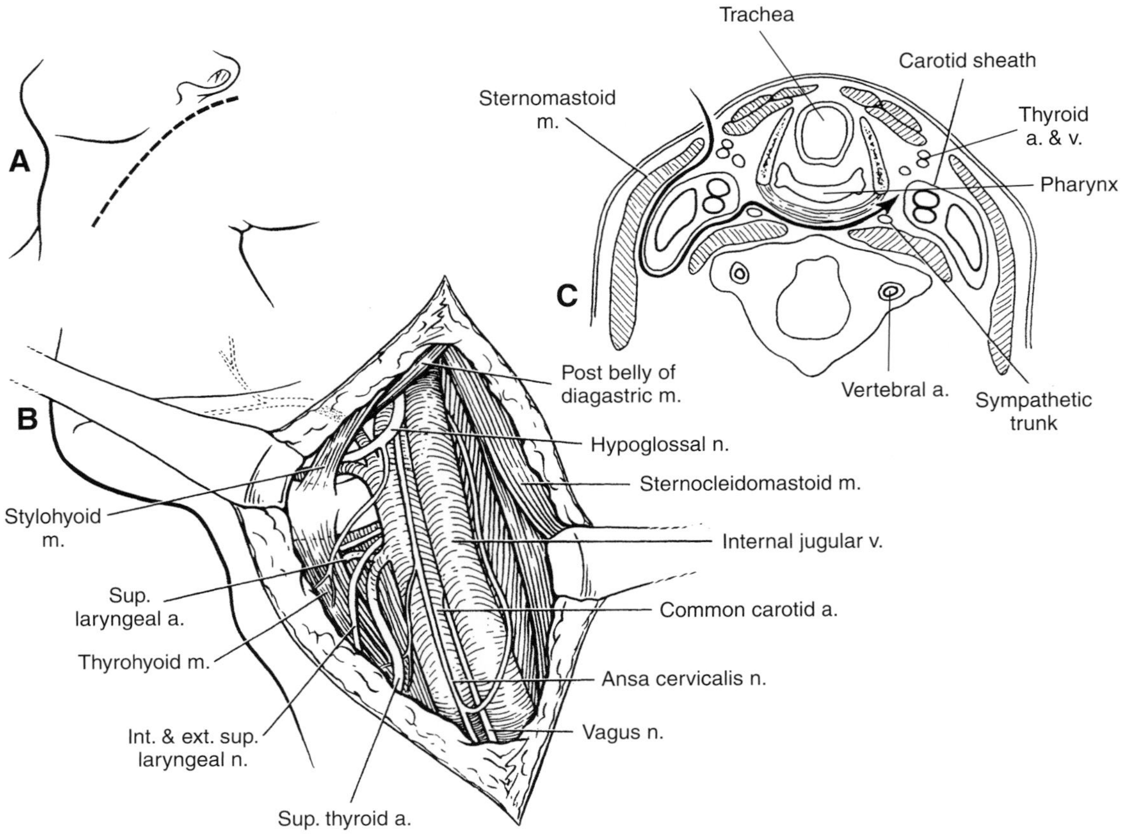

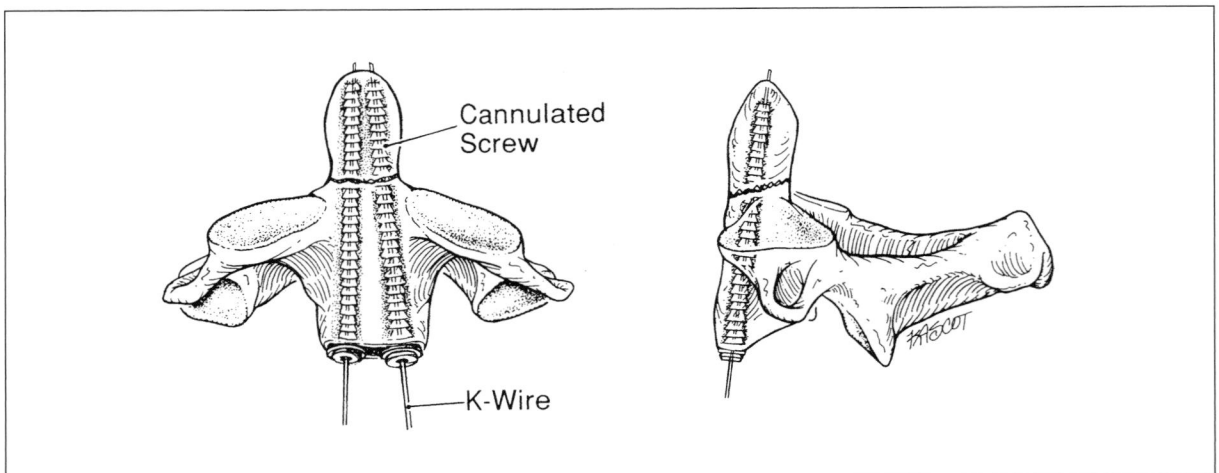

Figure 1.3-1. The anterolateral retropharyngeal approach (described by Whitesides and Kelly). (A) The skin incision is made from the mastoid, along the anterior aspect of the sternocleidomastoid. (B) The stenocleidomastoid and splenius capitus muscles are detached from the mastoid. (C) Dissection is posterior to the carotid contents leading to the transverse processes and anterior aspect of C1-3. (Reproduced with permission from An HS, Cotler JM: *Spinal Instrumentation.* Williams & Wilkins, 1992.)

Figure 1.3-2. Screw fixation technique, using cannulated screws. K-wire provides provisional stabilization and allows guided tapping and screw placement. (Reproduced with permission from An HS, Cotler JM: *Spinal Instrumentation.* Williams & Wilkins, 1992.)

ANTERIOR FUSION/FIXATION
OF THE UPPER CERVICAL (C1-C2) SPINE

SURGICAL CONSIDERATIONS

Description: Transoral odontoid excision: The **transoral approach** is indicated primarily to relieve ventral irreducible compression of the cervicomedullary junction due to extradural lesions involving the lower part of the clivus, C1 and C2 vertebral bodies. This approach provides direct access to the C1 anterior arch and odontoid process of C2. The anesthetized patient is positioned supine with 5-10 lbs of cervical traction. A Dingman retractor is used to facilitate surgical access. The soft palate is retracted upwards with stay sutures. Through a posterior midline incision over the pharyngeal wall, the C1 anterior arch and C2 vertebra are exposed (Fig 1.3-3). Using fluoroscopic guidance, bony decompression of the clivus, C1 anterior arch, odontoid process, and C2 vertebral body is performed. Instrumentation of C1-C2 may be performed with plate and screws. The wound is closed in two layers after securing hemostasis. As the procedure often results in significant instability at the craniovertebral junction, posterior occipitocervical fusion often is required.

Variants of the transoral procedure: Transpalatal exposure with removal of hard palate or a **tongue-splitting transmandibular approach** may be required for adequate exposure of the clivus or upper C-spine, respectively.

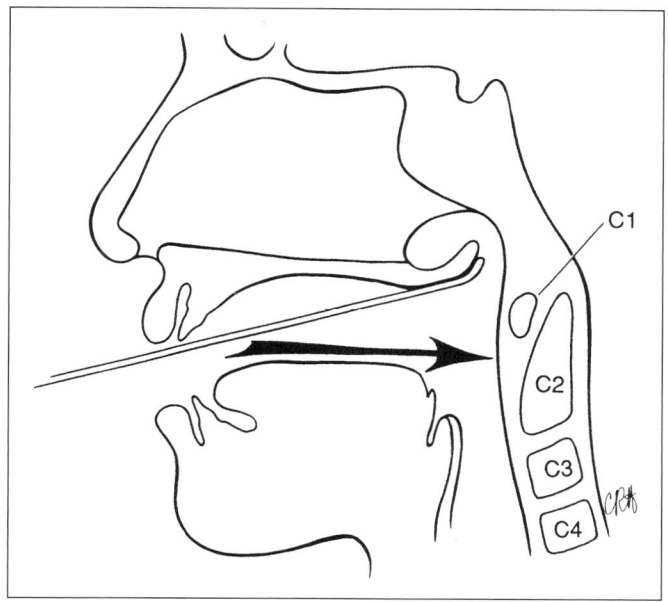

Figure 1.3-3. The transoral approach. (Reproduced with permission from An HS, Cotler JM: *Spinal Instrumentation*. Williams & Wilkins, 1992.)

High cervical odontoid excision: The **high cervical anterior retropharyngeal approach** provides wide bilateral access to C1-C2 vertebrae and avoids the potential contamination from the oral and pharyngeal cavities. It also allows access to the entire C-spine. This is a safe, effective alternative to the transoral approach as it permits neural decompression, fusion, and instrumentation of C1-C3 vertebrae, avoiding the need for an additional posterior procedure and maintaining occipitoatlanto mobility. The patient is positioned supine with a slight extension and 30° contralateral rotation of the neck. A horizontal skin incision is made 2 cm inferior and parallel to the mandible, and the platysma is incised in line with the skin incision (Fig 1.3-1A). The fascia between the digastric muscle and the hyoid bone is transected and the digastric muscle is retracted rostrally (Fig 1.3-1B). The fascia over the hyoid bone is incised along its course lateral to the carotid sheath, and the retropharyngeal space (Fig 1.3-1C) is opened to expose C1 and C2 vertebrae. The odontoid process and C2 body are removed. Iliac bone (auto or allograft) is used to achieve fusion between C1 and C3, and then stabilized with a plate and screws.

Transodontoid screw fixation: Fractures of the odontoid process of C2 account for 10-20% of all C-spine fractures and are classified (**Anderson and D'Alonzo**) into three types, based on anatomical location. **Type I fractures**, which occur at the tip of dens, are treated conservatively. **Type II fractures**, which occur through the waist of the odontoid process, are the most common and are often inherently unstable, requiring surgical treatment. **Type III fractures** occur through the body of C2 and are often treated by halo immobilization. Screw fixation is the ideal treatment for Type II fractures, as it provides immediate stability while preserving C1-C2 rotation.

The anesthetized patient is placed in a supine position with halo traction of 5-10 lbs. The mouth is kept open using a radiolucent jaw distractor. A horizontal skin incision is made at approximately C5 level, and the platysma is cut along the skin incision. The anterior C-spine is exposed by opening the natural plane between trachea and esophagus medially and carotid sheath laterally. Using a guide tube, a hole is drilled under I.I. through the body of C2, the odontoid process, and its apex, through the fracture. The drilled hole is tapped, and an appropriately sized screw is placed (Fig 1.3-2). At this point, fluoroscopy of the patient's neck in flexion and extension is done to exclude C1-C2 instability.

Usual Preop diagnosis: Basilar impression (telescoping of C-spine into posterior fossa); odontoid fracture; rheumatoid arthritis with atlantoaxial instability; traumatic irreducible atlantoaxial instability; Type II odontoid fractures (recent or remote)

SUMMARY OF PROCEDURES

	Transoral	High-Cervical	Transodontoid Screw Fixation
Position	Supine, head in mild extension with traction	⇐ + 30° rotation of head	Supine; head in mild extension with traction
Incision	Posterior oropharynx	Horizontal incision 2 cm below mandible (see Fig 1.3-1A)	Transverse skin incision in the anterolateral neck at C5 level
Special instrumentation	Operating microscope, I.I., Dingman retractor	Operating microscope, I.I., cervical plates/screws	K-wire, drill, odontoid screw instrumentation
Unique considerations	Requires ≥ 3 cm mouth opening; armored ETT must be taped securely away from surgical field. Tracheostomy is needed occasionally. Fiber optic intubation may be required.	Fiber optic intubation may be required.	Fiber optic intubation in patients with C1-C2 instability; biplanar fluoroscopy is mandatory.
Surgical time	2-3 h	3-4 h	2-3 h
Closing considerations	Extubation may be delayed due to lingual swelling.	Extubation may be delayed due to pharyngeal swelling.	Routine wound closure
EBL	25-200 ml	200-300 ml	25-200 ml
Postop care	ICU or close observation unit. Monitor airway for respiratory obstruction. ± Postop immobilization	⇐ May need enteral support × 1-2 wk. Halo device/hard cervical collar	PACU → room; cervical collar
Mortality	0-3%	< 1%	1%
Morbidity	All < 20%: CSF leak/dural tear Infection Neural injury Pharyngeal wound dehiscence	All < 10%: CSF leak/dural tear Neural injury (cord, root, recurrent laryngeal nerve) Transient dysphagia Esophageal/tracheal erosion Vascular injury (carotid vertebral) Pneumothorax	Overall: < 15% Hardware failure (screw pullout, screw fracture): 10% Nonunion: 5-10% Superficial wound infection: 2%
Pain score	3-5	3-5	3-5
PATIENT POPULATION CHARACTERISTICS			
Age range	18-85 yr (usually 20-60 yr)	⇐	15-90 yr (usually 20-60 yr)
Male:Female	1:2	⇐	1.5:1
Incidence	Rare	⇐	Common (10-20% of C-spine fractures)
Etiology	Neoplastic; traumatic; congenital; degenerative	⇐	Traumatic
Associated conditions	Rheumatoid arthritis	⇐	–

ANESTHETIC CONSIDERATIONS

See Anesthetic Considerations for Cervical Neurosurgical Procedures, p. 83.

References

1. Apelbaum RI, Lonser RR, Veres R, Casey A: Direct anterior screw fixation for recent and remote odontoid fractures. *J Neurosurgery (Spine 2)* 2000; 93:227-36.
2. Menezes AH: Transoral approach to the clivus and upper cervical spine. In *Neurosurgery*. Wilkins RH, Rengachary SS, eds. McGraw-Hill, New York: 1995, 306-13.
3. Crockard AH: Transoral approach to intra/extradural tumors. In *Surgery of Cranial Base Tumors*. Sekhar LN, Janecka ID, eds. Raven Press, New York: 1993, 225-34.
4. Vender JR, Harrison SJ, McDonnell DE: Fusion and instrumentation at C1-3 via the high anterior cervical approach. *J Neurosurgery (Spine 1)* 2000; 92:24-9.

POSTERIOR FUSION/FIXATION OF THE UPPER CERVICAL SPINE

SURGICAL CONSIDERATIONS

Description: Craniocervical (occipitocervical, craniovertebral) fusion/fixation or instrumentation involves stabilization of the occiput and upper three or four cervical vertebrae, while **atlantoaxial fusion/fixation** involves stabilization of the atlas (C1) and axis (C2). Instability may be caused by congenital, traumatic, degenerative, neoplastic, or infectious conditions resulting in compression of the lower brain stem or cervical spinal cord. Sx may include paresthesias and/or weakness of the upper and lower extremities.

Atlantoaxial techniques: Atlantoaxial (C1-C2) fusion is performed in the prone position, with skeletal traction. Through a posterior midline incision, the occiput and upper C-spine are exposed. A posterior iliac or rib graft is harvested and fashioned appropriately. The bone graft is secured with wire to the decorticated segments to be fused. Traditionally, the fixation has been performed with sublaminar wires; however, recent fixation techniques—such as **C1-C2 transarticular screw fixation** and **C1-C2 lateral mass bony plating** (lateral mass = bony column between facet joints)—are being used more often because they are biomechanically strong, permitting early ambulation with minimal orthotic support.

In **C1-C2 posterior wiring techniques**, the posterior arches of C1 and C2 laminae are exposed through a midline incision. Of the various wiring techniques used, **Gallie's** and **Brooks'** are the most widely accepted. In **Gallie's fusion** (Fig 1.3-4A, a wire loop or cable is passed underneath the C1 arch and brought over a bone graft wedged between C1 and C2 and then tightened over the C2 spinous process. In **Brook's technique** (Fig 1.3-4B), wires are passed beneath the C2 lamina and C1 posterior arch on each side and tightened over a bone graft placed between C1 and C2. The posterior aspects of C1 and C2 are decorticated to facilitate the bony fusion. Wiring techniques are simpler, but carry the risk of cord injury during wire placement.

C1-C2 transarticular screw fixation has become increasingly popular because of its greater biomechanical stability, higher fusion rates (87-100%), and superior fixation of atlantoaxial rotation.[1] The occiput and C1-3 vertebrae are exposed by a conventional posterior approach. Screws are placed from C2 toward the anterior tubercle of C1 under fluoroscopic guidance. The major risks of this technique include injury to the vertebral artery (4.1%), malposition of screws, or instrumentation failure. Twenty percent of patients will have an anomalous vertebral artery, demonstrated by radiographic studies, precluding use of this technique.

In C1-C2 plating, the C-spine is exposed subperiosteally from occiput to C3-4 vertebrae by a conventional posterior approach. In this technique, polyaxial screws are passed into the lateral mass of C1 and C2 pedicles and fixed to rods or plates under fluoroscopic guidance. If required, a reduction maneuver is carried out by repositioning the head or by direct manipulation of the C1 and C2 vertebrae. C1-2 interfacetal fusion or posterior fusion may be added as required. C1-2 plating can be combined with cervical decompression. Because of the superior and medial placement of C2 pedicle screws, the risks of injuring the vertebral artery are minimal.

Craniocervical techniques: Occipitocervical fusion involves a surgical exposure similar to that of atlantoaxial fusion, except that a more extensive exposure of the occipital bone is required. Fixation can be obtained by **Luque rectangle/ contoured rod and wiring** or plate and screws. An appropriately fashioned rib or iliac crest graft is wired in place. Postop immobilization by hard collar or halo device is required.

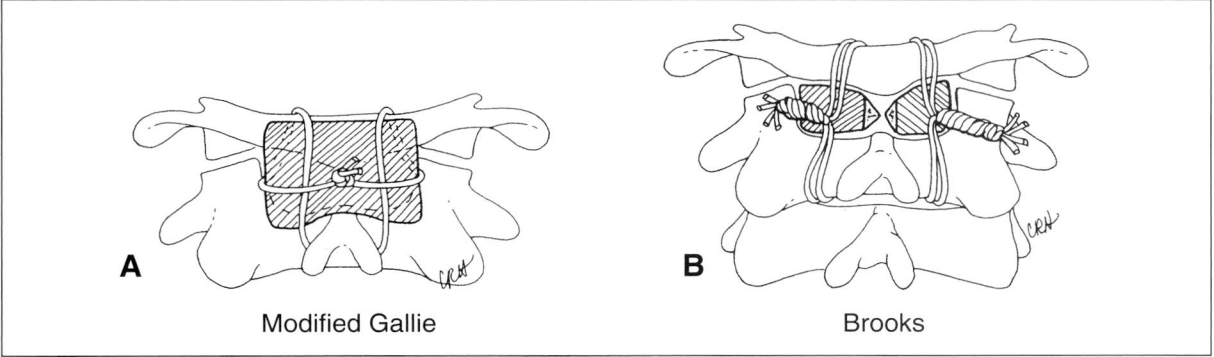

Modified Gallie

Brooks

Figure 1.3-4. Posterior wiring techniques. (A) Modified Gallie using an H-shaped bone graft form the iliac crest, contoured to fit over the posterior arches of C1 and C2. A double U-shaped 18- or 20-ga wire is passed under the arch of C1 from inferior to superior. (B) Brooks-type fusion with doubled-twisted 24-ga wires passed under the arch of C1 and then under the lamina of C2. Rectangular iliac crest bone grafts are fitted in the intervals between the arch of C1 and each lamina of the axis. (Reproduced with permission from An HS, Cotler JM: *Spinal Instrumentation.* Williams & Wilkins, 1992.)

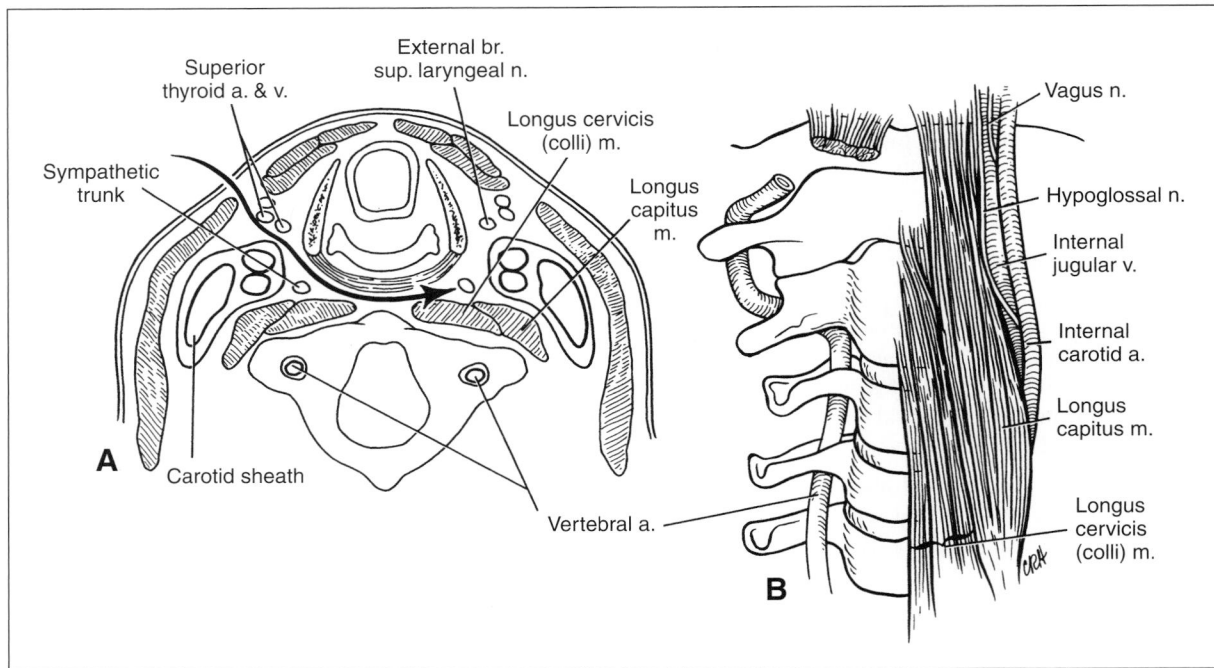

Figure 1.3-5. Upper C-spine. (A) Cross-section showing the anteromedial approach. (B) Anterior aspect, after stripping the longus collis muscle. (Reproduced with permission from An HS, Cotler JM: *Spinal Instrumentation*. Williams & Wilkins, 1992.)

In **occipitocervical contoured rod fixation**, the occiput and posterior C-spine are exposed through a posterior incision, and trephines are made 2.5 cm to either side of the midline and about 2 cm above the foramen magnum. Wires or cables are passed from these occipital holes through the foramen magnum on both sides. Sublaminar wires are passed beneath laminae of the atlas, axis, and C3 vertebrae on each side, and are tightened over a rod. Other cervical vertebrae may be included in the fixation as required. A tricorticate iliac or rib graft is fixed with wires over the occipitocervical region. Decortication of occipital bone and laminae of the atlas, axis, or C3 vertebrae is essential for bony fusion.

Occipitocervical plate fixation can be performed by using a T- or Y-shaped plate fixed by screws to the occiput and lateral masses of the cervical vertebrae. C1-C2 transarticular screws or wiring techniques can be added for additional stability. Plating techniques are biomechanically stable, often obviating the need for rigid postop immobilization; however, they are technically demanding. The major concerns include possible dural penetration by occipital screws and obtaining adequate contouring of the construct (Fig 1.3-5).

Usual preop diagnosis: Transoral odontoid resection; occipitoatlantal instability; atlantoaxial instability; odontoid fractures; spinal fractures; cervical instability; previous failed fusions

SUMMARY OF PROCEDURES

	Atlantoaxial (C1-C2) Fusion/Fixation	Occipitocervical Fusion/Fixation
Position	Prone, head in tong traction or pins	⇐
Incision	Posterior midline incision	⇐
Special instrumentation	Fluoroscopy; drills; wires/cables; lateral-mass plate and screws; transarticular screws	Fluoroscopy; drills; rods, wires/cables; plates and screws
Unique considerations	Iliac/rib autograft ± posterior ilium for graft. Fiber optic intubation and SSEPs	⇐
Surgical time	2-3 h	3-4 h
Closing considerations	Routine wound closure	Halo vest may be needed in selected cases.
EBL	100-500 ml	⇐
Postop care	PACU, then → room	⇐
Mortality	< 1%	⇐

	Atlantoaxial (C1-C2) Fusion/Fixation	Occipitocervical Fusion/Fixation
Morbidity	Vertebral artery injury: 4.1%	Neural injury
	CSF leak	⇐
	Instrumentation failure	⇐
	Nonunion	⇐
Pain score	5-9	5-10

PATIENT POPULATION CHARACTERISTICS

Age range	18-85 yr (usually 20-60 yr)
Male:Female	1:2
Incidence	Rare
Etiology	Neoplastic; traumatic; congenital; degenerative; infections; rheumatoid arthritis

ANESTHETIC CONSIDERATIONS

See Anesthetic Considerations for Cervical Neurosurgical Procedures, p. 83.

References

1. Harms J, Melcher R: Posterior C1-C2 fusion with polyaxial screw and rod fixation. *Spine* 26: 2001, 2467-71.
2. Sonntag VKH, Dickman CA: Posterior occipital C1-C2 instrumentation. In *Principles of Spinal Surgery*. Menezes AH, Sonntag VKH, eds. McGraw-Hill, New York: 1995, 1067-79.
3. Vangilder JC, Menezes AH: Craniovertebral abnormalities and their neurosurgical management. In: *Operative Neurosurgical Techniques*. Schmidek HH, Sweet WH, eds. WB Saunders, Philadelphia: 2000, 1934-45.
4. Wright N, Lauryssen C: Vertebral artery injury in C1-2 transarticular screw fixation: results of a survey of the AANS/CNS section on disorders of the spine and peripheral nerves. *J Neurosurg* 1998; 88:634-40.

ANTERIOR FUSION/FIXATION
OF THE MID AND LOWER CERVICAL SPINE

SURGICAL CONSIDERATIONS

Description: The first description of the anterior approach for excision of a cervical disc was made by Smith and Robinson in 1958. This approach permits easy and safe access to the entire C-spine below C2. **Anterior cervical discectomy** is commonly indicated for the removal of herniated discs or osteophytes compressing the spinal cord or nerve roots. Multisegmental cervical spondylosis (narrowing of spinal canal) may require single- or multilevel corpectomy (removal of a vertebral body). During anterior cervical discectomy, an approach from the left side of the neck is often preferred, as it minimizes the chances of injury to the recurrent laryngeal nerve. The dissection is carried along the avascular plane between the trachea and esophagus medially, and the carotid sheath laterally (Fig 1.3-6). The fascia is incised to expose the longus colli muscles and anterior C-spine. The disc level is confirmed using I.I. The annulus is incised, and the disc is removed in piecemeal fashion with the use of an operating microscope. **Fusion and instrumentation** are often performed after discectomy to maintain disc space height, restore normal cervical lordosis, prevent graft extrusion, facilitate early ambulation, and possibly prevent delayed deformity and pain due to collapse of the disc space. After discectomy, osteophytes are removed from the vertebral bodies, and an appropriately sized bone graft or carbon-fiber prosthesis is placed in the intervertebral space. Carbon-fiber cages can be used alone, without plating systems, as their tooth-like serrations provide support and restrict any displacement once locked in. These cages are radiolucent and allow good assessment of bony fusion. Fusion with instrumentation is often essential for immediate stability and early ambulation.

Anterior screw-plate fixation (with MRI-compatible titanium) is the preferred method of fixation for C2-7. It provides stable fixation after discectomy or corpectomy, prevents bone graft migration, improves fusion rate, corrects spinal deformities, and may restore anterior and middle column function following cervical trauma. Plates and screws are placed under fluoroscopic guidance to prevent dural penetration or malposition. Hemodynamic changes should be monitored closely during the procedure since ↓HR or ↓BP during the instrumentation may suggest cord compression.

Usual preop diagnosis: Cervical radiculopathy (nerve-root compression due to disc herniation or osteophytic compression); cervical myelopathy (spinal-cord compression by disc/osteophytes); cervical instability (ligamentous laxity or disruption)

Variant procedure: Cervical (vertebral) corpectomy and fusion are used to treat conditions in which there is anterior impingement of the spinal cord or narrowing of the spinal canal at the level of the vertebral body, including multisegmental cervical spondylitic compression, ossification of the posterior longitudinal ligament (OPLL), tumors, infections (e.g., TB, osteomyelitis), or C-spine injury. The surgical exposure is similar to that for anterior cervical discectomy. A transverse neck incision is preferred for corpectomy involving two or three vertebrae; however, a vertical skin incision along the anterior border of the sternomastoid is preferred if more than three vertebrae are involved. Before the removal of a vertebral body, adjacent discs are resected The posterior part of the vertebra and osteophytes at the posterior margins are excised. Reconstruction is accomplished with an autograft, allograft, or cages (metallic or carbon-fiber spacer spanning the vertebral bodies filled with allograft or autograft bone fragments). Supplemental fixation with plates and screws is essential to prevent graft extrusion, to facilitate fusion, and to permit early ambulation.

Usual preop diagnosis: Cervical myelopathy (spinal cord compression) 2° fracture of the C-spine (traumatic or pathologic); narrowing of the spinal canal due to congenital conditions; degenerative conditions, such as severe disc disease with osteophyte formation; OPLL; cervical instability (ligamentous laxity or disruption or destruction of bone due to tumor or infection); failed previous spinal fusion

SUMMARY OF PROCEDURES

	Cervical Discectomy ± Fusion and Plating	**Cervical Corpectomy ± Fusion and Plating**
Position	Supine, head extended on headrest	⇐
Incision	Transverse anterolateral	⇐ or vertical anterolateral
Special instrumentation	Operating microscope; anterior cervical plates	⇐
Unique considerations	Fiber optic intubation may be necessary; ± cervical traction	⇐
Antibiotics	Cefazolin 1 g	⇐
Surgical time	2-2.5 h	2.5-3 h for single level; add 20-30 min for each additional level.
Closing considerations	Cervical collar (soft)	Cervical collar (soft/hard)
EBL	25-250 ml	50-1000 ml
Postop care	PACU → room	⇐
Mortality	< 1%	0-5%
Morbidity	Esophageal perforation: < 1%	⇐
	Infection: < 1%	⇐
	Massive blood loss—carotid or jugular injury, epidural ooze: < 1%	⇐
	Myelopathy: < 1%	⇐
	Nerve injury:	
	Recurrent laryngeal nerve: 5%	⇐
	Root: < 1%	⇐
	Sympathetic chain: < 1%	⇐
	Postop instability: < 1%	⇐
	Instrument failure: < 1%	1-15%
	Slipped graft: < 1%	⇐
Pain score	3-5	3-5

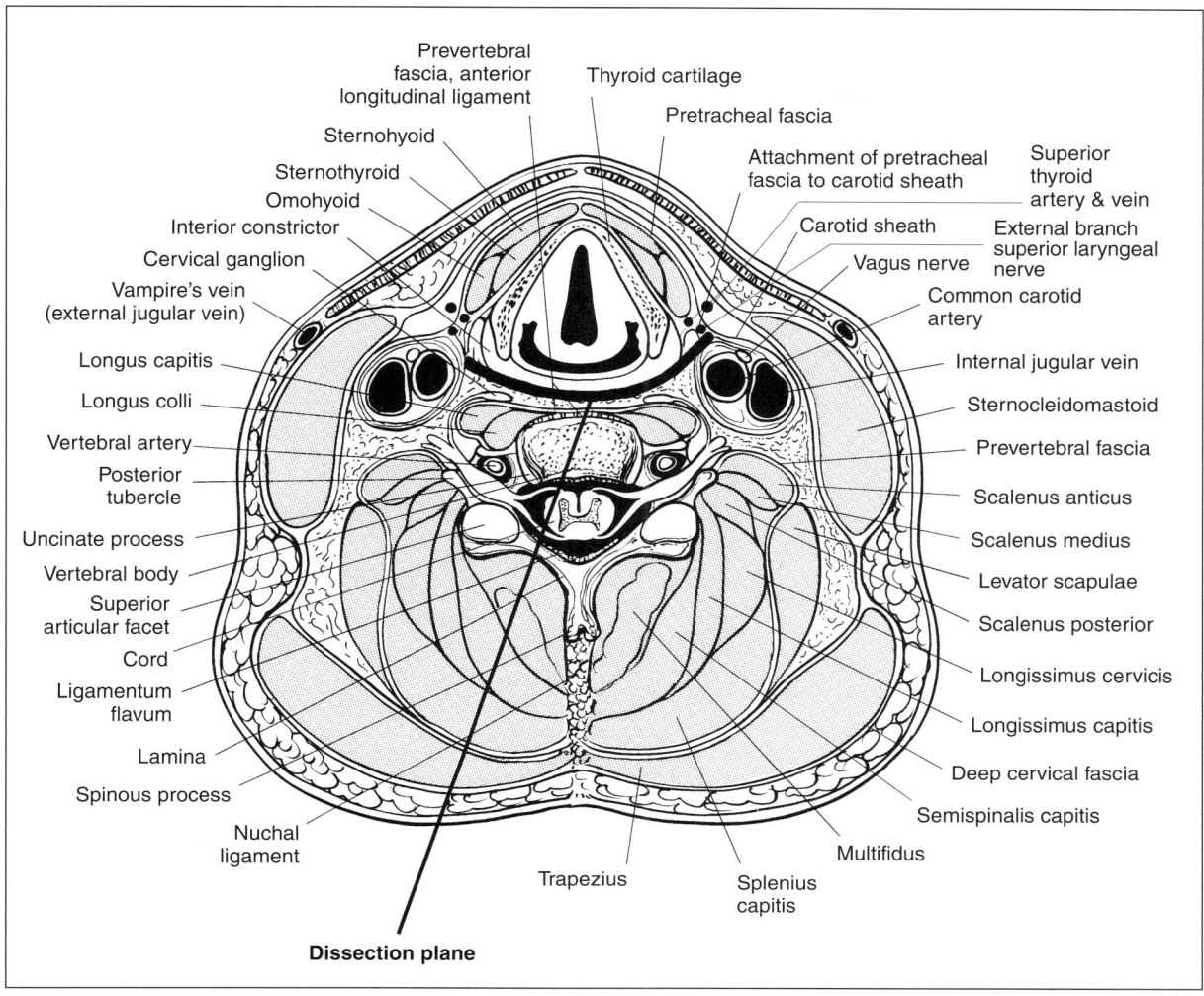

Prevertebral
fascia, anterior
longitudinal ligament
Thyroid cartilage
Pretracheal fascia
Sternohyoid
Sternothyroid
Omohyoid
Interior constrictor
Cervical ganglion
Vampire's vein
(external jugular vein)
Longus capitis
Longus colli
Vertebral artery
Posterior
tubercle
Uncinate process
Vertebral body
Superior
articular facet
Cord
Ligamentum
flavum
Lamina
Spinous process
Nuchal
ligament
Attachment of pretracheal
fascia to carotid sheath
Superior
thyroid
artery & vein
Carotid sheath
Vagus nerve
External branch
superior laryngeal
nerve
Common carotid
artery
Internal jugular vein
Sternocleidomastoid
Prevertebral fascia
Scalenus anticus
Scalenus medius
Levator scapulae
Scalenus posterior
Longissimus cervicis
Longissimus capitis
Deep cervical fascia
Semispinalis capitis
Multifidus
Trapezius
Splenius
capitis

Dissection plane

Figure 1.3-6. Cross-section of the C-spine at C5 level. Note the deep cervical fascia, the pretracheal fascia, and the prevertebral fascia. Note the relationship of the pretracheal fascia to the carotid sheath. Dissection plane is shown. (Modified with permission from Hoppenfeld S, deBoer P: *Surgical Exposures in Orthopaedics: The Anatomic Approach*, 2nd edition. Lippincott Williams & Wilkins, 1994.)

	Cervical Discectomy ± Fusion and Plating	Cervical Corpectomy ± Fusion and Plating
	PATIENT POPULATION CHARACTERISTICS	
Age range	18-85 yr (usually 20-60 yr)	⇐
Male:Female	1:2	⇐
Incidence	Rare	⇐
Etiology	Neoplastic; traumatic; congenital; degenerative; OPLL	⇐

ANESTHETIC CONSIDERATIONS

See Anesthetic Considerations for Cervical Neurosurgical Procedures, p. 83.

References

1. Brislin BT, Hilibrand AS: Avoidance of complications in anterior cervical spine revision surgery. *Curr Opin Orthop*, 2001; 12(3):257-64.
2. Dickman CA, Marciano FF: Principles and techniques of screw fixation of the cervical spine. In *Principles of Spinal Surgery.* Menezes AH, Sonntag VKH, eds. McGraw-Hill, New York: 1995, 123-39.

POSTERIOR FUSION/FIXATION
OF THE MID AND LOWER CERVICAL SPINE

SURGICAL CONSIDERATIONS

Description: Posterior cervical laminectomy (removal of lamina), **foraminotomy** (opening of the neural foramina), and **laminotomy** (removal of a portion of the lamina) are posterior procedures for decompression of the neural elements in the C-spine. These procedures are used to treat cervical radiculopathy 2° degenerative disc disease (e.g., herniated discs, osteophytes). The major advantage of **foraminotomy** over an anterior approach is that it does not require fusion and, thus, preserves the motion of the involved vertebral segments. It also permits decompression of multiple levels, if required. Disadvantages of foraminotomy include an increased incidence of neck pain and the fact that it is not an effective approach to midline disc herniation. **Decompressive laminectomy** can be used to treat cervical canal stenosis (congenital or degenerative) and for removal of intraspinal masses (tumors, AVMs, infective granulomas), which may be extradural, intradural, extramedullary, or intramedullary. Depending on the location of the tumor, the surgeon may need to open the dura and/or spinal cord. Obviously, the intradural intramedullary tumors involve more risk and are more delicate to remove. Many laminae may be removed to expose and excise the tumor. Surgical adjunctive tools (e.g., CUSA, laser, surgical microscope, etc.) may be used to aid in removal of the tumor. Intraop evoked potential monitoring may be used during these procedures to test the integrity of the dorsal columns. Once the tumor has been removed, the wound is closed in layers, as in a simple laminectomy.

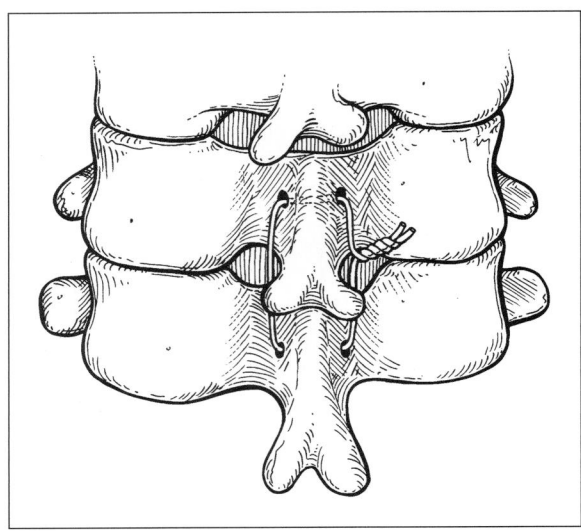

Figure 1.3-7. Intraspinous wiring. Wires passed through drilled holes in base of adjacent spinous processes and tightened. (Reproduced with permission from An HS, Cotler JM: *Spinal Instrumentation*, 2nd edition. Lippincott Williams & Wilkins, 1999.)

Surgery is performed in the prone or sitting position through a posterior midline incision over the involved vertebrae. The paraspinal muscles are dissected off the spinous processes, and lamina and bone are removed piecemeal. The extent of the procedure depends on the indications for treatment. Hemostasis is achieved with bipolar cautery, and raw bone surfaces are sealed with bone wax. Topical hemostatic agents are used to aid in hemostasis in the epidural gutters. If the patient has an intradural tumor or process such as syringomyelia, the dura is opened and the operating microscope is used for this portion of the procedure. Once the intradural procedure is complete, the dura is closed, and the surgeon may wish to test the integrity of the closure with a Valsalva-like maneuver (sustained inspiration to 30-40 cmH$_2$O). The wound is closed in layers, and a drain may be left in the epidural space. Multilevel laminectomies with foraminotomies (involving partial removal of cervical facet joints) can result in late-onset cervical kyphosis, an extremely difficult condition to treat. These patients are usually considered for concomitant posterior fusion and instrumentation, especially in the presence of cervical segmental instability.

Posterior cervical wiring techniques include: 1) **interspinous wiring** (Fig 1.3-7) (wires are passed through drilled holes in the base of adjacent spinous processes and then tightened); 2) **sublaminar wiring** (Fig 1.3-8) with Luque rods or rectangles (sublaminar wires are passed at each level on both sides and are tightened over the rods or rectangles); and 3) a **triple-wire technique** (Fig 1.3-9) with the first wire being passed through drill holes at the base of each spinous process, and the second and third wires passed through the same holes and then through drill holes in the previously placed bone grafts. This latter technique is biomechanically sound, as it places the bone grafts in compression. Wiring techniques, while stable in flexion, however, are less stable in extension and rotation, and they cannot be performed in patients with prior laminectomy or requiring laminectomy.

In the **posterior cervical lateral plating** technique, the C-spine is exposed through a midline incision over the involved vertebral segments. The lateral mass (bony column between facet joints) is identified, drilled, and tapped. Cortical screws are passed into the lateral mass and fixed with plates or rods. Adjacent facet joints are decorticated and bone grafts are placed. Lateral mass plating provides a rigid multisegmental fixation and can be performed in patients with prior laminectomy. The major risks involved with this procedure are nerve-root and vertebral artery injuries.

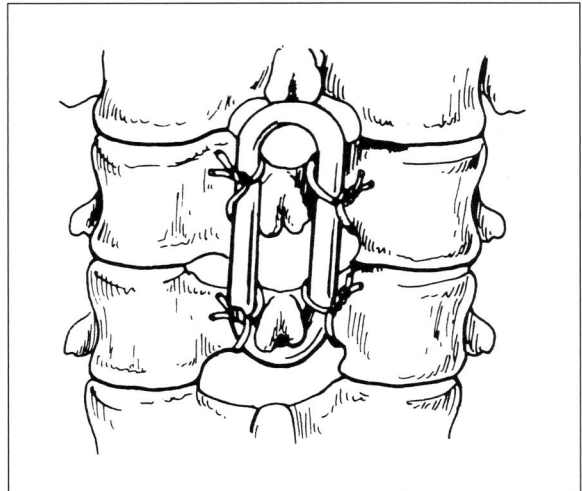

Figure 1.3-8. Luque loop fixation with sublaminar wires. (Reproduced with permission from Wilber RG, Peters JG, Likavec MJ: Surgical techniques in cervical spine surgery. In *Spinal Trauma*. Errico TJ, Bauer RD, Waugh T, eds. JB Lippincott, 1991.)

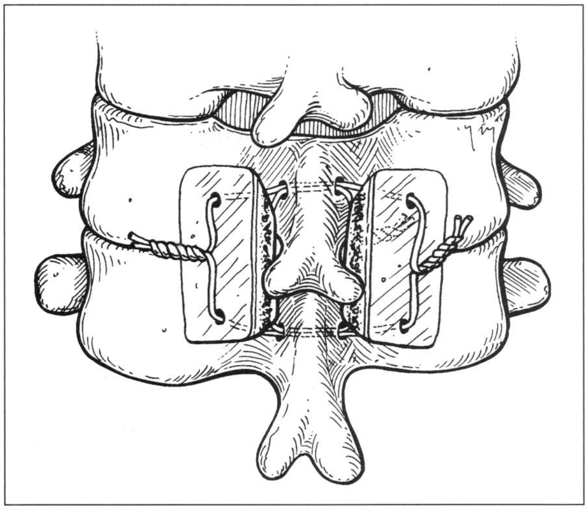

Figure 1.3-9. Triple-wire technique with interspinous process wires, compressing bone grafts to lamina. (Reproduced with permission from An HS, Cotler JM: *Spinal Instrumentation*, 2nd edition. Lippincott Williams & Wilkins, 1999.)

Cervical pedicle screw plate fixation is an effective alternative to lateral mass plating. In this technique, screws are passed under fluoroscopic guidance into the cervical pedicles and secured to plates or rods. This procedure is technically demanding, as the cervical pedicles are narrow and in close proximity to nerve roots, vertebral artery, and spinal cord. This technique is biomechanically stable and permits the correction of deformity by application of compression or distraction forces.

Usual preop diagnosis: Cervical radiculopathy (nerve-root compression); cervical myelopathy (spinal-cord compression); cervical disc disease (herniation or degeneration of one or more cervical discs); C-spine injury

Variant procedures: Patients with panvertebral disease (involving anterior and posterior elements of the spine) and three-column spinal instability often require **combined anterior and posterior decompression, reconstruction, and instrumentation.** Anterior screw plates provide a strong tension band to resist vertical/horizontal translation and neck extension; however, they are less able to resist flexion or rotation. By contrast, posterior cervical plates strongly resist flexion or rotation, but are less able to resist extension. Thus, in the presence of three-column spinal instability, combined anterior and posterior instrumentation often is required. This technique provides rigid fixation of spinal segments and avoids the need for rigid external orthotic devices.

Combined instrumentation techniques are challenging and require several special considerations. Patients with any unstable C-spine may require fiber optic intubation, intraop cervical traction, and electrophysiological monitoring. **Anterior and posterior cervical instrumentation** is usually carried out in a single surgical session. The transition between the anterior and posterior approaches requires a specialized operating table (e.g., Jackson spinal table or Stryker frame) and careful coordination among the entire OR team. The long duration of surgery may be associated with increased incidence of respiratory complications, blood loss, and prolonged ICU stays.

Usual preop diagnosis: C-spine injury causing three-column (severe, unstable) injuries; cervicothoracic junctional pathologies; correction of kyphotic deformities; panvertebral disorders involving C-spine (neoplasms, infection, spondylitic myelopathy); failed symptomatic anterior cervical fusions

SUMMARY OF PROCEDURES

	Cervical Laminectomy/ Foraminotomy	Cervical Laminectomy with Instrumentation	Combined Anterior/ Posterior Cervical Instrumentation
Position	Prone or sitting; pin fixation or horseshoe headrest	Prone; pin fixation or horseshoe headrest	⇐ + supine
Incision	Posterior midline neck	⇐	⇐ + transverse or longitudinal anterolateral

	Cervical Laminectomy/ Foraminotomy	Cervical Laminectomy with Instrumentation	Combined Anterior/ Posterior Cervical Instrumentation
Special instrumentation	Operating microscope for intradural procedures	⇐ + implants, pedicle screws with plates	Implants; anterior and posterior plates with screws
Unique considerations	Fiber optic intubation; I.I. to assess correct level	⇐ ; I.I. for screw placement	Implants; anterior and posterior plates with screws
Antibiotics	Cefazolin 1 g	⇐	⇐
Surgical time	1.5-2 h	⇐ Add 30-45 min/level of instrumentation	4-5 h
EBL	25-500 ml	⇐	250-600 ml
Postop care	PACU → room	⇐	⇐ ; sometimes needs short ICU stay
Mortality	0-3%	⇐	⇐
Morbidity	All < 5%: Neurological: Myelopathy Nerve-root injury CSF leak Postop instability Infection	⇐ Nerve-root injury 2° screws Instrumentation failure	5-10% Displacement of bone Infection Respiratory problems
Pain score	5-10	5-10	7-10

PATIENT POPULATION CHARACTERISTICS

Age range	18-85 yr (usually 20-60 yr)
Male:Female	1:2
Incidence	Rare
Etiology	Neoplastic; traumatic; congenital; degenerative; infections; rheumatoid arthritis

ANESTHETIC CONSIDERATIONS

See Anesthetic Considerations for Cervical Neurosurgical Procedures, p. 83.

Reference

1. Collias JC, Roberts MP: Posterior surgical approaches for cervical disk herniation and spondylitic myelopathy. In *Operative Neurosurgical Techniques.* Schmidek HH, ed. WB Saunders, Philadelphia: 2000, 2016-28.

ANTERIOR CERVICOTHORACIC SPINE SURGERY

SURGICAL CONSIDERATIONS

Description: The **anterior approach** to the **cervicothoracic junction** (CTJ–C7-T3) is performed for discectomy, stabilization of spinal fractures, tumor resection, spinal reconstruction, and instrumentation. Anterior approaches to the CTJ often are challenging, as this area represents a rapid transition from cervical lordosis to thoracic kyphosis, resulting in abrupt increase in the depth of the wound. The confluence of great vessels, and visceral (trachea, esophagus) and neural structures at the thoracic inlet makes them susceptible to injury. The **transsternal approach** involves a longitudinal incision along the anterior border of the sternomastoid, extended over the midline of the sternum to the xiphisternum. The sternum is divided using an oscillating saw and retracted to expose the anterior aspect of the CTJ. The wide exposure available with this approach permits vertebral resection, reconstruction, and instrumentation. The **transclavicular approach** involves a T-shaped incision over the clavicles, with a vertical limb extending down the midline of the sternum. Subplatysmal flaps are elevated; and the sternal and clavicular heads of the sternomastoid are detached from their origin and retracted supero-laterally. The medial third of the clavicle and manubrium are resected to provide an excellent direct anterior approach to the CTJ for vertebral decompression, reconstruction, and stabilization.

Variant procedure and approaches: Axillary thoracotomy and high transthoracic thoracotomy approaches permit an anterolateral exposure to CTJ. As these procedures involve entering the thoracic cavity, they typically require OLV during the procedure.

Usual preop diagnosis: C7-T3 disc disease, fracture, tumor, and deformity

SUMMARY OF PROCEDURES

	Transsternal Approach	Transclavicular Approach	Axillary/High Thoracotomy
Position	Supine	⇐	Lateral
Incision	Longitudinal incision along anterior border of sternomastoid	T-shaped incision over clavicles with a vertical limb down the midline of sternum	Lateral chest wall
Special instrumentation	Anterior cervical plates Special oscillating saw for sternal opening	⇐ Special blades for clavicular resection	⇐
Unique considerations	OLV not necessary	⇐	OLV necessary
Antibiotics	Cefazolin 1 g iv	⇐	⇐
Surgical time	3-4 h	⇐	⇐
Closing considerations	Soft cervical collar	⇐	⇐
EBL	200-500 ml	⇐	⇐
Postop care	PACU → room	⇐	⇐
Mortality	1-2%	⇐	⇐
Morbidity	Wound infection breakdown Injury to great vessels at thoracic inlet	⇐ ⇐ Cosmetic deformity	Respiratory problems ⇐
Pain score	7-10	7-10	7-10

PATIENT POPULATION CHARACTERISTICS

Age range	30-50 yr
Male:Female	1:1
Incidence	Uncommon
Etiology	Disc herniations; trauma; tumor; infections

Reference

1. Kim DH, Beck CE, Dietz DD, Fessler RG: Surgical approaches to the cervicothoracic junction. In *Operative Neurosurgical Techniques.* Schmidek HH, ed. WB Saunders, Philadelphia: 2000, 2107-21.

ANESTHETIC CONSIDERATIONS FOR CERVICAL NEUROSURGICAL PROCEDURES

(Procedures covered: anterior/posterior fusion/fixation of upper and mid/lower C-spine; anterior cervicothoracic spine surgery)

PREOPERATIVE

Surgery of the C-spine is common, primarily because of the frequency of herniation of a cervical intervertebral disc causing compression of the adjacent spinal nerve roots. Other, less frequent indications for cervical surgery include: acute or chronic instability of the neck requiring fusion; removal of a tumor of the spinal cord; or craniocervical decompression for Arnold-Chiari malformation (see p. 51).

Respiratory	Acute fractures of the C-spine may be associated with sufficient trauma to the spinal cord to cause acute respiratory insufficiency and inability to handle oropharyngeal secretions. If this occurs, immediate tracheal intubation is necessary. Before initiating intubation, the neck must be stabilized, preferably in Gardner-Wells tongs or a body jacket; lacking those, a tight neck collar with sandbags on each side of the head will suffice. The objective is to **not flex or extend the head or move it laterally** during the course of tracheal intubation. **Tests:** Consider ABG to substantiate degree of respiratory impairment, if present.
Cardiovascular	Acute fractures of the C-spine and associated spinal cord trauma may → loss of sympathetic tone, which, in turn, may cause peripheral vasodilation and bradycardia. Generally, this condition can be treated effectively with crystalloid and/or colloid infusion, and atropine to ↑HR. Rarely is it necessary to use vasopressors to maintain BP or HR. **Tests:** As indicated from H&P.
Neurological	Patients with herniation of a cervical disc generally complain first of pain in the neck, particularly with lateral rotation of the head. The pain may radiate down one or, rarely, both arms. As nerve compression continues, patients begin to develop weakness and atrophy of specific muscle groups in the arm. These Sx, however, are not specific to herniation of a disc and may be caused by a spinal cord tumor or cyst. Patients with acute fractures of the neck and attendant spinal cord trauma at T1 level will be paraplegic, while fractures above C5 may result in quadriplegia and loss of phrenic nerve function. Injuries between these two levels result in variable loss of motor and sensory functions in the upper extremities. A careful documentation of preop sensory and motor deficits is important. **Tests:** MRI has replaced myelography as the primary diagnostic test, because it distinguishes disc from tumor from cyst. Emergency CT is invaluable in the assessment of patients with acute neck injuries and suspected cervical fracture; if not available, A-P and lateral x-rays of the neck generally will reveal the site and extent of bony injury.
Hematologic	Antiplatelet agents should be stopped 10 d before surgery. **Tests:** Hct; others as indicated from H&P.
Laboratory	Other tests as indicated from H&P.
Premedication	Premedication is very useful in this patient population. Midazolam 2-4 mg iv and meperidine 20-40 mg iv in divided doses prior to entering the OR makes patients amnestic and tractable.

INTRAOPERATIVE

Anesthetic technique: GETA

Induction	For patients with a stable neck, orotracheal intubation using standard laryngoscopy is acceptable. If the operation is to be performed transorally or at C1-2; if the patient's neck is unstable; if the head is in tongs, a halo device, or a body jacket; or if the findings on the H&P suggest that tracheal intubation may be difficult, it is preferable to place the ETT using FOL under local anesthesia before induction of GA. (For details of fiber optic intubation, see p. B-6.) Consider using a wire-reinforced tube as it allows for maximal bending of the tube to remove it from the surgical field, and it will not be compressed by the Dingman retractor. Most importantly, it is vital to discuss the severity of the surgical lesion and the planned intubation with the surgeon before proceeding. Nasotracheal intubation is rarely needed for this type of surgery. Once the ETT is in place, anesthesia is induced with STP 3-5 mg/kg or propofol 1.5-2.5 mg/kg.
Maintenance	Standard maintenance (see p. B-3). Neuromuscular blockade with vecuronium 10 mg or rocuronium 50 mg is helpful for positioning the patient and insertion of the Dingman retractor. Once the retractor is in place and the operation is under way, further use of relaxants is usually not necessary.
Emergence	If a cervical fusion has been performed, and the patient is returned to a halo device or body jacket, it is desirable to leave ETT in place until patient is fully awake, responding to commands, and able to ★ manage his/her own airway. **NB:** Immediate airway obstruction 2° soft-tissue occlusion or superior laryngeal nerve damage may occur on extubation. A useful way to test for airway patency is to deflate the cuff of the tracheal tube and determine that patient is able to breathe around the tube as well as through it. If there is any question about adequacy of the airway after ETT removal, it is prudent to leave the ETT in place and spray lidocaine 4% 4 ml down the trachea using a laryngotracheal anesthesia device (LTA). This technique will usually prevent or minimize coughing or bucking on the ETT for about 15-30 min. One also should consider inserting an airway exchange catheter

Emergence, cont.		through the ETT tube before its removal. AECs are well tolerated, and can be left in place until one is confident that no further airway compromise will occur. So long as the AEC is not touching the carina, it will not induce coughing or bucking, and the patient can talk without difficulty. This catheter will provide a conduit for immediate reinsertion of an ETT if airway obstruction from early or delayed swelling, bleeding, or hematoma formation should occur.
Blood and fluid requirements	IV: 16-18 ga × 1 NS/LR @ 4-6 ml/kg/h	Blood transfusion is rarely needed for operations on the C-spine.
Monitoring	Standard monitors (see p. B-1). ± Arterial line ± CVP line ± Doppler ± Urinary catheter	If a standard BP cuff is to be used, consider placing it on a leg at the ankle. If placed on an arm, the surgeons tend to lean on the cuff, making it difficult to take consistent, reliable measurements. If a posterior surgical approach with patient in seated position is planned, an arterial catheter is useful for monitoring BP, and a CVP catheter is necessary for monitoring CVP and aspiration of air, if an air embolism occurs. If patient is seated, an ultrasonic Doppler flow probe also should be placed on the anterior chest wall, with confirmation of its performance by injecting 1 ml of agitated NS into CVP line and listening for the change in Doppler sound.
	SSEP	If SSEP monitoring is planned, the combination of sevoflurane, O_2, opiates (fentanyl or meperidine), and neuromuscular blockage (rocuronium) is the ideal anesthetic regimen for optimizing the potentials. N_2O and isoflurane make SSEP monitoring less satisfactory.
Positioning	Supine: ✓ and pad pressure points. ✓ eyes. Shoulder roll Cervical traction	For **anterior cervical discectomy** and/or fusion, patient is positioned supine with a roll under the shoulders, and the head is moderately hyperextended. A cervical strap is placed below the chin and behind the occiput, and attached to a weight of 5-10 lbs hung over the head of the bed. If patient is in a halo or tongs, 5-10 lbs of weight are attached to the device. Alternatively, the surgeon may request measured traction of 20-50 lbs intermittently during insertion of bone plugs for fusion. The surgical incision usually is made in the right side of the neck.
	Prone: ✓ and pad pressure points. ✓ eyes. ✓ genitalia. Sitting: ✓ and pad pressure points. ✓ eyes. VAE monitoring: ✓ ETT position.	A **posterior approach** is used if the operation is for spinal stenosis or craniocervical decompression. With this approach, patient is positioned either prone (on a Wilson frame or on bolsters), or sitting, with the head in 3-point fixation. There are advantages to the neurosurgeon, the anesthesiologist, and, thus, the patient as well, in using a seated position. Advantages for the neurosurgeon: (1) easier access to the lesion; (2) less blood loss, since both arterial and venous pressures are lower than if patient were prone;[2] (3) less interference from CSF, since it readily drains away from the operative site; and (4) lower incidence of postop neurological injury.[2] Advantages to the anesthesiologist are: (1) less chance that ETT and other arterial and venous catheters will become dislodged than with patient prone; (2) less chance for inadvertent pressure injury; (3) easier assessment and management of ventilation; and (4) easier access to patient for insertion of additional catheters, if necessary.
Complications	VAE	The major disadvantage of the sitting position is the risk of VAE, particularly paradoxical air embolism to the left side of the heart through a PFO (or, rarely, through the pulmonary circulation) → CNS or coronary emboli. Incidence

**Complications,
   cont.**

of VAE is 25-45% in patients operated on in the seated position.[2,3] VAE is easily detected using a combination of Doppler, ETCO$_2$, and ETN$_2$ analysis; and complications are rare.[1,2] If VAE is suspected (Sx = ↓ETCO$_2$, ↑ETN$_2$, ↓BP, dysrhythmias), notify the surgeon and aspirate the right atrial catheter using a 10 ml syringe. This generally will confirm the Dx as well as provide treatment. If VAE continues, and the surgeon has difficulty identifying the site of air entrainment, consider using PEEP ≤ 10 cmH$_2$O or bilateral jugular compression to increase CVP and cerebral venous pressure. Low levels of PEEP applied and released gradually will not promote paradoxical air embolism.[4,6]

Hypotension

↓BP caused by venous pooling, inadequate venous return to the heart, and ↓CO can be treated by wrapping lower extremities while patient is supine, infusing adequate fluid volume to maintain right heart filling pressure, and avoiding excessive depth of anesthesia.

POSTOPERATIVE

Complications

Airway obstruction, edema
Hematoma
Neurologic deficit

The cause of airway obstruction is usually from soft tissue falling back against the posterior pharyngeal wall, which cannot be corrected by forward displacement of the mandible because of the neck fusion or postop traction/stabilization device (halo or body jacket). May require oral or nasal airway.

Tension pneumothorax

Delayed respiratory insufficiency usually is caused by either development of a tension pneumothorax from entrainment of air via the surgical wound or an unsuspected oropharyngeal laceration during tracheal intubation, or from bleeding into the neck at the surgical site, with progressive compression and occlusion of the airway. If a tension pneumothorax is suspected and circulatory signs are stable, immediate CXR should confirm the Dx. If circulation is failing, an 18- or 20-ga needle catheter should be inserted immediately anteriorly at the 2nd intercostal space on the suspected side to relieve the pneumothorax. If the Dx is airway obstruction from bleeding into the neck, the wound should be opened immediately and clots and blood removed. This should be done **before attempting tracheal intubation**. Intubation of the airway is futile and wastes valuable time if the cause is airway compression by blood in the wound. It is sometimes difficult to distinguish airway obstruction from tension pneumothorax by physical signs. One useful way is to check for the 'puff sign.' With airway obstruction from any cause, what gas moves in and out of the airway does so very slowly because of the obstruction. In contrast, with tension pneumothorax, gas moves in and out of airway with great speed because of high intrapleural pressure. By applying positive pressure to airway and listening at patient's mouth for the sound of gas escaping as airway pressure is released, one hears either a puff or jet of air escaping (tension pneumothorax) or slow, gradual exit of air (airway obstruction).

Pain management   PCA (see p. C-3).

Tests

CXR
Hct

Repeat neurological exam prior to discharge from PACU.

References

1. Black S, Cucchiara RF, Nishimura RA, Michenfelder JD: Parameters affecting occurrence of paradoxical air embolism. *Anesthesiology* 1989; 71(2):235-41.
2. Black S, Ockert DB, Oliver WC Jr, Cucchiara RF: Outcome following posterior fossa craniectomy in patients in the sitting or horizontal positions. *Anesthesiology* 1988; 69(1):49-56.
3. Cucchiara RF, Nugent M, Seward JB, Messick JM: Air embolism in upright neurosurgical patients: Detection and localization by two-dimensional transesophageal echocardiography. *Anesthesiology* 1984; 60(4):353-5.
4. Pearl RG, Larson CP Jr: Hemodynamic effects of positive end-expiratory pressure during continuous venous air embolism in the dog. *Anesthesiology* 1986; 64(6):724-9.
5. Sonntag VKH, Hadley MN: Management of upper cervical spinal instability. In *Neurosurgery Update*, Vol II. Wilkins RH, Rengachary SS, eds. McGraw-Hill, New York: 1991, 222-33.
6. Zasslow MA, Pearl RG, Larson CP Jr, Silverberg G, Shuer LF: PEEP does not affect left atrial-right atrial pressure difference in neurosurgical patients. *Anesthesiology* 1988; 68(5):760-3.

ANTERIOR THORACIC SPINE SURGERY

SURGICAL CONSIDERATIONS

Description: The **anterior approach** to the mid and lower thoracic spine (T4-T12/L1) is performed for spinal fracture, scoliosis/kyphosis, tumor, and infection. The **anterior transthoracic approach** provides a wide and easy exposure of the thoracic spine from T4-T10. The patient is placed in a lateral decubitus position (right or left, based on spinal pathology). An incision is made over the involved vertebrae and extended rostrally one or two intercostal spaces. The muscles and ribs are retracted; and the pleura is opened and lungs retracted to expose the vertebral bodies. Discectomy, corpectomy, bony reconstruction, and stabilization can be performed as required under radiographic guidance. The risk of spinal cord injury depends on the extent of surgery and reconstruction.

The transition zone at the thoracolumbar (TL) spine (T11-L1) is somewhat difficult to expose and requires a combined transthoracic and retroperitoneal approach through the diaphragm (**thoracolumbar transdiaphragmatic approach**). A left-sided approach is preferred, since it is easier to retract the spleen and stomach than the liver. The skin incision is made over the 10th rib, down to thoracic muscles, and the rib is resected subperiosteally to provide wide exposure. Blunt dissection separates the peritoneum from the undersurface of the diaphragm and lateral and posterior abdominal walls. With gentle retraction of the lung and abdominal contents, the diaphragm is well visualized and is sectioned circumferentially from the chest wall. This provides an excellent exposure of the anterior aspect of the TL junction. Most procedures can be performed with minimal retraction of lung tissue at this level; thus, OLV is not typically required. Vertebral resection, reconstruction, and stabilization are performed with radiographic guidance.

Variant procedure or approach: An **11th rib extrapleural-retroperitoneal approach** offers an alternative approach to the TL junction. It provides excellent exposure without the need to incise the diaphragm, resulting in less morbidity and reduced risk of pulmonary complications. Since the pleural cavity is not entered, chest drains and OLV are not needed.

Thoracoscopic spine surgery, while less invasive, permits thoracic discectomy, corpectomy, deformity correction, and bony reconstruction with bone grafts or cages, and instrumentation can be performed as with open procedures. It has been used successfully in the management of spinal fractures, tumors, infections, and deformities, with excellent cosmetic and functional results. This procedure is performed in the lateral position with GA, using OLV. Four 10-15 mm portals are made, with the working portal centered over the target vertebrae. The optical (scope) portal is placed two or three intercostal spaces cranial to the target vertebrae. Separate portals anterior to the working channel allow suction/irrigation and retraction. When using **thoracoscopic instrumentation**, hardware is placed through the portals in the chest wall under fluoroscopic guidance. Since instrumentation requires a wide exposure of the spine, OLV is essential. Recently developed instruments greatly facilitate the endoscopic placement of hollow screws, which can be passed over a K-wire. They also permit the use of compression or distraction forces over the bone grafts. The major advantages of thoracoscopic surgery include minimal rib retraction; minimal blood loss, with consequent early removal of chest drain; reduced wound pain; early ambulation; and low morbidity. These factors combine to reduce hospital stays.

Usual preop diagnosis: Fractures (usually at the TL junction); scoliosis; primary and metastatic tumors of the spine; pyogenic and tuberculous osteomyelitis; Scheuermann`s kyphosis

SUMMARY OF PROCEDURES

	Transthoracic (T4-T10)	Transdiaphragmatic (T11-L1), 10th Rib	Thoracoscopic
Position	Lateral decubitus + axillary roll	⇐	⇐
Incision	Over involved vertebrae	Along 10th rib	3-4 portals (10-15 mm)
Special instrumentation	Z-plate; Kaneda instrumentation, etc.	⇐	Thoracoscopic spinal instrumentation; MACS-TL
Unique considerations	DLT ± OLV	⇐	DLT; OLV mandatory
Antibiotics	Cefazolin 1 g iv	⇐	⇐
Surgical time	2-6 h	⇐	⇐
Closing considerations	Transfer to bed before emergence. **NB:** sudden movement may dislodge grafts or implants. ★	⇐	⇐ + May need closure of diaphragm.
EBL	200-5000 ml; nontumor cases: 200-400 ml	⇐	⇐
Postop care	Chest tube to water seal Chest physiotherapy/incentive spirometer Short ICU stay is usual. Bleeding > 200 ml/h → re-exploration	⇐	⇐ Shorter period of chest drain/ ICU stay
Mortality	3-5%	⇐	⇐
Morbidity	Overall: 5-15% DVT Neurological Infection Vascular injury Sepsis Atelectasis Pneumonia	⇐ ⇐ ⇐ ⇐ ⇐ ⇐ ⇐ ⇐	Problems with OLV Conversion to open procedure: 4% – – – ⇐ ⇐ Neurological injury: 1-2%
Pain score	7-10	7-10	5-8

PATIENT POPULATION CHARACTERISTICS

Age range	12-30 yr (scoliosis surgery); > 40 yr (tumor and infection surgery)
Male:Female	1:1; except for > scoliosis surgery in females
Incidence	20,000/yr
Etiology	Scoliosis, idiopathic (50%); trauma (20%); scoliosis, neuromuscular (15%); infections, tumors (10%); scoliosis, congenital (5%)
Associated conditions	See Etiology, above.

ANESTHETIC CONSIDERATIONS

See Anesthetic Considerations for Thoracolumbar Neurosurgical Procedures, p. 97.

References

1. Francaviglia N, Maiello M: Anterolateral techniques for stabilization in the thoracic spine. In: *Operative Neurosurgical Techniques*. Schmidek HH, Sweet WH, eds. WB Saunders, Philadelphia: 2000, 2141-5.
2. Johnson MR, Murphy JM, Southwick OW: Surgical approaches to the spine. In *The Spine*. Herkowitz NH, Garfin RS, eds. WB Saunders, Philadelphia: 1999, 1463-1571.
3. Kim M, Nolan P, Finkelstein JA: Evaluation of 11th rib extrapleural-retroperitoneal approach to the thoracolumbar junction. *J Neurosurgery (Spine)* 2000; 93:168-74.
4. Kumar R, Dunsker SB: Surgical management of thoracic disc herniation. In *Operative Neurosurgical Techniques*: Schmidek HH, Sweet WH, eds. WB Saunders, Philadelphia: 2000, 2122-40.

5. Kurz LT, Pursel SE, Herkowitz HN: Modified anterior approach to the cervicothoracic junction. *Spine* 1991; 16(10 Suppl): S542-47.
6. Sundaresan N, Shah J, Feghali JG: A transsternal approach to the upper thoracic vertebrae. *Am J Surg* 1984; 148:473-7.
7. Sunderesan N, Shah J, Foley KM, et al: An anterior approach to upper thoracic vertebrae. *J Neurosurg* 1984; 61: 686-90.

POSTERIOR THORACIC SPINE SURGERY

SURGICAL CONSIDERATIONS

Description: Thoracic laminectomy (midline removal of the lamina) and **costotransversectomy** (off midline removal of the rib head and transverse process) are procedures for decompressing the neural elements of the thoracic spine via a posterior approach. (Commonly used approaches are shown in Fig 1.3-10.)

Thoracic laminectomy is used to treat spinal cord compression due to disc herniation, neoplasm, or trauma. It also is used to gain access to the spinal canal or spinal cord for various intradural mass lesions, including syringomyelia. Thoracic laminectomy is done through a posterior midline incision centered over the involved vertebrae. The paraspinal muscles are retracted subperiosteally from the spinous processes and laminae on both sides. Laminae are removed piecemeal with ronguers or drills. Extensive laminectomy involving several segments or requiring removal of facet joints may require stabilization with transpedicular screws or hooks. Intradural procedures are performed with an operating microscope and microneurosurgical instruments. After completion of the intradural procedure, watertight closure of the dura is obtained and tested with Valsalva maneuver (sustained inspiration at 30-40 cmH$_2$O).

A **transpedicular approach** may be indicated for removal of herniated discs, excision or decompression of tumors, and the treatment of infection involving vertebral bodies. This procedure is performed in the prone position through a posterior midline incision centered over the affected vertebrae. The paraspinal muscles are retracted subperiosteally on both sides to expose laminae and facet joints. Facet joints and the superior half of the involved pedicle are drilled out to expose the lateral limits of the thecal sac and the nerve roots. A laterally herniated disc can be removed in a piecemeal fashion. If required, total removal of the pedicle is done to facilitate adequate bony decompression. Posterior instrumentation by pedicle screws, sublaminar wiring with rods, or a hook-rod construct may be performed.

The **lateral extracavitary approach** is a modification of a **costotransversectomy** and provides access to the anterior and posterior elements of the spine, thereby avoiding the need for a thoracotomy. This approach is performed with the patient in the prone position. A midline skin incision is made three levels above and below the involved vertebrae. The lower part of the incision may be curved over the involved side, if needed. A myocutaneous flap is developed by dissecting the scapular muscles (trapezius, rhomboids, etc.) laterally. Paraspinal muscles are freed from the spinous processes and dorsal spinal elements to enable retraction, which exposes the entire rib cage and dorsal vertebral elements. Subperiosteal resection, from its costovertebral tip to the posterior bend of the appropriate rib is done. The parietal pleura is gently separated from the ribs and the vertebrae to expose the postero-lateral aspect of the vertebral bodies. The

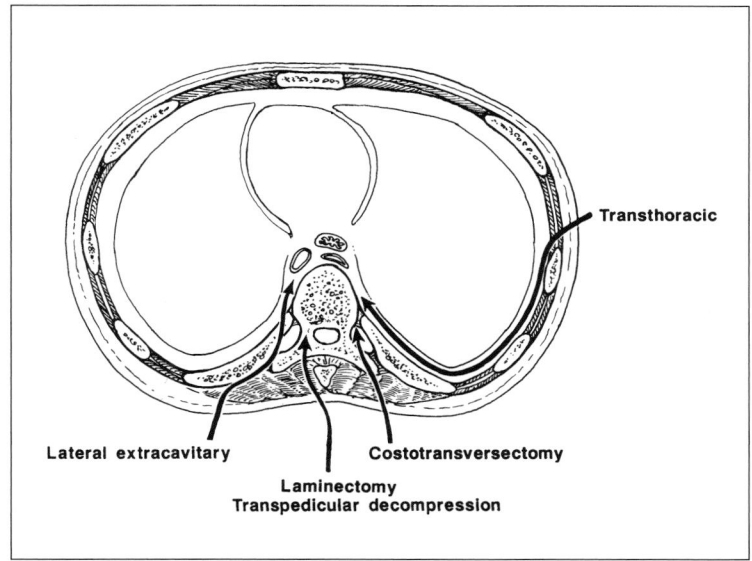

Figure 1.3-10. Surgical approaches to the thoracic spine. (Reproduced with permission from Tindall GT, Cooper PR, Barrow DL: *The Practice of Neurosurgery*, Vol. II. Williams & Wilkins, 1996.)

transverse process, pedicle, and laminae are removed, as required, to permit direct visualization of the cord during decompression of the vertebral body. Discectomy/corpectomy, vertebral reconstruction, and instrumentation are performed as required. At the end of the procedure, the operative field is filled with saline to check for any evidence of air leak. A small chest tube can be placed if an air leak is present. A layered wound closure (with Hemovac drain) is performed.

A **hook-rod construct** is used when the narrow pedicles in the upper and midthoracic region precludes the safe insertion of a pedicle screw. In this technique, hooks are placed to engage pedicles, laminae, or transverse processes, and then are fixed to rods by screws. Correction of scoliotic deformities or unstable fractures often require a combination of distraction and compression forces. To prevent construct failure, hook-rod instrumentation should extend at least three levels above and two levels below the involved vertebral level. A narrow spinal canal in the thoracic region prevents the use of laminar, but not pedicle or transverse-process, hooks. Rigid posterior thoracolumbar instrumentation techniques have largely replaced the **Harrington rod technique**.

Usual preop diagnosis: Thoracic radiculopathy (nerve-root compression); thoracic disc disease (herniation or degeneration of thoracic disc); thoracic myelopathy (spinal cord compression); thoracic canal stenosis (degenerative); infections (TB, pyogenic osteomyelitis) and tumors to spine (primary bone tumors or metastatic); intraspinal tumors; syringomyelia

SUMMARY OF PROCEDURES

	Thoracic Laminectomy	Transpedicular Approach	Lateral Extracavitary Approach
Position	Prone	⇐	⇐
Incision	Posterior midline	⇐	⇐ ; with hockey-stick extension
Special instrumentation	Operating microscope ± EP monitoring ± Pedicle screws/hooks	⇐	⇐ ± anterior and posterior spinal instrumentation
Unique considerations	I.I. localization	⇐	⇐
Surgical time	2-3 h	⇐ Add 30-45 min for bony/tumor decompression	4-7 h, based on need for anterior bony resection/reconstruction
Closing considerations	Often no cast	TL support/orthosis	⇐
EBL	100-1000 ml	200-1000 ml	300-3000 ml
Postop care	PACU → room	⇐	⇐ ± ICU
Mortality	0-5%	⇐	⇐
Morbidity	All < 5%	⇐	⇐
	Neurological: Myelopathy Nerve-root injury Massive blood loss CSF leak	⇐	⇐
Pain score	6-10	6-10	8-10

PATIENT POPULATION CHARACTERISTICS

Age range	18-85 yr (usually 20-60 yr)
Male:Female	1:2
Incidence	Rare
Etiology	Neoplastic; traumatic; congenital; degenerative

ANESTHETIC CONSIDERATIONS

See Anesthetic Considerations for Thoracolumbar Neurosurgical Procedures, p. 97.

References

1. Fessler RG: Lateral extracavitary and extrapleural approaches to the thoracic and lumbar spine. In *The Principles of Spine Surgery*. Menezes AH, Sonntag VKH, eds. McGraw-Hill, New York: 1995, 1279-91.

2. Kim DH, Beck CE, Dietz DD, Fessler RG: Surgical approaches to the cervicothoracic junction. In *Operative Neurosurgical Techniques*. Schmidek HH, Sweet WH, eds. WB Saunders, Philadelphia: 2000, 2107-21.
3. Kumar R, Dunsler SB: Surgical management of thoracic disc herniation. In *Operative Neurosurgical Techniques*. Schmidek HH, Sweet WH, eds. WB Saunders, Philadelphia: 2000, 2122-31.

ANTERIOR LUMBAR/LUMBOSACRAL SPINE SURGERY

SURGICAL CONSIDERATIONS

Description: The use of anterior procedures is steadily increasing among spine surgeons. Most procedures permit short-segment instrumentation of the spine, which often obviates the need for subsequent posterior fixation. The most significant disadvantage of these procedures involves the risk of injury to the great vessels; thus, these procedures are commonly done in association with a vascular or general surgeon. Anterior instrumentation systems generally fall into three categories: 1) **plating systems** (e.g., Z plating, anterior locking plates, and MACS-TL); 2) **rod systems** (e.g., Kostuik-Harrington, Kaneda, and Moss-Miami); and 3) **interbody devices** (e.g., cages and allografts).

An **anterior lumbar interbody fusion** can be done with cages or by threaded allograft bone dowels. After exposure of the disc space, the exact midline of the space is marked and verified with fluoroscopy. A spacing guide determines the exact position for pilot holes; and a partial discectomy is performed through these

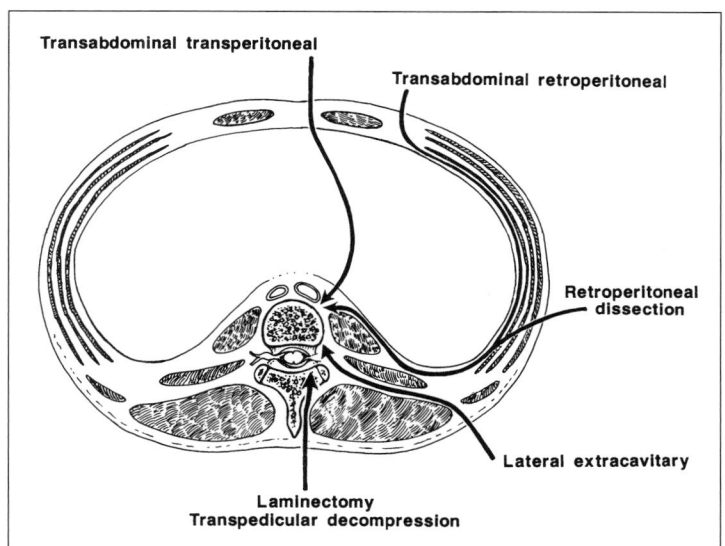

Figure 1.3-11. Surgical approaches to the lumbar spine. (Reproduced with permission from Tindall GT, Cooper PR, Barrow DL: *The Practice of Neurosurgery*, Vol. II. Williams & Wilkins, 1996.)

pilot holes, which are distracted and later reamed. A titanium cage or bone dowel is then attached to a specialized implant driver for insertion under fluoroscopic guidance. Harvested bone chips are placed into the cages or around the bone dowel. Anterior lumbar interbody fusion provides immediate mechanical stability and long-term load support, with the ability to heal through the disc space. Its primary disadvantages include bleeding and possible major vessel injury.

A **transperitoneal approach** involves laparotomy through a Pfannenstiel's or subumbilical vertical midline incision. After opening the peritoneum, intestines are retracted to expose the anterior aspect of lower lumbar and lumbosacral spine, an exposure that is often difficult to achieve with the retroperitoneal approach. Exposure of L4-5 disc spaces requires mobilization of the aorta and inferior vena cava, along with its bifurcations.

Variants of the transperitoneal approach: A laparoscopic transperitoneal approach often is used at the L5-S1 level. With the patient supine, Trendelenburg position is used to move the small intestine away from the operative field. The procedure is performed through one 10 mm portal for a 30° endoscope, two 5 mm portals for retraction, and one 20 mm working portal for instruments. For access to the L5-S1 level, the posterior peritoneum is incised at the base of the sigmoid mesocolon with endoscopic scissors. Median sacral vessels are clipped to expose the L5-S1 disc space. Laparoscopic interbody fusion and instrumentation is performed as required, using specially designed long-alignment tubes, distraction plugs, and a reamer, as in the open procedure. Finally, after insertion of cages or bone dowels, the peritoneum is closed with endoscopic sutures or clips. The major advantages of this technique are related to the minimal manipulation of abdominal viscera required and minimal trauma to the abdominal wall. Additionally, postop pain, recovery time, and length of hospitalization are often less, permitting an early return to the patient's normal activities.

A **retroperitoneal approach** provides an excellent exposure of the lumbar spine from L1-S1 through a flank incision. The procedure is performed in the lateral decubitus or partial decubitus position, with the affected side up. The upper hip and knee are flexed to relax the psoas muscle, facilitating exposure of the lumbar vertebral bodies. The skin incision is made from the lateral border of the paravertebral muscles at the midlumbar level to the lateral border of the rectus abdominis. The incision is angulated below the umbilicus for exposure of the lower lumbar and lumbosacral junction, and is carried down to the peritoneum. With blunt dissection, the peritoneum is peeled off the lateral and posterior abdominal walls, diaphragm, and iliopsoas, exposing the anterior aspect of the lumbar spine. Vertebral resection and reconstruction are carried out in the routine manner. During this procedure, the great vessels, ureter, and sympathetic trunk need to be protected. Monopolar cautery is avoided, as it can cause injury to the presacral plexus, which can result in retrograde ejaculation.

Variants of the retroperitoneal approach: The **supine retroperitoneal approach** is accomplished through a left paramedian incision, and the peritoneum and abdominal contents are retracted. Ligation of lumbar intersegmental arteries and tributaries of the iliac vein may be required to allow a direct anterior exposure from L3-S1. A **laparoscopic retroperitoneal approach** often is used for performing an anterior lumbar interbody fusion following discectomy in patients with lumbar segmental instability. This procedure is performed in the right lateral decubitus position. A 10-12 mm port is made in the posterior axillary line midway between the 12th rib and iliac crest, and a trochar is advanced into the peritoneum. Retroperitoneal dissection is accomplished by balloon inflation, with 1000 ml of air or saline, through a trochar. This procedure is carried out under direct vision through the laparoscope. Discectomy, fusion, or instrumentation require two additional working portals. Retroperitoneal insufflation with CO_2 may be required during the procedure.

Usual preop diagnosis: Degenerative disc disease; segmental instability; vertebral fractures; benign and neoplastic diseases of lumbar spine; vertebral osteomyelitis; TB

SUMMARY OF PROCEDURES

	Transperitoneal Instrumentation	Retroperitoneal Instrumentation	Endoscopic Approach
Position	Supine	Lateral decubitus	Right lateral decubitus
Incision	Pfannenstiel's/vertical subumbilical	Flank incision	3-4 ports
Special instrumentation	Z plates, Kaneda instrumentation, MACS-TL, femoral rings, cages; intervertebral disc replacements	⇐	Endoscopic instrumentation; balloon dissector
Unique considerations	NG tube, preop bowel prep	⇐	⇐
Antibiotics	Cefazolin 1 g iv	⇐	⇐
Surgical time	3-4 hrs	⇐	⇐
Closing considerations	Transfer to bed while anesthetized. Smooth emergence necessary to avoid graft/implant disruption.	⇐	Rapid closure of ports
EBL	200-600 ml	200-5,000 ml; nontumor cases: 200-400 ml	100-500 ml
Postop care	PACU → ward; patients with infections/tumors → ICU. Postop ileus common.	⇐	⇐
Mortality	Malignancy and sepsis: 1-2%	⇐ Elective: < 1%	– ⇐
Morbidity	Neurological injury: 2-6% Vascular injury: 2-15% Retrograde ejaculation: 5-35%	⇐ ⇐ < 5%	– – ⇐
Pain score	6-7	6-7	4-6

PATIENT POPULATION CHARACTERISTICS

Age range	Variable, infant-adult (usually 20-60 yr)
Male:Female	1:1 (usually)
Incidence	Uncommon
Etiology	Degenerative; lumbar segmental instability; neoplastic; traumatic; infectious

ANESTHETIC CONSIDERATIONS

See Anesthetic Considerations for Thoracolumbar Neurosurgical Procedures, p. 97.

References

1. Harrington FJ, Friehs G, Epstein MH: Surgical management of segmental spinal instability. In: *Operative Neurosurgical Techniques*. Schmidek HH, Sweet WH, eds. WB Saunders, Philadelphia: 2000, 2280-2302.
2. Kostuik JP, Carl A, Ferron S: Anterior Zielke instrumentation for spinal deformity in adults. *J Bone Joint Surg* [Am] 1989; 71(6):898-906.
3. Kozak JA, O'Brien JP: Simultaneous combined anterior and posterior fusion. An independent analysis of a treatment for the disabled low-back pain patient. *Spine* 1990; 15(4):322-8.
4. Leong JCY: Anterior interbody fusion. In *Lumbar Interbody Fusion*. Lin PM, Gill K, eds. Raven Press, New York: 1989,133-47.

POSTERIOR LUMBAR SPINE SURGERY

SURGICAL CONSIDERATIONS

Description: Lumbar laminotomy (partial removal of lamina) and **laminectomy** (complete removal of lamina) are procedures for decompressing the neural elements of the lumbar spine via a posterior approach. They can be used to treat lumbar radiculopathy 2° degenerative disc disease (e.g., herniated discs or osteophytes). **Decompressive laminectomy** can be used to treat compression of the cauda equina, usually 2° degenerative disease, congenital stenosis, neoplasm, and, occasionally, trauma. Lumbar laminectomy is also used to gain access to the spinal canal for dealing with intradural tumors, arteriovenous malformations (AVMs), and other spinal cord lesions.

Through a vertical midline incision, the lumbodorsal fascia is exposed, and then the paraspinal muscles are dissected off the spinous process and lamina of the segments intended for decompression. The level may need to be checked by intraop x-ray if the surgeon is not able to identify location based on visual confirmation of anatomic level. The bone landmarks are identified and ligamentous attachments are cut. The bone is removed piecemeal with either rongeurs, gouges, or power drills. Care is taken not to injure the underlying dura. If a dural tear is made, it must be repaired. The surgeon may want a Valsalva-like maneuver (sustained inspiration at 30-40 cmH$_2$O) performed to test the integrity of the repair. If disc is to be removed, the dura is retracted and the annulus incised. The disc is removed piecemeal with a series of curettes and disc-biting rongeurs. There is a risk of damage to retroperitoneal structures (e.g., great vessels or intestines) during this portion of the procedure. More commonly, there may be troublesome epidural bleeding, which may be difficult to control and will necessitate transfusion. Hemostasis is obtained prior to closure. The wound is closed in layers; and a drain may be left in the epidural space. The patient is rolled supine onto a bed at the completion of the procedure.

Variant procedure or approaches: Microendoscopic lumbar discectomy (MED) is performed through a 1.5 cm paramedian incision at the level of the affected disc. Under radiographic guidance, a series of soft dilators are inserted over a previously placed K-wire to create an operative corridor through the paraspinous musculature. A tubular retractor is inserted over the dilators and connected to a flexible support arm assembly. A 25° rod lens endoscope is inserted through the retractor and a laminotomy and discectomy are performed using the endoscopic instruments. As the retractor is withdrawn at the end of the procedure, the paraspinal muscles resume their normal anatomic position, obliterating the dead space. Skin margins are closed with subcuticular sutures.

Usual preop diagnosis: Lumbar radiculopathy (nerve-root compression); lumbar disc disease (herniation or degeneration of lumbar discs); lumbar canal stenosis; lateral recess stenosis; neurogenic claudication; herniated disc; metastatic tumor to spine; lumbar spine tumor; lumbar spondylosis (degeneration of lumbar spine); spondylolysis (structural defect in the pars interarticularis of the vertebra); spondylolisthesis (slipping of one vertebra over another)

SUMMARY OF PROCEDURES

	Laminectomy	Lumbar Laminotomy	MED
Position	Prone	⇐	⇐
Incision	Posterior midline	⇐	Paramedian port over disc
Special instrumentation	± Operative microscope	⇐	Endoscopic instrumentation
Unique considerations	I.I. localization to assess the correct level	⇐	⇐
Antibiotics	Cefazolin 1 g iv	⇐	⇐
Surgical time	1-2 h for single level; add 0.5-1 h/ additional level	2 h for single level; add 0.5 h/ additional level	⇐
EBL	25-500 ml	50-1,000 ml	⇐
Postop care	PACU → room	⇐	⇐
Mortality	0.5%	⇐	⇐
Morbidity	All < 5%:	⇐	⇐
	CSF leak	⇐	⇐
	Nerve root injury	⇐	⇐
	Infection	⇐	–
	Postop instability	–	–
	Massive blood loss	–	–
	Injury to retroperitoneal structures	⇐	⇐
Pain score	4-7	4-9	4-6

PATIENT POPULATION CHARACTERISTICS

Age range	15-85 yr (usually 30-60 yr)
Male: Female	3:2
Incidence	Common
Etiology	Degenerative; traumatic; neoplastic; infectious

ANESTHETIC CONSIDERATIONS

See Anesthetic Considerations for Thoracolumbar Neurosurgical Procedures, p. 97.

References

1. Foley KT, Smith MM, Raja Rampersaud Y: Microendoscopic discectomy. In *Operative Neurosurgical Techniques.* Schmidek HH, Sweet WH, eds. WB Saunders, Philadelphia: 2000, 2246-56.
2. Finneson BE, Schmidek HH: Lumbar disc excision. In *Operative Neurosurgical Techniques.* Schmidek HH, Sweet WH, eds. WB Saunders, Philadelphia: 2000, 2219-31.

POSTERIOR LUMBAR FUSION AND INSTRUMENTATION

SURGICAL CONSIDERATIONS

Description: Posterior lumbar spinal fusion may relieve low-back pain resulting from intervertebral movement. This surgery is often indicated for segmental lumbar instability, spondylolisthesis, or iatrogenic instability due to extensive laminectomy or facetectomy.

The **pedicle screw stabilization** technique provides rigid three-column spinal fixation and is the preferred mode of instrumentation in lumbar spinal surgery (Fig 1.3-12). Pedicle screws are passed after tapping the entry site, and are fixed with rods or plates on each side of each vertebral segment. The major risks with pedicle screw fixation include screw malposition and nerve-root injury. Pedicle screws may be combined with hooks to provide fixation of the lumbar/thoracolumbar spine, an approach that improves the stability of the construct and minimizes the risk of instrumentation failure.

Posterolateral fusion is performed through a posterior midline incision, with the paraspinal muscles retracted subperiosteally from the affected lumbar vertebrae. Decompressive laminectomy and discectomy are performed as needed. Posterolateral fusion is performed by decorticating the facet joints and transverse

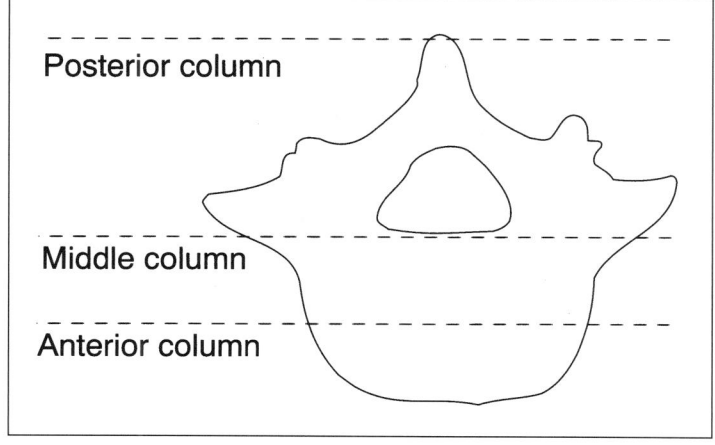

Figure 1.3-12. Spinal three-column model developed by F. Denis.[1] Disruption of elements of two or more columns renders the spine unstable. (Reproduced with permission from Tindall GT, Cooper PR, Barrow DL: *The Practice of Neurosurgery*, Vol. II. Williams & Wilkins, 1996.)

processes. Auto or allograft bone is then placed over the decorticated bone. Instrumentation with pedicle screws and plate/ rod constructs often is done for stability and to facilitate fusion.

Posterior lumbar interbody fusion (PLIF) consists of a bilateral laminectomy and removal of the inferior facet and the medial portion of the superior facet. The dural sac is retracted, and a total discectomy, together with the removal of cartilaginous end plates, is performed. The anterior half of the disc space is packed with autologous bone (harvested from the ilium or the laminectomy site). Appropriately sized rectangular bone grafts (auto or allografts) or cages are inserted into the posterior half of the disc space on both sides to provide structural support close to the center of rotation. This placement also allows radiographic assessment of the fusion anterior to the bone graft or cages. The nerve roots above and below the disc space should be visualized during the procedure to avoid excessive retraction. Instrumentation with pedicle screws and a rod/plate construct is often added to facilitate early fusion and ambulation, while preventing the extrusion of the graft. The major advantage of this procedure is that it provides the ability to achieve combined anterior and posterior spinal fusion, while avoiding the significant morbidity often associated with anterior lumbar surgery. Its major disadvantages include the potential risk of nerve-root injury and compromise of the structural integrity of both facet joints.

Transforaminal lumbar interbody fusion (TLIF) is a modification of the PLIF, using a unilateral posterolateral approach. A **hemilaminectomy** is performed and the facet complex is removed. A near total discectomy is performed and the first bone graft or cages are inserted across the disc space to the contralateral side. A second bone graft is inserted into the ipsilateral posterior disc space, and satisfactory placement of the bone grafts is confirmed by I.I.. Supplemental pedicle screw stabilization is indicated as in PLIF.

Usual Preop diagnosis: Lumbar segmental instability; spondylolisthesis; iatrogenic lumbar instability; spondylolysis; mechanical back pain syndrome

SUMMARY OF PROCEDURES

	Posterolateral Fusion	PLIF	TLIF
Position	Prone	⇐	⇐
Incision	Posterior midline	⇐	⇐
Special instrumentation	Drills, pedicle screws, or hooks	⇐; osteotomes, curettes, bone plugs, or cages	⇐; angled curettes, angled impactors
Unique considerations	I.I. localization and guidance	⇐	⇐
Antibiotics	Cefazolin 1 g iv	⇐	⇐
Surgical time	2 h for single level + 0.5 h/ additional level	3-4 h for single level + 1 h/ additional level	2-3 h for single level + 0.5-1 h/additional level
Closing considerations	No brace/lumbosacral corset	⇐	⇐
EBL	250-500 ml	250-1000 ml	250-750 ml

	Posterolateral Fusion	**PLIF**	**TLIF**
Postop care	PACU → room	⇐	⇐
Mortality	0-5%	⇐	⇐
Morbidity	Nonunion: 20-30%	10-20%	⇐
	Nerve-root injury	⇐	⇐
	CSF leak	⇐	⇐
	Infection	⇐	⇐
	Massive blood loss		
Pain score	6-10	6-10	6-10

PATIENT POPULATION CHARACTERISTICS

Age range	15-85 yr (usually 30-60 yr)
Male: Female	3:2
Incidence	Common
Etiology	Degenerative; traumatic; neoplastic; infectious

ANESTHETIC CONSIDERATIONS

See Anesthetic Considerations for Thoracolumbar Neurosurgical Procedures, p. 97.

COMBINED ANTERIOR AND POSTERIOR INSTRUMENTATION OF THE THORACIC AND LUMBAR SPINE

SURGICAL CONSIDERATIONS

Description: Patients with multilevel vertebral collapse, unstable three-column injuries, severe kyphosis or scoliosis, and/or neoplastic or infective conditions involving multiple spinal levels often require **combined anterior and posterior instrumentation**. This approach provides: 1) complete circumferential neural decompression, which facilitates maximal neuronal recovery; 2) rigid short-segment spinal fixation, which facilitates early ambulation with minimal orthotic support; and 3) maximal correction of deformities with low instrumentation failure and high fusion rates. The combined approach maximizes the possibility of complete resection of the neoplastic or infective process. Patients with major systemic disease or poor marrow reserve may require staged procedures. Combined instrumentation procedures are often lengthy, requiring 5-10 h of surgery. Major related morbidities include infection, wound breakdown, respiratory complications, and significant blood loss. The transition between anterior and posterior procedures should be performed carefully to minimize disruption of the instrumentation.

Usual preop diagnosis: Lumbar segmental instability; spondylolisthesis; iatrogenic lumbar instability; spondylolysis; mechanical back pain syndrome

SUMMARY OF PROCEDURE

Position	Prone + supine/lateral
Incision	Posterior midline skin incision + transverse
Special instrumentation	Anterior and posterior spinal implants and instrumentation sets
Unique considerations	OLV for anterior thoracic approaches; radiological localization; intraop EP monitoring (optional)
Antibiotics	Cefazolin 1 g
Surgical time	4-10 h
EBL	500-5,000 ml
Postop care	PACU → room; sometimes needs short ICU stay.
Mortality	0-3%

Morbidity	Respiratory problems: atelectasis, pneumonia
	Infection
	Bone graft dislodgement
Pain score	7-10

PATIENT POPULATION CHARACTERISTICS

Age range	15-85 yr (usually 30-60 yr)
Male:Female	3:2
Incidence	Not common
Etiology	Degenerative; traumatic; neoplastic; infectious

References

1. Denis F: The three column spine and its significance in the classification of acute thoracolumbar spinal injuries. *Spine* 1983; 8:817-31.
2. Harrington FJ, Friehs G, Epstein MH: Surgical management of segmental spinal instability. In *Operative Neurosurgical Techniques*. Schmidek HH, Sweet WH, eds. WB Saunders, Philadelphia: 2000, 2280-2302.
3. Leong JCY: Anterior interbody fusion. In *Lumbar Interbody Fusion*. Lin PM, Gill K, eds. Raven Press, New York: 1989,133-47.
3. Lowe TG, Tahernia D: Unilateral transforaminal posterior lumbar interbody fusion. *Clin Ortho* (and related research) 2002; 394:227-36.
4. Sundaresan N, Steinberger AA, Moore F, Arginteanu M: Surgical management of primary and metastatic tumors of the spine. In: *Operative Neurosurgical Techniques*. Schmidek HH, Sweet WH, eds. WB Saunders, Philadelphia: 2000, 2146-70.

ANESTHETIC CONSIDERATIONS
FOR THORACOLUMBAR NEUROSURGICAL PROCEDURES

(Procedures covered: anterior/posterior thoracic spine surgery; anterior lumbar/lumbosacral spine surgery; posterior lumbar spine surgery; posterior lumbar fusion and instrumentation; combined anterior/posterior instrumentation of the thoracic and lumbar spine)

PREOPERATIVE

Surgery of the lumbar or thoracic spine is common as a result of a variety of spinal disorders, including herniation of lumbar or thoracic intervertebral disks, causing compression of the adjacent spinal cord or nerve roots; spinal stenosis from bony overgrowth, causing compression of the nerve roots or spinal cord; spondylolisthesis; traumatic injury to the spine; and removal of a spinal tumor or placement of a shunt from a spinal cord cyst into the subarachnoid or peritoneal spaces. Since these diseases span a wide age range, the patients may be healthy, or they may have severe cardiovascular and/or respiratory disorders. Generally, the surgical incision is made in the thoracic or lumbar region, but occasionally the surgeon will elect to approach a lumbar disk retroperitoneally using an abdominal or flank incision. Sometimes both anterior and posterior approaches are used sequentially.

Neurologic	Patients with a herniated disk or spinal stenosis generally complain of pain, often in the pelvis or radiating down one or both legs. As nerve or spinal cord compression continues, patients develop motor weakness and atrophy of muscle groups in the legs. These changes also may result from a spinal cord tumor or cyst, so an MRI must be obtained to establish the cause. The MRI may be enhanced by the use of gadolinium or other contrast material.
	Tests: MRI
Hematologic	Blood loss may be substantial if the surgeon plans both an anterior and posterior approach in the same patient, or if the operation includes both spinal cord decompression and posterior spinal instrumentation. For these operations, at least 2 U autologous, directed-donor, or bank blood should be available. Many of these patient will have been taking aspirin or NSAIDs, which may have been stopped ≥ 2 wk before surgery, and bleeding can be excessive even if coag studies are normal.
Laboratory	Preop Hct if autologous donations made. Other tests as indicated from H&P.
Premedication	Adequate premedication is important. Many of these patients will have had prior back operations and dread having another one. Also, they often come to the preop suite complaining of pain because they were instructed not to take their daily analgesic medication. Midazolam 2-4 mg and sometimes meperidine 20-30 mg will increase their preop comfort level.

INTRAOPERATIVE

Anesthetic technique: GA is almost invariably used for these operations because it maximizes patient comfort, provides airway control, and permits use of controlled ↓BP. Spinal and epidural anesthesia are, in principle, excellent techniques for lumbar surgery, particularly for removal of a lumbar intervertebral disc, but they are seldom used because of the medicolegal concern that the regional anesthetic may be blamed for a new neurological deficit, if one should occur as a result of the surgery. Regional anesthesia is generally not suitable for lumbar fusion or removal of a spinal cord tumor or cyst because the duration of operation is usually unpredictable, and may be prolonged.

Induction	Standard induction (p. B-2). Use of a wire-reinforced tube should be considered to avoid tube kinking and occlusion when the patient is turned prone. If the surgeon elects to approach isolated disease of the thoracic spine through the chest, a DLT will be necessary to deflate the lung on the operative side For anterior approaches, regardless of whether the surgical approach is intra- or retroperitoneal, avoid N_2O to prevent bowel enlargement and impingement on the operative site.
Maintenance	Standard maintenance (see p. B-3). A combination of N_2O, opiate, sevoflurane or isoflurane, and NMB will provide adequate anesthesia. Once exposure is completed with the posterior approach, muscle relaxation is no longer needed. If an anterior and then a posterior approach are to be used in the same patient, one can either move the patient to a gurney after the anterior portion is completed, and then roll the patient onto the same operating table, or transfer the patient from one OR table to another. Another alternative is to perform the operation on a Jackson table, which allows the patient to be turned from supine to prone without having to move them. If this table is used, it is advisable for the anesthesiologist to disconnect all iv lines and electrical wires so they are not inadvertently pulled out during the 180° rotation. For anterior approaches, neuromuscular blockade must be maintained until the spine surgery is complete and closure is under way.
Emergence	Standard emergence (p. B-4), once the patient has been returned to the supine position on a bed or gurney. If the intubation was difficult, or the operation was prolonged and airway edema or respiratory depression is possible, it may be advisable to leave the patient's trachea intubated overnight.

Blood and fluid requirements	IV: 16-18 ga × 1 NS/LR @ 5 ml/kg/h	Blood transfusion is usually necessary only when there has been extensive bony decompression and fusion. Cell Saver is useful if large blood loss is anticipated.
Control of blood loss	Controlled hypotension	Modest decreases in BP are helpful to ↓ blood loss when extensive surgery is anticipated. This may be accomplished with combinations of sevoflurane or isoflurane and opiates, or by the use of α- and β-blockers (e.g., labetalol, esmolol) and SNP. BP values ~20% < the patient's lowest recorded pressure when awake are usually satisfactory, but should not be < mean BP of 60 mmHg in young adults or 80 mmHg in elderly patients. Once the bony dissection is complete, the benefit of controlled ↓BP wanes, and a more normal BP is advisable.
Monitoring	Standard monitors (see p. B-1). ± Arterial line ± CVP line	For simple back surgery, standard monitors are sufficient. If controlled ↓BP or an anterior and posterior approach are planned, an arterial catheter is essential to monitor BP, and a CVP catheter is recommended for infusion of vasoactive drugs and monitoring of CVP.
	± Urinary catheter	A urinary drainage catheter is also desirable if surgery is expected to last several h or substantial fluid shifts are anticipated.
Positioning	✓ and pad pressure points. ✓ eyes and ears frequently. ✓ breasts and genitals. ✓ free abdominal movement. Neutral C-spine	Except for syringoperitoneal shunts, which are performed with the patient in the lateral position, patients are positioned prone on a Wilson frame or on bolsters, or in the knee-chest position on an Andrews table. The head is placed in a neutral position using a foam pillow with cutouts for the eyes, nose, and chin (e.g., Andrews Gentle-Rest pillow). If the patient also has cervical disk disease, it is advisable to place a cervical collar before turning

Positioning, **cont.**		the patient prone. Other options are to use a horseshoe headrest or place the head in Gardner-Wells tongs or in a Mayfield headrest. Elbows, knees, feet, and any pressure points need padding.
Complications	↓BP Bowel or ureteral injury Hemorrhage	↓BP may be 2° abdominal compression and ↓venous return. ↑blood loss may occur 2° epidural vein engorgement, abdominal compression or vascular injury.

POSTOPERATIVE

Complications	↓BP Hemorrhage Nerve-root injury Blindness	If ↓BP persists despite vigorous blood and fluid administration, the anesthesiologist should suspect bleeding into the retroperitoneal space or abdomen. Alert the surgeon of this possibility and prepare for immediate exploration of the abdomen.
Pain management	PCA (p. C-3) Epidural opiate (p. C-2)	Some surgeons may place a mixture consisting of Duramorph, steroid, and Avitene hemostat into the epidural space before closing.
Tests	Hct; document neurological status.	If postop bleeding is suspected, serial Hct determinations are useful.

Reference

1. Sonntag VRH, Hadley MN: Surgical approaches to the thoracolumbar spine. In *Clinical Neurosurgery*, Vol 36. Williams & Wilkins, Baltimore: 1990, 168-85.

Surgeons

Gary K. Steinberg, MD, PhD (*Carotid endarterectomy*)
Robert L. Dodd, MD, PhD
Lawrence M. Shuer, MD (*Percutaneous procedures*)

1.4 EXTRACRANIAL NEUROSURGERY

Anesthesiologists

Richard A. Jaffe, MD, PhD
Stanley I. Samuels, MB, BCh, FFARCS
C. Philip Larson, Jr, MD, MS

CAROTID ENDARTERECTOMY

SURGICAL CONSIDERATIONS

Gary K. Steinberg and Robert L. Dodd

Description: Carotid endarterectomy (CEA) is frequently used to treat severe atherosclerotic occlusive disease involving internal carotid arteries at the common carotid artery bifurcation. Atherosclerotic carotid artery disease commonly causes thromboembolic or hemodynamic stroke and transient ischemic attacks (TIAs). Recent studies[4,9,10,14,24,26,28] proved the efficacy of this operation, compared with medical treatment for symptomatic high-grade stenosis (70-99%), symptomatic moderate stenosis (50-69%), and asymptomatic high-grade stenosis (≥ 60%).

The operation involves opening the common carotid arteries and the proximal internal carotid arteries in the neck (Fig 1.4-1), removing atherosclerotic plaque from the inside of the artery, and resuturing the wall of the arteries (media and adventitia). Opening the carotid artery (**arteriotomy**) requires temporary occlusion of the proximal common carotid artery, distal internal carotid artery, external carotid artery and, usually, its first branch, the superior thyroid artery. The entire procedure can be achieved under continued occlusion of these vessels, if the collateral blood flow to the territory supplied by the occluded internal carotid is deemed adequate (on the basis of intraop EEG monitoring, internal carotid artery

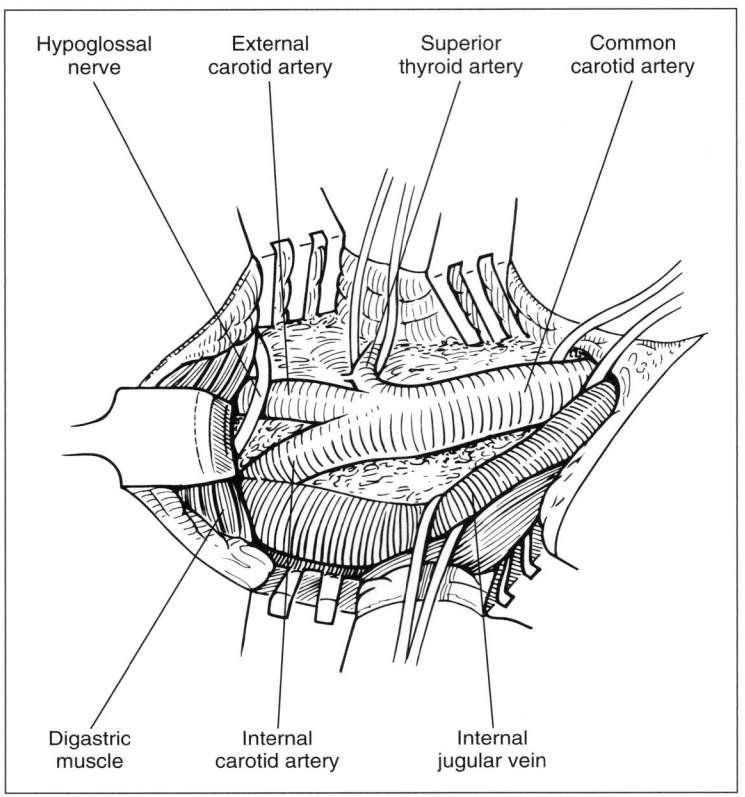

Figure 1.4-1. Exposure and control of carotid artery. (Reproduced with permission from Calne R, Pollard SG: *Operative Surgery*. Gower Medical Pub: 1992.)

back-bleeding, stump pressures, CBF studies, or angiography). Alternatively, an internal shunt between the proximal common carotid artery and distal internal carotid artery can be placed after the arteriotomy for use during the endarterectomy. Sometimes a synthetic graft (e.g., Dacron) or, occasionally, a vein graft, is used to reconstruct ('patch') the arteriotomy site and increase the luminal diameter.

Usual preop diagnosis: Stroke; TIAs; carotid artery stenosis; carotid artery dissection

SUMMARY OF PROCEDURE

Position	Supine
Incision	Anterolateral neck; occasionally, if 'patching' arteriotomy, may have to harvest portion of greater saphenous vein from leg.
Special instrumentation	Magnification loupes; vascular instruments ± shunt (Bard, Javid, Pruitt-Inahara)
Unique considerations	Techniques for monitoring collateral blood flow: EEG-spectral analysis or raw EEG, somatosensory evoked potentials (SEPs), back-bleeding or internal carotid artery stump pressure (> 50 mmHg), CBF measurements using Xenon, transcranial Doppler. Full anticoagulation with heparin (5,000-10,000 U iv) during arterial occlusion ± reversal with protamine (25-100 mg iv) at end of arteriotomy repair and 10 min after reopening of carotid arteries. Maintaining mild HTN during internal carotid artery occlusion (MAP 90-110). Use of intraop neuroprotective agents during internal carotid artery occlusion (e.g., iv STP 4-5 mg/kg).
Antibiotics	Cefazolin (1 g iv q 6 h)
Surgical time	2-2.5 h

Closing considerations	Avoid HTN or ↓BP (MAP 80-110); meticulous hemostasis.
EBL	50-150 ml
Postop care	Control of BP (MAP 80-100 mmHg); start aspirin on postop d 1; ICU or other monitored bed × 6 h.
Mortality	0.5-1%
Morbidity	Cranial nerve injury: Up to 39%
	Stroke: 1-2%
	MI: ≤ 1%
	Wound infection: Rare
Pain score	3

PATIENT POPULATION CHARACTERISTICS

Age range	50-80 yr
Male:Female	1:1
Incidence	150,000 CEAs/yr in U.S.
Etiology	Atherosclerosis; occasionally, traumatic (dissection)
Associated conditions	HTN; CAD; PVD; smoking; obesity; alcohol abuse; hyperlipidemia

ANESTHETIC CONSIDERATIONS

(Procedure covered: carotid endarterectomy—neurosurgery, vascular)

PREOPERATIVE

The incidence of occlusive or ulcerative lesions of the extracranial or intracranial vasculature increases with advancing years. Generally, these lesions are asymptomatic until the cross-sectional area of the vessel is decreased by at least 50%. This is because the cerebral vasculature has excellent collateral circulation, most importantly the Circle of Willis, but also the carotid-basilar anastomosis via the trigeminal artery and the extra- to intracranial collateral flow via the ophthalmic artery or branches of the vertebral artery. Patients presenting for CEA generally fall into one of three categories: (1) Those with TIAs, presenting with symptoms that may be focal or generalized. (2) Patients with completed stroke. If the stroke is recent (< 2-4 wk), some surgeons will not operate on the patient for fear of converting an ischemic infarct into a hemorrhagic infarct; however, if the infarct is small and clinical deficit minor, early surgery may be indicated. Angiographic evaluation usually demonstrates a stenotic and/or ulcerative lesion at the carotid bifurcation. (3) Patients with asymptomatic bruit, which usually is found during a routine physical examination of the neck. These are of concern because they may signal the development of carotid stenosis[36] and may benefit from surgical intervention.

Respiratory
If there is evidence of pulmonary infection, appropriate antibiotic therapy should be instituted. If secretions are excessive, preop pulmonary physiotherapy, including bronchodilator therapy, may be indicated. Patients should be asked to stop smoking prior to anesthesia, even if only the night before. While cessation of smoking for such a short time will not lessen the volume of secretions appreciably, or make the airways less irritable to a foreign body such as an ETT, it will provide sufficient time for the carbon monoxide levels in the blood to decrease, thereby enhancing O_2-carrying capacity. Any Hx of pulmonary disease should be evaluated with spirometry, ABGs, and CXR.
Tests: ABGs; spirometry; CXR, if indicated from H&P.

Cardiovascular
In addition to the usual measures taken in preop evaluation of any patient undergoing anesthesia, there are special considerations that relate to patients who are to undergo a CEA. Most important is a careful evaluation of cardiovascular status, including a detailed Hx of cardiovascular function and serial determinations of BP in both arms to establish the range of pressures that normally occur, and whether there are regional differences. If BP is different in the two arms, it should be measured intraop and postop in the arm with the higher values. Also, a preop ECG is mandatory. The reason for concern about cardiovascular function is twofold: (1) It is often necessary to administer vasoactive drugs to regulate BP during CEA, either to maintain it at a normal value, or sometimes to increase it as much as 20% above the highest resting pressure to maintain optimal collateral circulation during surgical carotid occlusion. (2) The incidence of perioperative MI in this surgical population is at least 1%, and represents the most common major postop complication in this operation. Except in the

Cardiovascular, cont.	case of emergencies, anesthesia and operation should not proceed in the face of severe, uncontrolled HTN, diabetes, or a MI within the last 3 mo. Antihypertensive medications should be continued up to the time of anesthesia. **Tests:** ECG; others as indicated from H&P.
Neurological	The Sx of cerebrovascular insufficiency are due to either critical stenosis or occlusion of cerebral vessels, combined with inadequate collateral circulation, or the development of ulcerative lesions at arterial branch points. The degenerative plaques or mural thrombi readily break off from the vessel wall and cause focal ischemic lesions. Manual occlusion of the carotid arteries is not an appropriate test of tolerance to temporary circulatory occlusion, as it may endanger the patient by precipitating embolization from an ulcerative lesion or by inducing bradycardia and ↓BP from activation of the carotid sinus reflex. It is desirable, however, to position the patient's head in the operative position as a test of the effect of that position on CBF. It is well documented that hyperextension and lateral rotation of the head may occlude vertebral-basilar flow between the scalenus anticus and longus coli muscles and, if sustained, contribute to postop cerebral ischemia. Sx of dizziness or diplopia will emerge with this maneuver if CBF is compromised. **Tests:** Carotid and cerebral angiography will identify type of lesion (ulcerative or stenotic), its location, and extent of collateral circulation. Other commonly used techniques include MR angiography, CT angiography, and duplex ultrasonography. As part of the preop evaluation, the anesthesiologist should examine the angiograms of the patient to become familiarized with the type, location, and extent of the lesion.
Hematologic	Aspirin or other anti-Plt therapy usually is begun preop to ↓ the risk of periop thromboembolic complications. **Tests:** PT; PTT
Laboratory	Tests as indicated from H&P.
Premedication	Use of premedication in patients undergoing CEA is controversial. Should a new TIA or stroke occur in the immediate preop period, its Sx may be difficult to distinguish from those associated with excessive responses to premedication. In this population, detailed discussion about the anesthetic and surgical plan, with appropriate reassurance, is usually enough. If medication is desired, midazolam 1-3 mg is preferable to opiates.

INTRAOPERATIVE

Anesthetic technique (regional): In the developmental stage of CEA, regional anesthesia—in the form of a superficial and deep cervical plexus block, supplemented as needed by a local field block—was used by most anesthesiologists and surgeons. It provided the opportunity to evaluate cerebral function during a trial occlusion of 2-3 min. If the patient showed no adverse effects, the operation was completed under regional anesthesia. If the patient developed neurological changes, a shunt was inserted or GA was induced and ET intubation performed, following which the operation was completed. Regional anesthesia, however, has several disadvantages: absence of cerebral protection, patients may tolerate occlusion for 10 min or more before suddenly losing consciousness or developing a Sz; and conversion to GETA may be technically difficult. Nevertheless, the technique still has some advocates among anesthesiologists and surgeons.[1,2,5,6,7,8,13,27,32] It is claimed that: it decreases the need for a surgical shunt and, thereby, avoids the complications of shunt insertion;[2,5,7] it decreases the length of stay in the ICU;[13] and, as an anesthetic technique, it is well accepted by some patients.[8]

Anesthetic technique (GETA): GETA offers both direct and indirect advantages for patients undergoing CEA: cerebral protection by decreasing $CMRO_2$ and redistributing flow toward the potentially ischemic area; greater patient comfort; and the ability to regulate PO_2, PCO_2, and MAP. Despite these arguments favoring GA, recent studies comparing regional and GA suggest that there is no clear outcome advantage of one technique over the other.[1,2,27]

Induction	Both STP (3-5 mg/kg) and propofol (1-2 mg/kg), when slowly administered, are suitable for induction agents, as arterial BP will generally remain at acceptable levels (± 20% of baseline) in normovolemic patients. These agents will ↓ $CMRO_2$, constrict normally reactive cerebral vessels, and → a redistribution of CBF toward potentially ischemic areas. Propofol has the additional advantages of antiemesis and prompt recovery. Etomidate (0.1-0.4 mg/kg) may be useful for induction of anesthesia in hemodynamically unstable patients. A muscle relaxant, such as vecuronium (0.15 mg/kg), cisatracurium (0.1-0.2 mg/kg), or rocuronium (0.5-0.6 mg/kg) is administered for tracheal intubation. An analgesic, such as meperidine (2-3 mg/kg), fentanyl (2-5 μg/kg), or remifentanil (0.05-2 μg/kg/min), may be given to minimize the cardiovascular responses to ET intubation. These opiates have minimal effects on CBF or $CMRO_2$.[36]

Maintenance	Isoflurane (up to 0.6%) or sevoflurane (up to 2.5%) inspired, either alone or in combination with N_2O 60% and/or remifentanil (0.05-0.2 μg/kg/min), is satisfactory. Just before cross-clamping of the carotid artery, an additional dose of STP sufficient to produce burst suppression on the EEG (usually 2-4 mg/kg) may be administered for its cerebral protective effects. Frawley, et al, have suggested that STP adequately protects the brain during CEA, and that a surgical shunt is obsolete and not needed.[12]	
Emergence	Upon removal of the carotid cross-clamps, total carotid occlusion time should be noted on the anesthetic record. Once bleeding from the arteriotomy site has been controlled, protamine (typically 0.5 mg/100 U heparin) is administered iv slowly over at least 10 min. If ↓BP occurs, rate of protamine administration is slowed. If vasopressors were used during operation, patient should be weaned from them during emergence, because HTN is likely as patient awakens from anesthesia. The need to control BP with a combination of esmolol and SNP is likely in the emergence phase. Antiemetic prophylaxis (e.g., ondansetron 4 mg iv 30 min before end of case) is appropriate.	
Blood and fluid requirements	IV: 18 ga × 2 NS/LR @ 5-10 ml/kg/h Hetastarch 6% < 20 ml/kg	Blood replacement is seldom an issue. Studies indicate that glucose may worsen the tolerance of brain to ischemia; thus, it is prudent to avoid glucose-containing solutions. Hetastarch stays in the intravascular compartment longer (2-3 d) than crystalloid solutions (1-3 h).
Monitoring	Standard monitors (see p. B-1). Arterial line UO	Marked fluctuations in BP may occur, necessitating hypertensive or hypotensive drug therapy. The arterial pressure transducer should be placed at the level of the head to accurately assess CPP. A CVP catheter is seldom necessary. Vasoactive drugs usually can be given safely through a cannula placed in the arm.
Cerebral perfusion monitoring	rCBF EEG	Regional CBF (rCBF) >24 ml/min/100 g brain is satisfactory, and < 18 ml/min/100 g indicates potential for cerebral ischemia; however, capability for making rCBF measurements is not generally available in OR. A variety of spectral compression EEG techniques permit computerized EEG analysis in OR. The major disadvantages of this analysis are: the EEG usually does not change until severe cerebral ischemia occurs, so it is not a good prodromal indicator of ischemia; the EEG may not identify small focal areas of ischemia; the depth of anesthesia and level of ventilation must be held stable or the EEG will not be interpretable; and there is a high incidence of false positives and negatives.
	Stump pressure	Stump pressure (pressure distal to the carotid clamp – also called 'back pressure') – is used to evaluate the adequacy of cerebral perfusion. Cerebral ischemia rarely occurs at stump pressures > 60 mmHg. The major criticism of stump pressure is the large number of false positives; that is, a stump pressure < 60 mmHg and a rCBF > 24 ml/min/100 g brain. This occurs in about a third of patients[21] and results in a shunt being placed when none is needed. The simplicity of the measurement and its validity when pressure > 60 mmHg still make it a useful clinical method for ensuring adequate perfusion.
	Cerebral oximetry	Cerebral oximetry has been used to evaluate cerebral perfusion during CEA.[31] Cerebral oximeters are placed on the forehead, where it is presumed they measure O_2 sat in the superficial distal cortex. With carotid occlusion, ipsilateral oximetric values may decrease. Oximetry values have been extremely variable among patients both before and during carotid occlusion, and no correlation with cerebral ischemia has been made.

Cerebral perfusion, cont.	SSEP	Monitoring of SSEPs has been advocated as a means of determining the adequacy of cerebral perfusion during temporary occlusion of a major cerebral artery, although its reliability as an indicator of cerebral ischemia has been questioned.
	Transcranial Doppler (TCD)	TCD scanning alone[14] or combined with EEG monitoring[11] is a useful method for detecting microemboli (air or particulate matter) during CEA. It also has been suggested that TCD can be used as a guide for regulating BP postop to minimize the occurrence of post endarterectomy cerebral hyperperfusion states.[11]
Control of BP	Keep MAP ≥ awake levels. Autoregulation Vasopressors	It is highly desirable to maintain MAP at or slightly above the patient's highest recorded resting pressure while awake. Surgical occlusion of the carotid artery often will decrease distal perfusion pressure (stump pressure) < 60 mmHg. Volatile anesthetics impair autoregulation; therefore, the higher the pressure, the more likely it is that cerebral perfusion will be adequate during surgical occlusion. A pure α-adrenergic agonist (e.g., phenylephrine) is ideal to support BP because it has minimal dysrhythmogenic potential. The modified V-5 lead usually will indicate if the ↓BP is causing myocardial ischemia. If hypertensive episodes occur during surgery, infusions of esmolol ± SNP work well.
Positioning	✓ and pad pressure points. ✓ eyes.	

POSTOPERATIVE

Complications	Circulatory instability	Circulatory instability is common.[34] ↓BP may be due to hypovolemia, depression of circulation by anesthetic or other drugs, dysrhythmias, or exposure of the baroreceptor mechanism to a new higher pressure, causing an exaggerated reflex response. Rx by volume expansion and pressors.
	HTN MI	HTN may be due to loss of the normal carotid baroreceptor mechanism. It may → excessive bleeding, increased myocardial O_2 consumption or dysrhythmias and MI, intracerebral hemorrhage and ↑ICP from cerebral edema.
	Loss of carotid body function	Chemoreceptor function is lost in most patients after CEA, as evidenced by a loss of ventilatory and circulatory responses to hypoxia and a modest increase in resting arterial $PaCO_2$.[34] These patients should be given supplemental O_2 postop. Special attention must be directed toward preventing atelectasis or other pulmonary or circulatory abnormalities that might cause hypoxemia, and to which the patient could only respond by further respiratory and circulatory depression and loss of consciousness.
	Respiratory insufficiency	Acute respiratory insufficiency may occur 2° hematoma formation with tracheal deviation, vocal cord paralysis from surgical traction on laryngeal nerves, or tension pneumothorax from dissection of air through the wound into the mediastinum and pleural space. Unexpected respiratory distress should immediately bring these 3 possibilities to mind, with appropriate Dx and therapy. A hematoma that causes respiratory distress always should be evacuated before reintubation is attempted.

| **Complications, cont.** | Tension pneumothorax | Likewise, if there is evidence of circulatory insufficiency, a tension pneumothorax should be relieved immediately by needle evacuation. |
| | Intimal flap → stroke | Should a patient emerge from anesthesia with a new neurological deficit, immediate surgical exploration of the operative site or immediate cerebral angiography should be performed to determine if an intimal flap has formed at the site of operation. This is a surgically correctable lesion and, if corrected immediately, may lessen the severity of the subsequent neurological deficit. |

| **Pain management** | Meperidine (10 mg iv prn) Codeine (30-60 mg im q 4 h) |
| **Tests** | Cerebral angiography |

References

1. Allen BT, Anderson CB, Rubin BG, Thompson RW, Flye MW, Young-Beyer P: The influence of anesthetic technique on perioperative complications after carotid endarterectomy. *J Vasc Surg* 1994; 19:834-42.
2. Anthony T, Johansen K: Optimal outcome for "high-risk" carotid endarterectomy. *Am J Surg* 1994; 167:469-71.
3. Archer DP, Tang TKK: The choice of anaesthetic for carotid endarterectomy: does it matter? *Can J Anaesth* 1995; 42: 566-70.
4. Barnett HJM, et al (North American Symptomatic Carotid Endarterectomy Trial Collaborators): Benefit of carotid endarterectomy in patients with symptomatic moderate or severe stenosis. *N Eng J Med* 1998; 339:1415-25.
5. Benjamin ME, Silva MB Jr, Watt C, McCaffrey MT, Burford-Foggs A, Flinn WR: Awake patient monitoring to determine the need for shunting during carotid endarterectomy. *Surgery* 1993; 114:673-9.
6. Chang BB, Darling RC, Shah DM, Paty PS, Leather RP: Carotid endarterectomy can be safely performed with acceptable mortality and morbidity in patients requiring coronary artery bypass grafts. *Am J Surg* 1994; 168:94-6.
7. Davies MJ, Mooney PH, Scott DA, Silbert BS, Cook RJ: Neurologic changes during carotid endarterectomy under cervical block predict a high risk of postoperative stroke. *Anesthesiology* 1993; 78:829-33.
8. Davies MJ, Murrell GC, Cronin KC, Meads A, Dawson AR: Carotid endarterectomy under cervical plexus block: a prospective clinical audit. *Anaesth Intensive Care* 1990; 18:219-23.
9. European Carotid Surgery Trialists' Collaborative Group: MCR European carotid surgery trial: interim results for symptomatic patients with severe (70-99%) or with mild (0-29%) carotid stenosis. *Lancet* 1991; 337:1235-43.
10. Executive Committee for the Asymptomatic Carotid Atherosclerosis Study: Endarterectomy for Asymptomatic Carotid Artery Stenosis. *JAMA* 1995; 273:1421-8.
11. Fiori L, Parenti G, Marconi F: Combined transcranial Doppler and electrophysiologic monitoring for carotid endarterectomy. *J Neurosurg Anesthesiol* 1997; 9:11-16.
12. Frawley JE, Hicks RG, Gray LJ, Niesche JW: Carotid endarterectomy without a shunt for symptomatic lesions associated with contralateral severe stenosis or occlusion. *J Vasc Surg* 1996; 23:421-7.
13. Gabelman CG, Gann DS, Ashworth CJ, Carney WI: One hundred consecutive carotid reconstructions: local versus general anesthesia. *Am J Surg* 1983; 145:477-82.
14. Gaunt ME, Ratliff DA, Martin PJ, Smith JL, Bell PR, Naylor AR: On-table diagnosis of incipient carotid artery thrombosis during carotid endarterectomy by transcranial Doppler scanning. *J Vasc Surg* 1994; 20:104-7.
15. Hobson RW II, Weiss DG, Fields WS, Goldstone J, Moore WS, Towne JB, Wright CB: Efficacy of carotid endarterectomy for asymptomatic carotid stenosis. The Veterans Affairs Cooperative Study Group. *N Engl J Med* 1993; 328(4):221-7.
16. Kearse LA Jr, Brown EN, McPeck K: Somatosensory evoked potentials sensitivity relative to electroencephalography for cerebral ischemia during carotid endarterectomy. *Stroke* 1992; 23:498-505.
17. Kearse LA Jr, Lopez-Bresnahan M, McPeck K, Zaslavsky A: Preoperative cerebrovascular symptoms and electroencephalographic abnormalities do not predict cerebral ischemia during carotid endarterectomy. *Stroke* 1995; 26:1210-14.
18. Kearse LA Jr, Martin D, McPeck K, Lopez-Bresnahan M: Computer-derived density spectral array in detection of mild analog electroencephalographic ischemic pattern changes during carotid endarterectomy. *J Neurosurg* 1993; 78:884-90.
19. Kraft SA, Larson CP Jr, Shuer LM, Steinberg GK, Benson GV, Pearl RG: Effect of hyperglycemia on neuronal changes in a rabbit model of focal cerebral ischemia. *Stroke* 1990; 21(3):447-50.
20. Kresowik TF, Khoury MD: Limitations of EEG monitoring in the detection of cerebral ischemia accompanying carotid endarterectomy. *J Vasc Surg* 1991; 13:439-43.
21. McKay RD, Sundt TM, Michenfelder JD, et al: Internal carotid artery stump pressure and cerebral blood flow during carotid endarterectomy: modification by halothane, enflurane, and Innovar®. *Anesthesiology* 1976; 45(4):390-9.
22. Michenfelder JD, Sundt TM, Fode N, Sharbrough FW: Isoflurane when compared to enflurane and halothane decreases the frequency of cerebral ischemia during carotid endarterectomy. *Anesthesiology* 1987; 67(3):336-40.

23. Mirko MK, Morasch MD, Burke K, Greisler HP, Littooy FN, Baker WH: The changing face of carotid endarterectomy. *J Vasc Surg* 1996; 23:622-7.
24. Moore WS: Carotid endarterectomy for prevention of stroke. *West J Med* 1993; 159:37-43.
25. Mutch WAC, White IWC, Donin N, Thomson IR, Rosenbloom M, Cheang M, West M: Haemodynamic instability and myocardial ischaemia during carotid endarterectomy: a comparison of propofol and isoflurane. *Can J Anaesth* 1995; 42: 577-87.
26. North American Symptomatic Carotid Endarterectomy Trial Collaborators: Beneficial effect of carotid endarterectomy in symptomatic patients with high-grade carotid stenosis. *N Engl J Med* 1991; 325(7):445-53.
27. Ombrellaro MP, Freeman MB, Stevens SL, Goldman MH: Effect of anesthetic technique on cardiac morbidity following carotid artery surgery. *Am J Surg* 1996; 171:387-90.
28. Penn AA, Schomer DF, Steinberg GK: Imaging studies of cerebral hyperperfusion after carotid endarterectomy: Case report. *J Neurosurg* 1995; 83:133-7.
29. Pulsinelli WA, et al: Moderate hyperglycemia augments ischemic brain damage: a neuropathologic study in the rat. *Neurology* 1982; 32(11):1239-46.
30. Ropper AH, Wechsler LR, Wilson LS: Carotid bruit and the risk of stroke in elective surgery. *N Engl J Med* 1982; 307(22): 1388-90.
31. Samra SK, Dorje P, Zelenock GB, Stanley JC: Cerebral oximetry in patients undergoing carotid endarterectomy under regional anesthesia. *Stroke* 1996; 27:49-55.
32. Shah DM, Darling RC, Chang BB, Bock DE, Paty PS, Leather RP: Carotid endarterectomy in awake patients: its safety, acceptability, and outcome. *J Vasc Surg* 1994; 19:1015-19.
33. Smith A, Hoff JT, Nielsen SL, Larson CP Jr: Barbiturate protection in acute focal cerebral ischemia. *Stroke* 1974; 5(1):1-7.
34. Wade, JG, Larson CP Jr, Hickey RF, Ehrenfeld WK, Severinghaus JW: Effect of carotid endarterectomy on carotid chemo-receptor and baroreceptor function in man. *N Engl J Med* 1970; 282(15):823-9.
35. Warner DS, Hindman BJ, Todd MM, Sawin PD, Kirchner J, Roland CL, Jamerson BD: Intracranial pressure and hemo-dynamic effects of remifentanil versus alfentanil in patients undergoing supratentorial craniotomy. *Anesth Analg* 1996; 83: 348-53.
36. Wolf PA, Kannel WB, Sorlie P, McNamara P: Asymptomatic carotid bruit and risk of stroke. The Framingham Study. *JAMA* 1981; 245(14):1442-5.

PERCUTANEOUS PROCEDURES FOR TRIGEMINAL NEURALGIA

SURGICAL CONSIDERATIONS

Lawrence M. Shuer

Description: Three percutaneous procedures are commonly used to treat trigeminal neuralgia (a well defined pain disorder of the face). Each involves placing a needle percutaneously from the cheek into the foramen ovale at the base of the skull under a light iv anesthetic. For the **glycerol injection**, it is necessary for the surgeon to verify that the needle is placed in the cistern of the trigeminal nerve or gasserian ganglion. This usually is done via I.I. or x-ray films, with contrast instilled into the cistern by the surgeon. There should be free flow of CSF through the needle. The patient is then placed in the seated position, with head flexed, and sterile glycerol is injected into the cistern (a potentially painful event). The patient is taken to the recovery room, with the head still flexed, for 1 h. The glycerol damages neurons in the ganglion, which usually causes mild sensory loss and relieves the tic pain in most cases. **Percutaneous balloon compression** of the ganglion is a procedure done in some centers for this condition. The needle is placed similarly to the above procedure, but, in this case, a balloon catheter is placed through the needle, and the balloon is inflated, once it is successfully located in the gassarian ganglion cistern. The patient may be kept sedated throughout this procedure. Compression of the ganglion will relieve the pain in many patients.

Radiofrequency (RF) rhizotomy is another percutaneous procedure used for trigeminal neuralgia. This procedure differs from glycerol injection in that a RF generator is used to place a thermal lesion in the appropriate portion of the gasserian ganglion. The needle is actually an insulated electrode with a portion of the tip exposed. The proper needle position is determined by applying stimulating current, with the patient awake, while assessing patient's responses. Multiple brief periods of anesthesia may be required to adjust needle position or to lesion the nerve. It is important for the patient to awaken quickly and be able to cooperate with the stimulus localization throughout this procedure.

Usual preop diagnosis: Trigeminal neuralgia; tic douloureux

SUMMARY OF PROCEDURES

	Glycerol Injection	Balloon Compression	RF Rhizotomy
Position	Supine	⇐	⇐
Incision	Needle placed lateral to mouth on cheek	⇐	⇐
Special instrumentation	I.I.	⇐	⇐ + RF generator
Unique considerations	Hypertensive response to needle placement	⇐	⇐ + Requirement for periodic deep sedation with rapid awakening for RF lesioning.
Antibiotics	Usually none	⇐	⇐
Surgical time	0.5 h	1 h	1-1.5 h
EBL	None	⇐	⇐
Postop care	Seated position with head flexed for 1 h	PACU	PACU
Mortality	< 1%	⇐	⇐
Morbidity	Usually < 5%: Infection Complete facial numbness (anesthesia dolorosa) Extraocular muscle paresis CSF leak Carotid puncture Facial hematoma	⇐	⇐
Pain score	3-7	2-4	2-4

PATIENT POPULATION CHARACTERISTICS

Age range	40-85 yr (usually 60-70 yr)
Male:Female	~2:3
Incidence	Relatively common neurosurgical procedure
Etiology	Vascular compression of a cranial nerve; multiple sclerosis plaque
Associated conditions	HTN; multiple sclerosis

ANESTHETIC CONSIDERATIONS

PREOPERATIVE

Trigeminal neuralgia, or tic douloureux, is a condition that develops in adults usually > 60 yr old. It is more common in women in whom an intermittent, severe, lancinating pain arises over the maxillary and/or mandibular divisions of the trigeminal nerve. The ophthalmic division of the trigeminal nerve is rarely involved. The pain is unilateral and often can be precipitated by stimulating a trigger point, such as by rubbing the cheek, mastication, or brushing the teeth. The cause of this condition is not known. Medical management consists of therapy with carbamazepine (Tegretol), an anticonvulsant and analgesic specific for this condition. Surgery is considered when medical management fails to control pain, or complications of drug therapy develop (anemia, bleeding disorders, dizziness, etc.). One of two types of percutaneous procedures is performed: either **glycerol injection** or **RF rhizotomy** of the symptomatic branches of the trigeminal ganglion. If these treatments fail, surgical exploration of the trigeminal ganglion is considered.

Respiratory	No special considerations, unless patient has a longstanding Hx of smoking and has COPD. **Tests:** As indicated from H&P.
Cardiovascular	Most patients have Hx of idiopathic HTN and take any one of a variety of antihypertensive medications. Good control of BP preop is important because most patients become hypertensive during the operative procedure. Intraop HTN is unavoidable because of the surgical need to have the patient awake during much of the procedure. **Tests:** As indicated by H&P.
Neurological	The presenting symptom is pain in the maxillary and/or mandibular division of the trigeminal nerve, unaccompanied by motor or sensory deficits.

Laboratory	As indicated from H&P.
Premedication	None, except for atropine 0.5 mg or glycopyrrolate 0.2 mg iv shortly before induction of anesthesia to minimize oral secretions while the surgeon is working in the mouth, positioning the needle.

INTRAOPERATIVE

Anesthetic technique: GA, regardless of which percutaneous technique is to be used. O_2 by nasal cannula should be administered before induction of anesthesia. To keep the cannula out of the surgeon's field, it must be taped above the eye on the side of operation.

Induction	Because the surgeon will want the patient awake as soon as the needle is in place to check for symptoms of pain, the induction drug must be potent, but short-acting. Either methohexital 1-1.5 mg/kg or propofol (1-2 mg/kg) alone or at a reduced dose in combination with remifentanil (0.5 µg/kg) are suitable for this purpose. The drug should be injected by bolus into a rapidly flowing iv to achieve a high concentration of drug in the brain quickly. Continuous infusion of the drug is not satisfactory, because it either fails to achieve a high brain concentration quickly, or its continuous administration prolongs the time before the patient is sufficiently arousable to communicate with the surgeon. In experienced hands, the needle is placed within a matter of 2-3 min. If difficulty is encountered in placing the needle, additional doses of induction drug may be needed. Patients invariably develop apnea for 1-2 min, followed by partial or total airway obstruction, while the surgeon has his hand in the mouth positioning the needle. Prior to induction of anesthesia, therefore, it is essential that the anesthesiologist optimize ventilation and oxygenation by asking patient to take a series of deep breaths through the nose with the mouth closed. This will ↑ the O_2 level and ↓ the CO_2 level in the lungs before induction. To maintain adequate spontaneous ventilation and oxygenation, it is usually necessary to institute forward displacement of the mandible while the surgeon inserts the needle. Another alternative is to insert a nasal airway.

If **glycerol injection** is used, needle position is verified by radiological imaging, using a radio-opaque dye. Patient is awakened and placed in a seated position with head flexed. The glycerol is injected, causing severe pain. Patient is then moved to recovery room still in seated position with the head forward to keep the glycerol localized to the region of the trigeminal ganglion.

If **RF rhizotomy** is performed, the patient is awakened and the position of the needle is verified by stimulating the ganglion with heat and determining the site of pain. The patient is then reanesthetized with a smaller bolus of the same drug to permit high-intensity heat stimulation for ~1 min. This procedure may be repeated several times. Each time, the patient needs less anesthetic, because of both the cumulative effects of the drug, and the fact that the trigeminal ganglion is becoming permanently damaged by the heat. |
Emergence	In the recovery room, patients are maintained in a seated position with an ice pack on the cheek at the site of needle insertion to minimize postop bleeding and swelling. Following glycerol injection, patients often complain of pain in the face, requiring opiate analgesics. Following RF rhizotomy, the face is usually numb, which is the end point for concluding the operation.
Blood and fluid requirements	IV: 18 ga × 1 NS/LR @ 4-6 ml/kg/h
Monitoring	Standard monitors (see p. B-1).
Control of BP	Clonidine patch Labetalol	Patients almost invariably become hypertensive during this therapy. Attempts to lessen these episodes with a clonidine patch preop or use of intermittent doses of labetalol prophylactically or therapeutically are only partially successful.
Positioning	Table turned 180° ✓ and pad pressure points. ✓ eyes.	Patient supine with head in the midline.
Complications	Failure of needle placement Bleeding Respiratory arrest	Major complications from this operation are uncommon, but include: (1) Failure to identify the foramen ovale, through which the needle must be inserted to reach the trigeminal

Complications, cont.

ganglion. If the needle cannot be placed within 30-40 min, the procedure usually is aborted until another day. (2) Bleeding into cheek from puncture of a branch of the facial artery. (3) Apnea from spillover of the neurolytic solution into circulating CSF, presumably affecting the respiratory center in the 4th ventricle.

POSTOPERATIVE

Pain management   Parenteral opiates (see p. C-2).

References

1. Percutaneous treatment of trigeminal neuralgia: advances and problems (Review). *Clin Neurosurg* 2000; 46:455-72.
2. Young RF: Stereotactic procedures for facial pain. In *Brain Surgery: Complication, Avoidance and Management*. Apuzzo MLJ, ed. Churchill Livingstone, New York: 1993, 2097-113.

Surgeons

Christopher J. Engelman, MD
Peter R. Egbert, MD
Weldon W. Haw, MD
Michael W. Gaynon, MD (*Retinal surgery*)

2.0 OPHTHALMIC SURGERY

Anesthesiologists

Stanley I. Samuels, MB, BCh, FFARCS
Richard A. Jaffe, MD, PhD

CATARACT EXTRACTION WITH INTRAOCULAR LENS INSERTION

SURGICAL CONSIDERATIONS

Description: Cataract—the leading cause of treatable blindness in the world—is defined as opacification of the crystalline lens. **Cataract surgery** is among the most common surgical procedures, with more than 1.3 million performed in the U. S. each year. Several approaches to cataract removal have evolved as a result of advances in both instrumentation and artificial intraocular lenses (IOL). Most modern cataract surgery is performed using the **extracapsular technique**, which involves removal of the crystalline lens through an opening made in the anterior lens capsule (known as a **capsulectomy**). Removal of the lens nucleus can then be accomplished intact, which requires an 8-10 mm corneal incision, or by **phacoemulsification** wherein ultrasound energy is used to fragment the lens, allowing aspiration of the lens material. The advantage to phacoemulsification is that the entire procedure can be performed through a much smaller, clear corneal incision (usually ~3 mm in length). With both approaches, the softer, more peripheral cortical lens material is then removed by aspiration, leaving the posterior capsular bag intact to support an IOL implant (Fig 2-1). If the lens capsule is torn or is for any reason unable to support an IOL, the lens can be fixated with sutures in the posterior chamber (behind the iris), or an anterior chamber IOL can be placed in front of the iris. Presently, the most popular

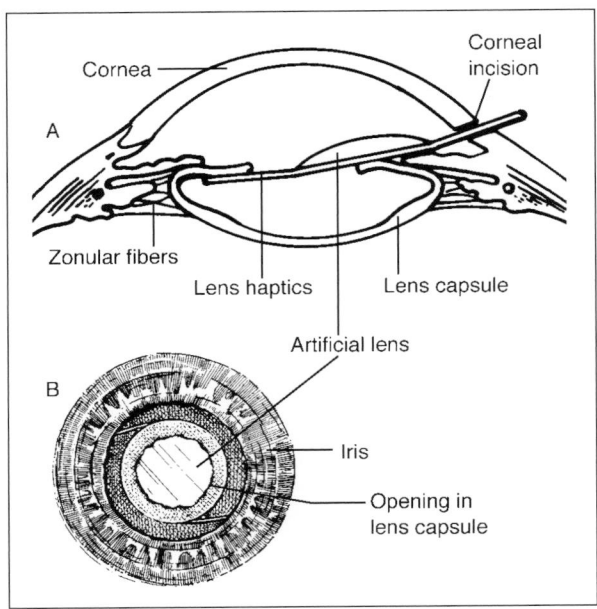

Figure 2-1. (A) Placement of intraocular lens into remaining capsular bag. (B) 'In-the-bag' insertion.

materials for IOL implants are polymethylmethacrylate, silicon, and acrylic. Only silicon and acrylic are foldable, which allows their insertion through a small corneal incision, and, therefore, are the most commonly used. The wound is closed with nylon or Vicryl suture (9-0 or 10-0) to achieve a watertight seal, although when small incisions are used, the wounds are often self-sealing and do not require sutures.

Variant procedure or approaches: **Intracapsular cataract extraction** involves removal of the crystalline lens with its surrounding capsular bag intact. To accomplish this, the zonules that normally stabilize and center the lens must be broken, and a cryoprobe often is used to remove the lens from the eye through a large incision. This procedure is performed infrequently, given the superior visual outcomes of extracapsular techniques. It may be indicated in situations where capsular bag support has been compromised by either trauma or inherited disorders.

Usual preop diagnosis: Cataract

SUMMARY OF PROCEDURE

Position	Supine, table rotated 90-180°
Incision	3 mm peripheral cornea (phacoemulsification) or 8-10 mm (corneoscleral junction)
Special instrumentation	Surgical microscope; phacoemulsification machine
Antibiotics	Subconjunctival cefazolin (50-100 mg) or gentamicin (20-40 mg) or a topical fluoroquinalone
Surgical time	20-60 min
EBL	None
Postop Care	Possible eye patch/shield for 24 h, topical medications
Mortality	Rare
Morbidity	Posterior capsule rupture: 3.1%
	Corneal edema: < 2%
	Macular edema: 1-2%
	Retinal detachment: < 1%
	Choroidal hemorrhage: 0.3%
	Endophthalmitis: < 0.2 %
Pain score	1-2

PATIENT POPULATION CHARACTERISTICS

Age range	3 mo-75 yr
Male:Female	1:1
Incidence	> 1,000,000/yr in U.S.
Etiology	Congenital; metabolic; traumatic; senile; medication-induced (steroids)
Associated conditions	Systemic diseases of elderly patients–common; cardiovascular disease; diabetes; HTN

ANESTHETIC CONSIDERATIONS

See Anesthetic Considerations for Ophthalmic Surgical Procedures under MAC (adult), p. 124, or for Pediatric Ophthalmic Surgery, p. 951.

References

See General References following Ophthalmic Surgery section, p. 137.

CORNEAL TRANSPLANT

SURGICAL CONSIDERATIONS

Description: **Corneal transplantation (penetrating keratoplasty [PKP])** involves replacing a portion of the host cornea with tissue from a donor eye (allograft). The primary goals of this procedure are to restore both the integrity of the cornea and to establish a clear visual axis. The ideal death-to-preservation time of the donor cornea is <18 h, and the donor cornea can be stored for up to 2 wks before transplantation. The procedure often begins with placement of a scleral fixation ring (Flieringa ring), just beyond the corneoscleral junction, which is secured with 7-0 Vicryl sutures. This provides additional scleral support that is especially helpful in children or patients who have undergone previous cataract surgery. The donor corneal button is removed from the surrounding corneoscleral rim with a trephine and kept in storage medium until the recipient bed is prepared. The host cornea is then trephined in a previously marked central location, using either manual or vacuum-assist techniques. Once the eye is opened, it is critical to avoid patient movement, coughing, bucking, or any Valsalva maneuvers, to prevent expulsion of the intraocular contents through the wound. The size of the donor button is generally cut ~0.25 mm larger than the host bed. The donor cornea is then sutured into place with 10-0 nylon sutures, which can be accomplished using 16 interrupted sutures, running sutures, or a combination, depending on a number of factors unique to each patient. Great care is taken during manipulation of the allograft to avoid trauma to the inner surface of the graft, as damage to the endothelial cells in this location can result in primary graft failure.

Variant procedure or approaches: PKP may be combined with **cataract extraction** or exchange of a previously placed intraocular lens (IOL). Additionally, PKP may be combined with **limbal stem-cell transplantation** (autograft from less injured eye) in cases where the most superficial corneal epithelial layer is unable to regenerate following damage (e.g., chemical burn injuries) to the limbal stem cells. **Partial-thickness transplants**, called **lamellar keratoplasty**, also can be performed in certain clinical situations.

Usual preop diagnosis: Persistent corneal edema; inherited corneal dystrophy; keratoconus; corneal scar

SUMMARY OF PROCEDURE

Position	Supine, table rotated 90-180°
Incision	Corneal
Special instrumentation	Surgical microscope
Unique considerations	Open-globe precautions: Avoid coughing, bucking, or Valsalva, to prevent expulsion of intra-ocular contents.
Antibiotics	Subconjunctival cefazolin (50-100 mg) or gentamicin (20-40 mg)
Surgical time	60-90 min
EBL	Minimal
Postop care	Patch/shield for 24 h, long-term topical immunosuppression to prevent graft rejection
Mortality	Rare
Morbidity	Graft rejection: ~5%
	Suprachoroidal hemorrhage: < 1% (higher for MAC: ~ 4%)
	Infection: < 1%
Pain score	2

PATIENT POPULATION CHARACTERISTICS

Age range	Any age
Male:Female	1:1
Incidence	> 40,000 cases/yr in U.S. and Canada
Etiology	Corneal opacity or decompensation resulting from endothelial failure; inherited dystrophy; keratoconus; scarring related to trauma/chemical burn/infection
Associated conditions	Congenital malformations; sleep apnea; atopic disease/asthma; Down syndrome

ANESTHETIC CONSIDERATIONS

See Anesthetic Considerations for Ophthalmic Surgical Procedures under MAC (adult), p. 124, or for Pediatric Ophthalmic Surgery, p. 951.

References

See General References following Ophthalmic Surgery section, p. 137.

TRABECULECTOMY

SURGICAL CONSIDERATIONS

Description: **Glaucoma** is a disorder characterized by progressive optic neuropathy in which elevated intraocular pressure (IOP) is the most modifiable risk factor. It is the second most common cause of blindness in the U.S. and accounts for more than 5.1 million cases of blindness throughout the world. **Trabeculectomy** is the most common surgical procedure used to reduce IOP and is often undertaken only after medical therapy has failed. In trabeculectomy, a drainage fistula is created from the anterior chamber to the subconjunctival space, allowing aqueous humor to drain from the eye. (Normal anatomy relevant for aqueous fluid production is shown in Fig 2-2). First, an incision is created in the conjunctiva and Tenon's layer, exposing the underlying bare sclera. A partial-thickness (4-5 mm) scleral flap, hinged at the limbus, is then created. Because scarring is the most common cause of surgical failure, antimetabolites, such as mitomycin-C or 5-fluorouracil, are often applied to the surgical site to slow or prevent fibroblast proliferation. Next, an incision into the anterior chamber is created at the base of the scleral flap and converted to a sclerotomy by removing an approximate

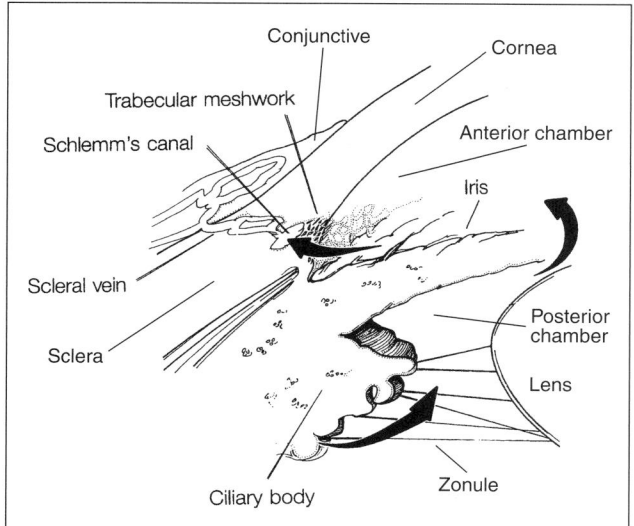

Figure 2-2. Ocular anatomy concerned with control of IOP. (Reproduced with permission from Barash PG, Cullen BF, Stoelting RK, eds: *Clinical Anesthesiology,* 4th edition. Lippincott Williams & Wilkins, 2001.)

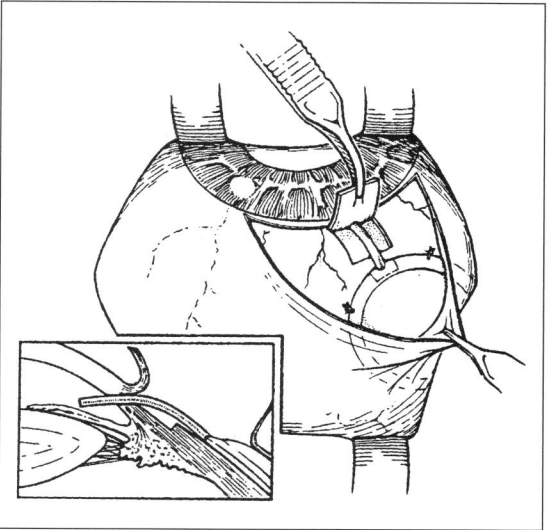

Figure 2-3. Basic technique of inserting Molteno implant. Silicone tube is inserted into anterior chamber via needle track and is connected to a subconjunctival acrylic plate that is attached to the sclera near the equator. (Reproduced with permission from Shields MB: *Textbook of Glaucoma,* 4th edition. Williams & Wilkins, Philadelphia, 1998.)

1 × 4 mm piece of corneoscleral tissue. To prevent the iris from entering the fistula as well as to protect against future angle closure, an **iridectomy** is performed, followed by closure of the overlying scleral flap with 10-0 nylon sutures. Before closure, it is important to avoid coughing, bucking, or Valsalva maneuvers, which might cause suprachoroidal hemorrhage or expulsion of intraocular content. The conjunctiva is then reapposed, using running 8-0 or 9-0 Vicryl suture.

Variant procedure or approaches: In patients for whom trabeculectomy has failed, a variety of **drainage implants** have been created to maintain the patency of the drainage fistula. These devices (e.g., **Ahmed, Molteno, Krupin, Baerveldt**) consist of plastic reservoirs that are placed in the sub-Tenon's space and are connected to a tube that enters the anterior chamber (Fig 2-3). These devices differ in implant size and whether or not there is an internal valve to prevent excessive drainage. Long-term IOP reduction with drainage implants is not as successful as trabeculectomy.

In infants and children with congenital glaucoma (see Pediatric Ophthalmic Surgery, p. 950), the anterior chamber angle, which normally allows outflow of aqueous, develops abnormally and often requires surgical intervention. **Goniotomy** (opening Schlemm's canal) is usually the initial procedure of choice. An alternative procedure is a trabeculotomy performed by exposing Schlemm's canal (the drainage system) in a corneoscleral cutdown. A trabeculotome is then threaded into this canal and is rotated, creating a tear in the trabecular meshwork and allowing direct communication between the anterior chamber and Schlemm's canal.

Usual preop diagnosis: Glaucoma

SUMMARY OF PROCEDURE

Position	Supine, table rotated 90-180°
Incision	Superior portion of eye
Special instrumentation	Surgical microscope
Unique considerations	Prevent coughing, bucking, Valsalva while globe is open, to prevent expulsion of intraocular contents.
Antibiotics	Subconjunctival cefazolin (50-100 mg) or gentamicin (20-40 mg)
Surgical time	30-60 min
EBL	Minimal
Postop care	Patch/shield × 24 h; long-term topical immunosuppression to reduce scarring. Scleral flap sutures can be cut with a laser postop to increase flow.
Mortality	Rare

Morbidity	Overfiltration causing hypotony
	Leaking bleb
	Fistula scarring
	Infection
Pain score	1-2

PATIENT POPULATION CHARACTERISTICS

Age range	Any age; more common in the elderly
Male:Female	1:1
Incidence	1.7% Caucasians; 5.6% African-Americans
Etiology	Cause of primary open angle unknown, but elevated IOP is the strongest risk factor. Many secondary causes, including angle closure, trauma, inflammation, neovascularization, and congenital abnormalities
Associated conditions	Diseases of the elderly, including cardiovascular disease, HTN, and diabetes. Children may have multiple congenital anomalies.

ANESTHETIC CONSIDERATIONS

See Anesthetic Considerations for Ophthalmic Surgical Procedures under MAC (adult), p. 124, or for Pediatric Ophthalmic Surgery, p. 951.

References

See General References following Ophthalmic Surgery section, p. 137.

ECTROPION REPAIR

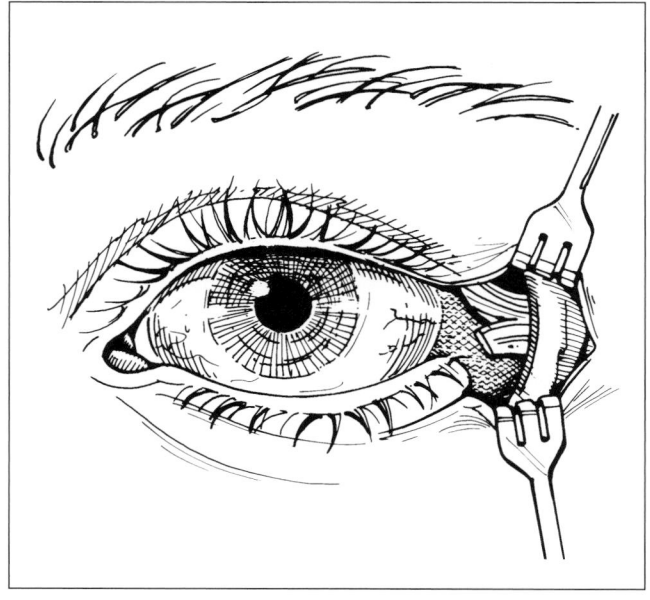

SURGICAL CONSIDERATIONS

Description: Ectropion is a malposition of the eyelid, in which the lid margin is everted away from the globe. The surgical approach depends on the underlying anatomic abnormality, which can be congenital, involutional, cicatricial (scarring), or due to mechanical traction from masses or facial nerve palsy. A lateral **tarsal strip procedure** is often used, with the lateral canthal tendon first released by performing a **lateral canthotomy and cantholysis** of the crus (Fig 2-4). A lateral portion of tarsus is then dissected free of overlying skin, muscle, and conjunctiva. This strip of tarsus is trimmed to the appropriate length and is secured to the periosteum of the lateral orbital rim with suture. Excess skin is removed and the defect is closed.

Figure 2-4. In the tarsal strip procedure, the lower eyelid is incised laterally. The entire lower crus of the canthal tendon must be severed. (Redrawn with permission from *Duane's Clinical Ophthalmology*, Vol. 5. Williams & Wilkins, Philadelphia, 2000.)

Variant procedure or approaches: Cicatricial ectropion from a contracting scar can sometimes be released with a Z-plasty incision that releases vertical skin tension. Alternatively, a full-thickness skin graft may be required, and can be harvested from the upper lid or the postauricular or supraclavicular regions.

Usual preop diagnosis: Ectropion of the eyelid

SUMMARY OF PROCEDURE

Position	Supine, table rotated 90-180°
Incision	Lateral canthal region or area of scarring
Special instrumentation	Surgical loupes
Antibiotics	None intraop
Surgical time	0.5-1 h
EBL	Minimal
Postop care	Topical antibiotic ointment
Mortality	Rare
Morbidity	Lid malposition
	Infection: Very rare
Pain score	1-2

PATIENT POPULATION CHARACTERISTICS

Age range	Any age
Male:Female	1:1
Incidence	Common
Etiology	Congenital; aging; malignancy; facial nerve palsy
Associated conditions	Systemic diseases of elderly patients common; cardiovascular disease; diabetes; HTN

ANESTHETIC CONSIDERATIONS

See Anesthetic Considerations for Ophthalmic Surgical Procedures under MAC (adult), p. 124, or for Pediatric Ophthalmic Surgery, p. 951.

References

See General References following Ophthalmic Surgery section, p. 137.

ENTROPION REPAIR

SURGICAL CONSIDERATIONS

Description: Entropion is a condition characterized by an inward rotation of the eyelid margin. The surgical approach depends on the underlying anatomic abnormality, which can be congenital, spastic, involutional, or cicatricial (scarring). For the more common involutional or age-related cases, the primary defect involves horizontal lid laxity, disinsertion of the lower lid retractors and/or an overriding orbicularis muscle. Correction often involves use of the **lateral tarsal strip procedure** (see description under Ectropion Repair, above) to achieve tightening of the lower lid. Reattachment of the eyelid retractor muscles/aponeurosis may also be used in certain cases, either alone or in addition to a tarsal strip procedure.

Variant procedure or approaches: **Cicatricial entropion** results from a contracting scar of the tarsus and/or conjunctiva pulling the lid margin inward. Correction requires release of this tension and either a **lid-splitting procedure** with tarsal advancement, rotational grafts, or free mucosal grafts harvested from hard palate. In the latter case, nasal intubation will be required to allow access to the graft site.

Usual preop diagnosis: Entropion of eyelid

SUMMARY OF PROCEDURE

Position	Supine, table rotated 90-180°
Incision	Lateral canthal region or area of conjunctival scarring. Mucosal graft may be harvested from hard palate.
Special instrumentation	Surgical loupes
Antibiotics	Non intraop
Surgical time	0.5-1 h
EBL	Minimal
Postop Care	Topical antibiotic ointment
Mortality	Rare
	Lid malposition
Morbidity	Infection: Very rare
Pain score	1-2

PATIENT POPULATION CHARACTERISTICS

Age range	Any age
Male:Female	1:1
Incidence	Common
Etiology	Congenital; aging; inflammation
Associated conditions	Cicatricial entropion can be associated with pemphigoid; Stevens-Johnson syndrome (a sometimes fatal form of erythema multiforme); chemical burns; trachoma.

ANESTHETIC CONSIDERATIONS

See Anesthetic Considerations for Ophthalmic Surgical Procedures under MAC (adult), p. 124, or for Pediatric Ophthalmic Surgery, p. 951.

References

See General References following Ophthalmic Surgery section, p. 137.

PTOSIS REPAIR

SURGICAL CONSIDERATIONS

Description: Ptosis (drooping of the upper eyelid margin) can be severe enough to obstruct the visual axis. Causes include congenital maldevelopment, mechanical traction, myogenic conditions (e.g., dystrophies, myasthenia gravis), neurogenic conditions (e.g., Horner's syndrome, cranial nerve III palsy), and aponeurotic dehiscence. The surgical approach depends primarily on the presence or absence of adequate levator muscle function that is responsible for elevating the upper eyelid. The most common etiology is age-related dehiscence or disinsertion of the levator aponeurosis from its normal attachment to the tarsus. Because levator muscle function is usually satisfactory in these patients, surgical correction involves reinserting the aponeurosis to the anterior tarsus alone or in combination with shortening of the aponeurosis by advancement or resection. Access is obtained by an incision in the upper eyelid crease. Removal of excess skin and orbicularis muscle (**blepharoplasty**) may be performed simultaneously. While several formulas have been devised to determine the amount of aponeurotic shortening, intraop measurement usually is performed to ensure that the appropriate lid position and contour are achieved. This requires that the procedure be performed under local anesthesia and that the patient be positioned and draped in a way that allows him/her to sit upright during surgery.

Variant procedure or approaches: In patients with levator muscle function that is not adequate to achieve eyelid elevation, a **frontalis sling procedure** is performed to elevate the upper eyelid (Fig 2-5). More commonly required in children with congenital ptosis, this allows the patient to open the eye by elevating the brow. A variety of materials can be used to accomplish this suspension, including silicon rods or fascia. In children < 3 yr, autologous fascia lata can be harvested from the outer thigh from hip to knee. The material is tunneled beneath the skin and muscle from the brow incisions to the anterior tarsal region of the eyelid using Wright needles. After appropriate contour and height are achieved, the sling is secured and incisions are closed. Frontalis suspension usually is performed under GA in both adults and children.

Usual preop diagnosis: Ptosis

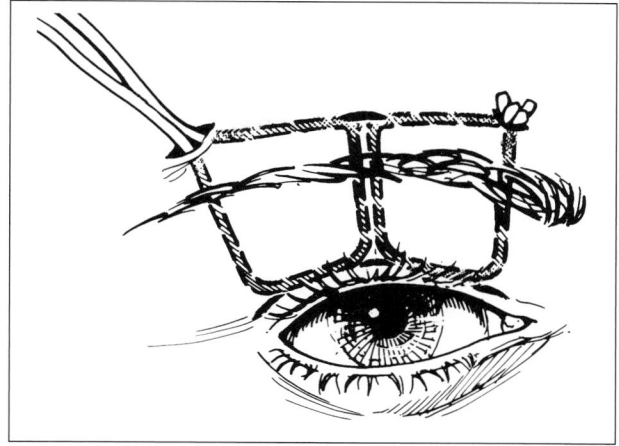

Figure 2-5. Frontalis sling (modified Crawford technique). Note location of brow and lid incisions and double rhomboid fascial slings. (Redrawn with permission from *Duane's Clinical Ophthalmology*, Vol. 5. Williams & Wilkins, Philadelphia, 2000.)

SUMMARY OF PROCEDURE

Position	Supine, table rotated 90-180°
Incision	Upper eyelid crease; brow; and lateral thigh (frontalis sling)
Special instrumentation	Surgical loupes
Antibiotics	Cefazolin 1 g iv
Surgical time	30-60 min
EBL	Minimal
Postop care	Topical antibiotic ointment; cool compresses
Mortality	Rare
Morbidity	Lid malposition
	Corneal exposure
	Infection: More common with silicone rods
Pain score	1-2

PATIENT POPULATION CHARACTERISTICS

Age range	Any Age
Male:Female	1:1
Incidence	Common
Etiology	Congenital; aponeurotic; neurogenic; myogenic; mechanical
Associated conditions	Neurogenic causes associated with myasthenia gravis; myogenic causes include chronic external ophthalmoplegia (can have dysrhythmias and SZ disorders); oculopharyngeal dystrophy

ANESTHETIC CONSIDERATIONS

See Anesthetic Considerations for Ophthalmic Surgical Procedures under MAC, p. 124.

References

See General References following Ophthalmic Surgery section, p. 137.

EYELID RECONSTRUCTION

SURGICAL CONSIDERATIONS

Description: Given the relatively small tissue area of the eyelids and their importance in both ocular health and cosmesis, excision of lid tumors often requires some form of reconstructive surgery. For lesions suspected of being malignant, **frozen-sections** are often performed prior to closing the defect. Additionally, **Moh's technique** (microscopically controlled serial excision) may be performed (usually by a dermatologist) to achieve clear margins, with reconstruction undertaken during a separate operation. During closure of full-thickness defects that involve the eyelid margin, attention is focused on aligning the lid in all dimensions (Fig 2-6), while avoiding exposed sutures on the conjunctival surface that might damage the cornea. For small lid defects involving < ¼ of the lid length, direct closure often can be accomplished with release of the lateral canthal tendon (**canthotomy and cantholysis**) to reduce wound tension, if necessary.

Variant procedure or approaches: Larger excisions often require **grafting techniques** that are designed to replace both the anterior (skin/orbicularis) and posterior (tarsus/conjunctiva) lamellae of the eyelid. This can be accomplished with rotational grafts, a tarsoconjunctival advancement flap or free grafts of cartilage, hard palate, cadaver sclera, or composite grafts as posterior lamellar replacement materials.

Usual preop diagnosis: Basal-cell carcinoma; squamous-cell carcinoma; melanoma; sebaceous carcinoma; or trauma

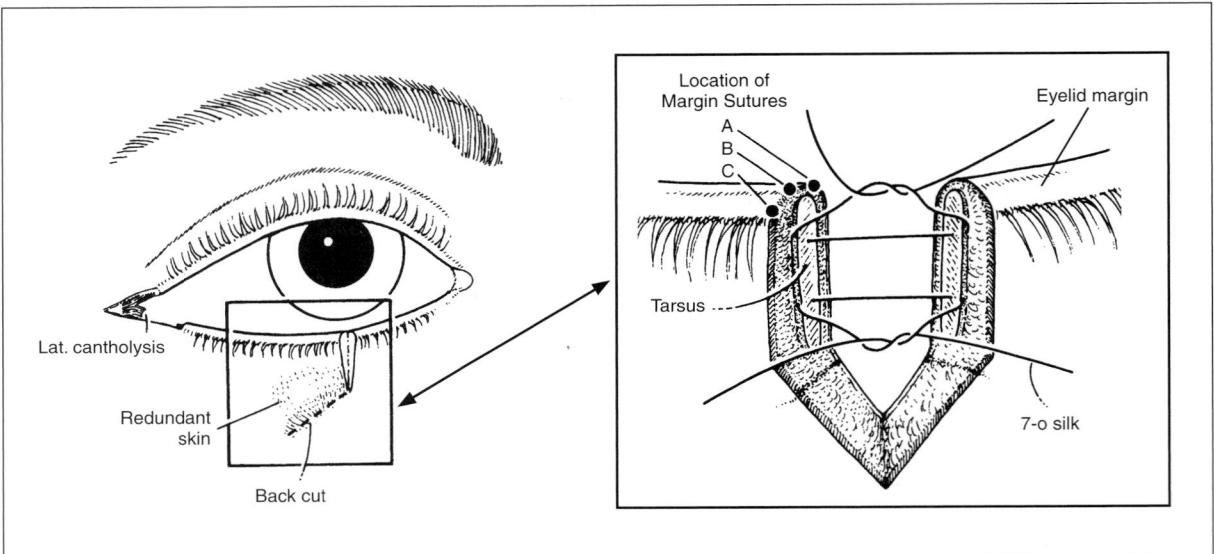

Figure 2-6. Closure of full-thickness defect in the lower lid. The tarsal sutures and half-thickness tarsus are placed first, with the secondary closures at points A, B, C, and the eyelid margin. (Reproduced with permission from McCord CD, Tanenbaum M, eds: *Oculoplastic Surgery*, 2nd edition. Raven Press, New York, 1987.

SUMMARY OF PROCEDURE

Position	Supine, table rotated 90-180°
Incision	Upper and/or lower eyelid. Postauricual, supraclavicular, or hard palate if graft harvesting required.
Special instrumentation	Surgical loupes
Antibiotics	Cefazolin 1 g iv
Surgical time	0.5-2 h
EBL	Minimal
Postop care	Topical antibiotic ointment; cool compresses; pressure dressing
Mortality	Rare
Morbidity	Graft failure
	Lid deformity
	Corneal exposure
	Infection: < 1%
Pain score	2-3

122

PATIENT POPULATION CHARACTERISTICS

Age range	Usually elderly
Male:Female	1:1
Incidence	Common
Etiology	Sun exposure-related malignancy
Associated conditions	Diseases of the elderly, including cardiovascular disease, HTN, and diabetes

ANESTHETIC CONSIDERATIONS

See Anesthetic Considerations for Ophthalmic Surgical Procedures under MAC, p. 124.

References

See General References following Ophthalmic Surgery section, p. 137.

PTERYGIUM EXCISION

SURGICAL CONSIDERATIONS

Description: Pterygia are fibrovascular growths that originate in the interpalpebral conjunctiva and grow into the superficial layer of the cornea. They often produce refractive changes and/or obstruct the central visual axis and, thus, require removal. While this procedure is often performed in the clinic or minor-procedure room, larger lesions may require an OR. In both settings, local anesthesia is applied both topically (tetracaine 0.5%) and subconjunctivally (lidocaine 2%). The lesion is dissected from the cornea and from the surrounding healthy conjunctiva, leaving a bed of bare sclera that may or may not be closed primarily (Fig 2-7).

Variant procedure or approaches: For larger excisions and to decrease the rate of recurrence, **conjunctival transposition** or **free-graft techniques** can be used to cover the area of bare sclera. Topical antimetabolites, such as mitomycin-C, also may be applied to prevent recurrence.

Preop diagnosis or indications: Pterygium

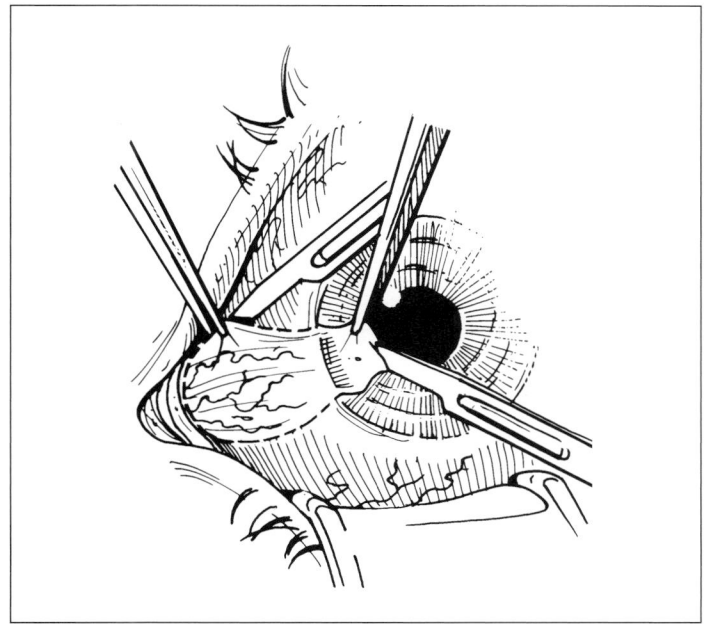

Figure 2-7. Bare sclera excision can be started from the corneal apex or by incising around the conjunctival body of the pterygium. (Redrawn with permission from *Duane's Clinical Ophthalmology*, Vol 6. Williams & Wilkins, Philadelphia, 2000.)

SUMMARY OF PROCEDURE

Position	Supine, table rotated 90-180°
Incision	Interpalpebral area adjacent to involved limbus
Special instrumentation	Operating microscope
Antibiotics	Topical postop
Surgical time	15-45 min
EBL	Minimal
Postop care	Topical antibiotic ointment
Mortality	Rare
Morbidity	Recurrence: 37%, without adjunctive therapy or grafting
	Extraocular muscle injury (higher risk in re-op eyes)
Pain score	1-2

PATIENT POPULATION CHARACTERISTICS

Age range	Usually young-to-middle age
Male:Female	1:1
Incidence	Common
Etiology	Related to sun exposure

ANESTHETIC CONSIDERATIONS FOR OPHTHALMIC SURGICAL PROCEDURES UNDER MAC

(Procedures covered: cataract extraction and other procedures; corneal transplant; trabeculectomy; ectropion-entropion repair; ptosis surgery; eyelid reconstruction; pterygium excision)

PREOPERATIVE

Ophthalmic procedures that are of relatively short duration and those that result in minimal blood loss are being performed increasingly more often on an outpatient basis, usually with topical or regional anesthesia (e.g., retrobulbar or peribulbar blocks) under MAC (see p. B-4). Both retrobulbar and peribulbar injections achieve excellent anesthesia and may also provide akinesia. Given the associated risk of inadvertent intrathecal injection of anesthetic, orbital hemorrhage, need for heavy sedation during injection, and delayed return of visual function postop, most cataract surgery is now performed using topical anesthesia. An additional benefit is that the bleeding risk is lower and the procedure can be performed safely in patients taking anticoagulants or with bleeding disorders. While satisfactory pain relief usually is achieved with this method, the lack of akinesia requires a highly cooperative patient to prevent sudden eye movements during surgery. Some surgeons will supplement topical anesthesia with intracameral lidocaine (injections into the anterior chamber) although this has not been proven better than topical anesthetics alone in terms of patient comfort and satisfaction. **Sub-Tenon's injection** is another anesthetic technique used by many surgeons as a compromise between topical application and orbital injections. After preop application of topical anesthetics, a small incision is made in the bulbar conjunctiva, exposing the sub-Tenon's space. A blunt cannula is inserted under direct visualization and local anesthetic injected into the retrobulbar space. The main benefit is that no sharp needle is used, thereby reducing the risk of intrathecal injection and orbital hemorrhage from vessel injury. The onset of akinesia, however, is often delayed, and this technique still has the disadvantage of delayed return of postop visual function.

Because the majority of ocular procedures are performed on elderly patients, multiple coexisting medical illnesses are often present. A thorough preop H&P, along with appropriate ancillary studies are mandatory even though local anesthesia/MAC is planned. Contraindications to regional anesthesia/MAC for ocular surgery may include bleeding diathesis, open-eye injuries, claustrophobia, chronic cough, inability to lie flat, or patient refusal.

Respiratory	Elderly patients have increased incidence of hiatal hernia and, therefore, are at increased risk for pulmonary aspiration. Assess the patient's ability to lie flat for the duration of the procedure. Patients with chronic cough may require GA.
	Tests: As indicated from H&P.
Cardiovascular	Hx of HTN, CAD, CHF, or poor exercise tolerance should prompt a thorough investigation into the patient's cardiac status, including efficacy of current medications and recent ECG (compared with previous ECGs). Consultation with a cardiologist may be appropriate to optimize the patient's condition before surgery.

Cardiovas., cont.	**Tests:** ECG; others (e.g., ECHO) as indicated from H&P.	
Diabetes	Diabetic patients are at increased risk for silent myocardial ischemia. Pulmonary aspiration 2° diabetic gastroparesis is also a risk in this population. Patients usually take 1/2 or 1/3 of their normal NPH insulin dose (on the morning of surgery); fasting blood sugar is checked; and an iv infusion of D5 LR is started if glucose < 90 mg/dl, or treated with regular insulin if glucose > 200 mg/dl. Blood sugar is checked intraop and postop.	
Musculoskeletal	Arthritic changes make lying flat difficult for some patients.	
Hematologic	✓ for recent aspirin/NSAID use, particularly in patients undergoing lid or orbital procedures. **Tests:** As indicated from H&P.	
Laboratory	Cr usual in patients > 64 yr; in other patients, as indicated from H&P.	
Premedication	Patients will benefit from a detailed explanation of events prior to surgery (including iv placement, application of monitors, performance of local block, ocular pressure, prepping eye and draping of the whole face, and provision of supplemental O_2) and the assurance that the anesthesiologist will always be nearby, monitoring them. Midazolam (0.5-1 mg iv) is often beneficial. For patients with increased risk of aspiration (e.g., with hiatal hernia or diabetic gastroparesis) and for obese and/or very anxious patients, metoclopramide 10 mg iv may enhance gastric emptying.	

INTRAOPERATIVE

Anesthetic technique: MAC (see p. B-4). Topical anesthesia typically is accomplished by the ophthalmologist, using 0.5% tetracaine, supplemented with 2% lidocaine, injected subconjunctivally. Placement of retrobulbar or peribulbar blocks may be painful and very short-acting agents (e.g., remifentanil 0.5-1 μg/kg, alfentanil 5-7 μg/kg, or propofol 30-50 mg) should be administered to minimize patient discomfort. Dose requirements vary significantly among patients, and the anesthesiologist should be prepared to treat ↓BP and apnea. Usually, further sedation is unnecessary and may interfere with patient cooperation during the surgery. Coughing should be avoided during the procedure, and the anesthesiologist must always be prepared to administer GA if necessary.

Retrobulbar block: Using a 25- or 27-ga needle (1.5"), the retrobulbar space is approached from the infratemporal quadrant of the orbit. The eye should be in a neutral or downward and medial position. Once the needle is positioned and there is no return of blood or CSF on aspiration, 3-5 ml of anesthetic solution is injected slowly. A facial nerve block is necessary to prevent eyelid movement. This can be accomplished by injecting 4-8 ml of anesthetic solution above and below the lateral aspect of the orbit. Typically, the anesthetic solution consists of a 50:50 mixture of 0.5% bupivacaine and 2% lidocaine with hyaluronidase.

Peribulbar block: Using a 25- or 27-ga needle (5/8"-1"), 5-6 ml of anesthetic solution is injected into the peribulbar space, entering just superior to the inferior rim of the orbit at the junction of the lateral and middle thirds of the lower lid. While perforation of the globe and hemorrhage are still possible, direct injury to the optic nerve and subdural injection are not likely due to the length and position of the needle. Peribulbar blocks generally have a slower onset than retrobulbar blocks and are more likely to cause conjunctival swelling, which may interfere with surgery.

Blood and fluid requirements	IV: 18 ga × 1 NS/LR @ 1.5-3 ml/kg/h	Excessive fluids → bladder distention → ↑BP.
Monitoring	Standard monitors (see p. B-1). Verbal response	It is important to remain in communication with the patient throughout the procedure. (Take care to avoid evoking head movement.)
Positioning	✓ and pad pressure points. ✓ nonoperated eye.	Place pillows under knees to relieve back strain.
Complications	Dysrhythmias, especially ↓HR	Usually 2° traction on ocular/periocular strabismus (see OCR, p. 951).
	↑BP	2° anxiety, pain, etc. Rx: labetalol 5 mg or hydralazine 4-mg increments, as appropriate.
	Retrobulbar hemorrhage (1-3%)	Rx: pressure bandage; usually cancel surgery.
	Globe perforation	If a needle perforation, usually no repair is necessary.
	Convulsions 2° iv local anesthetic	Supportive treatment with IPPV
	Respiratory arrest	2° subarachnoid injection. Rx: CPR.
	Oculocardiac reflex (OCR)→↓↓HR, ↓↓BP	Rx: Stop stimulation; use atropine (see OCR, p. 951).

POSTOPERATIVE

Complications   Myocardial ischemia   Rx: Provide O_2; ✓ BP; sublingual NTG; ✓ ECG; cardi-
                          Corneal abrasion   ology consultation.
                          Photophobia
                          N/V   Rx: Ganisetron 100 μg iv, metoclopramide 10 mg iv,
                          Diplopia   droperidol 0.625 mg iv, or ondansetron 4 mg iv.

Pain management   Acetaminophen 325-1000 mg po

Table 2-1. Commonly Used Ophthalmic Drugs and Their Systemic Effects	
Phenylephrine	An α-adrenergic agonist that causes mydriasis (pupillary dilation) and vasoconstriction to aid ocular surgery; however, it also can precipitate significant HTN and dysrhythmias.
Echothiophate	An irreversible cholinesterase inhibitor used in glaucoma treatment to cause miosis and ↓IOP. Its systemic absorption can reduce plasma cholinesterase activity and thereby prolong paralysis 2° to succinylcholine (usually not more than 20-30 min).
Timolol	A nonselective β-blocker that decreases production of aqueous humor → ↓IOP. Rarely, it may be associated with atropine-resistant bradycardia, asthma, CHF, and ↓BP.
Acetazolamide	A carbonic anhydrase inhibitor used to ↓IOP. It also can cause diuresis and a hypokalemic metabolic acidosis.
Betaxolol	A relatively oculospecific β-blocker used to ↓IOP. Effects may be additive to systemic β-blockers.
Cyclopentolate	A commonly used mydriatic with the potential for CNS toxicity, including Sz, psychotic reactions, and dysarthria.
Atropine	An anticholinergic that produces mydriasis to aid with ocular examination and surgery. It also can precipitate central anticholinergic syndrome. (Sx range from dry mouth, tachycardia, agitation, delirium, and hallucinations to unconsciousness.) Physostigmine 0.01-0.03 mg/kg will increase central acetylcholine and reverse the symptoms. (It may be repeated after 15-30 min.)

References

1. Friedman DS, Bass EB, Lubomski LH, et al: Synthesis of the literature on the effectiveness of regional anesthesia for cataract surgery. *Ophthalmology*; 108: 519-29.
2. McGoldrick KE, ed: *Anesthesia for Ophthalmic and Otolaryngologic Surgery*. WB Saunders, Philadelphia: 1992.
3. McGoldrick KE: Anesthesia and the eye. In *Clinical Anesthesia*, 4th edition. Barash PG, Cullen BF, Stoelting RK, eds. Lippincott Williams & Wilkins, Philadelphia: 2001, 969-88.

REPAIR OF RUPTURED OR LACERATED GLOBE

SURGICAL CONSIDERATIONS

Description: A ruptured globe involves a tear of either the corneal or scleral layers of the eye and can occur in the setting of blunt, penetrating, or perforating trauma. The primary goal of surgical repair is to replace extruded intraocular contents, close defects, and remove any foreign body. Orbital CT scans are performed preop to aid in the identification of the latter. To reduce the risk of causing further damage, complete examination of the eye is often delayed until the patient is in the controlled setting of the OR under GA. While anterior injuries are readily identifiable, posterior injuries may require extensive exploration that can require a 360° opening of the conjunctiva and isolation of each extraocular muscle to allow adequate inspection of the entire scleral surface. Corneal lacerations usually are closed with 10-0 nylon sutures while 8-0 nylon or Vicryl may be used for scleral tissue. It is crucial that, until these wounds are closed, Valsalva maneuvers, which may raise IOP, be avoided to prevent further extrusion of intraocular contents.

Variant procedures or approaches: After globe integrity has been established, other associated injuries may be addressed, including repair of conjunctival lacerations, extraocular muscle injuries/detachments, retinal detachments, or removal of a traumatic cataract.

Usual preop diagnosis: Ruptured globe

SUMMARY OF PROCEDURE

Position	Supine, table rotated 90-180°
Incision	Conjunctival peritomy (360° conjunctival incision) to allow exposure of posterior sclera
Special instrumentation	Operating microscope
Antibiotics	IV gentamicin (80 mg) and cefazolin (1 g); subconjunctival and topical antibiotics
Closing considerations	Avoid Valsalva maneuvers (coughing, bucking, etc.).
Surgical time	1-2 h
EBL	Minimal
Postop care	Hospital admission for iv antibiotics
Mortality	Rare
Morbidity	Wound leak
	Infection: Rate depends on injury
	Sympathetic ophthalmia: Rare
Pain score	4

PATIENT POPULATION CHARACTERISTICS

Age range	Usually < 40 yr
Male:Female	9:1
Incidence	Common
Etiology	Work- or sports-related injury; motor vehicle accidents
Associated conditions	Intoxication; orbital/facial trauma; head injury

ANESTHETIC CONSIDERATIONS

PREOPERATIVE

This is a generally healthy patient population; however, patients with penetrating eye injuries present the anesthesiologist with two special challenges: (1) They invariably have full stomachs, resulting in risk of aspiration. (2) They are at risk of blindness 2° ↑IOP and loss of ocular contents, which may be a result of coughing, crying, and/or struggling during induction. Normal IOP ranges from 10-22 mmHg, depending on the rate of formation and drainage of aqueous humor, choroidal blood volume, scleral rigidity, extraocular muscle tone, as well as extrinsic pressure on the eye (e.g., a poorly fitting mask or retrobulbar hematoma). Patient movement, coughing, straining, vomiting, hypercarbia, HTN, and ET intubation also may ↑ IOP as much as 40 mmHg or more.

Full-stomach precautions	Consider patient to have a full stomach if the injury occurred within 8 h of the last meal. Pain and anxiety due to trauma will delay gastric emptying. Goal is to minimize risk of aspiration pneumonitis by decreasing gastric volume and acidity. Consider premedication with metoclopramide (10-20 mg iv), antacids such as Na citrate (15-30 ml orally, immediately prior to induction), and H_2-histamine receptor antagonists (ranitidine [50 mg iv]). H_2-histamine receptor antagonists, however, have no effect on the pH of gastric secretions present in the stomach prior to administration and are, therefore, of limited value in patients presenting for emergency surgery. If patient has Hx of smoking or is an asthmatic, consider preop use of inhalers such as albuterol (2-4 puffs).
Laboratory	Tests as indicated from H&P.
Premedication	Patients often are very anxious and may benefit from benzodiazepines (e.g., for pediatric population, midazolam 0.5-0.75 mg/kg po in cola or apple juice, 15-30 ml). Avoid narcotic premedication, which may ↑ nausea and possibility of emesis.

INTRAOPERATIVE

Anesthetic technique: GETA. Regional anesthesia (e.g., retrobulbar block) is contraindicated in patients with open-eye injury because of ↑IOP, which may accompany injection of local anesthetic behind the globe. Thus, in spite of the increased risk of aspiration from a full stomach, GETA is recommended.

Induction	To protect the airway and prevent ↑IOP, a rapid-sequence induction with cricoid pressure and a smooth intubation are required. While the choice of induction agent is relatively straightforward—propofol 1-2 mg/kg or STP 3-5 mg/kg—the choice of neuromuscular blocking agents for facilitating intubation is controversial. Succinylcholine provides a rapid onset, short duration of action, and excellent intubating conditions, but it also transiently increases IOP. This ↑IOP is not always attenuated by pretreatment with a nondepolarizing agent (e.g., d-tubocurarine). Rocuronium (1 mg/kg) produces muscle relaxation in 1-2 min and may be a satisfactory alternative to succinylcholine; however, a premature attempt at intubation may significantly ↑ IOP as a result of coughing and straining. Of interest, there are no reports in the literature documenting exacerbation of eye injuries with the use of succinylcholine following pretreatment with a NMR. Given that the anesthesiologist's main concern is safe airway management, the following is a suggested induction plan:

(1) Preoxygenation, avoiding external pressure on the eye from face mask.

(2) Pretreatment with a nondepolarizing relaxant (e.g., d-tubocurarine 0.06 mg/kg), followed by iv lidocaine (1 mg/kg) and fentanyl (2-3 μg/kg) to blunt the cardiovascular response to laryngoscopy and intubation.

(3) Consider 5-10 mg labetalol, also to blunt cardiovascular response to laryngoscopy and intubation (if patient does not have reactive airway disease).

(4) 4 min later, with cricoid pressure, induce with propofol (1.5-2.5 mg/kg) and succinylcholine (1.5 mg/kg). Intubate with oral RAE tube. Note: for pediatric patients, it might be appropriate to induce with sevoflurane while maintaining cricoid pressure and intubating when the patient is deeply anesthetized. Trying to start an iv prior to induction may precipitate struggling and crying, leading to further eye injury.

Maintenance	Standard maintenance (see p. B-3). Avoid hypercapnia, which → ↑IOP. Muscle relaxation is mandatory until the eye is surgically closed. Humidify gases for pediatric patients.
Emergence	Decompress the stomach with OG tube. Goal is smooth emergence and extubation with patient awake with intact airway reflexes. IV lidocaine (1.5 mg/kg) 5 min before extubation; posterior pharyngeal suctioning with patient deeply anesthetized, combined with a small amount of narcotic (remifentanil 1-2 μg/kg), may blunt cough reflex prior to extubation. The common occurrence of PONV requires administration of intraop antiemetics (e.g., metoclopramide 10 mg iv, and/or granisetron 100 μg iv 30 min before end of surgery).

Blood and fluid requirements	IV: 18 ga × 1 (adult) 20 ga × 1 (child) NS/LR @ 5-10 ml/kg/h Warm fluids.	
Monitoring	Standard monitors (see p. B-1).	Neuromuscular blockade must be monitored closely and additional relaxant given as necessary to prevent patient movement during surgery.
Positioning	✓ and pad pressure points. ✓ nonoperated eye.	
Complications	↑IOP with extrusion of intraocular contents Aspiration of gastric contents	IOP (normal = ~10-22 mmHg) increased by: blink = 10-15 mmHg; forced closure = > 70 mmHg

POSTOPERATIVE

Complications	N/V Corneal abrasion Aspiration pneumonitis Photophobia Diplopia Hemorrhagic retinopathy	Rx: Metoclopramide 10 mg iv, droperidol 0.625, ondansetron 4 mg iv. Provide O_2 by face mask, if not intubated. Follow O_2 sat. ✓ CXR.
Pain management	Acetaminophen	Occasionally, parenteral opiates (see p. C-2).

References

1. Barash PG, Cullen BF, Stoelting RK, eds: *Clinical Anesthesia,* 4th edition. Lippincott Williams & Wilkins, Philadelphia: 2001.
2. McGoldrick KE, ed: *Anesthesia for Ophthalmic and Otolaryngologic Surgery.* WB Saunders, Philadelphia: 1992.

Also see General References following Ophthalmic Surgery section.

DACRYOCYSTORHINOSTOMY (DCR)

SURGICAL CONSIDERATIONS

Description: **Dacryocystorhinostomy (DCR)** is performed for patients with symptomatic obstruction of the nasolacrimal duct (NLD) and is commonly associated with chronic dacryocystitis. The procedure is designed to create a fistula from the common canaliculus to the nasopharynx, which bypasses the site of obstruction. DCR can be performed under GA or local anesthesia (subcutaneous and nasal cavity cocaine 4%). Intranasal phenylephrine and/or cocaine pledgets are often placed to decrease mucosal bleeding. A skin incision is made below the medial canthal tendon that is extended to the lacrimal fossa with blunt dissection. Bleeding can be excessive if the angular vessels are injured. The now exposed periosteum is incised and a 1.5 cm × 1.5 cm osteotomy is created with a burr and/or Kerrison punch, exiting at the level of the middle meatus. A Crawford lacrimal probe attached to silicone tubing is inserted into the superior punctum and advanced into the lacrimal sac, which is then opened along its medial wall. Following incision of the nasal mucosa through the osteotomy, the posterior flap of the lacrimal sac is sutured to the posterior nasal mucosa flap. The probe is advanced through the osteotomy and into the middle meatus, where it is retrieved through the nare. The second end of the probe is advanced along the same path but beginning through the inferior punctum. The ends of the silicone tubing are tied together in the nare and the anterior flaps of lacrimal sac and nasal mucosa are sutured together. Thrombin and gel foam can be used to control mucosal bleeding and the skin is reapproximated after ensuring hemostasis.

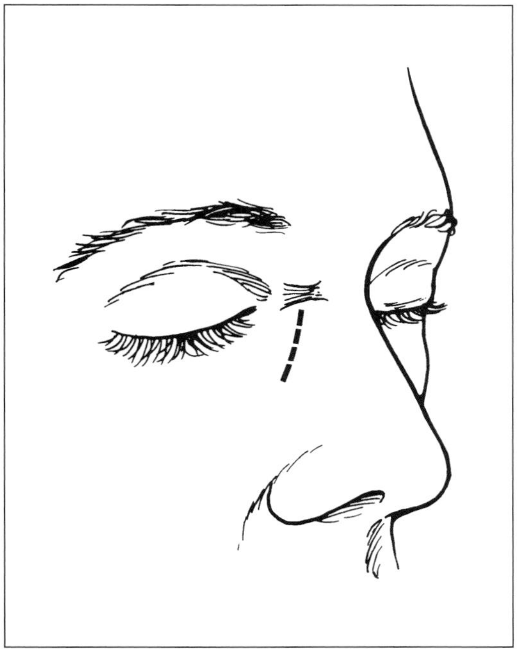

Figure 2-8. Linear skin incision for a standard DCR. (Reproduced with permission from Wright KW: *Textbook of Ophthalmology.* Williams & Wilkins, Philadelphia, 1997.)

Variant procedures or approaches: If the lacrimal obstruction is more proximal to the lacrimal sac, a **Jones tube** can be placed (Fig 2-9), creating an artificial lumen from the conjunctiva to the nasopharynx to bypass the entire nasolacrimal drainage system.

Usual preop diagnosis: NLD obstruction

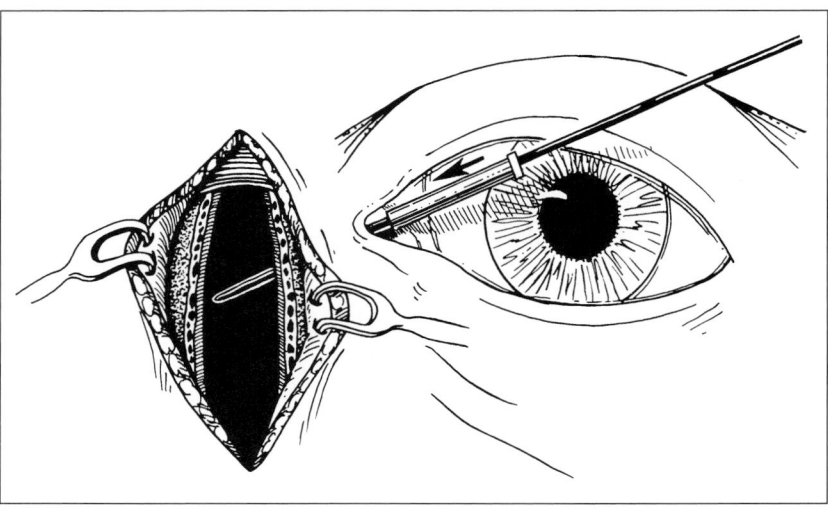

Figure 2-9. Insertion of a Pyrex Jone's tube. (Reproduced with permission from McCord CD, Tanenbaum M, Nunery WR: *Oculoplastic Surgery*. Raven Press, 1995.)

SUMMARY OF PROCEDURE

Position	Supine, table rotated 90-180°
Incision	15 mm, just below medial canthus (Fig 2-8)
Special instrumentation	Headlight; surgical loupes
Unique considerations	Nasal packing with phenylephrine/cocaine. Blood may drain into upper airway during surgery.
Antibiotics	Cefazolin 1 g iv
Surgical time	1-1.5 h
EBL	100-200 ml
Postop care	Outpatient
Mortality	Rare
Morbidity	Failure to drain
	Bleeding: 5%
	Infection: < 1%
Pain score	3-4

PATIENT POPULATION CHARACTERISTICS

Age range	30-70 yr
Male:Female	1:1
Incidence	Common
Etiology	Usually scarring from prior infection or trauma
Associated conditions	Deviated septum; nasal polyps; nasopharyngeal masses

ANESTHETIC CONSIDERATIONS

See Anesthetic Considerations for Ophthalmic Surgical Procedures under MAC, p. 124.

References

See General References following Ophthalmic Surgery section, p. 137.

ENUCLEATION

SURGICAL CONSIDERATIONS

Description: Enucleation involves removal of the entire globe and a portion of the optic nerve. It usually is performed for painful blind eyes or intraocular tumors (e.g., retinoblastoma, melanoma). The surrounding ocular adnexa, including the conjunctiva, Tenon's connective tissue, and extraocular muscles, are left in place to secure an orbital implant. The procedure begins with a 360° conjunctival incision (**peritomy**) at the limbus, allowing exposure of the underlying extraocular muscles and sclera. Each of the recti muscles is isolated with a muscle hook and secured with fixation sutures before disinsertion from the globe. The oblique muscles are cut and allowed to retract into the orbit (Fig 2-10). A curved clamp is closed across the optic nerve ~3-10 mm posterior to the globe, and the nerve is cut and the globe removed. After hemostasis has been ensured, an orbital implant (polymethylmethacrylate or hydroxyapetite) is placed into the socket. The overlying muscles, connective tissue, and conjunctiva are closed to improve motility and prevent extrusion.

Variant procedure or approaches: Evisceration involves removing all intraocular contents through a corneoscleral incision, leaving the scleral shell with the attached adnexa in place. This usually is performed in cases of endophthalmitis, but never if malignancy is suspected. **Exenteration** is

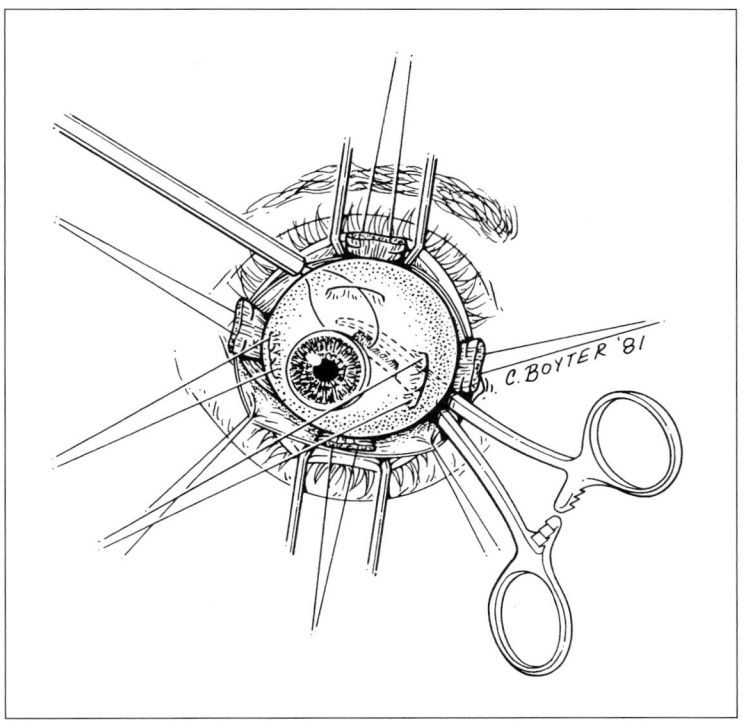

Figure 2-10. Each of the four recti is isolated with 6-0 Dexon suture. The superior oblique tendon is detached. The inferior oblique is sutured to the inferior border of the lateral rectus. 4-0 silk traction sutures are in place over the medial and lateral rectus stump. The globe is rotated laterally, while a curved clamp is introduced form the medial direction. Either a curved scissors or an enucleation snare may be used to transect the optic nerve. (Reproduced with permission form McCord, CD Jr, Tanenbaum M, Nunery WR: *Oculoplastic Surgery.* Raven Press, Philadelphia, 1995.)

a more extensive procedure for the management of aggressive malignant tumors or infections where all orbital tissue, often including surrounding orbital bone and adjacent sinuses, is removed.

Usual preop diagnosis: Painful blind eye; intraocular tumors; sympathetic ophthalmia

SUMMARY OF PROCEDURE

Position	Supine, table rotated 90-180°
Incision	360° conjunctival (peritomy)
Special instrumentation	Surgical loupes
Antibiotics	Irrigate socket with gentamicin postop
Surgical time	1 h
EBL	< 100 ml
Postop care	Outpatient
Mortality	Rare
Morbidity	Extrusion of implant
	Infection: < 1%
Pain score	3-4

PATIENT POPULATION CHARACTERISTICS

Age range	Any age
Male:Female	1:1
Incidence	Relatively common
Etiology	Trauma; infection; glaucoma; tumors; inflamation
Associated conditions	Diabetes mellitus

ANESTHETIC CONSIDERATIONS

See Anesthetic Considerations for Ophthalmic Surgical Procedures under MAC, p. 124.

References

See General References following Ophthalmic Surgery section, p. 137.

ORBITOTOMY—ANTERIOR AND LATERAL

SURGICAL CONSIDERATIONS

Description: Surgical access to the orbit is required for biopsy/excision of masses, drainage of orbital abscesses, removal of a foreign body, or repair of orbital fractures, among other procedures. The orbit may be divided into several compartments and the surgical approach will vary by the location and size of the lesion. In general, an **anterior orbitotomy** is used for small tumors in the anterior orbit and can be approached from a transconjunctival, transseptal, or transperiosteal incision. By contrast, a **lateral orbitotomy** allows for removal of larger masses located further posteriorly in the orbit, as well as those lesions involving the lacrimal gland. In this procedure, the skin incision can be placed just under the brow (**Stallard-Wright**), in the lid crease with lateral extension, or higher in the eyebrow (**coronal**). The dissection is carried down to the periosteum, which is then incised and reflected. The lateral orbital wall is exposed and an osteotomy is performed using an oscillating saw, after preplacing suture holes with a power drill. The section of bone is removed with a clamp and the periorbita is opened, allowing intraorbital dissection. After biopsy or removal of the mass, the periorbita is closed and the bone fragment replaced.

Variant procedures or approaches: A **medial orbitotomy** is often required to access lesions that are located medial to the optic nerve.

Usual preop diagnosis: Orbital mass; fractures; foreign body; abscess

SUMMARY OF PROCEDURE

Position	Supine, table rotated 90-180°
Incision	Variable (see above).
Special instrumentation	Surgical loupes
Antibiotics	Cefazolin 1 g iv
Surgical time	1-3 h
EBL	Usually minimal, unless vascular tumor
Mortality	Rare
Morbidity	Orbital hemorrhage
	Impaired ocular motility
	Secondary infection
	Loss of vision
	Infection: < 1%
Pain score	3-6

PATIENT POPULATION CHARACTERISTICS

Age range	Any age
Male:Female	1:1
Incidence	Fairly common
Etiology	Tumor, such as hemangioma, lymphangioma, lymphoma; lacrimal gland tumors; infection; fracture; foreign body

---

ANESTHETIC CONSIDERATIONS

(Procedures covered: dacryocystorhinostomy (DCR); enucleation; anterior and lateral orbitotomy.)

PREOPERATIVE

Patients presenting for DCR, enucleation, and orbitotomy represent a diverse population. These patients are generally healthy, aside from the infection, tumor, or trauma underlying their ocular or periocular pathology. Preop evaluation should focus on possible coexisting disease and the systemic manifestations of previous therapeutic interventions (e.g., chemotherapy and drugs used to treat glaucoma).

Laboratory	Tests as indicated from H&P.
Premedication	Standard premedication (see p. B-2).

INTRAOPERATIVE

Anesthetic technique: GETA.

Induction	Standard induction (see p. B-2). An oral RAE ETT may be preferred.	
Maintenance	Standard maintenance (see, p. B-3). Muscle relaxation is not required.	
Emergence	No special considerations. The common occurrence of PONV requires the administration of intraop antiemetics (e.g., metoclopramide 10 mg iv, and/or ganisetron 100 μg).	
Blood and fluid requirements	Blood loss variable IV: 18 ga × 1 NS/LR @ 4-6 ml/kg/h	
Monitoring	Standard monitors (see p. B-1).	
Positioning	Table rotated 90° ✓ and pad pressure points. ✓ nonoperated eye.	
Complications	Oculocardiac reflex (OCR) → $\downarrow\downarrow$HR	See discussion in Anesthetic Considerations for Strabismus Surgery, p. 951.

POSTOPERATIVE

Complications	PONV	Rx: Metoclopramide 10 mg iv, and/or ondansetron 4 mg iv.
Pain management	Acetaminophen	Occasionally parenteral opiates (see p. C-2).

RETINAL SURGERY

SURGICAL CONSIDERATIONS

Michael W. Gaynon

Description: Retinal surgery is performed for a wide variety of conditions (see Usual preop diagnoses, below). Most retinal detachments are due to one or more small tears in the retina caused by traction following a vitreous separation. Retinal detachments may be complicated by proliferative vitreoretinopathy (PVR), in which scar tissue grows along the surface of the retina, rendering it stiff and difficult to reattach. Less commonly, retinal detachments are induced by other forms of vitreoretinal traction, or by trauma involving an open globe. Care must be taken to avoid any increase in intraocular pressure (IOP) in an eye that may be ruptured. On rare occasion, retinal detachments are due to the formation of a giant retinal tear. Just as rarely, retinal surgery may be done on premature infants in an effort to prevent or repair retinal detachments. The ultimate aim of retinal surgery is the preservation or recovery of vision through the restoration of normal posterior segment anatomy. (Anatomy of the eye is shown in Fig 2-11.)

Retinal surgery may involve various procedures alone or in combination, including scleral buckling, vitrectomy, gas-fluid exchange, and injection of vitreous substitutes. **Scleral buckles** are silicone rubber appliances sutured to the sclera to indent the eye wall, thereby relieving vitreous traction and functionally closing retinal tears. This is an external procedure in which the eye may either not be entered at all or entered with a small needle puncture through the sclera for drainage of subretinal fluid.

Vitrectomy is an intraocular procedure in which three 19–25-ga openings are made into the vitreous cavity with a myringotomy blade 3-4 mm posterior to the limbus (junction of the cornea and sclera.) One of these openings in the inferotemporal quadrant is used for infusion of balanced salt solution via a sutured cannula. The remaining openings are at the 9:30 and 2:30 o'clock positions. One is used for a hand-held fiber optic light; the other, for insertion of a variety of manual and automated instruments, including suction cutters, scissors, and forceps, used to remove and section abnormal tissue within the vitreous cavity.

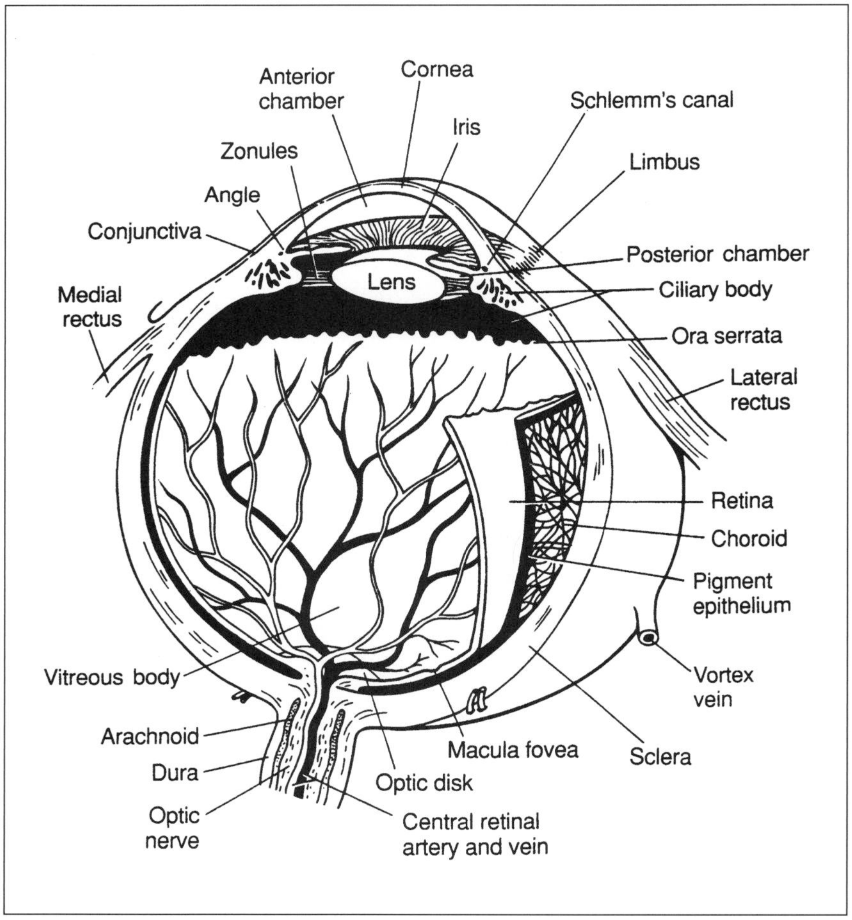

Visualization of the retina during vitrectomy is made possible by a contact lens, which is either sutured to the eye or held in position by an assistant. Some of these lenses provide a wide-field, inverted view of the retina, necessitating an image inverter on the microscope. Alternatively, a noncontact, wide-field lens may be positioned just above the cornea, suspended from the microscope. Balanced salt solution replaces the vitreous and other tissues removed during the operation. A bubble of gas is sometimes introduced into the vitreous cavity during a scleral buckle or a vitrectomy when the surgeon wants an internal tamponade of retinal tears that cannot be closed adequately by a scleral

Figure 2-11. Eye anatomy. (Reproduced with permission from Langston D, ed: *Manual of Ocular Diagnosis and Therapy*, 2nd edition. Little, Brown, Boston: 1985.)

buckle alone. N₂O must be discontinued before a gas-fluid exchange to avoid an intraop or postop change in gas bubble size, possibly accompanied by abnormal IOP.

In the case of a giant retinal tear, a **gas-fluid exchange** formerly was performed with the patient in the prone position toward the end of the operation. This required that the patient be on a Stryker frame, so that he or she could be moved from the supine to the prone position for the gas-fluid exchange. Perfluorocarbon liquids now obviate the need for a Stryker frame.

Liquid vitreous substitutes, such as perfluorocarbon liquids or silicone oil, are sometimes introduced into the vitreous cavity during a vitrectomy. Perfluorocarbon liquids are heavier than water and are used as an intraop tool to unfold the detached retina; they are removed at the end of the procedure. Perfluorocarbon liquids make possible repair of giant retinal tears in the supine position, thus eliminating the need for a Stryker frame. They also facilitate reattaching the retina when PVR is present, by allowing a relaxing retinotomy for those situations where the retina is too stiff and foreshortened to be reattached by less invasive measures. Silicone oil is used for complex detachments in which a long-term, internal tamponade of retinal tears is deemed necessary to prevent redetachment. It usually is removed a few months postop with a second operation. **Cryotherapy** or lasers are used frequently to establish chorioretinal adhesions around retinal tears. Cryotherapy is applied to the sclera; a laser is applied with a fiber optic cable introduced into the vitreous cavity during vitrectomy surgery, often in combination with a wide-field viewing system. It also can be administered with an indirect ophthalmoscope delivery system for those eyes not undergoing vitrectomy.

Simple detachments frequently can be repaired by a **pneumatic retinopexy**, in which retinal tears are treated with cryotherapy and/or laser, and an expanding gas is injected into the vitreous cavity. This technique usually is done in phakic eyes (eyes with intact lens) with tears between the 8 o'clock and 4 o'clock positions. Pneumatic retinopexy usually is done as an outpatient office procedure, with local anesthesia, or, less commonly, MAC. The other procedures discussed usually are done with MAC, although GA may be used, according to surgeon's preference and the patient's systemic condition. Some surgeons inject retrobulbar or subconjunctival bupivacaine at the end of a procedure done under GA to decrease postop pain.

Usual preop diagnosis: Simple and complex retinal detachment; diabetic retinopathy; vitreous hemorrhage or opacification; macular epiretinal membranes; other surgically correctable macular conditions, such as macular holes or macular degeneration with subfoveal choroidal neovascularization or hemorrhage; dislocated intraocular lenses; endophthalmitis; macular degeneration with posterior segment trauma, including repair of ruptured globes and removal of intraocular foreign bodies; retinopathy of prematurity (ROP)

SUMMARY OF PROCEDURE

Position	Supine
Incision	Transconjunctival
Special instrumentation	Vitrectomy machine; cryoprobe; laser; indirect ophthalmoscope; microscope
Unique considerations	Ruptured globe—avoid ↑IOP. Stop N₂O 5-10 min before a gas-fluid exchange.
Antibiotics	May use iv antibiotics at the start of surgery, in addition to subconjunctival antibiotics at conclusion of surgery.
Surgical time	Pneumatic retinopexy: 1 h Scleral buckle: 1-3 h Vitrectomy: 1-4+ h Giant tear: 2-4+ h
Closing considerations	Try to avoid postop bucking or vomiting.
EBL	None
Postop care	Prone positioning, if gas was injected.
Mortality	Extremely rare
Morbidity	Hemorrhage: < 5% Retinal detachment: < 5% Infection: < 1%
Pain score	6

PATIENT POPULATION CHARACTERISTICS

Age range	Usually adults; occasionally premature infants (ROP) and children (retinal detachment or trauma)
Male:Female	1:1
Incidence	1/20,000 phakic; 1/250 pseudophakic (postcataract extraction with placement of intraocular lens)
Etiology	Majority idiopathic; some related to systemic disease or induced by trauma

Associated conditions	Idiopathic: retinal detachment, epiretinal membrane, macular hole
	Diabetic retinopathy: vitreous hemorrhage or traction retinal detachment
	Prior eye surgery: retinal detachment
	Macular degeneration: subfoveal choroidal neovascularization or hemorrhage
	Trauma: vitreous hemorrhage, retinal detachment, ruptured globe
	Intraocular foreign body (IOFB)
	HTN: vitreous hemorrhage
	Extreme prematurity: ROP, retinal detachment

ANESTHETIC CONSIDERATIONS

PREOPERATIVE

Retinal detachments are classified as traction, exudative (not usually treated with surgery), or rhegmatogenous (rupture, tear). Children, especially those with ROP or trauma, may develop retinal detachments. In adults, retinal detachments are most frequently associated with diabetes, myopia, trauma, and previous cataract surgery. Rhegmatogenous retinal detachments (more common in adults) start off with a small retinal tear, which allows the vitreous to seep in between the retina and pigment epithelium, forcing retinal separation. Sx range from floaters and flashes to showers of black specks and, ultimately, to a dark shadow that impinges on the field of vision. Surgeons prefer a normotensive eye during retinal reattachment surgery and, therefore, patients may be given acetazolamide or mannitol to decrease IOP.

Cardiovascular	Mannitol decreases IOP by increasing plasma oncotic pressure relative to aqueous humor pressure. It usually is given just before or during surgery. Total dosage should not exceed 1.5-2 g/kg iv over a 30-60 min period. Rapid infusion of large doses of mannitol may precipitate CHF, pulmonary edema, electrolyte abnormalities, HTN, and, possibly, myocardial ischemia; hence, the importance of a thorough evaluation of the patient's renal and cardiovascular status prior to administering mannitol. **Tests:** As indicated from H&P.
Diabetes	Diabetic patients are at increased risk for silent myocardial ischemia. Pulmonary aspiration 2° diabetic gastroparesis is also a risk in this population. Patients usually take 1/2 or 1/3 of their normal NPH insulin dose (on the morning of surgery); fasting blood sugar is checked; and an iv infusion of D5 LR is started if glucose < 90 mg/dl, or treated with regular insulin if glucose > 200 mg/dl. Blood sugar is checked intraop and postop.
Renal	Acetazolamide, a carbonic anhydrase inhibitor, decreases secretion of aqueous humor. It also inhibits renal carbonic anhydrase, thereby facilitating the loss of HCO_3, Na^+, K^+, and water. Thus, patients on chronic therapy may be acidotic, hypokalemic, and hyponatremic. **Tests:** Electrolytes; others as indicated from H&P.
Hematologic	✓ for sickle-cell disease. Sickle-cell trait is not commonly associated with periop complications. Patients with sickle-cell anemia should be well hydrated and transfused preop, as necessary to increase HbA concentration > 40%.
Laboratory	Tests as indicated from H&P.
Premedication	Midazolam 0.5 mg po for pediatric patients and midazolam 1-2 mg iv incrementally for adults, to alleviate anxiety. Avoid excessive sedation (respiratory depression) in sickle-cell patients.

INTRAOPERATIVE

Anesthetic technique: Retinal detachment surgery may be performed under regional anesthesia; however, if the surgery is expected to be > 2 h, GETA may be preferable.

Induction	Standard induction (see p. B-2) is appropriate for these patients, with care being taken not to put pressure on the affected eye with the face mask.
Maintenance	Standard maintenance (see p. B-3). Ophthalmologists, however, may use expanding gases, such as sulfur hexafluoride (SF_6) or perfluoropropane (C_3F_8), for internal tamponade of the retinal tears and, if N_2O is used, the injected bubble may expand rapidly, causing a dramatic rise in IOP. This can impair retinal blood flow. N_2O, if used at all, should be D/C'd at least 15 min before gas injection. If patient needs a second surgery and GA after the first gas injection, N_2O should be avoided for 5 d after air injection, 10 d after SF_6 injection, and 15-30 d after C_3F_8. Nondepolarizing muscle relaxants may be advantageous, especially if N_2O is D/C'd.

Emergence	Use narcotics for pain control and iv lidocaine 1.0-1.5 mg/kg 5 min prior to extubation to provide smooth emergence. The common occurrence of PONV requires the administration of intraop antiemetics (e.g., metoclopramide 10 mg iv and granisetron 100 μg iv 30 min before the end of surgery).
Blood and fluid requirements	IV: 18 ga × 1 (adult) 20 ga × 1 (child) NS/LR @ 4-6 ml/kg/h
Monitoring	Standard monitors (see p. B-1).
Positioning	✓ and pad pressure points. ✓ and pad nonsurgical eye.
Complications	Oculocardiac reflex (OCR)	See Intraoperative Complications under Anesthetic Considerations for Strabismus Surgery, p. 951.

POSTOPERATIVE

Complications	PONV Corneal abrasion Vitreous hemorrhage Glaucoma Ptosis Diplopia Loss of vision Infection	Rx: Metoclopramide 10 mg iv or droperidol 0.625 iv; however, eye pain (e.g., 2° to corneal abrasion) may also cause N/V. If this is the case, treat pain (ophthalmology consult).
Pain management	Meperidine 0.5-1 mg/kg/h iv Retrobulbar anesthesia	
Tests	None routinely required.	

References for Retinal Surgery

1. Hamilton RC: Techniques of orbital regional anaesthesia. *Brit J Anaesth*. 1995; 75:88-92.
2. McGoldrick KE: *Anesthesia and the Eye*. In Clinical Anesthesia, 4th edition. Barash PG, Cullen BF, Stoelting RK, eds. Lippincott Williams & Wilkins, Philadelphia: 2001, 969-88.
3. McGoldrick KE, ed: *Anesthesia for Ophthalmic and Otolaryngologic Surgery*. WB Saunders, Philadelphia: 1992.
4. Ryan SJ, ed: *Retina*, 3rd edition. CV Mosby Co, St. Louis: 2001.

General Ophthalmic Surgery References

1. Albert DM, Jakobiec FA, eds. *Principles and Practice of Ophthalmology*. WB Saunders, Philadelphia: 2000,1463-76.
2. External Disease and Cornea. *Basic and Clinical Science Course*. The Foundation of the American Academy of Ophthalmology 1998; 8:411-36.
3. Greenbaum G, ed: *Ocular Anesthesia*. WB Saunders, Philadelphia: 1997.
4. Krachmer JH, Mannis MJ, Holland EJ: *Cornea*. Mosby-Year Book, St Louis: 1997.
5. Lens and Cataract. *Basic and Clinical Science Course*. The Foundation of the American Academy of Ophthalmology 2001;11:66-186.
6. Levine MR, ed: *Manual of Oculoplastic Surgery*, 2nd edition. Butterworth-Heinmann, New York: 1996.
7. Nesi FA, Smith BC, eds: *Ophthalmic Plastic and Reconstructive Surgery*, 2nd edition. Mosby-Year Book, St. Louis: 1997.
8. Phelps CD, Hansjoerg EJ, eds: *Manual of Common Ophthalmic Surgical Procedures*. Churchill Livingstone, New York: 1986.
9. Shields MB: *Textbook of Glaucoma*, 4th edition. Williams & Wilkins, Baltimore: 1998.
10. Waltman SR, Keates RH, Hoyt CS, Frueh BR, Herschler J, Carroll DM, eds: *Surgery of the Eye*. Churchill Livingstone, New York: 1988.

Surgeons

Willard E. Fee, Jr., MD
Winston C. Vaughan, MD (*Sinus surgery*)
Joseph B. Roberson, MD (*Skull base surgery*)
Jerome Hester, MD (*Sleep-disordered breathing*)
Robert J. Troell, MD (*Sleep-disordered breathing*)
Robert W. Riley, DDS, MD (*Sleep-disordered breathing*)
Nelson B. Powell, MD (*Sleep-disordered breathing*)
Kasey K. Li, DDS, MD (*Sleep-disordered breathing*)

3.0 OTOLARYNGOLOGY—HEAD AND NECK SURGERY

Anesthesiologists

Vladimir Nekhendzy, MD
Edward R. Baer, MD (*Skull base surgery*)
Michael W. Champeau, MD (*Sleep-disordered breathing*)

OTOLARYNGOLOGY—HEAD AND NECK SURGERY: INTRODUCTION—SURGEON'S PERSPECTIVE

Willard E. Fee, Jr.

AIRWAY COMPETITION

Induction and maintenance of anesthesia for surgery of the head and neck requires interdisciplinary cooperation. Thorough communication both preop and intraop is required for a satisfactory outcome. Of necessity, anesthesiologists cannot have control of the head for many of the cases and competition for the airway produces some anxiety on the part of both physicians. For many procedures, head movement is the norm and, unless the tube is properly secured, extubation can occur. Inflammatory or neoplastic lesions of the upper aerodigestive tract produce some degree of airway obstruction and may make intubation extremely difficult—in some cases impossible—necessitating tracheostomy under local anesthesia before induction of GA. Airway obstruction upon induction of anesthesia can occur even with seemingly simple procedures such as tonsillectomy. Communication between the surgeon and anesthesiologist is crucial to assure success.

PREMEDICATION

There are few areas in surgery that have as many functional and/or cosmetic consequences as surgery of the head and neck. The properly informed patient understands the consequences and comes to the OR with a certain degree of anxiety. For oral cavity procedures or endoscopy, a drying agent facilitates performance of the procedure, making a combination of morphine or meperidine and scopolamine the agents of choice for people < 70 yr old. A small percentage of patients > 70 yr will have a postscopolamine psychosis that is unpleasant for all concerned. For that reason, atropine or glycopyrrolate is substituted. Anxiolytics must be used with great caution to avoid airway compromise.

TUBES AND TUBE SIZE

Seldom is there a need for anything larger than a size 6.0 mm ETT. The surgeon may need to lift the tube to examine the larynx adequately, and having to move a larger tube around can be difficult. For procedures on the oral cavity and pharynx, or for endoscopy, a cuffed tube is required to prevent anesthesia blow-by or aspiration of blood into the tracheobronchial tree. If a mouth gag is utilized, an anode or armored tube should be used to prevent compression of the tube by the gag. Although rare, anode tube obstruction does occur, and constant vigilance is required. If intraoral or laryngeal surgery is performed with the laser, compatible ETTs must be used to prevent ignition of the tubes → intratracheal or laryngeal fires. Maintenance of anesthesia for laser cases should be performed without N_2O and with $FiO_2 < 0.3$. If FiO_2 must be raised beyond that for any reason, the laser should not be used until the $FiO_2 < 0.3$.

MUSCLE RELAXATION

In some cases, muscle relaxation is mandatory; in others, it is contraindicated. In the case of parotidectomy, visual or monitored facial muscle movements are required; thus, no muscle relaxant is indicated. In the case of rigid esophagoscopy, muscle relaxation is often helpful in passing through the cricopharyngeal muscle. As a matter of habit, it is best to ask, as there is nothing more frustrating than having to wait for muscle relaxation to wear off before proceeding.

PATIENT POSITIONING

It is rare that anything other than the supine position is used. Before induction, the shoulders should always be at the break in the table so that head and neck can be flexed and/or extended as required intraop. This is especially true for endoscopy. A reverse Trendelenburg position is used for esophagoscopy to prevent gastric contents from seeping into the esophagus and slowing down the performance of the procedure. For most major head and neck procedures, elevating the head to ~30° increases venous return, decreases blood loss, and expedites the procedure.

HYPOTENSIVE ANESTHESIA

Anything that can be done to reduce blood loss results in faster surgery and less morbidity to the patient. One-third of the anatomy of the entire body is concentrated in the head and neck, and most surgical procedures are designed to preserve function, making some dissections quite tedious. Anything that can be done to maintain relative hypotension is very much appreciated by the surgeon (SBP = 80-100 mmHg is desirable). True hypotensive anesthesia usually is required only for excisions of angiofibromas, AV malformations, hemangiomas, or glomus tumors.

INTRODUCTION—ANESTHESIOLOGIST'S PERSPECTIVE

Vladimir Nekhendzy

PATIENT POPULATION

Many ENT patients are smokers and/or elderly, and have a high incidence of CAD, HTN, chronic renal insufficiency, and COPD. Careful H&P must be performed to assure that the patient's functional status is optimized.

AIRWAY

ENT patients often present difficult airway management problems, including: (1) certain anatomic characteristics (e.g., ↓C-spine ROM, large tongue, receding jaw); (2) Hx of stridor and hoarseness (airway narrowing and possible vocal cord dysfunction); (3) Hx of neck surgery, trauma, or XRT; (4) Hx of difficult intubation; (5) infections (e.g., epiglottitis, retropharyngeal abscess, Ludwig's angina). Patients with head and neck cancer often have had previous surgery or radiation therapy, and these treatments may further compromise airway management by significantly decreasing tissue compliance and adversely affecting neck ROM and mouth opening. Meticulous airway examination must be performed, and abnormal findings should heighten the anesthesiologist's concern for difficult ventilation/intubation. There should be a low threshold for an awake fiber optic intubation (FOI) if the airway is questionable. If the anesthesiologist decides to proceed with conventional means of securing the airway, the patient's head positioning should be optimized carefully, and intubating aids (e.g. stylets, gum elastic bougie), as well as ETTs of different sizes, should be available. If some difficulty in securing the patient's airway is anticipated—but direct laryngoscopy is, for some reason, preferred—there must be a clear backup plan for alternative airway management, with all the corresponding airway equipment readily available.

For the majority of ENT surgical procedures, the patient's airway is not only shared with the surgeon, but immediate access to the airway is difficult because the patient is turned 90° or 180° away from the anesthesiologist. The ETT must be secured diligently (there may be limited space available to secure ETT on the patient's face) and its positioning should be monitored carefully during surgery. Insecure taping may cause the ETT cuff to migrate to the subglottic area and exert pressure on the recurrent laryngeal nerves. For certain procedures (e.g., excision of tongue-base tumors, excision of certain parotid tumors, tongue suspension for obstructive sleep apnea [OSA], etc.), nasal intubation may be desirable to facilitate surgical access, and the surgeon should be consulted before induction.

ANESTHETIC MANAGEMENT

The essential anesthesia requirements for ENT surgery are:

1. Assurance of good intraop and postop analgesia (most of the procedures are performed on highly reflexogenic areas).

2. Quiet surgical field (the operated areas are highly vascular). Controlled ↓BP (SBP < 100 mmHg and MAP = 60-70 mmHg) is widely employed, unless contraindicated 2° concomitant medical conditions.

3. Patient immobility. For certain procedures, profound muscle relaxation may be required, while for others, administration of NMRs is avoided.

4. Smooth emergence from anesthesia is often a challenging task for the anesthesiologist, and every attempt should be made to avoid or minimize patient reaction to the ETT. Straining, bucking, or coughing will cause an increase in venous pressure that may provoke postop bleeding, disruption of delicate suture lines (e.g., facial nerve repair), and/or tympanic graft dislodgement following tympanoplasty. Many ENT surgeons have their own 'list' of procedures where reaction to ETT should be completely avoided, and an anesthesiologist should be familiar with the surgeon's preferences.

With the exception of patients presenting for OSA surgery (see Anesthetic Considerations for Reconstructive Surgery for Sleep-Disordered Breathing, p. 196), **opioid-based techniques** are especially advantageous for achieving the previously stated anesthetic requirements. With these techniques, hemodynamic stability will be maintained more easily and patient reaction to the ETT will be blunted reliably. In addition, an opioid-based technique will facilitate emergence from anesthesia in a timely manner. Volatile anesthetics can be reduced safely (or DC'd) as the surgery approaches its end, without fear of patient reaction to the ETT. This is particularly beneficial for the many ENT procedures that are characterized by a minimal surgical closure. The choice of an opioid depends on the degree of surgical stimulation, anticipated postop pain, and duration of surgery. Highly-potent opioids (fentanyl: loading dose 4-10 μg/kg; sufentanil: loading dose 0.5-1.5 μg/kg; followed by either intermittent boluses or continuous infusion) are the author's preferred choice for major ENT surgery (e.g., neck dissection). For procedures that are characterized by minimal postop discomfort (e.g., laser surgery of the airway), short-acting opioids may be preferred (remifentanil: loading dose 0.5-1.0 μg/kg, infusion 0.1-0.25 μg/kg/

min; alfentanil: 20-40 μg/kg loading dose, infusion 0.25-1 μg/kg/min). Continuous infusions of opioids may offer potential advantages over intermittent boluses, resulting in ↓total dose, greater hemodynamic stability, more rapid recovery of consciousness, less pain in the immediate postop period, and ↓time to discharge.

Deliberate ↓BP usually is accomplished easily with a potent inhalational anesthetic and/or intermittent boluses of vasoactive agents (e.g., esmolol 0.3-1 mg/kg, labetalol 0.1-0.3 mg/kg, hydralazine 0.05-0.15 mg/kg). Infusion of NTG or SNP (0.25-1 μg/kg/min) is rarely necessary. Additional dose of a longer-acting α-blocker (e.g. labetalol) is frequently beneficial at the end of surgery to prevent patient hypertensive responses in the early postop period.

Antiemetic prophylaxis should be routine, and most commonly is achieved by iv administration of a 5-HT$_3$ blocker (e.g., granisetron 100 μg). The addition of metoclopramide (10 mg iv) may be beneficial for patients who have swallowed some blood (nasal or intraoral surgery).

GETA is most widely employed. Flexible LMAs have been used successfully in different ENT procedures, including adenotonsillectomy, ear and nasal surgery, as well as head and neck surgery. The main advantage of the LMA over the ETT for ENT patients is a less stimulating emergence, with significant reduction in the number of episodes of coughing, postremoval laryngospasm, laryngeal trauma, and clinically significant airway events. In particular, the incidence of coughing and laryngospasm on emergence is reduced by 30- and 3-fold, respectively. The safe use of LMA for selected ENT procedures is discussed below.

A **flexible LMA** is recommended for use in ENT anesthesia because it can be bent away from the surgical field to find the optimal angle for connection to the anesthesia circuit. Because of its flexibility, this type of LMA is not likely to get displaced during rotation of the patient's head. It is important to minimize the risk of esophageal insufflation if PPV is planned. Although it is difficult to predict the optimal size of the LMA for PPV, the largest size possible (#5 or #4) should be used to minimize leak and gastric insufflation. Gastric insufflation is further avoided by ↓ TV to 8-10 ml/kg and by keeping PIP < 20 cmH$_2$O. The absence of gastric insufflation should be documented in the anesthesia record after auscultating the stomach area. Maintaining neuromuscular blockade during PPV through a LMA is recommended to ↑ chest-wall compliance and to minimize reflux or regurgitation 2° inadvertent movement or reaction to the LMA in situ.

Use of LMA is associated with a very low patient morbidity, which most commonly manifests as feelings of 'fullness' (25%), transient dysphagia (4-24%), bacteremia (4%), and minor pharyngeal abrasions (2%). The single most limiting feature of the LMA is the potential for aspiration of stomach contents. The main contraindications to the LMA are patients at risk for aspiration ('full stomach', morbidly obese, etc.), with low lung/chest-wall compliance, and with high airway resistance. Relative contraindications are patients with pharyngeal pathology (abscess, hematoma, tissue disruption), with glottic or subglottic airway obstruction, and bleeding diatheses.

References

1. Asai T, Murao K, Yukawa H, Shingu K: Re-evaluation of appropriate size of the laryngeal mask airway. *Br J Anaesth* 1999; 83(3):478-9.
2. Bailey PL, Egan TD, Stanley TH: Intravenous opioid anesthetics. In *Anesthesia*. 5th edition. Miller RD, ed. Churchhill Livingstone, Philadelphia: 2000, 273-376.
3. Benumof J: Laryngeal mask airway and the ASA difficult airway algorithm. *Anesthesiology* 1996; 84(3):686-96.
4. Brimacombe JR: Positive pressure ventilation with the size 5 laryngeal mask. *J Clin Anesth* 1997; 9:113-7.
5. Brimacombe JR, Berry A: The incidence of aspiration associated with the laryngeal mask airway: a meta-analysis of published literature. *J Clin Anesth* 1995; 7:297-305.
6. Brimacombe JR, Brain AJ: *The Laryngeal Mask Airway: a Review and Practical Guide*. WB Saunders, London: 1997.
7. Brown BR: Anaesthesia for ear, nose, throat and maxillofacial procedures. In *International Practice of Anaesthesia*. Prys-Roberts C, Brown BR, eds. Butterworth-Heinemann, Oxford: 1996, 2-9.
8. Donlon JV: Anesthesia for eye, ear, nose, and throat surgery. In *Anesthesia*, 5th edition. Miller RD, ed. Churchhill Livingstone, Philadelphia: 2000, 2173-98.
9. Dougherty TB: The difficult airway in conventional head and neck surgery. In *Airway Management: Principles and Practice*. Benumof JL, ed. Mosby-Year Book, St. Louis: 1996, 686-97.
10. Gotta AW, Ferrari LR, Sullivan CA: Anesthesia for otolaryngologic surgery. In *Clinical Anesthesia*, 4th edition. Barash PG, Cullen BF, Stoelting RK, eds. Lippincott Williams & Wilkins, Philadelphia: 2001, 989-1004.
11. Illing L, Duncan PG, Yip R: Gastroesophageal reflux during anesthesia. *Can J Anesth* 1992; 39(5):466-70.
12. Joseph MM: Anesthesia for ear, nose, and throat surgery. In *Principles and Practice of Anesthesiology*, 2nd edition. Longnecker DE, Tinker JH, Morgan GE, eds. Mosby, St. Louis: 1998, 2200-22.
13. Kirk GA. Anesthesia for ear, nose, and throat surgery. In *Principles and Practice of Anesthesiology*. Rogers MC, Tinker JH, Covino BG, Longnecker DE, eds. Mosby-Year Book, St. Louis: 1993, 2257-74.
14. Nair MB, Bailey PM: Review of uses of the laryngeal mask in ENT anesthesia. *Anaesthesia* 1995; 50:898-900.
15. Ng A, Smith G: Gastroesophageal reflux and aspiration of gastric contents in anesthetic practice. *Anesth Analg* 2001; 93: 494-513.

TONSILLECTOMY AND/OR ADENOIDECTOMY

SURGICAL CONSIDERATIONS

Description: The dissection for **tonsillectomy** is carried out with the patient supine, shoulders elevated on a small pillow (Fig 3-1). A mouth gag is inserted; and, if an **adenoidectomy** is being done concurrently, adenoids are removed first, with a curette, and the nasopharynx packed. The tonsillectomy is accomplished by firmly grasping the upper pole of the tonsil and drawing it medially, allowing a mucosal incision to be made over the anterior faucial pillar. The tonsil is dissected from its bed and removed. A snare may be used to snip the dissected tonsil off at the lower pole. Hemostasis is secured with gauze packs and the use of electrocautery. Packs are removed from the nasopharynx and tonsillar beds before extubation. Tonsillectomy may be combined with **palatopharyngoplasty** in cases of obstructive sleep apnea (OSA) or stertorous breathing (see p. 193).

Variant procedure or approaches: Guillotine technique (rarely used)

Usual preop diagnosis: Chronic tonsillitis and/or adenoiditis (most common); OSA; asymmetric enlargement of tonsils (to r/o cancer); nasal airway obstruction; snoring; peritonsillar abscess

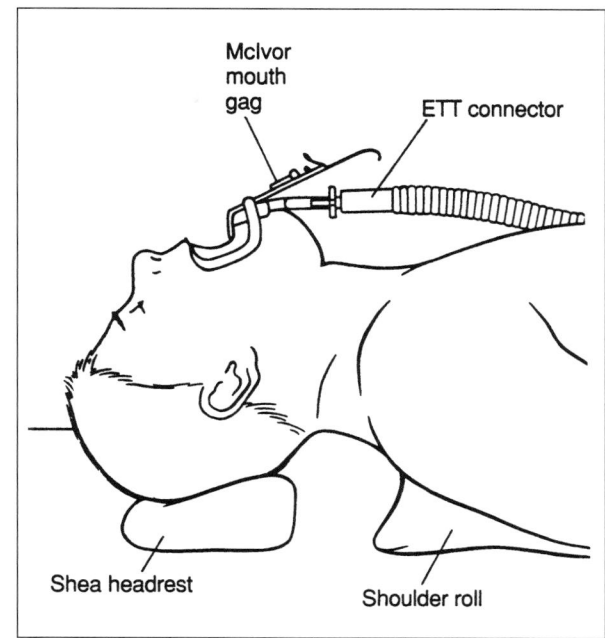

Figure 3-1. The 'Rose' position for tonsillectomy.

SUMMARY OF PROCEDURE

Position	'Rose' (supine, shoulder roll, head extended); surgeon at head of table (turned 90°-180°)
Incision	Intraoral mucosal
Special instrumentation	Mouth gag (McIvor)
Unique considerations	Use of armored ETT prevents compression of tube by mouth gag. Tube should be secured to lower lip in midline.
Antibiotics	Amoxicillin
Surgical time	30-60 min
Closing considerations	If patient has OSA, a heightened sensitivity to narcotics and sedatives may make emergence more difficult. Avoid hypercapnia on emergence to prevent vasodilation and resultant bleeding. Awake extubation will provide maximum airway protection.
EBL	25-200 ml. Monitor suction bottle contents and irrigation as an indication of blood loss.
Postop care	Lateral position; head down; gentle suctioning
Mortality	Rare
Morbidity	Bleeding: 4%[1]
	Infection: 4%
	Delayed bleeding: 3.2%
	Aspiration: Rare
	Tooth damage: Rare
Pain score	4-6

PATIENT POPULATION CHARACTERISTICS

Age range	2+ yr
Male:Female	1:1
Incidence	750,000 cases/yr in U.S.
Etiology	Chronic infection; OSA; peritonsillar abscess; snoring; cancer
Associated conditions	Nonspecific

ANESTHETIC CONSIDERATIONS

PREOPERATIVE

Most T/A patients are young and otherwise healthy; however, a subset of both pediatric and adult patients may present with Sx of OSA or URI. For many children, this is their first anesthetic; therefore, it is imperative to ✓ family Hx for anesthetic problems. Most adult and pediatric patients are discharged from the hospital on the day of surgery.

Airway	In patients with a Hx of snoring or OSA, the probability of difficult mask ventilation and/or intubation may be high, 2° airway characteristics peculiar to these patients (see Anesthesia for Reconstructive Surgery for Sleep-Disordered Breathing, p. 196). In children with short-stature syndrome, including achondroplastic dwarfism and selected cases of Down syndrome, atlantoaxial subluxation and stenosis of the spinal canal may be present, and neck extension in these patients should be avoided.
Respiratory	In patients presenting with Sx of acute URI (purulent sputum or nasal secretions, fever, etc.), the general recommendation is to postpone any elective procedure until symptoms have abated, usually within 7-14 d. The rationale for postponing surgery includes the possibility of progression from a URI to a lower respiratory tract infection, presence of secretions that may obstruct the ETT and plug small airways, predisposition to laryngospasm, and ↓respiratory reserve. **Tests:** As indicated from H&P.
Dental	The presence of chipped, loose, or broken teeth should be documented preop and the patient (or parents, if appropriate) should be informed that there is a possibility of further tooth damage/dislodgement during the procedure.
Cardiovascular	Rarely, chronic airway obstruction (e.g., OSA) with hypoxemia may → pulmonary HTN and right heart failure. Patients with Down syndrome may have concomitant CHD. **Tests:** As indicated from H&P.
Hematologic	✓ for recent aspirin use and Hx of excessive bleeding following minor trauma or tooth extraction.
Laboratory	CBC; other tests as indicated from H&P.
Premedication	Sedative premedication is routine, but should be avoided in OSA patients and patients with Sx of upper airway obstruction. Some surgeons request preop administration of an antisialagogue to achieve a dry surgical field.

INTRAOPERATIVE

Anesthetic technique: Balanced GETA is most commonly used in adults. (For pediatric anesthetic concentrations, see p. 957.) The essential surgical requirement is adequate muscle relaxation (propofol 100-150 μg/kg/min) to facilitate surgical exposure and prevent swallowing. Specific airway considerations include the possibility of difficult mask ventilation and/or difficult intubation 2° ↓pharyngeal space (e.g., tonsils/adenoids), as well as the possibility of obstructing the ETT with the mouth gag.

Induction	An **intravenous induction** with propofol (2 mg/kg) and fentanyl (2-3 μg/kg) is suitable for the majority of patients (consider avoiding STP for outpatient surgery). If difficulty with mask ventilation is encountered, an oral airway is preferred to a nasal airway, 2° the possibility of trauma to the hypertrophied adenoid tissue and the resultant brisk bleeding. **ET intubation** is facilitated by administration of either succinylcholine or an intermediate or short-duration NMR. Patients with peritonsillar abscess may have trismus, which usually resolves after induction of anesthesia and administration of a muscle relaxant. Careful **laryngoscopy** will avoid bleeding 2° inadvertent trauma to the enlarged tonsils. In patients with significant tonsillar hypertrophy, the **blind light-wand technique** of tracheal intubation should be avoided. A small (# 6.0) reinforced (anode) ETT or an oral RAE ETT is used, depending on the surgeon's preference. It is essential to verify tube positioning before and after Boyle-Davis mouth gag application (e.g., chest movement, bilateral and equal breath sounds, and normal PIP). The ETT may be obstructed, dislodged, kinked, or inadvertently advanced into a mainstem bronchus, or the patient's trachea can be prematurely extubated when the mouth gag is removed. Reinforced ETTs are more expensive than the RAE ETTs, but much less prone to obstruction by the mouth gag. In patients with peritonsillar abscess, great care must be exercised to prevent rupture of the abscess and soiling of the airway.
	It has been documented that the use of a **flexible LMA** instead of an ETT safely protects the airway during adenotonsillectomy and reduces the incidence of postextubation complications in adults and children. Its use for this procedure, however, has never become popular in the U.S.

Maintenance	Opening of a mouth gag and the tonsillectomy itself constitute powerful noxious stimuli; therefore, an adequate depth of anesthesia must be maintained. Moderate ↓BP is desirable but not obligatory; and judicious use of vasoactive drugs (see Introduction, p. 141) is preferred to very deep levels of anesthesia in achieving this objective.
	Remifentanil infusion, as part of either balanced or TIVA technique (propofol 100-150 μg/kg) may provide superior hemodynamic stability and facilitate smooth emergence from anesthesia. For the balanced inhalational technique, desflurane and sevoflurane are the preferred agents for these short surgical procedures.
	The mouth gag may be repositioned several times during the procedure and is removed only at the end of the case. Vigorous patient movement while the mouth gag is hooked on the Mayo stand may cause C-spine injury; thus, neuromuscular blockade should be maintained at a relatively deep level until the end of the procedure. Continuous muscle relaxation also will allow safe reduction of the inhalational anesthetic before the end of surgery to promote quick awakening. Prevention of PONV is of major importance. The stomach should be suctioned at the end of the case, and further emptying will be facilitated by iv administration of metaclopromide. Administration of 5-HT$_3$ blockers (see Introduction, p. 142), with or without steroids, will constitute adequate antiemetic prophylaxis.
Emergence	Removal of a throat pack (if used by the surgeon) should be verified before extubation. Care must be exercised while suctioning the oropharynx to avoid bleeding. Extubation should be smooth and performed after the patient is able to follow commands, since this usually signifies return of protective airway reflexes.
	If extubation is to be performed at deeper levels of anesthesia (e.g., in small children), the patient should be placed in the lateral decubitus, head-down position ('tonsillar position') to protect the airway from soiling 2° postop bleeding or aspiration of gastric contents. The patient should remain in this position until fully awake. This method of extubation is more time- and labor-consuming, and an adequate depth of anesthesia must be assured to prevent postextubation laryngospasm. With the head-down position, venous pressure in the surgical wound is increased, with the possibility of provoking postop bleeding. This method of extubation cannot be advocated for routine use in adults.
Blood and fluid requirements	IV: 18 ga × 1 (adult) 20 ga × 1 (child) NS/LR @ 4-6 ml/kg/h (adult) Blood loss typically averages 4 ml/kg, although it may be difficult to assess 2° drainage into stomach. Adequate hydration should continue in the immediate postop period.
Monitoring	Standard monitors (p. B-1)
Positioning	✓ and pad pressure points. ✓ eyes.
Complications	ETT damage/obstruction ETT dislodgement Bleeding ETTs of different sizes should be readily available. Blood loss sometimes may be difficult to assess 2° drainage into stomach, especially if a throat pack is not used. Careful observation of suction canisters and close communication with the surgeon are essential.

POSTOPERATIVE

Complications	Retention of throat pack	Manifested by immediate symptoms of upper airway obstruction. Under direct laryngoscopy, remove pack with Magill forceps.
	Laryngospasm	A relatively common complication, particularly in the pediatric population. Rx: 100% O$_2$ via mask ventilation with jaw thrust and CPAP. Rapid-sequence induction and direct laryngoscopy/intubation for persistent laryngospasm.
	Bleeding tonsil	Bleeding usually occurs at a slow pace; large volumes of blood may be swallowed and hypovolemia may occur before any bleeding is detected. Frequent swallowing should alert to the possibility of ongoing hemorrhage. ET intubation (RSI) may prove difficult due to poor visualization (effective suction must always be available) and upper airway edema. (See Pediatric section on Anesthesia for Tonsillectomy, p. 957.)

Complications, cont.	Postobstructive (negative pressure) pulmonary edema (POPE)	POPE is a rare complication; however, it may occur in patients with preexisting symptoms of severe upper airway obstruction. These patients may require reintubation and postop ventilatory support.
Pain management	Fentanyl (0.5-1 μg/kg iv) may be the preferred analgesic, especially if the patient will be discharged home from the recovery room.	If the patient's disposition is unclear, morphine or meperidine may be used more liberally.
Tests	Hct (if blood loss suspected).	Frequent swallowing may be a sign of ongoing hemorrhage.

References

1. Breson K, Diepeveen J: Dissection tonsillectomy—complications and follow-up. *J Laryngol Otol* 1969; 83(6):601-8.
2. Brimacombe JR, Keller C, Gunkel AR, Pühringer F: The influence of the tonsillar gag on efficacy of seal, anatomic position, airway patency, and airway protection with the flexible laryngeal mask airway: a randomized, cross-over study on fresh adult cadavers. *Anesth Analg* 1999; 89:181-6.
3. Brown BR: Anaesthesia for ear, nose, throat and maxillofacial procedures. In *International Practice of Anaesthesia*. Prys-Roberts C, Brown BR, eds. Butterworth-Heinemann, Oxford: 1996, 2-9.
4. Davis L, Cook-Sather SD, Schreiner MS: Lighted stylet intubation: a review. *Anesth Analg* 2000; 90:745-56.
5. Donlon JV: Anesthesia for eye, ear, nose, and throat surgery. In *Anesthesia*. 5th edition. Miller RD, ed. New York: Churchill Livingstone, 2000: 2173-98.
6. Dougherty TB: The difficult airway in conventional head and neck surgery. In *Airway Management: Principles and Practice*. Benumof JL, ed. Mosby-Year Book, St. Louis: 1996, 686-97.
7. Ebert TJ, Robinson BJ, Uhrich TD, Mackenthun A, et al: Recovery from sevoflurane anesthesia. A comparison to isoflurane and propofol anesthesia. *Anesthesiology* 1998; 89:1524-31.
8. Gotta AW, Ferrari LR, Sullivan CA: Anesthesia for otolaryngologic surgery. In *Clinical Anesthesia*. 5th edition. Barash PG, Cullen BF, Stoelting RK, eds. Lippincott Williams and Wilkins, Philadelphia: 2001, 989-1004.
9. Kirk GA: Anesthesia for ear, nose, and throat surgery. In *Principles and Practice of Anesthesiology*. Rogers MC, Tinker JH, Covino BG, Longnecker DE, eds. Mosby-Year Book, St. Louis: 1993, 2257-74.
10. Kokki H: Nonsteroidal anti-inflammatory drugs for postoperative pain: a focus on children. *Paediatr Drugs* 2003; 5(2): 103-23.
11. Pollard BJ: ENT surgery. In *Handbook of Clinical Anesthesia*. Goldstone JC, Pollard BJ, eds. Churchill Livingstone, New York: 1996, 301-13.
12. Randall DA, Hoffer ME: Complications of tonsillectomy and adenoidectomy. *Otolaryngol Head Neck Surg* 1998; 118(1): 61-8.
13. Sukhani R, Pappas AL, Lurie J, Hotaling AJ, Park A, Fluder E: Ondansetron and dolasetron provide equivalent postoperative vomiting control after ambulatory tonsillectomy in dexamethasone-pretreated children. *Anesth Analg* 2002; 95(5): 1230-5.
14. Webster AC, Morley-Forster PK, Dain S, Ganapathy S, et al: Anaesthesia for adenotonsillectomy: a comparison between tracheal intubation and the armored laryngeal mask airway. *Can J Anesth* 1993; 40(12):1171-7.
15. Windfuhr JP, Chen YS: Post-tonsillectomy and -adenoidectomy hemorrhage in nonselected patients. *Ann Otol Rhinol Laryngol* 2003; 112(1):63-70.

LARYNGOSCOPY/BRONCHOSCOPY/ESOPHAGOSCOPY

SURGICAL CONSIDERATIONS

Description: Laryngoscopy is used for visualization of the pharynx, hypopharynx, or larynx for diagnostic and/or therapeutic benefit. The patient is supine with cervical spine flexed and atlantoaxial joint extended (this position is best achieved with a headrest); and the teeth are protected with a mouth guard. The laryngoscope is introduced (Fig 3-2); then, with a lifting motion, a thorough examination of the oropharynx, hypopharynx, laryngopharynx, and larynx is carried out and biopsies can be taken. Any bleeding normally can be controlled easily with pressure. Laryngoscopy often is combined with esophagoscopy, bronchoscopy, or direct nasopharyngoscopy to survey the aerodigestive tract for malignancy. If the procedure is diagnostic, the surgeon may need to visualize the airway before intubation and/or muscle relaxation. If a laser is to be utilized, use of a special laser ETT, < 30% O_2 concentration, and avoidance of N_2O are required.

Usual preop diagnosis: Oropharyngeal, hypopharyngeal or laryngeal tumors

Bronchoscopy is used for visualization of the tracheo-bronchial tree for both diagnostic and therapeutic purposes. The patient is supine with head elevated and neck extended at the upper cervical level. The bronchoscope is directed along the right side of the tongue forward toward the midline to visualize the epiglottis. Next, the bronchoscope tip is used to lift the epiglottis and advance the bronchoscope through the vocal cords, into the trachea and bronchus (Fig 3-3). The scope can be directed for inspection of the carina, main bronchi, and, with the aid of telescopes, the segmental bronchi. This often is performed with direct laryngoscopy, esophagoscopy, or as part of **panendoscopy**.

Usual preop diagnosis: Head and neck squamous-cell carcinoma; foreign body (FB) in bronchus

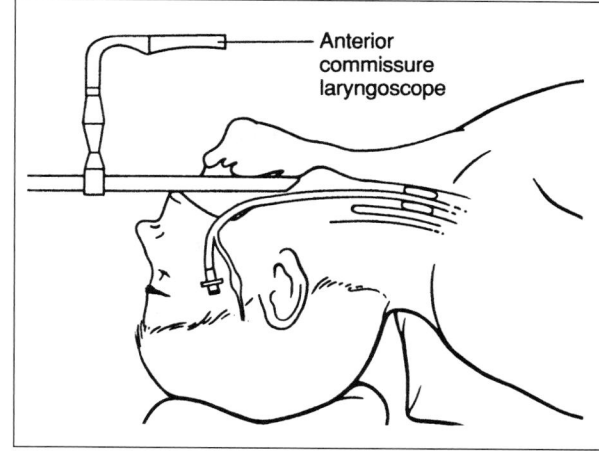

Figure 3-2. Placement of anterior commissure laryngoscope for laryngoscopy.

Esophagoscopy is used for visualization of the esophagus for either diagnostic or therapeutic benefit. The patient is supine with head elevated and neck extended at the upper cervical level. The esophagoscope (held in the right hand) is advanced through the mouth behind the arytenoids, gently using the left thumb. The bevel of the scope is then used to advance through the cricopharyngeal muscle (upper esophageal sphincter) with an upward lifting movement, entering the cervical esophagus. As the scope advances, the head may have to be lowered or the neck extended and the scope directed slightly toward the left. It should be advanced only when a visible lumen is seen all the way down to the cardia. A biopsy may be taken through the scope. Esophagoscopy also is often performed as part of **panendoscopy**.

Usual preop diagnosis: Head and neck squamous-cell carcinoma; FB ingestion

SUMMARY OF PROCEDURES

	Laryngoscopy	Bronchoscopy	Esophagoscopy
Position	Supine; table 90°	⇐	⇐ + reverse Trendelenburg or head up 30° to prevent gastric reflux.
Special instrumentation	Laser ETT; microscope (both used occasionally)	Rigid or flexible bronchoscopes of various sizes. If rigid scope used, an adaptor connects it to anesthesia tubing. If flexible scope used, accessory port adaptor should be connected to the ETT.	Rigid esophagoscope or flexible gastroscope
Unique considerations	Steroids (dexamethasone 4-12 mg) may be helpful if airway is compromised and extensive manipulation or therapeutic procedure required.	With laser ablation, keep O_2 < 30%; avoid N_2O. Bleeding following biopsy or removal of tumors is rare, but may require rescoping and suctioning to adequately ventilate the patient.	May need to deflate ETT cuff to introduce scope or retrieve FB.
Antibiotics	None	Usually none	None
Surgical time	10-90 min (diagnostic vs therapeutic)	10-60 min	⇐
EBL	Minimal	⇐	⇐
Postop care	Rarely, may require overnight ICU monitoring, if airway compromised and no tracheostomy performed.	Usually PACU. If surgery 2° airway obstruction, it may worsen immediately postop, requiring ICU observation.	PACU; may require overnight observation to r/o perforation.
Mortality	< 1%	⇐	< 0.1%

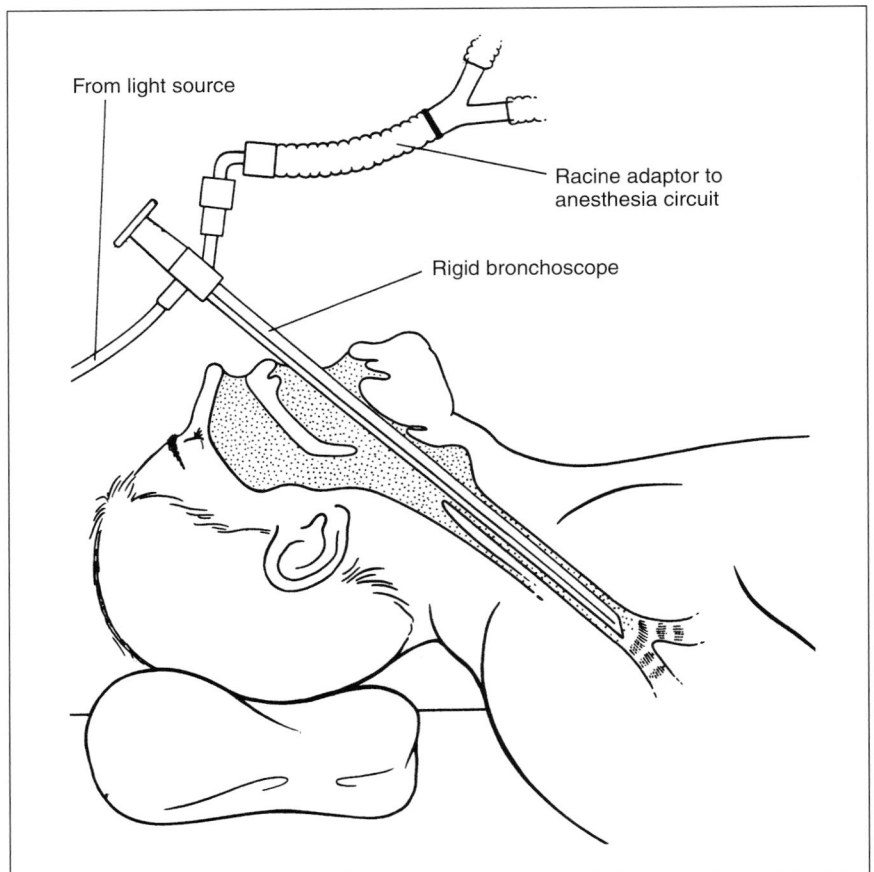

Figure 3-3. Rigid bronchoscopy showing adaptor (Racine) for anesthesia machine. Note neck flexion and head extension to align oropharyngeal and tracheal axes.

	Laryngoscopy	**Bronchoscopy**	**Esophagoscopy**
Morbidity	Laryngospasm: < 5%	–	⇐
	Airway obstruction upon induction: 1%	⇐	< 1%
	Damaged teeth: < 1%	1%	⇐
	Laryngeal edema requiring tracheostomy or reintubation: < 1%	Pneumonia: 1%	Perforation of esophagus: 1%
Pain score	1-2	1-2	1-2

PATIENT POPULATION CHARACTERISTICS

Age range	Newborn–old age	⇐	⇐
Male:Female	1:1	⇐	⇐
Incidence	Common	⇐	⇐
Etiology	Neoplasia; FB; congenital webs/ cysts	⇐	⇐

ANESTHETIC CONSIDERATIONS

(Procedures covered: direct laryngoscopy, bronchoscopy, esophagoscopy)

PREOPERATIVE

Many patients are elderly and have a Hx of smoking and drinking, with corresponding implications for intraop management. Patient nutritional status may be further compromised by preexisting cancerous disease. Meticulous attention to airway management is paramount in these procedures, and close communication with the surgeon is essential. Some patients presenting for esophagoscopy may have obstructing lesions of the esophagus, active GI bleeding, or require the removal of a FB, putting them at ↑risk of aspiration.

Airway	**Occult airway compromise** may be present in these patients; thus, a thorough preop airway assessment is essential, and a clear backup plan for securing the airway should be devised and discussed with the surgeon before induction of GA.
	Stridor at rest suggests an airway diameter ≤ 4.5 mm, although airway diameter can be seriously reduced even without stridor being present. Inspiratory stridor usually is associated with supraglottic lesions, while expiratory stridor suggests airway narrowing below the glottis.
	Subglottic lesions may be characterized by both inspiratory and expiratory stridor.
	Patients with **lesions in the mediastinum** may have involvement of the recurrent laryngeal nerve, with hoarseness and potential airway management problems (e.g., difficult mask ventilation, difficult intubation, ↑aspiration risk). (See Anesthetic Considerations for Mediastinoscopy, p. 232.)
Respiratory	These patients may have a high incidence of COPD and ↓respiratory reserve. The nature and characteristics of a productive cough must be noted. Wheezing on exam must be treated with bronchodilators before induction.
	Tests: CXR; other tests as indicated from H&P.
Dental	Physical exam should include a careful dental assessment and documentation. Patients (or parents, as appropriate) should be informed that loose teeth may be dislodged or damaged by surgical instrumentation of the mouth during the procedure.
Cardiovascular	Adrenergic responses during endoscopy may be associated with up to 4% incidence of myocardial ischemia. Look for Sx of CAD (e.g., angina) and CHF (e.g., orthopnea, PND, peripheral edema) in patients with cardiac risk factors (including age up to 40 yr, male, HTN, hypercholesteremia, long Hx of smoking, obesity, and family Hx). The volume status of debilitated patients who are unable to eat because of obstructing lesions of the esophagus should be assessed by measuring orthostatic BP changes.
	Tests: ECG. Orthostatic BP and HR changes >10 mmHg, ↓SBP, and/or 15 bpm ↑HR suggest significant (> 20%) hypovolemia. Other tests as indicated from H&P.
Neurologic	Some patients may have Hx of ETOH abuse, which may → increased anesthetic requirements because of hepatic enzyme induction. Symptoms of alcohol withdrawal (e.g., tremulousness, ↑sympathetic activity, and altered mental status), should be fully controlled prior to surgery.
Hematologic	Patients with malignancy or chronic disease may have evidence of anemia or coagulopathy.
	Tests: Consider CBC, PT, PTT, Plt.
Gastrointestinal	In some patients (e.g., with malignant tumors), significant electrolyte abnormalities may be present 2° malnutrition. Hypokalemia and hypomagnesemia should be corrected preop. In patients with Hx of ETOH abuse, liver disease and cirrhosis may be present.
	Tests: Electrolytes; BUN; Cr; LFT; coag studies, as indicated from H&P.
Premedication	A drying agent (e.g., glycopyrrolate 0.2 mg iv) frequently is givent to facilitate panendoscopy, especially in patients with a significant amount of secretions. Risks and benefits of an antisialagogue should be considered carefully in patients with preexisting cardiac disease, and the need for its use should be discussed with the surgeon. Sedative premedication is routine, but should be minimized in the elderly and avoided in patients with symptoms of upper airway obstruction.

INTRAOPERATIVE

Anesthetic technique: GETA. The challenge of airway management in these cases requires careful planning and continuous communication with the surgeon. The specific surgical requirements are: adequate muscle relaxation (movement, coughing, or bucking during endoscopy may have disastrous consequences) and immobile vocal cords for vocal cord surgery. Cardiovascular stability is important: laryngeal, tracheal, and carinal reflexes may provoke severe HTN and ↑HR, which can be detrimental in some patients. Adequate depth of anesthesia is essential, together with rapid awakening and return of laryngeal reflexes. β-blockers may be indicated to treat break-through adrenergic responses. Use of short-acting opioids, preferably by infusion to assure stable plasma concentration, is highly beneficial for these procedures. Endoscopy procedures and laser surgery of the airway, although highly stimulating, are characterized by minimal postop pain, and the majority of patients are discharged home from the recovery room.

Special considerations: These procedures involve a number of specific considerations involving panendoscopy, laser surgery of the airway, airway management for microsurgery of the larynx, and laser surgery of the airway.

Panendoscopy: Should **rigid bronchoscopy** be planned first, GA and complete muscle relaxation are induced, and the patient is turned over immediately to the surgeon, without securing an airway. Once the rigid bronchoscope is introduced into the patient's trachea, an anesthesia circuit is connected to it through the flexible side port adapter (Racine, Fig. 3-2), and an anesthesiologist ventilates the patient by hand. High flows usually are required because of the leak around the bronchoscope. Close communication with the surgeon is essential for adjusting ventilation when the bronchoscope is introduced into the mainstem bronchus to avoid high inflating pressures and assure complete exhalation. After rigid bronchoscopy is completed, care should be taken to ventilate the patient with 100% O_2 by mask before intubation, to assure good oxygenation and normocapnia. Patient's trachea is intubated either by the anesthesiologist or by the surgeon; ETT is secured; and the surgeon proceeds with **laryngoscopy** (or micro-direct laryngoscopy if the operating microscope is used) and **rigid esophagoscopy**. For these procedures, the ETT should be moved to the left side of the patient's mouth to facilitate introduction of the surgical instruments, and taped to the chin, rather than to the upper jaw, because full opening of the patient's mouth is required. If **flexible bronchoscopy/esophagoscopy** is planned, patient is intubated by the anesthesiologist immediately after induction of anesthesia, and then turned over to the surgeon.

Laser surgery of the airway: If laser surgery of the vocal cords is planned, cords must remain motionless during the laser firing. The CO_2 laser, which can precisely vaporize superficial tissue, is widely used for vocal cord surgery, while the Nd:YAG (neodymium-yttrium-aluminum-garnet) laser usually is employed for airway tumor debulking because of its ability to coagulate deeper lesions. The Nd:YAG can be used through the suction channel of the fiber optic bronchoscope, whereas the CO_2 laser must be aimed directly at the targeted tissue. Both the CO_2 and Nd:YAG wavelengths lie outside the visible spectrum, and a separate, lower energy visible beam is used for aiming. The patient's eyes must be protected with tape and moistened gauze, OR personnel must wear protective goggles, and the laser must be in a stand-by mode when not in use.

Airway management for microsurgery/laser surgery: In principal, airway management for microsurgery of the larynx and laser surgery of the airway can be accomplished in three ways: ET intubation, intermittent apnea technique, and jet ventilation.

For **ET intubation**, either a small-diameter (5.0-6.0 mm), cuffed regular ETT or long microlaryngeal tube (MLT) is used to facilitate visualization of the larynx. A reinforced ETT may be desirable for esophagoscopy to avoid possible compression of the ETT. For laser cases, precautions must be taken to prevent airway fire, including:

- Use the lowest possible FiO_2 (≤ 0.3-0.4), assuring adequate oxygenation (dilute O_2 with air, N_2, or helium) and avoid NO (high FiO_2 and FiN_2O support combustion).

- Use colored (methylene blue-tinged) NS in the ETT cuff (will immediately alert the surgeon in case of a laser hit).

- Place the ETT deep enough in the trachea for the cuff to be out of the operator's sight.

- Use special laser ETT (e.g., Mallinkrodt Laser-Flex, Xomed Laser Shield), although none of them provides 100% protection from all types of lasers.

An **intermittent apnea technique** involves hyperventilation, followed by intermittent tracheal extubation for 1-5 min, during which the laser is used. This approach is time-consuming and may be associated with a higher incidence of airway trauma and edema, due to the repeated ET intubation. A properly working pulse oximeter is essential for this technique.

Jet ventilation (Fig 3-4) may be necessary when an ETT cannot be used (e.g., some supraglottic and subglottic lesions). For supraglottic jet ventilation, a ventilating laryngoscope is most commonly used. The axis of the jet should be in line with the trachea, and full egress of air (complete chest deflation) should be assured between the jet ventilator 'puffs'. The jet should be triggered during pauses between laser firings to keep the vocal cords immobile. If jet ventilation is used for laser resection of papillomas, there is a risk of spreading the virus to OR personnel, and special face masks should be worn in the OR. Jet ventilation is associated with potentially severe complications, including barotrauma, pneumothorax, and gastric distension (risk of regurgitation), and is hindered by ↓chest-wall or lung compliance. Complete muscle relaxation is absolutely essential for the procedures performed during jet ventilation. High-frequency jet ventilation may be used safely through a catheter passed below the vocal cords, but this requires special equipment that is not widely available. Its advantages include excellent operating conditions, low risk of barotrauma (low airway pressures), less vocal cord motion, and improved cardiovascular stability.

Induction	Patients at risk for aspiration require RSI with cricoid pressure; otherwise, induction is performed in a standard manner. Fentanyl should be limited to 1-2 μg/kg (minimal postop discomfort). The author's preference is to completely omit fentanyl in favor of a short-acting opioid (see Introduction, p. 141), supplemented as necessary with bolus esmolol (0.5-1 mg/kg) to block the hemodynamic

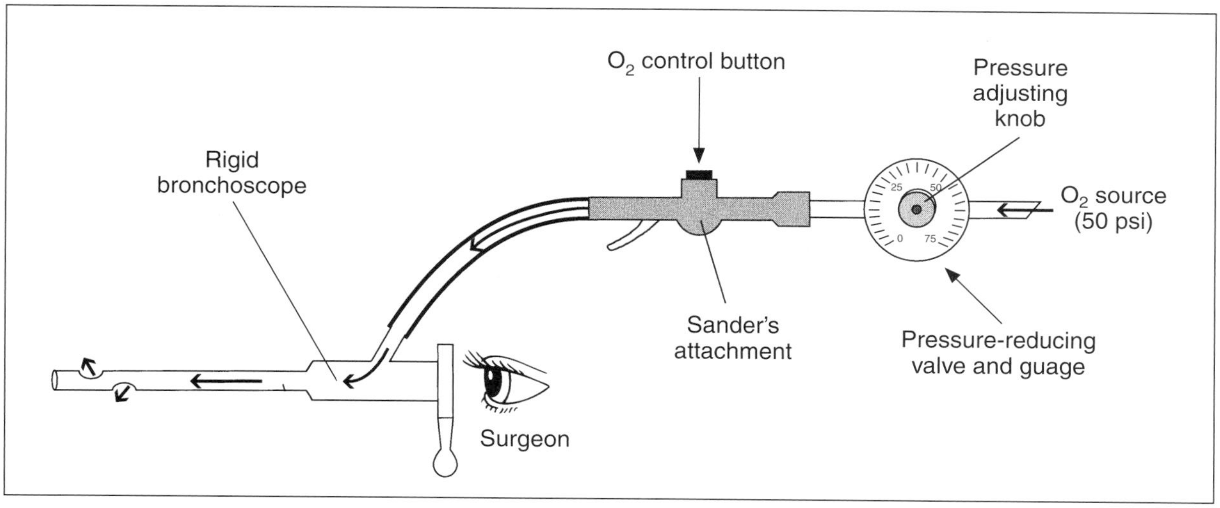

Figure 3-4. Rigid bronchoscope with modified Sanders jet ventilation technique. The wall oxygen supply at 50 psi is connected to a reducing valve that allows the pressure to be adjusted from 0 to 50 psi. The side port of the bronchoscope is used as the Venturi injector site, and the open end can be used for continuous viewing by the endoscopist.

Induction, cont.	responses to intubation. Propofol (1-2 mg/kg) is the ideal induction agent, given the short duration of these typically outpatient procedures. Full muscle relaxation is routine. Patients with soft-tissue supraglottic tumors (e.g., papillomatosis, epiglottic cancer, large vocal cord polyps) are at ↑risk for complete airway obstruction after induction of GA, with or without neuromuscular blockade. Anesthetic management of these patients requires careful planning and meticulous preparation. (For anesthetic management of a partially obstructed airway, see Anesthetic Considerations for Laryngectomy, p. 176.) The surgeon should be consulted about the extent of the disease and the potential need for a tracheostomy. The surgeon should be present during induction for the possible need to perform rigid bronchoscopy or emergent/semiemergent tracheostomy.
Maintenance	TIVA (propofol: 100-150 μg/kg/min; remifentanil 0.1-0.25 μg/kg/min or alfentanil 0.25-1 μg/kg/min) is used widely, especially when rigid bronchoscopy or jet ventilation/intermittent apnea techniques are planned. When an ETT is used throughout the case, delivery of anesthetic gases may be used instead of a propofol infusion. Desflurane and sevoflurane are the preferred agents because of their low blood:gas solubility; sevoflurane may be favored in patients with preexisting cardiac disease to minimize dose-dependent tachycardia. Break-through adrenergic responses can be managed safely by iv β-blockers or small boluses of a short-acting opioid (see Introduction, p. 141). With intermittent apnea or jet ventilation techniques, it may be difficult to avoid hypercapnia and hypoxemia, which may provoke intraop dysrhythmias.
	Vocal cord immobility is essential for microlaryngeal surgery, and prolonged neuromuscular blockade should be maintained. For laryngeal surgery, it may be more accurate to monitor the facial nerve (orbicularis oculi muscle), than the ulnar nerve (adductor pollicis muscle), since the recovery of the former better reflects the recovery of the laryngeal muscles. If this method is chosen, care should be taken to avoid prolonged complete neuromuscular blockade by coordinating administration of additional doses of muscle relaxants with the surgeon. As the surgery approaches its end, deepening the level of anesthesia is the preferred approach. A succinylcholine infusion (2-6 mg/min) can be used safely (maximum dose $\leq$ 4-6 mg/kg) to avoid phase 2 block in selected patients.
Emergence	Patient should have full return of protective airway reflexes prior to extubation. The patient's stomach should be decompressed following jet ventilation. Smooth emergence from anesthesia is obligatory to avoid additional trauma to the vocal cords. For this reason, some surgeons request deep extubation after the vocal cord surgery, which presents extra challenges to the anesthesiologist (see Emergence for Tonsillectomy, Adenoidectomy, p. 145).
Blood and fluid requirements	IV: GI bleeder: 14-16 ga × 2 Others: 20 ga × 1 NS/LR @ 2-3 ml/kg/h For esophagoscopy: NS/LR @ 4-6 ml/kg/h	Blood loss is usually minimal; however, in case of GI bleed, blood loss may be massive. T&C patient for 2 U PRBC, with blood immediately available in OR.

Monitoring	Standard monitors (p. B-1).	In case of potential hemorrhage, an arterial line is desirable.
Positioning	Table rotated 90° ✓ and pad pressure points. ✓ eyes.	Patient should have a shoulder roll with neck extension to facilitate endoscopy. For flexible fiber optic endoscopy, patient is usually in the lateral decubitus position.
Complications	Inadequate ventilation Loss of airway	Hypoxia and hypercarbia
	Perforation of airway Dysrhythmias Pneumothorax	Mechanical or laser perforation of the airway may → bronchospasm or uncontrollable hemorrhage. Dx: ↑RR, ↓BP, ↑CVP, wheezing, ↓O_2 saturation, ↑ PIP, SOB, chest pain, ↓breath sounds, ↓ECG amplitude, dullness on percussion, CXR. Rx: chest tube or needle aspiration, 100% O_2; ventilation and volume expansion.
	Eye trauma Bleeding post biopsy	Eye trauma from surgical instruments used during endoscopy may require ophthalmology consult.
Airway fire	Disconnect patient from anesthesia circuit. (Note: turning ventilator off is not sufficient, as fresh gas continues to be delivered.) Extinguish fire with NS. Remove ETT after deflating cuff. Extinguish and remove all burning material. Reestablish airway. Resume ventilation by face mask with 100% O_2. Reintubate trachea. ✓ airway for extent of damage and foreign bodies (fragments of ETT or packing materials). Save ETT for later examination.	This is an acute, life-threatening emergency. Rigid or flexible bronchoscopy is required to ✓ extent of damage and airway edema. All inhaled gases should be humidified. Patients with extensive airway burns should be kept intubated and monitored in the ICU.

POSTOPERATIVE

Complications	Dental trauma Massive bleeding Eye trauma	Dental trauma may result from surgical manipulation of the airway, and the anesthesiologist must check the teeth immediately after airway access is gained. If dental trauma is detected, promptly notify the surgeon for notation in the surgical summary.
	Postop airway compromise	Has a higher incidence than in general surgery patient population. Patients with T3 lesions and those with associated laryngeal biopsy (→ airway swelling) after panendoscopy may be at high risk for reintubation in PACU.
	Esophageal perforation	Complaints of painful swallowing postop may suggest an esophageal perforation.
	Pneumothorax Pneumomediastinum Hemothorax Aspiration	Pneumothorax, mediastinal air or hemothorax from esophageal perforation may present as ↓BP and cardiovascular collapse.
Pain management	Short-acting iv opiods (e.g., fentanyl, 25-50 μg iv prn) are usually sufficient.	
Tests	CXR Hct	For evidence of pneumothorax, hemothorax, mediastinal air.

References

1. Brown BR: Anaesthesia for ear, nose, throat and maxillofacial procedures. In *International Practice of Anaesthesia.* Prys-Roberts C, Brown BR, eds. Butterworth-Heinemann, Oxford: 1996:2-9.

2. Donati F, Meistelman C, Benoit P: Vecuronium neuromuscular blockade at the adductor muscles of the larynx and adductor pollicis. *Anesthesiology* 1991; 74:833-7.
3. Donlon JV: Anesthetic and airway management of laryngoscopy and bronchoscopy. In *Airway Management: Principles and Practice*. Benumof JL, ed. Mosby-Year Book, St. Louis: 1996:666-85.
4. Dougherty TB. The difficult airway in conventional head and neck surgery. In *Airway Management: Principles and Practice*. Benumof JL, ed. Mosby-Year Book, St. Louis: 1996, 686-97.
5. Gaumann DM, Tassonyi E, Fathi F, Griessen M: Effects of topical laryngeal lidocaine on the sympathetic response to rigid panendoscopy under general anesthesia. *J Otorhinolaryngol Relat Spec* 1992; 54(1):49-53.
6. Gotta AW, Ferrari LR, Sullivan CA: Anesthesia for otolaryngologic surgery. In *Clinical Anesthesia*, 5th edition. Barash PG, Cullen BF, Stoelting RK, eds. Lippincott Williams and Wilkins, Philadelphia: 2001, 989-1004.
7. Hill RS, Koltai PJ, Parnes SM: Airway complications from laryngoscopy and panendoscopy. *Ann Otol Rhinol Laryngol* 1987; 96(6):691-4.
8. Kirk GA: Anesthesia for ear, nose, and throat surgery. In *Principles and Practice of Anesthesiology*. Rogers MC, Tinker JH, Covino BG, Longnecker DE, eds. Mosby-Year Book, St. Louis: 1993, 2257-74.
9. Loré JM: *An Atlas of Head and Neck Surgery*, 3rd edition. WB Saunders, Philadelphia: 1988.
10. Lyon ST, Holinger LD: Endoscopic evaluation of the patient with head and neck cancer. *Clin Plast Surg* 1985; 12(3): 331-41.
11. Pollard BJ: ENT surgery. In *Handbook of Clinical Anesthesia*. Goldstone JC, Pollard BJ, eds. Churchill Livingstone, New York: 1996, 301-13.
12. Rampil IJ: Anesthetic considerations for laser surgery. *Anesth Analg* 1992; 74:424-35.
13. Sosis MB: Anesthesia for laser airway surgery. In *Airway Management: Principles and Practice*. Benumof JL, ed. Mosby-Year Book, St. Louis: 1996:698-735.

NASAL SURGERY

(RHINOPLASTY, SEPTOPLASTY, SEPTORHINOPLASTY)

SURGICAL CONSIDERATIONS

Description: Nasal surgery is performed for either cosmetic or functional restoration of the airway, or both. Functional restoration is usually performed for either congenital or posttraumatic deviations of the septum. The procedure varies in each case, although in all nasal surgery, the nasal cavity is first cocainized with 4% cocaine-soaked pledgets placed in each nostril for 5-10 min. **Septoplasty** (reconstruction of the nasal septum) usually can be carried out under sedation with local anesthesia, using 1% lidocaine with 1:100,000 epinephrine. **Rhinoplasty-septorhinoplasty** usually is carried out under local anesthesia, but if GA is used, a mouth pack is inserted. Local infiltration with 1% lidocaine with 1:100,000 epinephrine is used to ensure vasoconstriction and to minimize bleeding. Intranasal incisions are made and septal problems corrected. Generally, an anterior hemitransfixion incision is made down to the cartilage, and a submucoperichondrial flap is elevated the length of the septum. A similar flap may be elevated on the contralateral side. Bony deformities are resected with an osteotome, while cartilaginous deformities are either resected or weakened by morselizing, either in situ or after removal, and then replaced. The incision is closed with interrupted absorbable sutures. In **rhinoplasty**, tip remodelling, hump reduction, and bony osteotomies are performed to remodel the nasal contour. Surgery on the inferior turbinates in the form of intramural cautery, resection of turbinate bone, resection of turbinate mucosa or, in some cases, complete turbinectomy may be required to produce a satisfactory airway. After the surgery is complete, both nasal cavities are packed and external splints may be used for rhinoplasty and septorhinoplasty cases.

Usual preop diagnosis: Nasal deformity or deviation; deviated septum

SUMMARY OF PROCEDURE

Position	Head up 30° to ↓ bleeding. Table may be turned 90°-180°.
Incision	Intranasal, usually; extended only in open septorhinoplasty
Unique considerations	Nose initially cocainized; use of 1% lidocaine with 1:100,000 epinephrine to ↓ bleeding.
Antibiotics	Cefazolin 1 g iv; routinely used as long as nasal packs are in place.
Surgical time	1-2.5 h
Closing considerations	Nose often packed postop, necessitating oral airway after extubation.
EBL	50-100 ml (excessive blood loss rare)

Postop care	PACU
Mortality	Minimal
Morbidity	Septal perforation: 5%
	Bleeding: 4%
	Infection: 4%
Pain score	4-6

PATIENT POPULATION CHARACTERISTICS

Age range	Young teens–young adults
Male:Female	1:1
Incidence	Common
Etiology	Congenital/traumatic septal and/or nasal deviation

ANESTHETIC CONSIDERATIONS FOR NASAL SURGERY

PREOPERATIVE

These cases typically are performed on an outpatient basis. Most patients are young and otherwise healthy, but some who are presenting for septoplasty and turbinate reduction surgery may have OSA, with the corresponding implications for intraop management (see p. 197). Older patients may present for major reconstructive surgery following resections of a basal cell carcinoma of the nose. Patients presenting for closed reduction of nasal fractures may have suffered concomitant closed head trauma. If the nose injury is recent, blood may have been swallowed, and the patient should be considered 'full stomach'.

Respiratory	Some patients may present with a Hx of reactive airway disease; their status should be optimized preop. **Tests:** As indicated from H&P.
Cardiovascular	In patients with preexisting cardiac disease, cocaine use by the surgeon for topical anesthesia or control of bleeding may be contraindicated. **Tests:** ECG in older population; others as indicated from H&P.
Premedication	Standard premedication (p. B-3). Sedation should be avoided in patients with OSA.

INTRAOPERATIVE

Anesthetic technique: Septorhinoplasty may be performed under local anesthesia with MAC, although GA is used more commonly. The essential surgical requirements are: patient immobility; clear surgical field (nasal mucosa is extremely vascular); and smooth emergence from anesthesia to avoid postop hemorrhage. GETA or GA with flexible LMA and spontaneous or controlled ventilation can be used in this patient population (see Introduction, pp. 141-142).

Induction	Propofol (1-2 mg/kg) is an ideal induction agent (provides short duration and intrinsic antiemetic effect). Fentanyl, if used, should be limited to 1-2 μg/kg. For GETA, an oral RAE tube will facilitate surgical access.
Maintenance	A balanced inhalational or TIVA technique can be used safely. A moderate degree of ↓BP (see Introduction, p. 142) is essential. Propofol infusion (100-150 μg/min) may offer the advantage of ↓BP without compensatory ↑HR and ↓incidence of PONV. A low-dose remifentanil infusion (0.1-0.2 μg/kg/min) will improve hemodynamic stability and facilitate rapid and smooth emergence from anesthesia. Additional doses of fentanyl are usually not necessary.
Emergence	Emergence from anesthesia after nasal surgery presents significant challenges to the anesthesiologist. Nasal passages may be packed at the end of surgery, making the patients obligate mouth-breathers. The oropharynx should be suctioned carefully, and pressure on the surgical site with the face mask should be avoided. Full return of airway reflexes should occur before extubation, which must be accomplished smoothly, without excessive bucking and coughing. A flexible LMA may be superior to the ETT in this regard.
Blood and fluid requirements	Blood loss usually minimal IV: 20 ga × 1 NS/LR @ 2-3 ml/kg/hr	Blood loss controlled with surgical hemostasis and topical applications of vasoconstrictor (epinephrine), but also may include cocaine.
Monitoring	Standard monitors (p. B-1)	

Positioning	Head elevated 15-30°	Patient's arms usually tucked and carefully padded.
	Table turned 90-180°	
	✓ and pad pressure points.	
	✓ eyes.	For rhinoplasty, patient's eyes should be protected so as to allow for early recognition of an orbital injury. Use scleral shields with eye ointment.
Complications	Tachycardia, dysrhythmias	Usually related to use of vasoconstrictor agents and may present a problem in patients with CAD. Short-acting β-blocker (esmolol, 0.5-1 μg/kg in boluses) should be available to blunt these hemodynamic effects.

POSTOPERATIVE

| **Complications** | Occult postop bleeding | The patient may swallow large quantities of blood (↑ aspiration risk); and repacking the nostrils may be required. |
| **Pain management** | Short-acting iv opioids (e.g., fentanyl, 25-50 μg iv prn) are usually sufficient. | These patients typically have minimal immediate postop pain 2° local anesthetic in the surgical field. |

References

1. Niechajev I, Haraldsson PO: Two methods of anesthesia for rhinoplasty in outpatient setting. *Aesthetic Plast Surg* 1996; 20(2): 159-63.
2. Sheen JH: *Aesthetic Rhinoplasty*, 2nd edition. Sheen JH, Sheen AD, eds. CV Mosby, St. Louis: 1987.
3. Toriumi DM: Surgical correction of the aging nose. *Facial Plast Surg* 1996; 12(2):205-14.
4. Webster AC, Morley-Foster PK, Janzen V, Watson J, et al: Anesthesia for intranasal surgery: a comparison between tracheal intubation and the flexible reinforced laryngeal mask airway. *Anesth Analg* 1999; 88:421-5.

Also see General References for Nasal and Sinus Surgery, p. 160.

EXTERNAL SINUS SURGERY

SURGICAL CONSIDERATIONS

Winston C. Vaughan

Description: Sinus surgery is performed to eliminate infection, polyps, or neoplastic conditions that result in obstruction of the sinuses → secondary infection. Providing aeration of the sinuses so that mucous secretion can adequately drain into the nose and nasopharynx is the goal. The patient should be intubated orally and the pharynx may be packed. Nasal mucosa often is cocainized (4% cocaine), and a local injection of 1% lidocaine with 1:100,000 epinephrine is given before making incisions. **Endoscopic sinus surgery** (see p. 157) is carried out intranasally using endoscopes with a video monitor. Biting forceps are used to remove polyps, diseased mucosa, or biopsy material.

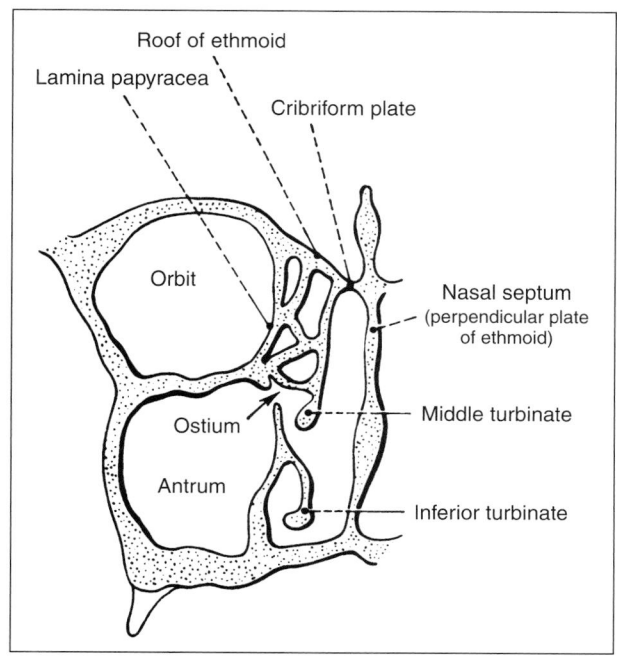

Figure 3-5. Diagrammatic representation of the relationships of the orbit, maxillary antrum, ethmoid labyrinth, and nasal cavity. Note that the medial wall of the ethmoid labyrinth is an upper extension of the attachment of the middle turbinate. The attachment of the upper extension separates the roof of the ethmoid and the cribriform plate. (Reproduced with permission from Montgomery WW: *Surgery of the Upper Respiratory System*, 3rd edition. Williams & Wilkins, 1996.)

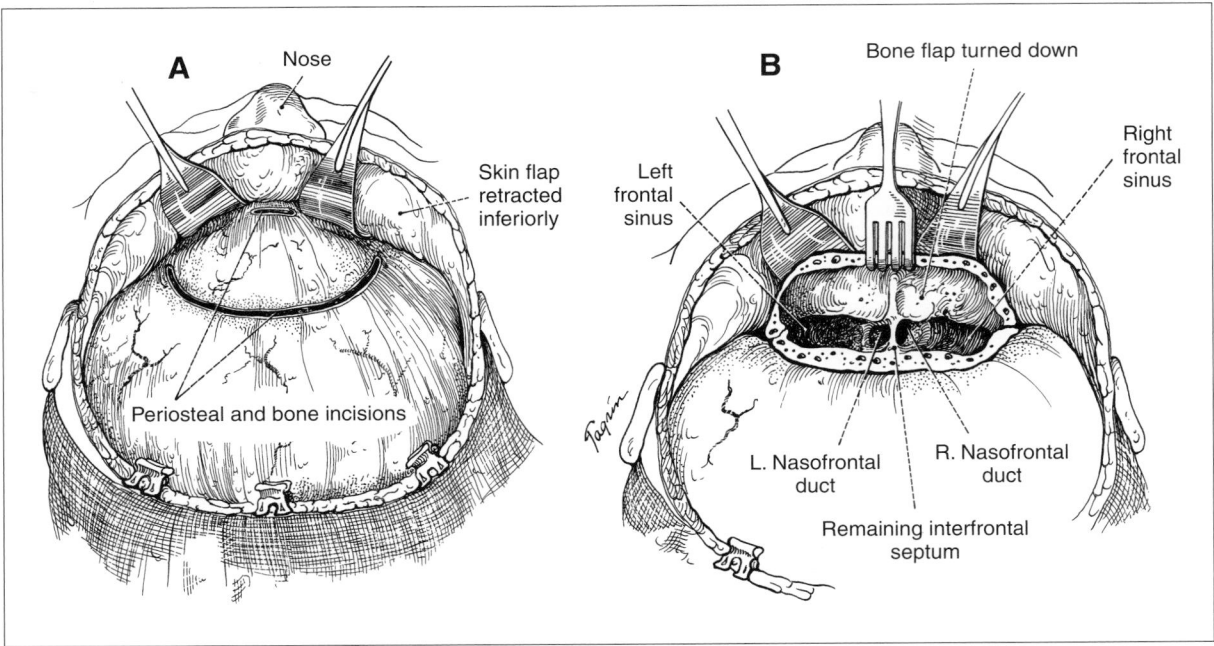

Figure 3-6. Bilateral osteoplastic operation. (A) Coronal flap has been reflected inferiorly. It is important for the periosteum and bone incisions to include the supraorbital rim medially and laterally on each side. (B) Osteoplastic flap has been elevated, exposing the contents of both frontal sinuses. (Reproduced with permission from Montgomery WW: *Surgery of the Upper Respiratory System*, 3rd edition. Williams & Wilkins, 1996.)

External approaches include: **Caldwell-Luc** (a sub-labial approach to the maxillary sinus), **transantral ethmoidectomy**, **external ethmoidectomy**, **transseptal sphenoidectomy**, and **frontal osteoplastic flap** via coronal or brow incision. These procedures accomplish the same end as endoscopic sinus surgery; however, they involve external incisions and tend to be done for persistent diseases that recur despite intranasal surgery. The **Caldwell-Luc** is performed through an intraoral incision in the gingival-buccal sulcus just posterior to the canine fossa. A submucoperiosteal flap is elevated superiorly, exposing the infraorbital nerve. The sinus is entered just inferior to this nerve using a small osteotome. The opening is widened with biting forceps, and the mucosal lining of the diseased sinus usually is exenterated. Typically, a nasoantral window is placed through the inferior meatus to allow additional drainage. The gingival-buccal incision is then closed with interrupted absorbable sutures. External methods also may be the preferred approaches to deal with neoplastic conditions. A craniofacial **combined neurosurgical-external sinus approach** occasionally is required to clear extensive neoplastic nasal and sinus disease. After endoscopic or external sinus surgery, the nose/sinus usually is packed; thus, an oral airway will aid postop mouth breathing on extubation until patient is fully awake.

Usual preop diagnosis: Infection; nasal polyps; neoplasia (benign or malignant)

SUMMARY OF PROCEDURE

Position	Head up 30° (minimizes bleeding). Table may be turned 90°-180°.
Incision	Endoscopic: intranasal. External: sublabial, medial orbital, or bicoronal.
Special instrumentation	Nasal endoscopes; video monitor setup; microscope (may be used for external approaches).
Unique considerations	Nose may be packed bilaterally, necessitating use of oral airway on emergence. 1% lidocaine with 1:100,000 epinephrine normally used to ↓ bleeding.
Antibiotics	Cefazolin 1 g iv
Surgical time	1-3 h
EBL	50-300 ml (excessive blood loss rarely anticipated). Watch suction bottle and measure irrigation.
Postop care	PACU
Mortality	Minimal
Morbidity	Bleeding: 4%
	Infection: 4%
Pain score	2-4 (4-6 for external approaches)

PATIENT POPULATION CHARACTERISTICS

Age range	Children–adults
Male:Female	1:1
Incidence	Common
Etiology	Infectious; allergic; neoplastic
Associated conditions	Asthma patients most often will benefit from sinus surgery, with reduction in the incidence and/or severity of asthmatic attacks. Rarely, surgery itself may precipitate an asthmatic attack on emergence or in the immediate postop period. Cystic fibrosis patients may be assisted by postop bronchoscopy at the termination of procedure to facilitate pulmonary toilet in the immediate postop period.

ANESTHETIC CONSIDERATIONS

See Anesthetic Considerations following Endoscopic Sinus Surgery, p. 158.

ENDOSCOPIC SINUS SURGERY

SURGICAL CONSIDERATIONS

Winston C. Vaughan

Description: Sinus surgery is performed most often for the management of chronic sinus disease, nasal polyps, and recurrent sinus infections, or for neoplastic conditions that may → obstruction of the sinus cavities. This includes either external procedures, through the skin or oral cavity, or endoscopic approaches, through the nostrils. The endoscopic approach—the preferred technique for most surgeons—is called **endoscopic sinus surgery (ESS)** or **functional endoscopic sinus surgery (FESS)**. Other surgical procedures—including septoplasty; turbinate reduction; and, occasionally, sleep apnea surgery involving the tonsils, palate, and oropharynx—may be combined with FESS.

Endoscopic Sinus Surgery: Providing openings (drainage, aeration) to the sinus cavities and obtaining tissue for pathological evaluation are the main aims of ESS. Patients are orally intubated and small sponges (throat pack) can be placed in the pharynx to decrease the amount of blood swallowed. Oral gastric tubes are recommended if more than minimal bleeding is expected. LMA also may be used in these procedures if no oropharyngeal surgeries are planned. Following induction of anesthesia, local medications are applied to the nasal cavity, including injection of 1% lidocaine with 1: 100,000 epinephrine and/or topical application of 4% cocaine. It is important that these local medications be noted in the anesthesia record, as complications (HTN, dysrhythmias, Sz) from local application have been reported. Patients with a Hx of illicit cocaine use should be warned of potential drug interactions, and the intraop use of vasoactive drugs should be limited to avoid unexpected cardiovascular events.

Intranasal endoscopes and endoscopic instruments are used to remove tissue and widen passages. Biopsies, cultures, irrigation, and suctioning of the sinus cavities are performed. At the end of the procedure, packing may be placed. It is imperative that the pharyngeal or throat pack be removed before the end of the procedure.

Sinus surgical procedures may use **image guidance or surgical navigation tools**. These computer-assisted techniques involve a preop CT or MRI scan to create a navigational map for the surgeon to localize disease, normal tissues, and the boundaries of the surgical dissection. Surrounding the sinuses are several vital structures, including the periorbital tissues (e.g., orbital muscles, lacrimal apparatus, and the optic nerve); the sphenopalatine artery; the ethmoid arteries and their branches; as well as the skull base (CSF leak, meningitis, pneumocephalus).

Variant procedure or approaches: For **external approaches** to sinus surgery, see External Sinus Surgery, p. 155.

Usual preop diagnosis: Nasal polyps; chronic sinusitis; recurrent acute sinus infections; benign and malignant tumors; inverting papilloma; management of previous surgical complications (e.g., repair of CSF leak, lacrimal duct injury, and persistent or remnant ethmoid cells, scar tissue formation)

SUMMARY OF PROCEDURE

Position	Head of bed elevated 10-30° (↓ bleeding); table turned 90-180°; arms tucked; TEDs and SCDs, if surgery > 2 h.
Incision	Intranasal with dissection between the middle turbinate and the sinonasal cavities. Some procedures may include both endoscopic and external approaches.
Special instrumentation	Nasal endoscopes; video monitors; recording equipment; occasionally, microscopes; surgical navigation system
Unique considerations	Nasal cavity may be packed (→ obligate mouth breathing). Injection of vasoconstrictor ± topical cocaine → ↑BP + dysrhythmias + Sz. If a stereotactic headset for surgical navigation is placed, it should be released at intervals to improve blood flow to the areas over which it is clamped.
Antibiotics	Cefazolin 1 g iv, especially in patients with valvular heart disease
Surgical time	1-5 h (depending on extent of disease)
EBL	50-500 ml
Postop care	PACU. ✓ eyes and vision. Discharge to home usually within 2 h. It is important that these patients are aware of the possibility of postop intracranial, orbital, or bleeding complications.
Morbidity	Bleeding: < 5%
	Infection: < 5%
	Meningitis
	Brain abscess
	Subdural hematoma
	Orbital/ocular trauma
Pain Score	1-2 (maxillary and ethmoid)
	4-6 (extensive ethmoid, frontal, and sphenoid sinus)
	6-8 (external surgical procedures)

PATIENT POPULATION CHARACTERISTICS

Age range	Children and adults
Male:Female	1:1
Incidence	~35 million Americans suffer from chronic sinus disease. Sinus surgical interventions are increasingly more common, second only to procedures for tonsils, adenoids, and PE tubes.
Etiology	Infectious; 'allergic'; neoplastic
Associated conditions	Asthma (20-30%); GERD; cystic fibrosis; Triad (Samter's) disease with aspirin allergy; nasal polyps. (Avoid NSAIDs and Toradol.)

ANESTHETIC CONSIDERATIONS FOR EXTERNAL AND FUNCTIONAL ENDOSCOPIC SINUS SURGERY

PREOPERATIVE

The majority of these procedures are performed on an outpatient basis. Patients with extensive polypoid disease or active infection, and those presenting for revision surgery, may have significant blood loss (> 400 ml). Many will have received a short preop course of steroid therapy to ↓ tissue swelling and reduce bleeding intraop. Routine intraop administration of Decadron 8-12 mg (to minimize postop edema) makes an additional stress-dose of glucocorticoids unnecessary.

Respiratory	Many patients with nasal polyposis have a high incidence of reactive airway disease (up to 26%) and hypersensitivity to aspirin, which can → bronchospasm (triad patients). In these patients, NSAIDs, including ketorolac, should be avoided. (In general, ketorolac administration for postop pain relief is not recommended in these patients because it may affect microvascular bleeding.) **Tests:** CXR, as indicated by H&P.
Cardiovascular	See Anesthetic Considerations for Nasal Surgery, p. 154.
Premedication	Standard premedication (p. B-2). Sedation should be avoided in patients with OSA.

INTRAOPERATIVE

Anesthetic technique: **FESS** can be performed under local anesthesia with sedation (MAC) or GA. The essential surgical requirements are similar to those for other types of nasal surgery (above), though more meticulous control of intraop BP is essential. Local anesthesia offers the advantage of reduced blood loss, but GETA is performed more frequently and may be associated with a ↓incidence of surgical complications. Patients with extensive sinus disease, Hx of multiple previous nasal and sinus surgeries, reactive airway disease, or labile HTN may not be candidates for MAC. Use of a flexible LMA instead of an ETT offers significant advantages (see Introduction), including ↓airway reactivity and ↑mucociliary clearance. As with other types of nasal surgery, immediate postop pain is minimal as the result of local anesthesia by the surgeon.

Induction	Same as for nasal surgery (p. 154). The patient's eyes should be protected in a manner that allows the surgeon to observe and palpate the eyes for signs of intraorbital hemorrhage (e.g., ecchymosis, chemosis, and proptosis).	
Maintenance	Same as for nasal surgery (p. 154). A propofol infusion may provide superior operating conditions, compared with inhalational anesthetics, especially in the ethmoid and sphenoid sinuses. β-blockade is preferred over SNP for maintaining ↓BP in the quality of the surgical field. Break-through adrenergic responses occur more frequently with FESS than with other types of nasal surgery, because many reflexogenic areas (e.g., skull base) cannot be blocked by local anesthetic injection. These responses can be effectively controlled by vasoactive agents (see Introduction, p. 142) or additional boluses of short-acting opioid (e.g. remifentanil 0.5-1.0 μg/kg). The anesthesiologist should observe the video monitor frequently for signs of possible complications, such as prolapse of periorbital fat (orbital injury) and 'wash-out' of blood in the surgical field (CSF leak).	
Emergence	See Anesthetic Considerations for Nasal Surgery (p. 154). If a dural injury has occurred, a smooth extubation is mandatory.	
Blood and fluid requirements	Blood loss generally 100-150 ml IV: 20 ga × 1 (low-risk) 18 ga × 1 (high-risk) NS/LR @ 3-4 ml/kg/h	Blood loss can be substantial in high-risk patients (as described above).
Monitoring	Standard monitors (p. B-1)	
Positioning	Head elevated 15-30° Table turned 90°-180° ✓ and pad pressure points, eyes.	Patient's arms usually tucked and carefully padded.
Complications	Dysrhythmias Tachycardia	Usually related to use of vasoconstrictor agents; may be a problem in patients with CAD. Short-acting β-blocker should be available to blunt these hemodynamic effects.

POSTOPERATIVE

Complications	Occult postop bleeding	The patient may swallow large quantities of blood; repacking the nostrils may be required.
Pain management	Short-acting iv opioids (e.g., fentanyl) are usually sufficient.	These patients typically have minimal immediate postop pain, 2° local anesthetic in the surgical field. Occasionally, pain after FESS may be significant. If external approaches to the sinuses were utilized, higher doses of opioids may be necessary.

References for Sinus Surgery

1. Anderhuber W, Walch C, Nemeth E, Semmelrock HJ, Berghold A, Ranftl G, Stammberger H: Plasma adrenaline concentrations during functional endoscopic sinus surgery. *Laryngoscope* 1999; 109(2 Pt 1):204-7.
2. Boezaart AP, Van der Merwe J, Coetzee A: Comparison of sodium nitroprusside- and esmolol-induced hypotension for functional endoscopic sinus surgery. *Can J Anesth* 1995; 42(5):373-6.
3. Gittelman PD, Jacobs JB, Skorina J: Comparison of functional endoscopic sinus surgery under local and general anesthesia. *Ann Otol Rhinol Laryngol* 1993; 102:289-93.
4. Kennedy DA, Senior BA: Endoscopic sinus surgery: a review. *Otolaryngol Clin North Am* 1997; 30(3):313-30.
5. Kinsella JB, Calhoun KH, Bradfield JJ, Hokanson JA, et al: Complications of endoscopic sinus surgery in a residency training program. *Laryngoscope* 1995; 105:1029-32.

6. May M, Levine HL, Mester SJ, Schaitkin B: Complications of endoscopic sinus surgery: analysis of 2108 patients—incidence and prevention. *Laryngoscope* 1994; 104:1080-3.

7. Pavlin JD, Colley PS, Weymuller EA, Norman GV, et al: Propofol vs isoflurane for endoscopic sinus surgery. *Am J Otolaryngol* 1999; 20(2):96-101.

8. Riegle EV, Gunter JB, Lusk RP, Muntz HR, Weiss KL: Comparison of vasoconstrictors for functional endoscopic sinus surgery in children. *Laryngoscope* 1992; 102(7):820-3.

General References for Nasal and Sinus Surgery

1. Abdulatif M: Sodium nitroprusside induced hypotension: haemodynamic response and dose requirements during propofol or halothane anaesthesia. *Anaesth Intens Care* 1994; 22:155-60.

2. Asai T, Murao K, Yukawa H, Shingu K: Re-evaluation of appropriate size of the laryngeal mask airway. *Br J Anaesth* 1999; 83(3):478-9.

3. Brimacombe JR: Positive pressure ventilation with the size 5 laryngeal mask. *J Clin Anesth* 1997; 9:113-7.

4. Brimacombe JR, Brain, AJ: *The Laryngeal Mask Airway: A Review and Practical Guide*. WB Saunders, London: 1997.

5. Brown B: Anaesthesia for ear, nose, throat and maxillofacial procedures. In *International Practice of Anaesthesia*. Prys-Roberts C, Brown BR, eds. Butterworth-Heinemann, Oxford: 1996, 2-9.

6. Illing L, Duncan PG, Yip R: Gastroesophageal reflux during anesthesia. *Can J Anesth* 1992; 39(5):466-70.

7. Kirk GA: Anesthesia for ear, nose, and throat surgery. In *Principles and Practice of Anesthesiology*. Rogers MC, Tinker JH, Covino BG, Longnecker DE, eds. Mosby-Year Book, St. Louis: 1993, 2257-74.

8. Nair MB, Bailey PM: Review of uses of the laryngeal mask in ENT anesthesia. *Anaesthesia* 1995; 50:898-900.

9. Ng A, Smith G: Gastroesophageal reflux and aspiration of gastric contents in anesthetic practice. *Anesth Analg* 2001; 93:494-513.

10. Pollard BJ: ENT surgery. In *Handbook of Clinical Anesthesia*. Goldstone JC, Pollard BJ, eds. Churchill Livingstone, New York: 1996, 301-13.

11. Rice DH, Schaefer SD: *Endoscopic Paranasal Surgery*. Raven Press, New York: 1988.

12. Rontal M, Rontal E, Anon JB: An anatomic approach to local anesthesia for surgery of the nose and paranasal sinuses. *Otolaryngol Clin North Am* 1997; 30(3):403-20.

13. Van Den Berg AA, Savva D, Honjol NM, Rama Prabhu NV: Comparison of total intravenous, balanced inhalational and combined intravenous-inhalational anaesthesia for tympanoplasty, septorhinoplasty and adenotonsillectomy. *Anaesth Intens Care* 1995; 23:574-82.

14. Vaughan, WC: Medical and surgical management of polypoid rhinosinusitis. *Opin in Otolaryngol, Head Neck Surg* 2000; 8:11-17.

15. Webster AC, Morley-Foster PK, Janzen V, Watson J, et al: Anesthesia for intranasal surgery: a comparison between tracheal intubation and the flexible reinforced laryngeal mask airway. *Anesth Analg* 1999; 88:421-5.

16. Williams PJ, Thompsett C, Bailey PM: Comparison of the reinforced laryngeal mask airway and tracheal intubation for nasal surgery. *Anaesthesia* 1995; 50:987-9.

EAR SURGERY

SURGICAL CONSIDERATIONS

Description: Surgery on the external ear is performed for reconstruction of a congenitally deformed ear or following trauma and, therefore, may involve multiple cosmetic procedures. More commonly, surgery is performed to restore hearing, eliminate infections, remove cholesteatoma, or for neoplastic conditions. The surgical approaches, techniques, and instrumentation are highly variable and individualized, according to the surgeon; however, anesthesia for ear surgery is relatively generic. Since the facial nerve travels in the temporal bone, most surgeons do not want the patient paralyzed, so that they can either observe or monitor facial nerve function intraop. If **tympanoplasty** (repair of the ear drum) or a **tympanomeatal flap** is being created (as in the case of **stapedotomy** or **stapedectomy**), N_2O is not used. This is to prevent pressurization of the middle ear space, which leads to displacement of either the tympanic membrane or the graft. There are many approaches to the **middle ear**, but, basically, the procedures are performed via a transcanal approach, using the microscope, or from a postauricular approach, through the mastoid. A myringotomy typically is made in radial fashion in the anterior/inferior quadrant of the tympanic membrane and fluid liberated with a suction. If long-term ventilation is indicated, a tympanostomy tube is placed with the flange on the medial and lateral surface of the tympanic membrane. In most cases, these procedures can be performed using mask GA. **Exploratory tympanotomy** begins with injection of 2% lidocaine, 1:20,000 of epinephrine, followed by a curved incision along the posterior external auditory canal. The canal skin and the tympanic membrane are elevated forward to expose the middle ear contents, which can be approached either through the canal, or by a postauricular approach. A tympanic membrane perforation can be repaired by placing a temporalis fascia graft, while abnormalities in the ossicular chain can be repaired with a prosthesis. Gelfoam is frequently placed in the middle ear, and the tympanic membrane is returned to its anatomic position. The external canal is likewise packed with Gelfoam. A postauricular approach usually is employed for a **simple mastoidectomy**. After gaining exposure of the mastoid cortex, a large

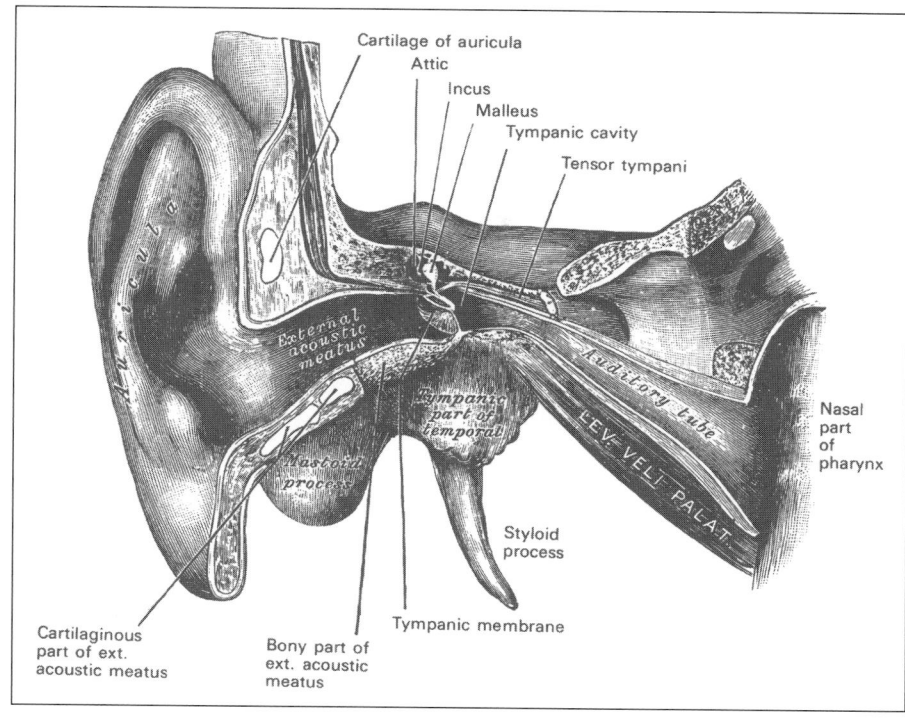

Figure 3-7. External and middle ear, opened anteriorly, right side. (Reproduced with permission from Clemente CD, ed: *Gray's Anatomy of the Human Body*, 30th American edition. Williams & Wilkins, 1985.)

burr is used to drill away the diseased mastoid air cells, exposing the facial nerve, the semicircular canals, and the middle ear space. The incision is closed and a mastoid dressing applied. A **modified radical mastoidectomy** is similar to a **simple mastoidectomy**, except that the posterior wall of the external auditory canal is removed, so that the mastoid can be visualized through the external canal during postop visits. Finally, a **radical mastoidectomy** includes not only removal of the posterior external canal, but of the tympanic membrane, malleus, and incus as well. This surgery is rarely performed. Glomus tumors may extend into the neck and require both a transmastoid and a transcervical approach. Removal of large glomus tumors may → rapid and profound blood loss (> 1000 ml) and require intraarterial monitoring and the ability to provide rapid transfusion. (Middle ear anatomy is shown in Fig 3-7.)

Usual preop diagnosis: Congenitally deformed ear; conductive hearing loss; chronic otitis media ± perforation of the tympanic membrane; cholesteatoma; neoplasia; trauma

SUMMARY OF PROCEDURE

Position	Supine
Incision	Postauricular, endaural, or transcanal
Special instrumentation	Ear instruments; microscope; occasionally laser; microdrill
Unique considerations	Facial nerve monitoring or observation; therefore, no muscle relaxation. D/C N_2O 30 min before laying down tympanic membrane graft.
Antibiotics	Varies with situation and type of surgery.
Surgical time	1.5-4 h
EBL	Negligible for most; the rare exception is excision of glomus tumors (mentioned above).
Mortality	Minimal
Morbidity	The incidence of these complications varies according to type of surgery and primary pathology: Infection Vertigo Sensorineural hearing loss Facial nerve paralysis Perilymph fistula
Pain score	2–6, depending on extent of surgery

PATIENT POPULATION CHARACTERISTICS

Age range	Infants–adults
Male:Female	1:1
Incidence	Common
Etiology	Infectious; traumatic; congenital; neoplastic

ANESTHETIC CONSIDERATIONS FOR EAR SURGERY

PREOPERATIVE

Patients presenting for ear surgery are generally young and healthy and most procedures are performed on an outpatient basis. Communicating with these patients may be difficult 2° ↓hearing ability. Myringotomy and pressure equalization tube insertion are very short procedures. In contrast, ossicular reconstruction and tympanic membrane reconstruction with facial nerve preservation may last several h. Patients presenting for external ear reconstructions may be associated with other congenital abnormalities, which should be considered preop.

Respiratory	Patients may present with Sx of concurrent URI (see Anesthetic Considerations for Tonsillectomy, Adenoidectomy, p. 144). **Tests:** As indicated from H&P.
Cardiovascular	No special considerations **Tests:** ECG in older population.
Laboratory	Tests as indicated from H&P.
Premedication	Standard premedication (p. B-2)

INTRAOPERATIVE

Anesthetic technique: GETA or GA through a LMA. The essential surgical requirements are absence of patient movement (muscle relaxation is frequently contraindicated 2° facial nerve monitoring), a clear surgical field, smooth emergence from anesthesia to avoid straining, and rapid awakening to assess facial nerve function. The incidence of PONV can be as high as 80% after tympanomastoid surgery if no antiemetic prophylaxis is given. Administration of 5-HT$_3$-blockers should be routine and may be enhanced by the addition of dexamethasone (see Anesthesia for Tonsillectomy, p. 144). LMA use in children undergoing myringotomy and PE tube placement may be associated with ↓incidence of intraop hypoxemia and better operating conditions compared with use of standard face mask technique. Use of LMA is beneficial for major ear surgery (minimizes risk of coughing, gagging, and straining on emergence, which may displace grafts). FLMA normally is used with PPV (see Introduction, for discussion of the safe use of LMA with PPV, p. 142). Postop pain is usually mild-to-moderate, but can be minimal (e.g., laser stapedectomy) or severe (e.g., mastoidectomy).

Induction	Opioid-based techniques (see Introduction, p. 141) are desirable for major ear surgery; induction and maintenance doses of opioids can be reduced safely if a FLMA is used. Propofol may be the preferred agent 2° its intrinsic antiemetic effect.
Maintenance	Both TIVA and inhalational agents can be used for maintenance. Compared to isoflurane, patients receiving propofol-based anesthetic (see Anesthetic Considerations for Nasal Surgery, p. 154) may recover faster and have ↓incidence of PONV. Moderate ↓BP (see Introduction, p. 142) is essential. Intermediate or long-acting muscle relaxants should be avoided if facial nerve monitoring is used. N$_2$O, if used, should not exceed 50% concentration and must be D/C'd at least 15 min before tympanic membrane graft placement.
Emergence	At the end of the procedure, the patient's head may be moved during dressing application → gagging or bucking. Smooth emergence from anesthesia is mandatory. If postextubation laryngospasm occurs, the use of CPAP may unseat the tympanic membrane graft or disrupt other repairs.
Blood and fluid requirements	IV: 18-20 ga × 1 NS/LR @ 3-4 ml/kg/h	Blood loss is usually minimal in these cases.
Control of bleeding	Head-up position (10-15°) Injection of epinephrine-containing solutions by surgeon Deliberate moderate ↓BP	These special considerations are applicable to microscopic surgical procedures, where even the smallest quantity of blood may interfere with visualization.

Monitoring	Standard monitors (p. B-1)	
Positioning	✓ and pad pressure points. ✓ eyes. ✓ opposite ear.	Surgeon may request unobstructed access to the head. Under those circumstances, a RAE or anode tube should be used to secure airway.

POSTOPERATIVE

Complications	PONV Facial nerve injury	Liberal prophylactic use of antiemetics is indicated.
Pain management	Fentanyl (outpatient) Morphine (inpatient)	The use of iv PCA may be appropriate in adults for selected cases.

References

1. Fujii Y, Toyooka H, Tanaka H: Prophylactic antiemetic therapy with a combination of granisetron and dexamethasone in patients undergoing middle ear surgery. *Br J Anaesth* 1998; 81(5):754-6.
2. Glasscock ME: *Surgery of the Ear*, 4th edition. Glasscock ME, Shambaugh GE, eds. WB Saunders, Philadelphia: 1990.
3. Goycoolea MV, Paparella MM, Nissen RL, eds: *Atlas of Otologic Surgery*. WB Saunders, Philadelphia: 1989.
4. Jellish WS, Leonetti JP, Fahey K, Fury P: Comparison of 3 different anesthetic techniques on 24-hour recovery after otologic surgical procedures. *Otolaryngol Head Neck Surg* 1999; 120(3):406-11.
5. Jellish WS, Leonetti JP, Murdoch JR, Fowles S: Propofol-based anesthesia as compared with standard anesthetic techniques for middle ear surgery. *Otolaryngol Head Neck Surg* 1995; 12(2):262-7.
6. Liu YH, Li MJ, Wang PC, Ho ST, et al: Use of dexamethasone on the prophylaxis of nausea and vomiting after tympanomastoid surgery. *Laryngoscope* 2001; 111:1271-4.
7. Munson SE: Transfer of nitrous oxide into body air cavities. *Br J Anaesth* 1974; 46:202-9.
8. Nair MB, Bailey PM: Review of uses of the laryngeal mask in ENT anesthesia. *Anaesthesia* 1995; 50:898-900.
9. Pollard BJ: ENT surgery. In *Handbook of Clinical Anesthesia*. Goldstone JC, Pollard BJ, eds. Churchill Livingstone, New York: 1996, 301-13.
10. Ruby RF, Webster AC, Morley-Forster PK, Dain S: Laryngeal mask airway in paediatric otolaryngologic surgery. *J Otolaryng* 1995; 24:288-91.
11. Wang JJ, Wang PC, Liu YH, Chien CC: Low-dose dexamethasone reduces nausea and vomiting after tympanomastoid surgery: a comparison of tropisetron with saline. *Am J Otol* 2002; 23(5):267-71.
12. Watcha MF, Garner FT, White PF, Lusk R: Laryngeal mask airway vs face mask and Guedel airway during pediatric myringotomy. *Arch Otolaryngol Head Neck Surg* 1994; 120:877-80.

PAROTIDECTOMY: SUPERFICIAL, TOTAL, RADICAL

SURGICAL CONSIDERATIONS

Description: A **superficial parotidectomy** (better called a **supraneural parotidectomy**) removes all of the parotid gland lateral to the facial nerve, dissecting and protecting the facial nerve (Fig 3-8). It usually is performed for a tumor, but occasionally is performed for infectious disorders or to enable the surgeon to approach tumors of the deep lobe. A **total parotidectomy** is performed for either infectious disorders or for tumors that arise in the parotid gland medial to the facial nerve. The integrity of the facial nerve is preserved during total parotidectomy, as long as it is not involved with malignancy. It may be combined with neck dissection (radical or functional) or with modified temporal bone resections when the tumor extends into the ear canal or middle ear or invades the facial nerve at the base of the skull.

A **radical parotidectomy** removes the total parotid gland, together with the facial nerve, which usually is reconstructed with a facial-nerve graft. The mastoid may have to be drilled to get a healthy proximal end of the facial nerve. **Microsurgical techniques** are then used to graft the resected nerve. The graft may be harvested from the opposite greater auricular nerve or the sural nerve may be used.

Usual preop diagnosis: Superficial parotidectomy: benign or malignant tumor of the superficial lobe of the parotid gland; infectious disorders. Total parotidectomy: malignant tumors or benign tumors of the deep lobe of the parotid gland. Radical parotidectomy: invasive malignant parotid tumors.

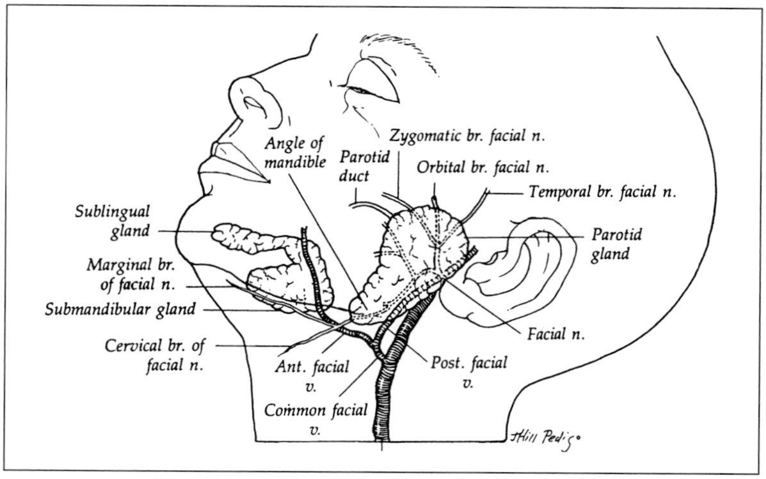

Figure 3-8. Relationship of parotid gland and neurovascular structures. (Reproduced with permission from Ballenger JJ: *Diseases of the Nose, Throat, Ear, Head & Neck.* Lea & Febiger, 1991.)

SUMMARY OF PROCEDURES

	Superficial	Total	Radical
Position	Supine; head turned slightly to opposite side	⇐	⇐
Incision	Preauricular, extending into neck; has many variations, including modified face-lift incision.	⇐	May require postaural extension for mastoid access.
Special instrumentation	Facial nerve stimulator, facial nerve monitor	⇐	⇐ + drill for mastoidectomy; microscope/microsurgical instruments and 9-0 nylon for nerve reanastomosis
Unique considerations	Muscle relaxation is not indicated 2° facial nerve identification. Tape oral ETT to the opposite side of the mandible.	Nasal intubation may be necessary to dislocate mandible anteriorly. Be certain that the ETT is well below vocal cords to allow for anterior dislocation → 1-2 cm of superior ascent of ETT.	⇐
Antibiotics	None or cefazolin 1 g	Cefazolin 1 g	⇐
Surgical time	1.5-2 h	2-4 h	4-6 h
EBL	25-200 ml	200-300 ml	500-700 ml for total parotidectomy, neck dissection, and modified temporal bone resection. Sudden, large blood losses do not occur; transfusion usually not necessary.
Mortality	Very rare	⇐	⇐
Morbidity	Dysesthesia or anesthesia of the greater auricular nerve: 100% (almost all will recover within 1 yr).	⇐	Facial nerve loss: With graft, function returns slowly over 1 yr.
	Facial nerve weakness (temporary): 20-50%	⇐	⇐
	Frey's syndrome: 35% will have measurable gustatory sweating, but only 5% will have clinical symptoms.	⇐	⇐

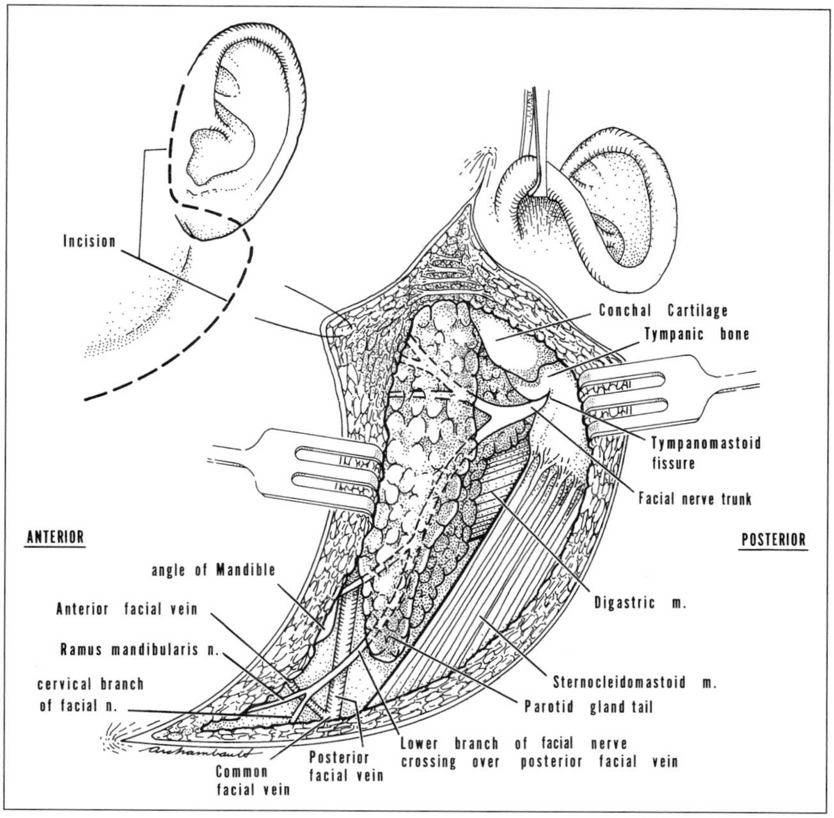

Figure 3-9. Inferior approach to facial nerve. The lower branch of the facial nerve is found immediately external to the posterior facial vein as it exits the lower pole of the parotid gland. The lower branch may divide into the ramus mandibularis and cervical branches before or after crossing the posterior facial vein. The lower branch of the facial nerve is dissected proximally to the facial-nerve trunk. The posterior facial vein should not be confused with the external jugular vein, as the facial vein runs deep to the sterno-cleidomastoid muscle, whereas the external jugular vein lies superficial to this muscle. Elevation of the tail of the parotid gland greatly facilitates this dissection, which must be accomplished in a plane between the posterior facial vein and the parotid gland. (Reproduced with permission from Montgomery WW: *Surgery of the Upper Respiratory System*, 2nd edition. Lea & Febiger, 1989.)

Figure 3-10. The parotid gland has been dissected from the trunk, divisions, and branches of the facial nerve. The anterior projection of the gland has been dissected free, and the parotid duct is being ligated. This dissection is conducted, for the most part, with a hemostat clamp. First, tunnels are created lateral to the branches; and the fascia between tunnels is incised as the gland is dissected forward. The facial-nerve stimulator is a useful adjunct to this dissection. (Reproduced with permission from Montgomery WW: *Surgery of the Upper Respiratory System*, 2nd edition. Lea & Febiger, 1989.)

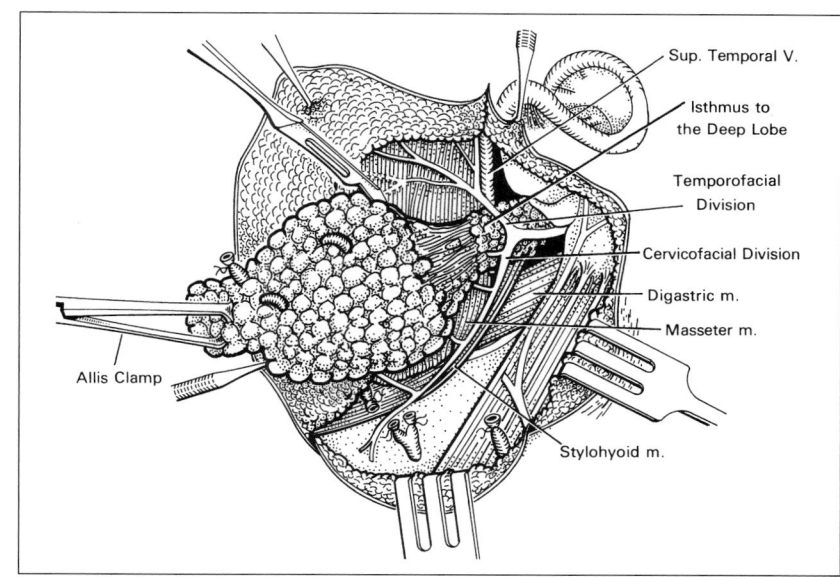

	Superficial	Total	Radical
Morbidity, cont.	Bleeding: 4%	⇐	⇐
	Infection: 4%	⇐	⇐
	Permanent facial nerve paralysis: < 1%		
Pain score	2-3	3-4	4-6

PATIENT POPULATION CHARACTERISTICS

Age range	Infants–old age
Male:Female	1:1
Incidence	Common
Etiology	Benign mixed tumor (pleomorphic adenoma) (75%); variety of low- to high-grade malignant cancers (25%); chronic sialoadenitis (results from ductal strictures and/or stones) (rare)
Associated conditions	Nonspecific

ANESTHETIC CONSIDERATIONS

See Anesthetic Considerations following Submandibular Gland Excision, p. 167.

References

1. Chan Y, Irish JC, Wood SJ, Rotstein LE, Brown DH, Gullane PJ, Lockwood GA: Patient education and informed consent in head and neck surgery. *Arch Otolaryngol Head Neck Surg* 2002; 128(11):1269-74.
2. Lee KJ, Fee WE Jr, Terris DJ: The efficacy of corticosteroids in postparotidectomy facial nerve paresis. *Laryngoscope* 2002; 112(11):1958-63.
3. Terris DJ, Fee WE: Current issues in nerve repair. *Arch Otolaryngol. Head Neck Surg* 1993; 119(7):725-31.
4. Terris DJ, Tuffo KM, Fee WE: Modified facelift incision for parotidectomy. *J Laryngol Otol* 1994; 108:574-8.
5. Thawley SE, Panje WR, eds: *Comprehensive Management of Head and Neck Tumors*. WB Saunders, Philadelphia: 1987.

SUBMANDIBULAR GLAND EXCISION

SURGICAL CONSIDERATIONS

Description: Removal of the submandibular gland is performed for either chronic sialoadenitis due to ductal strictures and/or stones or benign or malignant tumors of the submandibular gland. (General anatomy of the area is shown in Fig 3-11.) The patient lies supine with a pillow under the shoulder, and head turned slightly to the opposite side. A skin crease incision is made below the mandible and skin flaps elevated. The marginal mandibular nerve usually is identified carefully or may

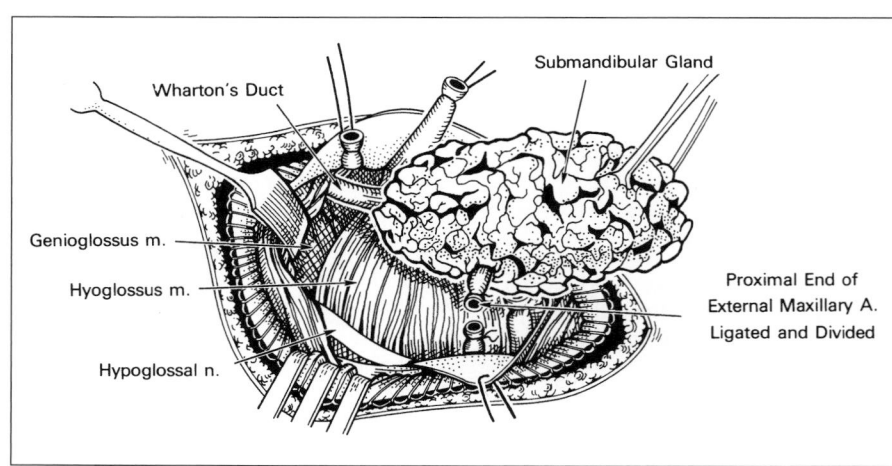

Figure 3-11. Exposure of the submandibular gland. (Reproduced with permission from Montgomery WW: *Surgery of the Upper Respiratory System*, 2nd edition. Lea & Febiger, 1989.)

be avoided by identifying the facial vein and dissecting deep to its plane, employing the **Hayes-Martin maneuver**. Dissection is carried out within the capsule of the submandibular gland, which is then excised and removed. Frozen section usually is performed; and, if necessary, further excision, including a neck dissection for high-grade malignancies, is done.

Variant procedure or approaches: Occasionally, it may be necessary to perform a **neck dissection** (radical or functional) in the case of high-grade malignancy.

Usual preop diagnosis: Chronic sialoadenitis; stones; benign or malignant tumors

SUMMARY OF PROCEDURE

Position	Supine
Incision	Upper neck skin crease
Special instrumentation	Occasionally, facial nerve stimulator
Unique considerations	If surgeon plans to use facial nerve stimulator, muscle relaxation is contraindicated.
Antibiotics	Usually not indicated
Surgical time	0.5-1 h
EBL	25 ml (400 ml if neck dissection is done)
Postop care	PACU → room or home
Mortality	Minimal
Morbidity	Marginal mandibular nerve paresis or paralysis: 20%
	Bleeding: 4%
	Infection: 4%
	Lingual dysesthesia: 1%
	XIIth nerve paresis or paralysis: < 1%
Pain score	2-4

PATIENT POPULATION CHARACTERISTICS

Age range	Unlimited
Male:Female	1:1
Incidence	Rare
Etiology	Chronic infection
	Neoplasia: ~60% of tumors are benign, with the remaining being low- and high-grade malignancies.
Associated conditions	Nonspecific

ANESTHETIC CONSIDERATIONS

(Procedures covered: parotidectomy, submandibular gland excision)

PREOPERATIVE

The majority of these patients are > 40 yr, and any coexisting medical conditions should be fully evaluated. Diseases of the parotid gland have been associated with the abuse of alcohol and with autoimmune disease (e.g., Mikulicz-Sjögren syndrome); therefore, Sx of these conditions should be sought.

Respiratory	Airway may be affected by impaired mouth opening or parotid gland enlargement. Patients with involvement of the masseter muscle may present with trismus.
	Tests: As indicated from H&P.
Neurological	Surgical approach to the parotid gland will place the facial nerve at jeopardy; any preop facial nerve deficits should be documented. Also see Preoperative Considerations for Laryngoscopy/Bronchoscopy/Esophagoscopy, p. 149.
	Tests: As indicated from H&P.
Hematologic	Submandibular and parotid malignancies may be associated with chronic debilitation and anemia.
	Tests: CBC; Hb
Laboratory	Other tests as indicated from H&P. Liver panel and coags in patients with Hx of chronic ETOH abuse.
Premedication	Standard premedication (p. B-2)

INTRAOPERATIVE

Anesthetic technique: GETA is most commonly used. Use of a FLMA also has been advocated, but does not represent the author's preference (distorted surgical anatomy 2° inflated FLMA cuff). The FLMA also may be displaced 2° surgical manipulations or intrusion into the submandibular space. These procedures involve meticulous surgical dissection and are characterized by 'layered' stimulation: alternation of (relatively long) stable level of surgical stimulation, with sudden adrenergic responses when surgery progresses into deeper layers. (For essential surgical requirements, see Introduction, p. 142.) Emergence should be rapid enough to allow patient cooperation for assessment of facial nerve function. The anesthesiologist should inquire about the surgeon's preference for muscle relaxation before induction. Patients after submandibular gland resection frequently are discharged home the same day, while patients who had parotidectomy are admitted to the ward.

Induction	Opioid-based techniques (see Introduction, p. 141) are beneficial. Propofol (1-2 mg/kg) can be used safely. ETT should be secured on the nonoperative side. Nasal intubation may be requested by the surgeon (inquire preop) to allow full manipulation of the patient's jaw.
Maintenance	Moderate ↓BP (see Introduction, p. 142) can be maintained by an inhalational agent and will greatly improve operating conditions. Anticipate ↑anesthetic requirements in patients with Hx of ETOH abuse. Neuromuscular blockade (if used) should be light-to-moderate to permit intraop reversal, if that becomes necessary.
Emergence	Smooth emergence and absence of reaction to the ETT is obligatory, if facial nerve repair has been performed.
Blood and fluid requirements	EBL typically ~200 ml 3rd spacing is usually minimal. IV: 18 ga × 1 NS/LR @ 3-6 ml/kg/h
Monitoring	Standard monitors (p. B-1)
Positioning	Table usually is rotated 90°-180°. ✓ & pad pressure points. ✓ eyes.

POSTOPERATIVE

Complications	Facial paralysis 2° surgical trauma Notify surgeons.
Pain management	Parenteral opiates (p. C-2) PCA (p. C-3)

References

1. Johns ME, Price JC, Mattox DE: *Atlas of Head and Neck Surgery*. BC Decker, Philadelphia: 1990.
2. Joseph MM: Anesthesia for ear, nose, and throat surgery. In *Principles and Practice of Anesthesiology*, 2nd edition. Longnecker DE, Tinker JH, Morgan GE, eds. Mosby, St. Louis: 1998, 2200-22.
3. Nair MB, Bailey PM: Review of uses of the laryngeal mask in ENT anesthesia. *Anaesthesia* 1995; 50:898-900.
4. Pollard BJ. Head and neck surgery. In *Handbook of Clinical Anesthesia*. Goldstone JC, Pollard BJ, eds. Churchill Livingstone, New York: 1996, 315-28.

NECK DISSECTION: FUNCTIONAL, MODIFIED RADICAL, RADICAL

SURGICAL CONSIDERATIONS

Description: A **radical neck dissection** consists of a complete **cervical lymphadenectomy**, together with the resection of the sternocleido-mastoid muscle, IJ vein, and cranial nerve XI. A **modified neck dissection** is a variation between a functional neck dissection and a radical neck dissection, and includes supraomohyoid neck dissection, posterior neck dissection, anterior neck dissection, etc. A **functional neck dissection** is a complete cervical lymphadenectomy, preserving the sternocleidomastoid muscle, IJ vein, and cranial nerve XI. Neck dissections are seldom performed as isolated surgical procedures; usually they are combined with resection of the primary lesion, which may involve the tongue, pharynx, larynx, etc.

Typically, the neck dissection is performed through one or two horizontal neck incisions—occasionally extending vertically to expose the neck from the mandible down to the clavicle. The procedure usually begins with transection of the sternocleidomastoid muscle at its sternal attachment, if this muscle is to be removed. The IJ vein is isolated, cut, and tied (again, if it is to be removed). The inferior portion of the dissection includes identification and preservation of the brachial plexus, the phrenic nerve, the vagus nerve, and carotid artery. As the dissection specimen is swept superiorly, cervical sensory branches are divided. The accessory nerve (XI) is identified and carefully preserved (Fig 3-12). When the digastric muscle is encountered, the submandibular portion of the dissection is complete. The hypoglossal nerve (XII) and lingual nerve are identified and preserved. The submental triangle may or may not be resected. The specimen is attached at the skull base and after retraction of the digastric muscle, the IJ vein is ligated and cut at the skull base. The sternocleidomastoid muscle is divided at the mastoid and the specimen is removed. Drains are placed posteriorly, and the wound is closed in layers.

Variant procedure or approaches: In a **composite resection** ('**commando**,' a radical neck dissection + partial mandibulectomy ± partial glossectomy), the neck dissection normally is done first, and an attempt is made to keep the neck specimen in continuity with the primary resection. Although the upper limb of the neck incision is commonly extended through the chin and lip to gain exposure to the oral cavity and oropharynx, this is not necessary. A combination of intraoral exposure and external approach

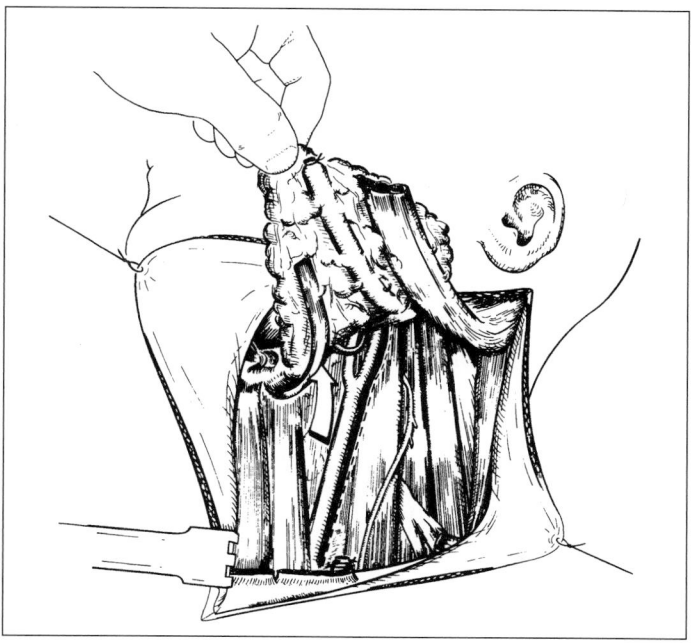

Figure 3-12. Completion of the dissection along the carotid artery elevating the associated lymphoareolar tissue, muscle, and vein. The dotted line marks the course of the vagus nerve, which helps to guide this portion of the dissection. (Reproduced with permission from Baker RJ, Fischer JE: *Mastery of Surgery*, Lippincott Williams & Wilkins, 2001.)

through the neck incision is sufficient to visualize the primary lesion and resect it, usually with a segment of mandible. The resultant defect is closed either primarily, with a split-thickness skin graft, or with a chest flap (pectoralis major or deltopectoral). More recently, free flaps may be brought in for closure and revascularized using the facial artery or superior thyroid artery. A **tracheostomy** is almost always performed as part of a composite resection.

Usual preop diagnosis: Cancer of the mouth, oropharynx or tonsil, with documented or suspected spread from a primary source to the cervical lymph nodes

SUMMARY OF PROCEDURES

	Functional	Modified Radical	Radical
Position	Supine; head turned to opposite side; pillow below shoulders	⇐	⇐
Incision	Various neck incisions (e.g., utility, McFee, lip split, etc.), depending on site of primary.	⇐	⇐
Unique considerations	If neck dissection performed on opposite side, significant laryngeal edema may ensue, necessitating tracheostomy.	If cranial nerve XI is dissected/preserved, nerve stimulator may be needed, so muscle relaxation is undesirable.	Rarely, carotid artery needs to be resected or resected/reconstructed, making vascular instruments desirable.
	Dissection around the carotid bulb may result in profound bradycardia, responsive to local anesthetic injection of the bulb and/or iv atropine.	⇐	⇐
Antibiotics	Cefazolin 1 g iv (+ metronidazole 500 mg if aerodigestive mucosa is involved).	⇐	⇐
Surgical time	Neck dissection: 1.5-3 h With resection of primary and reconstruction: 3-6 h	⇐	⇐

	Functional	**Modified Radical**	**Radical**
EBL	Neck dissection: 150-200 ml	⇐	⇐
	Postradiated patients: 200-400 ml	⇐	⇐
	If primary is also resected: 400-700 ml	⇐	⇐
	If flap reconstructions are required: 700-1200 ml	⇐	⇐ Uncontrolled bleeding of IJ vein at skull base (rare) can result in sudden large blood loss. Usually can be controlled by surgeon with digital pressure, allowing anesthesiologist to prepare for increasing fluid volume or transfusion.
Postop care	Routine ward care for neck dissection; tracheostomy care if opposite neck also dissected. ICU overnight if 6-8 h operating time.	⇐	⇐
Mortality	Rare	⇐	⇐
Morbidity	Bleeding	⇐	⇐
	Infection	⇐	Painful shoulder syndrome: 20%
	Cranial nerve injury	⇐	
	Chyle leak	⇐	
Pain score	4-6 (Depending on 1° site, pain score may be 6-8.)	6-8	6-8

PATIENT POPULATION CHARACTERISTICS

Age range	Adults
Male:Female	3:1
Incidence	Common
Etiology	Head and neck tumors
Associated conditions	COPD; atherosclerosis

ANESTHETIC CONSIDERATIONS

PREOPERATIVE

Most of these patients are older males with a long Hx of smoking and ETOH use and a high incidence of associated cardiopulmonary diseases (see Introduction, p. 141). Nutritional status may be poor and should be optimized before surgery. Neck dissections are lengthy, but are rarely associated with significant blood loss, except in patients who have undergone radiation therapy.

Airway	Airway management may be difficult as a result of limited head and neck mobility; decreased mouth opening; distorted airway; decreased pharyngeal space; and fixation of tissues 2° tumor expansion, radiation fibrosis, or previous surgeries.
	A clearly devised backup plan for airway management is essential; and a review of preop indirect and direct laryngoscopies and/or CT scans may be helpful in planning intubation. If a difficult intubation is foreseen, awake FOI or tracheostomy under local anesthesia may be the techniques of choice (see Anesthetic Considerations for Laryngectomy, p. 149). Emergent tracheostomy may be technically very difficult because of advanced disease, neck edema, previous surgeries, and distorted anatomy.
Respiratory	High incidence of chronic bronchitis and COPD. **Tests:** CXR; others as indicated from H&P. Preop ABG in patients with advanced COPD, CO_2 retention, and O_2 dependence. Flow-volume loops may be helpful in patients with Sx of partial airway obstruction.

Cardiovascular	Careful assessment of cardiac risk factors and functional status. Documenting asymptomatic neck bruits or existing carotid artery stenosis, as well as any Sx of compromised cerebral circulation is important (see Emergence, below). HTN must be controlled preop, especially in patients presenting for radical neck dissection and flap reconstruction. Uncontrolled HTN in these patients carries additional risk of exaggerated hemodynamic responses postop 2° the surgical denervation of the carotid sinus (discussed below). **Tests:** ECG. Consider carotid ultrasound, cardiac stress testing, and imaging studies, if indicated from H&P.
Neurologic	See Preoperative Considerations for Laryngoscopy/Bronchoscopy/Esophagoscopy, p. 148. **Tests:** As indicated from H&P.
Hematologic	In cases of malignancy or chronic disease, anemia or coagulopathies may be present. **Tests:** CBC; coag studies
Laboratory	Liver panel; electrolytes; albumin; BUN; Cr; others as indicated from H&P.
Premedication	Standard premedication (p. B-2). Avoid premedication in patients with symptoms of partial airway obstruction.

INTRAOPERATIVE

Anesthetic technique: GETA. Deep and superficial cervical plexus blocks, as well as a cervical epidural anesthesia, either alone or in combination with light GETA, have been used occasionally. The specific requirements for the anesthetic technique are outlined in the Introduction (p. 141). Straining or coughing/gagging on emergence is particularly undesirable in neck surgery (bleeding and swelling at the surgical site). Smooth emergence from anesthesia is essential, but a FLMA in major neck cancer surgery is dubious (see Anesthetic Considerations for Parotidectomy, Submandibular Gland Excision, p. 167).

Induction	Choice of induction technique will depend on the degree of airway compromise and anatomic location of the obstructing lesion. It is impossible to provide a universal 'recipe' for all clinical presentations: airway may need to be secured asleep, with the patient breathing spontaneously; awake (FOI), or tracheostomy may be necessary. With a normal airway, highly potent opioids (see Introduction, p. 141) can be used safely. The induction dose of a hypnotic agent frequently must be reduced due to the patient's age, preexisting medical condition, and hypoalbuminemia.
Maintenance	Choice of an inhalational agent will depend on the anesthesiologist's preference, patient's hemodynamic response, and concomitant medical conditions. Maintaining moderate ↓BP (see Introduction, p. 142) and aggressive treatment of the break-through adrenergic responses are necessary. In patients with flap reconstruction, ↑↑BP may overcome vasospasm, dislodging a small blood clot or poorly tied ligature → formation of flap hematoma. Muscle relaxation may or may not be contraindicated for the functional or modified radical neck dissection, depending on the surgeon's preference (inquire preop). All inspired gases should be humidified to minimize ↓T and mucous plugging. Venous air embolism (VAE) during radical neck surgery occurs rarely; maintaining adequate intravascular volume and PPV will ↓ incidence of this complication. If a large collection of air bubbles is observed by the surgeon in the internal jugular vein, the anesthesiologist should be notified immediately; these bubbles can be safely aspirated with a fine needle and discarded. Vagal reflexes from the carotid sinus may cause bradycardia and ↓BP. Prolongation of the QT interval during right radical neck dissection has been described and may progress to ventricular arrhythmias and even cardiac arrest. Tracheostomy can be performed as part of the radical neck dissection, with the same implications for anesthesia management (see Anesthetic Considerations for Tracheostomy, p. 184).
Emergence	Smooth emergence is essential. In situations when preop airway compromise has been present, and tracheostomy was **not** performed, consider extubating over a tube changer, with equipment prepared for possible reintubation. The majority of patients with microvascular flap reconstruction will have a tracheostomy placed, and will be continued on ventilatory support in the ICU. Other patients with the performed tracheostomy must be awakened in the OR to exclude possible embolic stroke (carotid atherosclerosis) before their transfer to the ICU or PACU. Up to 10% of patients may develop sustained hypertensive response (↑risk of stroke) early postop, probably 2° denervation of the carotid sinus; Rx agressively.
Blood and fluid requirements	IV: 16 ga × 1 NS/LR @ 5-7ml/kg/h Fluid warmer and humidifier	T&S for 2 U blood. Blood loss usually gradual. Sudden blood loss resulting from injury to the jugular vein or carotid artery usually can be controlled by the surgeon.

Control of blood loss	Surgical hemostasis Deliberate ↓BP Head-up tilt 30°	Continue aggressive Rx of ↑BP in the PACU.
Monitoring	Standard monitors (p. B-1) ± Arterial line	 A-line may be indicated in patients with severe cardio-pulmonary disease, CRI, symptoms of cerebrovascular insufficiency, location of tumor near the carotid artery, or in patients presenting for lengthy procedures, including microvascular flap reconstruction.
	± CVP line Foley catheter	CVP may be warranted in severely malnourished patients, those with severe COPD or CRI, and those presenting for microvascular flap reconstruction.
Positioning	Usually supine, head elevated 30° Table turned 180° ✓ and pad pressure points. ✓ and pad eyes.	
Complications	Vagal reflexes → ↓HR and ↓BP	2° carotid sinus stimulation. Rx: stop surgery; lidocaine infiltration of the carotid sinus by the surgeon; iv atropine.
	↑Q-T interval	Probably caused by interruption of cervical sympathetic outflow to heart (with right radical neck dissection).
	Dysrhythmias	Due to either the carotid sinus stimulation or the ↑Q-T interval
VAE	↓ETCO$_2$ ↑ETN$_2$ ↓BP ↑ST segment 'Mill wheel' murmur Dysrhythmias	With large veins open in the neck, VAE is possible and may account for unexplained ↓BP and/or dysrhythmia. Rx: notify surgeon (compress open neck veins); flood field with NS; left lateral decubitus/head-down position; aspirate CVP; 100% O$_2$ circulatory support (fluid, pressors, as required).

POSTOPERATIVE

Complications	HTN and ↑HR	May be 2° carotid sinus denervation or pain. Rx: aggressive pharmacological intervention
	Nerve injury Diaphragmatic paralysis	Facial nerve injury can cause facial droop. Recurrent laryngeal nerve injury can result in vocal cord dysfunction. The phrenic nerve also may pass in the surgical field and respiratory problems may develop if diaphragmatic paralysis occurs.
	Pneumothorax	Pneumothorax may occur with low neck dissection. Dx & Rx: See Postoperative Considerations for Laryngoscopy/Bronchoscopy/Esophagoscopy, p. 152.
	Agitation	Agitation → ↑PaCO$_2$, ↓PaO$_2$, ↑HR. Rx: ✓ restrictive neck dressings; evacuate hematoma; reestablish airway with ETT; 100% O$_2$; ventilate patient as required.
Pain management	PCA (p. C-3) Parenteral opiates (p. C-2)	
Tests	CXR	CXR for position of tracheostomy tube and evidence of pneumothorax.
	ECG	ECG for diagnosis of rhythm disturbances.

References

1. Bonner S, Taylor M: Airway obstruction in head and neck surgery. *Anaesthesia* 2000; 55:290-1.
2. Brown BR. Anaesthesia for ear, nose, throat and maxillofacial procedures. In *International Practice of Anaesthesia*. Prys-Roberts C, Brown BR, eds. Butterworth-Heinemann, Oxford: 1996, 112:2-9.
3. de Cassia Braga Ribeiro K, Kowalski LP, Latorre Mdo R: Perioperative complications, comorbidities, and survival in oral or oropharyngeal cancer. *Arch Otolaryngol Head Neck Surg* 2003; 129(2):219-28.

4. Dougherty TB, Nguyen DT: Anesthetic management of the patient scheduled for head and neck cancer surgery. *J Clin Anesth* 1994; 6:74-82.

5. Kirk GA: Anesthesia for ear, nose, and throat surgery. In *Principles and Practice of Anesthesiology*. Rogers MC, Tinker JH, Covino BG, Longnecker DE, eds. Mosby-Year Book, St. Louis: 1993, 2257-74.

6. Loré JM Jr: *An Atlas of Head and Neck Surgery*, 3rd edition. WB Saunders, Philadelphia: 1988, 626-9.

7. Mason RA, Fielder CP: The obstructed airway in head and neck surgery. *Anaesthesia* 1999; 54:625-8.

8. McGuirt WF, May JS: Postoperative hypertension associated with radical neck dissection. *Arch Otolaryngol Head Neck Surg* 1987; 113:1098-110.

9. Prasad KC, Shanmugam VU: Major neck surgeries under regional anesthesia. *Am J Otol* 1998; 19(3):163-9.

10. Rice JH, Gonzalez RM: Large visible gas bubbles in the internal jugular vein: a common occurrence during supine radical neck surgery? *J Clin Anesth* 1992; 4:21-4.

11. Rice M, Turner M, Carapiet D: The use of the laryngeal mask airway in maxillofacial surgery. *Anaesthesia* 2002; 57:826.

12. van Wilgen CP, Dijkstra PU, van der Laan BF, Plukker JT, Roodenburg JL: Shoulder complaints after neck dissection; is the spinal accessory nerve involved? *Br J Oral Maxillofac Surg* 2003; 41(1):7-11.

13. Wittich DJ, Berny JJ, Davis RK: Cervical epidural anesthesia for head and neck surgery. *Laryngoscope* 1984; 94:615-9.

14. Zacay G, Bedrin L, Horowitz Z, Peleg M, Yahalom R, Kronenberg J, Taicher S, Talmi YP: Syndrome of inappropriate antidiuretic hormone or arginine vasopressin secretion in patients following neck dissection. *Laryngoscope* 2002; 112(11): 2020-4.

LARYNGECTOMY: TOTAL, SUPRAGLOTTIC, HEMI

SURGICAL CONSIDERATIONS

Description: A **total laryngectomy** involves removal of the vallecula (or, if necessary, the posterior third of the tongue) to the first or second tracheal rings. An **apron flap incision** (Fig 3-13) allows exposure in a subplatysmal plane from the hyoid bone to the clavicle. A **tracheostomy** is performed and an anode tube placed. The strap muscles are divided inferiorly and the hyoid bone is skeletonized. The thyroid gland is resected away from the trachea, unless it is to be included in the specimen. Typically, the larynx is transected just above the hyoid bone, and the specimen is removed. The pharynx is closed in a T-shape and the trachea is brought out to the skin as an end-tracheostomy. No ET or tracheostomy tube is required.

A **supraglottic laryngectomy** (Fig 3-14) involves resection of the larynx from the ventricle to the base of tongue, leaving the true vocal cords. The exposure is similar to that for a total laryngectomy; however, the strap muscles are preserved intact. Once the thyroid cartilage is exposed, subperichondrial flaps are elevated off of the thyroid lamina and used later for reconstruction. Cuts are made either with a knife or saw through the midthyroid cartilage at a level just above the true cords and completed at the base of tongue. The specimen includes the false vocal cords and supraglottic larynx, the epiglottis and a portion of the base of tongue. Closure is obtained by approximating the thyroid perichondrium to the base of tongue and then the strap muscles, also to the base of tongue (Fig 3-15). A temporary tracheostomy is required.

A **hemilaryngectomy** (also called a **vertical partial laryngectomy**) involves removal of a unilateral true and false cord, retaining the epiglottis and opposite side true and false cord, with various methods of reconstruction. The exposure required for a hemilaryngectomy is similar to that for a supraglottic laryngectomy. A perichondrial flap is similarly raised; however, it is limited to the ipsilateral thyroid lamina. Cuts on the ipsilateral thyroid cartilage (Fig 3-16) are made with either a knife or saw and the anterior commissure is divided with Pott's scissors. After the tumor is resected, closure is obtained utilizing the thyroid perichondrium. Typically, the sternohyoid muscle is used to reconstruct the vocal cord. The wound is then closed in layers and drains are placed. Again, a tracheostomy is required.

A **near-total laryngectomy** involves removal of all of the larynx except for one arytenoid in constructing a phonatory shunt for speaking. All of the techniques involve creation of a temporary or permanent **tracheostomy**, and may be combined with **neck dissection** (radical or functional) and with partial or total **pharyngectomy**, which necessitates flap reconstruction.

Usual preop diagnosis: Cancer of larynx; intractable aspiration, with resultant pneumonia unresponsive to other techniques

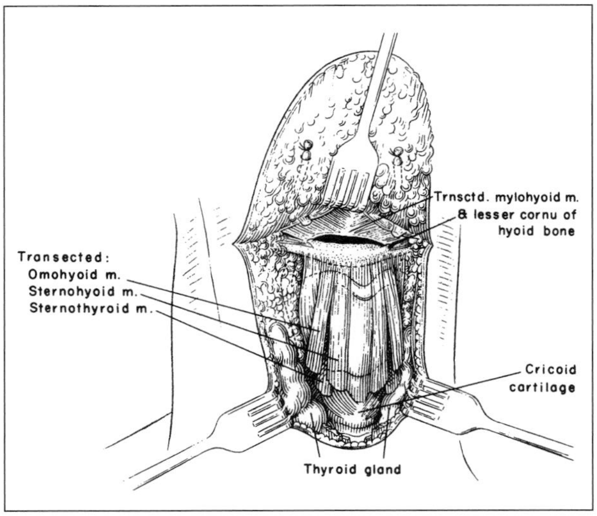

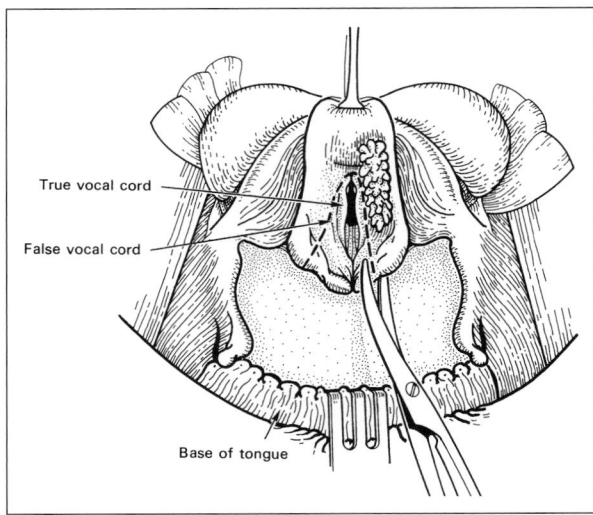

Figure 3-13. Via an apron flap incision, the sternohyoid, omo-hyoid, and sternothyroid muscles have been transected, expos-ing the thyroid gland on each side, the thyroid isthmus, and, occasionally, the cricoid cartilage. The suprahyoid musculature has been transected, along with the lesser cornu of the hyoid bone. (Reproduced with permission from Montgomery WW: *Surgery of the Upper Respiratory System*, 2nd edition. Lea & Febiger, 1989.)

Figure 3-14. The larynx is viewed from the midline, as seen by the surgeon standing at the head of the operating table. Unless the lesion extends posteriorly to the arytenoid, the ary-epiglottic fold is transected on each side by placing one blade of the dissecting scissors into the laryngeal ventricle or above the false vocal cord and the other blade in the pyriform sinus. The arytenoid on one side can be resected if the tumor extends posteriorly to involve this structure. (Reproduced with permis-sion from Montgomery WW: *Surgery of the Upper Respiratory System*, 2nd edition. Lea & Febiger, 1989.)

SUMMARY OF PROCEDURES

	Total	Supraglottic	Hemi
Position	Supine	⇐	⇐
Incision	Various neck incisions, depending on whether or not reconstruction is anticipated, and requirements of neck dissection.	Horizontal	⇐
Special instrumentation	Major head/neck set; head-lights; sterile anesthesia con-necting tubes; 6 Fr anode tube; No. 8 and No. 10 cuffed laryngectomy tubes	⇐	Newborn Finochetto rib retractor
Unique considerations	Tumors of the larynx necessarily produce distortion of the airway and, occasionally, a compromised airway prior to onset of anesthesia. A patient with compromised airway is probably best treated by tracheostomy under local anesthesia before the start of GA. Intubation can be exceedingly difficult.	⇐	⇐
Antibiotics	Cefazolin 1 g; metronidazole 500 mg	⇐	⇐
Surgical time	2-6 h	⇐	⇐ Rarely is neck dis-section necessary.
EBL	Total laryngectomy: 200-300 ml Total laryngectomy with neck dissection: 500-700 ml Total laryngectomy, pharyngectomy and flap reconstruc-tion: 700-1200 ml.	200-300 ml	25-100 ml
	Sudden large blood losses do not occur; transfusion usually is not necessary.	⇐	⇐
Postop care	Suctioning of tracheal secretions as in tracheostomy.	⇐	⇐
Mortality	< 1%	⇐	⇐
Morbidity	Fistula (radiation salvage): 20%	1%	⇐
	Fistula formation (unirradiated): 5%	–	–
	Bleeding: 4%	⇐	–
	Infection: 4%	⇐	–
Pain score	4-6	4-6	4-6

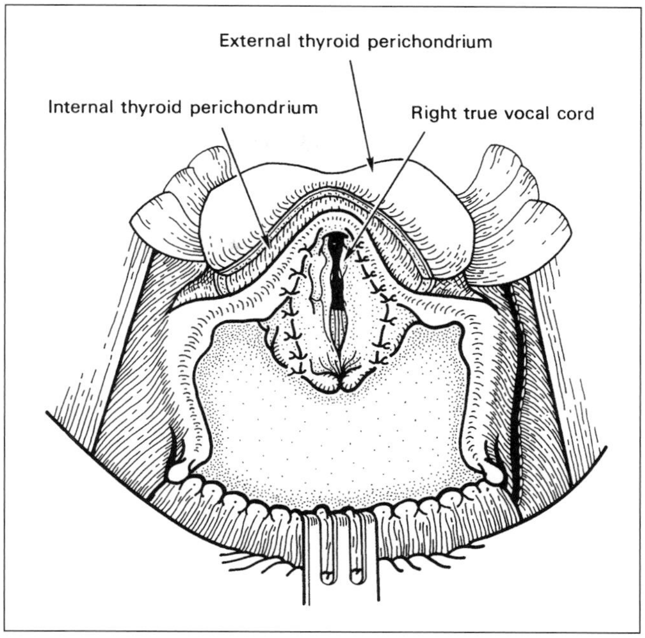

Figure 3-15. The repair following supraglottic partial laryngectomy begins by carefully approximating the margin of the mucous membrane of the pyriform sinus to the lateral margin of the laryngeal ventricle (right), or to the margin of resection above the false vocal cord (left). There is usually some distortion of the true vocal cord when the repair is accomplished, as is shown on the patient's right side. The repair is continued anteriorly by placing multiple interrupted No. 3-0 chromic catgut sutures. (Reproduced with permission from Montgomery WW: *Surgery of the Upper Respiratory System*, 2nd edition. Lea & Febiger, 1989.)

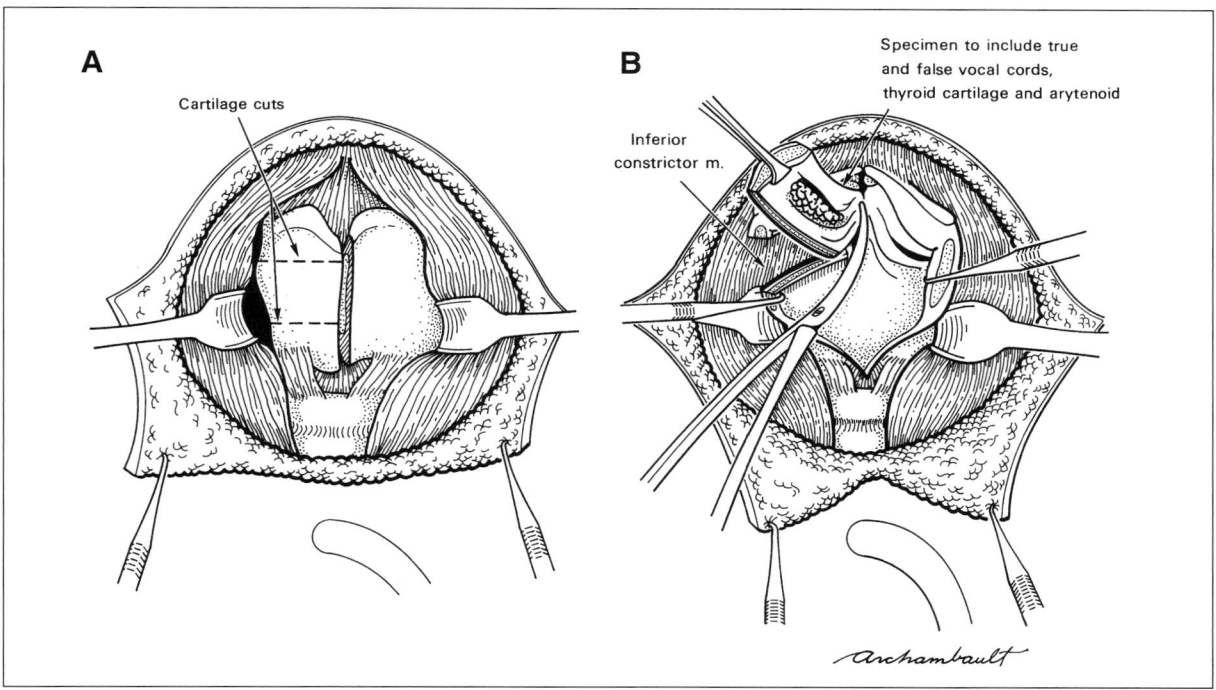

Figure 3-16. (A) Horizontal incisions, corresponding to the mucosal incision, are made through the thyroid lamina. (B) The specimen—including true and false vocal cords, the arytenoid, and a portion of the thyroid lamina—is resected en bloc. (Reproduced with permission from Montgomery WW: *Surgery of the Upper Respiratory System*, 2nd edition. Lea & Febiger, 1989.)

PATIENT POPULATION CHARACTERISTICS

Age range	40-80 yr
Male:Female	3:1
Incidence	Common
Etiology	Smoking; alcohol
Associated conditions	COPD; atherosclerosis

ANESTHETIC CONSIDERATIONS

PREOPERATIVE

See preop considerations for Neck Dissection, p. 170. Patients with airway obstruction (e.g., stridor, difficulty breathing, sleeping upright, use of accessory muscles on inspiration) will likely be difficult to ventilate and intubate. They may manifest baseline hypoxemia (± hypercarbia) 2° ↓airway diameter and atelectasis caused by ↓ability to effectively expectorate sputum.

INTRAOPERATIVE

Anesthetic technique: GETA. Although tracheostomy is performed universally in these patients, smooth emergence is still important 2° delicate suture lines. Full muscle relaxation is essential. Moderate ↓BP (see Introduction, p. 142) is desirable, but may be limited by concomitant cardiovascular disease.

Induction	There is no universal recipe for management of obstructed airway. One approach is outlined below. If stridor is **absent** and airway assessment is normal, standard induction followed by DL is appropriate. In patients with preexisting stridor, attempts to secure an airway while awake (including awake FOI) may precipitate complete upper airway obstruction. In patients with **moderate stridor**, in whom intubation is considered possible (larynx visible on preop nasal endoscopy, tumor not too large, absence of gross anatomical distortion, absence of fixed hemilarynx), inhalational induction, followed by gentle DL or asleep FOI, is the technique of choice. The ENT surgeon should be present in the OR, ready to perform rigid bronchoscopy or emergent tracheostomy. If the airway cannot be secured after 2-3 attempts, tracheostomy must be performed under controlled conditions, with the patient breathing spontaneously. In patients with **severe stridor** and low probability of successful intubation, a preliminary tracheostomy must be performed under local anesthesia. Other considerations are similar to those in Neck Dissection, p. 171.
Maintenance	See Neck Dissection, p. 171. After tracheostomy, a sterile anode ETT is inserted by the surgeon and connected to the sterile anesthesia breathing circuit. Proper ETT placement should be confirmed by presence of ETCO$_2$ waveform, equal bilateral breath sounds and normal airway compliance. Following tracheostomy, ↑ FiO$_2$ to at least 50%, because the surgeon will continue working around it, occasionally removing ETT for suture application. Position of ETT in the tracheostoma should be monitored closely to prevent ETT from slipping into the right mainstem bronchus.
Emergence	See Neck Dissection, p. 171.

For further discussion, see Intraop considerations for Neck Dissections, p. 171.

POSTOPERATIVE

See Postop considerations for Neck Dissections, p. 172.

References

1. Bonner S, Taylor M: Airway obstruction in head and neck surgery. *Anaesthesia* 2000; 55:290-1.
2. Dougherty TB, Nguyen DT: Anesthetic management of the patient scheduled for head and neck cancer surgery. *J Clin Anesth* 1994; 6:74-82.
3. Friedman M, ed: Laryngeal Surgery. *Operative Techniques in Otolaryngology/Head and Neck Surgery* 1990; 1(1):1-82.
4. Hilgers FJ, Ackerstaff AH, Van As CJ, Balm AJ, Van den Brekel MW, Tan IB: Development and clinical assessment of a heat and moisture exchanger with a multi-magnet automatic tracheostoma valve (Provox FreeHands HME) for vocal and pulmonary rehabilitation after total laryngectomy. *Acta Otolaryngol* 2003; 123(1):91-9.
5. Kirk GA: Anesthesia for ear, nose, and throat surgery. In *Principles and Practice of Anesthesiology*. Rogers MC, Tinker JH, Covino BG, Longnecker DE, eds. Mosby-Year Book, St. Louis: 1993, 2257-74.
6. Mason RA, Fielder CP: The obstructed airway in head and neck surgery. *Anaesthesia* 1999; 54:625-8.
7. McGuirt WF, May JS: Postoperative hypertension associated with radical neck dissection. *Arch Otolaryngol Head Neck Surg* 1987; 113:1098-110.
8. Orgill R, Krempl GA, Medina JE. Acute pain management following laryngectomy. *Arch Otolaryngol Head Neck Surg* 2002; 128(7):829-32.
9. Rice JH, Gonzalez RM: Large visible gas bubbles in the internal jugular vein: a common occurrence during supine radical neck surgery? *J Clin Anesth* 1992; 4:21-4.
10. Roberson JB, Fee WE: Conservation surgery for laryngeal carcinoma. *Ann Acad Med Singapore* 1991; 20(5):656-64.
11. Shah JP, Kamell LH, Hoffman HT, Ariyan S, Brown GS, Fee WE, Glass AG, Goepfert H, Ossoff RH, Fremgen A: Patterns of care for cancer of the larynx in the United States. *Arch Otolaryngol Head Neck Surg* 1997; 123:475-83.

GLOSSECTOMY

SURGICAL CONSIDERATIONS

Description: **Glossectomy**, either **partial** or **total**, is performed for neoplastic lesions of the tongue. During this procedure, nasal intubation is helpful, but not mandatory. On the other hand, complete relaxation is necessary. Additionally, a drying agent, such as scopolamine or glycopyrrolate, helps reduce oral secretions and facilitates surgery. A side-biting or Dingman mouth gag is used to gain adequate surgical exposure. The lesion is resected with electrocautery and usually can be closed primarily. Depending on the extent of resection, and location on the tongue, a **tracheostomy** may be indicated; or oral intubation alone may suffice for a period of 24-48 h. If neither is done, a short course of steroids helps reduce the lingual edema. A NG tube is placed for postop feeding. A **total glossectomy** is performed in similar fashion, but frequently is combined with a **laryngectomy** because of ensuing aspiration.

Variant procedure or approaches: Glossectomy can be done with a **neck dissection** or **mandibulectomy** and (on occasion) also can be combined with a **total laryngectomy**.

Usual preop diagnosis: Neoplastic disease of the tongue or adjacent structures (e.g., alveolus, floor of mouth) with involvement of the tongue

SUMMARY OF PROCEDURES

	Partial	Total
Position	Supine	⇐
Incision	Intraoral	⇐ + suprahyoid approach/neck approach
Special instrumentation	Dingman mouth gag	⇐
Unique considerations	Hypotensive anesthesia Nasal intubation Postop tracheostomy Steroids, if tracheostomy not performed.	⇐
Antibiotics	Cefazolin 1 g, metronidazole 500 mg	⇐
Surgical time	30 min-1 h	2-4 h
Closing considerations	Usually primary closure. May keep patient intubated 24-48 h if minimal tongue edema expected.	Flap repair required; laryngeal suspension usually required. Tracheostomy mandatory postop.
EBL	50-100 ml	200-400 ml
Postop care	Intubated 24-48 h	Tracheostomy care
Mortality	< 1%	⇐
Morbidity	Bleeding Infection Aspiration	Aspiration Bleeding Infection
Pain score	1-2	2-4

PATIENT POPULATION CHARACTERISTICS

Age range	Adults
Male:Female	3:1
Incidence	Uncommon
Etiology	Neoplasia
Associated conditions	Nonspecific

ANESTHETIC CONSIDERATIONS

PREOPERATIVE

For preop considerations, see Preoperative considerations for Neck Dissection, p. 170.

Airway	Thorough airway assessment is mandatory. Nasal intubation may or may not be required, depending on location of tumor (side vs base of tongue) and surgeon's preference (inquire preop).
Premedication	Preop administration of antisialagogue (e.g., glycopyrrolate 0.2 mg iv) may improve operating conditions.

INTRAOPERATIVE

Anesthetic technique: GETA. Complete muscle relaxation is an essential surgical requirement. For partial glossectomy, smooth extubation is desirable but not mandatory, unless skin graft was used for closure (graft hematomas are the primary cause of skin graft failure). Intraop infiltration with a local anesthetic effectively supplements intraop and postop analgesia.

Induction	With a normal airway, standard induction (p. B-2) is appropriate. Care should be taken on DL not to dislodge or fragment the tumor and provoke bleeding. Large immobile tumors may make conventional ET intubation extremely difficult or impossible. Awake nasal FOI may be a technique of choice in these cases but may prove difficult if the pharyngeal space is significantly decreased. In these patients, awake tracheostomy must be considered strongly before induction of GA.
Maintenance	During a partial glossectomy, surgical closure is quick, and short-acting inhalational agents (desflurane, sevoflurane) may be favored. Moderate ↓BP (see Introduction, p. 142), although desirable, is not mandatory for partial glossectomy. If tracheostomy is performed, the usual considerations apply (see Anesthetic Considerations for Laryngectomy, p. 150, and Tracheostomy, p. 184).
Emergence	Consider evaluating airway edema under direct vision (gentle DL) at the end of the case (as it may be impossible to reintubate the patient if postextubation airway obstruction occurs). Rapid recovery with full return of protective airway reflexes is essential in patients after partial glossectomy.
Complications	Vagal reflexes: ↓HR, ↓BP, mediated by surgical manipulation at base of tongue	Rare. Rx: notify surgeon; deepen anesthetic; iv atropine.

For further discussion, see Intraoperative Considerations for Neck Dissection, p. 171.

POSTOPERATIVE

Complications	Postop airway obstruction	May occur 2° ↑airway edema; emergent tracheostomy may be required. Prophylactic intraop steroids are beneficial.
Pain management	PCA (p. C-3) Parenteral opiates (p. C-2)	

For further discussion, see Neck Dissection, p. 172.

References

1. Dougherty TB, Nguyen DT: Anesthetic management of the patient scheduled for head and neck cancer surgery. *J Clin Anesth* 1994; 6:74-82.
2. Kirk GA: Anesthesia for ear, nose, and throat surgery. In *Principles and Practice of Anesthesiology*. Rogers MC, Tinker JH, Covino BG, Longnecker DE, eds. Mosby-Year Book, St. Louis: 1993, 2257-74.
3. Loré JM Jr: *An Atlas of Head and Neck Surgery*, 3rd edition. WB Saunders, Philadelphia: 1988, 626-9.
4. Morrison JD: *Anesthesia for Eye, Ear, Nose and Throat Surgery*, 2nd edition. Morrison JD, Mirakhur RK, Craig HJL, eds. Churchill Livingstone, New York: 1985.

MAXILLECTOMY

SURGICAL CONSIDERATIONS

Description: Maxillectomy is performed for benign or malignant neoplastic lesions of the maxillary sinuses. There are two basic types of this procedure: (1) **partial maxillectomy** and (2) **total maxillectomy**, with or without orbital exenteration, depending on tumor extent. Dental obturator usually is fitted immediately after the surgical resection. A Weber-Ferguson incision is made along the nasofacial groove and ala, exposing the face of the maxilla. An intraoral Caldwell-Luc incision is made and connected with the Weber-Ferguson incision. An **external ethmoidectomy** is usually performed at this time.

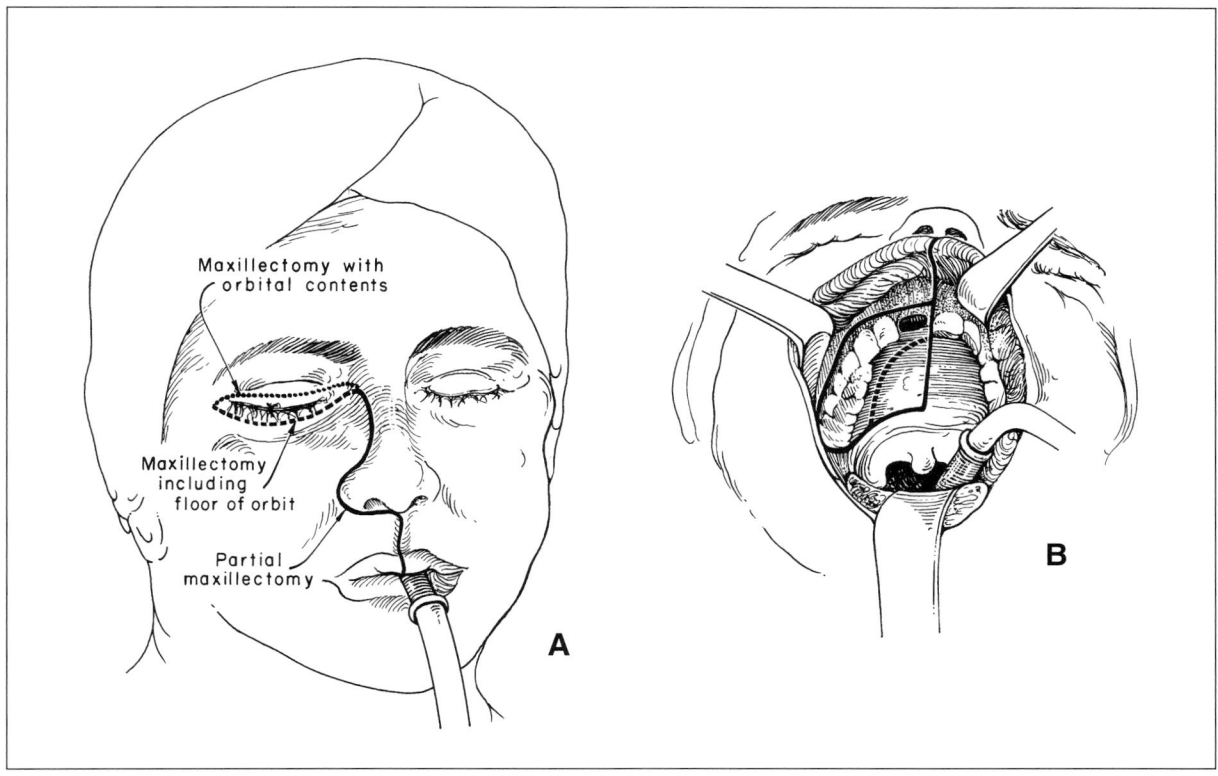

Figure 3-17. Maxillectomy incisions. (A) Incision begins midway between the inner canthus and nasal dorsum, and extends to the upper lip, which is split in the midline. (B) The buccal side of the upper lip is split vertically in the midline, and the mucosal incision incises the mucous membrane over the hard palate. At the junction of the soft and hard palate, the incision is directed laterally toward the posterior margin of the alveolar ridge, with the mucous membrane in the gingivobuccal sulcus being incised. The interrupted line indicates an alternate incision used when preserving the mucous membrane over the hard palate. (Reproduced with permission from Montgomery WW: *Surgery of the Upper Respiratory System*, 3rd edition. Williams & Wilkins, 1996.)

The proposed osteotomy sites are then outlined with electrocautery and the bone is exposed. A sagittal saw or osteotome is used to make the bony cuts through the palate, maxillary tuberosity, and maxilla at a point dictated by the tumor. Frequently, the specimen must be dissected away from the pterygoid musculature and the internal maxillary artery. After bleeding is controlled, the defect is lined with a split-thickness skin graft and packed with gauze, which is held in place by a dental obturator. For a partial or medial maxillectomy, the palate and lateral maxilla are preserved intact, so that a split-thickness skin graft and dental obturator are not necessary.

Variant procedure or approaches: Maxillectomy may be included in a **craniofacial en bloc resection**.

Usual preop diagnosis: Neoplastic disease of maxillary sinus or lateral wall of nose

SUMMARY OF PROCEDURES

	Partial Maxillectomy	**Total Maxillectomy**
Position	Supine, with head elevated 30°	⇐
Incision	Oral approach for partial palatal resections. Weber-Ferguson incision for medial maxillectomy.	Weber-Ferguson, with extension around eye-lids if orbital exenteration involved.
Special instrumentation	Power saw, drill; dermatome; nasal and curved Lambottes osteotomes; dental instruments for tooth extraction	⇐
Unique considerations	Hypotensive anesthesia during procedure to reduce blood loss	⇐
Antibiotics	Cefazolin 1 g + metronidazole 500 mg	⇐
Surgical time	1-2 h	2-4 h
Closing considerations	Nose may be packed, mandating oral airway upon extubation.	⇐

Figure 3-18. Maxillectomy: roof of ethmoid sinus. The medial wall of the orbit is exposed by retracting the orbital contents downward and laterally. (Reproduced with permission from Montgomery WW: *Surgery of the Upper Respiratory System*, 3rd edition. Williams & Wilkins, 1996.)

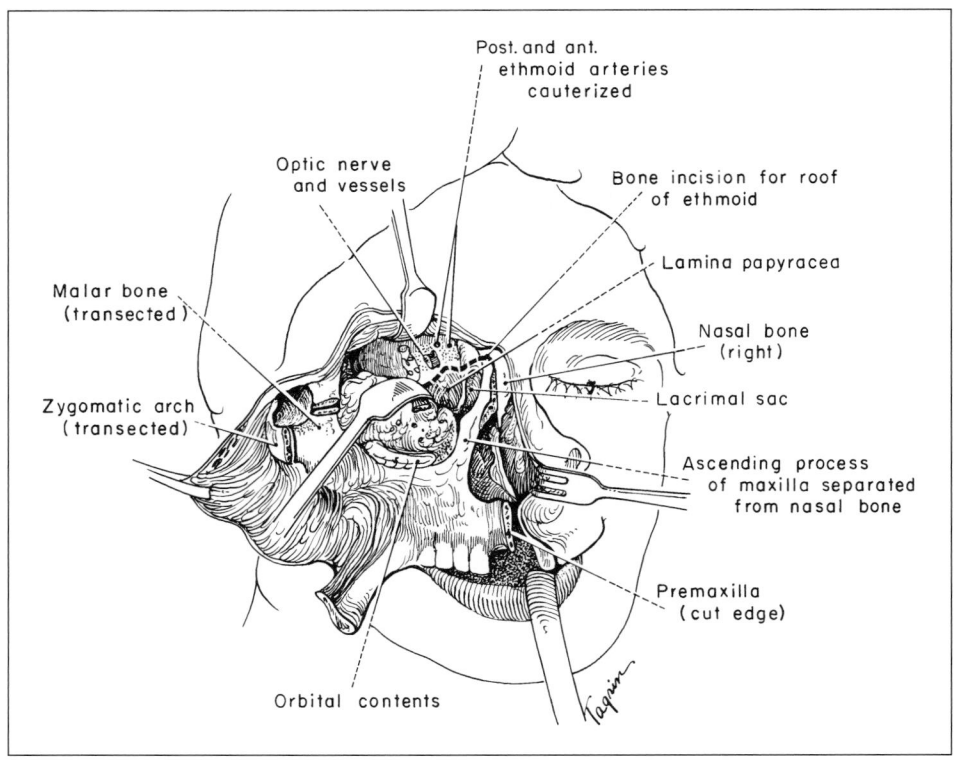

	Partial Maxillectomy	Total Maxillectomy
EBL	100-200 ml. Sudden brisk bleeding due to transection of internal maxillary artery occurs when posterior maxillary cut is made with curved osteotome. Control of this bleeding often cannot be achieved until specimen is removed. A 200-300 ml blood loss within 5 min is not unusual. Although not often needed, T&C for 1-2 U PRBCs. Watch suction bottle and measure irrigation.	200-700 ml
Postop care	Mist via face mask is helpful (especially if the nose is packed) to prevent drying of oral mucous membranes immediately postop.	⇐
Mortality	< 1%	⇐
Morbidity	Bleeding: 5%	⇐
	Diplopia (if eye saved): 5%	
	Infection: 4%	
Pain score	2-3	3-6

PATIENT POPULATION CHARACTERISTICS

Age range	Usually 6th-7th decade
Male:Female	3:1
Incidence	Common
Etiology	Benign and malignant paranasal sinus and nasal neoplasia; inverting papilloma

ANESTHETIC CONSIDERATIONS

PREOPERATIVE

Typically, these patients are older males who may have concomitant cardiopulmonary disease. Their nutritinal status is not usually affected.

Airway	A careful inspection is warranted, although it is unlikely that the disease process will → airway compromise. With large tumors, space available for laryngoscope blade manipulation may be reduced. XRT typically is done postop.
Cardiovascular	Preop evaluation should focus on suitability for controlled ↓BP: relatively contraindicated in patients with advanced cerebrovascular or cardiovascular disease. **Tests:** ECG; other tests as indicated from H&P.
Laboratory	Tests as indicated from H&P.
Premedication	Standard premedication (p. B-2)

INTRAOPERATIVE

Anesthetic technique: GETA. These procedures are very stimulating, and use of highly potent opioids (see Introduction, p. 141) is beneficial. The essential surgical requirement is ↓↓bleeding (see Introduction, p. 142). Intraop hemorrhage may be brisk and substantial (> 500 ml), and maintaining adequate circulating volume in anticipation of the osteotomy is essential. Promotion of rapid awakening with full return of protective airway reflexes presents additional challenges to the anesthesiologist.

Induction	Opioid-based technique, as outlined above (see Introduction, p. 141). Any iv induction agent can be safely used; ↓ dose in elderly and patients with significant cardiac disease. Oral ET intubation is performed with a small (#6.0) anode ETT to facilitate surgical manipulation inside patient's mouth. With large tumors, especially on the right side, special care is necessary when performing DL to avoid bleeding. ETT can be secured with a short piece of tape over the chin. Placement of a small esophageal T probe will not interfere with surgical field.
Maintenance	Moderate deliberate ↓BP (unless contraindicated) usually is accomplished by titration with an inhalational agent and/or iv β-blockers (see Introduction, p. 142). It is the author's preference to use desflurane for these procedures to rapidly adjust the anesthetic depth. After the specimen has been removed, surgical stimulation decreases and the inhalational anesthetic concentration should be reduced or even DC'd to promote rapid awakening. A throat pack is used routinely, and is removed before the end of surgery to permit placement of a dental prosthesis.
Emergence	The stomach should be suctioned at the end of the case (throat pack removed previously) and metoclopromide (10 mg iv) administered (promotes gastric emptying). Nasal passages may be packed, → obligate mouth breathing; oropharynx must be suctioned thoroughly and carefully. No dressing is applied postop; blood washed off patient's face may result in movement of the head and the ETT. If sufficient doses of opioids have been used, patient will tolerate this well, without coughing/gagging/straining, while breathing spontaneously. Extubation should be smooth, with full return of protective airway reflexes. Hemoptysis may occur after extubation and the patient's mouth should be covered with an O$_2$ mask.

Blood and fluid requirements	IV: 16-18 ga × 1-2 LR @ 5-7 ml/kg/h	Blood loss moderate-to-severe. It can be sudden and substantial.
Monitoring	Standard monitors (p. B-1) ± Arterial line	A-line usually not necessary, but may be indicated in patients with significant cardiovascular disease.
Positioning	Head elevated 30° Table may be turned 90°-180°. ✓ and pad pressure points. ✓ eyes.	
Complications	Dysrhythmias ↓BP	Dysrhythmias may occur 2° significant surgical stimulation and break-through adrenergic responses. ↓BP may be sudden 2° brisk blood loss.

POSTOPERATIVE

Complications	Occult postop bleeding	Postop bleeding may cause the patient to swallow large quantities of blood, which represent an aspiration risk and may manifest as ↓BP or PONV.
Pain management	PCA (p. C-3) Parenteral opioids (see p. C-2).	

References

1. Dougherty TB, Nguyen DT: Anesthetic management of the patient scheduled for head and neck cancer surgery. *J Clin Anesth* 1994; 6:74-82.
2. Kirk GA: Anesthesia for ear, nose, and throat surgery. In *Principles and Practice of Anesthesiology*. Rogers MC, Tinker JH, Covino BG, Longnecker DE, eds. Mosby-Year Book, St. Louis: 1993, 2257-74.
3. Le QT, Fu KK, Kaplan M, Terris DJ, Fee WE, Goffinet DR: Treatment of maxillary sinus carcinoma: a comparison of the 1997 and 1977 American joint committee on cancer staging systems. *Cancer* 1999; 86:1700-11.
4. Loré JM: *An Atlas of Head and Neck Surgery*. WB Saunders, Philadelphia: 1988.
5. Maniglia AJ, Phillips DA: Midfacial degloving for the management of nasal, sinus, and skull base neoplasms. *Otolaryngol Clin North Am* 1995; 28(6):1127-43.
6. Nibu K, Sugasawa M, Asai M, Ichimura K, Mochiki M, Terahara A, Kawahara N, Asato H: Results of multimodality therapy for squamous cell carcinoma of maxillary sinus. *Cancer* 2002; 94(5):1476-82.

TRACHEOSTOMY

SURGICAL CONSIDERATIONS

Description: Tracheostomy is performed either prophylactically in anticipation of upper airway obstruction 2° major head and neck surgery, or to establish an airway in acute infectious processes of the head and neck associated with airway obstruction. Other indications include laryngeal fractures, sleep apnea, inability to intubate for various reasons, and requirements for prolonged ventilatory assistance. A tracheostomy tube is placed; or a permanent tracheostomy can be fashioned by using interdigitating neck skin flaps and tracheal flaps. Rarely, an ETT may serve as a tracheostomy securing an airway. Tracheostomy under local anesthesia is the preferred technique for anyone with upper airway obstruction. After infiltrating the operative site with 1% lidocaine with 1:100,000 epinephrine, a horizontal incision is made 1 cm below the cricoid, exposing the strap muscles, which then are separated in the midline. The thyroid isthmus is encountered and divided with electrocautery. The pretracheal fascia is removed (Fig 3-19), and the cricoid cartilage identified. The trachea is entered, usually at the 2nd or 3rd ring, with either a horizontal or cruciate incision; or a segment of tracheal wall may be removed. In infants, a vertical incision is used with stay sutures attached to each flap. The tracheotomy tube is introduced and secured with trach ties and/or sutures.

Variant procedure or approaches: Cricothyroidotomy (incision placed just over the cricothyroid membrane into the subglottic larynx) is the preferred technique to obtain a rapid airway in an emergency. Conversion to a conventional tracheostomy should be performed either immediately or within the first 24 h to prevent development of cricoid cartilage chondritis with resultant subglottic stenosis.

Usual preop diagnosis: Acute upper airway obstruction; respiratory failure with ventilator dependence

SUMMARY OF PROCEDURES

	Tracheostomy	Cricothyrotomy
Position	Supine; head extended; sandbag under shoulder, if tolerated.	⇐
Incision	Transverse skin crease, midway between thyroid notch and suprasternal notch	Transverse skin crease between thyroid and cricoid cartilage
Special instrumentation	None	Cricothyrotome or minitracheostomy set
Unique considerations	Most often performed under controlled conditions, if possible with patient intubated. Can be performed under local anesthesia.	Usually performed in acute emergency situations and converted to standard tracheostomy when patient stabilized.
Antibiotics	None	⇐
Surgical time	3-20 min	3-5 min
EBL	5-25 ml	Minimal
Postop care	Warm mist to replace humidification, warm inhaled air. Hospitals should have full protocol for tracheostomy suctioning and cleaning.	⇐

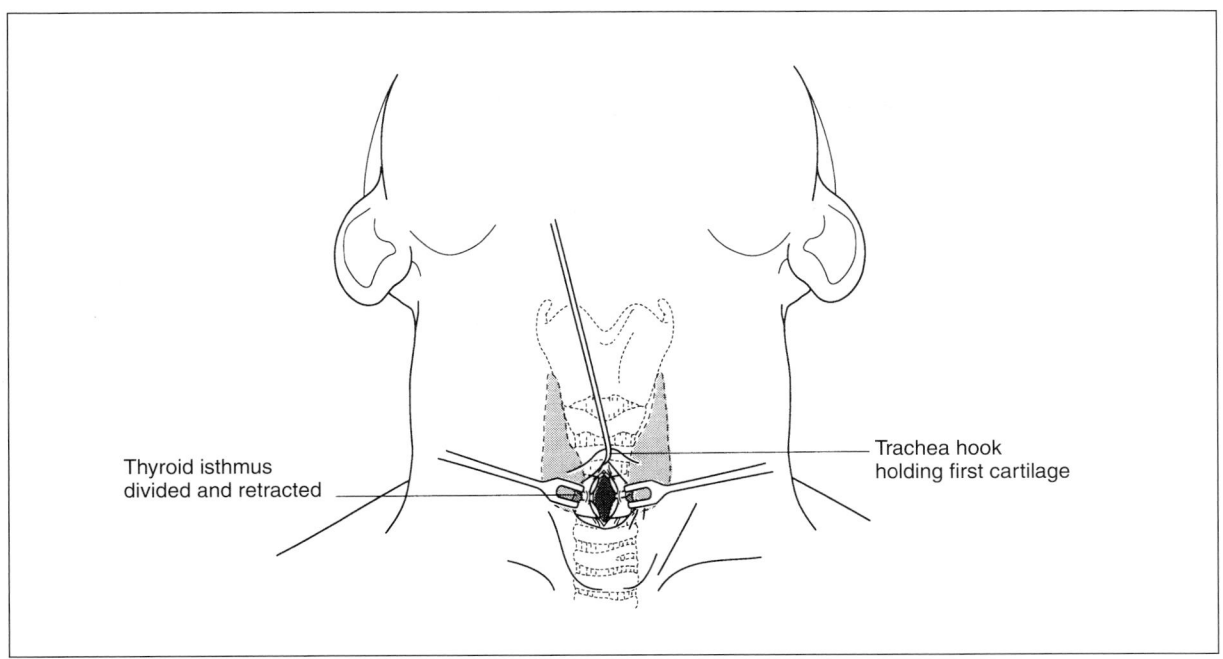

Thyroid isthmus
divided and retracted

Trachea hook
holding first cartilage

Figure 3-19. Standard tracheostomy using a vertical incision through the second and third tracheal rings. (Reproduced with permission from Greenfield LJ, et al, eds: *Surgery: Scientific Principles and Practice*, 2nd edition. Lippincott-Raven, 1997.)

	Tracheostomy	Cricothyrotomy
Mortality	< 1%	⇐
Morbidity	Bleeding: < 5%	⇐
	Infection: < 5%	Subglottic stenosis
	Tracheomalacia: 1%	
	Tracheostenosis: 1%	
Pain score	1-2	2-3

PATIENT POPULATION CHARACTERISTICS

Age range	Adults
Male:Female	2:1
Incidence	Common
Etiology	Upper airway obstruction; prolonged intubation; airway toilet

ANESTHETIC CONSIDERATIONS

PREOPERATIVE

Typically, there are three patient populations presenting for tracheostomy: (1) intubated patients in chronic respiratory failure or following major trauma; (2) patients for whom tracheostomy is part of a scheduled procedure (e.g., laryngectomy); and (3) patients with impending or total upper airway obstruction (e.g., Ludwig's angina, retropharyngeal abscess). Aside from an occasional otherwise healthy patient in the 3rd category, all patients presenting for tracheostomy are usually debilitated and have associated cardiac or pulmonary disease and neurological and metabolic abnormalities.

For features of the H&P that may be associated with a difficult airway, see Introduction, p. 141.

Respiratory   Patients in group 1 may have respiratory insufficiency, requiring mechanical ventilation with PEEP to maintain adequate oxygenation. The continued application of PEEP may be an important consideration during transport from ICU → OR. Patients in group 2 require a careful airway evaluation (see Anesthetic Considerations for Neck Dissection, p. 170, and Laryngectomy, p. 149). Based on the assessment, the anesthesiologist must decide whether to choose a direct laryngoscopy, an awake

Respiratory, cont.	FOI, or a tracheostomy under local anesthesia to secure the airway. Patients in group 3 will require semiemergent or emergent tracheostomy. Patients in all three groups should be evaluated for the effects of possible persistent aspiration. **Tests:** CXR; ABG, as indicated from H&P.
Cardiovascular	All of these patients may have significant cardiac risk factors, including smoking, alcohol abuse, male gender, ↑cholesterol, family Hx, and HTN. Some patients may have recently undergone other major surgery, and may be on pharmacological inotropic support, with full invasive monitoring, including PA line. **Tests:** ECG, and other tests as indicated, in patient with cardiac risk factors
Neurological	Preop neurological deficits should be documented fully.
Hematologic	In cases of malignancy or chronic disease, coagulopathies or anemia may be present. **Tests:** Hb; PT; PTT; CBC
Laboratory	Other tests as indicated from H&P.
Premedication	Standard premedication (p. B-2) in elective cases. Premedication is best avoided if airway is compromised or in emergencies.

INTRAOPERATIVE

Anesthetic technique: GETA (intubated or intubatable patients) or local anesthesia (in the presence of significant airway compromise or anticipated difficult intubation). Most tracheostomies are elective or semiurgent, and are performed under GA. Patients with ↑mucosal swelling (e.g., generalized edema, prolonged intubation) or ↑tissue fragility (e.g., chronic steroid therapy) are at risk of tracheal mucosal separation → creation of a false passage during tracheostomy. This will constitute a true emergency (see Postoperative Complications, below).

Induction	If already intubated, convert preexisting sedation to GA, using carefully titrated induction (e.g., etomidate 0.2-0.3 mg/kg iv) or inhalation agents. If not intubated and no airway problems are anticipated, a standard induction (p. B-2) may be appropriate. If airway problems are anticipated, an awake fiber optic intubation or tracheostomy performed under local anesthesia may be the techniques of choice (see Anesthetic Considerations for Neck Dissection, p. 171, and Laryngectomy, p. 150). In any event, the anesthesiologist should be prepared to deal with a failed intubation and have a surgeon immediately available to perform a tracheostomy if ventilation proves impossible.
Maintenance	Standard maintenance (see p. B-3). Full muscle relaxation is required. 100% O_2 usually is required before insertion of tracheostomy. This high O_2 concentration, combined with electrocautery may → airway fire (see Postop Complications, below). A cuffed ETT should be used to prevent O_2 from leaking into the surgical site. In order to avoid this 2° inadvertent ETT cuff puncture, consider advancing the ETT closer to the carina, before the trachea is opened. The trachea is usually opened above the cuff, and the ETT is retracted cephalad by the anesthesiologist, under direct vision by ★ the surgeon. (**NB:** Do not remove the ETT completely!) Sterile CO_2 tubing, extra ETTs, and anesthesia circuit should be readily available (see Maintenance for Laryngectomy. p. 150). Once the tracheostomy tube is secured, it should be suctioned and connected to the anesthesia circuit. Verify the CO_2 tracing and ✓ the inflation pressures.
Emergence	Considerations for groups 2 and 3 patients are described above. Patients in the first group will continue on ventilatory support in the ICU. The tracheostomy tube must be suctioned carefully and delivered O_2 should be humidified. Opioid sedation will minimize reaction to suctioning in the early postop period. Tracheostomy tubes should not be removed for at least the first 5 d, until a track is formed.

Blood and fluid requirements	IV: 18 ga × 1 NS/LR @ 2-3 ml/kg/h	Generally, EBL is minimal when tracheostomy is performed as an isolated procedure.
Monitoring	Standard monitors (p. B-1)	Avoid monitor placement in prepped area. Invasive monitoring may be appropriate, depending on patient condition.
Positioning	Shoulder roll ✓ and pad pressure points. ✓ eyes.	Generally, patient will have a shoulder roll with neck extension.
Complications	Pneumothorax Pneumomediastinum	Pneumothorax may occur with low neck dissection or if a false passage (see Postop Complications, below) has

Complications, cont.	Hemorrhage Aspiration of blood Difficult ETT insertion/reinsertion False tracheal passage/tracheal disruption	been created during the tracheostomy tube insertion. Dx & RX: See Anesthetic Considerations for Laryngoscopy/Bronchoscopy/Esophagoscopy, p. 152. This is an airway emergency, and must be quickly recognized (absent CO_2, ↑PIP, absent or very distant breath sounds). Reintroduction of the existing ETT from the proximal trachea should be attempted. Rigid bronchoscope should be available to reestablish airway in case of failed reintubation. An alternative approach is to insert a large-bore iv catheter into the tracheal lumen distal to the tracheostomy site and jet-ventilate the patient. Insertion of the airway exchange catheter through the bronchoscopy elbow adapter attached to the existing ETT has been advocated **prior** to tracheostomy tube insertion in patients at high risk for this complication.
	Airway fire	Tracheostomy fires are usually not catastrophic, possibly because tracheostomy acts as a vent. Rx: immediately disconnect patient from the anesthesia machine, extinguish the fire, and ventilate the lungs with room air, using a self-inflating bag. Removing or changing the existing ETT at this point may be more risky than leaving it in, if the patient was difficult to intubate or the airway has become edematous.

POSTOPERATIVE

Complications	Pneumothorax Pneumomediastinum Hemorrhage	See Anesthetic Considerations for Laryngoscopy/Bronchoscopy/Esophagoscopy, p. 152.)
	Occlusion of tracheostomy tube	Could be due to secretions, mucus plug, blood, or positioning of the tube against the tracheal wall.
	Tracheostomy tube displacement	Reintubate orally or through tracheostomy site.
Pain management	PCA (p. C-3)	IV opiates, as patient will remain npo postop.
Tests	CXR	For position of tracheostomy tube, evidence of pneumothorax or pneumomediastinum

References

1. Brown BR: Anaesthesia for ear, nose, throat and maxillofacial procedures. In *International Practice of Anaesthesia*. Prys-Roberts C, Brown BR, eds. Butterworth-Heinemann, Oxford: 1996, 112:2-9.
2. Chee WK, Benumof JL: Airway fire during tracheostomy: extubation may be contraindicated. *Anesthesiology* 1998; 89:1576-8.
3. Cheng E, Fee WE: Dilatational versus standard tracheostomy: a meta-analysis. *Ann Otol Rhinol Laryngol* 2000: 109:803-7.
4. Kirk GA: Anesthesia for ear, nose, and throat surgery. In *Principles and Practice of Anesthesiology*. Rogers MC, Tinker JH, Covino BG, Longnecker DE, eds. Mosby-Year Book, St. Louis: 1993, 2257-74.
5. Lotempio MM, Shapiro NL: Tracheotomy tube placement in children following cardiothoracic surgery: Indications and outcomes. *Am J Otolaryngol* 2002; 23(6):337-40.
6. McGuire G, El-Beheiry H, Brown D: Loss of the airway during tracheostomy: rescue oxygenation and re-establishment of the airway. *Can J Anesth* 2001; 48(7):697-700.
7. Morar P, Singh V, Makura Z, Jones A, Baines P, Selby A, Sarginson R, Hughes J, van Saene R: Differing pathways of lower airway colonization and infection according to mode of ventilation (endotracheal vs tracheotomy). *Arch Otolaryngol Head Neck Surg* 2002; 128(9):1061-6.
8. Peterson JL: Odontogenic infections. In *Otolaryngology–Head & Neck Surgery*, Vol 2, 2nd edition. Cummings CW, Schuller DE, eds. Mosby-Year Book, St Louis: 1993, 1199-1215.
9. Pollard BJ: ENT surgery. In *Handbook of Clinical Anesthesia*. Goldstone JC, Pollard BJ, eds. Churchill Livingstone, New York: 1996, 301-13.
10. Rogers ML, Nickalls RWD, Brackenbury ET, Salama FD, et al: Airway fire during tracheostomy: prevention strategies for surgeons and anaesthetists. *Ann R Coll Surg Engl* 2001; 83:376-80.

INTUBATION FOR EPIGLOTTITIS

ANESTHETIC CONSIDERATIONS

PREOPERATIVE

Epiglottitis is an acute inflammation and swelling of the epiglottis, associated with a generalized systemic toxicity, usually due to *Haemophilus influenza* Type B. It also can be caused by β-hemolytic streptococci, staphylococci, pneumococci, or unusual pathogens among immunocompromised individuals and drug/alcohol abusers. It occasionally results in total laryngeal obstruction and death 2° asphyxia. At one time, the typical patient was a previously healthy child 3-5 yr old; however, since the advent of the H-flu vaccine, epiglottitis is more common in adults (primarily males) than in children. The most common presenting symptoms are sore throat, dysphagia/odynophagia, fever, respiratory difficulty, and drooling. Pediatric patients may appear toxic on presentation.

Airway	Enlarged epiglottis seen frequently on neck x-ray. Neck tenderness or swelling also observed in some patients. Patients with stridor are at high risk for upper airway obstruction.
Respiratory	The patients, typically sitting upright, may display hoarseness, muffled voice, dyspnea, and chest-wall retractions. It is imperative to realize that total airway obstruction can occur suddenly and ★ without warning. **NB:** Rapid treatment should be instituted instead of performing time-consuming investigations. The sudden development of respiratory obstruction in the x-ray suite could have a disastrous outcome.
Hematologic	A high leukocyte count usually is found in these patients. **Tests:** Blood drawing before the airway is secured may be inadvisable.
Premedication	None

INTRAOPERATIVE

Anesthetic technique: GETA. Patients presenting with imminent or actual airway obstruction should be intubated immediately. Airway management for adults presenting with mild-to-moderate symptoms is controversial. Although prophylactic intubation of these patients may not be necessary, 18% subsequently may develop complete airway obstruction; thus, close monitoring is mandatory, if intubation is deferred. It is critical that an experienced anesthesiologist be present for this procedure. In the pediatric patient, it is critical that neither visualization of the epiglottis nor other maneuvers be attempted to confirm the Dx before anesthesia. In adults, it has been suggested that indirect laryngoscopy or FOB may be performed without the risk of precipitating complete airway obstruction, although this is controversial.

Induction	If an iv is in place, atropine 0.02 mg/kg may be given to the pediatric patient to prevent vagal reflexes and bradycardia from manipulation of the inflamed epiglottis. If no iv access is available, im administration should be avoided to prevent agitation, crying, and subsequent total airway obstruction (iv line is placed after induction of anesthesia). An experienced ENT surgeon, ready to perform an emergency tracheostomy, must be present at induction. Inhalation induction, with sevoflurane/halothane and 100% O_2, is used, with the patient in the sitting position. Early application of CPAP is essential. Induction may be prolonged and intubation extremely difficult. Different sizes of ETTs must be available.
Maintenance	Standard maintenance (see p. B-3).
Emergence	The patient will remain intubated for 24-48 h and should be kept sedated and restrained to prevent accidental extubation.

Blood and fluid requirements	Minimal blood loss
	IV: 18 ga (adult)
	    22-26 ga (child)
	NS/LR @ 4-7 ml/kg/h (adult)
	    @ 2-3 ml/kg/h (child)

Monitoring	Standard monitors (p. B-1)
Positioning	✓ and pad pressure points. ✓ eyes.
Complications	Pulmonary edema	A short-lived pulmonary edema occasionally occurs after relief of the obstruction (postobstructive pulmonary edema) and must be treated with IPPV.

POSTOPERATIVE

Complications	Accidental extubation ETT blockage	Accidental extubation and ETT blockage are serious complications that can prove fatal. The blockages are sometimes due to crusting of the ETT because of insufficient humidification.
Pain management	PCA (see p. C-3). IV opioids	Postop sedation and manual restraints

References

1. Brown BR. Anaesthesia for ear, nose, throat and maxillofacial procedures. In *International Practice of Anaesthesia*. Prys-Roberts C, Brown BR, eds. Butterworth-Heinemann, Oxford: 1996, 112:2-9.
2. Crockett DM, Healy GB, McGill TJ, Friedman EM: Airway management of acute supraglottitis at the Children's Hospital, Boston: 1980-1985. *Ann Otol Rhinol Laryngol* 1988; 97(2Pt1):114-19.
3. Dort JC, Frohlich AM, Tate RB: Acute epiglottis in adults: diagnosis and treatment in 43 patients. *J Otolaryngol* 1994; 23(4): 281-5.
4. Park KW, Darvish A, Lowenstein E: Airway management for adult patients with acute epiglottitis. *Anesthesiology* 1998; 88: 254-61.
5. Senior BA, Radkowski D, MacArthur C, Spredner RC, Jones D: Changing patterns in pediatric supraglottitis: a multi-institutional review, 1980 to 1992. *OHNS* 1994; 110(2):203-10.

SKULL BASE SURGERY

SURGICAL CONSIDERATIONS

Joseph B. Roberson

Description: The temporal bone is the gateway to the skull base, which comprises the undersurfaces of the cerebellum, temporal lobe, and the anterior and lateral surfaces of the brain stem. Access to these areas and to the associated vessels and nerves is the domain of the skull-base surgeon. **Posterior fossa craniotomy** (translabyrinthine, transcochlear, far lateral, or infratemporal fossa craniotomy) is carried out with the patient supine, rotated 180° from the anesthesiologist. The patient's head is rotated to the side to allow access to the cranium posterior and inferior to the ear. An incision is made from the supraauricular area into skin overlying the mastoid and, in some cases, into the neck. Bone is removed around, and sometimes including, the inner ear structures to allow access to the posterior cranial fossa and skull base. Continuous intraop monitoring of cranial nerves 5-12, SSEPs, and auditory EPs may be used; therefore, muscle relaxants should be avoided. The patient should be placed on the table and secured with two seat belts, as lateral rotation is necessary during the procedure. A CSF leak is produced, and then repaired with tissue (fat) taken from the abdomen during closure.

In contrast to the standard neurosurgical approach, the **translabyrinthine approach** to the posterior fossa remains extradural, avoiding direct retraction of the cerebellum or other brain structures. We believe the advantages include a decreased incidence of seizures, prolonged headaches, CSF leaks and aseptic meningitis. Most importantly, however, is the advantage of finding the facial nerve in a normal position and tracing it over the tumor. From the **suboccipital approach**, the facial nerve is on the opposite side of the tumor from the surgeon and may be difficult to locate. This can slow down the surgery and has been associated with abnormal facial nerve function. In the translabyrinthine approach, however, the facial nerve is identified in the mastoid and then followed (after removal of bone) back to the internal auditory canal. The nerve is then traced over the top of the tumor, permitting removal of the tumor without damaging the nerve.

Usual preop diagnosis: Vestibular schwannoma (acoustic neuroma); vestibular neuritis; Meniere's disease; cholesterol granuloma; meningioma; cholesteatoma; facial nerve paralysis; aneurysms; primary intracranial tumor; glomus tumors of the skull base

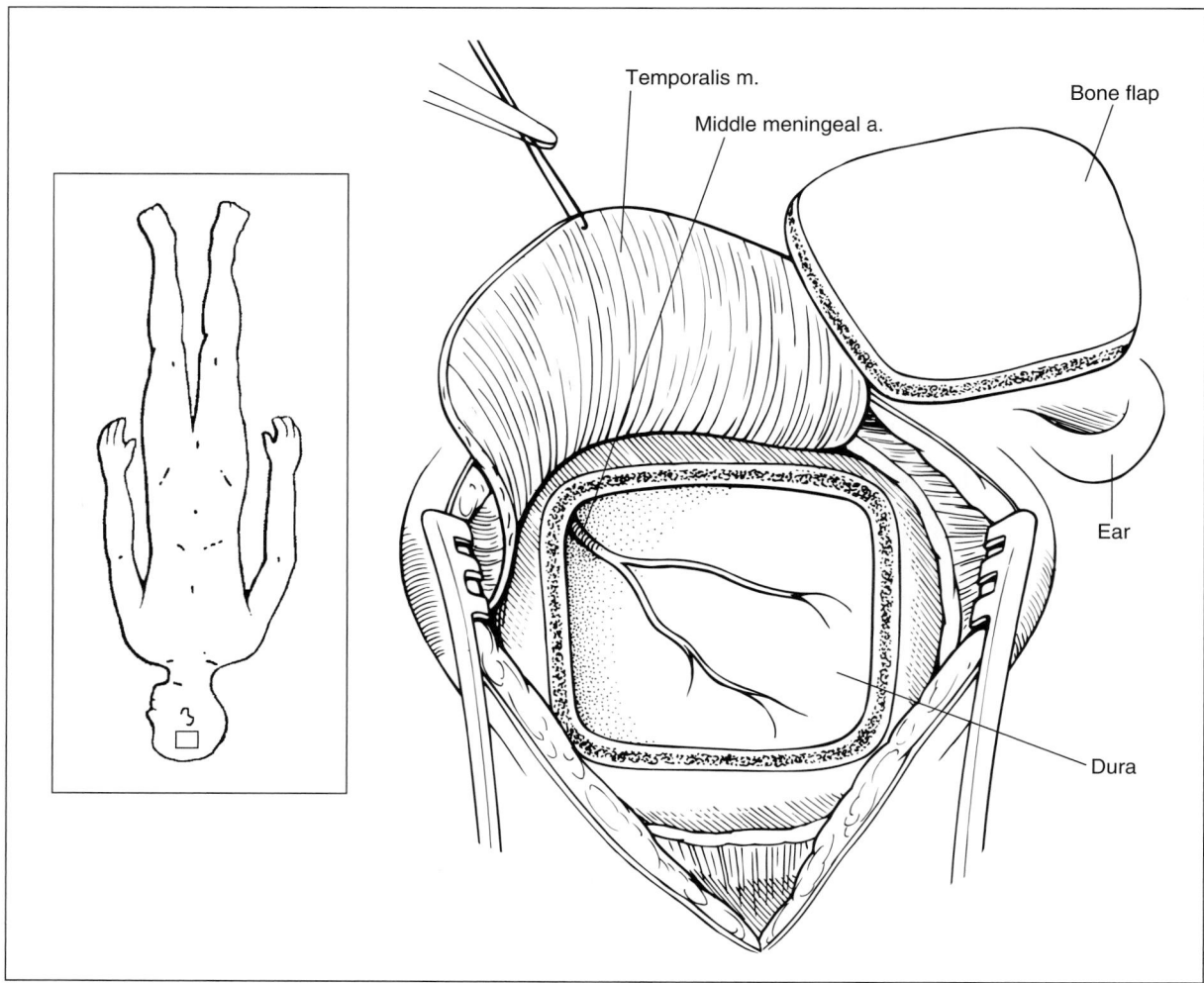

Figure 3-20. Right middle fossa approach: surgeon is looking down at patient's head, which is turned to the left. The temporalis has been reflected inferiorly and a square craniotomy has been performed. The dura is visible, with the middle meningeal artery visible on it.

Middle fossa craniotomy also is carried out with the patient supine, rotated 180° from the anesthesiologist. The head is turned to the side to allow access to the cranium superior to the ear. An incision is made from the pretragal area in a curved fashion onto the side of the head. A craniotomy of approximately 3" × 3" is performed superior to the ear (Fig 3-20). Elevation of the dura and placement of retractors allows exposure of the bone at the base of the skull. Bone is removed over the areas of interest to allow access to pathologic tissues for resection (Fig 3-21). Continuous intraop monitoring of cranial nerves 5-12, SSEPs and auditory EPs may be used. The patient should be placed on the table and secured with two seat belts, since lateral rotation is frequently necessary during this procedure. Trendelenburg and reverse Trendelenburg changes also are necessary during surgery to allow for exposure of critical structures. As in posterior fossa craniotomy, a CSF leak is produced, and then repaired with tissue (fat) taken from the abdomen during closure.

Usual preop diagnosis: Vestibular schwannoma (acoustic neuroma); vestibular neuritis; Meniere's disease; cholesterol granuloma; cholesteatoma; facial nerve paralysis; aneurysms in the cerebellar pontine angle and prepontine space

SUMMARY OF PROCEDURES

	Posterior Fossa Craniotomy	**Middle Fossa Craniotomy**
Position	Supine, table turned 180°, surgeon sitting to the side of the patient's head, with scrub nurse directly across and microscope in between (Fig. 3-22)	Supine, surgeon at head of table, table turned 180°, patient secured with 2 seat belts (Fig. 3-23).

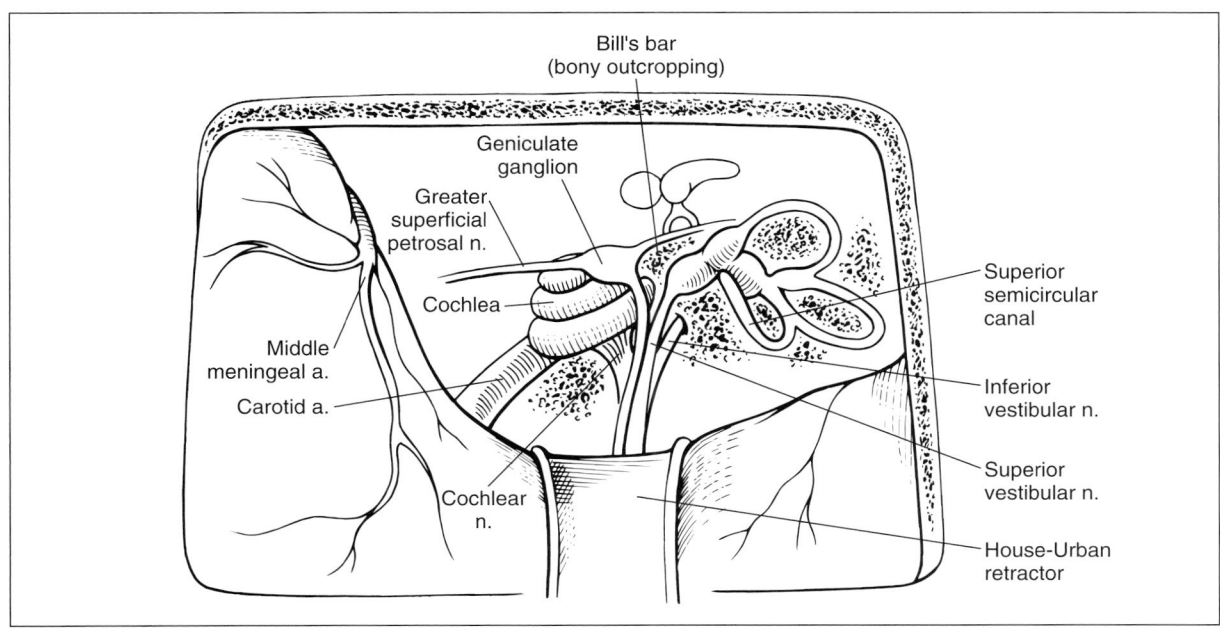

Figure 3-21. Right middle fossa approach with House-Urban retractor holding dura off the middle cranial fossa floor. The anatomic structures shown are under the floor and not visible, except for the greater superficial petrosal nerve and a prominent bony outcropping over the superior semicircular canal, which allows the location of the other structures to be calculated. Low pCO_2 and use of mannitol allow sufficient retraction of the dura and temporal lobe.

	Posterior Fossa Craniotomy	Middle Fossa Craniotomy
Incision	Temporal/mastoid ± neck extension	Pretragal to lateral temporal
Special instrumentation	Microscope, cranial nerve monitor, bipolar cautery, US aspirator, BAER computer	⇐
Unique considerations	TED hose, SCDs, Foley catheter, arterial line ± CVP monitoring. Lumbar drainage with some patients. Avoid muscle relaxants.	TED hose, SCDs, Foley catheter, arterial line ± CVP monitoring
Special medications	Dexamethasone 8 mg iv. (Note: hyperventilation and osmotic diuretic agents are usually not necessary with posterior fossa craniotomy.)	Mannitol 0.5-1.0 g/kg infusion, started after induction of anesthesia. Furosemide (10 mg iv); dexamethasone (8 mg iv).
Antibiotics	Vancomycin 1 g iv + ceftazidime 1 g iv q 8 h	Vancomycin 1 g iv, ceftazidime 1 g iv
Procedure time	3-12 h	3-6 h
Closing considerations	Sterile dressing placed after all drapes are removed (3-5 min application time). Attempt to minimize coughing and Valsalva to ↓ risk of intracranial bleeding. It is acceptable to use muscle relaxants after CSF leak repair.	Minimize coughing and Valsalva to ↓ risk of intracranial bleeding.
EBL	150-1000 ml (Have 1 U autologous blood available.)	150-500 ml (Have 1 U autologous blood available.)
Postop care	Direct transfer to ICU after extubation. Transport with ECG/O$_2$ sat/BP monitor. Establish level of consciousness and hemodynamic stability in ICU.	ICU
Mortality	Rare	⇐
Morbidity	Hearing loss: 5-100% (depending on approach)	30%
	Transient facial weakness: 20-30%	10-30%
	Permanent facial nerve weakness: ≤ 10%	⇐
	Postop CSF leak: ≤ 2%	⇐
	Infection: ≤ 2%	⇐

	Posterior Fossa Craniotomy	Middle Fossa Craniotomy
Morbidity, cont.	Delayed bleeding: 1-2%	⇐
	Meningitis: 1-2%	⇐
	Stroke: ≤ 1%	⇐
	Aspiration: Rare	⇐
Pain score	6	6

PATIENT POPULATION CHARACTERISTICS

Age range	Usually adults (occasional approaches of this type are used in children)	10+ yr
Male:Female	1:1	1:1
Incidence	1/20,000/yr in U.S.	1/40,000/yr in U.S.
Etiology	Neoplasm; chronic infection; recurrent dizziness; congenital lesions	Neoplasm; chronic infection; recurrent dizziness
Associated conditions	Hearing impairment in some patients (✓ for a hearing device, which should be removed after patient is asleep); balance disturbance	Hearing impairment

ANESTHETIC CONSIDERATIONS

Edward R. Baer

PREOPERATIVE

Typically, these patients are otherwise healthy, and ↑ICP occurs infrequently.

Respiratory	Elective surgery is contraindicated in patients with active respiratory tract infections.
Cardiovascular	HTN is a risk for periop bleeding and should be controlled before surgery. **Tests:** ECG; others as indicated from H&P.
Neurological	Any Sx of ↑ICP (e.g., HA, N/V, papilledema) warrant further evaluation. Some patients may have hearing aids, which may be removed after induction of anesthesia.
Hematologic	Recent use of an NSAID may force delay of elective surgery. ✓ family Hx for bleeding disorder. **Tests:** As indicated from H&P.
Laboratory	**Tests:** HCT and others, if indicated from H&P.
Premedication	In the absence of ↑ICP, midazolam 1-3 mg is used commonly.

INTRAOPERATIVE

Anesthetic technique: GETA, controlled ventilation. Use of cranial nerve monitors precludes use of muscle relaxants during most of the procedure.

Induction	Defasiculate with NMR. Induce anesthesia with STP (3-5 mg/kg) or propofol (1.5-2.5 mg/kg), an opiate (e.g., fentanyl 5 μg/kg), and succinylcholine (1.5 mg/kg). The airway will be inaccessible during surgery, so the ETT must be well secured. An alternative to taping the ETT is to secure the tube with a suture or dental floss. First tie the suture around the base of an incisor at the gingiva; then wrap and tie the suture around the ETT. This ensures that the ETT remains in place when the patient's head is turned or extended during surgery. A small dose of mivacurium may be used, if necessary, to facilitate placement of the CVP line and positioning of patient. Occasionally, a modified ETT and vocal cord electrode are required for cranial nerve monitoring (Xomed NIM-2 EMG ETT). After the table is turned 180°, the surgeon performs direct laryngoscopy and inserts the vocal cord electrodes. Intramuscular needle electrodes are placed before prep and drape for monitoring: CN7 (face), CN8 (hearing), CN9 (pharynx), CN10 (vocal cord), CN11 (trapezius), and CN12 (tongue).
Maintenance	Standard maintenance (p. B-3). Usually, a balanced technique combining low doses of an opiate, propofol, and a volatile agent ± N_2O. Dexamethasone 8 mg is given. Commonly, only mild hyperventilation for posterior fossa craniotomies. Middle fossa craniotomies, at surgeon's request,

Figure 3-22. OR configuration for posterior fossa and translabyrinthine craniotomies.

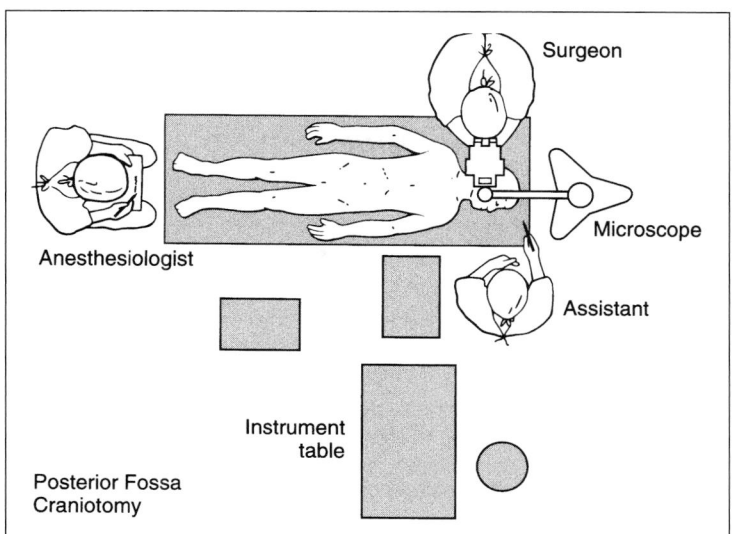

Figure 3-23. OR configuration for middle fossa craniotomy.

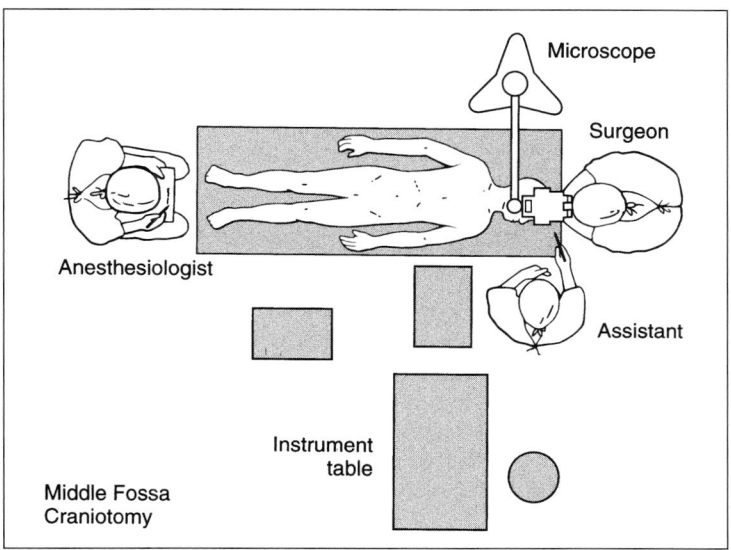

Maintenance, cont.	may require hyperventilation and mannitol (0.5-1 g/kg). Vasodilators (e.g., SNP) or β-blockers (e.g., labetalol, esmolol) may be necessary to prevent HTN.
Emergence	As the surgeon begins to close, the cranial nerve monitoring is D/C'd, and it is possible to add a low dose of intermediate-acting muscle relaxant (e.g., mivacurium 0.1 mg/kg or vecuronium 0.05 mg/kg) to the technique. Application of the surgical dressings takes several minutes and involves much manipulation of the head and neck. It is important to prevent coughing or Valsalva, which will ↑ ICP and ↑ BP. The use of a muscle relaxant prevents coughing, while allowing the patient to be rapidly awakened after the dressings are applied. If a vocal cord electrode has been used, it may be pulled out gently (without direct visualization) before the ETT is removed. The ETT is removed in the OR and the patient is taken to ICU. (If any significant neurologic injury is suspected, the ETT should not be removed.) A rapid-acting agent (e.g., SNP) should be available to treat HTN.
Blood and fluid requirements	IV: 18 ga × 1 NS @ 5-10 ml/h UO ≥ 0.5 ml/h

NS to maintain UO ≥ 0.5 ml/h. Avoid hypotonic fluids and glucose. Colloid may be used for volume. Maximum blood loss occurs with opening. Blood loss with glomus tumors can be brisk (100-300 ml over 5 min) during tumor resection. Transfusions usually not required, but patients with cardiovascular disease may fare better with an Hct ≥ 30.

Monitoring	Standard monitors (p. B-1) Arterial line CVP catheter UO	Cranial nerve monitoring typically performed by surgical team. Controlled ↓BP may be required.
Positioning	✓ & pad pressure points. ✓ eyes.	Consider covering the eyes with rigid shields. ✓ & pad pressure points with careful attention to arms. As the table is frequently tilted from side-to-side, the patient is secured with 2-4 belts.
Complications	Labile BP Pneumothorax (2° CVP)	Occasional BP lability during tumor resection for large lesions impacting the brain stem or involving the 9th and 10th nerve complex

POSTOPERATIVE

Complications	Neurologic deficits Intracranial bleeding Pneumothorax Peripheral nerve injury PONV	Uncontrolled HTN → intracranial bleeding. Occasional 9th or 10th nerve damage → smaller than usual glottic opening. (Fully awake patients can be extubated safely.) Stroke may be predicted with intraop monitoring techniques. Sx of depressed consciousness (2° intracranial bleeding or acute obstructive hydrocephalus) can occur several h following surgery. Follow level of consciousness closely in the immediate postop period. Patients who have resection of either the cochlear vestibular nerve or removal of the inner ear are expected to be vertiginous with strong nystagmus after awakening. This is also manifested as N/V in the immediate postop period. Nonsedating antiemetics are used as a first choice (e.g., ondansetron 4 mg iv or granisetron 100 μg iv). If required, promethazine (Phenergan) 12.5-25 mg or prochlorperazine (Compazine) 5-10 mg iv may be used.
Pain management	Fentanyl or morphine iv	
Tests	Neurological exam Hct CXR	If intracranial bleeding is suspected, a CT or MRI. To r/o pneumothorax and confirm that tip of the central venous line is outside the heart

---

References

1. Brackmann DE: Middle cranial fossa approach. In *Acoustic Tumors*, Vol. 2. House WF, Leutje C, eds. University Park Press, Baltimore: 1979, 15-41.
2. Brackmann DE, Green JD: Translabyrinthine approach. *Otolaryngol Clin North Am* 1992; 24:311-30.
3. Gantz BJ, Parnes LS, Harker LA, McCabe BF: Middle cranial fossa acoustic neuroma excision: results and complications. *Ann Otol Rhinol Laryngol* 1986; 95:454-9.
4. House WF, Hitselberger WE: The transcochlear approach to the skull base. *Arch Otolaryngol* 1976; 102:334-42.
5. House WF, Shelton C: Middle fossa approach for acoustic tumor removal. *Otolaryngol Clin North Am* 1992; 25:347-60.
6. Kawaguchi M, Sakamoto T, Ohnishi H, Karasawa J, Furuya H: Do recently developed techniques for skull base surgery increase the risk of difficult airway management? Assessment of pseudoankylosis of the mandible following surgical manipulation of the temporalis muscle. *J Neurosurg Anesthesiol* 1995;7(3):183-6.
7. Morrison AW: Translabyrinthine surgical approach to the internal acoustic meatus. *J R Soc Med* 1978; 71:269-73.
8. Sekhar LN, Estonillo R: Transtemporal approach to the skull base: an anatomical study. *Neurosurgery* 1986; 19:799-808.
9. Shelton C, Brackmann DE, House WF, Hitselberger WE: Middle fossa acoustic tumor surgery: results in 106 cases. *Laryngoscope* 1989; 99:405-8.
10. Stetchison MT: Neurophysiologic monitoring during cranial base surgery. *J Neurooncol* 1994; 20(3):313-25.
11. Tos M, Hashimoto S: Anatomy of the cerebellopontine angle visualized through the translabyrinthine approach. *Acta Otolaryngol* 1989; 108:238-45.

RECONSTRUCTIVE SURGERY
FOR SLEEP-DISORDERED BREATHING

SURGICAL CONSIDERATIONS

Jerome Hester, Robert J. Troell, Robert B. Riley, Nelson B. Powell, and Kasey K. Li

Description: The surgical approaches to the upper airway attempt to relieve obstruction occurring most commonly at the level of the palate, base of tongue, or pharynx. These fall into three categories: 1) classic procedures that directly enlarge the upper airway; 2) specialized procedures that directly enlarge the upper airway; and 3) tracheotomy to bypass the pharyngeal portion of the upper airway. The surgeon performs a preop evaluation, including complete head and neck exam, fiber optic examination of the upper airway, and cephalometric radiographs. This, together with the results of the polysomnogram, will enable the surgeon to determine what levels of the airway need to be surgically modified. Individuals with severe obstruction may require a multistage approach to treatment.

Uvulopalatopharyngoplasty (UPPP) (Fig 3-24) is a procedure that removes a rim of the soft palate, including the uvula. This shortens and tightens this tissue, thus preventing collapse during sleep. The tonsils, if present, are removed. The muscular crease of the palate is used as a landmark to prevent overly aggressive resection, which could → velopharyngeal insufficiency (VPI), an uncommon but serious complication. The wound is then closed, using interrupted absorbable sutures.

Uvulopalatal flap (UPF) (Fig 3-25) is a variation of UPPP, used for treating palatal obstruction. Rather than excising a rim of the soft palate, the mucosa of the anterior aspect of the uvula is removed, along with a corresponding area of the soft palate. The uvula is then reflected superiorly and sutured into place with absorbable suture. This procedure may be done in combination with a tonsillectomy. UPF is theoretically reversible if signs of VPI become evident. UPF also may be somewhat less painful than UPPP.

Uvulopalatopharyngoglossoplasty (UPPGP) is a rarely performed, intraoral procedure incorporating a modified UPPP, with limited resection of the base of tongue for both retropalatal and retrolingual collapse.

Laser midline glossectomy (LMG) is used to enlarge the retrolingual airway by excision of ~2.5 cm × 5 cm of midline tongue tissue through an intraoral approach. This also may require lingual tonsillectomy, reduction of the aryepiglottic folds, and partial epiglottectomy (Fig 3-26). LMG usually is combined with a tracheotomy for airway protection.

Lingualplasty (LP) is the same procedure as LMG, except that additional tongue tissue is extirpated posteriorly and laterally to that portion removed by LMG (Fig 3-26). It is usually combined with a tracheotomy (see below) for airway protection.

Inferior sagittal mandibular osteotomy and genioglossal advancement (MOGA) (Fig 3-27) is an intraoral approach designed to enlarge the retrolingual area. This procedure relies on the firm attachment of the genioglossus

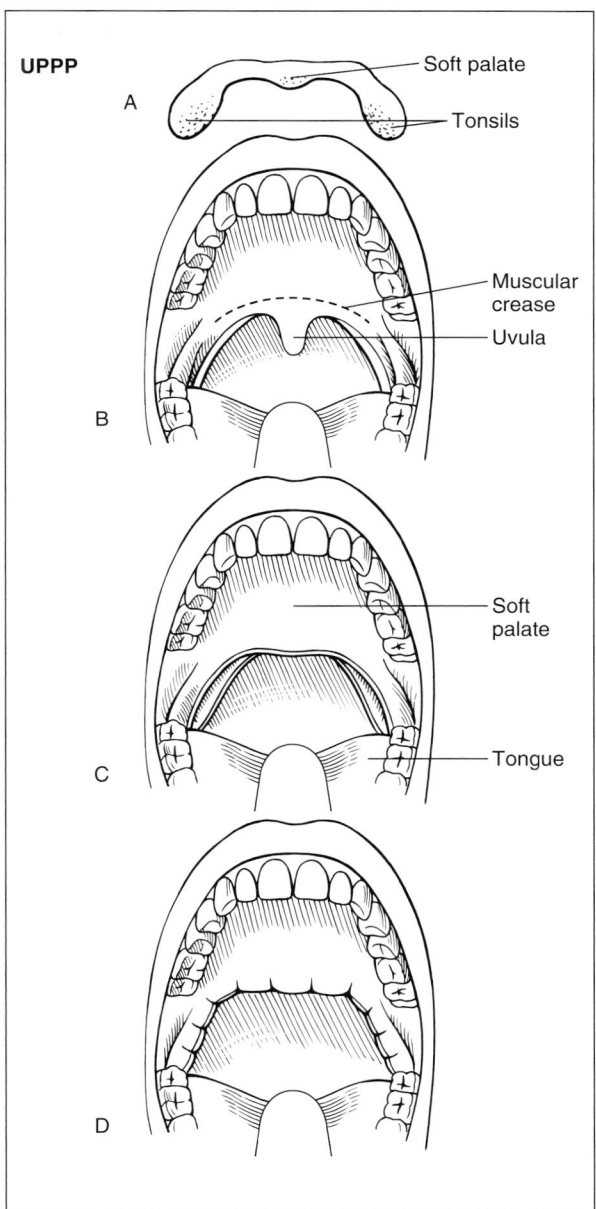

Figure 3-24. Uvulopalatopharyngoplasty (UPPP): (A&B) tonsils and redundant soft palate are excised.; (C) mucosal flaps are prepared for closure; (D) the soft palate is closed to itself, and the anterior and posterior tonsillar pillars are sutured to each other.

muscle to the geniotubercle, a bony protuberance on the medial (lingual) aspect of the mandible. A mucosal incision is made intraorally and soft tissue, including the mentalis muscle, is elevated off the mandible. Osteotomies, which include the geniotubercle on the inner cortex, are then performed. The segment is advanced and rotated to lock it in place. The outer cortex is removed and the fragment is fixated to the inferior mandible with a titanium screw. The advancement is limited by the width of the mandible and laxity in the genioglossus muscle.

Hyoid myotomy and suspension (HM) is a retrolingual procedure that alleviates obstruction by redundant lateral pharyngeal tissue or a retrodisplaced epiglottis. A horizontal cervical incision above the hyoid bone is performed, and the dissection is carried down to the suprahyoid musculature. The midline hyoid bone is isolated and then advanced over the thyroid ala. It is then immobilized with two medial and two lateral permanent sutures (Fig 3-28). The wound is closed, a drain placed and a pressure dressing applied.

Maxillomandibular osteotomy and advancement (MMO) prevents retropalatal collapse through stenting of the superior pharyngeal muscles and widening of the nasopharyngeal inlet. It also minimizes retrolingual obstruction by placing the genioglossus muscle under tension, providing more room in the oral cavity for soft tissues, and stenting the lateral pharyngeal wall. An outer-table cranial bone graft usually is performed, along with arch-bar placement (or orthodontic banding in an outpatient setting) prior to the osteotomies. A LeFort I maxillary osteotomy and bilateral sagittal-split mandibular osteotomy are performed. The skeletal arches are advanced forward ~10 mm and secured with the aid of a methylmethacrylate dental splint (Fig 3-29). Immobilization with wires, plates and screws

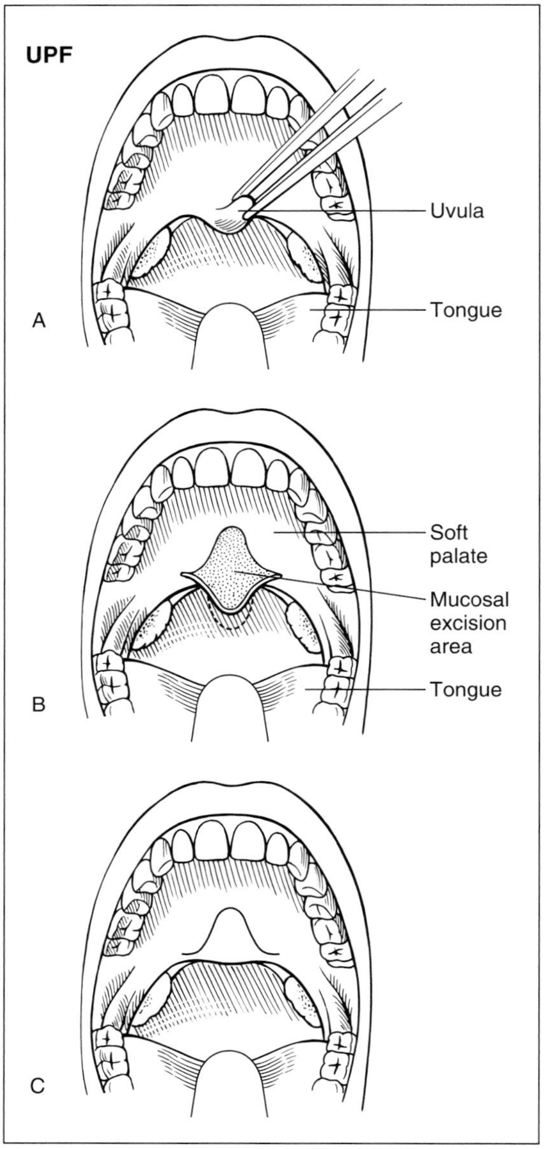

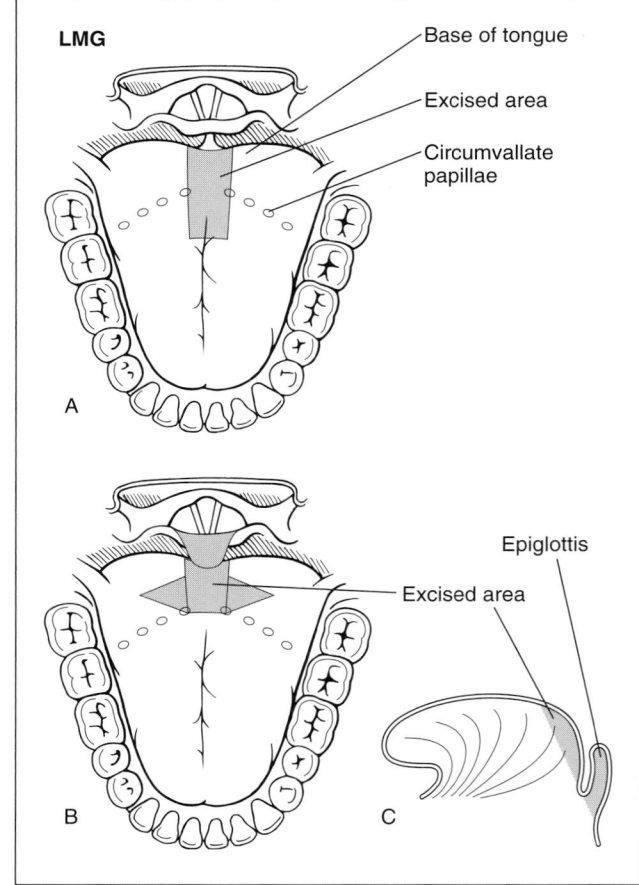

Figure 3-25. Uvulopalatal flap (UPF): (A) uvula is reflected back to the hard palate to identify the muscular crease; (B) mucosa on the oral side of the uvula and soft palate are removed, and part of the uvula is amputated; (C) mucosal incisions are closed with absorbable suture.

Figure 3-26. LMG/lingualplasty technique: (A) Excision of a midline segment of the base of the tongue is performed with a laser or electrocautery; this excision occasionally is carried lateral. (B) The remaining tongue muscle edges are reapproximated with absorbable suture. (C) Lateral view of tongue.

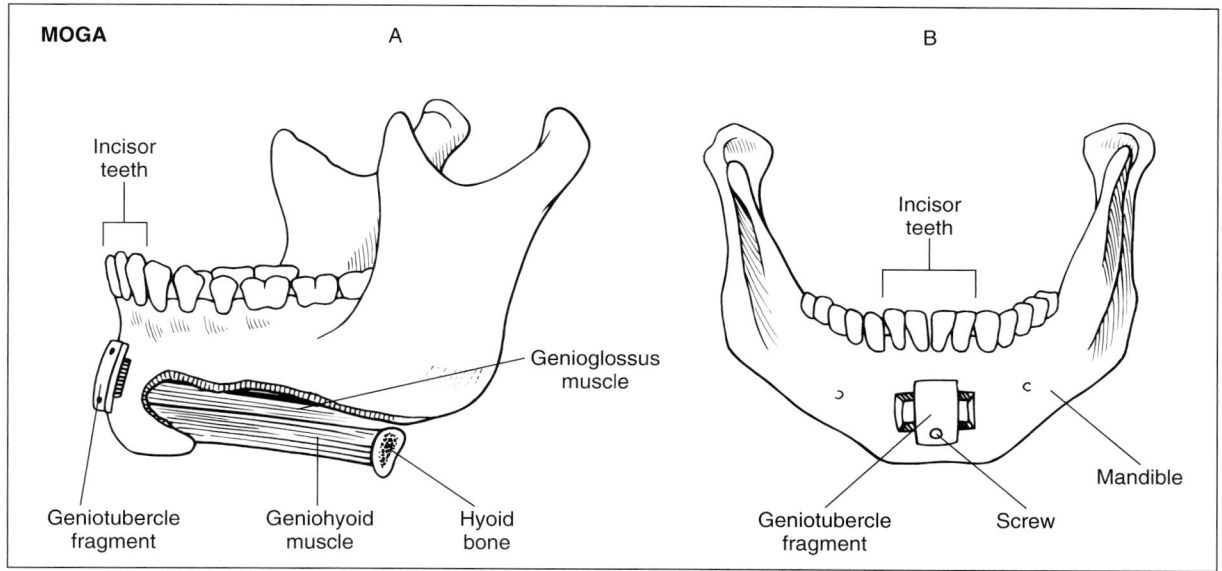

Figure 3-27. The mandibular osteotomy and genioglossus advancement (MOGA) technique: (A) Lateral view. (B) Anterior view. A rectangular anterior mandibular osteotomy below the incisor teeth is advanced, rotated, and immobilized.

follows, then wound closure, intermaxillary fixation, and pressure dressing application. This procedure usually is performed if previous upper airway procedures have not completely relieved the sleep-related obstruction.

Tracheotomy is a procedure performed to bypass pharyngeal obstruction. It is usually reserved for those individuals with severe OSA, and may be used to secure the airway before other procedures. Preop evaluation, including fiber optic examination, will help identify those individuals whose airways are so compromised that the tracheotomy should be done with the patient awake and under local infiltration anesthetic. A horizontal cervical incision is performed midway between the manubrium and the cricoid cartilage. Dissection is carried out in the midline down to the trachea, frequently transecting the thyroid gland; then, an opening in the superior trachea allows placement of a tracheotomy tube (Fig 3-19).

Radiofrequency (RF) probes use heat to cause reduction and tightening of tissue. This may be used to enable the airway at the level of the nose (by reduction of the turbinates), the palate, or the base of tongue. Whereas the nasal and palatal procedures are usually performed as outpatient under local anesthesia, the initial treatment of the base of tongue commonly is performed in the OR, either alone or in conjunction with other airway procedures. The area of the tongue just anterior to the circumvallate papillae is infiltrated with local anesthetic. A needle-like RF probe is then used to heat the tissue. There is usually little or no immediate edema, although the surgeon may admit the patient overnight for airway observation.

Usual preop diagnosis: Sleep disordered breathing, including upper airway resistance syndrome and obstructive sleep apnea (OSA) syndrome

SUMMARY OF PROCEDURES

Position	Supine
Incision	Intraoral (except HM–horizontal cervical above hyoid bone)
Special instrumentation	For osteotomy cases (MOGA, MMO), sagittal and reciprocating saws, drills
Unique considerations	When using a CO_2 laser (LMG, LP), a laser-safe ETT or, more commonly, a tracheotomy tube is required. MMO requires a nasal intubation. Tracheotomy may be performed with patient sitting with iv sedation and/or local infiltration. Dexamethasone 8 mg iv.
Antibiotics	Cefazolin 1 g iv
Surgical time	UPPP, UPF: 20-60 min
	UPPGP, LMG, LP: 1-3 h
	MOGA, HM: 30-60 min
	MMO: 3-5 h
EBL	UPPP, UPF, MOGA, HM: 0-100 ml
	UPPGP, LMG, LP: 50-250 ml
	MMO: 100-500 ml
Postop care	UPPP, UPF: PACU → ward
	Multiple procedures, MMO, labile HTN: ICU → ward
Mortality	Rare

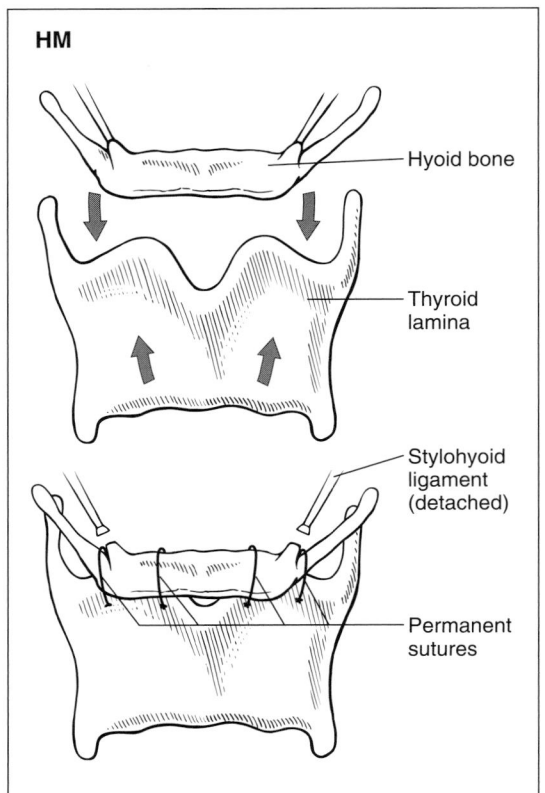

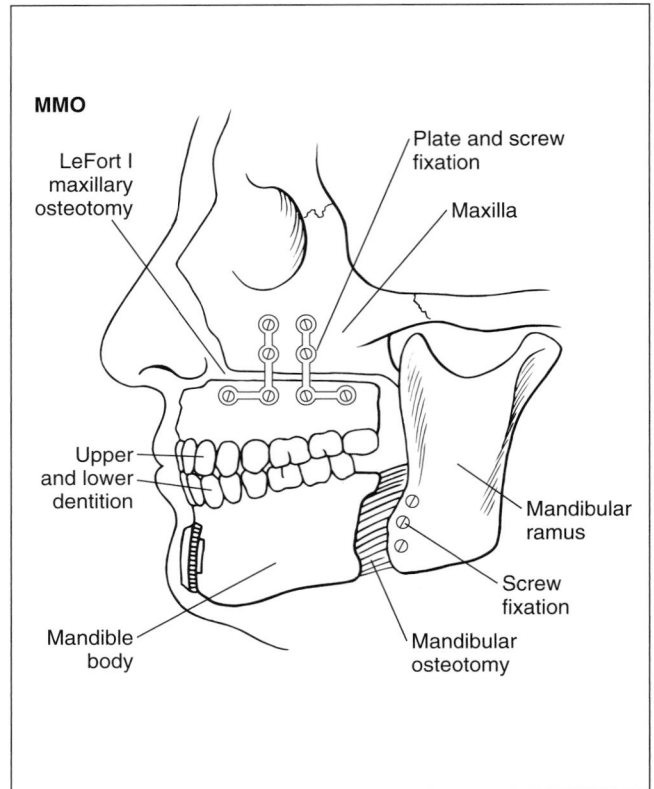

Figure 3-28. The hyoid myotomy (HM) and suspension technique: the hyoid is advanced over the thyroid lamina and immobilized.

Figure 3-29. Maxillomandibular osteotomy (MMO) and advancement surgery technique.

Morbidity	Paresthesias: 10%
	HTN: 5%
	Wound dehiscence: 5%
	Bleeding: 1-2%
	Infection: 1-2%
	Hematoma/seroma: 1-2%
	Upper airway obstruction: 1%
Pain score	UPPP, UPPGP, LMG, LP: 8-10
	UPF, MOGA, HM, MMO: 6-8

PATIENT POPULATION CHARACTERISTICS

Age range	Children, adolescents, adults
Male:Female	3-10: 1
Incidence	4-10% of adult males; 2-4% of adult females
Etiology	Upper airway collapse by frank obstruction or muscular relaxation
Associated conditions	Systemic and pulmonary HTN; CAD; cardiac arrhythmias; GERD; depression; obesity; polycythemia

ANESTHETIC CONSIDERATIONS

Michael W. Champeau

PREOPERATIVE

Patients with OSA often present with a variety of related medical conditions. These may range from chronic fatigue to an increased risk of sudden death. Some patients may have OSA associated with morbid obesity (see p. 401). Typically, these patients are exquisitely sensitive to sedative drugs. Preop evaluation should include their ability to tolerate the supine position without obstructing.

Respiratory   Chronic OSA → hypoxia/hypercarbia → pulmonary HTN → right heart failure. Careful assessment of the airway is essential (suitability for mask ventilation vs need for awake FOL or tracheostomy). Typically, 25% of patients will present with airway management problems that may require awake FOL (4%) or tracheostomy (3%). Preop evaluation should include a discussion with the surgeon of the results of preop fiber optic nasopharyngoscopy.
Tests: PFT; ABG and CXR, if indicated from H&P.

Cardiovascular   Patients are at ↑risk for systemic and pulmonary HTN (Sx: loud P_2, clubbing, ↑JVD, cyanosis, RVH, right-axis deviation), cardiac arrhythmias, cerebrovascular disease, and CAD. These patients may have dyspnea on exertion and at rest, making routine assessment of cardiovascular function and reserve difficult.
Tests: ECG; stress ECHO if abnormal ECG; others as indicated from H&P.

Neurologic   These patients may be chronically fatigued and irritable due to disrupted sleep patterns. Daytime sleepiness also may be associated with hypothyroidism or anemia, which should have been ruled out.
Tests: As indicated by H&P.

Hematologic   Chronic hypoxia → polycythemia (Sx: clubbing, cyanosis) → ↑risk of CVA.
Test: Hct

Gastrointestinal This patient population has a higher incidence of GERD and hiatal hernia; thus, full-stomach precautions (see p. B-5) may be required.

Laboratory   **Tests:** As indicated from H&P.

Premedication   Typically, sedative medications should be kept to a minimum in this patient population; however, if sedative premedication is to be given, the anesthesiologist **must** remain with the patient and be prepared to manage the airway.

INTRAOPERATIVE

Anesthetic technique: Typically GETA; however, patients undergoing UPF, MOGA, and HM may only require MAC.

Induction   Consideration must be given to securing the airway before induction of anesthesia if a difficult intubation is anticipated. Fiber optic intubation with minimal sedation is recommended for these patients (see Awake FOI, p. B-6); otherwise, standard induction with no muscle relaxant until ability to mask ventilate is assured. A short-acting (e.g., mivacurium 0.15 mg/kg) or intermediate-acting (e.g., vecuronium 0.1 mg/kg) muscle relaxant may be administered after mask ventilation is established. MMO requires nasal intubation.

Maintenance   Maintenance with N_2O, propofol, and narcotics, in conjunction with low-dose inhalational agents, will facilitate smooth emergence compared to maintenance with higher doses of inhalational agents. The use of propofol (75-150 μg/kg/min) and remifentanil (0.05-0.150 μg/kg/min) infusions has been particularly successful in providing the smooth, rapid emergence required for safe extubation of these patients. Anticipate ↑BP in response to surgical procedure, especially in patients with preexisting HTN, during UPPP, and with down-fracture of pterygoid plate in MMO. Resist temptation to treat ↑BP with ↑inhalational anesthetics alone, as emergence will be compromised. Labetalol (5-10 mg increments) and hydralazine (5 mg increments) usually are required, while esmolol and SNP infusions are needed occasionally. Dexamethasone 0.1-0.15 mg/kg is recommended to ↓ postop airway edema.

Emergence   The patient should remain intubated until sufficiently awake to respond to a series of commands. Premature extubation can cause complete loss of airway or laryngospasm. Airway is likely to be worse upon emergence than preop because of surgically induced edema. Extubation over a tube changer may be appropriate in some cases. Anticipate ↑BP during emergence, which will continue into first postop day. Antihypertensive agents usually required, as postop HTN can cause bleeding, particularly from osteotomy sites.

Blood and fluid IV: 16-18 ga × 1   Minimal-to-little blood loss with all except MMO. EBL
requirements   NS/LR @ 1-3 ml/kg/h   with MMO is 100-500 ml. Attempt to minimize fluids to reduce severity of postop airway edema (< 1000 ml of NS/LR for all except MMO; < 2000 ml for MMO).

Monitoring	Standard monitors (p. B-1)	
	Arterial line (MMO)	Arterial line also suggested for postop BP control in all patients with preexisting HTN and in any patient who displays labile BP intraop. Control of BP in the postop period is a high priority.
Positioning	✓ and pad pressure points.	Occasional requests for minimal Trendelenburg or sitting maneuvers.
	✓ eyes.	
Complications	ETT damage	ETT may be cut during MMO, necessitating rapid rein-
	Hemorrhage	tubation.

POSTOPERATIVE

Complications	Airway compromise	Airway compromise 2° hematoma, edema, excessive seda-
	Airway obstruction	tion, or underlying disease. Consider observation in ICU for patients having multiple procedures, MMO, or labile HTN.
	HTN	Postop HTN is extremely common and can contribute
	Aspiration	significantly to likelihood of postop airway obstruction 2° hematoma.
Pain management	Minimize iv narcotics.	Avoid excessive postop sedation. UPPP patients, in particular, should be warned preop of anticipated significant postop discomfort.

References

1. Burgess L, Derderian S, Morin G, et al: Postoperative risk following uvulopalatopharyngoplasty for obstructive sleep apnea. *Otolaryngol Head Neck Surg* 1992; 106:81-6.
2. Conway W, Fujita S, Zorick F, et al: Uvulopalatopharyngoplasty. One-year followup. *Chest* 1985; 88:385-7.
3. Escalamado RM, Glenn MG, McCulloch TM, Cummings CW: Perioperative complications and risk factors in the surgical treatment of obstructive sleep apnea. *Laryngoscope* 1989; 99:1125-9.
4. Fairbanks, DN: Snoring: Surgical vs nonsurgical management. *Laryngoscope* 1984; 94:1188-92.
5. Fujita S, Conway W, Zorick F, et al: Surgical correction of anatomic abnormalities in obstructive sleep apnea syndrome: Uvulopalatopharyngoplasty. *Otolaryngol Head Neck Surg* 1981; 89:923-34.
6. Johnson JT, Pollack GL, Wagner RL: Transoral radiofrequency treatment of snoring. *Otolaryngol Head Neck Surg* 2002; 127:235-7.
7. Li KK, Powell NB, Riley RW, et al: Radiofrequency volumetric tissue reduction for treatment of turbinate hypertrophy: A pilot study. *Otolaryngol Head Neck Surg* 1998; 119:569-73.
8. Li KK, Powell NB, Riley RW, Guilleminault C: Temperature controlled radiofrequency tongue base reduction for sleep-disordered breathing: Long term outcomes. *Otolaryngol Head Neck Surg* 2002; 127:230-3.
9. Mickleson SA, Rosenthal L: Midline glossectomy and epiglottidectomy for obstructive sleep apnea syndrome. *Laryngoscope* 1997; 107:614-9.
10. Powell N, Riley R, Guilleminault C, Troell R: A reversible uvulopalatal flap for snoring and sleep apnea syndrome. *Sleep* 1996; 19(7):593-9.
11. Riley R, Powell N, Guilleminault C: Obstructive sleep apnea and the hyoid: a revised surgical procedure. *Otolaryngol Head Neck Surg* 1994; 111:717-21.
12. Riley RW, Powell NP, Guilleminault C, Pelayo R, Troell RJ: Obstructive sleep apnea surgery: Risk management and complications. *Otolaryngol Head Neck Surg* 1997; 117(6):648-52.
13. Riley R, Powell N, Guilleminault C: Obstructive sleep apnea syndrome: a review of 306 consecutively treated surgical patients. *Otolaryngol Head Neck Surg* 1993; 108:117-25.
14. Sher A, Schechtman K, Piccirillo J: The efficacy of surgical modifications of the upper airway in adults with obstructive sleep apnea syndrome. *Sleep* 1996; 19(2):156-77.
15. Woodson BT, Fujita S: Clinical experience with lingualplasty as part of the treatment of severe obstructive sleep apnea. *Otolaryngol Head Neck Surg* 1992; 107:40-8.

Surgeons

Sabine C. Girod, MD, DDS, PhD
Stephen A. Schendel, MD, DDS, FACS

4.0 DENTAL SURGERY

Anesthesiologists

Richard A. Jaffe, MD, PhD
Stanley I. Samuels, MB, BCh, FFARCS

TEMPOROMANDIBULAR JOINT ARTHROSCOPY/ARTHROTOMY

SURGICAL CONSIDERATIONS

Description: Temporomandibular joint (TMJ) surgical procedures include closed surgical techniques (arthroscopy) and open surgical techniques (arthrotomy).

TMJ arthrotomy involves a preauricular, postauricular, or endaural incision to gain access to the joint compartment. It usually is performed for severe fibrous adhesion removal in the TMJ, bony or fibrous ankylosis, tumor resection, chronic dislocation, painful nonreducing disc dislocation, and severe osteoarthritis. **Open TMJ** surgery may range from discoplasty; discectomy; arthroplasty; and/or eminoplasty (reshaping of articular eminentia) to optimize the fit of the disc, condyle, and fossa; to total joint replacement utilizing costochondral grafts or vitallium metal implants.[1] For the open treatment of condylar fractures, extraoral approaches (e.g., preauricular, retromandibular, and submandibular) are used. All extraoral approaches to the TMJ have the risks of facial nerve dam-

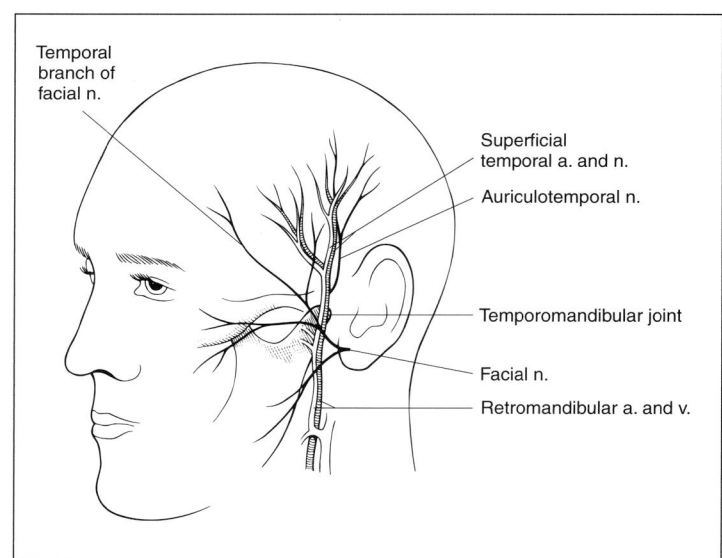

Temporal branch of facial n.

Superficial temporal a. and n.

Auriculotemporal n.

Temporomandibular joint

Facial n.

Retromandibular a. and v.

Figure 4-1. Anatomy for TMJ procedure.

age and the creation of visible scars. Due to those possible complications, endoscopically assisted transoral approaches for open reduction and miniplate fixation of condylar mandible fractures are used increasingly more often.[5]

TMJ Arthroscopy is a minimally invasive technique that has reduced the need for open surgery of the TMJ.[3] Arthroscopic TMJ surgery is indicated for treatment of internal derangements and intracapsular disorders. The major advantage is that it results in less periarticular tissue disruption and better preservation of vascular supply and lymphatic drainage of the joint. The procedure involves insertion of a TMJ miniscope through a preauricular puncture on the canthus-tragus line and insertion of an outflow needle. The joint compartment is continually lavaged with LR. A second cannula can be inserted; and arthroscopic procedures are performed using a triangulation technique. Arthroscopic TMJ procedures include lysis of adhesions and lavage, partial synovectomy, and abrasion arthroplasty. Sometimes a holmium: YAG laser is used to make intraarticular incisions anterior to displaced discs and to treat inflamed synovial tissue.[4] Usually, at the end of the procedure, 2 mg dexamethasone is injected into the joint space. Injection of 2 mL 0.5% bupivacaine mixed with 1 mL sterile saline solution has been shown to significantly reduce postop pain.[2] Arrhythmia, reflex bradycardia, and pulmonary edema have been reported as general complications in TMJ arthroscopy.[6]

Usual preop diagnosis: Internal derangement, subluxation, and ankylosis of TMJ

SUMMARY OF PROCEDURES

	Arthroscopy	Arthrotomy
Position	Supine	⇐
Incision	Preauricular	⇐
Special instrumentation	Arthroscope; laser	Power tools, endoscope, implant plates
Antibiotics	Cefazolin 1 g	⇐
Surgical time	0.5 h	1.5-3.5 h/side
EBL	Minimal	Minimal-moderate
Postop care	Outpatient procedure	24 h stay
Mortality	Minimal	⇐
Morbidity	VII nerve damage	⇐
	V nerve damage	⇐
	Hemorrhage	⇐
	Partial hearing loss	
	Ear fullness	
	Vertigo	
Pain score	5	5

200

PATIENT POPULATION CHARACTERISTICS

Age range	20-40 yr
Male:Female	1:9
Incidence	20% of adult population suffers from TMJ dysfunction (TMJD).
Etiology	TMJD possibly 2° muscle spasm, bruxism, osteoarthritis; idiopathic; trauma
Associated conditions	Psychiatric problems (typically depression); trismus; pain on opening mouth; stress

ANESTHETIC CONSIDERATIONS

See Anesthetic Considerations for Dental/Oral Surgery, p. 203.

References

1. Fricton JR, Look JO, Schiffman E, Swift J: Long-term study of temporomandibular joint surgery with alloplastic implants compared with nonimplant surgery and nonsurgical rehabilitation for painful temporomandibular joint disc displacement. *J Oral Maxillofac Surg* 2002; 60(12):1400-11.
2. Furst IM, Kryshtalskyj B, Weinberg S: The use of intra-articular opioids and bupivacaine for analgesia following temporomandibular joint arthroscopy: a prospective, randomized trial. *J Oral Maxillofac Surg* 2001; 59(9):979-83.
3. Indresano AT: Surgical arthroscopy as the preferred treatment for internal derangements of the temporomandibular joint. *J Oral Maxillofac Surg* 2001; 59(3):308-12.
4. Mazzonetto R, Spagnoli DB: Long-term evaluation of arthroscopic discectomy of the temporomandibular joint using the Holmium YAG laser. *J Oral Maxillofac Surg* 2001; 59(9):1018-23.
5. Schon R, Schramm A, Gellrich NC, Schmelzeisen R: Follow-up of condylar fractures of the mandible in 8 patients at 18 months after transoral endoscopic-assisted open treatment. *J Oral Maxillofac Surg*; 61(1):49-54.
6. Tsuyama M, Kondoh T, Seto K, Fukuda J: Complications of temporomandibular joint arthroscopy: a retrospective analysis of 301 lysis and lavage procedures performed using the triangulation technique. *J Oral Maxillofac Surg* 2000; 58(5):500-5.

ORAL SURGERY

SURGICAL CONSIDERATIONS

Description: The most common surgeries of the oral cavity are third-molar removal, surgical extractions, apicoectomies, orthodontic exposures of teeth, osseointegrated implants, bone grafting, treatment of oral pathologic conditions, and preprosthetic surgery. **Surgical extractions** of teeth involve intraoral exposure of the roots through a mucosal incision and removal of overlying bone with a surgical drill. Risks associated with removal of teeth in the mandible are damage to the inferior alveolar nerve (anesthetic numb lip), lingual nerve (anesthetic numb tongue),[1] and, rarely, mandibular fracture.[5] In the posterior maxilla, oroantral fistulas can occur and are closed with a mucoperiosteal flap. **Exposure of teeth** for orthodontic therapy involves creation of a mucoperiosteal flap and attachment of a bracket with a small gold chain, on which the orthodontist can pull to integrate the tooth into the dental arch. **Bone grafting** to the maxilla and mandible is done for augmentation of the atrophied alveolar ridge and the maxillary sinus[4] and in cases of cleft lip and palate.[2] A second team usually harvests the bone at the same time. Possible extraoral harvesting sites include the anterior or posterior iliac crest, the tibia, and the skull. **Preprosthetic surgery** of the oral soft tissue in preparation for dentures has been replaced largely by insertion of **osseointegrated implants** for retention of individual teeth and dentures.[3] Surgical treatment of **oral pathology** can range from removal of dentigerous cysts, with and without bone graft, to laser or surgical removal of mucosal lesions.

SUMMARY OF PROCEDURES

	Dental Surgery	Dental Implants	Oral Pathology	Bone Grafting
Position	Supine	⇐	⇐	Supine or prone
Incision	Intraoral	⇐	⇐	Intraoral and donor site

	Dental Surgery	**Dental Implants**	**Oral Pathology**	**Bone Grafting**
Special instrumentations	Surgical drill	Implant drill and kit	Surgical drill, laser	–
Antibiotics	None	Penicillin 1 g	Cefazolin 1 g	⇐
Unique considerations	Nasotracheal intuba-tion	⇐	⇐	⇐
	Throat pack	⇐	⇐	⇐
Surgical time	0.5 h/tooth	0.5 h/implant	1-3 h	2-3 h
EBL	Minimal	⇐	⇐	Moderate
Postop care	Outpatient	⇐	⇐ or 24 h stay	24 h stay
Mortality	Minimal	⇐	⇐	⇐
Morbidity	V nerve damage	⇐	⇐	Hemorrhage
	Aspiration of dental debris	⇐		
Pain score	3	2	3-5	5

PATIENT POPULATION CHARACTERISTICS

	Dental Surgery	**Dental Implants**	**Oral Pathology**	**Bone Grafting**
Age range	12-40 yr	> 16 yr	All ages	> 8 yr
Male:Female	1:1	⇐	⇐	⇐
Etiology	Idiopathic	Tooth loss	Various	⇐
Associated conditions	Craniofacial syndromes			

ANESTHETIC CONSIDERATIONS

See Anesthetic Considerations for Dental/Oral Surgery, p. 203.

References

1. Bataineh AB: Sensory nerve impairment following mandibular third molar surgery. *J Oral Maxillofac Surg* 2001; 59(9): 1012-7.
2. Bilkay U, Tokat C, Ozek C, Gundogan H, Gurler T, Tegsel Z, Songur E: Cancellous bone grafting in alveolar cleft repair: new experience. *J Craniofac Surg* 2002; 13(5):658-63.
3. Coulthard P, Esposito M, Worthington HV, Jokstad A: Interventions for replacing missing teeth: preprosthetic surgery versus dental implants (Cochrane Review). *Cochrane Database Syst Rev* 2002; (4):CD003604.
4. Kaufman E: Maxillary sinus elevation surgery. *Dent Today* 2002; 21(9):96-101.
5. Perry PA, Goldberg MH: Late mandibular fracture after third molar surgery: a survey of Connecticut oral and maxillofacial surgeons. *J Oral Maxillofac Surg* 2000; 58(8):858-61.

RESTORATIVE DENTISTRY

SURGICAL CONSIDERATIONS

Description: Multiple dental restorative procedures are performed under GA when there is rampant caries, and an extensive amount of dental work must be performed at one time. The second most common indication for GA is for procedures that need to be performed on mentally retarded patients who are not candidates for a local anesthetic. The actual amount of restorative dentistry is quite variable, depending on the individual case; thus, surgical time can be quite variable. Generally, blood loss is not a problem.

SUMMARY OF PROCEDURE

Position	Supine
Incision	Intraoral
Special instrumentation	Dental armamentarium
Unique considerations	Nasal intubation; throat pack
Antibiotics	Penicillin × 5 d po
Surgical time	0.5-3 h
EBL	Minimal
Postop care	PACU → home
Mortality	Minimal
Morbidity	Pain
	Aspiration of dental debris
	Swelling
Pain score	1-3

PATIENT POPULATION CHARACTERISTICS

Age range	2 yr - adult
Male:Female	1:1
Incidence	Unknown
Etiology	Idiopathic or congenital anomalies
Associated conditions	Mental retardation (majority); Down syndrome, seizures

ANESTHETIC CONSIDERATIONS FOR DENTAL/ORAL SURGERY

PREOPERATIVE

Most patients presenting for dental or oral surgery usually will require only local anesthesia provided by the dentist/oral surgeon. GA may be required, however, for several unique patient groups: (1) young children (some with systemic diseases such as CHD, hemophilia); (2) the mentally retarded; (3) those with poorly controlled seizure disorders; (4) those presenting for TMJ procedures; and (5) those with an oral septic focus, who may be quite ill. If the patient does not fall into one of these readily identifiable categories, the reasons for GA should be ascertained.

Airway	Patients presenting for TMJ procedures may have problems with mouth opening (2° pain, trismus, and arthritis), making airway examination difficult. Mouth opening may not improve with GA and muscle relaxation. Nasotracheal intubation using FOL (done awake in patients with difficult airways) should be planned. Examine nares for patency; check for loose teeth.
Respiratory	Surgery should be postponed (2 wk) in patients presenting with Sx of acute RTI (fever, coughing, purulent sputum, etc.). Sx of chronic respiratory disease should be sought and treated before surgery. **Tests:** As indicated from H&P.
Cardiovascular	Patients with dysrhythmias may be sensitive to the epinephrine used in local anesthetic solutions administered intraop. As with other types of elective surgery, preexisting cardiovascular problems should be treated before inducing anesthesia. Prophylactic antibiotics for endocarditis may be required in some patients. **Tests:** As indicated from H&P.
Neurological	Patients with seizure disorders should be on optimal medical therapy before surgery. Discuss precipitating factors and prodromal Sx with the patient. **Tests:** ✓ therapeutic levels of anticonvulsant (e.g., phenytoin = 10-20 μg/ml; carbamazepine = 3-12 μg/ml; phenobarbital = 10-40 μg/ml).
Musculoskeletal	In addition to TMJ problems, rheumatoid arthritis is associated with cricoarytenoid joint immobility and cervical spine immobility/instability that may complicate intubation.
Laboratory	Other tests as indicated from H&P.

Premedication	Standard premedication (see p. B-2) usually is appropriate, although in patients with limited airway access, sedation may be inappropriate. If FOL is planned, pretreatment with an antisialagogue (e.g., glycopyrrolate 4 μg/kg) is useful.

INTRAOPERATIVE

Anesthetic technique: GETA. Typically a nasotracheal intubation is required, using an ETT 0.5-1 mm smaller than for oral intubation. In patients with difficult airways, an awake nasal FOL is indicated. (See general discussion of Awake FOL, p. B-6.)

Induction	In patients with normal airways, a standard induction (see p. B-2) is appropriate. Following loss of consciousness, topical intranasal cocaine may be applied (4% on pledgets, 4 ml maximum) to shrink the nasal mucosa and for vasoconstriction. Side effects are rare, but may include ↑BP, ↑ or ↓HR, dysrhythmias, and Sz. Other topical vasoconstrictors (e.g., 0.05% oxymetazoline) may be used; however, they are associated with cardiovascular side effects. The well lubricated ETT is passed through the nose into the trachea, either blindly or assisted by McGill's forceps under direct laryngoscopy. ETT is often sewn to nasal septum. Alternatively, the successful use of a reinforced LMA in both adult and pediatric dental patients has been reported. (See Reference 8 for review.) Claimed advantages include no risk of epistaxis and airway protection without need of a throat pack.
Maintenance	Standard maintenance (see p. B-3).
Emergence	★ **NB:** No special considerations except that **throat packs must be removed prior to extubation**.
Blood and fluid requirements	IV: 18 ga × 1 NS/LR @ 4-6 ml/kg/h
Monitoring	Standard monitors (see p. B-1).
Positioning	✓ and pad pressure points. ✓ eyes.

POSTOPERATIVE

Complications	Airway obstruction 2° retained throat pack
	N&V — These patients may swallow blood, with consequent N&V. Rx: metoclopramide 10 mg iv.
Pain management	Oral analgesics (see p. C-2).

References for Dental/Oral Surgery

1. Dolwick MF, Kretzschmar DP: Morbidity associated with the preauricular and perimeatal approaches to the temporomandibular joint. *J Oral Maxillofac Surg* 1982; 40(11):699-700.
2. Finder RL, Moore PA: Adverse drug reactions to local anesthesia. *Dent Clin North Am* 2002; 46(4):747-57.
3. Girdler NM, Hill CMM: Sedation in Dentistry. John Wright, Oxford: 1998.
4. Indresano AT: Surgical arthroscopy as the preferred treatment for internal derangements of the temporomandibular joint. *J Oral Maxillofac Surg* 2001; 59(3):308-12.
5. Jackson DL, Johnson BS: Conscious sedation for dentistry: risk management and patient selection. *Dent Clin North Am* 2002; 46(4):767-80.
6. Jackson DL, Johnson BS: Inhalational and enteral conscious sedation for the adult dental patient. *Dent Clin North Am* 2002; 46(4):781-802.
7. Peterson LJ, Tucker MR, Ellis EI: Contemporary Oral and Maxillofacial Surgery. Mosby-Year Book, St. Louis: 1998.
8. Rosenblatt WH: Airway Management in Clinical Anesthesia, 4th edition. Barash PG, Cullen BF, Stoelting RK, eds. Lippincott Williams & Wilkins, Philadelphia: 2001, 602-5.
9. Webb MD, Moore PA: Sedation for pediatric dental patients. *Dent Clin North Am* 2002; 46(4):803-14, xi.
10. Zuniga JR: Guidelines for anxiety control and pain management in oral and maxillofacial surgery. *J Oral Maxillofac Surg* 2000; 58(10Supp2):4-7.

Surgeons

Richard I. Whyte, MD
Walter B. Cannon, MD
Jessica S. Donington, MD

5.0 THORACIC SURGERY

Anesthesiologists

John L. Chow, MD, MS
Jay B. Brodsky, MD

THORACIC SURGERY

INTRODUCTION—SURGEON'S PERSPECTIVE

AIRWAY AND LUNG ACCESS CONFLICTS

As in Head and Neck Surgery, induction and maintenance of anesthesia for thoracic surgery requires interdisciplinary cooperation. Perioperative communication between the surgeon and anesthesiologist is required for a satisfactory outcome. For example, during periods of OLV, significant hypoxia and hypotension may occur. Surgery may need to be stopped temporarily while the hypoxia is corrected by reinflation of the unventilated lung. Hypotension in the absence of bleeding can be corrected by less vigorous retraction of the lung and heart by the surgeon. Quick and timely communication between the anesthesiologist and the surgeon can be life-saving. Occasionally, during critical parts of the dissection, cessation of all respiration for short periods of time can make the surgeon's job much easier.

TUBES AND TUBE SIZES

Although the size of the ETTs may not be particularly critical for most patients, thoracic surgical procedures may be different. Fiber optic bronchoscopy (FOB) through the ETT is a common event. The standard FOB just fits through the 8.0 ETT. The fiber optic laryngoscope (FOL) used for difficult intubations will fit smaller ETTs and DLTs. Proper lubrication of the bronchoscope with a Carbowax ointment (rather than an aqueous jelly, which will dry out quickly) makes manipulation quite easy. The FOL can be used for correct positioning of the DLT. If the bronchial portion of the DLT cannot be advanced into the left main bronchus, the bronchoscope can be advanced through the bronchial side of the DLT into the left main bronchus. Then, through use of the bronchoscope as a stent, the DLT can be advanced over the bronchoscope into the left bronchus. The depth of the tube can be determined by bronchoscopic observation of the right main bronchus through the tracheal side of the DLT. If a laser is to be involved, have a laser-compatible ETT available, keep FiO_2 to < 0.3 and do not use N_2O.

PATIENT POSITIONING AND SURGICAL INCISIONS

Patient positioning for these procedures is dictated by the type of incision used. The incisions used most often by thoracic surgeons are the **posterolateral thoracotomy** (and its variations) (Fig 5-1A), the **median sternotomy** (Fig 5-1B), and the anterior thoracotomy (often bilateral) (Fig 5-1C). For procedures where excellent exposure of both lungs is mandatory (e.g., bipulmonary lung transplantation), the **'clamshell' incision** (Fig 5-2) has become popular. Generally, patients are in the **supine position** for anterior incisions (sternotomy, cervical, and anterior thoracotomy) and in the **lateral position** for lateral and posterolateral thoracotomies. Thoracoscopic procedures (VATS) typically are performed in the lateral position. (Note: A review of a recent CXR in the OR will help ensure that the thoracotomy is performed on the correct side.)

Patients undergoing surgery in the **lateral position** are initially placed on a bean bag. When GA is induced, the patient is rolled onto his/her side with the kidney rest being positioned at the level of the lower ribs. An axillary roll is placed to prevent axillary compression, and the table is flexed to assist in spreading the ribs. The head and neck must be aligned in a neutral position to avoid brachial plexus injuries. The lower arm can be either extended on an arm board or flexed and placed next to the patient's head (Fig 5-3A). The upper arm is then extended and held in position with either an airplane

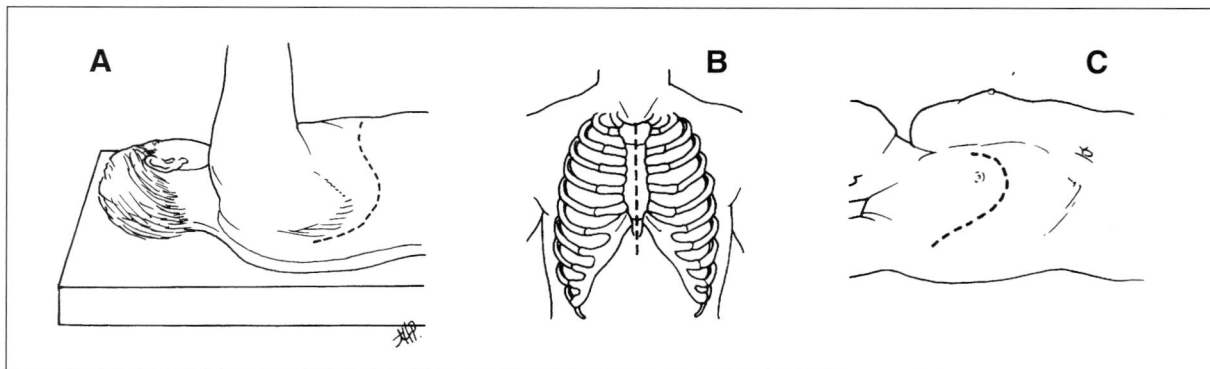

Figure 5-1. Primary incisions for thoracic surgery. (A) Posterolateral thoracotomy, in lateral position. The incision curves in an S shape, passing under the tip of the scapula over in the fifth interspace anteriorly. (B) Median sternotomy, in supine position, arms at side: the incision is made from the suprasternal notch to a point between the xiphoid process and umbilicus. (C) Anterior thoracotomy in supine position. (Reproduced with permission from Fry WA: Thoracic incisions. In *General Thoracic Surgery*, 5th edition. Shields TW, LoCicero J III, Ponn RB, eds. Lippincott Williams & Wilkins, 2000.)

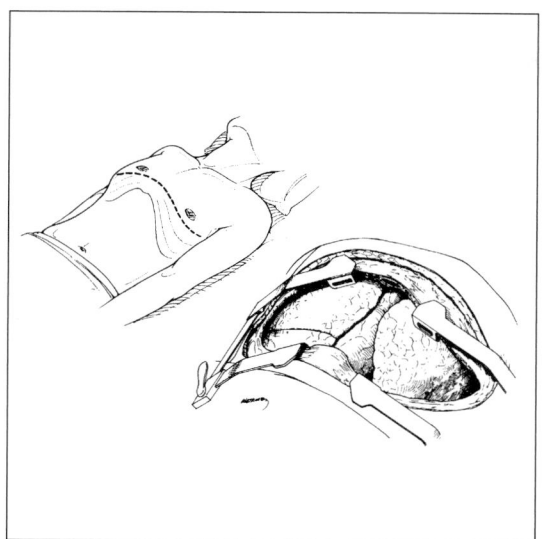

Figure 5-2. The 'clamshell' incision, in classic supine position, affords excellent exposure, especially for bilateral lung procedures. (Reproduced with permission from Fry WA: Thoracic incisions. In *General Thoracic Surgery*, 5th edition. Shields TW, LoCicero J III, Ponn RB, eds. Lippincott Williams & Wilkins, 2000.)

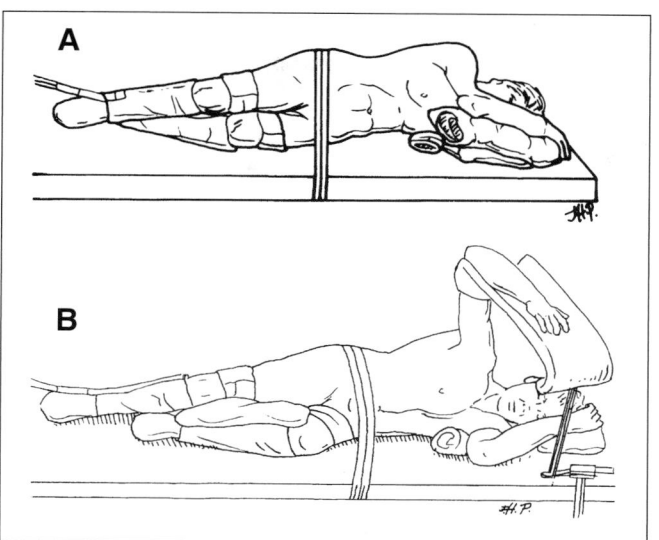

Figure 5-3. Lateral positioning for thoracic lateral and posterolateral procedures. (A) Patient on his side, with kidney rest, axillary roll, pillows between knees, and padding under elbows. Wide adhesive tape secures the position. (B) Upper arm abducted 90% on arm board. (Reproduced with permission from Fry WA: Thoracic incisions. In *General Thoracic Surgery*, 5th edition. Shields TW, LoCicero J III, Ponn RB, eds. Lippincott Williams & Wilkins, 2000.)

holder or an arm board with several pillows (Fig 5-3B). The lower leg should be flexed and the upper leg should be left extended and supported by pillows. The back is kept in a vertical position, while the beanbag is evacuated of air (bolsters of blankets may be placed next to the patient). Wide adhesive tape is placed across the hips to further secure the patient. A lower-body warming blanket (e.g., Bair Hugger) should be used to avoid hypothermia. To facilitate closure, the table can be returned to the flat position. Ideally, this is accompanied by inflation, and subsequent deflation, of the beanbag. The anesthesiologist may be asked to exert downward pressure on the patient's shoulder to diminish tension on the latissimus dorsi closure.

While the standard posterolateral thoracotomy involves division of the latissimus dorsi and serratus anterior muscles, **muscle-sparing incisions**—either transverse or vertical—are gaining in popularity because they are perceived to decrease pain and provide a more rapid recovery. Variations on the posterolateral thoracotomy all have position requirements similar to those of the standard posterolateral incision.

For an anterior incision, the patient is placed supine. A small roll placed under the shoulder blades will serve to extend the neck and facilitate access to the upper mediastinum. This is particularly important for an operation on the upper trachea, and improves visualization for cervical mediastinoscopy. In general, the arms should be tucked at the patient's sides. Having an arm extended during a sternotomy can place undue stretch on the brachial plexus → injury.

The probability of DVT in general thoracic cases is controversial, although the risks of prophylaxis are minimal. Given that patients undergoing thoracotomy often have protracted periods of immobility, both during and after surgery, and often have a Dx of a malignant disease (hypercoaguability), use of DVT prophylaxis is good practice. We use SCDs for all patients, except those undergoing short video-assisted procedures, and reserve subcutaneous heparin for those at higher than normal risk (e.g., with prolonged postop immobility).

POSTOPERATIVE ISSUES

The most common postop issues relevant to anesthesiologists are:

- The need for postop mechanical ventilation;
- Airway management;
- Hemodynamic instability; and
- Pain control.

The majority of patients undergoing thoracotomy can be extubated immediately postop. The most common exceptions are patients requiring preop mechanical ventilation, lung transplant patients, and those with 'difficult' airways. Patients undergoing prolonged surgery may require postop mechanical ventilation. With shorter procedures, and those performed using minimally invasive techniques, even patients undergoing lung-volume-reduction surgery for severe emphysema generally can be extubated at the conclusion of the procedure.

Since DLTs are larger than standard ETTs, there is greater potential for laryngeal trauma and airway edema → loss of airway following extubation. By exchanging the DLT for a single-lumen ETT over a tube changer, this potentially catastrophic complication can be avoided.

Hemodynamic instability following surgery may be 2° several causes, the most important being ongoing blood loss (or inadequate intraop fluid replacement) and cardiac dysfunction. Use of epidural anesthesia may accentuate ↓BP both intraop and postop.

With the use of epidural anesthesia and systemic analgesics (e.g., ketorolac) postop pain can be managed effectively. It is important for the anesthesiologist to communicate to the surgeon (and postop care team) as to which agents have been used, how the patient responded to them, and what types of hemodynamic, pulmonary, and neurological effects can be expected in the postop period.

LOBECTOMY, PNEUMONECTOMY

SURGICAL CONSIDERATIONS

Description: Surgery remains the most appropriate form of treatment for early-stage lung cancer. Other, less common indications include infection (particularly mycobacterial disease and bronchiectasis), developmental abnormalities, such as sequestrations, and trauma. Patients with Stage I or II non-small-cell lung cancer (disease confined to the lung, or those with intrapulmonary node involvement only) generally are offered surgery, unless their pulmonary function is prohibitively poor or their comorbidities pose an unacceptable risk. Patients with Stage IIIA disease often receive preop chemotherapy and/or radiation; and those with Stage IIIB or IV disease are rarely offered an operation.

Regardless of the underlying disease, preop evaluation should include an assessment of pulmonary function (Table 5-1). Spirometry is adequate for most patients with little or no functional impairment, but more elaborate tests—such as measurement of diffusion capacity, quantitative ventilation/perfusion scans, or formal exercise testing (Fig 5-5)—are appropriate for others.

Following induction of GA, many surgeons perform a preop bronchoscopy. In patients with more proximal tumors, this bronchoscopy may be important in determining whether the patient should undergo a lobectomy, sleeve lobectomy, or pneumonectomy. Most patients undergoing **lobectomy** or **pneumonectomy** are placed in the lateral decubitus position. This approach permits a lateral or posterolateral thoracotomy (Fig 5-1A)—the incision that provides optimal exposure of the pulmonary hilum. A more limited, **muscle-sparing incision** may be used; however, the exposure may be somewhat

Table 5-1. Spirometric Criteria for Pulmonary Resection		
Spirometry	**Operable**	**Further Study Suggested**
Forced vital capacity (FVC)	> 60% predicted	< 60% predicted
Forced expired volume in 1 sec (FEV$_1$)	> 60% predicted	< 60% predicted
FEV$_1$:FVC ratio	> 50%	< 50%
Maximum voluntary ventilation	> 50% predicted	< 50% predicted
Gas exchange		
Diffusing capacity for carbon monoxide	> 60% predicted	< 60% predicted
Arterial carbon dioxide tension	< 45 mmHg	> 45 mmHg

(Used with permission from Olson GN: Pulmonary physiologic assessment of operative risk. In *General Thoracic Surgery*, 5th edition. Shields TW, LoCicero J III, Ponn RB, eds. Lippincott Williams & Wilkins, 2000.)

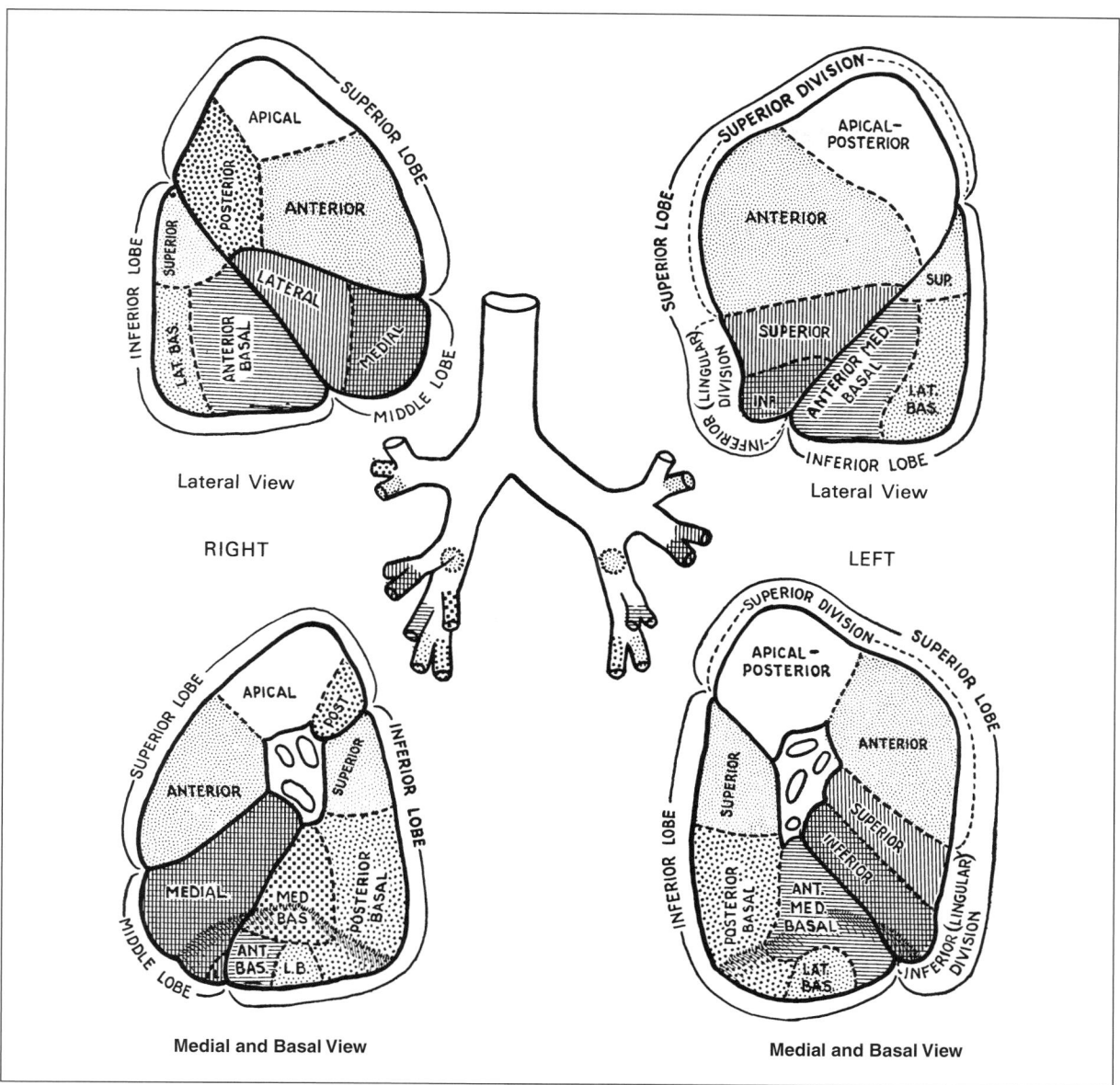

Figure 5-4. Segmental anatomy of the lungs. (Reproduced with permission from Clemente CD: *Gray's Anatomy*, 30th American edition. Williams & Wilkins, 1985.)

limited. Occasionally, a **median sternotomy approach** (Fig 5-1B) is used, when there is significant involvement of the anterior mediastinum by the tumor.

Following entry into the chest, the lung on the operative side is allowed to deflate. If the lung remains inflated, a flexible bronchoscope should be used to verify correct positioning of the ETT (Fig 5-6). Alternatively, the surgeon may be able to feel the tip of the ETT and guide it into the correct position. Once stable OLV has been obtained, the lung is mobilized and the bronchovascular structures are identified. Generally, the vascular structures are divided first, although when exposure is limited, it may be best to divide the bronchus first. Hypotension and arrhythmias may occur when the hilar structures or pericardium are retracted vigorously. Such aberrations generally resolve quickly on restoration of normal anatomic relationships. Entry into a branch of the pulmonary artery during dissection can result in rapid blood loss. Since these vessels are usually under low pressure, bleeding generally can be controlled with direct pressure on the bleeding site, while the anesthesiologist resuscitates the patient and the surgeon obtains more definitive vascular control. During a lobectomy, the surgeon will ask the anesthesiologist to reinflate the lung while the bronchus leading to the lobe that will be removed is occluded. This will ensure that the remaining lobes inflate appropriately. Thorough suctioning immediately before the lobectomy eliminates secretions as a cause of continued atelectasis. Once the lung or lobe has been resected, positive pressure is applied to the bronchial stump (and lobe) to check that there is no significant postop air leak. Large air leaks are best addressed at the time of surgery, rather than waiting for them to resolve postop.

Chest drainage is standard following lobectomy and involves placement of two 28-36 Fr chest tubes attached to underwater seal or suction. Placing the tubes to suction typically increases observed air leak, while extubating the patient in the supine position typically decreases the leak. Following pneumonectomy, chest drainage is not uniformly carried out; however, if a chest tube is to be placed, a balanced drainage system must be used or the mediastinum will shift to the operative side → adverse hemodynamic consequences. An alternative to drainage (after the patient is placed supine) is to aspirate air from the operative pleural space until a slight negative pressure is obtained.

Usual preop diagnosis: Carcinoma of the lung; infection; developmental abnormalities; trauma

SUMMARY OF PROCEDURES

	Lobectomy	Pneumonectomy
Position	Lateral/supine	⇐
Incision	Posterolateral/median sternotomy	⇐
Special instrumentation	DLT; SCD or TED hose	⇐
Antibiotics	Cefazolin 1 g	⇐
Surgical time	2-3 h	⇐
EBL	< 500 ml (more in redo or inflammatory cases)	⇐
Postop care	PACU ± IIC; careful attention to pulmonary toilet; chest tube output	⇐ + Special balanced drainage tube
Mortality	± 1%	± 5%
Morbidity	Dysrhythmias: 10-20%	30-40%
	DVT: 5-20%	⇐
	ARDS	⇐
	PE	⇐
	MI	⇐
	Bronchopleural fistula	⇐
	Chylothorax	⇐
	Subcutaneous emphysema	⇐
	Phrenic nerve injury	⇐
	Recurrent laryngeal nerve injury	⇐
Pain score	7-8	7-8

PATIENT POPULATION CHARACTERISTICS

Age range	0-80 yr
Male:Female	15:1
Incidence	Common thoracic procedure; increasing in females
Etiology	Smoking
Associated conditions	Cardiopulmonary disease; PVD

ANESTHETIC CONSIDERATIONS

PREOPERATIVE

Most patients presenting for these operations have either an infectious process or a lung neoplasm. They often have Hx of cigarette smoking with associated emphysema and/or chronic bronchitis. Selective lung isolation, with or without OLV (with a DLT or a BB), is essential for this procedure.

Respiratory   Question patient about dyspnea, productive cough and cigarette smoking. Examine patient for cyanosis, clubbing, RR, and pattern. Listen to chest for wheezes, rhonchi, rales. Morbidity and mortality following thoracotomy increased with preexisting pulmonary, cardiovascular, and neurologic disease. Timely cessation of smoking (> 8 wk), adequate management of bronchospasm with bronchodilator treatment ± steroids, and prompt treatment of preexisting lung infections are important to reduce postop pulmonary complications.

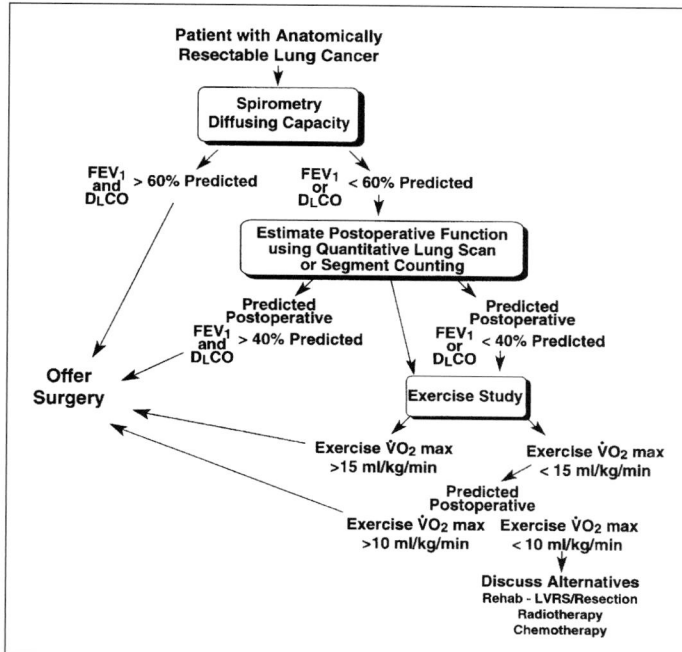

Figure 5-5. Physiologic assessment of patients with compromised lung function. (Reproduced with permission from Olson GN: Pulmonary physiologic assessment of operative risk. In *General Thoracic Surgery*, 5th edition. Shields TW, LoCicero J III, Ponn RB, eds. Lippincott Williams & Wilkins, 2000.)

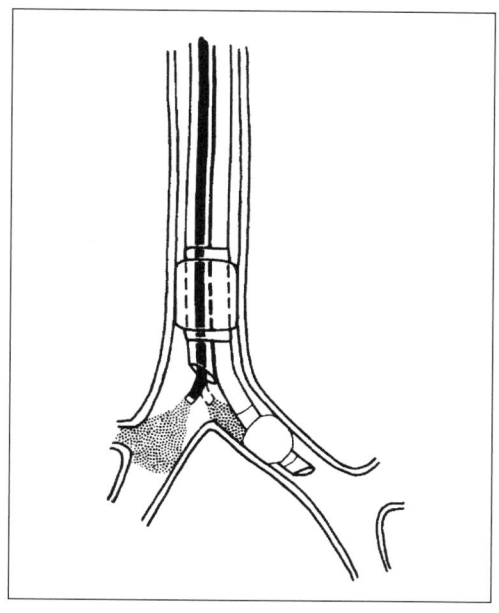

Figure 5-6. Use of a fiber optic bronchoscope to assure correct positioning of a left-side DLT. (Reproduced with permission from Ovasspian A: Conduct of anesthesia. In *General Thoracic Surgery*, 5th edition. Shields TW, LoCicero J III, Ponn RB, eds. Lippincott Williams & Wilkins, 2000.) with permission from Fry WA: Thoracic incisions. In *General Thoracic Surgery*, 5th edition. Shields TW, LoCicero J III, Ponn RB, eds. Lippincott Williams & Wilkins, 2000.)

Respiratory, cont.	**Tests:** PFT (see below and Table 5-2); CXR; if chest CT available, look for airway obstruction that could interfere with DLT placement; ABG (only if indicated from H&P).
Pulmonary function	Establish a baseline and identify patients with advanced pulmonary disease who are unable to tolerate planned operation. Obtain whole-lung tests (ABG, spirometry), and single-lung tests (split-function lung tests = V/Q studies) if pneumonectomy planned. A VC at least $3 \times$ TV is necessary for effective cough postop. A VC < 50% predicted or < 1500 ml, predicts ↑risk for postop complications following pulmonary resection. Operative risk for pneumonectomy increases if patient is hypercapnic ($PaCO_2$ > 45 mmHg) on room air, FEV_1/FVC < 50% of predicted, FEV_1 < 2 L, if > 60-70% blood flow is to diseased lung, and if mean PAP increases > 30 mmHg with occlusion of PA. Mimic post pneumonectomy conditions by temporary unilateral occlusion of main PA. Patient may show improvement in PFTs following bronchodilator therapy.
Cardiovascular	Prophylactic digitalization to ↓ risk of postop heart failure, or atrial fibrillation has not proven effective clinically. Consider subcutaneous heparin (5000 U) for DVT prophylaxis. **Tests:** ECG—look for evidence of RV hypertrophy, conduction problems, ischemia, and prior MI. ECHO to evaluate ventricular function; others as indicated from H&P.
Neurological	✓ Hx of previous back surgery, peripheral neuropathy. Examine thoracolumbar area for skin lesions, infection, deformities.
Musculoskeletal	Patients with lung cancer may have myasthenic (Eaton-Lambert) syndrome with resistance to depolarizing muscle relaxants and ↑sensitivity to NMRs. Monitor relaxation with peripheral nerve stimulator.
Hematologic	Transfuse patient with preop Hct < 25% or < 30% in patients with Hx of CAD. Adequate O_2-carrying capacity essential. T&C 2 U of blood, or obtain 1-2 U of autologous blood during the month before surgery; or consider erythropoietin in patients who are anemic. **Tests:** Hct; PT; PTT (if epidural anesthesia planned)

Table 5-2. Assessment of Risk of Postop Pulmonary Complications Following Thoracic and Abdominal Procedures

Category	Point
I. Expiratory Spirogram	
a. Normal (%FVC + %FEV$_1$/FVC >150)	0
b. %FVC + %FEV$_1$/FVC = 100-150	1
c. %FVC + %FEV$_1$/FVC < 100	2
d. Preop FVC < 20 ml/kg	3
e. Post-bronchodilator FEV$_1$/FVC < 50%	3
II. Cardiovascular System	
a. Normal	0
b. Controlled HTN, MI sequelae for more than 2 yr	0
c. Dyspnea on exertion, orthopnea, paroxysmal nocturnal dyspnea, dependent edema, CHF, angina	1
III. ABGs	
a. Acceptable	0
b. PaCO$_2$ >50 mmHg or PaCO$_2$ < 60 mmHg on room air	1
c. Metabolic pH abnormality > 7.50 or < 7.30	1
IV. Nervous System	
a. Normal	0
b. Confusion, obtundation, agitation, spasticity, discoordination, bulbar malfunction	1
c. Significant muscular weakness	1
V. Postop Ambulation	
a. Expected ambulation (minimum, sitting at bedside) within 36 h	0
b. Expected complete bed confinement for at least 36 h	1

0 Points = Low Risk; 1-2 Points = Moderate Risk; 3 Points = High Risk

Shapira BA, Harrison RA, Kacmarek RM, Cane RD: *Clinical Application of Respiratory Care*, 3rd edition. Year Book Medical Publishers, Chicago: 1985. (With permission.)

Laboratory   Other tests as indicated from H&P.

Premedication   Midazolam 1-2 mg iv if patient anxious. When epidural opioids are planned, avoid additional systemic opioid or sedative premedication that can potentiate postop respiratory effects of spinal opioids.

INTRAOPERATIVE

Anesthetic technique: Combined epidural (lumbar or thoracic) and inhalational agent. Anesthesia for lobectomy/pneumonectomy relies on OLV techniques to improve surgical exposure and minimize damage to the operative lung in the case of lobectomy or bilobectomy. The challenges to the anesthesiologist include maintaining adequate oxygenation in patients with poor pulmonary reserve and ensuring that the patient is comfortable, warm, and awake at the end of surgery.

Preinduction   A thoracic or lumbar epidural catheter is placed and advanced 4-6 cm past needle in epidural space; secure with tape. Administer test dose: 3 ml lidocaine (1.5%) + 1:200,000 epinephrine. If no evidence of inadvertent intravascular or intrathecal catheter placement, then administer 5-10 ml of 2% lidocaine with 1:200,000 epinephrine to elicit segmental block. Confirm functioning epidural catheter preop to ensure predictable periop analgesia. Giving local anesthetics through the epidural catheter intraop reduces the amounts of GA and muscle relaxants required. Post thoracotomy analgesia is excellent with thoracic or lumbar epidural opioids.

Induction   Standard induction (p. B-2). If flexible bronchoscopy is planned prior to lung resection, intubate with an ETT (≥ 8 mm), which will be replaced with DLT after bronchoscopy (see below). Otherwise, proceed to intubation with an appropriate sized DLT (e.g., adult male, 39 Fr; adult female, 37 Fr) after induction.

Maintenance   O$_2$ and isoflurane (1.0-1.5%); less anesthetic required when epidural local anesthetics used. Avoid N$_2$O, especially during OLV, since hypoxemia is unpredictable. Use FiO$_2$ = 1.0. A local anesthetic (e.g., 2% lidocaine with 1:200,000 epinephrine or 0.25% bupivacaine) can be infused or injected

Maintenance, cont.	hourly into a thoracic (3-5 ml) or lumbar (5-10 ml) epidural catheter. Continuous infusion of local anesthetic generally provides better hemodynamic stability than hourly bolus injection. To enhance the effect of epidural analgesia, a loading dose of opiate (e.g., hydromorphone 0.4-1 mg [thoracic] or 1-1.5mg [lumbar]) can be administered early in the surgery and at least 1 h before conclusion of the case. Epidural hydromorphone is preferred since, in equipotent doses, analgesia is equivalent to that with morphine, but with fewer side effects. Lung manipulation during surgery releases vasoactive substances that interfere with hypoxic pulmonary vasoconstrictive (HPV) reflex. Thus, clinically, the choice of anesthetic agent should not be influenced by experimental studies that indicated that the HPV reflex is maintained with iv agents, but may not be with inhalational agents. Inhalational anesthetics are potent bronchodilators and depress airway reflexes.	
Emergence	Before closing of chest, lungs are inflated gradually to 30 cmH_2O pressure to reinflate atelectatic areas and to ✓ for significant air leaks. Surgeon inserts chest tubes to drain pleural cavity and aid lung reexpansion. Patient is extubated in OR. If postop ventilation is required (rare), DLT exchanged for single-lumen ETT. Patient transferred in head-elevated position to PACU or ICU, breathing mask O_2. If hemodynamically unstable, monitor ECG, pulse oximetry, and arterial pressure during transfer.	
Blood and fluid requirements	IV: 18 ga x 1 + 14 or 16 ga × 1 Avoid hypervolemia. Blood: ± 1 U autologous blood if available; use vasopressor (ephedrine 5-10 mg iv bolus or phenylephrine 50-100 μg iv bolus) if hypotensive.	Postop, PVR is increased proportionate to the amount of lung tissue removed. An overhydrated patient is at risk of RV failure and pulmonary edema. Replace blood loss with crystalloid (1:3) or colloid (1:1). Third-space loss is negligible and need not be replaced. Use of epidural local anesthetics can cause ↓BP in a volume-restricted patient; vasopressor often needed.
Monitoring	Standard monitors (p. B-1) Arterial line Urinary catheter ± CVP line ± PA line	It is mandatory to follow oxygenation continuously during OLV. Typically, this can be done with pulse oximetry, although continuous intraarterial PO_2 monitoring is now commercially available. CVP and/or PA line optional for pneumonectomy and for patients with coexisting cardiac disease. During open thoracotomy, CVP monitoring may be inaccurate. A PA line, placed immediately preop in the operated PA, may interfere with pneumonectomy. Central volume monitoring is useful for postop management.
Positioning	Axillary roll, 'airplane' for upper arm Avoid hyperextending arms. ✓ and pad pressure points. ✓ eyes, ears, genitals.	✓ radial pulses to ensure correct placement of axillary roll (if misplaced, will compromise distal pulses). Placing the oximeter probe on the down arm may assist in monitoring perfusion adequately.
Fiber optic bronchoscopy	FOB performed immediately before thoracotomy to evaluate resectability of lesion. Patient intubated with large ETT (≥ 8 mm), replaced with DLT or BB following bronchoscopy (see Bronchoscopy, p. 235).	Use the largest plastic DLT that atraumatically passes through the glottis (typically, 39 Fr for men, 37 Fr for women).[2] DLT can be placed accurately by careful auscultation ± confirmation by FOB. If FOB is used, pass down tracheal lumen. Top of blue endobronchial cuff should be visible below carina in bronchus. For small children, the balloon of a Fogarty embolectomy catheter is used as a BB; for adults, either a BB or a Univent tube may be used if the proper size DLT cannot be placed. FOB always needed to confirm BB placement. With BB, operated lung cannot be reinflated, collapsed, and suctioned safely periodically during surgery.
Lung isolation	Separate lungs to prevent contralateral contamination (infection, pus, blood, tumor), allow selective ventilation and facilitate operation.	
OLV	Use large TV (10-12 ml/kg) during two-lung ventilation. When using OLV, reduce TV to keep $ETCO_2$ @ 35-45 mmHg and PIP < 35 cmH_2O.	Adequate TV during OLV prevents atelectasis of the dependent ('down,' ventilated) lung. Overdistension of the ventilated lung can → volutrauma and lung injury. Ventilation rate adjusted to avoid dynamic hyperinflation or hyperventilation. Compliance is reduced and resistance is increased

OLV, cont.

(1 lumen instead of 2). PIPs will be higher, and some auto-PEEP may be generated, depending on size of DLT. Intraop hypoxemia during OLV is less likely when $FiO_2 = 1.0$ and adequate TV used. If pulse oximetry < 95% or $PaO_2 < 100$, recheck position of DLT or BB. The DLT endobronchial cuff can obstruct the upper lobe bronchus of the ventilated lung or the DLT or BB balloon can herniate into the carina, obstructing both lungs. Hypoxemia may be 2° luminal }obstruction by blood or pulmonary secretions, requiring aggressive suctioning. PEEP to ventilated lung can be used, but with caution, since overdistention of alveoli will increase shunt to the 'up' lung, worsening hypoxemia. If hypoxemia persists, insufflate operated ('up,' collapsed) lung with 100% O_2 and apply CPAP (5-10 cmH$_2$O) to the 'up' lung to improve oxygenation without interfering with surgical field. The PA of the operated lung during pneumonectomy can be clamped completely, eliminating shunt.

Complications	Hypoxemia	Hypoxemia during OLV most commonly results from luminal obstruction (by blood or pulmonary secretions or malposition) of the DLT, and ↑shunting. Rx: suctioning the DLT; PEEP to ventilated lung (but may ↑ shunting); CPAP to nonventilated lung; return to double-lung ventilation; and ✓ DLT position. Temporary clamping of the PA (or inflating the balloon of the PA catheter, if available) may be necessary to improve shunting and, thus, oxygenation.
	Hypercarbia	Ensure adequate TV and RR.
	Arrhythmia	✓ for mechanical compression of heart or great vessels.
	Hypotension	✓ volume status and cardiac function. Consider neosynephrine for BP support if ↓BP is 2° epidural.
	Airway rupture	✓ integrity of intubated bronchus after reexpanding lung.
	DVT	Preventive measures using TED hose and SCD.

POSTOPERATIVE

Complications	Airway trauma from intubation, tracheobronchial rupture	Do not overdistend bronchial balloon or DLT cuffs. DLT bronchial cuff usually requires < 2 ml air for airtight seal, if an appropriate (large) DLT is used.
	Injuries related to lateral positioning	Pressure damage to ear, eye, nose, deltoid muscle, iliac crest, brachial plexus, and radial, ulnar, common peroneal, and sciatic nerves have all been reported.
	Structural injuries related to thoracotomy	Neurologic (phrenic and recurrent laryngeal nerves), thoracic duct, spinal cord; bronchopleural fistula, tracheobronchial disruption
	Surgical complications	Cardiac herniation, tension pneumothorax, bleeding, torsion of residual lobe, post pneumonectomy PE/ARDS
	Cardiopulmonary complications	Supraventricular dysrhythmias, SVT, acute RV failure, atelectasis, BPF, pneumonia, PE. For SVT, treat underlying cause and correct electrolyte abnormalities. Adenosine (e.g., 6 mg iv) may be effective. Most postop SVTs are 2° atrial fibrillation catecholamine surge and may resolve spontaneously. Hemodynamically unstable patients will require cardioversion. Beta blockers, amiodarone, Ca^{++} channel blockers, and over-drive cardiac pacing are effective in patients with unstable AF.
Pain management	Neuraxial opioids – epidural or intrathecal Parenteral opioids (iv, im, continuous iv, PCA [p. C-3])	Effective analgesia is essential for patient to cough, deep breathe, and ambulate early. Thoracic epidural often is recommended, but lumbar route is as effective and is safer. In immediate postop period, 0.2-0.3 mg/h of hydromor-

Pain management, cont.	Intercostal blocks	phone + local anesthetic infused through epidural. Fentanyl 50-100 μg bolus in 10 ml NS for breakthrough pain.
	Interpleural analgesia	
	Epidural local anesthetics	
	Cryoanalgesia	
	NSAID (ketorolac)	Ketorolac (30 mg) is helpful as adjunct analgesic.
Tests	Hct, CXR, ABG and others as indicated.	

References

1. Amar D: Perioperative atrial tachyarrhythmias. *Anesthesiology* 2002; 97(6):1618-23.
2. Baue AE, ed: *Glenn's Thoracic and Cardiovascular Surgery*, 6th edition, Volume II. Geha AS, Hammond GL, Laks H, Naunheim KS, assoc eds. Appleton & Lange, Norwalk, CT: 1996.
3. Brodsky JB, Fitzmaurice B: Modern anesthetic techniques for thoracic operations. *World J Surg* 2001; 25(2):162-6.
4. Brodsky JB, Macario A, Mark JBD: Tracheal diameter predicts double-lumen tube size: a method for selecting left double-lumen tubes. *Anesth Analg* 1996; 82: 861-4.
5. Chow JL, Alfille PH: Postpneumonectomy pulmonary edema. In *The Harvard Department of Anaesthesia Electronic Anesthesia Library (HEAL)* on CD-ROM. Bailin MT, ed. Lippincott Williams & Wilkins, Philadelphia: 2001.
6. Cohen E, Eisenkraft JB, Thys DM, et al: Oxygenation and hemodynamic changes during one-lung ventilation: Effects of $CPAP_{10}$, $PEEP_{10}$, $CPAP_{10}/PEEP_{10}$. *J Cardiothorac Anesth* 1988; 2 (1): 34-40.
7. Fry WA: Thoracic incisions. In *General Thoracic Surgery*, 5th edition. Shields TW, LoCicero J III, Ponn RB, eds. Lippincott Williams & Wilkins, Philadelphia; 2000, 367-748.
8. Kavanagh BP, Katz J, Sandler AN, et al: Pain control after thoracic surgery. A review of current techniques. *Anesthesiology* 1994; 81:737-59.
9. Neustein SM, Kahn P, Krellenstein DJ, Cohen E: Incidence of arrhythmias after thoracic surgery: thoracotomy versus video-assisted thoracoscopy. *J Cardiothorac Vasc Anesth* 1998; 12(6)659-61.
10. Olson GN. Pulmonary physiologic assessment of operative risk. In *General Thoracic Surgery*, 5th edition. Shields TW, LoCicero J III, Ponn RB, eds. Lippincott Williams & Wilkins, Philadelphia; 2000, 297-304.
11. Ovassapian A: Conduct of anesthesia. In *General Thoracic Surgery*, 5th edition. Shields TW, LoCicero J III, Ponn RB, eds. Lippincott Williams & Wilkins, Philadelphia; 2000, 327-44.
12. Sabiston DC Jr, Spencer FC: *Surgery of the Chest*, 6th edition, Vol II. WB Saunders, Philadelphia: 1995.
13. Slinger PD, Hickey DR: The interaction between applied PEEP and auto-PEEP during one-lung ventilation. *J Cardiothorac Vasc Anesth* 1998; 12(2):133-6.
14. Smetana GW: Preoperative pulmonary evaluation. *N Eng J Med* 1999; 340(1):937-44.

WEDGE RESECTION OF LUNG LESION

SURGICAL CONSIDERATIONS

Description: Wedge resection (removal of a mass and 1 cm margins in a manner that does not remove an entire anatomical pulmonary segment) may be carried out for a number of reasons. A known or suspected cancer may be removed by this limited resection. There is general agreement that this is an appropriate operation for patients with limited pulmonary reserve who are unable to withstand lobectomy. Wedge resection also is used for resection of single- or multiple-metastatic lesions from various primary neoplasms. A single metastasis may be removed through a limited thoracotomy incision. At the other extreme, a **median sternotomy** may be carried out to remove bilateral lesions. Wedge resection also is indicated for diagnostic and therapeutic purposes in lesions which defy diagnosis by less invasive techniques. Incisions vary with location, number of lesions, and technique used. **Limited thoracotomy, standard thoracotomy,** or **median sternotomy** may be used under different circumstances. **Stapling** (Fig 5-7), **clamp and suture** technique, or **excision and suture** technique

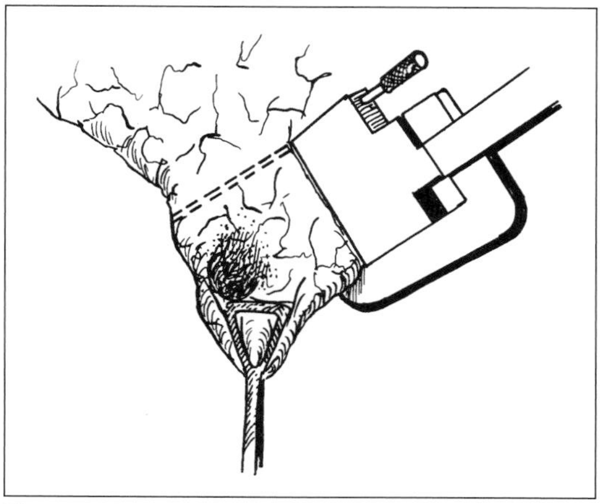

Figure 5-7. Stapler used to perform wedge incision. (Reproduced with permission from Scott-Conner CEH, Dawson DL: *Operative Anatomy*. Lippincott Williams & Wilkins, 2003.)

may be used for lesions in different locations. Wedge resection is best performed in the lateral position and with OLV. Small nodules on the edge of the lung and diagnostic biopsies for interstitial lung disease often can be performed with the thoracoscope, thereby avoiding a thoracotomy. In patients who cannot tolerate OLV (e.g., with ARDS), it may be necessary to keep the patient supine and ventilate both lungs. The wedge resection itself generally is carried out with a surgical stapling device (Fig 5-7) that simultaneously staples the lung parenchyma and cuts between staple lines. Alternatively, the lung tissue can be clamped and oversewn—a technique applicable to particularly indurated lung tissue that is too thick for a stapler. A final option is to perform a pneumonotomy, enucleate the nodule, and suture the lung closed. A single chest tube usually is placed for postop chest drainage.

Variant approach: Video-assisted thoracoscopy surgery (VATS) (see p. 240).

Usual preop diagnosis: Metastatic tumor to the lungs; primary lung cancer (typically, lobectomy); unknown pulmonary lesion

SUMMARY OF PROCEDURE

Position	Lateral or supine
Incision	Limited and related to location of solitary lesion; sternotomy for bilateral lesions
Special instrumentation	DLT
Antibiotics	Cefazolin 1 g (or as indicated from culture and sensitivity)
Surgical time	< 1-3 h, depending on number of lesions
EBL	< 500 ml
Postop care	PACU ± IIC; careful attention to pulmonary toilet, chest tube output
Mortality	Minimal
Morbidity	Air leaks
	Cardiac dysrhythmias
Pain score	2-6

PATIENT POPULATION CHARACTERISTICS

Age range	30-60 yr most common
Male:Female	1:1
Incidence	Common thoracic procedure
Etiology	Variable – neoplasm or inflammatory disease
Associated conditions	COPD; cardiovascular disease; malignancy; infection

ANESTHETIC CONSIDERATIONS

PREOPERATIVE

The anesthetic considerations for this procedure are very similar to those for lobectomy/pneumonectomy. Wedge resection of the lung often is reserved for patients with poor pulmonary reserve, e.g., an absolute $FEV_1 < 1.2$-1.4 L or 40% predicted.

Respiratory	PFTs similar to major thoracotomy. Further evaluation directed toward an underlying disease (e.g., immunocompromised patient for open-lung biopsy, patient with metastatic lesions, etc.). **Tests:** PFTs (see Lobectomy, Pneumonectomy, p. 211); CXR; if chest CT available, look for airway obstruction that could interfere with DLT placement; Hct; ABG, as indicated from H&P.
Cardiovascular	**Tests:** ECG—look for evidence of RV hypertrophy, conduction problems, ischemia, and previous MI.
Neurological	Hx of previous back surgery, peripheral neuropathy. Examine thoracolumbar area for skin lesions, infection, deformities. The placement of an epidural catheter in patient with neurologic problems is controversial.
Musculoskeletal	Patients with lung cancer may have myasthenic (Eaton-Lambert) syndrome with resistance to depolarizing muscle relaxants and ↑sensitivity to NMRs. Monitor relaxation with a peripheral nerve stimulator.
Hematologic	Patients are often anemic from primary disease. Consider preop blood transfusion or erythropoietin therapy. **Tests:** Hct

Laboratory	Other tests as indicated from H&P.
Premedication	Midazolam 1-2 mg iv if patient anxious. When epidural opioids are planned, avoid additional systemic opioid or sedative premedication, which can potentiate postop respiratory effects of central neuraxial opioids.

INTRAOPERATIVE

Anesthetic technique: GETA, often combined with epidural for thoracotomy approach. VATS approach does not require an epidural. DLT will be required for lung isolation.

Induction	STP 3-5 mg/kg iv or propofol 1-2 mg/kg iv, succinylcholine 1-1.5 mg/kg or vecuronium 0.1 mg/kg for tracheal intubation.	
Maintenance	**Balanced technique:** O_2, isoflurane, and iv opioids (usually fentanyl or remifentanil). N_2O used during two-lung ventilation, but D/C'd during OLV. Epidural catheter seldom used in thorascopic approach because pain from limited incision is treated easily by conventional analgesic therapy. If epidural used, follow same guidelines as for major thoracotomy (opioid dosage may be reduced). If an epidural is not utilized, a possible useful adjunct is intercostal block and/or local anesthetic given through the chest tube once the lung is inflated. Bupivacaine 0.25% with epinephrine, to a maximum of 0.5 ml/kg, is appropriate.	
Emergence	Extubate in OR, transfer in head-up position to PACU or ICU, breathing O_2 by mask.	
Blood and fluid requirements	IV: 16-14 ga × 1 NS/LR @ 2 ml/kg/h (maintenance fluid)	Replace blood loss with crystalloid (1:3) or colloid (1:3). Third-space loss is negligible and does not need to be replaced.
Monitoring	Standard monitors (p. B-1) ± Arterial line	Arterial line needed occasionally.
Positioning	Lateral decubitus or supine, with wedge under back on operated side. ✓ and pad pressure points. ✓ eyes, ears, genitals.	
Ventilation	ETT; DLT or BB generally needed; TV (12-15 ml/kg) during two-lung ventilation. Reduce TV to keep ETCO₂ 35-45 mmHg and PIP < 35 cmH₂O.	For OLV, see Anesthetic Considerations for Lobectomy/Pneumonectomy, p. 213.
Complications during OLV	See OLV under Intraop Anesthetic Considerations for Lobectomy/Pneumonectomy, p. 214.	

POSTOPERATIVE

Complications	Atelectasis Pneumonia Fluid overload	See Postop Complications for Lobectomy, Pneumonectomy (p. 214).
Complications during OLV	See OLV under Postop Anesthetic Considerations for Lobectomy/Pneumonectomy, p. 214.	
Pain management	Parenteral opioids (iv, im, continuous iv, PCA [p. C-3]). Epidural Intercostal blocks Interpleural analgesia NSAID (ketorolac 30 mg)	See Pain Management for Lobectomy, Pneumonectomy (p. 214).

References

1. Baue AE, ed: *Glenn's Thoracic and Cardiovascular Surgery*, 6th edition, Volume II. Geha AS, Hammond GL, Laks H, Naunheim KS, assoc eds. Appleton & Lange, Norwalk, CT: 1996.

2. Mitchell RL: The lateral limited thoracotomy incision: standard for pulmonary operations. *J Thorac Cardiovasc Surg* 1990; 99(4):590-5.
3. Sabiston DC Jr, Spencer FC: *Surgery of the Chest*, 6th edition, Vol II. WB Saunders, Philadelphia: 1995.
4. Shah JS, Bready LL: Anesthesia for thoracoscopy. *Anesthesiol Clin North Am* 2001; 19(1):153-71.
5. Slinger PD: Lung isolation. In *Cardiac, Vascular, and Thoracic Anesthesia*. Youngberg JA, Lake CL, Roizer MF, Wilson RS, eds. Churchill Livingstone, Philadelphia: 2000, 603-38.

CHEST-WALL RESECTION

SURGICAL CONSIDERATIONS

Description: Removal of portions of the thoracic cage may be required under several circumstances. Perhaps the most common indication is lung cancer that has invaded the chest wall. Chest-wall resection is also the treatment of choice for most primary chest-wall tumors, the exceptions being Ewing's sarcoma and rhabdomyosarcoma. Although preop chemotherapy is not standard treatment for chest-wall sarcomas, some patients may have received Adriamycin, which is associated with cardiotoxicity at high doses. If the tumor or other disease process involves the skin, an appropriate area of skin—typically, 4 cm around the tumor—must be resected along with the specimen. Underlying subcutaneous tissue and muscle should always be resected in continuity; however, the tumor itself must not be exposed. Wide skin flaps are frequently necessary as well. Resection of larger areas of the chest wall may require extensive reconstruction. Limited resection (1-5 cm segments of 1-3 ribs) generally requires limited chest-wall reconstruction (including the use of plastic mesh replacement with or without methylmethacrylate, rib grafts and muscle, or myocutaneous flaps). Extensive reconstruction of the chest wall (procedures that are often complex and time-consuming) is usually carried out in conjunction with plastic surgeons. Larger defects can be tolerated posteriorly without reconstruction, as the scapula provides chest-wall stabilization and prevents lung herniation. If a prosthesis is required, it must be covered by viable muscle so as to avoid erosion through the skin. Removal of anterolateral or anterior portions of the chest wall, particularly resections that include the sternum, are associated with greater postop instability than are resections of posterior portions of the chest wall, which are protected by the back muscles and scapula. Thus, anterior resections may require more extensive reconstruction with wide preparation and draping.

Usual preop diagnosis: Lung cancer with chest-wall attachment; primary tumor of the chest wall (bone, cartilage, or soft tissue); radiation necrosis

SUMMARY OF PROCEDURE

Position	Supine or lateral
Incision	Over mass to be resected
Special instrumentation	Bone instruments; Marlex (or other) mesh; methylmethacrylate
Antibiotics	Cefazolin 1 g (or as indicated by culture and sensitivity)
Surgical time	1-8 h
Closing considerations	May require help of plastic surgeon in extensive cases.
EBL	100-2000 ml
Postop care	PACU or ICU; some patients require temporary ventilatory support.
Mortality	< 5%
Morbidity	Paradoxical chest-wall motion (less in posterior resections)
	Pneumothorax
	Wound complications
Pain score	3-8

PATIENT POPULATION CHARACTERISTICS

Age range	Adults of all ages; children, rarely
Male:Female	1:1
Incidence	Relatively rare
Etiology	Unknown
Associated conditions	Lung cancer; metastatic disease; smoking-related diseases; cardiovascular disease

ANESTHETIC CONSIDERATIONS

See Anesthetic Considerations following Repair of Pectus Excavatum or Carinatum, p. 220.

References

1. Baue AE, ed: *Glenn's Thoracic and Cardiovascular Surgery*, 6th edition, Volume II. Geha AS, Hammond GL, Laks H, Naunheim KS, assoc eds. Appleton & Lange, Norwalk, CT: 1996.
2. Sabiston DC Jr, Spencer FC: *Surgery of the Chest*, 6th edition, Vol II. WB Saunders, Philadelphia: 1995.

REPAIR OF PECTUS EXCAVATUM OR CARINATUM

SURGICAL CONSIDERATIONS

Description: Standard bony and cartilaginous repair of a pectus excavatum (funnel chest) or carinatum (pigeon breast) is usually elective surgery to improve contour and body image. There is no documentation that these repairs have any positive effect on cardiopulmonary function, although some surgeons feel that it can be more than a cosmetic procedure. To **repair pectus excavatum**, enough pairs of costal cartilages—usually 4-6—must be removed to be able to mobilize and elevate the sternum. Depending on the severity of the defect and patient's age, fixation of the sternum in the corrected position may be necessary. **Repair of pectus carinatum** is somewhat more varied because the defects are more varied; however, removal of cartilages and correction of the position of the sternum are still the mainstays of treatment.

A midline incision provides the most satisfactory access to the cartilages and sternum. For cosmetic reasons, however, it may be important to use a curvilinear transverse incision, particularly in females. This incision requires extensive mobilization of subcutaneous and muscle flaps. The wound complication rate is somewhat greater after transverse incisions. The costal cartilages are moved by subperichondrial dissection. This may be tedious and time-consuming, especially since 4 or 5, or even more, pairs of cartilages need to be removed. The elevation of the sternum is usually fairly straightforward, and usually is accompanied by a transverse sternal osteotomy (Fig 5-8). Intercostal muscle bundles may be left attached to the sternum or may be detached and reattached for better positioning of the sternum. Sternal support normally is not used in infants, but may be used in older children. The most common method of support is the use of a transverse metal strut resting on the ribs, but beneath the sternum. This is removed at a later date. The final position of the sternum is easier to predict following repair of pectus carinatum than following repair of pectus excavatum. Because of the negative intrathoracic pressure, it is easier to hold the sternum down than up. Ideally, patients for repair of pectus excavatum are just under school age. Satisfactory repair, however, may be carried out at almost any time during childhood. As full growth is attained, results tend to be less favorable. Pectus carinatum generally has its onset during adolescence, and it is well to let the patient complete his or her growth spurt prior to undertaking repair. (Also see Repair of Pectus Excavatum/Carinatum in Pediatric General Surgery, p. 1029.)

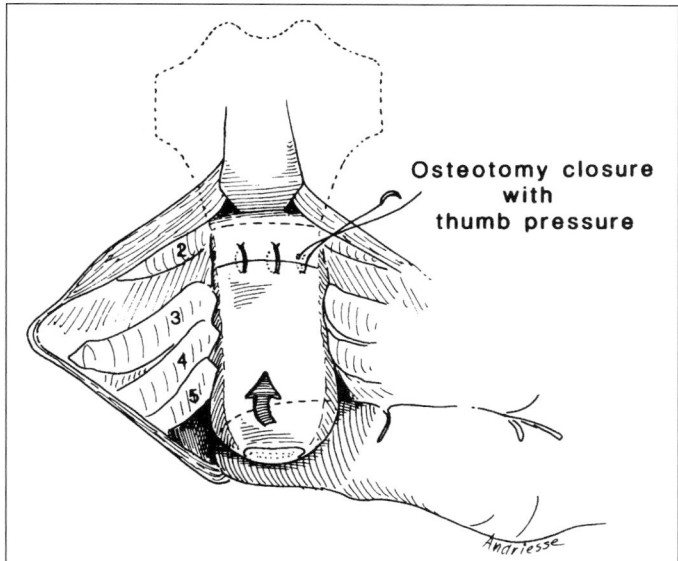

Osteotomy closure
with
thumb pressure

Figure 5-8. Correction of a pectus excavatum defect. After subperichodrial resection of the involved costal cartilages, a wedge osteomy permits anterior mobilization of the lower portion of the sternum. (Reproduced with permission from Shamberger RC: Chest wall deformities. In *General Thoracic Surgery*, 5th edition. Shields TW, LoCicero J III, Ponn RB, eds. Lippincott Williams & Wilkins, 2000.)

Variant procedure or approaches: In certain circumstances, particularly in teenage girls and patients who do not engage in strenuous sports, subcutaneous, custom-made implants may be placed to improve body contour without necessitating major bony and cartilaginous repairs. These are usually carried out by plastic surgeons.

Usual preop diagnosis: Pectus excavatum or carinatum

SUMMARY OF PROCEDURE

Position	Supine
Incision	Transverse or vertical
Special instrumentation	Bone instruments; sometimes metal struts or wires for reconstruction
Antibiotics	Cefazolin 1 g iv q 8 h × 36-48 h
Surgical time	2-3 h
Closing considerations	Pleural and wound drainage common
EBL	100-500 ml
Postop care	ICU
Mortality	Minimal
Morbidity	Pneumothorax: 5-10%
	Wound infection
	Sternum necrosis
	Immigration of strut
	Paradoxical chest-wall motion → hypoventilation/atelectasis
Pain score	4-5

PATIENT POPULATION CHARACTERISTICS

Age range	Usually children, 5-10 yr; teenagers, sometimes; adults, rarely
Male:Female	1:1
Incidence	Unusual
Etiology	Unknown
Associated conditions	Marfan syndrome; MVP

ANESTHETIC CONSIDERATIONS

(Procedures covered: chest-wall resection; repair of pectus excavatum/carinatum)

PREOPERATIVE

Patients for chest-wall resection often have extensive cancer and may be weak and debilitated. A very large resection may create a 'flail chest' situation, compromising postop ventilation.

Respiratory	Mild pectus seldom interferes with ventilation; no special studies indicated. Severe pectus deformity can be associated with ↓ in lung volumes, forced expiratory flow, and V/Q abnormalities. **Tests:** CXR; PFT, ABG, if indicated from H&P.
Cardiovascular	With severe pectus, the heart is displaced to the left and compressed, arrhythmias and RVOTO can occur 2° impaired filling, especially during exercise or in upright position. ECG may show right axis deviation, atrial and ventricular arrhythmias. A functional murmur may be detected. ECHO may reveal ↓SV with MVP. **Tests:** ECG; cardiac catheterization if indicated. Obtain ECHO if MVP suspected.
Hematologic	**Tests:** Hct
Musculoskeletal	Chest-wall resection performed for invasive or metastatic cancer; patient may be malnourished, anemic; pectus repair of chest-wall deformity for cosmetic, orthopedic, or cardiopulmonary indications; pectus deformity usually asymptomatic.
Laboratory	Other tests as indicated from H&P.
Premedication	Midazolam 1-2 mg iv if patient anxious. When epidural opioids are planned, avoid systemic opioid or sedative premedication, which can potentiate postop respiratory effects of central neuraxial opioids.

INTRAOPERATIVE

Anesthetic technique: GETA, occasionally combined with epidural for minimal chest-wall resection; however, epidural anesthesia is an excellent adjunct for extensive chest-wall resections or repair of pectus deformities.

Induction	Standard induction (see p. B-2). If severe RVOTO, high-dose opioid/O_2 technique (e.g., fentanyl 10-25 μg/kg and midazolam 1-2 mg/kg iv or etomidate [e.g. 0.3 mg/kg]) can be used. Avoid myocardial depressants.	
Maintenance	Standard maintenance (see p. B-3) or high-dose opioid technique (fentanyl 10-25 μg/kg) for patient with severe RVOTO. Patients with MVP will require prophylactic antibiotics for bacterial endocarditis.	
Emergence	Extubate in OR; if high-dose opioid → ICU for later extubation.	
Blood and fluid requirements	IV: 18-16 ga × 1 NS/LR @ 1-2 ml/kg/h	Usually minimal blood loss. Fluid restriction unnecessary as this is extrapulmonary operation.
Monitoring	Standard monitors (p. B-1) ± Arterial line	Close monitoring with arterial catheter may be required in patients with significant cardiopulmonary impairment.
Positioning	✓ and pad pressure points. ✓ eyes.	
Complications	Pneumothorax	Unintentional pleural tear can cause pneumothorax. Intraop deterioration with ↑ventilatory pressure suggests pneumothorax. D/C N_2O. Insert chest tube immediately following operation.

POSTOPERATIVE

Complications	Hypoventilation Flail chest Atelectasis	Although most patients do not require postop ventilatory support, with extensive chest-wall resection, patient may hypoventilate. Respiratory stimulants, such as doxapram hydrochloride, should be avoided as they may → deep inspirations that can → severe sternal retractions. Paradoxical chest-wall movement during spontaneous ventilation with flail chest; postop atelectasis from splinting. Obtain postop CXR.
Pain management	Depends on site and extent of chest wall resected. Parenteral or epidural opioids.	Epidural opioids and local anesthetics are particularly useful if flail chest present—reduces need for ventilatory support.

References

1. Baue AE, ed: *Glenn's Thoracic and Cardiovascular Surgery*, 6th edition, Volume II. Geha AS, Hammond GL, Laks H, Naunheim KS, assoc eds. Appleton & Lange, Norwalk, CT: 1996.
2. Garcia VF, Seyfer AE, Graeber GM: Reconstruction of congenital chest-wall deformities. *Surg Clin North Am* 1989; 69(5): 1103-18.
3. Ghory MJ, James FW, Mays W: Cardiac performance in children with pectus excavatum. *J Pediatr Surg* 1989; 24(8):751-5.
4. McBride WJ, Dicker R, Abajian JC, et al: Continuous thoracic epidural infusions for postoperative analgesia after pectus deformity repair. *J Pediatr Surg* 1996; 31(1): 105-7.
5. Nuss D, Croitoru DP, Kelly RE, et al: Review and discussion of the complications of minimally invasive pectus excavatum repair. *Eur J Pediatr Surg* 2002; 12(4):230-4.
6. Robicsek SA, Lobato EB: Repair of pectus excavatum. Anesthesia considerations. *Chest Surg Clin North Am* 2000; 10(2): 253-9.
7. Sabiston DC Jr, Spencer FC: *Surgery of the Chest*, 6th edition, Vol II. WB Saunders, Philadelphia: 1995.
8. Shamberger RC: Chest wall deformities. In *General Thoracic Surgery*, 5th edition. Shields TW, LoCicero J III, Ponn RB, eds. Lippincott Williams & Wilkins, Philadelphia: 2000, 535-62.

THORACOPLASTY

SURGICAL CONSIDERATIONS

Description: The objective of a **thoracoplasty** (removal of several ribs) is to permanently obliterate an existing pleural space or to collapse a portion of the lung. Formerly, this operation was used in the treatment of tuberculosis (TB); however, because of better drug therapy, appropriate pulmonary resection and the decrease in incidence of TB, thoracoplasty is now rare. The procedure also was used for obliterating empyema spaces and helping to close bronchopleural fistulas (BPFs). The use of **pedicled muscle flaps** (serratus anterior, pectoralis major, and latissimus dorsi are the most common) or an **omental transposition** have largely replaced thoracoplasty for filling empyema spaces and encouraging closing of BPFs. These operations are less deforming and better tolerated physiologically since they do not result in paradoxical motion of the chest wall.

For patients whose lungs will never expand to fill the space—such as those who have had a pneumonectomy or who have a permanently noncompliant lung—resection of multiple overlying ribs may be necessary (Fig 5-9). Thoracoplasty is accomplished by removing several ribs in a subperiosteal fashion, allowing the underlying chest wall to collapse. This collapse is aided by the normally negative intrapleural pressure. Since the periosteum is left intact, the ribs will regenerate, resulting in a permanent, bony collapse of the chest wall. If the objective of the thoracoplasty is to

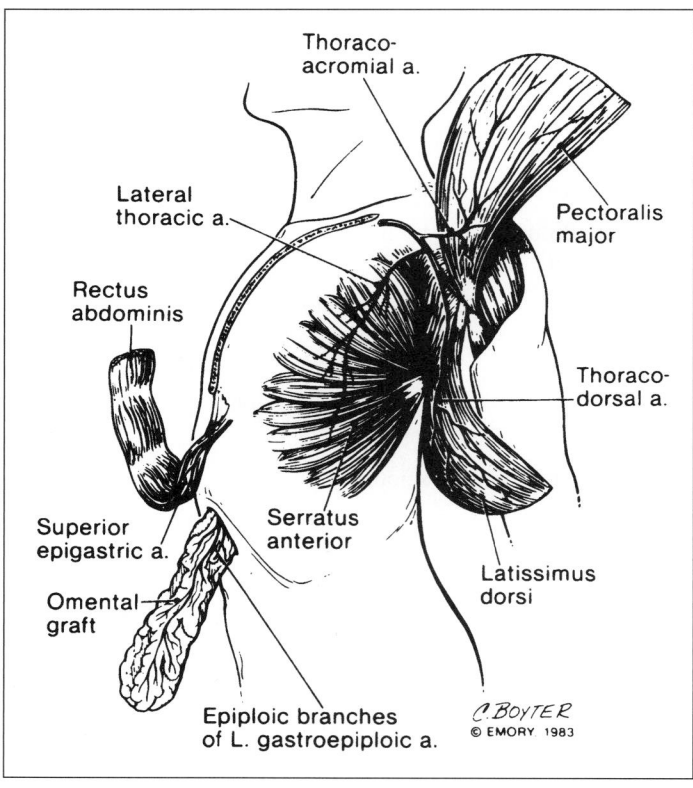

Figure 5-9. Extrathoracic muscle flaps that may be used to obliterate a postpneumonectomy empyema cavity. (Reproduced with permission from Miller JI Jr: Postsurgical empyema. In *General Thoracic Surgery*, 5th edition. Shields TW, LoCicero J III, Ponn RB, eds. Lippincott Williams & Wilkins, 2000.)

obliterate a relatively small space (meaning that segments of only 2-3 ribs need be removed), the procedure may be done in a single stage, with little postop physiologic impairment of respiration. If extensive thoracoplasty is necessary, however, the procedure may be done in stages to minimize postop chest-wall instability and resultant respiratory problems.

Usual preop diagnosis: Pulmonary TB; BPF; empyema

SUMMARY OF PROCEDURE

Position	Usually lateral
Incision	Along rib line
Special instrumentation	Bone instruments
Unique considerations	TB or fungal infection may be present
Antibiotics	As indicated by culture and sensitivity
Surgical time	2-3 h
EBL	500 ml or more
Postop care	ICU
Mortality	Minimal
Morbidity	Paradoxical chest-wall motion → atelectasis → hypoxemia: 10%
	Pneumothorax: Rare
Pain score	7-8

222

PATIENT POPULATION CHARACTERISTICS

Age range	Middle-aged or older adults
Male:Female	1:1
Incidence	Rare
Etiology	TB; pneumococcal infection; neoplasm; complication of pneumonectomy
Associated conditions	Immunosuppression

ANESTHETIC CONSIDERATIONS

See Anesthetic Considerations following Drainage of Empyema, p. 224.

References

1. Baue AE, ed: *Glenn's Thoracic and Cardiovascular Surgery*, 6th edition, Volume II. Geha AS, Hammond GL, Laks H, Naunheim KS, assoc eds. Appleton & Lange, Norwalk, CT: 1996.
2. Sabiston DC Jr, Spencer FC: *Surgery of the Chest*, 6th edition, Vol II. WB Saunders, Philadelphia: 1995.

DRAINAGE OF EMPYEMA

SURGICAL CONSIDERATIONS

Description: Empyema is infection within the pleural space, and the primary treatment for it is drainage. Patients may be acutely ill or they may have a Hx of prolonged infirmity. There are three phases of an empyema: exudative, fibrinopurulent, and organized. The most common cause of empyema is extraparenchymal extension of a pneumonia, although other causes include trauma, iatrogenic, and esophageal perforation. Therapy is dependent on the stage of the disease, as well as the underlying cause of infection. The early phase of an empyema usually is associated with fever, dyspnea, and a pleural effusion, with the Dx generally being made by thoracentesis. In more established infections, patients may complain of chronic symptoms, such as pain, dyspnea, and chest heaviness, and their medical Hx may include several previous courses of antibiotics.

Except in its earliest phase, chest tube drainage alone rarely provides adequate therapy. In the fibrinopurulent stage, thoracoscopic drainage with disruption of loculations and removal of the fine peel on the lung is enough to drain the infected fluid and allow the underlying lung to expand. This procedure typically is done with the patient in the lateral position and involves three thoracoscopy ports. Blood loss is generally small, although large volumes of irrigation fluid may be necessary to thoroughly debride the thoracic cavity.

As the empyema becomes more established, the peel becomes thicker and more difficult to remove thoracoscopically. In such cases, an **open thoracotomy** is necessary. Due to the extensive intrapleural inflammation, fluid losses may be substantial. To identify the correct plane between the lung and the thickened pleura, the lung may need to be reexpanded frequently throughout the procedure. Satisfactory drainage is accomplished when the infected fluid is removed and the lung expands freely. Because the peel is often intimately adherent to the underlying lung, there may be a moderate postop air leak.

In patients too ill to undergo thoracotomy, **rib resection** with subsequent open drainage tube will permit the underlying lung to expand over a period of several weeks. While this may be done under local anesthesia, a brief GA is often easier on the patient. In this operation, the patient is placed in the lateral position and an incision is made over the rib corresponding to the most dependent portion of the empyema cavity. A 6-cm length of the rib is excised and a large-diameter ($\geq$ 50 Fr) tube is inserted into the empyema cavity. More permanent open drainage is obtained by fashioning an **Eloesser flap**. In this procedure, a U-shaped flap of skin is rotated into the empyema cavity after rib resection. This creates a long-term, skin-lined tube that will last indefinitely. A variant of this procedure—the **Clagett procedure**—is carried out for empyema (with or without bronchopleural fistula) following **pneumonectomy**, since closed drainage rarely suffices in such a situation. The principal is the same: that is, an epithelial-lined, permanent opening to achieve drainage of an empyema. In the Clagett procedure, the opening is generally made anterolaterally and dependently so that drainage is effective and the patient can handle dressing changes without assistance. Segments of 2 or 3 ribs are removed and the skin is sutured to the parietal pleura, leaving a permanent opening for drainage and irrigation. Without an underlying lung, and with a relatively fixed mediastinum, this procedure is well tolerated physiologically. (For pediatric drainage of empyema, see p. 1027.)

Usual preop diagnosis: Nontuberculosis empyema (typically pneumococcal)

SUMMARY OF PROCEDURES

	Eloesser or Clagett	Tube Thoracostomy
Position	Usually lateral	Lateral
Incision	Over empyema pocket for Eloesser; low anterolateral for Clagett	Lateral
Special instrumentation	None	Large tubes
Unique considerations	Patient may have BPF	Local or GA
Antibiotics	As indicated by culture and sensitivity	$\Leftarrow$
Surgical time	1 h; occasionally more	< 1 h
Closing considerations	Wound left open	None
EBL	100 ml	Minimal
Postop care	PACU → room	$\Leftarrow$
Mortality	Minimal	$\Leftarrow$
Morbidity	Fluid drainage Bleeding: Rare	Air leak
Pain score	3-4	2-3

PATIENT POPULATION CHARACTERISTICS

Age range	Usually adults
Male:Female	1:1
Incidence	Decreasing
Etiology	Pneumonia; esophageal or bronchial leak; lymphatic or hematogenous spread of infection; posttrauma or thoracic surgery
Associated conditions	Bronchopleural fistula (BPF); sepsis; malnutrition

---

ANESTHETIC CONSIDERATIONS

(Procedures covered: thoracoplasty; drainage of empyema)

PREOPERATIVE

The guiding principle in the anesthetic management of empyema is to protect the nonaffected lung from soiling by the affected side. These patients are often chronically ill with sepsis and cachexia; and there is usually an underlying BPF (which may require awake intubation).

Respiratory	Patients usually have preexisting pulmonary disease. Preop pulmonary findings may include collapse of the ipsilateral lung, impaired hypoxic pulmonary vasoconstriction 2° infection, and mediastinal shift to the ipsilateral side. Procedure often is performed for empyema in the presence of BPF following lung resection (particularly pneumonectomy), penetrating injury to chest, or rupture of a cyst or bulla. When possible, surgeon should drain empyema under local anesthesia before induction, with patient sitting upright. If empyema is loculated, complete drainage may not be possible. **Tests:** Consider PFTs; ABG; obtain CXR to determine efficacy of preop chest drainage; if chest CT available, look for airway obstruction that could interfere with DLT placement.
Cardiovascular	There may be ECG changes because of mediastinal shift to the affected side. **Tests:** As indicated from H&P.
Neurological	✓ Hx of back surgery, peripheral neuropathy. Examine lumbar area for skin lesions, infection, deformities. Avoid placement of epidural catheter in patient with neurologic problems or if obviously bacteremic or septic.
Musculoskeletal	Patients with lung cancer may have myasthenic (Eaton-Lambert) syndrome with resistance to depolarizing muscle relaxant and ↑sensitivity to NMRs. Monitor relaxation with peripheral nerve stimulator.

Hematologic	Transfuse patients with preop Hct < 25% or Hct < 30% in patients with CAD. (Hb level necessary to maintain adequate O_2 content.) Obtain autologous blood during the month before surgery or consider preop erythropoietin therapy in anemic patients.
Laboratory	Other tests as indicated from H&P.
Premedication	Midazolam 1-2 mg iv if patient anxious. When epidural opioids are planned, avoid systemic opioid or sedative premedication, which can potentiate postop respiratory effects of central neuraxial opioids.

INTRAOPERATIVE

Anesthetic technique: GETA; combined with epidural anesthesia/analgesia if thoracotomy is indicated and patient is not bacteremic or septic.

Induction	Consider inhalational induction with inhalation agent (e.g., sevoflurane) if patient has significant BPF. Rapid-sequence induction with cricoid pressure is an alternative (p. B-5). Intubate with DLT; isolate lungs to protect from aspiration and tension pneumothorax. Use DLT with bronchial lumen to side opposite BPF. Contamination of the healthy lung from aspiration of pus is a major concern; thus, proper tube position should be verified by FOB, and adequate cuff inflation should be checked. Large DLT provides snug fit in bronchus and limits aspiration. Pus may appear in tracheal lumen (lumen to the diseased lung); suction frequently to avoid soiling good lung.
Maintenance	O_2 and isoflurane (1.0-1.5%); less required if epidural local anesthetics used. Avoid N_2O, especially during OLV, since hypoxemia during OLV is unpredictable. Use $FiO_2 = 1.0$. A local anesthetic (e.g., 2% lidocaine with 1:200,000 epinephrine or 0.25% bupivacaine) can be infused or injected hourly into a thoracic (3-5 ml) or lumbar (5-10 ml) epidural catheter. Continuous infusion of local anesthetic generally provides better hemodynamic stability than hourly bolus injection. To enhance the effect of epidural analgesia, a loading dose of opiate (e.g., hydromorphone 0.4-1 mg [thoracic] or 1-1.5mg [lumbar]) can be administered early in the surgery and at least 1 h before conclusion. Following intubation, isolate lung with DLT or BB. Chest tube is then removed while chest is prepped for operation. Ventilate only the healthy lung. Since BPF is an abnormal communication between bronchial tree and pleural cavity, if no chest tube present, conventional intubation with IPPV can produce tension pneumothorax. Keep unclamped and do not remove a functioning chest tube until lung is isolated and ventilation to diseased lung stopped. Once chest is opened, there is no chance of pneumothorax, but the large air leak through BPF may prevent satisfactory ventilation of that lung. High-frequency ventilation (HFV) is recommended by some, but studies show no benefit; in some patients the BPF is actually increased with HFV.
Emergence	Before closing the chest, lungs are inflated gradually to 30 cmH_2O pressure to reinflate atelectatic areas and to check for significant air leaks. The surgeon will insert chest tubes to drain pleural cavity and aid lung reexpansion. Patient is extubated while still in OR. If postop ventilation is required (rare), the DLT is exchanged for an ETT. If BPF is still open, consider selective ventilation postop through DLT. It may be necessary to ventilate each lung separately; use smaller TVs to lung with BPF. Alternatively, pressure-controlled ventilation may be used to avoid major air leaks through BPF.

Blood and fluid requirements	IV: 16-18 ga × 1 Avoid hypervolemia.	An overhydrated patient is at increased risk of right-heart failure and pulmonary edema. Replace blood loss with crystalloid (1:3) or colloid (1:1). Third-space losses are negligible and do not need to be replaced.
	Use vasopressor (ephedrine 5-10 mg iv bolus or phenylephrine 50-100 μg iv bolus) if hypotensive.	Use of epidural local anesthetics can cause ↓BP in a volume-restricted patient; vasopressor often needed.
Monitoring	Standard monitors (p. B-1) ± CVP and/or PA line ± Arterial line	It is mandatory to follow oxygenation continuously during OLV. Typically this is done with pulse oximetry, although continuous intraarterial PO_2 monitoring is now commercially available.
Positioning	Axillary roll, 'airplane' for upper arm Avoid hyperextending arms. ✓ and pad pressure points. ✓ eyes, ears, genitals.	Placing the oximeter probe on the down side may help detect inadequate perfusion from compression.

POSTOPERATIVE

Complications	Tension pneumothorax	Functioning chest tube necessary to prevent tension
	Aspiration pneumonia ('down' lung)	pneumothorax.
Pain management	Analgesic requirements minimal	See Pain Management under Anesthetic Considerations
	Parenteral opiods (iv, im, PCA [p. C-3)],	for Lobectomy, Pneumonectomy, p. 214.
	epidural, NSAID	

References

1. Baue AE, ed: *Glenn's Thoracic and Cardiovascular Surgery*, 6th edition, Volume II. Geha AS, Hammond GL, Laks H, Naunheim KS, assoc eds. Appleton & Lange, Norwalk, CT: 1996.
2. Benjaminsson E, Klain M: Intraoperative dual-mode independent lung ventilation of a patient with bronchopleural fistula. *Anesth Analg* 1981; 60(2):118-19.
3. Bishop MJ, Benson MS, Sato P, Pierson DJ: Comparison of high-frequency jet ventilation with conventional mechanical ventilation for bronchopleural fistula. *Anesth Analg* 1987; 66(9):833-8.
4. Langston HT: Thoracoplasty: the how and the why. *Ann Thorac Surg* 1991; 52(6):1351-53.
5. Miller JI Jr: Postsurgical empyema. In *General Thoracic Surgery*, 5th edition. Shields TW, LoCicero J III, Ponn RB, eds. Lippincott Williams & Wilkins, Philadelphia: 2000, 709-16.
6. Sabiston DC Jr, Spencer FC: *Surgery of the Chest*, 6th edition, Vol II. WB Saunders, Philadelphia: 1995.

TRACHEAL RESECTION

SURGICAL CONSIDERATIONS

Description: The primary indications for **tracheal resection** are benign stricture and primary tracheal neoplasm. Benign strictures often are related to previous intubation or tracheostomy; consequently, these patients often have a Hx of head and neck surgery. The preop assessment of patients with tracheal disease generally involves imaging with either CT or MRI. Important considerations include the length and position of the lesion and the caliber of the airway. While up to 50% of the trachea can be resected with a successful primary anastomosis, shorter segment resections are technically simpler and do not require special techniques to maximize tracheal mobility.

Stenoses of the upper and mid-trachea can be approached through the neck, while lesions of the lower trachea and carina must be approached through the right chest. When using the **cervical approach**, the patient is positioned with the neck extended. A transverse collar incision is used and subplatysmal planes are developed. The trachea is then extensively mobilized anteriorly and posteriorly. To minimize risk of devascularizing the trachea, only the region to be removed should be circumferentially dissected. During this portion of the operation, care is taken to avoid injury of the recurrent laryngeal nerves. The trachea is then opened, the oral ETT is withdrawn into the proximal trachea, and a sterile armored ETT is passed across the operative field. Fine, interrupted, absorbable sutures are placed but not tied. Once all sutures are in place, the armored tube is removed and the oral ETT is positioned across the anastomosis. The ends of the trachea are approximated with minimal tension and the sutures are tied (Fig 5-10). To provide minimal tension, it may be necessary to flex the neck for this portion of the procedure. A suture may be placed from the chin to the chest wall to maintain neck flexion for several days postop. At the end of the procedure, the patient should be extubated to minimize airway irritation and disruption of the anastomosis.

Lesions of the lower trachea must be approached thought the right chest, where the same techniques as discussed above are used. To facilitate exposure of the distal trachea, OLV using either a DLT or a single-lumen tube advanced into the left main bronchus is helpful.

As is apparent from the above discussion, all tracheal procedures require cooperation and frequent communication between the surgeon and anesthesiologist. Occasionally, special techniques, such as jet ventilation or CPB, may be necessary for tracheal surgery.

Usual preop diagnosis: Tracheal stenosis or tumor (adenoid cystic carcinoma or squamous cell carcinoma most common)

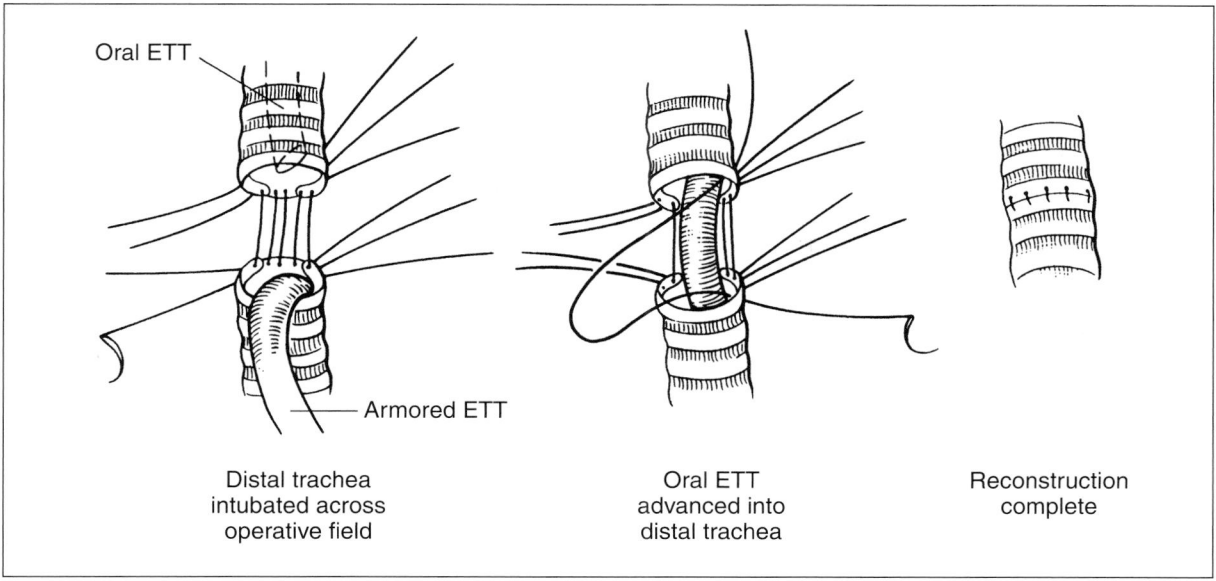

Figure 5-10. Stages of tracheal reconstruction. Note ETT in distal trachea. (Reproduced with permission from Grillo HC: *Current Problems in Surgery*. Year Book Medical Publishers, 1970.)

SUMMARY OF PROCEDURES

	Cervical Approach	Sternotomy	Right Thoracotomy
Position	Supine	⇐	Left lateral decubitus
Incision	Transverse low cervical	Cervical + sternotomy	Right thoracotomy
Antibiotics	Cefazolin 1 g	⇐	⇐
Surgical time	3 h	3-4 h	4 h
Closing considerations	Neck flexion (chin stitch)	⇐	⇐
EBL	200 ml	350 ml	350-500 ml
Postop care	ICU	⇐	⇐
Mortality	< 5%	5%	⇐
Morbidity	Retained secretions Dehiscence Recurrent stenosis Recurrent/superior laryngeal nerve injury Granuloma	⇐	⇐
Pain score	3-4	5-6	7-9

PATIENT POPULATION CHARACTERISTICS

Age range	Wide variation
Male:Female	1:1
Incidence	Rare
Etiology	Stenosis usually 2° to intubation or injury; tumor, either primary (e.g., smoking) or secondary (e.g., esophageal, lung, thyroid cancer)
Associated conditions	Carcinoid syndrome; cardiopulmonary disease; tracheoesophageal fistula (TEF)

ANESTHETIC CONSIDERATIONS

PREOPERATIVE

Respiratory   Initial presentation may involve Sx of airway obstruction (stridor, cough, dyspnea), which may be misdiagnosed as asthma or pneumonitis. A careful evaluation of the airway is usually followed by

Respiratory, cont.	bronchoscopy. Lesion should be identified by site and size. Using this information, estimate what size ETT will easily pass lesion site. **Tests:** PFTs; flow/volume loops; CT scan to determine extent of tracheal obstruction
Laboratory	Other tests as indicated from H&P.
Premedication	Patients with stridor or critical airway lesions should not receive preop sedation. It is probably best to avoid sedation in all patients.

INTRAOPERATIVE

Anesthetic technique: GETA, combined with epidural if thoracotomy approach is used.

Induction	Be prepared for airway emergency. Surgeon must be present and prepared for emergency rigid bronchoscopy and/or to perform tracheostomy below lesion. Mask inhalational induction or awake FOI with spontaneous ventilation; avoid iv drugs that could depress ventilation. Avoid muscle relaxants; if necessary, consider small doses of succinylcholine. Sevoflurane/O_2 is preferred for smooth induction with depression of cough reflex; avoid N_2O. High concentrations of sevoflurane may be necessary. Helium has been recommended to decrease resistance to flow past the obstruction; however, helium is not usually available.
	Have a variety of laryngeal blades and uncut ETTs of all sizes, including thin (5 mm) tubes. If ETT passes beyond lesion, can begin IPPV. If ETT cannot be passed, spontaneous ventilation with 100% O_2 and sevoflurane is required. Careful and gradual dilation of the sterotic lesion may be required, using different sizes of ETTs or rigid bronchoscopy to facilitate placement of an adequate size ETT for ventilation. For carinal resections, use a sterile armored ETT, which can be placed by surgeon directly into each bronchus during resection. An armored tube is preferable because it is constantly being removed while the surgeon works; also, there is less kinking and less chance of obstructing.
Maintenance	Standard maintenance (p. B-3). FiO_2 = 1.0 during apneic oxygenation; continuous monitoring with pulse oximetry mandatory. TIVA (p. B-3), with propofol and remifentanil, is an excellent alternative that avoids polluting the OR with inhalation agents when intermittent interruptions of ventilation are required or when the airway is open during surgery. A low-dose, longer-acting opioid (morphine 0.025-0.075 mg/kg), given 30-60 min before the end of the case, will provide adequate initial postop analgesia. Consider HFV through a small-diameter catheter if ETT interferes with operation. HFV will require iv anesthesia since inhalational agents cannot be delivered predictably; CPB can be used (rare).
Emergence	Early extubation; presence of ETT and IPPV can disrupt fresh suture line. Remove ETT as soon as patient is awake enough to protect airway and breathing spontaneously, but before bucking and coughing occur. Assess integrity of recurrent laryngeal nerve after extubation.
Blood and fluid requirements	IV: 16-18 ga × 1 (left arm) NS/LR @ 3 ml/kg/h	
Monitoring	Standard monitors (p. B-1) ± Arterial line	Left radial artery cannulation permits uninterrupted monitoring of BP during periods of innominate artery compression. Placement of iv in left arm allows unimpeded infusion. Right-extremity pulse oximetry will help detect innominate artery occlusion (which otherwise could lead to stroke.)
Positioning	✓ and pad pressure points. ✓ eyes.	
Airway management	ETT replaced with sterile ETT and circuit intraop.	Once the trachea is divided, the surgeon places a sterile ETT in the distal trachea. The original ETT is withdrawn above the surgical site. The surgeon attaches a sterile anesthesia circuit to distal ETT for ventilation. Then, the surgeon places a suture through the distal tip of the original ETT. Before reanastomosis of trachea, the distal trachea is suctioned to remove accumulated blood and secretions. After a posterior suture line is completed, the original ETT is pulled through the trachea and the distal tube (which is below the resection) is removed. Reattach and ventilate patient through original ETT.

| Complications | Tracheal edema | Corticosteroids (dexamethasone 6-8 mg iv) to ↓ tracheal edema. |
| | Injury to neck | Any structure in the neck can be damaged, including superior and recurrent laryngeal nerves, trachea, and thoracic duct. |

POSTOPERATIVE

Complications	Tracheal disruption	Neck swelling, subcutaneous emphysema, and inability to ventilate indicate loss of air-tight anastomosis. Immediate reexploration of neck is essential.
	Recurrent laryngeal nerve injury	Bilateral (occasionally unilateral) laryngeal nerve damage may → airway obstruction, necessitating reintubation. Mask ventilation may be ineffective.
Position	Airway edema Keep head flexed to reduce tension on tracheal suture line.	Place patient in head-up, neck-flexed position. Treat with nebulized racemic epinephrine if airway compromise occurs. Reintubation will be required, using a small (6 mm ID) uncuffed ETT under either direct laryngoscopy or fiber optic guidance to avoid disruption of the anastomosis.
Pain management	Parenteral opioids (p. C-2) ± Epidural	Once patient is fully awake.

References

1. Baue AE, ed: *Glenn's Thoracic and Cardiovascular Surgery*, 6th edition, Volume II. Geha AS, Hammond GL, Laks H, Naunheim KS, assoc eds. Appleton & Lange, Norwalk, CT: 1996.
2. Grillo HC, Mathisen DJ: Surgical management of tracheal strictures. *Surg Clin North Am* 1988; 68(3):511-24.
3. Perera ER, Vidic DM, Zivot J: Carinal resection with two high-frequency jet ventilation delivery systems. *Can J Anaesth* 1993; 40(1): 59-63.
4. Sabiston DC Jr, Spencer FC: *Surgery of the Chest*, 6th edition, Vol II. WB Saunders, Philadelphia: 1995.
5. Sandberg W: Anesthesia and airway management for tracheal resection and reconstruction. *Int Anesthesiol Clin* 2000; 38(1): 55-75.

EXCISION OF MEDIASTINAL TUMOR

SURGICAL CONSIDERATIONS

Description: Mediastinal tumors are characterized by their location (anterior, middle, and posterior) and their size. Common anterior mediastinal tumors include thymic tumors (benign or malignant thymoma and thymic carcinoma), germ-cell tumors, lymphoma, and substernal goiters. Typically, thymic and germ-cell tumors are resected, while lymphomas are biopsied. Substernal goiters usually can be resected through the neck. Tumors in the anterior mediastinum usually are removed through a **median sternotomy**, while tumors in the middle and posterior mediastinum usually are removed through a **lateral thoracotomy**. While middle and posterior mediastinal tumors usually do not present airway management problems, the issue of functioning neuroendocrine tissue must be considered. Mediastinal pheochromocytomas are uncommon middle mediastinal tumors. As with pheochromocytomas arising in other locations, appropriate preop adrenergic management is necessary. Some cysts or small tumors may be excised using **video thoracoscopy** (see Video-Assisted Thoracoscopy, p. 240).

Mediastinal tumors that are well encapsulated generally are removed in a straightforward fashion. If anterior mediastinal tumors are not well encapsulated and are attached to pericardium or lung on either side, appropriate portions of these attached structures may be removed in continuity with the tumor. If there is attachment to phrenic nerves on either side, one nerve may be sacrificed if necessary to remove the tumor completely. In patients with anterior mediastinal tumors, invasion of the major vascular structures, particularly the aorta and arch vessels, presents an even greater problem. Patients with large anterior mediastinal masses who have some evidence of intrathoracic obstruction (e.g., orthopnea, cough) may have airway obstruction at the time of induction. Although most mediastinal masses do not cause obstruction of the trachea or tracheobronchial tree, large mediastinal masses in the anterior mediastinum, in conjunction with muscle relaxation, can lead to complete obstruction of the airway with inability to ventilate the patient. Although rigid bronchoscopy may permit ventilation through the obstruction, it cannot be counted on to relieve the obstruction; therefore, only short-acting or no muscle relaxants (spontaneous ventilation) should be used in these patients.

In general, the surgical procedure is quite limited, involving a small anterior thoracotomy for a biopsy. Rarely is a large procedure undertaken for these masses as they are usually unresectable or are treated by other means. A DLT is often helpful if the tumor extends into the lung parenchyma; in which case, a **pulmonary wedge resection** (or even lobectomy) may be necessary. Posterior mediastinal tumors are usually benign. Even so, they may be densely adherent to the posterior chest-wall structures. On occasion, dissection can result in injury to an intercostal vessel. Mediastinal tumors sometimes cause tracheal compression, and special anesthetic techniques may be necessary to safely secure the airway. Close communication between the surgeon and anesthesiologist is essential.

Usual preop diagnosis: Thymoma; teratodermoid; ganglioneuroma; lymphoma; schwannoma; substernal goiter

SUMMARY OF PROCEDURE

Position	Supine or lateral
Incision	Median sternotomy or lateral thoracotomy
Special instrumentation	Sternal or rib retractors
Antibiotics	Cefazolin 1 g
Surgical time	≤ 2 h
EBL	< 500 ml
Postop care	Frequently ICU
Mortality	Minimal
Morbidity	Bleeding
Pain score	5-8

PATIENT POPULATION CHARACTERISTICS

Age range	All ages
Male:Female	1:1
Etiology	**Anterior mediastinum:** Thymoma; teratoma; pericardial cyst; lymphoma; parasternal (Morgagni) hernia; lipoma **Superior mediastinum:** Goiter; aneurysm; parathyroid tumor; esophageal tumor; angiomatous tumor **Middle mediastinum:** Lymphoma; lymph node inflammation; bronchogenic tumor; bronchogenic cyst **Posterior mediastinum:** Neurogenic tumor; aneurysm (enteric cyst); esophageal tumor; bronchogenic tumor
Associated conditions	SVC syndrome; myasthenia gravis; recurrent laryngeal nerve damage; airway obstruction; dyspnea; Horner's syndrome

ANESTHETIC CONSIDERATIONS

See Anesthetic Considerations following Mediastinoscopy, p. 232.

References

1. Baue AE, ed: *Glenn's Thoracic and Cardiovascular Surgery*, 6th edition, Volume II. Geha AS, Hammond GL, Laks H, Naunheim KS, assoc eds. Appleton & Lange, Norwalk, CT: 1996.
2. Lewer BM, Torrance JM: Anaesthesia for a patient with a mediastinal mass presenting with acute stridor. *Anaesth Intensive Care* 1996; 24(5):605-8.
3. Narang S, Harte HB, Body SC: Anesthesia for patients with a mediastinal mass. *Anesthesiol Clin North Am* 2001; 19(3):559-79.
4. Sabiston DC Jr, Spencer FC: *Surgery of the Chest*, 6th edition, Vol II. WB Saunders, Philadelphia: 1995.
5. Viswabathans S, Campbell CE, Cork RC: Asymptomatic undetected mediastinal mass: A death during ambulatory anesthesia. *J Clin Anesth* 1995; 7(2):151-5.

MEDIASTINOSCOPY

SURGICAL CONSIDERATIONS

Description: Mediastinoscopy is used for biopsy of mediastinal lymph nodes. The most common indication for this procedure is bronchogenic carcinoma, although lymphadenopathy associated with lymphoma, sarcoidosis, and infectious granulomatous diseases are also indications for mediastinoscopy. **Cervical mediastinoscopy** provides access to the pretracheal, paratracheal, and anterior subcarinal nodes (Fig 5-11), while **transthoracic mediastinoscopy** (also known as **anterior mediastinotomy** or **Chamberlain's procedure**) provides access to the aortopulmonary lymph nodes. Previous mediastinoscopy and radiation are relative contraindications to this procedure. If a thoracic aneurysm is present or SVC is obstructed, mediastinoscopy is contraindicated, as the anatomy is distorted and vessels can be punctured inadvertently by the mediastinoscope.

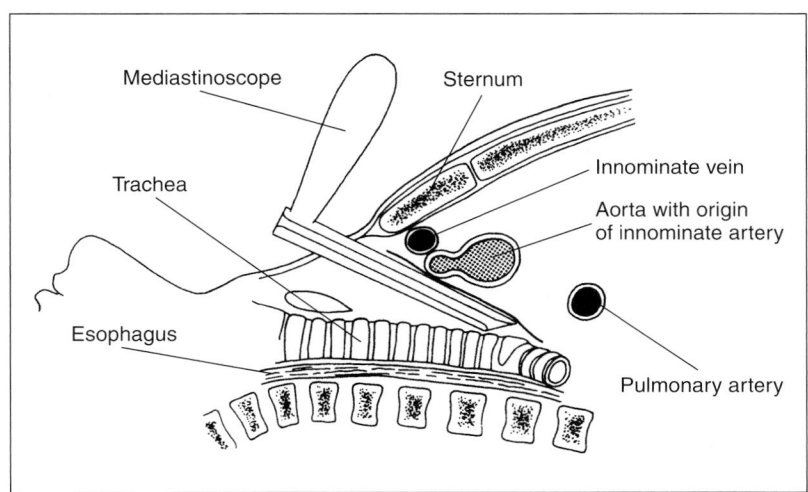

Figure 5-11. Mediastinoscope is inserted through a small cervical incision into the middle mediastinum, along the pretracheal plane. (Reproduced with permission from Baker RJ, Fischer JE: *Mastery of Surgery.* Lippincott Williams & Wilkins, 2001.)

Variant procedure or approaches: For nodes on the left side of the mediastinum, **transthoracic mediastinoscopy** is performed through a limited anterior thoracotomy. In the classic **Chamberlain's procedure**, the 3rd costal cartilage is resected and the mediastinum is explored without entering the pleural space. As with cervical mediastinoscopy, visualization is often limited and lymph nodes should be aspirated before biopsy. If the pleural space is entered during the course of the procedure, either a chest tube can be placed postop or the pleural space can be aspirated immediately before wound closure. Patients should be extubated at the end of the operation. Cervical mediastinoscopy is usually an outpatient procedure, while patients undergoing transthoracic mediastinoscopy are usually hospitalized overnight.

Usual preop diagnosis: Carcinoma of the lung with enlarged mediastinal nodes; mediastinal node enlargement 2° lymphoma, thymoma, or other

SUMMARY OF PROCEDURE

Position	Supine
Incision	For mediastinoscopy, suprasternal; usually left 2nd interspace for anterior mediastinotomy.
Special instrumentation	Mediastinoscope
Antibiotics	Cefazolin 1 g
Surgical time	≤ 1 h
EBL	Minimal (but risk of significant blood loss if major vascular injury occurs).
Postop care	PACU → room
Mortality	< 0.1%
Morbidity	Bleeding
	Pneumothorax: Rare
	Vocal cord paralysis: Rare
	Esophageal perforation: Rare
	Pleural tear: Rare
	Tracheal laceration: Rare
Pain score	2 (mediastinoscopy); 2-3 (anterior mediastinotomy)

PATIENT POPULATION CHARACTERISTICS

Age range	Adults, usually > 50 yr
Male:Female	Male > female
Incidence	Frequently part of evaluation for patients with lung cancer.
Etiology	Lung cancer; lymphoma; thymoma; retrosternal goiter
Associated conditions	Airway obstruction

ANESTHETIC CONSIDERATIONS

PREOPERATIVE

(Procedures covered: excision of mediastinal tumor; mediastinoscopy)

Typically, these patients can be divided into two populations, depending on the presence or absence of a significant mediastinal mass (with the potential for catastrophic airway obstruction or cardiovascular collapse on induction of anesthesia). The preop assessment must focus on the differentiation of these two populations. Close consultation with the surgeon is essential in formulating the anesthetic plan.

Respiratory	Question patient with anterior mediastinal mass about ability to lie supine and the presence of cough or dyspnea. Change in position may cause superior caval obstruction or cardiac and airway compression by mediastinal mass (which may be apparent only following induction or on emergence from anesthesia). On PE, ✓ for presence of cyanosis, wheezing, or stridor in the upright and supine positions. If significant airway compression or SVC obstruction is present, the surgeon may delay surgery for radiation or chemotherapy. Patients with SVC syndrome (edema; venous engorgement of head, neck, and upper body; supine dyspnea; ± headache; mental status change) may have significant airway edema. **Tests:** If airway compression is present, obtain PFTs with flow volume loops in upright and supine positions (Fig 5-14 shows flow volume loop). Airway obstruction is worsened during inspiration in patients with an extrathoracic mass and during expiration in patients with an intrathoracic mass. Order CT/MRI scan to determine airway distortion or compression and anatomic involvement with other intrathoracic structures.
Cardiovascular	Intrathoracic vascular structures (e.g., heart, PA, SVC) may be compressed → ↓BP, hypoxia, SVC syndrome. **Tests:** ECHO, CT/MRI if indicated by H&P.
Musculoskeletal	Patients with lung cancer may have myasthenic (Eaton-Lambert) syndrome with resistance to depolarizing agents and ↑ sensitivity to NMRs. Monitor relaxation with peripheral nerve stimulator.
Neurologic	Patient may have ↑ICP if SVC is obstructed. Consider neurology consultation. Patients with preexisting carotid disease are at risk for stroke if there is significant compression of the innominate artery during the procedure.
Laboratory	Other tests as indicated from H&P.
Premedication	Avoid sedation in patients with the potential for airway obstruction; otherwise, midazolam 1-2 mg iv may be appropriate.

INTRAOPERATIVE

Anesthetic technique: GETA, combined with epidural if thoracotomy is planned.

Induction	Consider awake FOB intubation (e.g., if symptomatic in supine position) or use short-acting muscle relaxant (e.g., succinylcholine) in clinically asymptomatic patients. A mask induction with sevoflurane/O_2 in a spontaneously breathing patient may be a safe alternative. Complete or partial airway obstruction by anterior mediastinal mass can be due to changes in lung and chest-wall mechanics associated with changes in the patient's position (sitting to supine during procedure) or to muscle relaxation. A surgeon familiar with rigid bronchoscopy should be in the OR ready to bypass obstruction.
Maintenance	O_2 (100%) and isoflurane (1-1.5%) or sevoflurane (1.5-2.5%). Avoid N_2O, especially during OLV. Short-acting muscle relaxant and opioid as required.
Emergence	Extubation in OR

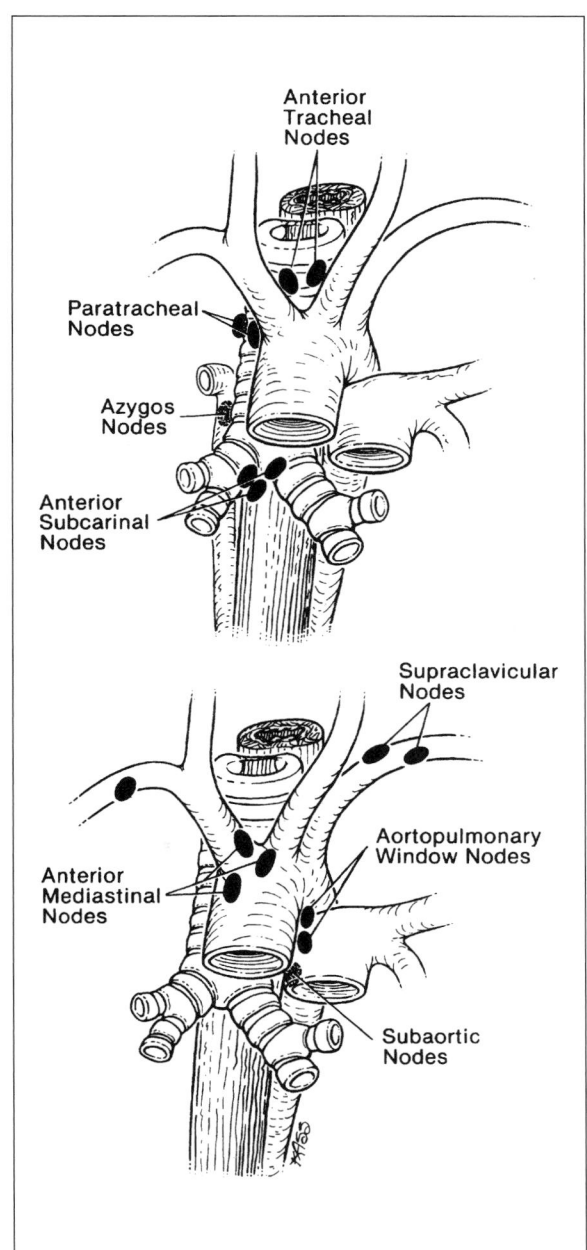

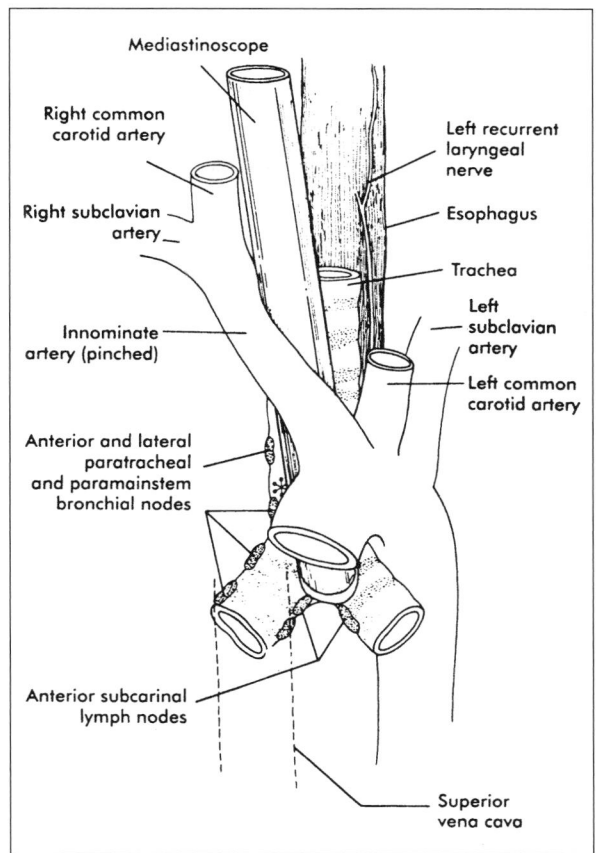

↑ **Figure 5-13.** Relationship of mediastinoscope to trachea and great vessels. (Reproduced with permission from Petty C: Right radial artery pressure during mediastinoscopy. *Anesth Analg* 1979; 58:428. Modified in Rogers MC: *Principles & Practices of Anesthesiology*. Mosby-Year Book, St. Louis: 1993.)

← **Figure 5-12.** Lymph node sites accessible to mediastinoscope biopsy. Many of these can be reached by standard cervical mediastinoscopy. Anterior and aortopulmonary window nodes, however, require extended or anterior mediastinoscopy, VATS, or needle biopsy. (Reproduced with permission from Bocage J-P, Mackenzie JW, Nosher JL: Invasive diagnostic procedures. In *General Thoracic Surgery*, 5th edition. Shields TW, LoCicero J III, Ponn RB, eds. Lippincott Williams & Wilkins, 2000.)

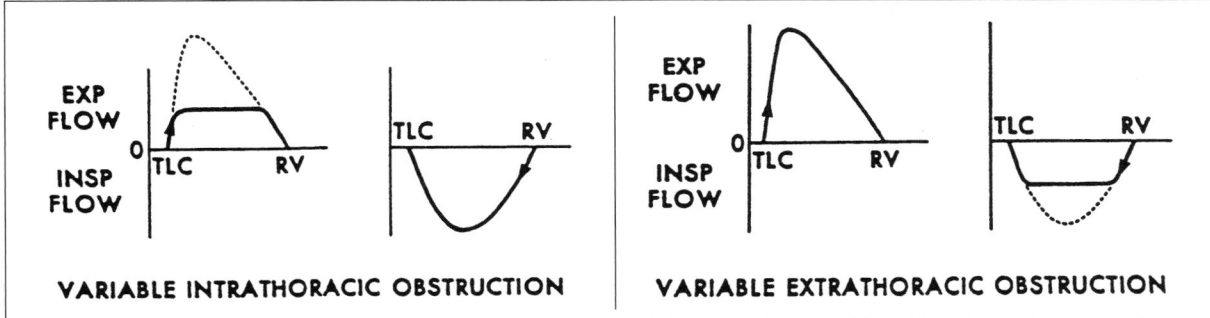

Figure 5-14. Flow volume loop: with variable extrathoracic lesion, the alteration in the flow volume loop is seen by flow limitation and a plateau on inspiration. The reverse occurs with variable intrathoracic lesions. (Reproduced with permission from Acres J, Kryger MH: Clinical significance of pulmonary function tests. *Chest* 1981; 80:207-11.)

Blood and fluid requirements	IV: 14-16 ga × 1 NS/LR @ 1-2 ml/kg/h Blood in OR	Have blood for transfusion available in OR prior to surgery. With venous bleeding, fluids given through an iv in upper limb may enter mediastinum through a tear in the vein. Patients with SVC syndrome may have impaired venous return from upper-limb iv's. A large-bore iv cannula should then be placed in lower limb for fluid and blood transfusions.
Monitoring	Standard monitors (p. B-1) ± Arterial line ± CVP/PA	Invasive monitors are appropriate in patients with large mediastinal masses. In the presence of SVC syndrome, CVP/PA catheters should be placed, using the femoral vein. BP cuff on left arm; radial artery line (if used) and pulse oximeter on right. Mass or mediastinoscope can compress innominate artery, causing reduction in right-radial pulse and right-arm BP. If only right-arm BP is measured, patients may be treated inappropriately for 'hypotension.' Suspect great vessel compression if right-arm pressure is lower than left, or if right-arm BP disappears in the presence of a normal ECG. Arterial compression can compromise cerebrovascular perfusion → cerebral ischemia → stroke.
Positioning	Head-up position ✓ and pad pressure points. ✓ eyes.	In patients with an anterior mediastinal mass, the head-up position reduces mass compression effect on airway and vascular structures, but may subject the patient to ↑risk, VAE if venous bleeding occurs during the procedure. Patients with SVC obstruction, if placed in head-down position with IPPV (further impedes venous return of thoracic cavity), are at ↑risk of airway edema and airway obstruction following extubation.
Complications	Bleeding	Surgical tamponade through mediastinoscope may be indicated. For major hemorrhage, emergency thoracotomy or median sternotomy may be required to stop bleeding. Can occur from laceration of mediastinal vein.
	Air embolism	Head elevation increases risk of embolism, particularly if patient breathes spontaneously. Monitor $ETCO_2$ and ETN_2.
	Airway rupture or obstruction Tracheal collapse	Requires immediate thoracotomy. Acute obstruction may require rigid bronchoscope to reopen airway.
	Recurrent laryngeal nerve injury	If recurrent laryngeal nerve injury is suspected, the vocal cords should be examined during spontaneous breathing at the time of extubation.

POSTOPERATIVE

Complications	Pneumothorax (see Postop Complications for Cervical Neurosurgical Procedures, p. 86). Phrenic/recurrent laryngeal nerve damage Bleeding	Bilateral laryngeal nerve damage may result in airway obstruction, necessitating reintubation. Mask ventilation may be ineffective.
Pain management	Parenteral opioids (p. C-2) ± Epidural	
Tests	CXR on all patients to r/o pneumothorax.	See Postop Complications for VATS, p. 242.

References

1. Barash PG, Tsai B, Kitahata LM: Acute tracheal collapse following mediastinoscopy. *Anesthesiology* 1976; 44(1):67-8.

2. Baue AE, ed: *Glenn's Thoracic and Cardiovascular Surgery*, 6th edition, Volume II. Geha AS, Hammond GL, Laks H, Naunheim KS, assoc eds. Appleton & Lange, Norwalk, CT: 1996.
3. Neuman GG, Weingarten AE, Abramowitz RM, et al: The anesthetic management of the patient with an anterior mediastinal mass. *Anesthesiology* 1984; 60(2):144-7.
4. Petty C: Right radial artery pressure during mediastinoscopy. *Anesth Analg* 1979; 58(5):428-30.
5. Pullerits J, Holzman R: Anesthesia for patients with mediastinal masses. *Can J Anaesth* 1989; 36(6):681-8.
6. Sabiston DC Jr, Spencer FC: *Surgery of the Chest*, 6th edition, Vol II. WB Saunders, Philadelphia: 1995.
7. Vaughan RS: Anesthesia for mediastinoscopy. *Anaesthesia* 1978; 33(2):195-8.
8. Vueghs PJ, Schurink GA, Vaes L, Langemeyer JS: Anesthesia in repeat mediastinoscopy: a retrospective study of 101 patients. *J Cardiothorac Vasc Anesth* 1992; 6(2):193-5.

BRONCHOSCOPY—FLEXIBLE AND RIGID

SURGICAL CONSIDERATIONS

Description: Bronchoscopy can be performed using either rigid or flexible instrumentation. **Flexible fiber optic bronchoscopy (FOB)** is used for the Dx and evaluation of a variety of pulmonary conditions and can be accomplished using topical anesthesia and sedation without an anesthesiologist. Transbronchial biopsies can be performed in sedated patients, although more extensive interventions—such as laser ablation of a tumor, stent placement, and balloon dilation—generally require GA. When performed under GA, the bronchoscope should be passed through a size 8 or larger ETT.

Rigid bronchoscopy is more appropriate for evaluating hemoptysis and for intrabronchial procedures, including mechanical dilation of tracheal or bronchial strictures, tumor debridement, and removal of foreign bodies (FBs) that cannot be extracted with basket forceps through a flexible bronchoscope. Rigid bronchoscopy is performed under GA, with the patient's head and neck extended. The eyes, teeth, and gums must be protected throughout the procedure. The bronchoscope is inserted into the posterior pharynx until the epiglottis is visualized. The epiglottis is lifted anteriorly, with care being taken not to use the patient's teeth as a fulcrum. The bronchoscope is then advanced into the trachea (Fig 5-15) and the diagnostic or therapeutic procedure is carried out. Ventilation is through the side-arm of the bronchoscope, as there is no cuff to prevent escape of anesthetic gases. High ventilatory volumes may be required. Because interventions (e.g., biopsy or tumor debridement) require removal of the bronchoscope viewing lens, the anesthesiologist must time ventilation appropriately. A Venturi ventilator may be useful when the viewing lens must be off for prolonged periods.

Laser bronchoscopy can be performed using either flexible or rigid bronchoscopes. The CO_2 laser is characterized by limited tissue penetration. As such, it is useful for superficial lesions of the upper airway. The Nd:YAG lasers use higher energies, can be directed by fiber optic light guides, and can be used for tumor ablation. As both of these types of lasers rely on thermal damage to tissues, precautions—particularly $FiO_2 \leq 40\%$—must be taken to prevent the devastating complication of airway fire. **Photodynamic therapy** uses visible light to activate a photosensitive compound into a locally toxic drug. Since no thermal energy is involved, airway fires are not an issue.

Usual preop diagnosis: Carcinoma of the lung, primary or recurrent; hemoptysis; obstruction; foreign body; benign tumor; respiratory papillomatosis

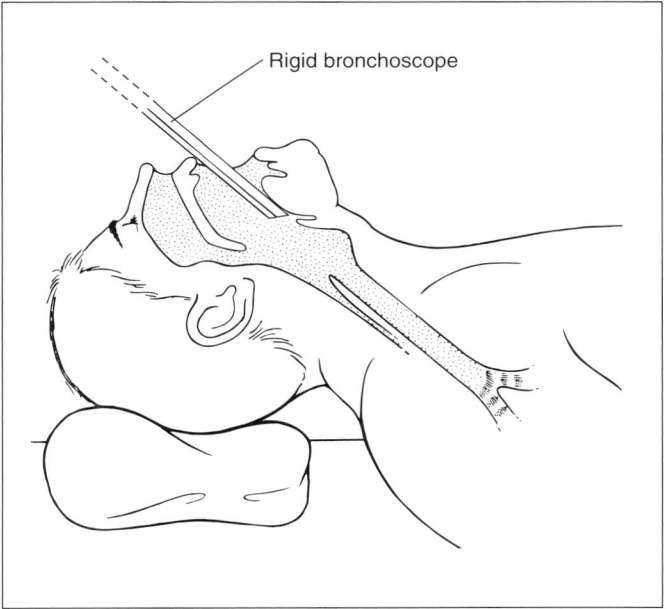

Figure 5-15. Patient positioning for rigid bronchoscopy.

SUMMARY OF PROCEDURES

	Fiber Optic Bronchoscopy	Rigid Bronchoscopy	Laser Bronchoscopy
Position	Supine	⇐	⇐
Special instrumentation	FOB and instruments	Rigid bronchoscope and instruments	Nd:YAG laser and bronchoscope
Unique considerations	None	Shared airway	⇐ + Keep $FiO_2 \leq 0.4$ during use of laser.
Antibiotics	Usually none	± Cefazolin 1 g	⇐
Surgical time	< 30 min	⇐	1 h
EBL	Minimal	⇐	⇐
Postop care	PACU → room	⇐	⇐
Mortality	Minimal	⇐	5%
Morbidity	Barotrauma	⇐	⇐
	Airway obstruction	⇐	Airway fire
	Pneumothorax	⇐	Hemorrhage
		Tooth damage	Perforation
		Tracheal laceration	
		Pneumomediastinum	
		Esophageal perforation	
Pain score	1	1	1

PATIENT POPULATION CHARACTERISTICS

Age range	Usually adults > 50 yr
Male:Female	1:1
Incidence	Common
Etiology	Smoking; hemoptysis; aspiration of foreign body
Associated conditions	Lung cancer or metastatic spread to tracheobronchial tree; airway obstruction 2° tumor or FB; lung infiltrates

ANESTHETIC CONSIDERATIONS

PREOPERATIVE

Patients presenting for bronchoscopy range from asymptomatic to those in severe respiratory distress. The fiber optic technique has virtually replaced rigid bronchoscopy for diagnostic procedures.

Respiratory   H&P to focus on underlying condition. Evaluate for acute and chronic pulmonary problems by H&P and lab and radiologic studies.
Tests: Consider ABG (indicated if patient has Hx of heavy tobacco use, has SOB at rest, or has poor exercise tolerance); PFT; CXR. Hypoxemia (PaO_2 < 70 mmHg) and/or hypercapnia ($PaCO_2$ > 45 mmHg) indicate significant respiratory impairment and predict increased risk.

Cardiovascular   Many patients have Hx of cardiac disease. Cardiology consultation should be obtained for acute change in cardiac status or for patient with poorly controlled chronic disease.
Tests: Consider ECG; others as indicated from H&P.

Musculoskeletal   Patients with lung cancer may have myasthenic (Eaton-Lambert) syndrome with resistance to depolarizing muscle relaxants and ↑sensitivity to NMRs. Monitor relaxation with peripheral nerve stimulator.

Hematologic   Blood T&C not necessary unless high risk of hemorrhage from biopsy (✓ with surgeon). Adequate O_2-carrying capacity important.
Tests: Hb/Hct

Laboratory   Other tests as indicated from H&P.

Premedication   Antisialagogue (prefer glycopyrrolate 0.2 mg iv, no central anticholinergic effects); atropine or scopolamine also can be used. Light sedation with midazolam 1-2 mg iv and/or fentanyl, 50-100 μg iv. Avoid heavy sedation that might impair postop ventilation.

INTRAOPERATIVE

Flexible bronchoscopy: Anesthetic technique for flexible FOB requires sedation or GA. Anxious patients and those with respiratory compromise may not tolerate sedation for awake FOB; and patients with Hx of gastric reflux or aspiration are not candidates for awake FOB.

Sedation with topical anesthesia	Sedate patient as necessary to ensure comfort and cooperation (midazolam 1-2 mg iv and/or fentanyl 50-100 μg iv). Spray palate, pharynx, larynx, vocal cords, and trachea with lidocaine (4%), using nebulizer, or have patient gargle viscous lidocaine (4%).
	Transtracheal local anesthesia: Pass needle through cricothyroid membrane, aspirate air into syringe, and then inject lidocaine (2%) 2 ml. Remove needle quickly since injection causes cough (spreads the anesthetic). Perform superior laryngeal nerve blocks. Insert needle anterior to superior cornu of thyroid cartilage. After resistance is felt, aspirate gently, then inject lidocaine (2%) 2 ml; repeat on other side. Alternatively, hold base of tongue forward and, using Krause's forceps, place pledgets soaked in local anesthetic in each pyriform fossa to block the internal branch of superior laryngeal nerve. Patient can hold a suction catheter in the mouth to remove oral secretions and waste anesthetic gases. A special face mask (Patil-Syracuse) incorporates a diaphragm through which the FOB can pass while patient breathes $FiO_2 = 1$. Use a special oral airway (Ovassapian) to guide FOB over back of tongue into trachea to prevent damage to FOB by teeth. Limit amount of suctioning by surgeon, since suctioning through FOB decreases FiO_2 and FRC, $\rightarrow \downarrow PaO_2$.

General anesthesia: Almost any anesthetic technique is acceptable. A large ETT has less resistance to air flow; minimum size is 8 mm (ID) for adult FOB. If patient requires ETT < 8 mm, use a pediatric FOB. FOB through ETT causes PEEP effect, which can $\rightarrow \downarrow$BP in hypovolemic patient.

Rigid bronchoscopy: Anesthetic technique utilizing rigid bronchoscopy provides superior visualization and improved suctioning, and allows introduction of biopsy forceps. Requires GA.

Induction	Preoxygenate to completely denitrogenate patient. Use only small amount of iv opioids, since postop analgesic requirements are minimal; consider remifentanil (1μg/kg). Postop respiratory depression should be avoided. STP 3-5 mg/kg, succinylcholine 1 mg/kg or mivacurium 0.2 mg/kg.
Maintenance	Isoflurane, or sevoflurane and 100% O_2; succinylcholine drip (1 g/250 ml NS, titrated to effect; be aware of onset of phase II block at doses > 5-6 mg/kg). Alternatively, a TIVA approach (p. B-3), using propofol (50-150 μg/kg/min) and remifentanil (0.1-0.5 μg/kg/min) infusions, is an excellent way to provide anesthesia without causing OR pollution by inhalation agents. Short-acting, nondepolarizing agents (atracurium, vecuronium, or mivacurium) also can be used. Manual IPPV through side-arm of rigid bronchoscope. High flow (up to 20 L/min) to compensate for leak. Hyperventilate patient in preparation for periods of apnea. Ventilation must be interrupted whenever surgeon removes eyepiece to suction or biopsy. Manually ventilate to compensate for compliance changes that occur when bronchoscope is in trachea (ventilating both lungs) and when it is in bronchus (ventilating one lung). O_2 flush is used to compensate for leak; bypasses anesthetic vaporizer. Frequent flushing lowers anesthetic concentration. **Sanders Injection System**—jet ventilation using Venturi effect—is an alternative. Uninterrupted ventilation is possible since the presence of eyepiece is not necessary for ventilation. Fewer interruptions may shorten length of procedure. Usually requires TIVA (p. B-3). Entrainment of air results in variable O_2 at distal tip. If total thoracic compliance is low, adequacy of ventilation is difficult to evaluate; patient easily hypoventilated. The greater need for muscle relaxation to move chest wall increases risk of residual weakness immediately postop.
Emergence	Reintubate with ETT after rigid bronchoscopy. Patient must be fully awake before extubation, with no residual neuromuscular blockade. Emergence can be 'stormy.' Patient may cough violently to clear secretions and blood. A smooth emergence may be facilitated by early suctioning of the airway, use of an antisialagogue and lidocaine (1 mg/kg iv) to decrease airway sensitivity. The sitting position improves breathing and clearance of secretions. Continue supplemental O_2.
Blood and fluid requirements	Blood usually not required. IV: 18 ga × 1 NS/LR @ 2 ml/kg/h	Transfusion unnecessary unless complicated by massive hemorrhage; be prepared for emergency thoracotomy. Usually restrict iv fluids to avoid fluid overload.
Monitoring	Standard monitors (p. B-1)	★ **NB:** ETCO$_2$ not accurate during rigid bronchoscopy because of dilution effect at sample port.

Positioning	✓ and pad pressure points. ✓ eyes. Shoulder roll for rigid bronchoscopy	
Complications	Hypoxemia	Monitor pulse oximetry continuously. If patient hypoxemic, surgeon must withdraw bronchoscope into trachea. If problem persists, remove bronchoscope and ventilate by mask or ETT.
	Hypercapnia	Common, due to hypoventilation. Ventricular dysrhythmias due to respiratory acidosis and 'light' anesthesia. Treat by hyperventilation (increased rate) which lowers CO_2 and deepens inhalational anesthesia; iv lidocaine for dysrhythmias.
	Bleeding Tracheobronchial injury Aspiration of debris	Requires frequent suctioning. For major hemorrhage, place uncut ETT down healthy bronchus and ventilate good lung. May require thoracotomy using DLT or BB to isolate and/or tamponade bleeding site.

POSTOPERATIVE

Complications	Hypoxemia	Rx: Supplemental O_2. Nebulized racemic epinephrine and steroids may ↓ airway edema. Humidified O_2 may ↓ airway irritation.
	Hypoventilation Dental damage Airway trauma Pneumothorax Hemorrhage	Incomplete reversal of muscle relaxants or opioid overdosage can cause hypoventilation. Obtain ABG if patient has difficulty breathing or is overly sedated. Be prepared to reintubate patient.
	Risk of aspiration Airway obstruction (bronchospasm, bleeding, dislodged tumor, FB)	If nerve blocks used to depress gag reflex, no eating or drinking for several h postbronchoscopy.
Pain management	Minimal pain; easily treated with iv opioids.	
Tests	CXR	Obtain CXR in recovery room to ✓ for atelectasis, pneumothorax, mediastinal emphysema.

References

1. Baue AE, ed: *Glenn's Thoracic and Cardiovascular Surgery*, 6th edition, Volume II. Geha AS, Hammond GL, Laks H, Naunheim KS, assoc eds. Appleton & Lange, Norwalk, CT: 1996.
2. Brimacombe J, Tucker P, Simons S: The Laryngeal mask airway for awake diagnostic bronchoscopy. A retrospective study of 200 consecutive patients. *Eur J Anaesthesiol* 1995; 12(4):357-61.
3. Fraioli RL, Sheffer LA, Steffenson JL: Pulmonary and cardiovascular effects of apneic oxygenation in man. *Anesthesiology* 1973; 39(6):588-96.
4. Graham DR, Hay JG, Clague J, et al: Comparison of three different methods used to achieve local anesthesia for fiber optic bronchoscopy. *Chest* 1992; 102(3):704-7.
5. Prakash N, McLeod T, Gao Smith F: The effects of remifentanil on haemodynamic stability during rigid bronchoscopy. *Anaesthesia* 2001; 56(6):576-80.
6. Sabiston DC Jr, Spencer FC: *Surgery of the Chest*, 6th edition, Vol II. WB Saunders, Philadelphia: 1995.
7. Wain JC: Rigid bronchoscopy: the value of a venerable procedure. *Chest Surg Clin North Am* 2001; 11(4):691-9.

ANESTHETIC CONSIDERATIONS FOR LASER RESECTION

PREOPERATIVE

Typically, these patients present with a long Hx of smoking and consequent pulmonary dysfunction, complicated by an airway mass (endobronchial, carinal, or tracheal) causing respiratory distress.

Respiratory	It is important to define the exact location and magnitude of any tracheal mass, in order to estimate an appropriate size for the ETT and the likelihood of obstruction on induction. CXR and CT scan should be studied. PFTs and flow volume loops may help characterize the lesion. **Tests:** PFTs; ABGs; CXR; CT scan (to determine site of airway obstruction)
Musculoskeletal	Although there may be no clinically detectable muscle weakness, some of these patients will have Eaton-Lambert syndrome →↑sensitivity to NMRs and ↑resistance to depolarizing muscle relaxants.
Hematologic	Transfuse patients with preop Hct < 25% (or < 30%, if CAD present). **Tests:** Hct
Laboratory	Other tests as indicated from H&P.
Premedication	Minimal; avoid respiratory depressants.

INTRAOPERATIVE

Anesthetic technique: GETA or local anesthesia with heavy sedation. Unexpected patient movement may be disastrous. Nd:YAG laser can be transmitted through a flexible quartz monofilament passed through either a rigid bronchoscope or FOB. Rigid bronchoscope provides improved visibility and better debris retrieval. It also maintains the airway with less chance of fire since metal is nonignitable (it can reflect the laser beam, however, causing tissue damage), although manual ventilation through the side-arm may be more difficult. FOB is used with local anesthesia or through ETT under GA. Laser-safe ETTs (required for surgery in the proximal trachea) include regular ETTs wrapped in metallic tape or commercially available 'laser' tubes (usually some combination of aluminum, stainless steel, Teflon, and/or silicon). Fill cuff with saline (± methylene blue to facilitate leak detection). Steps also must be taken to protect the OR staff from laser injury. These include safety glasses to avoid ocular damage and specially designed filter face masks to protect from inhalation of vaporized viral particles.

Induction	**Without airway obstruction:** Standard induction (see p. B-2). **With airway obstruction:** Awake FOB may precede intubation to determine the feasibility of tracheal intubation. In patients with less severe obstruction, an inhalation induction with spontaneous ventilation may be appropriate. Avoid muscle relaxants until the airway has been secured. For FOB resections, a large, red rubber ETT is preferred as it is less flammable, and fewer combustible toxic products are released if ignited, than if a plastic ETT is ignited. Special laser ETTs are not needed since Nd:YAG laser is fired distal to the tip of the ETT.
Maintenance	Use isoflurane, air (N_2) and O_2 mixture. Keep FiO_2 < 0.3. Avoid N_2O, which supports combustion. TIVA (p. B-3) with propofol (50-150 μg/kg/min) and remifentanil (0.1-0.5 μg/kg/mm) infusion is an excellent alternative to standard maintenance and avoids contamination of the OR with inhalational agents. Short-acting, nondepolarizing relaxant or succinylcholine infusion should be used, since it is essential that the operating field be stationary to avoid damage to tissue from a misdirected laser beam. If the patient becomes hypoxemic, ventilate the lungs with higher FiO_2 and ask the surgeon to stop.
Emergence	Following rigid bronchoscopy, the patient usually is reintubated until awake and breathing well and protective airway reflexes have returned. Emergence can be 'stormy,' with bleeding and secretion clearance a problem. Patient should be recovered in the sitting position.

Blood and fluid requirements	IV: 14-16 ga × 1-2 NS/LR @ 1-2 ml/kg/h	There is a potential for massive blood loss following inadvertent perforation of a major blood vessel.
Monitoring	Standard monitors (p. B-1)	Continuous pulse oximetry essential; monitor $ETCO_2$ to assess adequacy of ventilation. Keep alveolar O_2 < 40%.
Positioning	✓ and pad pressure points. ✓ eyes.	
Complications	Airway obstruction Hypoxemia/hypercarbia Bleeding Perforation of tracheobronchial tree	From tumor, blood, tissue debris, etc. From inadequate ventilation. Can be massive from perforation of blood vessel by laser. Apply topical epinephrine following laser photocoagulation to control bleeding. → pneumothorax/mediastinum → cardiac arrest.

Complications, cont.	Airway fire	Rx: stop ventilation, remove O_2 source, extubate trachea to decrease inhalation of toxic products. Suction all debris from airway. Ventilate patient by mask, then reintubate. Prior to extubation, perform bronchoscopy to reevaluate airway damage and suction debris.

POSTOPERATIVE

Complications	Airway edema	Only the surface of the affected tissue is visibly changed; there may be underlying edema formation. Patient may require emergency reintubation if airway obstruction 2° edema occurs. Steroids usually given (dexamethasone 6-8 mg iv). Nebulized racemic epinephrine is helpful. Complications such as hemorrhage or obstruction can be delayed up to 48 h.
Pain management	Minimal pain; rarely requires analgesic.	
Tests	Continuous pulse oximetry monitoring. Frequent ABGs.	

References

1. Baue AE, ed: *Glenn's Thoracic and Cardiovascular Surgery*, 6th edition, Volume II. Geha AS, Hammond GL, Laks H, Naunheim KS, assoc eds. Appleton & Lange, Norwalk, CT: 1996.
2. Blomquist S, Algotsson L, Karlsson SE: Anaesthesia for resection of tumours in the trachea and central bronchi using the Nd:YAG-laser technique. *Acta Anaesthiol Scand* 1990; 34(6):506-10.
3. Chan AL, Tharratt RS, Siefkin AD, et al: Nd:YAG laser bronchoscopy. Rigid or fiber optic mode? *Chest* 1990; 98(2):271-5.
4. Conacher ID, Pae LL, McMahon CC, et al: Anesthetic management of laser surgery for central airway obstruction, a 12-year case series. *J Cardiothorac Vasc Anesth* 1998; 12(2):153-6.
5. McCaughan JS Jr, Barabash RD, Penn GM, Glavan BJ: Nd:YAG laser and photodynamic therapy for esophageal and endobronchial tumors under general and local anesthesia. Effects on arterial blood gas levels. *Chest* 1990; 98(6):1374-8.
6. Sabiston DC Jr, Spencer FC: *Surgery of the Chest*, 6th edition, Vol II. WB Saunders, Philadelphia: 1995.
7. Vanderschueren RG, Westermann CJ: Complications of endobronchial neodymium:YAG (Nd:YAG) laser application. *Lung* 1990; 168 Suppl:1089-94.

VIDEO-ASSISTED THORACOSCOPY SURGERY (VATS)

SURGICAL CONSIDERATIONS

Description: **Video-assisted thoracoscopy surgery** (VATS) is used most often for assessment of pleural processes of unknown etiology (e.g., pleural effusion that has defied diagnosis). Its use is accepted for treatment of spontaneous pneumothorax 2° apical blebs, for biopsy of peripheral infiltrates or nodules, for talc pleurodesis, and for drainage of pleural effusions and other fluid collections. Accessible, small lung cancers may be removed using the videoscope (wedge resections). VATS also has been used for lung-volume reduction surgery (see p. 249). **Heller myotomy** and **upper dorsal sympathectomy** can be done using video thoracoscopy. Less well accepted procedures include **lobectomy**, **pneumonectomy** and **esophagectomy**. Use of a DLT to provide collapse of the ipsilateral lung is mandatory, since satisfactory visualization of the pleural cavity is impossible without this collapse of the lung. The patient is usually in the lateral position. Several small incisions are used—usually 3; sometimes 4 or more. The video thoracoscope is placed through the first incision and the pleural cavity is inspected. Other small incisions are then made for insertion of instruments. The position of the video thoracoscope and instruments may be interchanged, depending on the location of the problem.

Usual preop diagnosis: Pleural disease (e.g., effusions); recurrent empyema; recurrent pneumothorax; localized lung masses; achalasia; pulmonary infiltrates; hyperhidrosis; reflex sympathetic dystrophy (RSD)

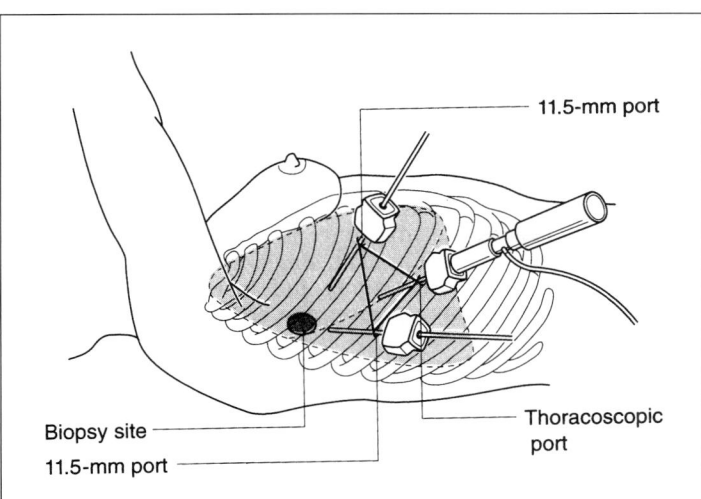

Figure 5-16. Example of thoracoscopic port placement. Positioning varies for individual need, but the principle of triangulation used for laparoscopic surgery is equally applicable in the thorax. (Reproduced with permission from Greenfield LJ, et al., eds: *Surgery: Scientific Principles and Practice.* Lippincott-Raven Publishers: 1997, 741.)

SUMMARY OF PROCEDURE

Position	Lateral
Incision	Usually 3 small incisions (portals) (Fig 5-16)
Special instrumentation	Video thoracoscope with thoracoscopy instruments; DLT required.
Antibiotics	Cefazolin 1 g
Surgical time	1-3 h
Closing considerations	Chest tube placed
EBL	Minimal, although there is a risk for major bleeding.
Postop care	Chest tube
Mortality	Minimal
Morbidity	Major vascular injury: Rare
	Conversion to open thoracotomy: 4%
	Pneumothorax/persistent air leak
Pain score	2-3

PATIENT POPULATION CHARACTERISTICS

Age range	All age groups
Male:Female	1:1
Associated conditions	Pleural effusions; lung mass; pneumothorax

---

ANESTHETIC CONSIDERATIONS

PREOPERATIVE

As VATS is used for both diagnostic and therapeutic purposes, this patient population is quite diverse in symptomatology; however, it has in common some intrathoracic/respiratory disease processes.

Respiratory	The preop evaluation should focus on the patient's ability to tolerate OLV, as well as the postop effects of the planned surgery. PFTs and ABG are useful prognostic tests. Question patient about dyspnea, productive cough, and cigarette smoking; examine for cyanosis, clubbing, RR, and pattern. Listen to chest for wheezes, rhonchi, and rales. Preop lung function may be improved by treating respiratory tract infections, stopping smoking, and treatment with bronchodilators and steroids, as indicated.
	Tests: PFT; CXR; if chest CT available, look for airway obstruction that could interfere with DLT placement; ABG.
Cardiovascular	Directed at any underlying disease process.

Laboratory	As indicated from H&P.
Premedication	Standard premedication (see p. B-2). Avoid heavy sedation that might impair postop respiratory function.

INTRAOPERATIVE

Anesthetic technique: GETA, typically with OLV, using DLT or BB (see OLV, pp. 213-214). Local or regional anesthetic technique ± sedation also may be used. The use of epidural with GETA is rarely required, unless the potential for converting from a VATS to an open thoracostomy approach is high.

Regional anesthesia: The incision site is infiltrated with local anesthetics, and intercostal nerve blocks are performed at the level of incision and at several levels above and below incision. Alternatively, thoracic epidural anesthesia may be used. When the chest is opened, air enters pleural cavity, causing partial pneumothorax. Most patients usually tolerate this if warned in advance about the potential for dyspnea and visceral discomfort. Thoracoscope in chest-wall incision prevents complete lung collapse.

General anesthesia: The patient is intubated with DLT or BB to selectively collapse operated lung. Anesthetic choice optional; but FiO_2 = 1 during OLV. GA allows IPPV with complete reexpansion of lung without pain, if pleurodesis performed.

Induction	Standard induction (see p. B-2). (Placement of DLT is discussed on p. 214.)
Maintenance	O_2 (100%) and isoflurane (1-1.5%). Avoid N_2O, especially during OLV. Short-acting muscle relaxant (e.g., mivacurium 0.01-0.1 mg/kg) and opioids as required. Consider remifentanil infusion (0.1-0.5 μg/kg/min).
Emergence	Extubation in OR
Blood and fluid requirements	IV: 16-18 ga × 1 NS/LR @ 2 ml/kg/h
Monitoring	Standard monitors (p. B-1) ± Arterial line	Arterial catheter generally not required, unless indicated by patient's medical condition.
Positioning	✓ and pad pressure points. ✓ eyes, ears, genitals.	See p. 213 for proper positioning.
Complications	Air leak from lung Hemorrhage Injury to intrathoracic structures Air embolism	Air leak observed on reexpansion of lung. Excessive blood drainage via chest tube; falling Hct Repair may require open thoracotomy.

POSTOPERATIVE

Complications	Tension pneumothorax	In the absence of chest tube, air leak can → pneumothorax that can progress to tension pneumothorax if not treated. This may manifest as wheezing, hyperresonance, ↓chest-wall movement, dyspnea, subcutaneous emphysema, tracheal shift, dysrhythmias, cardiovascular collapse, ↓PO_2, and ↓SaO_2. CXR diagnostic. Requires immediate decompression of tension pneumothorax with large-bore iv cannula through chest wall, followed by chest tube and continuous suction.
Pain management	IV opioids, ketorolac (30 mg) Intrapleural anesthesia	Analgesic requirements less than for lateral thoracotomy. Intrapleural local anesthetics (0.25% bupivacaine + 1:200,000 epinephrine 0.5 ml/kg) via thoracostomy drainage tube after lung is reinflated but before chest tube suction applied.
Tests	CXR postop	

References

1. Allen MS, Deschamps C, Jones DM, et al: Video assisted thoracic surgical procedures: the Mayo experience. *Mayo Clinic Proceedings* 1996; 71(4):351-9.

2. Baue AE, ed: *Glenn's Thoracic and Cardiovascular Surgery*, 6th edition, Volume II. Geha AS, Hammond GL, Laks H, Naunheim KS, assoc eds. Appleton & Lange, Norwalk, CT: 1996.

3. Bolotin G, Lazarovici H, Uretzky G, et al: The efficacy of intraoperative internal intercostal nerve block during video-assisted thoracic surgery on postoperative pain. *Am Thorac Surg* 2000; 70(6):1872-5.

4. Landreneau RJ, Hazelrigg SR, Ferson PF, et al: Thoracoscopic resection of 85 pulmonary lesions. *Ann Thorac Surg* 1992; 54(3):415-19.

5. Lin JC, Landreneau RJ: Instruments and techniques of video-assisted thoracic surgery. In *General Thoracic Surgery*, 5th edition. Shields TW, LoCicero J III, Ponn RB, eds. Lippincott Williams & Wilkins, Philadelphia: 2000, 439-54.

6. Mault JR, Harpole DH, Douglas JM: Thoracoscopic pulmonary resection. In *Atlas of laparoscopic surgery*. Pappas TN, Schwartz LB, Eubanks S, eds. *Current Medicine*, 1996; 26:10.

7. Miller, DL, Allen MS, Trastek VF, et al: Videothorascopic wedge excision of the lung. *Ann Thorac Surg* 1992; 54(3): 410-14.

8. Rusch VW, Mountain C: Thoracoscopy under regional anesthesia for the diagnosis and management of pleural disease. *Am J Surg* 1987; 154(3):274-78.

9. Sabiston DC Jr, Spencer FC: *Surgery of the Chest*, 6th edition, Vol II. WB Saunders, Philadelphia: 1995.

10. Shah JS, Bready LL: Anesthesia for thoracoscopy. *Anaesthesiol Clin North Am* 2001; 19(1):153-71.

THYMECTOMY

SURGICAL CONSIDERATIONS

Description: The two most common indications for **thymectomy are myasthenia gravis** and **thymoma**. The severity of myasthenia gravis can be classified using the Osserman scheme, which assigns Stage I to patients with ocular symptoms only, with Stages II-IV for progressive degrees of bulbar and systemic Sx. Indications for surgery vs medical management remain controversial, with some neurologists referring nearly all patients with myasthenia gravis for surgery, while others referring only those with the most refractory Sx. Patients referred for surgery often take a combination of pyridostigmine (Mestinon) and immunosuppressants (steroids and azathioprine). In cases of severe myasthenia gravis, preop plasmapheresis may be helpful in minimizing periop muscle weakness. Patients with thymoma may be asymptomatic, although ~10-20% have a Hx of myasthenic symptoms.

Thymectomy can be a performed through a **complete sternotomy**, an upper sternal split (manubrium only), or via a cervical approach. The value of a complete sternotomy is that it allows for removal of all anterior mediastinal tissue that may harbor small thymic rests. This is the most invasive approach, however, and the one associated with the greatest degree of intraop tissue injury. An **upper sternal split** is performed with the neck extended and a roll placed under the shoulder blades. Either a short vertical incision or a transverse incision at the level of the sternal angle may be used. Division of only the manubrium provides adequate exposure for identification, dissection, and removal of the thymus. Mobilization of the thymus can be accomplished without entering the pleural space. Care must be taken to avoid injuring the phrenic nerves. In contrast with the removal of anterior mediastinal tumors, thymectomy usually does not require OLV.

Transcervical thymectomy is performed through a collar incision similar to that used for thyroidectomy (Fig 7.11-3). The cervical extensions of the thymus are identified and the dissection is advanced progressively into the neck. Attachments of the gland are cauterized, and a clip is placed on the thymic vein (which drains directly into the innominate vein). Exposure is aided by a special retractor that elevates the sternum anteriorly and exposes the anterior mediastinum.

At the conclusion of the operation—whether it is done through the chest or the neck—the thymic bed is drained with a small suction drain. Preop medications should be resumed as soon as possible.

Usual preop diagnosis: Myasthenia gravis; thymoma

SUMMARY OF PROCEDURES

	Sternotomy	Cervical Approach
Position	Supine	⇐
Incision	Median sternotomy	Suprasternal
Special instrumentation	None	Special sternal retractor
Antibiotics	Cefazolin 1 g	⇐
Surgical time	1-2 h	⇐

	Sternotomy	**Cervical Approach**
EBL	< 500 ml	⇐
Postop care	ICU – special attention to muscle strength, related to respiratory function	⇐
Mortality	< 5%	⇐
Morbidity	Infection Pneumothorax Hemothorax	⇐
Pain score	5-7	2

PATIENT POPULATION CHARACTERISTICS

Age range	Usually young adults
Male:Female	Females > males
Incidence	Infrequent
Etiology	Unknown
Associated conditions	Myasthenia gravis; benign or malignant thymoma; other autoimmune diseases (e.g., rheumatoid arthritis)

ANESTHETIC CONSIDERATIONS

PREOPERATIVE

Patients presenting for thymectomy may have myasthenia gravis, an autoimmune disease of the neuromuscular junction characterized by muscle weakness and easy fatiguability. Thymomas (benign or malignant) also may be associated with myasthenia gravis. The anesthesiologist needs to be aware of the possible compression effects of the tumor (see Excision of Mediastinal Tumor, p. 229), the potential for respiratory failure, and the interaction of various treatment modalities.

Respiratory	Patient may have marked reduction in VC 2° muscle weakness; establish baseline spirometry values. Criteria necessary to predict need for postop ventilation include: duration of disease > 6 yr; chronic respiratory disease; pyridostigmine dose > 750 mg/d; VC < 2.9 L; preop use of steroids; and previous episode of respiratory failure. **Tests:** PFTs, others as indicated from H&P.
Cardiovascular	There is a rare association between myasthenia gravis and cardiomyopathy. Consider ECG and cardiac consult if indicated from H&P.
Neurological	Review neurological assessment. Patients often exhibit diplopia, ptosis, and easy fatiguability of muscles. Difficulties with swallowing and speaking are common. Review tests (EMGs, Tensilon) done by neurologist to evaluate the adequacy of drug therapy (steroids, anticholinesterases, azathioprine, and cyclosporin A). Azathioprine (Imuran) may actually antagonize neuromuscular blockade by inhibiting phosphodiesterase. Cyclosporin A is reserved for severe disease because of the side effects of renal insufficiency and HTN. It may prolong neuromuscular blockade. 10-50% of the patients with thymomas will have myasthenia gravis and >85% of myasthenics will have thymus abnormalities.
Musculoskeletal	Determine adequacy of anticholinesterase medication. Evaluate hand strength, inspiratory efforts and PFTs. Note that an excess of anticholinesterase agents can cause weakness and respiratory failure (cholinergic crisis) indistinguishable from myasthenia. A deleterious response to the Tensilon test (10 mg), as well as the presence of cholinergic side effects (e.g., pupil constriction), distinguish cholinergic from myasthenic crises. Plasmapheresis may offer temporary (days to weeks) improvement in symptoms. Typically, patients with worsening symptoms receive 4-8 treatments prior to surgery. There should be a 24-h delay between the last plasmapheresis and surgery to restore clotting factors and immunoglobulins. Plasmapheresis also may transiently decrease plasma cholinesterase, which could prolong the effects of succinylcholine, mivacurium, and ester-type local anesthetics.
Endocrine	Due to the autoimmune nature of myasthenia gravis, associated thyroid dysfunction may be seen in this patient population. Sx of thyroid dysfunction should be evaluated. **Tests:** TSH; evaluate screening test if indicated from H&P.

Laboratory	Other tests as indicated from H&P.
Premedication	Avoid premedication; for the anxious patient, give a small dose of midazolam (1-2 mg); avoid opioids or any other sedatives that may depress ventilation. Current recommendations for anticholinesterases suggest that, in mild disease without psychological dependence, the morning dose can be held or halved. Patients with severe disease or with marked anticholinesterase dependence should receive their regular morning dose. For patients on steroids—depending on dosage and duration of steroid therapy—hydrocortisone (up to 100 mg iv bolus) before induction, then 100 mg q 8 h × 24 h, may be helpful.

INTRAOPERATIVE

Anesthetic technique: GETA, combined with thoracic or lumbar epidural if transsternal thymectomy. DLT may be requested by surgeon.

Induction	Mask inhalational induction with sevoflurane to avoid muscle relaxants entirely; however, patients with profound muscle weakness are at risk for aspiration 2° inadequate airway protective mechanism. Alternatively, iv STP 2-4 mg/kg induction without muscle relaxants. Succinylcholine may be used to facilitate intubation; however, the response to succinylcholine is unpredictable (myasthenia → ↓sensitivity; anticholinesterases → ↑sensitivity).
Maintenance	Standard maintenance (see p. B-3). Patients with myasthenia gravis have ↑sensitivity to NMRs, which usually are not required (especially during cervical thymectomy). If relaxants are needed, titrate small amounts of drug, using a peripheral nerve stimulator to maintain single twitch. Cisatracurium (20-30 μg/kg q 15-20 min or infusion 1-3 μg/kg/min) is useful since it is rapidly eliminated. Alternatively, potent inhalation agents may provide adequate muscle relaxation, and avoid the need for any muscle relaxant. Avoid drugs with neuromuscular blocking effects (e.g., antidysrhythmics, diuretics, aminoglycosides). If the patient has normal ventilatory function, then spontaneous ventilation during cervical thymectomy may be appropriate. Patients undergoing sternotomy, and any patient with ↓pulmonary reserve, require mechanical ventilation.
Emergence	Criteria for extubation include: head lift (5 sec); MIF > –25 cmH$_2$O; TV > 5 ml/kg; and full reversal evidenced by twitch monitor. Extubate when fully awake; usually immediate postop ventilation is not necessary. Because of the variable response to muscle relaxation and delayed benefits of the surgery, some patients may require postop ventilation. Whether intubated or not, monitor patient for pulmonary function by measuring MIF and spirometry (TV). Avoid residual pharmacologic neuromuscular blockade, which will → hypoventilation and ↑ risk of gastric aspiration if protective airway reflexes are inadequate.
Blood and fluid requirements	IV: 18 ga × 1 NS/LR @ 1-2 ml/kg/h	
Monitoring	Standard monitors (p. B-1)	Avoid muscle relaxants if possible; if not, use neuromuscular twitch monitor.
Positioning	✓ and pad pressure points. ✓ eyes.	
Complications	Hemorrhage Dysrhythmia Compression of mediastinal structures Pneumothorax	

POSTOPERATIVE

Complications	Pneumothorax Respiratory failure Phrenic nerve damage Myasthenic or cholinergic crises	Pleura can be entered; if so, chest tube needed. (For Dx and Rx, see VATS, p. 242.)
Pain management	Parenteral opioids (p. C-2) Epidural opioids (p. C-2)	Avoid respiratory depression; parenteral opioids for cervical incision; epidural opioids for median sternotomy.
Drug management	Usually ↓anticholinesterase requirement in the immediate postop period.	Begin anticholinesterase drugs at half preop dose. Beware of 'cholinergic' crisis. Sx include ↑salivation, sweating, abdominal cramps, urinary frequency, fasciculations, and

Drug management, cont.		weakness 2° anticholinesterase overdose. Rx: intubation and mechanical ventilation may be necessary.
Tests	Tensilon (edrophonium)	Neurologists can perform Tensilon test to differentiate between myasthenic and cholinergic crises.
	Muscle strength	Determine muscle strength postop (grip strength and sustained head lift).
	Pupil exam	Pupil dilation (myasthenic crisis); pupil constriction (cholinergic crisis)

References

1. Baraka A: Anesthesia and critical care of thymectomy for myasthenia gravis. *Chest Surg Clin North Am* 2001; 11(2):337-61.
2. Baue AE, ed: *Glenn's Thoracic and Cardiovascular Surgery*, 6th edition, Volume II. Geha AS, Hammond GL, Laks H, Naunheim KS, assoc eds. Appleton & Lange, Norwalk, CT: 1996.
3. Burgess FW, Wilcosky B Jr: Thoracic epidural anesthesia for transsternal thymectomy in myasthenia gravis. *Anesth Analg* 1989; 69(4):529-31.
4. Naquib M, el Dawlatly AA, Ashour M, et al: Multivariate determinants of the need for postoperative ventilation in myasthenia gravis. *Can J Anaesth* 1996; 43(10):1006-13.
5. Sabiston DC Jr, Spencer FC: *Surgery of the Chest*, 6th edition, Vol II. WB Saunders, Philadelphia: 1995.
6. Smith CE, Donati F, Bevan DR: Cumulative dose-response curves for atracurium in patients with myasthenia gravis. *Can J Anaesth* 1989; 36(4):402-6.

EXCISION OF BLEBS OR BULLAE

SURGICAL CONSIDERATIONS

Description: Pulmonary blebs or bullae requiring surgical treatment may vary from small, apical blebs—most usually seen in young people with spontaneous pneumothorax—to expanding, giant bullae causing respiratory distress. The small blebs can be excised through **video thoracoscopy** (see p. 240), although some surgeons still prefer an open technique for this procedure. Giant bullae are generally removed by **open thoracotomy**, although these lesions also may be excised by VATS techniques. The goal is to resect the nonfunctional bullae and allow the compressed, yet relatively preserved lung tissue to reexpand and contribute to gas exchange. Our preference is for **stapling** across the base and excising the lesion. **Clamp and suture** techniques may be used as well. It is important to ensure an airtight closure if possible. Prolonged air leaks that can be very debilitating may occur postop, particularly in patients with giant bullae and emphysema. Patients undergoing operation for giant bullae frequently have limited pulmonary reserve and present formidable operative risks. Since the operation is planned to improve their pulmonary function, however, these patients frequently do well following operation. **Pleural abrasion** or, rarely, **pleurectomy** may accompany the excision of blebs or bullae. The blebs in young patients with recurrent spontaneous pneumothorax usually are located at the apex of the upper lobe. Bullae in patients with emphysema are usually in the upper lobe, but may be anywhere in the lung. Preop localization by CT scan is usually sufficient. If a thoracotomy is done, the approach is usually lateral.

Variant procedure or approaches: Patients with more generalized emphysema may be candidates for lung-volume reduction surgery (see p. 249).

Usual preop diagnosis: Spontaneous pneumothorax 2° ruptured blebs; giant bullae causing respiratory distress

SUMMARY OF PROCEDURE

Position	Usually lateral
Incision	Axillary
Special instrumentation	Staplers
Antibiotics	Cefazolin 1 g

Surgical time	1-3 h
EBL	< 500 ml
Postop care	PACU → room; ICU or IIC for giant bullae
Mortality	Minimal
Morbidity	Air leak: 20% or more in giant bullae
Pain score	5-7

PATIENT POPULATION CHARACTERISTICS

Age range	Young adults (blebs/small bullae); elderly (large bullae)
Male:Female	3:1
Incidence	Not uncommon
Etiology	Emphysema (usually 2° smoking); congenital; infectious
Associated conditions	Spontaneous pneumothorax; emphysema; long smoking Hx; α-antitrypsin deficiency

ANESTHETIC CONSIDERATIONS

PREOPERATIVE

Older patients with this disease have significant COPD, often with pulmonary HTN and RV failure. Young patients are usually otherwise healthy. The risk of rupture of a bleb on the nonoperated side, with resultant tension pneumothorax, must be considered throughout the procedure.

Respiratory	Cysts may be bronchogenic, postinfective, infantile, or emphysematous. Bullae usually result from destruction of alveolar tissue; they represent end-stage emphysematous disease associated with severe COPD. Patient may have incapacitating dyspnea. With blebs, elicit Hx of repeat pneumothoraces. Obtain PFTs and ABG for baseline. Patient may have little pulmonary reserve. CO_2 retention ± hypoxia may be present.
	Tests: CXR; presence of pneumothorax; if chest CT available, look for airway obstruction that could interfere with DLT placement and also bilateral disease; ABG, as indicated from H&P.
Cardiovascular	**Tests:** ECG
Neurological	✓ Hx for previous back surgery, peripheral neuropathy. Examine thoracolumbar area for skin lesions, infection, deformities.
Hematologic	Transfuse patient with preop Hct < 25% (Hct < 30% if patient has CAD). T&C 2 U of blood or obtain 1-2 U of autologous blood during the month before surgery, or consider erythropoietin therapy in patients who are anemic.
	Tests: Hct
Laboratory	Other tests as indicated from H&P.
Premedication	Midazolam 1-2 mg iv if patient anxious. When epidural opioids are planned, avoid systemic opioid or sedative premedication, which can potentiate postop respiratory effects of central neuraxial opioids.

INTRAOPERATIVE

Anesthetic technique: GETA—may be combined with epidural.

Induction	Awake intubation or GA with patient breathing spontaneously. Awake intubation with a Univent or DLT is appropriate in cases with severe bilateral bullous disease with a past Hx of rupture. Ventilate those patients by hand with small TVs and a long expiratory time, minimizing peak pressures until the chest is open. Rapid placement of a chest tube is essential should a bulla rupture. If muscle relaxants are used to facilitate tracheal intubation, patient will need IPPV. If cyst or bleb ruptures, a tension pneumothorax can result on the operated side or on the opposite side, if bilateral disease is present.
Maintenance	Patients with severe COPD may have significant auto-PEEP. To avoid dynamic hyperinflation of lung, treat bronchospasm aggressively, allow adequate expiratory time (↓ I:E ratio), limit PIP to 15-20 cmH_2O, and minimize the use of applied PEEP. IPPV with small TVs until chest is opened. Inhalational anesthesia supplemented with epidural, local anesthetics, or iv opioids. Avoid N_2O at all times, since bullae may be filled with air.

Emergence	Reexpand lung under direct vision to check for major air leaks. Extubate patient early. Post-bullectomy, unlike other thoracotomy, patients have greater functional lung tissue than preop.	
Blood and fluid requirements	IV: 16 ga × 1 NS/LR @ 1-2 ml/kg/h Use vasopressor (ephedrine 5-10 mg iv bolus or phenylephrine 50-100 μmg iv bolus) if hypotensive.	An overhydrated patient is at ↑risk of right heart failure. Use of epidural local anesthetics can ↓BP in a volume-restricted patient; vasopressor often needed.
Monitoring	Standard monitors (p. B-1) Precordial stethoscope (nonoperated side) Arterial line ± CVP and/or PA line	Optional CVP and/or PA line for patients with coexisting cardiac disease
Positioning	✓ and pad pressure points. ✓ eyes, ears, genitals. Axillary roll; 'airplane' for upper arm	See Positioning, p. 213.
Ventilation	DLT or BB needed to separate the lungs.	Allows IPPV of the 'good' lung. Use gentle IPPV with smaller, more frequent TVs than during routine thoracotomy. Inspiratory pressure should not exceed 10 cmH$_2$O, to reduce likelihood of rupture of bullae in opposite lung. Treat intraop hypoxemia with CPAP to 'up' lung. In extreme cases consider CPB (rare).
Complications	Tension pneumothorax	Can occur on either side during induction, only on non-operated side after chest is open, and again on either side postop. Presents with ↑ventilatory pressure, progressive tracheal deviation, wheezing, cardiovascular collapse. CXR to r/o tension pneumothorax. Rx: insertion of chest tube.
	Broncho-pleural-cutaneous fistula	Placement of a chest tube can create a broncho-pleural-cutaneous fistula. Rx: low TV; may require DLT.
	Hypoxia Hypercardia Dysrhythmias	✓ position of DLT, suction DLT, avoid hypoventilation.

POSTOPERATIVE

Complications	Hypoventilation Dental damage Airway trauma Pneumothorax Hemorrhage Risk of aspiration Airway obstruction (bronchospasm, bleeding, dislodged tumor, FB)	Incomplete reversal of muscle relaxants or opioid overdosage can cause hypoventilation. Obtain ABG if patient has difficulty breathing or is overly sedated. Be prepared to reintubate patient. If nerve blocks used to depress gag reflex, no eating or drinking for several h postbronchoscopy.
Pain management	Epidural opioids (see p. C-2). Parenteral opioids	Parenteral opioids or intrapleural local anesthetics (0.5% bupivacaine + 1:200,000 epinephrine, 0.5 ml/kg) are adequate if procedure performed through a thoracoscope.
Tests	CXR	ABG if indicated.

References

1. Barker SJ, Clarke C, Trivedi N, et al: Anesthesia for thorascopic laser ablation of bullous emphysema. *Anesthesiology* 1993; 78(1):44-50.
2. Baue AE, ed: *Glenn's Thoracic and Cardiovascular Surgery*, 6th edition, Volume II. Geha AS, Hammond GL, Laks H, Naunheim KS, assoc eds. Appleton & Lange, Norwalk, CT: 1996.
3. Benumof JL: Sequential one-lung ventilation for bilateral bullectomy. *Anesthesiology* 1987; 67(2):268-72.
4. Connolly JE, Wilson A: The current status of surgery for bullous emphysema. *J Thorac Cardiovasc Surg* 1989; 97(3):351-61.

5. Liu HP, Yim AP, Izzat MB, et al: Thoracoscopic surgery for spontaneous pneumothorax. *World J Surg* 1999; 23(111):1133-6.
6. Mulcaida T, Ardou A, Date H, et al: Thoracoscopic operation for secondary pneumothorax under local and epidural anesthesia in high risk patients. *Ann Thorac Surg* 1998; 65(4):924-6.
7. Normandale JP, Feneck RO: Bullous cystic lung disease. Its anesthetic management using high frequency jet ventilation. *Anaesthesia* 1985; 40(12):1182-5.
8. Ohta M, Nakahara K, Yasumitsu T, et al: Prediction of postoperative performance status in patients with giant bulla. *Chest* 1992; 101(3):668-73.
9. Sabiston DC Jr, Spencer FC: *Surgery of the Chest*, 6th edition, Vol II. WB Saunders, Philadelphia: 1995.

LUNG-VOLUME REDUCTION SURGERY

SURGICAL CONSIDERATIONS

Description: Lung-volume reduction surgery (LVRS) was reintroduced by Joel Cooper in 1995 for the treatment of severe emphysema. Typically, these patients are chronically ill, requiring steroids, bronchodilators, and supplemental O_2. With appropriate periop care, these patients survive surgery and demonstrate improved pulmonary function. Physiologically, reducing the volume of the lung by resecting diseased tissue improves elastic recoil and decreases airway resistance. The chest cavity also is reduced in size, thereby improving chest-wall and diaphragmatic function.

The procedure can be carried out either through a median sternotomy or endoscopically. The **open approach** begins with a median sternotomy. OLV is initiated following opening of the pleurae. Often the diseased portions of the lung remain inflated, while healthy areas develop absorption atelectasis. These diseased portions are resected with the aid of a linear stapler. The visceral pleura is very thin; the stapling is done with bovine pericardium to bolster the staple line; and high inspiratory pressures (> 20 cmH$_2$O) must be avoided. From 15-30% of the lung volume may be removed. Following careful examination for air leaks, the pleurae and chest wall are closed.

The **endoscopic approach** is carried out via minithoracotomies with instrumentation ports placed to facilitate manipulation of the lung. Diseased tissue will have been identified preop using V/Q and CT scans. Endoscopic forceps are used to guide this diseased tissue into the jaws of the stapler. Again, 15-30% of lung tissue may be removed by this means. At some centers, the anesthesiologist may be asked to measure inspiratory and expiratory volumes. Any difference between these volumes may represent an air leak requiring further exploration. Following this, access ports and the thoracotomy are closed, and chest tubes are placed. The patient is turned over to the opposite side, reprepped and redraped, and the surgery is repeated. Patients should be extubated in the OR so that no unnecessary ventilatory pressures are put on the lungs. There is usually no suction on the chest tubes and, thus, a water seal is the primary method of controlling the pleural cavity pressures. A small pneumothorax (≤ 10%) is acceptable if the patient is not in respiratory distress. A functional epidural catheter, early extubation, and the avoidance of chest tube suction are important to the success of this procedure, especially in the very ill patient. Pleural drainage consists of two chest tubes per side; in contrast with lobectomy, however, they are often left to water seal so as not to exert excessive negative pressure on the lung and disrupt the staple lines. Ideally, patients are extubated at the conclusion of the operation. Since their respiratory status is often tenuous, close monitoring, vigorous pulmonary toilet, and good pain control are essential in the postop period.

Usual preop diagnosis: COPD (emphysema)

SUMMARY OF PROCEDURES

	Open LVRS	Endoscopic LVRS
Position	Supine	Lateral decubitus
Incision	Sternotomy	Minilateral thoracotomy
Special instrumentation	Stapling devices; DLT	⇐ + Endoscopic instrumentation
Unique considerations	Bovine pericardium to bolster staple line	⇐
Antibiotics	Cefazolin 1 g	⇐
Surgical time	2 h	45-60 min/side
Closing considerations	Avoid high PIPs (> 20 cmH$_2$O)	⇐
EBL	Minimal	⇐
Postop care	Extubated in OR; avoid chest tube suction	⇐

	Open LVRS	Endoscopic LVRS
Mortality	≤ 5-10%	⇐
Morbidity	Pneumothorax	⇐
	Infection	⇐
	Tearing of suture line	⇐
	Wound healing problems	⇐
Pain score	6-8	4-6

PATIENT POPULATION CHARACTERISTICS

Age range	> 50 yr
Male:Female	Male > female
Incidence	Although the incidence of emphysema is high in the general population, only a fraction of these patients will be candidates for LVRS.
Etiology	Smoking; genetic factors
Associated conditions	CAD; pulmonary HTN; PVD; cerebrovascular disease

Table 5.3. Suggested Selection Criteria for LVRS	
Medical history	Severe COPD (emphysema rather than chronic bronchitis) Age < 75 yr No cigarette smoking for 6 mo Lowest effective prednisone dose No previous chest surgery
Pulmonary function	FEV_1 > 30-35% of predicted $PaCO_2$ < 50 mmHg TLC > 120% of predicted
Cardiac function	Mean PAP < 35 mmHg (if pulmonary HTN is suspected). No evidence of LV dysfunction on dobutamine stress testing (if Hx of angina or CHF is present)
Radiographic	Hyperinflation, flattened diaphragm (CXR) Decreased upper lobe perfusion (Ventilation-Perfusion scan) Emphysema, with upper lobe predominance (CT scan)
Relative exclusion criteria	Continued smoking Illness other than emphysema that may cause severe dyspnea (e.g., CAD; CHF, cancer; interstitial lung disease; bronchiectasis) Severe malnutrition Obliteration of pleural space (e.g., pleurodesis or pleurectomy) Previous thoracic surgery Morbid obesity Severe pulmonary HTN (mean PAP > 35) Chest-wall deformity with restrictive lung disease (e.g., kyphoscoliosis; severe pectus deformity; $PaCO_2$ > 55 mmHg)

ANESTHETIC CONSIDERATIONS

PREOPERATIVE

LVRS (also known as '**reduction pneumoplasty**') involves either laser thermal contraction or surgical resection of emphysematous lung tissue. Patients have advanced, severe COPD, often associated with other cardiorespiratory problems. These patients are a great challenge to the anesthesiologist, since it may be difficult to maintain relatively normal physiologic parameters intraop, and to have a comfortable, spontaneously breathing patient at the completion of surgery.

Respiratory	Patients for this procedure by definition have advanced pulmonary emphysema. Examine patient for cyanosis, clubbing, RR, and pattern. Listen to chest—breath sounds are often very distant or absent. Hx should include use of O_2 supplementation, recent infection, severe bronchospasm, prior surgery on the chest, and other associated diseases, such as CAD or CHF.

Respiratory, cont.	**Tests:** PFT (± bronchodilators). Hyperinflation usually is indicated by TLC and RV value > 120%; V/Q scan; CXR; chest CT scan; noninvasive exercise test (6-min walk); preop ABG—check for hypoxemia, hypercarbia.
Cardiovascular	These patients often have coexisting cardiac disease with pulmonary HTN. **Tests:** Right heart function can be evaluated by dobutamine stress test or selective right heart catheterization and measurement of PA pressures, as indicated from H&P.
Premedication	Avoid premedication with sedative or opioids—cannot have respiratory depressants—patients have severe COPD, often CO_2 retainers.

INTRAOPERATIVE

Anesthetic technique: GETA (with DLT or BB) ± thoracic/lumbar epidural anesthesia. Place and test lumbar or thoracic epidural catheter before surgery. (See Lobectomy, Pneumonectomy, pp. 213-214.)

Induction	Standard induction (see p. B-2). DLT or BB absolutely necessary during surgery to selectively ventilate each lung (See Lobectomy, Pneumonectomy, p. 213).
Maintenance	Inhalational agent and/or propofol. IV opioids and sedative agents should not be used. Anesthesia may be supplemented by continuous or bolus administration of epidural anesthetics. Mechanical ventilation with O_2 and inhalation agent only. During 2-lung ventilation, VT = 8-12 ml/kg, adjusted to limit PIP to < 25 cmH$_2$O. Respiratory rate and inspiratory flow should be adjusted to minimize air trapping. Beware of overinflation and 'breath stacking,' which can → pulmonary tamponade with severe ↓BP and ↑airways resistance. Use ABG to maintain PaCO$_2$ at preop level. During OLV, VT is decreased by 25%; monitor PIP closely since ventilated lung has bullous disease also. Avoid overdistention with hyperinflation (→ pneumothorax) on ventilated, nonoperated lung. Patients with severe COPD may have significant auto-PEEP. To avoid dynamic hyperinflation of lung, treat bronchospasm aggressively, allow adequate expiratory time (↓ I:E ratio), limit PIP to 15-20 cmH$_2$O, and minimize the use of applied PEEP. During OLV, moderate hypercapnia is tolerated, so long as there is no significant hemodynamic effect or hypoxemia. CPAP to nonventilated lung may be necessary to maintain oxygenation. Maintenance of hemodynamic stability may require pressor support (e.g., ephedrine, phenylephrine, dopamine). Lung hyperinflation during mechanical ventilation should be suspected if ↓BP with ↑PIP occurs.
Emergence	These patients should be extubated while deeply anesthetized to prevent coughing and straining, which can exacerbate any air leak. These patients benefit from good analgesia, head elevation, and suctioning to ↓ mucous plugging (can be catastrophic). Recovery from GA occurs in the OR and may take 1-2 h. Ventilatory assistance via face mask with supplemental O_2 is usually necessary. ABG and CXR may be necessary. When spontaneous ventilation and analgesia are satisfactory, the patient is transported to ICU. If postop mechanical ventilation is required, consider using pressure support ventilation with low levels of CPAP. The CPAP may help minimize the inspiratory work of breathing caused by lung hyperinflation. The pressure support mode of ventilation will permit control of airway pressure, while allowing patient control of PaCO$_2$. If postop intubation is anticipated, changing from DLT to ETT is required.
Blood and fluid requirements	IV: 14-16 ga × 1 LR @ 1-2 ml/kg/h Autologous PRBC	Fluid management to restore preop deficit and provide maintenance fluid. Replace blood loss with 3 ml of LR per ml blood. Transfuse autologous blood for Hct < 30.
Monitoring	Standard monitors (see p. B-1). Arterial line Urinary catheter CVP and/or PA line	(See Lobectomy, Pneumonectomy, p. 213.) ✓ABGs: baseline (preop) during sternotomy; 15 min after initiation of OLV; 15 min after initiation of OLV on the second lung; during closure of sternotomy; prior to extubation. Useful for postop fluid management.
Positioning	✓ and pad pressure points. ✓ eyes, ears, genitals.	Axillary roll and support for upper airway is necessary for the lateral decubitus position. (See Lobectomy, Pneumonectomy, p. 213.)

POSTOPERATIVE

Complications	Hypercarbia Hypoxemia

Complications, cont.	Air leak/pneumothorax Hemorrhage	
Pain management	Lumbar or thoracic epidural opioids ± local anesthetics (see p. C-2).	Essential that patient be comfortable. Begin infusion of epidural opioids and local anesthetics (see Lobectomy, Pneumonectomy, p. 214). Breakthrough pain treatment options include iv morphine (1-2 mg) and/or ketorolac (30 mg).

References

1. Brantigarn OC, Mueller E, Kress MB: A surgical approach to pulmonary emphysema. *Am Rev Respir Dis* 1959; 80:194-202.
2. Brodsky JB, ed: Thoracic anesthesia. In *Problems in Anesthesia*. JB Lippincott, Philadelphia: 1990.
3. Buettner AU, McRae R, Myles PS, et al: Anaesthesia and postoperative pain management for bilateral lung volume reduction surgery. *Anaesth Inten Care* 1999; 27(5):503-8.
4. Cooper JD, Trulock EP, Triantafillou AN, et al. Bilateral pneumonectomy (volume reduction). *J Thorac Cardiovasc Surg* 1995; 109:106-19.
5. Gedddes D, Davies M, Koyama H, et al: Effect of lung-volume-reduction surgery in patients with severe emphysema. *N Engl J Med* 2000; 343(4):239-45.
6. Miller JI, Lee RB, Mansour KA: Lung volume reduction surgery: lessons learned. *Ann Thorac Surg* 1996; 61:1464-9.
7. National Emphysema Treatment Trial Research Group: Patients at high risk of death after lung-volume-reduction surgery. *N Engl J Med* 2001;345(15):1075-83.
8. Pearson FG, et al: *Thoracic Surgery*. Churchill Livingstone, New York, 1995.
9. Tschernko EM: Anesthesia considerations for lung volume reduction surgery. *Anesthesiol Clin North Am* 2001; 19(3):591-609.
10. Wakabayashi A: Thoracoscopic laser pneumonectomy in the treatment of diffuse bullous emphysema. *Ann Thorac Surg* 1995; 60(4):936-42.

BRONCHOPULMONARY LAVAGE

SURGICAL CONSIDERATIONS

Description: It is our practice to perform **unilateral lavage** only, although single-session, bilateral lavage has been reported. After induction of GA, a DLT is placed, and the correct position is confirmed bronchoscopically. The lung is then lavaged in aliquots of 500-1000 ml NS or 0.5-1.0 L NS to dilute and wash out excess alveolar surfactant, pus, or mucus, and to obtain material for cytological and histochemical examination. Care should be taken not to overdistend the lung, and a running tally of fluid instilled and withdrawn should be performed to avoid overhydrating the patient. Frequently, 9-12 L of fluid are used, with the initial effluent being very cloudy and the final effluent being clear. Techniques that may improve the distribution of the lavage fluid include external chest percussion and tilting the operating table (laterally as well as in the craniocaudal directions).

Usual preop diagnosis: Pulmonary alveolar proteinosis; refractory asthma; cystic fibrosis; bronchiectasis; lipoid pneumonitis; silicosis; alveolar microlithiasis; inhalation of radioactive dust

SUMMARY OF PROCEDURE

Position	Supine or lateral decubitus
Special instrumentation	Bronchoscope; DLT; lavage fluids
Antibiotics	None
Surgical time	45 min/side
EBL	None
Postop care	PACU → home
Mortality	Rare
Morbidity	Aspiration of lavage fluid Pneumothorax/hydrothorax Atelectasis
Pain score	1-2

PATIENT POPULATION CHARACTERISTICS

Age range	17-35 yr
Male:Female	1:1
Incidence	Uncommon
Etiology	Pulmonary alveolar proteinosis; cystic fibrosis; bronchiectasis; lipoid pneumonitis; silicosis
Associated conditions	Asthma and other abnormalities of lung function

---

ANESTHETIC CONSIDERATIONS

PREOPERATIVE

Although whole-lung lavage is primarily a treatment for pulmonary alveolar proteinosis, it is also used as a therapeutic modality for many other lung-related conditions (see Usual preop diagnosis, above). Respiratory dysfunction of variable symptomatology is expected in these patients. Indications for whole-lung lavage include dyspnea on exertion, resting room air PaO_2 < 60 mmHg, or shunt fraction > 10-12%. Since the procedure requires GA with OLV, it is recommended that preop V/Q scans be obtained so that unilateral lung irrigation can be performed first on the more severely affected lung. If both lungs are equally diseased, lavage should be performed on the left lung initially to allow the larger right lung to be used for ventilation to provide better gas exchange. Patients then return in subsequent days or weeks for therapeutic lavage of the contralateral lung. A nonoperative treatment option for pulmonary alveolar proteinosis using granulocyte-macrophage colony-stimulating factor (GM-CSF), has shown promise for some patients with the acquired form of pulmonary alveolar proteinosis.

Respiratory	Patients with pulmonary alveolar proteinosis generally present with cough (nonproductive > productive), dyspnea, and fatigue. Physical findings consist of diffuse rales ± clubbing or cyanosis. CXR typically reveals diffuse bilateral patchy airspace consolidation. Pulmonary compliance is reduced 2° the restrictive disease pattern. PFTs show ↓TLC, ↓RV, ↓VC, and ↓DL_{CO}. Though nonspecific, baseline ABGs classically demonstrate respiratory alkalosis and hypoxemia, with a calculated elevation in A-a DO_2 gradient. Some patients may be O_2-dependent or have concomitant COPD 2° Hx of smoking. Secondary infections, especially in the respiratory tract, are well recognized risks in these patients. Cessation of smoking (> 6-8 wk) and prompt treatment of any underlying infections before whole-lung lavage may be prudent. **Tests:** CXR; PFT; ABG; V/Q scans; ± CT
Cardiovascular	Directed at any underlying disease process.
Laboratory	Abnormal elevation of serum LDH has been reported in some patients and has been shown to correlate with the severity of A-a DO_2. **Tests:** LDH; other tests as indicated from H&P.
Premedication	Standard premedication (see p. B-2). Avoid heavy sedation that might impair adequate gas exchange before induction. O_2 supplementation may be required after premedication.

INTRAOPERATIVE

Anesthetic technique: GETA is required with OLV (see pp. 213-214) using a DLT. In pediatric patients or small adults where appropriate sized DLT is not available, and in patients who cannot tolerate OLV, the use of partial venoarterial CPB, venovenous bypass, or even ECMO has been reported. In some cases, sequential lobar lavage with smaller volume of lavage fluid has been achieved under conscious sedation for those patients in whom OLV is not possible.

Induction	Standard induction (see p. B-2). Adequate preoxygenation and denitrogenation for 3-5 min before induction. The largest DLT should be used to facilitate infusion and drainage of the lavage fluid. (Placement of DLT is discussed on p. 214.) Due to the underlying impaired respiratory function in these patients, instituting OLV will further compromise gas exchange. It is imperative to avoid spillage of lavage fluid into the ventilated lung during the procedure. This is achieved by verifying the correct position of the DLT with FOB and confirming the competency of the cuff seal by testing it against pressures as high as 50 cmH_2O. Baseline individual lung compliance, airway pressures, and ABG should be ✓'d after DLT placement.
Maintenance	100% FiO_2 with inhalational agent (e.g., sevoflurane) or TIVA using propofol and remifentanil infusions. Muscle relaxation is necessary to avoid movement or coughing that can cause leakage of

Maintenance, cont.	lavage fluid into the ventilated lung. Since chest physiotherapy, including vibration and percussion, is required after each cycle of lavage filling, any deleterious change from baseline lung compliance decrease or airway pressure increase of the ventilated lung should prompt the anesthesiologist to look for evidence of spillage. Filling the nonventilated lung with lavage fluid can → ↓pulmonary shunting (→ improved O_2 sat) and ↑PVR (→ ↓CO). Draining the lavage fluid can → ↑pulmonary shunting (→ ↓O_2 sat) and ↓PVR (→ ↑CO). Accurate inflow and outflow volume of the lavage fluid should be recorded.	
Emergence	At the conclusion of surgery, the lavaged lung should be adequately suctioned to remove any residual fluid. Bilateral lung ventilation should be reinstituted. Since the compliance of the lavaged lung is greatly reduced, higher airway pressures are required to reexpand it, but at the risk of causing barotrauma to the nonlavaged lung. A brief period of OLV to the lavaged lung, using large TVs or ↑airway pressure, may be necessary to recruit the collapsed alveoli (higher pressure, including PEEP, is needed to counter the increase in surface tension after the removal of significant amounts of surfactant). The patient's trachea should be extubated after adequate reversal of muscle relaxation; however, if prolonged postop ventilation is anticipated (e.g., in those who aspirated lavaged fluid to the ventilated lung), changing the DLT to an ETT is indicated. DLT should be retained for patients in whom differential lung ventilation is required postop.	
Blood and fluid requirements	IV: 18 ga × 1 NS/LR @ 1-2 ml/kg/h	
Monitoring	Standard monitors (p. B-1) Arterial line	Although warm, heparinized saline is used, some patients may still become hypothermic after several h of lavage under GETA.
	± CVP line ± PA line	CVP or PA line only needed as indicated by comorbid conditions. PA line positioned to the lavaged lung. A PA catheter offers the additional advantage of improving pulmonary shunting during OLV by way of balloon inflation.
Positioning	Supine ✓ and pad pressure points. ✓ eyes.	Some prefer the lavaged lung to be dependent so that the risk of leakage to the nondependent lung is reduced. Others prefer the lavaged lung to be nondependent since, in this position, perfusion will more closely match ventilation in the dependent lung. As a compromise, we perform lavage with the patient supine.
Complications	Hypoxemia	Hypoxemia during OLV is most commonly 2° luminal obstruction (by blood or pulmonary secretions) of the DLT, worsening of shunting, or malposition of DLT. Rx: suctioning of the DLT; PEEP to ventilated lung (may ↑ shunting); return to two-lung ventilation; and ✓ DLT position. In extreme cases, temporarily inflating the balloon of the PA catheter (if available) may be necessary to improve shunting and, thus, oxygenation.
	Hypercarbia Aspiration	Ensure adequate TV and RR. ✓ DLT position. Turn patient to lavaged side down and head down, suction the ventilated lung, reinstitute bilateral lung ventilation with PEEP, after the lavaged lung is thoroughly drained and suctioned. Termination of procedure may be needed in severe cases. Patient may need to be kept intubated after the procedure.

POSTOPERATIVE

Complications	Pneumothorax Hydrothorax	Obtain CXR; conservative measures if small pneumothorax or hydrothorax. Otherwise, chest tube placement will be required.
	Atelectasis	Decrease in surfactant after lavage will → airspace collapse. Most patients will experience moderate coughing, which will help reexpand the atelectatic lung units.

Pain management	Parental opioids or NSAID (ketorolac 30 mg iv)	Some patients may experience chest pain due to vigorous intraop percussion.

References:

1. Bussieres JS: Whole lung lavage. *Anesthesiol Clin North America* 2001; 19(3):543-58.
2. Cohen E, Eisenkraft JB: Bronchopulmonary lavage: effects on oxygenation and hemodynamics. *J Cardiothorac Anesth* 1990; 4(5):609-15.
3. Rogers RM, Levin DC, Gray BA, et al: Physiologic effects of bronchopulmonary lavage in alveolar proteinosis. *Am Rev Respir Dis* 1978; 118(2):255-64.
4. Seymour JF, Presneill JJ: Pulmonary alveolar proteinosis: progress in the first 44 years. *Am J Respir Crit Care Med* 2002; 166(2):215-35.
5. Whitsett JA, Weaver TE: Hydrophobic surfactant proteins in lung function and disease. *N Eng J Med* 2002; 347(26)2141-8.

LUNG TRANSPLANT

SURGICAL CONSIDERATIONS

Description: The most common indications for lung transplantation include emphysema, pulmonary fibrosis, cystic fibrosis, and pulmonary HTN. Patients with the first three of these diagnoses have marked abnormalities in mechanical pulmonary function, while patients with pulmonary HTN often have normal lung mechanics but very abnormal cardiac function. Patients with emphysema and pulmonary fibrosis often receive single-lung transplants, and those with cystic fibrosis require double-lung transplants. The best operation for patients with pulmonary HTN continues to be debated, with options including single-lung, double-lung, and heart-lung transplantation (see p. 365). Although candidates for lung transplantation, by definition, have end-stage lung disease, their overall state of health and functional abilities varies considerably. Furthermore, while these patients all have poor pulmonary function, many with multisystem disease are eliminated during the preop screening process. Thus, the remaining patients are generally well motivated and free of significant cardiac, renal, and vascular disease.

Single-lung transplants generally are carried out through a thoracotomy incision. Patients with emphysema as the underlying disease rarely require CPB, while those with pulmonary fibrosis (↓pulmonary reserve and ↑incidence of pulmonary HTN) more commonly require bypass. Although the need for bypass can be assessed at the outset of the operation by instituting OLV, a CPB circuit and perfusionist should always be available. The route for vascular access for bypass (transthoracic or through the groin vessels) must be considered by the surgeon at the start of the case.

Double-lung transplants generally are done through bilateral anterior thoracotomies or a single bilateral 'clamshell' incision (Fig 5-2). Mobilization of the lung is facilitated by use of a DLT. If the patient does not tolerate OLV, CPB can be established using aortic and atrial cannulation. Some surgeons routinely use a single-lumen ETT, with a defined plan for using CPB.

The procedure for both single- and double-lung transplantation is the same for each side. The native lung is mobilized, and the bronchovascular structures are divided. Mediastinal adenopathy and extensive pleural adhesions are the rule, rather than the exception, for patients with cystic fibrosis. Such pneumonectomies take significantly longer than those for emphysema. Once the native lung is removed, the donor lung is brought into the surgical field. The bronchial anastomosis is created first, and the lung is allowed to fall into the posterior costovertebral gutter. The venous anastomosis (atrial cuff anastomosis) is fashioned next. The final sutures are placed but left untied for later deairing. The arterial anastomosis is created last. Upon removal of the arterial clamp, the lung is perfused and deaired. The venous sutures are then tied and the atrial clamp is removed. After ensuring that the vascular anastomoses are hemostatic and that there is no air leak at the bronchial site, the incision is closed or, in the case of double-lung transplant, attention is directed to the other side.

The anesthesiologist should be aware that ↓BP is not uncommon on reperfusion of the donor lung, but that it usually resolves spontaneously. Specific immunosuppression protocols vary from institution to institution, but iv administration of steroids immediately before lung reperfusion is a common practice. Lung transplant patients typically are left intubated following surgery; however, changing from a DLT to a single-lumen tube at the conclusion of the operation facilitates postop ET suctioning.

Usual preop diagnosis: COPD; pulmonary fibrosis; cystic fibrosis; pulmonary HTN; Eisenmenger's syndrome.

For Summary of Procedure and Anesthetic Management, see Surgery for Lung and Heart/Lung Transplantation, p. 367, and Anesthetic Considerations for Lung Transplantation, p. 370.

6.0 CARDIOVASCULAR SURGERY

Surgeons

R. Scott Mitchell, MD
Norman E. Shumway, MD, PhD

6.1   CARDIAC SURGERY

Anesthesiologists

J. Kent Garman, MD, MS, FACC
Lawrence C. Siegel, MD

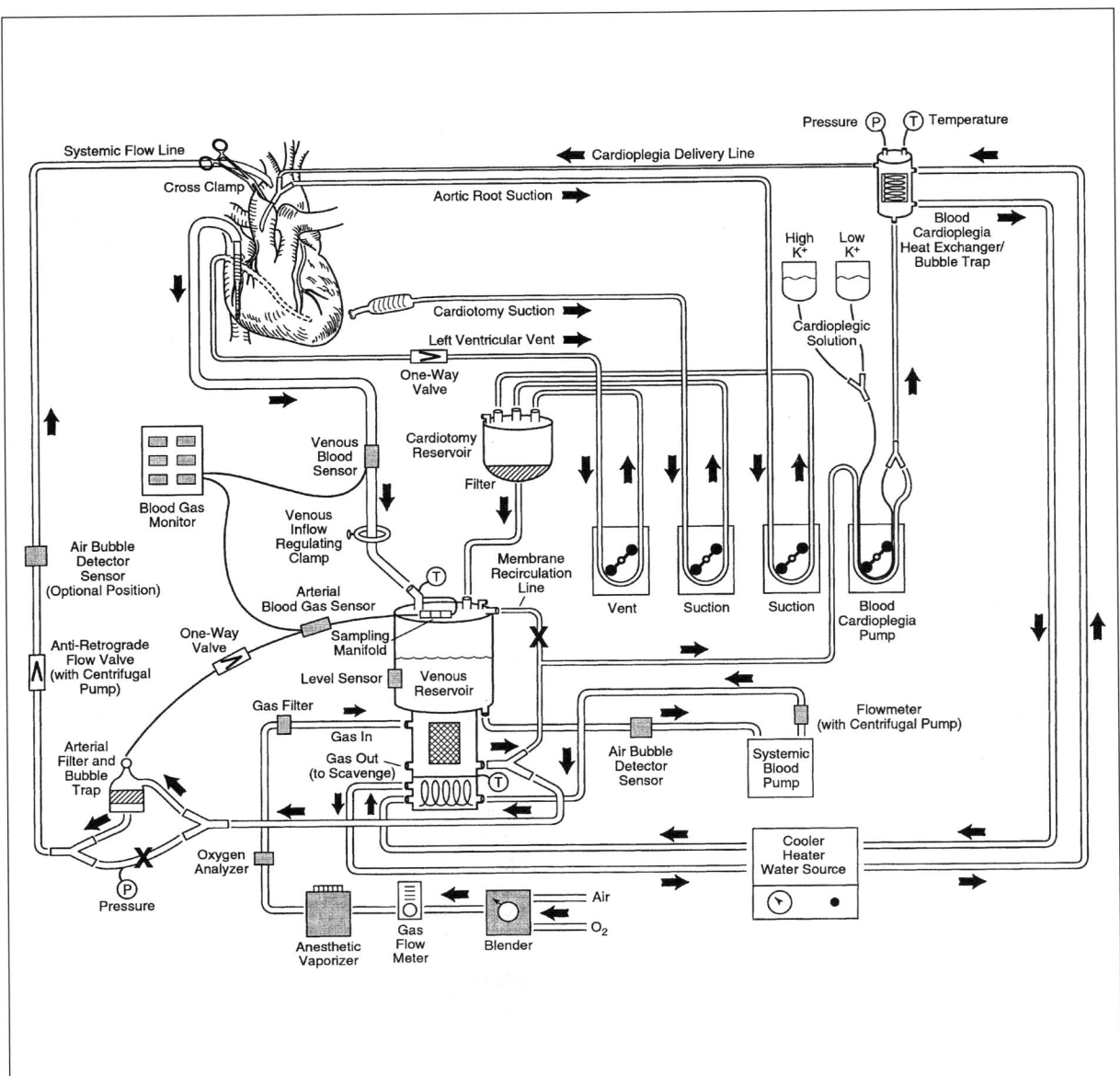

Figure 6.1-1. Detailed schematic of a typical CPB circuit with a membrane oxygenator that includes a heat exchanger sitting beneath an integral hard-shell venous reservoir (lower center) and an external cardiotomy reservoir. Venous cannulation is accomplished with a cavoatrial cannula, and arterial cannulation is in the ascending aorta. Systemic venous blood flows by gravity into the venous reservoir (on top of the membrane oxygenator in this figure). Cardiotomy suction and vent lines pass through roller pumps and then into the cardiotomy reservoir, from which the blood drains into the venous reservoir (sometimes the cardiotomy reservoir is physically incorporated into the venous reservoir). Venous blood is pumped out of this reservoir by the systemic blood pump (centrifugal or roller), through the systemic heat exchanger and membrane oxygenator (combined), and then back to the patient (usually through an arterial filter and bubble trap). Other components shown include the cardioplegia delivery system (on the right), which in this case is a one-pass system that mixes blood (from out of the membrane oxygenator) with cardioplegia solution before passing it through a heat exchanger and bubble trap; a cooler-heater water source that supplies water to the systemic and cardioplegia heat exchangers; and the gas source with air/O_2 blender and anesthetic vaporizer for the membrane oxygenator.

The air bubble detector may be placed on the line between the venous reservoir and systemic pump, between the pump and membrane oxygenator inlet, between the oxygenator outlet and arterial filter (not shown), or on the line after the arterial filter (optional position on drawing). One-way valves prevent retrograde flow. (Some circuits with a centrifugal pump also incorporate a one-way valve after the pump and within the systemic flow line.) Other safety devices include (1) an oxygen analyzer placed between the anesthetic vaporizer (if used) and the oxygenator gas inlet, and (2) a reservoir level sensor attached to the housing of the hard-shell venous reservoir (on the left). Arrows indicate direction of flow. Bold **X**s depict placement of tubing clamps. P and T denote pressure and temperature sensors, respectively. Hemoconcentrator is not shown. (Reproduced with permission from Gravlee GP, Davis RF, Kurusz M, eds: *Cardiopulmonary Bypass: Principles and Practice*, 2nd edition. Lippincott Williams & Wilkins, 2000.)

CARDIOPULMONARY BYPASS

SURGICAL CONSIDERATIONS

The development of cardiopulmonary bypass (CPB) technology has allowed the repair of many congenital and acquired lesions of the heart and great vessels. Designed to replace cardiac and pulmonary functions, full CPB requires a blood pump and oxygenator. The pump may be of the roller-head or centrifugal variety, with the latter producing less trauma to formed blood elements. The oxygenator may bubble gases (O_2 and CO_2) through a blood-filled reservoir (bubble oxygenator), or allow O_2 and CO_2 to diffuse through a thin membrane into the surrounding blood (membrane oxygenator). Utilization of any blood pump requires at least partial heparinization (ACT >180 sec), and introduction of an oxygenator mandates full heparinization (ACT > 400 sec).

Full CPB typically drains systemic venous return via the right atrium into a venous reservoir, from which the blood is pumped through an oxygenator and then returned to the aorta or femoral artery, completely bypassing the heart and lungs (Figs 6.1-1 and 6.1-2). **Partial CPB** usually supports only a portion of the body—typically the infradiaphragmatic portion—and may use the patient's lungs as an oxygenator (left atrium → femoral artery) or a mechanical oxygenator (femoral vein → femoral artery). Full CPB is utilized during a sternotomy for work on the heart, ascending aorta, and transverse arch. Partial CPB, in which some systemic venous blood returns to the heart and is ejected into the aorta, is normally used for work on the descending or thoracoabdominal aorta. Heparin-coated components, which partially eliminate the necessity for heparin, are available.

After exposure of the relevant organs (heart or descending thoracic aorta), and after heparinization, venous and arterial cannulae must be placed intraluminally. **Cannulation of the heart** usually involves venous drainage from the right atrium, with either two cannulae inserted through the atrium into the SVC and IVC (bicaval), or via a larger, dual-stage cannula draining the right atria and IVC. Bicaval cannulation reduces venous return (and rewarming) to the heart, and allows caval snares to be placed so that the right atrium can be opened without introducing air into the venous return. Occasionally, atrial manipulation for cannulation can depress CO, with resultant hypotension. This usually can be reversed with volume replacement. Aortic cannulation usually is not associated with any physiologic perturbation, although HTN must be avoided to minimize aortic complications. Once the cannulae are in place and connections are made to the bypass circuit, CPB may be instituted electively. Most cardiac operations are conducted under mild hypothermia (28°C), unless profound hypothermic circulatory arrest is to be utilized. In that case, a target temperature of 16-18°C is desirable. For operations on the descending thoracic aorta, normothermia is maintained.

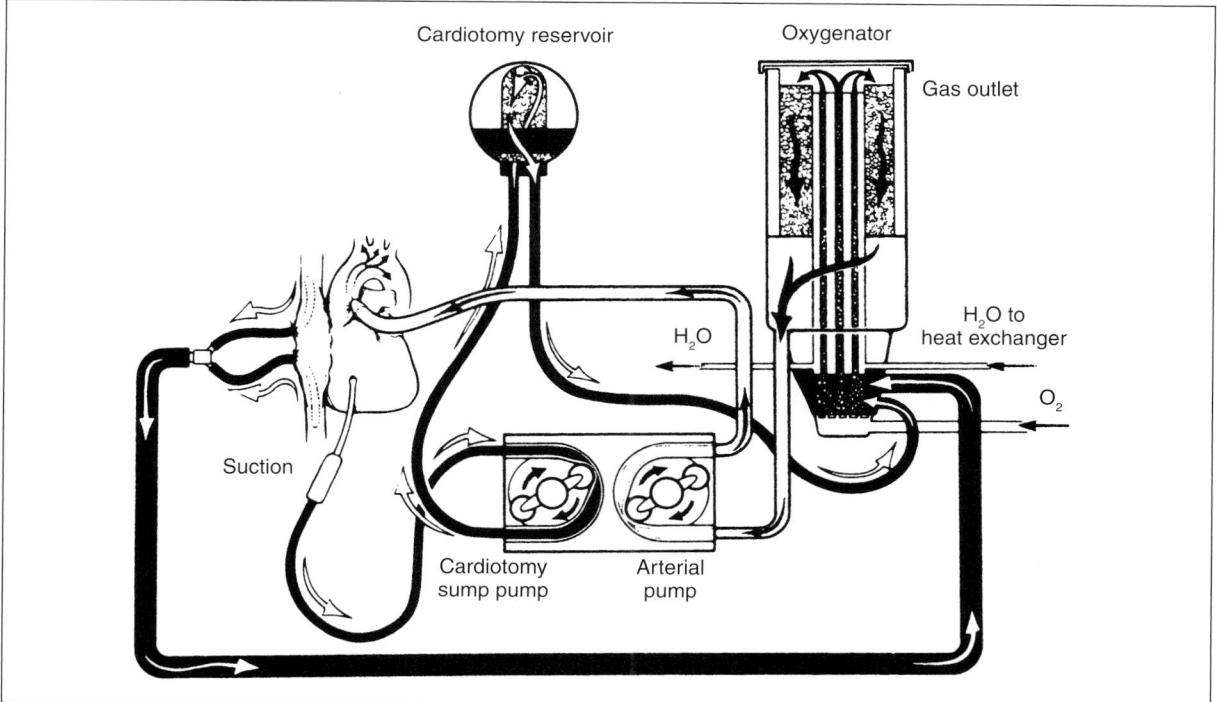

Figure 6.1-2. Schematic representation of the CPB circuit. (Reproduced with permission from Hardy JD: *Hardy's Textbook of Surgery*, 2nd edition. JB Lippincott: 1988.)

Cessation of CPB is accomplished by gradually decreasing pump flows, allowing for right heart filling, and gradually replenishing the circulating blood volume. Pulmonary and coronary vasodilation are mandatory during this phase, as there appears to be heightened vasoreactivity after periods of ischemia and hypothermia. For periods of cardiac arrest, during which the heart is deprived of its arterial blood supply, the metabolic demands of the myocardium must be minimized. This usually is accomplished by achieving diastolic arrest with a hyperkalemic cardioplegic solution, and also by lowering myocardial temperature to $< 15°C$. Frequent reinfusions of cardioplegia maintain hypothermia, prevent lactic acid accumulation, and deliver some minimally available dissolved O_2.

The **physiologic response to CPB** is complex, and is associated with a massive catecholamine release which resolves after its cessation. Subsequent changes include abnormal bleeding tendencies, increased capillary permeability, leukocytosis, renal dysfunction, and impairment of the immune response. Hemodilution, nonpulsatile flow, hypothermia, exposure of formed elements to nonendothelial surfaces, complement activation, protein denaturation, cascading effects within the coagulation and fibrinolytic system, and activation of the kallikrein-bradykinin cascade, all contribute to this unphysiologic state, and account for much of the morbidity and mortality after CPB.

Many physiologic variables are now controlled by the anesthesiologist, perfusionist, and surgeon, including systemic flow and perfusion pressure, arterial O_2 and CO_2, temperature, and Hct. Other physiologic parameters follow either directly or indirectly. Thus, physiologic monitoring for the anesthesiologist and perfusionist include, at a minimum, arterial pressure, CVP, ABG determination (preferably on-line during CPB), CO, UO, and ECG. Constant communication among surgeons, perfusionist, and anesthesiologist is mandatory for a smooth operation. Transesophageal echocardiography (TEE) is rapidly becoming standard practice for cardiac surgery.

Secondary effects of CPB demand some special considerations during the final stages of the procedure and chest closure. Adverse effects on coagulation have already been mentioned, and vigorous attention to maintenance and replacement of coagulation factors is essential. The capillary leak phenomenon results in interstitial myocardial and pulmonary edema. Decreased myocardial performance and compliance mandate an increased preload, especially during the physical act of chest closure, where a transient rise in intramediastinal pressure may depress systemic venous return. Similarly, decreased pulmonary compliance and gas exchange mandate vigilance over inspiratory pressures and lung volumes during chest closure, as mediastinal volume is physically decreased.

ANESTHETIC CONSIDERATIONS FOR CARDIOPULMONARY BYPASS (CPB)

This segment is not meant to be a definitive text on CPB, but rather a guide to the anesthetic management of bypass. Communication among surgeons, anesthesiologists, and pump technicians is of vital importance in carrying out this procedure.

PREPARATION FOR BYPASS

Prebypass/ anticoagulation   ✓ baseline ACT (normal = 90-130 sec). Heparin (3 mg[~300 U]/kg) is administered via a central vein (✓ back-bleeding to verify intravascular position) or by the surgeon directly into the atrium (preferred). ✓ ACT 3 min after heparin. It is essential to ensure adequate anticoagulation (ACT > 400 sec).

Aortic cannulation   Control MAP to ~70 mmHg for cannulation to ensure that the aortotomy does not extend. If needed, vasodilators may be used. The arterial line should be inspected for air bubbles.

Venous cannulation   Venous cannulation may be associated with atrial dysrhythmias. Blood loss can be excessive. Be prepared to infuse volume boluses, if necessary.

Pupils   Assess pupil symmetry for later comparison.

TRANSITION ONTO CPB

Stop ventilation   Commencing bypass is a dangerous period for the patient as a result of the many hemodynamic changes that occur. D/C ventilation once there is no pulmonary blood flow.

Withdraw PA catheter   Withdraw PA catheter 4-5 cm.

Stop infusions   Stop iv drugs and reduce iv fluid infusions to TKO.

Anticoagulation   ACT should be ✓'d after 5 min on CPB to ensure anticoagulation (ACT > 400 sec).

Oxygenation	Verify oxygenation by checking arterial inflow color and inline sensors and by ABG within 5 min of beginning CPB.
Flow	✓ for adequate venous drainage (CVP falls to a low level). Ensure adequate arterial inflow. Initial pressures may be very low, but usually will increase.
Anesthesia	Anesthetics (e.g., fentanyl and midazolam) may be needed. A repeat dose (e.g., 10 mg pancuronium) should be given to prevent movement or shivering (increases O_2 requirements).
Pupils	Assess pupils. Unilateral dilation may indicate arterial inflow into the innominate artery (unilateral carotid perfusion).

BYPASS PERIOD

Anticoagulation	ACT levels should be checked regularly (q 20-30 min) and kept at > 400. Add heparin (5,000-10,000 U), if needed.
Pressure/flow	There is controversy about safe flows and pressures. Generally, flows of 1.2-3 L/m²/min are used, with pressures of 30-80 mmHg. A MAP of 50-60 mmHg is probably best for cerebral perfusion and does not result in excessive noncoronary blood flow.
Acid-base status	Alpha-stat (ABG measured and interpreted at 37° regardless of actual patient temperature) regulation of acid-base status is preferred because of maintenance of normal cerebral flow and autoregulation on CPB.

Table 6.1-1. Difference Between α-Stat and pH-Stat Management During CPB

α-Stat (Temperature Corrected)	pH Stat (Temperature Uncorrected)
Plasma pH maintained at 7.4 (when measured at 37°C).	Plasma pH maintained at 7.4, regardless of temperature.
Arterial PCO_2 maintained at 40 mmHg (when measured at 37°C).	Arterial PCO_2 maintained at 40 mmHg, regardless of temperature.
Relative respiratory alkalosis during hypothermia	Requires addition of CO_2 to inspired gases.
Cerebral autoregulation preserved—CBF unchanged.	May result in loss of cerebral autoregulation—higher CBF.

Hct/Electrolytes	Generally, Hct will fall to ~20, which may be acceptable (however, Hct ≥ 25 is preferable) in most patients. Hypokalemia is common and should be corrected. A K^+ > 4.5 mEq/L is desirable.
UO	Keep UO >1 ml/kg/h. If needed, mannitol and/or furosemide should be given (assuming pump flow is adequate).
Temperature	During bypass, T is usually maintained at ~28°C.

TERMINATION OF BYPASS

Rewarming	Prior to discontinuing CPB, the patient should have a core temperature of at least 36.5°C.
Anesthesia/ relaxation	Patient awareness may be a problem during rewarming. Volatile agents ± benzodiazepine (e.g., diazepam 5-10 mg) ± a narcotic to prevent awareness. In addition, a muscle relaxant also should be given.
Acid-base/ electrolytes/Hct	✓ electrolytes, acid-base status, and Hct. Correct acidosis. K^+ 4.5-5.5, normal ionized Ca^{++}, and Hct ≥ 20 should be assured.
Air maneuvers	Air maneuvers (to remove intracardiac and intraaortic air) are carried out when the heart is opened. Ventilation is commenced once there is pulmonary blood flow and will aid in the evacuation of air. Pleural fluid should be removed.

WEANING FROM BYPASS

Prior to weaning	Prior to weaning from CPB, the aortic cross-clamp should have been off for 30 min to allow rewarming and reperfusion of the heart. Defibrillation is often needed and pacing may be required.

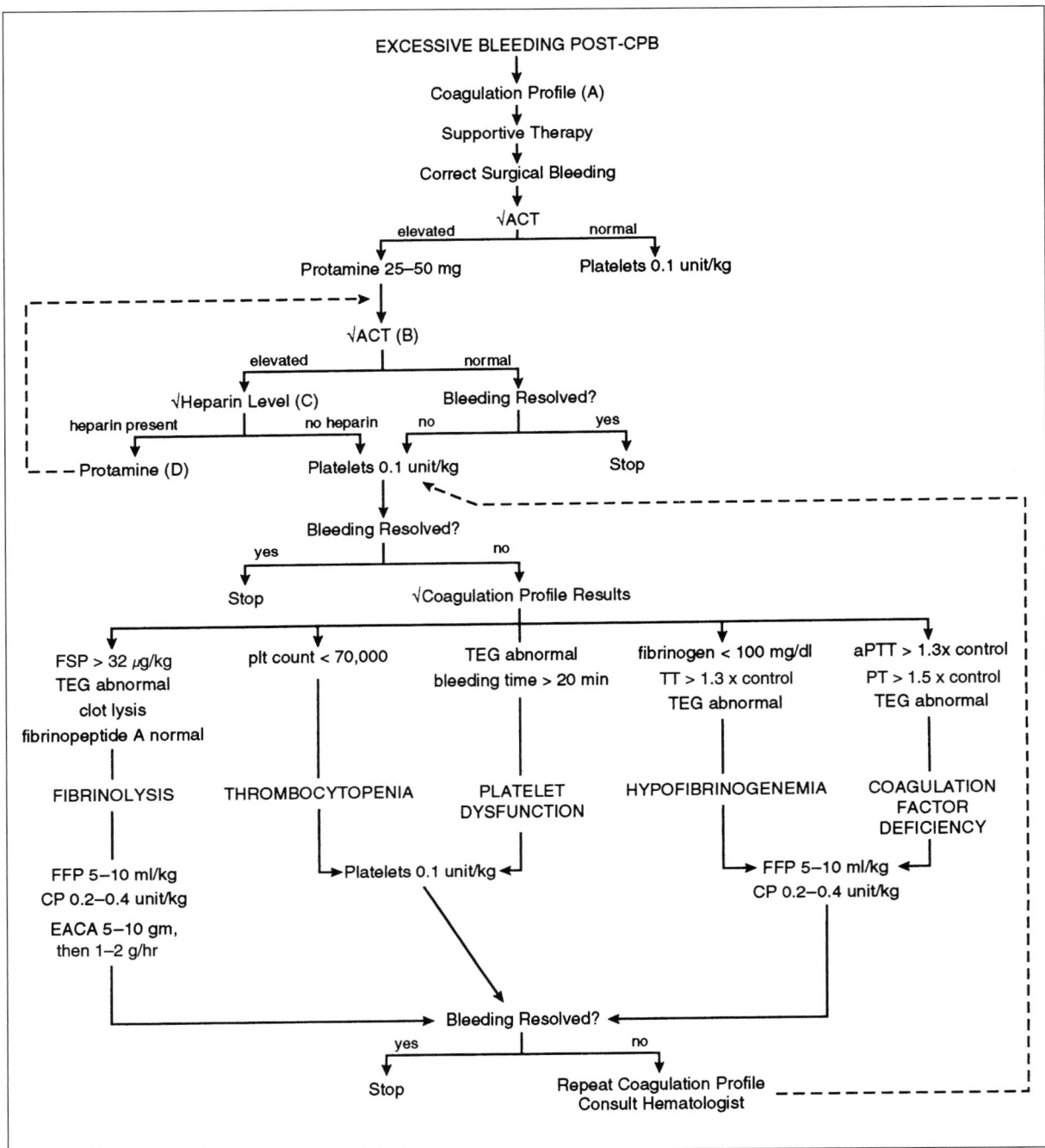

Figure 6.1-3. An algorithm for the treatment of patients bleeding excessively after CPB: (A) Commonly includes Plt count, PT, aPTT, TT, fibrinogen level, FSPs. Template bleeding time or TEG is desirable if available and feasible. (B) Heparin level may be checked at this step. (C) Most commonly by in vitro whole blood protamine titration (manual or automated); alternatively, by protamine-corrected TT. (D) Protamine dose determined by measured heparin level. Disseminated intravascular coagulation (DIC) is a rare cause of post CPB hemorrhage and, therefore, is not included in the outline of coagulation profile results and treatment of post CPB hemostatic abnormalities shown in the lower portion of the figure. It would be suspected on the occurrence of hypofibrinogenemia, thrombocytopenia, and elevated fibrinopeptides, in association with increased FSPs, clot lysis, or a TEG characteristic of fibrinolysis. The treatment of DIC includes identification and arrest of the inciting cause and coagulant replacement with FFP, CP, and platelets. EACA should not be administered to the patient with DIC and secondary fibrinolysis because of the risk of intravascular thrombosis.

ACT = activated coagulation time; aPTT = activated partial thromboplastin time; CP = cryoprecipitate; EACA = epsilon-aminocaproic acid; FFP = fresh frozen plasma; FSP = fibrin(ogen) split products; Plt count = platelet count; PT = prothrombin time; TEG = thromboelastogram; TT = thrombin time. (Reproduced with permission from Hensley FA Jr, Martin DE: *The Practice of Cardiac Anesthesia.* Little, Brown: 1990.)

Prior to weaning, cont.	NSR or AV pacing is preferred. Vasoactive drugs should be available. Once normal T, ventilation, cardiac rhythm, and reperfusion are established, bypass may be terminated. The heart is gradually volume-loaded (transfused from oxygenator) to adequate filling pressures and bypass flow slowly decreased over 15-45 sec until it is off. Return to bypass in the event of progressive cardiac distension or dysfunction. Assess CO and BP, and adjust vascular resistance as necessary. Inotropic agents often are required at this stage.
Reversal of anticoagulation	Once patient is off CPB, anticoagulation must be reversed with protamine (1-1.3 mg/100 U heparin), administered slowly over 10-20 min, since rapid administration can be associated with ↓BP. (Treat with α-agonists and volume.) Other reactions include pulmonary HTN and true allergic reactions. ✓ ACT to ensure that it has returned to control (90-130 sec).
BP management	Vasoactive support often is needed in the postbypass period; the need varies with surgical procedure, disease process, and underlying cardiac function. In general, SBP should be limited to 120 mmHg to avoid stress on the aortotomy site.

COAGULATION AND CPB

General	Bleeding is common post CPB and may be considerable. Both preop and intraop factors contribute to this. A knowledge of these factors and the tests involved will aid with the management of these patients (Fig 6.1-3).
Preop factors	Hx of previous bleeding during surgery is important. Many drugs may contribute to bleeding: aspirin/NSAIDs (Plt dysfunction), anticoagulants (heparin, Coumadin) and fibrinolytic agents. These should be stopped preop, if possible, or their action reversed. Other pathological processes (e.g., liver failure/congestion, renal failure, or hemophilia) also play a role. Preop testing is important and should include PT, PTT, Plt count and bleeding time, as a minimum.
Intraop factors	CPB is associated with ↓Plt count and function. Circulating clotting factors are decreased and fibrinolysis occurs. Many surgical teams routinely use either Amicar (5 g loading dose; 1 g/h, maintenance) or Aprotinin (1 ml, test dose; 1-2 million KIU, loading; 0.25-0.5 million KIU/h, maintenance) prophylactically during cardiac surgery to inhibit the fibrinolytic process. Aprotinin also has anti-inflammatory properties that may offset the inflammatory response to CPB.
Post CPB bleeding	The common causes of post CPB bleeding are: surgical causes, inadequate heparin reversal, ↓number of Plt and Plt dysfunction, ↓clotting factors, fibrinolysis, DIC, excessive BP, and hypothermia. Surgical causes and inadequate heparin reversal (✓ ACT) should be ruled out. If no surgical cause is found and ACT is normal, Plt (10 U) should be infused. PT, PTT, Plt count, TT, reptilase time, fibrinogen, and FSP should be checked. TEG may prove very useful. (See Fig 7.12-9 and Table 7.12-3 in Liver/Kidney Transplantation, pp. 557, 558.)

References

1. Ganapathy S, Murkin JM: Pathophysiology and management of cardiopulmonary bypass. In *Cardiac Anesthesia: Principles and Clinical Practice*, 2nd edition. Estafanous FG, Barash PG, Reves JG, eds. Lippincott Williams & Wilkins, Philadelphia: 2001, 415-46.
2. Hessel EA II: Cardiopulmonary bypass equipment. In *Cardiac Anesthesia: Principles and Clinical Practice*, 2nd edition. Estafanous FG, Barash PG, Reves JG, eds. Lippincott Williams & Wilkins, Philadelphia: 2001, 335-86.
3. McCloskey G: Termination of cardiopulmonary bypass and postbypass hemodynamic management: In *Cardiac Anesthesia: Principles and Clinical Practice*, 2nd edition. Estafanous FG, Barash PG, Reves JG, eds. Lippincott Williams & Wilkins, Philadelphia: 2001, 447-64.
4. Rosenkranz ER: Myocardial preservation. In *Cardiac Anesthesia: Principles and Clinical Practice*, 2nd edition. Estafanous FG, Barash PG, Reves JG, eds. Lippincott Williams & Wilkins, Philadelphia: 2001, 387-414.
5. Slaughter TF: The coagulation system and cardiac surgery. In *Cardiac Anesthesia: Principles and Clinical Practice*, 2nd edition. Estafanous FG, Barash PG, Reves JG, eds. Lippincott Williams & Wilkins, Philadelphia: 2001, 319-34.

CORONARY ARTERY BYPASS GRAFT SURGERY

SURGICAL CONSIDERATIONS

Description: **Coronary artery bypass grafting (CABG)** is the most frequently performed cardiac operation. Since the discovery that coronary thrombosis is the causative event for MI, many schemes have been devised to augment the restricted coronary blood flow (Fig 6.1-4), including collateral pericardial blood flow to epicardial arteries and implantation of the internal mammary artery (IMA) with unligated side branches into the LV muscle. With the discovery by Favalaro that saphenous veins can be anastomosed to the epicardial coronary arteries, a new era of myocardial revascularization began. Basically, the technique involves bypass to a narrowed or occluded epicardial coronary > 1 mm in diameter with a small-diameter conduit (usually reversed saphenous vein or IMA) distal to the narrowed segment, with the proximal arterial inflow source being the ascending aorta. The IMA may be mobilized from the chest wall, leaving its proximal origin with the subclavian artery intact (pedicled graft), or the IMA may be transected and its proximal end anastomosed to the aorta or saphenous vein as a 'free mammary graft.' An **'all-arterial revascularization,'** using the right IMA and nondominant RA, is being utilized with increasing frequency.

The heart is approached through a median sternotomy, with the patient supported on full **CPB** (see separate section on CPB, p. 261). Although various operative strategies may be used, the most common regimen is for all distal (epicardial) anastomoses to be performed during a single period of aortic cross-clamping and cardiac arrest. During that period of induced asystole, myocardial protection is achieved by hypothermia and occasional reperfusion via antegrade or retrograde cardioplegia. Cardiac standstill and a bloodless field are mandatory to allow these very demanding small-diameter anastomoses to be constructed, with no obstruction to flow, in a minimal amount of time. The cross-clamp is then removed and the heart allowed to resume beating. A partially occluding aortic cross-clamp can then be applied to allow construction of the proximal aortic anastomoses. After a sufficient period of resuscitation, the patient is weaned from CPB, and decannulation, heparin reversal, and chest closure are allowed to proceed as previously noted.

The choice of conduit depends on availability and durability. Historically, the saphenous vein was the first small vessel conduit with acceptable patencies; but with prolonged experience it appears that 50% of vein grafts will be significantly diseased or occluded at 10 yr. The IMA appears to have superior long-term performance, with ~90% 10-yr patency rates. Other arterial conduits, such as the left gastroepiploic artery, superficial epigastric artery, and the radial artery, are being investigated as to their long- and short-term durability. Typical target arteries include the distal right coronary and its major

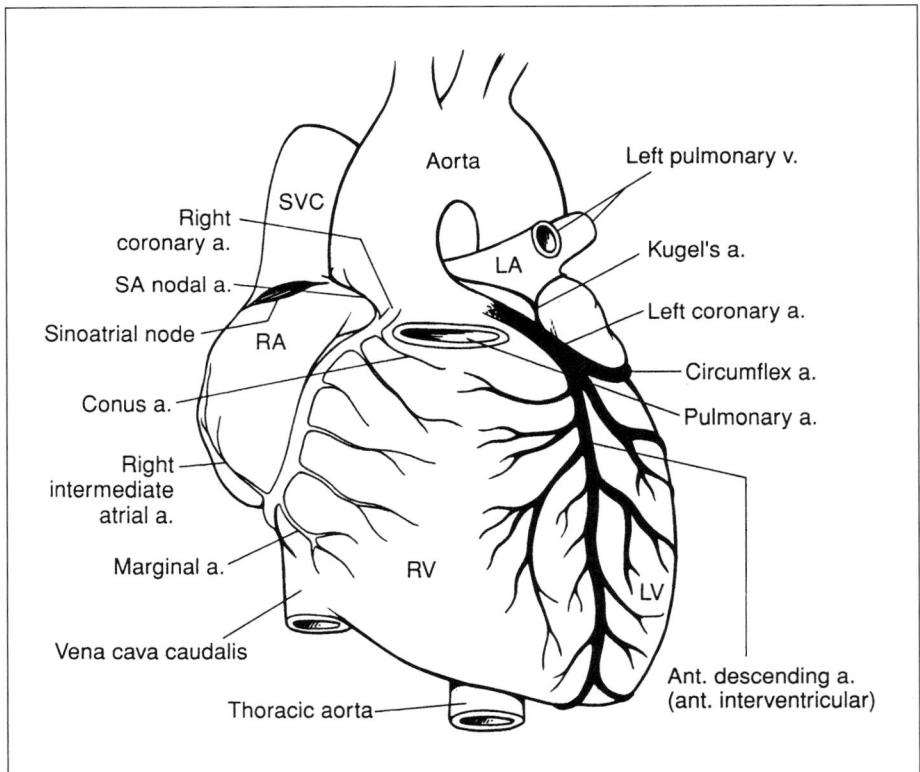

Figure 6.1-4. Coronary artery circulation—anterior view. (Reproduced with permission from Edwards EA, Malone PD, Collins JJ Jr: *Operative Anatomy of the Thorax*. Lea & Febiger, Philadelphia: 1972.)

terminal branch, the posterior descending artery. From the left circulation, the left anterior descending (LAD), with its diagonal and septal branches, is the most important, having been estimated to supply blood to 60% of the left ventricle.

The left circumflex coronary artery courses in the posterior atrioventricular groove, and is not easily accessible for bypass, which is usually performed to its obtuse marginal or posterolateral branches.

In a randomized study on coronary artery surgery (CASS),[5] coronary bypass was noted to be superior to medical management for relief of angina, and to prolong life in patients with left main CAD and in those with 3-vessel disease and impaired LV function. Other patients may receive bypass for intractable angina refractory to medical management.

Variant procedure or approaches: port access coronary artery revascularization (see p. 293); **off-pump and minimally invasive coronary artery bypass** (see p. 295).

Usual preop diagnosis: CAD with Class 3 or 4 angina (angina with minimal exertion or at rest)

SUMMARY OF PROCEDURE

Position	Supine
Incision	Median sternotomy with legs prepped for saphenous vein harvest
Special instrumentation	Complete hemodynamic monitoring; TEE
Unique considerations	CPB
Antibiotics	Cefamandole 1 g iv at induction
Surgical time	3.5-4.5 h
Closing considerations	Prevention of coagulopathy; maintenance of preload
EBL	500-600 ml
Postop care	ICU: 1-3 d, intubated 6-24 h.
Mortality	2-4%
Morbidity	Cognitive decline in patients > 60 yr: 26%[3]
	MI: 3-6%
	Pneumonia: 5%
	CVA/stroke: 2-4%[4]
	↓renal function
Pain score	7-8

PATIENT POPULATION CHARACTERISTICS

Age range	60-80 yr (mean = 74 yr)
Male:Female	2:1
Incidence	Common
Etiology	Coronary atherosclerosis
Associated conditions	LV failure; pulmonary HTN; ischemic mitral regurgitation; diabetes mellitus; obstructive pulmonary disease

ANESTHETIC CONSIDERATIONS

(Procedures covered: CABG; LV aneurysmectomy)

PREOPERATIVE

H&P and tests will divide these patients broadly into two groups: (1) high-risk, characterized by poor LV function (cardiac failure; EF < 40%; LVEDP > 18 mmHg; CI < 2.0 L/min/m^2; ventricular dyskinesia; 3-vessel disease; occlusion of left main or left main equivalent; valvular disease; recent MI; ventricular aneurysm; VSD; MI in progress; and old age); and (2) low-risk, characterized by good LV function. The type of monitoring chosen will depend on the patient's group.

Respiratory	Hx of smoking or COPD—patient should be encouraged to stop smoking at least 2 wk before surgery. Treat COPD and optimize therapy before surgery.
	Tests: CXR; PFTs; as indicated by H&P.
Cardiovascular	In the preop assessment, the following factors will affect patient management and surgical outcome:
	• Hx of angina (stable, unstable at rest, and precipitating factors)
	• Patient's exercise tolerance will provide a clue to LV functions and surgical outcome.

Cardiovascular, cont.	• The presence of CHF (Sx: SOB, PND, orthopnea, DOE, pulmonary edema, JVD, 3rd-heart sound). • Recent (< 6 mo) MI, dysrhythmias, HTN, vascular disease (particularly carotid stenosis, aortic disease). • Valvular disease (particularly MR or AS) or the presence of a VSD or LV aneurysm may portend increased risk of periop complications. **Tests:** 12-lead ECG: ✓ ischemia (area involved), LVH, previous MI, dysrhythmias. Exercise stress testing: ✓ effort tolerance, area of ischemia, maximal HR and BP before ischemia occurs, dysrhythmias. Thallium scan: ✓ component of reversible ischemia. ECHO (may be combined with stress ECHO): ✓ LV function, wall motion abnormalities, valvular disease, VSD. Cardiac catheterization: ✓ extent and location of disease, LV function, valvular pathology, VSD, LVEDP, LV aneurysm.
Postinfarction VSD	The development of a postinfarction VSD is associated with high operative morbidity and mortality because of the difficulty in repairing the lesion due to friable tissue, difficulty in obtaining hemostasis, emergent nature of the condition, and possible pulmonary edema. These patients effectively have poor LV function and should be considered as high risk. They often require support, including IABP, during induction, prebypass, and postbypass.
LV aneurysm	LV aneurysm is usually a late complication of infarction; however, it can occur early, when it usually is associated with cardiac rupture (and high mortality). These patients usually have poor myocardial function and should be anesthetized with full monitoring, including PA catheterization. Postbypass, the LV cavity is reduced in size and compliance. To ensure an adequate CO, maintain adequate preload, a higher than normal HR (A-V pacing if needed), and sinus rhythm, and consider the use of inotropes. LV aneurysms are often associated with dysrhythmias and may require cardiac mapping. Hemostasis is often difficult to obtain, and adequate iv access is a necessity. Treatment usually entails the use of blood and blood products.
Emergency revascularization	Emergency revascularization occurs in the setting of acute MI, often with acute LV failure or after failed PTCA, where the patient may be stable, suffering from acute ischemia and hemodynamically unstable, or even in full cardiac arrest. Factors to consider in these cases are: full stomach (and the need for rapid-sequence induction [p. B-5] in the face of ischemia); the prior use of fibrinolytic agents (with increased risk of hemorrhage); need for inotropes; antianginals; IABP; and dysrhythmias. These patients have a higher morbidity and mortality. In patients who have received fibrinolytic agents, consider postbypass use of antifibrinolytic agents (e.g., aminocaproic acid).
Neurological	Previous stroke or Hx/Sx of carotid artery disease should be documented and evaluated.
Endocrine	Diabetes is common and periop control of blood glucose is important. **Tests:** Blood glucose
Renal	✓ baseline renal function, as CPB places these patients at risk for renal failure. **Tests:** Cr; BUN; electrolytes (particularly K^+)
Hematologic	Patients are often on aspirin or other antiplatelet therapy, which may lead to increased intraop hemorrhage. These agents should be stopped 7-10 d before surgery, if possible. Some patients may be on anticoagulants (usually heparin in the immediate preop period). Heparin should be stopped 6-8 h preop; however, in some patients, heparin infusion is continued into the OR. Other patients may have received fibrinolytic agents that put them at increased risk for intraop hemorrhage. **Tests:** Consider Plt count, PTT, if indicated
Laboratory	Hb/Hct; other tests as indicated from H&P. T&C 2-4 U PRBCs.
Premedication	Patients should be instructed to continue all medications (e.g., nitrates, β-blockers; Ca^{++} antagonists, antidysrhythmics, and antihypertensives) before surgery, with the exception of diuretics on the day of surgery. Allaying anxiety may decrease the incidence of periop ischemia and help with the preinduction placement of lines. Typical preop sedation includes diazepam (10 mg po) or lorazepam (1-2 mg po) the night before and again 1-2 h before arrival in the OR, with the addition of morphine (0.1 mg/kg im) and scopolamine (0.3 mg im). Severely compromised patients will require less premedication.

INTRAOPERATIVE

Anesthetic technique: GETA. An arterial line should be inserted, using liberal amounts of local anesthetic, before induction. The presence of real-time BP monitoring can be critical in the care of these patients, especially during induction. Although it is helpful to have a CVP line before induction for preload monitoring and drug infusion, it is not essential. This line usually is inserted after the patient is intubated. If infused drugs are necessary before the CVP catheter is in place, they can be administered through a separate peripheral iv.

Induction	Generally, a moderate- to high-dose narcotic technique (e.g., fentanyl 10-100 μg/kg or sufentanil 2.5-20 μg/kg), supplemented by etomidate (0.1-0.3 mg/kg) or midazolam (50-350 μg/kg), is appropriate. As with all cardiac cases, the speed of induction and total drug dose depends on the patient's cardiac function and pathology. Muscle relaxation may be obtained using pancuronium (0.1 mg/kg), given slowly to avoid tachycardia, or vecuronium (possibility of bradycardia, especially if the patient is β-blocked). It is important to avoid the sympathetic response to laryngoscopy. The use of high-dose narcotics (see above), esmolol (100-500 μg/kg over 1 min, followed by 40-100 μg/kg/min infusion), SNP (0.5-3 μg/kg/min), lidocaine (1-2 mg/kg), or a combination of these agents, may decrease or ablate this response. NTG (0.5-2 μg/kg/min) also may be used during induction if evidence of ischemia occurs.
Maintenance	Usually narcotic (total: fentanyl 10-100 μg/kg or sufentanil 5-20 μg/kg) with midazolam (50-350 μg/kg) for amnesia. Patients with good LV function may benefit from the decreased myocardial O_2 demand associated with the use of volatile agents (2° $\downarrow$contractility). N_2O is generally avoided. Propofol infusion may be used while rewarming and postbypass.
Emergence	Transported to ICU, sedated, intubated, and ventilated. Extubate when able—often < 6 h if lower-dose narcotic technique used (fast-track).
Blood and fluid requirements	IV: 14 ga × 1-2 NS/LR @ 6-8 ml/kg/h UO 0.5-1 ml/kg/h Warm all fluids. Humidify gases.

Monitoring	Standard monitors (p. B-1) Arterial line	Standard monitors and A-line are placed before induction. ✓ BP in both arms. Right radial preferred if left IMA graft, because retraction of the sternum may compress the left subclavian.
	CVP or PA catheter	CVP (and/or PA line, if indicated), usually is placed after intubation. In the low-risk/good LV function group, CVP is adequate; in high-risk/poor LV function, a PA catheter is useful for hemodynamic monitoring, weaning from bypass, and vasoactive therapy. Some groups use routine PA catheterization for all patients undergoing CABG surgery.
	ECG TEE	5-lead monitoring II and V_5 (or area most at risk for ischemia). Will reflect regional wall motion abnormalities, papillary muscle dysfunction, and MR.

Myocardial O_2 Balance	Supply – Coronary blood flow:
	  Perfusion pressure (DBP-LVEDP)
	  Diastolic filling time (HR)
	  Blood viscosity (optimal Hct = 30)
	Coronary vasoconstriction:
	  Spasm
	  $PaCO_2$ (hypocapnia → constriction)
	  α-sympathetic activity
	Supply – O_2 delivery:
	  O_2 sat
	  Hct
	  Oxyhemoglobin dissociation curve
	Demand – O_2 consumption:
	  BP (afterload)
	  Ventricular volume (preload)
	  Wall thickness ($\downarrow$subendocardial
	   perfusion)
	  HR
	  Contractility
		The balance of myocardial O_2 supply vs demand is important in the management of these patients. The goal of anesthesia is to ensure that this balance remains in equilibrium and that no ischemia occurs, or, if it does, that it is treated promptly. Those patients with poor LV function or complicated disease will benefit from maintenance of contractility (avoid volatile agents) and a high FiO_2, whereas those with good LV function may benefit from mild cardiac depression ($\downarrow$demand associated with the addition of low-dose volatile agents). Certain events are associated with **increased risk of intraop ischemia**: intubation, incision, sternotomy, cannulation, tachycardia, $\uparrow$BP or $\downarrow$BP, ventricular fibrillation or distension, inadequate cardioplegia, emboli, spasm, or inadequate revascularization. Care should be taken to avoid these complications and to ablate responses to stimuli.

Detection of ischemia	ECG	ST segment depression or elevation or a new T-wave alteration may suggest ischemia. Monitoring 2 leads—one lateral (e.g., V_5) and one inferior (e.g., II)—give the best detection rate.
	PA catheter	Elevations of PCWP may be indicative of ischemia. A new V-wave on the PCWP trace is a better sign of possible ischemia (papillary muscle dysfunction).
	TEE	The appearance of a new regional wall motion abnormality is the most sensitive indicator of ischemia, but it requires constant monitoring.
Treatment of ischemia	Caused by tachycardia: Esmolol (100-500 μg/kg) ↑ anesthesia Verapamil (2.5-10 mg iv) Caused by ↑BP: NTG (0.5-4 μg/kg/min) ↑ anesthesia Caused by ↓BP: Phenylephrine (0.2-0.75 μg/ kg/min) ↑ preload Caused by ↓↓HR: A-V pacing	While avoidance of ischemia is the goal, when it does occur it should be treated aggressively. Treatment may include inotropic support (e.g., dopamine 1-5 μg/kg/min or dobutamine 0.5-30 μg/kg/min). If LV failure persists despite other therapy, an IABP may be inserted.
Positioning	✓ and pad pressure points. ✓ eyes.	

POSTOPERATIVE

Complications	Infarction Ischemia Tamponade Dysrhythmias Cardiac failure Coagulopathy Hemorrhage	Postop control of ischemia is important since hemodynamic instability may be associated with inadequate pain relief, awakening and ventilation.
Pain management	Parenteral opioids	Supplement with benzodiazepine for sedation.
Tests	ECG CPK CXR Electrolytes ABG Coag profiles	

References

1. Bondy RJ, Wynands JE, Dorman BH, Reves JG: Anesthesia for coronary artery bypass surgery. In *Cardiac Anesthesia: Principles and Clinical Practice*, 2nd edition. Estafanous FG, Barash PG, Reves JG, eds. Lippincott Williams & Wilkins, Philadelphia: 2001, 541-56.
2. Horrow JC, Hensley FA, Merin RG: Anesthetic management for myocardial revascularization. In *A Practical Approach to Cardiac Anesthesia*, 2nd edition. Hensley FA, Martin DE, eds. Little, Brown, Boston: 1995, 275-95.
3. Moller JT, Cluitmans P, Rasmussen LS, Houx P, Rasmussen H, Canet J, Rabbitt P, Jolles J, Larsen K, Hanning CD, Langeron O, Johnson T, Lauven PM, Kristensen PA, Biedler A, van Beem H, Fraidakis O, Silverstein JH, Beneken JE, Gravenstein JS: Long-term postoperative cognitive dysfunction in the elderly ISPOCD1 study. International Study of Post-Operative Cognitive Dysfunction. *Lancet* 1998; 351(9119):1888-9.
4. Roach GW, Kanchuger M, Mangano CM, Newman M, Nussmeier N, Wolman R, Aggarwal A, Marschall K, Graham SH, Ley C: Adverse cerebral outcomes after coronary bypass surgery. Multicenter Study of Perioperative Ischemia Research Group and Ischemia Research and Education Foundation Investigators. *N Engl J Med* 1996; 335(25):1857-63.
5. Rogers WJ, Coggin CJ, Green B, et al: 10-year followup of quality of life in patients randomized to receive medical treatment or coronary artery bypass graft surgery. *Circulation* 1990; 82(5):1647-58.

LEFT VENTRICULAR ANEURYSMECTOMY

SURGICAL CONSIDERATIONS

Description: Extensive MI may → large areas of myocardial necrosis, with subsequent aneurysm formation. LV failure may ensue as a result of continuous LV dilatation or mitral insufficiency 2° annular dilatation or involvement of papillary muscles. Indications for this surgery include worsening CHF and increased dysrhythmias.

Typically, apical dilatation with maintenance of basilar myocardial contractility allows for aneurysm resection and preservation of both myocardial contractility and chamber size to produce an adequate CO. Operation is commenced in the usual manner—by establishing CPB (see p. 261), cross-clamping the aorta, establishing myocardial protection, and then assessing the left ventricle. A thinned, dilated ventricular segment with full-thickness scar formation can be resected and ventricular continuity restored with improvement of ventricular geometry and myocardial energy demands. Coronary bypass can be performed during this same period. Then air is removed from the left side of the heart, the cross-clamp is removed, and coronary perfusion is reestablished. After a sufficient period of resuscitation and return of vigorous contractility, bypass is D/C'd, not infrequently with the assistance of intraaortic balloon pump (IABP) to augment forward output. Decannulation, protamine administration, and closure proceed as described in CPB, p. 261.

Usual preop diagnosis: LV aneurysm with CHF

SUMMARY OF PROCEDURE

Position	Supine
Incision	Median sternotomy, ± leg incision for saphenous vein harvest if coronary bypass is planned.
Unique considerations	Preparations (ECG leads) should be made for pre- or postop IABP or LV assist device (LVAD)
Antibiotics	Cefamandole 1 g iv at induction
Surgical time	Aortic cross-clamp: 40-100 min
	CPB: 70-130 min
	Total: 3-4 h
EBL	300-400 ml
Postop care	ICU × 1-3 d, intubated 6-24 h; usually requires inotropic support ± mechanical support (LVAD, IABP).
Mortality	5-7%
Morbidity	Overall: 8-10%
	Requirement for IABP: 10%
	Respiratory insufficiency: 5%
	CVA: 2-3%
Pain score	7-10

PATIENT POPULATION CHARACTERISTICS

Age range	50-70 yr
Male:Female	3:1
Incidence	Uncommon
Etiology	Usually the end result of MI 2° CAD
Associated conditions	Mitral insufficiency; pulmonary HTN; CAD

ANESTHETIC CONSIDERATIONS

See Anesthetic Considerations following Coronary Artery Bypass Graft Surgery, p. 267.

Reference

1. Mills NL, Everson CT, Hockmuth DR: Technical advances in the treatment of left ventricular aneurysm. *Ann Thorac Surg* 1993; 55:792-800.

AORTIC VALVE REPLACEMENT

SURGICAL CONSIDERATIONS

Description: Disease of the aortic valve may present as valvular stenosis, insufficiency, or a combination of the two. Valvular disease most commonly occurs as a result of rheumatic disease, but also may occur 2° calcific degeneration (aortic sclerosis) in the elderly. Congenitally bicuspid valves and endocarditis account for most of the remainder. Repair of the aortic valve is rarely possible, and most conditions require valve replacement. The three most commonly used **prostheses** are: porcine bioprostheses, especially in the older patient; mechanical prostheses, with the necessity for lifelong anticoagulation; and cryopreserved homografts, which, unfortunately, are expensive and in short supply. The operation, on full CPB, usually is performed through a median sternotomy. After routine bicaval and aortic cannulation, the patient is taken onto full CPB. Left heart drainage is through a pulmonary artery vent, and a left atrial vent usually is inserted through the right superior pulmonary vein. Because of the LV hypertrophy, myocardial protection is of utmost importance. Most centers favor hyperkalemic, hypothermic cardioplegic arrest, augmented by topical cooling, using either a continuous infusion of cold saline into the pericardial well or a cooling jacket. Cardioplegic administration can be achieved either antegrade into the coronary ostia or retrograde via the coronary sinus. Myocardial temperature is monitored continuously.

After the heart is arrested, the aorta is opened to expose the aortic valve. Continuous insufflation of the operative field with CO_2 reduces the amount of dislodged or trapped air. The rheumatic, stenotic valve, including aortic annulus, is frequently heavily calcified, and all Ca^{++} must be debrided to allow the prosthetic valve to be securely seated. This is frequently a tedious and time-consuming procedure, but one which then allows the remainder of the procedure to proceed in a timely fashion. After excision of the valve leaflets and debridement of the annulus, assuring that no particulate debris embolizes into the ventricle or coronary arteries, the annulus is measured to assure a proper match between prosthetic valve and annulus, and an appropriate valve prosthesis is selected. Interrupted sutures are placed through the annulus for its entire circumference, then passed through the sewing ring of the prosthesis. The prosthesis is lowered into the annulus and securely tied in place. Proper sizing and positioning are mandatory to prevent perivalve leaks or impingement on the coronary ostia. Systemic rewarming is initiated during the final stages of the valve implantation and the LV is allowed to fill during aortic closure. With the patient in the head-down position, all remaining air is vented from the left heart and aorta, and the cross-clamp is removed to allow myocardial perfusion. The heart is allowed to recover from this period of ischemia and, after sufficient resuscitation, with continuous venting of air from the aorta, the patient is weaned from CPB. Vasodilators are almost always utilized, as there appears to be excessive vasospasm present in both the coronary and pulmonary circulations after hypothermia. Decannulation and heparin reversal with protamine are then accomplished in the routine manner.

Usual preop diagnosis: Severe AS with syncope, chest pain or CHF; aortic insufficiency with CHF

SUMMARY OF PROCEDURES

	Valve Replacement with Prosthesis	Homograft Valve Replacement
Position	Supine	⇐
Incision	Median sternotomy	⇐
Special instrumentation	TEE; hemodynamic monitoring; CPB	TEE or surface ECHO
Unique considerations	ECHO assessment of valve function and regional wall motion intraop	ECHO assessment of annular size and intraop evaluation of valve function after implantation
Antibiotics	Cefamandole 1 g iv at incision	⇐
Surgical time	Aortic cross-clamp: 45 min	60 min
	CPB: 90 min	105 min
	Total: 3 h	⇐
EBL	300-400 ml	⇐
Postop care	ICU × 1-3 d, intubated 6-24 h; hypertrophied, noncompliant LV requiring high preload.	⇐
Mortality	5-8%	⇐
Morbidity	Pneumonia: 5-10%	⇐
	Neurological sequela:	⇐
	Transient: 3-7%	
	CVA: 1-2%	
	Permanent: 1-2%	
	Infection: 1%	⇐
Pain score	7-10	7-10

PATIENT POPULATION CHARACTERISTICS

Age range	Bicuspid valves – 50-60 yr; rheumatic – 55-80 yr (mean = 58 ± 13 yr)
Male:Female	3:1
Incidence	70-100 cases/yr in tertiary care center
Etiology	Postrheumatic (majority of patients); aortic sclerosis; progressive stenosis of a bicuspid aortic valve; endocarditis
Associated conditions	Poststenotic dilatation of the ascending aorta (may require separate surgical attention); rheumatic mitral valvular involvement; CAD; CHF

ANESTHETIC CONSIDERATIONS

PREOPERATIVE

Respiratory	Respiratory compromise may occur 2° pulmonary congestion (LV failure) and pleural effusion. An effusion, if significant, should be drained prior to surgery, as it may impair oxygenation and, with IPPV, may impair venous return → ↓CO + ↓myocardial perfusion. **Tests:** CXR
Cardiovascular	**Aortic stenosis (AS):** Sx are those of angina pectoris (if at rest may indicate concurrent CAD), syncope, and CHF (indicates severe disease with 2-yr life expectancy). The ejection murmur of AS is best heard at the 2nd right interspace. ECG shows LVH. Important points in the preop investigations include:

- Aortic orifice size: moderate AS = 0.7-0.9 cm^2; critical AS = < 0.5 cm^2 (normal = 2.6-3.5 cm^2)
- Aortic valvular gradient: severe = > 70 mmHg
- Ejection fraction (EF): ↓EF indicates evidence of LV failure (normal = > 0.6).
- Coronary angiography: associated CAD often demonstrated.
  AS → ↑LV work (↑pressure load) → LV concentric hypertrophy → ↓LV diastolic function + ↑risk for ischemia (MVO_2 + O_2 supply).
- Reliance on atrial 'kick': important to maintain NSR.
- Sensitivity to changes in SVR: ↓SVR → ↓↓BP → ↓myocardial perfusion + ↓CO → ↓↓↓BP.
- Sensitivity to volume changes: hypovolemia → ↓preload → ↓↓CO.
- Sensitivity to rate changes: tachycardia → ↓ejection time → ↓myocardial perfusion.
- LV wall tension + ↑duration of systole → ↑MVO_2.
- ↑LVEDP + ↑wall thickness and tension + ↓diastolic aortic pressure → ↓O_2 supply.

Aortic regurgitation (AR): Sx include DOE, orthopnea, PND, palpitations, and (less frequently) angina. Exercise tolerance may remain reasonably good, even with severe AR. Acute AR is very poorly tolerated. The pandiastolic murmur of AR is loudest over the sternum and left lower sternal border.

AR → chronic LV volume overload → LV eccentric hypertrophy → massive cardiomegaly → LV failure (CHF) → ↑LVEDP → ↑PA pressure and pulmonary congestion.

- Possibility of ischemia: ↑MVO_2 and ↓supply (↓diastolic pressure, ↑HR).
- Sensitivity to rate changes: ↓HR → ↑AR + ↓CO.
- Sensitivity to changes in SVR: ↑SVR → ↑regurgitation + ↓CO.

Tests: ECG: ✓ hypertrophy, LV strain, ischemia, rhythm. ECHO: ✓ LV function, valve area, regurgitant fraction. Angiography: ✓ LV function, right heart pressure, CAD, valve area, regurgitant fraction.

Hepatic	CHF may result in passive liver congestion with ↓liver function and possible coagulopathy. **Tests:** LFTs; PT; PTT
Neurological	Syncopal episodes may have resulted in neurologic deficits. These should be well documented.
Renal	Prerenal failure often is associated with AR 2° ↓CO. **Tests:** BUN; Cr, creatinine clearance, if indicated; electrolytes
Hematologic	**Tests:** Hb/Hct; clotting profile to investigate abnormalities. T&C for 8 U PRBCs.
Laboratory	✓ digitalis level and electrolytes; other tests as indicated from H&P.
Premedication	Beware of oversedation in patients with AS where ↓BP could be detrimental. Light premedication with an anxiolytic is usually sufficient. Digitalis and diuretics should be continued.

INTRAOPERATIVE

Anesthetic technique: GETA. An arterial line should be inserted, using liberal amounts of local anesthetic, before induction. The presence of real-time BP monitoring can be critical in the care of these patients, especially during induction. Although it is helpful to have a CVP line before induction for preload monitoring and drug infusion, it is not essential. This line usually is inserted after the patient is intubated. If infused drugs are necessary before the CVP catheter is in place, they can be administered through a separate peripheral iv.

Induction	**AS:** Typically, O_2 with moderate- to high-dose narcotic (e.g., fentanyl 10-100 μg/kg). Avoid sufentanil in AS because of ↓BP. Etomidate (0.1-0.3 mg/kg), midazolam (50-350 μg/kg) may be used to supplement the above. Paralysis with vecuronium or pancuronium (0.1 mg/kg, depending on desired HR). Induction is a critical period. CPB and surgeons should be available and ready to proceed. Danger is hypotension with a cycle of ischemia, further hypotension and more ischemia. Hypotension should be treated aggressively with fluid and α-adrenergic agonists (phenylephrine 50-100 μg iv bolus, infusion 0.1-0.75 μg/kg/min). Critical AS patients may benefit from the use of phenylephrine as an infusion during induction and prebypass. The avoidance of hypotension is even more critical in the presence of CAD. Drugs causing tachycardia should be avoided. Atrial fibrillation (AF) or SVT should be treated with cardioversion. β-blockers and other negative inotropes are generally contraindicated. Ventricular irritability should be treated early as ventricular fibrillation may be refractory to defibrillation. Beware of vasodilators, including NTG. **AR:** Again, O_2 with moderate- to high-dose narcotic (e.g., fentanyl 10-100 μg/kg or sufentanil 2.5-10 μg/kg). Etomidate (0.1-0.3 mg/kg) or benzodiazepines (e.g., midazolam 50-350 μg/kg) may be used to supplement the opiates. Muscle relaxation with pancuronium (0.1 mg/kg). These patients benefit from fluid augmentation, high normal HR (90 bpm) with afterload reduction (e.g., SNP 0.25-2 μg/kg/min) to improve forward flow.
Maintenance	Narcotic (e.g., total fentanyl 10-100 μg/kg). Low-dose volatile agent/air/O_2. Relaxant. (See Anesthetic Considerations for Cardiopulmonary Bypass, pp. 262-265.) The following table summarizes the goals of intraop management:

Parameter	AS	AR
LV preload	↑	Normal-to-↑
HR	Normal-to-slow ↓	Modest ↑
Rhythm	NSR	NSR
Contractility	Maintain	Maintain
SVR	Modest ↑	↓
PVR	Maintain	Maintain

Postbypass	**AS:** Postbypass, patients may be hyperdynamic and require vasodilators for HTN, although inotropes also may be needed. Because of the hypertrophied, noncompliant ventricle, filling pressure may be higher than normally required. **AR:** In the immediate postbypass period, patients with AR may require inotropic support (e.g., dopamine 3-10 μg/kg/min, dobutamine 5-10 μg/kg/min; epinephrine 25-100 ng/kg/min) is often needed. Maintain LV filling. Other supportive measures (e.g., IABP) may be necessary.
Emergence	Transport to ICU sedated, intubated (6-24 h), and ventilated. Early extubation may be possible if a lower-dose narcotic technique is used (fast-track).
Blood and fluid requirements	IV: 14 ga × 1-2 NS/LR @ 6-8 ml/kg/h UO 0.5-1 ml/kg/h Warm all fluids. Humidify gases. T&C 2-4 U blood
Monitoring	Standard monitors (p. B-1) Standard monitors and arterial line should be placed before Arterial line induction. CVP line CVP (and/or PA line, if indicated), usually is placed after PA catheter intubation. CVP may underestimate left-side pressures. In acute AR, PCWP may underestimate true LVEDP. ECG V_5 lead should be monitored for ischemia.

Monitoring, cont.	TEE Urinary catheter	TEE may be useful to estimate LV filling and regional wall motion abnormalities.
Positioning	✓ and pad pressure points. ✓ eyes.	

POSTOPERATIVE

Complications	Hemorrhage Tamponade Cardiac failure Dysrhythmias Ischemia	Inotropic and vasodilator therapy usually is continued into the postop period, and then weaned.
Pain management	Parenteral opioids for pain relief Benzodiazepine for sedation	
Tests	ECG CXR Electrolytes Coag profile HCT	

References

1. Fann JI, Miller DC, Moore KA, Mitchell RS, Oyer PE, Stinson EB, Robbins RC, Reitz RA, Shumway NE: Twenty-year clinical experience with porcine bioprostheses. *Ann Thorac Surg* 1996; 62:1301-12.
2. Frasco PE, de Bruijn NP: Valvular heart disease. In *Cardiac Anesthesia: Principles and Clinical Practice*, 2nd edition. Estafanous FG, Barash PG, Reves JG, eds. Lippincott Williams & Wilkins, Philadelphia: 2001, 557-84.
3. Jackson JM, Thomas SJ: Valvular heart disease. In *Cardiac Anesthesia*, 4th edition. Kaplan JA, ed. WB Saunders, Philadelphia: 1999, Ch 22.
4. Scott WC, Miller DC, Haverich A, Dawkins K, Mitchell RS, Jamieson SW, Oyer PE, Stinson EB, Baldwin JC, Shumway NE: Determinants of operative mortality for patients undergoing aortic valve replacement. Discriminant analysis of 1,479 operations. *J Thorac Cardiovasc Surg* 1985; 89(3):400-13.

MITRAL VALVE REPAIR OR REPLACEMENT

SURGICAL CONSIDERATIONS

Description: **Mitral valve repair or replacement** is utilized typically for the correction of postrheumatic mitral valvular stenosis or insufficiency, as well as mitral valve prolapse, degenerative mitral insufficiency, or repair after endocarditis. For mitral regurgitation (MR) 2° posterior leaflet abnormalities (myxomatous degeneration, torn chordae) or pure annular dilatation, most valves can be repaired. For severe rheumatic calcific mitral stenosis (MS), mitral valve replacement with preservation of subannular structures may be necessary.

The technique of mitral valve repair or replacement is similar regardless of the mitral valve pathology. After aortic and bicaval venous cannulation, CPB (see p. 261) is established, and the left heart is vented through the PA. After cross-clamping of the aorta, diastolic arrest is accomplished with cardioplegia administered via the aortic root, augmented with topical cooling with either continuous pericardial saline infusion or a cooling jacket. Exposure is accomplished via a vertical incision in the left atrium just posterior to atrial septum. If the left atrium is not large enough, access may be gained via an incision in the right atrium and then incising the atrial septum, with caval snares in place to prevent air entry into the venous cannulae.

After suitable exposure, the atrium, atrial appendage, and mitral valve are carefully inspected, and a decision is made to repair or replace the valve. Repair of regurgitant valves caused primarily by posterior leaflet problems is usually possible. Similarly, annular dilatation 2° LV enlargement is also usually possible by means of a ring annuloplasty. Regurgitation 2° anterior leaflet abnormalities are more problematic, requiring significant expertise, and may be less durable. Preop and postop evaluation are greatly facilitated by use of TEE. Valve replacement can be performed after excising the valve leaflets; or, the leaflets may be preserved in an attempt to maintain the benefits of the subvalvar apparatus to global ventricular performance. After appropriate excision and debridement, the annulus is rimmed with interrupted sutures, passed through the sewing ring of the valve prosthesis. The prosthesis is carefully positioned, and the sutures are tied. After filling both the LV and atrium with blood, the atrium is closed, air is evacuated from the left heart, and the cross-clamp is removed to allow coronary perfusion. After a satisfactory period of resuscitation, and after all air has been evacuated from the circulation, CPB may be D/C'd, usually with the assistance of vasodilator agents. TEE may be utilized at this stage to assess adequacy of mitral valve repair.

Variant procedure or approaches: **Mitral commissurotomy** may be done closed (e.g., during pregnancy).

Usual preop diagnosis: Class 3 or 4 CHF 2° mitral insufficiency or mitral stenosis

SUMMARY OF PROCEDURES

	Mitral Valve Replacement/Repair	Closed Commissurotomy
Position	Supine	Right lateral decubitus
Incision	Median sternotomy	Left lateral thoracotomy
Special instrumentation	TEE and epicardial ECHO to assess valve function and regional wall motion; CPB.	Performed without CPB.
Unique considerations	Special loading conditions may be used to estimate the amount of MR, which is frequently afterload-dependent.	⇐
Antibiotics	Cefamandole 1 g iv	⇐
Surgical time	Aortic cross-clamp: 45-150 min CPB: 90-200 min Total: 3-4 h	Total: 2 h
EBL	300-400 ml	200-400 ml
Postop care	ICU × 1-3 d, intubated 6-24 h; vasodilator therapy for reversal of pulmonary HTN and afterload reduction.	⇐
Mortality	5-8%	< 5%
Morbidity	Pneumonia: 10-15% CNS complications: Transient neurologic dysfunction: 5-10% CVA: 1-2% Infection: < 1%	⇐ ⇐ ⇐ ⇐
Pain score	7-10	7-10

PATIENT POPULATION CHARACTERISTICS

Age range	40-75 yr	20-40 yr
Male:Female	1:1	Almost exclusively pregnant females
Etiology	Postrheumatic: majority of cases; increased aging; myxomatous degeneration; ischemic etiologies (increasing)	⇐
Associated conditions	Aortic valvular involvement with rheumatic disease, CAD, pulmonary HTN, and tricuspid regurgitation	⇐

ANESTHETIC CONSIDERATIONS

PREOPERATIVE

Respiratory   Pulmonary congestion, edema, pleural effusions may be present, with an overall restrictive lung pattern. Pleural effusions should be drained before surgery if significant (↓oxygenation, ↓venous return with IPPV). ↑LA volume may compress the left recurrent laryngeal nerve → left vocal cord paralysis (Ortner's syndrome).
Tests: CXR; PFTs, if indicated

Cardiovascular	**Mitral Stenosis (MS):** Sx include exertional dyspnea and fatigue, progressing to pulmonary edema, atrial fibrillation (AF), and hemoptysis. Embolic events occur in 15% of patients. The opening snap and diastolic murmur of MS are best heard between apex and left sternal border. The ECG may show AF or wide-notched P-waves. It is important to grade the severity of MS by symptomatology and valve area: mild = 1.5-2 cm^2; moderate = 1-1.5 cm^2; and severe = < 1.0 cm^2 (nl = 4-6 cm^2). AF is often the factor precipitating deterioration in these patients.

Because of the decreased LV filling, these patients are sensitive to:
• Loss of atrial 'kick': maintain NSR.
• Volume changes: keep full.
• Rate changes: avoid ↑HR →↓diastolic filling time →↓CO.
Pathophysiology:
• MS →↓LVH filling →↓CO.
• MS →↑LA pressure → pulmonary edema + ↑PA pressure →↑PVR → RV failure + TR + left shift of iv septum →↓CO →↑LA pressure →↑LA volume → AF and thrombi.

Mitral Regurgitation (MR): May be acute (MI/endocarditis) or chronic (often associated with MS). Chronic Sx include: palpitations, DOE, PND, fatigue, and orthopnea. Acute MR may → sudden ↓↓CO and pulmonary edema. MR can be classified as mild (< 30% RF), moderate (30-60% RF), or severe (> 60% RF). The pansystolic murmur is loudest at the apex. The ECG may show LA and LV overload. MR patients are sensitive to:
• Changes in SVR: ↑SVR →↑RF →↓CO +↓BP.
                    ↓SVR →↓RF →↑CO + ↑BP.
• Change in HR: ↓HR → acute LA volume overload.
                    Mild ↑HR →↑CO.
Pathophysiology:
• Acute MR → ↑↑LA pressure →↓CO + ↓BP →↑HR →↑contractility →↑O$_2$ demand.
                    →↑LV diastolic volume →↑LVEDP →↑O$_2$ demand.
                    → Pulmonary edema.
• Chronic MR →↑LA volume + AF → pulmonary edema → RV failure.
                    → LV volume overload → LVH →↓CO + LV failure.
Tests: ECG: ✓ LVH, left and right atrial enlargement, rhythm. ECHO: ✓ RF, valve pressure gradients, LV function, valve pressure gradient and area.

Neurological	The large left atrium and AF may result in thrombus formation, with the possibility of embolism. Neurological deficits should be documented.
Gastrointestinal	Hepatic congestion may → decreased function, which may be reflected in coagulation problems. **Tests:** Consider LFTs; PT; PTT
Renal	↓CO may lead to renal failure. **Tests:** BUN; Cr; electrolytes
Hematologic	Because of the potential for thromboembolism, these patients may be on anticoagulants, which may be given up to the day before surgery. In the case of Coumadin, anticoagulant effects can be reversed by the use of FFP and vitamin K. **Tests:** Consider PT; PTT
Laboratory	T&C for 2-4 U PRBCs. Hb/Hct; coagulation profile; other tests as indicated from H&P.
Premedication	Premedication with an anxiolytic (e.g., lorazepam 1-2 mg po, midazolam 0.05-0.2 mg/kg im) or an analgesic (e.g., morphine 0.1-0.2 mg/kg); or a combination of these agents may be used, depending on patient status.

INTRAOPERATIVE

Anesthetic technique: GETA. An arterial line should be inserted, using liberal amounts of local anesthetic, before induction. The presence of real-time BP monitoring can be critical in the care of these patients, especially during induction. Although it is helpful to have a CVP line before induction for preload monitoring and drug infusion, it is not essential. This line usually is inserted after the patient is intubated. If infused drugs are necessary before the CVP catheter is in place, they can be administered through a separate peripheral iv.

Induction	Typically, moderate- to high-dose narcotic (fentanyl 10-100 μg/kg or sufentanil 2.5-20 μg/kg), supplemental midazolam (50-350 μg/kg) or etomidate (0.1-0.3 mg/kg). Use pancuronium (MR) or vecuronium (MS) (0.1 mg/kg), depending on the desired HR to facilitate intubation.

Induction, cont.

MS: ↓BP should be treated with fluid, but beware of precipitating pulmonary edema. Occasionally, phenylephrine may be needed to maintain SVR. Tachycardia should be avoided; if it occurs, it should be treated (↑ anesthesia, esmolol if ventricular function is preserved). Sinus rhythm should be maintained. New onset atrial flutter/AF should be treated with defibrillation. Avoid factors that may increase PVR (N_2O, acidosis, hypoxia, hypercarbia).

MR: Maintain or augment preload, depending on response to fluid load. Inotropic agents may be useful to maintain contractility. Afterload reduction will improve forward flow. Generally SNP (0.5-4 μg/kg/m) is used, but NTG (0.5-4 μg/kg/m) may be more appropriate in patients with ischemia-induced regurgitation. Avoid ↑PVR caused by N_2O, acidosis, hypoxia, or hypercarbia. IABP may be useful periop in patients with acute MR 2° MI (↓afterload, ↑coronary perfusion pressure).

Maintenance

Narcotic (total = fentanyl 10-100 μg/kg, or sufentanil 5-20 μg/kg) with benzodiazepine (e.g., midazolam 50-350 μg/kg) for amnesia; low-dose isoflurane; O_2/air.

The following table summarizes the goals of intraop management:

Parameter	MS	MR
LV preload	Normal-to-↑	Normal → ↑
HR	↓	↑
Rhythm	NSR	NSR
Contractility	Maintain	Maintain
SVR	Normal	↓
PVR	Avoid ↑	Avoid ↑

Postbypass

Although patients with MS generally do well after valve replacement, inotropes (e.g., dopamine, dobutamine) occasionally are necessary. This is especially true late in the disease when cardiomyopathy may be present.

Emergence

Transport to ICU, intubated and ventilated 6-24 h. Early extubation is possible if lower-dose narcotic technique is used (fast-track).

Blood and fluid requirements

IV: 14 ga × 1-2
NS/LR @ 6-8 ml/kg/h
Maintain UO 0.5-1 ml/kg/h.
Warm all fluids.
Humidify gases.

Monitoring

Standard monitors (p. B-1)
Arterial line
CVP line
PA catheter
Urinary catheter

TEE

Standard monitors and A-line are placed before induction. CVP (and/or PA line, if indicated), usually is placed after intubation. Care should be exercised with PA catheter insertion because the dilated PA may be susceptible to rupture with the catheter. In MS, PCWP may overestimate LV filling pressure because of stenosis.

TEE may help in volume management, regional wall motion abnormalities (postacute MI) and in assessing the success of mitral valve repair. Occasionally, the use of a valve ring during repair may cause systolic anterior motion of the valve leaflet, with resultant regurgitation, which may be seen on ECHO.

Positioning

✓ and pad pressure points.
✓ eyes.

POSTOPERATIVE

Complications

Hemorrhage
Tamponade
Cardiac failure
Dysrhythmias
Conduction defects
Atrioventricular disruption

Inotropic support or vasodilator therapy may be needed. IABP for mitral incompetence, especially in the presence of acute MR 2° infarction.

Pain management

Parenteral opioids for pain relief
Benzodiazepine for sedation

Tests	ECG
	CXR
	ABG
	Coag profile
	Electrolytes

References

1. Fann JI, Miller DC, Moore KA, Mitchell RS, Oyer PE, Stinson EB, Robbins RC, Reitz RA, Shumway NE: Twenty-year clinical experience with porcine bioprostheses. *Ann Thorac Surg* 1996; 62:1301-2.
2. Frasco PE, de Bruijn NP: Valvular heart disease. In *Cardiac Anesthesia: Principles and Clinical Practice*, 2nd edition. Estafanous FG, Barash PG, Reves JG, eds. Lippincott Williams & Wilkins, Philadelphia: 2001, 557-84.
3. Galloway AC, Colvin SB, Baumann FB, et al: A comparison of mitral valve reconstruction with mitral valve replacement: intermediate-term results. *Ann Thorac Surg* 1989; 47:655-62.
4. Jackson JM, Thomas SJ: Valvular Heart Disease. In *Cardiac Anesthesia*, 4th edition. Kaplan JA, ed. WB Saunders, Philadelphia: 1999, Ch 22.

TRICUSPID VALVE REPAIR

SURGICAL CONSIDERATIONS

Description: Insufficiency of the tricuspid valve is almost always 2° left-sided valvular disease, with tricuspid annular dilatation and resultant valvular insufficiency usually 2° pulmonary HTN. Some congenital conditions (e.g., Ebstein's deformity) may persist into early adulthood, when replacement is usually necessary. Tricuspid repair is normally possible in the absence of primary involvement of tricuspid leaflets. The procedure is usually accomplished on CPB (see p. 261), either with the heart fibrillating or during a brief period of aortic cross-clamping and diastolic arrest. After instituting CPB and snaring the venous cannulae to prevent air entry into the pump circuit, the tricuspid valve is exposed through an incision in the right atrium. In the absence of leaflet involvement by the rheumatic process, repair usually can be accomplished by a simple **annuloplasty**. After atrial closure, evacuation of air, and myocardial resuscitation, the patient is weaned from CPB with vasodilator agents. Temporary pacing wires usually are inserted and passed to the anesthesiologist in case inadvertent injury to the AV node or His bundle cause complete heart block.

Variant procedure or approaches: Tricuspid valve replacement

Usual preop diagnosis: Tricuspid regurgitation, 2° annular dilatation 2° pulmonary HTN and left-side failure

SUMMARY OF PROCEDURE

Position	Supine
Incision	Median sternotomy
Special instrumentation	Intraop ECHO; hemodynamic monitoring; CPB
Antibiotics	Cefamandole 1 g iv at induction
Surgical time	Aortic cross-clamp: 30-40 min
	CPB: 70-80 min
	Total: 3-4 h
EBL	400-800 ml (Long-standing tricuspid regurgitation may → impaired hepatic production of coagulation factors.)
Postop care	ICU × 1-3 d, intubated 6-24 h; vasodilator therapy for pulmonary HTN
Mortality	2-3%
Morbidity	Third-degree heart block: 10%
	RV failure: 2-3%
Pain score	7-10

PATIENT POPULATION CHARACTERISTICS

Age range	50-75 yr
Male:Female	1:1
Incidence	Rare
Etiology	Rheumatic; congenital (Ebstein's anomaly)
Associated conditions	Rheumatic involvement of left-side valves with pulmonary HTN

ANESTHETIC CONSIDERATIONS

PREOPERATIVE

Cardiovascular **Tricuspid regurgitation (TR)** usually is well tolerated and Sx (↓CO) may go unnoticed, masked by Sx associated with left-side valvular disease and pulmonary HTN. Occasionally, TR is 2° endocarditis and raises the suspicion of iv drug abuse. TR may be caused by pulmonary HTN → ↑RV afterload → RV dilation, ↑RV wall tension → dilation of tricuspid valve annulus and TR. Pathophysiology:

- TR → ↓CO 2° ↑RV size → shift of the intraventricular septum to the left → ↓LV size, ↓LV compliance → LV underloading due to ↓LV size and ↓RV stroke volume.
- TR → atrial fibrillation (AF) 2° ↑right atrial size. In isolated insufficiency, the ↑ in right atrial pressure may result in shunting across a patent foramen ovale (PFO), leading to paradoxical embolization with potentially disastrous consequences.

Tests: ECG: ✓ AF. ECHO: ✓ relative chamber size, contractility, PFO, valve lesions. Cardiac catheterization: ✓ contractility, CO, pulmonary pressures and their response to vasodilators, other valvular pathology.

Respiratory Pulmonary HTN (> 25 mmHg mean pressure), pulmonary edema, and effusions may be present.
Tests: CXR: ✓ pulmonary edema, pleural effusion.

Renal Chronic venous congestion may → prerenal failure.
Tests: BUN; Cr; electrolytes

Hepatic Hepatic congestion may → impaired synthetic function, particularly coag factors.
Tests: Consider PT; PTT

Hematologic **Tests:** Hb/Hct; other tests as indicated from H&P and Sx. Consider viral testing (HIV, hepatitis in isolated tricuspid endocarditis or in iv drug abusers). T&C 2-4 U PRBCs.

Laboratory Other tests as indicated from H&P.

Premedication Standard premedication (p. B-2) is usually appropriate.

INTRAOPERATIVE

Anesthetic technique: GETA. An arterial line should be inserted, using liberal amounts of local anesthetic, before induction. The presence of real-time BP monitoring can be critical in the care of these patients, especially during induction. Although it is helpful to have a CVP line before induction for preload monitoring and drug infusion, it is not essential. This line usually is inserted after the patient is intubated. If infused drugs are necessary before the CVP catheter is in place, they can be administered through a separate peripheral iv.

Induction Typically, O_2 and moderate- to high-dose narcotic (fentanyl 10-100 μg/kg or sufentanil 2.5-20 μg/kg) with etomidate (0.1-0.3 mg/kg) or midazolam (50-150 μg/kg). Muscle relaxation is obtained with a nondepolarizing agent (e.g., pancuronium 0.1 mg/kg, vecuronium 0.1 mg/kg).

Maintenance The choice of narcotic/benzodiazepine/O_2 or volatile agent and O_2 will be determined by the underlying lesion and ventricular function. Avoid N_2O (pulmonary HTN). Low-dose isoflurane may be used. Benzodiazepines (e.g., midazolam 50-300 μg/kg, diazepam 0.3-0.5 mg/kg) may be used for amnesia. Exact choice of agents for maintenance depends on underlying lesion, ventricular function, and coexisting disease. Management goals of TR are often those of coexisting valvular problems. The general principles, however, are: (1) Adequate preload (↓preload → ↓RV stroke volume); (2) HR: normal-to-increased; (3) Contractility: normal. May require inotropic support for ↑PVR, anesthetic myocardial depression or IPPV. (4) PVR: normal or decreased (high PVR → ↓RV stroke volume). (5) SVR: little effect unless it affects left-side pathology.

Emergence	To ICU intubated and ventilated × 6-24 h. Early extubation may be possible if a lower-dose narcotic technique is used (fast-track).	
Blood and fluid requirements	IV: 14 ga × 1-2 NS/LR @ 6-8 ml/kg/h UO 0.5-1 ml/kg/h Warm all fluids. Humidify gases. T&C 2-4 U PRBC.	Because of the possibility of PFO and R→L shunt, ensure that all venous lines are clear of air.
Monitoring	Standard monitors (p. B-1) Arterial line CVP or PA catheter Urinary catheter	Standard monitors and A-line are placed before induction. CVP (and/or PA line, if indicated), usually is placed after intubation. CVP may be a poor indicator of RV or LV filling. PA catheter may be helpful in the management of fluid balance, CO, and management of pulmonary HTN, but may be difficult to place and will require removal while valve or annular ring is placed.
	TEE	Because RV distention may affect LV filling and stroke volume, TEE may be useful in judging filling and relative LV size.

Pulmonary HTN	↑PVR can result from:
	  ↓PaO_2
	  ↑$PaCO_2$
	  ↓pH
	  N_2O
	  α-agonists
	  Inadequate anesthesia
		In TR, control of PVR is important because ↑PVR may result in ↓CO. Hypoxia, hypercarbia, acidosis, N_2O, or α-agonists may ↑PVR. PVR may be reduced with hypocarbia, inotropic support with dobutamine (5-10 μg/kg/min), isoproterenol (10-50 ng/kg/m), or amrinone (loading 0.75 mg/kg, infusion 2-20 μg/kg/min), and by using pulmonary vasodilators—NTG (1-4 μg/kg/min), SNP (0.5-4 μg/kg/min), prostaglandin E_1 (0.05-0.4 μg/kg/min), or NO (0.1-100 ppm inhaled).

Positioning	✓ and pad pressure points. ✓ eyes.	
Complications	Coagulopathy Hemorrhage RV failure	Coagulopathy 2° prolonged bypass time for multiple valve replacements. RV failure 2° ↑PVR (previously, RV decompressed by tricuspid incompetence). Rx includes inotropes: dobutamine (5-10 μg/kg/min), isoproterenol (25-100 ng/kg/min), amrinone (loading 0.75 mg/kg, infusion 2-20 μg/kg/min), epinephrine (25-100 ng/kg/min), avoidance of factors causing ↑PVR, and the use of pulmonary vasodilators.

POSTOPERATIVE

Complications	Hemorrhage Coagulopathy Dysrhythmias RV failure Infection Renal impairment Methemoglobinemia	Inotropic support and pulmonary vasodilators will need to be continued. Avoid those factors which ↑PVR. Measure metHb levels during NO therapy.
Pain management	Parenteral opioids	Supplement with benzodiazepine for sedation.
Tests	ECG Coag profile Renal panel: BUN, Cr ABG Electrolytes	

References

1. Frasco PE, de Bruijn NP: Valvular heart disease. In *Cardiac Anesthesia: Principles and Clinical Practice*, 2nd edition. Estafanous FG, Barash PG, Reves JG, eds. Lippincott Williams & Wilkins, Philadelphia: 2001, 557-84.
2. Jackson JM, Thomas SJ: Valvular heart disease. In *Cardiac Anesthesia*, 4th edition. Kaplan JA, ed. WB Saunders, Philadelphia: 1999, Ch 22.

SEPTAL MYECTOMY/MYOTOMY

SURGICAL CONSIDERATIONS

Description: Patients with asymmetric septal hypertrophy usually present with symptoms 2° LV outflow tract obstruction (LVOTO), increased diastolic dysfunction and stiffness, or a combination of the two, manifested as syncope, CHF, or severe chest pain. The systolic hemodynamic abnormality is caused by anterior leaflet of the mitral valve being drawn into the LV outflow tract (LVOT), and abutting the asymmetrically hypertrophied intraventricular septum, narrowing the LVOT, and producing a large intracavitary gradient. Additionally, severe mitral insufficiency may result. The most common surgical procedure for asymmetric septal hypertrophy is **septal myectomy/myotomy**. After institution of CPB, aortic cross-clamping, and cardioplegic arrest, the aorta is opened, and visualization of the subvalvar ventricular septum is attained. Bimanual palpation, as well as TEE visualization, can localize the asymmetric hypertrophy. Using the right coronary orifice as a landmark, the ventricular septum is longitudinally incised with two parallel incisions ~1 cm apart, with care being taken to avoid injury of the papillary muscle or mitral valve chordae. A trough of the hypertrophied septum is then excised, alleviating the LVOTO. Removal of a portion of the asymmetrically hypertrophied myopathic septum also usually reduces the systolic anterior motion (SAM) of the anterior mitral leaflet, and reduces the intracavitary gradient and mitral regurgitation (MR). Infrequently, mitral valve replacement may be necessary for persistent MR.

Usual preop diagnosis: Asymmetric septal hypertrophy with CHF, chest pain, and/or syncope

SUMMARY OF PROCEDURE

Position	Supine
Incision	Median sternotomy
Special instrumentation	TEE; hemodynamic monitoring; CPB
Unique considerations	Because of LV hypertrophy, maintenance of adequate preload is essential. Afterload also must be maintained to prevent LVOTO. Temporary pacing wires ususally are placed at the start of the procedure.
Antibiotics	Cefamandole 1 g iv at induction
Surgical time	2.5 h
EBL	150 ml
Postop care	ICU, intubated on ventilator 6-24 h
Mortality	3-4%
Morbidity	Complete heart block: 5%
	Persistent MR: 5%
	New aortic insufficiency: 2-5%
	CVA: < 1%
	VSD: < 1%
Pain score	6-10

PATIENT POPULATION CHARACTERISTICS

Age range	20-80 yr (mean = 45 yr)
Male:Female	1:1
Incidence	10/yr at Stanford University Medical Center
Etiology	Asymmetric septal hypertrophy

ANESTHETIC CONSIDERATIONS

PREOPERATIVE

Respiratory Affected only 2° to cardiac failure.

Cardiovascular Patients with idiopathic hypertrophic subaortic stenosis (IHSS) often present with Sx of syncope, angina pectoris (CAD), CHF, and palpitations. The main feature of IHSS is dynamic LVOTO 2° to septal hypertrophy and a possible venturi effect that draws the anterior mitral valve leaflet into the outflow tract. LVOTO → ↑LV hypertrophy → ↓compliance and ↓diastolic function → ↑LVEDP, making diastolic filling dependent on preload and atrial contraction. Obstruction is worsened by decreased preload or afterload, increased contractility or HR. IHSS also results in ↑MVO$_2$ and ↓coronary perfusion, especially to the septum and subendocardium, which increases the risk of ischemia. Hypertrophy occurs throughout the whole myocardium and may lead to further dysfunction. MR, caused by a venturi suction effect, is often present and is exacerbated by the same conditions that increase LVOTO. (Note that ↓afterload → ↑MR, unlike the usual [nonventuri-suction] form of MR.) Patients are often on β-blockers or Ca^{++} antagonists. These should be continued to day of surgery.
Tests: ECG: ✓ Q-waves (indicative of septal hypertrophy); short PR interval with slurred QRS complex; supraventricular tachycardia; LV hypertrophy.
ECHO: ✓ septal hypertrophy; MR; LV hypertrophy, myocardial dysfunction.
Cardiac catheterization: ✓ LVOT pressure gradient, which may increase with provocation (e.g., Valsalva maneuver); obliteration of the LV cavity; MR; CAD.

Neurological Document syncope and any neurological deficits.

Laboratory Hb/Hct; electrolytes; other tests as indicated from H&P.

Premedication Avoid activation of the sympathetic nervous system since this will cause ↑HR and ↓inotropy → ↓CO + ↓BP. Thus, adequate anxiolysis is essential and can be obtained by premedication with a benzodiazepine (e.g., midazolam 0.05-0.2 mg/kg im, lorazepam 1-2 mg po, or diazepam 5-10 mg po). Avoid ↓SVR, and maintain β-blockade and Ca^{++} channel blocker therapy.

INTRAOPERATIVE

Anesthetic technique: GETA. An arterial line should be inserted, using liberal amounts of local anesthetic, before induction. The presence of real-time BP monitoring can be critical in the care of these patients, especially during induction. Although it is helpful to have a CVP line before induction for preload monitoring and drug infusion, it is not essential. This line usually is inserted after the patient is intubated. If infused drugs are necessary before the CVP catheter is in place, they can be administered through a separate peripheral iv.

Induction Typically, moderate- to high-dose narcotic (fentanyl 10-100 μg/kg; avoid sufentanil due to vasodilation). Supplement with etomidate (0.1-0.3 mg/kg), midazolam (50-350 μg/kg), or STP (2-4 mg/kg). Ketamine should be avoided due to the activation of the sympathetic nervous system. Introduction of a volatile agent prior to intubation may be helpful. Vecuronium (0.1 mg/kg) for muscle relaxation. Use pancuronium with caution (tachycardia) and avoid d-tubocurarine (↓BP).

Maintenance O$_2$ and narcotic (total fentanyl 10-100 μg/kg) + volatile agent—most commonly, halothane because of decreased contractility and preservation of SVR. Halothane, however, may lead to loss of NSR. Isoflurane is relatively contraindicated (↓SVR). Midazolam (50-350 μg/kg) can be used for amnesia. The cornerstone of anesthesia for IHSS is to avoid factors which will increase LVOTO: (1) ↓preload, (2) ↓afterload, (3) ↑contractility, (4) loss of NSR, and (5) ↑HR.

Emergence To ICU intubated and ventilated × 6-24 h. Early extubation is possible if a lower-dose narcotic technique is used (fast-track).

Blood and fluid requirements IV: 14 ga × 1-2
NS/LR @ 6-8 ml/kg/h
Maintain UO 0.5-1 ml/h
Warm fluids.
Humidify gases.

Monitoring Standard monitors (p. B-1)   Standard monitors and A-line are placed before induction.
Arterial line
PA catheter   CVP (and/or PA line, if indicated), usually is placed after
Urinary catheter   intubation. A PA catheter is useful for assessment of LV

Monitoring, cont.		filling (keep high normal PCWP) and for monitoring SVR (normal-to-high). A pacing or pace port PA catheter may be useful for conduction problems occurring postop.
	TEE	TEE is useful to judge LV filling, LV contractility, LVOTO, MR, and VSD.
Intraoperative problems	↓Preload	Rx: volume, phenylephrine
	↓Afterload	Rx: phenylephrine
	↑Contractility	Rx: esmolol, halothane
	↑HR	Rx: esmolol
	Loss of NSR	Rx: cardioversion, verapamil
	Complete heart block	Should have reliable means of pacing available, including temporary ventricular leads.
	VSD	Septum may be damaged, → VSD (diagnosed by TEE). If present, it should be repaired.
Position	✓ and pad pressure points.	
	✓ eyes.	

POSTOPERATIVE

Complications	Hemorrhage	Dx: from chest tube drainage. Rx with blood and factors as needed. ✓ coag status. May require reexploration.
	Complete heart block	Pacing should be available. Occasionally, inotropes of vasodilators required. β-blockers and Ca^{++} antagonists usually D/C'd.
	Late VSD	Late VSD, indicated by development of a murmur, will require repair.
	Tamponade	Dx: by raising filling pressure, equalization of CVP, and PADP, ↓CO, ↓UO, and by ECHO. Rx: reexploration and drainage.
Pain management	Parenteral opioids	Supplement with benzodiazepine for sedation.
Tests	ECG: ✓ conduction problems.	
	ABG	
	ECHO: ✓ LVOTO; VSD.	
	Coag profile	
	Electrolytes	

References

1. Frasco PE, de Bruijn NP: Valvular heart disease. In *Cardiac Anesthesia: Principles and Clinical Practice*, 2nd edition. Estafanous FG, Barash PG, Reves JG, eds. Lippincott Williams & Wilkins, Philadelphia: 2001, 557-84.
2. Jackson JM, Thomas SJ: Valvular Heart Disease. In *Cardiac Anesthesia*, 4th edition. Kaplan JA, ed. WB Saunders, Philadelphia: 1999, Ch 22.
3. Maron BJ, Bonow RO, Cannon RO III, Leon MB, Epstein SE: Hypertrophic cardiomyopathy. Interrelations of clinical manifestations, pathophysiology, and therapy. *N Engl J Med* 1987; 316(13):780-89; 316(14):844-52.

PACEMAKER INSERTION

SURGICAL CONSIDERATIONS

Description: **Pacemaker insertion** may be required for relief of abnormalities of the conduction system. A transvenous pacemaker lead may be placed via the subclavian vein, through the tricuspid valve into the RV (single-chamber pacing); or two leads may be placed, one into the right atrium and the other into the RV (dual-chamber pacing). Typically, 2nd- or 3rd-degree heart block is the diagnostic indication, although sick sinus syndrome (SSS) and other abnormalities also may be found. Access to the subclavian veins usually is attained percutaneously, although a cut-down may be used to expose the cephalic vein in the deltopectoral groove. Passage of a guide wire into the RV may cause frequent premature ventricular beats, which usually subside spontaneously with repositioning of the guide wire or lead. After ventricular and/or atrial lead placement, the pacing lead will have to be tested for sensing threshold, pacing threshold, depolarization amplitude, and lead resistance. After satisfactory placement of the pacing leads, the actual pacemaker generator unit is connected and then placed in a subcutaneous pocket at the site of percutaneous lead placement.

Usual preop diagnosis: Abnormalities of S-A nodal function (SSS) or A-V nodal function (heart block)

SUMMARY OF PROCEDURE

Position	Supine
Incision	Left subclavicular; mostly percutaneous
Special instrumentation	Fluoroscopy with fluoro-table
Unique considerations	Patient usually awake with mild sedation
Antibiotics	Cefamandole 1 g iv at induction
Surgical time	1 h
EBL	Minimal
Postop care	PACU → CCU; ECG monitoring × 2-4 h; chest radiograph to document lead configuration.
Mortality	0-1%
Morbidity	Lead displacement: 1-2%
	Pneumothorax: 1-2%
Pain score	2

PATIENT POPULATION CHARACTERISTICS

Age range	50-80 yr
Male:Female	2:1
Incidence	Infrequent
Etiology	CAD; cardiac valve repair/replacement
Associated conditions	Complete heart block with syncope; SSS; paroxysmal tachycardia; SVT

Table 6.1-2. Five-Position Pacemaker Code (ICHD)

Position	I	II	III	IV	V
Category	Chamber(s) paced	Chamber(s) sensed	Mode of response(s)	Programmable functions	Special tachyarrhythmia functions
Letters used	V - Ventricle	V - Ventricle	T - Triggered	P - Programmable (rate and/or output)	B - Bursts
	A - Atrium	A - Atrium	I - Inhibited	M - Multiprogrammable	N - Normal rate competition
	D - Double	D - Double	D - Double O - None		S - Scanning
		O - None	R - Reverse	O - None	E - External
Manufacturer's designation only	S - Single chamber	S - Single chamber			

ANESTHETIC CONSIDERATIONS

PREOPERATIVE

The indications for permanent pacemaker insertion are usually bradydysrhythmias (e.g., 3rd-degree heart block, sinus node dysfunction, etc.) or, less commonly, tachycardia (e.g., atrial flutter not responsive to medical therapy). There are many different types of pacemakers, which are classified according to the chamber paced, chamber sensed, response to sensing, programmability, and antitachyrhythmia functions. The anesthesiologist should be aware of the type of pacemaker to be implanted and the means for external control.

Cardiovascular	Evaluate patient for associated disease, including CAD (~50%), HTN (~20%), cardiomyopathy, CHF, valvular defect, and for any symptoms or recent changes related to the conduction problems (syncope, CHF). It is important to know the reason for pacemaker implantation and the patient's escape rhythm. These patients are often on antidysrhythmics, diuretics, cardiac glycosides, and a variety of other cardiovascular agents, which should be continued up to the day of surgery. **Tests:** Exercise tolerance by Hx. ECG: ✓ rate, ischemic changes, rhythm. Other tests as indicated by H&P. ✓ serum digoxin and other antidysrhythmic levels.
Pacemaker	If a permanent pacemaker is already in place, its type and present functional state should be assessed. (Sx of problems include chest pain, palpitations, syncope, and weakness.) If no permanent pacemaker, a temporary transvenous pacemaker should be placed before surgery, except in unusual circumstances. **Tests:** ECG: ✓ Valsalva maneuver or carotid sinus massage—may slow the heart sufficiently to allow the permanent pacemaker to fire and allow assessment of function. A rate lower than the set rate may indicate battery failure. CXR: ✓ lead continuity.
Hematologic	Hct or Hb
Laboratory	✓ K+ level, which can affect pacing threshold, → loss of pacemaker capture, if low, or ventricular tachycardia, if high. Other tests as indicated from H&P.
Premedication	Standard premedication (p. B-2)

INTRAOPERATIVE

Anesthetic technique: Permanent pacemakers commonly are placed via the transvenous route, requiring only local anesthesia and MAC with sedation. For epicardial pacemaker placement, GETA is required. These patients should be monitored during transport to OR. Care is taken to avoid dislodging temporary pacing electrodes. The function of the temporary pacemaker should be checked prior to induction.

General anesthesia:

Induction	Usually anesthesia can be induced with STP (3-5 mg/kg) or etomidate (0.2-0.3 mg/kg), in combination with an opiate (e.g., fentanyl 1-2 μg/kg), to attenuate the response to intubation. Vecuronium or pancuronium (0.1 mg/kg) will provide adequate muscle relaxation.	
Maintenance	Standard maintenance (p. B-3). Avoid excessive hyperventilation (→ ↓K+) and use volatile agents with caution, as they may increase A-V conduction time.	
Emergence	Generally, patient is extubated at the end of the case.	
Blood and fluid requirements	Minimal fluid requirements IV: 16 ga × 1 NS/LR @ 4-6 ml/kg/h	
Monitoring	Standard monitors (p. B-1) Urinary catheter	Rarely, arterial line if patient disease indicates.
Electrocautery interference	Minimize by: • Using bipolar cautery, if possible; • Grounding pad on leg; • Limiting cautery output; • Limiting cautery use.	The use of electrocautery may interfere with pacemaker function and → dysrhythmias or failure of the pacemaker. Monitor ECG and pulse (since electrical activity does not mean CO) for interference. Have a magnet available to convert the pacemaker to asynchronous mode (check that this is possible and will not change the programming of the pacemaker).
Complications	Dysrhythmias Air embolism Cardiac tamponade Hemo/pneumothorax Hemorrhage	Availability of temporary pacing is important because complete heart block or dislodgement of leads may occur. In addition, pharmacologic agents (atropine, 0.5-2 mg; isoproterenol 10-100 ng/kg/min) to increase HR should be available.

POSTOPERATIVE

Complications	Dislodging of electrodes Dysrhythmias

Complications, cont.	Pneumothorax
	Tamponade
Pain management	Parenteral opioids for pain relief
	Benzodiazepine for sedation
Tests	ECG
	CXR
	Electrolytes

References

1. Matthews EL, Atlee JL, Luck JC, Martin DE: Anesthesia for patients with electrophysiologic disorders. In *A Practical Approach to Cardiac Anesthesia*, 2nd edition. Hensley FA, Martin DE, eds. Little, Brown, Boston: 1995, 392-415.
2. Rosenfeld LE, Elefteriades JA: Surgical and device therapy for cardiac arrhythmias. In *Cardiac Anesthesia: Principles and Clinical Practice*, 2nd edition. Estafanous FG, Barash PG, Reves JG, eds. Lippincott Williams & Wilkins, Philadelphia: 2001, 617-36.

PERICARDIECTOMY

SURGICAL CONSIDERATIONS

Description: Constrictive pericarditis, either acute or chronic, interferes with ventricular filling, reducing stroke volume and depressing the cardiac index (CI). Although there are many possible etiologies (infectious, nephrogenic, postradiation), the cause remains unknown for a majority of patients. Typically, patients present with a progressive Hx of breathlessness, fatigability, or peripheral or abdominal swelling, often months to years after the inciting event. The Dx may be confirmed by cardiac catheterization, with equalization of end diastolic pressures, although volume loading may be necessary to demonstrate this in the patient under medical management. The differentiation between constrictive pericardial disease and restrictive myocardial disease may be difficult, if not impossible, and may coexist in a single patient. Once this Dx has been confirmed, surgical **pericardiectomy** should be undertaken, since the outlook without surgical relief is one of gradual, but persistent deterioration. Although surgical mortality remains in the 10-15% range, long-term relief for survivors is good. Since these patients are usually significantly compromised hemodynamically, intensive monitoring is indicated. Approach may be through a **median sternotomy** or left **anterolateral thoracotomy.** Removal of both visceral and parietal pericardium is essential for relief, but dense adhesions of these layers to underlying muscle may make this dissection very difficult, tedious, and bloody, especially if the visceral pericardium and epicardium are involved in the constrictive process. CPB (see p. 261) may be utilized for hemodynamic instability, but it obviously increases bleeding complications. Complete excision from both ventricular surfaces is mandatory. Most periop difficulties evolve from cardiac failure.

Variant procedure or approaches: A limited **pericardial window**, draining fluid into the left hemithorax, may relieve tamponade, but will be of no benefit for a true constrictive process.

Usual preop diagnosis: Constrictive pericarditis

SUMMARY OF PROCEDURES

	Median Sternotomy	Anterolateral Thoracotomy
Position	Supine	Supine, with elevation of left hemithorax
Incision	Midline	Fifth interspace
Special instrumentation	TEE; full hemodynamic monitoring; CPB standby	⇐
Antibiotics	Cefamandole 1 g iv at induction	⇐
Surgical time	2-5 h, depending on tenacity of visceral peel	⇐

	Median Sternotomy	**Anterolateral Thoracotomy**
Closing considerations	Avoid volume overload and cardiac distention. Chronically depressed hearts may require inotropic or mechanical support (i.e., IABP) postop.	⇐
EBL	100-500 ml	⇐
Postop care	ICU; intubated × 4-6 h. Hemodynamic monitoring. Low CO state may persist postop.	⇐
Mortality	5-15%, predominantly from cardiac failure	⇐
Morbidity	Persistent CHF: 5%	⇐
	Transient phrenic nerve dysfunction: < 1%	
Pain score	7-10	7-10

PATIENT POPULATION CHARACTERISTICS

Age range	10-80 yr (median = 45 yr)
Male:Female	2:1
Incidence	3-4 patients/yr at tertiary referral center
Etiology	Majority unknown. Infectious, radiation, prior cardiac operation, rheumatic pericarditis, amyloid deposition.
Associated conditions	Restrictive myocardial diseases

ANESTHETIC CONSIDERATIONS

PREOPERATIVE

Pericardiectomy is performed most commonly for patients with constrictive pericarditis, while pericardial window procedures are used for patients with cardiac tamponade.

Respiratory   Restrictive disease may be present 2° fibrosis (e.g., post TB) or pleural effusions. This may impair oxygenation and, if the effusions are significant, may ↓ venous return on institution of IPPV → rapid decompensation (↓CO). Drain prior to surgery.
Tests: CXR: ✓ active disease, fibrosis, effusions, pericardial calcification. Consider ABG, PFT, as indicated by CXR and Sx and if time permits.

Cardiovascular   Of importance is the presence or absence of a pericardial effusion. A large effusion that develops slowly (chronic pericarditis) may cause little or no Sx. Conversely, a small and rapidly forming effusion may → cardiac tamponade. While the cardiovascular signs for both tamponade and constriction are similar (pulsus paradoxus, venous HTN, exaggerated venous pulsations, ↓BP, tachycardia), it is important to differentiate between them, as it may affect intraop management. Constrictive pericarditis can be differentiated from cardiac tamponade by ECHO, by pulsus paradoxus (frequent, with tamponade; rare, with constrictive pericarditis). Kussmaul's sign (distention of the jugular veins on inspiration) is rare with tamponade and common with constrictive pericarditis. Electrical alternans is present with tamponade and absent in constrictive pericarditis. Examination of the RV pressure wave form is unchanged in tamponade, but shows a dip and prominent Y descent in constrictive pericarditis. Anesthetic management is influenced by the planned procedure, the underlying process (constriction or tamponade) and its severity. Clues to severity are the physical symptoms and the degree of tachycardia, ↓BP, and the filling pressure. (While it is not possible to give exact figures, a HR of >100 bpm, systolic BP < 100 mmHg, and a filling pressure > 15 mmHg are probably significant.) In addition, it is important to assess concurrent cardiac problems: cardiomyopathy, CAD, or valvular disease (especially in constrictive disease associated with TB, radiation therapy, or in rheumatoid diseases, such as lupus).
Tests: ECG: ✓ low-voltage complexes, electrical alternans. ECHO: ✓ pericardial effusion, calcification of pericardium, valvular lesions, myocardial function.

Gastrointestinal   Chronic hepatic congestion may → ↓synthetic function (↓procoagulants). Development of ascites may → ↑intraabdominal pressure. Because of this and the fact that these are sometimes emergency procedures, consider possible full stomach.
Tests: Consider LFTs; PT; PTT

Renal	Renal failure may cause pericarditis and, conversely, pericarditis may cause renal failure (2° prerenal factors: ↑venous pressure, ↓perfusion pressure). This may affect the choice of drugs used for anesthesia that depend on renal clearance (particularly muscle relaxants). **Tests:** BUN; Cr; consider creatinine clearance; electrolytes.
Hematologic	Some renal or hepatic conditions may be associated with coagulation disorders. These include both procoagulant and Plt problems. If possible, any coagulopathy should be corrected before surgery with FFP, Plt, or both. Consult with a hematologist, if necessary. **Tests:** Hb/Hct; PT; PTT; Plt count
Laboratory	Other tests as indicated from H&P.
Premedication	Little or no premedication may be indicated; otherwise, a benzodiazepine (e.g., midazolam 0.05-0.2 mg/kg im) may be used. Consider full-stomach precautions: H_2-antagonists (e.g., ranitidine 50 mg iv), metoclopramide (10 mg iv), antacids (e.g., Na citrate 0.3 M 30 ml po).

INTRAOPERATIVE

Anesthetic technique: GETA. An arterial line should be inserted, using liberal amounts of local anesthetic, before induction. The presence of real-time BP monitoring can be critical in the care of these patients, especially during induction. Although it is helpful to have a CVP line before induction for preload monitoring and drug infusion, it is not essential. This line usually is inserted after the patient is intubated. If infused drugs are necessary before the CVP catheter is in place, they can be administered through a separate peripheral iv. Consider pericardiocentesis or pericardial window under local anesthesia prior to induction, as drainage of even a small amount of fluid may improve the patient's status dramatically. The considerable manipulation of the heart, extensive dissection, blood loss, dysrhythmias, and unrelieved tamponade make pericardiectomy cases a challenge.

Induction	Typically, ketamine 1-2 mg/kg or etomidate 0.2-0.3 mg/kg ± narcotic (fentanyl 2-30 μg/kg), depending on patient status. Consider maintaining spontaneous ventilation in tamponade patients until drained, as institution of IPPV may result in rapid decompensation and cardiac arrest due to ↓↓venous return. Otherwise, succinylcholine (1 mg/kg) with cricoid pressure (full stomach) or pancuronium (0.1 mg/kg) for muscle relaxation.
Maintenance	Narcotic (total fentanyl 5-50 μg/kg), low-dose volatile agent, midazolam (50-350 μg/kg), or a combination of these agents in 100% O_2. CO is dependent on maintaining a high preload to ensure adequate cardiac filling, avoiding and treating bradycardia and preserving myocardial contractility. The use of inotropes (dobutamine, isoproterenol, or epinephrine) may be necessary; α-agonists should be avoided but, on occasion, may be needed to increase coronary perfusion. These anesthetic considerations apply to both tamponade and constrictive disease.
Emergence	In general, plan for extubation in the OR in the case of pericardial window and transport to ICU for postop ventilation 4-24 h following pericardiectomy.

Blood and fluid requirements	IV: 14 ga (or 7 Fr) × 1-2 UO: 0.5-1 ml/kg/h Warm fluids and humidify gases. T&C 2-4 U for pericardiectomy.	During pericardiectomy, anticipate rapid blood loss (a major cause of mortality). For this reason, CPB should be available on standby for all pericardiectomy procedures.
Monitoring	Standard monitors (p. B-1) Arterial line CVP line PA catheter TEE Urinary catheter	Standard monitors and A-line are placed before induction. CVP (and/or PA line, if indicated), usually is placed after intubation. PA catheters aid the management of filling pressures, CO and afterload. TEE may be useful to gauge filling volume and degree of relief of pericardial constriction.
Complications	Cardiac tamponade Dysrhythmias Hemorrhage Coagulopathy Heart failure	Intrathoracic pressure associated with IPPV may produce a ↓↓CO in these patients (because of ↓venous return). Spontaneous ventilation, therefore, is preferred until the tamponade is drained. Hemorrhage is not usually a problem unless penetrating trauma is the cause of the tamponade. Once constriction is relieved, myocardial function does not return to normal quickly. Inotropes are often needed. Due to

Complications, cont.

Positioning   ✓ and pad pressure points.
✓ eyes.

extensive dissection and hemorrhage, coagulopathies may develop and should be treated aggressively.

POSTOPERATIVE

Complications

Hemorrhage
Coagulopathy
Ventricular hypofunction
Dysrhythmias
Ischemia

Following pericardial window surgery, patients improve with the relief of the tamponade. Postpericardiectomy patients, however, may have a continuation of intraop dysrhythmias and myocardial depression. Inotropes (e.g., dopamine 5-10 μg/kg/min) may be needed for 24-48 h. Normal cardiac function can take 4-6 wk to return.

Pain management   Parenteral opioids

Supplement with benzodiazepine for sedation.

Tests

ECG
CXR
ABG
Coag profile
Electrolytes

Reference

1. Savage RM, Aronson S, Shanewise JS, Mossad EB, Licina MG: Intraoperative echocardiography. In *Cardiac Anesthesia: Principles and Clinical Practice*, 2nd edition. Estafanous FG, Barash PG, Reves JG, eds. Lippincott Williams & Wilkins, Philadelphia: 2001, 237-94.

Surgeon

James I. Fann, MD

6.2 MINIMALLY INVASIVE CARDIAC SURGERY

Anesthesiologist

Lawrence C. Siegel, MD

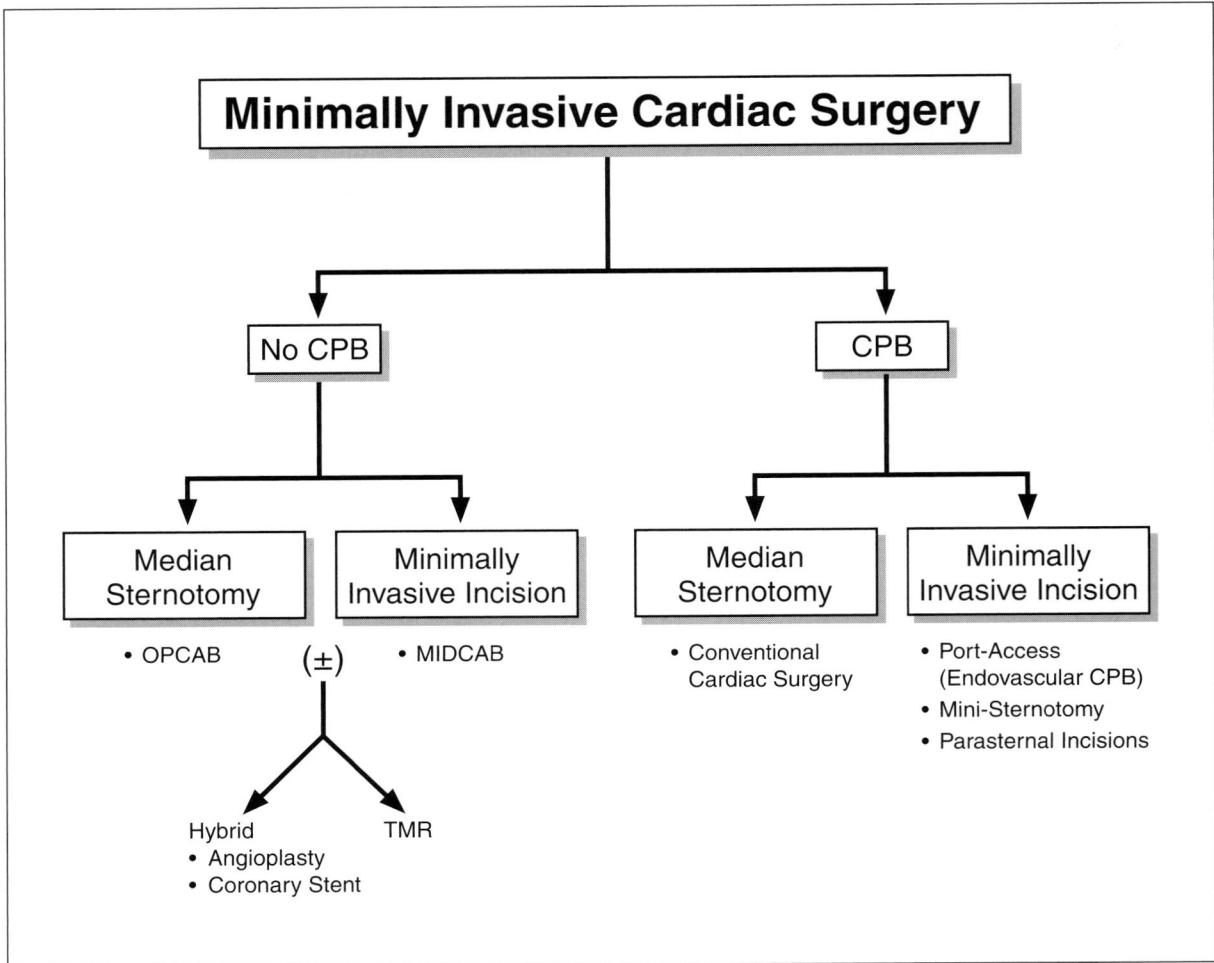

Figure 6.2-1. Variations in coronary artery bypass and valvular heart surgery, with minimally invasive techniques. CPB = cardiopulmonary bypass. OPCAB = off-pump coronary artery bypass. MIDCAB = minimally invasive direct coronary artery bypass. TMR = transmyocardial revascularization. (Redrawn with permission from Estafanous FG, Barash PG, Reves JG: *Cardiac Anesthesia: Principles and Clinical Practice*, 2nd edition. Lippincott Williams & Wilkins, 2001.)

Table 6.2-1. Common Abbreviations Used in Minimally Invasive Cardiac Surgery

Abbreviation	Definition
MICS	Minimally invasive cardiac surgery
MICAB	Minimally invasive coronary artery bypass (includes OPCAB, MIDCAB, port-access, and mini-sternotomy techniques)
OPCAB	Off-pump coronary artery bypass ('beating heart surgery'; median sternotomy)
MIDCAB	Minimally invasive direct coronary artery bypass (direct vision, no sternotomy, CPB, or cardioplegia)
MIDCABG	Minimally invasive direct coronary artery bypass graft (same as MIDCAB)
MITACAB	Minimally invasive thoracoscopically assisted coronary artery bypass
VADCAB	Video-assisted direct coronary artery bypass
LAST	Left anterior small thoracotomy
PACAB	Port-access coronary artery bypass (also called Port-CAB, Port-CABG)

PORT-ACCESS CORONARY REVASCULARIZATION

SURGICAL CONSIDERATIONS

Description: Advances in videoscopic technology have led to less invasive approaches in the treatment of many general and thoracic surgical disorders. The development of less invasive surgery has resulted in alternative and novel approaches to cardiac surgery, including **port-access cardiac surgery** and **off-pump coronary revascularization** (see p. 295). Using a port-access approach, the surgeon can perform cardiac operations (e.g., CABG) and valve surgery in a motionless, bloodless field through small chest incisions (avoiding a median sternotomy). This approach typically relies on peripheral CPB (**femoral artery and femoral vein cannulation**, Fig 6.2-2). The femoral artery is cannulated with a 19-23 Fr Y-shaped cannula, which permits arterial inflow and insertion of the endoaortic clamp. Venous drainage is provided by the 22-25 Fr cannula, introduced through a femoral vein. Drainage may be augmented by 20-40%, using vacuum-assisted venous drainage or a centrifugal venous drainage pump placed between the venous cannula and the reservoir. The port-access system includes a 10.5 Fr endoaortic 'clamp' (EAC), a triple-lumen catheter with an inflatable balloon at its distal end. This clamp is positioned in the ascending aorta using fluoroscopy and TEE guidance. The lumen used for balloon inflation is connected to a manometer to monitor balloon pressure. Cardioplegic solution is delivered through a central lumen, which also acts as an aortic root vent after cardioplegia delivery. A third lumen serves as an aortic root pressure monitor. Additionally, a percutaneous PA venting catheter, placed via the jugular approach, helps in ventricular decompression. The left internal mammary artery (IMA) is harvested under direct vision (Fig 6.2-3) or with video-assisted thoracoscopy (VAT) (Fig 6.2-4). After peripheral CPB is achieved, the EAC provides aortic occlusion and cardioplegic arrest. Exposure of the lateral and posterior aspects of the heart is accomplished easily in the arrested heart, thereby permitting two- and three-vessel coronary revascularization. Notably, if the ascending aorta is accessible, a newly developed dual-armed, Y-shaped cannula can be placed directly into the ascending aorta with one arm of the cannula connected to the arterial inflow of the CPB circuit and the other arm as a conduit for introducing the EAC.

Usual preop diagnosis: CAD

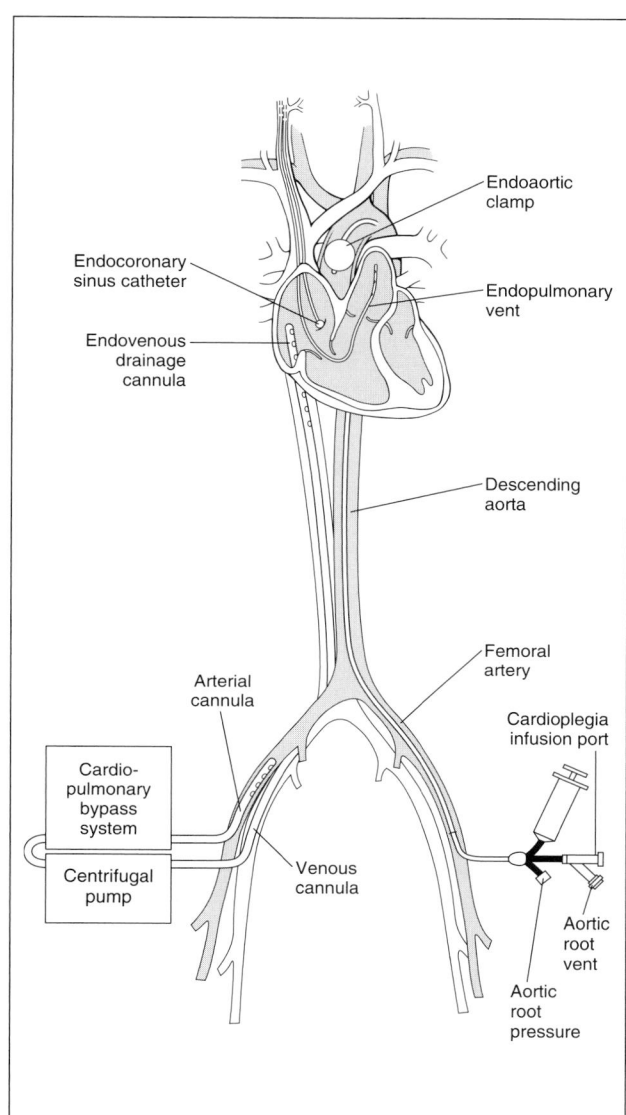

Figure 6.2-2. The port-access cardiopulmonary bypass (CPB) system. Femoro-femoral (fem-fem) CPB is utilized, and a centrifugal pump augments venous drainage. The endoaortic balloon occlusion catheter is inflated in the ascending aorta, and antegrade cardioplegia is delivered through the central lumen. The endopulmonary vent assists in ventricular decompression. (Redrawn with permission from Fann JI, et al: Port-access cardiac surgery with cardioplegic arrest. *Ann Thorac Surg* 1997; 63:S35-9.)

SUMMARY OF PROCEDURE

Position	Supine
Incision	4th interspace, left anterior thoracotomy for CABG; may need to resect 4th rib; may need thoracoscopy for IMA harvest.
Special instrumentation	TEE and fluoroscopy

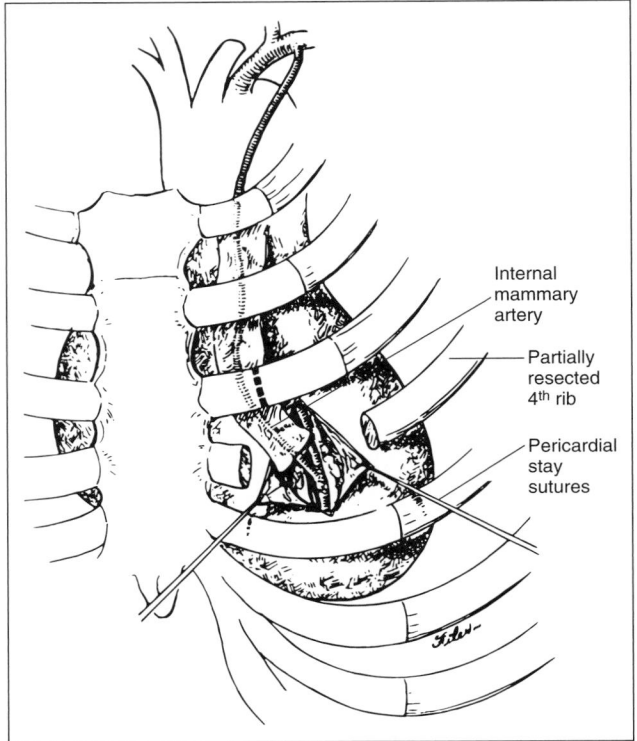

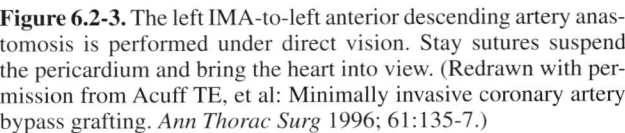

Figure 6.2-3. The left IMA-to-left anterior descending artery anastomosis is performed under direct vision. Stay sutures suspend the pericardium and bring the heart into view. (Redrawn with permission from Acuff TE, et al: Minimally invasive coronary artery bypass grafting. *Ann Thorac Surg* 1996; 61:135-7.)

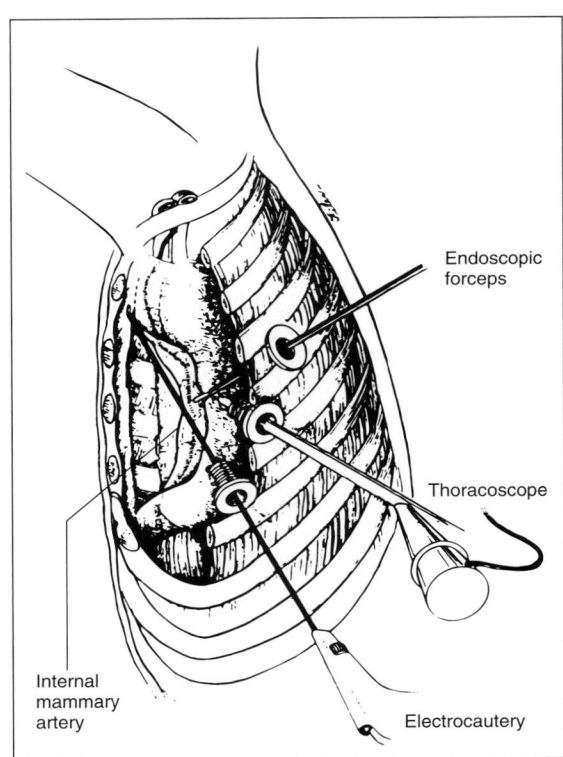

Figure 6.2-4. Dissection and harvesting of the left IMA using a thoracoscopic approach. (Redrawn with permission from Acuff TE, et al: Minimally invasive coronary artery bypass grafting. *Ann Thorac Surg* 1996; 61:135-7.)

Unique considerations	CPB used with peripheral femoral cannulation; percutaneous insertion of PA vent and retrograde cardioplegic catheter.
Antibiotics	Cefazolin 1-2 g iv at induction
Surgical time	3-5 h
Closing considerations	Assess chest wall for hemorrhage; chest tube insertion. Bupivacaine for field block.
EBL	250-500 ml
Postop care	ICU monitoring; early extubation; may require inotropic support.
Mortality	1-3%, depending on comorbidities
Morbidity	Arrhythmias (including atrial fibrillation): 10%
	Conversion to sternotomy: 4%
	MI: 0-4%
	Reoperation for bleeding: 3%
	Stroke: 2%
	Thrombosis of graft (graft failure): Rare
	Fem-fem bypass complications (e.g., arterial dissection): Rare
Pain score	1-4

PATIENT POPULATION CHARACTERISTICS

Age range	40-80 yr
Male:Female	3:2
Incidence	< 50,000/yr in U.S.
Etiology	Multifactorial for atherosclerosis
Associated conditions	LV dysfunction; COPD; PVD; HTN; diabetes mellitus; cigarette smoking

ANESTHETIC CONSIDERATIONS

See Anesthetic Considerations for Port-Access Procedures, p. 301.

References

1. Dogan S, Graubitz K, Aybek T, Khan MF, Kessler P, Moritz A, Wimmer-Greinecker G: How safe is the port access technique in minimally invasive coronary artery bypass grafting? *Ann Thorac Surg* 2002; 74:1537-43.
2. Fann JI, Pompili MF, Stevens JH, Siegel LC, StGoar FG, Burdon TA, Reitz BA: Port-access cardiac surgery with cardioplegic arrest. *Ann Thorac Surg* 1997; 63:S35-9.
3. Groh MA, Sutherland SE, Burton HG 3rd, Johnson AM, Ely SW: Port-access coronary artery bypass grafting: technique and comparative results. *Ann Thorac Surg* 1999; 68:1506-8.
4. Grossi EA, Groh MA, Lefrak EA, Ribakove GH, Albus RA, Galloway AC, Colvin SB: Results of a prospective multicenter study on port-access coronary bypass grafting. *Ann Thorac Surg* 1999; 68:1475-7.
5. Stevens JH, Burdon TA, Peters WS, Siegel LC , Pompili MF, Vierra MA, StGoar FG, Ribakove GH, Mitchell RS, Reitz BA: Port-access coronary artery bypass grafting: A proposed surgical method. *J Thorac Cardiovasc Surg* 1996; 111:567-73.

Also see references for Port-Access Procedures, pp. 305-306.

OFF-PUMP AND MINIMALLY INVASIVE CORONARY ARTERY BYPASS GRAFTING

SURGICAL CONSIDERATIONS

Description: Although coronary artery bypass grafting (CABG) without CPB was originally proposed more than 5 decades ago, development and advances in CPB resulted in the abandonment of off-pump cardiac surgery by most cardiac centers until the 1990s. The resurgence of **off-pump coronary revascularization** was due in part to reported adverse effects of CPB, increased comorbidities in an aging population, medical economics, and the development of mechanical stabilization devices (Fig 6.2-5). From the standpoint of terminology, **off-pump coronary artery bypass grafting** (**OPCAB**), applies to all cases of coronary revascularization not using the CPB circuit; and, while it does not refer directly to the surgical approach, most are via conventional median sternotomy. **Minimally invasive direct coronary artery bypass grafting** (**MIDCAB**) refers to off-pump coronary revascularization via a small anterolateral thoracotomy incision. Challenges of off-pump coronary revascularization include accurate vascular anastomosis, while minimizing hemodynamic perturbations during the procedure. Interrupting flow to the target artery can → regional ischemia, arrhythmias, and hemodynamic instability; displacing the heart to expose lateral or posterior arteries may → ventricular compression and profound hemodynamic compromise. Pharmacologic interventions to decrease HR and ischemic preconditioning may facilitate the anastomosis. Though not fully defined, ischemic preconditioning results

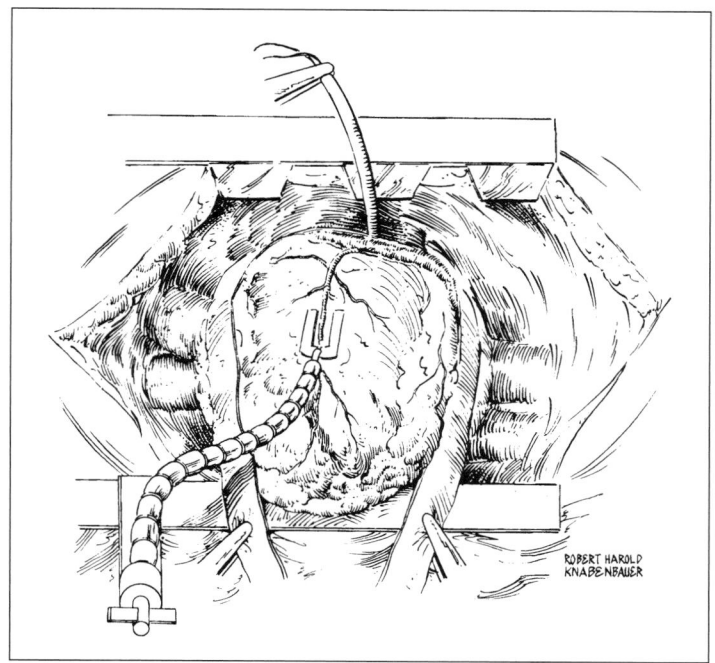

Figure 6.2-5. Manipulation of the heart and placement of a pressure-plate mechanical stabilizer is performed in preparation for OPCAB. (Reproduced with permission from Estafanous FG, Barash PG, Reves JG: *Cardiac Anesthesia: Principles and Clinical Practice*, 2nd edition. Lippincott Williams & Wilkins, 2001.)

from exposure to transient myocardial ischemia and is an endogenous adaptation that may mitigate the effects of subsequent prolonged myocardial ischemia. Thus, mechanically occluding the coronary artery for a brief period may confer some protection from ischemic injury associated with coronary occlusion during the anastomosis. Important preop considerations include the number and suitability of distal-target coronary arteries, cardiac and pulmonary status, and other medical comorbidities. The presence of cardiomegaly may limit the degree of intraop cardiac manipulation. The perfusionist is present during the procedure so that rapid conversion to conventional on-pump CABG can be achieved if there is hemodynamic compromise, unsuitable distal target, inability to expose lateral or posterior target vessels, or regional myocardial ischemia.

For **OPCAB**, a standard median sternotomy is made (Fig 6.2-6). If the internal mammary artery (IMA) is to be used as a graft, it is harvested in the usual fashion. The patient is partially heparinized, and an intravenous bolus of lidocaine is given. A sternal retractor with attachments for coronary stabilization is placed (Fig 6.2-5). If vein grafts are used, the proximal anastomoses may be performed at this point or later, after the completion of the distal anastomoses, using a partial side-biting aortic cross-clamp. During the period of partial aortic clamping, BP typically is lowered to reduce potential complications associated with the use of the clamp. The goal of the operation is to establish adequate perfusion of the most critical vascular bed first. Provided it is a target vessel, the LAD artery is often approached first because an IMA graft (or vein graft) can provide immediate perfusion and requires minimal cardiac manipulation to construct the anastomosis. Mechanical coronary artery stabilizers, based on local myocardial compression (Fig 6.2-5) or vacuum suction (Fig 6.2-7) and attached to the retractor, provide stable local epicardial motion restraint, thereby facilitating the anastomosis. After stabilization, the artery is occluded (following a period of ischemic preconditioning), and an arteriotomy is made. Equipment that minimizes blood in the operative site includes standard suction attachments, temporary intracoronary shunts, vessel occluders, and 'blower-misters' that displace blood by delivering a combination of gas (CO_2) and heparinized saline. The distal anastomosis is

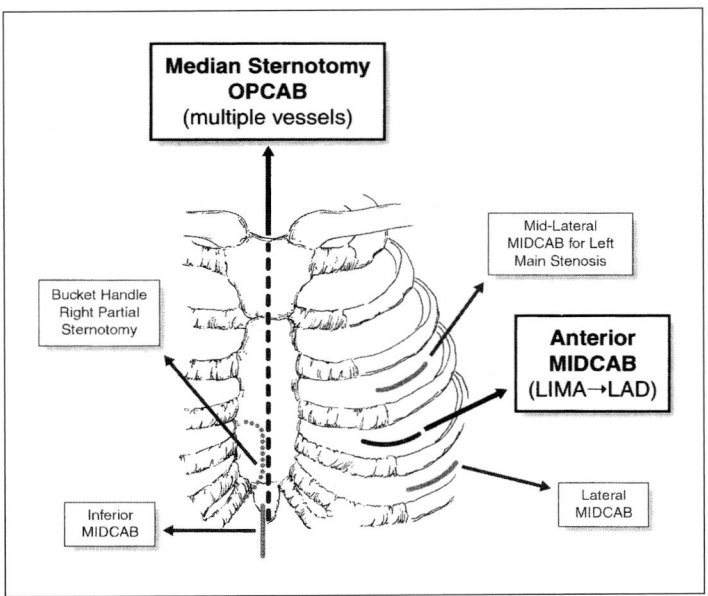

Figure 6.2-6. Incision sites for access to various target coronary arteries in MICAB. (Reproduced with permission from Estafanous FG, Barash PG, Reves JG: *Cardiac Anesthesia: Principles and Clinical Practice*, 2nd edition. Lippincott Williams & Wilkins, 2001.)

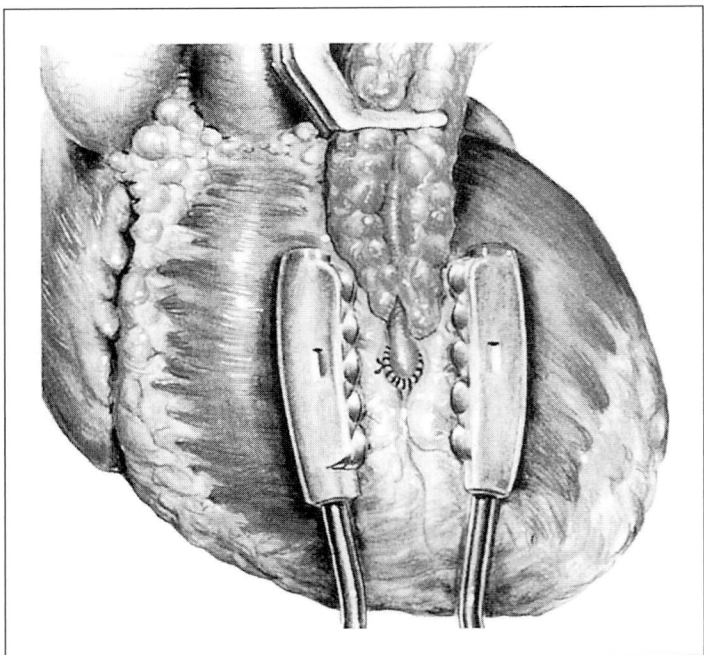

Figure 6.2-7. The Octopus 2 (Medtronic, Minneapolis MN) uses a series of suction cups on two fixed arms that adhere to the epicardial surface and reduce myocardial motion at the anastomotic site during OPCAB. (Reproduced with permission from Estafanous FG, Barash PG, Reves JG: *Cardiac Anesthesia: Principles and Clinical Practice*, 2nd edition. Lippincott Williams & Wilkins, 2001.)

then performed. The patient is monitored closely at this point for any signs of myocardial ischemia and/or hemodynamic instability. To expose the lateral and posterior target vessels, manipulation of the heart is necessary and may not be well tolerated. During lateral and posterior pericardial suture placement, the surgeon displaces and compresses the heart, result-

Figure 6.2-8. OR configuration for MICAB. (Reproduced with permission from Estafanous FG, Barash PG, Reves JG: *Cardiac Anesthesia: Principles and Clinical Practice*, 2nd edition. Lippincott Williams & Wilkins, 2001.)

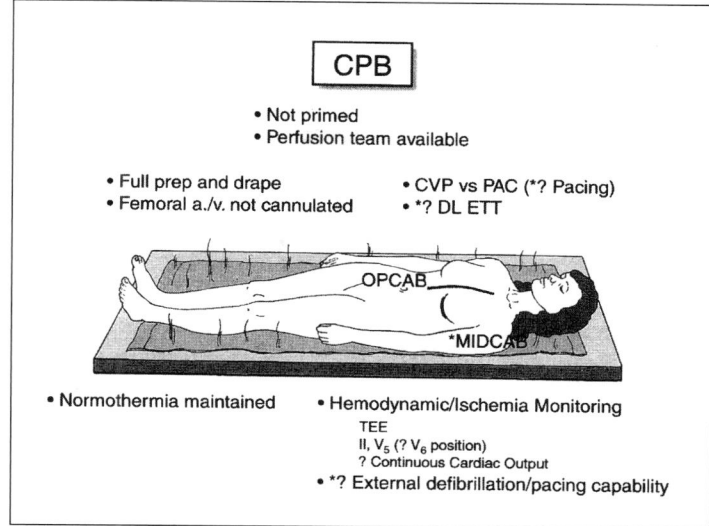

ing in temporary hemodynamic compromise. Ventilation may need to be stopped temporarily to facilitate this maneuver. Additional exposure techniques include Trendelenburg position and tilting the operating table to the right, release of right pericardial stay sutures, opening of the right pleura, incising the right pericardium, lifting of the right sternal edge to create space for the right heart, and placement of laparotomy sponges. The target vessel is stabilized again, ischemic preconditiong is carried out, and the artery is opened. After construction of the distal anastomosis, the graft is flushed to eliminate any residual air before securing the sutures and releasing the target vessel occluders. Graft flow is assessed using Doppler ultrasound.

SUMMARY OF PROCEDURE

Position	Supine (Fig 6.2-8)
Incision	Median sternotomy (OPCAB); alternatively, limited left anterolateral thoracotomy (MIDCAB) (Fig 6.2-6)
Antibiotics	Cefazolin 1 g iv
Surgical time	3-4 h
Closing considerations	No special considerations. Patients often can be intubated in OR.
EBL	200-400 ml (consider using Cell-Saver)
Postop care	ICU for cardiac monitoring ± ventilator management; less volume required than with conventional CABG.
Mortality	0-5% (higher with increasing age)
Morbidity	AF: 2-30%
	Pulmonary insufficiency: 3-5%
	Reoperation for bleeding: 1-4%
	Cardiac (e.g., myocardial infarction): 0-4%
	Mediastinal infection: 1-2%
	Neurologic (cerebrovascular accident): 1-2%
	Renal dysfunction: 1-2%
	IABP use: 0-2%
Pain score	4-6

PATIENT POPULATION CHARACTERISTICS

Age range	40 - > 90 yr
Male:Female	3:2
Incidence	150,000/yr in U.S.
Etiology	Multifactorial for atherosclerosis
Associated conditions	HTN; diabetes; PVD; COPD; cigarette smoking

ANESTHETIC CONSIDERATIONS FOR MICAB/OPCAB

PREOPERATIVE

Preop assessment is similar to that used for standard CABG patients (see p. 267). Relative contraindications for MICAB include: low EF, morbid obesity, previous cardiac surgery, AF, and COPD.

Premedication	Adequate control of preop anxiety using midazolam (titrated to effect) may reduce the dose of β-blocker required intraop for rate control.

INTRAOPERATIVE

Anesthetic technique: GETA. DLT or Univent ETT. Unlike CABG on CPB, the anesthetic demands for OPCABG are somewhat different, as CPB will not be providing hemodynamic support. Positioning of the heart for access to the target vessel, as well as mechanical stabilization of the heart to immobilize the vessel for accurate anastomosis tend to produce hemodynamic compromise. In particular, elevation of the LV apex to allow access to lateral and posterior wall vessels can limit LV filling and obstruct RV outflow tract. Additionally, ↓TV may be necessary to prevent obstruction of visualization. Snares may be placed around the coronary target vessel to create a dry operative field; however, this may provoke regional ischemia. Many of these changes are assessed by intraop TEE, and they may require resuscitative measures with volume loading and inotropic support (e.g., dobutamine). Interventions on the RCA are particularly prone to arrhythmias, and appropriate antiarrhythmics should be available. For further discussion, see Intraoperative considerations for CABG, p. 268.

Induction	As for CABG surgery (see p. 269). For MICAB, these patients will undergo a small anterior thoracotomy, and the aim is to extubate them at the end of the procedure or shortly thereafter. Thus, the dose of narcotic should be moderate (e.g., fentanyl 5-15 μg/kg). Long-acting muscle relaxants should be avoided for the same reason. Consider spinal narcotics (e.g., morphine 0.3-0.5 mg).	
Maintenance	Since early extubation is planned, volatile agents or propofol should be used and the overall dose of narcotic reduced.	
Emergence	For further discussion, see Postoperative Considerations for CABG, p. 270. If the patient is not suitable for extubation in the OR, a DLT may be exchanged for a conventional ETT (over a tube changer) before transport to ICU.	
Blood and fluid requirements	See CABG surgery (p. 269).	Without the use of CPB, hemodilution from the pump prime is avoided.
Monitoring	See CABG surgery (p. 269).	PA catheters are useful for detecting ischemia in patients with poor LV function. If a continuous CO thermodilution catheter is used, consideration must be given to the large delays in data display.
	TEE	Useful for detecting ischemia and LV dysfunction.
Special considerations	Temporary occlusion → ischemia Vessel immobilization → ↓CO Need for ↓HR	During grafting, the vessel is temporarily occluded by surgeon to avoid flooding the field with blood. The myocardium distal to this may become ischemic. ✓ ECG, TEE. In addition, the surgeon will place instruments to immobilize the vessel being grafted. Pressure from these instruments may impair cardiac function. TEE imaging will be affected by surgical mechanical manipulation of the heart. It may be necessary to ↓HR to facilitate the anastomosis. This is done with esmolol (titrated to effect), diltiazem (5-25 mg over 10 min), adenosine (6 mg), or a combination of these drugs.
Positioning	✓ and pad pressure points. ✓ eyes.	

POSTOPERATIVE

Complications	See CABG surgery (p. 270). Premature extubation	
Pain management	Same as CABG surgery (p. 270).	Intrathecal narcotics or intercostal blocks placed at the end of surgery may aid in early extubation.
Tests	See CABG surgery (p. 270).	

References – Surgeon's

1. Baumgartner FJ, Gheissari A, Capouya ER, et al: Technical aspects of total revascularization in off-pump coronary bypass via sternotomy approach. *Ann Thorac Surg* 1999; 67:1653-8.

2. Calafiore AM, Di Giammarco G, Teodori G, et al: Midterm results after minimally invasive coronary surgery (LAST operation). *J Thorac Cardiovasc Surg* 1998; 115:763-71.

3. Cartier R, Brann S, Dagenais F, et al: Systematic off-pump coronary artery revascularization in multivessel disease: Experience of three hundred cases. *J Thorac Cardiovasc Surg* 2000; 119:221-9.

4. Hirose H, Amano A, Takahashi A: Off-pump coronary artery bypass grafting for elderly patients. *Ann Thorac Surg* 2001; 72:2013-9.

5. Lund O, Christensen J, Holme S, et al: On-pump versus off-pump coronary artery bypass: Independent risk factors and off-pump graft patency. *Eur J Cardiothorac Surg* 2001; 20:901-7.

6. Mack M, Bachand D, Acuff T, et al: Improved outcomes in coronary artery bypass grafting with beating-heart techniques. *J Thorac Surg* 2002; 124:598-607.

7. Novitsky D, Bowen TE, Larsen A, et al: Aiming towards complete myocardial revascularization without cardiopulmonary bypass: A systematic approach. *Heart Surg Forum* 2002; 5:214-20.

8. Plomondon ME, Cleveland JC Jr, Ludwig ST, et al: Off-pump coronary artery bypass is associated with improved risk-adjusted outcomes. *Ann Thorac Surg* 2001; 72:114-9.

9. Puskas JD, Thourani VH, Marshall JJ, et al: Clinical outcomes, angiographic patency, and resource utilization in 200 consecutive off-pump coronary bypass patients. *Ann Thorac Surg* 2001; 71:1477-84.

10. Sabik JF, Gillinov AM, Blackstone EH, et al: Does off-pump coronary surgery reduce morbidity and mortality? *J Thorac Cardiovasc Surg* 2002; 124:698-707.

11. Subramanian VA, McCabe JC, Geller CM: Minimally invasive direct coronary artery bypass grafting: Two-year clinical experience. *Ann Thorac Surg* 1997; 64:1648-55.

References – Anesthesiologist's

1. Arom K, Flavin T, Emery R, et al: Safety and efficacy of off-pump coronary artery bypass grafting. *Ann Thorac Surg* 2000; 69:704-10.

2. Calafiore AM, Di Giammarco G, Teodori G, et al: Midterm results after minimally invasive coronary surgery (LAST operation). *J Thorac Cardiovasc Surg* 1998; 115:763-71.

3. Diegeler A, Matin M, Kayser S, et al: Angiographic results after minimally invasive coronary bypass grafting using the minimally invasive direct coronary bypass grafting (MIDCAB) approach. *Eur J Cardiothoracic Surg* 1999; 15:680-4.

4. Gayes JM, Emery RW: The MIDCAB experience: A current look at evolving surgical and anesthetic approaches. *J Cardiothorac Vasc Anesth* 1997; 11:625-8.

5. Gayes JM, Emery RW, Nissen M: Anesthetic considerations for patients undergoing minimally invasive coronary bypass surgery: ministernotomy and minithoracotomy approaches. *J Cardiothorac Vasc Anesth* 1996; 10:531-5.

6. Greenspun HG, Adourian UA, Fonger JD, Fann JS: Minimally invasive direct coronary artery bypass (MIDCAB): surgical techniques and anesthetic considerations. *J Cardiothorac Vasc Anesth* 1996; 10(4):507-9.

7. Gundry SR, Romano MA, Shattuck OH, et al: Seven-year follow-up of coronary artery bypasses performed with and without cardiopulmonary bypass. *J Thorac Cardiovasc Surg* 1998; 115:1273-8.

8. Kessler P, Neidhart G, Bremerich DH, Aybek T, Dogan S, Lischke V, Byhahn C: High thoracic epidural anesthesia for coronary artery bypass grafting using two different surgical approaches in conscious patients. *Anesth Analg* 2002; 95:791-7.

9. Mack MJ, Magovern JA, Acuff TA, et al: Results of graft patency by immediate angiography in minimally invasive coronary artery surgery. *Ann Thorac Surg* 1999; 68:383-90.

10. Maslow AD, Park KW, Pawlowski J, Haering JM. Cohn WE: Minimally invasive direct coronary artery bypass grafting: changes in anesthetic management and surgical procedure. *J Cardiothorac Vasc Anesth* 1999; 13:417-23.

11. Nierich AP, Diephuis J, Jansen EWL, et al: Embracing the heart: Perioperative management of patients undergoing off-pump coronary artery bypass grafting using the Octopus tissue stabilizer. *J Cardiothorac Vasc Anesth* 1999; 13:123-9.

12. Pfister AJ, Zaki MS, Garcia JM, et al: Cornary artery bypass without cardiopulmonary bypass. *Ann Thorac Surg* 1992; 54:1085-91.

13. Place DG, Peragallo RA, Carroll J, Cusimano RJ, Cheng DC: Postoperative atrial fibrillation: a comparision of off-pump coronary artery bypass surgery and conventional coronary artery bypass graft surgery. *J Cardiothorac Vasc Anesth* 2002; 16:144-8

14. Roosens C, Heerman J, De Somer F, Caes F, Van Belleghem Y, Poelaert JI: Effects of off-pump coronary surgery on the mechanics of the respiratory system, lung, and chest wall: Comparison with extracorporeal circulation. *Crit Care Med* 2002; 30:2430-7.

15. Siegel LC, Hennessy MM, Pearl RG: Delayed time response of the continuous cardiac output pulmonary artery catheter. *Anesth Analg* 1996; 83:1173-7.

16. Straka Z, Brucek P, Vanek T, Votava J, Widimsky P: Routine immediate extubation for off-pump coronary artery bypass grafting without thoracic epidural analgesia. *Ann Thorac Surg* 2002; 74:1544-7.

17. Tasdemir O, Vural KM, Karagoz H, et al: Coronary artery bypass grafting on the beating heart without the use of extracorporeal circulation: Review of 2052 cases. *J Thorac Cardiovasc Surg* 1998; 116:68-73.

LIMITED THORACOTOMY AND PORT-ACCESS
APPROACH TO MITRAL VALVE SURGERY

SURGICAL CONSIDERATIONS

Description: Although the field of mitral valve surgery has seen marked advances in biomaterials and innovative repair techniques since the early 1960s, the **conventional median sternotomy approach** to access and expose the mitral valve has not changed substantially. Because of the progress in video-assisted surgery, a less invasive approach to cardiac surgery has been proposed, and various techniques of mitral valve surgery through **limited thoracotomy** or **upper sternotomy** incisions and a **port-access technique** to achieve cardioplegic arrest are now used in the clinical setting.

Limited thoracotomy: The right thoracotomy incision is a less invasive approach (compared to median sternotomy) for mitral valve procedures (Fig 6.2-9). Utilizing hypothermic fibrillatory or cardioplegic arrest, the mitral valve, annulus, and subvalvular apparatus can be visualized directly and the valve procedure carried out. The addition of video-assisted thoracoscopy (VAT) to mitral valve surgery has resulted in even smaller thoracotomy incisions for these procedures.

Chitwood, et al, reported a **'micro-mitral' approach** to mitral valve replacement, using VAT through a limited thoracotomy. Peripheral cardiopulmonary bypass (fem-fem) is used, and a catheter is placed in the coronary sinus for retrograde cardioplegia delivery. An external aortic cross-clamp is introduced through a separate incision in the chest.

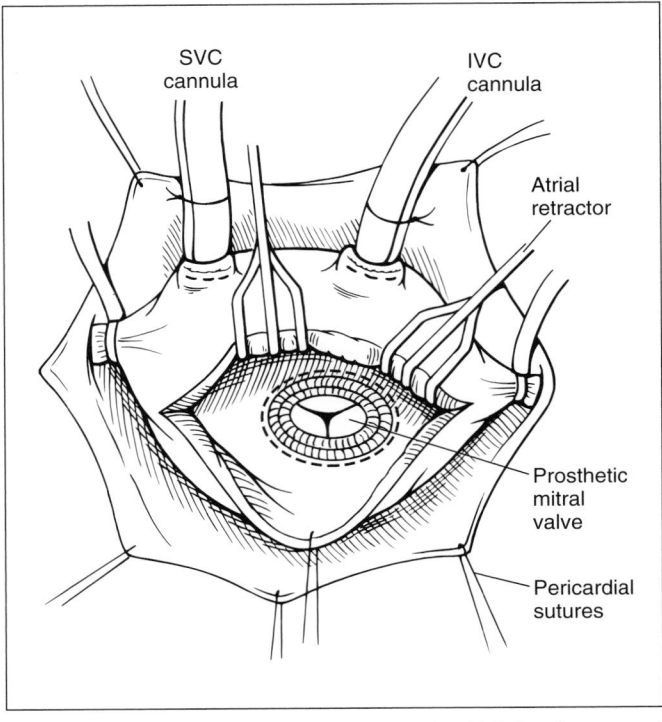

Figure 6.2-9. The right thoracotomy approach with left atriotomy and exposure of the mitral valve area with prosthetic valve in place. (Reproduced with permission from Tribble, et al: Anterolateral thoracotomy as an alternative to repeat median sternotomy for replacement of the mitral valve. *Ann Thorac Surg* 1987; 43:380-2.)

After achieving cardioplegic arrest, the mitral valve is replaced with thoracoscopic assistance. Proposed advantages of the micro-mitral approach include the avoidance of a sternotomy, with decreased chest-wall trauma and patient discomfort.

Arom and Emery have described an alternative **partial sternotomy approach** to mitral and aortic valve surgery. The 7-cm partial sternotomy permits aortic and right atrial cannulation for CPB. The external aortic cross-clamp is positioned and a left ventricular vent is placed through the right superior pulmonary vein. Mitral valve exposure is achieved through the dome of the left atrium.

Port-access mitral valve surgery: The port-access system has been used successfully in mitral valve surgery. To facilitate dissection and to provide adequate exposure of the left atrium, DLT intubation for OLV is used. Under fluoroscopic and TEE guidance, a retrograde cardioplegia catheter is directed into the coronary sinus via an introducer placed in the jugular vein; a PA-venting catheter is inserted through another jugular vein introducer. A limited right thoracotomy is made, with or without dividing the fourth rib, followed by the placement of a soft-tissue retractor. A separate port is placed in the 6th interspace for introduction of a thoracoscope, if necessary. The pericardium is opened anterior to the phrenic nerve. After systemic heparinization, the femoral artery and vein are cannulated. The endoaortic clamp is introduced through the side limb of the femoral arterial cannula and its tip positioned in the ascending aorta. CPB is initiated and systemic hypothermia achieved. The balloon of the endoaortic clamp is inflated, achieving effective aortic occlusion. Cold blood cardioplegia is delivered using the distal port of the endoaortic clamp; retrograde cardioplegia is administered via the coronary sinus catheter. A left atriotomy is made, and an atrial retractor is placed through a separate port. Valve repair or replacement is carried out using specially designed instruments. Before completion of atriotomy closure, deairing maneuvers are accomplished. These include temporarily discontinuing pulmonary and aortic root venting, inflating the lungs to displace residual air, and increasing the patient's blood volume from the venous reservoir. Also, the patient is placed in a Trendelenburg and left lateral decubitus position for further deairing. The balloon of the endoaortic catheter is deflated, and the catheter is left in place for further deairing through the aortic vent lumen. Temporary ventricular pacing wires are placed. After being weaned from CPB, the patient is decannulated and the anticoagulation reversed.

The overall safety and efficacy of less invasive mitral valve surgery await long-term evaluations and followup.

Usual preop diagnosis: Mitral valve disease

SUMMARY OF PROCEDURES

	Port-Access	Limited Thoracotomy
Position	Supine, with right side slightly elevated	⇐
Incision	4th interspace right thoracotomy; ports for possible thoracoscopy; port for atrial retractor.	⇐ ± port for aortic cross-clamp
Special instrumentation	Specially designed retractors; TEE and fluoroscopy for guiding placement of endopulmonary vent, retrograde cardioplegia catheter, and endoaortic clamp	Specially designed instruments ± thorascopic instruments
Unique considerations	CPB is achieved with peripheral femoral cannulation; placement of endopulmonary vent; placement of retrograde cardioplegia catheter; may require conversion to open procedure.	CPB via femoral artery and vein
Antibiotics	Cefazolin 1-2 g iv at induction	⇐
Surgical time	3-5 h	⇐
Closing considerations	Assess chest wall for hemorrhage.	⇐
EBL	250-500 ml	⇐
Postop care	ICU monitoring; early extubation; may require inotropic support.	⇐
Mortality	1-6%, depending on comorbidities (lower for mitral valve repairs).	⇐
Morbidity	AF: 10-20%	⇐
	Chest-wall hemorrhage: 2-9%	–
	Stroke: 1-3%	–
	Conversion to sternotomy: 2%	–
	Vascular injury: Rare	–
	Pneumonia	⇐
	Renal failure	–
Pain score	1-4	4-7

PATIENT POPULATION CHARACTERISTICS

Age range	40-70 yr
Male:Female	1:1
Incidence	< 20,000/yr in U.S.
Etiology	Myxomatous mitral valve; rheumatic valve disease; endocarditis; ischemic (papillary muscle dysfunction); mitral annular calcification
Associated conditions	Pulmonary HTN; atrial arrhythmias; CAD; aortic valve disease; tricuspid regurgitation

ANESTHETIC CONSIDERATIONS FOR PORT-ACCESS PROCEDURES

PREOPERATIVE

As with all anesthetic procedures, the use of the port-access system should not be attempted without appropriate training. Catheter placement and monitoring relies on TEE and/or fluoroscopy. The evaluation of the patient for port-access cardiac surgery should parallel that of patients having conventional cardiac surgery. (For mitral valve surgery, see p. 277; for CABG surgery, see p. 267.) There are, however, a number of specific conditions which preclude the use of the port-access system:

1. Aortic regurgitation (AR): While mild-to-moderate AR is not a contraindication, it may make the delivery of antegrade cardioplegia via the endoaortic clamp catheter (EAC) problematic; therefore, insertion of the endocoronary sinus catheter (ESC) is very important. Severe AR is a contraindication.

2. Atherosclerotic disease of the aorta: Perfusion may be associated with embolization of atheromatous plaques (particularly pedunculated lesions).

3. PVD: Femoral bypass may be associated with retrograde arterial dissection. PVD and tortuous femoral and iliac vessels are contraindications to use of femoral arterial cannulation.

4. Thoracic aortic aneurysm/Marfan syndrome: Port-access procedures require passage of the EAC into the thoracic aorta and inflation of the EAC balloon; therefore, aneurysms or a weakened aortic wall are contraindications.

5. Scarring of the pleural cavity (e.g., chest trauma, previous thoracotomy) may make surgical access difficult.

6. Inability to obtain TEE or fluoroscope imaging, since monitoring and placement of catheters relies on imaging.

Preop evaluation should focus on the underlying pathophysiology (valvular disease vs CAD). In addition, the following aspects should be considered:

Respiratory	OLV is used to facilitate surgical exposure; thus, evaluation of patients with severe lung disease may include CXR, ABG, PFTs (see Thoracic Surgery, p. 213-214).
Cardiovascular	The vascular system should be evaluated with respect to insertion of the catheters and cannulae for endovascular CPB. Severity of arterial occlusive or atherosclerotic disease should be evaluated (embolization/dissection risk). The possible presence of a persistent left SVC should be considered. **Tests:** CXR; aortography; iliofemoral arteriography; vascular MRI/MRA; vascular ultrasound; TEE
Premedication	As for the underlying condition. Usually, a mild anxiolytic (e.g., midazolam 1-3 mg iv) is sufficient.

INTRAOPERATIVE

Anesthetic technique: GETA (DLT or BB). Anesthetic technique depends on the underlying pathophysiology (e.g., valvular disease vs CAD). Early extubation and postop pain relief can be facilitated by using intrathecal narcotics (e.g., Duramorph 10 μg/kg intrathecal) injected before induction.

Induction	Typically, induction can be accomplished with etomidate (0.1-0.3 mg/kg), propofol (0.5-2 mg/kg) or STP (2-4 mg/kg), with fentanyl (5-20 μg/kg) and pancuronium or vecuronium (0.1 mg/kg). The overall length of port-access procedures is similar to or slightly longer than conventional approaches, so that a long-acting muscle relaxant can be used. Intubation is accomplished with a DLT, and its placement is checked by auscultation or bronchoscopy.
Maintenance	With the goal of early extubation, it is important to avoid oversedation. The use of volatile agents or a propofol infusion (25-100 μg/kg/min) before, during, and after CPB will facilitate early extubation. During dissection of the IMA or exposure of the left atrium, OLV is needed.
Emergence	At the end of the procedure, intercostal blocks with ropivacaine or bupivacaine may be placed, and infiltration of the skin incision also may be helpful. Extubation in the OR may be appropriate for stable patients. Alternatively, the patient may be transported to ICU and ventilated. The DLT may be exchanged for a single-lumen tube when postop mechanical ventilation is required.
Special considerations: Placement/ monitoring of endocardio-pulmonary system	The port-access system consists of CPB with venous drainage via an endovenous drain (EVD) and an aortic or femoral arterial return cannula, which is Y-ed to accept the EAC. These are placed by the surgeon with the aid of fluoroscopy and/or TEE. Additional drainage of the right side of the heart is accomplished via an endopulmonary vent (EPV) placed by the anesthesiologist. Immediately after intubation and before CVP insertion, a TEE exam should be performed to exclude any contraindication to endo-CPB (e.g., severe AR, aortic atheromatous disease, aortic aneurysm); the size of the ascending aorta should be measured (aids the surgeon in inflation of the aortic balloon); and the coronary sinus should be identified to aid placement of the ESC (coronary sinus catheter). The right IJ vein is then cannulated with 2 sheaths (9 Fr for EPV and 11 Fr for the ESC). Cardioplegia is delivered in an anterograde fashion via the EAC or retrograde via an ESC, also placed by the anesthesiologist (Fig. 6.2-2).
Placement of ESC	The ESC can be placed with fluoroscopy and/or TEE. The coronary sinus is identified on TEE (transverse view of the right atrium or longitudinal bicaval view). Prior to placement, the patient should be partially anticoagulated with 70 U/kg of heparin. The ESC is placed through the 11 Fr sheath. Once the tip of the catheter engages the coronary sinus, the catheter is advanced either directly or over a guiding wire until the occlusion balloon is 2-4 cm inside the sinus. Position is

Placement of ESC, cont.	confirmed by inflating the balloon and obtaining ventricularization of the pressure tracing. Careful note should be taken of the volume of fluid required to occlude the coronary sinus (1-2 ml) so that overinflation and possible coronary sinus trauma do not occur. Contrast injection will define the correct positioning of the ESC in the coronary sinus. Care should be taken to avoid injecting contrast too quickly, thus pushing the ESC out of the coronary sinus. A time limit (20-30 min) should be set to pass this catheter, as repeated attempts increase the risk of cardiac injury (e.g., cardiac perforation).
Placement of EPV	The EPV (pulmonary vent) is positioned by advancing the catheter, using balloon flotation with pressure monitoring (as with a Swan-Ganz catheter). Fluoroscopy and/or TEE also may be used.
Placement of EVD	The EVD (venous drain) cannula is placed via the femoral vein into the right atrium over a guide wire. Fluoroscopy or TEE is used to ensure that the wire enters the SVC before advancing the EVD into position. The tip of the EVD should be at the SVC/RA junction or just inside the SVC.
Placement of arterial cannula	The aorta may be cannulated with a 'Y' cannula with an incising introducer. For femoral arterial cannulation, a guide wire is advanced under fluoroscopy and no resistance to its passage should be felt. The guide wire is advanced into the descending aorta and its intraluminal position confirmed on TEE prior to advancing the aortic return cannulation into its final position. The perfusionist should confirm normal line pressures with a test bolus of fluid and ✓ that normal arterial pulsation is present. These precautions will decrease the likelihood of arterial dissection.
Placement of EAC	The EAC (endoaortic clamp) may be advanced via the 'Y' arterial cannula. For a femoral arterial cannula, the EAC is advanced over a guide wire with imaging into the ascending aorta so that the tip of the catheter is just proximal to the sinotubular ridge (2-3 cm above the aortic valve). Position is confirmed by contrast injection and/or TEE. It is also useful to identify the takeoff of the innominate artery in relation to the balloon. Migration of the balloon proximally or distally can occur and, thus, its position needs to be monitored. Monitoring of the pressure in the aortic root via this catheter should show that the mean aortic root pressure is the same as mean radial artery pressure prior to the initiation of bypass.
Sequence of events during endo-CPB	After initiation of bypass, the anesthesiologist should observe the descending aorta to exclude aortic dissection and open the EPV to allow venting. EPV pressures during bypass should be negative (positive pressures may indicate inadequate decompression of the heart or kinking of the EPV). Once adequate CPB is established and the heart is drained, the EAC balloon can be inflated (balloon pressure = 250-350 mmHg). Occlusion of the aorta is confirmed by a differential between the radial and aortic root pressures and by an aortic root contrast injection. Antegrade cardioplegia is delivered via the EAC with careful monitoring to ensure that the balloon is not displaced distally, thus occluding the innominate artery (see Monitoring of endo-CPB: regional perfusion, below). After cardioplegic arrest, retrograde cardioplegia may be delivered via the ESC, and the left side of the heart may be vented via the EAC. Avoid overventing, high systemic pressures, or high CPB flow, which could displace the EAC toward the aortic valve. Initiation of retrograde cardioplegia should begin with a low flow to avoid displacing the ESC, followed by inflation of the ESC balloon until the pressure in the coronary sinus just starts to rise, indicating coronary sinus occlusion. No further inflation of the balloon should take place. Normal coronary sinus perfusion pressure is < 40 mmHg. After retrograde cardioplegia is delivered, the ESC balloon is deflated. Once the surgery is completed, the EAC balloon is deflated (after deairing procedures, as needed); the heart is reperfused; and the EAC is removed. Prior to weaning from CPB, mobility of the ESC and EPV should be assessed in mitral procedures to ensure that they have not been incorporated in the atrial suture line. Weaning from bypass is routine. The ESC should be removed prior to heparin reversal and the EPV can be replaced with a pulmonary artery catheter, if needed.

Blood and fluid requirements	As for underlying condition:
	  For mitral valve surgery, see
	  p. 275+.
	  For CABG, see p. 266+.

Monitoring	As for underlying condition: Special monitoring considerations for port-access are dis-
	  For mitral valve surgery, see cussed below. External defibrillator pads should be placed
	  p. 278. on all patients.
	  For CABG, see p. 269.

Positioning	Supine Roll under left chest for CABG and under right chest for mitral valve.	
Monitoring of endo-CPB	Regional perfusion	Distal migration of the EAC (innominate artery occlusion →↓cerebral blood flow) is possible, especially while cardioplegia is being delivered when pressure in the aortic root exceeds that in the systemic arterial system. Monitoring for regional perfusion includes: (1) Right-sided arterial pressure—radial, brachial, or axillary. The pump-induced artifact may be of use if roller heads are being used. (2) Bilateral arterial lines—right-sided, plus a second line in the left radial or in the femoral vessels to allow comparison. (3) TEE—EAC visible in the ascending aorta proximal to the innominate artery. (4) Transcranial or carotid artery Doppler. (5) Fluoroscopy
	Proximal EAC balloon migration	Most likely to occur during aortic root venting when the systemic pressure exceeds aortic root pressure. Monitored by TEE.
	Cardiac decompression	TEE can be useful in monitoring for adequate decompression of the heart.
	EAC balloon pressure	This is usually monitored by the perfusionist and ranges from 250-550 mmHg. Decreases in pressure may be 2° proximal migration of the balloon into a wider area of the ascending aorta, rupture of the balloon, or prolapse into the left ventricle. Loss of balloon occlusion is indicated by blood in the surgical field, return of cardiac activity, cardiac distension, increased root venting, and TEE evidence.
	Aortic root pressure	< 80 mmHg while giving cardioplegia; 0-10 mmHg, during venting. Overventing should be avoided, as should venting when the left side of the heart is open, to avoid drawing air into the aortic root.
	Intracardiac air	TEE is very useful for determining that adequate deairing of the heart has occurred.
Complications of endo-CPB	Retrograde aortic dissection Coronary sinus damage EAC balloon migration EAC balloon rupture Retained EPV in atrial suture line Chest-wall hemorrhage Limb ischemia	 Especially 2° sutures placed in the mitral valve annulus. It is important that the surgeon ✓ the chest wall before closure. May follow femoral cannulation.

POSTOPERATIVE

Complications	As for the primary procedure Low CO Chest-wall hemorrhage Problems associated with peripheral cannulation (e.g., dissection, embolization) Perivalvular leak Heart block	See mitral valve surgery (p. 278) or CABG (p. 270).

Pain management	Parenteral narcotics	Pain control is important to facilitate early extubation. Intrathecal narcotics and/or intercostal blocks with wound infiltration may be useful.
	NSAIDs	
Tests	ECG	
	Electrolytes	
	ABG	

References for Port-Access Procedures–Surgeon's

1. Arom KV, Emery RW: Minimally invasive mitral operations (let). *Ann Thorac Surg* 1997; 63:1219-20.
2. Chaney MA, Durazo-Arvizu RA, Fluder EM, Sawicki KJ, Nikolov MP, Blakeman BP, Bakhos M: Port-access minimally invasive cardiac surgery increases surgical complexity, increases operating room time, and facilitates early postoperative hospital discharge. *Anesthesiology* 2000; 92:1637-45.
3. Chitwood WR, Elbeery JR, Chapman WHH, Moran JM, Lust RL, Wooden WA, Deaton DH: Video-assisted minimally invasive mitral valve surgery: The "micro-mitral" operation. *J Thorac Cardiovasc Surg* 1997; 113:413-4.
4. Dogan S, Aybek T, Andressen E, Byhahn C, Mierdl S, Westphal K, Matheis G, Mortia A, Wimmer-Greinecker G: Totally endoscopic coronary artery bypass grafting on cardiopulmonary bypass with robotically enhanced telemanipulation: report of forty-five cases. *J Thorac Cardiovasc Surg* 2002; 123:1029-30.
5. Fann JI, Pompili MF, Burdon TA, Stevens JH, StGoar FG, Reitz BA: Minimally invasive mitral valve surgery. *Semin Thorac Cardiovasc Surg* 1997; 9(4):320-30.
6. Glower DD, Siegel LC, Frisshmeyer KJ, Galloway AC, Ribakove GH, Grossi EA, Robinson NB, Ryan WH, Colvin SB: Predictors of outcome in a multicenter port-access valve registry. *Ann Thorac Surg* 2000; 70:1054-9.
7. Groh MA, Sutherland SE, Burton HG, Johnson AM, Ely SW: Port-access coronary artery bypass grafting: Technique and comparative results. *Ann Thorac Surg* 1999; 68:1506-8.
8. Grossi EA, Galloway AC, LaPietra A, Ribakove GH, Ursomanno P, Delianides J, Culliford AT, Bizekis C, Esposito RA, Baumann FG, Kanchuger MS, Colvin SB: Minimally invasive mitral valve surgery: a 6-year experience with 714 patients. *Ann Thorac Surg* 2002; 74:660-4.
9. Schroeyers P, Wellens F, DeGeest R, Degrieck I, VanPraet F, Vermeulen Y, Vanerman H: Minimally invasive video-assisted mitral valve surgery: Our lessons after a 4-year experience. *Ann Thorac Surg* 2001; 72:S-1050-4.
10. Stevens JH, Burdon TA, Peters WS, Siegel LC , Pompili MF, Vierra MA, StGoar FG, Ribakove GH, Mitchell RS, Reitz BA: Port-access coronary artery bypass grafting: A proposed surgical method. *J Thorac Cardiovasc Surg* 1996; 111:567-73.

References for Port-Access Procedures–Anesthesiologist's

1. Applebaum RM, Colvin SB, Galloway AC, Ribakove GH, Grossi EA, Tunick PA, Kronzon IK: The role of transesophageal echocardiography during port-acess minimally invasive cardiac surgery: A new challenge for the echocardiographer. *Echocardiography* 1999; 16:595-602.
2. Burfeind WR, Glower DD, Davis RD, Landolfo KP, Lowe JE, Wolfe G: Mitral surgery after prior cardiac operation: port-access versus sternotomy or thoracotomy. *Ann Thor Surg* 2002; 74:S1323-5.
3. Clements F, Wright S, deBruijn NP: Coronary sinus catheterization made easy for port-access minimally invasive cardiac surgery. *J Cardiothorac Vasc Anesth* 1998; 12:96-101.
4. Galloway AC, Shemin RJ, Glower DD, Boyer JH, Groh MA, Kuntz RE, Burdon TA, Ribakove GH, Reitz BA, Colvin SB: First report of the port-access international registry: *Ann Thorac Surg* 1999; 67:51-8.
5. Glower DD, Komtebedde J, Clements FM, deBruijn NP, Stafford-Smith M, Newman MF: Direct aortic cannulation for port-access mitral or coronary artery bypass grafting. *Ann Thorac Surg* 1999; 68:1878-80.
6. Glower DD, Landolfo K, Clements F, deBruijn NP, Stafford-Smith M, Smith PK, Duhaylongsod F: Mitral valve operation via port access versus median sternotomy. *Eur J Cardiothorac Surg* 1998; 14:S143-7.
7. Glower DD, Siegel LC, Galloway AC, Ribakove G, Grossi E, Robinson N, Ryan WH, Colvin S, Shemin R: Predictors of operative time in multicenter port-access valve registry: institutional differences in learning. *Heart Surg Forum* 2001; 4: 40-6.
8. Grocott HP, Stafford-Smith M, Glower DD, Clements F: Endovascular aortic balloon clamp malposition during minimally invasive cardiac surgery: detection by transcranial Doppler monitoring. *Anesthesiology* 1998; 88:1396-9.
9. Grossi EA, Zakow PK, Ribakove GH, Kallenbach K, Ursomano P, Gradek CE, Baumann FG, Colvin SB, Galloway AC: Comparison of post-operative pain, stress response, and quality of life in port access vs. standard sternotomy coronary bypass patients. *Euro J Cardiothorac Surg* 1999; 16(Suppl 2):S39-42.
10. Peters WS, Siegel LC, Stevens JH, StGoar FG, Pompili MF, Burdon TA: Closed-chest cardiopulmonary bypass and cardioplegia for less invasive cardiac surgery. *Ann Thorac Surg* 1997; 63:1748-54.
11. Plotkin IM, Collard CD, Aranki SF, Rizzo RJ, Shernan SK: Percutaneous coronary sinus cannulation guided by transesophageal echocardiography. *Ann Thorac Surg* 1998; 66:2085-7.
12. Reichenspurner H, Boehm DH, Gulbins H, Schulze C, Wildhirt S, Welz A, Detter C, Reichart B: Three-dimensional video and robot-assisted port-access mitral valve operation. *Ann Thorac Surg* 2000; 69:1176-82.

13. Schwartz DS, Ribakove GH, Grossi EA, Buttenheim PA, Schwartz JD, Applebaum RM, Kronzon IK, Baumann FG, Colvin SB, Galloway AC: Minimally invasive mitral valve replacement: port-access techniques, feasibility, and myocardial functional preservation. *J Thorac Cardiovasc Surg* 1997; 113:1022-31.

14. Schwartz DS, Ribakove GH, Grossi EA, Stevens JH, Siegel LC, StGoar FG, Peters WS, McLaughlin P, Baumann FG, Colvin SB, Galloway AC: Minimally invasive cardiopulmonary bypass and cardioplegic arrest: a closed chest technique with equivalent myocardial protection. *J Thorac Cardiovasc Surg* 1996; 111:556-66.

15. Siegel LC, StGoar FG, Stevens JH, Pompili MF, Burdon TA, Reitz BA, Peters WS: Monitoring considerations for port-access cardiac surgery. *Circulation* 1997; 96:562-8.

16. Toomasian JM, Peters WS, Siegel LC, Stevens JH: Extracorporeal circulation for port-access cardiac surgery. *Perfusion* 1997;12:83-91.

Surgeons

James I. Fann, MD
R. Scott Mitchell, MD
Stephen T. Kee, MD (*Endovascular stent-grafting*)
Michael D. Dake, MD (*Endovascular stent-grafting*)

6.3 VASCULAR SURGERY

Anesthesiologist

Pieter Van der Starre, MD, PhD

CAROTID ENDARTERECTOMY (VASCULAR)

SURGICAL CONSIDERATIONS

Description: Carotid endarterectomy (CEA) is one of the most commonly performed vascular surgery procedures in the U.S. Because of presumed microemboli from stenotic/ulcerated plaques at the carotid bifurcation, CEA has been championed as an effective procedure to reduce the risk of subsequent stroke. The NASCET Collaborators determined, in a prospective, randomized, blinded trial, that CEA is more effective than medical therapy for symptomatic patients with internal carotid artery narrowing between 60-90%.[3] Symptoms are usually hemispheric (contralateral, upper or lower extremity paresis or numbness) or retinal (unilateral monocular blindness). Symptoms may be transient (TIA or reversible ischemic neurological deficit [RIND]) or permanent (CVA). The Asymptomatic Carotid Atherosclerosis Study (ACAS) has shown benefit from prophylactic CEA in asymptomatic patients with > 60% stenosis of the internal carotid artery. Although some surgeons routinely prefer local anesthesia, most prefer GA with careful hemodynamic monitoring because of the frequent concomitant CAD.

The carotid artery is approached through an oblique neck incision along the anterior border of the sternocleidomastoid muscle. After division of the common facial vein, the carotid sheath is opened and the carotid artery is exposed, avoiding injury to the phrenic, vagus, ansa hypoglossi, and hypoglossal nerves (Fig 6.3-1). After controlling the internal, external, and common carotid arteries, heparin is administered, and the internal, external, and common carotid arteries are clamped sequentially. To maintain carotid perfusion, an indwelling shunt may be utilized (Fig 6.3-2B), at the discretion of the surgeon. An endarterectomy plane is established proximally (Fig 6.3-2C), and developed distally into both the external

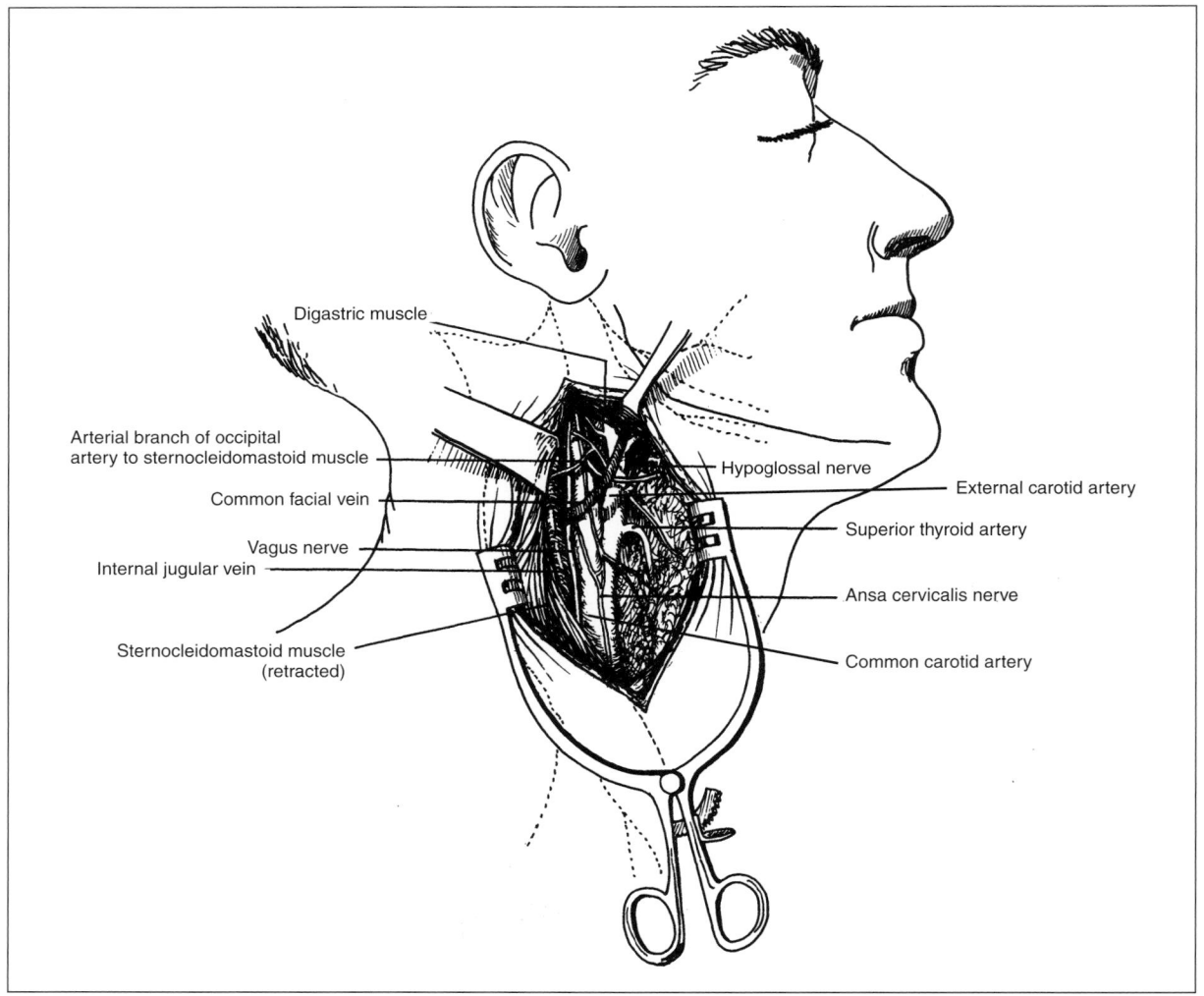

Figure 6.3-1. Exposure of the carotid bifurcation. (Reproduced with permission from Scott-Conner CEH, Dawson DL: *Operative Anatomy*, 2nd edition. Lippincott Williams & Wilkins, Philadelphia, 2003.)

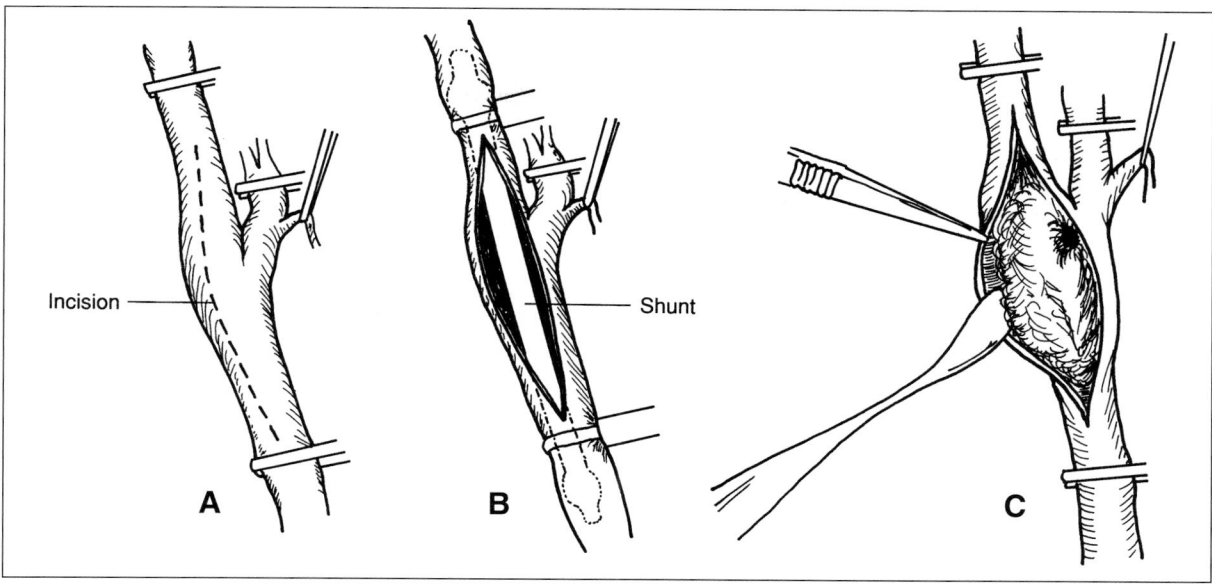

Figure 6.3-2. Carotid endarterectomy: (A) Following occlusion of the superior thyroid and internal, external, and common carotid arteries, an arteriotomy is performed opposite the external carotid take off. (B) A shunt may be placed to restore internal carotid flow. (C) Plaque is separated from the artery wall. (Reproduced with permission from Scott-Conner CEH, Dawson DL: *Operative Anatomy*, 2nd edition. Lippincott Williams & Wilkins, 2003.)

and internal branches, with establishment of a fine tapered end point. After removal of all thrombus, loose smooth-muscle fibers, and endothelium, the arteriotomy is closed, with or without a patch, the artery flushed, and flow restored. The incision is closed, after meticulous hemostasis has been assured.

Usual preop diagnosis: Carotid artery disease

SUMMARY OF PROCEDURE

Position	Supine, with neck extended and turned away from the side of the lesion
Incision	Anterior to sternocleidomastoid from earlobe to base of neck, or curvilinear in a skin crease over the carotid bifurcation
Special instrumentation	EEG monitors; ± shunt
Unique considerations	Capability to measure stump pressure may be needed. This can be accomplished by a high-pressure arterial line passed off the field to a pressure transducer. Avoid ↓BP durring carotid cross-clamping. An indwelling shunt may be utilized to restore carotid perfusion. Heparin 5,000-10,000 U 5 min prior to cross-clamping, and protamine may be given after restoration of flow.
Antibiotics	Cefazolin 1 g iv at induction of anesthesia
Surgical time	Carotid cross-clamp: 30 min Total operating time: 90 min
Closing considerations	In order to assess the patient's neurologic status, it is best to be able to awaken and extubate the patient at the conclusion of the procedure. Avoidance of HTN is also critical during this period, since the endarterectomy tissues are thin and friable.
EBL	100-200 ml
Postop care	ICU × 12-24 h; BP control; cardiac monitoring
Mortality	1%

Morbidity	MI: Major cause of postop mortality
	Cranial nerve injury (recurrent and superior laryngeal nerves): 39%
	Restenosis
	  Asymptomatic: 9-12%
	  Symptomatic: < 3%
	Neurologic complications: < 2%
	Hemorrhage: 1%
	False aneurysm: < 0.5%

Pain score	3-5

PATIENT POPULATION CHARACTERISTICS

Age range	55-80 yr
Male:Female	3:1
Incidence	Second most common vascular surgical procedure (after AAA repair)
Etiology	Arteriosclerosis; fibromuscular dysplasia
Associated conditions	Significant CAD coexists with carotid artery disease in at least 30% of patients, necessitating careful cardiac and hemodynamic monitoring.

ANESTHETIC CONSIDERATIONS

See Anesthetic Considerations for Carotid Endarterectomy (Neurosurgical) in Extracranial Procedures, p. 103.

References

1. Gates PC, Eliasziw M, Algra A, Barnett HJ, Gunton RW: Identifying patients with symptomatic carotid artery disease at high and low risk of severe myocardial infarction and cardiac death. *Stroke* 2002; 33:2413-6.
2. Moore WS, Barnett HS, Beebe HG, et al: Guidelines for carotid endarterectomy. A multidisciplinary consensus statement from the Ad Hoc Committee, American Heart Association. *Circulation* 1995; 91:566-79.
3. NASCET Collaborators: *N Engl J Med* 1991; 325:445-53.
4. Young B, Moore WS, Robertson JT, et al: An analysis of perioperative surgical mortality and morbidity in the Asymptomatic Carotid Atherosclerosis Study. ACAS Investigators. *Stroke* 1996; 27:2216-24.

REPAIR OF THORACIC AORTIC ANEURYSMS

SURGICAL CONSIDERATIONS

Description: Repairs of aneurysms of the ascending, transverse arch, and descending thoracic aorta are performed to repair expanding or leaking aneurysms or prophylactically to prevent rupture. Patients with Sx of rapid expansion or aneurysm leaking may require urgent repair. Each surgical type—ascending, arch, and descending—is considered separately, as follows. Aneurysms of the **ascending aorta** may arise 2° the degenerative changes of atherosclerosis (exacerbated by old age, HTN, tobacco use); from inborn errors of metabolism (Marfan syndrome); or from poststenotic dilatation and continued expansion of a chronic dissection. Diseases of the entire aorta, including the sinuses of Valsalva, as in Marfan syndrome and annuloaortic ectasia, require replacement of the entire aorta with a composite, valved conduit, while acquired diseases usually allow replacement of the aorta distal to the sinotubular ridge. Repair of the ascending aorta is usually accomplished on full CPB with an aortic cross-clamp placed just proximal to the innominate artery and arterial inflow through the femoral artery. The aneurysmal ascending aorta is replaced with a Dacron tube graft from the sinotubular ridge to the innominate artery. Dilatation of the sinuses of Valsalva mandates replacement with a valved conduit sewn proximally to the aortic annulus and distally to the aorta at the innominate, with coronary ostia reimplanted in the side of the tube graft.

Aneurysms of the **aortic arch** are the least common of the thoracic aorta. Because of the need for concomitant replacement of the arch vessels, however, they are the most complex to repair. Total CPB is utilized, and cerebral protection is accomplished either by CPB perfusion of one or all cerebral vessels, or by profound hypothermic circulatory arrest at 15-18°C. Repair can originate from the aortic annulus and extend distally to the mid descending thoracic aorta at the level of the carina. Routine caval cannulation is accomplished via a median sternotomy, and arterial access is gained via the femoral artery. If circulatory arrest is to be used, the patient is cooled to 15-18°C, the heart is arrested and, with no distal cross-clamp, distal anastomosis is accomplished, followed by implantation of the head vessels attached to an island of aorta. Perfusion is then reinstituted, the graft clamped proximal to the innominate artery, and the proximal anastomosis performed, while the patient is being rewarmed. Alternatively, if one elects to perfuse the cerebral vessels, the innominate and left carotid arteries can be individually cannulated and perfused via a 'Y' connection from the femoral arterial perfusion line. The necessity for profound hypothermic circulatory arrest is thus avoided. After completion of the distal aortic, arch vessel island and proximal aortic anastomoses, weaning from CPB and subsequent steps proceed in a routine fashion.

Repair of aneurysms of the **descending thoracic aorta** is usually performed for symptomatic and leaking aneurysms, enlarging aneurysms, and aneurysms of sufficient size to warrant prophylactic repair. **Aneurysm repair** is accomplished through a left posterolateral thoracotomy on partial CPB. After entry into the left thorax, venous drainage for CPB may be obtained from the PA or the femoral vein, and arterial return is via the femoral artery. If partial bypass without an oxygenator is elected, thus minimizing the amount of heparin necessary, venous access can be gained via the pulmonary veins or left atrium, and arterial return via the femoral artery or distal thoracic aorta. After institution of bypass, the aorta is cross-clamped above and below the aneurysm, the aorta is divided, a tube graft is interposed, and clamps are removed. The patient is weaned from bypass, and the operation is terminated in the routine fashion.

Usual preop diagnosis: Enlarging or symptomatic aortic aneurysm

SUMMARY OF PROCEDURES

	Ascending Aorta	Transverse Arch	Descending Aorta
Position	Supine	⇐	Lateral decubitus with left side up
Incision	Median sternotomy	⇐	Left posterolateral thoracotomy with access to femoral artery and vein
Special instrumentation	CPB, if used.	Complete hemodynamic monitors; CPB	⇐ + DLT; lower extremity BP monitor
Unique considerations	Routine CPB hemodynamic monitoring	If profound hypothermic arrest is utilized, neuroprotective adjuncts, including local hypothermia, barbiturates, and steroids, should be used.	OLV; partial CPB
Antibiotics	Cefazolin 1 g iv	⇐	⇐
Surgical time	Aortic cross-clamp: 40-120 min CPB: 70-150 min Total: 2.5-5 h	Aortic cross-clamp: 75-120 min Circulatory arrest: 30-45 min CPB: 3-4.5 h Total: 4-6 h	Aortic cross-clamp: 25-45 min CPB: 30-60 min Total: 2.5-4.5 h
Closing considerations	Aggressive management of coagulopathy, if a long pump run is necessary.	Aggressive management of coagulopathy	Replacement of DLT with single-lumen tube
EBL	300-400 ml	400-700 ml	200-300 ml
Postop care	ICU, intubated 5-20 h, depending on preop condition	ICU, intubated 6-24 h	ICU, intubated 5-24 h
Mortality	5-10%	10-15%	⇐
Morbidity	Renal failure: 5-10% CVA: 4-6% Respiratory failure: 3-5% MI: 2-5%	– 2-5% 10% ⇐	10-15% 2-4% 10-15% 2-4%
Pain score	7-10	7-10	9-10

PATIENT POPULATION CHARACTERISTICS

Age range	23-80 yr (mean = 55 yr)	50-75 yr	34-79 yr (mean = 65 yr)
Male:Female	3:1	2:1	2.5:1
Incidence	15-20/yr at tertiary center	10-15/yr at tertiary center	10-20/yr at tertiary center
Etiology	Degenerative disease Atherosclerotic disease	⇐ ⇐ Chronic dissections	⇐ ⇐ ⇐
Associated conditions	CHF (50%); angina (30%); HTN (30%); COPD (15%)	Aortic valve disease (30%); COPD (20%); CAD (15%)	HTN (65%); CAD (50%); COPD (30%); CHF (10%)

ANESTHETIC CONSIDERATIONS

PREOPERATIVE

Typically, patients with thoracic aortic aneurysms have atherosclerosis and HTN. A subset of patients will have a connective tissue disorder (e.g., Marfan syndrome). In contrast with thoracic aortic dissections, thoracic aortic aneurysms may be of a more chronic and asymptomatic nature. A ruptured or leaking aneurysm, however, may have a more precipitous presentation.

Cardiovascular	**Arch and ascending aneurysms** (60-70% of aneurysms): commonly associated with HTN, cystic medial necrosis, connective tissue disorder (e.g., Marfan syndrome), atherosclerosis, or syphilis. CHF may occur 2° to dilation of the aortic annulus and aortic incompetence (AR). Aneurysmal compression or intrinsic disease of the coronary arteries may result in myocardial ischemia. **Descending** (30%): usually associated with HTN, cystic medial necrosis, Marfan syndrome, atherosclerosis. **Tests:** ECG: ✓ for LVH, ischemia. ECHO: ✓ for valvular disease, size and extent of aneurysm, LV function. Angiography: ✓ exact extent of aneurysm (allows planning of procedure and sites for arterial monitoring), coronary artery anatomy and degree of occlusion.
Respiratory	Recurrent laryngeal nerve palsy may → hoarseness (ascending/arch aneurysms). Tracheal deviation ± stridor or dyspnea may be present 2° tracheal or bronchial compression (✓ CT scan). Hemoptysis or a hemorrhagic pleural effusion suggest aneurysmal leakage or rupture. The implications include the possibility of compromised oxygenation, risk of massive hemorrhage on thoracotomy, increased intrathoracic pressure, and consequent decreased venous return (especially when IPPV is instituted). **Tests:** CXR: ✓ for widened mediastinum, distortion of trachea and left main bronchus (because it may affect the placement of DLT); MRI/CT with contrast: ✓ anatomic relation of aneurysm to surrounding structures (e.g., trachea/bronchi); others as indicated from H&P.
Neurologic	Any deficit should be well documented as neurologic sequelae (e.g., paraplegia/paraparesia) may occur after surgery.
Renal	Renal problems may occur 2° to AR (↓CO) and heart failure, HTN, or involvement of renal arteries in the aneurysm. **Tests:** BUN; Cr; consider Cr clearance; electrolytes
Gastrointestinal	Descending aneurysms that involve the celiac or superior mesenteric arteries may → bowel ischemia. **Tests:** Consider ABG: ✓ persistent metabolic acidosis (2% bowel ischemia). If indicated by H&P, consider abdominal CT/x-ray: ✓ ileus.
Hematological	If time permits, consider autologous blood donation; preexisting coagulopathy increases risk of the procedure. **Tests:** PT; PTT; Hct/Hb
Musculoskeletal	✓ Marfanoid appearance; others as indicated from H&P.
Laboratory	Others as indicated from H&P.
Premedication	Pain and anxiety may significantly contribute to HTN and should be treated (e.g., morphine 0.1 mg/kg iv ± midazolam 0.025-0.1 mg/kg iv); but avoid obtundation. Since many of these patients present emergently, consider full-stomach precautions—H_2 antagonists (e.g., ranitidine 50 mg iv), metoclopramide (10 mg iv), and antacids (e.g., Na citrate 0.3 M 30 ml po).

INTRAOPERATIVE

Anesthetic technique: The anesthetic management of patients with aortic dissections and aortic aneurysms are similar in many respects. For intraop and postop management of these conditions, see Anesthetic Considerations for Repair of Acute Aortic Dissections and Dissecting Aneurysms, p. 318.

References

1. Cammarata BJ: Anesthesia for surgery of the thoracic aorta. In *Anesthesia for Cardiac Surgery,* 2nd edition. DiNardo JA, ed. Appleton & Lange, Stamford: 1998, 259-76.
2. Estrera AL, Miller CC III, Huynh TT, Porat EE, Safi HJ: Replacement of the ascending and transverse aortic arch: determinants of long-term survival. *Ann Thorac Surg* 2002; 74:1058-65.

3. Estrera AL, Rubenstein FS, Miller CC: Descending thoracic aortic aneurysm: surgical approach and treatment using the adjuncts cerebrospinal fluid drainage and distal aortic perfusion. *Ann Thorac Surg* 2001; 72:481-6.
4. Fann JI: Descending thoracic and thoracoabdominal aortic aneurysms. *Coron Artery Dis* 2002; 13:93-102.
5. Fann JI, Miller DC: Descending thoracic aortic aneurysms. In *Glenn's Thoracic and Cardiovascular Surgery*, 6th edition. Baue AE, Geha AS, Hammond GL, Laks H, Naunheim KS, eds. Appleton & Lange, Stamford: 1996, 2255-72.
6. Hagel C, Ergin MA, Galla JD, Lansman SL, McCullough JN, Speilvogel D, Sfeir P, Bodian CA, Griepp RB: Neurologic outcome after ascending aorta-aortic arch operations: effect of brain protection technique in high-risk patients. *J Thorac Cardiovasc Surg* 2001; 121:1107-21.
7. Okita Y, Ando M, Minatoya K, Tagusari O, Kitamura S, Nakajima N, Takamoto S: Early and long-term results of surgery for aneurysms of the thoracic aorta in septuagenarians and octogenarians. *Eur J Cardiothorac Surg* 1999; 16:317-23.
8. Pressler BA, McNamara JJ: Thoracic aortic aneurysm. Natural history and treatment. *J Thorac Cardiovasc Surg* 1980; 79: 489-98.
9. Skeehan TM, Cooper JR Jr: Anesthetic management for thoracic aneurysms and dissections. In *The Practice of Cardiac Anesthesia*. Hensley FA Jr, Martin DE, eds. Little, Brown and Co, Boston: 1990, 461-92.
10. Svenson LG: Progress in ascending and aortic arch surgery: minimally invasive surgery, blood conservation, and neurologic deficit prevention. *Ann Thora Surg* 2002; 74:1786-8.

ENDOVASCULAR STENT-GRAFTING OF AORTIC ANEURYSMS

SURGICAL CONSIDERATIONS

Description: The standard treatment for descending **thoracic aortic aneurysm** is surgical resection of the aneurysm and replacement with a segment of prosthetic graft material. While resection of aneurysms often can be performed without the need for extracorporeal circulation, the procedure has a reported mortality rate of up to 50% in emergency cases and 12-15% in elective cases. Transluminal endovascular stent-grafting offers an alternative treatment that is less invasive, less hazardous, and potentially less expensive than standard operative repair.

In the initial workup, all patients have contrast-enhanced spiral CT scans of the thorax and thoracic aortography to assess the dimensions of the aneurysms. The most important features to consider in evaluating an aortic aneurysm for endovascular stent-graft treatment is the presence of an adequate proximal and distal neck. A minimum neck length of at least 1.5 cm is required to allow secure anchoring of most stent-grafts. The distance from the origins of the left subclavian artery and celiac axis to the aneurysm should be at least 1.5-3 cm to ensure that the stent-graft does not inadvertently block these arteries. In an effort to reduce the incidence of paraplegia, and to limit exclusion of intracostal arteries, the overall length of the stent-graft is kept to a minimum.

Another important anatomic consideration is the size of the proposed conduit vessels (e.g., iliac) for introduction of the stent-graft to ensure that they are adequate for accommodation of the device-introducer system, which usually requires at least an 8-mm-diameter vessel. Where the pelvic vessels are less than 8 mm, either a retroperitoneal iliac or retroperitoneal aortic approach is utilized. The stent is the metallic framework to which the graft material is applied. Various balloon-expandable or self-expanding stents are available. For application in the thoracic aorta, stents of 30-40 mm in diameter (mean 35 mm) are required.

Typically, thoracic aortic aneurysm stent-graft procedures are performed in the cath lab (although some may be performed in the OR, depending on equipment availability and local politics), with the patient intubated and under GA. The cath lab is prepared for aortic surgery, with the patient placed on the table in a shallow right decubitus position. The patient's thorax may be prepped and draped for a left thoracotomy. For an approach via the common femoral artery, the groin area is prepped for a femoral artery cutdown. When the iliac arteries are of insufficient size, the left lower abdomen is prepped for a retroperitoneal approach to either the aorta or the common iliac artery. High-quality fluoroscopic equipment is essential to assure accurate placement of the device, and a portable C-arm with digital subtraction capability is moved into position and centered over the thorax. When the iliac vessels are of sufficient size, a cutdown is performed on a femoral artery, the artery is punctured, and a guide wire is advanced into the thoracic aorta. A pigtail catheter is placed and an aortogram is performed. The patient is then anticoagulated with iv heparin (100 IU/kg). A long, stiff guide wire is placed, and the 24 Fr sheath and dilator assembly is advanced over the wire until the sheath tip is proximal to the proximal aneurysm neck. The dilator and guide wire are withdrawn, and the stent-graft is introduced into the sheath from its loading cartridge using the Teflon pusher. The device is pushed through the sheath until the stent-graft approaches the tip of the sheath.

In order to reduce the likelihood of inadvertent downstream deployment of the stent-graft caused by the force of blood flow during initial delivery, the arterial BP may be lowered to a mean of 50-60 mmHg using SNP. Holding the pusher firmly in position, the sheath is rapidly withdrawn, and the stent-graft expands into position. Rapid deployment helps to minimize distal migration of the stent-graft. Immediately following deployment, the SNP is discontinued, allowing the BP to normalize. Repeat aortogram is performed, and any early leakage of contrast into the aneurysm is treated either with balloon angioplasty of the stent-graft or further stent-graft placement. Occasionally a faint, persistent leak of contrast is caused by leakage through the graft material. This typically ceases when the patient's coagulation status returns to normal. Following removal of the delivery sheath, heparin is reversed with protamine sulfate and the arteriotomy is repaired surgically. For stent placement through the retroperitoneal aorta, the procedure has a more extensive surgical component; however, the technique is similar.

The basic concept of **abdominal aortic aneurysm (AAA)** repair via an endovascular route is similar to the preceding section on thoracic aneurysm repair, with some notable exceptions. AAAs commonly arise inferior to the renal arteries, and 80-90% of cases involve either one or both iliac arteries. For this reason, stent-grafts that can accommodate this more complicated anatomy are required. The superior aneurysm neck needs to be of sufficient length (1.5-2 cm) inferior to the most inferior renal artery to provide for stable anchoring. Inferiorly the stent-graft must accommodate either or both iliac arteries. The procedure is performed in a two-stage fashion. Initially an aorta-to-single-iliac-artery device is placed from the infrarenal aortic neck into one of the iliac vessels. A contralateral femoral artery puncture is then performed and a catheter and guide wire are used to access an open stump of the stent-graft from the contralateral limb. At this stage, a modular section of stent-graft is placed from the aortic component into the contralateral limb; in this way, an aorta-to-bi-iliac graft is placed.

Usual preop diagnosis: Aortic aneurysm

SUMMARY OF PROCEDURES

	Thoracic Aortic Aneurysms	**Abdominal Aortic Aneurysms**
Position	Supine/slight right decubitus	Supine
Incision	Femoral artery cutdown	Bilateral femoral artery cutdowns
Special instrumentation	Catheters, guide wires, sheaths, dilators and stent-grafts	⇐
Unique considerations	May require adjunctive procedure (e.g., brachial artery catheterization, balloon angioplasty, possible left subclavian-to-common carotid artery bypass procedure); iv heparin 300 IU/kg	⇐
Antibiotics	Cefazolin 1 g iv	⇐
Surgical time	1-3 h	⇐
Closing considerations	None	⇐
EBL	Usually minimal; however, can be up to 2-3 U	⇐
Postop care	ICU × 1 d	⇐
Mortality	3-5%	2-3%
Morbidity	Paraplegia: 2-3%	Acute rupture: < 1%
	Infection: 1%	⇐
	Surgical conversion: < 1%	⇐
Pain score	3-4	3-4

PATIENT POPULATION CHARACTERISTICS

Age range	30-90 yr	40-90 yr
Incidence	1/10,000 of the population in U.S.	1/1000 of the population in U.S.
Etiology	Atherosclerosis; HTN; trauma; aortic dissection; infection	Atherosclerosis; infection
Associated conditions	CAD; aneurysmal disease elsewhere	⇐

ANESTHETIC CONSIDERATIONS

The anesthetic considerations for thoracic and abdominal stent-grafting are similar since the surgical techniques, complications, patient concurrent disease, and stent-graft deployment techniques are similar. Patients may be asymptomatic; most will have coexisting CAD, PVD, and/or cerebrovascular disease.

PREOPERATIVE

Preop considerations for these patients are the same as for any patient undergoing repair of a descending thoracic aneurysm, abdominal aortic aneurysm, or aortobifemoral aneurysm. Many of these patients, however, are not suitable for conventional repair via a thoracotomy because of respiratory disease (e.g., $FEV_1 < 1$ L, severe COPD, $PaCO_2 > 60$ mmHg), CAD, renal failure, CHF, or a combination of these factors. As such, they generally are at very high risk for periop morbidity and mortality. Before surgery the anesthesiologist should consult with the surgical and radiological teams to decide what will be done should a complication such as penetration or rupture of the aneurysm occur during surgery (typically, an emergency thoracotomy or laparotomy performed in the cath lab).

INTRAOPERATIVE

Anesthetic technique: Usually GETA (OLV may be required for emergency thoracotomy 2° ruptured thoracic aneurysm). Abdominal stent-grafts may be placed under epidural anesthesia. Rarely, stent-grafting may be carried out with local anesthesia or MAC in patients unable to tolerate GA or epidural. In that case, the patient will come to the OR for removal of the introducer system and repair of the femoral artery.

Induction	Since these patients are typically extubated, the dose of fentanyl (5-10 μg/kg) is limited to that which will suppress the hypertensive response to intubation, while still allowing for early extubation. The same considerations apply to the use of muscle relaxants (e.g., vecuronium [0.1 mg/kg]). A DLT or a Univent ETT should be used, unless the team decides that a thoracotomy will not be performed under any circumstance.	
Maintenance	Usually a balanced anesthetic technique of O_2/air/isoflurane, supplemented with fentanyl (or remifentanil infusion) as needed. Hemodynamic control of BP (esmolol, SNP, NTG) to avoid HTN and myocardial ischemia is important. **Anesthetic management during stent-graft deployment:** During stent-graft deployment, the aorta is momentarily occluded. Formerly, this resulted in a rapid $\uparrow$ BP → stent-graft being moved from its intended position. The newer generations of stent-grafts, using thermal or mechanical means for rapid deployment, cause minimal hemodynamic change, eliminating the need for aggressive BP control.	
Emergence	Extubation is desirable, although hypothermia ($< 34°$ C) may prevent this. Otherwise, aim for early extubation in the ICU. DLT (if used) may be replaced with a standard ETT at end of procedure if the patient is not extubated in the cath lab. Recovery is usually in the ICU.	
Blood and fluid requirements	IV: 14-16 ga × 1 NS/LR @ 4-8 ml/kg/h PRBC available	Although usually minimal, blood loss can be considerable.
Monitoring	Standard monitors (p. B-1) Arterial line CVP catheter Urinary catheter TEE	Arterial line placement should be on the right as the radiologists may require access to the left brachial artery. CVP monitoring is usually sufficient. Central access for vasoactive drugs may be needed. TEE is used to aid in the identification of the thoracic aneurysm necks, to monitor deployment of the stent-graft and to identify any continued flow of blood into the aneurysmal sac after deployment (endoleak).
	CSF pressure/drainage	CSF drainage → $\downarrow$CSF pressure may be necessary to minimize spinal cord ischemia (anterior spinal artery syndrome).
Positioning	✓ and pad pressure points. ✓ eyes.	Supine ± slight right lateral decubitus
Complications	Hemorrhage	Hemorrhage at the groin site can be considerable and may be concealed.
	Vessel damage	Damage to the vessels (femoral, iliac, or abdominal aorta) during passage of the insertion system can occur with attendant massive hemorrhage.
	Rupture of aorta	Rupture or penetration of the thoracic aneurysm also can occur, necessitating rapid conversion to open thoracotomy.

| Complications, cont. | Deployment failure/incorrect position | The stent-graft may deploy in an incorrect position or fail to fully deploy. This may require positioning of further stent-grafts, balloon expansion of the stent-graft, or conversion to thoracotomy. |
| | Hypothermia | Hypothermia can be a problem as a circulating-water warming blanket cannot be used on the operating table (use of fluoroscopy). Much of the patient's body is exposed (upper-body Bair-Hugger usually ok) and a lower-body warming blanket cannot be used as the lower limbs may be ischemic during insertion of the stent-graft. |

POSTOPERATIVE

Complications	Aortic perforation/rupture	Emergency surgery
	Migration of grafts	→loss of distal pulses, mesenteric ischemia, acute renal insufficiency.
	Femoral artery dehiscence	Requires prompt return to OR.
	Distal embolization	✓ pulses; angiography/surgical intervention.
	Paraplegia	✓ reflexes; prompt return to OR.
Pain management	Minimal analgesic requirements	If groin incision, local anesthetic infiltration may be used.
Tests	As indicated by patient condition.	CT scan, angiogram prior to discharge and at regular intervals following discharge

References

1. Baker B: Anesthesia for endovascular surgery. *Probl Anesthesiol* 1999; 11:179-92.
2. Chuter TA, Malina M, Brunkwall J, Lindh M, Ivancev K, Lindblad B, Risberg B: A telescopic stent-graft for aortoiliac implantation. *Eur J Vasc Endovasc Surg* 1997; 13(1):79-84.
3. Dake MD, Miller DC, Semba CP, Mitchell RS, Walker PJ, Liddell RP: Transluminal placement of endovascular stent-grafts for the treatment of descending thoracic aortic aneurysms. *N Engl J Med* 1994: 331(26):1729-34.
4. Fann JI, Miller DC: Results of endovascular stent-grafting in patients with descending thoracic aortic aneurysm. In: *Progress in Vascular Surgery*. Yao JST, Pearce WH, eds. Appleton and Lange, Stamford: 1997, 241-54.
5. Fleck T, Hutschala D, Weissl M, Wolner E, Grabenwöger M: Cerebrospinal fluid drainage as a useful treatment option to relieve paraplegia after stent-graft implantation for acute aortic dissection type B. *J Thorac Cardiovasc Surg* 2002; 123: 1003-05.
6. Herold U, Piotrowski J, Baumgart D, Eggebrecht H, Erbel R, Jakob H: Endoluminal stent graft repair for acute and chronic type B aortic dissection and atherosclerotic aneurysm of the thoracic aorta: an interdisciplinary task. *Eur J Cardiothorac Surg* 2002; 22:891-7.
7. Kahn RA, Moskowitz DM: Endovascular aortic repair. *J Cardiothorac Vasc Anesth* 2002; 16:218-33.
8. Mitchell RS: Stent grafts for the thoracic aorta: a new paradigm? *Ann Thorac Surg* 2002; 74:1818-20.
9. Mitchell RS, Dake MD, Semba CP, Fogarty TJ, Zarins CK, Liddel RP, Miller DC: Endovascular stent-graft repair of thoracic aortic aneurysms. *J Thorac Cardiovasc Surg* 1996; 111(5):1054-62.
10. Moon MR, Mitchell RS, Dake MD, Zarins CK, Fann JI, Miller DC: Simultaneous abdominal aortic replacement and thoracic aortic stent-graft placement for multilevel aortic disease. *J Vasc Surg* 1997; 25:332-40.
11. Rapezzi C, Rocchi G, Fattori R, Caldarera I, Ferlito M, Napoli G, Pierangeli A, Branzi A: Usefulness of transesophageal echocardiographic monitoring to improve the outcome of stent-graft treatment of thoracic aortic aneurysms. *Am J Cardiol* 2001; 87:315-9.
12. Schütz W, Gauss A, Meierhenrich R, Pamler R, Görich J: Transesophageal echocardiographic guidance of thoracic aortic stent-graft implantation. *J Endovasc Ther* 2002; 9:14-19.
13. Semba CP, Kato N, Kee ST, Lee GK, Mitchell RS, Miller DC, Dake MD: Acute rupture of the descending thoracic aorta: repair with use of endovascular stent-grafts. *J Vasc Interv Radiol* 1997; 8(3):337-42.
14. Taylor PR: Vascular stents and stent-grafts: a vascular surgeon's view. *Cardiovasc Intervent Radiol* 1997; 20(1):1-4.
15. Wain RA, Marin ML, Ohki T, Sanchez LA, Lyon RT, Rozenblit A, Suggs WD, Yuan JG, Veith FJ. Endoleaks after endovascular graft treatment of aortic aneurysms: classification, risk factors, and outcome. *J Vasc Surg* 1998; 27:69-80.

REPAIR OF ACUTE AORTIC DISSECTIONS AND DISSECTING ANEURYSMS

SURGICAL CONSIDERATIONS

Description: Repair of **acute aortic dissection** is performed to prevent life-threatening complications such as hemorrhage, tamponade, and heart failure 2° acute aortic valvular insufficiency and to redirect flow into the true lumen. Emergent repair of acute ascending dissections is generally accepted therapy to prevent rupture of the aortic root with exsanguination or pericardial tamponade. Mortality for acute ascending dissection is estimated at 1% per h, for the first 48 h. The management of descending thoracic aortic dissections remains controversial, but surgical intervention probably should be recommended only for younger patients, patients with uncontrolled pain or evidence for continued expansion or extravasation, and those with branch-vessel compromise.

Ascending dissections typically produce sharp, tearing retrosternal pain that penetrates straight through to the subscapular area. The presentation, however,

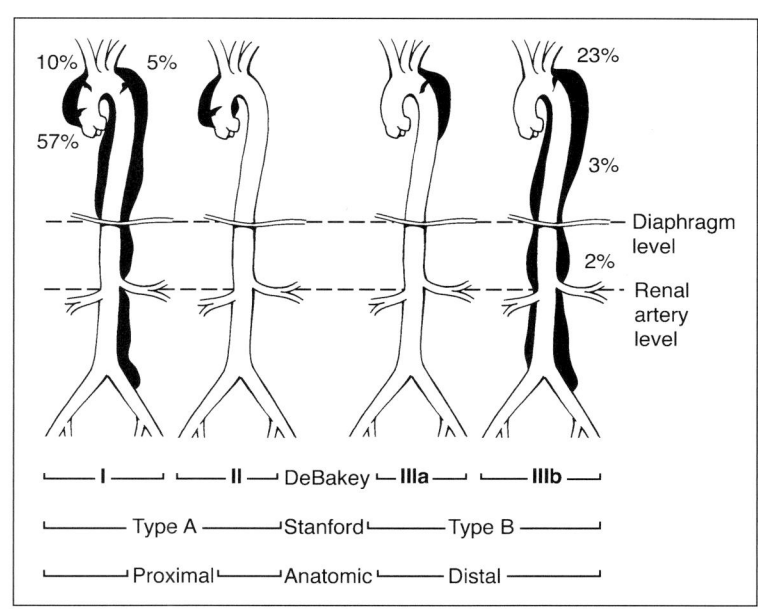

Figure 6.3-3. The three classification systems of aortic dissection and the distribution of the intimal tear.

is so frequently variable that any patient in extremis, especially with migratory pain or vacillating findings, and even asymptomatic patients with valvular aortic regurgitation (AR), should be considered for the diagnosis. With a suggestive Hx, a new murmur, or a pulse deficit, an enlarged mediastinal shadow on chest radiography should prompt further diagnostic efforts. CT scanning, MRI, and aortography may all be diagnostic, but no diagnostic modality has 100% sensitivity. TEE appears to be highly sensitive in detecting a mobile intimal flap in the ascending or descending aorta. In addition, TEE can provide useful information regarding AR, periaortic hematoma and flow within a false channel. It is usually available at the bedside or in the emergency ward and does not subject the patient to a contrast load.

Once diagnosed, these patients are transported immediately to the OR. Through a median sternotomy, venous access is gained via the right atrium, and arterial inflow is supplied through a femoral artery. CPB is established, the patient cooled to 18°C, and circulatory support discontinued. During a period of profound circulatory arrest, the ascending aorta is opened and the tear localized. The repair is carried distally into the arch, if the entire dissection can be resected, and the distal aortic layers are reapproximated with a Teflon felt strip supporting the medial and adventitial layers. The distal graft anastomosis is then completed, the graft clamped, the bypass pump restarted and systemic warming commenced. Proximally, the aortic root is reconstructed, again using Teflon felt to support the medial and adventitial layers and to resuspend the aortic valve, which can be salvaged in approximately 85% of cases. The heart is then cleared of air, and the cross-clamp removed to allow reperfusion of the coronary circulation. After a sufficient period of resuscitation, the patient is weaned from CPB. Aggressive management of an acquired coagulopathy is not unusual prior to chest closure.

Repair of **dissections** involving the **descending thoracic aorta** is accomplished through a left thoracotomy utilizing partial CPB. Venous drainage is usually via the femoral vein, although the PA or pulmonary vein may be used. Arterial access is via the femoral artery. After institution of CPB, the dissected aorta above and below the most damaged area is cross-clamped and the aorta transected. After oversewing patent intercostal arteries, the medial and adventitial layers are buttressed with Teflon felt, and an interposition Dacron graft is sewn into place. After evacuation of air, clamps are removed, and the patient weaned from CPB. Heparin reversal, decannulation, and closure are accomplished in the usual manner.

Usual preop diagnosis: Acute dissection of the aorta (See Fig 6.3-3 for types of dissection.)

SUMMARY OF PROCEDURES

	Ascending Aorta	Descending Aorta
Position	Supine	Lateral decubitus, left side up
Incision	Median sternotomy	Left lateral thoracotomy
Unique considerations	Full hemodynamic monitoring, with provisions for circulatory arrest, profound hypothermia, barbiturates and steroids; TEE	DLT; CPB; TEE; lumbar drain
Antibiotics	Cefazolin 1 g iv	⇐
Surgical time	Cross-clamp: 30-50 min	30-60 min
	Circulatory arrest: 20-30 min	–
	CPB: 60-100 min	35-60 min
	Total: 3-5 h	⇐
Closing considerations	Aggressively treat coagulopathy (frequently 2° ↓Plt).	Replace DLT with single-lumen ETT.
EBL	400-800 ml	600-800 ml
Postop care	ICU: 1-2 d, intubated	⇐
Mortality	10-25%	⇐
Morbidity	Bleeding: 3-8%	Paraplegia: 5%
	Respiratory insufficiency: 2-5%	CVA: 1-2%
	CVA: 2-4%	MI: 1-2%
Pain score	7-10	9-10

PATIENT POPULATION CHARACTERISTICS

Age range	40-70 yr
Male:Female	3:2
Incidence	10/100,000
Etiology	Degenerative aortic disease
Associated conditions	HTN; secondary AR; bicuspid aortic valve; Marfan syndrome

ANESTHETIC CONSIDERATIONS

PREOPERATIVE

Sx are usually of sudden onset and depend on the site of dissection and specific organ involvement. Aortic dissections are divided into 2 types, depending on the site of intimal tear: **Type A**—ascending and aortic arch, and **Type B**—descending aorta (Fig 6.3-3). Initial treatment involves the use of antihypertensive medications (e.g., SNP) to control BP and β-blockers (e.g., esmolol) to ↓ contractility. Type A dissections usually require urgent surgery. Patients presenting electively for thoracotomy (descending aorta) may have a thoracic epidural catheter placed the night before surgery. These patients are only heparinized during the procedure.

Respiratory   ✔ for recurrent laryngeal nerve palsy with chronic aneurysmal dilation. Tracheal and left main bronchus compression → difficult intubation, atelectasis; hemoptysis 2° rupture into lung; hemothorax → compromised oxygenation, ↑intrathoracic pressure →↓ venous return, especially with IPPV.

Tests: CXR: ✔ for widened mediastinum, tracheal or left main bronchus compression and distortion (affects DLT placement), atelectasis, pleural effusion (or hemothorax 2° rupture).

Cardiovascular   Aortic dissections may be associated with chronic HTN, cystic medial necrosis, or other connective tissue disorder (e.g., Marfan syndrome) and trauma. Dissection may result in cardiac tamponade, acute aortic valve incompetence, acute cardiac failure, angina, MI, or rupture of the aorta. Dissection of major arteries may result in ↓ or absent peripheral pulses, which may affect the placement sites for intraarterial monitoring and central venous access. Pain and anxiety may result in HTN, while rupture or leakage may result in ↓BP and shock.

Tests: ECG: ✔ for Sx of LVH, ischemia or infarction, low voltage (tamponade). ECHO: ✔ for site of dissection, valvular competence, LV function, pericardial effusion or tamponade. Angiography: ✔ for site of dissection (Type A or B), valvular function, involvement of coronary and other major arteries, sites of rupture, LV function. CT scan: ✔ site and extent of dissection.

Neurological	Deficits are not uncommon, especially with Type B dissections where the blood supply to the spinal cord may be jeopardized. Document carefully.
Renal	Renal failure 2° renal artery involvement in dissection, shock, or cardiac failure. UO should be monitored closely during initial medical therapy. **Tests:** UO; BUN; Cr; electrolytes
Gastrointestinal	Compromised blood supply to the bowel or liver may result in ischemia → metabolic acidosis and ↓liver function. **Tests:** Consider ABG: ✓ persistent metabolic acidosis; LFTs, if indicated by H&P.
Hematologic	Coagulopathy may be present 2° massive hemorrhage or liver involvement, and can increase risk of the surgery. **Tests:** PT; PTT; Hct/Hb
Laboratory	Other tests as indicated from H&P.
Premedication	Since many of these patients present emergently, consider full-stomach precautions: H_2-antagonists (ranitidine 50 mg iv), metoclopramide (10 mg iv), antacids (Na citrate 0.3 M 30 ml po). Alleviate anxiety and pain, which may worsen HTN, but avoid obtundation (e.g., morphine 0.1 mg/kg im, ± midazolam 0.025-0.1 mg/kg iv or 0.05-0.2 mg/kg im).

INTRAOPERATIVE

Anesthetic technique: GETA ± thoracic epidural. Preinduction control of BP and contractility (NTG or SNP to SBP = 105-115 and esmolol to HR = 60-80) is important in preventing extension of the dissection or rupture of the aneurysm. Fluid resuscitation may be necessary prior to induction. If present, cardiac tamponade should be relieved by pericardiocentesis.

Induction	Control of hypertensive response to laryngoscopy and intubation is important and may be accomplished with moderate-dose narcotic (fentanyl 10-15 μg/kg or sufentanil 1-2 μg/kg) and etomidate (0.1-0.3 mg/kg), esmolol (5-10 mg iv bolus), or SNP (25-50 μg bolus). Pretreatment with lidocaine (1.5 mg/kg) also may be required to further control the hypertensive response to laryngoscopy. Muscle relaxation may be obtained using vecuronium (0.1 mg/kg), rocuronium (1-2 mg/kg), or pancuronium (0.1 mg/kg). Remember the possibility of a full stomach in this patient population. Hence, a modified rapid-sequence induction (cricoid pressure with manual ventilation and NMR) may achieve the two goals of relatively rapid induction and intubation and tight control of BP. Usually a left DLT is used in patients with descending lesions to improve surgical access; however, it may be difficult to place due to aneurysmal compression of the trachea and left mainstem bronchus, and it is associated with a small risk of aneurysmal rupture. For these reasons, a right DLT may be preferred. FOB is mandatory to verify ET placement.
Maintenance	O_2/narcotic/benzodiazepine: low-dose volatile agent (isoflurane [0.3-0.5%] or sevoflurane [0.5-1%]) may be used to control BP (MAP = 60-80), although infusion of vasopressors, vasodilators, or inotropes may be necessary. Control HR (< 80; anesthesia, esmolol) and contractility (β-blockade or inotropes, depending on circumstances). Benzodiazepines may be used for amnesia (midazolam 100 μg/kg). If thoracic epidural in place, fentanyl (20-30 μg/kg) or sufentanil (4-6 μg/kg) may be used. Most Type A aneurysms and ascending/arch aneurysms require hypothermic CPB (see Anesthetic Considerations for Cardiopulmonary Bypass, p. 262). Intraop anesthetic considerations are governed primarily by the site of the aortic pathology. These considerations are discussed below.
Emergence	Transported to ICU, sedated, intubated, and ventilated × 24-48 h. Following repairs of the descending aorta (thoracotomy incision), weaning from ventilator may be aided by epidural narcotics after documentation of normal spinal cord function and coagulation.
Blood and fluid requirements	Anticipate large blood loss. IV: 14 ga - 7 Fr × 2 NS/LR @ 6-8 ml/kg/h Warm all fluids. Humidify gases. Cross-match 6-8 U of blood. UO 0.5-1 ml/kg/h	In Type A dissections and arch aneurysms, if possible, avoid iv placement in the left arm or left IJ/subclavian veins because of the possibility of innominate vein ligation. Mannitol (0.5 g/kg iv) should be given if renal perfusion is compromised by dissection or before cross-clamping. Consider normovolemic hemodilution if the patient is stable and the Hct > 35. After unclamping: furosemide (1 mg/kg), if hemodynamically stable.
Monitoring	Standard monitors (p. B-1). Arterial line CVP, PA catheter (optional)	Arterial line site is dependent on type of surgery and location of the lesion. Because the right subclavian artery may be compromised in patients with ascending lesions, the left

Monitoring, cont.	Urinary catheter	radial or femoral arteries may need to be used. Aortic arch lesions may involve the vascular supply to both upper extremities; hence, femoral artery catheterization may be necessary. In ascending lesions, two artery lines may be required—right radial (above clamp pressure) and left femoral (below clamp pressure). Consult with surgeon as to best site.
	TEE	TEE is useful to assess cardiac function, regional wall motion abnormalities, valvular pathology, aortic valvular repair (if required as part of a Type A repair). Probe passage may increase compression of the trachea, impeding ventilation. Caution should be used in the presence of aneurysmal compression of the esophagus.
	Temperature	Monitor both core (esophageal/bladder) and tympanic membrane T (as indicative of brain T)—important in deep hypothermic arrest.
	EEG/EP (arch/ascending lesions)	EEG/EP may help in assessing effectiveness of cerebral protection or adequacy of cerebral perfusion.
	SSEPs/MEPs (descending lesions)	SSEPs may detect posterior spinal perfusion problems, while MEPs may detect anterior cord dysfunction. Both EEG and EPs may require expert help to set up, monitor, and interpret.
Complications	Hemorrhage Coagulopathy	Both are common. Hemorrhage should be treated with crystalloid, colloid, or blood products, as indicated.
Ascending lesions	CPB AR Coronary arteries	Usual site of cannulation for CPB is the ascending artery or femoral artery. Aortic valve replacement may be necessary. Patients may have myocardial ischemia 2° coronary artery occlusion; may require CABG or reimplantation of vessels.
	Deep hypothermic arrest	Cerebral protective measures and selective perfusion of cerebral vessels may be required. (See below.)
Arch lesions	CPB Deep hypothermic arrest	Usual site of cannulation for CPB is femoral or axillary artery. Cerebral protection relies on hypothermia (15-18°C) and drugs (methylprednisolone [Solu-Medrol] 1 g, mannitol 0.5 g/kg, STP 15-30 mg/kg) to reduce $CMRO_2$ and neuronal injury. The head is surface cooled (protect eyes and ears from cold injury). EEG may be monitored to ensure absence of brain electrical activity. Monitor tympanic membrane T as an indication of brain T. Avoid hyperglycemia and maintain normal pH and $PaCO_2$ when measured at 37°C (alpha stat). Maintain muscle relaxation.
Descending lesions	Pre cross-clamping	Mannitol (0.5 g/kg) should be given before clamp application to provide renal protection, even if a shunt is placed. Hypothermia (32-34°C) may protect spinal cord.
	Shunt	A heparin-bonded shunt may be used from the aortic arch to the femoral artery to provide distal perfusion.
	Partial bypass	Partial CPB may be used to provide distal perfusion. In this arrangement, the heart perfuses the head and upper extremities, while CPB is used to perfuse and oxygenate the lower body. Venous drainage is from the femoral vein, PA, or left atrium and returned via the femoral artery. Distal and proximal pressures are altered by controlling cardiac filling, pump flow, and vasodilators.
	Cross-clamping	Application of clamp may → acute HTN with ischemia and LV failure. This may be controlled by partial bypass, shunting or use of vasodilators (SNP 0.5-4 μg/kg/min, NTG 0.5-4 μg/kg/min). During cross-clamping, monitor

Descending lesions, cont.		UO and ✓ metabolic acidosis (renal or bowel ischemia) with serial ABGs. Cross-clamp time should be < 30 min to reduce incidence of paraplegia. The surgeons often request that a lumbar CSF drain be inserted to ↓ CSF pressure (to ≤ CVP) and, thus, improve spinal cord blood flow.
	Unclamping	Unclamping may result in severe ↓BP and myocardial depression. Hypovolemia, acidosis, vasoactive factors, and reactive hyperemia have been implicated as the cause. Prior to unclamping, ensure adequate volume status (PCWP 2-5 mmHg above patient's normal); treat acidosis; have vasopressors available; and the clamp should be released slowly over 1-2 min. Use of partial bypass or a shunt to ensure distal perfusion will mitigate unclamping shock. When hemodynamically stable, give furosemide (1 mg/kg iv). Inotropes (dopamine) may be needed to support circulation.
Positioning	✓ eyes. ✓ and pad pressure points. Arch and ascending: supine, shoulder roll Descending: lateral decubitus, axillary roll, pillow between knees	

POSTOPERATIVE

Complications	Myocardial ischemia, CHF Dysrhythmias Hemorrhage Coagulopathy Renal failure Bowel ischemia Respiratory failure Paraplegia	A DLT may be required in lesions of the descending aorta, if hemorrhage continues from left lung; otherwise, the tube may be replaced at the end of procedure by a single-lumen ETT. BP should be controlled to MAP 60-80 and HR < 100 to decrease the likelihood of repeat dissection, bleeding, or graft dehiscence. Anterior spinal artery syndrome
Pain management	PCA (p. E-2) Epidural (p. E-3)	Thoracic epidural catheter may be used in patients following thoracotomy if coagulation status normal.
Tests	ECG: ischemia, infarction, dysrhythmias CXR: line and ETT placement; pulmonary contusion Coagulation profile Renal: BUN, Cr ABG: Respiratory, gut ischemia CT scan: CNS or spinal neurologic deficits Electrolytes	

References

1. Brodkin IA, Murkin, JM: Protection of the brain during cardiac surgery. In *The Practice of Cardiac Anesthesia*, 2nd edition. Hensley FA Jr, Martin DE, eds. Little, Brown: 1995, 581-602.
2. Cammarata BJ: Anesthesia for surgery of the thoracic aorta. In *Anesthesia for Cardiac Surgery,* 2nd edition. DiNardo JA, ed. Appleton & Lange, Stamford: 1998, 259-76.
3. Dong CCJ, MacDonald DB, Janusz MT: Intraoperative spinal cord monitoring during descending thoracic and thoracoabdominal aneurysm surgery. *Ann Thorac Surg* 2002; 74:S1873-6.
4. Fann JI, Smith JA, Miller DC, et al: Surgical management of aortic dissection over a 30-year period. *Circulation* 1995; 92(II):113-21.
5. Khan IA, Nair CK: Clinical, diagnostic, and management perspectives of aortic dissection. *Chest* 2002; 122:311-28.
6. Karmy-Jones R, Aldea G, Boyle EM Jr: The continuing evolution in the management of thoracic aortic dissections. *Chest* 2002; 117:1221-3.
7. Klompas M: Does this patient have an acute thoracic aortic dissection? *JAMA* 2002; 287:2262-72.
8. Kwitka G, Kidney SA, Nugent M: Thoracic and abdominal aortic aneurysm resections. In *Vascular Anesthesia*. Churchill-Livingstone, New York: 1991, 363-94.

9. Ling E, Arrellano R: Systematic overview of the evidence supporting the use of cerebrospinal fluid drainage in thoracoabdominal aneurysm surgery for prevention of paraplegia. *Anesthesiology* 2000; 93:1115-22.

10. Lips J, de Haan P, de Jager S, Vanicky I, Jacobs MJ, Kalkman CG: The role of transcranial motor evoked potentials in predicting neurologic and histopathologic outcome after experimental spinal cord ischemia. *Anesthesiology* 2002; 97:183-91.

11. Penco M, Paparoni S, Dagianti A: Usefulness of transesophageal echocardiography in the assessment of aortic dissection. *Am J Cardiol* 2000; 86:53G-56G.

12. Willens HJ, Kessler KM: Transesophageal echocardiography in the diagnosis of diseases of the thoracic aorta: Part 1. Aortic dissection, aortic intramural hematoma, and penetrating atherosclerotic ulcer of the aorta. *Chest* 1999; 116:1772-9.

REPAIR OF ANEURYSMS OF THE THORACOABDOMINAL AORTA

SURGICAL CONSIDERATIONS

Description: Aneurysms of the thoracoabdominal aorta (TAAA) may occur because of degenerative aortic disease (atherosclerosis), as a consequence of hereditary disorders of metabolism (Marfan syndrome), or as a sequela of chronic aortic dissections. These aneurysms are classified into four types (Fig 6.3-4) that occur with equal frequency: Type I consists of aneurysms that involve most of the descending thoracic and upper abdominal aorta. Type II involves most of the descending thoracic aorta and most or all of the abdominal aorta. Type III involves the distal thoracic and varying segments of the abdominal aorta. Type IV involves most or all of the abdominal aorta, including the origins of the visceral vessels.

Repair of these aneurysms is an extensive, difficult, and demanding procedure, as blood flow to the entire body below the neck is interrupted, with resultant renal and visceral ischemia. Additionally, the blood supply to the spinal cord may arise from lumbar and/or intercostal vessels in the affected aortic segment, producing critical cord ischemia during cross-clamping and postop paraplegia.

Almost all thoracoabdominal aneurysm repairs are performed through a thoracoabdominal incision (Fig 6.3-5) using the **inclusion technique** (Fig 6.3-6) as advocated by **Crawford**, et al.[4] After opening the chest, the incision is extended across the costal cartilage onto the abdomen. The diaphragm is radially incised to the aortic hiatus, and the retroperitoneal

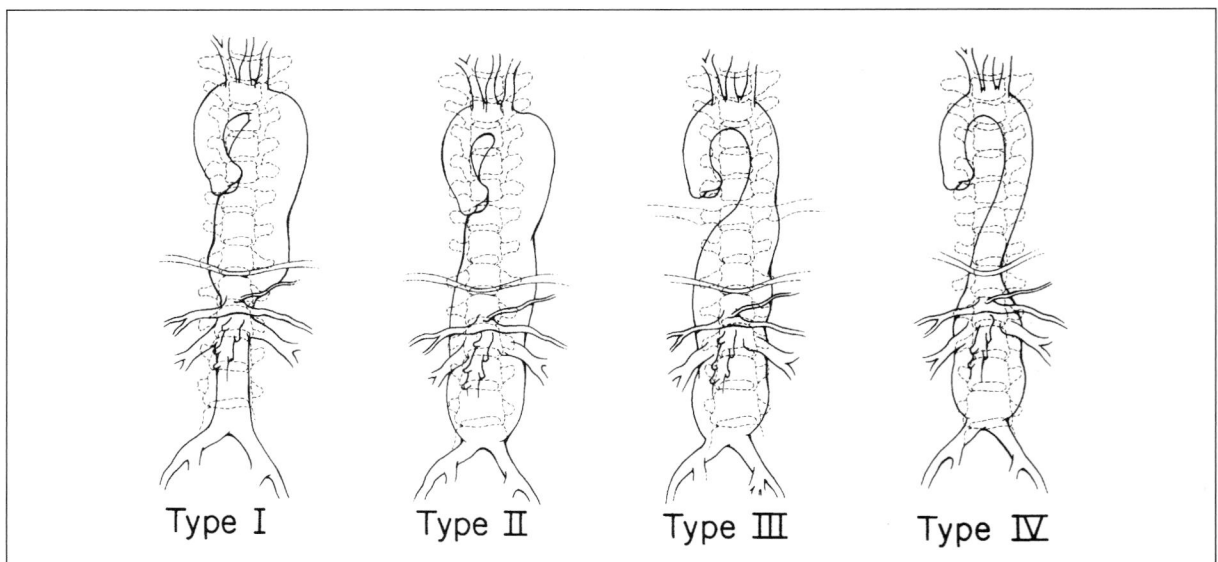

Figure 6.3-4. Crawford's classification of thoracoabdominal aortic aneurysms (TAAA). (Reproduced with permission from Baker RJ, Fischer JE: *Mastery of Surgery*, Vol. 2. Lippincott Williams & Wilkins, 2001.)

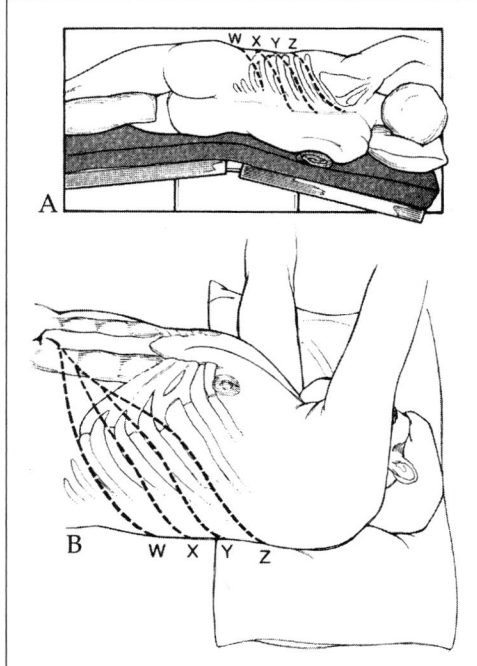

Figure 6.3-5. Lateral (A) and frontal (B) views of the thoracoabdominal incisions used for repair of type IV (W,X), type III (Y,Z), and types I and II (Z) TAAAs. (Reproduced with permission from Baker RJ, Fischer JE: *Mastery of Surgery*, Vol. 2. Lippincott Williams & Wilkins, 2001.)

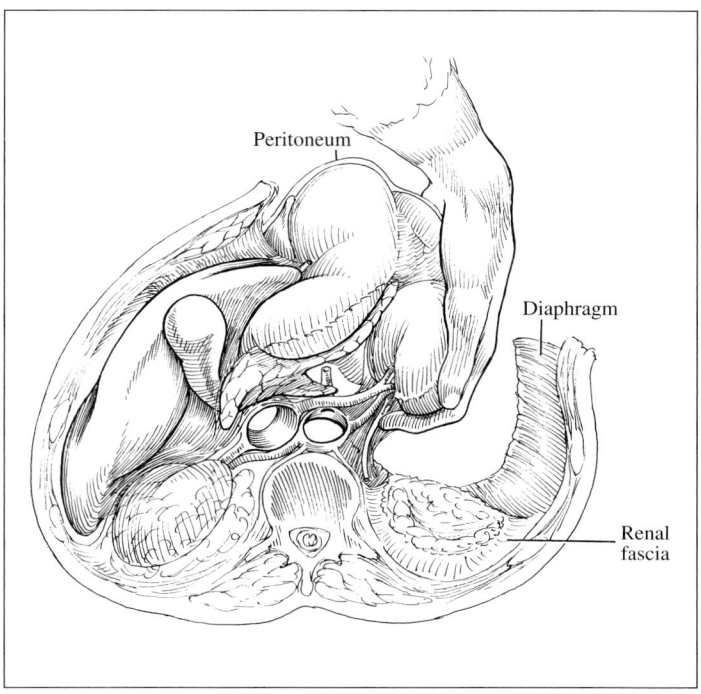

Figure 6.3-6. During the inclusion technique, the anterior renal fascia is opened and the kidney is mobilized, along with the upper abdominal organs (on the left). (Reproduced with permission from Wind GG, Valentine RJ: Anatomic Exposures in Vascular Surgery. Williams & Wilkins, Baltimore, 1991.)

dissection plane established anterior to the psoas musculature. All intraabdominal contents, as well as the left kidney, are reflected anteriorly (Fig 6.3-6). Only proximal aortic control is established. After minimal heparinization, OLV is established to allow collapse of the left lung, the proximal aorta at the aneurysm neck is cross-clamped, and the aneurysm is incised. Back-bleeding from patent intercostal, mesenteric, and renal vessels can be controlled by balloon catheters; and aggressive blood salvage with autotransfusion devices is mandatory. The repair entails suturing a tube graft proximally to the divided aorta, and then sewing islands of aortic tissue containing intercostal visceral vessels onto appropriate sized holes in the side of the tube graft. This allows reperfusion of important intercostal, celiac axis, superior mesenteric, renal arteries and, finally, the distal aorta or iliac arteries. Since there is obligate visceral ischemia during the period of cross-clamping (which must be limited to < 60-75 min), the operation must proceed expeditiously.

Alternatively, in an effort to afford both spinal cord and visceral protection through hypothermia, the operation may be performed on CPB during a period of profound hypothermic circulatory arrest, which, unfortunately, may exacerbate hemorrhagic complications.

After aortic cross-clamping, the aneurysm is opened and the repair performed from within the aneurysm, sewing on-lay patches of the intercostal, mesenteric, and renal vessels to openings created in the tube graft. This no-clamp technique allows reasonable management of these very extensive aneurysms, but results in an obligatory and ongoing blood loss through back-bleeding of visceral vessels until the anastomoses are complete.

Usual preop diagnosis: Expanding, painful, or large thoracoabdominal aneurysm

SUMMARY OF PROCEDURE

Position	Right lateral decubitus; hips rotated posteriorly to 45° and left arm draped forward over an airplane sling. Axillary roll placed. (See Fig 6.3-5A.)
Incision	Posterolateral thoracotomy incision, in appropriate interspace, extended across the costal margin to midline, then extended inferiorly as a midline abdominal incision (Fig 6.3-5). The incision is one of the largest incisions in surgery, necessitated by the absolute need for exposure in this difficult area, and is, unfortunately, associated with a lot of postop pain.
Special instrumentation	DLT; CPB; NG tube; Cell Saver; rapid-infusion device

Unique considerations	OLV with collapse of left lung necessary for most cases. Cold LR may be injected into renal or visceral arteries for organ preservation. Alternatively, operation can be performed under profound hypothermic circulatory arrest for spinal cord protection in patients with chronic dissections. Frequently, operation is performed with only proximal cross-clamping; so there may be an obligate ongoing blood loss.
Antibiotics	Cefazolin 1 g iv
Surgical time	6 h. Proximal aortic cross-clamping until completion of visceral revascularization may extend to 60 min. Longer cross-clamp times may be anticipated in patients with chronic aortic dissections for which profound hypothermic circulatory arrest is frequently utilized.
Closing considerations	OR → ICU, intubated × 24-72 h.
EBL	Ongoing back-bleeding from visceral and iliac vessels results in substantial volume loss during cross-clamping, approaching 5-7 L. Most red-cell volume may be salvaged and returned through a RBC salvage system.
Postop care	ICU, intubated and ventilated × 24-72 h. Rewarming, hemodynamic monitoring and volume resuscitation are often required in ICU.

	Aneurysm Group:	**Type I**	**Type II**	**Type III**	**Type IV**
Mortality	Overall: 9%	–	10-25%	–	5%
Morbidity	Paraplegia/spinal cord ischemia	6%	15%	3%	2%
	Other neurological complications	6%	12%	2%	1%
	Renal insufficiency	–	2-5%	–	–
	Respiratory failure	–	10%	–	–
	Hemorrhage	Common	⇐	⇐	⇐
	Graft infection	–	1-6%	–	–
	MI	Rare	⇐	⇐	⇐
	Graft failure	–	Rare	–	–
	False aneurysm	Rare	⇐	⇐	⇐
	Embolization	Rare	⇐	⇐	⇐
	Bowel ischemia	–	2-10%	–	–
	Impotence	Rare	⇐	⇐	⇐
	Ureteral injury	Rare	⇐	⇐	⇐
Pain score	6-10				

PATIENT POPULATION CHARACTERISTICS

Age range	Non-Marfan: 55-75 yr; Marfan: 35-55 yr
Male:Female	3:1
Incidence	< 5 cases/yr in most hospitals, except major referral centers
Etiology	Predominantly atherosclerotic. Patients with Marfan syndrome may present with a progressive dilatation of a chronic dissection.
Associated conditions	HTN (75%); CAD (30%); COPD (30%); renal insufficiency (15%)

ANESTHETIC CONSIDERATIONS

PREOPERATIVE

Sx are usually of sudden onset and depend on the site of dissection and specific organ involvement. Initial treatment involves the use of antihypertensive medications (e.g., SNP) to control BP, and β-blockers (e.g., esmolol) to ↓ contractility. Patients presenting electively for thoracotomy (descending aorta) may have a thoracic epidural catheter placed the night before surgery. These patients are only heparinized during the procedure.

Respiratory	Chronic pulmonary disease is associated with postop morbidity. Preop preparation with bronchodilators, cessation of smoking, incentive spirometry, and chest physiotherapy may decrease the risk of postop problems.
	Tests: CXR: ✓ for distortion of the left mainstem bronchus, which may affect placement of the DLT. May need PFTs, ABG to determine severity of pulmonary disease.
Cardiovascular	CAD is the most frequent cause of periop and late death in elective thoracoabdominal aortic aneurysm repair. It is commonly associated with HTN.
	Tests: ECG: ✓ for LVH and ischemia.

Neurological	Increased risk of spinal cord ischemia with cross-clamping of the aorta; therefore, any preop neurologic deficits should be well documented. The use of CSF drainage and/or deep hypothermic circulatory arrest may be used in patients with chronic aortic dissections.
Renal	Preop renal dysfunction increases the potential for postop renal problems. Aneurysmal involvement of the renal arteries also may occur. **Tests:** BUN; Cr. Consider creatinine clearance.
Gastrointestinal	Aneurysmal involvement of the inferior mesenteric and superior mesenteric arteries may cause visceral ischemia. **Tests:** Consider abdominal x-ray (ileus) and ABG (metabolic acidosis).
Hematologic	Preexisting coagulopathy increases risk. Many patients have been on aspirin preop. Excessive alcohol use is associated with anemia, thrombocytopenia, and low production of vitamin K-dependent factors. Rarely, a DIC process may occur within the lumen of the aneurysm. **Tests:** PT; PTT; Plt count; Hct
Laboratory	Electrolytes; radiologic assessment of aneurysm (ultrasonography, CT, and arteriography)
Premedication	Anxiety and pain may contribute to HTN and risk of aneurysmal rupture. Rx: morphine 0.1 mg/kg iv and midazolam 1-5 mg iv. Full-stomach precautions for emergent procedures (e.g., metoclopramide 10 mg iv, ranitidine 50 mg iv, Na citrate 30 ml po).

INTRAOPERATIVE

Anesthetic technique: GETA. The goals of anesthesia for this procedure are to: (1) preserve myocardial, renal, pulmonary, CNS and visceral organ function; (2) maintain adequate intravascular volume so that CO is not impaired; (3) control BP so that the transmural pressure across the aneurysm does not increase, which would increase the risk of rupture; and (4) provide good perfusion of other organs. CPB is used to accomplish deep hypothermic circulatory arrest. The rationale for this use is controversial. Deep hypothermic cardiac arrest (DHCA) may confer spinal cord protection and is usually reserved for patients with chronic dissections. In addition, removal of CSF has been proposed as another means of protecting the spinal cord against ischemic injury. CPB also may be used for distal perfusion of organs and afterload protection of the left ventricle. Partial CPB usually is reserved for suprarenal or supraceliac aneurysms to perfuse bowel and kidneys. (See Anesthetic Considerations for Cardiopulmonary Bypass, p. 262, and Repair of Acute Aortic Dissections, p. 318, for more discussion on CPB and DHCA.)

Induction	Prevent hypertensive response to laryngoscopy and intubation with moderate-dose narcotic technique (fentanyl 10-20 μg/kg or sufentanil 1-2 μg/kg) in combination with STP (2-4 mg/kg) or propofol (1-2 mg/kg). Esmolol 100-500 μg/kg over 1 min, NTP 0.5-3 μg/kg, or lidocaine administered either by topical spray or an iv dose of 1.5 mg/kg also will decrease the cardiovascular response to intubation. Muscle relaxation for intubation may be achieved with vecuronium (beware of ↓HR), rocuronium (1 mg/kg), or pancuronium (0.1 mg/kg). Etomidate (0.1-0.3 mg/kg) is useful in unstable patients for emergent repair following rupture or ongoing dissection. A modified rapid-sequence induction may be necessary in emergent cases. A DLT is mandatory for this procedure; however, it may be difficult to position due to distorted anatomy. FOB is mandatory to verify position of DLT.
Maintenance	O$_2$/air/narcotic, ± low-dose volatile agent. Benzodiazepines may be used for amnesia (e.g., midazolam 100 μg/kg). When epidural catheter in place, sufentanil (loading dose 25-50 μg, followed by 4-6 μg/h) may provide adequate additional analgesia. In hemodynamically unstable patients, scopolamine (400 μg) provides amnesia. Maintain CO and control of BP at preop levels. These patients may have increased hemodynamic variability on cross-clamping aorta, 2° bleeding, and coexisting disease. Keeping the patient warm may be difficult due to large incision and visceral exposure.
Emergence	Deferred to ICU. Postop ventilation 24-72 h. DLT may need to be maintained postop 2° to facial, oral, and airway edema.
Blood and fluid requirements	Anticipate large blood loss. IV: 14 ga or 7 Fr × 2 Rapid infuser Cell Saver T&C 8-10 U PRBCs. Warm fluids and humidify gases. Maintain UO 0.5-1 ml/kg/h.	Large incision and visceral exposure requires administration of large volumes of fluid. Consider use of mannitol or furosemide if concerned about renal function and UO.

Monitoring	Standard monitors (p. B-1) CVP ± PA catheter ± ST segment analysis Arterial line UO	✓ for ↑ PA pressures and PCWP, ↓ in CO, TEE wall motion abnormalities, and changes in SV. Consult with surgeon regarding placement of cross-clamp so arterial line will not be affected.
	TEE	TEE is a good monitor for ventricular filling and myocardial ischemia.
	Core temperature	Monitor core T (esophageal, bladder). Tympanic membrane T (indicative of brain T) is monitored for circulatory arrest cases.
	± EEG, SSEP, MEP	EEG and EPs may be useful in assessment of cerebral protection (SSEP) and spinal cord perfusion problems (MEP ± SSEP).
Cross-clamping	Clamping	Application of cross-clamp at supraceliac level probably produces the greatest hemodynamic stress experienced by surgical patients. Application of the clamp may → HTN and ischemia. Preload, afterload, and HR can be controlled with SNP (0.25-5 μg/kg/min) and esmolol (100-500 μg/kg/min) infusions. Bolus dose NTG (100 μg) may be useful to terminate an acute hypertensive episode.
	Unclamping	Ensure adequate volume; replace blood loss. Just before removal of the cross-clamp, filling volumes are allowed to rise gradually, avoiding the occurrence of myocardial ischemia. Dilators are D/C'd. ↓ BP may occur with removal of cross-clamp 2° hypovolemia, reactive hyperemia, acidosis, ↑ K$^+$, or myocardial dysfunction. BE > -5 should be connected before unclamping. If necessary, surgeon can reclamp or occlude the aorta.
Positioning	Right axillary roll ✓ and pad pressure points. ✓ eyes.	Right lateral decubitus with hips rotated posteriorly. Left arm placed in airplane sling or supported by pillows.
Complications	Myocardial ischemia HTN Coagulopathy Hemorrhage Hemostasis Hypothermia Other organ ischemia	Coagulopathy due to dilutional and consumptive processes. Hypothermia may exacerbate coagulopathy, cause dysrhythmias, and depress cardiac contractility.

POSTOPERATIVE

Complications	Myocardial ischemia Neurologic deficits 2° cerebral or spinal cord ischemia Renal failure Respiratory failure	BP should be closely controlled postop to decrease bleeding from graft site and raw surfaces.
Pain management	Epidural narcotics (p. C-2)	In selected patients, a thoracic epidural catheter may be placed the night before surgery; otherwise, an epidural is placed only after normal neurologic and coagulation status is determined.
Tests	CXR: line and ETT placement Coagulation profile ABG analysis	

References

1. Arisan Ergin M, Galla JD, Lansman SL, Quintana C, Bodian C, Griepp RP: Hypothermic circulatory arrest in operations on the thoracic aorta. *J Thorac Cardiovasc Surg* 1994; 107:788-99.

2. Cambria RP, Clouse WD, Davison JK, Dunn PF, Corey M, Dorer D: Thoracoabdominal aneurysm repair: results with 337 operations performed over a 15-year interval. *Ann Surg* 2002; 236:471-9.
3. Coselli JS, Lemaire SA, Miller CC, Schmittling ZC, Koksoy C, Pagan J, Curling PE: Mortality and paraplegia after thoracoabdominal aortic aneurysm repair: A risk factor analysis. *Ann Thorac Surg* 2000; 69:408-14.
4. Dong CCJ, MacDonald DB, Janusz MT: Intraoperative spinal cord monitoring during descending thoracic and thoracoabdominal aneurysm surgery. *Ann Thorac Surg* 2002; 74:S1874-76.
5. Fann JI: Descending thoracic and thoracoabdominal aortic aneurysms. *Coron Artery Dis* 2002; 13:93-102.
6. Gharagozloo F, Larson J, Dausman MJ, Neville RF, Gomes MN: Spinal cord protection during surgical procedures on the descending thoracic and thoracoabdominal aorta. *Chest* 1996; 109:799-809.
7. Kazama S, Masaki Y, Maruyama S, Ishihara A: Effect of altering cerebrospinal fluid pressure on spinal cord blood flow. *Ann Thorac Surg* 1994; 58(1):112-5.
8. Ling E, Arrellano R: Systematic overview of the evidence supporting the use of cerebrospinal fluid drainage in thoracoabdominal aneurysm surgery for prevention of paraplegia. *Anesthesiology* 2000; 93:1115-22.
9. Lips J, de Haan P, de Jager S, Vanicky I, Jacobs MJ, Kalkman CG: The role of transcranial motor evoked potentials in predicting neurologic and histopathologic outcome after experimental spinal cord ischemia. *Anesthesiology* 2002; 97:183-91.
10. Moore W: *Vascular Surgery*, 5th edition. WB Saunders Co, Philadelphia: 1998.
11. O'Connor CJ, Rothenberg DM: Anesthetic considerations for ascending thoracic aortic surgery. *J Cardiothorac Vasc Anesth* 1995; 9:581-8.
12. Roizen MF, Beaupre PN, Alpert RA, et al: Monitoring with two-dimensional transesophageal echocardiography. Comparison of myocardial function in patients undergoing supraceliac, suprarenal-infraceliac, or infrarenal aortic occlusion. *J Vasc Surg* 1984; 1:300-5.

SURGERY OF THE ABDOMINAL AORTA

SURGICAL CONSIDERATIONS

Description: Operations on the abdominal aorta are generally performed for aneurysmal or occlusive diseases. Although **aortic aneurysms** may involve the suprarenal aorta, the majority are infrarenal in origin, and may extend into the iliac arteries (Fig 6.3-7). Most (> 95%) are asymptomatic, and are discovered incidentally during investigation of another medical problem. Because of the associated increased risk for rupture as the aneurysm increases in size, most vascular surgeons recommend prophylactic repair for aneurysms > 5 cm in cross-section dimension. Repair also is indicated for painful aneurysms, those that have been associated with atheroembolism, and when there is documented recent increase in size or evidence of leak or rupture. CAD coexists in 30-40% of these patients, and should be assessed preop.

The operative repair may be either **transperitoneal** or **retroperitoneal** (Fig 6.3-8). After

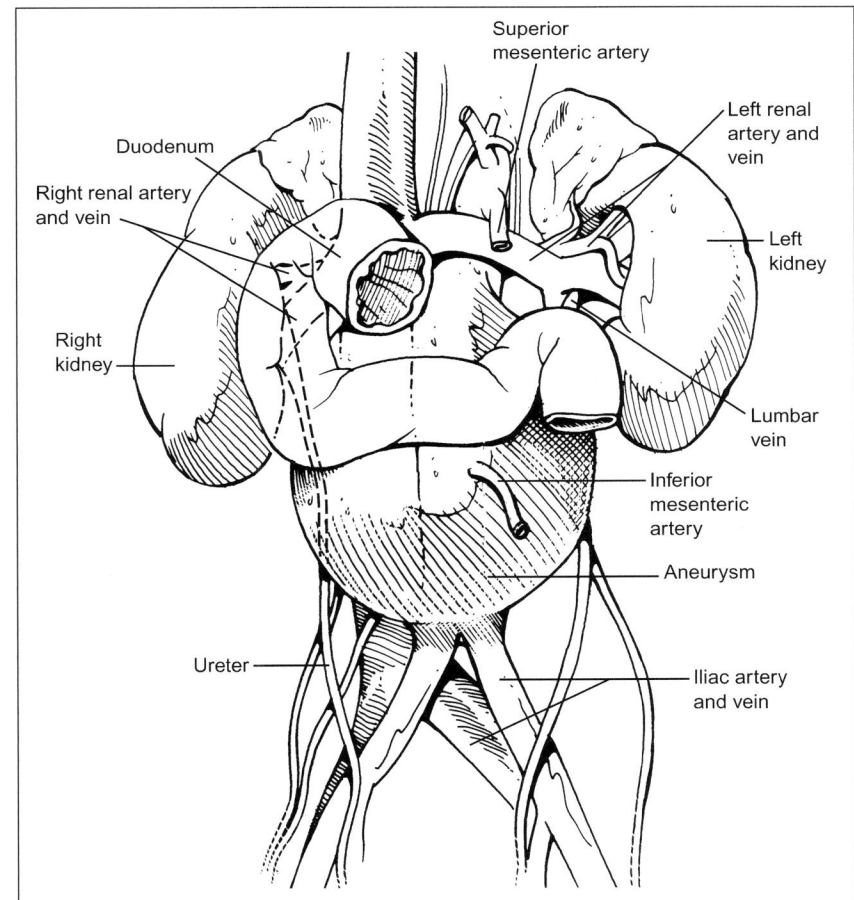

Figure 6.3-7. Aneurysm of the abdominal aorta.

exposure of the abdominal aorta from the level of the renal vein distally to the iliac arteries, the aorta is cross-clamped, distally at first to prevent atheroembolism, and then proximally. Graft origin is usually from the infrarenal aorta, but may arise from the inframesenteric aorta or even the supraceliac aorta. Graft termination may be to the distal aorta above the bifurcation (tube graft), to the common or external iliac arteries (Y graft), or the femoral arteries. Immediately prior to cross-clamping, vasodilators are increased to reduce afterload, which is significantly increased with application of the aortic cross-clamp. The aorta is then incised, lumbar vessels oversewn, and the aorta transected to allow an interposition graft to be sewn into place. The retroperitoneal approach has many advocates, as it may require less volume intraop, may be associated with less temperature loss, and may result in a shorter period of postop

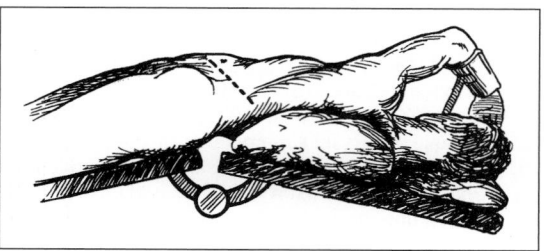

Figure 6.3-8. Retroperitoneal approach to the aorta: the incision is extended from the tip of the 11th rib or 10th intercostal space laterally toward the midhypogastrium. (Reproduced with permission from Scott-Conner CEH, Dawson DL: *Operative Anatomy*, 2nd edition. Lippincott Williams & Wilkins, Philadelphia, 2003.)

adynamic ileus. In a randomized, prospective study, however, no significant differences could be detected between these two approaches for blood loss or postop recovery time.

Aortoiliac occlusive disease can be a significant cause of lower extremity arterial insufficiency. Although the operative approach may be similar to that for aneurysmal disease, there exists a significant intraop difference in that there are not such profound changes associated with aortic clamping, since there is already some element of increased afterload 2° the occlusive disease. Nevertheless, hemodynamic monitoring is mandatory to allow for rapid volume shifts, and to assure adequate preload and sufficient afterload reduction, especially during the period of aortic cross-clamping.

Variant procedure or approaches: In the rare patient with COPD severe enough to preclude weaning from the ventilator postop, extraanatomic grafts (e.g., axillofemoral, iliofemoral, and fem-fem bypass) can be constructed under local anesthesia.

Usual preop diagnosis: Abdominal aortic aneurysm (AAA); severe aortoiliac stenosis sufficient to cause debilitating buttock, thigh, or calf claudication; isolated-inflow (aortoiliac) disease (rarely the sole cause for ischemic symptoms at rest or for tissue loss, except as a result of embolic complications)

SUMMARY OF PROCEDURES

	Transperitoneal Approach	Retroperitoneal Approach
Position	Supine	Supine with mild elevation of left flank
Incision	Midline abdominal	Left subcostal, left oblique, along 10th rib toward umbilicus (See Fig 6.3-8.)
Special instrumentation	Self-retaining retractor; TEE; If suprarenal change: SMA + renal artery perfusion catheters.	⇐
Unique considerations	Will need pharmacologic manipulation to ↓ afterload or ↑ preload coincident with clamping or unclamping of aorta.	⇐ (The retroperitoneal approach is not used for emergency cases.)
Antibiotics	Cefazolin 1 g iv	⇐
Surgical time	3-5 h	⇐
EBL	500 ml	⇐
Postop care	ICU 8-16 h, often extubated. Requires aggressive volume administration to allow for 3rd-space loss in 1st 12 h postop. Patient comfort and respiratory management markedly improved by epidural catheter for postop analgesia. Careful cardiac monitoring.	⇐
Mortality	2-5% elective; 50% emergent	⇐
Morbidity	MI: 10-15% (3% fatal)	⇐
	Respiratory insufficiency/pneumonia: 5-10%	
	Lower extremity ischemia: 2-5%	
	Renal insufficiency: 2-5%	
	Bowel complications: 3-4%	
	Hemorrhage: 2-4%	
	CVA: < 1%	
	Infection: < 1%	
	Paraplegia: < 0.4%	
Pain score	8-10	7-10

PATIENT POPULATION CHARACTERISTICS

Age range	55 yr +
Male:Female	4:1
Incidence	3% of males > 55 yr; > 5% of patients > 50 yr in a general cardiology clinic; 30-66/1000
Etiology	Atherosclerosis; Marfan syndrome; Ehlers-Danlos syndrome; dissection; infection, including syphilis
Associated conditions	HTN; CAD; COPD; cerebrovascular disease; renal insufficiency

---

ANESTHETIC CONSIDERATIONS

PREOPERATIVE

Patients presenting for AAA repair are typically older males with multiple coexisting diseases (e.g., CAD, HTN, PVD, COPD). Most commonly these patients are asymptomatic and the Dx is made as an incidental finding during routine exams or other medical procedures; however, some patients may present with severe ↓BP following aneurysm rupture. These patients require prompt resuscitation (SBP goal: 90-100 mmHg) and emergent aortic cross-clamping. For anesthetic considerations, see Abdominal Trauma: Vascular Injuries (p. 585).

Respiratory	Many patients have COPD and a long Hx of smoking. Preop preparation—including bronchodilators, cessation of smoking, incentive spirometry, and chest physiotherapy—will ↓ risk of postop complications. **Tests:** CXR. May need PFTs and ABG to determine severity of pulmonary disease.
Cardiovascular	CAD is the most common cause of morbidity and mortality in this patient population. HTN increases risk of aneurysmal rupture; hence, preop control of BP is essential. ✓ BP in both arms to determine placement of arterial line intraop (arterial line should be placed in arm with higher BP). **Tests:** Radiologic assessment of aneurysm using ultrasonography, CT, arteriography, and MRI. ECG: ✓ for evidence of ischemia, infarction, and LVH.
Renal	Chronic renal insufficiency occurs frequently in this patient population 2° HTN, diabetes mellitus (DM), and atherosclerotic renovascular disease. Hypovolemia 2° radiographic dye studies and bowel prep → renal failure. **Tests:** BUN, Cr; consider creatinine clearance; electrolytes
Hematologic	Preop coagulation disorders should be corrected. Many patients are on aspirin, which should be D/C'd 7 d preop. Alcohol abuse can be associated with anemia, thrombocytopenia, and ↓ vitamin K-dependent factors. **Tests:** PT; PTT; Hct; Plt
Laboratory	Other tests as indicated from H&P.
Premedication	Anxiety and pain may cause HTN and ↑ risk of aneurysmal rupture. Sedatives and analgesics should be used as indicated (p. B-2). Full-stomach precautions for emergent procedures (p. B-5).

INTRAOPERATIVE

Anesthetic technique: GETA or combination of epidural and GA. The goals of anesthesia are to: (1) preserve myocardial, renal, pulmonary, and CNS perfusion; (2) maintain adequate intravascular volume and CO; (3) anticipate the surgical maneuvers that will affect BP and blood volume; and (4) control BP to minimize risk of rupture, while ensuring perfusion of other organs.

Induction	If it is planned to extubate the patient postop, anesthesia should be induced using fentanyl (4-6 μg/kg) in conjunction with STP (2-4 mg/kg) or etomidate (0.2-0.4 mg/kg). If an epidural will be used for postop pain relief, no further iv doses of narcotic should be given intraop. Patients with an epidural typically receive morphine (2-4 mg), fentanyl (150-200 μg), or sufentanil (50 μg) in 10 ml. Local anesthetics may cause hemodynamic instability after unclamping 2° sympathectomy. Muscle relaxants are chosen to minimize tachycardia or ↓BP (e.g., vecuronium 0.1 mg/kg or rocuronium 1 mg/kg). Anesthesia is deepened before intubation by mask ventilation with 1% sevoflurane. If there is a hemodynamic response to oral airway insertion, tracheal lidocaine or further anesthetic is given before gentle laryngoscopy and intubation. Etomidate is useful for induction in hemodynamically unstable patients. Full-stomach precautions may be necessary.

Maintenance	O_2/air/narcotic and volatile agent. N_2O can be used, but it may cause bowel distention. Combining epidural and GA offers good abdominal relaxation. Patients receiving epidural local anesthesia may require phenylephrine to treat $\downarrow$BP 2° sympathetic blockade. Epidural catheter placement before systemic anticoagulation is a safe technique. Narcotic epidural analgesia should be given within 1 h of skin incision if morphine 3-8 mg is used. If hydromorphone (0.5-0.8 mg) is given epidurally, it is given within 1 h of abdominal closure. Patient may become hypothermic 2° large incision with visceral exposure and prolonged operation.	
Emergence	Normothermic (> 35.5°C) patients who have had uneventful surgery, especially utilizing a retroperitoneal approach, are frequently extubated in the OR, or shortly after arrival in the ICU. Patients with severe cardiac or pulmonary disease generally are mechanically ventilated for 24-48 h. Prevention of HTN and tachycardia during emergence may require titration of ß-adrenergic-blocking drugs (e.g., esmolol 50-300 μg/kg/min) and/or vasodilators (e.g., SNP 0.25-5.0 μg/kg/min) or NTG (0.25-5.0 μg/kg/min). Epidural morphine (2-4 mg) or hydromorphone (0.5-0.8 mg) is given ~60 min before the end of surgery. It is important to assure full reversal from neuromuscular blockade.	
Blood and fluid requirements	Major blood loss IV: 14 ga (or 7 Fr) × 2 4 U PRBC UO 0.5-1 ml/kg/h Warm all fluids. Humidify all gases.	Use of rapid infusion and blood-salvaging devices helpful. Consider acute normovolemic hemodilution. Hemorrhage should be treated with crystalloid, colloid, or blood products as appropriate. Low-sider, upper-body Bair-Hugger.
Monitoring	Standard monitors (p. B-1)	Monitor for cardiac ischemia. Automated ST segment analysis is useful.
	CVP line	The measurement of CVP may be sufficient in patients with good ventricular function and exercise tolerance.
	PA catheter	In patients with recent MI, Hx of CHF, Hx of unstable angina, multisystem disease, or in those presenting emergently (without the benefit of a complete workup), however, a PA catheter is appropriate.
	TEE	TEE is invaluable for assessing cardiac changes 2° cross-clamping and unclamping the aorta.
	Arterial line Urinary catheter	The arterial line is generally placed in the radial artery of the arm having the higher BP (if difference exists).
Cross-clamping	$\uparrow\uparrow$ Afterload $\rightarrow$ HTN $\downarrow$ Preload $\uparrow$ Filling pressures $\pm\downarrow$ Spinal cord perfusion $\pm\downarrow$ Renal perfusion $\downarrow$ Perfusion to viscera below the clamp ABGs/electrolytes regularly	Application of aortic cross-clamp causes HTN proximal to the clamp. In a healthy heart, this is well tolerated, with minimal increase in filling pressure. In hearts with poor ventricular function, filling pressures generally rise. Control of preload, afterload, and HR can be accomplished with vasodilators and β-blockers. Negative inotropic agents (e.g., β-blockers, inhalational anesthetics) are used cautiously. Occlusion of infrarenal aorta $\downarrow$ renal blood flow. Ensure adequate intravascular volume and CO. Administer mannitol (0.5 g/kg) before clamping to maintain UO.
Aortic unclamping	$\downarrow\downarrow$ Afterload Volume loading Lactate washout $\pm$ Phenylephrine	Immediately before unclamping, D/C dilators and negative inotropic agents. Gradually increase filling pressures (volume loading) to avoid myocardial ischemia. $\downarrow\downarrow$BP may occur with removal of cross-clamp 2° to hypovolemia, reactive hyperemia, or myocardial dysfunction. Reperfusion of lower limbs and washout of lactate does not usually require use of HCO_3. Patients with an epidural sympathetic block often require phenylephrine support during unclamping. The surgeon can reclamp or occlude the aorta, if $\downarrow\downarrow$BP persists. If hemodynamically stable with $\downarrow$UO, consider furosemide 40-80 mg.
Positioning	✓ and pad pressure points. ✓ eyes.	

Complications	Myocardial ischemia	Hypothermia may cause dysrhythmias, depress contrac-
	HTN	tility, and exacerbate coagulopathy.
	Hemorrhage	
	Coagulopathy	
	Hypothermia	
	Organ ischemia	

POSTOPERATIVE

Complications	Myocardial ischemia	
	Renal failure	
	Respiratory failure	
Pain management	Epidural narcotics (p. C-1)	
Tests	CXR to ✓ line and ETT placement	BP should be closely controlled postop to decrease bleed-
	ABG	ing from graft site and raw surfaces.
	Coagulation profile	
	BUN; Cr	

References

1. Adams van der Vliet J, Boll APM: Abdominal aortic aneurysms. *Lancet* 1997; 349:863-6.
2. Arko FR, Lee WA, Hill BB, Olcott C IV, Dalman RL, Harris EJ Jr, Cipriano P, Fogarty TJ, Zarias CK. Aneurysm-related death: primary endpoint analysis for comparison of open and endovascular repair. *J Vasc Surg* 2002; 36:297-304.
3. Boccara G, Jaber S, Eliet J, Mann C, Colson P: Monitoring of end-tidal dioxide partial pressure changes during infrarenal aortic cross-clamping: a non-invasive method to predict unclamping hypotension. *Acta Anesthesiol Scand* 2001; 45:188-93.
4. Brimacombe J, Berry A: A review of anaesthesia for ruptured abdominal aortic aneurysm with special emphasis on pre-clamping fluid resuscitation. *Anaesthes Intensive Care* 1993; 21(3):311-23.
5. Dunn E, Prager RL, Fry W, Kirsh MM: The effect of abdominal aortic cross-clamping on myocardial function. *J Surg Res* 1977; 22:463-8.
6. Falk JL, Rackow EC, Blumenberg R, et al: Hemodynamic and metabolic effects of abdominal aortic cross-clamping. *Am J Surg* 1981; 142:174-7.
7. Gold MS, DeCrosta D, Rizzuto C, Ben-Itarari RR, Ramanathan S: The effect of lumbar epidural and general anesthesia on plasma catecholamines and hemodynamics during abdominal aortic aneurysm repair. *Anesth Analg* 1994; 78(2):225-30.
8. Gooding JM, Archie JP Jr, McDowell H: Hemodynamic response to infrarenal aortic cross-clamping in patients with and without coronary artery disease. *Crit Care Med* 1980; 8:382-5.
9. Patra P, Chaillou P, Bizouarn P: Intraoperative autotransfusion for repair of unruptured aneurysms of the infrarenal abdominal aorta. *J Cardiovasc Surg* 2000; 41:407-13.
10. Sprung J, Abdelmalak B, Gottlieb A, Mayhew C, Hammel J, Levy PJ, O'Hara P, Hertzer NR: Analysis of risk factors for myocardial infarction and cardiac mortality after major vascular surgery. *Anesthesiology* 2000; 93:129-40.
11. Thompson RW, Geraghty PJ, Lee JK: Abdominal aortic aneurysms: Basic mechanisms and clinical implications. *Curr Probl Surg* 2002; 39:110-230.

INFRAINGUINAL ARTERIAL BYPASS

SURGICAL CONSIDERATIONS

Description: Due to the limited durability of distal bypass procedures, bypass to the infrainguinal arteries is indicated only for salvage of the severely ischemic lower extremity, as manifest by gangrene, ischemic ulceration, or ischemic rest pain. Less frequently, it is used to alleviate functional ischemia of claudication, or leg discomfort with exercise. Its use is predicated on the preexistence of adequate inflow to the level of the groin or femoral artery. Other necessary components include an adequate target vessel, preferably in continuity with runoff into the plantar arch of the foot, and an adequate conduit, preferably autologous saphenous vein. Long-term patency rates of nonautologous conduits to the below-knee arteries is distinctly inferior to that of saphenous vein and should be avoided whenever possible. This population, almost by definition, includes patients with diabetes mellitus (DM), CAD, and cerebrovascular disease, all of which must be assessed preop.

The operative repair usually involves incisions at the groin and distal bypass sites to expose the donor and recipient arteries and to harvest leg or arm venous conduit. The operative approaches are rather similar. An unobstructed inflow source—usually the common femoral, superficial femoral, or deep femoral artery—is exposed in the groin. The target distal artery, usually at the level of the knee or below, can be approached through a medial incision. More distally, the peroneal and anterior tibial arteries can be approached laterally at the midtibial level. At the level of the malleolus, both the dorsalis pedis and posterior tibial arteries can be revascularized. After control of donor and recipient vessels, an anatomic tunnel is created, and the bypass conduit (saphenous vein, prosthetic graft) is passed through its length. After administration of 10,000 U of heparin, the distal anastomosis is constructed first, followed by the proximal anastomosis. A completion arteriogram confirms unobstructed flow. Heparin is then partially reversed and meticulous hemostasis obtained, and the wounds are closed.

Although conventional wisdom has held that the anesthetic and operative risks for patients undergoing distal reconstructions are low, there may be little difference in postop morbidity and mortality when compared with patients undergoing a major inflow procedure within the abdomen.[6]

Usual preop diagnosis: Severe peripheral vascular disease (PVD); CAD; DM; HTN; obstructive PA disease. (These are almost ubiquitous comorbidities.)

SUMMARY OF PROCEDURE

Position	Supine
Incision	Groin, medial knee, ± distal leg incisions; + incision to harvest venous conduit
Antibiotics	Cefazolin 1 g iv at induction of anesthesia
Surgical time	2-5 h
Closing considerations	Optimization of coagulation status
EBL	200-300 ml
Postop care	Possible ICU × 24 h; patients are at risk for myocardial ischemia.
Mortality	2-4%
Morbidity	MI: 5-12%
	Respiratory insufficiency: 5%
	Infection: 2-5%
	Amputation: 2-4%
	CVA: < 1%
Pain score	4-6

PATIENT POPULATION CHARACTERISTICS

Age range	> 55 yr (mean age = > 70 yr)
Male:Female	4:1
Incidence	Claudication fairly common in elderly; however, 75% will remain untreated, but stable, over 2-5 yr, with < 5% requiring amputation.
Etiology	Arteriosclerosis (primarily); chronic embolic disease (rare); vasculitis; popliteal artery entrapment; cystic adventitial disease of popliteal artery
Associated conditions	CAD; cerebrovascular disease; DM; HTN; COPD

ANESTHETIC CONSIDERATIONS

**(Procedures covered: infrainguinal arterial bypass; arterial embolectomy;
lumbar sympathectomy; venous thrombectomy or vein excision)**

PREOPERATIVE

Patients presenting for peripheral vascular surgery may suffer from major systemic diseases, including CAD, HTN, and DM. Three types of occlusive vascular disease have been described: Type 1—isolated to the aortic and iliac bifurcations; is not associated with CAD. Type 2—diffuse pattern involving coronary and cerebral circulations; associated with a higher incidence of DM and HTN. Type 3—involves small vessels, especially of the lower limbs; associated with higher postop morbidity and mortality.

Respiratory	Vascular patients frequently have Hx of smoking and COPD. Preop evaluation of pulmonary function helps to determine whether regional vs GA is appropriate, while providing baseline values for postop comparison. **Tests:** CXR; consider PFTs; ABG

Cardiovascular	Vascular surgery of the lower extremities is often associated with ↑morbidity and mortality 2° ↑incidence of CAD and HTN in this patient population. **Tests:** ECG: ✓ for LVH and ischemia; other tests as indicated from H&P.
Neurological	↑incidence of cerebrovascular disease. Careful neurological assessment is necessary to document existing deficits.
Endocrine	↑incidence of DM, which may be associated with peripheral and autonomic neuropathies (silent MI, labile BP) and delayed gastric emptying. Insulin requirements for most diabetic patients can be managed by administering one-half the usual a.m. dose of insulin, once a dextrose-containing iv (e.g., D5LR) has been established. Frequent blood glucose measurements should be made periop.
Renal	There is a higher incidence of renal artery disease and renal insufficiency in this patient population. **Tests:** BUN; Cr; consider creatinine clearance; electrolytes; UA
Hematologic	Many patients presenting for this surgery are taking anticoagulant/anti-Plt medications. Inquire as to bleeding or bruising tendency. **Tests:** Hct; Plt; consider PT, PTT.
Laboratory	As indicated from H&P.
Premedication	Continue usual medications up to time of surgery. Anxiety can contribute to HTN and tachycardia. Premedicate conservatively (midazolam 0.5-2 mg iv) for elderly patients. If ischemic pain is present, a narcotic such as fentanyl (25-50 μg iv) can be given. Avoid im administration in patients on anticoagulant therapy.

INTRAOPERATIVE

Anesthetic technique: Either regional anesthesia or GETA may be used. For **infrainguinal arterial bypass**, there is evidence that regional anesthesia is superior for promoting graft survival. To date, no study has shown a difference in patient mortality between these anesthetic techniques. **Lumbar sympathectomy** may be accomplished with regional or GA. For **thrombectomy**, GETA with IPPV may reduce the risk of pulmonary emboli.

General anesthesia:

Induction	Hemodynamic stability is important; therefore, a slow, gradual induction is carried out. Preoxygenation is followed by smooth iv induction, using small, incremental doses of fentanyl (1-3 μg/kg); then STP is given in divided doses (50-75 mg at a time) until the patient is asleep. A full dose of muscle relaxant is given and ventilation is controlled. Muscle relaxation is not necessary during the procedure, but muscle relaxant is given to facilitate intubation. The muscle relaxant is chosen to avoid undesirable effects on HR. Alternatively, if the LV function is poor, and the depressant effects of STP cannot be tolerated, etomidate (0.2 mg/kg iv) in combination with fentanyl (100-200 μg) is appropriate.
Maintenance	Standard maintenance (p. B-3) with fentanyl (1-2 μg/kg/h). Continued muscle relaxation is usually unnecessary. These surgical procedures are associated with minimal hemodynamic instability.
Emergence	Tracheal extubation should be based on standard criteria, such as adequacy of ventilation, return of airway reflexes and reversal of muscle relaxation. Control of BP is accomplished with vasodilators (e.g., NTG 0.1-4.0 μg/kg/min or SNP 0.25-5.0 μg/kg/min). Esmolol can be given in incremental doses of 10 mg or by infusion (50-200 μg/kg/min).

Regional anesthesia: Patients presenting for regional anesthesia must have a normal coagulation profile; also, they cannot be on heparin (including low molecular weight), urokinase, or streptokinase. The important goals in regional anesthesia are to achieve hemodynamic stability while establishing an adequate block. An epidural or spinal catheter (multiorifice) is frequently used to infuse local anesthetic for a gradual onset and to prevent an excessively high block. Hemodynamic stability can be improved by infusing 500-1000 ml of crystalloid before performing the block. The patient may be placed in the lateral decubitus position (with operative side down), which may provide a denser and more prolonged block on that side. Achieving a T8-T10 level is optimal. Overzealous hydration may → CHF in this patient population, when the vasodilation 2° regional sympathectomy dissipates. The use of regional anesthesia in patients receiving intraop anticoagulation is controversial. We feel it is a relatively safe procedure and have not had a complication with this technique. If blood is aspirated after placement of an epidural, we remove the catheter and then replace it at a different interspace. Patients on minidose heparin should have a normal PTT before use of regional anesthesia.

Spinal	**One-shot spinal:** 1% hyperbaric tetracaine (6-10 mg) or 0.75% bupivacaine (10-15 mg). Add epinephrine 0.2 mg (generally increases duration of block about 50%) or phenylephrine 5 mg (generally increases duration of block about 100%). Do not add vasoconstrictor if patient is diabetic. Large doses of hyperbaric local anesthetic should be avoided as they may cause postop cauda equina syndrome.	
	Continuous spinal: A 20-ga catheter is placed via an 18-ga Tuohy needle. 0.5% hyperbaric tetracaine or 0.75% bupivacaine is titrated to desired anesthetic level (T8-T10). Catheters should be redosed every 60-80 min or as soon as BP trends upward. The risk of spinal headache is very low with continuous spinals.	
Epidural	Lidocaine 2% with 1:200,000 epinephrine or 0.5% bupivacaine is used. Titrate to desired anesthetic level (T8-T10).	
Blood and fluid requirements	IV: 14 or 16 ga × 1 NS/LR @ 3-5 ml/kg/h Warm fluids. Humidify gases. Maintain UO 0.5-1 ml/kg/h.	Minimal-to-moderate blood loss. Use forced-air warmer (e.g., Bair-Hugger).
Monitoring	Standard monitors (p. B-1) Arterial line ST-segment analysis	An arterial line is most often used in patients with severe cardiopulmonary disease or brittle diabetics. Blood sampling for ABGs, electrolytes, glucose, and Hct is facilitated by the use of an arterial line.
	± CVP/PA catheters	CVP and PA catheters are not used routinely because large changes in intravascular volumes are uncommon. Patients with poor LV function, recent MI, or severe valvular disease may need PA monitoring.
Positioning	✓ and pad pressure points. ✓ eyes.	Diabetic patients may be at risk of skin ischemia due to poor positioning or inadequate padding of limbs, etc.
Complications	HTN Ischemic reperfusion syndrome (post-embolectomy) Hypothermia Hemorrhage	Reperfusion of an ischemic limb → ↓ pH, ↑ K^+, and release of myoglobin from injured muscle → ATN.

POSTOPERATIVE

Complications	CHF Hypothermia Graft occlusion	Infrainguinal bypass: Avoid overhydration; when epidural sympathectomy fades, these patients are at increased risk for CHF. Maintain normovolemia so that peripheral vasoconstriction (which may limit outflow to the graft) does not occur. Hypothermia causes vasoconstriction and also may limit outflow to the graft.
Pain management	Epidural/spinal opiates (p. C-1) PCA	Epidural (or spinal) catheter may be used for postop analgesia (p. C-2).
Tests	CXR if central line placed Hct	

References

1. Bernards CM: Epidural and spinal anesthesia. In *Clinical Anesthesia,* 3rd edition. Barash PG, Cullen BF, Stoelting RK, eds. Lippincott-Raven, Philadelphia: 1997, 645-68.
2. Byrne J, Darling RC, Chang BB, Paty PS, Kreienberg PB, Lloyd WE, Leather RP, Shah DM: Inguinal arterial reconstruction for claudication: Is it worth the risk? An analysis of 409 procedures. *J Vasc Surg* 1999; 29:259-67.
3. Damask MC, Weissman C, Barth A, et al: General vs epidural—which is the better anesthetic technique for femoral-popliteal bypass surgery? *Anesth Analg* 1986; 65:539.
4. Darling RC, Reddy BP, Chang BB, Paty PS, Kreienberg PB, Maharaj D, Shah DM: Long-term results of revised infrainguinal arterial reconstructions. *J Vasc Surg* 2002; 35:773-8.

5. Denny N, Masters R, Pearson D, Rend J, Sihota M, Selander D: Postdural puncture headache after continuous spinal anesthesia. *Anesth Analg* 1987; 66(8):791-4.
6. Krupski WC, Layug EL, Reilly LM, Rapp JH, Mangano DT: Comparison of cardiac morbidity between aortic and infrainguinal operations. Study of Perioperative Ischemia (SPI) Research Group. *J Vasc Surg* 1992; 15(2):354-65.
7. Rosenfeld BA, Beattie C, Christopherson R, Norris EJ, Frank SM, Breslow MJ, Rock P, Parker SD, Gottlieb SO, Perler BA, Williams GM, Seidler A, Bell W: Perioperative Ischemia Randomized Anesthesia Trial Study Group: The effects of different anesthetic regimens on fibrinolysis and the development of postoperative arterial thrombosis. *Anesthesiology* 1993; 79:435-43.

ARTERIAL EMBOLECTOMY

SURGICAL CONSIDERATIONS

Description: The etiology of acute arterial insufficiency is often the result of thromboembolism, which is usually of cardiac origin. Patients at high risk for embolization are those with MI, mitral stenosis, or atrial fibrillation (AF), all of which increase the risk of intracardiac thrombus formation. Noncardiac causes include thoracic and abdominal aortic pathology, such as aneurysms, severe atherosclerotic disease, and paradoxical embolus via a patent foramen ovale (PFO). The emboli usually become lodged at tapering regions and branch sites and most commonly involve the extremities; the cerebrovascular and mesenteric vasculature also may be involved. In the lower extremities, emboli frequently lodge at the iliac, femoral, or popliteal arteries; the common femoral artery is involved in up to 50% of all embolic events. Emboli to the upper extremities typically affect the brachial artery. Because the collateral circulation may not be well developed in patients without underlying peripheral vascular disease, muscle necrosis can appear within 4-6 h after onset, although this time frame is highly variable. Patients are heparinized at time of diagnosis. Therapy directed at the specific etiology is critical to achieve a successful outcome. Revascularization after 8-12 h of ischemia usually is less effective. If the underlying source of the emboli is not adequately treated, recurrence is likely and is associated with poor prognosis. The surgical approach to femoral embolectomy is a groin incision and isolation of the common, superficial, and deep femoral arteries. Both the superficial and deep femoral systems are explored, and small embolectomy catheters are passed into the distal lower extremity. In addition to passage of embolectomy catheters, angioscopy may be helpful. Residual thrombus on intraop arteriogram requires distal surgical exposure and exploration.

Usual preop diagnosis: Peripheral artery embolism

SUMMARY OF PROCEDURE

Position	Supine
Incision	Limited groin, medial knee, possible distal leg incisions
Antibiotics	Cefazolin 1 g iv
Surgical time	Variable, 1-4 h
Closing considerations	Ischemia-reperfusion syndrome with acidosis and hyperkalemia, renal tubular necrosis from myoglobinuria
EBL	100-300 ml
Postop care	May need ICU for cardiac monitoring; monitor metabolic disturbances, neurovascular status, and for compartment syndrome
Mortality	10-40% (~80% cardiac); older age; acute onset →↑ risk.
Morbidity	Arterial reocclusion or thrombosis: 20%
	Wound hematoma: 10-20%
	Recurrent emboli: 6-45% (less with anticoagulation)
	Amputation: 5-10%
	Metabolic complications: Frequent
	Compartment syndrome: Occasional
Pain score	4-6

PATIENT POPULATION CHARACTERISTICS

Age range	30-90 yr
Male:Female	3:2
Incidence	50/100,000 admissions
Etiology	Cardiac origin (AF accounts for 50-75% of patients; less frequent, LV thrombus from MI) or noncardiac origin (mural thrombus from thoracic or abdominal aortic pathology)
Associated conditions	Rheumatic heart disease and mitral stenosis, mitral or aortic valve prosthesis, CAD and MI, CHF, endocarditis, peripheral vascular and cerebrovascular disease.

ANESTHETIC CONSIDERATIONS

See Anesthetic Considerations following Infrainguinal Arterial Bypass, p. 332.

References:

1. Brewster DC: Acute peripheral arterial occlusion. *Cardiol Clin* 1991; 9:497-513.
2. Dregelid EB, Stangeland LB, Eide GE, Trippestad A: Patient survival and limb prognosis after arterial embolectomy. *Eur J Vasc Surg* 1987; 1:263-71.
3. Lau LS, Blanchard DG, Hye RJ: Diagnosis and management of patients with peripheral macroemboli from thoracic aortic pathology. *Ann Vasc Surg* 1997; 11:348-53.
4. Panetta T, Thompson JE, Talkington CM, Garrett WV, Smith RL: Arterial embolectomy: A 34 year experience with 400 cases. *Surg Clin North Am* 1986; 66:339-53.
5. Tawes RL, Harris EJ, Brown WH, Shoor PM, Zimmerman JJ, Sydorak GR, Beare JP, Scribner RG, Fogarty TJ: Arterial thromboembolism. A 20 year perspective. *Arch Surg* 1975; 120:595-9.
6. Varty K, Johnston JA, Beets G, Campbell WB: Arterial embolectomy. A long-term perspective. *J Cardiovasc Surg* 1992; 33: 79-84.

LUMBAR SYMPATHECTOMY

SURGICAL CONSIDERATIONS

Description: The role of **lumbar sympathectomy** is not well defined.[5] The procedure is used selectively in patients with causalgia, inoperable lower limb ischemia with rest pain or toe gangrene, symptomatic vasospastic disorders (e.g., Raynaud's phenomenon, frostbite), and sometimes as an adjunct to distal revascularization procedures.[1,5] Causalgia responds well to lumbar sympathectomy, especially if performed early in the clinical course. There may be some benefit of the procedure in 50-60% of patients with rest pain or ischemic ulceration.[4] Sympathectomy may increase collateral blood flow and local skin blood flow. Scleroderma with impending 'minor' amputation may benefit from sympathectomy with improved wound healing. Sympathetic denervation involves the division of preganglionic fibers along their segmental origins and resection of corresponding relay ganglia.[5] For most clinical indications, L2 and L3 **ganglionectomy** sufficiently sympathectomizes the lower extremity (Fig 6.3-9).

The **anterolateral retroperitoneal approach** (**Flowthow**) is most commonly performed because of the adequate exposure and a relatively well tolerated incision.[5] For this approach, an oblique incision is made through the abdominal musculature, extending from the lateral border of the rectus abdominus to the anterior axillary line. Cephalad and caudad blunt dissection is performed between the transversalis fascia and peritoneum. The dissection is continued in a retroperitoneal fashion. The psoas muscle is identified, with care being taken to leave the ureter and gonadal vessels attached to overlying peritoneum. The sympathetic chain is identified between the psoas muscle and the vertebra (medial to psoas and overlying the transverse process of lumbar vertebra). On the left side, the sympathetic chain is lateral to the abdominal aorta; on the right, the sympathetic chain is beneath the IVC. The sympathetic chain is dissected free from surrounding tissue, clipped proximally and distally, and resected. Hemostasis is achieved and the abdominal wall is closed in layers.

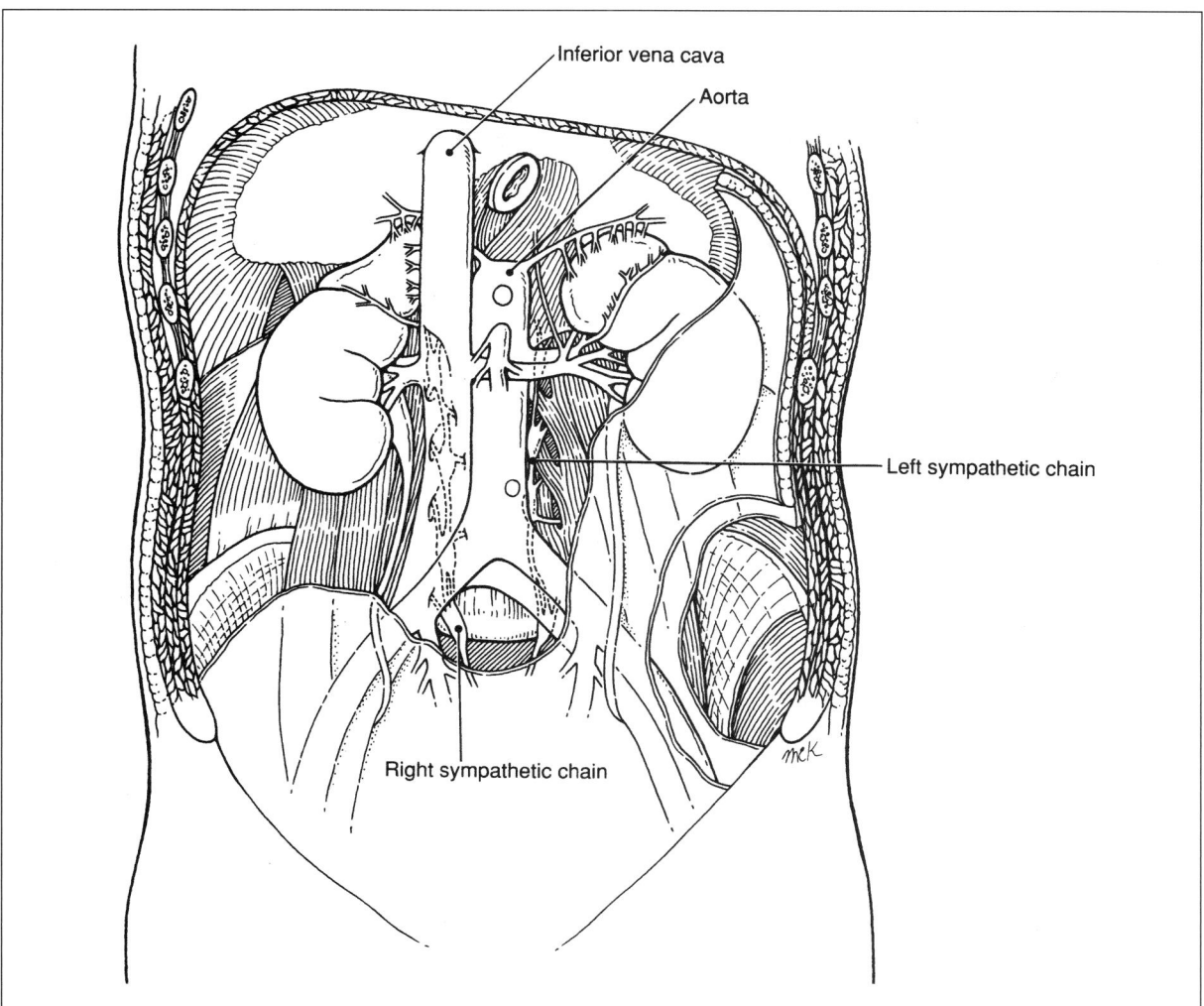

Figure 6.3-9. Surgical anatomy for lumbar sympathectomy. (Reproduced with permission from Scott-Conner CEH, Dawson DL: *Operative Anatomy*, 2nd edition. Lippincott Williams & Wilkins, 2003.)

A **posterior approach** (**Royle**) is used less often because of significant postop paraspinous muscle spasms. In this approach, a transverse lumbar incision is made, and the paraspinous muscles are partially divided and retracted to expose the vertebra. The sympathetic chain is identified and resected as described. The **anterior/transperitoneal approach** is performed in conjunction with an abdominal aortic or intraperitoneal procedure. Dissection is carried to the psoas muscle; the retroperitoneum is entered and the sympathetic chain is isolated in the groove between the psoas and the vertebra. The sympathetic chain is clipped proximally and distally and resected. **Adson's anterior transperitoneal approach** is used when combined with an abdominal aortic or other intraperitoneal procedure.

Usual preop diagnosis: Causalgia; inoperable arterial occlusive disease with limb-threatening ischemia causing rest pain, ulceration, or superficial digital gangrene; symptomatic vasospastic disorders (e.g., Raynaud's phenomenon or frostbite)

SUMMARY OF PROCEDURES

	Anterolateral (Flowthow)	Posterior (Royle)	Anterior (Adson)
Position	Supine (flank slightly raised); widen distance between costal margin and iliac crest.	Prone	Supine
Incision	Oblique (lateral edge of rectus to ribs at anterior axillary line)	Posterior transverse over mid-lumbar region	Transverse or midline abdominal
Special instrumentation	Self-retaining retractor	⇐	⇐

	Anterolateral (Flowthow)	**Posterior (Royle)**	**Anterior (Adson)**
Unique considerations	May use frozen section to confirm specimen.	⇐	⇐
Antibiotics	Cefazolin 1g iv	⇐	⇐
Surgical time	2-3 h	3 h	4 h
Closing considerations	Flex table to facilitate abdominal wall closure; occasionally drain is placed.	⇐	⇐
EBL	50-100 ml (unless complicated)	50-100 ml	⇐
Postop care	PACU → ward. (May require cardiac and hemodynamic monitoring in high-risk patients, or if combined with distal revascularization.)	⇐	⇐
Mortality[1,3,4]	Minimal	⇐	⇐
Morbidity	Postsympathectomy neuralgia: 50%	~50%	⇐
	Sexual derangement—retrograde ejaculation (usually bilateral L1 sympathectomy): 25-50%	~25-50%	⇐
	Wound hematoma: 10%	~10%	⇐
	Wound infection: 1-3%	~1-3%	⇐
		Paraspinous muscle spasms	
Pain score	5	5	5 (related to primary procedure)

PATIENT POPULATION CHARACTERISTICS

Age range	38-91 yr; younger patients with vasospastic disease; older patients with PVD
Male:Female	2:1
Incidence	Unknown. Approximately 30 cases/yr at Stanford University Medical Center, mainly for inoperable lower extremity ischemia or as an adjunct to revascularization procedures.
Etiology	PVD (rest pain and tissue loss); vasospastic disorders; causalgia
Associated conditions	PVD (rare); vasospastic disorders (rare)

ANESTHETIC CONSIDERATIONS

See Anesthetic Considerations following Infrainguinal Arterial Bypass, p. 332.

References

1. Abu Rahma AF, Robinson PA: Clinical parameters for predicting response to lumbar sympathectomy in patients with severe lower limb ischemia. *J Cardiovasc Surg* 1990; 31(1):101-6.
2. Bandyk DF, Johnson BL, Kirkpatrick AF, Novotney ML, Back MR, Schmacht DC: Surgical sympathectomy for reflex sympathetic dystrophic syndromes. *J Vasc Surg* 2002; 35:269-77.
3. Claeys LG: The use of lumbar sympathectomy for peripheral vascular disease. *World J Surg* 1999; 23:981-3.
4. Repelaer van Driel OJ, van Bockel JH, van Schilfgaarde R: Lumbar sympathectomy for severe lower limb ischaemia: results and analysis of factors influencing the outcome. *J Cardiovasc Surg* 1988; 29(3):310-14.
5. Rutherford RB: Role of sympathectomy in the management of vascular disease. In *Vascular Surgery*, 5th edition. Moore WS, ed. WB Saunders, Philadelphia: 1998, 349-60.

UPPER EXTREMITY SYMPATHECTOMY

SURGICAL CONSIDERATIONS

Description: **Upper extremity sympathectomy** is the surgical treatment for hyperhidrosis, reflex sympathetic dystrophy (RSD), posttraumatic pain syndromes, and certain vasospastic disorders affecting the hands and digits.[3,4] Palmar hyperhidrosis is especially responsive to surgical sympathectomy.[4] The results achieved with sympathectomy for upper extremity ischemic and posttraumatic pain syndromes are less favorable. It is recommended that T2 and T3 ganglia be excised and the stellate ganglion spared. Manipulation of the stellate ganglion is associated with increased incidence of Horner's syndrome.[4] The **supraclavicular approach** was introduced in 1935 and is still used commonly. The **axillary, extrapleural approach** of **Atkins** was designed to provide an anatomic approach to the sympathetic chain. **Roos'** modification of the Atkins technique includes an extrapleural approach to the sympathetic chain after resection of the first rib. This is very useful for identifying the exact level of the sympathetic chain, and is associated with less postop pain because rib retraction is unnecessary. The **anterior thoracic approach** involves a limited thoracotomy through the third interspace, which provides excellent exposure. It is, however, associated with the morbidity and mortality of a thoracotomy. Part of the sympathetic chain below the stellate ganglion may be excised more readily via this approach. All of these methods have intrinsic advantages and disadvantages, but only the supraclavicular and axillary methods are widely used.

Variant procedure or approaches: The **thoracoscopic technique** for sympathectomy has largely replaced open surgical techniques because of its less invasive nature and technical simplicity. **CT-guided phenol sympathetic block** is a nonsurgical alternative.

Usual preop diagnosis: Hyperhidrosis; RSD; ischemia; posttraumatic pain syndromes; vasospastic disorders; various forms of arteritis

SUMMARY OF PROCEDURES

	Supraclavicular	Axillary Transthoracic Or Extrapleural	Anterior Transthoracic
Position	Supine	Lateral decubitus (arm supported to avoid brachial plexus traction)	Supine (slight lateral decubitus)
Incision	Above medial 1/3 of clavicle	For **transthoracic:** transverse lower axilla (enter thorax at 2nd or 3rd interspace); for **extrapleural:** transverse axillary (resect 1st rib)	Anterior thoracotomy (enter thorax at 3rd interspace and divide 3rd-costal cartilage)
Special instrumentation	DLT	⇐	⇐
Antibiotics	Cefazolin 1 g iv	⇐	⇐
Surgical time	3-4 h	⇐	⇐
Closing considerations	May need drain.	Chest tube placed and connected to water seal for transthoracic approach.	Chest tube placed and connected to water seal.
EBL	100-200 ml	⇐	⇐
Postop care	PACU → ward	⇐	⇐
Mortality	Minimal	⇐	⇐
Morbidity	Postsympathectomy neuralgia: Common	⇐	⇐
	Pleurotomy: 10%	–	–
	Pleural effusion: 7%	~7%	⇐
	Gustatory sweating: 6%	~6%	⇐
	Horner's syndrome: 4%	~4%	⇐
	Pneumonia: 3%	~3%	⇐
	Atelectasis: 2%	~2%	⇐
	Phrenic nerve injury: 2%	–	–
	Pneumomediastinum: 2%	–	–
	Subclavian artery injury: 2%	–	–
	Lymphocele: 1%	–	–
	Wound hematoma: 1%	–	–
	Chylous fistula: Rare	⇐	–
	Winged scapula: Rare	⇐	–
Pain score	4	5	5

PATIENT POPULATION CHARACTERISTICS

Age range	11-45 yr
Male:Female	1:1
Incidence	Hyperhidrosis ≤ 1% of the population (palmar hyperhidrosis in 0.15-0.25%)
Etiology	Hyperhidrosis (strong family Hx); vasospasm and arteritides (idiopathic); ischemia—PVD, trauma, autoimmune disease
Associated conditions	PVD; trauma; autoimmune disease

ANESTHETIC CONSIDERATIONS

PREOPERATIVE

Patients are often young and generally healthy, although they may have associated autoimmune diseases and PVD.

Respiratory	Patients may require OLV during surgery. ✓ for Hx of asthma, pneumonia, respiratory disease, and recent Sx of dyspnea or productive cough. **Tests:** PFT and CXR, if indicated from H&P.
Musculoskeletal	Avoid BP cuff and iv placement in affected limb.
Laboratory	Other tests as indicated by H&P.
Premedication	Midazolam 1-2 mg iv

INTRAOPERATIVE

Anesthetic technique: GETA ± epidural. A thoracic epidural is beneficial for postop pain management.

Induction	Standard induction (p. B-2). DLT placement may be requested (see discussion of OLV, pp. 213-214).	
Maintenance	Standard maintenance (p. B-3)	
Emergence	No special considerations	
Blood and fluid requirements	Minimal blood loss IV: 18 ga × 1	
Monitoring	Standard monitors (p. B-1)	Arterial line needed occasionally.
Positioning	✓ and pad pressure points. ✓ eyes.	Avoid brachial plexus traction.
Complications	Pneumothorax Subclavian artery injury	

POSTOPERATIVE

Complications	Atelectasis Pneumothorax Pneumomediastinum Pleural effusion Chylous effusion Phrenic nerve injury Horner's syndrome	
Pain management	Epidural PCA (p. C-3)	Local anesthetic opioid (p. C-2)
Tests	CXR Hct	As indicated

References

1. Ahn SS, Wieslander CK, Ro KM: Current developments in thoracoscopic sympathectomy. *Ann Vasc Surg* 2000; 14:415-20.
2. D'Haese J, Camu F, Noppen M, Herregodts P, Claeys MA: Total intravenous anesthesia and high-frequency jet ventilation during transthoracic endoscopic sympathectomy for treatment of essential hyperhidrosis palmaris: a new approach. *J Cardiothorac Vasc Anesth* 1996; 10(6):767-71.

3. Hartrey R, Poskitt KR, Heather BP, Durkin MA: Anaesthetic implications for transthoracic endoscopic sympathectomy. *Eur J Surg* (Suppl) 1994; (572):33-6.

4. Hashmonai M, Kopelman D, Kein O, Schein M: Upper thoracic sympathectomy for primary palmar hyperhidrosis: long-term follow-up. *Br J Surg* 1992; 79(3):268-71.

5. Moore WS: *Vascular Surgery,* 5th edition. WB Saunders, Philadelphia: 1998.

6. Rutherford RB. Role of sympathectomy in the management of vascular disease. In *Vascular Surgery*, 5th edition. Moore WS, ed. WB Saunders, Philadelphia: 1998, 349-60.

7. Zacherl J, Imhof M, Huber ER, Plas EG, Herbst F, Jakesz R, Fugger R: Video assistance reduces complication rate of thoracoscopic sympathectomy for hyperhidrosis. *Ann Thorac Surg* 1999; 68:1177-81.

VENOUS SURGERY—THROMBECTOMY OR VEIN EXCISION

SURGICAL CONSIDERATIONS

Description: Standard therapy for acute DVT consists of anticoagulation, bed rest, and elevation of the extremity.[2,4] Surgical thrombectomy for acute iliofemoral DVT remains controversial. **Venous thrombectomy** is recommended for patients with threatened limb loss or venous gangrene caused by massive DVT associated with high compartment pressures and arterial insufficiency (phlegmasia cerulea dolens).[2,4] Venous thrombectomy requires exposure of the femoral vein via a groin cut-down. The common femoral vein is isolated (located medial or posteromedial to the femoral artery) and controlled proximally and distally. The patient is given iv heparin at this stage, if not already heparinized. A transverse venotomy is followed by extraction of the thrombus, using forceps and Fogarty embolectomy catheters (Fig 6.3-10). Distal thrombi are expressed through the same incision with the aid of an Esmarch bandage placed on the extremity.[2] After complete removal of the thrombus, the venotomy is closed with nonabsorbable sutures, and flow through the femoral vein is reestablished. The femoral incision is closed in layers. A plastic/Silastic drain may or may not be used. The best results of thrombectomy are obtained in young patients with the first episode of proximal (iliofemoral) thrombosis.

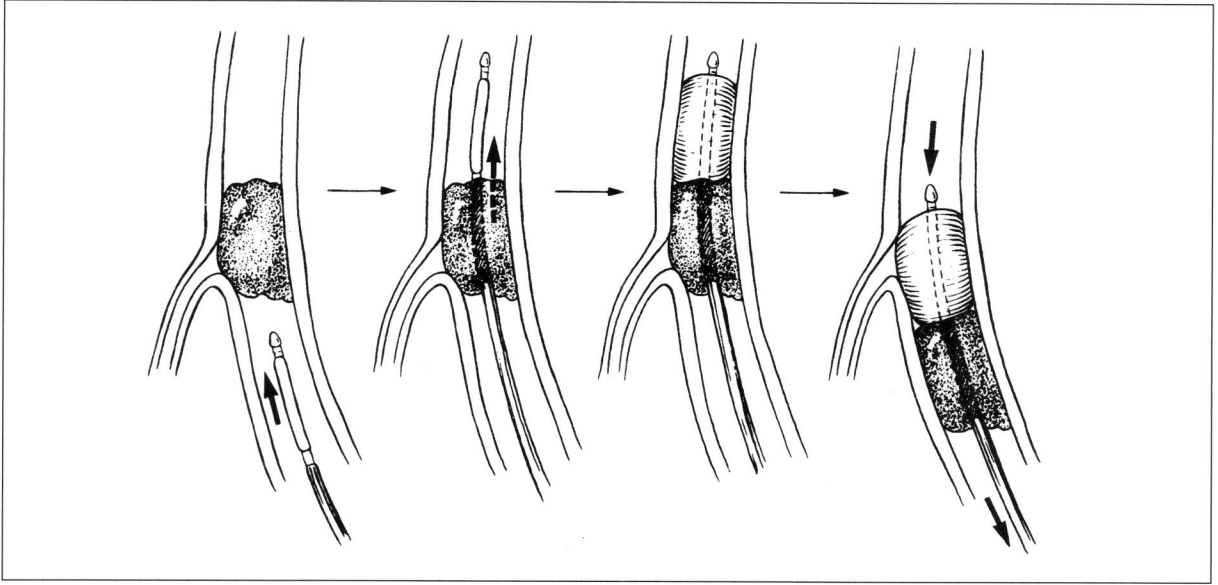

Figure 6.3-10. Fogarty catheter embolectomy with catheter insertion in the distal vessel. (Reproduced with permission from Baker RJ, Fischer JE: *Mastery of Surgery*, Vol. 2. Lippincott Williams & Wilkins, 2001.)

Nonsuppurative thrombophlebitis of the superficial veins may develop due to local trauma, prolonged inactivity, fungal infection, or the use of oral contraceptives.[2] Suppurative thrombophlebitis may occur as a complication of iv line placement or iv drug abuse. Underlying varicose veins may predispose to thrombophlebitis. Migratory superficial thrombophlebitis may be associated with chronic ischemia of the extremities in Buerger's disease, or it may develop in patients with a malignancy.[2] Conservative management with hot compresses, nonsteroidal anti-inflammatory medications, and elevation of the extremity is effective in most cases. Rarely, **excision** of the acutely thrombosed greater saphenous vein is indicated to prevent progression of thrombosis to the saphenofemoral junction and into the deep venous system.[2] Vein excision is simply approached by a longitudinal incision directly over the affected vein. The phlebitic vein is dissected from the surrounding tissue, ligated proximally and distally, and removed. The surrounding fibrotic tissue is debrided gently. The wound is irrigated and packed open with moist gauze. Suppurative phlebitis is treated with iv antibiotics and complete excision of the involved vein segment through multiple small incisions.

Usual preop diagnosis: Lower-limb venous thrombosis threatening viability; femoral thrombosis < 10 d; iliac thrombosis < 3 wk; floating thrombi at hip level; acute deep or superficial venous thrombosis; suppurative thrombophlebitis

SUMMARY OF PROCEDURES

	Thrombectomy	Vein Excision
Position	Supine	⇐
Incision	Ipsilateral longitudinal or oblique groin incision	Multiple small incisions along the course of vein to be excised
Special instrumentation	Fogarty embolectomy catheters; RBC salvage system	None
Unique considerations	IPPV during thrombectomy may decrease chance of PE 2° ↓venous return → more complete extraction of the thrombus.	None
Antibiotics	Cefazolin 1 g iv. If the patient has septic thrombus, antibiotic is dependent on blood culture.	Dependent on culture of aspirate. Usually a septic patient is on broad-spectrum antibiotics (guided by culture).
Surgical time	2-3 h	1-3 h
Closing considerations	None	Wound packed open for drainage
EBL	50-250 ml	⇐
Postop care	PACU → ward; ICU in high-risk patients; heparin administered before and after procedure, followed by Coumadin for 1-6 mo.[4]	PACU → ward; support stockings
Mortality	Minimal (depending on underlying illness)	Minimal
Morbidity	Postthrombotic syndrome: < 10-44%[4] Venous stasis Nonpitting edema Brawny induration Aching pain	Minimal
Pain score	3	2

PATIENT POPULATION CHARACTERISTICS

Age range	Young adult–elderly
Male:Female	1:2
Incidence	6-7 million in U.S. have adverse effects from chronic venous stasis[5]; 500,000 have complications of leg ulceration.
Etiology	Chronic primary varicose veins; defective venous valves; impaired pumping action of muscles in leg; previous iliofemoral thrombophlebitis; obstruction of venous return
Associated conditions	Multifactorial: varicose veins; underlying malignancy; altered coagulation status (hypercoagulability, acquired or congenital); Hx of DVT/thrombophlebitis

ANESTHETIC CONSIDERATIONS

See Anesthetic Considerations following Infrainguinal Arterial Bypass, p. 332.

References

1. Angle N, Bergan JJ: Varicose veins: Chronic venous insufficiency. In *Vascular Surgery*, 5th edition. Moore WS, ed. WB Saunders, Philadelphia: 1998, 800-7.
2. Gloviczki P, Merrell SW: Surgical treatment of venous disease. *Cardiovasc Clin* 1992; 22(3):81-100.
3. Greenfield LJ: Venous thromboembolic disease. In *Vascular Surgery,* 5th edition. Moore WS, ed. WB Saunders, Philadelphia: 1998, 787-99.
4. Lord RS, Chen FC, et al: Surgical treatment of acute deep venous thrombosis. *World J Surg* 1990; 14(5):694-702.
5. Wakefield TW: Treatment options for venous thrombosis. *J Vasc Surg* 2000; 31:613-20.

SURGERY FOR PORTAL HYPERTENSION

SURGICAL CONSIDERATIONS

Description: Alcoholic liver disease is the major cause of portal HTN; and end-stage liver disease (ESLD) with cirrhosis is the 10th leading cause of death in the U.S. (exceeding 23,000/yr). Of patients with portal HTN, 15-20% have variceal hemorrhage during the first yr of diagnosis (additional 5-10 % incidence of bleeding per yr); and the initial episode of variceal hemorrhage is associated with 50% mortality. Portal HTN (>15 mmHg) develops when splanchnic venous flow to the right heart becomes impeded.[1,2] Medical and surgical therapeutic interventions are directed not at portal HTN per se, but at its complications—notably bleeding esophageal varices. Intractable ascites and hypersplenism are less common indications for operative therapy. Presinusoidal portal HTN, unlike sinusoidal or postsinusoidal obstruction, is not associated with severe hepatocellular disease; thus, the prognosis for patients with presinusoidal block is better than for those with sinusoidal or postsinusoidal disease. Surgical approaches can be divided into shunt and nonshunt procedures. **Shunt procedures** can be classified as either **total** (decompression of the portal venous system) or **selective** (decompression of only the varix-bearing area).[11] It should be noted, however, that surgery for portal HTN has been replaced largely by the TIPS procedure (see p. 1169).

SHUNT PROCEDURES

There are two general types of total shunt (**portosystemic shunt**) procedures. The **end-to-side portacaval shunt** (Fig 6.3-11A) is technically simpler and may be more appropriate in emergency situations. It is associated with immediate control of hemorrhage in the majority of cases. The portacaval shunt, however, does eliminate portal perfusion of the liver and does not decompress the hepatic sinusoids. Alternatively, the **functional side-to-side shunt** (Fig 6.3-11B) allows decompression of hepatic sinusoids and may preserve some degree of portal perfusion of the liver. Also, it is more effective in controlling ascites. Variations of the side-to-side shunt include: **portacaval**, **splenorenal**, **mesocaval** (**Clatworthy**), and **portarenal** (rarely used).

For the **end-to-side** and **side-to-side portacaval shunts**, the approach is via an extended right subcostal incision. **Cholecystectomy** usually is not performed because of the likelihood of profuse bleeding from the liver bed. The hepatoduodenal ligament is identified, and the portal vein is exposed from the hilum of the liver to the pancreas. The gastroduodenal and right gastric branches may be divided to provide additional exposure of the portal vein. The IVC is exposed by incising the peritoneum just beneath the hepatic triad. Proximal and distal control of the portal vein is achieved; and a side-biting clamp is placed on the IVC. In order to perform an end-to-side portacaval shunt, the portal vein is divided and oversewn proximally; the end-to-side anastomosis is performed from the portal vein to the IVC. The alternative is to perform a side-to-side anastomosis of the portal vein to the IVC without division of the portal vein.

The **proximal splenorenal shunt** is approached through a left thoracoabdominal or transabdominal incision. The spleen is isolated and removed, and the distal splenic vein is mobilized from the distal pancreatic bed. The left renal vein is exposed and controlled. The distal splenic vein is then anastomosed in an end-to-side fashion to the mid renal vein. The **mesocaval shunt** (Fig 6.3-11C) is indicated in cases of ascites, periportal fibrosis, portal vein thrombosis, and Budd-Chiari syndrome.[1] The mesocaval shunt is approached through a vertical midline incision. The colon is retracted cephalad and the superior mesenteric vein (SMV) is identified at the root of the mesentery. A length of the SMV is isolated and encircled. A **Kocher maneuver** (mobilization of the duodenum) is performed and the IVC is exposed anteriorly and laterally. A side-biting clamp partially occludes the IVC and a 14-20 mm dacron graft is anastomosed in an end-to-side fashion to the IVC. The graft is clamped and the side-biting clamp removed from the IVC, thereby restoring flow via the IVC. The

SMV is clamped and an end-to-side anastomosis is created from the graft to the SMV. Flow is thus reestablished from the SMV through the graft to the IVC.

Selective shunts are designed to decompress esophageal varices, while some portal perfusion of the liver is maintained.[7] The hallmark example of this approach is the **distal splenorenal shunt** (**Warren**) (Fig 6.3-11D), which is seldom used in emergency situations. The principal feature of this shunt is disconnection of the splenic and superior mesenteric venous drainage systems. The distal splenorenal shunt is approached through a left chevron or extended left subcostal incision. The lesser sac is entered after division of the gastroepiploic vessels and mobilization of the splenic flexure of the colon. The stomach is retracted cephalad and the peritoneum overlying the inferior aspect of the pancreas is incised. The splenic vein is identified and controlled proximally and distally. The inferior mesenteric vein is divided. The splenic vein is divided proximally and the proximal stump is oversewn. Then the splenic vein is mobilized from the pancreatic bed. The left renal vein is identified and 5-7 cm of the vein is isolated. The splenic vein is anastomosed in an end-to-side fashion to the renal vein. The coronary vein is ligated close to its origin. The distal splenorenal shunt decompresses the stomach, distal esophagus, and spleen and controls variceal hemorrhage in 85% of patients.[7]

Variant procedure or approaches: **Total shunt** (e.g., portacaval, proximal splenorenal, mesocaval); **selective shunt** (e.g., **Warren**); **non-shunt procedures** (e.g., **Sugiura, Hassab,** and **esophageal transection with stapling**)

Usual preop diagnosis: Bleeding esophageal varices (as a result of portal HTN); ascites; hypersplenism

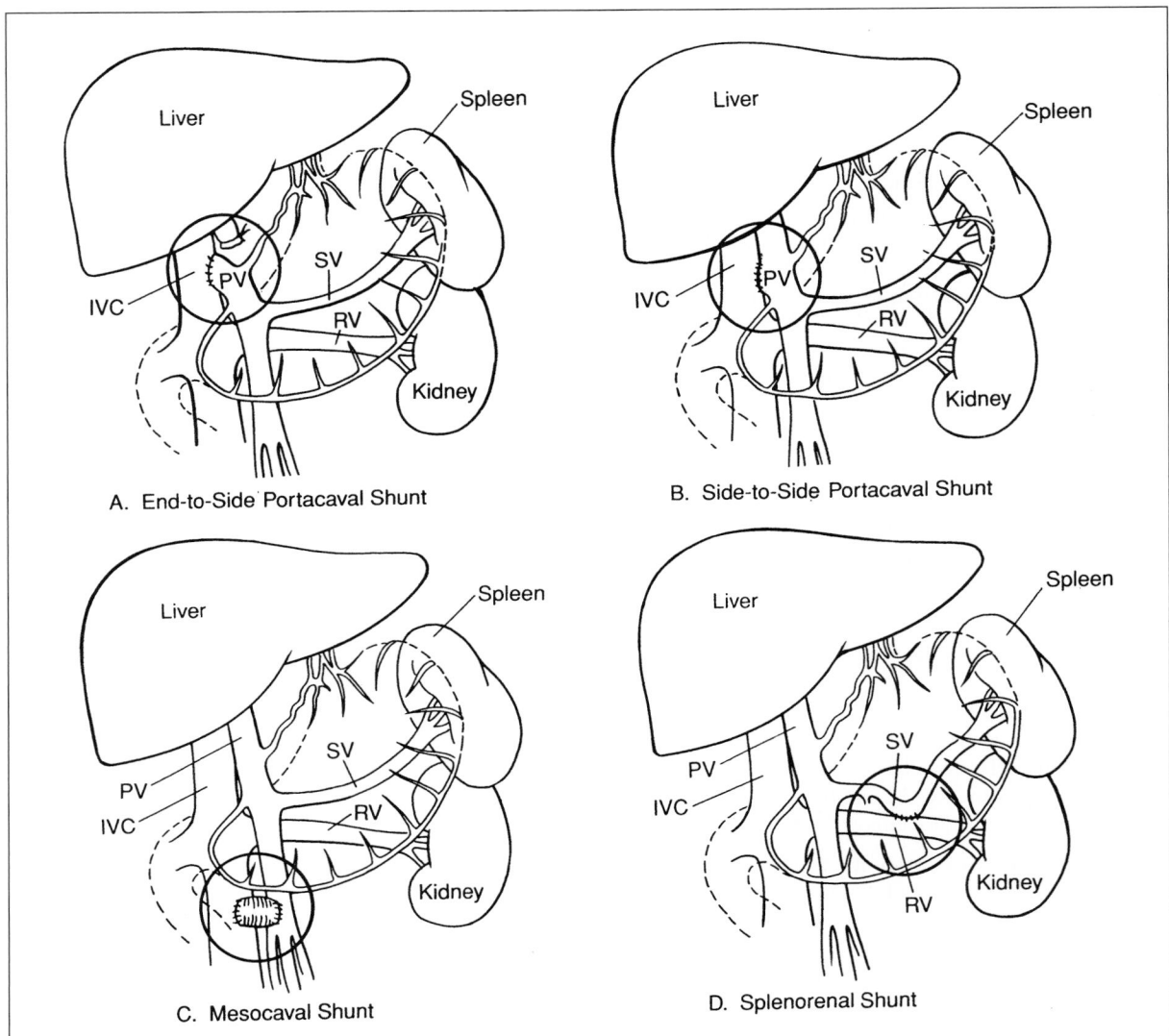

Figure 6.3-11. Types of shunts: (A) End-to-side portacaval; (B) side-to-side portacaval; (C) mesocaval shunt; (D) distal spleno-renal. (Reproduced with permission from Hardy JD: *Hardy's Textbook of Surgery*, 2nd edition. JB Lippincott, 1988.)

SUMMARY OF PROCEDURES (TOTAL AND SELECTIVE SHUNTS)

	Portacaval	Proximal Splenorenal	Mesocaval (Clatworthy)	Distal Splenorenal (Warren)
Position	Supine	Supine ± left flank elevated	Supine	Supine, left side elevated slightly
Incision	Extended right subcostal—may be lengthened or converted to left thoracoabdominal.	Left thoracoabdominal or left subcostal, or vertical midline	Vertical midline abdominal	Left chevron or left subcostal with midline extension
Special instrumentation	Self-retaining retractor	⇐	⇐	⇐
Unique considerations	May need FFP; consider Cell Saver.	⇐	⇐	⇐
Antibiotics	Cefazolin 1 g iv	⇐	⇐	⇐
Surgical time	4-6 h	⇐	⇐	⇐
Closing considerations	None	⇐	⇐	⇐
EBL	1000-2000 ml	⇐	⇐	⇐
Postop care	Patient → ICU; careful fluid management; consider Na restriction; may require PA catheter.	⇐	⇐	⇐
Mortality [1,2,7,11,14,16]	Emergency: 38% Elective: 3% Child's A: 0-15%* Child's B: 1-43%* Child's C: 6-58%*	5-10%	⇐	1-16%
Morbidity [1,8,11]	Late liver failure: 50%	~50%	⇐	–
	Encephalopathy: 32% Child's A: 8%* Child's B: 20%* Child's C: 30%*	~32%	⇐	5-47% (overall) 5% at 2 yr 12% at 3-6 yr 27% at 10 yr
	Early rebleeding: 0-19%	~0-19%	⇐	–
	Shunt thrombosis: 1-10%	20%	9-30% Duodenal obstruction Erosion through bowel wall	Loss of selectivity: 60% (@ 2 yr) Recurrent variceal hemorrhage (shunt occlusion): 3-19% Portal vein thrombosis: 4-10%
Pain score	6	6	6	6

Note: In addition to the shunt procedure itself, other factors that determine postop morbidity and mortality include: severity of hepatocellular disease, degree of hepatic reserve, and urgency of the procedure. Although the specific numbers may vary, several comparative series have shown no difference in operative mortality rate or long-term survival rate among the various shunt procedures.[11]

*See p. 1170 for description of Child's Classification.

NONSHUNT PROCEDURES

Nonshunt procedures are designed to devascularize the esophagogastric region, thus eliminating acute variceal hemorrhage. Procedures of this type include: **portazygous disconnection**; **splenectomy**; **coronary vein ligation**; and **transesophageal** or **transgastric varix ligation**.

The **Sugiura operation**, approached via abdominal and thoracic incisions, includes esophageal transection and devascularization, splenectomy, and pyloromyotomy. This procedure is usually performed in two operative stages, sometimes with a delayed second stage. The **Hassab procedure** involves devascularization of the upper half of the stomach and splenectomy, thus effectively disconnecting the esophageal varices.[6] (This operation has been reserved in some centers for the failures of sclerotherapy.) Finally, **esophageal transection**, using a stapling device, disconnects the varices in the lower esophagus. This is accomplished by placing a row of staples at the esophagus just above the esophagogastric junction.[2,8,9,15] Because portal perfusion of the liver is maintained after the nonshunt procedures, hepatic function is preserved.[2]

SUMMARY OF NONSHUNT PROCEDURES

	Sugiura (2 Stages)	Hassab	Esophageal Transection
Position	Supine, left side elevated	Supine	⇐
Incision	Abdominal stage: midline; thoracic stage: left thoracotomy	Vertical midline	⇐
Special instrumentation	Self-retaining retractor	⇐	⇐
Antibiotics	Cefazolin 1 g iv	⇐	⇐
Surgical time	4-6 h for both stages	4 h	⇐
EBL	1000-2000 ml	⇐	⇐
Postop care	ICU; careful hemodynamic monitoring; PA catheterization	⇐	⇐
Mortality[1,5,11,15]	Overall: 5-14% Emergent: 14% (≤ 60%) Elective: 3%	12-38% 10%	10-83%
Morbidity[5,15]	Recurrent hemorrhage: 2-50% Esophagopleural leak: 6% Encephalopathy: 3% Ascites: 2% Wound infection: 2%	7% – 1-25% 4% –	0-50% 3% 33% 11% 11%
Pain score	6	5	5

PATIENT POPULATION CHARACTERISTICS FOR SHUNT AND NONSHUNT PROCEDURES

Age range	11-72 yr (mean age = 48 yr); depending on etiology: pediatric (e.g., congenital hepatic fibrosis) to adult (e.g., alcoholic liver disease)
Male:Female	2-8:1
Incidence	Rare
Etiology	Alcoholic liver disease (alcoholic hepatitis, chronic alcoholism, cirrhosis); postnecrotic cirrhosis; portal vein thrombosis; splenic vein occlusion; hematologic diseases; hepatic vein occlusion; schistosomiasis; congenital hepatic fibrosis; sarcoidosis; sinusoidal occlusion (vitamin A toxicity, Gaucher's disease); venoocclusive disease
Associated conditions	Alcohol dependency; cirrhosis/liver failure; poor nutritional status; coagulopathy; encephalopathy

ANESTHETIC CONSIDERATIONS

(Procedures covered: shunt and nonshunt procedures for portal HTN surgery)

PREOPERATIVE

Respiratory — Hypoxemia may be present 2° ascites, V/Q mismatch, ↑R→L pulmonary shunting, atelectasis, pulmonary infections and ↓pulmonary diffusing capacity.
Tests: Consider ABG; PFTs, as indicated; CXR

Cardiovascular — Patients presenting with portal HTN often have a hyperdynamic circulatory state with ↑plasma volume, ↑CO, and ↓SVR, with a decreased ability to ↑ SVR or ↑ HR in response to stimuli. Ventricular performance may be abnormal (CHF), especially in patients with alcoholic liver disease. Ascites →↑intrathoracic pressure, ↓FRC, ↓venous return, and ↓CO. Older patients in this population usually have CAD.
Tests: ECG. If LV function in question, ECHO or angiography.

Hepatic	The physical manifestations of hepatic disease include palmar erythema, caput medusae, spider angiomas, and gynecomastia. Albumin and other products of liver synthesis (e.g., coagulation factors) may be decreased. Encephalopathy may be present 2° impaired ammonia metabolism. **Tests:** Bilirubin; albumin; PT; SGOT; SGPT; ammonia; alkaline phosphatase
Gastrointestinal	Portal HTN eventually → esophageal and gastric varices. Patients may present emergently with profuse GI bleeding. Ascites occurs in ~80% of patients with portal HTN and splenomegaly is invariably present. As a result of elevated intraabdominal pressure from ascites, and slow gastric emptying, a rapid-sequence induction with full-stomach precautions will be necessary (see p. B-5).
Renal	Portal HTN → ↓GFR and ↓renal blood flow → renal failure. **Tests:** Consider UA; creatinine clearance as indicated from H&P
Hematologic	These patients are often anemic as a result of poor nutrition, malabsorption, and intestinal tract blood loss. Hypersplenism may be present (Plt count < 50,000 and WBC < 2,000). Synthesis of all coagulation factors is decreased except factor VIII and fibrinogen. A low-grade DIC may be present. T&C for 8-10 U PRBC. **Tests:** CBC; Plt count; PT; PTT; consider DIC screen.
Pharmacologic	The liver is the major site of drug biotransformation; however, the effects of hepatic dysfunction on drug elimination and disposition are inconsistent.
Laboratory	These patients may have significant electrolyte disturbances (e.g., ↓↓Na^+, ↓K^+). **Tests:** Electrolytes and others as indicated from H&P.
Premedication	If premedication is appropriate, small doses of anxiolytic, such as midazolam (0.5-1 mg iv), are preferable. Avoid im medications in patients with possible coagulopathy. Full-stomach precautions are necessary. Metoclopramide (10 mg iv) and ranitidine (50 mg iv) may be given 60 min before surgery.

INTRAOPERATIVE

Anesthetic technique: GETA. Preservation of intravascular volume and myocardial stability can be a challenge in these patients.

Induction	Rapid-sequence induction with STP (3-5 mg/kg) and succinylcholine (1-2 mg/kg) should be used. Replace blood loss and ensure normovolemia before induction (if possible). Etomidate (0.2 mg/kg) or ketamine (1 mg/kg) may be preferable for induction in hemodynamically unstable patients.
Maintenance	High-dose narcotic technique with fentanyl (50-100 μg/kg) or sufentanil (10-15 μg/kg) and low-dose isoflurane. Midazolam (0.1-0.2 mg/kg) often is given in conjunction with the narcotic to ensure amnesia during times of hemodynamic instability when isoflurane cannot be tolerated. N_2O is avoided to prevent bowel distention. Muscle relaxation is needed (e.g., vecuronium 0.1 mg/kg or less, titrated using a nerve stimulator).
	★ **NB:** After drainage of ascitic fluid, there may be a precipitous drop in BP requiring rapid volume replacement ± vasopressor.
Emergence	Generally deferred to ICU due to large fluid shifts and transfusion requirements. Patients who have undergone uneventful and nonemergent surgery may be candidates for extubation.
Blood and fluid requirements	Anticipate large blood loss. IV: 14 ga × 2 or 7 Fr × 2 Rapid infuser RBC salvage device 8-10 U PRBC Warm all fluids. Humidify all gases. Warming blanket Bair-Hugger warmer	FFP, Plt, and cryoprecipitate should be available to treat coagulopathy.
Monitoring	Standard monitors (p. B-1) Arterial line CVP or PA catheter	Arterial and central pressure monitoring are essential. A PA catheter is useful in this setting because most patients are cirrhotic and may have excessive blood loss and large fluid shifts.

Monitoring, cont.	UO	In these procedures, prevention of hypothermia is important. UO is measured and is helpful as a monitor of renal perfusion. Mannitol (0.25-1 g/kg iv) may be needed to maintain UO. In patients with large varices, avoid esophageal placement of T probes or stethoscopes.
	ABGs	Serial ABGs to determine adequacy of ventilation and normal acid base status should be done.
	Hct, coags, Ca^{++}	Hct, coagulation, and Ca^{++} should be measured following replacement of large blood volumes.
	Electrolytes	Electrolytes and glucose also should be monitored.
	Blood glucose	Glucose metabolism in liver disease may be impaired → ↓glucose.
Positioning	✓ and pad pressure points. ✓ eyes.	
Complications	Coagulopathy Hemorrhage Hypothermia	

POSTOPERATIVE

Complications	Coagulopathy Hypothermia Encephalopathy Renal failure	
Pain management	PCA (p. C-3) Parenteral opiates	
Tests	CXR: line placement Hct Electrolytes Glucose	DIC screen, if continued bleeding.

References

1. Collini FJ, Brener B: Portal hypertension. *Surg Gynecol Obstet* 1990; 170(2):177-92.
2. Gelabert HA: Portal hypertension. In *Vascular Surgery*, 5th edition. Moore WS, ed. WB Saunders, Philadelphia: 1998, 754-86.
3. Gelman S, Fowler KC, Smith LR: Liver circulation and function during isoflurane and halothane anesthesia. *Anesthesiology* 1984; 61:726-30.
4. Gusberg RJ: Selective shunts in selected older cirrhotic patients with variceal hemorrhage. *Am J Surg* 1993; 166(3):274-8.
5. Haberer JP, Schoeffler P, Couderc E, Duraldestin P: Fentanyl pharmacokinetics in anesthetized patients with cirrhosis. *Br J Anaesth* 1982; 54:1267.
6. Hassab MA: Nonshunt operations in portal hypertension without cirrhosis. *Surg Gynecol Obstet* 1970; 131(4):648-54.
7. Henderson JM: The distal splenoral shunt. *Surg Clin North Am* 1990; 70(2):405-23.
8. Hoffmann J: Stapler transection of the oesophagus for bleeding oesophageal varices. *Scand J Gastroenterol* 1983; 18(6):707-11.
9. Huizinga WK, Angorn IB, Baker LW: Esophageal transection versus injection sclerotherapy in the management of bleeding esophageal varices in patients at high risk. *Surg Gynecol Obstet* 1985; 160(6):539-46.
10. Jenkins RL, Gedaly R, Pomposelli JJ, Pomfret EA, Gordon F, Lewis WD: Distal splenorenal shunt: role, indications, and utility in the era of liver transplantation. *Arch Surg* 1999; 134:416-20.
11. Langer B, Taylor BR, Greig PD: Selective or total shunts for variceal bleeding. *Am J Surg* 1990; 160(1):75-9.
12. Martella AT, Levine BA: Portal hypertension: Nonshunting procedures. In *Current Surgical Therapy*, 5th edition. Cameron JL, ed. Mosby-Year Book, St Louis: 1995, 305-8.
13. Orozco H, Mercado MA, Takahashi T, Hernandez-Ortiz J, Capellan JF, Garcia-Tsao G: Elective treatment of bleeding varices with the Sugiura operation over 10 years. *Am J Surg* 1992; 163(6):585-9.
14. Smith GW: Use of hemodynamic selection criteria in the management of cirrhotic patients with portal hypertension. *Ann Surg* 1974; 179(5):782-90.
15. Takasaki T, Kobayashi S, Muto H, Suzuki S, Harada M, Nakayama K: Transabdominal esophageal transection by using a suture device in cases of esophageal varices. *Int Surg* 1977; 62(8):426-8.
16. Turcotte JG, Lambert MJ III: Variceal hemorrhage, hepatic cirrhosis, and portacaval shunts. *Surgery* 1973; 73(6):810-17.

ARTERIOVENOUS ACCESS FOR HEMODIALYSIS

SURGICAL CONSIDERATIONS

Description: **Peripheral subcutaneous arteriovenous (AV) fistula,** or **prosthetic graft,** is the current procedure of choice for patients requiring permanent hemodialysis access.[2] The blood flow in the autogenous AV fistula increases with time, and the resulting vein wall thickening prevents venous tears and infiltration during dialysis.

The standard AV fistula is usually constructed by anastomosing the cephalic vein to the radial artery at the wrist level (**Brescia-Cimino fistula**) (Fig 6.3-12). Other locations include the 'snuff box,' or antebrachium. Vascular access using vascular substitutes or prosthetic grafts is performed when there is a lack of suitable veins in patients who have had failed-access procedures, peripheral vein sclerosis, or severe arterial disease involving the upper extremity. Forearm grafts are constructed as a direct communication between the radial or ulnar artery and the antecubital or brachial vein, or as a 'loop' between the brachial artery and these veins (Fig 6.3-13). Similarly, an access can be constructed in the upper arm as a communication between the brachial artery above the elbow and the basilic or axillary vein in a straight fashion.[2] The polytetrafluoroethylene (Teflon) graft has become the mainstay for hemodialysis access in patients who are not candidates for Brescia-Cimino fistula placement. These grafts are associated with a primary patency rate of 50-60% at 2-3 yr.

Variant procedure or approaches: **Loop or straight graft,** using vascular substitute in forearm; **upper-arm straight graft**

Usual preop diagnosis: End-stage renal failure requiring graft hemodialysis

SUMMARY OF PROCEDURES

	Forearm AV Fistula	Forearm Loop or Straight Graft	Upper-Arm Straight Graft
Position	Supine, arm abducted	⇐	⇐
Incision	Longitudinal or transverse at wrist, or 'snuff box'	Transverse at antecubital fossa and/or at wrist; counterincision in forearm	Transverse or longitudinal in upper arm
Special instrumentation	Arm/hand table (for arm abduction); Doppler flow probe may be used.	⇐	⇐
Unique considerations	Local anesthesia; consider brachial plexus block (increased incidence of hematoma); heparinization	⇐	⇐
Antibiotics	None	Vancomycin 1 g iv	⇐
Surgical time	1-2 h	⇐	⇐
Closing considerations	Use of Doppler to ✓ shunt patency	⇐	⇐
EBL	25-50 ml	25-100 ml	⇐
Postop care	Hemodynamic monitoring for poor-risk patients; can be done as outpatient.	⇐	⇐
Mortality	Minimal, depending on associated risk factors	⇐	⇐
Morbidity	Thrombosis: 20%	8-32%	~8-32%
	Technical failure: 10-15%	⇐	⇐
	Arterial steal: Rare	⇐	⇐
	Cardiac failure: Rare	⇐	⇐
	Infection: Rare	10%	⇐
	No venous outflow: Rare	6%	~6%
	Seroma: Rare	⇐	⇐
	Venous aneurysm: Rare	⇐	⇐
	Venous HTN: Rare	⇐	⇐
Pain score	1	2	2

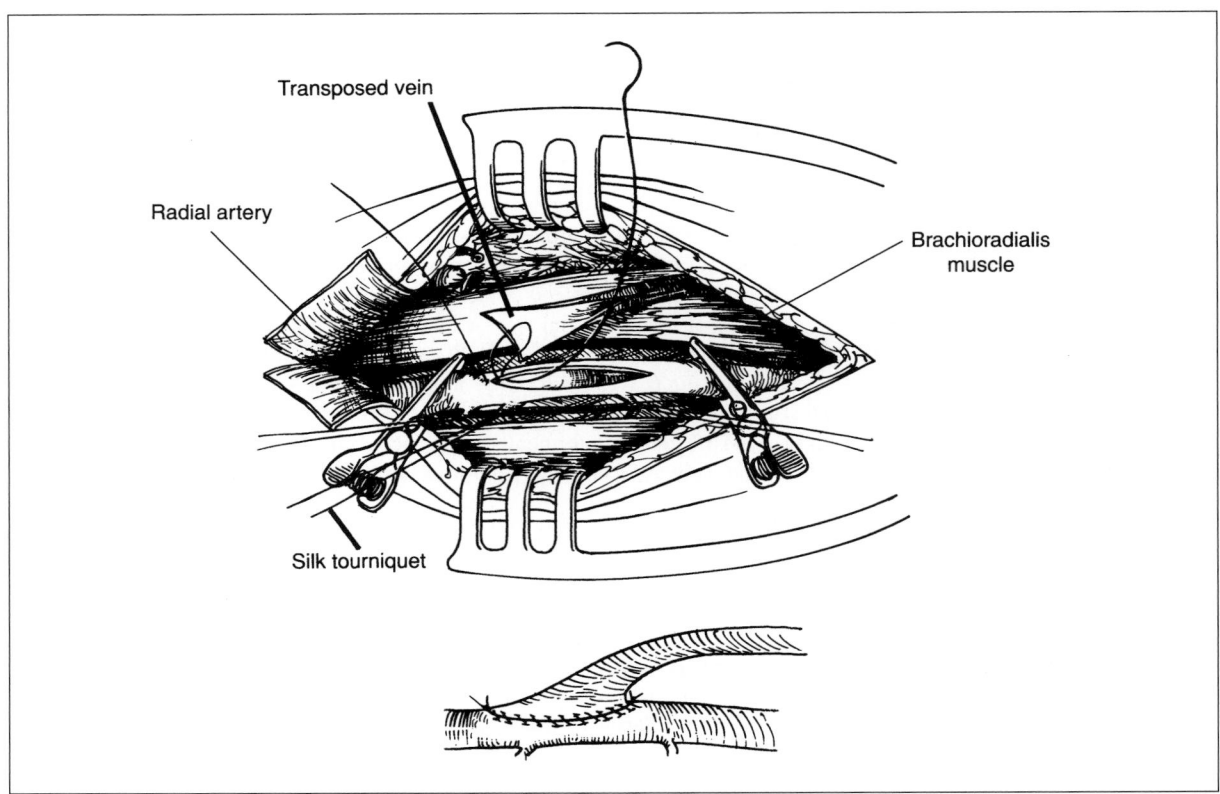

Figure 6.3-12. Brescia-Cimino fistula (side-to-end anastomosis). (Reproduced with permission from Scott-Conner CEH, Dawson DL: *Operative Anatomy*, 2nd edition. Lippincott Williams & Wilkins, Philadelphia, 2003.)

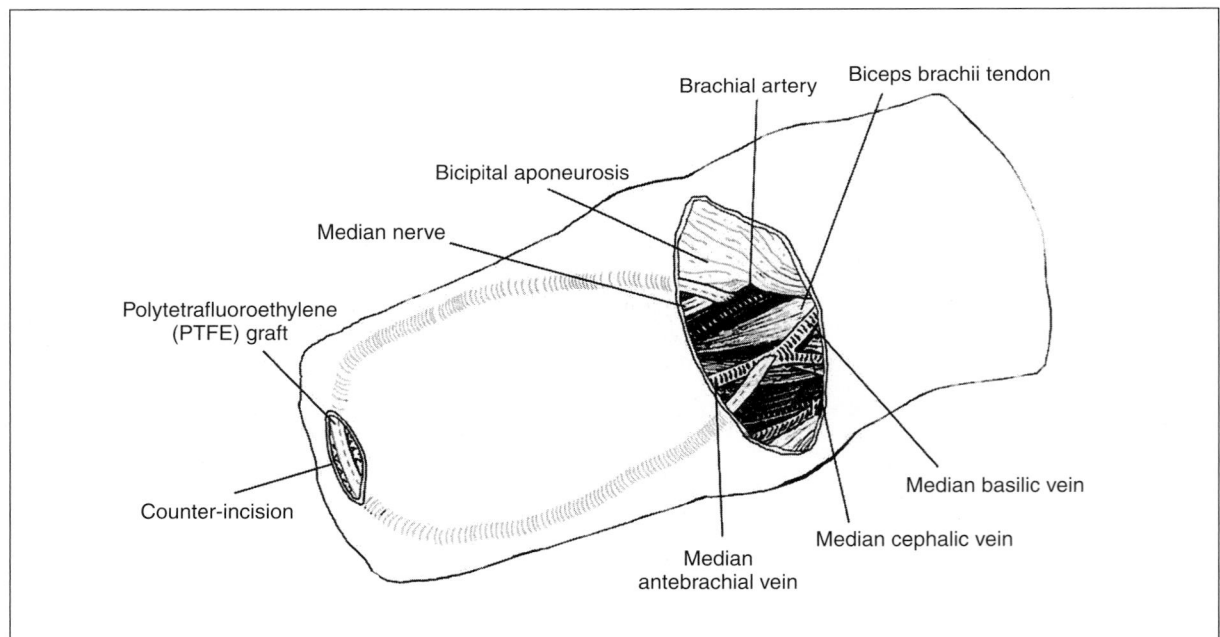

Figure 6.3-13. In arteriovenous hemodialysis access with prosthetic graft, the brachial artery and the median antebrachial, median basilic, and median cephalic veins are exposed via a horizontal incision below the antecubital joint crease. (Reproduced with permission from Scott-Conner CEH, Dawson DL: *Operative Anatomy*, 2nd edition. Lippincott Williams & Wilkins, Philadelphia, 2003.)

PATIENT POPULATION CHARACTERISTICS

Age range	Pediatric and adult population
Male:Female	1:1
Incidence	Hemodialysis access is one of the most commonly performed procedures by vascular surgeons.
Etiology	Glomerulonephritis; diabetes; HTN; pyelonephritis
Associated conditions	Diabetes mellitus; PVD/CAD

ANESTHETIC CONSIDERATIONS

See Anesthetic Considerations following Permanent Vascular Access, p. 352.

References

1. Allon M, Robbin ML: Increasing arteriovenous fistulas in hemodialysis patients: Problems and solutions. *Kidney Int* 2002; 62:1109-24.
2. Bennion RS, Wilson SE: Hemodialysis and vascular access. In *Vascular Surgery*, 5th edition. Moore WS, ed. WB Saunders, Philadelphia: 1998, 626-47.
3. Khosla N, Ahya SN: Improving dialysis access management. *Semin Nephrol* 2002; 22:507-14.

PERMANENT VASCULAR ACCESS

SURGICAL CONSIDERATIONS

Description: Silastic or plastic catheters are placed in patients who require venous access for chronic antibiotic therapy, TPN, chemotherapy, or hemodialysis. **Hickman, Broviac,** and **Groshong catheters** are made of silicone rubber or plastic with a cuff near the skin exit site, which (in theory) serves as a barrier to infection. Access is generally achieved via subclavian, IJ, or femoral vein puncture. These catheters are available in various sizes and in single- or double-lumen configurations. Larger diameter (13 Fr) Hickman or **Permacath DL** catheters have been introduced for hemodialysis. **Mediport** and **Portacath devices** have a metallic or plastic reservoir connected to the catheters and are intended for complete subcutaneous implantation. These catheters are used in chronically ill patients, particularly those requiring chemotherapy. The implantable access ports have been associated with improved patient comfort and reduced infection rates. Long-term catheter survival is limited by infection. Removal and replacement of the catheter is the only way to eradicate the infection.

Variant procedure or approaches: Two major distinctions: Hickman/Broviac catheters (no reservoir) vs Mediport/Portacath catheters (subcutaneous with reservoir). Subclavian, IJ, or femoral vein puncture is selected, depending on vein status, previous operations, and patient comfort.

Usual preop diagnosis: Chronic antibiotic therapy; TPN; chemotherapy; end-stage renal failure

SUMMARY OF PROCEDURES

	Hickman/Broviac/Groshong	Mediport/Portacath
Position	Supine, slight Trendelenburg	⇐
Incision	Puncture site (subclavian, IJ, or femoral vein); subcutaneous tunnel for passage of catheter. Alternative: cephalic or IJ vein cut-down to achieve access.	Puncture site (subclavian, IJ, or femoral vein); subcutaneous pocket for port. Alternative: cephalic or IJ vein cut-down to achieve access.
Special instrumentation	I.I. or fluoroscope	⇐
Unique considerations	Local anesthesia; may need iv sedation; monitor for ectopy during placement.	⇐
Antibiotics	Cefazolin 1 g iv	⇐

	Hickman/Broviac/Groshong	Mediport/Portacath
Surgical time	30-90 min	45-90 min
EBL	10-25 ml	25-50 ml
Postop care	CXR in recovery room; may be outpatient.	⇐
Mortality[5]	Minimal	⇐
Morbidity[1,3,6]	Catheter thrombosis: 25%	4%
	Skin exit site infection: 13%	–
	Poor flow: 10-13%	~10-13%
	Catheter sepsis: 5-8%	2%
	Arterial puncture: 6%	~6%
	Local bleeding: 5%	–
	SVC thrombosis: 5%	~5%
	Catheter displacement: 3%	~3%
	Subclavian thrombosis: 2%	~2%
	Pneumothorax 1-2%	~1-2%
	Failed attempt: 1%	~1%
	Infection: 3-5/1000 cath days	–
		Pocket hematoma: 2%
		Pocket infection: 3%
		Catheter leakage: 1%
Pain score	1	2

PATIENT POPULATION CHARACTERISTICS

Age range	Pediatrics and adults, 8-80 yr
Male:Female	1:1
Incidence	Depending on underlying disease
Etiology	Access for chemotherapy; infections; hemodialysis; chronic TPN
Associated conditions	Malignancy; chronic illness/infection; renal failure

ANESTHETIC CONSIDERATIONS FOR VASCULAR ACCESS

(Procedures covered: arteriovenous access for hemodialysis; permanent vascular access)

PREOPERATIVE

The patient populations presenting for vascular access surgery are extremely diverse. Patients requiring vascular access for chemotherapy, TPN, and chronic antibiotic therapy frequently can be done with MAC (p. B-4). Also presenting for these procedures are end-stage renal failure patients who need arteriovenous access for hemodialysis (generally involving the upper extremity). These patients return to the OR frequently for revising or replacing of fistulas. They are often ASA III & IV patients who may require GA or an upper extremity block. Anesthetic considerations for the chronic renal patient are discussed below.

Respiratory	Pulmonary edema may be present from fluid overload. CHF and uremic pleuritis can occur. Pneumonia occurs more frequently in these patients due to depressed immune systems. Hemodialysis contributes to hypoxemia due to V/Q mismatch and hypoventilation. **Tests:** CXR; consider ABG.
Cardiovascular	Often have HTN related to hypervolemia and a disorder of the renin-antiogensin system. May have LVH 2° to HTN. Cardiomyopathy, pericarditis, and pericardial effusion occur with uremia. Hypervolemia and hypoalbuminemia can contribute to CHF. Uremic patients often have defective aortic and carotid body reflex arcs. Ejection murmurs are common. **Tests:** ECG; others as indicated from H&P.
Renal	A comprehensive preop evaluation should include an assessment of renal function and adequacy of recent dialysis therapy. Ascertaining the patient's usual and recent weights is useful. Dialysis is usually advisable shortly before anesthesia and surgery. The symptoms of uremia (Plt dysfunction, electrolyte/fluid abnormalities, CNS, and GI disturbances) improve with dialysis. If a transfusion is needed, it is best done during dialysis so intravascular volume can be controlled. **Tests:** Serum BUN; Cr. If patient produces urine, consider creatinine clearance, UA.

Hematologic	Chronic anemia with Hct ranging from 15-21 g/dL. Normochromic, normocytic anemia present 2° bone marrow depression, lack of erythropoietin, nutritional deficiency, and diminished red-cell survival time. Patients adjust to chronic anemia through ↑CO and ↑2,3-DPG levels. Accumulation of waste products inhibit Plt function. Defects do occur in the coagulation cascade, but PT and PTT are usually normal. **Tests:** CBC; Plt; PT; PTT
Gastrointestinal	Uremic patients commonly have hiccups, anorexia, N/V, and diarrhea. They are very prone to developing GI bleeds. Renal failure causes ↓gastric emptying. Premedication with metoclopramide (10 mg po) and ranitidine (150 mg po) will ↓ gastric volume and pH.
Nervous system	CNS Sx of uremia range from malaise to Sz to coma. Fatigue and intellectual impairment commonly occur. Peripheral and autonomic neuropathies exist. Peripheral neuropathy presents as itching and paresthesia of the lower extremities. Autonomic dysfunction can cause postural ↓BP. Document deficits carefully.
Endocrine	Diabetes frequently may be the cause of renal failure, with its attendant problems. **Tests:** Glucose
Immune system	Often depressed. Patients prone to sepsis. Hepatitis and HIV infections from blood products may exist.
Metabolic and biochemical	Accumulation of K⁺ urea, parathyroid hormone (hypercalcemia), Mg, aluminum (neurotoxicity), acid metabolites, and phosphate occurs. Knowing hyperkalemia exists is of importance because of the potential for fatal cardiac dysrhythmias. Shift of the oxyhemoglobin curve to the right occurs due to the metabolic acidosis and ↑2,3-DPG (improves tissue oxygenation). Hyponatremia is a common electrolyte disturbance in chronic renal failure.
Premedication	If warranted, it is best to use light premedication with sedatives or opioids due to the possibility of exaggerated effects (p. B-2).

INTRAOPERATIVE

Anesthetic technique: GA, upper extremity block, or MAC.

Regional anesthesia: May be advantageous due to decreased number of drug effects. See section on upper extremity blocks (Anesthetic Considerations for Wrist Procedures, p. 740). If the patient was very recently dialyzed, there may be a residual heparin effect. Regional anesthesia is contraindicated if coagulopathy is present.

General anesthesia: The duration of action and elimination of many anesthetic drugs is altered in the patient with renal failure.

Induction	Renal failure reduces protein binding; therefore, highly protein-bound drugs may produce prolonged and exaggerated effects. Acidemia increases the proportion of agent existing in the nonionized, unbound state, which increases its availability to effector sites (e.g., brain). In addition, renal failure patients require a lower dose of STP for induction due to the increased permeability of the blood-brain barrier 2° uremia. Because ketamine and benzodiazepines are less heavily protein-bound than barbiturates, the induction dose does not need to be decreased as much. Ketamine may exaggerate preexisting HTN. Succinylcholine is not associated with greater than normal increases in K⁺ in renal-failure patients. It should be avoided, however, if the K⁺ > 5.5 mEq/L. Repeated doses of succinylcholine do not prolong muscle relaxation, since serum cholinesterase levels are normal in renal failure. NMRs, such as pancuronium and d-tubocurarine, have delayed excretion and increased duration of action. Cisatracurium elimination is not significantly affected in renal failure. Similarly, vecuronium does not have a significantly increased duration of action.
Maintenance	Inhalation anesthetics (isoflurane, sevoflurane) offer the advantage of not requiring renal elimination. Biotransformation may produce some inorganic fluoride (nephrotoxin); however, this is not an issue in dialysis patients. Opioids can produce an increased magnitude and duration of effect. Increased accumulation of morphine glucuronides → prolonged respiratory depression. An accumulated metabolite of meperidine (normeperidine) can cause Sz. Fentanyl and remifentanil are good choices, 2° rapid tissue redistribution (fentanyl) or rapid metabolism (remifentanil).
Emergence	Prolonged effect of anticholinesterases (e.g., neostigmine and edrophonium) effectively offsets prolongation of blockade. Other factors affecting reversal of nondepolarizers should be taken into account. These include acid-base status, depth of blockade, temperature and use of drugs such as diuretics or antibiotics, which can potentiate blockade.

Blood and fluid requirements	IV: 18-20 ga × 1 NS @ 1-2 ml/kg/h	IV access may be difficult; avoid iv placement in operated arm. Minimize fluids in renal-failure patients.
Monitoring	Standard monitors (p. B-1)	Avoid BP cuff placement on operated arm.
Positioning	✓ and pad pressure points. ✓ eyes.	
Complications	Local anesthetic toxicity	

POSTOPERATIVE

Complications	Nerve damage Hematoma	These are rare complications of brachial plexus blocks.
Pain management	PO analgesics	

References

1. Bour ES, Weaver AS, Yang HC, Gifford RR: Experience with the double lumen Silastic catheter for hemoaccess. *Surg Gynecol Obstet* 1990; 171(1): 33-9.
2. Don HF, Dieppa RA, Taylor P: Narcotic analgesics in anuric patients. *Anesthesiology* 1975; 42:745.
3. Kaufman BS, Contreras J: Preanesthetic assessment of the patient with renal disease. *Anesth Clin North Am* 1990; 8:677.
4. Monk J: Hemodialysis catheters and ports. *Semin Nephrol* 2002; 22:211-20.
5. Monk TG, Weldon BC: The renal system and anesthesia for urologic surgery. In *Clinical Anesthesia,* 3rd edition. Barash PG, Cullen BF, Stoelting RK, eds. Lippincott-Raven, Philadelphia: 1997, 941-74.
6. Murphy GJ, White SA, Nicholson ML: Vascular access for hemodialysis. *Br J Surg* 2000; 87:1300-15.
7. Silberman H, Berne TV, Escandon R: Prospective evaluation of a double-lumen subclavian dialysis catheter for acute vascular access. *Am Surg* 1992; 58:443-5.

VENOUS SURGERY—VEIN STRIPPING AND PERFORATOR LIGATION

SURGICAL CONSIDERATIONS

Description: Chronic venous insufficiency results from static blood flow in the deep, superficial, and perforating veins of the lower extremities.[5] Clinical manifestations include pathologic changes in the skin and subcutaneous tissues, such as pigmentation, dermatitis, induration, and ulceration around the lower portion of the leg.[2] The condition is most commonly caused by defective venous valves, and less often by obstruction to the venous return or impaired pumping action of the muscles in the leg.[5] The disorder is sometimes the residual of previous iliofemoral thrombophlebitis. Varicose veins of the primary type, particularly those of long duration, are a common cause of chronic venous insufficiency of milder degrees.[5] Most symptoms respond well to conservative management, which includes compression stockings, elevation of the extremity, and topical treatment of ulcerations. Failure of medical management is an indication for surgical intervention. Split-thickness skin grafting is indicated for large ulcers to accelerate healing and shorten hospitalization time.[2,5] **Ligation of perforators** is best performed when the ulcer has completely healed. The classic approach of **Linton** is rarely used today. If the quality of the skin overlying the perforators prevents a direct approach, **subfascial ligation** of the perforators may be performed through a short, posterior midline incision. The incompetent greater or lesser saphenous veins are resected only if patency of the deep system is confirmed. Venous ulcers recur in 30% of patients after surgical therapy, and ulcerations persist for prolonged period in 15% of patients.[2] Adjunctive procedures include: **valvuloplasty, vein transposition,** and **venous valve transplant.**

Usual preop diagnosis: Chronic deep venous insufficiency

SUMMARY OF PROCEDURE

Position	Supine
Incision	**Vein stripping:** longitudinal or oblique groin incision and transverse incision at medial malleolus; transverse incision over posterior lower leg for lesser saphenous vein stripping.
	Perforator ligation: longitudinal incision along medial aspect of tibia to posterior medial malleolus
Special instrumentation	Vein stripper
Antibiotics	If patient has an associated venous ulcer, preop antibiotics should be based on culture results; generally, cefazolin 1 g iv, if culture results are not available.
Surgical time	3 h
EBL	50-250 ml
Postop care	PACU → ward; antiembolism stockings and SCDs
Mortality	Minimal
Morbidity[5]	Persistence of nonhealing ulcer: 20-53%
Pain score	3

PATIENT POPULATION CHARACTERISTICS

Age range	Young adult–elderly (generally older adults, although present in younger patients as well)
Male:Female	1:2
Incidence	6-7 million people in U.S. have adverse effects from chronic venous stasis;[5] 500,000 have complications of leg ulceration.
Etiology	Chronic primary varicose veins; defective venous valves; impaired pumping action of muscles in leg; previous iliofemoral thrombophlebitis; obstruction of venous return
Associated conditions	Varicose veins; Hx of DVT/thrombophlebitis

ANESTHETIC CONSIDERATIONS

See Anesthetic Considerations following Varicose Vein Stripping, p. 356.

References

See references for Venous Surgery—Thrombectomy or Vein Excision, p. 358.

VARICOSE VEIN STRIPPING

SURGICAL CONSIDERATIONS

Description: In patients with primary varicose veins, no definite cause has been identified, although age, female sex, pregnancy, obesity, and positive family Hx are predisposing factors. The causes of secondary varicosity include incompetence or obstruction of the deep veins as a result of previous DVT, tumor, trauma, or congenital or acquired arteriovenous fistulas. Usual indications for operative therapy include aching, swelling, heaviness, cramps, itching, cosmesis, stasis dermatitis, pigmentation, burning, and ulcers. Surgical treatment is contraindicated in: pregnant patients; elderly patients who are considered high risk; and patients with arterial insufficiency of the lower extremities, lymphedema, skin infection, or coagulopathy.

There are two principal approaches: the **stab avulsion technique** and **high ligation and stripping.** With **stab avulsion,** the varicosities are marked preop. Small transverse or longitudinal incisions are made directly over these varicosities, which are dissected from the surrounding subcutaneous tissue (with undermining of the skin) and bluntly removed or avulsed. Firm pressure over the region being operated on will achieve hemostasis. After removal of all marked varicosities, sterile dressings are placed and a compression bandage wrapped around the affected leg. The patient is instructed to keep the leg elevated as much as possible while convalescing at home. The chief advantage of the stab avulsion technique is preservation of the saphenous vein when it is not directly involved with varicosities.

If there is valvular incompetence of the saphenous vein, the treatment of choice is **stripping (avulsion)** of the incompetent portion of the greater and lesser saphenous veins, together with avulsion of the superficial varicose veins of the thigh and calf. **High ligation and stripping** refers to the removal of the greater saphenous vein from the level of medial malleolus to the saphenofemoral junction. A small transverse incision is made at the level of the ankle and the saphenous vein is dissected free. A longitudinal or oblique incision at the groin permits isolation of the saphenous vein at the saphenofemoral junction. The greater saphenous vein is ligated proximally and distally. After a **venotomy,** a plastic or metallic vein stripper is passed and the vein is removed or stripped in a distal-to-proximal fashion. Sterile dressings are applied, followed by a compressive dressing.

If all varicose veins are removed and the incompetent segment of the saphenous vein is stripped, 85% of the patients will have good-to-excellent results at late follow-up. These procedures can be performed with regional or GA.

Usual preop diagnosis: Varicose veins; symptoms of venous insufficiency; cosmetic considerations

SUMMARY OF PROCEDURES

	Stab Avulsion Technique	High Ligation and Stripping
Position	Supine	⇐
Incision	Varicosities marked preop; short stab incisions made and veins avulsed with small forceps.	Varicosities marked preop; small transverse incision over saphenous vein proximal to medial malleolus; proximal saphenous vein exposed via groin incisions and stripper passed.
Special instrumentation	None	Vein stripper
Unique considerations	May be facilitated by tourniquet.	⇐
Antibiotics	None	⇐
Surgical time	2-3 h	⇐
Closing considerations	Leg compressed with elastic wrap	⇐
EBL	50-250 ml	50-150 ml
Postop care	PACU → ward; support stockings	⇐ + Elevate foot of bed 10°; short periods of ambulation.
Mortality	Minimal	⇐
Morbidity	Recurrence: < 10%	⇐
	Hematoma: Rare	⇐
	Infection: Rare	⇐
	Lymph fistula: Rare	⇐
	Nerve injury: Rare	⇐
	Postop DVT: Rare	5%
	Femoral artery injury: Nil	Very rare
Pain score	2	2

PATIENT POPULATION CHARACTERISTICS

Age range	Wide range, young adult–elderly (average = 48 yr)
Male:Female	1:3
Incidence	24,000 in U.S.
Etiology	Primary varicose veins: no definite cause (Predisposing factors include age, female sex, pregnancy, obesity, and positive family Hx.)
	Secondary varicose veins: incompetence or obstruction of the deep veins from DVT, tumor, trauma, or high venous pressures due to congenital or acquired arteriovenous fistulas
Associated conditions	Older age; pregnancy; obesity; DVT; tumor; trauma

ANESTHETIC CONSIDERATIONS

(Procedures covered: vein stripping and perforator ligation; varicose vein stripping)

PREOPERATIVE

Patients presenting for varicose vein surgery are a generally healthy patient population (ASA I & II). Preop considerations and tests, therefore, should be guided by the H&P.

Hematologic	If regional anesthesia planned, check patient's coagulation status. **Tests:** Plt count; Hct
Laboratory	Tests as indicated from H&P.
Premedication	If necessary, standard premedication (p. B-2).

INTRAOPERATIVE

Anesthetic technique: General, regional, or local anesthesia, ± sedation, are all appropriate anesthetic techniques. Choice depends on factors such as extent of surgery, patient physical status, and patient and surgeon preference.

Regional anesthesia:

Spinal	**Single-shot vs continuous:** Patient in sitting or lateral decubitus position (operative site down) for placement of hyperbaric subarachnoid block. Doses of local anesthetics are as follows for T10-T12 level: 0.75% bupivacaine in 8% dextrose 7-10 mg; 0.5% tetracaine in 5% dextrose 10-12 mg. For continuous spinal (multiorifice catheter), titrate local anesthetic to desired surgical level (T12). Large doses of hyperbaric local anesthetic should be avoided as they may cause postop cauda equina syndrome.
Epidural	Patient in sitting or lateral decubitus position for placement of epidural catheter. After locating the epidural space, administer a test dose (e.g., 3 ml of 1.5% lidocaine with 1:200,000 epinephrine) to elucidate whether the catheter is subarachnoid or intravascular. Titrate local anesthetic until desired surgical level is obtained (3-5 ml at a time) usually < 15 ml.
Local	Requires gentle surgical technique. Surgical field block, plus ilioinguinal and iliohypogastric nerve blocks using 0.5% bupivacaine with 1:200,000 epinephrine. Usually done by surgeon.

General anesthesia:

Induction	LMA/mask vs ETT: Standard induction (p. B-2). LMA or mask GA may be suitable for many patients.
Maintenance	Standard maintenance (p. B-3)
Emergence	No special considerations
Blood and fluid requirements	Minimal blood loss IV: 18 ga × 1 NS/LR @ 5-8 ml/kg/h
Monitoring	Standard monitors (p. B-1)
Positioning	✓ and pad pressure points. ✓ eyes.

POSTOPERATIVE

Complications	Cauda equina syndrome	The diagnosis of cauda equina syndrome (urinary and fecal incontinence, paresis of lower extremities, perineal hypoesthesias) should be sought in the postop period in patients who have received large doses of intrathecal local anesthetic during continuous spinal techniques. ✓ patients for bowel or bladder dysfunction and perineal sensory deficits. If present, consider a neurology consultation and continue followup of the patient's neurologic dysfunction.
	Urinary retention common with regional anesthesia	Patients with urinary retention may require intermittent catheterization until urinary function resumes.
Pain management	PO analgesics: Acetaminophen and codeine (Tylenol #3 1-2 tab q 4-6 h) Oxycodone and acetaminophen (Percocet 1 tab q 6 h)	Regional anesthesia should provide sufficient analgesia postop.

References

1. Mackenzie RK, Paisley A, Allan PL, Lee AJ, Ruckley CV, Bradbury AW: The effect of long saphenous vein stripping on quality of life. *J Vasc Surg* 2002; 35:1197-1203.
2. Merchant RF, DePalma RG, Kabnick LS: Endovascular obliteration of saphenous reflux: A multicenter study. *J Vasc Surg* 2002; 35:1190-6.
3. Vloka JD, Hadzic A, Mulcare R, Lesser JB, Kitain E, Thys DM: Femoral and genitofemoral nerve blocks versus spinal anesthesia for outpatients undergoing long saphenous vein stripping surgery. *Anesth Analg* 1997; 84(4):749-52.

Surgeons

James I. Fann, MD
Bruce A. Reitz, MD

6.4   HEART/LUNG TRANSPLANTATION

Anesthesiologists

J. Kent Garman, MD, MS, FACC
Lawrence C. Siegel, MD

SURGERY FOR HEART TRANSPLANTATION

SURGICAL CONSIDERATIONS

Description: Although heart transplantation has been practiced since 1967, it has had its greatest expansion since the early 1980s with the introduction of cyclosporine and its more recently introduced formulations (e.g., Gengraf). Currently, there are approximately 150 transplant centers and 2,200 heart transplant procedures performed yearly in the U.S. Indications for heart transplantation range from hypoplastic left heart syndrome (HLHS) in the neonate to cardiomyopathy and ischemic heart disease in the adult. Recipients usually have end-stage heart disease manifested by CHF and a prognosis of less than 1-yr survival. Many patients are on inotropic drugs or on some type of additional mechanical assist, such as the use of an intraaortic balloon pump (IABP) or an implanted LV-assist device. Current immunosuppressive protocols consist of a combination of cyclosporine with prednisone and azathioprine. Immunosuppression begins either immediately preop or perioperatively and will continue throughout the life of the patient. Current 1-yr survival averages 85% in most centers, with 5-yr survival of > 60%.

In **adult heart transplantation**, following median sternotomy, the pericardium is opened, with care being taken to preserve the phrenic nerve. The aorta and vena cava are cannulated, the aorta is cross-clamped, and caval tapes (tourniquets to prevent VAE) are applied. The aorta and PA are then transected. This is followed by an incision through the atria, and the recipient heart is removed. The donor heart is prepared by opening the left atrium through the pulmonary veins, separating the aorta and PA. The donor heart is attached by a long, continuous suture line around the left atrium, followed by a similar suture line around the right atrium. Alternatively, the donor SVC is anastomosed to the recipient SVC and the donor and recipient IVCs are anastomosed. Next, the PA and aorta are anastomosed to their respective recipient vessels. Multiple deairing maneuvers are followed by aortic unclamping and rewarming and resuscitation of the heart. NSR is established and CPB D/C'd. Heparin is reversed, hemostasis is secured, and the chest is closed in a routine manner. (See pp. 361+ for discussion of CPB.)

Neonatal heart transplantation differs in that the PA is cannulated if the ductus arteriosus is patent. Reconstruction of the aortic arch in the patient with HLHS requires CPB with deep hypothermia (< 18°C) and circulatory arrest. The heart is then excised and the transverse aortic arch is opened beyond the ductus arteriosus to minimize risk of late coarctation. The donor heart is prepared, with special attention given to trimming the transverse aortic tissue for subsequent reconstruction. The left and right atrium, PA, and aorta are sutured in place. The new ascending aorta and right atrium are cannulated and CPB with rewarming is reinstituted. Chest closure is routine.

Usual preop diagnosis: Cardiomyopathy; CAD with ischemic cardiomyopathy; CHD (e.g., HLHS or anomalous left coronary artery); end-stage valvular heart disease

SUMMARY OF PROCEDURES

	Adult Heart Transplantation	**Neonatal Heart Transplantation**
Position	Supine	⇐
Incision	Median sternotomy	⇐
Special instrumentation	Ascending aortic, SVC, and IVC cannulae	Ascending aortic and right atrial cannulae
Unique considerations	Due to complete excision of the heart, use of a PA catheter is usually not feasible.	Deep hypothermia with circulatory arrest
Antibiotics	Erythromycin 500 mg + cefamandole 1 g iv	Erythromycin 5-10 mg/kg + cefamandole 10-30 mg/kg iv
Surgical time	Cross-clamp: 45-60 min Surgery: 3-4 h	Circulatory arrest: 45-60 min Surgery: 3-4 h
Closing considerations	Temporary AV pacing wires are usually placed. A PA catheter may be advanced, especially with concerns about residual pulmonary HTN and donor right heart function. An isoproterenol infusion is started intraop to keep HR = 100-110 and help improve right heart function and ↓ PVR. Inhaled NO may be used to further ↓ PVR.	Temporary ventricular pacing wire is usually placed. Temporary transthoracic left atrial line may be placed. Extensive aortic suture line requires avoidance of postop hypertensive episodes.
EBL	500-1500 ml	50-100 ml
Postop care	Cardiac ICU: 1-2 d of assisted ventilation; 2-3 d stay.	Pediatric ICU × 1-2 d of assisted ventilation; 4-5 d stay, with attention to pulmonary care.
Mortality	< 5%	⇐

360

	Adult Heart Transplantation	**Neonatal Heart Transplantation**
Morbidity	Early acute rejection episodes from 10-21 d: 50%	$\Leftarrow$
	Infection, particularly pulmonary: 10%	Respiratory problems: 20%
	Pulmonary HTN with right heart dysfunction: < 10%	Infection: 10%
	Dysrhythmias with nodal rhythms: 5%	Pulmonary vasospasm with right heart dysfunction: < 10%
	Bleeding: 2-4%	Bleeding: 2-4%
	Hyperacute rejection: Rare (< 1%)	
	Intracoronary air emboli	
Pain score	8-10	8-10

PATIENT POPULATION CHARACTERISTICS

Age range	18-65 yr (average 45-50 yr)	1 d-2 mo
Male:Female	7:3	1:1
Incidence	2200/yr (U.S.)	Rare
Etiology	Cardiomyopathy (50%); CAD with multiple previous infarcts (48%); other (2%)	No apparent correlation with any specific genetic disorder. Cardiomyopathy (49%); CHD (42%); other (7%)
Associated conditions	CHF	Other congenital anomalies

ANESTHETIC CONSIDERATIONS

PREOPERATIVE

Patients scheduled for heart transplantation are terminally ill, typically with CHF, which is associated with a mortality of >50% in 2 yr. (Studies have shown that patients with severe CHF have a mortality of 50% in 6 mo.) The progression of cardiovascular disease is usually well documented in these patients. A Hx of recent exacerbation of cardiac dysfunction should be sought and all data should be interpreted in light of interval changes.

Respiratory	The presence of pulmonary HTN and $\uparrow$PVR may be disclosed by catheterization. The severity of the abnormality and the responsiveness to specific vasodilators must be determined.
	Tests: Right heart catheterization
Cardiovascular	Indicators to consider include: hemodynamic status; LV EF (mortality is rapid in patients with EF < 10% and is worse for patients with EF of 10-20%, as compared with those with EF > 20%); myocardial structure and morphology, symptoms, and functional capacity; neuroendocrine status; serum sodium; and dysrhythmia. Unfortunately, while these measures show trends with mortality, they are not individually strong enough to predict a particular patient's course. Low maximum O_2 consumption (< 10 ml/kg/min) is associated with poor survival. Normal O_2 consumption is 40 ml/kg/min. In practice, however, this measure is too severe, as many patients awaiting heart transplantation have maximum O_2 consumption of 20 ml/kg/min. Dysrhythmia is a major cause of death, and electrophysiology studies of these patients may not be helpful because dysrhythmia tends to be noninducible in them. This phenomenon frustrates efforts to select and test antidysrhythmic drug therapy. The effectiveness of past antidysrhythmic therapy should be reviewed.
	Tests: ECG; cardiac catheterization; ECHO
Hematologic	Patients with dilated cardiomyopathy or previous cardiac surgery are frequently treated with anticoagulants to reduce the risk of thrombus formation, although the efficacy of this therapy has not been studied. Hepatic dysfunction may result from RV failure and may reduce synthetic function. Mild hepatic dysfunction and chronic anticoagulation may contribute to postop bleeding. The anticoagulant effect of warfarin should be reversed with FFP.
	Tests: Hct; PT; PTT; fibrinogen; Plts
Endocrine	Neuroendocrine abnormalities are often present in severe CHF cases. The cardiomyopathy produces low CO → compensatory sympathetic activation and renin-angiotensin activity. The result is excessive vasoconstriction with salt and H_2O retention, which further impair myocardial performance. Markedly

Endocrine, cont.	worse survival is seen in CHF patients with serum sodium < 130. This may indicate the importance of neuroendocrine pathophysiology, or may simply be evidence of the severity of the CHF. It may also simply indicate that patients with more severe CHF are treated with more diuretics. When patients are treated with an angiotensin-converting enzyme inhibitor such as enalapril, the serum sodium is normalized and survival chances are improved because of the slowing of the progression of CHF, not from alteration in the incidence of sudden death. **Tests:** Electrolytes; Cr
Laboratory	Evidence of renal and hepatic dysfunction should be sought by H&P and lab studies. Hypokalemia is generally not treated in view of the K^+ in the graft.
Premedication	Although anxious, these patients are usually well informed and psychologically prepared to undergo heart transplantation. They respond well to the reassurance of the preop visit, and pharmacologic premedication usually is not necessary. O_2 therapy should commence prior to transport of the patient to the OR. Reassuring the family of a patient who suffers from rapidly progressive cardiac dysfunction also is valuable. The patient may be at increased risk for pulmonary aspiration of gastric contents because of the unscheduled nature of the surgery and use of oral cyclosporine immediately preop. Ranitidine (50 mg) and metoclopramide (10 mg) may be administered iv, most efficiently accomplished in the OR.

INTRAOPERATIVE

Anesthetic technique: GETA. After the patient is placed on the operating table, O_2 and noninvasive monitors are applied. Dyspnea (a complication of the supine position) can be treated by raising the back of the table. As infection is a much-feared complication in the immunosupressed transplant patient, aseptic technique is extremely important. Airway equipment is presterilized, and a disposable circle system and bacterial filters are used. Aseptic technique is used in inserting and securing all vascular catheters. The anesthesia machine should be equipped with a supply of air to control the FiO_2.

Induction	An arterial line for BP and blood gas monitoring should be inserted, using liberal amounts of local anesthetics before induction. There are rare exceptions to this rule, but the presence of real-time BP monitoring can be critical during induction. If infusion drugs (e.g., dopamine) are necessary before insertion of the CVP catheter, they can be infused temporarily through a separate peripheral iv. In patients who have a ↓EF, it is often helpful to infuse dopamine 3-10 μg/kg/min during induction to avoid ↓HR and ↓CO. Anesthesia is not induced until the team harvesting the graft reports that the donor heart appears to be normal. The patient is denitrogenated (FiO_2 = 1.0), and cricoid pressure is applied just before induction. Induction agents include fentanyl (5-20 μg/kg) or sufentanil (1-4 μg/kg). Etomidate (0.1-0.2 mg/kg) is useful in permitting rapid control of the airway and for assuring lack of patient awareness. Midazolam also may be used. Vecuronium (0.15 mg/kg), pancuronium (0.1 mg/kg), or a combination of these two agents, should be administered immediately to permit airway control. Care must be taken to avoid bradycardia, which often results in low CO in these patients. Immediate control of the airway is crucial, as hypercarbia and hypoxia must be avoided. The patient can be expected to have a low CO, resulting in a delayed induction of anesthesia, which must be anticipated to avoid anesthetic overdosage. Low CO and a volume-contracted condition make the patient initially very sensitive to anesthetics. High preload is often necessary, and iv fluid often is administered to compensate for the vasodilating effect of anesthetic-mediated sympatholysis. Inotropic support may be necessary when induction is poorly tolerated. Patient should be ventilated by mask and cricoid pressure released only after the airway has been secured with a cuffed ETT. The usual aids for managing the unexpectedly difficult airway should be readily available. Antibiotics are administered, and additional monitors (urinary catheter with thermistor, nasopharyngeal temperature probe, TEE, or esophageal stethoscope) are set up. If there is a delay in the anticipated arrival of the graft, the recipient should be covered and kept warm and skin prep should be delayed. Additional narcotics should be administered only in immediate anticipation of the commencement of surgery.
Maintenance	Typical cumulative anesthetic doses for the entire intraop course are: fentanyl 50 μg/kg or sufentanil 10-15 μg/kg; midazolam 0.2 mg/kg; vecuronium 0.3 mg/kg or pancuronium 0.2 mg/kg; scopolamine 0.07 mg/kg.
Termination of CPB	Junctional rhythm is common in the denervated transplanted heart. Isoproterenol 10-75 ng/kg/min is used to achieve a HR of 100-120 bpm. Isoproterenol is also useful in providing inotropic support

Termination of CPB, cont.	and pulmonary vasodilation (see below). When sinus rhythm is achieved, it is common to observe 2 P-waves. The original atrial tissue produces nonconducting P-waves. Responses mediated by vagal tone will be observed in the rate of the original atrial tissue and have no clinical importance beyond the ease with which the ECG is interpreted. Atropine and neostigmine do not affect HR. HTN does not produce reflex bradycardia. The graft atrium produces normally conducted P-waves. The graft-conductive tissue contains adrenergic receptors and responds normally to norepinephrine, epinephrine, and isoproterenol.	

Inotropic support with dopamine (2-10 μg/kg/min), isoproterenol (10-150 ng/kg/min), and epinephrine (20-100 ng/kg/min) may be necessary, especially if pulmonary HTN promotes RV failure. A PA catheter may be helpful in guiding the use of inotropes and vasodilators.

After termination of CPB, TEE may be of particular value in assessing RV dysfunction and guiding appropriate fluid therapy, pharmacologic support, and mechanical support as necessary. RV failure may be produced by the presence of air in the RCA. Visual inspection may demonstrate this problem, and one should wait for the passage of the air and the resolution of ischemia before terminating CPB. SNP (0.2-2.0 μg/kg/min) is used for afterload reduction. NO, prostaglandin E$_1$ (PGE$_1$) (20-100 ng/kg/min), and NTG (0.2-2.0 μg/kg/min) may be used for pulmonary vasodilation, especially if a preop catheterization study demonstrates responsiveness of the pulmonary circulation. Isoproterenol infusion (10-100 ng/kg/min) may provide appropriate pulmonary vasodilation, chronotropy, and inotropy. IV fluid and vasodilators must be given with particular care, as the flow produced by the denervated heart is quite sensitive to preload.

Postbypass hemorrhage	Postbypass bleeding is a common problem brought on by the preop use of anticoagulants, the depressed synthetic function of the liver in chronic heart failure, and the trauma of CPB. Following administration of protamine, infusion of Plts, FFP, and RBCs may be necessary. Cryoprecipitate is needed occasionally, especially for patients with previous chest surgery. The use of aprotinin, epsilon amino caproic acid (EACA), or tranexamic acid may be appropriate in some cases.
Immuno-suppression	Methylprednisolone 500 mg is given after bypass is terminated.
Diuresis	There may be little urine production, especially if patient received high-dose diuretics preop. Cyclosporine may exacerbate renal dysfunction. Mannitol and furosemide may be needed to induce diuresis.
Transport	A Jackson-Rees system is used in transporting the patient to the ICU.

Blood and fluid requirements	Possible severe bleeding IV: 14-16 ga × 1-2 NS/LR @ 4-6 ml/kg/h	Bleeding is often a major problem after termination of CPB. A second iv catheter is inserted in patients with previous chest surgery.
Monitoring	Standard monitors (see p. B-1). Arterial line CVP/PA catheter UO	Although it may be helpful to have a triple-lumen CVP line before induction for preload monitoring and infusion of potent infusion drugs, it is not essential. This line is usually inserted after the patient is intubated to avoid patient dyspnea and discomfort. A PA catheter is usually not inserted before bypass since it must be removed during surgery. An 8.5 Fr introducer is used in anticipation that a PA catheter may be necessary to manage right heart failure following the transplantation. The left IJ vein is the preferred site of cannulation, which leaves the right IJ unscarred for repeated endomyocardial biopsy of the transplanted heart.
	TEE	TEE is used to optimize fluid therapy, inotropic agents, vasodilators, and chronotropic agents.
Positioning	✓ and pad pressure points. ✓ eyes. Arms padded at sides Chest roll	

POSTOPERATIVE

Complications	RV dysfunction	RV failure may occur in patients with pulmonary HTN and high RV afterload (see pulmonary HTN, below).

Complications, cont.	Pulmonary HTN	Maneuvers which exacerbate pulmonary HTN should be avoided. These include hypoxia, hypercarbia, acidosis, and extremes of lung volume. NO can be used to treat pulmonary HTN (0.1-100 ppm inspired concentration); however, it must be used with caution in patients with severe heart failure. Efforts to treat pulmonary HTN with vasodilator therapy may be complicated by impaired V/Q matching with hypoxemia and by systemic ↓BP producing poor coronary perfusion and RV ischemia. Inotropic support of the RV may be necessary. Isoproterenol infusion (10-150 ng/kg/min) is attractive because it combines inotropy, pulmonary vasodilation, and chronotropy.
	Oliguria Drug side effects: • Cyclosporine: HTN, nephrotoxicity, hepatotoxicity • Corticosteroids: glucose intolerance, HTN, obesity, hyperlipidemia, aseptic necrosis of hip, bowel perforation, infection • Azathioprine: anemia, thrombocytopenia, leukopenia, hepatotoxicity	Preexisting impairment may → chronic ↓UO state. Other renal problems may be related to cyclosporine toxicity, diuretic toxicity, or CPB. Rx by optimizing hemodynamics. Consider reduction or elimination of nephrotoxins and continuing use of diuretics. Cyclosporine nephrotoxicity occurs in most patients. A functional toxicity with ↓GFR occurs at low dose and is reversible. Tubular toxicity with morphologic changes occurs at high doses and is generally clinically unimportant and reversible. The most serious damage is vascular interstitial toxicity, which occurs over months at high doses and is not reversible.
Pain management	PCA (see p. C-3) after weaning from mechanical ventilation.	
Tests	Cr Hct	

References

1. Ashary N, Kaye AD, Hegazi AR, Frost EAM: Anesthetic considerations in the patient with a heart transplant. *Heart Dis* 2002 4(3):191-8.
2. Baumgartner WA, Reitz BA, Achuff SA, eds: *Heart and Heart-Lung Transplantation.* WB Saunders, Philadelphia: 1990.
3. Bennett LE, Keck BM, Hertz MI, Trulock EP, Taylor DO: Worldwide thoracic organ transplantation: A report from the UNOS/ISHLT International Registry for Thoracic Organ Transplantation. *Clin Transpl* 2001; 25-40.
4. Bigham M, Dickstein ML, Hogue, CW Jr: Cardiac and lung transplantation. In *Cardiac Anesthesia: Principles and Clinical Practice*, 2nd edition. Estafanous FG, Barash PG, Reves JG, eds. Lippincott Williams & Wilkins, Philadelphia: 2001, 637-62.
5. Boucek RJ, Boucek MM: Pediatric heart transplantation. *Curr Opin Pediatr* 2002; 14:611-19.
6. Cannon DS, Rider AK, Stinson EB, Harrison DC: Electrophysiologic studies in the denervated transplanted human heart. II. Response to norepinephrine, isoproterenol and propranolol. *Am J Cardiol* 1975; 36(7):859-66.
7. Cirella VN, Pantuck CB, Lee YJ, Pantuck EJ: Effects of cyclosporine on anesthetic action. *Anesth Analg* 1987; 66(8):703-6.
8. Costard A, Hill I, Schroeder J, Fowler M: Response to nitroprusside-predictor of early post transplant mortality. *J Am Coll Cardiol* 1989; 14:62A.
9. Demas K, Wyner J, Mihm FG, Samuels S: Anesthesia for heart transplantation. A retrospective study and review. *Br J Anaesth* 1986; 58(12):1357-64.
10. Hunt SA: Current status of cardiac transplantation. *JAMA* 1998; 280(19):1692-8.
11. Keogh AM, Freund J, Baron DW, Hickie JB: Timing of cardiac transplantation in idiopathic dilated cardiomyopathy. *Am J Cardiol* 1988; 61(6):418-22.
12. Keon WJ: Heart transplantation in perspective. *J Card Surg* 1999; 14(2):147-51.
13. Kieler-Jensen N, Ricksten SE, Stenqvist O, Bergh CH, Lindelov B, Wennmalm A, Waagstein F, Lundin S: Inhaled nitric oxide in the elevated pulmonary vascular resistance. *J Heart Lung Transplant* 1994; 13:366-75.
14. Loh E, Stamler JS, Hare JM, Loscalzo J, Colucci WS: Cardiovascular effects of inhaled nitric oxide in patients with left ventricular dysfunction. *Circulation* 1994; 90:2780-85.
15. Ouseph R, Stoddard MF, Lederer ED: Patent foramen ovale presenting as refractory hypoxemia after heart transplantation. *J Am Soc Echocardiogr* 1997; 10:973-6.
16. Propst J, Siegel L, Feeley T: Aprotinin reduces transfusions during repeat sternotomy for heart transplantation. *Anesthesia Analgesia* 1993; 76(25):5337.
17. Ryffel B, Foxwell BM, Gee A, Greiner B, Woerly G, Mihatsch MJ: Cyclosporine – relationship of side effects to mode of action. *Transplantation* 1988; 46(2 Suppl):90S-96S.

18. Schulte-Sasse Y, Hess W, Tarnow J: Pulmonary vascular response to nitrous oxide in patients with normal and high pulmonary vascular resistance. *Anesthesiology* 1982; 57(1):9-13.

19. Starling RC, Cody RJ: Cardiac transplant hypertension. *Am J Cardiol* 1990; 65(1):106-11.

20. Waterman PM, Bjerke R: Rapid-sequence induction technique in patients with severe ventricular dysfunction. *J Cardiothorac Anesth* 1988; 2:602-6.

SURGERY FOR LUNG AND HEART/LUNG TRANSPLANTATION

SURGICAL CONSIDERATIONS

Description: With the availability of cyclosporine, the ability to successfully transplant the heart and both lungs was proven in monkeys and then successfully applied in a patient in March, 1981. Subsequently, single-lung transplantation was successfully performed in 1984 and an en bloc, double-lung transplant in 1986. Clinical lung transplantation of these various types has increased markedly in the last few years, and, currently, approximately 700 single-lung transplants, 200 bilateral lung transplants, and 60 heart/lung transplants are performed in the U.S. each year.

Current indications for heart/lung transplantation are primarily those of combined heart and lung disease, including Eisenmenger's syndrome due to a congenital heart defect with irreversible pulmonary HTN. Certain types of diffuse lung disease, such as cystic fibrosis and primary pulmonary HTN without significant heart failure, also are treated in some centers by heart/lung transplantation. Recipients for single-lung transplant usually have end-stage pulmonary disease without significant sepsis. This includes patients with interstitial fibrosis, emphysema, and lymphangioleiomyomatosis. Some patients with pulmonary vascular disease, such as primary pulmonary HTN or pulmonary HTN associated with an ASD, have undergone single-lung transplantation, with or without cardiac repair. Bilateral lung transplantation is now performed usually as a sequential single-lung transplant, with the major indications being septic lung disease, such as cystic fibrosis, chronic bronchiectasis, severe bullous emphysema, or pulmonary vascular disease, with or without cardiac repair. Current immunosuppressive protocols consist of a combination of cyclosporine with prednisone and azathioprine, with or without early induction therapy, using a cytolytic agent, such as antithymocyte globulin. Immunosuppression may begin preop and continue throughout the life of the patient. Current 1-yr survival rates average 60% for heart/lung transplants and 70-80% for lung transplants.

Heart/lung transplants usually are performed through a median sternotomy, although occasionally bilateral, transsternal thoracotomy has been used. **Single-lung transplants** (usually left side) and **bilateral sequential lung transplants** use a lateral thoracotomy or transsternal bilateral thoracotomy. Single- and double-lung transplants are greatly facilitated with OLV, which is essential for these procedures. If this type of ventilation is not feasible, a bronchial-blocker must be inserted through the operative field during pneumonectomy and reimplantation. CPB is routinely used for heart/lung transplantation, and is used for either single- or bilateral-lung transplantation, depending on the stability of the patient during OLV and/or clamping of the PA. Patients with severe pulmonary HTN undergoing single- or double-lung transplantation will almost always require CPB to reduce PA pressure during clamping. For combined transplants, the recipient heart is removed as for standard heart transplantation (see Surgery for Heart Transplantation, p. 360). A portion of the PA near the ligamentum arteriosum, however, is left intact in order to preserve the recurrent laryngeal nerve. Next, each recipient lung is excised and the trachea is transected above the carina. For single-lung transplant, usually the left recipient lung is excised, leaving a bronchial stump and vascular pedicles for the PA and veins (left atrium). For bilateral-lung transplants, both recipient lungs are removed, the trachea transected just above the carina, and the main PA and left atrium prepared for subsequent anastomosis.

Implantation of the grafts involves a tracheal anastomosis, aortic and right atrial anastomosis for heart/lung transplants, and a bronchial anastomosis with PA and pulmonary venous anastomosis for single-lung transplantation. **Bilateral sequential lung transplants** are performed as if they were single-lung transplants. CPB requires heparinization and protamine reversal. Prior to closure, extensive exploration for potential bleeding sites within the posterior mediastinum is carried out with placement of right and left pleural and mediastinal drainage. Thoracotomies are closed in standard fashion with routine chest tube drainage.

Usual preop diagnosis: End-stage heart and lung disease, such as Eisenmenger's syndrome; cystic fibrosis; primary pulmonary HTN; emphysema; bronchiectasis; lymphangioleiomyomatosis; interstitial pulmonary fibrosis; sarcoidosis; other unusual forms of lung disease

SUMMARY OF PROCEDURES

	Heart/lung Transplantation	Single-Lung Transplantation	Bilateral-Lung Transplantation
Position	Supine	Lateral thoracotomy	Supine (arm above head)
Incision	Median sternotomy, usual; bilateral anterior thoracotomy, occasionally	Posterolateral thoracotomy	Transsternal bilateral thoracotomy
Special instrumentation	Ascending aortic, SVC, and IVC cannulae	Occasional need for BB to be inserted through the operative field.	± Aortic, SVC, and IVC cannulation; occasional need for BB.
Unique considerations	CPB. If recipient has had previous thoracotomies, mediastinal collaterals may cause troublesome bleeding. Some patients with cystic fibrosis have severe bilateral scarring, requiring extensive dissection to remove the recipient lung.	± CPB. Patient may become severely hypoxic or hypercarbic during OLV, requiring CPB. During right thoracotomy, cannulation can be performed through the thorax, but left thoracotomy may require femoral artery and vein cannulation.	CPB. Thoracotomy usually is performed on left side first, with implantation of lung on this side, followed by completion of right-side thoracotomy and right-lung transplantation. If patient becomes unstable, cannulation in the thorax is usually possible to facilitate transplantation.
Antibiotics	Continue specific antibiotic regime. Coverage for pseudomonas is suggested in patients with cystic fibrosis.	Cefazolin 1 g iv	⇐ With appropriate coverage for pseudomonas in patients with cystic fibrosis.
Surgical time	4-5 h	2-3 h	5-6 h
Closing considerations	Temporary pacing wire applied and isoproterenol infusion is usually started intraop to keep HR between 100-110, as with a cardiac transplant.	Ventilation with as low an FiO_2 as possible to maintain a PO_2 > 90. Minimize iv fluids.	⇐
EBL	500-2000 ml	< 500 ml (more if CPB is used)	500-2000 ml
Postop care	Cardiac ICU: 3-7 d; 1-2 d assisted ventilation	⇐	⇐
Mortality	10-15%	10%	10-15%
Morbidity	Early acute rejection episodes from 10-21 d: 75%	–	–
	Infection, particularly pulmonary: 30-40%	⇐	⇐
	Pulmonary interstitial edema: 20%	Bleeding: 2-4%	⇐
	Return for bleeding: 4-6%	Bronchial leak or stenosis: 2-4%	⇐
	Hyperacute rejection: Rare		
Pain score	8-10	8-10	8-10

PATIENT POPULATION CHARACTERISTICS

	Heart/lung Transplantation	Single-Lung Transplantation	Bilateral-Lung Transplantation
Age range	3 mo-55 yr (average 30-40 yr)	1-65 yr	⇐
Male:Female	1:1	⇐	⇐
Incidence	60/yr (U.S.) 200/yr (worldwide)	600/yr (U.S.) 1000/yr (worldwide)	200/yr (U.S.) 400/yr (worldwide)
Etiology	Eisenmenger's syndrome; CHD; cystic fibrosis; pulmonary HTN; other lung diseases	Acquired chronic lung disease; pulmonary HTN	Cystic fibrosis; interstitial fibrosis; emphysema
Associated conditions	Severe cyanosis and polycythemia; diabetes in patients with cystic fibrosis; sinus infections in patients with cystic fibrosis	Right heart dysfunction; pulmonary valve insufficiency and tricuspid valve insufficiency	Diabetes mellitus; sinus infections in patients with cystic fibrosis

ANESTHETIC CONSIDERATIONS FOR HEART/LUNG TRANSPLANTATION

PREOPERATIVE

Patients scheduled for heart/lung transplantation are terminally ill, although they may still be able to maintain limited activity. Indications include primary pulmonary HTN, Eisenmenger's syndrome, cystic fibrosis, and combined cardiac and pulmonary disease. The standard preanesthetic evaluation is supplemented with considerations particular to these patients. The progression of disease is usually well documented.

Respiratory   Patients with severe pulmonary HTN (80/50 mmHg) have enlarged PAs. Vocal cord dysfunction (Sx: hoarseness, inability to phonate "e") may occur when the left recurrent laryngeal nerve is stretched by an enlarged PA, making these patients at increased risk for pulmonary aspiration. Appropriate precautions to avoid aspiration should be taken (see Induction, below).
Tests: ABG; cardiac catheterization

Cardiovascular   Hx of recent exacerbation of symptoms should be sought and cardiac catheterization data interpreted in light of interval changes. The severity of pulmonary HTN and the responsiveness to specific vasodilators during catheterization should be reviewed.
Tests: ECG; cardiac catheterization; ECHO

Neurological   R → L intracardiac shunting may be present in patients with pulmonary HTN, and Hx of embolic episodes should be sought. Extra care should be used to avoid injection of even small quantities of intravenous air.

Hematologic   The medication schedule should be verified with particular attention to the recent use of anti-coagulants.
Tests: Hct; PTT; PT (special tubes required if severe polycythemia present $2°$ ↓plasma volume); Plt count; fibrinogen

Laboratory   Evidence of renal and hepatic dysfunction should be sought by H&P and lab studies. Hypokalemia is generally not treated because the heart/lung graft is preserved with K^+ and implantation will reverse hypokalemia.

Premedication   Although anxious, these patients are usually well informed and psychologically prepared. They respond well to the reassurance of the preop visit, and pharmacologic premedication usually is not necessary. O_2 therapy should commence prior to transport of patient to the OR. Patient may be at increased risk for pulmonary aspiration of gastric contents because of the unscheduled nature of the surgery, the use of oral cyclosporine immediately preop and the presence of recurrent laryngeal nerve damage. Ranitidine (50 mg) and metoclopramide (10 mg) may be administered iv preop.

INTRAOPERATIVE

Anesthetic technique: GETA. Infection is a much feared complication in the immunosupressed transplant patient; thus, aseptic technique is important. Airway equipment is presterilized; a disposable circle system and bacterial filters are used; and aseptic technique is used in inserting and securing all vascular catheters. The anesthesia machine should be equipped with a supply of air to permit control of the FiO_2; and anesthesia is not induced until the team harvesting the graft reports that it appears to be normal to direct inspection.

Induction   In the OR, the patient should be placed on the operating table and O_2 and noninvasive monitors applied. An arterial line for BP and blood gas monitoring should be inserted, using liberal amounts of local anesthetics before induction. There are rare exceptions to this rule, but the presence of real-time BP monitoring can be critical during induction. A patient who is dyspneic in the supine position may be treated by raising the back of the table. Cricoid pressure must be used when the patient is at risk for aspiration of gastric contents. A major goal of anesthetic induction is the avoidance of further increases in PVR by guarding against respiratory acidosis, hypoxia, N_2O, light anesthesia, and extremes of lung volume. When hemodynamically tolerated, fentanyl (30 μg/kg) is useful in blunting the pulmonary vascular response to intubation.
Etomidate (0.1-0.2 mg/kg) may be used when hypotension limits administration of narcotics. Vecuronium (0.15 mg/kg), pancuronium (0.1 mg/kg), or a combination of the two, should be administered early to permit rapid airway control. Midazolam and scopolamine produce amnesia. N_2O is not used because it exacerbates pulmonary HTN, reduces FiO_2, and expands intravascular air bubbles. Patient should be ventilated by mask, and cricoid pressure released only after the airway has been secured with a cuffed ETT. Excessive pressure of the cuff on the trachea should be avoided. An ETT of internal diameter of 8.0 mm will facilitate FOB postop.

Maintenance	Typical total anesthetic doses for the entire intraop course are: fentanyl 50 μg/kg or sufentanil 10-15 μg/kg; midazolam 0.2 mg/kg; vecuronium 0.3 mg/kg or pancuronium 0.2 mg/kg; scopolamine 0.07 mg/kg.
Termination of CPB	After tracheal anastomosis is complete, lungs are ventilated with FiO_2 = 0.21 at 5 breaths/min and a TV of 6 ml/kg. When bladder temperature reaches 36°C, ventilation is increased to 10 breaths/min and TV of 12 ml/kg. TV should be adjusted to eliminate atelectasis and to achieve a peak inflation pressure of 25-30 cmH$_2$O with the chest open. The FiO_2 is increased to 0.4 and may be altered in response to pulse oximetry and blood gas data. FiO_2 is limited in the hope of curtailing free radical injury. PEEP may be used to enhance oxygenation and is adjusted with an appreciation of the effect of lung volume on PVR. Hypoxemia must be avoided. Hyperkalemia may be treated with Ca^{++} (e.g., 3-5 ml 10% CaCl q 30 min), glucose (50 g), insulin (10 U), and diuresis.
	Junctional rhythm is common in the denervated transplanted heart. Isoproterenol (10-75 ng/kg/min) is used to achieve a HR of 100-120. When sinus rhythm is achieved, it is common to see two P-waves. The residual atrial tissue produces nonconducting P-waves. Responses mediated by vagal tone will be seen in the rate of the original atrial tissue and have no clinical importance beyond the ease with which the ECG is interpreted.
	In the denervated heart, atropine and neostigmine will not affect HR, and HTN will not produce reflex bradycardia. The graft atrium produces normally conducted P-waves. The transplanted heart contains adrenergic receptors and responds normally to norepinephrine, epinephrine, and isoproterenol.
	The CO of the denervated heart is quite sensitive to preload; thus, iv fluid and vasodilators must be given with particular care. SNP is used for afterload reduction. TEE may be of particular value in assessing RV dysfunction and guiding appropriate fluid therapy, pharmacologic support, and mechanical support as necessary. NO, PGE$_1$ (20-100 ng/kg/min), isoproterenol, and NTG (0.2-2.0 μg/kg/min) also may be used for pulmonary vasodilation. Inotropic support with dopamine (2-10 μg/kg/min), isoproterenol, and epinephrine (20-100 ng/kg/min) may be necessary, especially if pulmonary HTN and RV failure occur.
Immuno-suppression	Methylprednisolone 500 mg iv is given after bypass is terminated.
Diuresis	There may be little urine production, especially if patient received high-dose diuretics preop. Cyclosporine may exacerbate renal dysfunction. Mannitol and furosemide may be needed to induce diuresis.
Transport	A sterile, disposable Jackson-Rees system is used in transporting the patient to the ICU.
Blood and fluid requirements	Anticipate large blood loss. IV: 14-16 ga × 2	Bleeding is often a major problem after termination of CPB. Patients with intracardiac defects are at increased risk for cerebral embolic events. Care must be taken to remove all air bubbles from intravascular lines.
Control of blood loss	Postbypass bleeding is a common problem.	Postbypass bleeding is exacerbated by preop use of anticoagulants, depressed synthetic liver function, trauma of CPB, and/or previous chest therapy.
	Coagulation therapy necessary.	Coagulation therapy may include: protamine (30 mg/kg); Plts; FFP; RBCs; EACA (300 mg/kg); DDAVP; aprotinin (500,000 U/h after loading dose).
	Possible severe bleeding	Severe bleeding prompts further therapy: cryoprecipitate, factor IX concentrate.
Monitoring	Standard monitors (see p. B-1). Arterial line CVP/PA catheter UO	Typically, invasive monitors are placed prior to induction; however, if patient is very dyspneic in the supine position, it may be advantageous to insert the CVP catheter following anesthetic induction. An introducer permits the rapid insertion of a PA catheter when necessary. The left IJ vein is the preferred site of cannulation, leaving the right IJ unscarred for repeated endomyocardial biopsies of the transplanted heart.

Monitoring, cont.	TEE	TEE is used to optimize the selection of fluid therapy, inotropic agents, vasodilators, and chronotropic agents.

POSTOPERATIVE

Complications	Oliguria	Diuresis may be induced with mannitol and furosemide.
	Pulmonary edema	Given the lack of lymphatic drainage in the transplanted lung, pulmonary edema may occur. Diuresis and restriction of iv fluid may be required.
	RV dysfunction	RV failure may occur in patients with pulmonary HTN and high RV afterload (see pulmonary HTN Rx, below).
	Pulmonary HTN	Maneuvers which exacerbate pulmonary HTN should be avoided. These include hypoxia, hypercarbia, acidosis, and extremes of lung volume. NO can be used to treat pulmonary HTN (0.1-100 parts per million inspired concentration); however, it must be used with caution in patients with severe heart failure. Efforts to treat pulmonary HTN with vasodilator therapy may be complicated by impaired V/Q matching with hypoxemia and by systemic hypotension producing poor right coronary perfusion and RV ischemia. Inotropic support of the RV may be necessary. Isoproterenol is attractive because it combines inotropy, pulmonary vasodilation and chronotropy.
	Rejection	Monitor rejection Sx with transvenous endomyocardial
	Infection	biopsy and transbronchial biopsy.
	Drug side effects:	
	• Cyclosporine: HTN, nephrotoxicity, hepatotoxicity	Cyclosporine nephrotoxicity occurs in most patients. A functional toxicity with reduced GFR occurs at low dose and is reversible. Tubular toxicity with morphologic changes occurs at high doses and generally is clinically unimportant and reversible. The most serious damage is vascular interstitial toxicity, which occurs over months at high doses and is not reversible.
	• Corticosteroids: glucose intolerance, HTN, obesity, hyperlipidemia, aseptic necrosis of hip, bowel perforation, infection	
	• Azathioprine: anemia, thrombocytopenia, leukopenia, hepatotoxicity	
Pain management	PCA (see p. C-3).	

References

1. Baumgartner WA, Reitz BA, Achuff SA, eds: *Heart and Heart-Lung Transplantation.* WB Saunders, Philadelphia: 1990.
2. Bigham M, Dickstein ML, Hogue, CW Jr: Cardiac and lung transplantation. In *Cardiac Anesthesia: Principles and Clinical Practice*, 2nd edition. Estafanous FG, Barash PG, Reves JG, eds. Lippincott Williams & Wilkins, Philadelphia: 2001, 637-62.
3. Cirella VN, Pantuck CB, Lee YJ, Pantuck EJ: Effects of cyclosporine on anesthetic action. *Anesth Analg* 1987; 66(8):703-6.
4. Peterson KL, DeCampli WM, Feeley TW, Starnes VA: Blood loss and transfusion requirements in cystic fibrosis patients undergoing heart-lung or lung transplantation. *J Cardiothorac Vasc Anesth* 1995; 9:59-62.
5. Propst JW, Siegel LC, Feeley TW: Effect of aprotinin on transfusion requirements during repeat sternotomy for cardiac transplantation surgery. *Transplant Proc* 1994; 26:3719-21.
6. Pucci A, Forbes RD, Berry GJ, Rowan RA, Billingham ME: Accelerated post-transplant coronary arteriosclerosis in combined heart-lung transplantation. *Transplant Proc* 1991; 23(1P+2):1228-9.
7. Reitz BA, Wallwork JL, Hunt SA, Pennock JL, Billingham ME, Oyer PE, Stinson EB, Shumway NE: Heart-lung transplantation: successful therapy for patients with pulmonary vascular disease. *N Engl J Med* 1982; 306(10):557-64.
8. Shaw JH, Kirk AJ, Conacher ID: Anesthesia for patients with transplanted hearts and lungs undergoing non-cardiac surgery. *Br J Anesth* 1991; 67:772-8.
9. Waddell TK, Bennett L, Kennedy R, Todd TR, Keshavjee SH: Heart-lung or lung transplantation for Eisenmenger syndrome. *J Heart Lung Transplant* 2002; 21:731-7.
10. Whyte RI, Robbins RC, Altinger J, Barlow CW, Doyle R, Theodore J, Reitz BA: Heart-lung transplantation for primary pulmonary hypertension. *Ann Thorac Surg* 1997; 67:937-41.

ANESTHETIC CONSIDERATIONS FOR LUNG TRANSPLANTATION

PREOPERATIVE

The patient presenting for lung transplantation typically has end-stage pulmonary fibrosis or emphysema, although other diseases, such as pulmonary HTN, also may be treated by single-lung transplantation. Double-lung transplantation can be used to treat cystic fibrosis and bronchiectasis. The progression of the disease is usually well documented; however, Hx of recent exacerbation of symptoms should be sought.

Respiratory Assess the patient's ability to undergo OLV by review of the V/Q scan. If little perfusion of the nonoperative lung is present, anticipate the need for CPB.[10] The extent of the restrictive lung disease and diffusion abnormality must be assessed preop. For example, room-air $PaO_2 < 45$ mmHg predicts the need for CPB.
Tests: PFT; V/Q scan; ABG

Airway Patients with severe pulmonary HTN (80/50 mmHg) have enlarged pulmonary arteries. Vocal cord dysfunction (Sx: hoarseness, inability to phonate "e") may occur when the left recurrent laryngeal nerve is stretched by an enlarged PA, making these patients at increased risk for pulmonary aspiration; therefore, appropriate precautions to avoid aspiration should be taken (see Induction, below).

Cardiovascular Evidence of RV dysfunction with tricuspid regurgitation should be sought by physical exam, ECHO, and cardiac catheterization. RV ejection fraction (EF) may be estimated with radionuclide ventriculography (normal EF = > 50%). Pulmonary HTN is considered to be severe and may produce RV failure when pressure is > 2/3rds of systemic arterial pressure. Note response to specific vasodilators recorded during catheterization.
Tests: Preview cardiac catheterization data; ECG; mean PAP > 40 mmHg and PVR > 5 mmHg/min/L may predict the need for partial CPB.

Neurological R→L intracardiac shunting may be present in patients with pulmonary HTN, and Hx of embolic episodes should be sought. Extra care should be used to avoid injection of even small quantities of intravenous air.

Musculoskeletal Chronic cachexia precludes the procedure.

Hematologic Polycythemia 2° chronic hypoxemia is common. Autologous blood is collected as CPB is initiated.
Tests: Hct; coagulation studies require special blood tubes to correct for low plasma volume in patients with severe polycythemia.

Laboratory Other tests as indicated from H&P.

Premedication Patients awaiting lung transplantation are generally well informed about the planned perioperative course. These patients respond well to the reassurance of the preop visit, and pharmacologic premedication usually is not necessary. O_2 therapy, with the usual home O_2 regimen, should commence prior to transport to the OR. Patient may be at ↑risk for pulmonary aspiration of gastric contents because of the unscheduled nature of the surgery, the use of oral cyclosporin immediately before surgery, and the presence of recurrent laryngeal nerve damage. Ranitidine (50 mg) and metoclopramide (10 mg) may be administered iv before surgery.

INTRAOPERATIVE

Anesthetic technique: GETA. Typically, OLV through a DLT is required for single-lung transplants. Consider ETT/BB in cystic fibrosis patients with tenacious sputum. Infection is a much feared complication in the immunosuppressed transplant patient; thus, aseptic technique is important. Airway equipment is presterilized; a disposable circle system and bacterial filters are used; and aseptic technique is used in inserting and securing all vascular catheters.

Induction An arterial line for BP and blood gas monitoring should be inserted, using liberal amounts of local anesthetics before induction. There are rare exceptions to this rule, but the presence of real-time BP monitoring can be critical during induction. Typically, fentanyl 30 mg/kg (incremental doses) after invasive monitors placed, ± etomidate 0.1-0.2 mg/kg when rapid control of the airway is desirable; vecuronium 0.15 mg/kg or pancuronium 0.1 mg/kg (avoid succinylcholine 2° ↓HR); midazolam 0.1 mg/kg or scopolamine 0.005 mg/kg for amnesia. Cricoid pressure must be used when the patient is at risk for aspiration because of the unscheduled nature of the surgery, use of preop oral cyclosporin, and possible vocal cord dysfunction associated with stretch injury of the recurrent laryngeal nerve. Avoid

Induction, cont.	further increases in PVR by guarding against hypoxemia, acidosis, hypercarbia, light anesthesia, and extremes of lung volume.	
Maintenance	Typically, narcotic/O_2/air/± isoflurane (in absence of hypoxemia and right heart failure). Typical total anesthetic doses for the entire intraop course: fentanyl 50-75 μg/kg or sufentanil 10-15 μg/kg, midazolam 0.2 mg/kg, vecuronium 0.3 mg/kg, or pancuronium 0.2 mg/kg or pipecuronium 0.2 mg/kg, scopolamine 0.07 mg/kg.	
Emergence	Prior to closure of the chest, lungs are inflated to 35 cmH_2O to reinflate atelectatic areas and check adequacy of bronchial closure. At the conclusion of surgery, both lumens of the DLT should be aspirated and the tube replaced with a single-lumen 8.0 mm ETT. The patient is transported to the ICU intubated and ventilated.	
Blood and fluid requirements	IV: 14 or 16 ga × 1-2 NS/LR @ 4 ml/kg/h	Patients with intracardiac defects are at increased risk for cerebral embolic events; take care to remove all air bubbles from intravascular lines.
Monitoring	Standard monitors (see p. B-1). Arterial line PA catheter Urinary catheter with thermistor	ECG leads should be covered with tape to insure that electrical contact is not degraded by prep solution or blood. An 8.5 Fr introducer and a thermodilution PA catheter are inserted after induction of anesthesia. Mixed venous oximetry may be desirable during OLV, and with partial CPB. Be careful of air embolization during catheter insertion. Patients who are profoundly dyspneic (→ high negative intrathoracic pressure) are at high risk for VAE; consider inserting the catheter after GA and IPPV have been instituted. Oxygenation must be watched closely. Blood gases are sampled at 10-min intervals.
	TEE	RV EF measurement may be useful for evaluating RV function (normal EF = 0.5-0.7).
OLV	DLT: 41 Fr (men); 39 Fr (women) Use large TV (12-15 ml/kg) during regular and OLV.	A DLT is inserted in the left mainstem bronchus to permit surgical access. Verification of tube position by auscultation may be difficult due to the severity of the lung disease. FOB is used to verify proper tube placement. Positioning of the bronchial cuff in the proximal left mainstem bronchus does not interfere with surgical access to the bronchus. The position of the DLT should be verified after the patient is moved to the lateral position. Finally, verify ventilation and proper functioning of the tube, then eliminate volatile anesthetic or vasodilators which may blunt hypoxic pulmonary vasoconstriction. Apply O_2 with CPAP at 5 cmH_2O to the nondependent lung. Further adjustment of CPAP may enhance oxygenation. The nondependent lung may be reinflated with O_2, if necessary, to achieve adequate oxygenation. If adequate oxygenation cannot be achieved, CPB should be initiated.
	Frequent suctioning	Frequent suctioning is necessary in patients with tenacious secretions.
PA clamping	Improve V/Q mismatch. Improve oxygenation. PAP ↑↑→ RV failure	Clamping of the PA will improve V/Q mismatch and oxygenation; however, severe pulmonary HTN and RV failure may develop. Vasodilators, such as NTG (0.2-2 μg/kg/min), SNP (0.2-10 μg/kg/min) or PGE$_1$ (20-100 ng/kg/min), should be used to treat pulmonary HTN and ↓ RV afterload; however, care must be taken to avoid systemic hypotension. Inotropic support for the RV may be necessary (dopamine [2-10 μg/kg/min] or epinephrine [20-100 ng/kg/min]). The right atrial pressure should be monitored for evidence of tricuspid regurgitation associated with RV dilation.

PA unclamping	PIP: 20-25 cmH$_2$O O$_2$ sat: 95-100% PEEP: 5-10 mmHg	Temporary unclamping of the PA may be necessary to allow further pharmacologic therapy. If RV failure cannot be controlled pharmacologically, CPB should be initiated. The PA should not be unclamped until ventilation is possible to the transplanted lung. Perfusion without oxygenation of the transplanted lung would produce profound shunt and hypoxemia. TV should be adjusted to eliminate atelectasis and to achieve a PIP of 20-25 cmH$_2$O with the chest open. The FiO$_2$ (0.35) is limited in the hope of curtailing free radical injury. PEEP may be used to enhance oxygenation.
Positioning	For single-lung: • Supine to lateral decubitus • Axillary roll • Airplane splint • Avoid hyperextension (> 90°). For double-lung: • Supine with arms above head for bilateral subcostal incision ✓ and pad pressure points. ✓ eyes.	Verify correct position of DLT or BB after moving patient to the lateral position. Difficult access to airway after patient positioned. ★ **NB:** potential for kinking of iv and arterial lines

POSTOPERATIVE

Complications	Pulmonary edema Infection: bacterial, viral, fungal, or protozoan Side effects of immunosuppressive agents: • Cyclosporine: hepatotoxicity, HTN, nephrotoxicity, Sz • Corticosteroids: HTN, osteoporosis, glucose intolerance, hyperlipidemia • Azathioprine: anemia, thrombocytopenia, leukopenia	Given the lack of lymphatic drainage in the transplanted lung, pulmonary edema may occur. Diuresis and restriction of iv fluid may be required. Mannitol and furosemide can be used to induce diuresis. Immunosuppression drugs typically include: cyclosporine, azathioprine, and corticosteroids. Polyclonal antilymphocyte globulin or monoclonal antilymphocyte antibodies also may be used.
Pain management	Epidural narcotics (see p. C-2) Parenteral narcotics (see p. C-2)	Postop analgesia may be provided by infusion of narcotics through an epidural catheter. If CPB is used, the insertion of the epidural catheter should be delayed until normal coagulation function is documented in the ICU.

References

1. Adatia I, Lillehei C, Arnold JH, Thompson JE, Palazzo R, Fackler JC, Wessel DL: Inhaled nitric oxide in the treatment of postoperative graft dysfunction after lung transplantation. *Ann Thorac Surg* 1994; 57:1311-18.
2. Benumof JL, Partridge BL, Salvatierra C, Keating J: Margin of safety in positioning modern double-lumen endotracheal tubes. *Anesthesiology* 1987; 67(5):729-38.
3. Bigham M, Dickstein ML, Hogue, CW Jr: Cardiac and lung transplantation. In *Cardiac Anesthesia: Principles and Clinical Practice*, 2nd edition. Estafanous FG, Barash PG, Reves JG, eds. Lippincott Williams & Wilkins, Philadelphia: 2001, 637-62.
4. Carere R, Patterson GA, Liu P, Williams T, Maurer J, Grossman R: Right and left ventricular performance after single and double lung transplantation. The Toronto Lung Transplant Group. *J Thorac Cardiovasc Surg* 1991; 102(1):115-23.
5. Chetham PM: Anesthesia for heart or single or double lung transplantation in the adult patient. *J Card Surg* 2000; 15(3): 167-74.
6. Della Rocca G, Pugliese F, Antonini M, Coccia C, Pompei L, Vizza CD, Rendina EA, Ricci C, Cortesini R: Hemodynamics during inhaled nitric oxide in lung transplant candidates. *Transplant Proc* 1997; 29:3367-70.
7. DeMajo WAP: Pulmonary transplantation. In *Thoracic Anesthesia*, 2nd edition. Kaplan J, ed. Churchill Livingstone, New York: 1991, 555-62.
8. Gasparetto A: Intraoperative inhaled nitric oxide during anesthesia for lung transplant. *Transpl Int* 1997; 10:439-45.

9. Hurford WE, Kolker AC, Strauss W: The use of ventilation/perfusion lung scans to predict oxygenation during one-lung anesthesia. *Anesthesiology* 1987; 67(5):841-4.

10. Kramer MR, Marshall SE, McDougall IR, Kloneck A, Starnes VA, Lewiston NJ, Theodore J: The distribution of ventilation and perfusion after single-lung transplantation in patients with pulmonary fibrosis and pulmonary hypertension. *Transplant Proc* 1991; 23(1 P+2):1215-16.

11. Limbos MM, Chan CK, Kesten S: Quality of life in female lung transplant candidates and recipients. *Chest* 1997; 112: 1165-74.

12. Macdonald P, Mundy J, Rogers P, Harrison G, Branch J, Glanville A, Keogh A, Spratt P: Successful treatment of life-threatening acute reperfusion injury after lung transplantation with inhaled nitric oxide. *J Thorac Cardiovasc Surg* 1995; 110:861-3.

13. Mair P, Balogh D: Anaesthetic and intensive care considerations for patients undergoing heart or lung transplantation. *Acta Anaesthesiol Scand* Suppl 1997; 111:78-9.

14. Marshall SE, Lewiston NJ, Kramer MR, Sibley RK, Berry G, Rich JB, Theodore J, Starnes VA: Prospective analysis of serial pulmonary function studies and transbronchial biopsies in single-lung transplant recipients. *Transplant Proc* 1991; 23(1 P+2):1217-19.

15. Maurer JR, Winton TL, Patterson GA, Williams TR: Single-lung transplantation for pulmonary vascular disease. *Transplant Proc* 1991; 23(1 P+2):1211-12.

16. Patterson GA: Indications. Unilateral, bilateral, heart-lung, and lobar transplant procedures. *Clin Chest Med* 1997; 18:225-30.

17. Siegel LC, Brodsky JB: Choice of anesthetic agents for intrathoracic surgery. In *Thoracic Anesthesia*, 2nd edition. Kaplan JA, ed. Churchill Livingstone, New York: 1991.

18. Smith CM: Patient selection, evaluation, and preoperative management for lung transplant candidates. *Clin Chest Med* 1997; 18:183-97.

19. Williams EL, Jellish WS, Modica PA, Eng CC, Tempelhoff R: Capnography in a patient after single lung transplantation. *Anesthesiology* 1991; 74(3):621-2.

7.0 GENERAL SURGERY

Surgeon

Richard I. Whyte, MD

7.1   ESOPHAGEAL SURGERY

Anesthesiologist

John L. Chow, MD, MS

ESOPHAGOSTOMY

SURGICAL CONSIDERATIONS

Description: Esophagostomy is performed to divert oral secretions away from the esophagus to a stoma pouch in certain types of esophageal perforation. In addition, it may be utilized for feeding purposes when the patient cannot swallow due to obstructive lesions of the pharynx. Through a left cervical incision, the sternocleidomastoid muscle and carotid sheath are retracted laterally and the thyroid medially, exposing the cervical esophagus (Fig 7.1-1). The esophagus is mobilized, with care being taken not to injure the recurrent laryngeal nerve. The esophagus is brought to the skin surface as a loop or end stoma and sutured to the skin with absorbable sutures.

Variant procedure or approaches: The procedure is usually performed via a left cervical approach; the right side is an alternative.

Usual preop diagnosis: Esophageal perforation; nasopharyngeal cancer

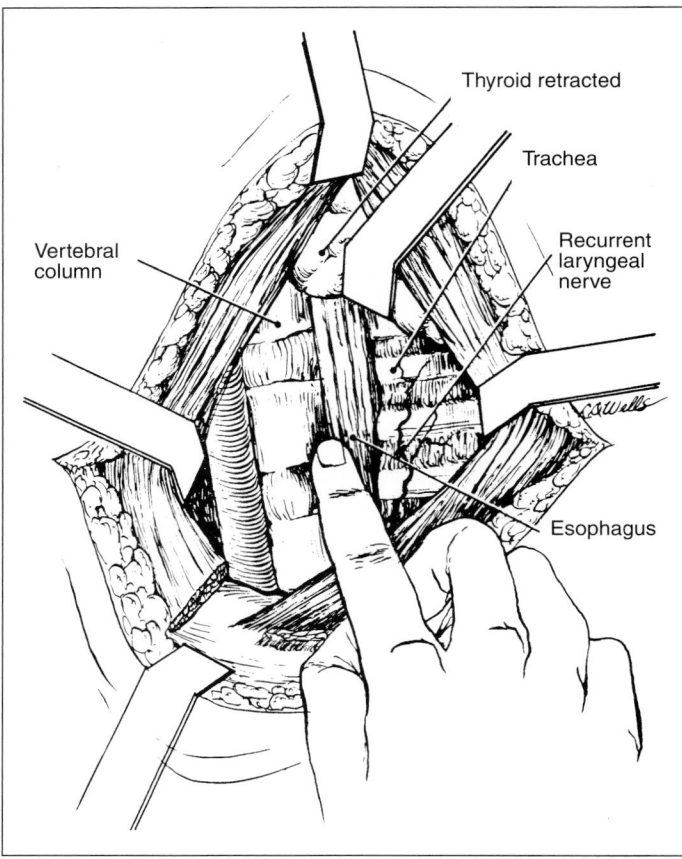

Figure 7.1-1. Surgical anatomy for cervical esophagostomy. (Reproduced with permission from Nora PF, ed: *Operative Surgery Principles and Techniques*. WB Saunders, 1990.)

SUMMARY OF PROCEDURE

Position	Supine, with head rotated to right
Incision	Cervical
Antibiotics	Cefazolin 1 g iv 30 min preop
Surgical time	45 min
EBL	25-50 ml
Postop care	Stoma pouch to collect saliva; PACU → room
Mortality	< 0.1%
Morbidity	Skin irritation: 15-20%
	Saliva leakage: 5-10%
	Wound infection: < 5%
Pain score	5-7

PATIENT POPULATION CHARACTERISTICS

Age range	Variable: 20-60 yr
Male:Female	1:1
Incidence	Not uncommon
Etiology	Surgically created
Associated conditions	Esophageal perforation; pharyngeal cancer

ANESTHETIC CONSIDERATIONS

See Anesthetic Considerations for Esophageal Surgery following Esophagectomy, p. 387.

Reference

1. Jones WG, Ginsberg RJ: Esophageal perforations: a continuing challenge. *Ann Thorac Surg* 1992; 53:534.

ESOPHAGEAL DIVERTICULECTOMY

SURGICAL CONSIDERATIONS

Description: Esophageal diverticula are divided into three anatomic types: **pharyngoesophageal (Zenker's), midesophageal,** and **epiphrenic**. Pharyngoesophageal diverticula account for 60-65% of all cases. These diverticula originate in Killian's triangle, a weak point in the posterior esophagus, just proximal to the transverse fibers of the cricopharyngeal muscle (Fig. 7.1-2) and are associated with incomplete, or discoordinate, upper esophageal sphincter relaxation. The resultant increased hypopharyngeal pressure produces a narrow-mouthed posterior diverticulum. These usually are present in the seventh decade and are 2-3 times more common in men. Symptoms depend on the stage of the disease. Early on, patients may complain of vague pharyngeal sensations, dysphagia, cough, and excess salivation. Later, more severe symptoms—such as severe (or frequent) dysphagia, regurgitation of food, halitosis, voice changes, aspiration, and odynophagia (painful swallowing)—may occur.

Surgery is the only effective therapy for Zenker's diverticulum. Respiratory (aspiration) or nutritional (weight loss) deficiencies may be directly attributable to the diverticulum and should not be contraindications to surgery. Multiple different operative approaches have been advocated: diverticulectomy alone, cricopharyngeal myotomy, diverticulectomy with myotomy and myotomy with suspension of the diverticulum. **Myotomy** alone, which corrects the underlying physiologic

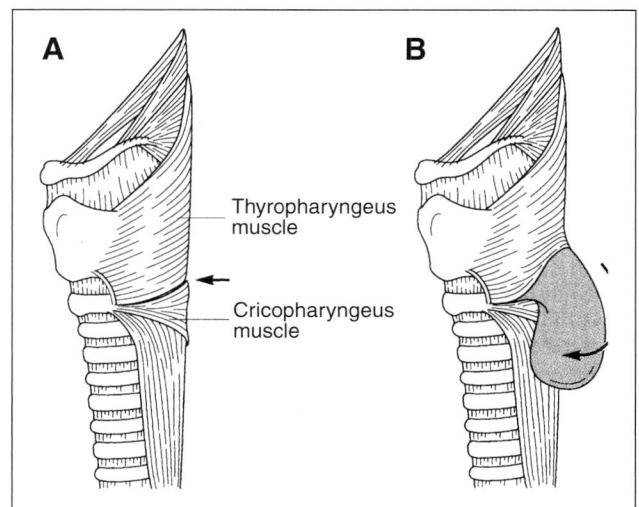

Figure 7.1-2. Formation of Zenker's diverticulum. (A) Herniation of the pharyngeal mucosa and submucosa occurs at the point of potential weakness (Killian's triangle [arrow]) between the oblique fibers of the thyropharyngeus muscle and the more horizontal fibers of the cricopharyngeus muscle. (B) As the diverticulum enlarges, it drapes over the cricopharyngeus sphincter and descends into the superior mediastinum in the prevertebral space. (Reproduced with permission from Greenfield LJ, et al, eds: *Surgery: Scientific Principles and Practice*, 3rd edition. Lippincott Williams & Wilkins, 2001. After Orringer MB: Diverticula and miscellaneous conditions of the esophagus. In *Textbook of Surgery*, 13th edition. Sabiston DC Jr, ed. WB Saunders, 1986.)

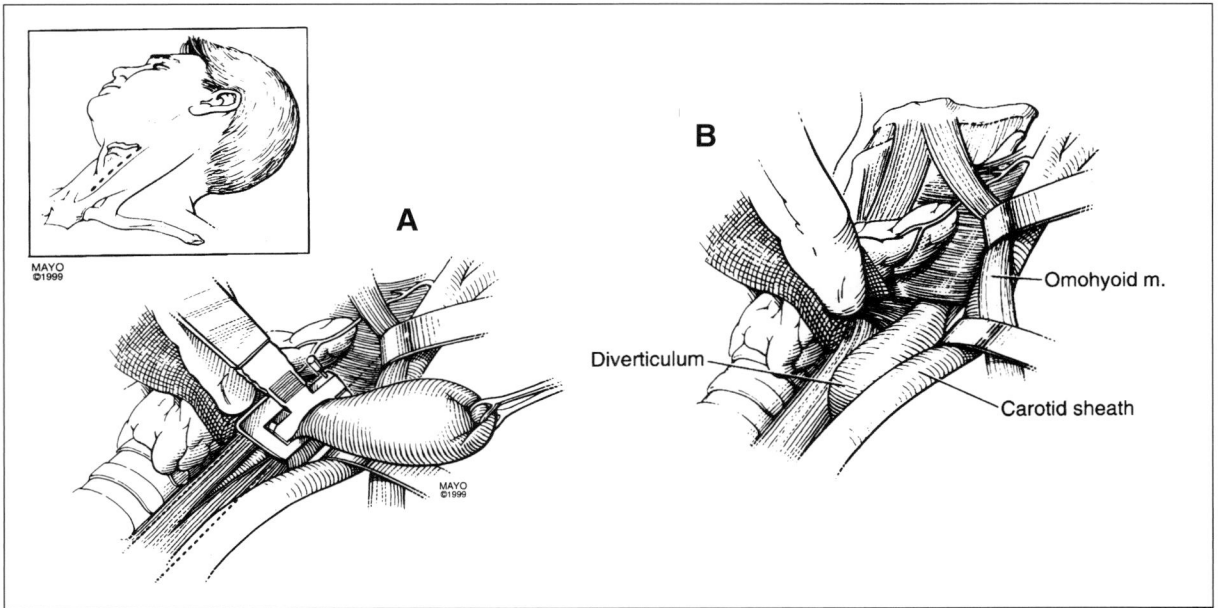

Figure 7.1-3. Zenker's diverticulum approached through a left cervical incision (inset). (A) The diverticulum is grasped and a cricopharyngeal myotomy is extended onto the upper esophagus. (B) The base of the diverticulum is stapled and the diverticulum is resected. (Reproduced with permission from Shields TW, LoCicero J III, Ponn RB: *General Thoracic Surgery*, 5th edition. Lippincott Williams & Wilkins, 2000.)

abnormality, is up to 78% effective and may be considered for patients with small (< 2 cm) diverticula. **Diverticulectomy** or **suspension** should be added if the diverticulum itself is large or dependant. Both procedures are performed via a left cervical incision (Fig. 7.1-3 inset) and are associated with a low rate of recurrence and complications. The upper esophagus is exposed by retracting the sternocleidomastoid muscle and carotid sheath laterally and the thyroid gland medially. The diverticulum is located in the prevertebral space. Care is taken not to injure the recurrent laryngeal nerve. Following excision of the diverticulum, a **myotomy** may be performed, starting on the upper esophagus and curving across the cricopharyngeal muscle near the neck of the diverticulum.

Recent emphasis has been placed on endoscopic treatment of Zenker's diverticulum (**Dohlman procedure**). In this procedure, a modified laryngoscope and endoscopic stapler are used to divide the common wall between diverticulum and true esophageal lumen.

Midesophageal diverticula, by definition, occur in the middle third of the esophagus. These 'true' diverticula, usually found within 4-5 cm of the carina, comprise an estimated 10-17% of all esophageal diverticula. Most midesophageal diverticula are asymp-

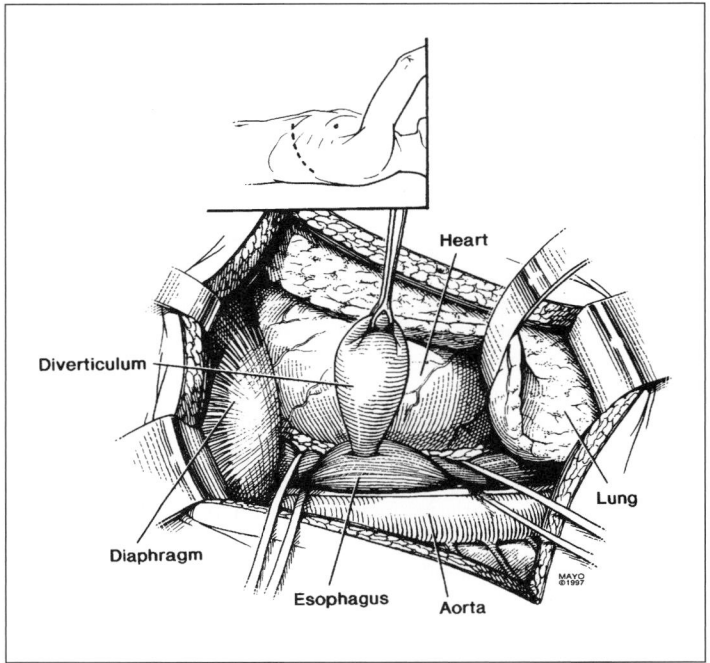

Figure 7.1-4. Epiphrenic diverticulum. Through a left thoracotomy, the diverticulum is mobilized and resected. A contralateral myotomy is then created and extended distally to the stomach to eliminate any functional obstruction secondary to the preexistent dysmotility. (Reproduced with permission from Shields TW, LoCicero J III, Ponn RB: *General Thoracic Surgery*, 5th edition. Lippincott Williams & Wilkins, 2000.)

tomatic and do not require surgical intervention. In cases that require resection, the approach is through a right thoracotomy with excision of the inflammatory mass. Primary closure of the fistula and the interposition of viable tissue should be performed.

Epiphrenic diverticula arise in the distal 10 cm of the esophagus and are thought to be related to an underlying esophageal motility disorder. Most commonly present in the sixth decade, the clinical presentation is variable, with most patients presenting with symptoms related to their dysmotility syndrome: dysphagia, chest pain, or regurgitation. Most patients with epiphrenic diverticula are asymptomatic, and there appears to be no relation between size of the diverticulum and symptoms. Surgery for epiphrenic diverticula typically consists of **diverticulectomy with myotomy** through a left thoracotomy (Fig. 7.1-4). After the esophagus is mobilized and encircled, the diverticulum is mobilized and excised. A **myotomy** should be performed opposite the diverticulectomy and should extend proximally above the diverticulum and distally onto the stomach. Because there is, by definition, an underlying motility disorder, the myotomy should be carried onto the stomach and a nonobstructing fundoplication may be added to prevent significant postop reflux.

Variant procedure or approaches: Laparoscopic diverticulectomy and myotomy has been described, and reported outcomes are similar to those obtained with the open procedure. The surgical approach is similar to that used during laparoscopic fundoplication (see p. 456). Dissection of the diverticula may be facilitated by the passage of a bougie or video endoscope. After the diverticulum is amputated using an endoscopic stapler, a myotomy is performed opposite the diverticula and a partial fundoplication is fashioned.

Usual preop diagnosis: Esophageal diverticulum

SUMMARY OF PROCEDURES

	Hypopharyngeal	Epiphrenic
Position	Supine	Right lateral decubitus
Incision	Left or right cervical	Left thoracotomy
Special instrumentation	None	Chest retractor
Unique considerations	Care not to injure recurrent laryngeal nerve	10 cm myotomy
Antibiotics	Cefazolin 1 g iv preop	⇐

	Hypopharyngeal	**Epiphrenic**
Surgical time	1-2 h	⇐
Closing considerations	Inspect for perforation	⇐
EBL	50-100 ml	100-200 ml
Postop care	PACU	ICU × 1-2 d
Mortality	< 1%	⇐
Morbidity	Recurrent nerve paralysis: < 5%	Atelectasis: 5-10%
	Temporary phonetic problems: < 5%	Esophageal stricture: < 5%
	Esophageal stricture: < 3%	Esophageal perforation: < 2%
	Esophageal fistula: < 2%	–
Pain score	6-7	7-9

PATIENT POPULATION CHARACTERISTICS

Age range	38-92 yr (50% of patients > 70 yr)
Male:Female	2:1
Incidence	Uncommon
Etiology	Uncoordinated cricoesophageal muscle and lower esophageal sphincter (100%); weakness of esophageal wall (100%)
Associated conditions	Cachexia (25-30%); hiatus hernia with or without reflux (25%); chronic pulmonary infection (15-20%); aspiration (30-40%)

ANESTHETIC CONSIDERATIONS

See Anesthetic Considerations for Esophageal Surgery following Esophagectomy, p. 387.

Reference

1. Deschamps C, Trastek V: Esophageal diverticula. In *General Thoracic Surgery*, 5th edition. Shields TW, LoCicero J III, Ponn RB, eds. Lippincott Williams & Wilkins, Philadelphia: 2000.
2. Rice TW, ed: *Seminars in Thoracic and Cardiovascular Surgery* 1999; 11(4):325.

MANAGEMENT OF ESOPHAGEAL PERFORATION

SURGICAL CONSIDERATIONS

Description: **Esophageal perforation** may be spontaneous, instrumental, traumatic, or 2° intrinsic esophageal disease. **Spontaneous perforations** commonly occur in the lower third of the esophagus. **Instrumental perforations** may occur at any level, but are most common just above the cardia and in the cervical esophagus. The level of **traumatic perforation** depends on the location of the penetrating wound. Sx of esophageal perforation at the cricopharyngeal sphincter include neck pain, fever, and crepitations in the substernal and neck areas. Perforation in the mediastinum may result in hydropneumothorax, mediastinitis, fever, and substernal pain. Cervical perforations are managed with antibiotics and drainage in the cervical area. Therapy for intrathoracic perforation generally requires emergent operation. Surgical options include **primary repair, drainage and diversion**, and **esophageal resection**. The optimal choice depends on the nature and duration of the perforation as well as the clinical condition of the patient. Spontaneous, or barogenic, perforations are often amenable to primary repair—either through the abdomen or the left chest. Patients suffering from iatrogenic perforation incurred during dilation of a malignant stricture may require urgent esophagectomy. Patients with delayed recognition of a perforation may be hemodynamically unstable and may only tolerate drainage and diversion (generally through a cervical esophagostomy).

Variant procedure or approaches: Cervical or right thoracic drainage are indicated when the perforation occurs in the neck or high in the mediastinum.

Usual preop diagnosis: Esophageal perforation

SUMMARY OF PROCEDURES

	Left Thoracotomy	Cervical or Thoracic Drainage
Position	Right lateral decubitus	Supine or right lateral decubitus
Incision	Left thoracotomy	Cervical or right chest
Antibiotics	Cefazolin 1 g iv	⇐
Surgical time	2-4 h	1 h
Closing considerations	Chest drain	Cervical or thoracic drain
EBL	100-200 ml	50-100 ml
Postop care	Chest tube to suction; PACU → room	⇐
Mortality	5-10%	2-5%
Morbidity	Pneumonia: 5-10%	–
	Esophageal leak: 2-5%	10%
	Pericarditis: 1-3%	–
Pain score	8-10	8-10

PATIENT POPULATION CHARACTERISTICS

Age range	Variable: 20-80 yr
Male:Female	1:1
Incidence	1 in 8,000 admissions
Etiology	Instrumental (endoscopy, dilatation, intubation); traumatic (penetrating, foreign body, caustic agents); intrinsic disease (carcinoma, peptic ulceration); spontaneous
Associated conditions	Esophageal stricture (75%); cancer (25%)

ANESTHETIC CONSIDERATIONS

See Anesthetic Considerations for Esophageal Surgery following Esophagectomy, p. 387.

References

1. Fell SC: Esophageal perforation. In *Esophageal Surgery*. Pearson FG, Cooper JD, Deslauriers J, Ginsberg RJ, Hiebert C, Patterson GA, Urschel HC Jr, eds. Churchill Livingstone, New York: 2002, 615-36.
2. Orringer MB: The mediastinum. In *Operative Surgery*, 3rd edition. Nora PF, ed. WB Saunders, Philadelphia: 1990, 370-3.

ESOPHAGOMYOTOMY

SURGICAL CONSIDERATIONS

Description: **Esophagomyotomy** is performed for achalasia and other motility disorders to facilitate esophageal emptying into the stomach. It consists of incising the muscular layer of the distal esophagus and continuing down across the gastroesophageal junction for at least 1 cm (**Heller's myotomy**).[2] The muscle is dissected back from the mucosa so that roughly 180° is exposed (Fig 7.1-5). The distal esophagus is mobilized either from below the diaphragm or via a left thoracic approach. Care is taken not to injure the vagus nerve.

When approached from the abdomen, the esophagus is exposed by incising the gastroesophageal ligament. The distal esophagus is mobilized and pulled downward to perform the myotomy.

Variant procedure or approaches: The procedure usually is performed through a left thoracotomy, but some surgeons prefer a **transabdominal approach**. More recently, laparoscopic or thoracoscopic approaches are being employed to perform esophagomyotomy (see p. 458).

Usual preop diagnosis: Achalasia; diffuse esophageal spasm; nutcracker esophagus

Figure 7.1-5. Surgical anatomy for esophagomyotomy. (Reproduced with permission from Hardy JD: *Hardy's Textbook of Surgery*, 2nd edition. JB Lippincott, 1988.)

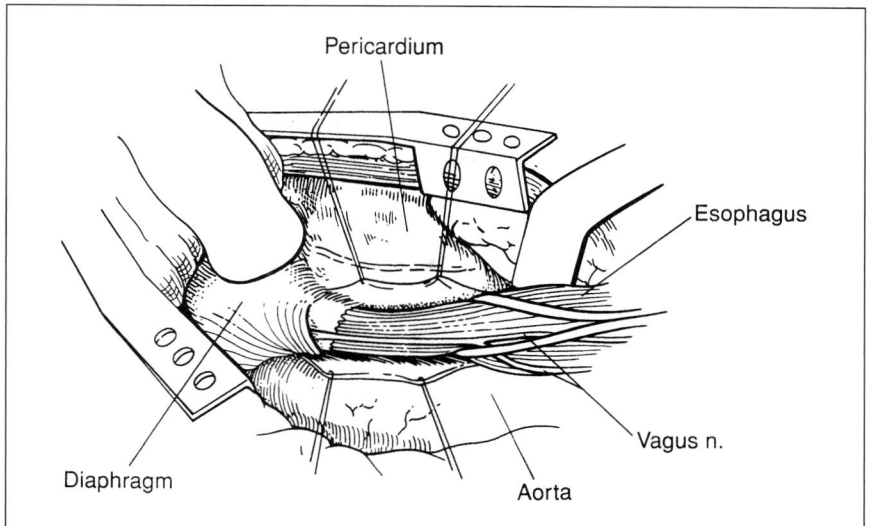

SUMMARY OF PROCEDURES

	Thoracic Approach	Abdominal Approach
Position	Right lateral decubitus	Supine
Incision	Left thoracotomy in 6th interspace	Midline upper abdomen
Special instrumentation	Chest retractor	Denier retractor
Unique considerations	Care should be taken to avoid extending gastric myotomy too far to prevent esophageal reflux.	⇐
Antibiotics	Cefazolin 1-2 g iv 30 min preop	⇐
Surgical time	1-2 h	⇐
Closing considerations	✓ for perforation. Consider fundoplication to prevent esophageal reflux.[2]	⇐
EBL	150-200 ml	100-150 ml
Postop care	ICU × 1-2 d	PACU → room
Mortality	< 0.5%	⇐
Morbidity	Esophagitis: ≤ 20%	⇐
	Transient dysphagia/reflux: 5%	⇐
	Esophageal leak: 1-2%	⇐
Pain score	7-9	6-8

PATIENT POPULATION CHARACTERISTICS

Age range	30-50 yr
Male:Female	1:1
Incidence	0.6/100,000
Etiology	Neuromuscular disorder of unknown etiology often characterized by absence of ganglion cells of Auerbach's plexus (100%)
Associated conditions	Predisposition to development of carcinoma (1-20%); pulmonary complications 2° aspiration (5-10%)

ANESTHETIC CONSIDERATIONS

See Anesthetic Considerations for Esophageal Surgery following Esophagectomy, p. 387.

References

1. Ellis FH Jr, Crozier RE, Watkins E Jr: Operation for esophageal achalasia. Results of esophagomyotomy without an antireflex. *J Thorac Cardiovasc Surg* 1984; 88(3):344-51.
2. Pellegrini C, Wetters LA, Palti M, et al: Thorascopic esophagomyotomy. *Ann Surg* 1992; 216:29.
3. Stuart RC, Hennessy TP: Primary motility disorders of the esophagus. *Br J Surg* 1989; 76:111.

ESOPHAGOGASTRIC FUNDOPLASTY

SURGICAL CONSIDERATIONS

Description: **Esophagogastric fundoplasty** represents a variety of operations designed to prevent esophageal reflux by wrapping the fundus of the stomach around a 3-4 cm segment of the lower esophagus. This fundal wrapping acts to reinforce the lower esophageal sphincter. Surgery may be performed transabdominally, transthoracically, or laparoscopically, depending on surgeon's preference. The most commonly used is the open or laparoscopic **Nissen fundoplication**, utilizing both the anterior and posterior walls of the stomach. They are sutured together around the lower esophagus with nonabsorbable sutures (Fig 7.1-6A). This is accomplished by incising the gastrosplenic ligament and ligating 3 or 4 short gastric vessels. Care must be taken not to injure the spleen or vagus nerves during the repair.

Variant procedure or approaches: Modifications of the Nissen fundoplication include the **Toupet procedure**, a posterior partial fundoplication, and the **Hill procedure**,[3] in which the gastroesophageal junction is sutured to the median arcuate ligament of the diaphragm or to the preaortic fascia (Fig 7.1-6B). Another modification is the **Belsey Mark IV**[1] repair, in which there is a 240° semifundoplication between the stomach and esophagus, making it easier for the patient to overcome the resistance of the wrap. There are proponents of each repair, although the Nissen fundoplication remains the procedure most widely used. The laparoscopic approach is being used with increasing frequency (see p. 456).

Usual preop diagnosis: Sliding hiatus (hiatal) hernia or free reflux

SUMMARY OF PROCEDURES

	Nissen (Toupet) Fundoplication	Hill Procedure	Belsey Mark IV
Position	Supine	⇐	Right lateral decubitus
Incision	Midline abdominal or laparoscopic ports	⇐	Left posterolateral thoracotomy
Special instrumentation	#40-50 Hurst dilators; NG tube	NG tube	Chest retractor; NG tube
Unique considerations	Fundoplication should be loose; parietal cell vagotomy performed if peptic ulcer disease present. Fundoplication may be limited to 180-280° posterior wrap (Toupet)	⇐	⇐
Antibiotics	Cefazolin 1-2 g iv 30 min preop	⇐	⇐
Surgical time	1-2 h	⇐	⇐
Closing considerations	Inspect spleen for bleeding	⇐	⇐
EBL	100-150 ml	⇐	100-200 ml
Postop care	PACU → room	⇐	ICU × 1-2 d
Mortality	< 0.5%	⇐	⇐
Morbidity	Recurrent hernia: 20%	⇐	⇐
	Gas-bloat syndrome: 10-20%	< 5%	⇐
	Temporary dysphagia: 5-10%	5%	2%
	Gastric fistula: < 2%	⇐	⇐
Pain score	6-8	7-8	7-9

PATIENT POPULATION CHARACTERISTICS

Age range	46-60 yr
Male:Female	1:2
Incidence	Not uncommon
Etiology	Esophagogastric reflux (100%); esophageal hiatus hernia (80-90%)
Associated conditions	Diverticulosis of colon (30-35%); cholelithiasis (25-30%)

ANESTHETIC CONSIDERATIONS

See Anesthetic Considerations for Esophageal Surgery following Esophagectomy, p. 387.

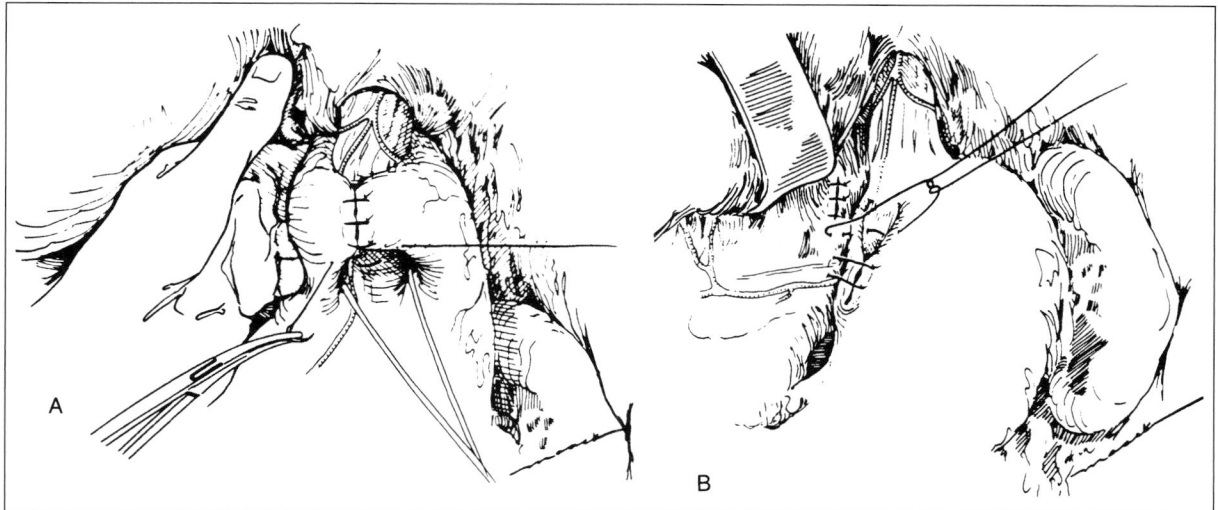

Figure 7.1-6. (A) Nissen fundoplication may be performed via either the transabdominal or transthoracic approach; (B) Hill repair is performed through the abdomen. (Reproduced with permission from Hardy JD: *Hardy's Textbook of Surgery*, 2nd edition. JB Lippincott, 1988.)

References

1. Belsey R: Mark IV repair of hiatal hernia by the transthoracic approach. *World J Surg* 1977; 1(4):475-81.
2. Cuschieri, A: Laparoscopic antireflux surgery and repair of hiatal hernia. *World J Surg* 1993; 17(1):40-5.
3. Hill LD: Progress in the surgical management of hiatal hernia. *World J Surg* 1977; 1(4):425-36

ESOPHAGECTOMY

SURGICAL CONSIDERATIONS

Description: Esophagectomy is most commonly performed for malignant disease of the middle and lower thirds of the esophagus and gastric cardia. This procedure also may be indicated for intractable benign stricture, **Barrett's esophagus** with high-grade dysplasia, and end-stage achalasia. There are several surgical options for esophageal resection, including the **Ivor Lewis approach**, which involves a laparotomy and right thoracotomy; the transhiatal approach, whereby the esophagus is mobilized through abdominal and neck incisions, and the **left thoracoabdominal approach** (Fig. 7.1-7). While there are advantages and disadvantages to each, the final result is to use a portion of the stomach to replace the esophagus. In all approaches, the stomach is mobilized while preserving its blood supply from the right gastroepiploic and gastric arteries. The stomach is then transposed into the chest and a gastroesophageal anastomosis is fashioned either in the chest (Ivor Lewis and left chest approaches) or in the neck (transhiatal approach). To avoid delayed gastric emptying, a **pyloroplasty** or **pyloromyotomy** is usually added, as is placement of a temporary jejunal feeding tube.

The above variants of esophagectomy all involve use of the **stomach** as an esophageal replacement. When the stomach is not available (as with prior resection or caustic injury), the **colon** can be used as an esophageal substitute. Both the left and right colon can be used, with the vascular supply to the grafts based on either the ascending branch of the left colic artery or the right colic artery. Colon interpositions typically have higher complication rates than esophagectomies using gastric conduits.

Usual preop diagnosis: Carcinoma of esophagus or gastroesophageal junction; Barrett's esophagus; benign strictures

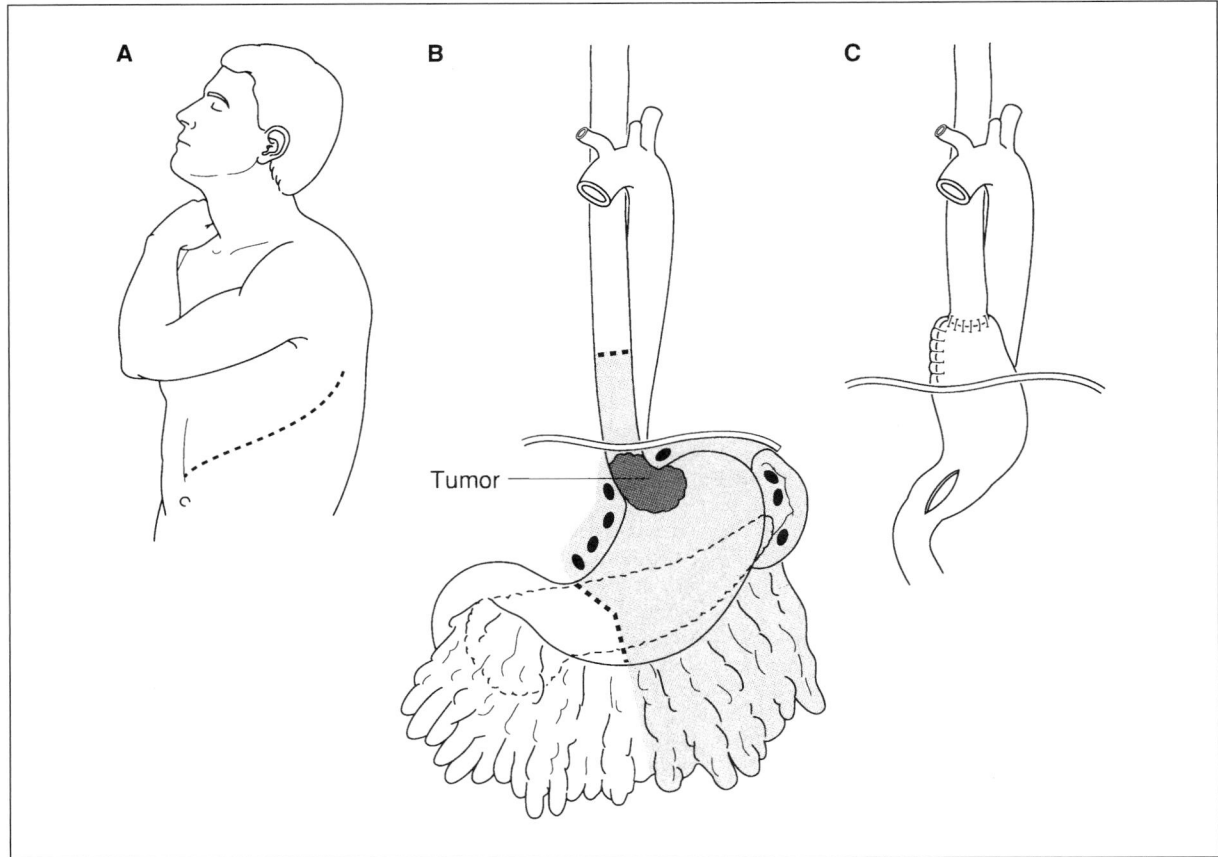

Figure 7.1-7. Standard thoracoabdominal esophagosgastrectomy for carcinomas of the distal esophagus and cardia. (A) Thoracoabdominal incision. (B) Tissue to be resected (darker area). (C) Completed reconstruction after intrathoracic esophagogastric anastomosis and either pyloromyotomy or pyloroplasty to prevent postvagotomy pylorospasm. (Reproduced with permission from Greenfield LJ, et al, eds: *Surgery: Scientific Principles and Practice*, 3rd edition. Lippincott Williams & Wilkins, 2001. After Ellis FH Jr: Treatment of carcinoma of the esophagus and cardia. *Mayo Clin Proc* 1960.)

SUMMARY OF PROCEDURES

	Esophagectomy	Transhiatal Esophagectomy	Esophago-gastrectomy	Total Esophagectomy + Colonic Interposition
Position	Supine and left lateral decubitus	Supine	Left lateral decubitus	Supine and right lateral decubitus
Incision	Midline abdominal + right or left chest and/or cervical incisions	Cervical and midline abdominal	Thoracoabdominal across costal margin	Midline + right thoracic and cervical
Special instrumentation	Chest retractor ± EEA stapler	Denier retractor	Chest retractor ± EEA stapler	Chest retractor
Unique considerations	DLT	None	DLT	⇐
Antibiotics	Cefazolin 2 g iv preop	⇐	⇐	⇐
Surgical time	3-4 h	4-5 h	3-4 h	5-6 h
Closing considerations	Lung reexpansion	Pneumothorax	Lung reexpansion	Vascular integrity of colonic interposition
EBL	300-800 ml	⇐	⇐	⇐
Postop care	ICU × 1-2 d	⇐	⇐	ICU × 2-3 d
Mortality	5-10%	⇐	⇐	10%
Morbidity	Respiratory complications: 15-20%	⇐	⇐	⇐

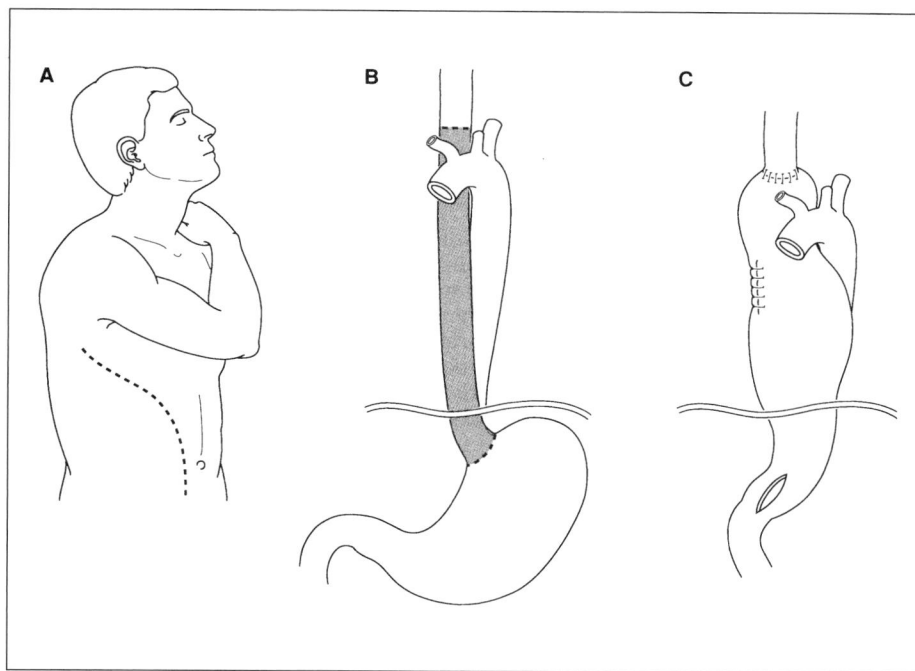

Figure 7.1-8. Standard thoracoabdominal esophagogastrectomy for tumors of the upper and middle thirds of the thoracic esophagus. (A) Either a continuous thoracoabdominal incision or separate thoracic and abdominal incisions are used. (B) Portion of esophagus to be resected (darker area). (C) Completed reconstruction with high intrathoracic esophagogastric anastomosis and gastric drainage procedure. (Reproduced with permission from Greenfield LJ, et al, eds: *Surgery: Scientific Principles and Practice*, 3rd edition. Lippincott Williams & Wilkins, 2001. After Ellis FH Jr: Treatment of carcinoma of the esophagus and cardia. *Mayo Clin Proc* 1960.)

	Esophagectomy	**Transhiatal Esophagectomy**	**Esophagogastrectomy**	**Total Esophagectomy + Colonic Interposition**
Morbidity, cont.	Anastomotic leakage: < 5%	5-10%	< 5%	10%
	Anastomotic stricture: < 5%	⇐	⇐	10%
	Wound infection: < 5%	⇐	⇐	⇐
Pain score	7-9	6-8	7-9	7-9

PATIENT POPULATION CHARACTERISTICS

Age range	4-80 yr
Male:Female	2:1 for carcinoma
Incidence	1-2% of malignant disease
Etiology	Alcohol and tobacco; dietary factors – hot spicy foods; lye burns
Associated conditions	Barrett's esophagus; hiatus hernia; reflux esophagitis; radiation esophagitis; caustic burns

Reference

1. Orringer MB: Resection of the esophagus. In *General Thoracic Surgery*, 5th edition. Shields TW, LoCicero J III, Ponn RB, eds. Lippincott Williams & Wilkins, Philadelphia: 2000, 1697-1722.

ANESTHETIC CONSIDERATIONS FOR ESOPHAGEAL SURGERY

(Procedures covered: esophagostomy; esophageal diverticulectomy; closure of esophageal perforation; esophagomyotomy; esophagogastric fundoplasty; esophagectomy)

Patients presenting for esophageal surgery typically are those with carcinoma, motility disorders, strictures, hiatal hernia, reflux esophagitis, diverticula, and/or perforation. Some forms of esophageal disorders will predispose the patient to aspiration pneumonitis.

PREOPERATIVE

Respiratory   Hx of gastric reflux suggests the possibility of recurrent aspiration pneumonia: ↓pulmonary reserve and ↑risk of regurgitation/aspiration during anesthetic induction. (See Premedication, below.) If thoracic approach is planned, patient should be evaluated to ensure that OLV can be tolerated (see below). Determine if patient has been exposed to bleomycin, which may cause pulmonary toxicity (above a total dose of 300 U/m²); toxicity may be made worse by high concentrations of O_2. Many patients with esophageal cancer have a long Hx of smoking, with consequent respiratory impairment. Mediastinal lymphadenopathy → tracheal compression.
Tests: Consider PFTs (FEV_1, FVC), ABG, if indicated by H&P. They can be helpful in predicting likelihood of periop pulmonary complications and the probability that patient may require postop mechanical ventilation. Patients with baseline hypoxemia/hypercarbia on room air will have a higher likelihood of postop complications and need for postop ventilatory support. Severe restrictive or obstructive lung disease also will increase the chance of pulmonary morbidity in the periop period. A-P, lateral CXR (if suggestive of tracheal compression → MRI/CT).

Cardiovascular   Elderly patients may have coexisting CAD. Patients may be hypovolemic and malnourished from dysphagia or anorexia. Preop chemotherapy treatment with agents such as doxorubicin may cause acute dysrhythmias and chronic cardiomyopathy (seen in 10% of patients if total dose is > 550 mg/m²). Chronic alcohol abuse also may produce a toxic cardiomyopathy. CHF, if present, may be refractory to treatment; however, preop optimization of cardiac function is essential.
Tests: ECG to r/o dysrhythmias, myocardial ischemia, or prior MI. ECHO or dobutamine stress ECHO will provide important functional information about the heart at rest or under stress, respectively.

Hematologic   **Tests:** CBC with differential

Laboratory   Tests as indicated from H&P.

Premedication   Midazolam titrated to effect. Consider H_2-antagonists (e.g., ranitidine 50 mg iv), metoclopramide (10 mg iv 1 h preop), and Na citrate (30 ml po 10 min preop). Patients with esophageal motility disorders may not tolerate premedication with Na citrate.

INTRAOPERATIVE

Anesthetic technique: GETA (with or without epidural for periop analgesia). If patient is clinically hypovolemic, restore intravascular volume before epidural placement and induction of GA. Surgeries involving only the cervical or endoscopic approach typically do not require epidural analgesia. If epidural analgesia is planned, placement and testing of the catheter before anesthetic induction is recommended. This is accomplished by injecting 5-10 ml of 2% lidocaine with 1:200,000 epinephrine via the epidural catheter and eliciting a segmental block. If a thoracic or thoracoabdominal approach is performed, placement of a DLT is indicated to provide OLV for optimal surgical conditions. (For additional discussion of DLT placement and OLV, see Anesthetic Considerations in Lobectomy, Pneumonectomy in Thoracic Surgery, p. 213+.)

Induction   Patients with esophageal disease are often at risk for pulmonary aspiration; therefore, the trachea should be intubated after rapid-sequence induction with cricoid pressure or with the patient awake. Awake intubation: (1) **Blind nasal:** topical vasoconstrictor to nose (1% phenylephrine or 4% cocaine on cotton-tipped applicators). Advance ETT until at laryngeal inlet; when patient inspires, advance ETT into trachea. Manipulation of ETT or head may be necessary for successful placement. (2) **Fiber optic intubation** (see p. B-6).

Maintenance   Standard maintenance (p. B-3), with or without N_2O (for OLV). Alternatively, a combined technique may be used. A local anesthetic (e.g., 2% lidocaine with 1:200,000 epinephrine or 0.25% bupivacaine) can be infused or injected into a thoracic (3-5 ml) or lumbar (5-10 ml) epidural catheter to provide both anesthesia and optimal surgical conditions (contracted bowel and profound muscle relaxation). Continuous infusion of local anesthetic generally provides better hemodynamic stability than hourly bolus injections. To enhance the effect of epidural analgesia, loading dose of opiates (e.g., hydromorphone 0.4-1 mg [thoracic] or 1-1.5 mg [lumbar]) can be administered early during the surgery and at least 1 h before conclusion of the case. Esophagectomy procedures can cause significant third-space losses; thus, adequate replacement of fluid and close monitoring of BP and UO are important to avoid hypovolemia. Esophageal procedures involving transient compression of the myocardium (i.e., thoracic approach for esophagomyotomy or esophagectomy) can induce dysrhythmias and/or ↓BP. Close monitoring of BP with an arterial catheter is recommended. Systemic sedatives (droperidol,

Maintenance, cont.	opiates, benzodiazepines, etc.) should be minimized during epidural opiate administration, as they may increase the likelihood of postop respiratory depression and aspiration.	
Emergence	Generally, tracheal extubation should be anticipated at the end of the case. The decision to keep the patient intubated postop depends on cardiopulmonary status and the extent of the surgical procedure. Patients with significant intraop fluid shift may develop airway edema that can → airway obstruction if extubated prematurely. For those who may require prolonged postop ventilation, the DLT should be exchanged to a single-lumen ETT (use an airway exchange catheter) before transport to ICU. Weaning from mechanical ventilation should begin when patient is awake and cooperative, able to protect the airway, hemodynamically stable, and have adequate return of pulmonary function (as measured by VC > = 10 ml/kg; MIF of –30 cmH$_2$O; rapid, shallow breathing index of ≤100 [RR÷TV(L)]; respiratory rate < 25; and ABG that demonstrates adequate gas exchange).	
Blood and fluid requirements	IV: 14-16 ga × 1 NS/LR @ 8-12 ml/kg/h Fluid warmer T&C for 4 U PRBC.	Plt, FFP, and cryoprecipitate (if required) should be administered according to lab tests (Plt count, PT, PTT, DIC screen, thromboelastography [TEG]).
Monitoring	Standard monitors (p. B-1) Urinary catheter ± Arterial line ± CVP	CVP cannulation site determined by surgical approach. Attempt to prevent hypothermia during long operations. Consider forced-air warmer, heated humidifier, warming blanket, warming room T, keeping patient covered until ready for prep, etc.
Positioning	If lateral decubitus position, use axillary roll, airplane arm holder. ✓ pressure points, including ears, eyes, and genitals. ✓ radial pulses to ensure correct placement of axillary roll (if misplaced, will compromise distal pulses).	Problems that can arise include brachial plexus injuries, damage to soft tissues, ears, eyes, genitals from malpositioning. Check down eye at frequent intervals. Placing the oximeter probe on the down arm may assist in monitoring adequacy of perfusion.
Complications	Hypoxemia	Hypoxemia during OLV most commonly results from luminal obstruction (by blood or pulmonary secretions) of the DLT, worsening of shunting, or malposition of DLT. Rx: suction DLT and ✓ position; PEEP to ventilated lung (but may ↑ shunting); CPAP to nonventilated lung; return to double-lung ventilation. Temporary clamping of the PA (or inflate the balloon of the PA catheter, if available) may be necessary to improve shunting and oxygenation.
	Hypercarbia Dysrhythmia ↓BP DVT	Ensure adequate TV and RR. ✓ for mechanical compression of heart or great vessels. ✓ volume status and cardiac function. Consider neosynephrine for BP support if ↓BP 2° to epidural anesthetic. Preventive measures using TED hose and SCD

POSTOPERATIVE

Complications	Aspiration Atelectasis Hemorrhage Pneumothorax Hemothorax Hypoxemia Hypoventilation Recurrent laryngeal nerve injury Esophageal anastomotic leak DVT	For patients at risk for atelectasis or aspiration, recover in the Fowler position (lateral). For hemorrhage, ✓ coags; replace factors as necessary. Dx for pneumothorax and hemothorax: wheezing, coughing, ↓PO$_2$, ↑PCO$_2$. Confirm by CXR. Rx: chest tube drainage as necessary. In emergency (e.g., tension pneumothorax), use needle aspiration. Supportive Rx: O$_2$, vasopressors, volume, ± ETT and IPPV. For hypoxemia and hypoventilation, adequate analgesia, minimize sedation, supplemental O$_2$, may require IPPV. For laryngeal nerve injury, indirect visualization of vocal cords; patient usually will be hoarse. Surgical repair for esophageal anastomotic leak

Complications, cont.	SVT/AFib	Treat underlying cause and correct electrolyte abnormalities. Adenosine (6 mg iv, push and repeat to 12 mg iv) may be used for SVT. Most postop SVTs are 2° catecholamine surge. AFib may resolve spontaneously. Hemodynamically unstable patients will require cardioversion. β-blockers, amiodarone, Ca^{++} channel blockers, and overdrive cardiac pacing are effective in patients with stable AFib.
Pain management	Lumbar-thoracic epidural analgesia: hydromorphone (0.5-1.5 mg load, 0.1-0.3 mg/h infusion) + local anesthetic PCA (p. C-3) NSAID	Patient should recover in ICU or hospital ward that is accustomed to treating side effects of epidural opiates (e.g., respiratory depression, breakthrough pain, nausea, pruritus). Ketorolac is helpful as adjuvant therapy for postop pain management.
Tests	CBC ABG CXR (r/o pneumothorax, atelectasis).	

References

1. Amar D: Cardiopulmonary complications of esophageal surgery. *Chest Surg Clin N Am* 1997; 7(3):449-56.
2. Belsey R: Reconstruction of the esophagus with left colon. *J Thorac Cardiovasc Surg* 1965; 49:33-55.
3. Eisenkraft JB, Cohen E, Neustein SM: Anesthesia for thoracic surgery. In *Clinical Anesthesia*, 3rd edition. Barash, PG, Cullen BF, Stoelting RK eds. JB Lippincott Co, Philadelphia: 1997, 769-804.
4. Kahn L, Baxter FJ, Dauphin A, et al: A comparison of thoracic and lumbar epidural techniques for post-thoracoabdominal esophagectomy analgesia. *Can J Anaesth* 1999; 46(5 Pt 1):415-22.
5. Kolker AC: Esophageal surgery. In *Cardiac, Vascular, and Thoracic Anesthesia*. Youngberg JA, Lake CL, Roizen MF, Wilson RS, eds. Churchill Livingstone, Philadelphia: 2000, 688-702.
6. Nagawa H, Kobori O, Muto T: Prediction of pulmonary complications after transthoracic oesophagectomy. *Br J Surg* 1994; 81(6):860-2.
7. Orringer MB: Tumors, injuries, and miscellaneous conditions of the esophagus. In *Surgery: Scientific Principles and Practice*, 2nd edition. Greenfield LJ, Mulholland M, Oldham KT, Zelenock GB, Lillemoe KD, eds. Lippincott-Raven Publishers, Philadelphia: 1997, 694-734.
8. Orringer MB, Orringer JS: Esophagectomy without thoracotomy: a dangerous operation? *J Thorac Cardiovasc Surg* 1983; 85(1):72-80.
9. Slinger PD, Hickey DR: The interaction between applied PEEP and auto-PEEP during one-lung ventilation. *J Cardiothorac Vasc Anesth* 1998; 12(2):133-6.
10. Smetana GW: Preoperative pulmonary evaluation. *N Eng J Med* 1999; 340(1):937-44.

Surgeons

H. Ward Trueblood, MD
Myriam J. Curet, MD (*Open operations for morbid obesity*)

7.2 STOMACH SURGERY

Anesthesiologists

Kevin A. Malott, MD
Jay B. Brodsky, MD (*Open operations for morbid obesity*)

GASTRIC RESECTIONS

SURGICAL CONSIDERATIONS

Description: **Total gastrectomy** is performed most commonly for gastric cancer, and may include **omentectomy, lymph node dissection,** and/or **splenectomy**, depending on the extent of the tumor, condition of the patient, and surgeon's preference. Occasionally, it is performed for uncontrollable symptoms due to Zollinger-Ellison syndrome. Rarely, this procedure may be used for control of hemorrhage from diffuse gastritis. Even more rarely, patients with intractable post-gastrectomy symptoms may eventually require total gastrectomy.

In a gastric resection, the abdomen is entered through an upper midline incision and the lateral segment of the left lobe of the liver is retracted to the patient's right, exposing the esophagogastric junction. The omentum is taken off of the colon and left attached to the greater curvature of the stomach. The spleen may be removed if crowded by tumor or nodes. The vessels to the stomach are individually ligated and divided. The short gastric vessels high on the greater curvature are difficult to reach and are a source of potential blood loss. Resection of the left gastric artery and the nodes at the celiac artery is another point of potential unexpected blood loss. In tumors of the middle or lower third of the stomach, it may be reasonable to preserve the upper stomach as the site of anastomosis. In most instances of gastric cancer, the antrum and pylorus are resected. Rarely is a **Billroth I connection** done for cancer. The upper stomach or esophageal resection line is often stapled, with care being taken to avoid entrapment of the NG tube. The jejunum is divided just beyond the Ligament of Treitz, and the distal end is brought up through a hole in the mesentery of the colon and anastomosed to the esophagus. The duodenum is closed with either sutures or staples. Intestinal continuity is established by anastomosing the end of the proximal limb of the jejunum to a Roux limb of jejunum, approximately 60 cm distal to the anastomosis with the esophagus. A drain is then placed. Occasionally, following total gastrectomy, the surgeon may choose to create a jejunal reservoir to simulate a stomach. This does not add appreciably to the duration, difficulty, or morbidity of the operation, but its efficacy is not widely accepted. An NG tube is advanced across the esophagojejunal anastomosis, and the abdomen is closed. Total gastrectomy traditionally has been associated with a morbidity and mortality out of proportion to the operation's apparent magnitude. This is most likely a consequence of the patient's underlying condition, which often includes advanced malignancy and, almost invariably, some degree of malnutrition.

Variant procedure or approaches: Exposure for a **hemigastrectomy** is similar to, but less extensive than that required for a total gastrectomy. The abdomen is entered through an upper midline or right subcostal incision, but the lateral segment of the left lobe of the liver is simply retracted superiorly. If the resection is performed for cancer, an **omentectomy** may still be performed; however, it would be unusual to intentionally perform a **splenectomy**. The blood supply to the distal stomach is divided, and the duodenum is divided just beyond the pylorus. The body of the stomach is divided, using either clamps and sutures or staples, at a level appropriate for the pathology. If the resection is for cancer, an adequate proximal margin will dictate the proximal line of resection; if for a benign gastric ulcer, approximately half of the distal stomach is resected (preferably excising the ulcer itself). Reconstruction may be either to the duodenum (**Billroth I**), loop of jejunum (**Billroth II**) (Fig 7.2-1), or to a **Roux-en-Y loop of jejunum**. The anastomoses may be stapled or sewn; then the abdomen is closed.

Tumors (usually adenocarcinoma) of the gastroesophageal (GE) junction are increasing in frequency and may be of either gastric or esophageal origin. Resection frequently requires a team of thoracic, general, and laparoscopic surgeons. If the tumor is associated with Barrett's esophagus (intestinal metaplasia in the esophagus, seen on endoscopy), surgery consists of either an **Ivor Lewis** (combined abdominal and transthoracic approach) or **transhiatal esophagectomy** (see p. 385) with gastroesophageal anastomosis in the neck. Bulky GE junction tumors that encompass the upper stomach will limit the extent of esophageal resection if stomach pull-up is used. Postop pain can be severe, and most patients will benefit from continuous epidural analgesia.

Usual preop diagnosis: Total gastrectomy: gastric malignancy; Zollinger-Ellison syndrome (hypergastrinemia, gastric hypersecretion, PUD); hemorrhage 2° diffuse gastritis; Hemigastrectomy: gastric cancer; gastric ulcers

SUMMARY OF PROCEDURES

	Total Gastrectomy	Hemigastrectomy
Position	Supine	⇐
Incision	Upper midline or bilateral subcostal	Upper midline or right subcostal
Special instrumentation	Upper-hand or other self-retaining costal retractor	Upper-hand or other costal retractor
Antibiotics	Cefotetan 1 g iv	⇐
Surgical time	2-4 h	1.5-2 h

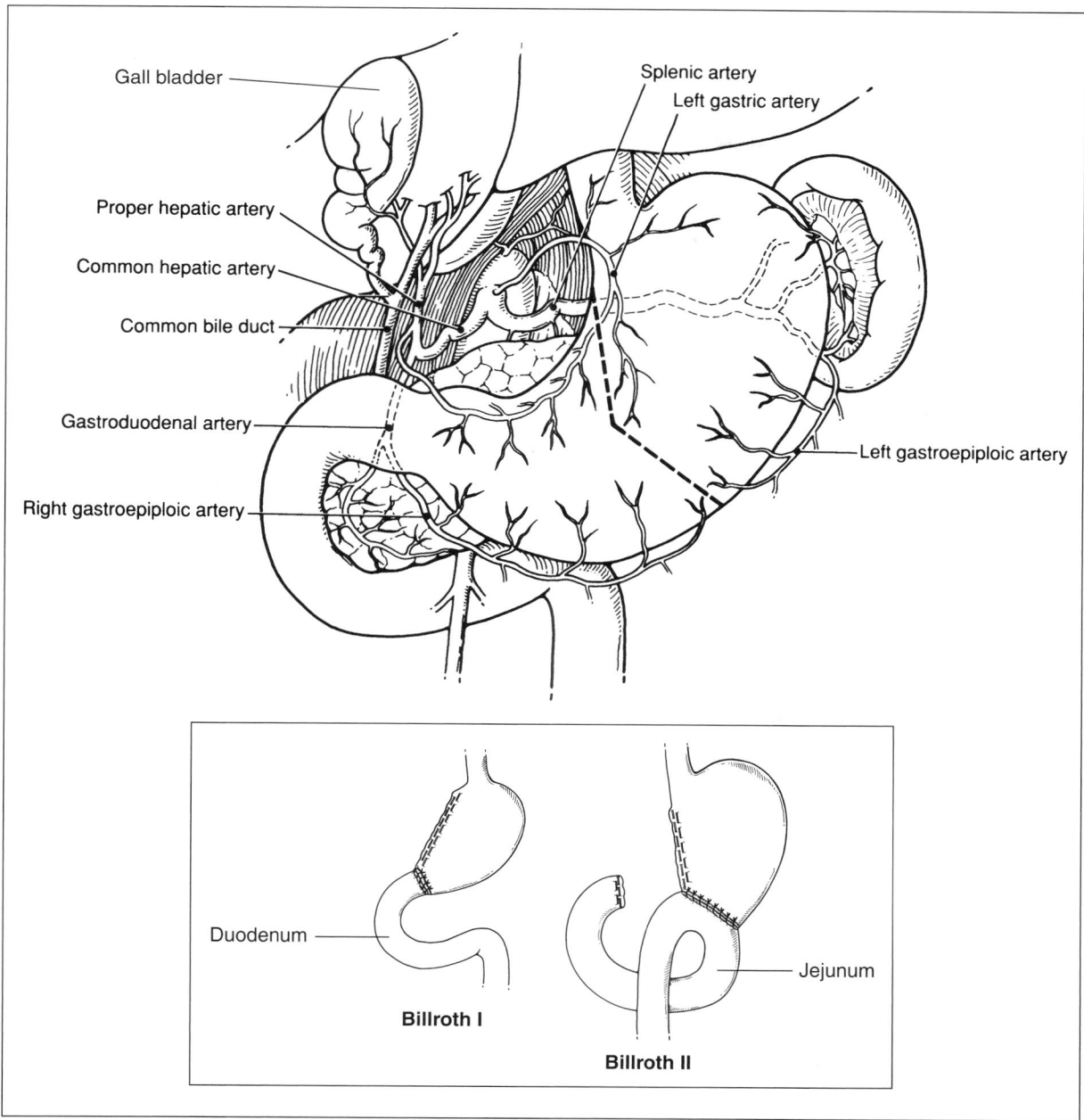

Figure 7.2-1. Anatomy of duodenostomy (Billroth I) and gastrojejunostomy (Billroth II). (Reproduced with permission from Scott-Conner CEH, Dawson DL: *Operative Anatomy*, 2nd edition. Lippincott Williams & Wilkins, 2003.)

	Total Gastrectomy	**Hemigastrectomy**
Closing considerations	Muscle relaxation required; NG suction	⇐
EBL	500+ ml, with potential for significantly more	100-500 ml
Postop care	PACU → ward	⇐
Mortality	0-22%	0-1.8% (may be >10% if emergency)
Morbidity	Pulmonary complications: 15%	Anastomotic leak
	Reoperation: 0-5%	Wound infection
	Esophagojejunal leak	Cardiopulmonary complications
	Sepsis	
	Late anastomotic stricture	
	Cardiac complications	
Pain score	7-8	7-8

PATIENT POPULATION CHARACTERISTICS

Age range	Mostly elderly
Male:Female	Male predominance
Incidence	Declining, due to declining incidence of gastric cancer and gastric ulcer and improved medical treatment for Zollinger-Ellison syndrome
Etiology	Gastric cancer and ulcer associated with: advanced age, alcohol and tobacco use, geographic location
Associated conditions	Weight loss (common); anemia (common); malnutrition (common); Zollinger-Ellison syndrome (rare)—avoid H$_2$-antagonists preop, if intraop gastric pH monitoring is planned by surgeon.

ANESTHETIC CONSIDERATIONS

See Anesthetic Considerations following Operations for Peptic Ulcer Disease, p. 397.

References

1. Adachi Y, Kitano S, Sugimachi K: Surgery for gastric cancer: 10-year experience worldwide. *Gastric Cancer* 2001; 4(4): 166-74.
2. Bozzetti F: Principles of surgical radicality in the treatment of gastric cancer. *Surg Oncol Clin N Am* 2001; 10(4):833-54, ix.
3. Dent DM, Madden MB, Price SK: Randomized comparison of R1 and R2 gastrectomy for gastric carcinoma. *Br J Surg* 1988; 75(2):110-12.
4. Herrington LL Jr: Vagotomy and antrectomy. In *Surgery of the Stomach, Duodenum and Small Intestine*, 2nd edition. Scott HW Jr, Sawyers JL, eds. Blackwell Scientific Publications, Boston: 1992, 524-39.
5. Mulholland MW: Duodenum ulcer. In *Surgery: Scientific Principles and Practice*, 3rd edition. Greenfield LJ, et al, eds. Lippincott Williams & Wilkins, Philadelphia: 2001, 750-66.
6. Mulholland MW: Gastric neoplasms. In *Surgery: Scientific Principles and Practice*, 3rd edition. Greenfield LJ, et al, eds. Lippincott Williams & Wilkins, Philadelphia: 2001, 774-86.

OVERSEW GASTRIC OR DUODENAL PERFORATION

SURGICAL CONSIDERATIONS

Description: Oversew operations are usually emergencies, and patients usually have peritonitis at presentation. Closure of the perforation alone, as opposed to performance of a definitive ulcer operation, is performed based on the surgeon's assessment of the patient's ability to tolerate a more extensive operation and the risk of recurrent ulceration.

In the younger patient with duodenal perforation (and where there is no delay in the diagnosis), a **highly selective vagotomy** may be added to closure of the perforation. Stomach or duodenum perforation is almost always a consequence of peptic ulcer disease, although on rare occasion, it may be caused by penetrating trauma. While perforation of the duodenum is almost never a consequence of malignant ulceration, perforation of the stomach due to malignant ulceration must always be considered. For this reason, the preferred treatment of a perforated gastric ulcer includes **resection**. If the general condition of the patient is poor or local inflammation is present, a biopsy of the ulcer, followed by closure, may be prudent. Biopsy of a perforated duodenal ulcer, on the other hand, is seldom necessary. In patients who are not systemically ill at the time of operation, and who do not have severe peritonitis, some surgeons prefer to do a definitive ulcer operation, such as a **vagotomy and pyloroplasty** or **highly selective vagotomy**, at the time of closure of the perforation. Under other circumstances, closure of the perforation alone may be appropriate.

For closure of perforations, an upper midline incision commonly is used, although a right subcostal incision may be appropriate. The liver is retracted superiorly and the area of perforation identified. An NG tube will have been placed preop and should remain on suction throughout the case to minimize ongoing leakage from the perforation. Perforation of the stomach may be handled either by resection (see Gastric Resections, p. 392) or by biopsy and simple suture closure. Perforation of the duodenum is usually repaired by simple suture of the site. Omentum often is used to buttress the area of closure of the stomach or duodenum. Closed suction drains are placed near the area of perforation and the abdomen is irrigated. Abdominal closure is routine, and the skin may be closed either primarily or packed open, depending on surgeon's preference.

Variant procedure or approaches: In certain patients, **nonoperative management** of perforated ulcer may be appropriate. In general, this has a relatively high likelihood of success in otherwise healthy patients with sealed duodenal perforation, but is much less reliable in frailer patients. While this may be a reasonable approach in some patients, there are no data to suggest that it is safer than traditional operative treatment.

Usual preop diagnosis: Perforated peptic ulcer

SUMMARY OF PROCEDURE

Position	Supine
Incision	Midline
Special instrumentation	Costal retractor
Unique considerations	Patients usually have peritonitis.
Antibiotics	Cefazolin or cefotetan 1 g iv
Surgical time	1 h
Closing considerations	Muscle relaxation required for closure; NG suction
EBL	Minimal
Postop care	PACU → ward
Mortality	5-15%, largely dependent on patient population
Morbidity	Pneumonia
	Intraabdominal abscess
	Sepsis
	Wound infection
	Reperforation
Pain score	7

PATIENT POPULATION CHARACTERISTICS

Age range	Adult, increasingly elderly, especially women
Male:Female	Previous heavy male predominance still exists for duodenal ulcer, but large increase in incidence in gastric perforation in women > 65.
Incidence	Fairly common. Stable incidence, but with change in distribution, especially more elderly women.
Etiology	Peptic ulcer disease (PUD); nonsteroidal medications; malignancy (if gastric)
Associated conditions	Malignancy (if perforation is gastric); nonsteroidal medications; steroid use, especially during pulse therapy; other risk factors for PUD (e.g., alcoholism, smoking, etc.)

ANESTHETIC CONSIDERATIONS

See Anesthetic Considerations following Operations for Peptic Ulcer Disease, p. 397.

References

1. Aoki T, Takayama S: Subtotal gastrectomy for gastric cancer. In *Mastery of Surgery*, 4th edition. Baker RJ, Fischer JE, eds. Lippincott Williams & Wilkins, Philadelphia: 2001, 982-96.
2. Brennan MF: Total gastrectomy for carcinoma. In *Mastery of Surgery*, 4th edition. Baker RJ, Fischer JE, eds. Lippincott Williams & Wilkins, Philadelphia: 2001, 997-1006.
3. Debas HT, Mulvihill SJ: Complications of peptic ulcer: In *Maingot's Abdominal Operations*, 10th edition, Vol. I. Zinner MJ, Schwartz SI, Ellis H, eds. Appleton & Lange, Stamford, CT: 1997, 981-998.
4. Johnston D, Martin I: Duodenal ulcer and peptic ulceration. In *Maingot's Abdominal Operations*, 10th edition, Vol. I. Zinner MJ, Schwartz SI, Ellis H, eds. Appleton & Lange, Stamford, CT: 1997, 941-970.
5. Kasakura Y, Ajani JA, Fujii M, Mochizuki F, Takayama T: Management of perforated gastric carcinoma: a report of 16 cases and review of world literature. *Am Surg* 2002; 68(5):434-40.
6. Mulholland MW: Duodenal ulcer. In *Surgery: Scientific Principles and Practice*, 3rd edition. Greenfield LJ, et al, eds. Lippincott Williams & Wilkins, Philadelphia: 2001, 750-66.
7. Sawyers JL: Acute perforation of peptic ulcer. In *Surgery of the Stomach, Duodenum and Small Intestine*. Scott HW Jr, Sawyers JL, eds. Blackwell Scientific Publications, Boston: 1992, 566-72.
8. Svanes C: Trends in perforated peptic ulcer: incidence, etiology, treatment, and prognosis. *World J Surg* 2000; 24(3):277-83.

OPERATIONS FOR PEPTIC ULCER DISEASE

SURGICAL CONSIDERATIONS

Description: Gastric ulcers are commonly associated with advanced age, and patients often have other medical problems, particularly cardiovascular and pulmonary. Two recent discoveries have transformed peptic ulcer disease (PUD) from a common surgical problem to a rare surgical emergency (e.g., perforation and bleeding typically in the chronically ill, hospitalized patient). These discoveries are: 1) inhibitors of gastric acid secretion, and 2) the role of gastric overgrowth by *Helicobacter pylori*. The first antisecretory drugs were H_2-receptor antagonists (e.g., cimetidine, ranitidine); however, proton pump inhibitors (PPIs) have proven to be more effective. The treatment of *H. pylori* consists of 14 d of a PPI, plus antibiotic therapy. The medical management of PUD has so revolutionized the treatment of this disease that few current graduating chief residents have seen or done the surgical procedures described below. All operations for PUD require exposure of the upper abdomen and may be performed using either an upper midline or a long, right subcostal incision. The

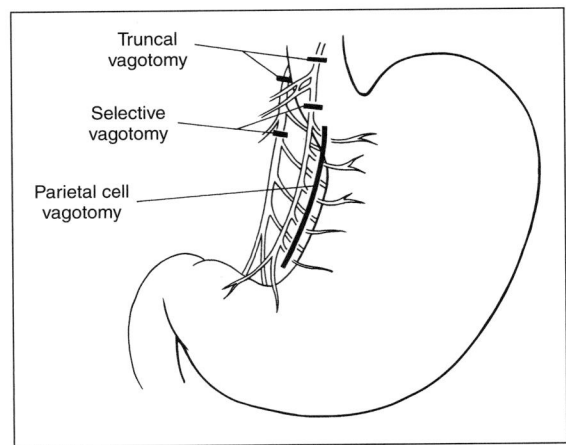

Figure 7.2-2. Types of vagotomy. Heavy lines indicate where vagal trunks are cut.

choice of surgical procedure depends on a number of considerations, including whether it is performed as an emergency or electively; the reason for performing the procedure (common factors include bleeding, perforation, intractability, or gastric outlet obstruction); duration of symptoms; condition of the patient; and experience of the surgeon.

Vagotomy and antrectomy (V&A): This is the most extensive of the operations performed for PUD, and generally is reserved for healthy patients with intractable symptoms. The esophageal hiatus is exposed either by taking down the lateral segment of the left lobe of the liver and reflecting it to the patient's right, or by retracting this segment of the liver superiorly to gain exposure. The phrenoesophageal ligament is divided and the anterior and posterior vagus nerves (there may be more than one of each) are identified by feel. Division of all vagal trunks at the esophageal hiatus is performed, and specimens of the nerves are sent for pathology. The blood supply to the antrum is then divided, usually by dividing the right gastric and gastroepiploic vessels first. The gastrohepatic ligament is divided and the stomach elevated off of its attachments to the transverse colon. The gastric antrum is resected, leaving the duodenum just beyond the pylorus and dividing the stomach just above the junction of the body with the antrum. Reconstruction may be as a **Billroth I** (stomach-to-duodenum) or **Billroth II** (stomach-to-jejunal loop) (Fig 7.2-1). The anastomosis may be stapled or hand-sewn. Drains are not commonly used if a Billroth I is performed, but may be used in Billroth II because of the concern for a leak from the duodenal stump.

Vagotomy and pyloroplasty (V&P): This is the most commonly performed operation for PUD in the U.S. and is especially common for emergency operations. It is generally accepted to be simpler and safer to perform than V&A, but not as effective at preventing recurrence of ulcer disease. The abdominal incision and exposure of the hiatus to perform a vagotomy is the same as for V&P. After division of both vagal trunks (Fig 7.2-2), a longitudinal incision is made through the pylorus. The incision is then sutured together transversely, completing the pyloroplasty.

Parietal cell vagotomy (PCV): This operation requires even more meticulous exposure of the esophageal hiatus than that needed for a truncal vagotomy. The hiatus is exposed as above, and the main vagal trunks supplying the stomach are identified, but not divided. The stomach is retracted downward, and it is often helpful to divide a portion of the gastrocolic omentum to facilitate grasping the stomach. Branches supplying the body of the stomach (Fig 7.2-2), are individually divided and ligated with fine ligatures. Because the nerve fibers run with the blood vessels to the stomach, this necessarily involves division of the blood supply to the proximal lesser curvature of the stomach. This dissection is carried to the region of the 'crow's foot' of the stomach, which is preserved. By denervating only the acid-producing portion of the stomach, while preserving innervation to the antrum, gastric acidity is diminished without significantly impairing gastric motility or emptying. A pyloroplasty is, therefore, not necessary. The operation is relatively tedious compared to the other procedures, and usually is performed electively or, rarely, urgently if there is a recent perforation and minimal soilage. It can be recommended only for duodenal ulcer disease, not gastric ulcer. Side effects of this operation are generally less than with other ulcer operations.

Variant procedure or approaches: **Laparoscopic approaches** to the treatment of gastroduodenal ulcer are also being used.

Usual preop diagnosis: V&P: complications of duodenal ulcer disease (bleeding, perforation, and gastric outlet obstruction). V&A: duodenal and prepyloric ulcer disease. PCV: isolated duodenal ulcer disease; recent perforation and minimal peritoneal soilage

SUMMARY OF PROCEDURES

	V&P	**V&A**	**PCV**
Position	Supine	⇐	⇐
Incision	Midline or long subcostal	⇐	Midline
Special instrumentation	Costal margin retractor	⇐	⇐
Antibiotics	Cefotetan 1 g iv	⇐	Cefazolin 1 g iv
Surgical time	1-2 h	1.5-3 h	1.5-2.5 h
Closing considerations	Muscle relaxation required for closure; NG suction	⇐	⇐
EBL	<250 ml; greater for emergency surgeries	250-500 ml	< 250 ml
Postop care	PACU → ward	⇐	⇐
Mortality	0-2% (most series include emergencies)	0-1.6% (most series do not include emergencies)	0-0.4%
Morbidity	Dumping and diarrhea: 6-20% Recurrence: 4.9-12.3%	17-27% 0-2%	— 5-15% Impaired gastric emptying: 0.3% Necrosis, lesser curve: < 0.3% PE: rare
Pain score	6	6	6

PATIENT POPULATION CHARACTERISTICS

Age range	Adults
Male:Female	Male > female
Incidence	Declining
Etiology	Acid hypersecretion; abnormal mucosal permeability and repair mechanisms; *H. pylori*
Associated conditions	Gastrinoma (rare); hyperparathyroidism (rare)

ANESTHETIC CONSIDERATIONS

(Procedures covered: gastric resections; oversew gastric/duodenal perforation operations for peptic ulcer disease; duodenotomy)

PREOPERATIVE

Patients presenting for gastric surgery generally comprise two groups: (1) those presenting for emergency surgery following GI bleeding or perforation, and (2) those presenting with gastric carcinoma or elective treatment of PUD. Patients in the first group are often hemodynamically unstable and require rapid preop assessment and appropriate fluid resuscitation. It is prudent to consider full-stomach precautions in both patient groups (see p. B-5).

Respiratory	Patients with GI bleeding are at ↑ risk for aspiration of blood and gastric contents. If this has occurred, patient may have significant respiratory insufficiency (in urgent need of tracheal intubation for 'protection' of airway). **Tests:** CXR; consider ABG.
Cardiovascular	Hypovolemia may be severe due to N/V, diarrhea, poor po intake, or GI blood loss. Sx include ↓skin turgor, ↑HR, ↓BP, ↓UO. Correct hypovolemia prior to inducing anesthesia. **Tests:** Orthostatic vital signs; ECG, if indicated from H&P.
Renal	GI fluid loss can lead to renal and electrolyte abnormalities. **Tests:** Consider electrolytes; BUN; Cr.

Hematologic	Misleading ↑Hct 2° GI fluid loss may be present; patients with GI bleeding will likely be anemic and may have a coagulopathy. Correct coagulopathy and anemia before induction, if possible. **Tests:** CBC with Plts
Laboratory	Other tests as indicated from H&P.
Premedication	Standard premedication (p. B-2) for elective procedures. Consider H₂-antagonist (ranitidine 50 mg iv slowly), metoclopramide (10 mg iv 1 h preop), and Na citrate (30 ml po 10 min preop). Prophylactic antibiotics should be considered if the patient has been rendered achlrohydric.

INTRAOPERATIVE

Anesthetic technique: GETA ± epidural for postop analgesia (if hemodynamically stable and no coagulopathy). If postop epidural analgesia is planned, insertion of catheter prior to anesthetic induction is helpful to establish correct placement in the epidural space (accomplished by injecting 5-7 ml of 1% lidocaine via the epidural catheter, eliciting a segmental block).

Induction	The patient with gastric disease or upper GI bleeding is often at risk for pulmonary aspiration, and the trachea should be intubated with the patient awake or after rapid-sequence induction with cricoid pressure (see p. B-5). If patient is clinically hypovolemic, restore intravascular volume (colloid, crystalloid, or blood) prior to induction, and titrate induction dose of sedative/hypnotic agents.
Maintenance	Standard maintenance (p. B-3) without N₂O (to avoid bowel distension). Balanced anesthesia with inhalational agents or propofol infusion (100-150 μg/kg/min) and narcotics. Maintain muscle relaxation based on nerve stimulator response. Discuss with surgeon the need for postop NG tube. If not needed, place OG tube to evacuate stomach contents intraop. **Combined epidural/GA:** A local anesthetic (2% lidocaine with 1:200,000 epinephrine) can be injected into a thoracic (3-5 ml) or lumbar (5-10 ml q 60 min) epidural catheter to provide both anesthesia and optimal surgical exposure (contracted bowel and profound muscle relaxation). A continuous infusion of local anesthetic (e.g., 2% lidocaine or 0.25% bupivacaine at 5-10 ml/h [lumbar]; 5 ml/h [thoracic]), may enhance hemodynamic stability, compared to an intermittent bolus. Be prepared to treat ↓BP with fluid and vasopressors. GA is administered to supplement regional anesthesia and for amnesia. Systemic sedatives should be minimized during epidural opiate administration as they increase the likelihood of postop respiratory depression. Treat ↓BP with fluid and vasopressors. If epidural opiates are used for postop analgesia, a loading dose (e.g., hydromorphone 1.0 mg [lumbar]; 0.5 mg [thoracic]) should be administered at least 1 h before conclusion of surgery.
Emergence	The decision to extubate at the end of surgery depends on the patient's underlying cardiopulmonary status and extent of the surgical procedure. Patient should be hemodynamically stable, warm, alert, cooperative, and fully reversed from any muscle relaxants prior to extubation.
Blood and fluid requirements	Anticipate large third-space losses. IV: 14-16 ga × 1 NS/LR @ 8-12 ml/kg/h Fluid warmer	T&C for 4 U PRBC. Plts, FFP, and cryoprecipitate should be administered according to lab tests (Plt count, PT, PTT, DIC screen, thromboelastography). Expect higher fluid requirements if epidural used (2° sympathectomy → vasodilation).
Monitoring	Standard monitors (p. B-1) UO ± Arterial line ± CVP catheter	+ others as indicated by patient's status. Prevent hypothermia: Consider heated humidifier, forced air warmer, warming blanket, warming room temperature, keeping patient covered until ready for prep, etc.
Positioning	✓ and pad pressure points. ✓ eyes.	
Complications	Acute hemorrhage Hypoxemia	2° abdominal packs → ↓FRC

POSTOPERATIVE

Complications	Atelectasis Hemorrhage Ileus Hypothermia
Pain management	Epidural analgesics (p. C-2) PCA (p. C-3)
Tests	CXR if CVP placed periop.

References

1. Gorey TF, Lennon F, Heffernan SJ: Highly selective vagotomy in duodenal ulceration and its complications. A 12-year review. *Ann Surg* 1984; 200(2):181-4.
2. Hoffmann J, Jensen HE, Christiansen J, Olesen A, Loud FB, Hauch O: Prospective controlled vagotomy trial for duodenal ulcer. Results after 11-15 years. *Ann Surg* 1989; 209(1):40-5.
3. Johnston D, Martin I: Duodenal ulcer and peptic ulceration: In *Maingot's Abdominal Operations*, 10th edition, Vol. I. Zinner MJ, Schwartz SI, Ellis H, eds. Appleton & Lange, Stamford, CT: 1997, 941-70.
4. Jordan PH Jr, Thornby J: Twenty years after parietal cell vagotomy or selective vagotomy antrectomy for treatment of duodenal ulcer: final report. *Ann Surg* 1994; 220(3): 283-93.
5. Kauffman GL Jr: Duodenal ulcer disease: treatment by surgery, antibiotics, or both. *Adv Surg* 2000; 34:121-35.
6. Nyhus LM: Selective vagotomy, antrectomy, and gastroduodenostomy for the treatment of duodenal ulcer. In *Mastery of Surgery*, 4th edition. Baker RJ, Fischer JE, eds. Lippincott Williams & Wilkins, Philadelphia: 2001, 921-32.
7. Passaro EP Jr, Stabile BE: Gastric ulcers: In *Maingot's Abdominal Operations*, Vol. I, 10th edition. Zinner MJ, Schwartz SI, Ellis H, eds. Appleton & Lange, Stamford, CT: 1997, 971-80.
8. Practice Guidelines for preoperative fasting and the use of pharmacologic agents to reduce the risk of pulmonary aspiration: Application to healthy patients undergoing elective procedures . A report by the American Society of Anesthesiologists Task Force on Preoperative Fasting. *Anesthesiology* 1999; 90:896.
9. Sawyers JL, Richards WO: Selective vagotomy and pyloroplasty. In *Mastery of Surgery*, 4th edition. Baker RJ, Fischer JE, eds. Lippincott Williams & Wilkins, Philadelphia: 2001, 933-41.
10. Soybel DI, Zinner MJ: Complications following gastric operations: In *Maingot's Abdominal Operations*, Vol. I, 10th edition. Zinner MJ, Schwartz SI, Ellis H, eds. Appleton & Lange, Stamford, CT: 1997, 1029-56.
11. Zittel TT, Jehle EC, Becker HD: Surgical management of peptic ulcer disease today—indication, technique and outcome. *Langenbecks Arch Surg* 2000; 385(2)84-96.

OPEN OPERATIONS FOR MORBID OBESITY

SURGICAL CONSIDERATIONS

Description: Open procedures for morbid obesity have been largely replaced by the laparoscopic approach (see p. 477). In selected patients (e.g., those with previous upper abdominal surgery or BMI > 60 [see p. 401]), however, open procedures may be more appropriate. Open techniques devised to promote weight loss are of two fundamental types: (1) **gastric partitioning procedures**, which work by decreasing the size of the gastric pouch, thereby limiting the amount of food that can be consumed at one time; and (2) **malabsorptive procedures**, which work by bypassing most of the small bowel and creating a state of chronic malabsorption. Of these two general types of procedures, the partitioning procedures are generally less effective at promoting weight loss than are the malabsorptive procedures, but are much more popular because they are associated with far fewer serious side effects.

The partitioning procedure most commonly used today is the **vertical banded gastroplasty (VBG)**. The abdomen is entered through an upper midline incision, and the esophagogastric junction is exposed either by retracting the liver superiorly or by taking down the ligamentous attachments of the lateral segment of the left lobe of the liver and retracting this down and to the patient's right. The vessels to the lesser curvature are taken down for a short distance near the esophagogastric junction, and the posterior attachments of the stomach are taken down. A large bougie is passed by the anesthesiologist into the stomach and a circular stapler is used to create a hole in the stomach adjacent to the bougie near the esophagogastric junction. Through this, a special stapler with thick, strong staples is passed and is fired up along the esophagus, creating a pouch of approximately 30 ml in volume (Fig 7.2-3). This leaves an outlet to the remainder of the stomach of only 1-2 cm,

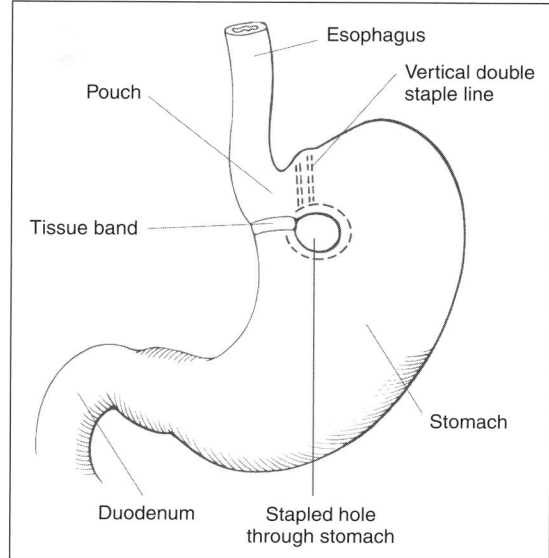

Figure 7.2-3. Vertical banded gastroplasty.

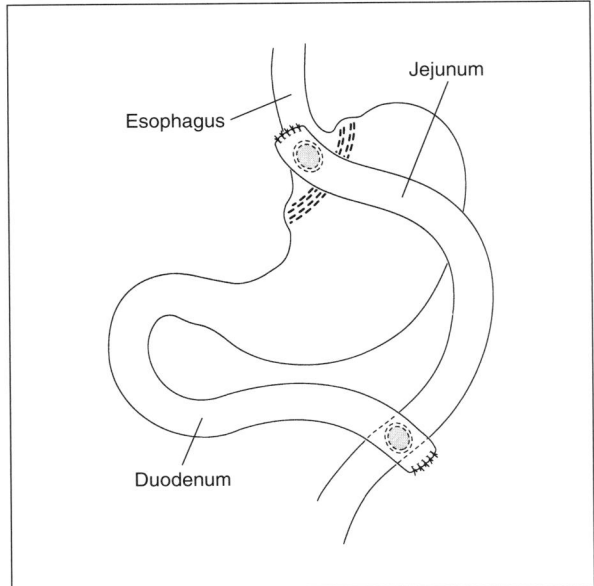

Figure 7.2-4. Proximal Roux-en-Y gastric bypass. (Reproduced with permission from Greenfield LJ, et al, eds: *Surgery: Scientific Principles and Practice*, 3rd edition. Lippincott Williams & Wilkins, Philadelphia, 2001.)

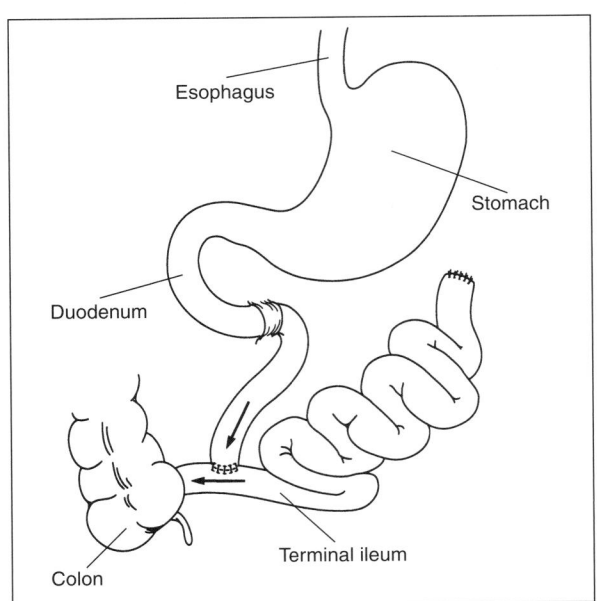

Figure 7.2-5. Schematic representation of jejunoileal bypass. (Reproduced with permission from Greenfield LJ, et al, eds: *Surgery: Scientific Principles and Practice*, 3rd edition. Lippincott Williams & Wilkins, Philadelphia, 2001.)

which is reinforced with a band of mesh. An NG tube is placed through the gastroplasty into the distal stomach and the abdomen is closed without drains.

Perhaps more commonly performed today than the gastroplasty is the **Roux-en-Y gastric bypass** (Fig 7.2-4). Exposure is similar to that for a VBG. The upper stomach is mobilized and two rows of staples are used to partition the stomach into a small proximal and large distal pouch. A Roux segment of jejunum is then anastomosed to the small proximal pouch to provide drainage of it. An NG tube is placed and the abdomen is closed without drains.

Variant procedure or approaches: An alternative open procedure is the **jejunoileal (JI) bypass** (Fig. 7.2-5), in which the proximal jejunum is anastomosed to the terminal ileum. This procedure has been largely abandoned because of the many associated complications, including cirrhosis, osteoporosis, kidney stones, and intractable diarrhea.

Usual preop diagnosis: Morbid obesity (> 100 lbs above ideal body weight, 100% over ideal body weight, or BMI > 36), generally in combination with some medical condition felt to be worsened by the obesity (e.g., osteoarthritis, diabetes, respiratory insufficiency, CHF).

SUMMARY OF PROCEDURE

Position	Supine (Fig 7.2-6)
Incision	Midline
Special instrumentation	Large OR tables; heavy-duty retractors; special stapling devices
Unique considerations	Prophylactic cholecystectomy often advocated. Pneumatic compression boots may not be large enough; heparin (5,000 U sc 2 h before surgery, then q 12 h) used commonly. ↑↑aspiration risk + potentially difficult airway.
Antibiotics	± Cefazolin 1 g iv
Surgical time	2-3 h
Closing considerations	Anticipate 1+ h closure time; NG suction
EBL	< 500 ml
Postop care	Postop ventilation may be necessary; DVT precautions.
Mortality	0.5-1.6%
Morbidity	Wound infection: 4-8%
	Anastomotic leak: 3%
	Dehiscence: 1.6%
	PE: 1-1.6%
Pain score	7

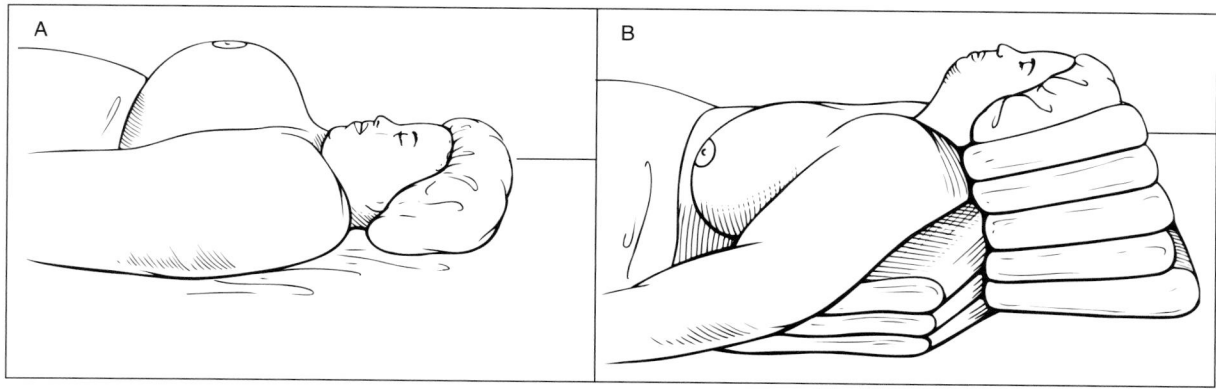

Figure 7.2-6. (A) In standard supine position, the atlantooccipital gap of morbidly obese patient is obliterated by fat, and access for laryngoscope is hindered by large breasts. (B) By elevating the shoulders and occiput so that head is in the 'sniffing' position, airway access is greatly facilitated.

PATIENT POPULATION CHARACTERISTICS

Age range	Adult
Male:Female	< 1:1
Incidence	4.9% of males and 7.2% of females in U.S. population considered morbidly obese
Etiology	Multifactorial
Associated conditions	Sleep apnea ± CO_2 retention; CAD/CHF/cardiomyopathy; pulmonary HTN/systemic HTN; diabetes; unusually high risk of DVT and PE; GERD

ANESTHETIC CONSIDERATIONS

PREOPERATIVE

Morbid obesity is variably defined (i.e., >100 lbs over ideal body weight, 2 times ideal body weight, or BMI > 36 [BMI = weight (kg) ÷ height^2 (m)]), and is associated with increased periop mortality/morbidity. Obstructive sleep apnea (OSA) is common in the morbidly obese patient.

Respiratory	Increased O_2 consumption and CO_2 production (e.g., ↑basal metabolic rate). ↓chest-wall compliance (↓20-60%) with normal lung compliance. ↓ERV and FRC; so tidal breathing may fall within the range of closing capacity → V/Q abnormalities. Supine position further ↓ FRC → worsening hypoxemia. ↑MV is required to remain normocarbic. There is a normal response to CO_2 unless patient develops the obesity hypoventilation (pickwickian) syndrome (↑$PaCO_2$, ↓PaO_2, loss of hypercarbic drive, sleep apnea, hypersomnolence, polycythemia, pulmonary HTN, CHF). Tracheal intubation may be difficult. **Tests:** CXR; PFTs (FVC, FEV_1, $MMEF_{25-75}$ ± bronchodilators; room-air ABG)
Cardiovascular	Blood volume and CO ↑ with increasing weight. HTN is very common (use correct size BP cuff). LV dysfunction may be present; patient unable to increase CO or tolerate ↑blood volume. Pulmonary HTN may be present in OSA. Obesity is a risk factor for CAD and sudden death. Anticipate problems with vascular access. Although phentermine/fenfluramine were removed from the market in 1997, patients with a Hx of treatment with these drugs should be evaluated for valvular disease. **Tests:** ECG; others as indicated from H&P. (Patient with SOB may require MUGA scan and ECHO for LV function, as SOB can have a cardiac or pulmonary etiology.)
Endocrine	Glucose intolerance and diabetes mellitus (DM) common. **Tests:** Fasting glucose
Hepatic	Liver function is often abnormal and drug metabolism may be significantly affected. Combined with altered pharmacokinetics, many drugs (e.g., midazolam and vecuronium) may have unpredictably prolonged action.
Gastrointestinal	↑intraabdominal pressure, gastric volume, and acidity, with ↑incidence of hiatal hernia, make this patient population at risk for pulmonary aspiration of gastric contents.

Airway	Obese patients may have greater airway problems. Careful airway examination (e.g., mouth opening, Mallampati classification, thyromental distance, neck ROM) is paramount. Awake fiber optic intubation should be considered if difficult airway access is anticipated. Establish availability of OR table large enough to accommodate morbidly obese patient (typical OR table capacity=500 lbs).
Hematologic	Polycythemia may occur 2° chronic hypoxemia. **Tests:** CBC
Laboratory	Other tests as indicated from H&P.
Premedication	Sedatives are best avoided for patients with OSA. A small dose of iv midazolam (0.5-1.0 mg) may be appropriate for the especially anxious patient. In the bariatric patient, intramuscular medications can be erroneously injected into adipose tissues. Consider anticholinergics if performing awake fiber optic intubation (glycopyrrolate 0.2 mg iv 30 min preop). Take full-stomach precautions (p. B-5): metoclopramide (10 mg iv 60 min preop); H_2-antagonist (ranitidine 50 mg iv); nonparticulate antacid (3 M Na citrate) 30 ml, 10 min prior to induction.

INTRAOPERATIVE

Anesthetic technique: GETA ± epidural for postop analgesia in open surgeries. If using a combined anesthetic approach, placement of an epidural catheter should be accomplished before induction, with the patient in the sitting position. A bilateral sensory block (using 5-7 ml 2% lidocaine) will help confirm correct placement of the catheter within the epidural space. Verification of placement is particularly important in this population since regional anesthesia in the obese patient is technically more difficult.

Induction	Patients are at risk for aspiration of gastric contents and should be intubated either awake (p. B-6) or after rapid-sequence induction with cricoid pressure. Mask ventilation and ET intubation may be difficult. Following successful intubation and induction of anesthesia, an OG/NG tube should be placed and the stomach contents suctioned. Lipophilic drugs (e.g., STP) will have a greater volume of distribution, necessitating increased dosage.
Maintenance	Standard maintenance (p. B-3). N_2O is best avoided to minimize bowel distention. Obese patients metabolize volatile anesthetics to a greater extent than their nonobese counterparts. **Combined epidural/GA:** A local anesthetic (2% lidocaine with 1:200,000 epinephrine) can be injected into a thoracic (3-5 ml) or lumbar (5-10 ml q 60 min) epidural catheter to provide both anesthesia and improved surgical exposure (contracted bowel and profound muscle relaxation). A continuous infusion of local anesthetic (e.g., 2% lidocaine or 0.25% bupivacaine at 5-10 ml/h [lumbar], 5 ml/h [thoracic]) may enhance hemodynamic stability. The dose of local anesthetic given via epidural catheter should be decreased to 75% of normal dose. Be prepared to treat ↓BP with fluid and vasopressors (ephedrine 5-10 mg iv, phenylephrine 50-100 µg iv). GA is administered to supplement regional anesthesia and for amnesia. Sedative drugs (opiates, benzodiazepines, etc.) should be minimized in the presence of epidural opiates, as they increase the likelihood of postop respiratory depression. If epidural opiates are used for postop analgesia, a loading dose (e.g., hydromorphone 0.5-1.0 mg) should be administered 1-2 h before end of surgery.
Emergence	The decision to extubate at the end of open surgery depends on patient's underlying cardiopulmonary status and the extent of the surgical procedure. Patients should be hemodynamically stable, warm, alert, cooperative, and fully reversed from any muscle relaxants before extubation. Elective ICU admission for postop care may be appropriate. Following laparoscopic surgery, in contrast, patients typically are extubated and admitted to PACU.
Blood and fluid requirements	Anticipate large fluid loss. IV: 14-16 ga × 1-2 NS/LR @ 10-15 ml/kg/h Warm all fluids. Humidify gases.	Third-space losses greatly exceed blood loss. Guide fluid management by UO, filling pressure. T&S for 2 U PRBCs.
Monitoring	Standard monitors (p. B-1) UO ± Arterial line	Invasive monitoring as clinically indicated. Arterial line if noninvasive BP unreliable 2° extremity size.
Positioning	Supine position = ↓FRC ✓ and pad pressure points. ✓ eyes. ★ **NB:** Avoid Trendelenburg.	Supine positioning → ↓lung volumes, which may ↑ V/Q, resulting in hypoxemia. This is exacerbated by use of the Trendelenburg position, which usually is not well tolerated by morbidly obese patients.

Complications	Hypoxemia 2° ↓FRC	100% O_2 → absorption atelectasis

POSTOPERATIVE

Complications	Hypoxemia Hypercarbia DVT PE Atelectasis	Recover patient in sitting position to improve ventilatory mechanics. Give supplemental O_2. Verify DVT prophylaxis preop.
Pain management	Epidural analgesia: hydromorphone (0.8-1.5 mg load; 0.2-0.3 mg/h infusion) PCA (p. C-3)	If epidural is used for postop analgesia, the Acute Pain Service should follow.
Tests	ABG CXR	Others as clinically indicated. CXR for line placement

References

1. Brodsky JB, Lemmens HJM, Brock-Utne JG, et al: Morbid obesity and tracheal intubation. *Anesth Analg* 2002; 94:732-6.
2. Brolin RE: Bariatric surgery and long-term control of morbid obesity. *JAMA* 2002; 288(22):2793-6.
3. Buchwald H, Buchwald JN: Evolution of operative procedures for the management of morbid obesity 1950-2000. *Obes Surg* 2002; 12(5):705-17.
4. Choban PS, Jackson B, Poplawski S, Bistolarides P: Bariatric surgery for morbid obesity: Why, who, when, how, where, and then what? *Cleve Clin J Med* 2002; 69(11):897-903.
5. Clegg AJ, Colquitt J, Sidhu MK, Royle P, Loveman E, Walker A: The clinical effectiveness and cost-effectiveness of surgery for people with morbid obesity: a systematic review and economic evaluation. *Health Technol Assess* 2002; 6(12):1-153.
6. Dubois F: New surgical strategy for gastroduodenal ulcer: Laparoscopic approach. *World J Surg* 2000; 24(3):270-6.
7. Flickinger DG, Pories WJ: Gastric bypass and other gastric restrictive procedures for morbid obesity. In *Surgery of the Stomach, Duodenum, and Small Intestine*, 2nd edition. Scott HW, Sawyers JL, eds. Blackwell Scientific Publications, Boston: 1992, 638-52.
8. Klein S: Medical management of obesity. *Surg Clin North Am* 2001; 81(5):1025-38, v.
9. Linner JH: Comparative effectiveness of gastric bypass and gastroplasty: a clinical study. *Arch Surg* 1982; 117(5):695-700.
10. Livingston EH: Obesity and its surgical management. *Am J Surg* 2002; 184(2):103-13.
11. Ogunnaike BO, Jones SB, Jones DB, Provost D, Whitten CW: Anesthetic considerations for bariatric surgery. *Anesth Analg* 2002; 95(6):1793-805.
12. Perilla V, Sollazzi L, Bozza P, et al: The effects of the reverse Trendelenberg position on respiratory mechanics and blood gases in morbidly obese patients during bariatric surgery. *Anesth Analg* 2000; 91:1520-5.
13. Sachdev M, Miller WC, Ryan T, Jollis JG: Effect of fenfluramine-derivative diet pills on cardiac valves: a meta-analysis of observational studies. *Am Heart J* 2002; 144(6):1065-73.
14. Shenkman Z, Shir Y, Brodsky JB: Perioperative management of the obese patient. *Brit J Anaesth* 1993; 70:340-59.
15. Sugarman HJ, DeMaria EJ: Gastric surgery for morbid obesity. In *Mastery of Surgery*, 4th edition. Baker RJ, Fischer JE, eds. Lippincott Williams & Wilkins, Philadelphia: 2001, 1026-36.

GASTROSTOMY PLACEMENT

SURGICAL CONSIDERATIONS

Description: A **gastrostomy** is a tube placed through the abdominal wall directly into the stomach. Such tubes can be used for gastric decompression or for feeding, and they may be permanent or temporary. Patients undergoing gastrostomy placement often have neurologic impairment that compromises their ability to handle oral secretions and increases their risk of aspiration. **Percutaneous endoscopic gastrostomy (PEG)**, in contrast to the other techniques, most commonly is performed using iv sedation and local anesthesia.

Variant procedure or approaches: The traditional **Stamm gastrostomy** usually is placed at the time of a laparotomy performed for another purpose; or it may be performed through a separate, small laparotomy incision in patients in whom endoscopic placement is not possible for technical reasons. The incision may be upper midline or transverse directly over the stomach. The anterior wall of the stomach is identified, and two pursestring sutures are placed in the stomach around the site where the tube will enter. The gastrostomy tube is introduced through the abdominal wall directly over the intended site of entry into the stomach. A small hole is made in the stomach in the center of the pursestring sutures, the tube is introduced into the stomach, and the pursestrings are tied securely around the tube. The wound is then closed. GA usually is preferred, but the operation may be performed under local anesthesia in thin patients.

The **Janeway gastrostomy**, a technical modification, also requires a laparotomy. The greater curvature of the stomach is identified and a stapler placed across a portion of this, creating a tube that arises from the main body of the stomach. The staple line may be oversewn, and then the end of the tube is brought through the abdominal wall and matured to the skin as a small stoma. This allows for permanent access to the stomach with removal of the tube between feedings, and is useful in patients with long-term dependence on gastrostomy access. The Janeway gastrostomy is rarely used, though young patients with neurologic impairment, who are expected to need lifetime gastrostomy feeding, are good candidates.

In **PEG**, the stomach is intubated endoscopically and the gastric and abdominal walls punctured under endoscopic guidance. The gastrostomy tube is introduced through the mouth and passed through the stomach and abdominal wall from inside out. In most centers, this has become the most common technique of gastrostomy placement due to its simplicity and because, in the majority of patients, it can be performed under local anesthesia with MAC. Previous gastric operations may make endoscopic placement difficult or dangerous, as may some obstructing lesions of the esophagus or pharynx. To avoid damage to the back wall of the stomach, the anesthesiologist may be asked to inject air forcefully into the stomach.

Usual preop diagnosis: Temporary gastrostomies often are used after major abdominal surgery as an alternative to NG suction. Percutaneous gastrostomies often are placed in patients with advanced malignancy and intestinal obstruction or inadequate oral intake, and in patients with neurologic impairment and difficulty in eating.

SUMMARY OF PROCEDURES

	Stamm	Janeway	PEG
Position	Supine	⇐	⇐
Incision	Midline or transverse	⇐	Puncture
Special instrumentation	None	⇐	Endoscope, percutaneous gastrostomy kit
Antibiotics	± Cefazolin 1 g iv	⇐	⇐
Surgical time	45 min	1 h	0.5-1 h
Closing considerations	Muscle relaxation for closure	⇐	None
EBL	Minimal	⇐	⇐
Mortality	Minimal	⇐	⇐
Morbidity	Wound infection: 2.1-9%	⇐	–
	Hemorrhage: 0.9-1.1%	⇐	⇐
	Aspiration pneumonia: 2.2%	⇐	1.6%
	Failure to function: 2.2%	⇐	–
Pain score	4-5	5	1-2

PATIENT POPULATION CHARACTERISTICS

Age range	All ages, though with peaks in infancy and the elderly
Male:Female	~1:1
Incidence	Common
Etiology	See Preop Diagnosis, above.
Associated conditions	Gastrostomy placed at time of laparotomy, when NG drainage is anticipated for prolonged period. For feeding in the neurologically impaired or in those with complex upper digestive difficulties. Advanced malignancy (for either feeding or palliative decompression).

ANESTHETIC CONSIDERATIONS

See Anesthetic Considerations for Ostomy Procedures in Intestinal Surgery, p. 411.

References

1. Grant JP: Comparison of percutaneous endoscopic gastrostomy with Stamm gastrostomy. *Ann Surg* 1988; 207(5):598-603.
2. Jesseph JM: Open gastrostomy. In *Mastery of Surgery*, 4th edition. Baker RJ, Fischer JE, eds. Lippincott Williams & Wilkins, Philadelphia: 2001, 888-93.
3. Ozmen MN, Akhan O: Percutaneous radiologic gastrostomy. *Eur J Radiol* 2002; 43(3):186-95.
4. Pennington C: To PEG or not to PEG. *Clin Med* 2002; 2(3):250-5.
5. Ponsky JL: Percutaneous endoscopic gastrostomy. In *Mastery of Surgery*, 4th edition. Baker RJ, Fischer JE, eds. Lippincott Williams & Wilkins, Philadelphia: 2001, 894-9.

Surgeon

Harry A. Oberhelman, MD, FACS

7.3 INTESTINAL SURGERY

Anesthesiologist

Kevin A. Malott, MD

DUODENOTOMY

SURGICAL CONSIDERATIONS

Description: A duodenotomy is performed to ligate a bleeding vessel at the base of a duodenal ulcer or to perform some procedure on the ampulla of Vater or the duct of Santorini. It is important, therefore, to be familiar with the anatomy of the proximal duodenum in relation to the major and minor pancreatic duct orifices (Fig 7.3-1). The duodenotomy may be made longitudinally or transversely, depending on the surgeon's preference. A transverse opening allows one to close the duodenotomy without tension; however, it must be made very accurately for the purpose of exposure. Bleeding vessels at the base of an ulcer must be secured with suture ligatures.

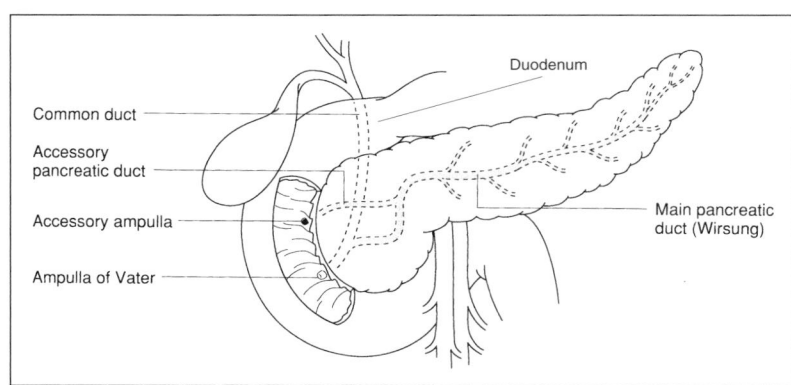

Figure 7.3-1. Anatomy of pancreatic ductal system. In 30% of patients, the accessory duct ends blindly. (Reproduced with permission from Greenfield LJ, et al: *Surgery: Scientific Principles and Practice*, 3rd edition. Lippincott Williams & Wilkins, 2001.)

Care must be taken to avoid perforating the duodenum when performing a sphincterotomy.

Usual preop diagnosis: Duodenal ulcer; impacted common duct stone; chronic pancreatitis 2° alcoholism, gallstones, pancreatic divisum, or other obstruction of the main pancreatic duct

SUMMARY OF PROCEDURE

Position	Supine
Incision	Midline abdominal or subcostal
Unique considerations	Magnifying glasses, if operation involves lesser pancreatic sphincter
Antibiotics	Cefazolin 1 g iv preop
Surgical time	1-2 h
Closing considerations	Secure closure of duodenum without tension
EBL	Minimal
Postop care	NG decompression
Mortality	< 0.5%
Morbidity	Duodenal leak: < 5%
	Postop pancreatitis: < 3%
Pain score	6-8

PATIENT POPULATION CHARACTERISTICS

Age range	Any age
Male:Female	1:1
Incidence	Not uncommon
Etiology	Duodenal ulcer; impacted common duct stone; villous tumors of ampulla; chronic pancreatitis, pancreatic divisum
Associated conditions	Bleeding duodenal ulcer (50-60%); chronic pancreatitis (20-25%); impacted common duct stones (10-15%)

ANESTHETIC CONSIDERATIONS

See Anesthetic Considerations following Operations for Peptic Ulcer Disease, Stomach Surgery, p. 397.

Reference

1. Nora PF: *Operative Surgery: Principles and Techniques*, 3rd edition. WB Saunders, Philadelphia: 1990.

OPEN APPENDECTOMY

SURGICAL CONSIDERATIONS

Description: Open appendectomy is performed for appendicitis or suspected appendicitis; however, it has been largely replaced by the laparoscopic approach (see p. 472). The negative laparotomy rate has been reduced by the judicious use of ultrasonography, laparoscopy, barium enema, and CT examination. Through a RLQ (**McBurney**) or right paramedian incision, the cecum is exposed and pulled into the wound (Fig 7.3-2). The appendix is then delivered through the wound; and the mesoappendix is clamped, cut, and ligated. The appendix is removed by crushing, ligating, and then transecting the base. The appendiceal stump may be invaginated into the wall of the cecum or left alone. In some instances it may be easier to divide the base of the appendix before delivering the appendix into the wound. The wound should be left open and soft drains used in cases of perforated appendix. In children, the appendix may be inverted and allowed to slough off internally.

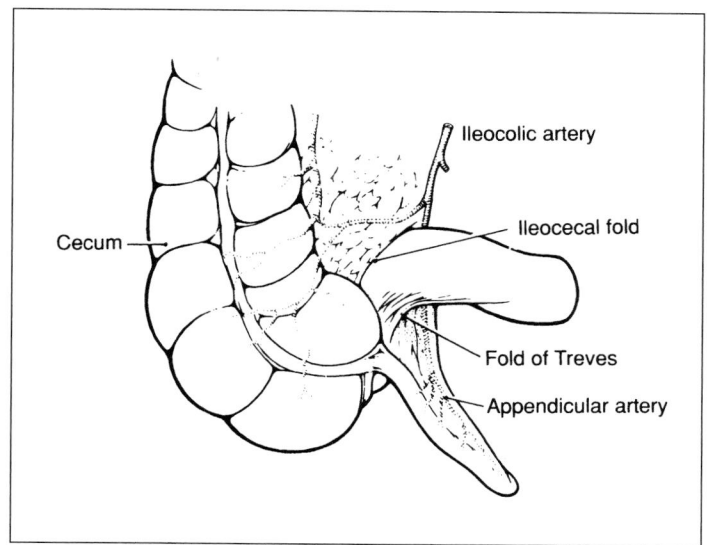

Figure 7.3-2. Relevant anatomy for appendectomy. (Reproduced with permission from Scott-Conner CEH, Dawson DL: *Operative Anatomy*, 2nd edition. Lippincott Williams & Wilkins, 2003.)

Variant procedure or approach: Laparoscopic appendectomy (see p. 472).

Usual preop diagnosis: Appendicitis

SUMMARY OF PROCEDURE

Position	Supine
Incision	RLQ (McBurney's) or right paramedian
Unique considerations	Variation in stump closure; NG tube if prolonged ileus expected.
Antibiotics	Cefazolin 1 g preop
Surgical time	1 h
Closing considerations	Skin wound should not be closed when appendix is perforated. Drain in presence of well defined abscess cavity.
EBL	< 75 ml
Postop care	Wound care when left open
Mortality	Perforated: 2%
	Nonperforated: < 0.1%
Morbidity	Pelvic, subphrenic, or intraabdominal abscess (perforation): 20%
	Wound abscess: < 5%
	Fecal fistula: < 1%
	Wound hematoma: < 0.5%
	Ileus: Variable
Pain score	5-7

PATIENT POPULATION CHARACTERISTICS

Age range	Any age
Male:Female	1:1
Incidence	1/15 persons
Etiology	Obstruction (80-90%); fecaliths (75%); carcinoid tumors (< 5%)
Associated conditions	None

ANESTHETIC CONSIDERATIONS

See Anesthetic Consideration following Excision of Meckel's diverticulum, below.

References

See References following Excision of Meckel's diverticulum, p. 410.

EXCISION OF MECKEL'S DIVERTICULUM

SURGICAL CONSIDERATIONS

Description: Meckel's diverticulum is a true congenital diverticulum, usually arising within two feet of the ileocecal valve. It was first described by Meckel in 1809. Excision of a Meckel's diverticulum is indicated for bleeding, obstruction, perforation, inflammation, intussusception, and when there is a palpable mass near the base of the diverticulum. Ectopic mucosa is present in roughly 50% of symptomatic patients, with gastric mucosa the most frequent. After entering the peritoneal cavity, the distal ileum, along with the diverticulum, is delivered into the wound. The diverticulum is excised and the wound is closed in two layers. Following excision of the diverticulum, care must be taken not to narrow the bowel lumen during closure. If a diagnosis can be made preop, a laparoscopic approach may be used (see Laparoscopic Bowel Resection p. 469).

Usual preop diagnosis: Meckel's diverticulum

SUMMARY OF PROCEDURE

Position	Supine
Incision	Midline abdominal or RLQ (McBurney's)
Antibiotics	Cefazolin 1-2 g iv preop
Surgical time	1-1.5 h
EBL	< 100 ml
Mortality	< 0.5%
Morbidity	Wound infection: 5%
	Pulmonary complication: < 5%
	Anastomotic leak: < 1%
Pain score	6-8

PATIENT POPULATION CHARACTERISTICS

Age range	< 40 yr
Male:Female	3:1
Incidence	0.3%-2.5%
Etiology	Congenital
Associated conditions	Exomphalos; esophageal atresia; anorectal atresia; gross malformations of CNS or CV system

ANESTHETIC CONSIDERATIONS

(Procedures covered: open appendectomy; excision of Meckel's diverticulum)

PREOPERATIVE

This patient population is generally fit and healthy, apart from their acutely presenting illness. Full-stomach precautions are appropriate in these patients. Surgery for appendicitis is one of the most common nonobstetric procedures performed on the pregnant patient (~1/1500 pregnancies). These patients often are more ill at the time of diagnosis, as early symptoms may be attributed to pregnancy, and the gravid uterus may hinder an accurate abdominal exam. Anesthesia management for the gravid appendicitis patient mirrors that of the nongravid patient (full-stomach precautions), with consideration of the maternal physiologic changes of pregnancy and the effects of anesthesia on the fetus and uteroplacental perfusion (See Anesthetic Considerations for Cervical Cerclage, Obstetric Surgery, p. 675.)

Respiratory	Respiratory impairment can occur 2° acute abdominal pain and splinting. Tachypnea and hyperpnea can be heralding Sx of appendiceal perforation and sepsis. Patients with acute abdomen should be treated as if they have full stomachs. Consider administration of metoclopramide (10 mg iv), H_2-antagonist (ranitidine 50 mg iv), and Na citrate 0.3 M 30 ml po. **Tests:** As indicated from H&P.
Cardiovascular	May be dehydrated from fever, emesis, and decreased oral intake, ↑HR 2° pain (↑BP), or ↓BP (sepsis, hypovolemia). Assess volume status with vital signs in the supine, standing, and sitting positions (if possible) and hydrate adequately prior to proceeding with anesthetic induction. **Tests:** ECG, if indicated from H&P.
Gastrointestinal	Patient typically has abdominal pain, with N/V. Muscular resistance to palpation of abdominal wall frequently parallels the severity of the inflammatory process. With spreading peritoneal irritation (as with perforation), patient will develop abdominal distension and paralytic ileus. Electrolyte abnormalities are common 2° N/V. **Tests:** Electrolytes
Hematologic	Moderate leukocytosis (10,000-18,000) with moderate left shift. Hemoconcentration is probable, if patient is dehydrated. **Tests:** CBC
Laboratory	Other tests as indicated from H&P.
Premedication	Full-stomach precautions (see p. B-5). Opiate premedication (morphine 0.03-0.15 mg/kg iv) is indicated after patient is scheduled for surgery. If surgical intervention is still in question, administration of opiates may mask Sx of appendicitis.

INTRAOPERATIVE

Anesthetic technique: GETA, with rapid-sequence iv induction, followed by ET intubation (see full-stomach precautions, p. B-5). If systemic sepsis absent, hydration adequate, patient cooperative, and high abdominal exploration unlikely, then regional anesthesia can be considered.

Induction	Rapid-sequence induction of anesthesia (see p. B-5). Restore intravascular volume prior to anesthetic induction if patient is clinically hypovolemic.
Maintenance	Standard maintenance (see p. B-3), without N_2O. Evacuate stomach with OG or NG tube. Maintain muscle relaxation based on nerve stimulator response.
Emergence	Patient should be extubated awake after return of airway reflexes.
Blood and fluid requirements	IV: 16-18 ga × 1 NS/LR @ 5-8 ml/kg/h
Monitoring	Standard monitors (see p. B-1). Others, as indicated by patient's status.
Positioning	✓ and pad pressure points. ✓ eyes.
Complications	Sepsis

POSTOPERATIVE

Complications	Sepsis (possible with appendiceal rupture) Adequate antibiotic coverage
	Paralytic ileus Atelectasis Adequate pain control, incentive spirometry, early ambulation
Pain management	PCA (see p. C-3).
Tests	As indicated clinically.

References

1. McBurney C: Experience with early operative interference in cases of disease of the vermiform appendix. *NY Med J* 1889; 50:676-84.
2. Meckel JF: Ulcer die divertikel an darmkanal. *Arch Physiol* 1809; 9:421-53.
3. Merritt WT: Anesthesia for gastrointestinal surgery. In *Principles and Practice of Anesthesiology,* 2nd edition. Longnecker DE, et al, eds. Mosby-Year Book, St. Louis: 1998, 1881-1903.
4. Morgan EG, Mikhail MS, Murray MJ: *Clinical Anesthesiology,* 3rd edition. Lange Medical Books, Stamford, CT: 2002.
5. Rosen MA: Management of anesthesia for the pregnant surgical patient. *Anesthesiology* 1999; 91:1159-63.
6. Söderlund S. Meckel's diverticulum. A clinical and histologic study. *Acta Chir Scand* 1959; Suppl 248:13-233.
7. Way LW, Doherty GM, eds: *Current Surgical Diagnosis Treatment.* Appleton & Lange, Stamford, CT: 1994; 610-13, Appendix.

ENTEROSTOMY

SURGICAL CONSIDERATIONS

Description: Enterostomy is performed for stenting the small intestine with a long tube, for feeding purposes, for bypassing small or large bowel obstructions, and following total proctocolectomy. An intestinal tube is either purse-stringed into the small bowel and brought through the abdominal wall, or the intestine itself is brought to the exterior and fashioned into a stoma. Different tubes are used for feeding, according to surgeon's preference. After purse-stringing the tube in the bowel, the seromuscular layer of the jejunum is sutured over the tube for a distance of 3-4 cm before exiting through the abdominal wall. The **Brooke ileostomy** is created by bringing a 2" segment of ileum through an abdominal wall stab wound. The ileum is folded back on itself and sutured to the skin edge or dermis (Fig 7.3-3). Some surgeons secure the ileum to the underlying peritoneum and/or fascia, but this is not necessary.

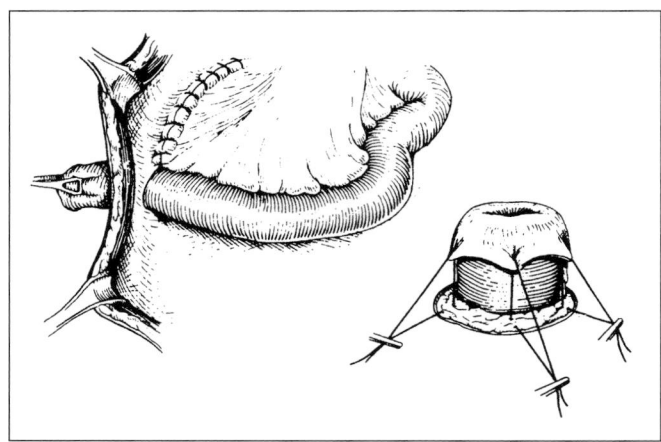

Figure 7.3-3. Brooke ileostomy. (Reproduced with permission from Hardy JD: *Rhoad's Textbook of Surgery,* 5th edition. JB Lippincott: 1977.)

Variant procedure or approaches: There are various intestinal or drainage tubes that may be inserted into the bowel, depending on the function required. For example, certain tubes are used for feeding, while others may be used for drainage or decompression.

Usual preop diagnosis: Intestinal obstruction due to extensive adhesions; following removal of the large intestine (including the rectum); for enteral feedings

SUMMARY OF PROCEDURES

	Enterostomy	Ileostomy
Position	Supine	⇐
Incision	Midline abdominal	⇐
Antibiotics	Cefazolin 1-2 g iv preop	⇐
Surgical time	1-1.5 h	⇐
Closing considerations	Securing tube to abdominal wall	Viable stoma
EBL	< 100 ml	⇐
Postop care	Tube irrigation	Stoma care
Mortality	< 0.5%	⇐

	Enterostomy	Ileostomy
Morbidity	Ileus: 60-70%	⇐
	Wound infection: < 5%	⇐
		Stoma necrosis: < 2%
Pain score	5-6	5-6

PATIENT POPULATION CHARACTERISTICS

Age range	20-65 yr
Male:Female	1:1
Incidence	Common
Etiology	Intestinal obstruction (60-70%); diseases resulting in total proctocolectomy (10-15%); inability to eat (5-10%)
Associated conditions	Inflammatory bowel disease (IBD); intestinal adhesions; inability to eat orally

ANESTHETIC CONSIDERATIONS FOR OSTOMY PROCEDURES

(Procedures covered: enterostomy; continent ileostomy; gastrostomy; gastrojejunostomy)

PREOPERATIVE

This patient population is very diverse and includes those with IBD or cancer, or those presenting post-CVA following trauma. Thus, the population ranges from the otherwise healthy to the critically ill. Many of these patients will have abnormal protective airway reflexes and are at risk of aspiration of gastric contents.

Respiratory	Patients post-CVA or head trauma may have abnormal laryngeal reflexes and difficulty swallowing, making them prone to aspiration of gastric contents and associated pneumonitis (evaluate gag reflex). Decreased pulmonary reserve and hypoxemia can be seen in patients with pulmonary infections. **Tests:** Consider CXR to r/o pneumonia. Consider ABG.
Cardiovascular	Patients are likely to be hypovolemic 2° chronically poor po intake and malnutrition. **Tests:** ECG; orthostatic vital signs
Musculoskeletal	Patients often sick and debilitated (e.g., post-CVA).
Gastrointestinal	Patients often malnourished and prone to electrolyte abnormalities 2° poor po intake. **Tests:** Electrolytes; BUN; Cr
Laboratory	CBC with differential; others as indicated from H&P.
Premedication	Depends on patient status. Titrate small doses of benzodiazepines (midazolam 0.25-0.5 mg iv) or opiate (fentanyl 25-50 μg iv). Consider H_2-antagonists (e.g., ranitidine 50 mg iv, 60 min preop) and metoclopramide (10 mg iv 20 min preop).

INTRAOPERATIVE

Anesthetic technique: MAC with local anesthesia to area of incision typical for gastrostomy; otherwise, GA is appropriate for ostomy procedures.

Induction	Patient may be at risk for pulmonary aspiration. If GA is planned, the trachea should be intubated while patient is awake or after rapid-sequence induction with cricoid pressure. If patient is hypovolemic, volume status should be restored before induction, and doses of sedative/hypnotic should be titrated to effect.
Maintenance	**MAC:** Titration of sedatives (e.g., propofol 50-100 μg/kg/min) and analgesics (fentanyl 25-50 μg iv). **GA:** Standard maintenance (see p. B-3).
Emergence	Trachea should be extubated after return of protective laryngeal reflexes, if patient at risk for aspiration of gastric contents.

Blood and fluid requirements	Minimal blood loss IV: 16-18 ga × 1 NS/LR @ 5-8 ml/kg/h	
Monitoring	Standard monitors (see p. B-1).	Others as clinically indicated.
Positioning	✓ and pad pressure points. ✓ eyes.	

POSTOPERATIVE

Complications	Atelectasis Aspiration Hypoxemia Hypercarbia
Pain management	PCA (see p. C-3).

Reference

1. Zinner MJ, Schwartz SI, Ellis H, eds: *Maingot's Abdominal Operations*, 10th edition, Vol. I. Appleton & Lange, Stamford, CT: 1997, 427-51.

CONTINENT ILEOSTOMY POUCH (KOCK)

SURGICAL CONSIDERATIONS

Description: A **Kock pouch**[2] consists of an internal reservoir fashioned from the distal ileum and an intussuscepted nipple valve used to provide continence. Approximately 45 cm of small bowel are required for construction of the pouch and valve. After suturing two limbs of the ileum together over a distance of 15 cm, the distal segment is intussuscepted over itself to form the nipple valve. The pouch is then sutured closed and mounted beneath the abdominal wall stoma site (Fig 7.3-4). The stoma is made flush with the skin for cosmetic reasons and left intubated for 1 mo with a special plastic catheter. The pouch remains decompressed for 1 mo before intermittent catheterization is initiated. The continent ileostomy reservoir has been modified by **Barnett**[1] to include the construction of an isoperistaltic valve with an intestinal collar around its base to prevent deintussusception and valve prolapse. These procedures are typically performed following total proctocolectomy or to replace conventional ileostomies.

Usual preop diagnosis: Inflammatory bowel disease; familial polyposis or malfunctioning ileostomies

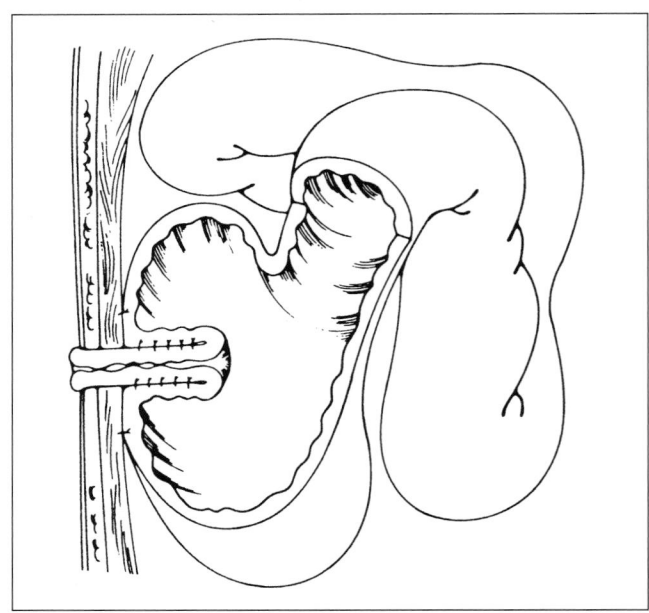

Figure 7.3-4. Continent ileostomy or Kock pouch. (Reproduced with permission from Hardy JD: *Hardy's Textbook of Surgery*, 2nd edition. JB Lippincott, 1988.)

SUMMARY OF PROCEDURE (KOCK OR BARNETT POUCH)

Position	Supine
Incision	Midline abdominal
Special instrumentation	GIA or TA staplers
Antibiotics	Usual bowel prep with antibiotics; cefazolin 1 g iv preop
Surgical time	3-4 h
Closing considerations	Valve vascularity
EBL	200-300 ml
Postop care	Maintain pouch decompression
Mortality	< 1%
Morbidity	Intestinal ileus: 5%
	Wound infection: < 5%
	Intestinal obstruction: 2-3%
	Pouch fistula: 1-3%
	Valve necrosis: < 0.5%
Pain score	6-8

PATIENT POPULATION CHARACTERISTICS

Age range	18-80 yr
Male:Female	1:1
Incidence	Common
Etiology	Ileostomy (50%); proctocolectomy (5%)
Associated conditions	Extracolonic inflammatory bowel manifestations (10%)

ANESTHETIC CONSIDERATIONS

See Anesthetic Considerations for Ostomy Procedures, p. 411.

References

1. Barnett WO: Modified techniques for improving the continent ileostomy. *Am Surg* 1984; 50(2):66-9.
2. Becker JM, Stuchni AF: Ulcerative colitis. In *Surgery: Scientific Principles and Practice,* 3rd edition. Greenfield LJ, et al, eds. Lippincott Williams & Wilkins, Philadelphia: 2001, 1070-89.
3. Little UR, Barboors RN, Shrock TR, Welton ML: The continent ileostomy—Long-term durability and patient satisfaction. *J Gastrointest Surg* 1999; 3:625-32.
4. Practice guidelines for preoperative fasting and the use of pharmacologic agents to reduce the risk of pulmonary aspiration: Application to healthy patients undergoing elective procedures. A report by the American Society of Anesthesiologists Task Force on Preoperative Fasting. *Anesthesiology* 1999; 90:896.

SMALL-BOWEL RESECTION WITH ANASTOMOSIS

SURGICAL CONSIDERATIONS

Description: Resection of the small bowel is performed for a number of diseases (listed below). After entering the peritoneal cavity, the involved small bowel is delivered into the wound and the lesion resected between bowel clamps (Fig 7.3-5). Varying amounts of mesentery are included, depending on the diagnosis. More extensive resections are indicated for malignant disease, including regional lymph nodes. Reanastomosis may be accomplished by various suturing techniques or stapling. The peritoneal cavity may be accessed through vertical or transverse incisions. Operative techniques include **open end-to-end**, **closed end-to-end**, **side-to-side**, or **stapled, functional end-to-end anastomoses**.

Figure 7.3-5. Block-Potts bowel clamps are applied from the antimesenteric to mesenteric border to avoid twisting. A Kocher clamp is applied on the specimen side, and the bowel is transected with a scalpel. (Reproduced with permission from Baker RJ, Fischer JE, eds: *Mastery of Surgery*, Vol II, 4th edition. Lippincott Williams & Wilkins, 2001.)

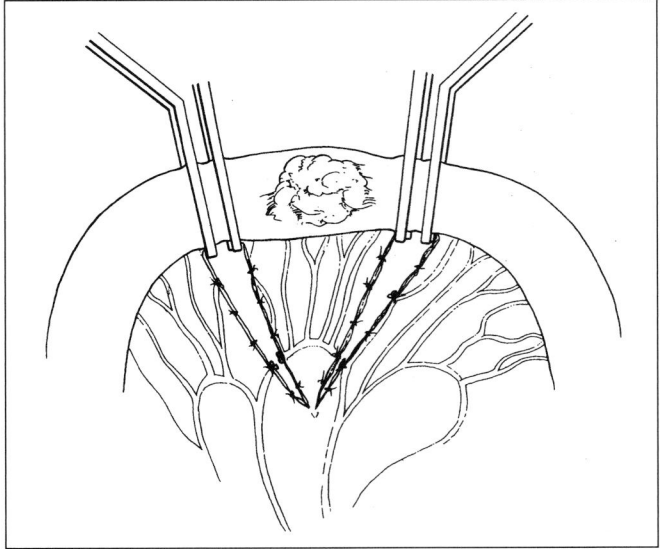

Variant procedure or approaches: Laparoscopic small-bowel resections are being performed more frequently (see p. 469).

Usual preop diagnosis: Intestinal obstruction, complicated by intestinal gangrene due to adhesions, internal hernia, volvulus, intussusception, mesenteric vascular occlusion, Crohn's disease, radiation enteritis, intestinal fistulae, small bowel tumors, and trauma[1]

SUMMARY OF PROCEDURE

Position	Supine
Incision	Vertical or transverse
Unique considerations	Adequate fluid resuscitation; NG tube
Antibiotics	Cefazolin 1-2 g iv preop
Surgical time	1-3 h
EBL	50-100 ml
Postop care	NG or long intestinal tube decompression
Mortality	Varies according to etiology: 1-5%
Morbidity	Atelectasis: < 10%
	Intestinal ileus: < 10%
	Wound infection: < 5%
	Intestinal leak, fistula: < 3%
Pain score	7-9

PATIENT POPULATION CHARACTERISTICS

Age range	20-90 yr
Male:Female	1:1
Incidence	Common
Etiology	Interference with blood supply (obstruction, strangulated hernia, volvulus, mesenteric thrombosis); trauma; tumors; Crohn's disease
Associated conditions	Multiple, depending on etiology (see Preop diagnosis, above).

ANESTHETIC CONSIDERATIONS

See Anesthetic Considerations for Intestinal and Peritoneal Procedures, p. 416.

Reference

1. Zollinger RM Jr, Zollinger RM: *Atlas of Surgical Operations*, 7th edition. MacMillan, New York: 1993.

ENTEROLYSIS

SURGICAL CONSIDERATIONS

Description: Enterolysis consists of separating loops of bowel adhesed to other loops or the abdominal wall by sharp dissection, and by excising adhesive bands. Care must be taken to avoid producing enterotomies. In recurrent cases of intestinal obstruction, small bowel plication or intraluminal tube stenting may be utilized. Plication is achieved by suturing the bowel or its mesentery so that the small bowel is aligned in an orderly manner without kinks. This also can be accomplished by threading a long intraabdominal tube orally or via a jejunostomy down through the small intestine.[1] This has the effect of holding the bowel in a nonobstructed position while new adhesions form. Covering potential adhesion sites with a hyaluronic carboxymethylcellulose membrane may lessen the formation of intraperitoneal adhesions.

Usual preop diagnosis: Intraabdominal adhesions; intestinal obstruction

SUMMARY OF PROCEDURE

Position	Supine
Incision	Midline abdominal
Special instrumentation	A long intestinal tube may be necessary for decompression and fixation of bowel loop.
Unique considerations	Bowel decompression
Antibiotics	Cefazolin 1 g iv preop
Surgical time	1-4 h
Closing considerations	Adequate decompression to permit wound closure
EBL	150-500 ml
Postop care	PACU; continued intestinal decompression 2-5 d
Mortality	1-3%
Morbidity	Wound abscess: 15-20%
	Prolonged ileus: 10-20%
	Fistula formation: < 10%
	Pulmonary complications: 5-10%
	Recurrent intestinal obstruction: 5-8%
Pain score	5-7

PATIENT POPULATION CHARACTERISTICS

Age range	Any age
Male:Female	1:1
Incidence	Common
Etiology	Previous intraabdominal operative procedure (> 90%); malignant tumors (15-20%); hernias (10-15%); volvulus (5-10%); inflammatory bowel disease (5%); gallstone ileus (< 5%); intussusception (< 5%)

ANESTHETIC CONSIDERATIONS

See Anesthetic Considerations for Intestinal and Peritoneal Procedures, p. 416.

References

1. Brolin RE, Krasna MJ, Mast BA: Use of tubes and radiographs in the management of small bowel obstruction. *Ann Surg* 1987; 206:126.
2. Close MB, Christensen NM: Transmesenteric small bowel plication or intraluminal tube stenting. Indications and contraindications. *Am J Surg* 1979; 138(1):89-96.
3. Vrijland WW, Tseng LN, Eijkman HJ, et al: Fewer intraperitoneal adhesions with use of hyaluronic acid-carboxymethylcellulose membrane: a randomized clinical trial. *Ann Surg* 2002; 235(2):193-9.

CLOSURE OF ENTERIC FISTULAE

SURGICAL CONSIDERATIONS

Description: Enteric fistulae may occur between the bowel and abdominal wall (enterocutaneous), between loops of the intestine (enteroenteric or enterocolic), or between the bowel and bladder or vagina (enterovesical or enterovaginal). Surgical repair is usually reserved for fistulae to the abdominal wall, bladder, and vagina, and consists of excising the fistula and repairing the bowel and the other organ separately. Most fistulae are characterized by the adherence of the two visceral organs with a communication between their lumens.

The organs involved are separated by blunt-sharp dissection and repaired locally after excision of the indurated margins of the defect. In the case of both the small and large intestines, it may be necessary to resect a segment of bowel with the defect and to perform an end-to-end anastomosis. If the repair sites involved lie close together, it is important to interpose tissue, such as the omentum, between the viscera to minimize chance of recurrence. Occasionally, a fistula may be bypassed rather than surgically resected.

Usual preop diagnosis: Enteric fistula

SUMMARY OF PROCEDURE

Position	Supine
Incision	Midline abdominal
Unique considerations	Preop nutritional support and fistula wound care
Antibiotics	Cefazolin 2 g iv preop
Surgical time	2-4 h
Closing considerations	Separation of repairs by interposition of omentum and other tissue
EBL	50-300 ml
Postop care	NG decompression until bowel function returns; TPN support
Mortality	0-5%
Morbidity	Ileus: 60-70%
	Pulmonary complications: 10%
	Recurrent fistula: 5-10%
	Wound infection: 5-10%
Pain score	6-8

PATIENT POPULATION CHARACTERISTICS

Age range	Any age
Male:Female	1:1
Incidence	Common
Etiology	Anastomotic leaks (60-70%); carcinoma (10-15%); Crohn's disease (5-10%); iatrogenic bowel injury (5-10%); perforative diverticulitis (5-10%); radiation enteritis (5%); foreign body perforation (< 5%)
Associated conditions	Malnutrition (30%); inflammatory bowel disease (25%); cancer (15%)

ANESTHETIC CONSIDERATIONS
FOR INTESTINAL AND PERITONEAL PROCEDURES

(Procedures covered: small-bowel resection; enterolysis; closure of enteric fistulae; excision of intraabdominal and retroperitoneal tumor; drainage of subphrenic abscess)

PREOPERATIVE

Patients requiring exploratory laparotomy present both electively and emergently for a very wide range of disorders. As a result of their abdominal pathology, these patients are often at high risk for the pulmonary aspiration of gastric contents. Precautions to prevent this are necessary to help assure safe patient outcome (see p. B-5).

Respiratory	Respiratory insufficiency can be present due to intraabdominal pathology (e.g., ascites, large tumor, free blood, bowel distension, pain); $\downarrow$FRC $\rightarrow$ $\uparrow$A-a gradient and arterial hypoxemia; diaphragmatic impairment and splinting $\rightarrow$ $\uparrow$respiratory insufficiency. **Tests:** Consider CXR; ABG.

Cardiovascular	Patients for emergency surgery are likely to be critically ill and should be evaluated for presence of hypovolemia (hypotension, tachycardia) and should receive adequate volume replacement before anesthetic induction. Elective patients may be hypovolemic 2° bowel prep. **Tests:** ECG; orthostatic vital signs
Musculoskeletal	Abdominal rigidity may be present; abdominal pain is common.
Gastrointestinal	Diarrhea, vomiting, and prolonged npo status can lead to electrolyte abnormalities. **Tests:** Electrolytes
Renal	Renal insufficiency/failure may be present, especially in elderly and/or chronically ill patients, and in those who are hypovolemic. **Tests:** Consider BUN; Cr; electrolytes.
Laboratory	CBC with differential; Plt count
Premedication	Standard premedication (see p. B-2). Consider H_2-antagonists (e.g., ranitidine 50 mg iv 1 hr preop), metoclopramide (10 mg iv 30 min preop; although contraindicated in bowel obstruction/perforation), and Na citrate (30 ml po 10 min preop).

INTRAOPERATIVE

Anesthetic technique: GETA ± epidural for postop analgesia. If postop epidural analgesia is planned, placement of catheter prior to anesthetic induction is helpful to establish correct placement in the epidural space (accomplished by injecting 5-7 ml of 2% lidocaine via the epidural catheter, eliciting a segmental block).

Induction	The patient with abdominal pathology is often at risk for pulmonary aspiration and the trachea should be intubated with patient awake or after rapid-sequence iv induction with cricoid pressure. (See Rapid-Sequence Induction, p. B-5.) If patient is clinically hypovolemic, restore intravascular volume (colloid, crystalloid, or blood) prior to induction and titrate induction dose of sedative/hypnotic agents.
Maintenance	**Balanced anesthesia** without N_2O (see Standard Maintenance Techniques, p. B-3): Maintain neuromuscular blockade based on nerve stimulator response. Place OG or NG tube to evacuate stomach contents. **Combined epidural and GA:** Local anesthetic (2% lidocaine with 1:200,000 epinephrine 5-10 ml q 60 min) can be injected into the epidural catheter to provide both anesthesia and optimal surgical exposure (contracted bowel and profound muscle relaxation). A continuous infusion of local anesthetic (e.g., 2% lidocaine or 0.25% bupivacaine) at 5-10 ml/h. Be prepared to treat hypotension with fluid and vasopressors. GA is administered to supplement regional anesthesia and for amnesia. If epidural opiates are used for postop analgesia, a loading dose (e.g., hydromorphone 1.0 mg) should be administered at least 1 h before the conclusion of surgery. Systemic sedatives (droperidol, opiates, benzodiazepines, etc.) should be minimized during this type of anesthetic as they increase the likelihood of postop respiratory depression. An NG tube should be kept on intermittent suction.
Emergence	The decision to extubate at the end of surgery depends on the patient's underlying cardiopulmonary status and the extent of the surgical procedure. Patients should be hemodynamically stable, warm, alert, cooperative, and fully reversed from any muscle relaxants prior to extubation. If the above criteria are not met, patient should remain intubated and transported to ICU for further care.
Blood and fluid requirements	Anticipate large fluid shift. IV: 14-16 ga × 1-2 T&C for 4 U RBCs. NS/LR @ 10-15 ml/kg/h Fluid warmer	Plts, FFP, and cryoprecipitate should be administered according to lab tests (Plt count, PT, PTT, DIC screen, thromboelastography [TEG]).
Monitoring	Standard monitors (see p. B-1). UO ± Arterial line ± CVP/PA catheter	Invasive monitors, as indicated by patient's status. Prevent hypothermia: consider heated humidifier, forced-air warmer, warming blanket, warm room temperature, keeping patient covered until ready for prep, etc.
Positioning	✓ and pad pressure points. ✓ eyes.	
Complications	Hemorrhage Sepsis	Acute septic shock may require PA catheter and aggressive hemodynamic support.

POSTOPERATIVE

Complications	Sepsis Hemodynamic instability Atelectasis Hypoxemia Hemorrhage Ileus	Pulmonary function abnormalities may persist for 1 wk postop (↓vital capacity and ↓FRC).
Pain management	Epidural analgesia (see p. C-2). PCA (see p. C-3).	Patient should be recovered in ICU or ward accustomed to treating the side effects of epidural opiates (e.g., respiratory depression, breakthrough pain, nausea, pruritus).
Tests	CBC; CXR (if central line placed); electrolytes; glucose	Others as directed by intraop course.

References

1. Aguirre A, Fischer JE, Welch CE: The role of surgery and hyperalimentation in the therapy of gastrointestinal-cutaneous fistulae. *Ann Surg* 1974; 180(4):393-401.
2. Merritt WT: Anesthesia for gastrointestinal surgery. In *Principles and Practice of Anesthesiology*, 2nd edition. Longnecker DE, et al, eds. Mosby-Year Book, St. Louis: 1998, 1881-1903.
3. Practice guidelines for preoperative fasting and the use of pharmacologic agents to reduce the risk of pulmonary aspiration: Application to healthy patients undergoing elective procedures. A report by the American Society of Anesthesiologists Task Force on Preoperative Fasting. *Anesthesiology* 1999;90:896.
4. Zinner MJ, Schwartz SI, Ellis H, eds: *Maingot's Abdominal Operations*, 10th edition, Vol. I. Appleton & Lange, Stamford, CT: 1997, 593-616.

Surgeons

Andrew A. Shelton, MD
Mark Lane Welton, MD

7.4 COLORECTAL SURGERY

Anesthesiologist

Afshin Abdollahi, MD

LAPAROSCOPIC COLORECTAL SURGERY

Laparoscopic surgery has changed the face of general surgery with the widespread use of laparoscopic cholecystectomy, appendectomy, and other surgical procedures. While most colorectal surgery continues to be done in the standard open fashion, laparoscopic techniques are being used more and more for procedures on the colon and rectum. All of the following procedures can be done, and have been done, laparoscopically. Advantages to the patient include smaller incisions, less postop discomfort, and, possibly, a slight decrease in hospital stay, with early return to work and normal activity. Steep positional changes are often used to facilitate retraction of the small bowel out of the operative field. The patient is often placed on a beanbag to prevent movement. The term 'laparoscopic-assisted' may be more appropriately used for colorectal procedures since the colon often is mobilized laparoscopically. A small incision is then made, through which the bowel is exteriorized, the mesentery divided, and an anastomosis created.

References

1. Braga M, Vignali A, Zuliani W, Radaelli G, Gianotti L, Toussoun G, Carlo V: Training period in laparoscopic colorectal surgery. *Surgical Endoscopy* 2002; 16(1):31-5.
2. Duepree HJ, Senagore AJ, Delaney CP, Brady KM, Fazio VW: Advantages of laparoscopic resection for ileocecal Crohn's disease. *Dis Colon Rect* 2002; 45(5):605-10.
3. Dwivedi A, Chahin F, Agrawal S, Chau WY, Tootla A, Tootla F, Silva YJ: Laparoscopic colectomy vs. open colectomy for sigmoid diverticular disease. *Dis Colon Rect* 2002; 45(10):1309-14; discussion 1314-5.
4. Ky AJ, Sonoda T, Milsom JW: One-stage laparoscopic restorative proctocolectomy: an alternative to the conventional approach? *Dis Colon Rect* 2002; 45(2):207-11.
5. Lacy AM, Garcia-Valdecasas JC, Delgado S, Castells A, Taura P, Pique JM, Visa J: Laparoscopy-assisted colectomy versus open colectomy for treatment of non-metastatic colon cancer: a randomised trial. *Lancet* 2002; 359(9325):2224-9.
6. Scheidbach H, Schneider C, Konradt J, Barlehner E, Kohler L, Wittekind Ch, Kockerling F: Laparoscopic abdominoperineal resection and anterior resection with curative intent for carcinoma of the rectum. *Surg Endo* 2002; 16(1):7-13.
7. Weeks JC, Nelson H, Gelber S, Sargent D, Schroeder G: Clinical Outcomes of Surgical Therapy (COST) Study Group. Short-term quality-of-life outcomes following laparoscopic-assisted colectomy vs open colectomy for colon cancer: a randomized trial. *JAMA* 2002; 287(3):321-8.

TOTAL PROCTOCOLECTOMY

SURGICAL CONSIDERATIONS

Description: A total proctocolectomy involves the removal of the entire colon, rectum, and anus (Fig 7.4-1). Indications for this operation include ulcerative colitis (UC), Crohn's disease (CD), and familial adenomatous polyposis (FAP). Inflammatory bowel disease (IBD) can be diagnosed at any age, but there are peaks in diagnosis in the teens and twenties and the sixties and seventies. The most common indication for total proctocolectomy in the setting of UC or CD is intractable symptoms despite maximal medical therapy. Patients are commonly chronically or acutely ill, and may be malnourished or anemic. They are often on high-dose steroids and other immune suppressants, such as 6-mercaptopurine or Imuran. FAP is an autosomal-dominant disease resulting in hereditary colon cancer. Patients develop hundreds to thousands of adenomatous polyps throughout their colon and rectum, as well as elsewhere in the GI tract. Colorectal cancer is inevitable unless proctocolectomy is performed. This is typically done in the late teens or twenties. In contrast to patients with CD or UC, patients with FAP are usually healthy without other medical comorbidities.

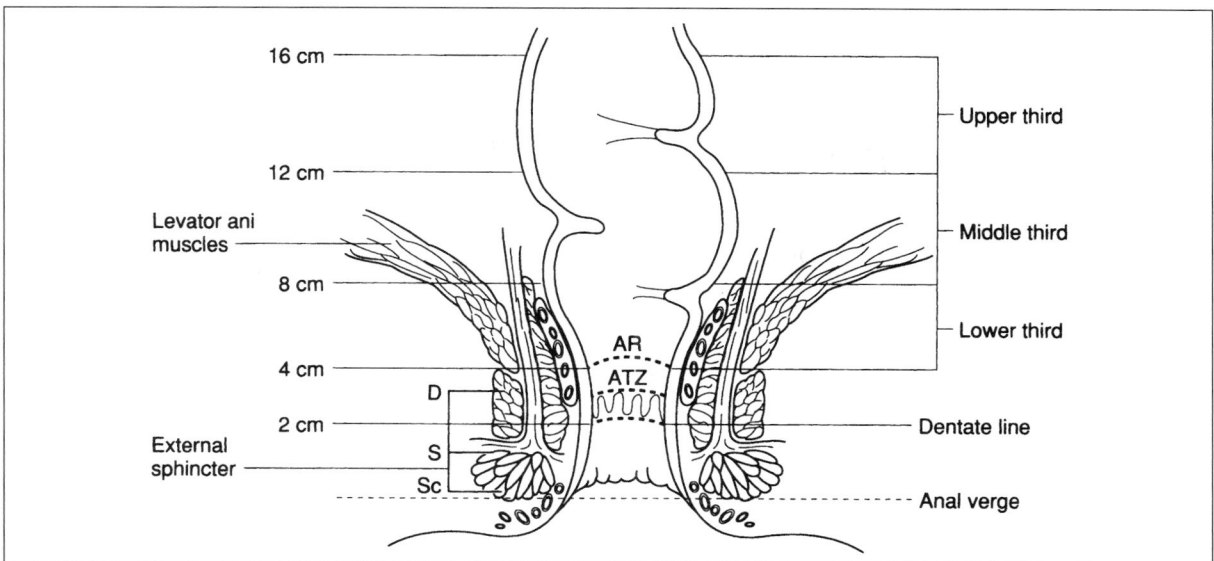

Figure 7.4-1. Anorectal anatomy with important landmarks. Approximate measurements are relative to the anal verge. D = deep; S = superficial; Sc = subcutaneous; AR = anorectal ring; ATZ = anal transition zone. (Reproduced with permission from Yahanda AM, Chang AE: Colorectal cancer. In *Surgery: Scientific Principles and Practice*, 3rd edition. Greenfield LJ, Mulholland MW, Oldham KT, Zelenock GB, Lillemoe KD, eds. Lippincott Williams & Wilkins, 2001.)

Patients usually are given a preop bowel preparation. The bacterial load of the colon is diminished by mechanical cleansing, which may be accomplished by cathartics, or nonabsorbed lavage solutions. As a result of this preparation, patients are often hypovolemic and hypokalemic. Sequential compression stockings are used for thromboprophylaxis. Patients with CD and UC are at ↑risk for the development of DVT and are often given subcutaneous heparin. Patients on chronic steroids are given stress-dose steroids before the procedure. Broad-spectrum antibiotics covering gram-negative rods and anaerobes are given prior to the incision.

Total proctocolectomy with end ileostomy, total proctocolectomy with **continent ileostomy (Koch pouch),** and **restorative proctocolectomy** with **ileal pouch anal anastomosis (IPAA)** all involve complete removal of the colon and rectum, down to the level of the pelvic floor or levator ani muscles. They differ in the fate of the anal canal, creation of a stoma, or construction of an anastomosis. The patient is placed in a lithotomy position in padded Allen stirrups. A Foley catheter is placed. The procedure is performed through a midline incision. The abdomen is explored for evidence of unexpected malignancy or, in the case of FAP, for desmoid tumors. The right colon is mobilized first, and then the small bowel mesentery is mobilized to allow for creation of an ileostomy. The transverse colon may be mobilized by separating it from the greater omentum, or the greater omentum may be resected along with the specimen. The sigmoid and descending colon are mobilized and the splenic flexure is taken down. At this point, the ileum is divided flush with the cecum. The vessels in the colon mesentery are ligated. At this point, the entire abdominal colon has been resected. An avascular fascial envelope surrounds the rectum and its mesentery, the mesorectum. It is possible to circumferentially dissect the rectum down to the level of the pelvic floor without ligating any vessels. There may be significant blood loss if an inadvertent injury to the spleen occurs during mobilization of the splenic flexure. Massive blood loss may occur if the presacral venous plexus is entered during posterior rectal mobilization.

Total proctocolectomy with ileostomy: For patients with CD, elderly patients with UC, or FAP patients with low rectal cancer, complete removal of the colon, rectum, and anus is the procedure of choice. After completing the abdominal mobilization of the colon and rectum, the perineal phase of the operation begins. Ideally, two teams of surgeons participate in the operation simultaneously. The abdominal surgeon can create the ileostomy and close the abdomen, while the perineal surgeon finishes removal of the rectum and anus. A circumferential incision is made at the anal verge and the intersphincteric plane is identified. The dissection proceeds cephalad until the abdominal dissection is encountered, and the specimen is removed. The levator ani muscle, external anal sphincter, and skin are closed. While this is being done, the abdominal surgeon makes a circular incision over the previously marked ileostomy site. A muscle-splitting incision is carried through the rectus fascia. The terminal ileum is then brought through this site. After the fascial and skin are closed, the ileostomy is matured.

Total proctocolectomy with continent ileostomy (Koch pouch): Removal of the colon, rectum, and anus is accomplished exactly as described above. Instead of creating an end ileostomy, for which the patient must wear an appliance, however, a reservoir and nipple valve are created out of the terminal ileum, and a 'continent' stoma is created. This is accomplished by anastomosing two limbs of ileum together in a side-to-side fashion. The nipple valve is constructed by intussuscepting the ileum into itself and the reservoir. An ileostomy is created, but the patient does not wear an appliance. Liquid ileostomy effluent collects in the reservoir that the patient then empties with periodic catheterization. Because of frequent complications and the development of alternative procedures (see below) this procedure is rarely performed today.

Restorative proctocolectomy with ileal pouch anal anastomosis (IPAA): IPAA is the procedure most commonly performed for patients with FAP and UC. In this operation, the colon and rectum are removed, down to the level of the pelvic floor; however, the anal canal and anal sphincter complex are preserved. The rectum is stapled and divided at the level of the surgical anal canal, ~1-1.5 cm above the dentate line. An ileal reservoir is constructed by anastomosing the distal 30 cm of ileum in a side-to-side fashion, creating a J-pouch. The apex of the pouch is then anastomosed to the anal canal using a circular stapling device. Rarely, a hand-sewn anastomosis is created. A temporary diverting loop ileostomy may or may not be created, depending on the clinical situation.

Usual preop diagnosis: Ulcerative colitis; familial adenomatous polyposis; Crohn's colitis

SUMMARY OF PROCEDURES

	Total Proctocolectomy With End Ileostomy	Total Proctocolectomy With Continent Ileostomy	IPAA
Position	Modified lithotomy	⇐	⇐
Incision	Long midline	⇐	⇐
Special instrumentation	2-table setup (separate abdominal and perineal instruments); deep pelvic instruments	2-table setup; long, noncutting linear staplers; Kock catheters; deep pelvic instruments	2-table setup; anal retractors; spinal needle; 1:200,000 epinephrine; deep pelvic instruments
Unique considerations	Patients frequently on chronic high-dose corticosteroids	⇐	⇐+ Epinephrine solutions injected under the rectal mucosa to facilitate dissection and reduce bleeding.
Antibiotics	Cefotetan 2 g iv	⇐	⇐
Surgical time	3-4 h	3-7 h	⇐
Closing considerations	Ileostomy completed after skin closed (15-30 min).	None	Temporary ileostomy commonly used, completed after skin closure.
EBL	300-1000 ml (most blood loss during pelvic and perineal dissections)	⇐	⇐
Postop care	Transient inability to void common.	Maintain patency of catheter draining pouch; transient inability to void common.	Small bowel mesentery lengthened by dissection around duodenum. This frequently necessitates use of postop NG tube. Transient inability to void common.
Mortality	2-5% (older patients and those with underlying medical problems)	0-2%	⇐
Morbidity	Dyspareunia: 30%	⇐	5-10%
	Stoma complications: 20%	–	–
	SBO: 10-15%	⇐	⇐
	Impotence: 2-4%	⇐	⇐
		Nipple valve failure: 20-50%	–
		Persistent perineal wound: 30%	–
		Pouchitis: 20-30%	⇐
		Intraabdominal sepsis: 5%	–
		Pouch incontinence 5%	–
			Nocturnal incontinence: 20%
			Poor function: 5%
			Pelvic sepsis: 0-4%
Pain score	8	8	8

PATIENT POPULATION CHARACTERISTICS

	Ulcerative colitis	Familial adenomatous polyposis
Age range	3rd-5th decade	2nd-4th decade
Male:Female	1:1	⇐
Incidence	6-10/100,000	100-150 cases/yr
Etiology	Unknown	Genetic
Associated conditions	Cushing's syndrome; anemia; malnutrition; colorectal cancer; sclerosing cholangitis	Colorectal cancer; desmoid tumors; adenomas or cancers of the duodenum and small intestine; brain tumors (Turcot's syndrome); adrenal adenomas; osteomas

ANESTHETIC CONSIDERATIONS

See Anesthetic Considerations for Large Bowel Surgery, p. 427.

References

1. Bertario L, Arrigoni A, Aste H, Fracasso P, Ponz de Leon M, Tonelli F, Heonaine A: Recommendations for clinical management of familial adenomatous polyposis. *Tumori* 1997; 83(5):800-3.
2. Ghosh S, Shand A, Ferguson A: Ulcerative colitis. *BMJ* 2000; 320(7242):1119-23.
3. Guy TS, Williams NN, Rosato EF: Crohn's disease of the colon. *Surg Clin North Am* 2001; 81(1):159-68, ix.
4. Katz JA: Medical and surgical management of severe colitis. *Sem Gastrointest Dis* 2002; 11(1):18-32.
5. King JE, Dozois RR, Lindor NM, Ahlquist DA: Care of patients and their families with familial adenomatous polyposis. *Mayo Clinic Proceedings* 2000; 75(1):57-67.
6. Litle VR, Barbour S, Schrock TR, Welton ML: The continent ileostomy: long-term durability and patient satisfaction. *J Gastrointest Surg* 1999; 3(6):625-32.
7. Michelassi F, Hurst R: Restorative proctocolectomy with J-pouch ileoanal anastomosis. *Arch Surg* 2000; 135(3):347-53.
8. Vasen HF, van Duijvendijk P, Buskens E, Bulow C, Bjork J, Jarvinen HJ, Bulow S: Decision analysis in the surgical treatment of patients with familial adenomatous polyposis: a Dutch-Scandinavian collaborative study including 659 patients. *Gut* 2001; 49(2):231-5.

SEGMENTAL (PARTIAL) COLECTOMY

SURGICAL CONSIDERATIONS

Description: Segmental colectomy involves removal of a portion of the colon (Fig 7.4-2) with the creation of an anastomosis or a stoma. The most common indications for the operation in the western world are colon cancer and diverticulitis. Less common indications include gastrointestinal hemorrhage, ischemic colitis, volvulus, and inflammatory bowel disease (IBD). Both colon cancer and diverticular disease occur most commonly in patients > 50 yr. Patients may have any of the comorbid medical conditions associated with aging, as well as complications related to the disease requiring colon resection. **Free perforation** of the colon can occur from a variety of conditions, including diverticulitis, cancer, and ischemia. Patients may be hypovolemic and have systemic sepsis. Emergent laparotomy should follow a period of resuscitation and administration of antibiotics. The involved segment of bowel is resected, the abdomen is irrigated, and a stoma is created.

Colon cancer is the second most common cancer in the U.S., with 130,000 new cases diagnosed annually. Patients may be completely asymptomatic with the Dx being made only as the result of a screening exam. Because of the large caliber of the colon and the liquid nature of stool, patients with cancers of the right colon are more likely to present with large cancers and anemia. The caliber of the left colon is smaller, and the stool more solid. Symptoms of obstruction and change in bowel habits predominate for left-sided lesions.

Colonic diverticula occur in up to 60-70% of people > 50 yr in the U.S. A colonic diverticulum is a herniation of the mucosa and submucosa through the relative weakening that occurs in the muscular wall of the bowel at the site of penetrating blood vessels. This occurs predominately in the sigmoid colon. The majority of people with colonic diverticula are completely asymptomatic and will never experience any complications related to diverticulosis. Diverticulitis occurs when a microscopic or macroscopic perforation of a colonic diverticulum occurs, resulting in a pericolonic inflammatory and infectious process. The severity of the attack depends on the degree of perforation and how well the body is able to wall it off. This ranges from minor inflammation around the sigmoid colon that can be managed with antibiotics, to an intraabdominal or pelvic abscess requiring percutaneous drainage, to free perforation with purulent or feculent peritonitis requiring emergency surgery. Repeated bouts of diverticulitis eventually can result in fibrosis of the colon, stricture formation, and obstruction.

Ideally, surgery on the colon is performed in an elective setting; however, perforation with peritonitis or complete obstruction of the colon may require emergency surgery. Most patients presenting for elective colon resection undergo preop bowel preparation that consists of mechanical cleaning of the colon. As a result, they are frequently hypovolemic and hypokalemic when they

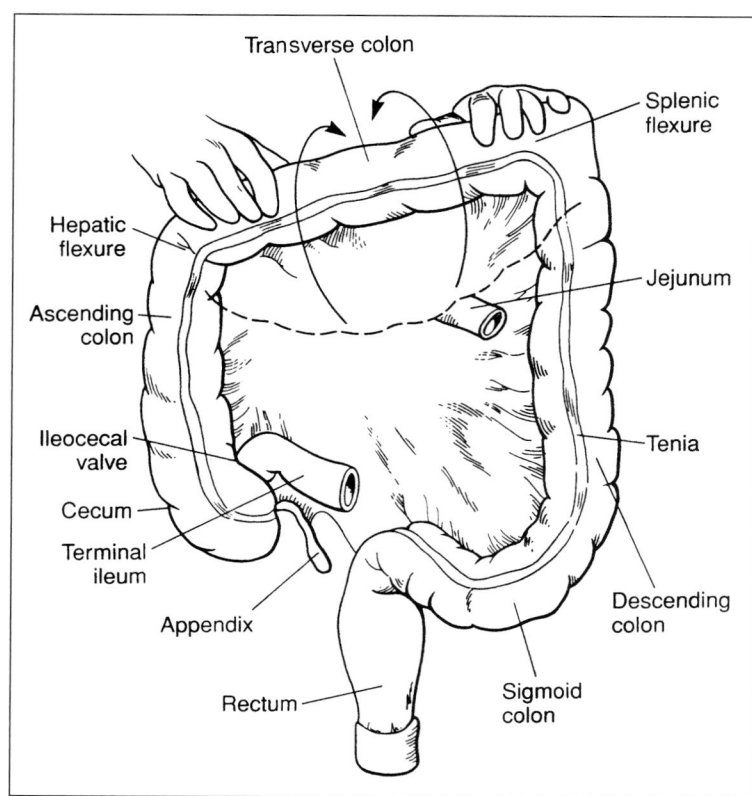

Figure 7.4-2. Anatomy of the colon. (Reproduced with permission from Hardy JD: *Hardy's Textbook of Surgery*, 2nd edition. JB Lippincott, 1988.)

come to the OR. The patient is positioned either supine, or in the modified lithotomy position, depending on the segment of colon to be removed. Sequential compression stockings are used for thromboprophylaxis. Intravenous antibiotics covering gram-negative rods and anaerobes should be given prior to the incision.

Segmental colectomy: Segmental resection of the colon may be performed via midline or transverse abdominal incisions, depending on the underlying disease, portion of the colon to be resected, and the surgeon's preference. In general, midline incisions are preferred when: a high-lying splenic flexure must be mobilized, IBD is present, or the extent of the colon resection is not known preop. Transverse incisions are most commonly reserved for resections of the right colon.

The most commonly performed **partial colon resections** are: right hemicolectomy, sigmoid colectomy, left hemicolectomy, and abdominal colectomy with an ileorectal anastomosis. The sequence of steps in partial colectomy are the same for all parts of the colon. The right colon and left colon are retroperitoneal structures, while the transverse colon and sigmoid colon are primarily intraperitoneal. The first step is mobilization of the colon and its mesentery. Care must be taken not to injure the left ureter during mobilization of the sigmoid colon or the duodenum during mobilization of the right colon. Proximal and distal sites for resection are selected and the intervening mesentery is divided. The anastomosis may be hand-sewn or stapled, a decision based primarily on surgeon preference. There is no clear advantage to either anastomotic technique. Creation of a colostomy rather than an anastomosis may be necessary in patients who are hemodynamically unstable, or when intraabdominal conditions, such as inflammation, carcinomatosis, or unprepped bowel, make an anastomosis unsafe. There may be significant blood loss if an inadvertent injury to the spleen occurs during mobilization of the splenic flexure. Excessive traction of the hepatic flexure can result in difficult-to-control venous bleeding.

Obstruction of the colon most commonly occurs as a result of cancers of the sigmoid colon or repeated bouts of diverticulitis. Patients present with abdominal distention, obstipation, N/V. Patients are treated with NG tube decompression and correction of hypovolemia. An attempt may be made to stent the obstructing lesion endoscopically preop to allow decompression and preparation of the colon. If this is not possible, surgical options include segmental resection with a colostomy, segmental resection with primary anastomosis and an on-table colonic lavage, or subtotal colectomy with an ileorectal anastomosis.

Usual preop diagnosis: Colon cancer; diverticular disease; Crohn's disease; ulcerative colitis; trauma; ischemic colitis; lower GI hemorrhage; intractable constipation; colon volvulus

SUMMARY OF PROCEDURE

Position	Supine or modified lithotomy
Incision	Transverse or vertical midline
Unique considerations	Bowel prep, or underlying disease may → dehydration, electrolyte abnormalities or anemia.
Antibiotics	Cefotetan 2 g iv
Surgical time	1-3 h
Closing considerations	Colostomy or ileostomy matured after wound is closed (requires 10-20 min).
EBL	100-300 ml (500-2000 ml if splenic injury, loss of major vascular pedicle, or repeat operation for cancer, Crohn's disease)
Postop care	ICU for underlying disease; NG tube for distention or vomiting. Avoid use of long-lasting anticholinergics (e.g., Phenergan).
Mortality	0.5-2% (mostly related to underlying disease)
Morbidity	SBO: 5-10%
	Wound infection: 4-10%
	For anastomosis-anastomotic leak: 2-4%
	Wound dehiscence: 1-2%
	Bleeding: 1%
	Splenic injury: 1%
Pain score	8

PATIENT POPULATION CHARACTERISTICS

	Crohn's Disease	Colon cancer	Trauma	Diverticula
Age range	2nd-4th decade	5th-7th decade	2nd-4th decades	> 40 yr
Male:Female	1:1	1.3:1	3:1	1:1
Incidence	1-6/100,000	30/100,000	1-2/100,000	10/100,000
Etiology	Unknown	Genetic: 5%	Trauma	Western countries: low-fiber diet
Associated conditions	Malnutrition; anemia; intraabdominal sepsis; intestinal fistulae; perianal disease; nephrolithiasis; sclerosing and ankylosing spondylitis	Iron deficiency; colonic obstruction; colonic perforation	Liver fracture; spleen fracture; rib fracture; closed-head injury; penetration of viscera adjacent to colon injury	Hemorrhoids; chronic constipation

ANESTHETIC CONSIDERATIONS

See Anesthetic Considerations for Large Bowel Surgery, p. 427.

References

1. Arnaud JP, Bergamaschi R: Emergency subtotal/total colectomy with anastomosis for acutely obstructed carcinoma of the left colon. *Dis Colon Rect* 1994; 37(7):685-8.
2. Blair NP, Germann E: Surgical management of acute sigmoid diverticulitis. *Am J Surg* 2002; 183(5):525-8.
3. Colquhoun PH, Wexner SD: Surgical management of colon cancer. *Curr Gastroenterol Rep* 2002; 4(5):414-9.
4. Deans GT, Krukowski ZH, Irwin ST: Malignant obstruction of the left colon. *Brit J Surg* 1994; 81(9):1270-6.
5. DeFriend D, Hill J: A review of emergency colonic surgery. *Br J Hosp Med* 1996; 56(7):326-9.
6. Koperna T, Kisser M, Reiner G, Schulz F: Diagnosis and treatment of bleeding colonic diverticula. *Hepato-Gastroenterol* 2001; 48(39):702-5.
7. Kumar SK, Goldberg RM: Adjuvant chemotherapy for colon cancer. *Curr Oncol Rep* 2001; 3(2):94-101.
8. Lavery IC, Lopez-Kostner F, Pelley RJ, Fine RM: Treatment of colon and rectal cancer. *Surg Clin North Am* 2000; 80(2): 535-69, ix.
9. Maggard MA, Chandler CF, Schmit PJ, Bennion RS, Hines OJ, Thompson JE: Surgical diverticulitis: treatment options. *Am Surgeon* 2001; 67(12):1185-9.
10. Makela J, Kiviniemi H, Laitinen S: Prevalence of perforated sigmoid diverticulitis is increasing. *Dis Colon Rect* 2002; 45(7):955-61.

STOMA CLOSURE OR
PERISTOMAL HERNIA REPAIR

SURGICAL CONSIDERATIONS

Description: A temporary colostomy or ileostomy can be made for a variety of staged procedures. An **end colostomy** is often created after resection of obstructing or perforated lesions of the left colon. A **proximal loop ileostomy or colostomy** is often created to protect a 'high-risk' anastomosis, such as a low pelvic colorectal or ileoanal anastomosis. A patient with a permanent stoma may develop a hernia at the stoma site. This may result in complications, such as obstruction or strangulation of the bowel, or problems with appropriate fitting of the stoma appliance. The extent of procedure depends on the type of stoma created.

Closure of loop stoma: Closure of a loop stoma is performed through a circular incision, placed just outside the muco-cutaneous junction of the stoma and the skin. The proximal and distal ends of the bowel are separated from the subcutaneous tissue and anterior fascia, and then the posterior fascia. The bowel is cleaned of adherent skin, and the previously opened antimesenteric border of the bowel is simply closed with sutures. Alternatively, the previously exteriorized portion of bowel is resected and the two ends are anastomosed with sutures or staples. On rare occasions, it is necessary to extend the incision transversely through the abdominal wall to safely effect an anastomosis. The fascia is closed in the standard fashion.

Closure of end stoma: Closure of an end stoma usually requires a midline abdominal incision. After entering the peritoneal cavity, the stoma is freed from the abdominal wall. Adhesions are lysed and the dysfunctional distal bowel is identified. It may be necessary to mobilize the proximal bowel to provide a tension-free anastomosis. An anastomosis can then be created using either hand-sewn or stapled techniques.

Paracolostomy hernia repair: The abdomen may be entered via a midline or a peristomal incision. The stoma is freed from the abdominal wall and hernia sac. The stoma is then moved to an alternate site and the defect in the abdominal wall is closed. Alternatively, the stoma may be left in its original site and the fascia closed around the bowel.

Usual preop diagnosis: Stomal stenosis; retraction; parastomal hernia; fistula

SUMMARY OF PROCEDURES

	Closure of Loop Stoma	Closure of End Stoma	Repair of Parastomal Hernia
Position	Supine	Supine or modified lithotomy*	Supine
Incision	Circumstomal	Midline or transverse abdominal	Midline or circumstomal
Special instrumentation	Anastomotic staplers	Endoscope for closure of Hartmann's procedure	Prosthetic mesh
Antibiotics**	Cefotetan 2 g iv	⇐	⇐
Surgical time	1-1.5 h	1-3 h	⇐
Closing considerations	Requires only a few fascial sutures; skin may be left open.	None	Stoma matured after abdomen closed.
EBL	< 100 ml	100-500 ml	< 100 ml
Mortality	1%	2-4%	1%
Morbidity	Anastomotic leak	⇐	Recurrent hernia
	SBO	⇐	Peristomal infection
	Wound infection	⇐	Stomal ischemia
Pain score	5	8	6

PATIENT POPULATION CHARACTERISTICS

Age range	Variable
Male:Female	1:1
Incidence	Not uncommon

* The modified lithotomy position is used for closure of a Hartmann's procedure when an endoscope or stapling device may need to be passed through the anus.

** Bowel prep consists of mechanical cleaning of the colon, accomplished with cathartics or lavage solutions, as well as oral antibiotics. A commonly used regimen is: neomycin 1 g po and erythromycin base 1 g po, given at 1 pm, 2 pm and 10 pm on the night before surgery.

Etiology	Protection or avoiding an insecure anastomosis; traumatic injuries to the colon; complete colonic obstruction; colonic infections, such as diverticulitis; inflammatory processes, such as Crohn's disease or ulcerative colitis; after-emergency resection for ischemic colitis
Associated conditions	Multiple trauma; inflammatory bowel disease (IBD); colon cancer; gut ischemia

References

1. Amin SN, Memon MA, Armitage NC, Scholefield JH: Defunctioning loop ileostomy and stapled side-to-side closure has low morbidity. *Ann Royal Coll Surgeons England* 2001; 83(4):246-9.
2. Cheung MT, Chia NH, Chiu WY: Surgical treatment of parastomal hernia complicating sigmoid colostomies. *Dis Colon Rect* 2001; 44(2):266-70.
3. Doberneck RC: Revision and closure of the colostomy. *Surg Clin North Am* 1991; 71(1):193-201.
4. Edwards DP, Chisholm EM, Donaldson DR: Closure of transverse loop colostomy and loop ileostomy. *Ann Royal Coll Surgeons England* 1998; 80(1):33-5.
5. Ghorra SG, Rzeczycki TP, Natarajan R, Pricolo VE: Colostomy closure: impact of preoperative risk factors on morbidity. *Am Surgeon* 1999; 65(3):266-9.
6. Kald A, Landin S, Masreliez C, Sjodahl R: Mesh repair of parastomal hernias: new aspects of the onlay technique. *Tech Coloproctol* 2001; 5(3):169-71.
7. Khoury DA, Beck DE, Opelka FG, Hicks TC, Timmcke AE, Gathright JB Jr: Colostomy closure. Ochsner Clinic experience. *Dis Colon Rect* 1996; 39(6):605-9.
8. Londono-Schimmer EE, Leong AP, Phillips RK: Life table analysis of stomal complications following colostomy. *Dis Colon Rect* 1994; 37(9):916-20.
9. Rubin MS, Schoetz DJ Jr, Matthews JB: Parastomal hernia. Is stoma relocation superior to fascial repair? *Arch Surg* 1994; 129(4):413-9.

ANESTHETIC CONSIDERATIONS FOR LARGE BOWEL SURGERY

(Procedures covered: total proctocolectomy; partial colectomy with anastomosis; colostomy; stoma closure and peristomal hernia repair)

PREOPERATIVE

Patients presenting for this group of surgical procedures have in common an increased risk for pulmonary aspiration. In addition, patients with bowel obstruction must be treated urgently as the obstruction may rapidly progress to bowel necrosis, perforation, and septic shock. Patients with IBD (e.g., ulcerative colitis, Crohn's disease) may have extracolonic manifestations of the disease (e.g., ankylosing spondylitis, liver disease, anemia), requiring modification of their anesthetic plan.

Respiratory	Patients may have respiratory insufficiency 2° pulmonary metastases (colon cancer) or acute abdominal process (e.g., pain, splinting, sepsis, metabolic acidosis) and bowel distention limiting diaphragmatic excursion (↓TV, ↓FRC). Arthritis associated with IBD → ↓neck ROM → difficult intubation. **Tests:** Consider CXR, ABG.
Cardiovascular	Hemodynamic instability 2° sepsis or pain (↑HR, ↓BP). Hypovolemia 2° poor po intake, vomiting, diarrhea, and bowel prep. Should restore intravascular volume and hemodynamic stability before induction of anesthesia. **Tests:** Orthostatic VS; ECG
Renal	Electrolyte abnormalities (hypokalemic hypochloremic metabolic alkalosis from vomiting or NG suctioning, hyperchloremic metabolic acidosis from diarrhea) are common and may be worsened by bowel prep. **Tests:** Electrolytes
Gastrointestinal	A NG tube is usually in place and the stomach should be emptied before induction of anesthesia. IBD may be associated with impaired liver function and altered drug metabolism.
Hematologic	Hemoconcentration due to GI fluid loss; anemia due to acute/chronic GI bleeding **Tests:** CBC with Plt
Laboratory	Other tests as indicated from H&P.
Premedication	Light standard premedication (p. B-2) is usually appropriate. For aspiration prophylaxis, ranitidine 50 mg iv 1 h before induction, followed by Na citrate (30 ml, 0.3 M po) 10 min before induction,

Premedication, cont.	will significantly decrease the acidity of gastric contents. Metoclopramide is contraindicated in patients with bowel obstruction or perforation. Patients with IBD on chronic steroid therapy should receive their usual daily dose of steroids throughout the periop period and may require full stress-dose steroids. (Glucocorticoid-dependent, critically ill patients requiring vasopressors should be tested for adrenocortical insufficiency and started on 100 mg iv hydrocortisone immediately.)

INTRAOPERATIVE

Anesthetic technique: GETA ± epidural for postop analgesia. Thoracic epidural is associated with improved postop pain control, earlier return of bowel function, intake of food, and out-of-bed mobilization. Placement of catheter before anesthetic induction is helpful to establish correct placement in the epidural space (accomplished by injecting 5-7 ml of 1% lidocaine via the epidural catheter, eliciting a segmental block).

Induction	The patient with an acute abdominal process is at risk for pulmonary aspiration; trachea should be intubated with patient awake or after rapid-sequence induction with cricoid pressure (p. B-5). A NG tube does not interfere with cricoid pressure and may be left in place. If patient is clinically hypovolemic, restore intravascular volume (colloid, crystalloid, or blood), before induction and titrate induction dose of sedative/hypnotic agents.	
Maintenance	Standard maintenance (p. B-3) without N_2O. **Combined epidural/GA:** local anesthetic (1.5-2% lidocaine with 1:200,000 epinephrine (5-10 ml q 60-90 min) can be injected into the epidural catheter to provide both anesthesia and optimal surgical exposure (contracted bowel and profound muscle relaxation). A continuous infusion of local anesthetic (e.g., 0.25% or 0.125% bupivacaine at 4-8 ml/h may enhance hemodynamic stability compared to bolus technique. A loading dose of epidural opiate (e.g., hydromorphone 0.4-0.8 mg) should be administered at least 1 h before conclusion of surgery for optimal results. Patients receiving epidural opiates should be monitored for development of delayed postop respiratory depression and systemic sedatives (e.g., opiates, benzodiazepines) should be minimized.	
Emergence	The decision to extubate at the end of surgery depends on the patient's underlying cardiopulmonary status and extent of surgical procedure. Patient should be hemodynamically stable, warm, alert, and cooperative, and fully reversed from any muscle relaxants before extubation, and have adequate return of pulmonary function (as measured by VC of 15 ml/kg, MIF of -25 cmH_2O, RR < 25 and ABG that approaches patient's baseline).	
Blood and fluid requirements	Anticipate large 3rd-space losses. IV: 14-16 ga × 1 NS/LR @ 10-15 ml/kg/h Fluid warmer T&C for 4 U PRBCs.	Plt, FFP, and cryoprecipitate should be administered according to lab tests (Plt count, PT, PTT, DIC screen). NS preferable to LR for fluid replacement in patients with metabolic alkalosis.
Monitoring	Standard monitors (p. B-1) UO ± Arterial line ± CVP Temperature	Arterial line and CVP, as indicated by patient's status. Hypothermia may delay healing and predispose patients to wound infections. Avoid hypothermia with forced-air warmer, heated humidifier, warming blanket, warming room temperature, keeping patient covered until ready for prep.
Positioning	✓ and pad pressure points. ✓ eyes.	
Complications	Septic shock	Hemodynamic instability 2° sepsis, hemorrhage, especially during manipulation of necrotic bowel.

POSTOPERATIVE

Complications	Hypoxemia Hemodynamic instability Sepsis	Patients with metabolic alkalosis receiving opiates are especially prone to hypoxemia/hypoventilation. Patients may have considerable 3rd-space losses, require invasive monitoring, ICU admission, vasopressors.

Pain management	Epidural analgesia (p. C-2)
	PCA (p. C-3)
Tests	CBC; CXR (if central line placed);
	electrolytes; glucose

References

1. Brown CJ, Buie W: Perioperative stress dose steroids: Do they make a difference? *J Am Coll Surg* 2001; 193(6):678-86.
2. Carli F, Mayo N, Klubien K, Schricker T, Trudel J, Belliveau P: Epidural analgesia enhances functional exercise capacity and health-related quality of life after colonic surgery: Results of a randomized trial. *Anesthesiology* 2002; 97(3):540-9.
3. Carli F, Trudel J, Belliveau P: The effect of intraoperative thoracic epidural anesthesia and postoperative analgesia on bowel function after colorectal surgery: A prospective, randomized trial. *Dis Colon Rect* 2001; 44(8):1083-9.
4. Kurz A, Sessler D, Lenhardt R: Perioperative normothermia to reduce the incidence of surgical-wound infection and shorten hospitalization. *New Eng J Med* 1996; 334(19):1209-15.

OPERATIONS FOR RECTAL PROLAPSE

SURGICAL CONSIDERATIONS

Description: Rectal prolapse (procidentia) is intussusception of the full thickness of the rectal wall beyond the anal canal. It must be distinguished from rectal mucosal prolapse, caused by elongation of the mucosal attachments to the underlying sphincter muscle, and internal intussusception, where the upper rectum folds into the lower rectum, but does not descend through the sphincter mechanism. Rectal mucosal prolapse is treated as part of the spectrum of hemorrhoidal disease, and mild-to-moderate intussusception does not benefit from surgery. Procidentia is associated frequently with anal incontinence. The surgical approaches to procidentia are determined by patient age, concurrent medical disease, sphincter function, and operative Hx.

Surgical treatment of procidentia may be undertaken through an abdominal or a perineal approach. The **abdominal approaches** have a lower recurrence rate and, because they do not diminish the capacity of the rectal reservoir, are generally preferable for maintaining fecal continence. **Rectopexy** is an abdominal approach in which the rectum is mobilized in the posterior plane from the sacral promontory to the levator muscles. The rectum is then pulled cephalad and sutured to the presacral fascia with multiple nonabsorbable sutures. Many surgeons routinely perform **sigmoid resection** along with rectopexy. They contend that removal of the redundant sigmoid further diminishes the chance of late recurrence and may alleviate constipation. The rectum also may be suspended by use of a sling attached to the rectum and secured to the presacral fascia. A number of approaches have been described, the most popular being the **Ripstein procedure**. **Sling procedures** have equivalent recurrence rates but higher complication rates. As in rectopexy, the rectum is mobilized along the presacral plane down to the level of the levators. A band of Marlex mesh is sewn to the presacral fascia at the sacral promontory, upward traction is placed on the rectum, and the mesh is sutured to the rectum.

In patients with significant comorbidities, prolapse may be repaired via a **perineal approach**. The most common of these is **perineal rectosigmoidectomy** (or **Altmeir procedure**). The prolapsed rectum is withdrawn through the anal canal to its full extent, and a circumferential incision is made in the outer tube of the prolapsed bowel just proximal to the dentate line. This exposes the inner tube of prolapsed bowel and mesentery. Redundant bowel is mobilized from the distal end, up to the point that no additional bowel can be delivered into the operative field. The redundant bowel is transected and a primary anastomosis is fashioned between the cut ends of the inner and outer bowel. Prior to anastomosis, the levator muscles are often approximated in the midline in an effort to aid continence. When the volume of prolapsed tissue is small or a previous abdominal approach makes blood supply to the rectum questionable, the **Delorme procedure** often is performed. During this procedure, the mucosa is stripped off the prolapsed rectum, and the prolapsed rectal muscle is foreshortened by plication until it resides above the sphincters.

Usual preop diagnosis: Full-thickness rectal prolapse (procidentia)

SUMMARY OF PROCEDURES

	Rectopexy	Rectopexy with Sigmoid Resection	Perineal Recto-sigmoidectomy	Delorme Procedure
Position	Lithotomy	⇐	Prone jackknife; lithotomy	⇐
Incision	Low transverse; low midline	⇐	No external incision	⇐
Special instrumentation	Deep pelvic instruments; mesh if sling planned	Deep pelvic instruments	Hip-roll for jackknife position; anastomosis may be created with EEA stapler.	Hip-roll for jackknife position
Unique considerations	Presacral venous plexus bleeding may occur; bowel prep may cause dehydration or hypokalemia.	⇐	Epinephrine solutions may be used to diminish bleeding; bowel prep may cause dehydration or hypokalemia.	⇐
Antibiotics	Cefotetan 2 g iv	⇐	⇐	⇐
Surgical time	1-2 h	⇐	⇐	⇐
EBL	< 100 ml; more if reoperation	100-300 ml; more if reoperation	100-200 ml	100 ml
Postop care	No rectal probes or medications	⇐	⇐	⇐
Mortality	0-2%	0-4%	1-4%	0-1%
Morbidity	Rectal stricture (with sling): 5-10%	–	–	–
	Recurrent prolapse: 2-8%	2-5%	20-40%	5-10%
	Pelvic infection: 5%	–	–	–
		Anastomotic leak: 2-4%	–	–
Pain score	7	7	2	2

PATIENT POPULATION CHARACTERISTICS

Age range	Women: peak incidence in 6th-7th decade; men: evenly distributed through age range
Male:Female	1:4
Incidence	Unknown
Etiology	Decreased pelvic muscular support; congenital deficiency of rectal support; pudendal neuropathy; chronic constipation and straining; multiparity; myelomeningocele; spina bifida; cystic fibrosis (children); acute parasitic diarrheal illness (children)
Associated conditions	Fecal incontinence; urinary stress incontinence; rectocele; cystocele

ANESTHETIC CONSIDERATIONS

See Anesthetic Considerations following Operations for Fecal Incontinence, p. 436.

References

1. Hayashi S, Masuda H, et al: Simple Technique for repair of complete rectal prolapse using a circular stapler with Thiersch procedure. *Eur J Surg* 2002; 168(2):124-7.
2. Lechaux JP, et al: Prosthetic rectopexy to the pelvic floor and sigmoidectomy for rectal prolapse. *Am J Surg* 2001; 182:465-9.
3. Liberman H, Hughes C, et al: Evaluation and outcome of the Delorme procedure in the treatment of rectal outlet obstruction. *Dis Colon Rectum* 2000; 43(2):188-92
4. Schultz I, et al: Long-term results and functional outcome after Ripstein rectopexy. *Dis Colon Rectum* 2000; 43: 35-43.
5. Solomon MJ, Young CJ, et al: Randomized clinical trial of laparoscopic versus open abdominal rectopexy for rectal prolapse. *Br J Surg* 2002; 89(1):35-9.
6. Zbar AP, Takashima S, et al: Perineal rectosigmoidectomy (Altemeier's procedure): a review of physiology, technique and outcome. *Tech Coloproctol* 2002; 6(2):109-16.

RECTAL SURGERY

SURGICAL CONSIDERATIONS

Description: Many lesions within the distal two-thirds of the rectum can be excised through a **transanal approach**. The most common benign tumors treated by local excision are adenomas. Lesions such as carcinoid tumor, endometrioma, and solitary rectal ulcer also may be locally excised. **Transanal excision** of benign lesions may be performed in the submucosal plane, while suspected malignancies are excised by removing the entire thickness of the rectal wall. A full antibiotic and mechanical bowel prep is given. Transanal excision usually is performed in the prone jackknife position, although the lithotomy position may be used when the lesion is located on the posterior rectal wall. A local anal block, usually 0.25% bupivacaine, with 1:200,000 epinephrine, is performed to relax the sphincter mechanism and minimize sphincter injury, aid in hemostasis, and diminish postop pain. An anoscope is inserted into the anal canal. Stay sutures may be placed adjacent to the area of resection. On occasion, lesions may be prolapsed all the way through the anus and excised outside of the body. Generally, the dissection starts at the distal end of the lesion and proceeds proximally. The proctotomy may be closed with running or interrupted sutures. These sutures are then grasped and used for further traction. When the specimen is removed, a few final sutures are needed to close the proximal-most incision. **Rigid proctoscopy** is performed to confirm preservation of an adequate lumen.

Variant procedure or approaches: The **transsacral (Kraske)**[1] **approach** to rectal tumors offers wider exposure than the transanal approach, but is more painful and has a substantially greater likelihood of complications (wound infection, fecal fistula, incontinence). A transsacral approach may be advantageous when the lesion is located behind the rectum (retrorectal tumors) and when resection of the lower sacrum or coccyx is anticipated. Transsacral resection generally is performed in the prone jackknife position. An incision is made from the posterior commissure of the anus to the base of the sacrum. The sphincter muscles are spared, but the levator muscles are divided to expose the posterior wall of the rectum. The coccyx may be disarticulated and removed to improve exposure. It is also possible to remove the lower sacral segments through this approach, but increasing morbidity accrues as the sacral nerve roots are sacrificed. For a posterior-wall lesion, the posterior wall of the rectum is opened and the lesion, along with a full-thickness disc of rectal wall, is excised. If the lesion is on the anterior wall, two proctotomy incisions are necessary. The proctotomy incisions are closed with standard anastomotic techniques. The levator muscles are reapproximated and the skin is closed. A drain may be placed within the retrorectal space before closing. The transsacral approach may be combined with an abdominal approach (**abdominal-transsacral resection**) in some cases of low rectal cancer.

The **transsphincteric (Mason)**[12] **approach** to rectal lesions also gives wider exposure than does the transanal approach, but at the expense of a substantially greater risk of fecal incontinence. Transsphincteric excision is performed with the patient in the prone jackknife position. An incision is made at the posterior commissure of the anus and is extended along the lateral border of the coccyx and sacrum. The external sphincter, internal sphincter and levator ani muscles are sequentially transected in the posterior midline. As each muscle is cut, the cut edges are tagged with sutures to facilitate accurate reapproximation. The rectal wall is incised and the lesion is excised. The proctotomy incision is closed via standard anastomotic suturing techniques, and the individual components of the sphincter muscle are reapproximated with interrupted sutures. The overlying skin is closed in a standard fashion.

Usual preop diagnosis: Villous adenoma; tubular adenoma; adenocarcinoma; carcinoid tumor; endometrioma; solitary rectal ulcer; retrorectal tumors (in decreasing frequency)

SUMMARY OF PROCEDURES

	Transanal Excision	Transsacral Excision	Transsphincteric Excision
Position	Prone jackknife or lithotomy	Prone jackknife	⇐
Incision	Intrarectal	Anus-to-lateral sacral wall	⇐
Special instrumentation	Rigid proctoscope; headlight and/ or fiber optic retractors; Foley catheter	Gigli or power saw if sacral resection contemplated; headlight and/or fiber optic retractors; Foley catheter	Headlight and/or fiber optic retractors; Foley catheter
Unique considerations	Bowel prep may → dehydration and hypokalemia.	⇐	⇐
Antibiotics	Cefotetan 2 g iv	⇐	⇐
Surgical time	15-120 min	1-2 h	⇐
EBL	< 100 ml	< 100 ml (500 ml if sacral resection)	⇐

	Transanal Excision	Transsacral Excision	Transsphincteric Excision
Postop care	No rectal temperatures, suppositories, or enemas	⇐	⇐
Mortality[1,2,9,11]	0-2%	⇐	⇐
Morbidity[1,2,9,11]	Tumor recurrence: 5-50%	50%	5-50%
	Urinary retention: 10-20%	⇐	⇐
	Bleeding: 2-5%	⇐	⇐
	Pelvic sepsis: 0-4%	⇐	⇐
	Ureteral injury: < 1% (minimized by use of Foley)	⇐	⇐
		Fecal fistula: 10-30%	–
		Fecal incontinence: 5-10%	10-40%
Pain score	3	7	7

PATIENT POPULATION CHARACTERISTICS

Age range	Rectal adenomas – 5th-7th decades; rectal adenocarcinoma – 6th-9th decades; endometrioma – 2nd-4th decades; solitary rectal ulcer syndrome – 4th-8th decades; carcinoid tumors – 5th-8th decades
Male:Female	1:1
Incidence	Varies with disease; not uncommon
Etiology	Varies with disease
Associated conditions	Preexisting anorectal pathology, such as fecal incontinence, may require concurrent treatment

ANESTHETIC CONSIDERATIONS

See Anesthetic Considerations following Operations for Fecal Incontinence, p. 436.

References

1. Bleday R, Breen E, et al: Prospective evaluation of local excision for small rectal cancers. *Dis Colon Rectum* 1997; 40(4): 388-92.
2. Chapuis P, Bokey L, Fahrer M, Sinclair G, Bogduk N: Mobilization of the rectum: anatomic concepts and the bookshelf revisited. *Dis Colon Rect*; 2002; 45(1):1-9.
3. Demartines N, von Flue MO, et al: Transanal endoscopic microsurgical excision of rectal tumors: indications and results. *World J Surg* 2001; 25(7):870-5.
4. Dorudi S, Steele RJ, McArdle CS: Surgery for colorectal cancer. *Brit Med Bull* 2002; 64:101-18.
5. Glimelius BL: The role of preoperative and postoperative radiotherapy in rectal cancer. *Clin Colorect Can* 2002; 2(2): 82-92.
6. Gould TH, Grace K, Thorne G, Thomas M: Effect of thoracic epidural anaesthesia on colonic blood flow. *Brit J Anaesth* 2002; 89(3):446-51.
7. Kanemitsu T, Kojima T, et al: The trans-sphincteric and trans-sacral approaches for the surgical excision of rectal and pre-sacral lesions. *Surg Today* 1993; 23(10):860-6.
8. Kapiteijn E, van de Velde CJ: Developments and quality assurance in rectal cancer surgery. *Euro J Cancer* 2002; 38(7): 919-36.
9. Mendenhall WM, Morris CG, et L: Local excision and postoperative radiation therapy for rectal adenocarcinoma. *Int J Cancer* 2001; 96(Suppl): 89-96.
10. Minsky BD. Adjuvant therapy of resectable rectal cancer. *Cancer Treat Rev* 2002; 28(4):181-8.
11. Moore HG, Guillem JG: Local therapy for rectal cancer. *Surg Clin North Am* 2002; 82(5):967-81
12. Paty PB, Nash GM, et al: Long-term results of local excision for rectal cancer. *Ann Surg* 2002; 236(4):522-30.
13. Rothenberger DA, Garcia-Aguilar J: Role of local excision in the treatment of rectal cancer. *Semin Surg Oncol* 2000; 19(4): 367-75.
14. Schrag D, Panageas KS, Riedel E, Cramer LD, Guillem JG, Bach PB, Begg CB: Hospital and surgeon procedure volume as predictors of outcome following rectal cancer resection. *Ann Surg* 2002; 236(5):583-92.
15. Sengupta S, Tjandra JJ: Local excision of rectal cancer: what is the evidence? *Dis Colon Rectum* 2001; 44(9):1345-61.
16. Visser BC, Varma MG, et al: Local therapy for rectal cancer. *Surg Oncol* 2001; 10(1-2):61-9.

ANAL FISTULOTOMY/FISTULECTOMY

SURGICAL CONSIDERATIONS

Description: The majority of perianal fistulae are 2° infection in the anal glands within the rectal wall that communicates with crypts located at the dentate line (cryptoglandular fistula). Fistulae also may be the result of trauma, Crohn's disease, inflammatory processes within the peritoneal cavity, neoplasms, or as a consequence of radiation therapy. The ultimate treatment of fistula-in-ano is determined by the etiology and the anatomic course of the fistula. The principle behind treatment of cryptoglandular fistulae is to ablate the offending gland and lay open the tract. Fistulae that track above the majority of the sphincter mechanism must be treated by procedures that either do not cut the overlying sphincter, cut the sphincter and repair it, or cut the sphincter very gradually (**seton**, see below). A fistula may be treated at the time of drainage of a perianal abscess or as a separate, elective operation. The route of a fistula tract is best determined by exploration at the time of operation. While local anesthesia is acceptable for most fistulae, a few fistula operations require regional or general anesthesia because the ultimate route and depth of the fistula is unknown. Special consideration is given to fistulae that arise in the setting of Crohn's disease. Poor wound healing and the importance of sphincter function in patients with chronic diarrhea dictate that only the most superficial fistulae be laid open. The primary goal is palliation; specifically, abscess drainage and recurrence prevention. This is often accomplished by placing a Silastic seton (a ligature around sphincter muscles) around the fistula tract and leaving it in place indefinitely. In the absence of active Crohn's disease in the rectum and anus, attempts at fistula cure may be undertaken.

Variant procedure or approaches: Fistulotomy involves cutting all tissues superficial to a fistula so that the fistula tract is brought to the skin level. The opened, fibrotic fistula wall is often sewn to the skin edge (marsupialized). **Fistulectomy** involves excision of the entire fistula tract. When conventional fistulotomy would cause incontinence, a **seton** may be used. Other approaches that may be used to avoid fecal incontinence are **complete fistulotomy with immediate reconstruction** of the sphincter and excision of the internal opening by an **endorectal advancement flap** technique.

Usual preop diagnosis: Fistula-in-ano

SUMMARY OF PROCEDURES

	Fistulotomy or Fistulectomy	Fistulotomy with Seton	Endorectal Advancement Flap
Position	Prone jackknife; rarely lithotomy	⇐	Prone jackknife
Incision	Perianal	⇐	⇐
Antibiotics	Cefotetan 2 g iv	–	Cefotetan 2 g iv
Surgical time	10-30 min	⇐	60-90 min
EBL	< 50 ml	⇐	⇐
Mortality	Minimal	⇐	⇐
Morbidity	Fecal incontinence: 0-30% Nonhealing, or recurrent fistula: 5%	10-30% 10-20%. (This procedure used only in complex fistulae, so complication rate appears higher.)	0-10% 10-40%. (This procedure used only in complex fistulae, so complication rate appears higher.)
Pain score	6	6	6

PATIENT POPULATION CHARACTERISTICS

Age range	2nd-7th decades
Male:Female	2:1
Incidence	Common
Etiology	Infection within anal glands located at dentate line (cryptoglandular fistula); trauma; Crohn's disease; inflammatory processes within the peritoneal cavity; neoplasms; consequence of radiation therapy

ANESTHETIC CONSIDERATIONS

See Anesthetic Considerations following Operations for Fecal Incontinence, p. 436.

References

1. Garcia-Aguilar J, et al: Patient satisfaction after surgical treatment for fistula-in-ano. *Dis Colon Rectum* 2000; 43:1206-12.

2. Hasegawa H, et al: Long-term results of cutting seton fistulotomy. *Acta Chir Iugosl* 2000; 47(S):19-21.
3. Ho YH, et al: Marsupialization of fistulotomy wounds improves healing (RCT). *Br J Surg* 1998; 85:105-7.
4. Knoefel WT, Hosch SB, et al: The initial approach to anorectal abscesses: fistulotomy is safe and reduces the chance of recurrence. *Dig Surg* 2000; 17(3):274-8.
5. Ortiz H, Marzo J: Endorectal flap advancement repair and fistulectomy for high trans-sphincteric and suprasphincteric fistulas. *Br J Surg* 2000; 87(12):1680-3.
6. Zimmerman DD, et al: Anocutaneous advancement flap repair of transsphincteric fistulas. *Dis Colon Rectum* 2001; 44: 1474-80.

HEMORRHOIDECTOMY

SURGICAL CONSIDERATIONS

Description: Hemorrhoids are normally occurring vascular tissues, located in discrete aggregations, known as hemorrhoidal cushions, within the distal rectum and anus. Thought to play a role in the fine control of enteric continence, they are only treated if they cause a symptom that persists after conservative therapy. Hemorrhoids may bleed, prolapse, and cause mucous drainage, itching, or pain (when thrombosed). The primary pathophysiologic event in the development of symptomatic hemorrhoids is thought to be mucosal prolapse 2° degeneration of the fibroelastic tissue that tethers vascular cushions and overlying mucosa to the submucosa. Many modern treatments diminish prolapse by fixing the mucosa to the submucosa with scar tissue. Hemorrhoids are classified as internal (when above the dentate line) or external (when below). Internal hemorrhoids are further classified by symptoms: I–bleed; II–bleed, prolapse, and spontaneously reduce; III–bleed, prolapse, and require manual reduction; IV–bleed, prolapse, and cannot be reduced. The most common symptom from external hemorrhoids is severe pain caused by thrombosis. Surgical treatment involves excision of the thrombosed hemorrhoid, often under local anesthetic, in the office. Internal hemorrhoids may be treated by nonexcisional or excisional techniques. Nonexcisional techniques generally are used in the office or outpatient clinic. They do not require an anesthetic because their use is limited to the insensate tissues above the dentate line. Nonexcisional treatments include **rubber-band ligation**, **infrared coagulation**, **sclerotherapy**, and **cryotherapy**.

Surgical hemorrhoidectomy may be performed in the lithotomy or prone jackknife position. An anoscope is placed in the anal canal and a hemorrhoid column is grasped and tented up into the lumen. A suture is placed at the internal apex of the complex. An incision is started at the external apex of the hemorrhoidal complex and a plane is developed deep to the hemorrhoidal tissue and superficial to the sphincter muscles. When the internal sphincter is identified, the dissection proceeds in the avascular space along its lumenal surface. The dissection is continued up into the rectum to the transfixing suture. Lateral incisions along the redundant tissue are completed to excise the hemorrhoid. Care is taken to leave healthy bridges of mucosa between adjacent hemorrhoidal columns. Hemostasis is obtained with cautery and the mucosal defect may be closed with a running, absorbable suture. It also is acceptable to leave the mucosal wound open. The procedure is repeated over the other enlarged, symptomatic hemorrhoidal complexes, removing redundant tissue and leaving long, vertical scars to prevent further mucosal prolapse.

Variant procedure or approaches: The **Whitehead hemorrhoidectomy (circumferential hemorrhoidectomy)** and **Lord procedure (sphincter stretch)** have been largely abandoned. **Lasers** have not been shown to improve results in the treatment of hemorrhoids.

Rubber-band ligation requires no anesthesia because the band is placed on the insensate, distal rectal mucosa. An anoscope is inserted into the anal canal to visualize a hemorrhoid column. The most proximal area of redundant mucosa is grasped with a clamp and pulled into the barrel of the ligation gun. A rubber band is placed on the base of the tented-up hemorrhoid tissue. The encompassed tissue sloughs over 4-7 d, and a scar is formed between the mucosa and the underlying muscle.

Usual preop diagnosis: Symptomatic hemorrhoids; bleeding, and/or prolapse

SUMMARY OF PROCEDURE

Position	Prone jackknife, lithotomy or left lateral decubitus
Incision	Series of vertical incisions from anal verge to top of hemorrhoid columns
Special instrumentation	Headlight or lighted anoscope; operating anoscope
Antibiotics	None
Surgical time	30-90 min
EBL	< 100 ml
Postop care	Sitz baths, oral fluids, fiber supplements
Mortality	Rare
Morbidity	Urinary retention: 15-30%
	Incontinence: 1-6%
	Bleeding: 2-5%
	Stricture: 2-5%
	Infection: 1-2%
Pain score	9

PATIENT POPULATION CHARACTERISTICS

Age range	Peak prevalence 45-65 yr
Male:Female	1:1
Incidence	Prevalence 75/1,000
Etiology	Low-fiber diet; genetic; pregnancy
Associated conditions	Constipation

ANESTHETIC CONSIDERATIONS

See Anesthetic Considerations following Operations for Fecal Incontinence (p. 436).

References

1. Correa-Rovelo JM, et al: Stapled rectal mucosectomy vs. closed hemorrhoidectomy (RCT). *Dis Colon Rectum* 2002; 45: 1367-75.
2. Gabrielli F, Chiarelli M, et al: Day surgery for mucosal-hemorrhoidal prolapse using a circular stapler and modified regional anesthesia. *Dis Colon Rectum* 2001; 44:842-4.
3. Gencosmanoglu R, et al: Hemorrhoidectomy: open or closed technique? (RCT). *Dis Colon Rectum* 2002; 45:70-5.
4. Hetzer FH, Demartines N, et al: Stapled vs excision hemorrhoidectomy: long-term results of a prospective randomized trial. *Arch Surg* 2002; 137(3):337-40.
5. Hussein AM: Ligation-anopexy for treatment of advanced hemorrhoidal disease. *Dis Colon Rectum* 2001; 44:1887-90.
6. Khan S, Pawlak SE, et al: Surgical treatment of hemorrhoids: prospective, randomized trial comparing closed excisional hemorrhoidectomy and the Harmonic Scalpel technique of excisional hemorrhoidectomy. *Dis Colon Rectum* 2001; 44: 845-9.
7. Konsten J, Baeten CG: Hemorrhoidectomy vs. Lord's method: 17-year follow-up. *Dis Colon Rectum* 2000; 43:503-6.
8. Moore BA, Fleshner PR: Rubber band ligation for hemorrhoidal disease can be safely performed in select HIV-positive patients. *Dis Colon Rectum* 2001; 44:1079-82.

OPERATIONS FOR FECAL INCONTINENCE

SURGICAL CONSIDERATIONS

Description: In the majority of patients, fecal incontinence is caused by a combination of pudendal neuropathy and atrophy of pelvic floor muscles. Only when an anatomic defect in the sphincter mechanism can be identified, is surgery likely to be beneficial. **Sphincteroplasty** is performed in the prone jackknife position after a full mechanical bowel prep. An incision is made at the anal verge, centered over the area of injured sphincter, and extended sufficiently around the anus to reach the retracted, cut edges of the sphincter. The anoderm and rectal mucosa are dissected off of the internal surface of the sphincter. The external surface of the sphincter mechanism is then dissected free to the level of the pelvic diaphragm. Care must be taken not to injure the inferior hemorrhoidal nerves during dissection around the posterior-lateral sphincter. The fibrotic portion linking the two ends of sphincter is cut, and the ends are overlapped and secured in place with two layers of interrupted horizontal mattress sutures. In women with obstetric injuries, the transverse perineal muscles are reapproximated. The skin may be reapproximated at the anal verge and along the reconstructed perineum or left open. The remainder of the skin is closed as completely as possible.

Variant procedure or approaches: The surgical options for patients without anatomic defects in their sphincters are generally unsuccessful. The **posterior anoplasty of Parks** was designed to passively enhance continence by increasing the normally occurring angle between the rectum and the anal canal, and to increase the mechanical efficiency of weak sphincter muscle by shortening the fiber length. Lack of efficacy has limited its use, although some surgeons still perform it in the setting of continued incontinence after abdominal repair of rectal prolapse. The operation is performed in the prone jackknife position after a standard bowel prep. A hemispherical incision is placed at the level of the intersphincteric groove over the posterior half of the anus. The plane between the internal and external anal sphincters is identified and developed proximally to above the puborectalis musculus. The puborectalis fibers are 'reefed,' or pulled together, as far as possible with nonabsorbable suture. The external sphincter is plicated together in the midline with a series of nonabsorbable sutures that start at the deep external sphincter and progress to the subcutaneous sphincter. Skin is closed with absorbable sutures.

The **Thiersch operation (pinch graft)** has a high complication rate and should be considered pimarily in debilitated patients with symptomatic rectal prolapse or fecal incontinence. As originally described, the anal canal was encircled with a silver wire, which served as a passive obstacle to prolapse or defecation. In more recent years, an elastic sheet of Dacron-impregnated Silastic mesh has been used. Two small incisions are made on opposite sides of the anal verge. A pathway around the anal canal is created by blunt dissection and a 1.5 cm-wide piece of mesh is led around the anal canal. The ends of the mesh are overlapped in one of the incisions and either sutured or stapled together at an appropriate level of tension. The wounds are irrigated with antibiotic solution and the incisions are closed.

Usual preop diagnosis: Fecal (enteric) incontinence

SUMMARY OF PROCEDURES

	Overlapping Sphincteroplasty	Parks Repair	Modified Thiersch Procedure
Position	Prone jackknife	⇐	Prone jackknife or lithotomy
Incision	Circumanal	⇐	2 small incisions lateral to the anus
Special instrumentation	Headlight	⇐	Headlight; Silastic mesh
Unique considerations	Urinary catheter preop; standard bowel prep	⇐	None
Antibiotics	Cefotetan 2 g	⇐	⇐
Surgical time	1-2 h	1 h	30-45 min
EBL	< 100 ml	⇐	⇐
Postop care	Early: Sitz baths	⇐	⇐
	Late: fiber supplement, stool softener	⇐	⇐
Mortality	Rare	⇐	⇐
Morbidity	Unimproved incontinence: 20%	60-80%	20%
	Improved, but minor incontinence: 30%	–	Erosion of prosthesis: 30-60%
	Prolonged wound healing: 20%	–	Obstructed defecation: 20-40%
	Infection: 1-2%	–	Infection
Pain score	8	7	6

PATIENT POPULATION CHARACTERISTICS

Age range	Bimodal: 3rd-5th decades for obstetric injury, fistulotomy, and perineal trauma; 6th-8th decades for pudendal neuropathy/pelvic floor atrophy
Male:Female	1:4
Incidence	Not uncommon
Etiology	Pudendal neuropathy; pelvic floor atrophy; obstetric injury; injury during anal surgery (fistulotomy, sphincterotomy, hemorrhoidectomy); perineal trauma; neurologic disease; congenital anomalies
Associated conditions	Urinary incontinence; chronic constipation; multiparity

ANESTHETIC CONSIDERATIONS

(Procedures covered: excision or repair of rectal prolapse; rectal surgery; anal fistulotomy/fistulectomy; anal sphincterotomy/sphincteroplasty; hemorrhoidectomy; operations for fecal incontinence)

PREOPERATIVE

Respiratory	A careful evaluation of patient's respiratory status is important. If patient has ↓ reserve, the lithotomy position may be better tolerated than the prone or jackknife positions. **Tests:** As indicated from H&P.
Musculoskeletal	Pain is likely to be present at the surgical site and should be considered when positioning patient for anesthetic induction (e.g., if patient has pain while sitting, perform regional anesthesia in the lateral decubitus position). Evaluate bony landmarks if regional anesthetic is planned.
Hematologic	Patients rarely anemic from chronic GI bleeding **Tests:** CBC
Laboratory	Other tests as indicated from H&P.
Premedication	Standard premedication (p. B-2)

INTRAOPERATIVE

Anesthetic technique: GA, spinal, or epidural techniques may be used.

General anesthesia:

Induction	**General (LMA vs ETT):** Standard induction (p. B-2). Procedures done in the prone or jackknife position may require ET intubation for airway control if regional anesthesia is not performed.
Maintenance	Standard maintenance (p. B-3)
Emergence	No special considerations

Regional anesthesia:

Spinal	Patient in either sitting, lateral decubitus, prone, or jackknife position for placement of a subarachnoid block. Doses of local anesthetics should be adequate to provide a high lumbar level (L1-2) of sensory anesthesia (e.g., lidocaine 5%, 50-75 mg; tetracaine 10-14 mg; bupivacaine 8-12 mg). Patients should remain in relative head-up or head-down position when using hypobaric or hyperbaric solutions to maintain restricted spread of block. Large doses of local anesthetic should be avoided as they may cause postop cauda equina syndrome.
Epidural	Patient in sitting or lateral decubitus position for placement of epidural catheter. A test dose (e.g., 3 ml of 1.5% lidocaine with 1:200,000 epinephrine) is administered and patient is observed for development of a subarachnoid block or symptoms of an intravascular injection. Then titrate 2% lidocaine with epinephrine (3-5 ml at a time) until desired level (usually L1-2 adequate) is obtained.
MAC	Should be performed only on selective patients who are highly motivated and with surgeons experienced in performing procedure with infiltration of local anesthesia (usually 2% lidocaine with 1:200,000 epinephrine and 0.5% bupivacaine mixture). Injection of local anesthetic may be quite painful and very short-acting agents (e.g., propofol 30-50 mg or alfentanil 4-7 μg/kg) should be administered to minimize patient discomfort. As doses vary significantly in patients, they should be administered in small increments. Deep sedation and apnea must be avoided, especially in patients in prone or jackknife positions. A bed must be immediately available to turn patients supine and the anesthesiologist should always be prepared to administer GA if necessary.

Blood and fluid requirements	IV: 16-18 ga × 1 NS/LR @ 5-8 ml/kg/h	Blood not likely to be required.
Monitoring	Standard monitors (p. B-1)	Others as clinically indicated.
Positioning	✓ and pad pressure points. ✓ eyes.	Chest support or bolsters to optimize ventilation in the jackknife position; care in positioning the patient's extremities and genitals after turning into jackknife position. Avoid pressure on eyes and ears after turning patient.
Complications	Peroneal nerve injury	Lithotomy position can → damage to peroneal nerve, resulting in foot drop. Laryngospasm will occur if inadequate depth of anesthesia during anal dilation.

POSTOPERATIVE

Complications	Urinary retention	Catheterize until return of urinary function.
	Cauda equina syndrome	Cauda equina syndrome is characterized by varying degrees of urinary/fecal incontinence, sensory loss in the perineal area, and lower extremity motor weakness.
	Poor wound healing	
	Atelectasis	
Pain management	PCA (p. C-3)	PO analgesics may be suitable: acetaminophen and codeine (Tylenol #3 1-2 tab q 4-6 h) or oxycodone and acetaminophen (Percocet 1 tab q 6 h).
	Epidural analgesia (p. C-2)	
Tests	As indicated by patient status.	

References

1. Bachoo P, Brazelli M, et al: Surgery for faecal incontinence in adults. *Cochrane Database Syst* Rev:(2):CD001757.
2. Barisic G, Krivokapic Z, et al: The role of overlapping sphincteroplasty in traumatic fecal incontinence. *Acta Chir Iugosl* 2000; 47(4 Suppl 1):37-41.
3. Bernard C: Epidural and spinal anesthesia. In *Clinical Anesthesia*, 3rd edition. Barash PG, Cullen BF, Stoelting RK, eds. Lippincott-Raven, Philadelphia: 1997, 645-65.
4. Habr-Gama A: Results of surgical treatment for faecal incontinence. *Tech Coloproctol* 2001; 5(2):118.
5. Malouf AJ, Norton CS, et al: Long-term results of overlapping anterior anal-sphincter repair for obstetric trauma. *Lancet* 2000; 355(9200):260-5.
6. Matsuoka H, Mavrantonis C, et al: Postanal repair for fecal incontinence—is it worthwhile? *Dis Colon Rectum* 2000; 43(11): 1561-7.
7. Parks AG: Anorectal incontinence. President's Address. *Proc R Soc Med* Meeting 27. 1975; 68(11):681-90.
8. Rigler ML, Drasner K, Krejcie TC, Yelich SJ, Scholnick FT, DeFontes J, Bohner D: Cauda equina syndrome after continuous spinal anesthesia. *Anesth Analg* 1991; 72(3):275-81.
9. Wong WD, Congliosi SM, et al: The safety and efficacy of the artificial bowel sphincter for fecal incontinence: results from a multicenter cohort study. *Dis Colon Rectum* 2002; 45(9):1139-53.

Surgeons

Samuel K. S. So, MD, FACS
Harry A. Oberhelman, MD, FACS

7.5 HEPATIC SURGERY

Anesthesiologist

Hendrikus J. M. Lemmens, MD, PhD

HEPATIC RESECTION

SURGICAL CONSIDERATIONS

Samuel K. S. So

Description: Liver resections usually are performed to remove primary tumors or metastatic tumors to the liver. The most common malignant primary liver tumor is hepatocellular carcinoma (HCC), usually caused by chronic hepatitis B or C. Liver resection also is performed for an enlarging hepatic adenoma, a benign primary tumor that is susceptible to rupture. The most common secondary tumors removed are metastases from colorectal cancer. In rare cases, it may be necessary to resect a devitalized area of the liver following trauma. The mortality and morbidity following liver resection depends on the extent of the surgery, experience of the surgeon, and the patient's hepatic function. In general, the risk of resection is higher in patients with primary HCC, where the uninvolved part of the liver frequently is cirrhotic or diseased from chronic hepatitis B or C. Cirrhotic patients with Plt counts < 80,000, portal HTN with varices, ascites, albumin < 3.5 g/L, and prolonged PT are generally unsuitable candidates for major liver resection because of the high risk of postop liver failure.

Intraop blood loss is the most important predictor of short-term survival. Bleeding is largely from intrahepatic branches of portal and hepatic veins injured during the dissection, potentially leading to massive blood loss within minutes. Liver resection often is performed without blood transfusions (Cell Saver should not be used when operating on cancer patients). The mortality rate of liver resection should be < 2-5%. Many patients do not require postop ICU care and are discharged within 4-5 d. Improved outcomes result from better surgical exposure and strategies, and the standard adoption of the CUSA ultrasonic dissector, combined with newer and more effective coagulating devices (e.g., TissueLink dissecting sealer). Intraop ultrasound is very helpful in planning the line of resection and mapping out its relationship with the large intrahepatic portal and hepatic veins.

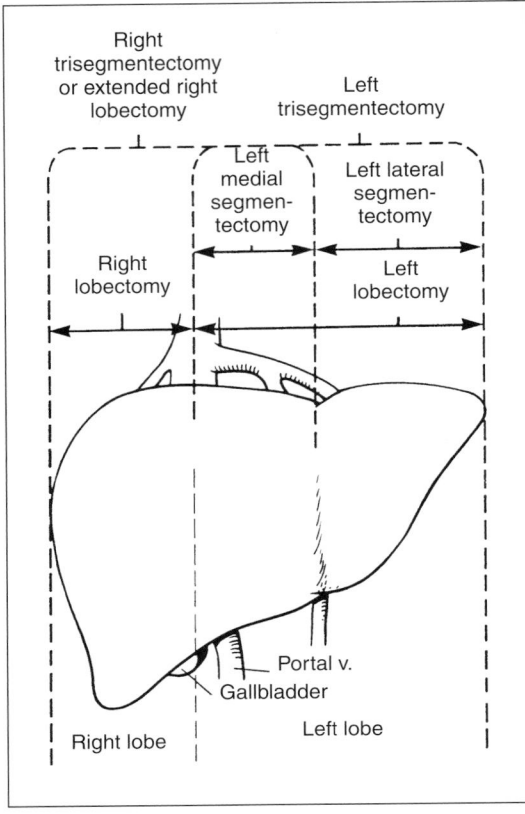

Figure 7.5-1. Types of liver resection. (Reproduced with permission from Hardy JD: *Hardy's Textbook of Surgery*, 2nd edition. JB Lippincott: 1988.)

Anatomic vs nonanatomic liver resection: Until the last decade, most liver surgeons performed anatomic liver resections in which the porta hepatitis is dissected and the corresponding extrahepatic branches of the hepatic artery, portal vein, bile duct, and hepatic vein are mobilized and ligated before resection of the liver parenchyma (Fig 7.5-1). In nonanatomic resection, only the tumor with a margin of 1-2 cm is removed instead of the entire anatomic lobe or segment. This approach is particularly appropriate in patients with cirrhosis or chronic hepatitis, in whom removing too much of the liver will predispose them to hepatic decompensation, and in patients with liver metastases where the risk of recurrence remains high. When nonanatomic resection is performed, dissection of the porta hepatis is unnecessary. Instead, branches of the vessels and hepatic ducts are ligated and resected as they are encountered during the resection of the liver parenchyma.

Temporary occlusion of the hepaticoduodenal ligament that contains the main portal vein, hepatic artery, and common bile duct (**Pringle maneuver**) can be used in resection to minimize blood loss. Most patients will tolerate this maneuver 15-20 min. In some patients, it may be necessary to repeat the maneuver once or twice to complete a major resection.

Usual preop diagnosis: Benign and malignant primary or metastatic tumors of the liver

SUMMARY OF PROCEDURES

	Right/Left Lobectomy/ Trisegmentectomy	**Partial Right Lobectomy**	**Left Lateral Segmentectomy**
Position	Supine	⇐	⇐
Incision	Upper midline, extending to right subcostal	⇐	Upper midline

440

	Right/Left Lobectomy/ Trisegmentectomy	Partial Right Lobectomy	Left Lateral Segmentectomy
Special instrumentation	Thompson liver retractor; CUSA; TissueLink dissecting sealer; argon beam laser; intraop ultrasound	⇐	⇐
Unique considerations	Maintain normal core T. Most intrahepatic bleeding can be controlled temporarily by compression. Note the duration of Pringle maneuver, if applied.	⇐	⇐
Antibiotics	Vancomycin/cefazolin 1 g iv on induction	⇐	⇐
Surgical time	4-8 h	2-4 h	⇐
Closing considerations	Secure meticulous hemostasis; place 1-2 perihepatic Jackson Pratt flat bulb suction drains.	⇐	⇐
EBL	Variable (100-800 ml)	100-500 ml	100-300 ml
Postop care	PACU → room	⇐	⇐
Mortality	< 2-5%	⇐	< 1%
Morbidity	Ascites: 20-30%	10-20%	< 10%
	Wound infection: 5-10%	⇐	⇐
	Liver failure: < 5%	⇐	< 2%
	Bile leak: < 5%	< 2-5%	⇐
	Postop bleeding: < 2-5%	⇐	⇐
Pain score	7-8	7-8	7

PATIENT POPULATION CHARACTERISTICS

Age range	19-85 yr
Male:Female	4:1 in primary HCC
	2:1 in liver metastases
Incidence	Metastatic colorectal cancer is the most common disease treated with liver resection in the U.S. The incidence of primary HCC is rising 2° the prevalence of chronic hepatitis C; however, because of delayed Dx and associated hepatitis C cirrhosis, many are not suitable resection candidates. Primary HCC is a common cancer in Asian Americans because of the high incidence of chronic hepatitis B. Many young Asians (30-50 yr) with HCC 2° chronic hepatitis B may not have cirrhosis.
Associated conditions	Cirrhosis; chronic hepatitis; and, rarely, hemachromatosis. Hx of colorectal surgery in patients with liver metastases

ANESTHETIC CONSIDERATIONS

See Anesthetic Considerations following Hepatorrhaphy, p. 442.

References

1. Oberfield RA, Steele G Jr, Gollan JL, Sherman D: Liver cancer. *CA Cancer J Clin* 1989; 39(4):206-18.
2. Parker GA, et al: Intraoperative ultrasound of the liver affects operative decision making. *Ann Surg* 1989; 209(5):569-77.
3. Sitzman RJV, et al: Preoperative assessment of malignant hepatic tumors. *Am J Surg* 1990; 159(1):137-42.

HEPATORRHAPHY

SURGICAL CONSIDERATIONS

Harry A. Oberhelman

Description: Although most liver lacerations have stopped bleeding by the time a surgeon sees them, others require suturing or partial liver resection to control bleeding. Various techniques are available to control hemorrhage, including packing, suturing, inflow occlusion, and resection. Small lacerations that have stopped bleeding require no specific therapy other than possible drainage. Lacerations that continue to bleed usually can be sutured and drained. Extensive tears of the liver that are actively bleeding may require temporary occlusion of the porta hepatis, containing the hepatic artery, portal vein, and bile duct (**Pringle maneuver**) to excise deviated parenchyma and control bleeding with sutures, clips, coagulators, etc. Occasionally, the hepatic vein draining the involved lobe will require clamping to control back-bleeding. When the bleeding cannot be controlled, it is expedient to pack the wound, drain the abdomen, and close. The pack can be removed without much risk of rebleeding within 48-72 h.

Usual preop diagnosis: Trauma with CT evidence of hepatic laceration

SUMMARY OF PROCEDURE

Position	Supine
Incision	Midline abdominal
Special instrumentation	Denier retractor
Antibiotics	Cefazolin 1 g iv
Surgical time	1-2 h
EBL	~300-2000 ml
Mortality	1-2%
Morbidity	Continued bleeding: 2-3%
	Biliary fistula
	Perihepatic abscess
	Intrahepatic hematoma
	Arteroportal fistula
	Hepatic and renal failure
Pain score	7-9

PATIENT POPULATION CHARACTERISTICS

Age range	Variable
Male:Female	1:1
Incidence	Rare
Etiology	Trauma (blunt vs penetrating); surgical; hepatic adenomas; needle biopsies of liver

ANESTHETIC CONSIDERATIONS FOR HEPATIC PROCEDURES

(Procedures covered: hepatic resection; hepatorrhaphy)

PREOPERATIVE

Patients presenting for hepatic surgery may have primary or metastatic tumors from GI and other sources. Liver function may be entirely normal in these patients. HCC is seen commonly in males > 50 yr, and is associated with chronic active hepatitis B and cirrhosis. The preop considerations listed below describe patients without cirrhosis. (See Preoperative Considerations for Surgery for Portal Hypertension, p. 346+) for evaluation of patients with cirrhosis).

Respiratory	Respiratory function is typically normal; however, patients with ascites may have respiratory compromise. **Tests:** CXR; others as clinically indicated.
Cardiovascular	Patients may be hypovolemic, and volume status should be carefully assessed before induction of anesthesia (skin turgor, UO, orthostatic BP, HR, etc). Tumors may surround major vascular structures and impede venous return. Consider evaluation with CT/MRI scan.
Hepatic	Liver resection can be indicated for hemangiomas, hydatid cysts, and tumors. It is important to determine the size of the tumor and involvement of vascular structures preop so as to be adequately prepared for major intraop blood and fluid losses. **Tests:** LFTs; albumin; ultrasound/CT/MRI
Hematologic	The liver produces all clotting factors except VIII, and the degree of hepatic insufficiency determines the extent of any coagulopathy. T&C 4 U PRBCs. **Tests:** CBC; PT; PTT; Plt count; others as indicated from H&P.
Laboratory	★ Tests as indicated from H&P. **NB:** For elective cases, if abnormal LFTs are present on preop labs, it is important to perform a complete medical workup. This can include reviewing old lab data, hepatitis serology, and an abdominal ultrasound to r/o cholestatic causes of liver dysfunction. Surgery and anesthesia in the presence of acute hepatitis is associated with a high mortality.

Premedication	Standard premedication (p. B-2). Consider administering vitamin K (e.g., 10 mg iv/sc) if PT is prolonged. (Beneficial results from vitamin K usually occur within 24 h. Consider FFP for rapid correction of PT.)

INTRAOPERATIVE

Anesthetic technique: GETA. For major liver resections, the surgeon may attempt to reduce blood loss by applying intermittent vascular inflow occlusion or total vascular exclusion. As the result of ischemia induced by vascular occlusion and the loss of liver mass during resection, liver function may be significantly abnormal in the postop period. Coagulation abnormalities may exist; consequently, an epidural catheter for postop pain relief may be associated with ↑risk of hematoma formation.

Induction	Standard induction (p. B-2). Restore intravascular volume before induction. Trauma patients or those with ascites require rapid-sequence induction (p. B-5) with cricoid pressure until intubation has been confirmed. If patient is hemodynamically unstable, consider etomidate (0.2-0.4 mg/kg) or ketamine (1-3 mg/kg) in place of STP.	
Maintenance	Standard maintenance (p. B-3); N_2O can be used if bowel distention will not impede surgical exposure/closure.	
	If total vascular occlusion is used, elevate CVP to at least 12 mmHg by rapid fluid administration before cross-clamping. Have neosynephrine and epinephrine infusions ready to treat ↓BP. After major resections, significant hemodynamic changes occur. CO and HR increase, and systemic vascular resistance decreases.[3]	
Emergence	For major hepatic resections, the patient will be best cared for in an ICU. After major blood loss, consider keeping the patient mechanically ventilated.	
Blood and fluid requirements	Anticipate large blood loss. IV: 14-16 ga × 2 NS/LR @ 10-20 ml/kg/h Fluid warmer Humidify gases. Consider utilizing rapid-transfusion device.	Blood loss can be significant; keep at least 2 U PRBC ahead. Lobectomies often are associated with more blood loss than wedge resections. Massive transfusions may be required and appropriate blood products should be available (e.g., 2 FFPs + 6 Plt per 10 U PRBC). If procedure does not involve cancer, blood salvage devices can be used.
Control of blood loss	Surgical control Pringle maneuver Total vascular exclusion	Surgical occlusion of the main blood vessels entering the hilar area (Pringle maneuver), or total vascular occlusion. Total vascular exclusion is accomplished by complete occlusion of liver inflow and outflow.
Monitoring	Standard monitors (p. B-1) UO CVP Arterial line Possibly, TEE	Others as clinically indicated. If the extent of the resection is not known at the beginning of surgery, appropriate monitoring (CVP, arterial line, additional iv's) should be established prior to beginning resection. Forced-air warmer.
Positioning	✓ and pad pressure points. ✓ eyes.	
Complications	Massive hemorrhage	Ensure adequate vascular access. Consider rapid-transfusion device.

POSTOPERATIVE

Complications	↓liver function Hemorrhage Electrolyte imbalance Hypoglycemia Hypothermia, shivering DIC Pulmonary insufficiency	Patients with normal liver function preop may have significant postop impairment of liver function 2° loss of liver mass or ischemia induced by vascular occlusion. > 90% of patients will develop some form of respiratory complication (atelectasis, effusion, pneumonia).
Pain management	Epidural analgesia (p. C-1) PCA (p. C-3)	Patient should be recovered in ICU or hospital ward that is accustomed to treating the side effects of epidural opiates (e.g., respiratory depression, breakthrough pain, nausea, pruritus).

Tests	ABG; CXR; others as clinically indicated.

References

1. Feliciano DV, Jordan GL Jr, Bitondo CG, Mattox KL, Burch JM, Cruse PA: Management of 1000 consecutive cases of hepatic trauma. *Ann Surg* 1986; 204:438-45.
2. Merritt WT, Gelman S: Anesthesia for liver surgery. In *Principles and Practice of Anesthesiology*. Longnecker DE, Tinker JH, Morgan GE, eds. Mosby-Year Book, St Louis: 1998, 1904-47.
3. Niemann CU, Roberts JP, Ascher NL, Yost CS: Intraoperative hemodynamics and liver function in adult to adult living liver donors. *Liver Transpl* 2002; 8:1126-32.

Surgeon

Mark A. Vierra, MD

7.6 BILIARY TRACT SURGERY

Anesthesiologist

Hendrikus J.M. Lemmens, MD, PhD

OPEN CHOLECYSTECTOMY

SURGICAL CONSIDERATIONS

Description: With the advent of laparoscopic cholecystectomy, the traditional **open cholecystectomy** has become a rarity, generally reserved for gallbladders that are expected to be difficult to remove due to inflammation, previous operations and adhesions, or because of other medical problems, such as coagulopathy or cirrhosis. In most institutions, fewer than 10% of cholecystectomies will be begun as open procedures, and perhaps 5% of laparoscopic cholecystectomies will be converted to open cholecystectomies during the course of the operation due to technical difficulties, complications, or unexpected findings. The open cholecystectomy of the 90s is, in general, a substantially more challenging operation for both surgeon and anesthesiologist than it was in previous decades.

The **open cholecystectomy** usually is performed through a right subcostal or midline incision. Upward traction is applied to the liver or gallbladder, while downward traction on the duodenum exposes the region of the cystic duct and artery and common duct. Depending on local conditions and the surgeon's preference, the gallbladder may be removed from the top down, excising the gallbladder from the liver bed and isolating the cystic duct and artery as the final stage of the operation. The cystic duct and artery may be isolated and divided first, and the gallbladder removed retrograde from the gallbladder bed as the final step of the procedure. The anatomy of the biliary tree is quite variable, and few surgeons always remove the gallbladder in exactly the same way every time. (Fig 7.6-1 shows exposure of the gallbladder.)

Cholangiography may be performed in either laparoscopic or open cholecystectomy, and is performed at the discretion of the surgeon. Some surgeons perform it in all patients and others perform it only in patients in whom there is some clinical evidence of choledocholithiasis. The cystic duct is opened and a catheter placed into the duct and secured with a ligature, tie, or special cholangiogram clamp. Dye is injected into the biliary tree via the catheter, and x-rays are taken. If stones are found, a common duct exploration may be performed. Alternatively, an endoscopic retrograde cholangiogram (ERCP) with stone extraction may be carried out postop. Cholangiography usually adds about 10-15 min to the procedure.

Choledochotomy, or **'common duct exploration,'** is the opening and exploration of the common duct for the purpose of extracting stones. The need for this may be anticipated preop or performed based on findings at operation, particularly the finding of common duct stones by cholangiography. A longitudinal incision ~1 cm long is made in the duct and exploration is carried out through this incision. The duct may be irrigated with NS, balloon catheters may be passed, and various instruments introduced to grasp, remove, or crush retained stones. The duct may be biopsied by this approach, and **choledochoscopy**—the direct visualization of the duct's interior using a small flexible scope—can be performed. Depending on the complexity of the findings, a common duct exploration can be expected to add from 30 min to > 1 h to the cholecystectomy. In general, the mortality of patients undergoing common duct exploration is ~2-5 times that of a simple cholecystectomy. This difference can be explained by the fact that patients undergoing common duct exploration tend to be older and sicker—the opening of the duct itself is not necessarily a significant physiologic insult. **Common bile duct exploration** and **sphincterotomy** for extraction of common bile duct stones have become rare procedures with the advent of **ERCP, endoscopic common bile duct stone removal**, and **endoscopic sphincterotomy.**

Variant procedure or approaches: Cholecystectomy remains the mainstay of treatment for symptomatic biliary stone disease. **Nonsurgical treatment** of cholelithiasis, particularly by **oral dissolution** and/or **lithotripsy**, have very limited usefulness and are rarely used in clinical practice. **Laparoscopic cholecystectomy** (see p. 459) has largely replaced the open approach.

Usual preop diagnosis: Symptomatic cholelithiasis; acute cholecystitis; choledocholithiasis

SUMMARY OF PROCEDURES

	Cholecystectomy	Cholecystectomy/ Common Duct Exploration
Position	Supine	⇐
Incision	Right subcostal or midline	Midline
Special instrumentation	Costal margin retractor ± cholangiogram catheter	Choledochotomy instruments
Unique considerations	Requires intraop x-ray for cholangiogram.	May include choledochoscopy.
Antibiotics	Ampicillin, piperacillin, or mezlocillin, 1-3 g iv ± gentamicin; or cefotetan 1-2 g iv	⇐
Surgical time	45-90 min	1-2.5 h
Closing considerations	Muscle relaxation	⇐
EBL	< 250 ml	⇐

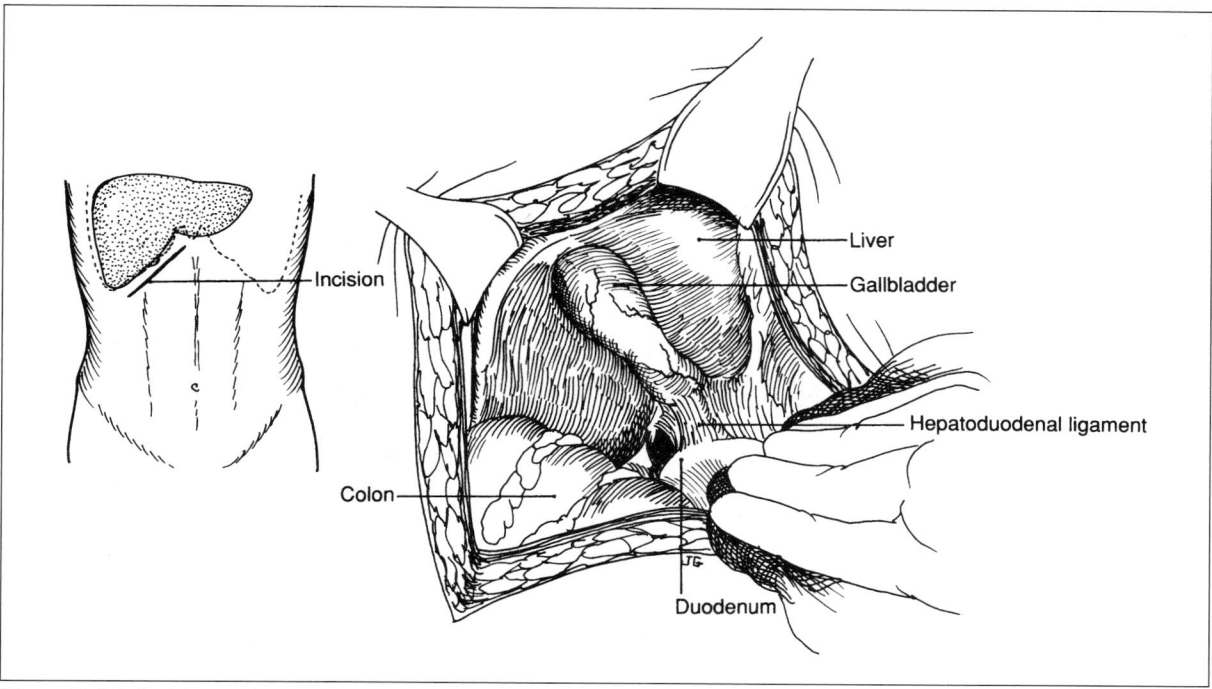

Figure 7.6-1. Incision and exposure of the gallbladder. (Reproduced with permission from Scott-Conner CEH, Dawson DL: *Operative Anatomy*, 2nd edition. Lippincott Williams & Wilkins, 2003.)

	Cholecystectomy	Cholecystectomy/ Common Duct Exploration
Postop care	PACU	⇐
Mortality	0.7%	0-1.5% < 60 yr; ≤ 5% in advanced age
Morbidity	Postop bile leak: 0-9%	⇐
	Pancreatitis: 0-4.6%	2-5%
	Bile duct injury: 0-0.25%	
	Cardiac and respiratory complications: Rare, but leading cause of death	
	Hemorrhage: Rare	
Pain score	6	6-7

PATIENT POPULATION CHARACTERISTICS

Age range	Mostly adult; increases with age
Male:Female	1:2-3
Incidence	600,000/yr in U.S.; 90+% performed laparoscopically.
Etiology	See Associated Conditions, below.
Associated conditions	Ileal disease; cirrhosis; hemolytic disorders; choledocholithiasis; cholangitis or active pancreatitis

ANESTHETIC CONSIDERATIONS

See Anesthetic Considerations for Biliary Tract Surgery, p. 452.

References

1. Brooks JR: Acute and chronic cholecystitis. In *Current Surgical Therapy*, Vol III. Cameron J, ed. BC Decker, Philadelphia: 1989, 257-62.
2. Cuschieri A, Dubois F, Mouiel J, Mouret P, Becker H, Buess G, Trede M, Troidl H: The European experience with laparoscopic cholecystectomy. *Am J Surg* 1991; 161(3):385-7.

3. McSherry CK, Glenn F: The incidence and causes of death following surgery for nonmalignant biliary tract disease. *Ann Surg* 1980; 191(3):271-5.
4. Peters JH, Ellison EC, Innes JT, Liss JL, Nichols KE, Lomano JM, Roby SR, Front ME, Carey LC: Safety and efficacy of laparoscopic cholecystectomy. A prospective analysis of 100 initial patients. *Ann Surg* 1991; 213(1):3-12.
5. Voyles CR, Petro AB, Meena AL, Haick AJ, Koury AM: A practical approach to laparoscopic cholecystectomy. *Am J Surg* 1991; 161(3):365-70.

BILIARY DRAINAGE PROCEDURES

SURGICAL CONSIDERATIONS

Description: Biliary drainage procedures may be performed for malignant and nonmalignant indications, and the type of drainage procedure performed depends on factors such as the nature of the biliary obstruction, the patient's overall condition and prognosis, the need for other surgical procedures, and institutional expertise. **Endoscopic** and **transhepatic techniques** are increasing in use and, today, most drainage procedures of the biliary tree are performed with these techniques. There remain a significant number of patients, however, for whom a traditional surgical procedure is the most appropriate. In general, the complexity of the different operations that may be performed and the morbidity attendant to these has more to do with the indications for operation than with the procedure that is performed.

All of these operations are performed under GA through an upper midline or right subcostal incision. Self-retaining retractors are used to retract the liver superiorly to expose the region of the porta hepatis. If the gallbladder will not be used for the bypass procedure (**cholecystojejunostomy**), then it usually is removed as the first step in the procedure (see Open Cholecystectomy, p. 446). If the patient has had previous upper right quadrant surgery, the complexity and duration of the procedure and blood loss may increase significantly. Any associated hepatic cirrhosis may make the procedure particularly demanding.

Transduodenal sphincteroplasty usually is performed for benign obstruction of the ampulla of Vater or for extensive choledocholithiasis. **Endoscopic sphincterotomy** is the most commonly performed technique for opening the ampulla, and usually is performed by gastroenterologists outside of the OR with iv sedation. **Open sphincteroplasty** is usually reserved for patients in whom endoscopic retrograde cholangiopancreatogram (ERCP) has been unsuccessful or in whom a laparotomy is required for other reasons. For these open procedures, the second portion of duodenum is incised over the region of the ampulla, and the ampulla is cannulated. A longitudinal incision is made over the course of the ampulla, and the mucosa of the ampulla is sutured to the mucosa of the duodenum with fine interrupted sutures, with care being taken not to compromise the pancreatic duct. The duodenum is closed with suture, a small closed suction drain is placed, and the wound is closed. A postop stay of 5-7 d can be expected.

Cholecystojejunostomy usually is performed as palliation for malignant obstruction of the distal bile duct. Its advantage is that it does not require dissection of the portal triad, but the long-term results are less reliable than with the other two drainage procedures. This is partly because the gallbladder may not drain as well as the common duct, and partly because the tumor may grow to occlude the junction of the common and cystic ducts. The abdomen is opened as described above, and the region of the porta hepatis examined to ensure that the cystic duct is not imminently compromised by tumor. The jejunum is then brought up to the gallbladder, usually bypassing the jejunum through the transverse mesocolon. The anastomosis may be performed either to an intact loop of jejunum (**loop cholecystojejunostomy**) or to a Roux-en-Y loop of jejunum (**Roux-en-Y cholecystojejunostomy**), and is carried out with one or two layers of sutures, depending on surgeon's preference. If a Roux-en-Y is created, a second jejunojejunal anastomosis must be performed.

In **choledochoduodenostomy** or **choledochojejunostomy**, an anastomosis is fashioned between the common duct and the duodenum, or the common duct and Roux loop of jejunum. This is often a relatively more demanding operation than cholecystojejunostomy because it requires dissection deep in the porta hepatis to gain access to the common duct. Long-term results are more reliable, however, and these are preferred for benign disease. Exposure of the biliary tree is the same as for the above procedures. The gallbladder is always removed (if it is still present). The common duct is dissected free from the surrounding structures in the porta hepatis and an anastomosis is constructed between the common duct and the duodenum or jejunum. If the jejunum is used, it is almost always brought up as a Roux-en-Y, requiring a second jejunojejunal anastomosis.

Variant procedure or approaches: Endoscopic or transhepatic placement of temporary or permanent **biliary stents** is an increasingly common alternative to surgical drainage in patients with incurable pancreatic or biliary tract disease.

Usual preop diagnosis: Transduodenal sphincteroplasty: extensive choledocholithiasis, often after failed attempt at ERCP; rarely, malignant disease. Cholecystojejunostomy: malignant obstruction of distal common bile duct, usually due to pancreatic cancer. Choledochojejunostomy or choledochoduodenostomy: benign strictures of the distal bile duct; longstanding stone disease; pancreatitis; iatrogenic injury; Oriental cholangiohepatitis; after resection of some tumors of the pancreas or distal bile duct.

SUMMARY OF PROCEDURES

	Cholecysto-jejunostomy	Choledocho-jejunostomy	Choledocho-duodenostomy	Transduodenal sphincteroplasty
Position	Supine	⇐	⇐	⇐
Incision	Midline or right subcostal	⇐	⇐	⇐
Special instrumentation	Costal retractor	⇐	⇐	⇐
Unique considerations	Consider usual prep for patients with obstructive jaundice.	⇐	⇐	⇐
Antibiotics	Ampicillin, piperacillin or mezlocillin, 1-3 g iv ± gentamicin; or cefotetan 1-2 g iv	⇐	⇐	⇐
Surgical time	1 h; may be significantly longer if resection of tumor is considered.	1.5-3 h	⇐	⇐
Closing considerations	Muscle relaxation; NG suction	⇐	⇐	⇐
EBL	< 250 ml (greater if tumor resection performed, or in presence of portal HTN).	250-500 ml (greater if tumor resection performed, or in presence of portal HTN).	⇐	< 250 ml (transfusion rarely needed).
Postop care	PACU	⇐	⇐	⇐
Mortality[1,3,5]	≤ 35% in advanced pancreatic cancer; otherwise, < 10%	≤ 29%, with pancreatic cancer; 0.5% for benign disease	0-5.4%[1,2,5] (usually for benign disease)	0-7%
Morbidity[3,5]	Sepsis	⇐	⇐	Pancreatitis: Rare
	Respiratory complications	⇐	⇐	Recurrent cholangitis: Rare
	Renal failure	⇐	⇐	
	Hemorrhage	⇐	⇐	
	Wound infection	⇐	⇐	
	Breakdown of biliary anastomosis	⇐	⇐	
	Thrombotic complications	⇐	⇐	
Pain score	7	7	7	6

PATIENT POPULATION CHARACTERISTICS

Age range	5th-7th decade; may be younger for sphincterotomy
Male:Female	1.1:2.1
Incidence	Procedure-related incidence not available, but clearly declining in favor of techniques by interventional gastroenterology and radiology.
Etiology	See Usual Preop Diagnosis, above.
Associated conditions	Jaundice (very common); fat-soluble vitamin deficiencies; malignancy, especially pancreatic (common); malnutrition (common)

ANESTHETIC CONSIDERATIONS

See Anesthetic Considerations for Biliary Tract Surgery, p. 452.

References

1. Baker AR, Neoptolemos JP, Carr-Locke DL, Fossard DP: Sump syndrome following choledochoduodenostomy and its endoscopic treatment. *Br J Surg* 1985; 72(6):433-5.
2. Birkenfeld S, Serour F, Levi S, Abulafia A, Balassiano M, Krispin M: Choledochoduodenostomy for benign and malignant biliary tract diseases. *Surgery* 1988; 103(4):408-10.
3. Hines LH, Burns RP: 10 years' experience treating pancreatic and periampullary cancer. *Am Surg* 1976; 42(6):441-7.
4. Karan JA, Roslyn JJ: Cholelithiasis and cholecystectomy. In *Maingot's Abdominal Operations*, 10th edition. Zinner MJ, Schwartz SI, Ellis H, eds. Appleton & Lange, Stamford CT: 1997, 1717-38.
5. Sarr MG, Cameron JL: Surgical palliation of unresectable carcinoma of the pancreas. *World J Surg* 1984; 8(6):906-18.
6. Thompkins RK: Choledocholithiasis and cholangitis. In *Maingot's Abdominal Operations*, 10th edition. Zinner MJ, Schwartz SI, Ellis H, eds. Appleton & Lange, Stamford, CT: 1997, 1739-54.
7. Weber S, Fong Y: Biliary Neoplasms. In *Surgery: Scientific Principles and Practice*, 3rd edition. Greenfield LJ, et al, eds. Lippincott Williams & Wilkins, Philadelphia: 2001, 1033-45.

EXCISION OF BILE DUCT TUMOR

SURGICAL CONSIDERATIONS

Description: Primary tumors of the extrahepatic bile ducts, including the hepatic bifurcation (Klatskin tumors) are uncommon malignancies, with the only curative treatment for them being surgical excision. Such tumors are usually classified as being proximal bile duct tumors, involving the hepatic bifurcation and above; middle bile duct tumors, involving the midportion of the common hepatic and common bile duct; and distal bile duct tumors, which involve the distal bile duct, including the intrapancreatic or intraduodenal portion of the bile duct (Fig 7.6-1). The gallbladder usually will be removed in any such operation.

Distal bile duct tumors, which carry a significantly higher cure rate than either proximal bile duct or pancreatic tumors, may be treated by **pancreaticoduodenectomy**. (See p. 490 for discussion of this operation.)

Mid bile duct tumors usually are excised by removing a generous portion of the mid bile duct, resecting the ducts up to the hepatic bifurcation, and sometimes performing a pancreaticoduodenectomy. Biliary drainage usually is established by anastomosing the proximal bile duct to a Roux loop of jejunum. For proximal bile duct tumors, most of the extrahepatic bile ducts are excised and biliary drainage is established by anastomosis of the right and left hepatic ducts to a Roux loop of jejunum. These are often technically demanding operations with the potential for major blood loss. It may be necessary to perform a major hepatic resection at the same time, and the possibility of this should always be assumed when an operation of this sort is carried out.

Surgical exposure for any of these operations usually is achieved through a long midline or transverse subcostal incision and the use of self-retaining retractors. Often, a transhepatic catheter will have been placed radiographically preop to provide relief of jaundice and to facilitate identification of the bile ducts. The liver and gallbladder are retracted superiorly while downward traction is placed on the duodenum. If the gallbladder is still in place, a cholecystectomy is performed (see p. 446). For proximal bile duct tumors and mid bile duct tumors not requiring pancreaticoduodenectomy, the bile duct is divided distally, just above the duodenum, and the pancreatic portion of the bile duct is oversewn. The bile duct is then resected proximally to the level of the bifurcation of the hepatic ducts. A Roux-en-Y loop of jejunum is anastomosed to the hepatic ducts to establish biliary drainage. Drains are placed and most surgeons place a NG tube for such cases.

Variant procedure or approaches: **Endoscopic** or **transhepatic stenting** of areas of stricture often is used as a palliative alternative to surgical excision. These are usually performed radiographically and do not require GA. They may be used as an alternative to resection or in preparation for surgery.

Usual preop diagnosis: Cholangiocarcinoma (common); benign strictures of the bile ducts (infrequent); sclerosing cholangitis (rare)

SUMMARY OF PROCEDURE

Position	Supine
Incision	Midline or subcostal
Special instrumentation	Costal retractor
Unique considerations	Many cases prove unresectable at operation. Intraop radiation therapy may be used.
Antibiotics	Ampicillin, piperacillin, or mezlocillin, 1-3 g iv, ± gentamicin; or cefotetan 1-2 g iv
Surgical time	3-8 h
Closing considerations	Muscle relaxation required for closure; NG suction.
EBL	500-5000 ml, depending on need for liver resection and presence of portal HTN.
Postop care	ICU postop
Mortality	5-10%
Morbidity	Sepsis; hemorrhage; anastomotic leakage; wound infection; liver failure; PE
Pain score	7-8

PATIENT POPULATION CHARACTERISTICS

Age range	50s-70s
Male:Female	Male > female
Incidence	4500 cases of bile duct cancer/yr in U.S.
Etiology	Multifactorial
Associated conditions	Ulcerative colitis; sclerosing cholangitis; typhoid carrier state; clonorchis sinensis; choledochal cyst; Caroli's disease; gallstones

ANESTHETIC CONSIDERATIONS

See Anesthetic Considerations for Biliary Tract Surgery, p. 452.

References

1. Yeo CJ, Cameron JL: Tumours of the gallbladder and bile ducts. In *Maingot's Abdominal Operations*, 10th edition. Zinner MJ, Schwartz SI, Ellis H, eds. Appleton & Lange, Stamford, CT: 1997, 1835-54.
2. Zinner MJ: Bile duct tumors. In *Current Surgical Therapy*, Vol III. Cameron JL, ed. BC Decker, Philadelphia: 1989, 289-91.

CHOLEDOCHAL CYST EXCISION OR ANASTOMOSIS

SURGICAL CONSIDERATIONS

Description: This rare congenital anomaly includes various types of dilatation of the biliary tree, and patients may present with cholangitis, pancreatitis or, rarely, malignancy. Although four types of cysts are commonly recognized, the vast majority consist of fusiform dilatation of much or most of the extrahepatic biliary tree. While the traditional description of choledochal cyst is that of an infant with a palpable abdominal mass and jaundice or cholangitis, this is a relatively rare presentation today. Today, many cysts are found in adults undergoing evaluation for symptoms thought to be due to gallbladder disease. These patients may present with biliary colic, pancreatitis, or cholangitis. Recommended treatment consists of **excision of the cyst**, when technically safe. **Cyst-enteric bypass**, usually to a Roux loop of jejunum, is almost never performed today because of the small, but real risk of developing malignancy in these cysts. Only in an elderly patient under unusual technical circumstances would this be appropriate.

The operation is performed through a midline or right subcostal incision. The liver is retracted superiorly and the duodenum inferiorly, exposing the biliary tree. The gallbladder is excised, along with as much of the cyst as possible. The duct is divided as distally as possible, just above the duodenum, and the cyst reflected superiorly. It usually is excised to the hepatic bifurcation; and an anastomosis is performed at this level, often between the common orifice of the right and left hepatic ducts and a Roux loop of jejunum.

Reoperative cases are not uncommon; most follow a cyst-enteric bypass. These cases may be significantly more difficult than first-time operations.

Variant procedure or approaches: There is an increasing tendency among gastroenterologists to perform **endoscopic sphincterotomy** in these patients, rather than to refer them for surgical resection, particularly in older patients. It remains to be seen if these patients will develop cancer in the retained cysts.

Usual preop diagnosis: Choledochal cyst, the most common type involving fusiform enlargement of the entire extrahepatic biliary tree

SUMMARY OF PROCEDURE

Position	Supine
Incision	Midline or right subcostal
Special instrumentation	Costal retractor
Antibiotics	Ampicillin, piperacillin, or mezlocillin, 1-3 g iv ± gentamicin; or cefotetan 1-2 g iv
Surgical time	2-4 h
Closing considerations	NG suction
EBL	250 ml, with potentially greater blood loss in reoperations
Postop care	PACU
Mortality	Very rare
Morbidity	Anastomotic leak
	Wound infection
	Pulmonary complications
	Pancreatitis
Pain score	5-7

PATIENT POPULATION CHARACTERISTICS

Age range	Classically, 60% < 10 yr of age, although this may be changing; also adults of all ages
Male:Female	1:3
Incidence	Rare in U.S.; more common in Japan
Etiology	Unclear
Associated conditions	Jaundice; pancreatitis; malignancy within the cyst

References

1. Crittenden SL, McKinley MJ: Choledochal cyst–clinical features and classification. *Am J Gastroenterol* 1985; 80(8):643-7.
2. Lippsett PA, Yeo CJ: Choledochal cysts. In *Maingot's Abdominal Operations*, 10th edition. Zinner MJ, Schwartz SI, Ellis H, eds. Appleton & Lange, Stamford, CT: 1997,1701-16.
3. Nagorney DM, McIlrath DC, Adson MA: Choledochal cysts in adults: clinical management. *Surgery* 1984; 96(4):656-63.

ANESTHETIC CONSIDERATIONS FOR BILIARY TRACT SURGERY

(Procedures covered: open cholecystectomy; cholangiography; choledochotomy; biliary drainage procedures; transduodenal sphincterotomy or sphincteroplasty; cholecystojejunostomy; excision of bile duct tumor; choledochal cyst excision/anastomosis)

PREOPERATIVE

Patients presenting for biliary tract surgery are an extremely diverse group, ranging from the otherwise healthy to the extremely ill. With the increasing popularity of laparoscopic surgery, open cholecystectomies will be performed rarely, or when it is not possible to complete the laparoscopic procedure. Cirrhosis, even of a mild degree, substantially increases the risk of cholecystectomy, with hemorrhage being the greatest danger. Patients with bile duct tumors are usually jaundiced at presentation and have undergone transhepatic and/or endoscopic studies for diagnostic purposes. Often an external transhepatic biliary drain may be present and jaundice may have been relieved in this way. Rarely, a hepatic resection may be performed as part of the procedure. Prior operation or the presence of portal HTN may substantially increase the duration, complexity, and blood loss of the procedure.

Respiratory	Pain 2° an acute abdominal process may impair respiratory function ($\downarrow$FRC, hypoventilation, atelectasis). For patients undergoing laparoscopic cholecystectomy, intraabdominal CO_2 insufflation may $\rightarrow$ atelectasis, $\downarrow$FRC, $\uparrow$PIP, and $\uparrow PaCO_2$. Studies comparing patients undergoing open vs laparoscopic cholecystectomy reveal that respiratory function is less impaired and function is recovered more quickly in those undergoing laparoscopic cholecystectomy. Tachypnea, hyperpnea, and acute respiratory alkalosis can be signs of sepsis, or due solely to pain associated with inflammation of the gallbladder. **Tests:** Consider CXR and others as indicated from H&P.
Cardiovascular	Patients may be dehydrated from fever, vomiting, and decreased oral intake; assess hemodynamic status by evaluating BP and HR in the supine and standing positions. Fluid resuscitate if patient shows Sx of orthostatic $\downarrow$BP until hemodynamic status improves. Patients undergoing laparoscopic cholecystectomy may experience hemodynamic compromise 2° positioning (reverse Trendelenburg $\rightarrow$ excessive intraabdominal pressure with subsequent impairment of venous return). Epigastric discomfort is common with biliary tract disease and can mimic symptoms of myocardial ischemia. **Tests:** ECG; others as indicated from H&P.
Renal	In patients with obstructive jaundice, preop administration of bile salts po may prevent renal insufficiency following surgery.[1] **Tests:** UA and others as indicated from H&P.
Gastrointestinal	Patients with peritonitis will exhibit guarding and may develop abdominal distention and paralytic ileus. Therefore, full-stomach precautions are warranted. Laparoscopic approach is contraindicated in these patients. **Tests:** Bilirubin; AST (SGOT); ALT (SGPT); alkaline phosphatase; albumin
Hematologic	Leukocytosis is often present with a moderate left shift. ✓ coags. Administer vitamin K as needed (10 mg iv/sc). **Tests:** CBC, with differential and Plt
Laboratory	Other tests as indicated from H&P.
Premedication	Meperidine (0.5-0.6 mg/kg iv) is thought to cause less sphincter of Oddi spasm than other opiates. Sphincter spasm can interfere with intraop cholangiograms and cause pain; reverse opiate-induced spasm with naloxone in 40 μg increments. Atropine (0.4-0.6 mg im or iv) or glycopyrrolate (0.2-0.3 mg im or iv) may help decrease spasm of the sphincter and can be given in combination with the opiate. Parenteral vitamin K is indicated if PT is prolonged (10 mg/d im for 3 d). Administer H_2-antagonists (ranitidine 50 mg iv); metoclopramide (10 mg iv) may be given if patient is at risk for gastric aspiration.

INTRAOPERATIVE

Anesthetic technique: GETA. In patients at risk for aspiration, ET intubation should be accomplished following a rapid-sequence iv induction (see p. B-5).

Induction	Standard induction (see p. B-2) if no aspiration risk. In patients at risk of aspiration, a rapid-sequence induction should be performed (see p. B-5).	
Maintenance	Standard maintenance (see p. B-3). Muscle relaxants facilitate surgery and are indicated.	
Emergence	If there is a risk for aspiration of gastric contents, patient should be extubated awake after return of protective airway reflexes; otherwise, no special considerations.	
Blood and fluid requirements	Minimal blood loss Possible 3rd-space loss IV: 16-18 ga × 1 NS/LR @ 5-8 ml/kg/h	Blood products usually not required. Anticipate that patient may be dehydrated and require generous iv hydration (e.g., 10-15 ml/kg) before anesthetic induction.
Monitoring	Standard monitors (see p. B-1).	Others as clinically indicated.
Positioning	✓ and pad pressure points. ✓ eyes.	A steep, reverse Trendelenburg position may be required, causing cardiorespiratory impairment: $\downarrow$venous return $\rightarrow \downarrow$CO.
Complications	Atelectasis 2° surgical retraction $\downarrow$BP	These complications are unique to laparoscopic procedures.

POSTOPERATIVE

Complications	Ventilatory impairment Pneumothorax Atelectasis PONV Subcutaneous emphysema	Monitor patients for hypoxemia in the postop period. Administer supplemental O_2, and consider a portable CXR to aid in the diagnosis.
Pain management	PCA (p. C-3)	Intercostal nerve blocks, intrapleural analgesia, or epidural analgesia are also useful techniques. Prolonged PCA meperidine is associated with ↑normeperidine → CNS disorder.
	Shoulder pain	2° subdiaphragmatic gas trapping

References

1. Cahill CJ: Prevention of postoperative renal failure in patients with obstructive jaundice–the role of bile salts. *Br J Surg* 1983; 70(10):590-5.
2. Marco AP, Yeo CJ, Rock P: Anesthesia for a patient undergoing laparoscopic cholecystectomy. *Anesthesiology* 1990; 73(6): 1268-70.
3. Strasberg S, Drebin J: Calculous biliary disease. In *Surgery: Scientific Principles and Practice*, 3rd ediition. Greenfield LJ, et al, eds. Lippincott Williams & Wilkins, Philadelphia: 2001, 1011-32.
4. Taylor E, Feinstein R, White PF, Soper N: Anesthesia for laparoscopic cholecystectomy. Is nitrous oxide contraindicated? *Anesthesiology* 1992; 76(4):541-3.
5. Venu RP, Geenen JE, Hogan WJ, Dodds WJ, Wilson SW, Stewart ET, Soergel KH: Role of endoscopic retrograde cholangio-pancreatography in the diagnosis and treatment of choledochocele. *Gastroenterology* 1984; 87(5):1144-9.

Surgeon

Myriam J. Curet, MD

7.7 LAPAROSCOPIC GENERAL SURGERY

Anesthesiologists

Sunita G. Sastry, MD
Brendan Carvalho, MBBCh, FRCA (*Laparoscopy in pregnancy*)
Sheila E. Cohen, MB, ChB, FRCA (*Laparoscopy in pregnancy*)

LAPAROSCOPIC ESOPHAGEAL FUNDOPLICATION

SURGICAL CONSIDERATIONS

Description: Approximately 40% of Americans suffer from heartburn, and most cases are treated medically. Indications for **esophageal fundoplication** (to ↑ lower esophageal sphincter pressure) include complications of GERD, such as stricture, respiratory problems, esophageal ulcerations, and Barrett's esophagus (a premalignant condition). Other indications include failure of medical management or an unwillingness to submit to a lifetime of medication. Most patients with GERD are treated laparoscopically; those undergoing laparoscopic fundoplication have the benefits of a minimally invasive approach—decreased pain, earlier return of GI function, earlier ambulation, earlier discharge, and quicker return to normal activities. The most common fundoplication is the **Nissen (360°) wrap**; and its variations include the Rossetti modification, a Toupet (270° posterior) wrap, and the Dor (anterior) wrap. Before surgery, patients with GERD should have documented esophageal hyperacidity (by either pH probe or by esophagitis revealed on upper endoscopy), and also should have a hypotensive sphincter (demonstrated on manometry). Typically, they will have been treated with proton pump inhibitors (e.g., lansoprazole) and sometimes with prokinetic agents (e.g., metoclopramide). The patient is placed supine in a low lithotomy position, with the surgeon standing between the legs. The abdomen is entered ~2 cm above the umbilicus with either a closed (**Veress needle:** blind placement) or open (**Hasson trocar:** direct visual placement) technique. A total of five trocars are inserted—two in the LUQ, two in the RUQ, and one at the umbilicus. The stomach should be decompressed either with a OG tube or with a gastroscope. The liver is elevated with a liver retractor, and the gastroesophageal (GE) junction and both diaphragmatic crura are dissected out. The hiatus should be closed with one or two sutures. The esophagus is encircled (Fig 7.7-1A), and the vagal nerves are identified and preserved. The short gastrics are then taken down to decrease tension on the wrap. The fundus is brought in through the retroesophageal window (Fig 7.7-2). An esophageal dilator (56-60 Fr) generally is placed (often by the anesthesiologist) to calibrate the wrap. Passage of the dilator is possibly the most hazardous part of the procedure, as it may cause perforation of the esophagus at the GE junction. As the dilator approaches the stomach, it is important to watch the junction on the video monitors to ensure that it is not being held at an angle that will risk perforation. The dilator is then withdrawn. An NG tube may be placed at this time.

Variant procedure or approaches: Open surgery (see Esophageal Surgery, p. 384) may be indicated if the patient has had previous gastric surgery or if there is a complication with an ongoing laparoscopic procedure. In the **Rossetti modification,** the short gastrics are not taken down, which decreases operative time. The **Dor fundoplication** is an anterior hemifundoplication in which the fundus is wrapped and sutured to the left and right sides of the esophagus and to the left and right crura, but anteriorly. A **Toupet procedure** (Fig 7.7-1B) is a posterior hemifundoplication in which the two walls of the fundus do not actually meet. The stomach is sewn to the left and right walls of the esophagus and then are anchored to the right and left crura. In the past, these proceudres were performed commonly in patients with a high risk of postop dysphagia (e.g., those who have impaired esophageal peristalsis or a preop stricture). Now, because of their higher failure rate, they are seldom performed. These procedures are identical to the Nissen fundoplication except for the wrap itself.

Usual preop diagnosis: GERD, with or without esophagitis, esophageal stricture, or Barrett's esophagus

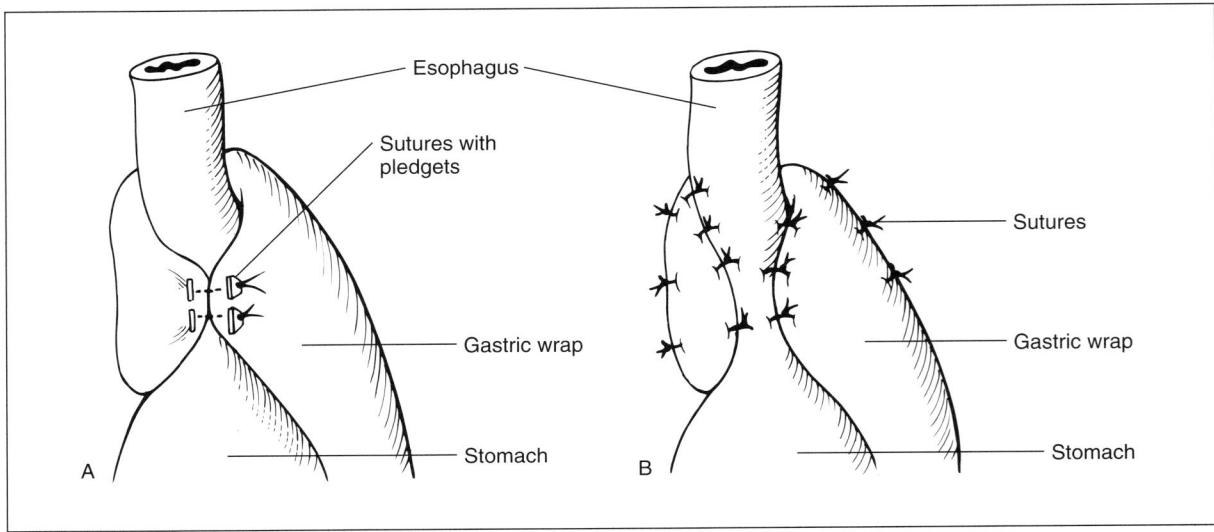

Figure 7.7-1. (A) Nissen fundoplication. (B) Partial fundoplication (Toupet procedure).

SUMMARY OF PROCEDURE

Position	Supine low lithotomy
Incision	5 ports, upper abdomen
Special instrumentation	Harmonic Scalpel; bipolar cautery or endoscope. Esophageal dilators should be available.
Antibiotics	Cefazolin 1 g
Surgical time	1.5-2.5 h
Closing considerations	Port closures only; muscle relaxation may be needed for fascial closure
EBL	< 75 ml
Postop care	1-2 d hospital stay; liquids on POD 1
Mortality	< 0.1%
Morbidity	Overall: 8% Atelectasis: Common Esophageal or gastric perforation: Rare (most commonly associated with passage of NG tube or esophageal dilator) Hemorrhage from short gastrics or splenic tear Pneumothorax (does not usually require treatment) Postop dysphagia
Pain score	4

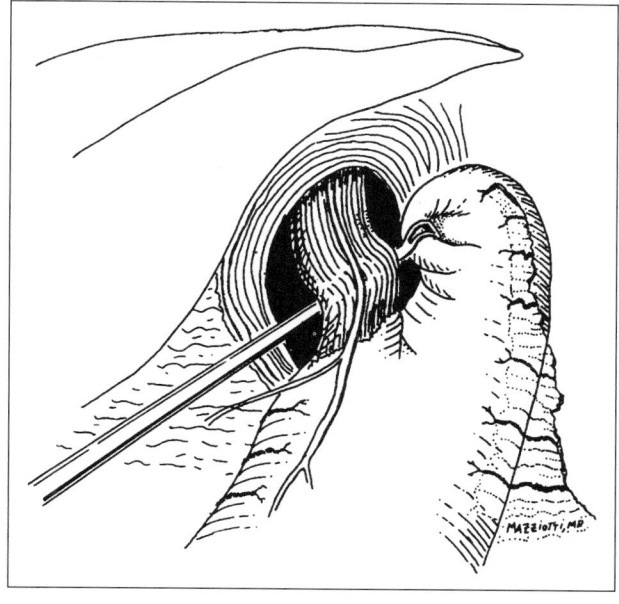

Figure 7.7-2. Gastric fundus is pulled posteriorly and to the right of the esophagus, with the fundus itself used as a retractor, reaching from right to left behind the esophagus to grasp the fundus and retract it back to the right side behind the esophagus. Placing caudad traction on the wrapped fundus, the GE junction and distal esophagus can be brought further into the abdominal cavity. (Reproduced with permission from Baker RJ, Fischer JE: *Mastery of Surgery*, Lippincott Williams & Wilkins, 2001.)

PATIENT POPULATION CHARACTERISTICS

Age range	All ages (indcidence ↑ with age). May be performed in infants; next peak occurs in adulthood; rare in children and adolescents.
Male:Female	1:1
Incidence	1% (increasing significantly over past 5 yr)
Etiology	Unknown
Associated conditions	Aspiration risk; reactive airway disease; occasionally, respiratory problems associated with chronic aspiration

ANESTHETIC CONSIDERATIONS

See Anesthetic Considerations following Laparoscopic Cholecystectomy, p. 461.

References

1. Amaral JF: Laparoscopic Nissen fundoplication with laparosonic coagulating shears. In *Atlas of Laparoscopic Surgery*. Ballantyne GH, ed. WB Saunders, Philadelphia: 2000, 102-18.
2. Champion JK, McKernan JB: Laparoscopic Toupet fundoplication. In *Surgical Laparoscopy*, 2nd edition. Zucker KA, ed. Lippincott Williams & Wilkins, Philadelphia: 2001, 401-8.
3. Dallemagne B: Laparoscopic Nissen Fundoplication. In *Atlas of Laparoscopic Surgery*. Ballantyne GH, ed. WB Saunders, Philadelphia: 2000, 92-101.
4. Hughes SG, Chekan EG, Ali A, Reintgen KL, Eubanks WS: Unusual complications following laparoscopic Nissen fundoplication. *Surg Laparosc Endosc Percutan Tech* 1999; 9(2):143-7.
5. Zucker KA: Laparoscopic Nissen Fundoplication Technique. In *Surgical Laparoscopy*, 2nd edition. Lippincott Williams & Wilkins, Philadelphia: 2001, 375-400.

LAPAROSCOPIC HELLER'S MYOTOMY
± ANTIREFLUX PROCEDURE

SURGICAL CONSIDERATIONS

Description: Laparoscopic and thoracoscopic esophageal myotomies have become much more common over the last 5 yr as confidence in laparoscopic esophageal surgery—particularly antireflux surgery—has increased. These procedures are performed for achalasia, an uncommon condition in which the lower esophageal sphincter fails to relax with swallowing, and in which the body of the esophagus simultaneously loses its peristalsis and dilates. Patients typically complain of dysphagia with chest pain and may experience regurgitation. The etiology of this condition remains unknown.

Treatment options consist of pneumatic dilation, botulinum toxin injection of the lower esophageal sphincter, or surgical myotomy. **Pneumatic dilation** remains the most common procedure performed for achalasia, and is effective in ~60% of patients. Many gastroenterologists are reluctant to perform this procedure, however, because of the risk of esophageal perforation, which is generally considered to be ~3-5%, but may be as high as 10%. **Botulinum toxin injection** is a newer technique that is effective to some degree in most patients, but the duration of its effectiveness is short. Most patients require retreatment within 1½ yr, and the efficacy of retreatment may diminish over time. In many centers, **surgical myotomy (Heller's operation)** has become the procedure of choice for the treatment of achalasia.

The patient is positioned as for a laparoscopic antireflux procedure—supine in the lithotomy position with reverse Trendelenburg. The abdomen is usually entered with a Veress needle or Hasson trocar at the umbilicus, and five laparoscopic ports are placed across the upper abdomen—two beneath the left costal margin, two beneath the right costal margin, and one in the midline either at the umbilicus or midway between the umbilicus and the xiphoid. The liver is elevated, and the ligamentous attachments anterior to the esophagus are divided. The esophagus is not usually encircled; and, as hiatal hernias are uncommon with achalasia, crural repair is seldom necessary.

The myotomy is begun at the gastroesophageal junction using monopolar cautery, bipolar scissors, or a Harmonic Scalpel. It is carried proximally until normal musculature is encountered. Some surgeons perform intraop esophagoscopy to ensure that the myotomy has been carried proximally enough and that there has not been a mucosal perforation. Generally, a myotomy of 5-8 cm is adequate, although sometimes a longer myotomy may be necessary. Some surgeons then perform a very loose, partial fundoplication to prevent reflux. This can be performed as an anterior or posterior fundoplication, bringing the fundus either anterior (our preference) or posterior to the esophagus. The stomach is secured to the esophageal wall and crural with sutures, and an NG tube may be passed. The ports are removed and port closure carried out.

Variant procedure or approaches: While most of these procedures are being performed laparoscopically, they also can be performed by thoracoscopy or thoracotomy. If a thoracoscopy or thoracotomy is performed, a DLT is required to allow collapse of the left lung.

Usual preop diagnosis: Achalasia

SUMMARY OF PROCEDURE

Position	Supine lithotomy, reverse Trendelenburg
Incision	5 ports, upper abdomen
Special instrumentation	Laparoscopic instrumentation ± gastroscope
Antibiotics	Cefazolin 1 g
Surgical time	1.5-2 h
Closing considerations	None
EBL	Minimal
Postop care	2 d hospital stay; liquids on POD 1
Mortality	Rare
Morbidity	Insignificant atelectasis: Common
	Esophageal or gastric perforation: Rare
	Pneumothorax (does not usually require treatment)
	Gastroesophageal reflux: > 15%
Pain score	4

PATIENT POPULATION CHARACTERISTICS

Age range	20-40 yr
Male:Female	1:1

Incidence	Uncommon but not rare
Etiology	Unknown
Associated conditions	None. Chagas' disease may produce identical esophageal findings.

ANESTHETIC CONSIDERATIONS

See Anesthetic Considerations following Laparoscopic Cholecystectomy, p. 461.

References

1. Balaji NS, Peters JH: Minimally invasive surgery for esophageal motility disorders. *Surg Clin North Am* 2002; 82(4):763-82.
2. Esposito PS: Laparoscopic management of achalasia. *Am Surg* 1997; 63(3):221-3.
3. Holzman MD: Laparoscopic surgical treatment of achalasia. *Am J Surg* 1997; 173(4):308-11.
4. Sharp KW, Khaitan L, Scholz S, Holzman MD, Richards WO: 100 minimally invasive Heller myotomies: lessons learned. *Ann Surg* 2002; 235(5):631-9.

LAPAROSCOPIC CHOLECYSTECTOMY, ± COMMON DUCT EXPLORATION

SURGICAL CONSIDERATIONS

Description: This operation typically is performed for symptomatic gallstones or acute cholecystitis. A laparoscopic approach is preferred over an open cholecystectomy because of its minimally invasive nature, which allows earlier recovery and return to normal activities. Laparoscopic cholecystectomy is not indicated for patients with prior upper abdominal surgery, severe COPD, or severe cardiac disease (unable to tolerate ↑intraabdominal pressure). The operation begins with access to the abdominal cavity at the umbilicus, either with a Veress needle (closed technique: blind placement) or a **Hasson trocar** (open technique: ↓risk of vascular, bowel, and bladder injury). If a **Veress needle** is to be used, the patient will need an OG tube and a Foley catheter to decompress the stomach and bladder before proceeding. CO_2 is insufflated to an intraabdominal pressure of 15 mmHg. If the patient develops ventilatory or hemodynamic problems, consider decreasing the intraabdominal pressure to 10-12 mmHg. A total of four trocars are used—one at the umbilicus and three in the RUQ. The cystic artery and cystic duct (with hepatic duct = triangle of Calot) are clipped and cut (Fig 7.7-3). The gallbladder is then dissected off the liver with monopolar cautery, placed in a bag, and brought out, usually through the umbilical cord site. Hemostasis is then achieved, the area is irrigated with NS, and the 10 mm trocar sites are closed. The rate of conversion to an open operation is ~5% for elective gallbladder surgery and ~15% for acute cholecystitis. Should this occur, the patient is then placed in reverse Trendelenburg position and rotated to the left to move the stomach, duodenum, and transverse colon away from the operative field. Surgery then proceeds as for an open cholecystectomy (see p. 446).

Cholangiography can be added easily to the laparoscopic cholecystectomy. A clip is placed high on the cystic duct; then a small incision is made in the duct just beneath the clip. A cholangiocatheter may be introduced and dye injected into the biliary tree. X-rays—either fluoroscopy or, more commonly, hard copy—are used to assess the biliary anatomy and to look for stones within the ductal system. Cholangiography carries few risks, generally adds about 10-15 min to the procedure, and can be used to identify the important anatomy ~85% of the time. Some surgeons perform it routinely during all cholecystectomies; others perform it selectively and only if there is evidence that the patient has had common duct stones or if the anatomy is in question.

In rare circumstances, **laparoscopic common duct exploration** may be carried out to treat common duct stones. A number of techniques have been used, most employing a thin fiber optic choledochoscope passed through the cystic duct into the common duct. This procedure is performed in only a relatively few centers. More commonly, **endoscopic retrograde cholangiopancreatography (ERCP)** will be used, either preop or postop to demonstrate the presence or absence of stones and to remove any stones that are found.

Variant procedure or approaches: Open cholecystectomy (p. 446) remains the major alternative to laparoscopic cholecystectomy, either because the cholecystectomy is predicted to be technically difficult or because of the illness of the patient. About 5% or less of laparoscopic cholecystectomies are converted to open cholecystectomy intraop because of difficulties with the procedure. **ERCP** remains the most common means of treating choledocholithiasis in the industrialized world, with laparoscopic techniques used in a relatively small number of centers and by a small number of surgeons. **Open common duct exploration** is occasionally necessary for stones not retrievable by ERCP (generally < 5%).

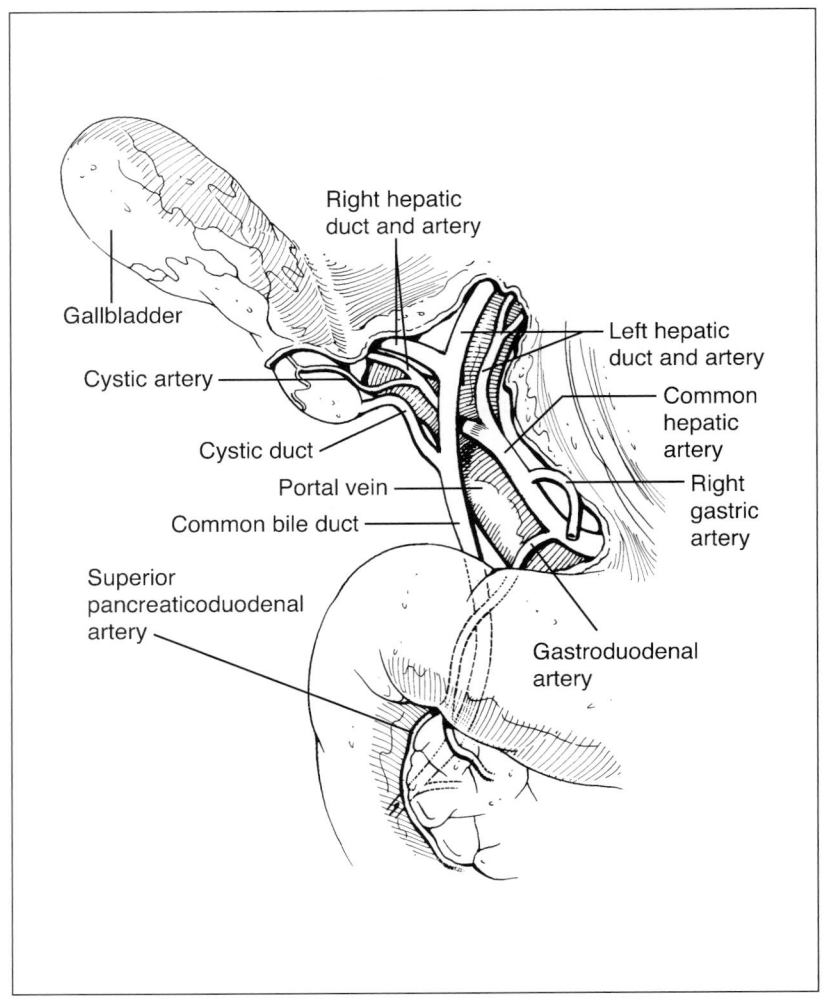

Figure 7.7-3. Surgical anatomy for laparoscopic cholecystectomy and common duct exploration.

Usual preop diagnosis: Acute or chronic cholecystitis, usually with cholelithiasis, with or without choledocholithiasis

SUMMARY OF PROCEDURE

Position	Supine
Incision	4 upper abdominal ports
Special instrumentation	Routine laparoscopic instruments. May require fluoroscopy and choledochoscopes for cholangiography, common duct exploration; OG tube
Antibiotics	Cefazolin 1 g
Surgical time	0.5-2 h; may be longer for common duct exploration.
Closing considerations	Muscular relaxation helpful for closure of umbilical port site
EBL	Minimal
Postop care	Usual discharge within 24 h
Mortality	< 1/1000
Morbidity	Bile leak: 1%
	Common duct injury: 0.5%
	Hemorrhage (requiring transfusion)
	Infection
	Injury to bowel
	Major vascular injury: Uncommon
Pain score	3

PATIENT POPULATION CHARACTERISTICS

Age range	Typically adult, increasing with age
Male:Female	Female > Male
Incidence	Common
Etiology	Stone disease. Risk factors = female gender, age, parity, obesity.
Associated conditions	Hemolytic anemia for pigmented stones

ANESTHETIC CONSIDERATIONS

(Procedures covered: laparoscopic esophageal fundoplication; laparoscopic Heller's myotomy and antireflux surgery; laparoscopic cholecystectomy)

PREOPERATIVE: LAPAROSCOPIC FUNDOPLICATION/HELLER'S MYOTOMY

In general, this patient population is healthy, with the exception of those with GERD. Patients often present with intractable heartburn, which is the reason for undergoing these surgical procedures.

Respiratory	Patients may have Hx of recurrent aspiration with subsequently impaired pulmonary function or chronic pneumonitis. Intraabdominal CO_2 insufflation → atelectasis, ↓FRC, ↑PIP, ↑$PaCO_2$ and ↓PaO_2; therefore, laparoscopic procedures may be contraindicated in patients with severe respiratory impairment. These patients are at risk for aspiration of gastric contents during anesthetic induction and emergence. **Tests**: Consider PA & lateral CXR; consider PFTs if Sx of impaired pulmonary function.
Cardiovascular	Cardiovascular changes caused by the pneumoperitoneum include ↓venous return → ↓CO and ↑SVR. Decreased blood flow to the splanchnic and renal circulations (→ ↓UO) may result from high intraabdominal pressures. Heartburn may mimic angina, and a cardiac origin for the pain should have been excluded prior to scheduling surgery. **Tests**: ECG (r/o MI as cause of pain); others as indicated from H&P.
Laboratory	As indicated from H&P.
Premedication	These patients are at risk for aspiration and should be treated with full-stomach precautions. H_2 antagonists (e.g., ranitidine 50 mg iv, metoclopramide 10 mg iv, both 30 min before induction of anesthesia). Na citrate 30 ml po immediately before induction.

PREOPERATIVE: LAPAROSCOPIC CHOLECYSTECTOMY

The preop evaluation of patients undergoing open cholecystectomy is discussed under Anesthetic Considerations for Biliary Tract Surgery, p. 452. Laparoscopic cholecystectomy is being performed much more commonly than the open procedure and can be accomplished quickly and safely, even in very sick patients.

Respiratory	Intraabdominal CO_2 insufflation → atelectasis, ↓FRC, ↑PIP, ↑$PaCO_2$ and ↓PaO_2; therefore, laparoscopic procedures may be contraindicated in patients with severe respiratory or cardiovascular disease. Postop respiratory function, however, is less impaired (e.g., ↓FRC 30% vs 50%) and is recovered more quickly (24 h vs 72 h) in patients undergoing laparoscopic cholecystectomy then in the open procedure.
Laboratory	CBC; others as indicated from H&P.
Premedication	See Anesthetic Considerations for Biliary Tract Surgery, p. 452.

INTRAOPERATIVE

Anesthetic technique: GETA

Induction	**Laparoscopic fundoplication** and **Heller's myotomy**: Given the patient's risk for aspiration, the trachea should be intubated after rapid-sequence induction with cricoid pressure (p. B-5). **Laparoscopic cholecystectomy**: Standard induction (p. B-2).
Maintenance	Standard maintenance (p. B-3) without N_2O, to prevent distension of the bowel. Continue muscle relaxation. Intraabdominal CO_2 insufflation will → ↑intraabdominal pressure, which will predispose to passive regurgitation of gastric contents. In addition, intraabdominal pressure > 15 mmHg → ↓venous

Maintenance, cont.	return + ↑SVR →↓CO. Controlled ventilation will minimize the possibility of hypercarbia from absorbed CO_2. N_2O can diffuse into CO_2 containing intraabdominal space and ↑distension, as well as risk of explosion.[11,13]	
Emergence	Given the high incidence of N/V (~50%), prophylactic antiemetics (e.g., metoclopramide 10 mg iv) are recommended and should be given 30-60 min before the end of the case.	
Blood and fluid requirements	IV: 16-18 ga × 1 NS/LR @ 8-12 ml/kg/h Fluid warmer	Blood loss should be minimal, although assessment may be difficult 2° concealed bleeding.
Monitoring	Standard monitors (see p. B-1). Urinary catheter NG tube	Others as clinically indicated. Prevent hypothermia (forced-air warmer, heated and humidified gases, warming blanket, warm OR, etc.).
Positioning	✓ and pad pressure points. ✓ eyes.	Initially in Trendelenburg position (↑venous return, ↓lung volumes, potential for mainstem intubation) for trocar placement; then reverse Trendelenburg (↓venous return, ↑lung volumes) during subsequent portions of the surgical procedure. Maintain adequate MAP to ensure cerebral perfusion in reverse Trendelenburg.

Complications	Respiratory:
	  Pneumoperitoneum
	  Hypercarbia/hypoxemia
	  Pneumothorax, pneumomediastinum
	  Endobronchial intubation
		Pneumoperitoneum with CO_2 allows the surgeon to operate laparoscopically. This creates cephalad displacement of the diaphragm with ↓FRC, ↓pulmonary compliance, and atelectasis. This can manifest as ↑PIP, ↓PO_2 and ↑PCO_2. Ventilation should be controlled during the operation to minimize the effects of pneumoperitoneum and hypercarbia. An increase in MV is appropriate. Pneumothorax can occur 2° retroperitoneal dissection of insufflated CO_2. Pneumothorax will manifest as ↓PO_2, ↑PIP, hemodynamic instability (↑HR, ↓BP), and possibly subcutaneous emphysema. The position of the ETT may change with altered patient position → endobronchial intubation.

	Cardiovascular:
	  ↓BP
	  Hemorrhage
	  Dysrhythmias
		↓BP can occur 2° patient positioning (reverse Trendelenburg) and from ↓venous return 2° pneumoperitoneum (↑intraabdominal pressure > 15 mmHg). Hemorrhage can result from inadvertent injury to blood vessels (during trocar placement). Vascular injection of CO_2 (air embolism) can cause ↓BP, dysrhythmias, and even cardiovascular collapse. If cardiopulmonary compromise occurs, the pneumoperitoneum can be released to allow for differential diagnosis and treatment.

	Visceral injury	Injury to the viscera may necessitate an open procedure or may go undiagnosed and → other postop complications, depending on the organ that is injured.
	Hypothermia	2° dry gas insufflation
	Subcutaneous emphysema	Dx: Sudden ↑$ETCO_2$ + subcutaneous crepitation (abdomen/chest wall). Rx: Stop insufflation of CO_2, D/C N_2O, ↑ventilation. Prevention: Keep CO_2 insufflation pressure < 12 mmHg.

POSTOPERATIVE

Complications	N/V (common) Shoulder pain Respiratory	Metoclopramide (10 mg iv), ondansetron (4 mg iv) From pneumoperitoneum; usually self-limited Respiratory complications can be seen in the postop period as well. See list in Intraop Complications, above.
Pain management	PCA (see p. C-3). Percocet 2 tabs po q 6 h	Shoulder pain responds to ketorolac (15-30 mg iv), provided no contraindications to this drug.[10]
Tests	As indicated from H&P.	

References

1. Callery MP, Strasberg SM, Soper NJ: Complications of laparoscopic general surgery. *Gastrointest Endosc Clin N Am* 1996; 6(2):423-44.
2. Cooperman A: Laparoscopic cholecystectomy. In *Atlas of Laparoscopic Surgery*. Ballantyne GH, ed. WB Saunders, Philadelphia: 2000, 36-48.
3. Cunningham AJ, Brull SJ: Laparoscopic cholecystectomy: anesthetic implications. *Anesth Analg* 1993; 76: 1120-33.
4. Feteiha MS, Curet MJ: Laparoscopic cholecystectomy. In *Surgical Laparoscopy*, 2nd edition. Zucker KA, ed. Lippincott Williams & Wilkins, Philadelphia: 2001, 121-32.
5. Gadaca TR: Update on laparoscopic cholecystectomy, including a clinical pathway. *Surg Clin North Am* 2000; 80:1127-50.
6. Gurbuz AT, Peetz ME: The acute abdomen in the pregnant patient. Is there a role for laparoscopy? *Surg Endosc* 1997; 11(2):98-102.
7. Hein HA: Hemodynamic changes during laparoscopic cholecystectomy in patients with severe cardiac disease. *J Clin Anesth* 1997; 9(4):261-5.
8. Joris JL: Anesthetic management of laparoscopy. In *Anesthesia*. Miller RD, ed. Churchill Livingstone, New York: 1994, 2011-29.
9. Lew JKL, Gin T, Oh TE: Anaesthetic problems during laparoscopic cholecystectomy. *Anaesthes Intens Care* 1992; 20:91-2.
10. Michaeliakou C, Chung F, Sharma S: Preoperative multimodal analgesia facilitates recovery after ambulatory laparoscopic cholecystectomy. *Anesth Analg* 1996; 82:44.
11. Neuman GG: Sidebotham G, Negorianu E, et al: Laparoscopic explosion hazards with nitrous oxide. *Anesthesiology* 1993; 78:875.
12. Safran DB: Cholecystectomy following the introduction of laparoscopy; more, but for the same indication. *Am Surg* 1997; 63(6):506-11.
13. Taylor E, Feinstein R, White PF, et al: Anesthesia for laparoscopic cholecystectomy: Is nitrous oxide contraindicated? *Anesthesiology* 1992; 76:541.

LAPAROSCOPIC SPLENECTOMY

SURGICAL CONSIDERATIONS

Description: Laparoscopic-assisted splenectomy is best suited for normal or slightly enlarged spleens (e.g., idiopathic thrombocytopenic purpura [ITP]). Laparoscopic splenectomy usually is contraindicated in patients who have cancer, large hilar lymph nodes, and portal hypertension. At present, the only absolute contraindication to the procedure is massive splenomegaly, with spleens > 30 cm in the longitudinal axis. There is a high conversion rate (to open surgery) if the size of the spleen is between 20-30 cm. Occasionally, a hand-assisted approach may be helpful for spleens in this size range. Conversion rates are higher in patients with perisplenitis and morbid myeloproliferative disorders. For the procedure, patients should be placed on a beanbag in a 45° lateral decubitus position or a full lateral decubitus position. The advantage of the 45° lateral decubitus position is that it is easy to rotate the table and place the patient in

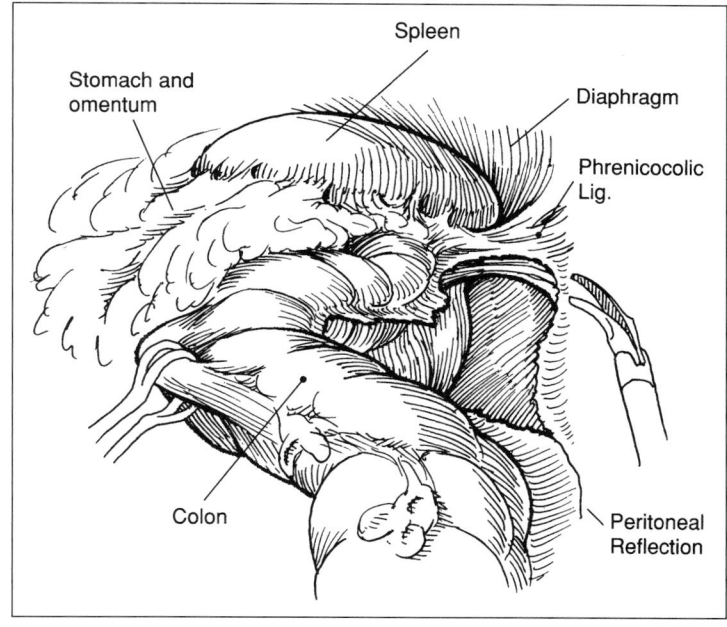

Figure 7.7-4. Anatomy of the spleen. (Reproduced with permission from Wind GG: The spleen. In *Applied Laparoscopic Anatomy: Abdomen and Pelvis*. Williams & Wilkins, Baltimore, 1997.)

a supine position if there is an urgent need for conversion. With the 45° lateral decubitus or the full lateral decubitus position, the kidney rest should be elevated and the OR table should be flexed to increase the area between the costal margin and the superior iliac crest. All pressure points should be padded, and the patient should be secured firmly to the table. The first trocar site is generally in the LUQ. Access can be with a closed (Veress needle or Optiview trocar) or open (Hasson trocar) approach. The initial approach may be to the hilum, short gastrics, or inferior pole. Most surgeons use the Harmonic Scalpel to take down the various ligaments and to dissect out the hilum, which generally is stapled with an endo GIA. The short gastrics are taken down either with the Harmonic Scalpel or are stapled. The lateral and superior attachments are taken down last. The spleen is then placed in a bag. Removal of the spleen can be done in several ways. Some surgeons remove it with a morcellizer placed through one of the trocar sites. Others enlarge one trocar site slightly and remove the spleen in chunks. For very large spleens, some surgeons make a Pfannenstiel incision and extract it through the pelvis.

Variant procedure or approaches: Open splenectomy (described on p. 499). A **hand-assist device** can be used for larger spleens. In such a case, a larger incision (~5 cm) is made either in the midline or the pelvis and a hand is inserted to assist in retracting and dissecting the spleen, while improving visualization.

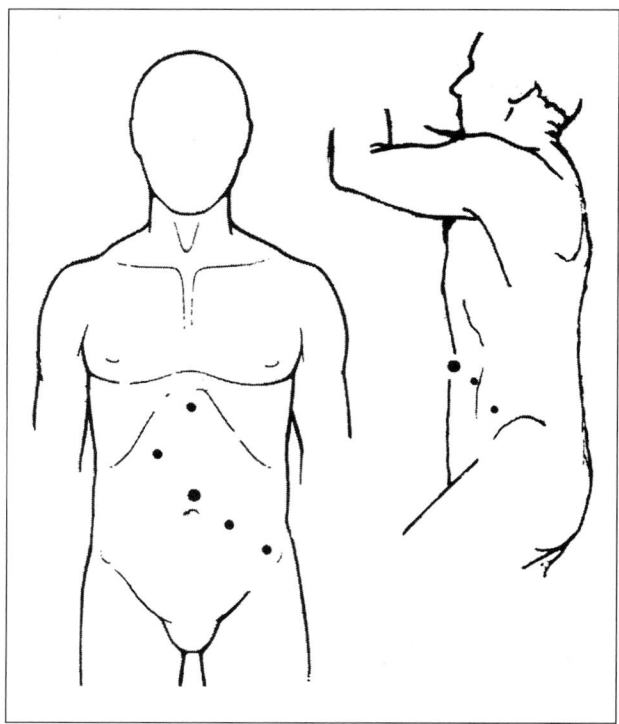

Figure 7.7-5. Trocar location for splenectomy. (Reproduced with permission from Scott-Conner CEH, Dawson DL: *Operative Anatomy*, 2nd edition. Lippincott Williams & Wilkins, 2003.)

Usual preop diagnosis: Idiopathic thrombocytopenic purpura (ITP) (60%); hereditary spherocytosis (10%); hemolytic anemia (5%); thrombotic thrombocytopenic purpura (TTP) (5%); lymphoma (5%); hypersplenism (5%)

SUMMARY OF PROCEDURE

Position	Usually decubitus, flexed or beanbag
Incision	3-5 trocar ports; 1 enlarged to extract spleen
Special instrumentation	Vascular staplers; Harmonic Scalpel; bipolar instruments
Unique considerations	Patients should have received vaccinations (pneumococcal, meningococcal, *Haemophilus influenzae*) preop. DVT prophylaxis; ± stress steroids; ± Plt transfusion.
Antibiotics	Cefazolin 1 g
Surgical time	1-3 h
Closing considerations	Rapid closure not requiring muscle relaxation (following search for accessory spleen)
EBL	< 100 cc; if significant enough to require transfusion, may require conversion to laparotomy.
Postop care	PACU → ward. Generally begin liquids POD 1 and discharge POD 2.
Mortality	0.1% (predominately related to underlying disease)
Morbidity	5%
	Hemorrhage
	Pulmonary
	Injury to pancreas, stomach or splenic flexure of colon
Pain score	5-6

PATIENT POPULATION CHARACTERISTICS

Age range	All ages; more common in adults
Male:Female	1:1
Incidence	Uncommon
Etiology	Hematologic disorders (e.g., ITP, TTP); tumor of the spleen (e.g., Hodgkin's disease); hypersplenism
Associated conditions	Steroid dependence; neutropenia; thrombocytopenia; hemolytic anemias

ANESTHETIC CONSIDERATIONS

PREOPERATIVE

Patients present for laparoscopic splenectomy with a variety of diseases, including ITP,[6] lymphomatous disease (Hodgkin's and non-Hodgkin's), autoimmune hemolytic anemia, TTP, hereditary spherocytosis, Evans's syndrome, hairy-cell leukemia, hypersplenism $2°$ portal HTN, sarcoidosis, polycythemia vera, and myelofibrosis. Open splenectomy is usually reserved for traumatic laceration of the spleen. Previous upper abdominal surgery does not absolutely mitigate against the laparoscopic procedure. Laparoscopic cases tend to take longer than open splenectomies.[3] Patients who have been treated with chemotherapeutic drugs will require careful preop exam to evaluate for potentially toxic side effects. (See Anesthetic Considerations for Splenectomy, p. 497.) Patients should receive pneumococcal, meningococcal, and H. influenza vaccinations at least 1 wk preop.

Respiratory	Patients who present with splenomegaly may have a degree of left lower-lobe atelectasis, which should be evaluated by physical exam. Intraabdominal CO_2 insufflation $\rightarrow$ further atelectasis, $\downarrow$FRC, $\uparrow$PIP, $\uparrow$PaCO$_2$ and $\downarrow$PaO$_2$; therefore, laparoscopic procedures may be contraindicated in patients with severe respiratory disease.
	Tests: Consider P/A & lateral CXR; ABG; PFTs, if clinically indicated.
Cardiovascular	Cardiovascular changes caused by the pneumoperitoneum include $\downarrow$venous return $\rightarrow$ $\downarrow$CO and $\uparrow$SVR. Decreased blood flow to the splanchnic and renal circulations ($\rightarrow$ $\downarrow$UO) may result from high intraabdominal pressures.
Hematologic	Cytopenias are very common.
	Tests: CBC & Plt count
Laboratory	As indicated from H&P.
Premedication	Standard premedication (see p. B-2).

INTRAOPERATIVE

Anesthetic technique: GETA

Induction	Standard induction (see p. B-2).	
Maintenance	Standard maintenance (see p. B-3) without N_2O, to prevent distension of bowel.	
Emergence	No special considerations. Prophylactic antiemetics (e.g., metoclopramide 10 mg) are appropriate.	
Blood and fluid requirements	IV: 16-18 ga × 1 NS/LR @ 8-12 ml/kg/h Fluid warmer	Blood loss should be < 1 U. If Plt transfusion is necessary, it should be given after ligation of splenic vessels ($\downarrow$sequestration). Be prepared to obtain more iv access if bleeding is excessive.
Monitoring	Standard monitors (see p. B-1). Urinary catheter NG tube	Others as indicated by patient status. Prevent hypothermia (forced-air warmer, heated and humidified inspired gases, warming blanket, warm OR, etc.).
Positioning	✓ and pad pressure points. ✓ eyes.	Careful positioning and padding of patient is essential.

Complications	Respiratory:
	  Pneumoperitoneum
	  Hypercarbia/hypoxemia
	  Pneumothorax, pneumomediastinum
	  Endobronchial intubation
	Cardiovascular:
	  $\downarrow$BP
	  Hemorrhage
	  Dysrhythmias
	Visceral injury
	Hypothermia
	Subcutaneous emphysema
	Bleeding
		The complications of laparoscopy are discussed in Anesthetic Considerations for Laparoscopic Cholecystectomy, p. 462.
		
		Typically, when blood loss > 750-1000 ml, convert to open splenectomy. Plt transfusion may be necessary.

POSTOPERATIVE

Complications	PONV	Metoclopramide (10 mg iv), ondansetron (4 mg iv)
	Shoulder pain	2° pneumoperitoneum; usually self-limited. Ketorolac (30 mg iv)
	Atelectasis	Usually left lower lobe
Pain management	PCA (see p. C-3).	
Tests	As indicated by patient status.	

References

1. Diaz J, Eisenstat M, Chung R: A case-controlled study of laparoscopic splenectomy. *Am J Surg* 1997; 173:348-50.
2. Farab RR: Comparison of laparoscopic and open splenectomy in children with hematologic disorders. *J Pediatr* 1997; 131(1):41-6.
3. Gigot JF, Etienne J, Lengele B, Kestens PJ: Elective laparoscopic splenectomy: Personal experience and literature review. *Semin Laparosc Surg* 1996; 3(1):34-43.
4. Katkhouda N, Mavor E: Laparoscopic splenectomy. *Surg Clin North Am* 2000: 80:1285-98.
5. Leggett PL: Laparoscopic splenectomy. *Ann Surg* 1997; 226(1):111-12.
6. Pace DE, Chiasson PM, Schlachta CM, Mamazza J, Poulin EC: Laparoscopic splenectomy for idiopathic thrombocytopenic purpura. *Surg Endosc* 2002; 40 (online publication).
7. Park AE: Lateral approach to laparoscopic splenectomy. In *Surgical Laparoscopy*, 2nd edition. Zucker KA, ed. Lippincott Williams & Wilkins, Philadelphia: 2001, 625-34.
8. Tsiotos G: Laparoscopic splenectomy for immune thrombocytopenic purpura. *Arch Surg* 1997; 132(6):642-46.

LAPAROSCOPIC ADRENALECTOMY

SURGICAL CONSIDERATIONS

Description: Laparoscopic adrenalectomy typically is performed for a variety of adrenal problems, such as Conn's disease, functioning adenoma, pheochromocytoma, Cushing's disease, hyperplasia, virilizing or feminizing tumors, and an enlarging, nonfunctioning adenoma. Contraindications to laparoscopic surgery include invasive malignancy, malignant pheochromocytoma, and an uncorrectable coagulopathy. Urologists generally use a retroperitoneal approach, while other surgeons use a transabdominal approach. The patient should be on a beanbag in the full lateral decubitus position. The kidney rest should be elevated and the table should be flexed to open up the area between the costal margin and iliac crest. A left adrenalectomy is typically easier than a right adrenalectomy. On the left side, three trocars are required along the costal margin. Surgery begins by immobilizing the spleen and the colon laterally, which allows the spleen to fall away completely from the adrenal gland. The adrenal is then seen behind the hilum of the spleen. Care should be taken to minimize manipulation of a pheochromocytoma, to prevent sudden, unexpected HTN during the operation. In general, most surgeons prefer to clip and cut the adrenal vein first. Once the adrenal is completely mobilized, it is removed through one of the port sites. For a right-sided approach, four trocars generally are required along the costal margin. The fourth trocar is used to retract the liver. The first step on the right side is to mobilize the lateral attachments of the liver to expose the adrenal. An enlarged right adrenal may be difficult to mobilize enough to see the adrenal vein, since the right adrenal vein empties directly into the IVC. Most surgeons recommend using an endo GIA stapler to divide the right adrenal vein.

Variant procedure or approaches: Open procedure (p. 530), or retroperitoneal approach

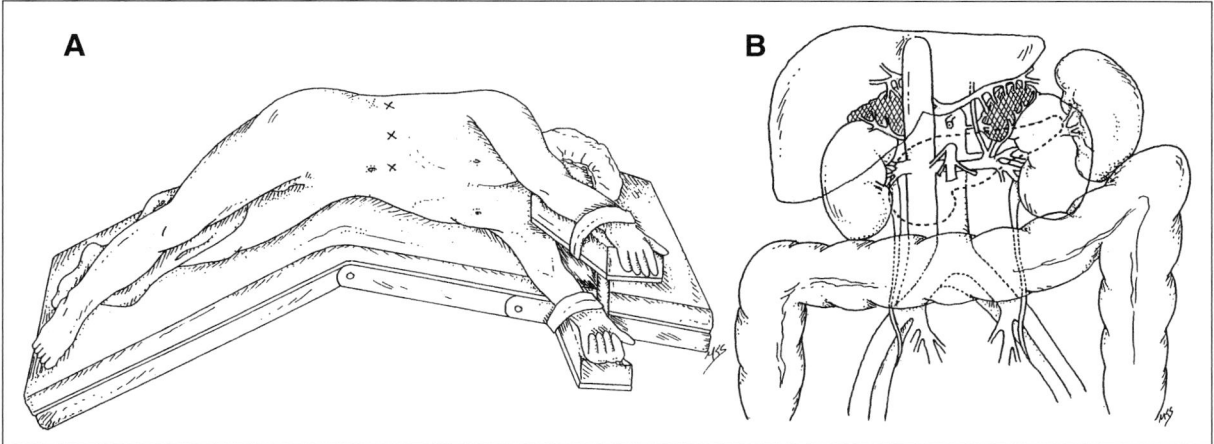

Figure 7.7-6. Laparoscopic adrenalectomy. (A) Patient positioning and port locations. (B) Anatomic relationships of adrenals (sutured) to adjunct and overlying structures. (Reproduced with permission from Scott-Conner CEH, Dawson DL: *Operative Anatomy*, 2nd edition. Lippincott Williams & Wilkins, 2003.)

Usual preop diagnosis: Indeterminate adrenal mass (nonfunctional adenoma); also can be performed for functional adenomas, rarely for pheochromocytoma. Contraindicated for known carcinoma.

SUMMARY OF PROCEDURE

Position	Lateral decubitus. A patient with bilateral disease may need repositioning between sides; or surgeon may use a supine approach.
Incision	3 ports on left side; 4 ports on right side
Antibiotics	Cefazolin 1 g iv
Surgical time	1-2 h
Closing considerations	Brief closure; muscle relaxation helpful for fascial repair
EBL	< 75 ml, although occasionally significant blood loss may occur.
Postop care	Patient usually discharged on POD 1 or 2, depending on BP control.
Mortality	< 0.1%
Morbidity	Hemorrhage/hematoma
	Injury to pancreas or kidney
	UTI
	DVT
Pain score	4

PATIENT POPULATION CHARACTERISTICS

Age range	All ages
Male:Female	1:1
Incidence	Varies with underlying disorder
Etiology	Pheochromocytoma (25%); nonfunctioning adenomas, aldosteronoma (21%); cortisol-producing adenoma (15%); Cushing's disease (8%)
Associated conditions	Depending on function of tumor (e.g., HTN for aldosteronoma, Cushing's disease)

ANESTHETIC CONSIDERATIONS

PREOPERATIVE

The preop evaluation of patients undergoing laparoscopic adrenalectomy is discussed under Anesthetic Considerations for (open) Adrenalectomy, p. 533.

Cardiovascular Cardiovascular changes caused by the pneumoperitoneum include ↓venous return → ↓CO and ↑SVR. Decreased blood flow to the splanchnic and renal circulations (→ ↓UO) may result from high intraabdominal pressures.

INTRAOPERATIVE

Anesthetic technique: GETA. An epidural should not be necessary for postop analgesia if the procedure is performed laparoscopically. If the surgical team feels that there is a high likelihood of conversion to an open procedure, consider placement of an epidural catheter for postop analgesia.

Induction	See induction under (open) Adrenalectomy, p. 534.	
Maintenance	See maintenance under (open) Adrenalectomy, p. 534.	
Emergence	See emergence under (open) Adrenalectomy, p. 534. Case is likely to take longer if performed laparoscopically, but usually has a less painful postop course. Prophylactic antiemetics (e.g., metoclopramide 10 mg with dolasetron 12.5 mg/ondansetron 4 mg iv) are appropriate.	
Blood and fluid requirements	IV: 14-16 ga × 1 NS/LR @10-15 ml/kg/h	Warming techniques important (forced-air warmers, fluid warmers, humidified inspired gases, etc.).
Monitoring	Standard monitors (see p. B-1). UO Arterial line ± PA catheter TEE	A PA catheter is useful in the management of patients with pheochromocytoma. TEE may be needed to evaluate cardiac function and filling.
Positioning	✓ and pad pressure points. ✓ eyes.	Careful support and padding of extremities and torso is very important.
Complications: laparoscopic	Respiratory: 　Pneumoperitoneum 　Hypercarbia/hypoxemia 　Pneumothorax, pneumomediastinum 　Endobronchial intubation Cardiovascular: 　↓BP 　Hemorrhage 　Dysrhythmias Visceral injury Subcutaneous emphysema Hypothermia	The complications of laparoscopy are discussed in Anesthetic Considerations for Laparoscopic Cholecystectomy, p. 565.
Complications: endocrine	Pheochromocytoma: 　BP lability 　Myocardial dysfunction Conn's syndrome: 　CHF 2° hypervolemia 　↓BP 　Electrolyte disturbances 　Hyperglycemia Cushing's syndrome: 　↓↓BP 　Acute adrenal insufficiency	Rx: intraop HTN with SNP or phentolamine (2.5-5 mg q 5 min); ↑HR with esmolol; ↓BP with phenylephrine or dopamine. (See Anesthetic Considerations for Adrenalectomy, p. 533.) See Anesthetic Considerations for Adrenalectomy, p. 533. Continue replacement steroids. (See Anesthetic Considerations for Adrenalectomy, p. 533.)

POSTOPERATIVE

Complications	PONV Shoulder pain Other	Metoclopramide (10 mg iv), ondansetron (4 mg iv). 2° pneumoperitoneum; usually self-limited. Ketorolac (30 mg iv).
Pain management	PCA (see p. C-3).	See Anesthetic Considerations for Adrenalectomy, p. 535.
Tests	As indicated	

References

1. Arca MJ, Gagner M: Laparoscopic management of adrenal lesions. In *Surgical Laparoscopy*, 2nd edition. Zucker KA, ed. Lippincott Williams & Wilkins, Philadelphia: 2001, 635-42.
2. Chapuis Y: Bilateral laparoscopic adrenalectomy for Cushing's disease. *Br J Surg* 1997; 84(7):1009.
3. Gagner M: Laparoscopic adrenalectomy. In *Atlas of Laparoscopic Surgery*. Ballantyne GH, ed. WB Saunders, Philadelphia: 2000, 280-99.
4. Hasan R, Harold KL, Matthews BD, Kercher KW, Sing RF, Heniford BT: Outcomes for laparoscopic bilateral adrenalectomy. *J Laparoendosc Adv Surg Tech A* 2000; 12(4):233-6.
5. Horgan S, Sinan M, Helton WS, Pellegrini CA: Use of laparoscopic techniques improves outcome from adrenalectomy. *Am J Surg* 1997; 173:371-4.
6. Raeburn CD, McIntyre RC Jr: Laparoscopic approach to adrenal and endocrine pancreatic tumors. *Surg Clin North Am* 2000; 80:1427-42.
7. Staren ED: Adrenalectomy in the era of laparoscopy. *Surgery* 1996; 120(4):706-9.
8. Vargas HI, Kavoussi LR, Bartlett DL, et al: Laparoscopic adrenalectomy: A new standard of care. *Urology* 1997; 49:673-8.

LAPAROSCOPIC BOWEL RESECTION

SURGICAL CONSIDERATIONS

Description: The surgical community has not uniformly embraced **laparoscopic bowel surgery**. It is technically very difficult because the surgeon has to maneuver in several quadrants during the operation. In benign diseases (e.g., ulcerative colitis, Crohn's disease, diverticular disease, and polyps) there are clear advantages to a laparoscopic approach to bowel resection, including decreased pain, earlier return of GI function, earlier ambulation, and earlier discharge from the hospital. Although these advantages also apply to the patient with cancer, there are still reservations about whether cure and survival rates are the same. Preliminary data from several ongoing multicenter trials indicate that the length of the specimen and the number of lymph nodes removed are the same with both approaches. Data regarding 2-yr survival will be available soon.

For a left-sided colon resection, the patient is placed in a low lithotomy position, while in other bowel resections, a supine position is used. The patient's arms should be tucked to improve access to all four quadrants. Generally, 4-5 ports are required, one in each quadrant. For a **laparoscopic-assisted approach**, one of these ports will be enlarged slightly for removal of the specimen. Very often the operating table will need to be tilted or rotated throughout the course of the procedure to help move the small intestines away from the surgical dissection site. The procedure typically begins with localization of the pathology. This may require an intraop sigmoidoscopy if the lesion has not already been marked on colonoscopy or if it is not grossly apparent. The involved section of the intestine is then mobilized. Often, division of the mesentery is done intracorporeally. Occasionally, surgeons will exteriorize the bowel and do extracorporeal division of the mesentery and extracorporeal

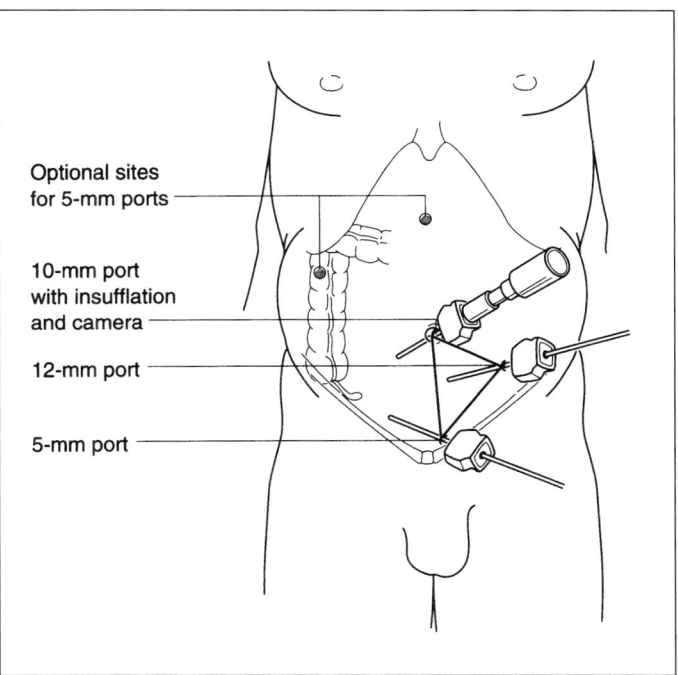

Figure 7.7-7. Trocar placement for a right colectomy. The general principle is to place the camera port so that the surgeon's visual axis is parallel to the telescope, and to place the working ports so that the operative site is at the apex of an isosceles triangle. (Reproduced with permission from Greenfield LJ, et al, eds: *Surgery: Scientific Principles and Practice*, 2nd edition. Lippincott-Raven Publishers, Philadelphia: 1997.)

Optional sites for 5-mm ports

10-mm port with insufflation and camera

12-mm port

5-mm port

division of the bowel. For right-sided lesions, the anastomosis typically is done extracorporeally; however, for left-sided lesions, once the bowel is removed, the extraction site will be closed. The pneumoperitoneum will be reinsufflated and the anastomosis will be performed intracorporeally with an end-to-end stapler placed through the anus.

Unipolar and bipolar cautery, the Harmonic Scalpel, and many different surgical staplers may be used during these procedures. These generally require longer operative times than the corresponding open procedures but, typically, they are associated with shorter hospitalization stays and earlier return to work than traditional laparotomy.

Variant procedure or approaches: Open surgery (see p. 413), laparoscopic-assisted, or totally laparoscopic procedures. Some surgeons also have recommended a hand-assisted procedure where a pneumoperitoneum is still used, but the port site of extraction is enlarged at the beginning of the operation. The surgeon's hand can be placed through a special sleeve that maintains pneumoperitoneum, but also allows the surgeon to retract and dissect manually. Occasionally, the specimen is removed via the anus or through a vaginotomy.

Usual preop diagnosis: Intestinal obstruction; inflammatory conditions (e.g., diverticulitis, bleeding, neoplasms); cancer (controversial)

SUMMARY OF PROCEDURE

Position	Usually supine; sometimes lithotomy for left-sided procedures
Incision	4-5 trocar sites, one in each quadrant. One site will be enlarged for specimen removal and/or anastomosis in laparoscopic-assisted procedures.
Special instrumentation	Harmonic Scalpel, various laparoscopic stapling instruments
Unique considerations	The operating table will be moved quite frequently to help with visualization.
Antibiotics	Cefotetan 1 g
Surgical time	1.5-2 h (small bowel resection); 3-4 h (colonic resection). Surgical times will ↑ in the presence of acute inflammation and as the bowel resection becomes more extensive.
Closing considerations	Usually requires closure of several port sites; muscle relaxation helpful.
EBL	< 200 ml
Postop care	NG tube seldom used. Most patients begin regular diet within 48 h; discharge, generally 3-4 d.
Mortality	< 0.1%

Morbidity	< 5% (similar in magnitude to those seen with open operations)
	Complications include:
	  Hemorrhage
	  Infection
	  Anastomotic leak
	  Intestinal obstruction

Pain score	6-7

PATIENT POPULATION CHARACTERISTICS

Age range	All ages (increases with age)
Male:Female	1:1
Incidence	Varies with disease process.
Etiology	Diverticulitis; polyps; inflammatory bowel disease (IBD)
Associated conditions	None

ANESTHETIC CONSIDERATIONS

PREOPERATIVE

For respiratory, cardiovascular, musculoskeletal, gastrointestinal, and renal considerations, see Anesthetic Considerations for Intestinal and Peritoneal Procedures, p. 416.

Cardiovascular	Cardiovascular changes caused by the pneumoperitoneum include ↓venous return → ↓CO and ↑SVR. Decreased blood flow to the splanchnic and renal circulations (→ ↓UO) may result from high intraabdominal pressures.
Premedication	Standard premedication (see p. B-2). If patient is at risk for a full stomach, administration of metoclopramide (10 mg iv) and H_2 blocker (ranitidine 50 mg iv), as well as Na citrate 0.3 M 30 ml po. Metoclopramide should not be used in patients with bowel obstructions or perforations.

INTRAOPERATIVE

Anesthetic technique: GETA

Induction	Standard induction (see p. B-2). Standard rapid-sequence induction if at risk for aspiration (see p. B-5).	
Maintenance	Standard maintenance (see p. B-3) without N_2O, to prevent distension of the bowel.	
Emergence	No special considerations unless the patient is at risk for aspiration; extubation should then occur after the patient is fully awake and has protective airway reflexes.	
Blood and fluid requirements	IV: 16-18 ga × 1 NS/LR @ 8-12 ml/kg/h Fluid warmer	Blood loss should be < 1 U.
Monitoring	Standard monitors (see p. B-1). Urinary catheter NG tube to decompress the stomach	Others as indicated by patient status. Prevent hypothermia (forced-air warmer, heated humidified gases, warming blanket, warm room, etc).
Positioning	✓ and pad pressure points. ✓ eyes.	

Complications	Respiratory:
	  Pneumoperitoneum
	  Hypercarbia/hypoxemia
	  Pneumothorax, pneumomediastinum
	  Endobronchial intubation
	Cardiovascular:
	  ↓BP
	  Hemorrhage
	  Dysrhythmias
	Visceral injury
	Hypothermia
	Subcutaneous emphysema
		These complications (associated with the preperitoneal approach), as well as the general complications of laparoscopy, are discussed in Anesthetic Considerations for Laparoscopic Cholecystectomy, p. 462.

POSTOPERATIVE

Complications	PONV Shoulder pain	Metoclopramide (10 mg iv), ondansetron (4 mg iv) 2° pneumoperitoneum. Usually self-limited. Ketorolac (30 mg iv).
Pain management	PCA (see p. C-3).	
Tests	As indicated by patient status.	

References

1. Ballantyne GH, ed: *Atlas of Laparoscopic Surgery*. WB Saunders, Philadelphia: 2000, 300-404.
2. Bohm B, Milsom JW, Fazio VW: Postoperative intestinal motility following conventional and laparoscopic intestinal surgery. *Arch Surg* 1995; 130:415-19.
3. Bokey EL: Morbidity and mortality following laparoscopic-assisted right hemicolectomy for cancer. *Dis Colon Rectum* 1996; 39(10):S24-S28.
4. Callery MP, Strasberg SM, Soper NJ: Complications of laparoscopic general surgery. *Gastrointest Endosc Clin N Am* 1996; 6:423-44.
5. Fleshman JW, Nelson H, Peters WR, Kim HC, Larach S, Boorse RR, Ambroze W, Leggett P, Bleday R, Stryker S, Christenson B, Wexner S, Senagore A, Rattner D, Sutton J, Fine AP: Early results of laparoscopic surgery for colorectal cancer. Retrospective analysis of 372 patients treated by Clinical Outcomes of Surgical Therapy (COST) Study Group. *Dis Colon Rectum* 1996; 39(10 Suppl):S53-S58.
6. Goh YC: Early postoperative results of a prospective series of laparoscopic vs. open anterior resections for rectosigmoid cancers. *Dis Colon Rectum* 1997; 40(7):776-80.
7. Laparoscopic repair of incisional hernia: Retrospective study of 159 patients. *Surg Endosc* 2002; 16(2):345-8.
8. Milsom JW, Hammerhofer KA, Bohn B, Marcello P, Elson P, Fazio VW: Prospective randomized trial comparing laparoscopic vs. conventional surgery for refractory ileocolic Crohn's disease. *Dis Colon Rectum* 2001; 44(1):1-8.
9. Paik PS: Laparoscopic colectomy. *Surg Clin North Am* 1997; 77(1):1-13.

10. Potenti FM, Wexner SD: Laparoscopy for benign colonic disease. In *Surgical Laparoscopy*, 2nd edition. Zucker KA, ed. Lippincott Williams & Wilkins, Philadelphia: 2001, 255-74.

11. Wexner SD: Laparoscopic colectomy in diverticular and Crohn's disease. *Surg Clin North Am* 2000; 80:1299-1320.

12. Wichmann MW, Meyer G, Angele MK, Schildberg FW, Rau HG: Recent advances in minimally invasive colorectal cancer surgery. *Onkologie* 2002; 25(4):318-23.

LAPAROSCOPIC APPENDECTOMY

SURGICAL CONSIDERATIONS

Description: Appendectomy generally is performed for suspected appendicitis.[5] The patient is placed in the supine position with the left arm tucked. An OG tube should be inserted to decompress the stomach. Access is obtained at the umbilicus, either through a closed (**Veress needle**) technique or open (**Hasson trocar**) technique. If a Veress needle is used, a Foley catheter should be inserted. Two additional trocars are inserted—one suprapubic and the other in the LLQ. The port in the LLQ is a 10/12 mm trocar to allow passage of an endo GIA stapler. Occasionally, a fourth trocar may be placed in the RUQ to help with mobilization and retraction. The table will then be rotated to the left side and the surgeon may ask for it to be placed in Trendelenburg or reverse Trendelenburg position, depending on the location of the cecum. The base of the cecum is identified and the appendix is mobilized (Fig 7.7-8B). This may require dissection of the peritoneal edge along the right gutter. Once the appendix is mobilized, a window is created in the mesoappendix, and the base of the appendix is stapled with an endo GIA. The mesoappendix is then stapled with a vascular-cartridge endo GIA. The appendix generally is placed in a bag prior to delivering it, or it may be brought directly through the 10/12 mm trocar. The umbilical fascia is closed and the skin is loosely approximated. When unexpected pathology is identified, it can be dealt with by laparoscopy or by laparotomy, with incision placement dependent on findings.

Variant procedure or approaches: Open appendectomy (see p. 407) via RLQ or midline incision

Usual preop diagnosis: Acute abdomen; possible acute appendicitis

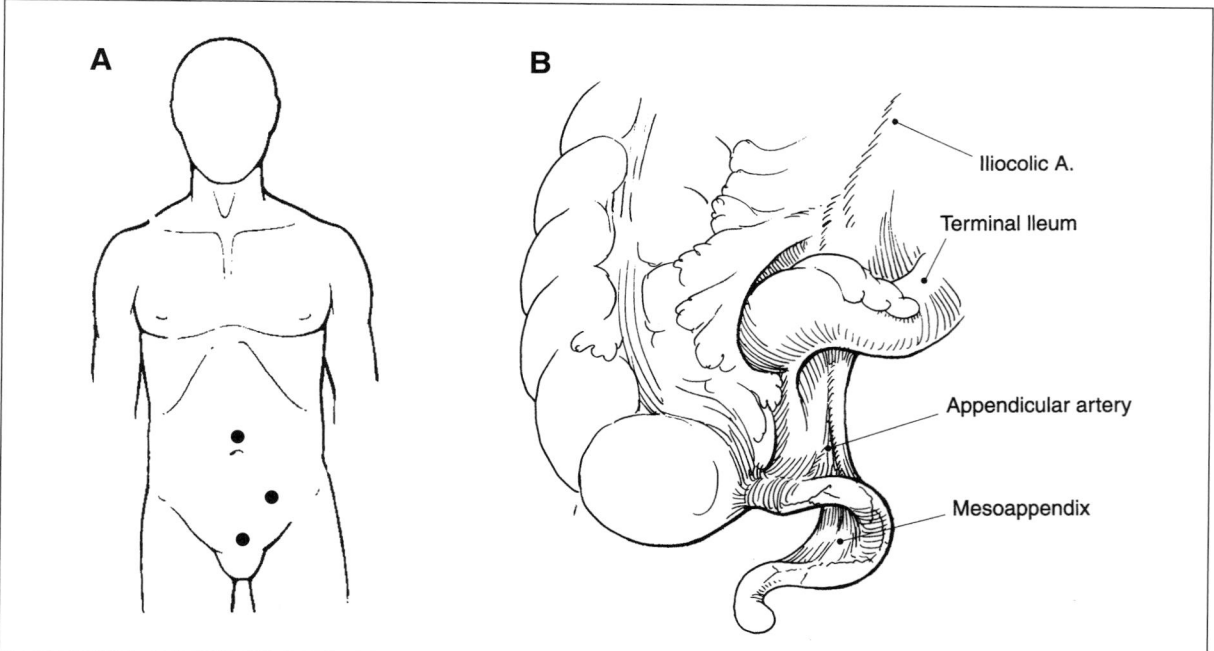

Figure 7.7-8. Setup and initial view for laparoscopic appendectomy. (A reproduced with permission from Scott-Conner CEH, Dawson DL: *Operative Anatomy*, 2nd edition. Lippincott Williams & Wilkins, 2003. B reproduced with permission from Wind GG: The spleen. In *Applied Laparoscopic Anatomy: Abdomen and Pelvis*. Williams & Wilkins, Baltimore, 1997.)

SUMMARY OF PROCEDURE

Position	Supine
Incision	3-4 ports (see Fig 7.7-8A)
Antibiotics	Cefazolin 1 g
Surgical time	60-90 min
Closing considerations	Muscular relaxation helpful for umbilical closure; NG tube if prolonged ileus suspected.
EBL	< 75 ml
Postop care	Patients are hospitalized for varying lengths of time, depending on their need for antibiotics. Many with simple acute appendicitis can go home within 24 h.
Mortality	Perforated: 2-5% (nonperforated: < 0 .1%); increased in elderly patients and infants.
Morbidity	Overall: 3% if nonperforated; 20-50% with perforation
	Intraabdominal abscess
	Hematoma
	Ileus
	Risk of intraabdominal abscess, mostly dependent on pathology (e.g., early acute inflammation vs perforation)
	Hemorrhage
	Infection
	Stump leak: exceedingly rare
	Conversion to open procedure: dependent on pathology and experience of surgeon
Pain score	4

PATIENT POPULATION CHARACTERISTICS

Age range	All ages; commonly, 19-25 yr
Male:Female	1:1
Incidence	Common (7%)
Etiology	Acute appendicitis; etiology unknown
Associated conditions	Consider other pelvic pathology in women of childbearing age.

ANESTHETIC CONSIDERATIONS

PREOPERATIVE

This patient population is generally fit and healthy, apart from their acutely presenting illness. Full-stomach precautions (see p. B-5) are appropriate in these patients.

Respiratory	Respiratory impairment can occur 2° acute abdominal pain and splinting. Tachypnea and hyperpnea can be heralding Sx of appendiceal perforation and sepsis. Patients with acute abdomen should be treated as if they have full stomachs. **Tests:** As indicated from H&P.
Cardiovascular	Cardiovascular changes caused by the pneumoperitoneum include ↓venous return → ↓CO and ↑SVR. Decreased blood flow to the splanchnic and renal circulations (→ ↓UO) may result from high intraabdominal pressures. May be dehydrated from fever, emesis, and decreased oral intake. Assess volume status with VS in the supine and standing positions (if possible) and hydrate adequately before anesthetic induction. **Tests:** ECG, if indicated from H&P.
Gastrointestinal	Patient typically has abdominal pain with N/V. Muscular resistance to palpation of abdominal wall frequently parallels the severity of the inflammatory process. With spreading peritoneal irritation (as with perforation), patient will develop abdominal distension and paralytic ileus. **Tests:** Electrolytes
Hematologic	Moderate leukocytosis (10,000-18,000) with moderate left shift. Hemoconcentration is probable, if patient is dehydrated. **Tests:** CBC
Laboratory	Others as indicated from H&P.

Premedication	Patients with acute appendicitis should be treated as if they have full stomachs. Consider administration of metoclopramide (10 mg iv) and H_2 blocker (ranitidine 50 mg iv), as well as Na citrate 0.3 M 30 ml po. Opiate premedication (morphine 0.08-0.15 mg/kg im) is indicated after patient is scheduled for surgery. If surgical intervention is still in question, administration of opiates may mask Sx of appendicitis.

INTRAOPERATIVE

Anesthetic technique: GETA, with rapid-sequence iv induction.

Induction	Preoxygenate patient and have an assistant apply cricoid pressure. Etomidate 0.1-0.4 mg/kg, STP 3-5 mg/kg + succinylcholine 1.5 mg/kg, for intubation.	
Maintenance	Standard maintenance (see p. B-3), without N_2O.	
Emergence	Extubate when the patient is awake and with active laryngeal protective reflexes.	
Blood and fluid requirements	IV: 16-18 ga × 1 NS/LR @ 5-8 ml/kg/h	
Monitoring	Standard monitors (see p. B-1). Urinary catheter NG tube	Others as indicated by patient status. Prevent hypothermia (forced-air warmer, heated humidified gases, warming blanket, warm room, etc.)
Positioning	✓ and pad pressure points. ✓ eyes. Secure or tuck arms.	Trendelenburg position with elevation of the right side of the abdomen improves surgical exposure.

Complications	Respiratory:
	  Pneumoperitoneum
	  Hypercarbia/hypoxemia
	  Pneumothorax, pneumomediastinum
	  Endobronchial intubation
	Cardiovascular:
	  Hypotension
	  Hemorrhage
	  Dysrhythmias
	Visceral injury
	Hypothermia
	Subcutaneous emphysema
		These complications (associated with the preperitoneal approach), as well as the general complications of laparoscopy, are discussed in Anesthetic Considerations for Laparoscopic Cholecystectomy, p. 462.

POSTOPERATIVE

Complications	PONV Urinary retention	Metoclopramide (10 mg iv), ondansetron (4 mg iv) Straight catheterization of the bladder
Pain management	PCA (see p. C-3). Oral opiates Ketorolac	 Tylenol #3 – 2 po q 6 h or Percocet – 2 po q 6 h 30 mg iv
Tests	As indicated by patient status.	

References

1. Amos JD, Schorr SJ, Norman PF, et al: Laparoscopic surgery during pregnancy. *Am J Surg* 1996; 171:425-37.
2. Callery MP, Strasberg SM, Soper NJ: Complications of laparoscopic general surgery. *Gastrointest Endosc Clin North Am* 1996; 6:423-44.
3. Caushaj PF: Laparoscopic appendectomy. In *Atlas of Laparoscopic Surgery*. Ballantyne GH, ed. WB Saunders, Philadelphia: 2000, 300-7.
4. Chiarugi M: Laparoscopic compared with open appendectomy for acute appendicitis: a prospective study. *Eur J Surg* 1996; 162(5):385-90.
5. Fogli L, Brulatti M, Boschi S, De Domenico M, Papa V, Patrizi P, Capizzi F: Laparoscopic appendectomy for acute and recurrent appendicitis: retrospective analysis of a single-group 5-year experience. *J Laparosc Adv Surg Tech A* 2002; 12(2): 107-10.
6. Josloff RK, Zucker KA: Laparoscopic appendectomy. In *Surgical Laparoscopy*, 2nd edition. Zucker KA, ed. Lippincott Williams & Wilkins, Philadelphia: 2001, 229-36.

7. Kumar R, Erian M, Sirrot S, Knoesen R, Kinde R: Laparoscopic appendectomy in modern gynecology. *J Am Assoc Gynecol Laparosc* 2002; 9(3):252-63.
8. Laine S: Laparoscopic appendectomy—is it worthwhile? A prospective, randomized study in young women. *Surg Endosc* 1997; 11(2):95-7.

LAPAROSCOPIC INGUINAL HERNIA REPAIR

SURGICAL CONSIDERATIONS

Description: Laparoscopic hernia repair is clearly preferred in patients with recurrent or bilateral hernias. In patients with first-time unilateral hernias, there are no clear advantages in terms of operative time, postop pain, time to discharge, or time to return to normal activities, compared with tension-free open repair (see p. 504). There are three types of laparoscopic hernia repairs. The first, **ONLAY**, generally has been discarded because of high recurrence rates. The other two are the **totally extraperitoneal (TEP)** and the **transabdominal preperitoneal (TAPP)** techniques. Of these, the TEP is somewhat more difficult to learn, but is associated with lower recurrence rates and complications than is the TAPP. For both the TEP and the TAPP, the patient is placed in the supine position with both arms tucked. Some surgeons insert a Foley, but many do not. A small incision is made at the umbilicus. For a **TEP**, this incision only goes to the preperitoneal space, and a balloon is then used for dissection. Two additional ports are placed in the midline—one suprapubic and one halfway between the umbilicus and the suprapubic port. Further dissection is required to identify the hernia defects, which are then reduced. The cord structures are completely freed and any cord lipomas are dissected. Mesh is placed to cover the

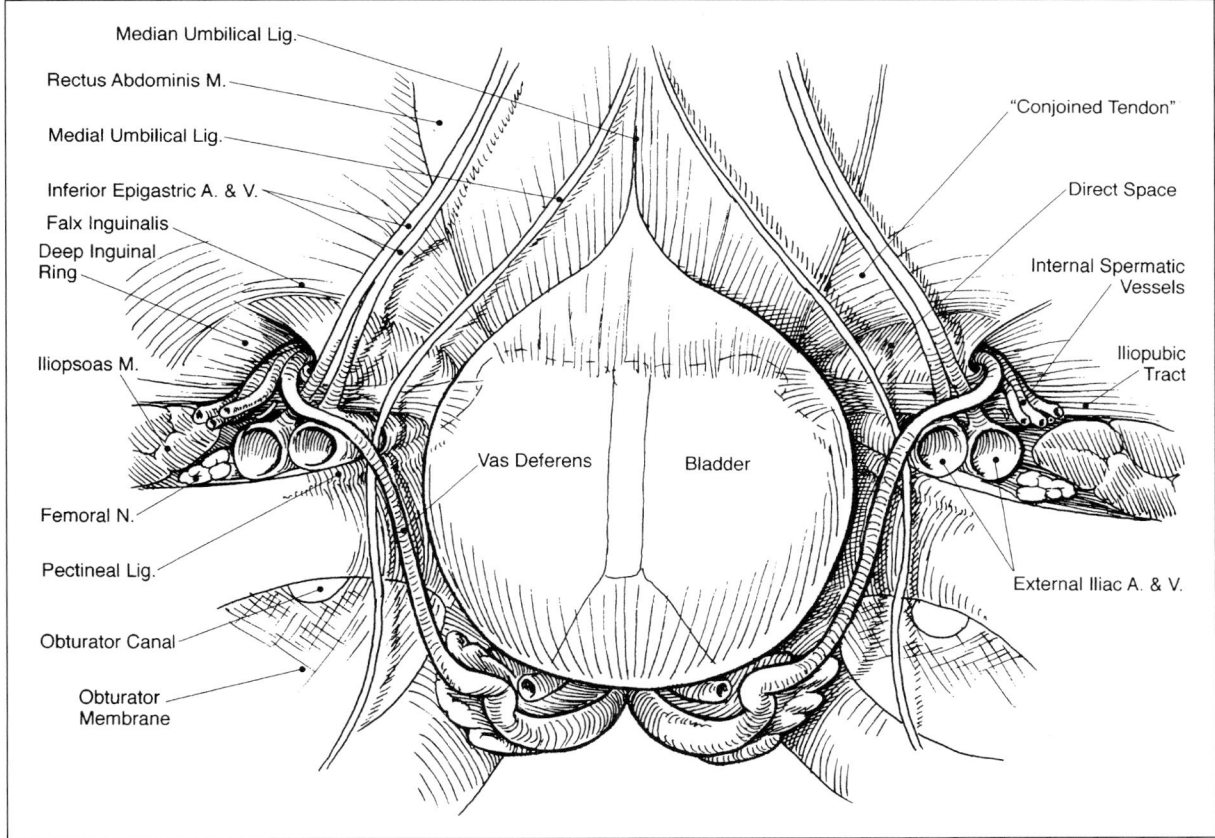

Figure 7.7-9. The inguinal region. (Reproduced with permission from Wind GG: The inguinal region. In *Applied Laparoscopic Anatomy: Abdomen and Pelvis.* Williams & Wilkins, Baltimore, 1997.)

entire area and is tacked to Cooper's ligament. For a **TAPP** repair, the umbilical incision extends into the abdomen. Two additional ports are placed at the level of the iliac crest—one in the RLQ and one in the LLQ. A peritoneal flap over the hernia defect is created and the preperitoneal space is entered. The rest of the dissection and the placement of the mesh are the same as with the TEP repair. At the end of the TAPP procedure, the peritoneal flap is placed over the mesh and tacked into place to prevent exposure of the bowel to the mesh.

Variant Procedure or approaches: Open hernia repair (see Inguinal Herniorrhaphy, p. 504).

Usual preop diagnosis: Inguinal hernia

SUMMARY OF PROCEDURE

Position	Supine, arms tucked
Incision	3 ports—1 at the umbilicus; 2 either in the midline or RLQ or LLQ, depending on the laparoscopic approach.
Special instrumentation	Balloon dissector for TEP repair
Antibiotics	Cefazolin 1 g
Surgical time	1-2 h
Closing considerations	Minimal time; muscle relaxation may be helpful.
EBL	< 50 ml
Postop care	1-2 h in PACU/holding area → home
Mortality	< 0.1%
Morbidity	2%
	Orchialgia, neuralgia
	Recurrence of hernia: Rare in experienced hands
	Bowel obstruction
	Bladder injury: Rarely reported
Pain score	3-4

PATIENT POPULATION CHARACTERISTICS

Age range	Mostly adults
Male:Female	Male > Female
Incidence	Common
Etiology	Most hernias congenital; chronically increased intraabdominal pressure (e.g., chronic cough, obesity)
Associated conditions	None important

ANESTHETIC CONSIDERATIONS

PREOPERATIVE

The preop evaluation of patients undergoing laparoscopic hernia repair is discussed in Anesthetic Considerations for Inguinal Hernia, p. 508. Patients presenting for this procedure are generally healthy. Laparoscopic repair of inguinal hernia is usually associated with less pain and earlier return to preop function when compared to the open procedure. Patients with strangulated or incarcerated hernias usually require open procedures.

Cardiovascular	Cardiovascular changes caused by the pneumoperitoneum include ↓venous return → ↓CO and ↑SVR. Decreased blood flow to the splanchnic and renal circulations (→ ↓UO) may result from high intraabdominal pressures.
Laboratory	Hb/Hct (healthy patients); otherwise, as indicated from H&P.
Premedication	Standard premedication (see p. B-2).

INTRAOPERATIVE

Anesthetic technique: GETA

Induction	Standard induction (see p. B-2).

Maintenance	Standard maintenance (see p. B-3), without N_2O, to prevent distension of the bowel.	
Emergence	No special considerations except to minimize coughing on emergence. Consider 1 mg/kg iv lidocaine.	
Blood and fluid requirements	IV: 18 ga × 1 NS/LR @ 5-8 ml/kg/h Fluid warmer	Blood loss should be minimal.
Monitoring	Standard monitors (see p. B-1). Urinary catheter NG tube	Others as indicated by patient status. Prevent hypothermia (forced-air warmer, heated and humidified gases, warming blanket, warm OR, etc.).
Positioning	✓ and pad pressure points. ✓ eyes.	Careful positioning and padding of the patient is essential.
Complications	Hemorrhage from trocar insertion. Subcutaneous emphysema	These complications (associated with the preperitoneal approach), as well as the general complications of laparoscopy, are discussed in Anesthetic Considerations for Laparoscopic Cholecystectomy, p. 462.

POSTOPERATIVE

Complications	PONV Urinary retention	Metoclopramide (10 mg iv), ondansetron (4 mg iv) Straight catheterization of the bladder
Pain management	Oral opiates Ketorolac	Tylenol #3 – 2 po q 6 h or Percocet – 2 po q 6 h. 30 mg iv
Tests	As indicated by patient status.	

References

1. Cooper SS: Laparoscopic inguinal hernia repair: is the enthusiasm justified? *Am Surg* 1997; 63(1):103-6.
2. Corbitt J: Laparoscopic transabdominal preperitoneal patch hernia repair. In *Atlas of Laparoscopic Surgery*. Ballantyne GH, ed. WB Saunders, Philadelphia: 2000, 502-15.
3. Crawford DL, Philips EH: Totally extraperitoneal laparoscopic herniorrhaphy. In *Surgical Laparoscopy*, 2nd edition. Zucker KA, ed. Lippincott Williams & Wilkins, Philadelphia: 2001, 571-84.
4. Cunningham AJ: Laparoscopic surgery—anesthetic implications. *Surg Endosc* 1994; 8(11):1272-84.
5. De La Torre R, Scott JS: Endoscopic total extraperitoneal hernia repair with balloon dissection. In *Atlas of Laparoscopic Surgery*. Ballantyne GH, ed. WB Saunders, Philadelphia: 2000, 516-25.
6. Kozal R, Lange PM, Kosir M, et al: A prospective, randomized study of open vs laparoscopic inguinal hernia repair. *Arch Surg* 1997; 132:292-5.
7. Liem MS: Comparison of conventional anterior surgery and laparoscopic surgery for inguinal-hernia repair. *N Engl J Med* 1997; 336(22):1541-7.

LAPAROSCOPIC BARIATRIC SURGERY

SURGICAL CONSIDERATIONS

Description: Morbid obesity is increasing in the American population. Many of these patients have associated comorbidities, such as HTN, diabetes, and sleep apnea, which they have been unable to correct by dieting and exercise. Surgical treatment has been shown to result in weight loss of approximately 2/3 of their excess body weight, most with consequent correction of their comorbidities. Operations for morbid obesity are classified as either restrictive, such as the **vertical banded gastroplasty**; malabsorptive, such as a **jejunoileal bypass**; or a combination, such as the **Roux-en-Y gastric bypass**. The 1991 NIH consensus statement indicated that the Roux-en-Y bypass was the best surgical treatment

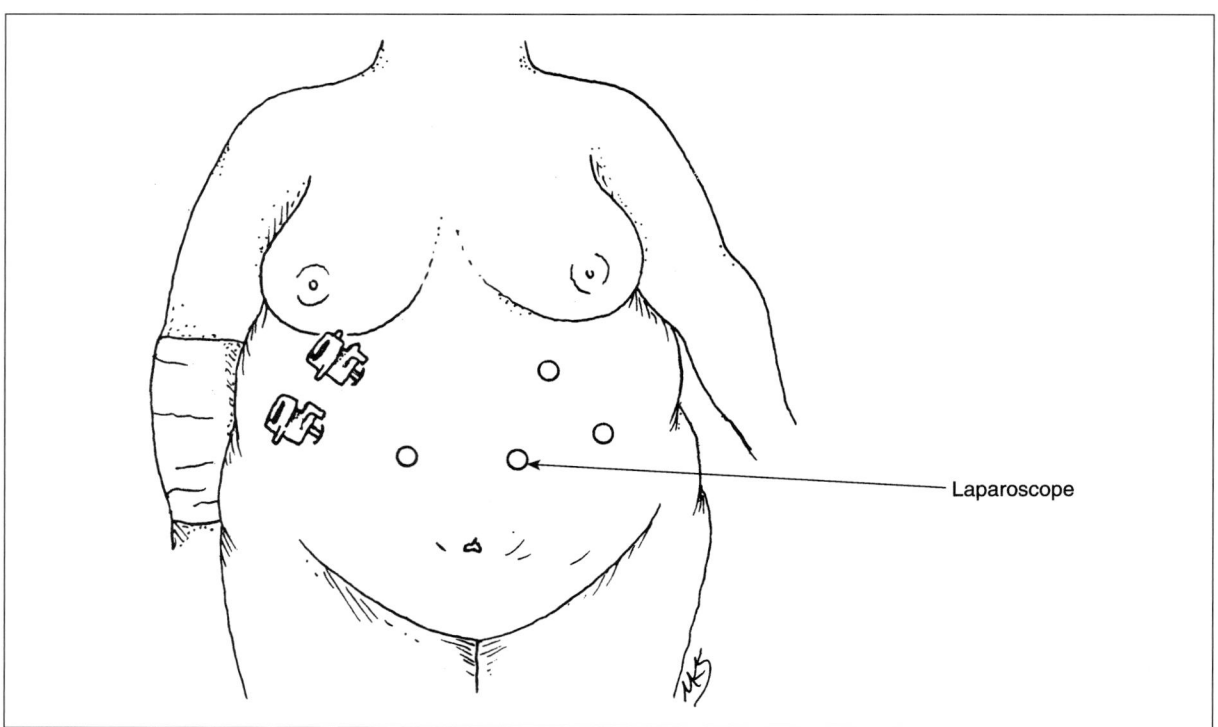

Figure 7.7-10. Patient position and trocar position for bariatric laparoscopic surgery. (Reproduced with permission from Scott-Connors CEH, Dawson, DL: *Operative Anatomy*, Lippincott Williams & Wilkins, Philadelphia, 2003.)

for morbid obesity. In general, this operation is approached laparoscopically in most patients because of the decreased pain, earlier ambulation, earlier discharge from the hospital, quicker return to regular activity, and decreased wound complication rates, as compared with an open approach. Open approaches are undertaken in patients who have had previous upper abdominal surgery; patients who may not tolerate an increased intraabdominal pressure (e.g., CHF, severe CAD, severe pulmonary disease); and, occasionally, in patients who fall into a super morbidly obese group (BMI > 60 kg/m^2). Surgery is indicated in patients with a BMI of 35-40 kg/m^2, if they have associated comorbidities, or > 40 kg/m^2, if they have no associated comorbidities.

In these procedures, the patient generally is placed in a supine position. Some surgeons prefer a split-leg table, with the surgeon standing between the legs. For a laparoscopic Roux-en-Y bypass, the first incision is made in the midline, ~halfway between the umbilicus and the xyphoid; 4-5 additional ports are then placed in the LUQ and the midline. Most surgeons begin by performing a jejunojejunostomy. During this time, the patient is placed in a reverse Trendelenburg position to drop the small intestines into the pelvis. The omentum is placed in the upper abdomen and the ligament of Treitz is identified. The jejunum is divided with an endo GIA stapler ~15 cm from the ligament of Treitz. A Roux limb of 100 cm is then measured. (Occasionally, this Roux limb may be 150 cm, if the patient's BMI is > 50 kg/m^2.) The jejunojejunostomy is created with a stapler and the enterotomy is closed. Some surgeons prefer a **retrocolic approach**, wherein a passage is made through the transverse mesocolon. Other surgeons prefer an **antecolic approach**, in which the omentum is divided to allow for a place where the Roux limb can pass without tension. Other surgeons prefer a **retrogastric approach**, but most bring the Roux limb through the gastrocolic ligament. At this point, the liver retractor is placed and the gastric pouch is created. Before the stomach stapling, everything in the stomach, including temperature probes, OG tubes, and calibrating tubes, should be removed. The gastric pouch is then stapled and cut. Often a calibrating tube is placed after the first two staple firings to help maintain the size of the pouch and the anastomosis. Some surgeons staple the anastomosis and place the anvil of the end-to-end anastomotic stapler through the mouth. A hand-sewn anastomosis generally is associated with longer operative times (+1 h). At the end, the gastrojejunostomy typically is tested by inflating air into the gastric pouch, either through an OG tube, the sizing tube, or a gastroscope. Generally, the NG or OG tube is removed at the end of the procedure. Often, at this point, surgeons will close the defect of the transverse mesocolon.

Variant procedure or approaches: Open bypass (see p. 399).

Usual preop diagnosis: Morbid obesity (100 lbs above ideal body weight, or 100% over ideal body weight), generally in combination with some medical condition felt to be worsened by the obesity (e.g., osteoarthritis, diabetes, respiratory insufficiency, CHF)

SUMMARY OF PROCEDURE

Position	Supine or split leg (See Fig 7.2-6 in Open Operations for Morbid Obesity, p. 401 for suggested positioning.)
Incision	5-6 port sites
Unique considerations	Patients are at high risk for aspiration, and airway management may be very difficult.
Antibiotics	Cefazolin 1 g iv
Surgical time	2-4 h
Closing considerations	Typically, fascial defects are not closed.
EBL	< 50 ml
Postop care	Most patients receive an upper GI study the next day. Clear liquids are begun if the study is normal, and most patients are discharged within 48 h.
Mortality	< 1%
Morbidity	Overall: 10%
	Stricture: 10%
	Leak: 1-2%
	DVT
	PE
	Pneumonia
	Hemorrhage
	Hernia
	Obstruction
	Infection
Pain score	5-6

PATIENT POPULATION CHARACTERISTICS

Age Range	Generally, between 18-60 yr
Male:Female	Female > Male
Incidence	5%
Etiology	Genetic; environmental
Associated conditions	Sleep apnea; HTN; diabetes; GERD

ANESTHETIC CONSIDERATIONS

See Anesthetic Considerations for Open Operations for Morbid Obesity, p. 401.

References

1. Higa KD, Boone KB, Ho T, Davies OG: Laparoscopic Roux-en Y gastric bypass for morbid obesity: technique and preliminary results of our first 400 patients. *Arch Surg* 2001; 135:1029-33.
2. Nguyen NT, Wolfe BM: Laparoscopic bariatric surgery. *Adv Surg* 2002; 36:39-63.
3. Nguyen NT, Wolfe BM: Laparoscopic versus open gastric bypass. *Semin Laparosc Surg* 2002; 9(2):86-93.
4. Schaier PR, Ikramuddin S: Laparoscopic surgery for morbid obesity. *Surg Clin North Am* 2001; 81:1145-79.
5. Schirmer BD: Laparoscopic bariatric surgery. *Surg Clin North Am* 2000; 80:1253-68.

ANESTHESIA FOR LAPAROSCOPY IN PREGNANCY

ANESTHETIC CONSIDERATIONS
PREOPERATIVE

Approximately 0.75-2% of pregnant woman require nonobstetric surgery, and 10-20% of those will require intraabdominal surgery (diagnostic or therapeutic), most commonly for cholecystectomy, appendectomy, or gynecological indications. If surgery cannot be avoided, it is best carried out in the 2nd trimester. Warn patients about possible fetal loss (12% in 1st trimester) and premature labor (5-8% in 2nd and 25-40% in 3rd trimesters). Anesthesia and surgery are associated with increased spontaneous abortion, growth retardation, and perinatal mortality; however, no increase in congenital abnormalities has been found.[4] Rates of fetal loss, premature labor, and maternal mortality are higher among sicker patients. It is unclear whether adverse outcomes after surgery relate to the disease process itself, disturbances in nutrition, the surgical procedure, exposure to radiation, or drugs. No correlation has been found between outcome and any specific anesthetic technique or agent (including N_2O).

Laparoscopy is the procedure of choice for many surgeries in nonpregnant patients; however, its use in pregnancy remains controversial, although significant experience now supports its safety and efficacy.[5] Advantages of laparoscopy include more rapid recovery, shorter hospital stays, less postop narcotic use ($\rightarrow \downarrow$fetal depression) and lower risk of wound infection.[3] No differences in fetal outcome or incidence of preterm labor have been found.[7] Risks of laparoscopy include difficult surgical access and potential uterine injury with Veress needles or trocars. Current recommendations suggest an open technique (e.g., Hasson cannula) for obtaining laparoscope access.[8]

Note that acute appendicitis and cholecystitis often present with advanced or complicated disease because of difficulty diagnosing the 'acute abdomen' and a reluctance to use radiation-based diagnostic tests in pregnancy.

Respiratory	Pregnant patients have $\uparrow$MV with respiratory alkalosis (PCO_2 = 32-34 mmHg) and are subject to the rapid onset of hypoxemia if ventilation is compromised ($\downarrow$FRC [$\downarrow$20%] and $\uparrow O_2$ consumption). Uptake of and sensitivity to inhalational anesthetics is enhanced ($\downarrow$FRC, $\downarrow$MAC, and hyperventilation). During laparoscopy, peritoneal insufflation and head-down positioning may further compromise lung function ($\downarrow$FRC and $\downarrow$lung compliance). Mucosal capillary engorgement in upper airways may necessitate a smaller ETT and mandates careful airway suctioning to avoid bleeding. Airway management is more difficult (7-10 ×) in this patient population. **Tests:** As indicated from H&P.
Cardiovascular	Pregnancy $\rightarrow \uparrow$CO, $\downarrow$MAP, $\uparrow$HR, $\uparrow$blood volume, and $\downarrow$oncotic pressure $\rightarrow \uparrow$risk of pulmonary edema. Supine hypotensive syndrome: To minimize aortocaval compression and $\rightarrow \downarrow\downarrow$BP (> 20 wk gestation), the supine position should be modified by the use of a left lateral pelvic tilt to displace the uterus. Moderate abdominal insufflation pressures (8-12 mmHg) should be used to minimize further caval compression and $\downarrow$uterine blood flow. **Tests:** As indicated from H&P.
Hematologic	WBC count is elevated during pregnancy (8,000-12,000/mm^2) and may delay diagnosis of concurrent infections (e.g., appendicitis). Iron deficiency anemia often is superimposed on the dilutional anemia of pregnancy (Hct 33%). Pregnant patients are hypercoagulable, and antiembolic compression devices should be used. **Tests:** Hb/Hct. T&S if significant blood loss is anticipated. Coag studies and Plt count if + PIH.
Gastrointestinal	Emergency surgery, $\downarrow$gastric motility, $\uparrow$GERD, $\uparrow$intragastric pressure and gastric hyperacidity $\rightarrow \uparrow$risk of aspiration pneumonitis. All pregnant patients must be considered to have full stomachs and should receive a nonparticulate antacid (e.g., 0.3 M Na citrate 30 ml) immediately before GA, as well as iv metoclopramide 10mg and ranitidine 50 mg 30-60 min before surgery.
Renal	Pregnancy $\rightarrow \uparrow$renal blood flow and creatinine clearance and $\downarrow$serum creatinine and $\downarrow$BUN. Dependent edema results from increased water and sodium retention. **Tests:** As indicated from H&P.
Laboratory	Others tests as indicated from H&P.
Premedication	Full-stomach precautions (see Gastrointestinal, above); midazolam (1-2 mg) given as appropriate to decrease anxiety.

INTRAOPERATIVE

Anesthetic technique: After 16 wk gestation, anticipate $\uparrow$risks of aspiration and difficult intubation. Plan ahead for management of a difficult airway (see pp. 463-464). GA is the preferred technique, since laparoscopy and abdominal surgery are poorly tolerated under regional anesthesia. A lead shield should be used to protect the fetus during fluoroscopy. Obtain preop obstetric consultation with baseline fetal heart rate (FHR) and uterine contraction readings. After ~24 wk gestation, consider continuous monitoring of FHR during surgery (transvaginal Doppler) and develop a management plan for evaluation and action if a nonreassuring trace develops.

General anesthesia: If difficult intubation is anticipated, an awake fiber optic intubation (see p. B-6) is recommended. In any event, emergency airway management equipment (e.g., LMA, transtracheal jet ventilator), must be immediately accessible in the OR. Communication with the surgeon and obstetrician regarding maternal and fetal condition is essential.

Induction	Tilt table or elevate left hip to displace uterus. Standard rapid-sequence induction (see p. B-5), as appropriate. To optimize intubation, place patient in maximal 'sniff' position with elevation of shoulders if necessary (obese patients) (see Fig 7.2-6, p. 401). If tracheal intubation is unsuccessful, follow the difficult intubation/ventilation drill (see pp. 463-464, B-5). Once ETT is secured, pass OG tube and decompress stomach to minimize injury from the Veress needle or trocar.	
Maintenance	0.8-1% isoflurane or sevoflurane in air/O_2 (50%) mixture. Avoid $N_2O \to$ distention of bowel, PONV. Administer an opioid (e.g. fentanyl 50-200 μg iv) and/or midazolam (1-2 mg) to $\downarrow$ volatile requirements and $\downarrow$ maternal awareness. Administer muscle relaxants (e.g., vecuronium 0.1 mg/kg). Control ventilation, avoiding hypocapnia ($PCO_2 < 30$ mmHg) $\to \downarrow$umbilical blood flow, and hypercapnia ($PCO_2 > 36$ mmHg) $\to$ fetal acidosis. Maintain $ETCO_2$ or $PaCO_2$ at 32-36 mmHg by $\uparrow$ MV. Use low insufflation cut-off pressure (8-12 mmHg, not 15 mmHg as for nonpregnant patient).[8]	
Emergence	Reverse muscle relaxation with neostigmine 0.05 mg/kg and glycopyrrolate 0.01 mg/kg or atropine 0.02 mg/kg. Anticholinergics (glycopyrrolate/atropine) given before neostigmine may minimize possible $\uparrow$uterine tone 2° neostigmine. Delay extubation until patient is fully awake and muscle strength has returned to normal. O_2 by mask and transport in the lateral position. Metoclopramide (10 mg iv) and/or ondansetron (4 mg iv) may be needed for PONV.	
Blood and fluid requirements	IV: 16-18 ga × 1 NS/LR 4-6 ml/kg/hr	Laparoscopy is associated with minimal blood loss; however, inadvertent vascular injury may occur.
Monitoring	Standard monitors ± Arterial line (major surgery) FHR monitor	 Continuous FHR monitoring is appropriate after 24 wk gestation.
	Uterine contraction monitor	Uterine contraction monitoring is usually not possible intraop; however, ✓ preop and postop. Maternal and neonatal outcome good, and severe acidosis absent when maternal ventilation controlled by $PaCO_2$ or $ETCO_2$ measurement. Clinical experience indicates no long-term adverse neonatal effects [2].
Positioning	✓ and pad pressure points. ✓ eyes.	Changes in position have marked effects on respiration ($\downarrow$compliance/$\uparrow$pressure, hypoxemia) and hemodynamics. Head-up position + GA + peritoneal insufflation $\to$ 50% $\downarrow$CO in the nonpregnant patient and even greater decrease in late pregnancy.[9] **Position changes should be gradual** to minimize adverse effects.[10]
	± left uterine displacement	If > 20 wk gestation, left uterine displacement to avoid aortocaval compression.
CO_2 peritoneum: Maternal effects	$\downarrow$ventilation $\downarrow$BP Reflux CO_2 absorption	Impairs ventilation $\to$ hypoxemia and respiratory acidosis. $\downarrow$venous return $\to \downarrow$BP. $\uparrow$GI reflux ($\uparrow$abdominal pressure) Absorption of $CO_2 \to \uparrow$MAP & $\uparrow$SVR.
CO_2 peritoneum Fetal effects	$\downarrow$uterine blood flow $\uparrow$preterm labor Fetal acidosis Fetal $\uparrow$HR/$\uparrow$BP	Up to 60% in animal studies $\to$ fetal hypoxia. 2° $\uparrow$abdominal pressure 2° absorbed CO_2
Complications	Uterine injury Bowel/organ injury	

Complications, cont.	Venous air embolism	Dx: ↓ETCO$_2$ hypoxemia, hypotension. Rx: 100% O$_2$, stop insufflation immediately, volume and pressors, attempt CVP air aspiration.
	Thromboembolism/PE	Prevention: Pneumatic compression devices. Rx: Supportive
	Pneumothorax	Dx: ↑Airway pressure, ↓breath sounds, and hyperresonance. Rx: 100% O$_2$, stop insufflation, tube thoracostomy.

POSTOPERATIVE

Pain management	Standard pain management (see p. C-2)	Avoid NSAIDS (e.g. ibuprofen) → pulmonary and CV fetal effects (closure of ductus venosus).
Tests	HCT/CBC	
	Others as indicated by operative course.	

References:

1. Cohen SE: Nonobstetric surgery during pregnancy. In *Obstetric Anesthesia: Principles and Practice*, 2nd edition. Chestnut DH, ed. CV Mosby, St. Louis: 1999.
2. Curet MJ: Special problems in laparoscopic surgery. *Surg Clin North Am* 2000; 80(4):1093-1110.
3. Curet MJ, Allen D, Josloff RK, Pitcher DE, Curet LB, Miscall BG, Zucker KA: Laparoscopy During Pregnancy. *Arch Surg* 1996; 131:546-51.
4. Czeizel AE, Pataki T, Rockenbauer M: Reproductive outcome after exposure to surgery under anesthesia during pregnancy. *Arch Gynecol Obstet* 1998; 261(4):193-9.
5. Fatum M, Rojansky N: Laparoscopic Surgery During Pregnancy. *Obstet Gynecol Survey* 2001; 56(1):50-9.
6. Goodman S: Anesthesia for nonobstetric surgery in the pregnant patient. *Semin Perinatol* 2002; 26(2):136-45.
7. Reedy MB, Kallen B, Kuehl TJ: Laparoscopy during pregnancy: A study of five fetal outcome parameters with use of the Swedish Health Registry. *Am J Obstet Gynecol* 1997; 177(3):673-9.
8. SAGES Guidelines for laparoscopic surgery during pregnancy. *Surg Endosc* 1998; 12:189-90.
9. Steinbrook RA, Bhavani-Shankar K: Hemodynamics During Laparoscopic Surgery in Pregnancy. *Anesth Analg* 2001; 93:1570-1.
10. Steinbrook RA, Brooks DC, Datta S: Laparoscopic cholecystectomy during pregnancy. Review of anesthetic management, surgical considerations. *Surg Endosc* 1996; 10:511-5.

Surgeon

J. Augusto Bastidas, MD

7.8 PANCREATIC SURGERY

Anesthesiologist

Martin Angst, MD

OPERATIVE DRAINAGE FOR PANCREATITIS

SURGICAL CONSIDERATIONS

Description: Surgical treatment for pancreatitis is indicated for drainage or debridement of infected peripancreatic tissue or pancreatic necrosis. Pancreatic abscesses usually develop in the lesser sac, but may spread to the subphrenic spaces or into the pericolic gutters. Fistulization into adjacent organs, particularly the transverse colon, is common. Severe intraabdominal hemorrhage from erosion into major arteries lying adjacent to the pancreas is uncommon, but may occur prior to, during, or after operative drainage. Intraop, exploration of the peritoneal cavity is performed before opening the lesser sac. Areas lateral to the left and right sides of the colon, as well as the base of the transverse mesocolon and the subhepatic areas, should be palpated to identify fluid or abscess collections. The gastrocolic ligament is then incised to approach the pancreas through the lesser sac. There are different operative approaches, depending on location of involved tissue and surgeon's preference. Upper midline or transverse abdominal incisions are used most often. Posterior drainage through the bed of the 12th rib, or retroperitoneal lateral approaches, may be used (Fig 7.8-1).

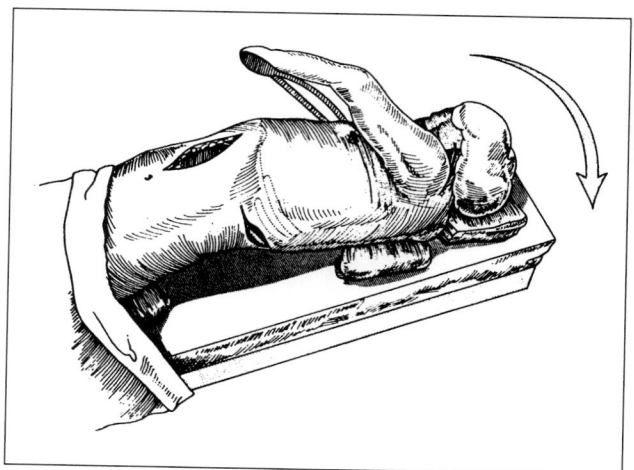

Figure 7.8-1. Incision for anterior and posterior drainage in pancreatitis. Note that bed or table is rotated until patient is almost supine. (Reproduced with permission from Berne TV, Donovan AJ: Synchronous anterior and posterior drainage of pancreatic abscess. *Arch Surg* 1981; 116:527-33. Copyright 1981, American Medical Association.)

Usual preop diagnosis: Severe pancreatitis 2° to gallstones, alcohol, or post ERCP

SUMMARY OF PROCEDURE

Position	Supine or rotated slightly (Fig 7.8-1) for posterior approach
Incision	Midline, transverse, flank, or synchronous anterior and posterior
Unique considerations	Must perform adequate debridement of necrotic tissue and provide adequate drainage of abdomen; NG tube; jejunal feeding tube
Antibiotics	Cefotetan 1-2 g 30 min preop, or antibiotic directed at cultured organisms
Surgical time	1-2 h
Closing considerations	Adequate drainage of pancreatic bed and fluid resuscitation of patient
EBL	300-750 ml
Postop care	Routine wound and drain care; usually ICU and intubated; often, subsequent operative procedures are required.
Mortality	8-30%
Morbidity	Fistulae formation: 18-55%
	Delayed gastric emptying: 50%
	Unremitting sepsis: 10-30%
	Atelectasis: 5-10%
	Respiratory deterioration: 5%
	Hemorrhage
	Bowel perforations
Pain score	7-9

PATIENT POPULATION CHARACTERISTICS

Age range	30-60 yr
Male:Female	1:1
Incidence	10-30% of patients with pancreatitis
Etiology	Alcoholism (30-50%); postop pancreatitis (15-40%); biliary tract disease (20-30%); idiopathic pancreatitis (15-20%)
Associated conditions	Malnutrition; glucose intolerance; multiorgan dysfunction

484

ANESTHETIC CONSIDERATIONS

See Anesthetic Considerations for Pancreatic Surgery, p. 491.

References

1. Bradley EL: Fifteen-year experience with open drainage for infected pancreatic necrosis. *Surg Gynecol Obstet* 1993; 177(3): 215-22.
2. Berne TV: Pancreatic abscesses. *Probl Gen Surg* 1984; 1:569-82.
3. Feranandez-del Castillo C, Rattner DW, Makary MA, et al: Debridement and closed packing for the treatment of necrotizing pancreatitis. *Ann Surg* 1998; 228:676-84.
4. Gotzinger P, Sautner T, Kriwanek S, et al: Surgical treatment for severe acute pancreatitis: Extent and surgical control of necrosis determine outcome. *World J Surg* 2002; 474-8.
5. Villazon A, Villazon O, Terrazas F, Rana R: Retroperitoneal drainage in the management of the septic phase of severe acute pancreatitis. *World J Surg* 1991; 15:103-8.

DRAINAGE OF PANCREATIC PSEUDOCYST

SURGICAL CONSIDERATIONS

Description: Internal drainage of a pancreatic pseudocyst may be accomplished by anastomosing the cyst to the stomach, duodenum, or other small bowel via a Roux-en-Y loop of jejunum. The procedure of choice for internal decompression depends on the location of the pseudocyst in relation to the portion of the GI tract that will provide maximal dependent

drainage of the cyst. Operation is reserved for patients with refractory symptoms. At operation, the abdomen is entered via a midline incision. If the pseudocyst lies behind the stomach (or duodenum), it is approached anteriorly, through the posterior wall of the stomach (or duodenum). A portion of the posterior wall is excised, allowing entry into the cyst cavity, which is then drained. An anastomosis is created between the cyst and stomach (or duodenum). The anterior wall of the stomach (or duodenum) is then closed. If the cyst presents inferior to the stomach, it is anastomosed in a similar fashion to a Roux-en-Y loop of jejunum (Fig 7.8-2). Drains are placed and external drainage is sometimes necessary, especially in the setting of infection. Spontaneous resolution of pancreatic pseudocyst may be expected in most patients.[5] If infection of the pseudocyst occurs with clinical signs of sepsis, percutaneous drainage under CT guidance can be performed, although subsequent operative drainage is often necessary.

Usual preop diagnosis: Pancreatic pseudocyst 2° to acute pancreatitis refractory to medical management

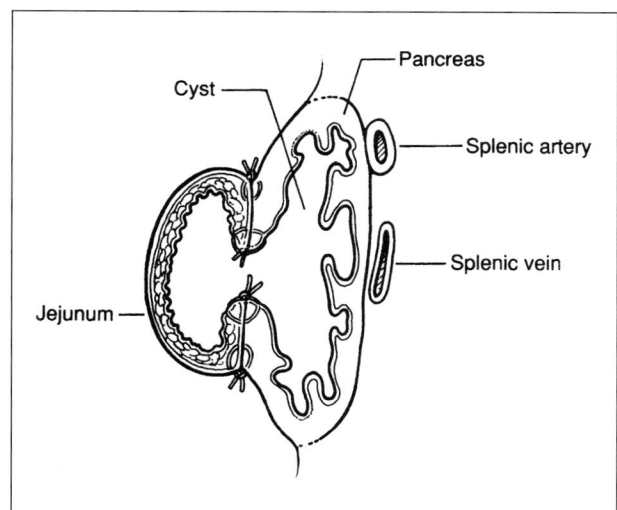

Figure 7.8-2. Roux-en Y drainage of a pseudocyst. (Reproduced with permission from Scott-Conner CEH, Dawson DL: *Operative Anatomy*, 2nd edition. Lippincott Williams & Wilkins, 2003.)

SUMMARY OF PROCEDURE

Position	Supine
Incision	Midline abdominal or transverse
Unique considerations	Location of pseudocyst in relation to GI tract; NG tube
Antibiotics	Cefazolin 1 g 30 min preop
Surgical time	1-2 h

Closing considerations	Adequate drainage
EBL	100-300 ml
Postop care	NG decompression
Mortality[3]	5-10%
Morbidity[3]	Bleeding: 5-7%
	Sepsis: < 5%
	Recurrence: 2-3%
Pain score	6-8

PATIENT POPULATION CHARACTERISTICS

Age range	15-80 yr
Male:Female	1:1
Incidence	Rare
Etiology	Acute pancreatitis; trauma
Associated conditions	Acute pancreatitis: 90%; gallstones; alcohol use; chronic pain

ANESTHETIC CONSIDERATIONS

See Anesthetic Considerations for Pancreatic Surgery, p. 491.

References

1. Criad E, Destefano AA, et al: Long-term results of percutaneous catheter drainage of pancreatic pseudocysts. *Surg Gynecol Obstet* 1992; 175:293.
2. Neff R: Pancreatic pseudocysts and fluid collections. *Surg Clin North Am* 2001; 81(2):399-403.
3. Vitas GJ, Sarr MG: Selected management of pancreatic pseudocysts: Operative versus expectant management. *Surgery* 1992; 11(2):123-30.
4. Warshaw AL, Rattner DW: Timing of surgical drainage for pancreatic pseudocyst: clinical and chemical criteria. *Ann Surg* 1985; 202(6):720-4.
5. Yeo CJ, Bastidas JA, Lynch-Nyhan A, et al: The natural history of pancreatic pseudocysts documented by CT. *Surg Gyn Obstet* 1990; 170:411.

PANCREATICOJEJUNOSTOMY

SURGICAL CONSIDERATIONS

Description: **Pancreaticojejunostomy,** as described by **Puestow,**[3] consists of a longitudinal opening of the pancreatic duct, which is then anastomosed to a Roux-en-Y loop of jejunum (Fig 7.8-3). This approach is necessary to ensure adequate drainage of a duct with multiple strictures and dilatations. Through a midline or transverse abdominal incision, the pancreas is exposed by mobilizing the duodenum (**Kocher maneuver**), exposing the head of the pancreas, and opening the lesser sac to visualize the body and tail. The pancreatic duct may be aspirated to identify its location, then it is incised longitudinally. A Roux-en-Y loop of jejunum is then brought up to the pancreas and anastomosed to the opened duct. A drain is left along the anastomosis; and the wound is closed in the usual fashion.

Variant procedure or approaches: A **Whipple resection** (**pancreaticoduodenectomy**; see p. 490) is an alternative surgical treatment for chronic pancreatitis confined to the head of the gland. Rarely, subtotal pancreatectomy is indicated.

Usual preop diagnosis: Abdominal pain with chronic pancreatitis and dilated pancreatic duct

Figure 7.8-3. Operative management of chronic pancreatitis with onlay Roux-en-Y pancreaticojejunostomy (Puestow). (Reproduced with permission from Hardy JD: *Hardy's Textbook of Surgery.* JB Lippincott, 1988.)

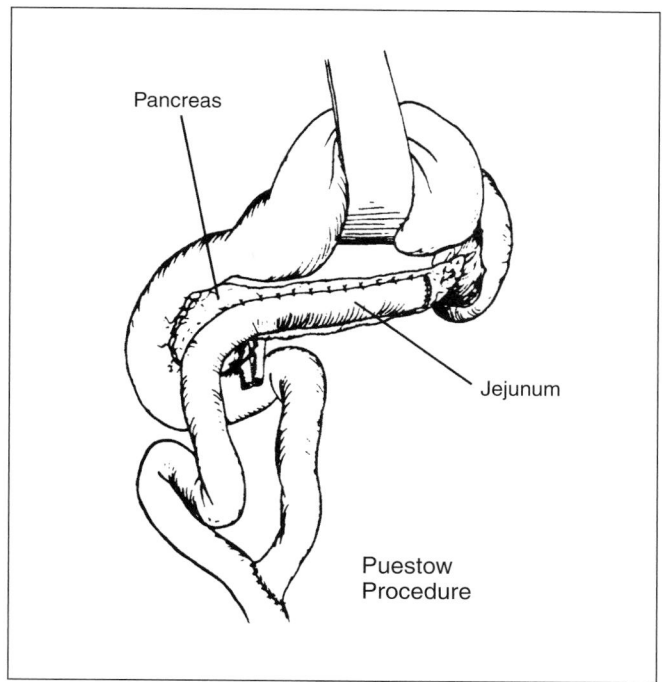

SUMMARY OF PROCEDURE

Position	Supine
Incision	Midline abdominal or transverse
Antibiotics	Cefazolin 1 g 30 min preop
Surgical time	2-3 h
Closing considerations	Adequate drainage
EBL	300-400 ml
Postop care	Monitor for glucose intolerance
Mortality	1-4%
Morbidity	Failure to relieve pain: 25-50%
	Pancreatic leak: 5-10%
	Wound infection: 5%
Pain score	6-8

PATIENT POPULATION CHARACTERISTICS

Age range	17-72 yr
Male:Female	2.5:1
Etiology	Alcoholism; biliary tract disease; idiopathic; trauma; familial pancreatitis
Associated conditions	Biliary tract disease (25-50%); hyperparathyroidism (< 5%); chronic pain; narcotic dependency

ANESTHETIC CONSIDERATIONS

See Anesthetic Considerations for Pancreatic Surgery, p. 491.

References

1. Harrison JL, Prinz RA: Surgical management of chronic pancreatitis: Pancreatic duct drainage. *Adv Surg* 1999; 32:1.
2. Howard VM, Zhaug Z: Pancreaticodenectomy (Whipple resection) in the treatment of chronic pancreatitis. *World J Surg* 1990; 14:77-82.
3. Puestow CB, Gillesby WJ: Retrograde surgical drainage of the pancreas for chronic relapsing pancreatitis. *Arch Surg* 1958; 76:898-907.

PANCREATECTOMY

SURGICAL CONSIDERATIONS

Description: **Distal pancreatectomy** is performed for tumors in the distal half of the pancreas (Fig 7.8-4). After entering the lesser sac, the gastrosplenic ligament is divided, ligating the short gastric vessels and the left gastroepiploic vessel. The peritoneum is incised along the inferior surface of the pancreas, with care being taken to avoid injury to the middle colic vessels. Following mobilization of the spleen, the splenic artery is ligated near its origin. The inferior mesenteric vein is ligated sometimes at the inferior border of the pancreas, and the splenic vein is ligated at the proposed point of transection. The transected pancreas (Fig 7.8-5) is usually stapled and drained, although some surgeons suture the cut end and ligate the duct. The spleen may be preserved when operating for benign disease.

Variant procedure or approaches: **Subtotal pancreatectomy** usually implies resecting the pancreas from the mesenteric vessels distally, leaving the head and uncinate process intact. This procedure may be performed for tumor or chronic pancreatitis. **Child's procedure** (near-total pancreatectomy) consists of removing all of the pancreas except a rim of tissue along the lesser curvature of the duodenum (Fig 7.8-6); preserving the duodenum makes it unnecessary to reconstruct the bile duct. This procedure is usually reserved for patients with chronic pancreatitis.

Usual preop diagnosis: Carcinoma of pancreas; islet cell tumors; cystic neoplasms; chronic pancreatitis

SUMMARY OF PROCEDURES

	Distal Pancreatectomy	Subtotal Pancreatectomy	Child's Procedure
Position	Supine	⇐	⇐
Incision	Midline abdominal or transverse	⇐	⇐
Unique considerations	NG tube	⇐	Preservation of vasculature of duodenum
Antibiotics	Cefazolin 1 g 30 min preop	⇐	⇐
Surgical time	2-3 h	⇐	3-4 h
Closing considerations	Adequate drainage	⇐	⇐
EBL	300-500 ml	500-750 ml	500-1000 ml
Postop care	NG decompression; PACU	⇐	⇐
Mortality	< 5%	⇐	⇐
Morbidity	Diabetes: 5%	⇐	⇐
	Wound infection: 5%	⇐	⇐
	Pancreatic fistula: < 5%	⇐	90%
	Common bile duct injury	⇐	⇐
	Hemorrhage	⇐	⇐
	Duodenal necrosis	⇐	⇐
	Pancreatic leakage	⇐	⇐
	Pancreatic insufficiency	⇐	⇐
Pain score	6-8	6-8	6-8

PATIENT POPULATION CHARACTERISTICS

Age range	30-60 yr
Male:Female	1:1
Incidence	~ 26,000/yr in U.S.
Etiology	Adenocarcinoma; chronic pancreatitis; islet cell tumors
Associated conditions	Alcoholism and biliary tract disease with chronic pancreatitis (90%); other endocrine disorders (3-5%)

ANESTHETIC CONSIDERATIONS

See Anesthetic Considerations for Pancreatic Surgery, p. 491.

Reference

1. Murayama KM, Joehl RJ: Chronic pancreatitis. In *Surgery: Scientific Principles and Practice*, 3rd edition. Greenfield LJ, et al, eds. Lippincott Williams & Wilkins, Philadelphia: 2001, 873-85.

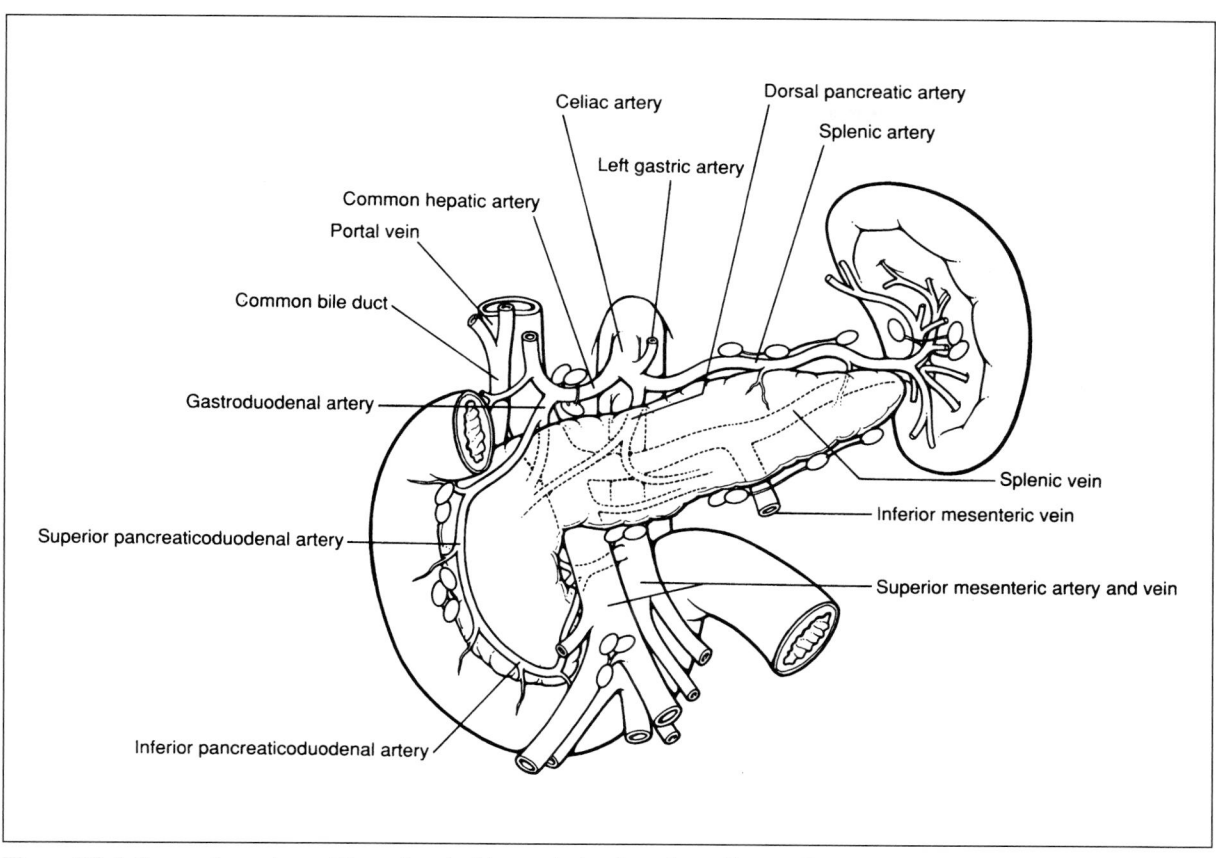

Figure 7.8-4. Pancreatic anatomy. (Reproduced with permission from Scott-Conner CEH, Dawson DL: *Operative Anatomy*, 2nd edition. Lippincott Williams & Wilkins, 2003.)

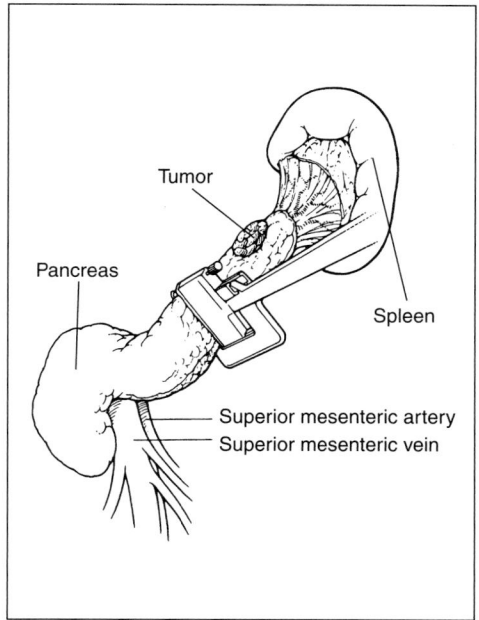

Figure 7.8-5. Resection of distal pancreas. (Reproduced with permission from Scott-Conner CEH, Dawson DL: *Operative Anatomy*, 2nd edition. Lippincott Williams & Wilkins, 2003.)

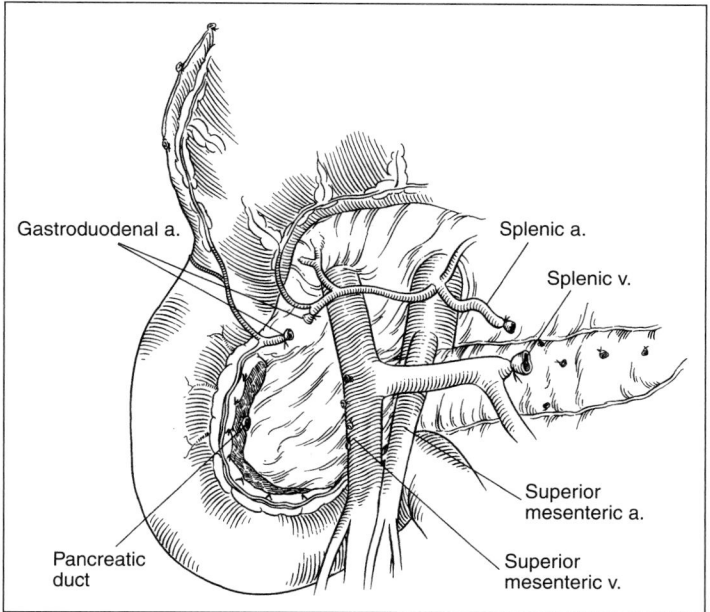

Figure 7.8-6. Near-total pancreatectomy. Shown is the operative field at the conclusion of the procedure. (Reproduced with permission from Baker RJ, Fischer JE: *Mastery of Surgery*, 4th edition. Lippincott Williams & Wilkins, 1997.)

WHIPPLE RESECTION

SURGICAL CONSIDERATIONS

Description: A **Whipple resection** consists of a **pancreaticoduodenectomy**, followed by a pancreaticojejunostomy, a **hepaticojejunostomy** and a **gastrojejunostomy** (Fig 7.8-7). On entering the peritoneal cavity, the resectability of the pancreatic lesion is determined. Contraindications to standard resection include: liver or peritoneal metastases; involvement of the superior mesenteric vessels; infiltration by tumor into root of the mesentery; and extension into the porta hepatis, with involvement of the hepatic artery. If the tumor is deemed resectable, further mobilization of the head of the pancreas is performed. The common duct is transected above the cystic duct entry and the gall bladder is removed. Once the superior mesenteric vein is freed from the pancreas, the latter is transected, with care being taken not to injure the splenic vein. The stomach is transected at the antral-body junction, or beyond the pylorus if uninvolved by tumor. The jejunum is transected beyond the ligament of Treitz and the specimen is removed by severing the vascular connections with the mesenteric vessels. Reconstitution is achieved by anastomosing the pancreatic stump, bile duct, and stomach into the jejunum. Drains are placed adjacent to the pancreatic anastomosis.

Variant procedure or approaches: There are several variants that consist of extensions of the Whipple procedure: **total pancreatectomy**; **regional pancreatectomy**, involving resection and reconstruction of the retropancreatic superior mesenteric vein and/or artery; and the pylorus-preserving **pancreaticoduodenectomy**. In addition, the distal pancreatic stump may be anastomosed to the posterior wall of the stomach.

Usual preop diagnosis: Carcinoma of the pancreas; malignant cystadenomas; chronic pancreatitis

SUMMARY OF PROCEDURES

	Whipple[3]	Total Pancreatectomy[5]	Regional Pancreatectomy[5]
Position	Supine	⇐	⇐
Incision	Midline abdominal or transverse (chevron)	⇐	⇐
Unique considerations	Large-bore iv lines	⇐	⇐
Antibiotics	Cefazolin 1 g preop	⇐	⇐
Surgical time	4-5 h	4-6 h	5-6 h
Closing considerations	Adequate drainage	⇐	⇐
EBL	500-750 ml	750-1000 ml	750-1500 ml
Postop care	NG decompression; PACU/ICU	NG decompression; diabetes management	⇐
Mortality	5-10%	12%	15%
Morbidity	Delayed gastric emptying: 25%	⇐	⇐
	Pancreatic fistula: 10-20%	NA	10-20%
	Sepsis: 5-15%	5%	25%
	Hemorrhage: 5%	< 5%	5%
	MI: 1-3%	⇐	< 5%
	Biliary fistula: < 2%	< 1%	< 2%
Pain score	7-9	7-9	7-9

PATIENT POPULATION CHARACTERISTICS (for cancer of pancreas[6])

Age range	50-80 yr
Male:Female	1:1
Incidence	10th most common cancer in U.S. – 29,000/yr
Etiology	Familial and genetic factors (probably most important); tobacco; diabetes; alcohol; diet; pancreatitis
Associated conditions	See Etiology, above.

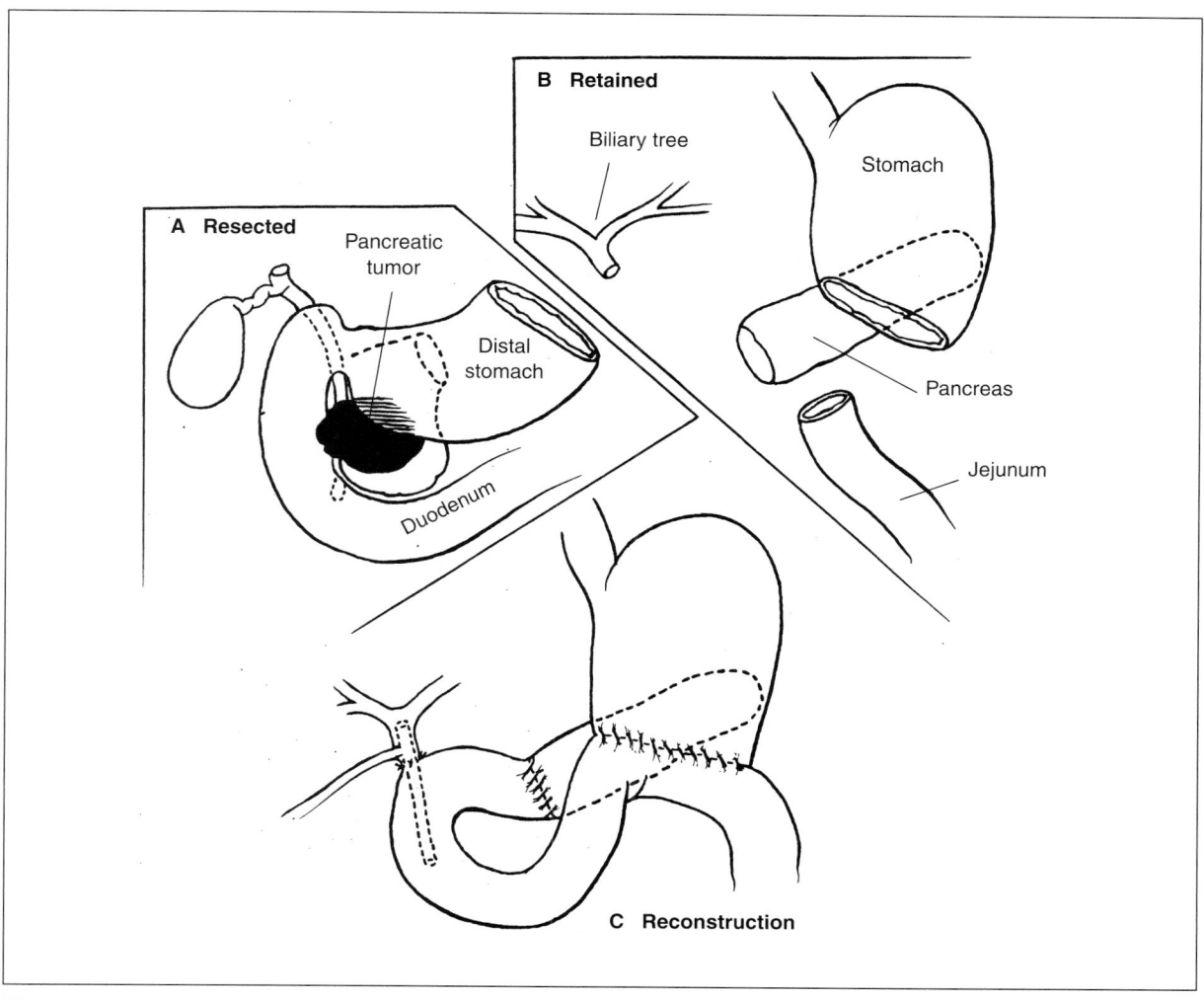

Figure 7.8-7. Standard pancreaticoduodenectomy. **(A)** Structures resected, including distal stomach, entire duodenum, head and neck of pancreas with tumor, gallbladder, and distal extrahepatic biliary tree. **(B)** Structures retained, including proximal stomach, body and tail of pancreas, proximal biliary tree, and jejunum distal to ligament of Treitz. **(C)** Reconstruction: proximal pancreaticojejunostomy, hepaticojejunostomy over T tube, and distal gastrojejunostomy. (Reproduced with permission from Hardy JD: *Hardy's Textbook of Surgery*, 2nd edition. JB Lippincott, 1988.)

ANESTHETIC CONSIDERATIONS FOR PANCREATIC SURGERY

(Procedures covered: drainage for pancreatitis; drainage of pancreatic pseudocyst; pancreaticojejunostomy; pancreatectomy; Whipple resection)

PREOPERATIVE

Patients presenting for pancreatic surgery can be divided into four groups: (1) those with acute pancreatitis, who failed medical treatment and may be extremely ill, presenting for operative excision or drainage of necrotic or infected foci; (2) patients with adenocarcinoma of the pancreas; (3) patients with neuroendocrine active (60-70%) or inactive islet cell tumors (mainly insulinoma and gastrinoma; rarely VIP-oma and glucagonoma); and (4) patients suffering from the sequelae of chronic pancreatitis (e.g., pseudocyst or abscess).

Respiratory   Respiratory compromise—such as pleural effusions, atelectasis, and ARDS, progressing to respiratory failure—may occur in up to 50% of patients with acute pancreatitis. Postop mechanical ventilation may be needed for these patients.
Tests: Consider CXR; ABG; as indicated from H&P.

Cardiovascular   Patients with acute pancreatitis may suffer from severe intravascular volume depletion 2° plasma exudation and in severe cases 2° hemorrhage (erosion of blood vessels). Aggressive volume resuscitation with crystalloids, colloids, and blood may be required during surgery. Hypocalcemia is often present (arrhythmias and ↓myocardial contractility). Serum K^+ may be elevated (2° acidosis or renal failure associated with acute pancreatitis) or decreased (2° watery diarrhea associated with gastrinoma, VIP-oma, prolonged NG suction), and should be corrected before surgery. Hypokalemia resistant to K^+ replacement may point to ↓Mg^{++} and warrants replacement.
Tests: ECG; electrolytes; others as indicated from H&P.

Gastrointestinal   Jaundice and abdominal pain are common presenting Sx in this group of patients. The presence of ileus (common in acute pancreatitis) or intestinal obstruction should mandate full-stomach precautions and rapid-sequence induction. Electrolyte abnormalities are common and may be 2° metabolic acidosis (K^+↑, 2° acute pancreatitis) or alkalosis and intestinal losses (K^+↓ and Mg^{++}↓, 2° diarrhea, NG suction). Acute pancreatitis is associated with ↓Ca^{++} (omental fat saponification) and ↑Na^+ (dehydration). Gastrinoma (Zollinger-Ellison syndrome) is associated with diarrhea, severe peptic ulcer, and GERD. VIP-oma often causes massive watery diarrhea (up to 20 L/d). Electrolyte abnormalities should be treated preop.
Tests: Electrolytes; glucose; LFTs; CA^{++}; amylase; others as indicated from H&P.

Renal   Patients should be evaluated for renal insufficiency predominantly 2° dehydration, with anesthetic plan adjusted accordingly.
Tests: BUN; creatinine; others as indicated from H&P.

Endocrine   Many patients with acute pancreatitis have diabetes 2° loss of islet cells. Endocrine tumors of the pancreas are linked (10-30%) with multiple endocrine syndrome type I (MEN I), featuring adenoma of the pituitary, parathyroid, and/or pancreas. Endocrine tumors also can secrete parathyroid hormone-related peptide, growth hormone RH, and corticotrophin-RH and adrenocorticotrophin, and may be associated with ↑Ca^{++}, acromegaly, and Cushing syndrome. Insulinoma is the most common endocrine tumor of the pancreas and can result in severe hypoglycemia, necessitating frequent periop blood glucose measurements (up to every 15 min has been suggested). Surgical manipulation of the insulinoma may result in massive release of insulin. VIP-oma is associated with mild diabetes and ↑Ca^{++}.
Tests: Electrolytes; glucose; others as indicated from H&P.

Hematologic   Hct may be falsely elevated, 2° hemoconcentration, or low, 2° hemorrhage. Coagulopathy may be present (DIC).
Tests: CBC with differential; Plt; consider PT, PTT, fibrinogen.

Laboratory   Other tests as indicated from H&P.

Premedication   Standard premedication (see p. B-2). Note: full-stomach precautions in patients with intestinal obstruction (see p. B-5): ranitidine 50 mg iv and 0.3 M Na citrate (30 ml po 10 min preop).

INTRAOPERATIVE

Anesthetic technique: GETA ± epidural for postop analgesia. If postop epidural analgesia is planned, establishing correct catheter placement in the epidural space can be accomplished by injecting 1-2% lidocaine (50-100 mg) via the catheter to elicit a segmental block.

Induction   The patient with bowel obstruction or ileus is at risk for pulmonary aspiration, and rapid-sequence induction with cricoid pressure is indicated (see p. B-5). If the patient is clinically hypovolemic, restore intravascular volume (colloid, crystalloid, or blood) prior to induction and titrate induction dose of sedative/hypnotic agents. Etomidate (0.2-0.4 mg/kg iv) or ketamine (1-3 mg/kg iv) may provide less hemodynamic depression on induction of anesthesia.

Maintenance   Standard maintenance (see p. B-3). Consider avoiding N_2O to minimize bowel distension. **Combined epidural/GA:** The epidural catheter ideally is placed at the level of a dermatome corresponding to the surgical site (generally mid-to-low thoracic spine). This allows the use of both lipophilic and hydrophilic drugs at the lowest possible dose, adding flexibility to the anesthesiologist's drug selection and minimizing the likelihood of side effects. A continuous infusion (after an initial bolus) is the preferred mode of administering local anesthetics via the epidural catheter. This minimizes fluctuations in analgesic/anesthetic effects as well as the occurrence of hemodynamic instability. Lower concentrations (e.g., bupivacaine 0.125-0.25%) are used to provide supplemental analgesia, while higher concentrations (e.g., bupivacaine 0.5%) generally provide optimal surgical conditions

Maintenance, cont.	(i.e., a complete sensory and motor block). The infusion rate is contingent on the desired segmental spread, but often ranges between 5-10 ml/h. Long-acting opioids (hydromorphone 0.4-0.8 mg or morphine 2-4 mg for epidural placement at the lower thoracic spine) can be given epidurally, along with an initial bolus of local anesthetics. Be prepared to treat ↓BP with fluids and vasopressors (e.g., ephedrine 5-10 mg iv). In patients undergoing a surgical procedure with a significant risk for major bleeding, it is prudent to delay administration of epidural local anesthetics until the critical part of surgery has been completed. **Low-dose ketamine:** If the placement of an epidural catheter is not an option, the use of a low-dose ketamine iv infusion may be considered as an adjuvant analgesic regimen (0.5 mg/kg bolus before surgical incision, followed by an infusion of 0.2 mg/kg that is stopped 30 min before the end of surgery). There is growing evidence that a low-dose ketamine infusion provides opioid-sparing effects, reduces postop wound hyperalgesia, and may decrease development of chronic pain after surgery.	
Emergence	The decision to extubate a patient at the end of surgery depends on the patient's underlying cardiopulmonary status. Patients undergoing extensive surgery with major fluid shifts may require prolonged intubation until sufficient reduction of soft tissue edema (compromised airway) is achieved.	
Blood and fluid requirements	Anticipate large fluid loss. IV: 14-16 ga × 2 NS/LR @ 10-15 ml/kg/h Warm all fluids. Humidify inhaled gases.	Blood loss can be significant, and blood should be immediately available. Procedures tend to be long and extensive, leading to hypothermia and large 3rd-space fluid loss. If procedure does not involve cancer or infection, cell-saving devices can be utilized. Guide fluid management by UO, filling pressures, CO.
Monitoring	Standard monitors (see p. B-1). UO Arterial line ± CVP or PA catheter	Most pancreatic surgery is associated with major fluid shifts and fluid loss. Invasive monitoring is usually required. In patients with cardiopulmonary compromise, a PA catheter may prove helpful for intraop fluid management. Use forced-air warmer to maintain normothermia.
Positioning	✓ and pad pressure points. ✓ eyes.	
Complications	Hypocalcemia Hypovolemia Severe hypoglycemia Sepsis	Release of pancreatic lipase → omental fat saponification. Extensive 3rd-spacing, major hemorrhage during pancreatic dissection. Uncontrolled insulin release from insulinoma Manipulation of infected tissue → cardiovascular instability, respiratory deterioration, DIC.

POSTOPERATIVE

Complications	Hyperglycemia Electrolyte imbalance Hypovolemia Hypothermia Hypocalcemia	Total pancreatectomy is associated with a brittle diabetes that can be very difficult to control. Subtotal resections lead to variable hyperglycemia.
Pain management	Continuous epidural analgesia (see p. C-2). PCA (see p. C-3).	Patient should be recovered in an ICU or hospital ward that is accustomed to treating the side effects of epidural opiates (e.g., respiratory depression, breakthrough pain, nausea, pruritus). Postop pain control with an epidural rather than a PCA regimen is superior in patients undergoing major abdominal surgery. Particularly in high-risk patients, an epidural regimen may reduce the incidence of respiratory failure. The improvement of other major clinical outcomes (e.g., cardiovascular) has not yet been demonstrated convincingly in patients undergoing nonvascular abdominal surgery.
Tests	CXR (if CVP placed); ABG; Hct	Electrolytes; Ca^{++}; glucose; Plts—as indicated for postop management.

References

1. Aldridge MC: Islet cell tumours: surgical treatment. *Hosp Med* 2000; 61:830-3.
2. De Kock M, Lavand'homme P, Waterloos H: Balanced analgesia in the perioperative period: is there a place for ketamine? *Pain* 2001; 92:373-80.
3. Longmire WP Jr: Cancer of the pancreas: palliative operation, Whipple procedure, or total pancreatectomy. *World J Surg* 1984; 8(6):872-9.
4. Merritt WT: Anesthesia for gastrointestinal surgery. In *Principles and Practice of Anesthesiology*. Longnecker DE, Tinker JH, Morgan GE, eds. Mosby-Year Book Inc, St Louis: 1998, 1881-1903.
5. Moossa AR, Scott MH, Lavelle-Jones M: The place of total and extended total pancreatectomy in pancreatic cancer. *World J Surg* 1984; 8(6):895-9.
6. Nakeeb A, Lillemoe KD, Yeo CJ, Cameron JL: Neoplasms of the exocrine pancreas. In *Surgery: Scientific Principles and Practice*, 3rd edition. Greenfield LJ, et al, eds. Lippincott Williams & Wilkins, Philadelphia: 2001, 885-98.
7. Park WY, Thompson JS, Lee KK: Effect of epidural anesthesia and analgesia on perioperative outcome: a randomized, controlled Veterans Affairs cooperative study. *Ann Surg* 2001; 234:560-9.
8. Rigg JR, Jamrozik K, Myles PS, Silbert BS, Peyton PJ, Parsons RW, Collins KS: Epidural anaesthesia and analgesia and outcome of major surgery: a randomized trial. *Lancet* 2002; 359:1276-82.
9. Taheri S, Meeran K: Islet cell tumours: diagnosis and medical management. *Hosp Med* 2000; 61:824-9.
10. Yeo CJ: Neoplasms of the endocrine pancreas. In *Surgery: Scientific Principles and Practice*, 3rd edition. Greenfield LJ, et al, eds. Lippincott Williams & Wilkins, Philadelphia: 2001, 899-914.

Surgeon

Harry A. Oberhelman, MD, FACS

7.9 PERITONEAL SURGERY

Anesthesiologist

Martin Angst, MD

EXPLORATORY OR STAGING LAPAROTOMY

SURGICAL CONSIDERATIONS

Description: Exploratory laparotomy is indicated primarily in patients suffering abdominal trauma or other acute abdominal castastrophies. It is important that a thorough and systematic intraabdominal examination be carried out to prevent missing significant injuries (e.g., ruptured duodenum or transected pancreas). Any active bleeding should be controlled prior to a systematic examination. Other indications for laparotomy include certain patients with fever of undetermined origin or those in whom a specific diagnosis cannot be made, or for staging of selected patients with Hodgkin's disease. A **staging laparotomy** (Fig 7.9-1) consists of **splenectomy**, **wedge** and **needle biopsies** of both lobes of the liver, and biopsies of the periaortic, celiac, mesenteric and portahepatic lymph nodes. In young women, sutur-

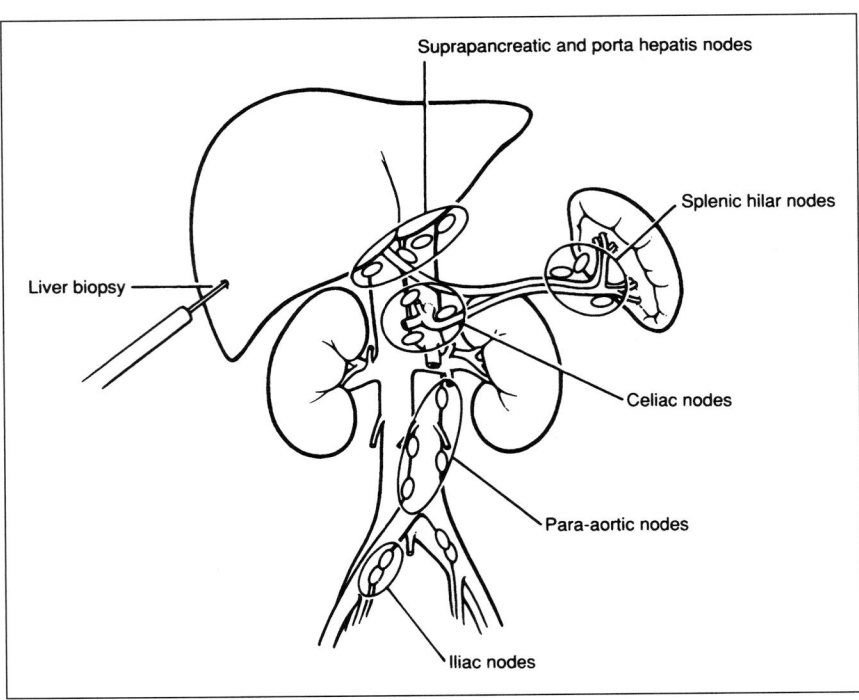

Figure 7.9-1. Biopsy of the iliac crest bone. (Reproduced with permission from Scott-Conner C.E.H., Dawson DL: *Operative Anatomy*, 2nd edition. Lippincott Williams & Wilkins, 2003.)

ing (pexing) the ovaries in the midline protects them from radiation. Indications for staging in Hodgkin's disease and lymphomas vary from institution to institution.

Basically, the procedure begins with a midline abdominal incision; then the abdomen is explored, and both needle and wedge biopsies of the liver may be performed. The spleen may be removed by incising the lateral peritoneal attachment and delivering the spleen into the wound. The short gastric vessels are cut and ligated and the splenic vessels exposed. These are cut individually and ligated, and the spleen is removed. Paraaortic nodes are exposed through a left paraaortic incision in the retroperitoneum, and removed for biopsy. Lymph channels are clipped to prevent lymphatic leakage. The nodes dissected extend to the inferior margin of the duodenum. It may be necessary to cross the aorta and biopsy any enlarged nodes on the right side. More recently, laparoscopy is being performed for staging of certain intraabdominal malignancies (e.g., pancreatic cancer).

Usual preop diagnosis: Abdominal trauma; Hodgkin's disease or other lymphomas

SUMMARY OF PROCEDURES

	Staging Laparotomy	Exploratory Laparotomy
Position	Supine	⇐
Incision	Midline abdominal	⇐ or transverse
Special instrumentation	Abdominal retractor	⇐
Unique considerations	Ovarian pexy	Careful monitoring of VS in trauma patients
Antibiotics	Cefazolin iv 1 g preop	Cefazolin iv 1 g preop; 1-2 g iv in trauma patients
Surgical time	1.5-2 h	Variable, 1-2 h+
Closing considerations	Splenic bed hemostasis	Hemostasis
EBL	100-200 ml	Variable, 200-500 ml

	Staging Laparotomy	**Exploratory Laparotomy**
Postop care	NG decompression; PACU → room	ICU for trauma patients
Mortality	< 1%	2-5%
Morbidity	Prolonged ileus: 10-15%	⇐ + In trauma patients:
	Pulmonary complications: 5-10%	Atelectasis: 5-10%
	Wound infection: 2-3%	Wound infection: 5-10%
	Small bowel obstruction: 1%	Hemorrhage: 1-3%
	Intraperitoneal bleeding: < 1%	Pneumonia: < 1%
Pain score	6-8	6-8

PATIENT POPULATION CHARACTERISTICS

Age range	15-60 yr	15-75 yr
Male:Female	1:1.5	1:1
Incidence	Common	⇐
Etiology	Unknown	Trauma
Associated conditions	Hodgkin's disease (95%); lymphoma (5%)	Other visceral or vascular injuries in trauma

ANESTHETIC CONSIDERATIONS

(Procedures covered: exploratory/staging laparotomy; splenectomy)

PREOPERATIVE

Typically, non-gynecologic patients presenting for **staging laparotomy** (which may include **splenectomy**) have Hodgkin's disease or other lymphomatous disorder. Apart from the primary disease, these patients are in reasonably good health and will not have had radiation or chemotherapy before the staging laparotomy. Patients presenting for **splenectomy** may be divided into two less healthy groups: (1) trauma patients (whose management is described in Trauma Surgery, p. 586+) and (2) a more complex group with myeloproliferative disorders, other varieties of hypersplenism, etc. These two groups may present complicated periop management problems. The latter group may have received chemotherapy and/or radiation therapy, which may affect a variety of organs and systems. It is incumbent upon the anesthesiologist to be aware of the periop implications of these adjunctive treatments. The actual extent of a staging or exploratory laparotomy can vary substantially. A good understanding of the surgeon's plan and its inherent risks (e.g., removing tumor in close proximity to a major blood vessel) is crucial for providing adequate anesthesia care.

Respiratory	Patients who have splenomegaly may have a degree of left lower lobe atelectasis and compromised ventilation 2° intraabdominal pathology: $\downarrow$FRC → $\uparrow$A-a gradient + $\downarrow$PaO$_2$. This should be evaluated by physical exam. Some may have been treated with bleomycin, a chemotherapeutic drug that causes pulmonary fibrosis at total doses > 200 mg/m^2. Methotrexate, cyclophosphamide, busulfan, chlorambucil, thiotepa, mitomycin, and cytarabine, among others, also may cause pulmonary toxicity. Toxic drug effects are potentiated by smoking, XRT, and high FiO$_2$. **Tests:** CXR; others as clinically indicated
Cardiovascular	Patients with systemic disease requiring splenectomy may be chronically ill or hypovolemic, and have $\downarrow$cardiovascular reserve. Patients who have received doxorubicin (Adriamycin) at doses > 550 mg/m^2, may have a dose-dependent cardiotoxicity that can be worsened by XRT. Other cardiotoxic agents include daunorubicin and busulfan. Manifestations include $\downarrow$QRS amplitude, CHF, pleural effusions, and dysrhythmias. **Tests:** ECG; consider ECHO or MUGA scan to determine LV function, if indicated.
Neurological	Patients may have neurological deficits from receiving chemotherapeutic agents (e.g., vinblastine and cisplatin can cause peripheral neuropathies; and 5-fluorouracil, mithramycin, and L-asparaginase may be CNS toxic). Any evidence of neurologic dysfunction should be documented in the preop evaluation.
Hematologic	Patients are likely to present with splenomegaly 2° hematologic disease (Hodgkin's disease, non-Hodgkin's lymphoma, reticulum cell sarcoma, chronic leukemia, Felty's syndrome, myeloid metaplasia, thrombotic thrombocytopenic purpura, idiopathic thrombocytopenic purpura, idiopathic autoimmune hemolytic anemia, sickle cell disease, thalassemia, hereditary elliptocytosis, hereditary

Hematologic, cont.	spherocytosis). Cytopenia is very common. Myelosuppression should be anticipated in all patients receiving active chemotherapy. **Tests:** CBC with differential; Plt count
Hepatic	Some chemotherapeutic agents (e.g., methotrexate, 6-mercaptopurine, thioguanine, L-asparaginase, and mithramycin) may be hepatotoxic. Evaluation of LFTs should be considered in patients deemed to be at risk. **Tests:** LFTs, if indicated from H&P
Renal	Some chemotherapeutic drugs (e.g., methotrexate, cisplatin) are nephrotoxic; therefore, patients exposed to such agents can present with renal insufficiency. **Tests:** Consider UA, electrolytes, BUN, creatinine, others as indicated from H&P.
Laboratory	Other tests as indicated from H&P
Premedication	Standard premedication (see p. B-2). Consider H_2-antagonists (e.g., ranitidine 50 mg iv) and metoclopramide (10 mg iv, which is contraindicated in bowel obstruction or perforation), both 1 h preop, and Na citrate (30 ml po) 10 min preop in patients at risk for pulmonary aspiration. Administer supplemental dose of steroids (e.g., 25-100 mg hydrocortisone) if patient receives them as part of chemotherapeutic regimen or in those who have received steroids within the last 12 mo.

INTRAOPERATIVE

Anesthetic technique: GETA ± epidural for postop analgesia. If postop epidural analgesia is planned, placement of catheter prior to anesthetic induction is helpful to establish correct placement in the epidural space (accomplished by injecting 1-2% lidocaine (50-100 mg) via the epidural catheter to elicit a segmental block).

Induction	Standard induction (see p. B-2) except in patients at risk for pulmonary aspiration, who require a rapid-sequence induction (see p. B-5).
Maintenance	Standard maintenance (see p. B-3). High inspired O_2 concentrations (>30%) may aggravate chemotherapy-induced (e.g., bleomycin) lung injuries. **Combined epidural/GA:** The epidural catheter ideally is placed at a level corresponding to the surgical site (generally, low thoracic). This allows the use of both lipophilic and hydrophilic drugs at the lowest possible dose, adding flexibility to the anesthesiologist's choice of agents, while minimizing the likelihood of side effects. A continuous infusion (after initial bolus) is the preferred mode of administering epidural local anesthetics to maintain stable BP and satisfactory analgesia. Lower concentrations of bupivacaine (0.125-0.25%) can be infused to provide supplemental analgesia, while higher concentrations (0.5%) may improve surgical conditions (complete motor block). The infusion rate is contingent on the desired segmental spread, but often ranges between 5-10 ml/h. Long-acting opioids (hydromorphone 0.4-0.8 mg or morphine 2-4 mg for an epidural placement at the lower thoracic spine) can be given, along with the initial bolus of local anesthetic. Be prepared to treat ↓BP with fluids and vasopressors (e.g., ephedrine 5-10 mg iv). In patients undergoing a surgical procedure with a significant risk for major bleeding, it is prudent to delay administration of epidural local anesthetics until the critical part of surgery has been completed. Systemic sedatives (droperidol, opiates, benzodiazepines, etc.) should be minimized as they increase the likelihood of postop respiratory depression. **Low-dose ketamine:** If the placement of an epidural catheter is not an option, the use of a low-dose ketamine iv infusion may be considered as an adjuvant analgesic regimen (0.5 mg/kg bolus before surgical incision, followed by an infusion of 0.2 mg/kg/h that is stopped 30 min before the end of surgery. There is growing evidence that low-dose ketamine infusion provides opioid-sparing effects, reduces wound hyperalgesia in the postop period, and may decrease the development of chronic pain after surgery.
Emergence	Most patients can be extubated at the end of surgery. Patients undergoing extensive surgery with major fluid shifts may require prolonged intubation until cardiovascular stability and sufficient reduction of soft-tissue edema (compromised airway) is achieved.

Blood and fluid requirements	IV: 14-16 ga × 1-2 NS/LR @ 10-15 ml/kg/h T&C for PRBC Fluid warmer Airway humidifier	Potential for major blood loss. In patients with difficult iv access, postinduction placement of additional access may be prudent. In splenectomy patients, Plt transfusions should be given after ligation of splenic vessels (↓sequestration).

Monitoring	Standard monitors (see p. B-1). ± Arterial line ± CVP UO (Foley catheter)	Others as indicated by patient's status. To prevent hypothermia during long operations, consider heated humidifier, warming blanket, warming room temperature, keeping patient covered until ready for prep, etc. Place an arterial line in patients with hemodynamic instability or those at risk for significant intraop bleeding. Consider CVP for guiding fluid management, particularly in patients with concomitant cardiovascular disease. Monitoring UO is mandatory.
Positioning	✓ and pad pressure points. ✓ eyes.	
Complications	Unexpected bleeding	Plt transfusion may be necessary.

POSTOPERATIVE

Complications	Bleeding Atelectasis (usually left lower lobe)	Patient should be recovered in ICU or hospital ward that is accustomed to treating side effects of epidural opiates (e.g., respiratory depression, breakthrough pain, nausea, pruritus).
Pain management	Epidural analgesia PCA (see p. C-3).	Epidural analgesia provides superior postop pain control, compared to other analgesic modalities. In high-risk patients, epidural analgesia may ↓ incidence of respiratory complications, but beneficial effects on other systems have not yet been demonstrated in patients undergoing nonvascular abdominal surgery.
Tests	CXR, if CVP placed perioperatively; CBC and Plt count.	

References

1. Brown CJ, Buie WD: Perioperative stress dose steroids: Do they make a difference? *J Am Coll Surg* 2001; 193:678-86.
2. DeKock M, Lavand'homme P, Waterloos H: Balanced analgesia in the perioperative period: Is there a place for ketamine? *Pain* 2001; 92(3):373-80.
3. Ellis H: Exploratory Laparotomy. In *Maingot's Abdominal Operations*, Vol. 1, 10th edition. Zinner MS, et al, eds. Appleton & Lange, Stamford, CT: 1997, 629-32.
4. Merritt WT: Anesthesia for gastrointestinal surgery. In *Principles and Practice of Anesthesiology,* 2nd edition. Longnecker DE, Tinker JH, Morgan GE, eds. Mosby-Year Book, St Louis: 1998, 1881-1903.
5. Park WY, Thompson JS, Lee KK: Effect of epidural anesthesia and analgesia on perioperative outcome: a randomized, controlled Veterans Affairs cooperative study. *Ann Surg* 2001; 234:560-9.
6. Rigg JR, Jamrozik K, Myles PS, Silbert BS, Peyton PJ, Parsons RW, Collins KS: Epidural anaesthesia and analgesia and outcome of major surgery: a randomised trial. *Lancet* 2002; 359:1276-82.
7. Taylor MA, Kaplan HS, Nelsen TS: Staging laparotomy with splenectomy for Hodgkin's disease: The Stanford experience. *World J Surg* 1985; 9(3):449-60.
8. Warshaw AL, Tepper JE, Shipley WV: Laparoscopy in the staging and planning for pancreatic cancer. *Am J Surg* 1986; 151:76.

SPLENECTOMY

SURGICAL CONSIDERATIONS

Description: Through a midline abdominal or left subcostal incision, the spleen is mobilized by dividing the lateral peritoneal attachments while the spleen is retracted medially. (Relevant anatomy is shown in Fig 7.9-2.) Once delivered into the operative wound, the short gastric vessels are clamped, cut, and ligated. The splenic artery and vein are then exposed, with care being taken not to injure the tail of the pancreas. By keeping the splenic hilum between the operator's fingers

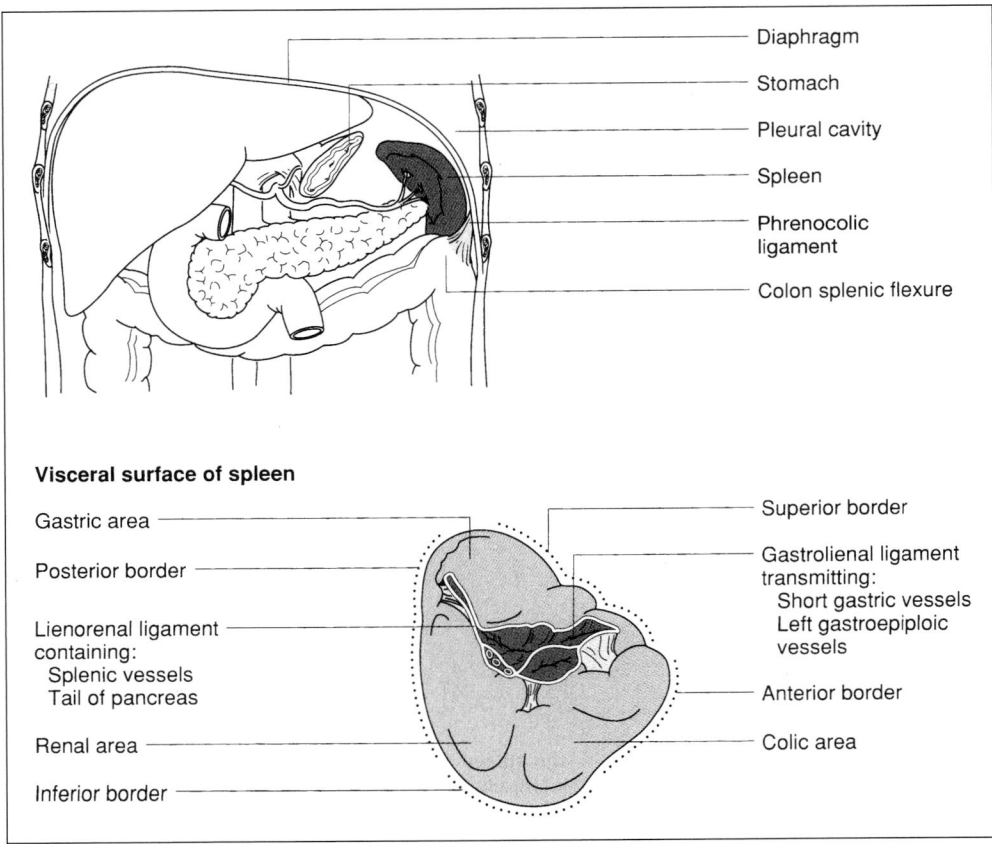

Figure 7.9-2. Anatomic relation of the spleen to the liver, diaphragm, pancreas, colon, and kidney. The stomach is sectioned to illustrate the anatomic relations in situ. (Reproduced with permission from Greenfield LJ, et al, eds: *Surgery: Scientific Principles and Practice*, 3rd edition. Lippincott Williams & Wilkins, 2001.)

and thumb, inadvertent bleeding can be controlled easily. Accessory spleens (incidence, 15-30%) also should be looked for if the splenectomy is being done for a hematologic disorder. They are found along the cephalad and caudad edges of the pancreas behind the stomach and in the area of the gastrohepatic ligament, greater omentum, and the splenic hilum. All patients undergoing splenectomy should receive polyvalent pneumococcal and H-influenza vaccines. Children may also require vaccination against meningococcus.

Variant procedure or approaches: Following trauma, efforts at splenic salvage (**splenorrhaphy**) may be made, if possible, to preserve all or part of the spleen. This may be accomplished by the use of local hemostatic techniques (electrocoagulation, argon beam coagulator, Surgicel or Gelfoam soaked in thrombin, microfibrillar collagen, and the use of fine sutures or mattress sutures with Teflon felt pledgets). Recently, splenectomy has been performed laparoscopically if the spleen is near normal size (see Laparoscopic Splenectomy, p. 463).

Usual preop diagnosis: Staging laparotomy results; trauma; immune thrombocytopenic purpura; hereditary spherocytosis; other hereditary hemolytic anemia types; or a variety of myeloproliferative disorders

SUMMARY OF PROCEDURES

	Splenectomy	**Splenorrhaphy**
Position	Supine	⇐
Incision	Midline or left subcostal	⇐
Special instrumentation	Suitable abdominal retractors	⇐
Unique considerations	Potential for major blood loss during procedure; avoid splenic laceration and damage to tail of pancreas.	⇐
Antibiotics	Cefazolin 1 g preop	⇐

	Splenectomy	**Splenorrhaphy**
Surgical time	1-2 h	1-2 h
Closing considerations	Adequate hemostasis	⇐
EBL	50-100 ml	200-500 ml
Postop care	NG decompression; PACU (nontrauma)	⇐
Mortality	0-3%	⇐
Morbidity[2]	Thrombocytosis: > 1,000,000 → DVT	⇐ (Overall complication rate: 11.8%[1])
	Pulmonary complications: 3-23%	
	Pancreatitis and/or pancreatic fistula: 1.5-7.7%	
	Subphrenic abscess: 0-6%	
	Bleeding: 1-5%	
	Overwhelming sepsis:[5]	
	Adults – 0.3-1.8%	
	Children – ≤ 4%	
Pain score	5-7	5-7

PATIENT POPULATION CHARACTERISTICS

Age range	Any age
Male:Female	1:1
Incidence	Common
Etiology	See Usual preop diagnosis, above.
Associated conditions	Blood dyscrasia (30-50%); abdominal or thoracic trauma (25%); Hodgkin's disease (5-10%); tumors (5%)

ANESTHETIC CONSIDERATIONS

See Anesthetic Considerations following Exploratory or Staging Laparotomy, p. 497.

References

1. Brunt LM, et al: Comparative analysis of laparoscopy versus open splenectomy. *Am J Surg* 1996; 172:596–601.
2. Davidson RN, Wall RA: Prevention and management of infection in patients without a spleen. *Clin Microbiol Infect* 2001; 12:657–60.
3. Feliciano DV et al: A four-year experience with splenectomy versus splenorrhaphy. *Ann Surg* 1985; 201(5):568-75.
4. Fraker DL: Spleen. In *Surgery: Scientific Principles and Practice*, 3rd edition. Greenfield LJ, et al, eds. Lippincott Williams & Wilkens, Philadelphia: 2001, 1236-59.
5. Pate JW, Peters TG, Andrews CR: Postsplenectomy complications. *Am Surg* 1985; 51(8):437-41.

EXCISION OF INTRAABDOMINAL, RETROPERITONEAL TUMORS

SURGICAL CONSIDERATIONS

Description: Intraabdominal and retroperitoneal tumors, other than those of visceral origin, consist primarily of sarcomas (liposarcoma, fibrous histiocytomas, mesenteric fibromas, and gastrointestinal stromal tumors). They are usually approached through a long midline incision for adequate exposure and to assess their resectability. Resection of such lesions may require excision of adjacent or involved small bowel or large intestine or other involved abdominal viscera. Care must be taken not to injure the ureters or major vessels, particularly at the root of the mesentery to the small bowel. It may be prudent to have ureteral stents placed to avoid injury to the ureters. If residual tumor remains, IORT may be indicated. In certain tumors, the patient may still benefit from 'tumor debulking' (removing as much tumor as possible and treating the remaining tumor with radiation and/or chemotherapy). Operative approaches are dictated by location of tumor. Although most operative approaches are transabdominal, some retroperitoneal tumors may be approached retroperitoneally via oblique incision on either side of the abdomen.

Usual preop diagnosis: Intraabdominal or peritoneal tumor

SUMMARY OF PROCEDURE

Position	Supine
Incision	Midline abdominal or transverse
Unique considerations	Availability of blood
Antibiotics	Cefazolin 1-2 g iv preop
Surgical time	3-4 h
Closing considerations	Hemostasis
EBL	300-1000 ml
Mortality	1-3%
Morbidity	Respiratory problems: 5-10%
	Wound infection: 2-4%
	Hemorrhage: 1-3%
Pain score	8-10

PATIENT POPULATION CHARACTERISTICS

Age range	Variable, 20-75 yr
Male:Female	1:1
Incidence	Common
Etiology	Unknown
Associated conditions	Partial bowel obstruction (10-15%); hydronephrosis (10-15%)

ANESTHETIC CONSIDERATIONS

See Anesthetic Considerations for Intestinal and Peritoneal Procedures, p. 416, and for Exploratory or Staging Laparotomy, p. 497.

Reference

1. *Color Atlas of Demonstrations in Surgical Pathology*, Vol 1. Royal College of Surgeons of Edinburgh. Williams & Wilkins, Baltimore: 1983, 530-43.

DRAINAGE OF SUBPHRENIC ABSCESS

SURGICAL CONSIDERATIONS

Description: Abscesses may occur in subphrenic spaces, including the right subphrenic, right subhepatic, left subphrenic, lesser sac, or bare area of the liver (Fig 7.9-3), following peritonitis, abdominal surgery or trauma. It is important to know the anatomy of these spaces for making a correct diagnosis and for treatment.

Drainage is accomplished by a **posterior** or **anterior extraperitoneal approach** or by a **transpleural approach**, depending on location of the abscess. Lesser sac abscesses are best approached by an **anterior transperitoneal route**. Abscesses in the bare area of the liver are drained posteriorly. Once the abscess is localized, the cavity is entered by finger dissection and drained. Loculations are broken up and the cavity thoroughly irrigated with NS or a suitable antibiotic solution. Appropriate drains are placed and the wound is closed in a conventional manner. Cultures are routinely obtained.

Variant procedure or approaches: Percutaneous approaches have become more popular as experience is gained by interventional radiologists. This technique should be reserved for unilocular collections, where sterile cavities are not penetrated and a safe route is available.

Usual preop diagnosis: Subphrenic abscess

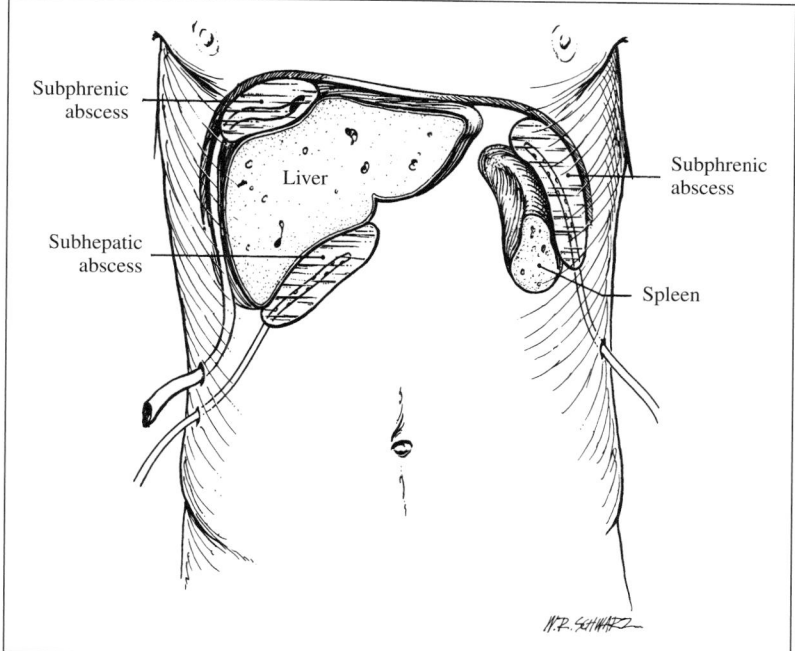

Figure 7.9-3. Anatomy of subphrenic abscess. (Reproduced with permission from Baker RJ, Fischer JE: *Mastery of Surgery*, Vol. I, Lippincott Williams & Wilkins, 2001.)

SUMMARY OF PROCEDURES

	Subphrenic Abscess Drainage	Percutaneous Approach
Position	Supine or lateral decubitus, right or left	⇐
Incision	Subcostal or oblique abdominal	None
Special instrumentation	Drainage tubes	Special catheters; CT guidance
Antibiotics	Cefazolin 1-2 g preop	⇐
Surgical time	1-1½ h	⇐
EBL	50-100 ml	10-25 ml
Postop care	Maintain patency of the drainage tubes	⇐
Mortality	< 5%	⇐
Morbidity	Inadequate drainage: 5-10%	⇐
	Pulmonary complications: 5-10%	
	Bowel perforation: < 2%	
Pain score	7-9	4-5

PATIENT POPULATION CHARACTERISTICS

Age range	Variable, 15-80 yr
Male:Female	1:1
Incidence	Common
Etiology	Postop (70-80%); peritonitis (25-30%); trauma (5-10%)
Associated conditions	See Etiology, above.

ANESTHETIC CONSIDERATIONS

See Anesthetic Considerations for Intestinal and Peritoneal Procedures, p. 416.

References

1. Baker RJ, Fischer JE: *Mastery of Surgery*, 4th edition. Lippincott Williams & Wilkins, Philadelphia: 2001, 1075-80.
2. Doherty GM, Way LW: Peritoneal cavity. In *Current Surgical Diagnosis and Treatment*, 11th edition. Way LW, Doherty GM, eds. Appleton & Lange, Stamford, CT: 2003, 517-32.

INGUINAL HERNIORRHAPHY

SURGICAL CONSIDERATIONS

Description: Groin hernias are defects in the transverse abdominis layer, where a direct hernia comes through the posterior wall of the inguinal canal and an indirect hernia comes through the internal inguinal ring. Surgical approach can be either anterior or posterior. In general, an **anterior approach** (Bassini, McVay's, Shouldice, or mesh repair) is used for primary repair of an indirect or direct inguinal hernia. The **Bassini repair** consists of ligation of the hernia sac and suturing the conjoint tendon to the shelving edge of Poupart's ligament. **McVay's repair** sutures the conjoint tendon to Cooper's ligament and usually is reserved for direct inguinal hernias. **Shouldice** emphasizes the closing of the transverse fascia and transversus abdominal muscle layers. Currently, the interposing of Marlex mesh or insertion of a Marlex plug between the conjoint tendon, the internal oblique muscle, and the inguinal ligament is commonly used. Other modifications are indicated in special situations.

A **posterior approach** is used by some surgeons for the repair of femoral hernias and recurrent inguinal hernias[3] and for treating incarcerated and strangulated hernias. The **posterior preperitoneal approach** is normally performed by suturing the transversus abdominis arch on the superior aspect of the hernia defect to Cooper's ligament and the iliopubic tract on the inferior aspect of the defect.

The **laparoscopic approach** is indicated for the repair of recurrent or bilateral inguinal hernias and utilizes a **preperitoneal patch repair** and results in less postop pain and an earlier return to normal physical activity (see Laparoscopic Inguinal Hernia Repair, p. 475).

Usual preop diagnosis: Groin pain or lump

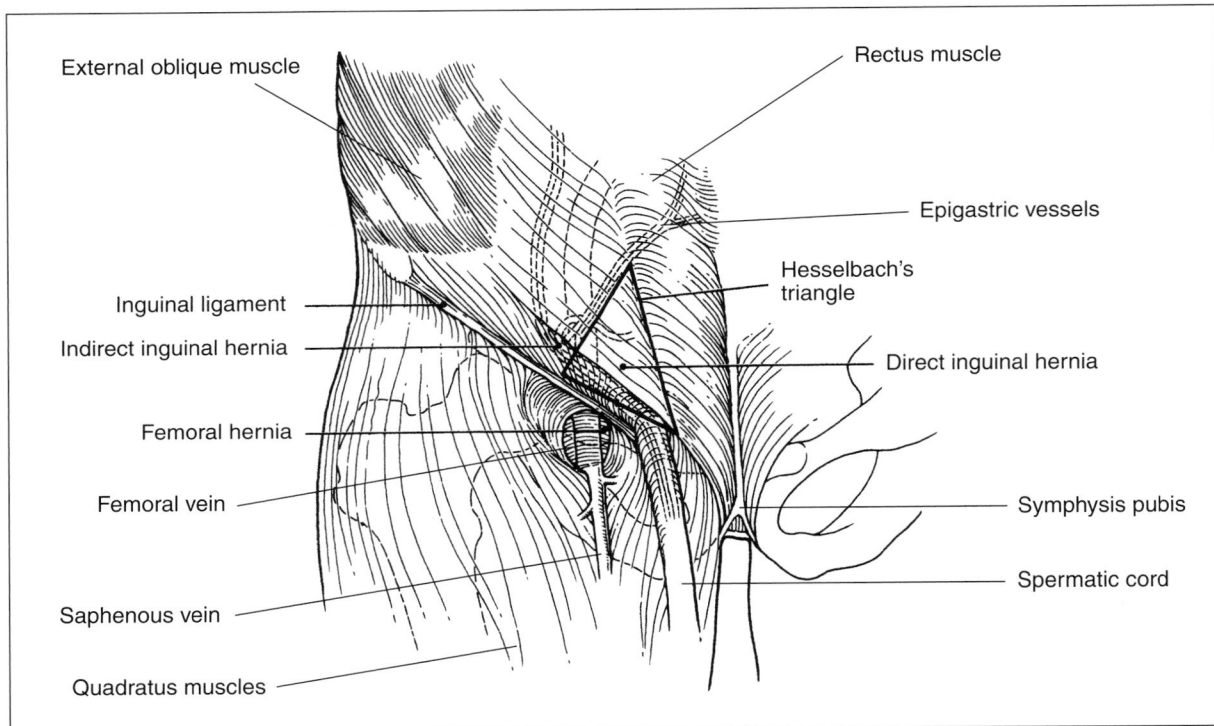

Figure 7.9-4. Inguinal anatomy. (Reproduced with permission from Scott-Conner CEH, Dawson DL: *Operative Anatomy*, 2nd edition. Lippincott Williams & Wilkins, 2003.)

SUMMARY OF PROCEDURE

Position	Supine
Incision	Oblique or transverse
Unique considerations	Avoid damage to nerve structure and spermatic cord. Avoid interfering with blood supply to testes.

Antibiotics	None or cefazolin 1 gm
Surgical time	1-1.5 h
Postop care	PACU → room
EBL	25-50 ml
Mortality	3/100,000
Morbidity	Wound abscess: < 3%
	Wound hematoma: < 2%
Pain score	4-5

PATIENT POPULATION CHARACTERISTICS

Age range	1-90 yr
Male:Female	85:15
Incidence	15/1000
Etiology	Congenital variants; reduced collagen synthesis in adults
Associated conditions	Chronic cough; urinary retention; chronic constipation

ANESTHETIC CONSIDERATIONS

See Anesthetic Considerations following Repair of Abdominal Dehiscence, p. 508.

References

1. Abrahamson J: Hernias. In *Maingot's Abdominal Operations*, 10th edition. Zinner MJ, Schwartz SI, Ellis H, eds. Appleton & Lange, Stamford CT: 1997, 479-580.
2. EU Hernia Trialists Collaboration. *Ann Surg* 2002; 235:322–32.
3. Read RC: Preperitoneal herniorrhaphy: a historical review. *World J Surg* 1989; 13(5):532-40.

FEMORAL HERNIORRHAPHY

SURGICAL CONSIDERATIONS

Description: The hernia sac is exposed as it exits the preperitoneal space through the femoral canal (Fig 7.9-5). If the hernia cannot be reduced, the possibility of strangulation needs to be kept in mind. The peritoneal sac in most cases should be opened proximal to the femoral canal in order to gain control of the intestine before it reduces itself into the peritoneal cavity. If the bowel is ischemic, it may require resection. The repair consists of suturing the iliopubic tract to Cooper's ligament, taking care not to compromise the femoral vein.[2]

Usual preop diagnosis: Bulging of tissues over femoral canal

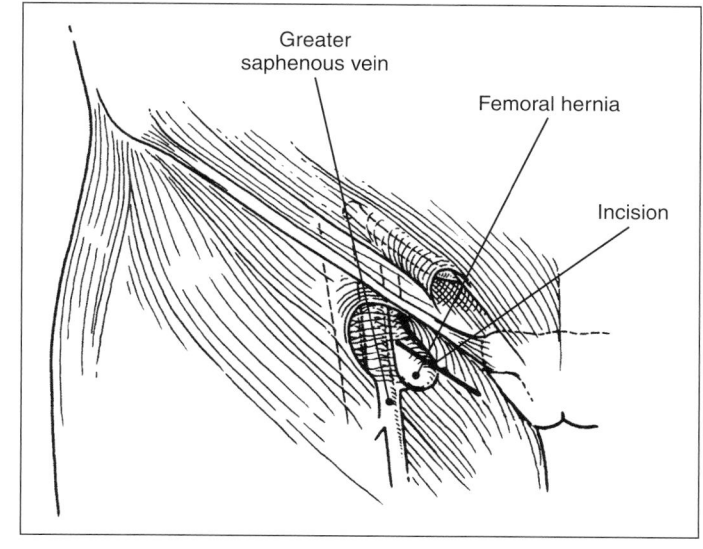

Figure 7.9-5. Femoral hernia repair. (Reproduced with permission from Scott-Conner CEH, Dawson DL: *Operative Anatomy*, 2nd edition. Lippincott Williams & Wilkins, 2003.)

SUMMARY OF PROCEDURE

Position	Supine
Incision	Oblique
Antibiotics	Cefazolin 1 g iv
Surgical time	1-1.5 h
EBL	25-50 ml
Postop care	PACU → room
Mortality	< 1% (6-20%, if strangulated)
Morbidity	Recurrence: 6%
Pain score	5-6

PATIENT POPULATION CHARACTERISTICS

Age range	Adults; rare in children
Male:Female	1:4
Incidence	1.5% of all groin hernias
Etiology	Failure of preformed peritoneal sac to obliterate; muscle atrophy in older age group

ANESTHETIC CONSIDERATIONS

See Anesthetic Considerations following Repair of Abdominal Dehiscence, p. 508.

References

1. Abrahamson J: Hernias. In *Maingot's Abdominal Operations*, 10th edition. Zinner MJ, Schwartz SI, Ellis H, eds. Appleton & Lange, Stanford CT: 1997, 479-580.
2. Richards AT, Quinn TH, Fitzgibbons RJ: Abdominal wall hernias. In *Surgery: Scientific Principles and Practice*, 3rd edition. Greenfield LJ, Mulholland MW, Oldham KT, Zelenock GB, Lillemoe KD, eds. Lippincott Williams & Wilkins, Philadelphia: 2001, 1200-15.

REPAIR OF INCISIONAL HERNIA

SURGICAL CONSIDERATIONS

Description: Incisional hernias can occur after any abdominal incision, but are most common following midline incisions. Factors leading to herniation are: wound infection, trauma, inadequate suturing, and ischemia. Following skin incision, the skin edges and subcutaneous fat are retracted and the dissection is carried down to the hernia defect. The redundant hernia sac is excised and the fascia is freed up on both sides of the wound. Primary closure is preferred, if possible.

Variant procedure or approaches: In addition to primary repair, the latter may be reinforced by an onlay mesh prosthesis, or the prosthesis may be used to fill the hernial defect or placed behind the muscle layer. In the repair of incisional hernias, laparoscopic tacking of mesh is gaining in popularity.

Usual preop diagnosis: Incisional hernia

SUMMARY OF PROCEDURE

Position	Supine
Incision	Vertical or transverse
Special instrumentation	Mesh prosthesis (when indicated)
Antibiotics	Cefazolin 1 g iv preop
Surgical time	1-2 h
Closing considerations	Retention sutures

EBL	100-200 ml
Postop care	NG decompression; abdominal binder; PACU → room
Mortality	< 1%
Morbidity	Ileus: 5-10%
	Respiratory complications: 5-10%
	Wound infection: 1-2%
Pain score	5-6

PATIENT POPULATION CHARACTERISTICS

Age range	20-70 yr
Male:Female	1:1
Incidence	3-5% of midline abdominal incisions
Etiology	Wound infection; trauma; inadequate suturing; weak tissues
Associated conditions	Obesity; malnutrition

ANESTHETIC CONSIDERATIONS

See Anesthetic Considerations following Repair of Abdominal Dehiscence, p. 508.

References

1. Condon RE: Ventral abdominal hernia. In *Mastery of Surgery*, Vol II, 4th edition, Baker RJ, Fischer JE, eds. Lippincott Williams & Wilkins, Philadelphia: 2001, 1983-8.
2. Liberman HA, Rosenthal RJ, Phillips EH: Laparoscopic ventral and incisional hernia repair: A simplified method of mesh placement. *J Am Coll Surg* 2002; 194:93-5.

REPAIR OF ABDOMINAL DEHISCENCE

SURGICAL CONSIDERATIONS

Description: Dehiscence implies a 'splitting apart' or 'bursting open' of a wound. A complete dehiscence is a separation of all layers of the abdominal wall and often is associated with an extrusion of abdominal viscera. If incomplete, the separation of fascial and muscular layers results in an incisional hernia or an obstruction of a herniated loop of intestine. The earliest sign of a wound dehiscence is the presence of a serosanguineous drainage from the wound. Minimal disruptions may be treated conservatively with occlusive dressings and an abdominal binder. Major dehiscence requires operative repair using retention sutures.

Variant procedure or approaches: Variations in the type of closure depend on surgeon's preference. Interrupted, nonabsorbable sutures and skin bridges are often used.

Usual preop diagnosis: Wound dehiscence

SUMMARY OF PROCEDURE

Position	Supine
Incision	Closure of previous incision
Unique considerations	Adequate muscle relaxation essential
Antibiotics	Cefazolin 1-2 g preop
Surgical time	1-2 h
EBL	50-100 ml
Postop care	Abdominal binder to relieve tension on suture line; PACU → room
Mortality	5-10%

Morbidity	Recurrent incisional hernia: 5-10%
	Wound infection: < 5%
	Wound ischemia: 1-2%
Pain score	4-5

PATIENT POPULATION CHARACTERISTICS

Age range	25-90 yr
Male:Female	1:1
Incidence	1.3% in patients < 45 yr
	5.4% in patients > 45 yr
Etiology	Wound infection; excessive coughing or sneezing; excessive abdominal distention; weak tissue; poor nutrition; hematoma formation; poor surgical technique with tissue ischemia
Associated conditions	Malnutrition (25-30%); ascites (20-25%); hypoproteinemia (20%); chronic anemia (5-10%); vitamin C deficiency (< 5%)

ANESTHETIC CONSIDERATIONS

Procedures covered: inguinal herniorrhaphy; femoral herniorrhaphy; incisional hernia repair; repair of abdominal dehiscence

PREOPERATIVE

Predisposing factors for hernia often include increased abdominal pressure 2° chronic cough, bladder outlet obstruction, constipation, pregnancy, vomiting, and acute or chronic muscular effort. These factors should be controlled preop to avoid postop recurrence. The patient population may range from premature infants to the elderly, who have the potential for presenting with multiple medical problems.

Musculoskeletal	Pain is likely to be present in area of hernia; evaluate bony landmarks if regional anesthesia is planned.
Gastrointestinal	Hernias may become incarcerated, obstructed, or strangulated, requiring emergency surgery. Fluid and electrolyte imbalance is likely. **Tests:** Electrolytes, if indicated from H&P
Hematologic	For regional anesthesia, ✓ patient's coagulation status, if indicated from H & P. **Tests:** As indicated from H&P
Laboratory	Other tests as indicated from H&P
Premedication	If necessary, standard premedication (see p. B-2).

INTRAOPERATIVE

Anesthetic technique: GA, regional, or local anesthesia ± sedation (MAC) are all appropriate anesthetic techniques for uncomplicated cases (e.g., without incarceration or obstruction). Choice depends on factors such as site of incision, patient physical status, and preference of both patient and surgeon. Profound muscle relaxation may be necessary to facilitate exploration and repair.

Regional anesthesia:

Spinal	**Single-shot vs continuous:** Patient in sitting or lateral decubitus position (operative site down) for placement of hyperbaric subarachnoid block. Doses of local anesthetics are as follows for T4-T6 level: 0.75% bupivacaine in 8.25% dextrose (10-15 mg); 0.5% tetracaine in 5% dextrose (12-16 mg). For continuous spinal, titrate local anesthetic (e.g., 2.5-5 mg increment for bupivacaine) to desired surgical level (e.g., T6).
Epidural	Patient in sitting or lateral decubitus position for placement of epidural catheter. After locating the epidural space, administer a test dose (e.g., 3 ml of 1.5% lidocaine with 1:200,000 epinephrine) to elucidate whether the catheter is subarachnoid or intravascular. Titrate local anesthetic (e.g., 0.5% bupivacaine, ropivacaine, or levobupivacaine) until desired surgical level is obtained (5-7 ml at a time), usually < 20 ml.
Local	Requires gentle surgical technique. Surgical field block, plus ilioinguinal and iliohypogastric nerve blocks, using 0.5% bupivacaine with 1:200,000 epinephrine. Usually done by surgeon.

General anesthesia:

Induction	**LMA vs ETT:** Standard induction (see p. B-2). Mask may be suitable for the patient who presents with a simple chronic hernia. If there is obstruction, incarceration, or strangulation, however, a rapid-sequence induction (see p. B-5) with ET intubation is indicated. GETA also may be indicated in the patient with wound dehiscence.
Maintenance	Standard maintenance (see p. B-3). Muscle relaxants may be necessary to facilitate surgical repair.
Emergence	Consider extubating the trachea while patient is still anesthetized to prevent coughing and straining. Patients who are at risk for pulmonary aspiration and require awake intubation or rapid-sequence induction (see p. B-5) are not candidates for deep extubation.
Blood and fluid requirements	Minimal blood loss IV: 16-18 ga × 1 NS/LR @ 5-8 ml/kg/h
Monitoring	Standard monitoring (see p. B-1).
Positioning	✓ and pad pressure points. ✓ eyes.
Complications	↓↓HR + ↓BP Vagal reflex evoked by bowel traction.

POSTOPERATIVE

Complications	Cauda equina syndrome	The diagnosis of cauda equina syndrome (urinary and fecal incontinence, paresis of lower extremities, perineal hyperesthesia) should be sought in the postop period in patients who have received large doses of intrathecal local anesthetic during continuous spinal techniques. ✓ patients for bowel or bladder dysfunction and perineal sensory deficits. If present, consider a neurology consultation and continue followup of the patient's neurologic dysfunction.
	Urinary retention, common with regional anesthesia	Patients with urinary retention may require intermittent catheterization until urinary function resumes.
	Wound dehiscence with coughing/straining	
Pain management	PO analgesics: Acetaminophen and codeine (Tylenol #3 1-2 tab q 4-6 h) or oxycodone and acetaminophen (Percocet 1 tab q 6 h)	Surgical field block or regional anesthesia should provide sufficient analgesia postop.

References

1. Cousins MJ, Bridenbaugh PO, eds: *Neural Blockade Pain Management*, 3nd edition. Lippincott-Raven Publishers, Philadelphia: 1998.
2. Ellis H: Incisions, closures and management of the wound. In: *Maingot's Abdominal Operations*, Vol. I, 10th edition. Zinner MJ, ed. Appleton & Lange, Stamford, CT: 1997, 395-426.
3. Horlocker TT, McGregor DG, Matsushige DK, Chantigian RC, Schroeder DR, Besse JA: Neurologic complications of 603 consecutive continuous spinal anesthetics using macrocatheter and microcatheter techniques. Perioperative Outcomes Group. *Anesth Analg* 1997; 84(5):1063-70.
4. Horlocker TT, McGregor DG, Matsushige Dk, Schroeder DR, Besse JA: A retrospective review of 4767 consecutive spinal anesthetics: central nervous system complications. Perioperative Outcomes Group. *Anesth Analg* 1997; 84(3):578-84.

Surgeons

Irene L. Wapnir, MD, FACS
Stefanie S. Jeffrey, MD, FACS

7.10 BREAST SURGERY

Anesthesiologist

Lindsey Vokach-Brodsky, MBChB, FFARCSI

BREAST BIOPSY

SURGICAL CONSIDERATIONS

Description: Description: Breast biopsy, or **lumpectomy**, is the surgical removal of breast tissue for histopathological examination. Many biopsies are done percutaneously as office procedures. Two approaches are used: **fine-needle aspiration cytology** and **core needle biopsy**. Ultrasound-guided biopsies, mammographically-guided, stereotaxic core biopsies, and MRI-guided biopsies are used as preop diagnostic procedures. **Open breast biopsies** are performed primarily in the OR for palpable or nonpalpable abnormalities. **Palpable lesions** include masses, nodules, or areas of asymmetric breast thickening. Breast pathology can manifest as a skin change—specifically, edema, redness, brawny discoloration, or ulceration—mandating biopsy of the involved skin and underlying breast tissue. The term **excisional biopsy** usually is applied to benign entities and implies the complete removal of the lesion in question (e.g., excision of a fibroadenoma). The term **lumpectomy** is used to characterize cancerous lesions that are removed with a rim of normal breast tissue to achieve tumor-free margins.

Another common reason for excisional biopsy is the occurrence of bloody or pathological **nipple discharge**. The underlying cause of this abnormality is, in most instances, a benign intraductal papilloma or, infrequently, carcinoma. **Ductoscopy** may be used to explore breast ducts that produce abnormal discharge fluid. The ductoscope is a 0.9 mm fiber optic microendoscope. It is inserted into the duct(s) following progressive dilatation with lacrimal probes. Once the intraductal lesion is visually identified, the surgeon injects methylene blue to further guide the duct excision and breast biopsy.

Nonpalpable lesions are usually discovered on routine screening mammography. Microcalcifications, masses, densities, and architectural distortion fall into the category of potentially malignant lesions. Similarly, ultrasound can identify complex cystic or solid masses and MRI areas of abnormal enhancement. In all these instances, the breast usually feels and looks normal. Typically, the radiologist places a percutaneous hook-wire in close proximity to the lesion, using local anesthesia. The surgeon uses this guide to identify the area of abnormality; therefore, these procedures are referred to as **wire localization, needle localization**, or **hook-wire localization** breast biopsies. In the OR, the surgeon removes the breast tissue surrounding the wire and confirms the removal of the wire and target lesion on specimen radiography and/or ultrasound.

Breast biopsies, or lumpectomies, are done under local anesthesia ± conscious sedation. In some cases, breast biopsies or lumpectomies are done under GA, either because of the size of the lesion, patient preference, or concerns of implant injury for patients who have subglandular implants. Alternatively, regional or paravertebral blocks can be used.

Usual preop diagnosis: Breast mass; nipple discharge; mammographic, sonographic, or MRI abnormality

SUMMARY OF PROCEDURES

	Breast Biopsy/Lumpectomy	Wire Localization Breast Biopsy
Position	Supine, with ipsilateral arm abducted. Table may be banked to center breast.	⇐
Incision	Over breast mass or circumareolar	⇐ + Incision may or may not incorporate skin entry site of wire.
Special instrumentation	Ductoscope; ultrasound	⇐
Antibiotics	Cefazolin 1 g iv (optional)	⇐
Surgical time	0.5-1 h	1-1.5 h, depending on time needed to get results of specimen radiograph.
Closing considerations	Steri-Strips, gauze, or transparent bandage.	⇐ + Specimen radiograph result must be obtained before completion of operation.
EBL	< 25 ml	⇐
Postop care	PACU → home	⇐
Mortality	Minimal	⇐
Morbidity	Seroma: Very common	⇐
	Ecchymosis or hematoma: < 10%	
	Infection: 1.20%	+ Target lesion is missed (2° misplacement or dislodging of wire).
		Wire cut; traverses or migrates into chest.
Pain score	2-5	2-5

PATIENT POPULATION CHARACTERISTICS

Age range	25-90	35-90 yr
Male:Female	Mainly female	⇐
Incidence	Common	⇐
Etiology	Unknown	⇐

ANESTHETIC CONSIDERATIONS

See Anesthetic Considerations for Breast Biopsy and Sentinel Lymph Node Biopsy, p. 514.

SENTINEL LYMPH NODE BIOPSY

SURGICAL CONSIDERATIONS

Description: Sentinel lymph node biopsy is a technique applied to patients with small, invasive breast cancers who do not have clinically pathologic lymph nodes. The sentinel lymph node is the first node to drain afferent lymphatics from the particular region of the breast where the cancer is located. The sentinel node is not necessarily the lowest lymph node in the axilla; it usually is located somewhere in the axilla, but may be situated in the internal mammary chain or other unusual sites. Because the sentinel lymph node is the first to drain the lymphatics from a breast cancer, it is the most likely lymph node to harbor metastatic tumor. Early studies suggest that absence of tumor metastasis on histological examination of sentinel nodes accurately predicts the histological status of nonsentinel nodes. The goal of this approach is to avoid conventional Level I and Level II axillary node dissection in node-negative patients. The technique has been validated in several large institutional and multicenter studies. Surgeons should perform ~10-30 sentinel node biopsies with complete axillary node dissections to ensure that their sentinel node identification rate approximates 90% and demonstrate tumor-positive sentinel nodes in node-positive axillas. **Completion axillary dissection** is currently recommended for patients outside clinical trials with tumor-positive sentinel nodes. Results of large, randomized clinical trials aimed at determining long-term outcomes of survival after sentinel node biopsy in lymph node-negative patients are pending.

Two **types of agents** have been principally tested and are now widely used for sentinel node identification procedures: **isosulfan blue vital dye** (Lymphazurin 1%) and **99^m-technetium-labeled sulfur colloid (TSC)** (unfiltered or filtered). Differences and controversy exist regarding ideal injection sites of these agents—peritumoral or around biopsy cavity, dermal, subareolar, or in combination. The first method instills 3-5 ml of isosulfan blue subareolar or at 3, 6, 9, and 12 o'clock surrounding the lesion. The breast is massaged and the axilla is incised 3-7 min later, depending on the distance of the tumor to the axilla. Typically, blue afferent lymphatics and blue nodes are identified below the clavipectoral fascia. The surgeon should inform the anesthesiologist when injecting the dye because a transient drop in the pulse oximeter reading of 2-5% is seen frequently. Patients may retain a bluish hue for a few h or longer and will excrete blue-tinged urine, stool, or emesis. Allergic reactions, consisting of 'blue hives' to full-blown, life-threatening anaphylactic shock, have been reported following the injection of isosulfan blue.

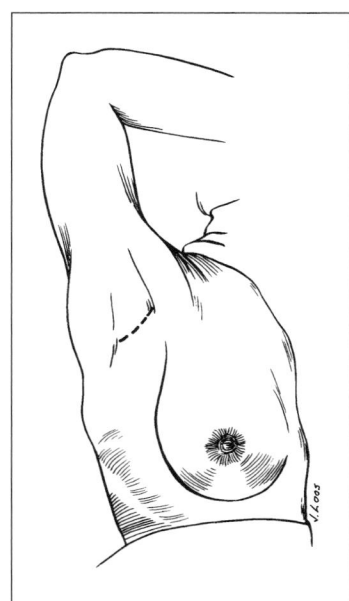

Figure 7.10-1. Arm may be draped into field and positioned on arm board at 90° or suspended over head, as shown. Incision site for lymph node biopsy is indicated by dotted line. (Reproduced with permission from Baker RJ, Fischer JE: *Mastery of Surgery*, 4th edition. Lippincott Williams & Wilkins, 2001.)

Another method utilizes **TSC** (~1 mCi), which can be injected, according to surgeon's preference, around the tumor or biopsy cavity, intradermal, or subareolar locations. Only parenchymal injections appear to track to extra-axillary sites. The tracer has very low radioactivity and is safe to handle, with no special protection required in handling specimens. TSC is injected 30 min-24 h before surgery. Post-injection **lymphoscintigraphy** is considered optional. After induction of GA or regional anesthesia, the operative field (chest and lymph node-bearing areas) is surveyed with a hand-held gamma probe (a slim rod, similar to a Geiger counter). The 'hot' spot(s), denoting accumulated tracer in lymph nodes, are identified and an incision is made in the overlying skin. It is customary to have a pathologist examine the sentinel node intraop, using touch-prep cytology or frozen section. The purpose is to identify node-positive cases and proceed with standard axillary dissection during the course of the same operative procedure.

Combination of blue dye and TSC yield the highest sentinel node identification rates. Whenever the sentinel node cannot be identified, a conventional axillary dissection should be performed. Larger clinical trials are under way to determine whether sentinel lymph node biopsy will eventually replace standard axillary lymph node dissection in node-negative patients.

Usual preop diagnosis: Invasive breast cancer

SUMMARY OF PROCEDURE

Position	Supine
Incision	Small axillary incision
Special instrumentation	Hand-held gamma-detection probe
Unique considerations	Radiation exposure negligble. Avoid BP cuff or iv in ipsilateral arm. Possible need to avoid muscle relaxants. Isosulfan blue vital dye → allergic reaction (1-2/100).
Antibiotics	Cefazolin 1 g iv (optional)
Surgical time	10-30 min, up to 1.5 h for axillary lymph node dissections
EBL	Minimal
Postop care	PACU → home
Mortality	Rare
Morbidity	Discoloration of urine and stool up to 48 h
	Permanent tattooing of skin with blue dye
	Transient blue tinging of skin
	Allergic dye or radioisotope reaction: ~1-2%
	Anaphylaxis 1/2000
Pain score	2-5

PATIENT POPULATION CHARACTERISTICS

Age range	20-90 yr; typically > 30 yr
Incidence	~1/8 American women will develop breast cancer.
Etiology	Unknown in most cases; familial history may be related to genetic mutation (BCRA 1&2).

ANESTHETIC CONSIDERATIONS FOR BREAST BIOPSY AND SENTINEL LYMPH NODE BIOPSY

PREOPERATIVE

Breast masses may vary in size and depth, which will, in part, determine what type of anesthetic is most suitable for the procedure in these otherwise healthy patients. Typically, these excisional biopsies can be accomplished with MAC/sedation and local anesthesia; however, patient wishes must be considered in the anesthetic plan. The suitability of local vs GA may be best addressed by preop discussion with the surgical team.

Psychosocial	Patients are likely to be very anxious concerning the possibility of breast malignancy, and should be counseled and premedicated appropriately.
Laboratory	CBC; other tests as indicated from H&P.
Premedication	Standard premedication (see p. B-2).

INTRAOPERATIVE

Anesthetic technique: GA or local anesthesia ± sedation are both appropriate techniques. Choice of anesthetic technique depends on the size and depth of lesion and the wishes of the patient. Often done on an outpatient basis.

MAC	Propofol infusion (25-100 μg/kg/min), combination of analgesics (e.g., fentanyl/remifentanil) and anxiolytics (e.g., midazolam), titrated to effect, are most commonly used. The surgeon may choose to add Na bicarbonate to 1% lidocaine (1:10) to reduce injection pain. The anesthesiologist may give remifentanil 0.5-1 μg/kg 90 sec before initial injection of local anesthetic in the skin.

Induction	Standard induction (see p. B-2). Mask or LMA anesthetic may be appropriate.	
Maintenance	Standard maintenance (see p. B-3). Muscle relaxants are not necessary for surgical procedure.	
Emergence	No special considerations	
Blood and fluid requirements	Minimal blood loss IV: 18-20 ga × 1 NS/LR @ 3-5 ml/kg/h	
Monitoring	Standard monitors (see p. B-1). Maintain verbal contact with patient if MAC.	Other monitors as clinically indicated. Isosulfan blue vital dye → artifactual $\downarrow O_2$ sat as low as 92-94%.
Positioning	✓ and pad pressure points. ✓ eyes.	
Complications	Inadequate analgesia	May have to supplement surgical field block with local anesthetic or convert to GA.
	Isosulfan dye reaction	Pruritus, localized swelling, blue hives. Rx: diphenhydramine (10-50 mg iv). $\downarrow$BP may require epinephrine.

POSTOPERATIVE

Complications	No specific complications anticipated.	Inform patients that urine, vomit, or stool may be blue for 24-48 h.
Pain management	PO analgesics (see p. C-2).	
Tests	As clinically indicated.	

References

1. Albertini JJ, Lyyman GH, Cox C, et al: Lymphatic mapping and sentinel node biopsy in the patient with breast cancer. *JAMA* 1996; 276:1818-22.
2. Albo D, Wayne JD, Hunt K, Rahlfs TF, Singletary SE, Ames FC, Feig B, Ross MI, Kuerer HM: Anaphylactic reactions to isosulfan blue dye during sentinel node biopsy for breast cancer. *Am J Surg* 1995; 182:393-8.
3. Alex JC, Krag DN: The gamma-probe guided resection of radiolabeled primary lymph nodes. *Surg Oncol Clin N Am* 1996; 5:33-41.
4. Birdwell RL, Smith KL, Betts BJ, Ikeda DM, Strauss HW, Jeffrey SS: Breast cancer: variables affecting sentinel lymph node visualization at preoperative lymphoscintigraphy. *Radiology* 2001; 220:47-53.
5. Bland KI, Copeland EM III, eds: *The Breast: Comprehensive Management of Benign and Malignant Diseases*. WB Saunders, Philadelphia: 1998.
6. Dooley WC: Routine operative breast endoscopy for bloody nipple discharge. *Ann Surg Oncol* 2002; 9(9):920-3.
7. Giuliano AE, Jones RC, Brennan M, Statman R: Sentinel lymphadenectomy in breast cancer. *J Clin Oncol* 1997; 15:2345-50.
8. Harris JR, Lippman ME, Morrow M, Hellman S, eds: *Diseases of the Breast*. Lippincott Williams & Wilkins, Philadelphia: 2000.
9. Hietala S-O, Hirsch JI, Faunce HF: Allergic reaction to Patent Blue Violet during lymphography. *Lymphology* 1977; 10: 158-60.
10. Hirsch JI, Tisnado J, Cho S-R, Beachley MC: Use of isosulfan blue for identification of lymphatic vessels: experimental and clinical evaluation. *Am J Roentgenol* 1982; 139:1061-4.
11. Krag D, Weaver D, Ashikaga T, et al: The sentinel node in breast cancer: A multicenter study. *N Eng J Med* 1998; 339:941-6.
12. Larsen VH, Freudendal-Pedersen A, Fogh-Andersen N: The influence of Patent Blue V on pulse oximetry and haemoximetry. *Acta Anaesthesiol Scand* 1995; 39(Suppl 107):53-5.
13. Longnecker SM, Gussardo MM, Van Voris LP: Life-threatening anaphylaxis following subcutaneous administration of isosulfan blue 1%. *Clin Pharm* 1985; 4:219-21. (Case Report)
14. Montgomery LL, et al: Isosulfan blue dye reactions during sentinel lymph node mapping for breast cancer. *Anesth Analg* 2002; 95:385-8.
15. Saito S, Fukura H, Shimada H, Fijita T: Prolonged interference of blue dye "patent blue" with pulse oximetry readings. *Acta Anaesthesiol Scand* 1995; 39:268-9.
16. Vokach-Brodsky L, Jeffrey SS, Lemmens HJM, Brock-Utne JG: Isosulfan blue affects pulse oximetry. *Anesthesiology* 2000; 93:102-3.
17. Zelcer J, White PF: Monitored anesthesia care. In *Anesthesia*, 4th edition. Miller RD, ed. Churchill Livingstone, New York: 1994, 1465-80.

BREAST-CONSERVING SURGERY AND MASTECTOMY ± RECONSTRUCTION

SURGICAL CONSIDERATIONS

Description: The treatment of invasive breast cancer has evolved greatly in the last 30 yr. The **radical mastectomy**, which removes the breast, the underlying pectoral muscles, and the axillary lymph nodes, has been replaced by the **modified radical mastectomy** or **lumpectomy (partial mastectomy)** with **axillary dissection**. Modified radical mastectomy entails removal of the breast and axillary lymph nodes. Lumpectomy or re-excision lumpectomy and axillary dissection are normally done through separate incisions. Postop adjuvant radiation therapy is routinely recommended in breast-conserving surgery and is administered following the completion of adjuvant chemotherapy.

In an **axillary dissection**, Levels I and II axillary lymph nodes—those that lie behind and lateral to the edge of the pectoralis minor muscle—are removed. The Level III, or highest group of axillary lymph nodes, are medial to the pectoralis minor muscle. For prognostic and treatment purposes, no advantage can be shown in removing Level III lymph nodes. As part of the axillary dissection, the surgeon preserves the thoracodorsal nerve (innervates the latissimus dorsi muscle) and the long thoracic nerve (innervates the serratus anterior muscle), as well as the blood and nerve supply to the pectoral muscles. The intercostobrachial nerves (sensory to the upper arm) course through the axillary contents. Preservation of some or all of these nerves usually can be accomplished so that permanent dysesthesias are averted.

A **total mastectomy** (also known as a **simple mastectomy**) removes only the breast. It is done mainly for treatment of extensive duct carcinoma in situ. There is no formal axillary dissection involved.

Immediate breast reconstruction is an option for most women undergoing mastectomy. Postop chest radiation may be a relative, but not absolute, contraindication to immediate reconstruction. Two approaches are commonly used: (1) prosthetic reconstruction with a temporary tissue expander or a saline-filled implant placed behind the pectoral muscles; and (2) autologous myocutaneous flaps (see Breast Reconstruction, p. 915). Truly excellent cosmetic results are possible with mastectomy techniques that preserve much of the breast skin and even, in some instances, the nipple-areolar complex **(skin-sparing mastectomy)**.

Usual preop diagnosis: Invasive or in situ breast cancer

SUMMARY OF PROCEDURES

	Modified Radical Mastectomy	Total Mastectomy	Lumpectomy, Axillary Lymph Node Dissection
Position	Supine, with ipsilateral arm abducted and prepped on field. May require repositioning (latissimus dorsi reconstruction).	⇐	⇐
Incision	Elliptical oblique or elliptical transverse to include nipple/areola and previous biopsy; periareolar, or 'tennis-racquet.'	⇐	Incision over breast mass or previous biopsy site. Separate transverse or oblique incision in axilla.
Unique considerations	Avoid iv and BP cuff on ipsilateral arm.	⇐	⇐
Antibiotics	Cefazolin 1 g iv (optional)	⇐	⇐
Surgical time	1.5-3 h (+ 1-7 h, if immediate breast reconstruction performed)	1-2 h (+ 1-7 h, if immediate breast reconstruction performed)	1-3 h
Closing considerations	Gauze bandage over incision	⇐	⇐
EBL	150-500 ml, depending on whether scalpel or electrocautery is used.	⇐	25-100 ml
Postop care	PACU → room × 2 d	PACU → room × 1-2 d, or occasionally → home	PACU → home
Mortality	Rare	⇐	⇐
Morbidity	Lymphedema: 5-30% (depending on extent of axillary dissection)	–	Lymphedema: 5-30% (depending on extent of axillary dissection)
	Seroma: 25%	⇐	⇐

	Modified Radical Mastectomy	Total Mastectomy	Lumpectomy, Axillary Lymph Node Dissection
Morbidity, cont.	Infection: 2-10%	⇐	⇐
	Flap necrosis: < 5%	⇐	–
	Hematoma: < 5%	⇐	< 10%
	Injury to axillary neurovascular structures: Rare	–	–
	Pneumothorax: Rare (may occur with attempts to obtain hemostasis of intercostal per-forating vessels)	⇐	⇐
Pain score	4-8	4-6	4-8

PATIENT POPULATION CHARACTERISTICS

Age range	20-90 yr (generally > 40 yr)
Incidence	Over their lifetime, ~1/8 of American women develop breast cancer; in 2002, 205,000 new cases of female breast cancer were diagnosed in the U.S.
Etiology	Unknown in most cases; familial Hx may be related to genetic mutation (BCRA 1/2).

ANESTHETIC CONSIDERATIONS

PREOPERATIVE

Patients often have no other underlying medical problems. Some consideration, however, should be given to the anesthetic implications of metastatic spread to bone, brain, liver, lung, etc.

Respiratory	Respiratory compromise can be present if patient has received XRT to the thorax as part of treatment.
	Tests: CXR (✓ for pleural effusion and rib or vertebral lesions). If patient shows any signs of respiratory compromise, obtain room air ABG. Consider PFTs (FVC, FEV_1, $MMEF_{25-75}$) if CXR or ABG abnormal. This will help predict pulmonary reserve and patient tolerance to GA. Patients who show signs of impaired pulmonary function might require postop care in an ICU for various reasons (e.g., mechanical ventilation, aggressive pulmonary toilet, close observation, etc.).
Cardiovascular	Chemotherapeutic agents (e.g., doxorubicin at doses > 550 mg/m^2) also cause severe cardio-myopathies. If patient was exposed to this type of drug, cardiac dysfunction may be present, and a cardiac consultation to evaluate ventricular function may be necessary.
	Tests: Consider ECHO or MUGA scan; ECG.
Neurological	Breast cancer often metastasizes to the CNS and can present with focal neurologic deficits, ↑ICP, or altered mental status. If patient has altered mental status, full workup should proceed without delay; postpone surgery until cause is found.
	Tests: CT/MRI scan should be recommended, if indicated from H&P.
Hematologic	Patient may be anemic 2° chronic disease or chemotherapeutic agents.
	Tests: CBC, with differential and Plt count
Laboratory	Routine lab exam; other tests as indicated from H&P.
Premedication	Standard premedication (see p. B-2).

INTRAOPERATIVE

Anesthetic technique: GETA or GA with LMA. Regional anesthesia (paravertebral block [PVB]) in breast surgery is associated with less PONV, less postop pain, and earlier discharge from the hospital.

General anesthesia:

Induction	Standard induction (see p. B-2).
Maintenance	Standard maintenance (see p. B-3). The use of muscle relaxants during axillary dissection should be avoided to permit surgical identification of nerves by nerve stimulator or if electrocautery is used in the axilla.
Emergence	Pressure dressings may be applied with the patient anesthetized and 'sitting up' at the end of the procedure. Discuss with surgeons whether they intend to apply this type of dressing, to enable

Emergence, cont.	appropriate timing of emergence. Prophylactic antiemetics (e.g., metoclopramide 10 mg + granisetron 100 μg iv 30 min before end of case) required because of high incidence of PONV in breast surgery.	

Regional anesthesia: Unilateral multiple level PVB provides satisfactory anesthesia for modified radical mastectomy and lumpectomy with axillary lymph node dissection. A block from C7-T6 is required. 0.5% bupivacaine or 0.5% ropivacaine with 1:300,000 epinephrine are suitable local anesthetics (4-5 ml/level). Sedation is useful during block placement and is continued intraop. (See Anesthetic Considerations for Breast Biopsy, p. 514.) PVB is contraindicated for the following reasons: (1) patient refusal; (2) local anesthetic allergy; (3) pathology or previous surgery → anatomic distortion of paravertebral space; and/or (4) infection at sites of injection.

Blood and fluid requirements	Minimal-to-moderate blood loss IV: 16-18 ga × 1 (avoid operative side) NS/LR @ 3-5 ml/kg/h	
Monitoring	Standard monitors (see p. B-1).	Others as indicated by patient status. BP cuff on arm opposite surgical site.
Positioning	✓ and pad pressure points. ✓ eyes.	
Complications	Pneumothorax	Deep surgical exploration may cause inadvertent pneumothorax; monitor patient for Sx (e.g., ↑PIP, ↓PaCO$_2$, asymmetric breath sounds, hyperresonance to percussion over the affected side, hemodynamic instability). Dx: CXR. Rx: Chest tube, 100% O$_2$.
Complications 2° PVB	Inadequate block (10%) Pleural puncture Horner's syndrome Inadvertent epidural	May result in pneumothorax.

POSTOPERATIVE

Complications	Pneumothorax Psychological trauma	If index of suspicion for pneumothorax is high, maintain oxygenation (100% FiO$_2$) and ventilation; inform surgeons of the likelihood of the Dx. If patient is hemodynamically unstable (suggesting a tension pneumothorax), place a 14-ga iv catheter in the 2nd intercostal space, while the surgeons set up for placement of a chest tube. If patient is hemodynamically stable and not hypoxemic, a portable CXR may aid in diagnosis.
Pain management	PCA (see p. C-3). PO analgesics (see p. C-2).	
Tests	Postop portable CXR, if pneumothorax is a consideration.	

References

1. Boerner TF, Gonzales RM, Policare R: How common are nausea and vomiting after breast surgery? *Anesth Analg* 1996; 82: 838.
2. Greengrass RA: Regional anesthesia for ambulatory surgery. *Anesth Clin North Am* 2000; 18(2):858-61.
3. Greengrass RA, O'Brien F, Lyerly K, et al: Paravertebral block for breast cancer surgery. *Can J Anaesth* 1996; 143(8):858-61.
4. Harris JR. Lippman ME, Morrow M, Hellman S, eds: *Disease of the Breast.* Lippincott Williams & Wilkins, Philadelphia: 2000.
5. Hunt KK, Baldwin BJ, Strom EA, et al: Feasibility of postmastectomy radiation after TRAM flap reconstruction. *Ann Surg Oncol* 1997; 4:377-84.
6. Karmakar MK: Thoracic paravertebral block. *Anesthesiology* 2001; 95:771-80.
7. Klein SM, Bergh A, Steele SM, et al: Thoracic paravertebral block for breast surgery. *Anesth Analg* 2000; 90:1402-5.
8. Rothschild J, Majchorzak J: Breast surgery is a high risk procedure for development of nausea and vomiting. *Anesthesiology* 1993; 79:A1095.
9. Singletary SE: Skin-sparing mastectomy with immediate reconstruction: the MD Anderson Cancer Center experience. *Ann Surg Oncol* 1996; 3:411-16.

Surgeons

Mark Koransky, MD
Ralph Greco, MD

7.11   ENDOCRINE SURGERY

Anesthesiologist

Frederick G. Mihm, MD

EXCISION OF THYROGLOSSAL DUCT CYST

SURGICAL CONSIDERATIONS

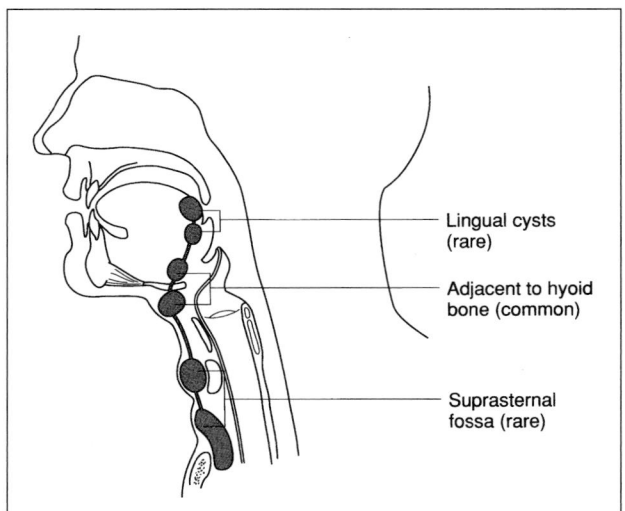

Figure 7.11-1. Location of thyroglossal duct cysts. (Reproduced with permission from Greenfield LJ, et al: *Surgery: Scientific Principles and Practice.* Lippincott Williams & Wilkins, 2001.)

Description: Thyroglossal duct cysts typically are located in the midline at or below the hyoid bone (Fig 7.11-1). Differential diagnoses after initial physical exam include epidermoid cysts or lymph nodes. Cysts should be removed because of an associated high risk of infection with oral flora and a slight (< 1%) risk of either squamous-cell or papillary-thyroid cancer developing in the cyst itself. A transverse skin incision is made over the cyst; and, if the cyst was previously infected and sinus tracts through the skin are present, the skin should be removed along with the cyst. The cyst is identified and followed cephalad to the hyoid bone (Fig 7.11-2). Then, the mid-portion of the hyoid bone is resected to minimize recurrence. There may be many small tracts associated with the cyst that tend to attenuate beyond the hyoid bone. The base of the tract or tracts is resected up to the level of the floor of the mouth at the foramen cecum and ligated with absorbable suture (**Sistrunk procedure**). The wound is irrigated copiously and closed in layers. The wings of the hyoid bone are not reapproximated.

Usual preop diagnosis: Thyroglossal duct cyst

SUMMARY OF PROCEDURE

Position	Supine, with neck in hyperextended position
Incision	Transverse skin incision
Unique considerations	Surgeon may request assistance, by placing finger at base of tongue to identify the cephalad extent of the needed dissection.
Antibiotics	Cefazolin 1 g iv
Surgical time	1-1.5 h
Closing considerations	Careful hemostasis. Coughing may be associated with venous congestion and hematoma formation.
EBL	5-10 ml
Mortality	< 0.1%
Morbidity	Bleeding: < 5%
	Infection: < 5%
Pain score	3-4

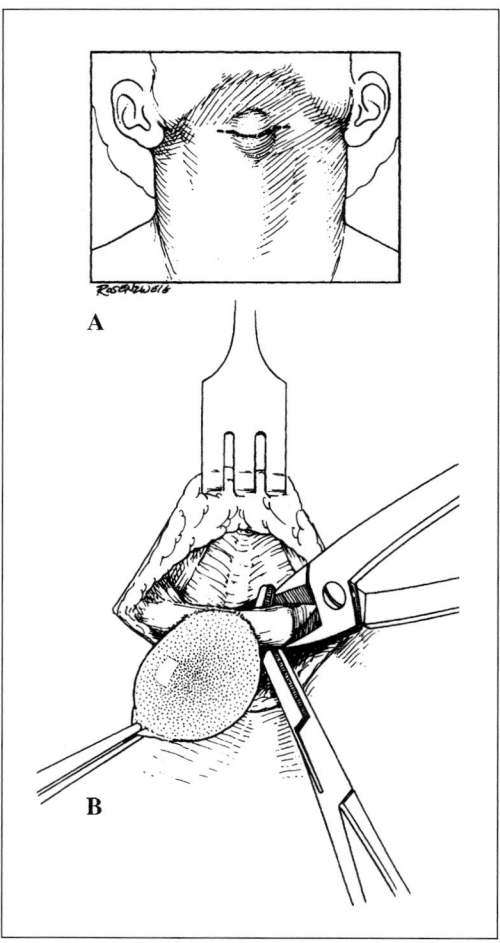

Figure 7. 11-2. Thyroglossal duct cyst excision. (A) Incision placed over presenting cyst; no skin excised. (B) Cyst has been dissected from surrounding tissues, and hyoid is exposed after division of sternohyoid and thyrohyoid muscles at insertion. The bone is encircled with a short right-angle clamp 1 cm from its midpoint, where it is divided with a bone cutter or cautery. (Reproduced with permission from Baker RJ, Fischer JE: *Mastery of Surgery*, 4th edition. Lippincott Williams & Wilkins, 2001.)

PATIENT POPULATION CHARACTERISTICS

Age range	6 mo-30 yr (40% present @ < 10 yr)
Male:Female	1:1
Incidence	~1:3000.
Etiology	Persistence of undifferentiated epithelial cells in area of hyoid bone that later become squamous-cell epithelium or glandular tissue

ANESTHETIC CONSIDERATIONS

See Anesthetic Considerations following Thyroidectomy, p. 523.

Reference

1. Organ GM, Organ CH: Thyroid gland and surgery of the thyroglossal duct: Exercise in applied embryology. *World J Surg* 2000; 24(8):886-90.
2. Waldhausen JHT, Tapper D: Head and neck sinuses and masses. In *Pediatric Surgery*, 3rd edition. Ashcraft KW, et al, eds. WB Saunders, Philadelphia: 2000, 987-99.

THYROIDECTOMY

SURGICAL CONSIDERATIONS

Description: **Thyroidectomy** is performed through a transverse neck incision (Fig 7.11-3) (**Kocher**), usually 6-8 cm long. **Minimally invasive approaches,** including a totally endoscopic approach, have been described, but they remain controversial, as the gland must be removed intact for adequate histological analysis. In the traditional approach, the platysma muscle is divided sharply and subplatysmal flaps are developed superiorly and inferiorly. The two large anterior jugular veins must be avoided and are occasionally a source of blood loss, although rarely of any hemodynamic significance. When the flaps are adequately developed, a large thyroid retractor may be placed to expose the midline prethyroid fascia (median raphe). This is sharply divided in the midline, exposing the strap muscles, which can then be mobilized off the thyroid gland.

Once the thyroid gland is exposed, resection can proceed. Resection may be total, subtotal (lobe + isthmus ± partial remaining lobe), or lobar. Degree of resection depends on diagnosis and may be modified based on operative findings.

During this portion of the operation, hemostasis is critical to maintain adequate visualization. Resection of a lobe usually begins with ligation of the middle thyroid veins along the mid-lateral aspects of the thyroid (Fig 7.11-4). The superior and inferior poles are then mobilized and ligated, with care being taken to identify the superior and inferior parathyroid glands. When the lateral aspects of the thyroid are mobilized, the medial portions may be dissected. Special care must be taken medially along the tracheal-esophageal groove to prevent damage to the recurrent laryngeal nerve, especially in reoperation. As soon as the gland is mobilized to the degree that it is only adherent to the trachea, it may be fully resected, using a knife to prevent cautery injury to the trachea. Any enlarged or suspicious lymph nodes should be excised and sent for pathological examination. After excision, hemostasis is secured. Closure involves the use of absorbable sutures to repair the midline fascia and the platysma. The skin may be closed with running

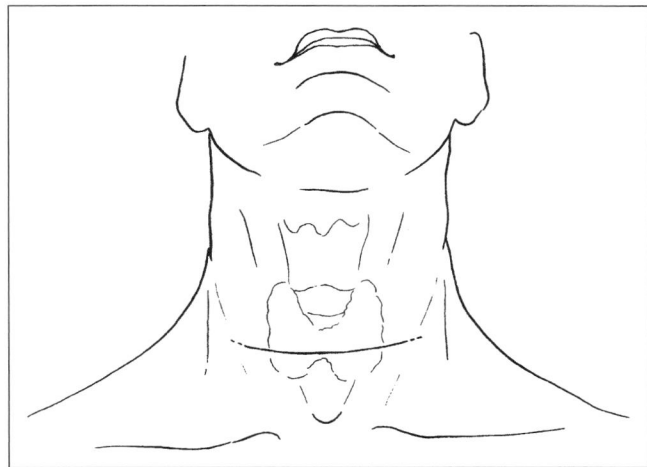

Figure 7.11-3. Transverse incision at base of neck for thyroidectomy. (Reproduced with permission from Baker RJ, Fischer JE: *Mastery of Surgery*, 4th edition. Lippincott Williams & Wilkins, 2001.)

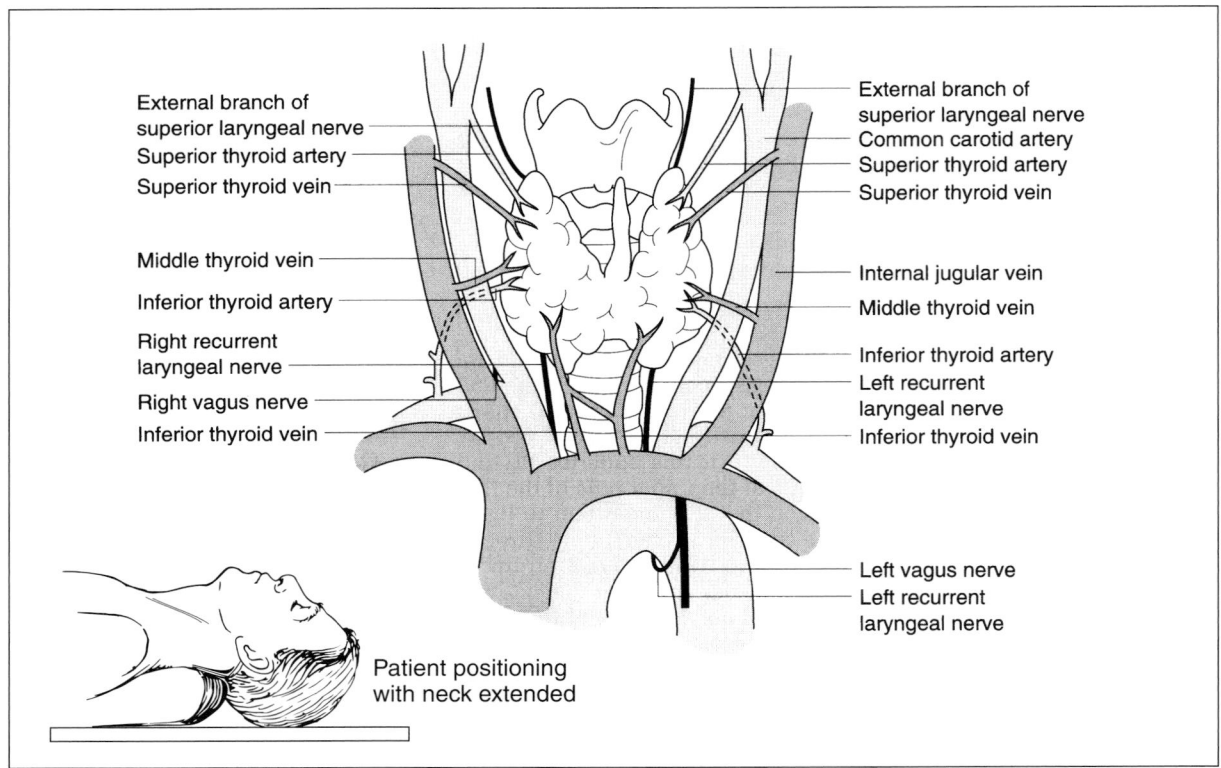

Figure 7.11-4. Vascular relationships to the thyroid gland. (Reproduced with permission from Greenfield LJ, et al: *Surgery: Scientific Principles and Practice* Lippincott Williams & Wilkins, 2001.) Inset shows patient positioning with neck extended.

monofilament suture or staples. The use of drains remains controversial and has not been shown to decrease the rate of hematoma formation.

Usual preop diagnosis: FNA findings of definite/suspicious/inconclusive for malignancy; goiter; thyroid cancer (papillary, follicular, medullary, anaplastic); thyroid nodule; hyperthyroidism; Grave's disease

SUMMARY OF PROCEDURE

Position	Supine with head elevated to 30° and neck extended (Fig 7.11-4, inset)
Incision	Transverse cervical.
Unique considerations	Patients with uncontrolled hyperthyroidism are at ↑risk for developing thyroid storm during surgery. Hyperthyroidism may be controlled preop with either β-adrenergic blockade or propylthiouracil. Preop iatrogenic hypothyroidism may be associated with ↓ BP and circulatory collapse during induction of anesthesia.
Antibiotics	None routinely used**.**
Surgical time	1-2 h
Closing considerations	Adequate hemostasis; minimize coughing
EBL	50-75 ml
Postop care	Observe for postop respiratory problems 2° recurrent laryngeal nerve injury (bilateral), hematoma, or ↓ Ca^{++}. Admit × 24 h. ✓ Ca^{++} the night of surgery and the following a.m. Same-day surgery remains controversial 2° delayed discovery of hematoma (16 h) and hypocalcemia.
Mortality	< 0.5%
Morbidity	Hypoparathyroidism (↓ Ca^{++}): 3-5%
	Hematoma: 1-2%
	Thyroid storm (usually in association with Graves' disease)
	Wound infection: 0.2-0.5%
	Recurrent laryngeal nerve damage
	Unilateral (hoarseness): 0.77%
	Bilateral (aphonia, respiratory obstruction): 0.39%
Pain score	3-4

PATIENT POPULATION CHARACTERISTICS

Age range	15-80 yr
Male: Female	Overall: 1:8
	Cancer: papillary (1:2); follicular (1:3); medullary; anaplastic; lymphoma (1:1)
Incidence	Cancer (Uncommon)
	Benign (Relatively common)
Etiology	Cancer (50%): papillary (80%); follicular (10%); medullary (5%); anaplastic (1%); lymphoma (1%)
	Benign lesions (50%): non-toxic goiter (20%); thyrotoxicosis (10%); thyroiditis (5%); benign nodules (5%); other (10%)
Associated conditions	Other endocrine disorders (e.g., pheochromocytoma in association with medullary thyroid carcinoma in patients with MEN 2A and 2B)

ANESTHETIC CONSIDERATIONS

(Procedures covered: excision of thyroglossal duct cyst; thyroidectomy)

PREOPERATIVE

Hyperthyroidism may be 2° Graves' disease (common), toxic multinodular goiter, thyroid adenomas, TSH-secreting tumor (rare), or overdosage of thyroid hormone. Common Sx are fatigue, sweating, intolerance to heat, ↑appetite, ↑HR, ↑BP, ↑pulse pressure, ↑T, weight loss or gain, thyroid goiter, and exophthalmos. Some older patients exhibit apathetic thyrotoxicosis, which is often mistaken for 'hypo'-thyroidism. CHF and AF are common with these patients. Hypothyroidism may be iatrogenic or 2° autoimmune thyroiditis. Common Sx are intolerance to cold, anorexia, fatigue, weight gain or loss, constipation, ↓HR, ↓pulse pressure, ↓DTR, ↓T, ↓mentation. Patients presenting for thyroidectomy usually are made euthyroid before surgery and may be taking one or more of the following medications: propylthiouracil, methimazole, potassium iodide, glucocorticoids, or β-blockers. An important aspect of the preop visit is to ensure that the patient is in a physiologically euthyroid state (✓ T, HR, pulse pressure, reflexes).

General:

Respiratory   Beware of tracheal compression with large goiters → tracheal deviation, stridor.
Tests: CXR; consider preop CT scan of neck to evaluate possible tracheal involvement, especially in patients with large goiters.

Endocrine	T4	T3ru	T3	TSH
Hyperthyroid	↑	↑	↑	Normal or ↓
1° hypothyroid	↓	↓	↓ or normal	↑
2° hypothyroid	↓	↓	↓	↓

Tests: Thyroid function; Ca⁺⁺; Mg; phosphate; alkaline phosphatase; glucose

Hyperthyroidism:

Respiratory   ↑BMR → ↑VO₂ → rapid desaturation on induction.

Cardiovascular   ↑HR, AF (10-40% incidence), palpitations, CHF. A normal resting HR is helpful in determining whether the patient is ready for surgery. If the situation calls for it (e.g., emergency surgery), the patient can be treated with β-blockers to blunt the sympathomimetic effects of the hyperthyroid state. β-blocker therapy can be problematic in patients with CHF (titrate while monitoring CO).
Tests: ECG; consider ECHO for evaluation of LV function.

Neurological   Warm, moist skin, nervousness, anxiety (may require generous sedation), tremor, ↑reflexes

Musculoskeletal   Higher incidence of myasthenia gravis and skeletal muscle weakness (↑sensitivity to muscle relaxants), clubbing of the fingers, weight loss, myopathy
Tests: CK, urine myoglobin

Hematologic   Mild anemia, thrombocytopenia
Tests: CBC

Gastrointestinal	Weight loss and diarrhea **Tests:** As indicated from H&P.
Laboratory	Other tests as indicated from H&P.
Premedication	Midazolam 0.025-0.05 mg/kg iv. Continue antithyroid medications preop. Hyperthyroid patients must be made euthyroid before elective surgery and may be on the following drugs: propylthiouracil, methimazole, potassium iodide, β-blockers, and glucocorticoids.
Thyroid storm	A life-threatening exacerbation of hyperthyroidism occurring during periods of stress, which is manifested by hyperthermia (> 40°C), tachycardia, anxiety, altered mental state → psychosis → coma, and myopathy (rhabdomyolysis in 50%; severe in 4%). (Thyroid storm has been mistaken intraop for malignant hyperthermia, sepsis, anaphylaxis, and other hypermetabolic reactions.) This is a condition most often associated with Graves' disease that has been incompletely treated prior to surgery. **General Rx:** ↑ FiO_2; fluid resuscitation; electrolyte replacement/correction (↑Ca); cooling blankets; acetaminophen; maintain diuresis if rhabdomyolysis; treat precipitating event (infection, CHF, DKA, pregnancy). **Specific Rx:** propylthiouracil (block synthesis) (200-250 mg po q 4 h); sodium iodide (block release) (1-2.5 g iv); steroids (mechanism unclear)—hydrocortisone (100 mg iv q 8 h), or dexamethasone (4 mg iv q 24 h); β-blockers (use with caution in patients with reactive airway disease, AV block, or CHF)—propranolol (20-120 mg po q h or 0.25-1.0 mg iv q 5 min), and/or esmolol (50-300 μg/kg/min). Note that synthesis should be blocked (1 h is adequate), before giving iodides to block release; otherwise, 'iodine escape' will occur.

Hypothyroidism:

Respiratory	Beware of tracheal compression with large goiters → tracheal deviation, stridor. ↓ventilatory response to ↑CO_2 and ↓O_2 (beware of opioids and sedatives). **Tests:** CXR; consider preop CT scan of neck to evaluate possible tracheal involvement, especially in patients with large goiters.
Cardiovascular	Bradydysrythmias, diastolic HTN, pericardial effusions, ECG → ↓voltage, ST-T wave Δs, ↑QT, occasional VT (torsades de pointe—pause-dependent). This type of VT is treated with $MgSO_4$, cardioversion; then isuprel or pacing to shorten QT. Thyroid replacement must be weighed against the risk of precipitating myocardial ischemia in patients with known CAD. Diastolic dysfunction, ↓LV compliance → sensitivity to fluid overload. **Tests:** ECG; consider ECHO for evaluation of LV systolic/diastolic function, pericardial effusion/tamponade.
Endocrine	Addison's disease occurs in 5-10% of patients with severe hypothyroidism; some patients may receive a 'stress dose' of steroids (hydrocortisone 100 mg iv q 8 h × 3) in the periop period. **Tests:** Cortisol stim test
Neurological	↓BMR → slow mentation and movement, cold intolerance, ↓reflexes with 'hangup'
Musculoskeletal	Arthralgias and myalgias
Renal	Impaired renal function 2° amyloidosis, urinary retention, oliguria **Tests:** Consider BUN; Cr; Na^+ (50% incidence of ↓Na^+)
Hematologic	Coagulation abnormalities, anemia **Tests:** CBC
Gastrointestinal	GI bleeding, constipation, ileus **Tests:** As indicated from H&P.
Laboratory	Other tests as indicated from H&P.
Premedication	Midazolam 0.025-0.05 mg/kg iv. (None in the patient who is clinically hypothyroid and requires emergent surgery.) Hypothyroid patients can undergo surgery if they have mild-to-moderate disease. Clinically hypothyroid patients (↓HR, ↓T, ↓pulse pressure, ↓DTRs) should be given thyroid replacement before elective surgery.
Myxedema coma	Severe hypothyroidism constituting a medical emergency, with mortality of > 50%. Manifestations include stupor or coma; hypothermia (24-32°C), which correlates inversely with mortality; hypoventilation with hypoxemia; bradycardia; hypotension; apathy; hoarseness; and hyponatremia. **Supportive measures:** early intubation and mechanical ventilation; treat ↓BP with cautious volume expansion (pulmonary edema), inotropes (arrhythmias), pacing (carefully, 60-70 b/min) and r/o pericardial effusion; passive rewarming only, especially if ↓BP (active warming for T < 30°C);

Myxedema coma, cont.	correct ↓ Na carefully; correct ↓ glucose. **Specific Rx:** L-thyroxine (T_4) (400-500 μg iv loading dose, 50-200 μg iv q d maintenance dose); or tri-iodothyronine (T_3) (12.5 μg iv q 6-12 h); hydrocortisone (100-300 mg iv q d). T_4 onset is slow (6 h after iv administration) and has to be converted peripherally (slowed in hypothyroid state) to biologically active T_3. Also, T_4 may be converted in some critically ill patients to biologically inactive rT_3. ↓TSH level is the earliest sign of response.

INTRAOPERATIVE

Anesthetic technique: Normally, GETA; infrequently, under local anesthesia. For inadequately treated hyperthyroid patients, it is important to establish an adequate depth of anesthesia to prevent an exaggerated sympathetic response to surgical stimulation. Avoid agents that stimulate the sympathetic nervous system (e.g., ketamine, pancuronium, meperidine). Hypothyroidism may be associated with ↑sensitivity to anesthetic agents and muscle relaxants.

Induction	Standard induction for euthyroid patients (p. B-2). If the patient has airway compromise 2° a large thyroid goiter, consider an awake fiber optic intubation (p. B-6).	
Maintenance	Standard maintenance (p. B-3). Maintain muscle relaxation.	
Emergence	Airway obstruction 2° recurrent laryngeal nerve damage, tracheomalacia, or hematoma can occur. Consider visualizing vocal cord function before extubation.	
Blood and fluid requirements	Minimal blood loss IV: 18 ga × 1 NS/LR @ 5-8 ml/kg/h Head-up position	Slight head-up position can help make for a bloodless surgical field without substantially increasing the risk of VAE.
Monitoring	Standard monitors (see p. B-1).	+ others as indicated by patient's status. Maintain temperature, especially in hypothyroid patients.
Positioning	✓ and pad pressure points. ✓ eyes.	Supine, with head slightly hyperextended, allows for surgical exploration of the neck.
Complications	Cardiorespiratory depression	In hypothyroid patients, marked ↓BP and ↓RR may occur with minimal anesthetic doses.

POSTOPERATIVE

Complications	Recurrent laryngeal nerve damage	Bilateral: patient will be unable to speak and will require reintubation. Unilateral: characterized by hoarseness.
	Tracheomalacia or hematoma with airway compromise	Acute airway obstruction may occur immediately postop, and rapid reintubation may be life-saving. If airway compromise is 2° hematoma, reopen incision and drain remaining blood; if patient still requires artificial airway, consider CPAP or awake reintubation.
	Acute hypoparathyroid state (hypocalcemia)	Acute hypocalcemia can present as laryngeal stridor (24-48 h postop), although it most often presents with tingling in the fingertips and in the lips. If untreated and severe, this can progress to tetany and seizures. Administering 1 amp Ca^{++} gluconate given iv over 20 min usually alleviates symptoms. Rx: measure Ca^{++}; replace if necessary. CPAP is effective for airway compromise.
	Thyroid storm	Can mimic MH (see Rx above).
Pain management	PCA morphine (see p. C-3).	
Tests	Vocal cord function	Ability to phonate 'e' implies continued vocal cord function.

References

1. Abbas G, Dubner S, Heller KS: Re-operation for bleeding after thyroidectomy and parathyroidectomy. *Head Neck* 2001; 23(7):544-6.
2. Bergamaschi R, Becouarn G, Ronceray J, Arnaud JP: Morbidity of thyroid surgery. *Am J Surg* 1998; 176(1):71-5.
3. Bhattacharyya N, Fried MP: Assessment of the morbidity and complications of total thyroidectomy. *Arch Otolaryngol Head Neck Surg* 2002; 128(4):389-92.
4. Efron, G: Thyroid cancer. In *Current Surgical Therapy*, 7th edition. Cameron JL, ed. Mosby Inc, St. Louis: 2001, 645-52.

5. Farling PA: Thyroid disease. *Br J Anaesth* 2000; 85:15-28.
6. Gaz, RD: Hyperthyroidism. In *Current Surgical Therapy*, 7th edition. Cameron JL, ed. Mosby Inc, St. Louis: 2001, 653-7.
7. Miccoli P: Minimally invasive surgery for thyroid and parathyroid diseases. *Surg Endosc* 2002; 16(1):3-6.
8. Ober KP: Endocrine emergencies. *Med Clin North Am* 1995; 79, No. 1.
9. Schwartz JJ, Rosenbaum SH, Graf GJ: Anesthesia and the endocrine system. In *Clinical Anesthesia*, 4th edition. Barash PG, Cullen BF, Stoelting RK, eds. Lippincott Williams & Wilkins, Philadelphia: 2001, 1119-39.
10. Udelsman R: Thyroid gland. In *Surgery: Scientific Principles and Practice*, 3rd edition. Greenfield LJ, et al, eds. Lippincott Williams & Wilkins, 2001, 1261-84.
11. Zeiger, MA: Nontoxic goiter. In *Current Surgical Therapy*, 7th edition. Cameron JL, eds. Mosby Inc, St. Louis: 2001, 642-4.

PARATHYROIDECTOMY

SURGICAL CONSIDERATIONS

Description: The traditional approach for primary hyperparathyroidism requires **four-gland visualization** with removal of any abnormally large glands. Newer methods of localization and confirmation of adenomas have ushered in an era of minimally invasive parathyroid surgery, using either a **minimally invasive approach,** with a small skin incision and focused operative dissection, or an **endoscopic technique,** with trocar ports and CO_2 insufflation.

For the standard open operation, an incision in the lower neck (Fig 7.11-5) is made and the platysma is divided. Flaps are created below the platysma superiorly and inferiorly to allow increased working space and expose the prethyroid fascia.

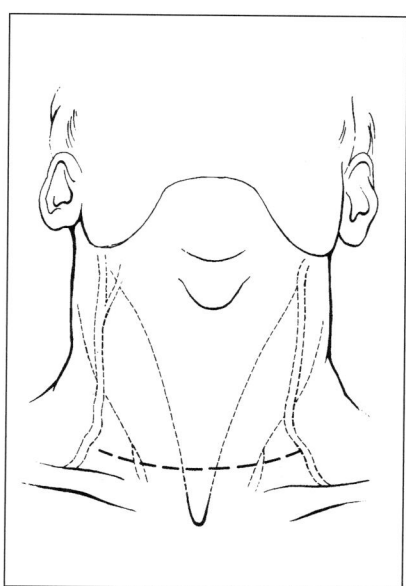

Figure 7.11-5. Skin incision for parathyroid exploration, made 1-2 finger-breadths superior to sternal notch, as far lateral as the external jugular veins on both sides. (Reproduced with permission from Baker RJ, Fischer JE: *Mastery of Surgery*, 4th edition. Lippincott Williams & Wilkins, 2001.)

The midline between the strap muscles is identified and divided, exposing the thyroid gland. The superior parathyroids are located behind the upper pole, in association with the superior thyroid artery, which often must be taken to locate the parathyroid. The inferior glands are located near the junction of the inferior thyroid artery and the recurrent laryngeal nerve (Fig 7.11-6). Hemostasis is crucial to maintain adequate visualization in the surgical field. For the traditional approach, all four glands are located, and biopsies are sent for confirmation of parathyroid tissue. Abnormal glands are removed. If four-gland hyperplasia is found (multiple endocrine neoplasia [MEN] 1 or 2A [secondary or tertiary hyperparathyroidism], then all four glands are removed and some tissue is saved for reimplantation in the forearm.

With preop localization studies, dissection may be limited to the area of suspicion, and the abnormal gland or glands removed. Confirmation of successful resection may be made by observing a 50% decrease in the parathormone level, 5 min after removal, as compared with the preop level. This very sensitive assay is rapidly becoming the standard of care in the treatment of primary hyperparathyroidism. The addition of preop methylene blue or radioactive tracers may lend additional assurances that the parathyroid tissue has been identified. If the parathyroid adenoma cannot be found, the surgeon should investigate other areas of the neck, including the retroesophageal space, carotid sheath, posterior triangle, and below the thyroid. Unilateral thyroid lobectomy may be performed when three normal glands have been found and the fourth gland is missing, as the adenoma may be in the thyroid substance. Mediastinal exploration should not be done on primary exploration.

Variant procedure or approaches: Initial studies of the endoscopic approach have suggested morbidity and rates of cure similiar to those of standard

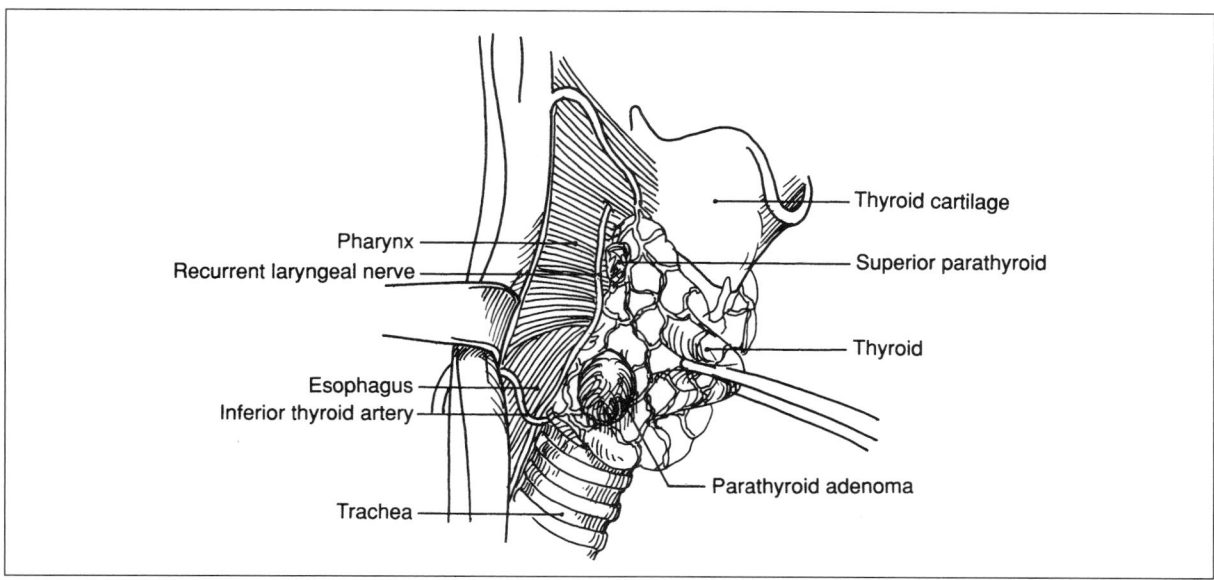

Figure 7.11-6. Identification of upper parathyroid gland on right side. (Reproduced with permission from Scott-Conner CEH, Dawson DL: *Operative Anatomy*, 2nd edition. Lippincott Williams & Wilkins, 2003).

procedures, with better cosmetic results. Larger series of randomized trials need to be completed before this approach can be applied broadly.

Usual preop diagnosis: Parathyroid adenoma (multiple in 2-3% of cases); hyperparathyroidism (secondary or tertiary); parathyroid carcinoma

SUMMARY OF PROCEDURE

Position	Supine; shoulder roll; reverse Trendelenberg or 30° tilt; head rest (gel donut)
Incision	Transverse cervical (4-8 cm) (Fig 7.11-5)
Unique considerations	Methylene blue (7.5 mg/kg in 500 mL of NS) may be administered in the preop holding area 30 min before surgery → spurious $\downarrow$SpO$_2$. Radioactive technetium sestimibi (20mCi) may be administered 60-90 min before operation. Methylene blue and radioactive tracers may be used independently or simultaneously to aid in identification of parathyroid tissue.
Antibiotics	Cefotetan 1 g iv preop
Surgical time	1-2 h
Closing considerations	Coughing may be associated with venous congestion and hematoma formation.
EBL	25-50 ml
Postop care	Monitor serum Ca^{++} (nl = 8.5-10.5 mg% total Ca; 1-1.3 mM ionized Ca^{++}). Patients typically admitted for 24 h observation to ✓ serum Ca^{++} levels and monitor for hematoma/airway compromise.
Mortality	< 0.5%
Morbidity	Hypocalcemia: < 15%
	Hypoparathyroidism: < 5%
	Hematoma: 1%
	Infection: 1%
	Recurrent laryngeal paralysis: < 1%
Pain score	3-4

PATIENT POPULATION CHARACTERISTICS

Age range	Increases with age
Male:Female	4:1
Incidence	50-100/100,000 (1.5/100 in elderly)
Etiology	Single adenoma (85%); double adenoma (2-3%); hyperplasia (10-15%); cancer (< 1%)
Associated conditions	Bone disease (5-15%); duodenal ulcer (5-10%); renal calculi (60-70%); MEN-1 (parathyroid + hyperplasia + pituitary adenoma + pancreatic neuroendocrine tumor); MEN-2A (parathyroid hyperplasia + medullary thyroid cancer + pheochromocytoma); HTN (20-50%)

ANESTHETIC CONSIDERATIONS

PREOPERATIVE

These patients typically present with hypercalcemia (hyperparathyroidism), which must be controlled before surgery. Although 25-50% of cases are asymptomatic, many will present with a variety of Sx, including fatigue, muscle weakness, depression, anorexia, nausea, constipation, abdominal and bone pain, HTN, renal stones, and polydipsia. Differential diagnosis for the hypercalcemic patient includes: metastatic disease, multiple myeloma, milk-alkali syndrome, vitamin D intoxication, sarcoidosis, hyperthyroidism, thiazide diuretics, adrenal insufficiency, Paget's disease, immobilization, or an exogenous parathyroid hormone-producing tumor.

Respiratory	Hyperparathyroidism is associated with ↓clearance of secretions from the tracheobronchial tree → postop atelectasis. Avoid respiratory or metabolic acidosis, which will ↑ the free fraction of Ca → hypercalcemia (↑BP, ↑muscle weakness, ↑HR). **Tests:** As indicated from H&P.
Cardiovascular	HTN (usually resolves with treatment; if severe, r/o pheochromocytoma); ECG may show tachycardia with ↓PR and ↓QT intervals. Patients may be hypovolemic (2° anorexia, N/V, and polyuria) and have ↑sensitivity to digitalis, resistance to catecholamines. **Preop management** includes correction of intravascular volume and electrolyte abnormalities. Preop treatment of hypercalcemia includes aggressive expansion of intravascular volume, followed by diuresis, to ↑ renal Ca^{++} excretion, usually accomplished with iv NS, and then furosemide. Calcium channel blockers (verapamil, nifedipine, diltiazem) can be used. Hypophosphatemia can impair myocardial contractility and should be corrected; hemodialysis or peritoneal dialysis can be used to lower dangerously elevated serum Ca^{++} levels. Mithramycin, plicamycin, calcitonin, bisphosphonates, cisplatin, or steroids are not useful for acute Rx of ↑Ca^{++} (too slow). ↓BP may result from polyuria → hypovolemia. **Tests:** ECG; electrolytes; others as indicated from H&P.
Neurological	Patient may present with Sz, hyporeflexia, mental status changes (somnolence, depression, memory loss, psychosis, coma), or peripheral neuropathy. Significant improvement may follow correction of hypercalcemia.
Musculoskeletal	These patients may have muscle atrophy and weakness, osteopenia, arthralgia, pathologic fractures (careful laryngoscopy and positioning), osteitis fibrosa cystica. Response to NMBs may be enhanced 2° ↑Ca^{++} → muscle weakness.
Hematologic	Patients also tend to be hypophosphatemic and may show Sx of hemolysis, Plt dysfunction, impaired ventricular contractility, and leukocyte dysfunction. **Tests:** CBC with Plt count, PO_4
Endocrine	Primary hyperparathyroidism is most commonly due to benign parathyroid adenoma (90%), or hyperplasia (9%) and rarely to carcinoma. It may be associated with MEN syndrome. MEN-1 consists of tumors of the parathyroid, pancreatic islets, and pituitary. MEN-2 consists of pheochromocytoma, ★ mucosal neuromas, parathyroid tumors, and medullary thyroid carcinoma. **NB: Anesthetizing a patient with an unrecognized pheochromocytoma could result in a fatality.** **Tests:** As indicated from H&P.
Renal	Patients may have renal dysfunction 2° nephrolithiasis, nephrocalcinosis, renal tubular disorders, and glomerular disorders. Polyuria 2° ↑Ca^{++} → electrolyte disturbances. **Tests:** Cr; BUN; electrolytes
Gastrointestinal	These patients may have constipation, anorexia, N/V, epigastric pain.
Laboratory	Serum Ca^{++} < 12 mg/dL, likely asymptomatic, but depends on rate of change; 12-14 mg/dL, mild symptoms; >16 mg/dL, life-threatening). Albumin (↑albumin by 1 g/dL will ↑total serum Ca^{++} by 0.8 mg/dL); electrolytes; Mg; phosphate (usually low).
Premedication	All medications to lower hypercalcemia should be continued unless Ca^{++} levels have normalized. If patient has been treated with steroids in the preop period, administer a stress dose (hydrocortisone 100 mg iv q 8 h × 24 h) before induction of anesthesia and continue into the early postop period. Standard premedications (p. B-2) are usually appropriate in this patient group, unless patient has mental status changes.

INTRAOPERATIVE

Anesthetic technique: GETA, with head slightly hyperextended, allows for surgical exploration of the neck. Cervical plexus blocks may be appropriate in selected patients; however, phrenic nerve block → respiratory compromise.

Induction	Standard induction (p. B-2). If patient is clinically hypovolemic, restore intravascular volume before induction and titrate induction dose of sedative/hypnotic agents.	
Maintenance	Standard maintenance (p. B-3), with muscle relaxant titrated to effect, using peripheral nerve stimulator. Avoid hyperventilation or hypoventilation (acidosis will ↑Ca^{++} levels, while alkalosis will ↓ Ca^{++} levels). Maintain adequate hydration and UO throughout the procedure.	
Emergence	No special considerations (see postop complications, below).	
Blood and fluid requirements	Minimal blood loss IV: 18 ga × 1 NS @ 5-8 ml/kg/h	Avoid Ca^{++}-containing iv solution (e.g., LR).
Monitoring	Standard monitors (p. B-1)	Others as indicated by patient status.
Positioning	✓ and pad all pressure points. ✓ eyes.	Patients should be positioned carefully as they tend to be osteopenic and are prone to pathologic bone fractures. Slight head-up position may ↓ blood loss and improve surgical visibility without significantly ↑ risk of VAE.
Complications	Hypocalcemia	See postop complications (below).

POSTOPERATIVE

Complications	Hypocalcemia
	  Hypocalcemic tetany
	  Sz
	  Laryngospasm
	  Hypophosphatemia
		Hypocalcemia may occur in the immediate postop period. Sx include parathesias, muscle spasm, tetany, laryngospasm, bronchospasm, and apnea. Rx: includes 10-20 ml Ca^{++} gluconate 10% over 10 min. Follow levels and repeat therapy until the clinical signs of hypocalcemia are controlled. CPAP is effective for airway obstruction.

	Recurrent laryngeal nerve injury Laryngeal edema 2° surgical trauma Stridor Hematoma with airway compromise	Recurrent laryngeal nerve dysfunction can be monitored by having the patient vocalize the letter 'e.' Unilateral vocal cord dysfunction results in hoarseness, while bilateral vocal cord dysfunction results in aphonia. CPAP is effective for airway obstruction.
	Pneumothorax	Dx: pleuritic chest pain, dyspnea, ↑RR, ↓breath sounds, ↑resonance, hypoxemia; ✓ CXR. Rx: O_2; chest tube and reintubation as necessary.
Pain management	PCA (p. C-3)	

Tests	Serial measurements of:
	  Ca^{++}
	  Phosphate
	  Mg
	  Others as clinically indicated
	CXR to rule out pneumothorax
		The lowest Ca^{++} level usually is seen after 4-5 d postop. Follow clinical Sx of hypocalcemia: Trousseau's sign (carpopedal spasm in response to application of a BP cuff at a pressure > SBP for 3 min); Chvostek's sign (contracture of the facial muscles produced by tapping on the facial nerve).

References

1. Abbas G, Dubner S, Heller KS: Re-operation for bleeding after thyroidectomy and parathyroidectomy. *Head Neck* 2001; 23(7):544-6.
2. Flynn MB, Bumpous JM, Schill K, McMasters KM: Minimally invasive radioguided parathyroidectomy. *J Am Coll Surg* 2000; 191(1):24-31
3. Gauger PG and Thompson NW: Persistent or recurrent hyperparathyroidism. In *Current Surgical Therapy*, 7th edition. Cameron JL, eds. Mosby Inc, St. Louis, 2001, 668-71.
4. Kessler MR, Eide T, Humayun B, Poppers PJ: Spurious pulse oximeter desaturation with methylene blue injection. *Anesthesiology* 1986; 65(4):435-6.
5. Miccoli P: Minimally invasive surgery for thyroid and parathyroid diseases. *Surg Endosc* 2002; 16(1):3-6.

6. Mihai R, Farndon JR: Parathyroid disease and calcium metabolism *Br J Anaesth* 2000; 85:29-43.

7. Schwartz JJ, Rosenbaum SH, Graf GJ: Anesthesia and the endocrine system. In *Clinical Anesthesia*, 4th edition. Barash PG, Cullen BF, Stoelting RK, eds. Lippincott Williams & Wilkins, Philadelphia: 2001, 1119-39.

8. Udelsman, R: Primary hyperparathyroidism. In *Current Surgical Therapy*, 7th edition. Cameron JL, eds. Mosby Inc, St. Louis: 2001, 662-7.

ADRENALECTOMY

SURGICAL CONSIDERATIONS

Description: Adrenalectomy can be performed via a number of different approaches, each with its own merits. Traditionally, the adrenal glands have been removed with an open incision through either the transperitoneal or extraperitoneal (flank) approach (Fig 7.11-8). With some exceptions (see below), laparoscopic approaches are becoming the favored methods. Indication in malignant disease or metastasis remains controversial and is currently being evaluated. Relative contraindications include large adrenal adenocarcinomas (> 5 cm), malignant pheochromocytoma, invasive adrenal mass, large adrenal mass (> 8-10 cm), or other contraindications to abdominal laparoscopic surgery (e. g., multiple previous abdominal surgeries). Each approach is discussed individually, but their basic principles remain the same. The anatomy of the retroperitoneum is shown in Fig 7.11-7.

Open transperitoneal approach: This approach allows for easy access to both adrenals and is preferred for large tumors. A midline or bilateral subcostal incision (Fig 7.11-8) is used, with the patient in the supine position. The left adrenal is accessed by incising the lateral peritoneal attachments of the spleen The spleen and tail of the pancreas are rotated medially, exposing Gerota's fascia, which is then incised at the upper pole of the kidney, exposing the adrenal gland. A combination of blunt and sharp dissection is used to mobilize the gland and expose the adrenal vein, which is ligated between ties, and the gland is removed. The right gland is exposed by retracting the liver cephalad and depressing the hepatic flexure inferiorly. The peritoneum is then incised lateral to the duodenum and the inferior vena cava (IVC) is exposed. The right kidney is pulled down and the right adrenal vein entering the IVC is identified. The adrenal vein is ligated and the gland is removed.

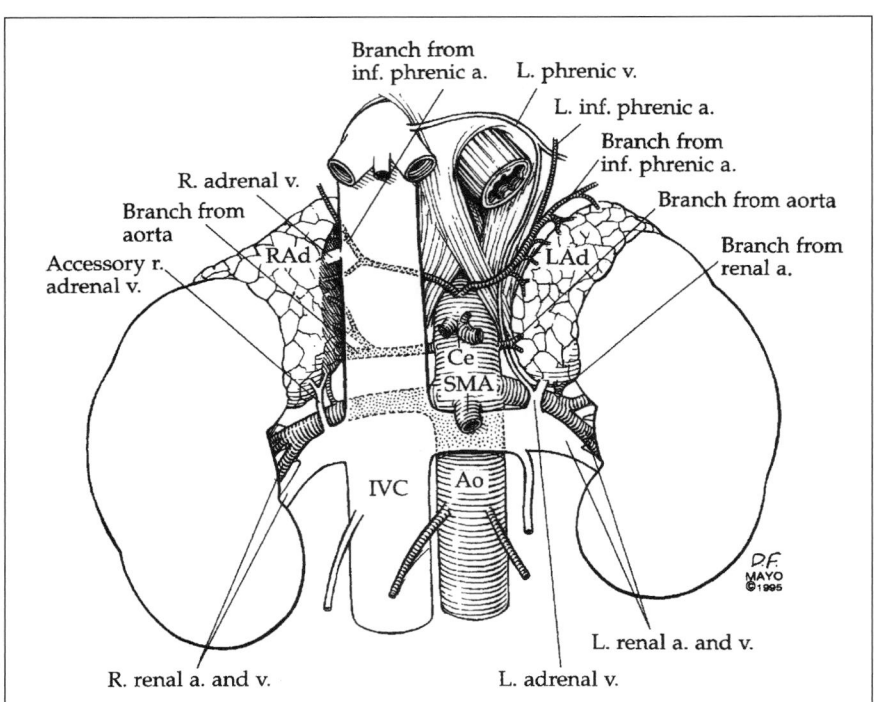

Figure 7.11-7. Anatomic relationships of the adrenal glands. Note the origins of the three main arteries: inferior phrenic, aortic, and renal branches. Note also the single draining veins (except for a small accessory right adrenal vein): the right-located superior and medial, and the left-found inferior and medial. (Ao=aorta; Ce=celiac; LAd=left adrenal gland; RAd=right adrenal gland). (Reproduced with permission from Baker RJ, Fischer JE: *Mastery of Surgery*, 4th edition. Lippincott Williams & Wilkins, 2001.)

Open extraperitoneal approach (flank): Before the advent of laparoscopic surgery, this approach was favored to minimize pain and improve postop recovery of adrenalectomy through use of smaller incision size and by remaining extraperitoneal. In general, this approach is best used for unilateral, smaller tumors. The patient is placed in the prone jackknife position and a dorsal curved flank incision is made, exposing the 12th rib. The rib is resected and Gerota's fascia is identified and incised, and the adrenal gland is resected.

Laparoscopic anterior transperitoneal approach: This approach may be used for bilateral adrenalectomy with the patient in the supine position. The surgical plan is similar to that of the transabdominal open approach, but is associated with longer operating times and additional trocar sites for placement of more retractors to mobilize the intraabdominal organs.

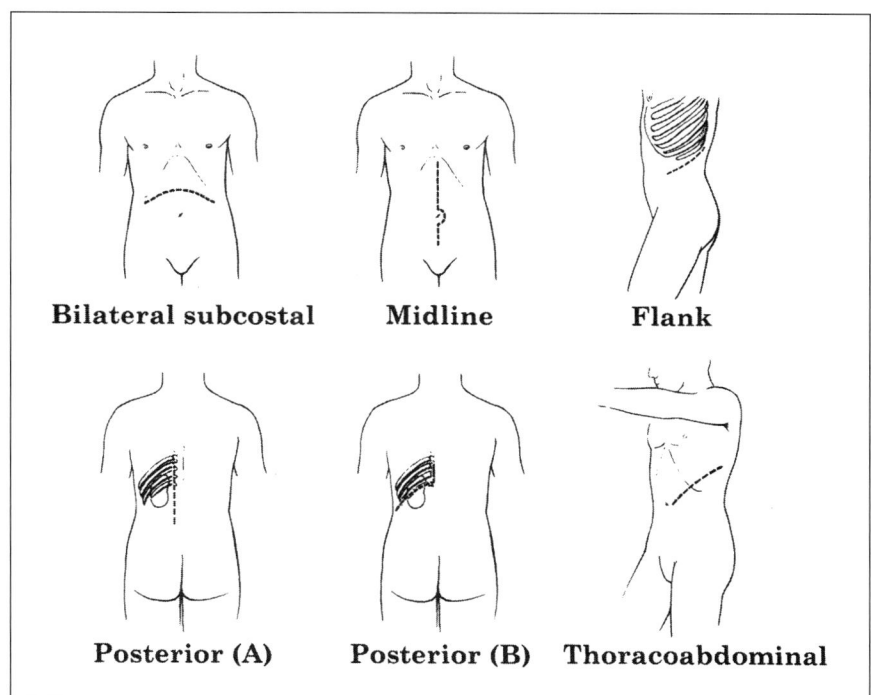

Bilateral subcostal   Midline   Flank

Posterior (A)   Posterior (B)   Thoracoabdominal

Figure 7.11-8. Potential incisions for adrenalectomy. (Reproduced with permission from Baker RJ, Fischer JE: *Mastery of Surgery*, 4th edition. Lippincott Williams & Wilkins, 2001.)

Laparoscopic lateral transperitoneal approach: This is the preferred approach for adrenalectomy in most centers. The patient is positioned in the lateral decubitus position with the operative site up, and is immobilized with a carefully placed beanbag to minimize nerve compression injuries. The patient is prepped for either an open or laparoscopic approach (so that conversion to an open procedure may be done swiftly, if necessary). If both adrenal glands are to be removed, the right is done first, as there is a slightly higher risk of converting to an open procedure because of the proximity of the adrenal vein to the IVC.

For **right adrenalectomy**, pneumoperitoneum (15 mmHg) is established, with a Veress needle placed in the midclavicular line below the right costal margin. A 5 mm liver retractor is placed, as are two operating trocar sites (usually a 5 mm and a 10 mm or 12 mm port) (Fig 7.11-9). The liver is retracted cephalad and the retroperitoneum incised with hook cautery. The right renal vein is dissected out carefully and ligated with clips. Dissection of the gland then proceeds from medial to lateral and inferior to superior. The gland is removed through a laparoscopic retrieval bag.

The **left adrenal gland** is approached in a similar fashion, with the Veress needle being placed in the left midclavicular line just below the costal margin. After placement of additional trocars, the peritoneum lateral to the spleen and the splenorenal ligament are incised. With the patient in the decubitis position, gravity will help pull the spleen medially, exposing the anterior surface of the kidney (Fig 7.11-10). The inferior and medial edges of the gland are dissected first, and the left adrenal vein is identified. Once the vein is clipped, the remainder of the gland may be dissected free and the gland removed as above.

Usual preop diagnosis: Hyperaldosteronism; hypercortisolism; pheochromocytoma; metastatic tumor; metastasis; lymphoma; angiomyolipoma; adrenal adenoma; adenocarcinoma

SUMMARY OF PROCEDURES

	Open Adrenalectomy	Laparoscopic Adrenalectomy
Position	Transperitoneal–supine; extraperitoneal–prone jackknife	Transperitoneal anterior–supine; transperitoneal lateral—decubitus
Incision	Transperitoneal–midline or bilateral subcostal (Fig 7.11-8); extraperitoneal–dorsal flank oblique or curved posterior	Transperitoneal anterior–4-5 trocar incisions (Fig 7.11-9); transperitoneal lateral–3-4 trocar incisions
Special instrumentation	Transperitoneal–Denier or Bookwalter retractor; extraperitoneal–none	Transabdominal anterior/lateral–video set-up

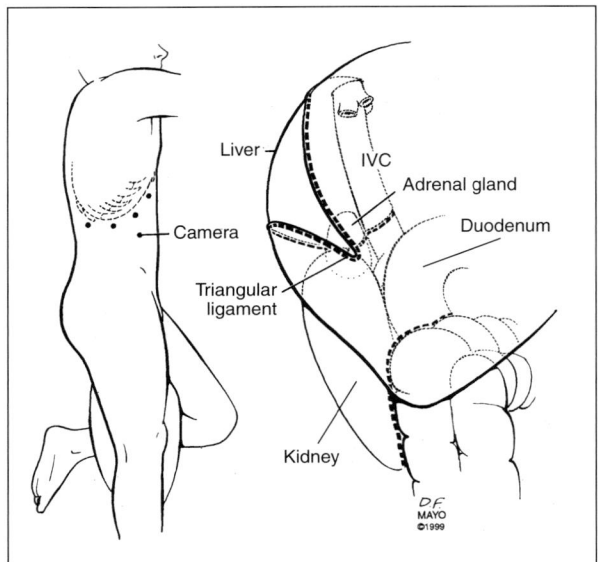

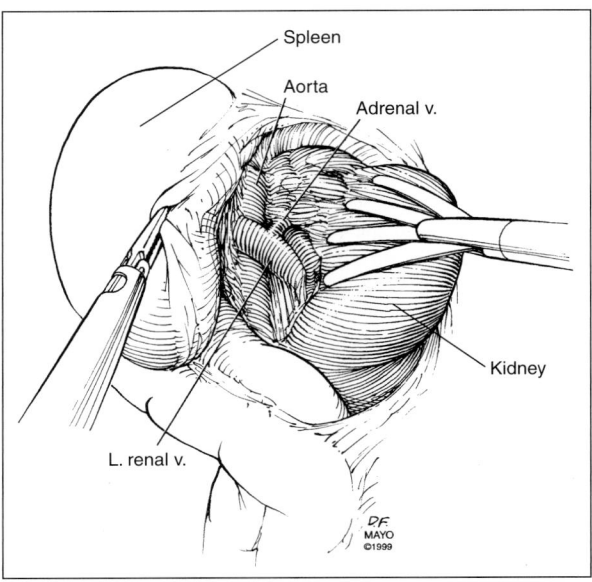

Figure 7.11-9. Port placement for laparoscopic right adrenalec- tomy. Relevant anatomy is displayed through the right lobe of the liver. (Reproduced with permission from Baker RJ, Fischer JE: *Mastery of Surgery*, 4th edition. Lippincott Williams & Wilkins, 2001.)

Figure 7.11-10. Exposure of left adrenal after mobilization of the spleen. (Reproduced with permission from Baker RJ, Fischer JE: *Mastery of Surgery*, 4th edition. Lippincott Williams & Wilkins, 2001.)

	Open Adrenalectomy	**Laparoscopic Adrenalectomy**
Unique considerations	BP monitoring essential for pheochromocytoma patients	⇐
Antibiotics	None	⇐
Surgical time	1-2 h	1-3 h
Closing considerations	Hemostasis; hemodynamic stability	⇐
EBL	100-250 ml	⇐
Postop care	Continue monitoring BP; PACU → room; ± ICU, based on hemodynamic stability	⇐
Mortality	< 0.5%	⇐
Morbidity	Overall: 1-12%	⇐
	Bleeding: < 10%	⇐
	Pancreatic fistula: < 1%	⇐
	DVT: 0.8%	⇐
	PE: 0.5%	⇐
	Renovascular HTN: < 1%	⇐
	Peroneal nerve palsy:< 1%	⇐
	Venous thrombosis with embolism (Cushing's): 2%	⇐
Pain score	6-8	5-6

PATIENT POPULATION CHARACTERISTICS

Age range	13-75 yr
Male:Female	1:2.8
Incidence	Pheochromocytoma: 0.4-2% of all hypertensive patients
	Primary hyperaldosteronism: ~4% of all hypertensive patients
	Cushing's syndrome: 6/1 million
Etiology	Adenoma or adenocarcinoma (90%); ectopic ACTH (15% of patients with Cushing's); Cushing's syndrome (hyperadrenocorticism) (10-15%); Conn's syndrome (hyperaldosteronism). Idiopathic hyperplasia is usually treated medically.
Associated conditions	HTN (75-80%); diabetes mellitus (10-15%)

ANESTHETIC CONSIDERATIONS
PREOPERATIVE

Cushing's syndrome: Hyperadrenocorticism can be due to adrenal hyperplasia, adrenal carcinoma, pituitary hypersecretion (Cushing's disease), hypersecretion from exogenous tumor, or exogenous steroid administration (most common). Adrenalectomy is the traditional treatment for hyperadrenocorticism 2° adrenal carcinoma. These typically moon-faced patients present with one or more of the following: HTN 2° glucocorticoids, renin (usually not severe); renal calculi; osteoporosis; glucose intolerance; personality changes; and myopathy. In addition, a fragile vasculature predisposes these patients to easy bruising and difficult vascular access.

Pheochromocytoma: Tumors of chromaffin tissue origin release massive amounts of catecholamines (norepinephrine > epinephrine) and are responsible for the patient's clinical presentation. The tumor usually is found unilaterally in one of the adrenal glands, but also can be found anywhere in the body that chromaffin tissue arises (e.g., urinary bladder, sympathetic chain). These patients require extensive preop preparation, consisting of α-blockade (phenoxybenzamine 40-400 mg/d × 1-2 wk) and concomitant volume expansion. Patients with tachydysrhythmias may require β-blockade only after institution of the α-blockers to prevent serious hypertensive sequelae. Adrenergic blockade and volume expansion may take up to 2 wk prior to surgical removal of the tumor. Inadequate preop preparation will increase the periop morbidity of patients with pheochromocytomas. The adequacy of medical therapy is assessed by the absence of symptoms of catecholamine excess, BP of ≤ 160/90 on 2 measurements in the 36 h preceding surgery, SBP dropping ≥ 15% on standing, but not less than an absolute BP of 80/45; no ST-T wave changes for 2 wk prior to surgery. There is an increased incidence of pheochromocytoma in certain diseases (e.g., multiple-endocrine neoplasia II, neurofibromatosis, tuberous sclerosis, Sturge-Weber syndrome, von Hippel-Lindau disease).

Conn's syndrome: Hyperaldosteronism can be primary (Conn's syndrome–adrenal adenoma or hyperplasia) or secondary (caused by excess renin secretion related to renal dysfunction). These patients are typically hypokalemic and alkalotic → muscle weakness, parathesias, tetany, and polyuria. They may also be hypervolemic (→ CHF), hypernatremic, and hypertensive (diastolic).

Respiratory	Cushing's syndrome: patient may be obese, with all attendant problems (see Preoperative Considerations in Operations for Morbid Obesity, p. 401). Conn's syndrome: respiratory muscle weakness **Tests:** As indicated from H&P.
Cardiovascular	Cushing's syndrome: HTN, hypervolemia, dysrhythmias 2° hypokalemia Pheochromocytoma: paroxysmal HTN, tachydysrhythmias, orthostatic hypotension, hypovolemia, myocardial dysfunction, cardiomyopathy, ventricular ectopy, ↓intravascular volume, ↓sensitivity of α-receptors to normal levels of catecholamines, CHF Conn's syndrome: HTN, dysrhythmias, ↓T wave, + U wave **Tests:** ECG; orthostatic VS; consider ECHO or MUGA scan to evaluate LV function, if indicated from H&P.
Renal	Cushing's syndrome: excess steroid production → Na^+ retention, K^+ excretion, and glucose intolerance (hyperglycemia). Conn's syndrome: renal HTN, polyuria, polydipsia, ↓K^+, ↑Na^+. Correction of hypokalemia requires > 24 h supplemental K^+ infusion (e.g., 5-20 mEq/h). Pheochromocytoma: HTN from excess catecholamine state may damage kidneys; hyperglycemia. **Tests:** UA; creatinine; glucose; urine concentrations of catecholamine metabolites; others as appropriate
Neurological	Cushing's syndrome: psychiatric changes, HA Pheochromocytoma: tremulousness, HA, anxiety, nervousness, paresthesia in arms, hypertensive retinopathy, dilated pupils
Musculoskeletal	Cushing's syndrome: striae, muscular wasting, buffalo hump, truncal obesity, thin skin, easy bruisability, osteopenia (compression fractures), weakness Pheochromocytoma: weight loss, weakness, fatigue Conn's syndrome: muscle weakness, tetany, ↑sensitivity to muscle relaxants, osteoporosis
Hematologic	Cushing's syndrome: polycythemia Pheochromocytoma: polycythemia (due to hemoconcentration)
Laboratory	Tests as indicated from H&P.
Premedication	Conn's syndrome: spironolactone often given to inhibit excess aldosterone effects. Midazolam (0.025-0.05 mg/kg); hydrocortisone 100 mg q 8 h

Premedication, cont.	Pheochromocytoma: midazolam (0.025-0.05 mg/kg iv). Preop steroid replacement if bilateral adrenalectomy is contemplated.

INTRAOPERATIVE

Anesthetic technique: GETA (± epidural for postop analgesia). If postop epidural analgesia is planned, placement of catheter before anesthetic induction is helpful in establishing correct placement in the epidural space and assuring a bilateral block (accomplished by placing 5-7 ml of 1% lidocaine via the epidural and eliciting a segmental block). Epidurals cannot be used for a posterior approach since they are in the operative field.

Induction	Gentle iv induction (titration to effect with STP or etomidate) and muscle relaxation (vecuronium 0.1 mg/kg). Patient should be adequately anesthetized before any stimulation. Unopposed parasympathetic response to laryngoscopy can occur, with resultant bradycardia/asystole.
Maintenance	Volatile anesthetic (isoflurane), opiate, muscle relaxant. N_2O can cause bowel distention and is best avoided. Local anesthetic (2% lidocaine **without** epinephrine [pheochromocytoma] [5-10 ml q 60 min]) can be injected into the epidural catheter to provide both anesthesia and optimal surgical exposure (contracted bowel and profound muscle relaxation). A continuous infusion of local anesthetic (e.g., 2% lidocaine or 0.25% bupivacaine) at 5-10 ml may enhance hemodynamic stability. Some anesthesiologists will not use the epidural catheter intraop because chemical 'sympathectomy' is more difficult to reverse. If epidural opiates are used for postop analgesia, a loading dose (e.g., hydromorphone 1.0 mg) should be administered at least 1 h before the conclusion of surgery. Systemic sedatives (droperidol, opiates, benzodiazepines, etc.) should be minimized during this type of anesthetic, as they increase the likelihood of postop respiratory depression. Intraop HTN in pheochromocytomic patients is best treated with SNP, tachycardia with esmolol, and ↓BP with phenylephrine or dopamine. Good communication with surgical team is very important, especially when the adrenal gland is being mobilized.
Emergence	Depends on ease of the surgical procedure and the hemodynamic stability of the patient intraop. If patient is hemodynamically unstable, hypothermic, or has a large 3rd-space fluid requirement, consider postop ventilation.
Blood and fluid requirements	Anticipate large fluid loss. IV: 14-16 ga × 2 NS/LR @ 10-15 ml/kg/h Warm all fluids. Humidify inhaled gases. Cell Saver	As blood loss can be significant, blood should be immediately available. If procedure does not involve cancer, cell-saving devices can be utilized. Guide fluid management by UO, filling pressures, CO.
Monitoring	Standard monitors (p. B-1) UO Arterial line CVP/PA catheter ± TEE	Others as clinically indicated (e.g., PA catheter for patients with pheochromocytoma). Forced-air warmer useful for maintaining body temperature. Use of TEE may be helpful in establishing fluid status and other hemodynamic parameters.
Complications	Labile HTN Dysrhythmias ↓BP (postexcision)	Surgical manipulation of the adrenal may cause ↑↑BP and dysrhythmias. Rx: Alert surgeon and control BP with esmolol/SNP. ↓BP not uncommon after removal of tumor. Rx: phenylephrine/dopamine infusions.
Positioning	✓ and pad pressure points. ✓ eyes.	Strict attention to patient positioning, padding, and taping are important in patients with glucocorticoid excess because of osteopenia and thin, easily traumatized skin.

POSTOPERATIVE

Complications	Pneumothorax (incidence approaches 20%) Hypoglycemia Hypoadrenocorticism after tumor resection	Dx: pleuritic chest pain, dyspnea, ↑RR, ↓breath sounds, hypoxemia. ✓ CXR. Rx: O_2; chest tube and reintubation as necessary. Consider glucocorticoid and mineralocorticoid replacement—hydrocortisone 100 mg q 8 h.

Complications, cont.	Cushing's syndrome:
	    Hypoventilation 2° to obesity
	    (hypoxemia, hypercarbia)
	    HTN
	Pheochromocytoma:
	    BP lability
	    Myocardial dysfunction	

Pain management	Epidural analgesia (p. C-2) PCA (p. C-3)	Patient should be recovered in an ICU or ward accustomed to treating the side effects of epidural opiates (e.g., respiratory depression, breakthrough pain, nausea, pruritus).
Tests	CXR; ECG; electrolytes; glucose	

References

1. Brunt, LM: Laparoscopic adrenalectomy. In *Current Surgical Therapy*, 7th edition. Cameron JL, eds. Mosby Inc., St. Louis: 2001, 1460-7.
2. Christopherson R, Parris WCV: Anesthesia for endocrine surgery. In *Principles and Practice of Anesthesiology*, 2nd edition. Longnecker DE, Tinker JH, Morgan GE Jr, eds. Mosby-Year Book, Inc, St. Louis: 1998, 1948.
3. Cousins MJ, Rubin RB: The intraoperative management of pheochromocytoma with total epidural sympathetic blockade. *Br J Anaesth* 1974; 46(1):78-81.
4. Hull CJ: Phaeochromocytoma—diagnosis, preoperative preparation and anaesthetic management. *Br J Anaesth* 1986; 58: 1453-68.
5. Kazaryan AM, Mala T, Edwin B: Does tumor size influence the outcome of laparoscopic adrenalectomy? *J Laparoendosc Adv Surg Tech* 2001; 11(1):1-4.
6. Kebebew E, Siperstein AE, Clark OH, Duh QY: Results of laparoscopic adrenalectomy for suspected and unsuspected malignant adrenal neoplasms. *Arch Surg* 2002; 137(8):948-53.
7. O'Riordan JA: Pheochromocytomas and anesthesia. *Int Anesth Clin* 1997; 35:99-127.
8. Prys-Roberts C: Phaeochromocytoma—recent progress in its management. *Br J Anaesth* 2000; 85:44-57.
9. Roizen MF: Pheochromocytoma. In *Anesthesia*. Miller RD, ed. Churchill Livingstone, New York: 2000, 924-7.
10. Sieber FE: Evaluation of the patient with endocrine disease and diabetes mellitus. In *Principles and Practice of Anesthesiology*, 2nd edition. Longnecker DE, Tinker JH, Morgan GE Jr, eds. Mosby-Year Book, Inc, St Louis: 1998, 303-22.
11. Smith CD, Weber CJ, Amerson JR: Laparoscopic adrenalectomy: New gold standard. *World J Surg* 1999; 23(4):389-96.
12. Witteles RM, Kaplan EL, Roizen MF: Safe and cost-effective preoperative preparation of patients with pheochromocytoma. *Anesth Analg* 2000; 91:302-4.

Surgeons

Stéphan Busque, MD, MSc, FRCSC (*Kidney, pancreas transplantation*)
Maria T. Millan, MD (*Kidney, pancreas transplantation*)
Dev M. Desai, MD (*Liver transplantation*)
Carlos O. Esquivel, MD, PhD (*Liver transplantation*)

7.12   LIVER/KIDNEY TRANSPLANTATION

Anesthesiologists

Timothy Angelotti, MD, PhD (*Kidney, pancreas transplantation, multiorgan procurement*)
Hendrikus J.M. Lemmons, MD, PhD (*Liver transplantation*)

KIDNEY TRANSPLANTATION—CADAVERIC AND LIVE-DONOR

SURGICAL CONSIDERATIONS

Description: Kidney transplantation offers patients with end-stage renal disease (ESRD) freedom from dialysis. The source of the renal graft may be a cadaveric donor, a relative (e.g., parent, sibling) or a genetically unrelated, but emotionally related individual (e.g., spouse).

After induction of anesthesia, a 3-way Foley catheter is placed into the bladder, and the kidney allograft is placed in the extraperitoneal iliac fossa. A curvilinear incision is made in the right or left lower quadrant. The dissection is maintained in the extraperitoneal space by retracting the peritoneum medial and cephalad, and a self-retaining retractor is usually placed. The external iliac artery and vein are identified, surrounding lymphatics are divided after ligation, and the vessels are mobilized for several centimeters. The external iliac vein is clamped first and the renal-vein-to-iliac-vein anastomosis is performed. Then the external iliac-artery-to-renal-artery anastomosis is performed, and the clamps are released (Fig 7.12-1). The patient should be euvolemic at this point; mannitol and/or furosemide can be given. The bladder is filled with an antibiotic irrigation solution to allow reimplantation of the ureter, which is performed after the detrusor muscle of the bladder has been dissected away from the mucosa. The wound is closed, normally leaving native kidneys intact.

Variant procedure or approaches: Cadaveric or live-donor transplantation

Usual preop diagnosis: ESRD

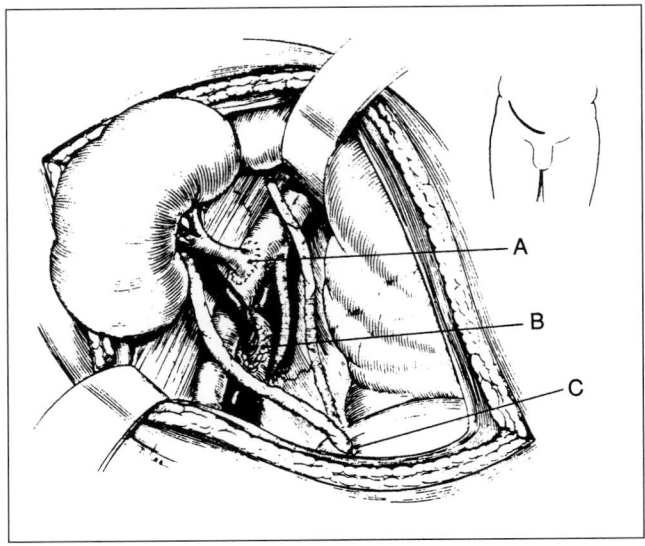

Figure 7.12-1. Kidney transplantation, showing anastomoses of: (A) renal artery to external iliac artery; (B) renal vein to iliac vein; and (C) ureter to bladder. To increase exposure of bladder for a ureteroneocystostomy, antibiotic solution is used to fill the bladder. Lower quadrant curvilinear incision is shown in inset. (Reproduced with permission from Hardy JD: *Hardy's Textbook of Surgery*, 2nd edition. JB Lippincott: 1988.)

SUMMARY OF PROCEDURES

	Cadaveric Kidney	Live-Donor Kidney
Position	Supine	⇐
Incision	Lower quadrant curvilinear (Fig 7.12-1 inset)	⇐
Special instrumentation	Self-retaining retractor; vascular instruments; CVP; Foley catheter (3-way)	⇐
Unique considerations	CVP 10-12 mmHg; mannitol 12.5-25 g; intraop immunosuppression before reperfusion (steroids, antilymphocyte preparation); potassium-free iv fluid; protection of shunt or fistula important.	⇐
Antibiotics	Cefazolin 1 g, 1 h preop	Cefazolin 1 g, 1 h preop
Surgical time	1.5-3 h	2-3 h
EBL	250 ml	⇐
Postop care	Replace UO ml/ml; may have delayed graft function 2° prolonged cold storage; ICU selectively	Fluid replacement; delayed graft function unlikely; ICU selectively
Mortality	1-2%	⇐
Morbidity	Lymph or serous leak/stenosis: 3-5%	⇐
	Postop bleeding: 3-5%	1-2%
	MI: 2-3%	⇐
	Ureteral leak/stenosis: 2-3%	⇐
	Wound infection: 2-3%	⇐

538

	Cadaveric Kidney	Live-Donor Kidney
Morbidity, cont.	Arterial thrombosis: 1-2%	⇐
	Venous thrombosis: 1-2%	⇐
	Wound hematoma: 1-2%	⇐
	Other infectious complications: 15-40%	⇐
Pain score	5	5

PATIENT POPULATION CHARACTERISTICS

Age range	3-70 yr
Male:Female	1:1
Incidence	60/1,000,000
Etiology	Glomerulonephritis (25%); HTN (25%); diabetes mellitus (25%); polycystic disease and others (25%)
Associated conditions	CAD (40%); HTN (25%); uremic and/or diabetic neuropathy (25%); hyperparathyroidism (15-20%)

ANESTHETIC CONSIDERATIONS

See Anesthetic Considerations following Cadaveric Kidney/Pancreas Transplantation, p. 541.

References

1. Flye MW, ed: *Atlas of Organ Transplantation.* WB Saunders, Philadelphia: 1995.
2. Kahan BD, Ponticelli C: *Principles and Practice of Renal Transplantation.* Martin Dunitz, Ltd. London: 2000.
3. Morris PJ: *Kidney Transplantation.* WB Saunders, Philadelphia: 2001.
4. Morris PJ: Renal transplantation: a quarter century. *Semin Nephrol* 1997; 17:188-95.
5. Odorico JS, Sollinger HW: Technical and immunosuppressive advances in transplantation for insulin-dependent diabetes mellitus. *World J Surg* 2002; 26:194-211.

CADAVERIC KIDNEY/PANCREAS TRANSPLANTATION

SURGICAL CONSIDERATIONS

Description: Pancreas transplantation: Combined kidney and pancreas transplantation not only provides kidney replacement for the Type I diabetes patient with end-stage renal disease (ESRD), but also controls diabetes. Eighty percent or more of pancreas transplants are performed in combination with kidney transplantation from the same donor (**simultaneous kidney/pancreas transplant [SPK]**). Pancreas transplantation also can be performed for patients who have received a previous kidney transplant (**pancreas after kidney [PAK]**). Less commonly, pancreas transplantation is done for patients with brittle diabetes or with impending complications while they still enjoy normal or near-normal kidney function. Immunosuppression regimen for pancreas transplantation is generally more aggressive than that used for kidney transplantation, and induction therapy with antilymphocyte preparation (ATG, IL-2 blockers, OKT3) is commonly used. The pancreas transplant is placed in the right iliac fossa and the kidney transplant in the left iliac fossa. This can be done through a transperitoneal lower midline incision or with two separate extraperitoneal lower-quadrant incisions in the same manner as kidney transplantation. The graft is prepared first on the back table. For arterial in-flow, a Y-graft is fashioned, using the donor iliac artery bifurcation. The graft duodenal segment is shortened on the back table. The iliac extension vascular graft is anastomosed to the recipient external or common iliac artery. The portal vein is anastomosed to the external iliac vein. The donor duodenum is anastomosed to a loop of small bowel or to the urinary bladder to drain the exocrine excretions (Fig 7.12-2A). With pancreas transplantation, there may be significant blood loss if the graft mesenteric vessels are not occluded properly. Once the pancreas is transplanted, the kidney transplant is placed into the opposite iliac fossa (as described in Kidney Transplantation, p. 538).

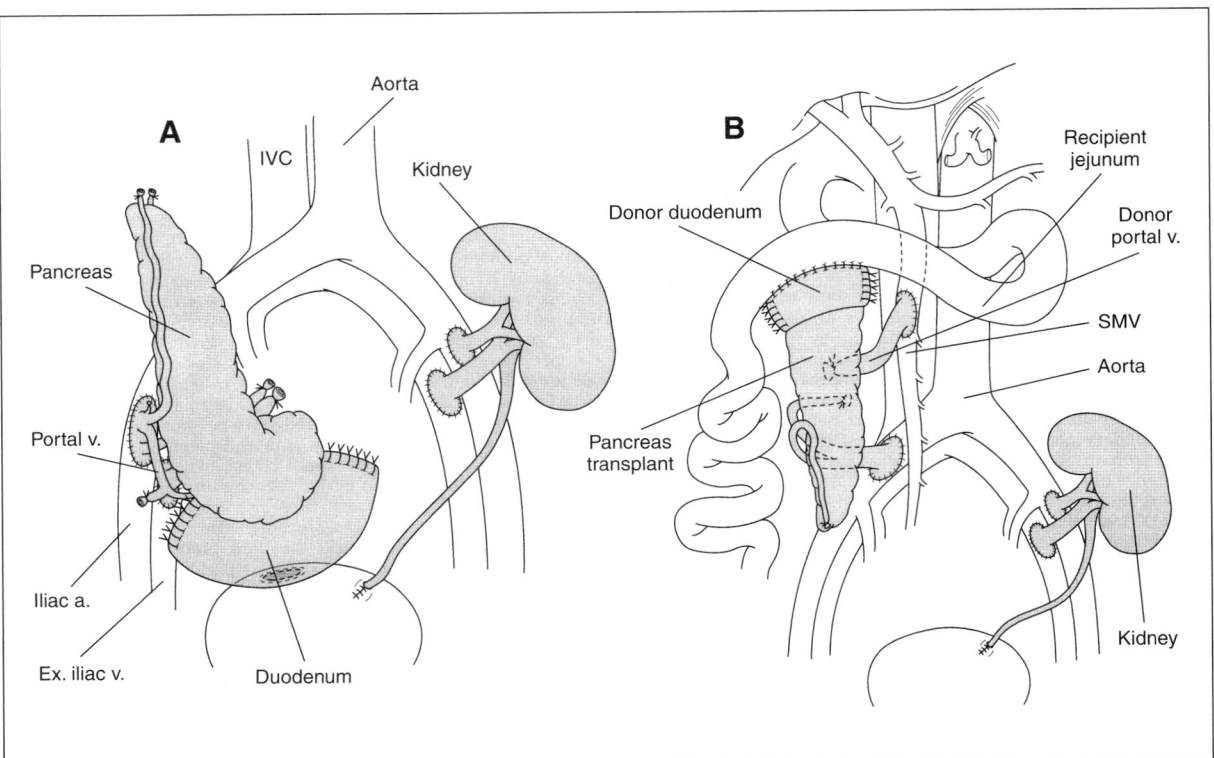

Figure 7.12-2. (A) SPK transplantation, with drainage of pancreatic exocrine secretions into the bladder. Note that portal vein drains into iliac vein (systemic venous [SV] drainage). In normal individuals, 50% of secreted insulin is extracted from the circulation in the first pass through the liver. Transplant recipients with SV have peripheral insulin levels 2-2½ × higher than normal. (B) SPK transplantation with drainage of pancreatic exocrine secretions into the proximal jejunum (enteric drainage [ED]). This technique has been adopted for SPK by most transplant centers in the U.S. For solitary pancreas transplantation, most centers still utilize ED to allow monitoring of the urinary amylase. Note that donor portal vein drains into the recipient superior mesenteric vein (portal venous [PV] drainage), preventing peripheral hyperinsulinemia. This technique appears to be associated with a lower incidence of rejection. Most centers continue to place the pancreas in the pelvis, combining ED and SV, which requires enteric anastomosis to a more distal segment of jejunum or ilium. (Reproduced with permission from Greenfield LJ, et al, eds: *Surgery: Scientific Principles and Practice*, 3rd edition. Lippincott Williams & Wilkins, 2001.)

Variant procedure or approaches: The pancreas may be placed in the upper abdomen with the portal vein anastomosed to the superior mesenteric vein. The exocrine secretions are bowel-drained. This more physiologic approach, however, is associated with a higher technical failure rate and requires a long upper midline incision (Fig 7.12-10). Pancreatic islet cells may be infused via a **portal vein approach,** a procedure that usually is performed in the radiology/angio suite.

Usual preop diagnosis: ESDR 2° diabetes mellitus (DM)

SUMMARY OF PROCEDURE

Position	Supine; cushion heels
Incision	Midline or bilateral lower quadrant
Special instrumentation	Thompson retractor; vascular instruments; Foley catheter; NG tube; CVP; arterial line
Unique considerations	Do not correct hyperglycemia < 300 mg/dL. Maintain adequate hydration, CVP 10-12 mmHg; mannitol 0.25-0.5 g/kg on unclamping; intraop immunosuppression before reperfusion (125-250 mg methylprednisolone, monoclonal or polyclonal preparation [e.g., ATG, Zenepax, OKT3, Simulect]).
Antibiotics	Piperacillin (Zosyn) 3.375 g iv q 6 h × 5 d; fluconazole 200-400 mg (nl creatine clearance)
Surgical time	4-6 h
EBL	250-500 ml
Postop care	ICU × 1-2 d, hourly monitoring of glucose; serum glucose should decline by 50 mg/dL each h and remain < 200 mg/dL.
Mortality	2%

Morbidity	Thrombosis of graft: 5-10%
	Postop bleeding: 5-10%
	Wound infection: 2-6%
	Pancreatitis: 2-4%
	Anastomotic leak: 1%
Pain score	7

PATIENT POPULATION CHARACTERISTICS

Age range	15-55 yr
Male:Female	1:1
Incidence	15-20% of all patients with ESRD
Etiology	Type I diabetes
Associated conditions	Retinopathy (100%); uremic and/or diabetic neuropathy (50%); CAD (25-50%); gastropathy (25%); hyperparathyroidism (15-20%)

ANESTHETIC CONSIDERATIONS
FOR KIDNEY AND KIDNEY/PANCREAS TRANSPLANTATION

PREOPERATIVE

Typically, patients presenting for renal transplantation fall into two patient populations: (1) the young and relatively healthy (following dialysis), or (2) an older, more chronically ill group. Rarely, patients will present for transplant surgery without adequate preparation (e.g., $\uparrow K^+$, $\downarrow pH$, hypervolemia). Patients presenting for pancreas transplantation are usually severe diabetics with many of the associated problems, such as CAD, autonomic neuropathy, gastroparesis, and stiff-joint syndrome (difficult intubation).

Respiratory	Pleuritis and pleural effusions may occur in this patient population. Increased susceptibility to infection is common in the patient with chronic uremia.
Cardiovascular	Pericarditis (acute or constrictive), HTN, CHF, dysrhythmias, pericardial effusion are common, especially in the undialyzed patient. Diabetes, a common cause of ESRD, is often associated with PVD, CAD, and autonomic neuropathy.
	Tests: ECG (rhythm, electrolyte abnormalities, pericarditis, LVH). Other tests (ECHO, stress, etc.) as indicated from H&P.
Gastrointestinal	Gastroparesis may occur, especially in diabetic patients with autonomic neuropathy. It is safer to assume that these patients will require full-stomach precautions. Ranitidine (50 mg iv) and metoclopramide (10 mg iv) should be given 60 min preop to aid gastric emptying and $\downarrow$ acidity. Na citrate (30 ml, 0.3 M po) should be given immediately before induction.
Renal	Patients are usually on dialysis. Postdialysis goals include: $K^+ = 4\text{-}5$ mEq/L, BUN < 60 mg%, creatinine < 10 mg%. Metabolic acidosis, hypocalcemia, and hypermagnesemia may be present, and require preop correction. Patient may be hypovolemic following dialysis; ✓ pre- and post-dialysis weight (> 2 kg loss is significant). Rapid correction of severe hyperkalemia can be achieved by giving iv 50 ml of 50% glucose, together with 12 U regular insulin and 50 mEq NaHCO. Further correction can be obtained by coadministration of an inhaled β-agonist (e.g., albuterol) (5-10 puffs).
	Tests: Cr; BUN; creatinine clearance; electrolytes
Hematologic	These patients are typically anemic (Hct = 18-24%). Usually it is not necessary to correct this anemia (unless $< 18\%$). A coagulation disorder may be present with abnormal Plt function (improved by dialysis) and possibly thrombocytopenia, resulting in a prolonged bleeding time. There is a high incidence of posttransfusion hepatitis in this patient population.
	Tests: Hct; PT; PTT; Plt count; bleeding time; hepatic screen
Neurologic	Peripheral neuropathy may occur and specific deficits should be documented. Autonomic neuropathy can → cardiac problems (e.g., orthostatic hypotension, $\uparrow HR$, or $\downarrow HR$), silent MI, and GI problems.
Premedication	Patients should continue their routine medications up to the time of surgery. A small dose of midazolam is usually a safe premedication for Rx anxiety. Consider the possibility of a full stomach and use full-stomach precautions (see p. B-5).

INTRAOPERATIVE

Anesthetic technique: GETA. Epidural anesthesia may be considered for some cases of renal transplantation.

Induction	Rapid-sequence induction (see p. B-5). ET intubation is aided by succinylcholine (1 mg/kg), if $K^+ < 5.5$ mEq/L; otherwise, use cisatracurium (0.2-0.5 mg/kg) or rocuronium (1.2 mg/kg). Fentanyl (2-5 μg/kg) may be used to suppress the cardiovascular response to intubation.	
Maintenance	Standard maintenance (see p. B-3). Maintain muscle relaxation with cisatracurium or rocuronium, titrated to effect using a nerve stimulator. Avoid meperidine (accumulation of normeperidine may cause CNS toxicity). Anticipate prolonged drug effects, and avoid agents that are primarily excreted by the kidney.	
Emergence	Usually extubated in the OR after protective laryngeal reflexes have returned. Pancreatic transplant patients (e.g., brittle diabetics, hemodynamically unstable) are sent to the ICU.	
Blood and fluid requirements	IV: 14 ga × 1 NS qs CVP = 10-15 mmHg Warm fluids. Humidify gases.	Preop fluid status is highly variable. Fluids should be given to maintain CVP 10-15 mmHg. It is important to maintain adequate vascular volume and BP. Mannitol (0.25-1 g/kg), furosemide (5-20 mg), and low-dose dopamine are often given with reperfusion of the kidney.
Monitoring	Standard monitors (see p. B-1). Arterial line CVP/PA line	Arterial pressure is often monitored. Avoid the side of AV fistulae. Axillary artery is a useful alternative. CVP is essential and a PA line is needed occasionally (severe cardiac disease). CVP is kept at 10-15 mmHg, especially after the new kidney is reperfused, to ensure adequate renal blood flow.
	Hct, K^+, and glucose	In pancreatic transplant patients, glucose should be checked q 30 min and then q 10 min for the first h following reperfusion. Keep glucose < 300 mg% prior to reperfusion, but do not fully correct to < 150 mg %.
	Neuromuscular	Monitor neuromuscular block to avoid excessive use of neuromuscular relaxants.
Positioning	✓ and pad pressure points. ✓ eyes.	
Complications	Hemorrhage Low UO Reperfusion injury (pancreas transplant)	

POSTOPERATIVE

Complications	Respiratory depression Femoral neuropathy Hemorrhage Electrolyte abnormalities	Monitor UO. Dialysis may be needed until renal function returns. Sudden cardiac arrest can complicate pancreatic transplantation (due to autonomic neuropathy).
Pain management	PCA (see p. C-3).	
Tests	Hct Electrolytes Cr, BUN Amylase Glucose	A rise in amylase and blood glucose may indicate failure of the pancreatic transplant.

References

1. Graybar GB, Deierhoi MH: Anesthesia and pancreatic transplantation. *Anesth Clin North Am* 1989; 7(3):515-49.
2. Sprung J, Kapural L, Bourke DL, O'Hara JF Jr: Anesthesia for kidney transplant surgery. *Anesth Clin North Am* 2000; 18(4): 919-51.
3. Sutherland DE: State of the art in pancreas transplantation. *Transplant Proc* 1994; 26:316-20.

LIVE-DONOR NEPHRECTOMY—LAPAROSCOPIC AND OPEN

SURGICAL CONSIDERATIONS

Description: Use of a kidney donated by a healthy genetically or emotionally related donor greatly increases the number and quality of available kidneys for transplantation. Kidney transplantation from living donors is associated with a better patient and graft survival rate. A **laparoscopic (LSC) approach** to kidney donation was introduced in 1995 as an alternative that would reduce postop pain, wound morbidity, and recovery time associated with open nephrectomy. The LSC approach is becoming more popular and was the procedure of choice for more than 50% of the live kidney donations in the U.S. in 2001. Initial concerns regarding ureteral complications and longer warm ischemic time have mostly subsided with the improvement of the surgical technique and greater experience. The left kidney is preferred for the LSC approach, as its renal vein is longer. Some centers use the LSC approach for the right kidney with comparable results.

The patient is positioned in lateral decubitus over a cushioned beanbag, the kidney rest is slightly elevated, and pillows and an axillary roll are used to prevent compression injury. Three or four ports are used. The pneumoperitoneum is kept < 15 mmHg to avoid decreased perfusion to the kidney. Aggressive hydration and intermittent use of iv mannitol help improve kidney perfusion. On the left side, the descending colon and spleen are mobilized medially; the renal vessels are exposed; the adrenal, lumbar, and gonadal veins are clipped and sectioned; the ureter is mobilized en bloc, along with the gonadal vein, up to the pelvic inlet. The artery is freed from surrounding lymphatic and neural tissue as is comes off the aorta (Fig 7.12-3). Gerota's fascia is mobilized to completely free the kidney. The ureter is sectioned distally. A 6 cm suprapubic incision is made, the peritoneum is exposed in the midline, and an 18 mm port is used to insert a 15 mm Endocatch retrieval bag. The kidney is placed in the bag as it continues to be perfused, avoiding warm ischemia. The patient is fully heparinized. An endo GIA vascular stapler is used to section and staple the artery close to the aorta and the vein close to the vena cava. The retrieval bag is brought to the suprapubic incision and gently extracted. The kidney is immediately immersed in the cold slush solution, and staple lines are cut off the renal artery and vein. The kidney is perfused with preservation solution in the usual manner. The heparin is reversed with protamine, the suprapubic incision is closed, and homeostasis is verified before extracting the ports. For a right nephrectomy, the right colon and duodenum are mobilized medially and the liver is retracted upward. The remainder of the operation is as described for the left kidney. The surgeon's hand may be inserted in the abdomen to help with the stapling of the vessels and kidney retrieval.

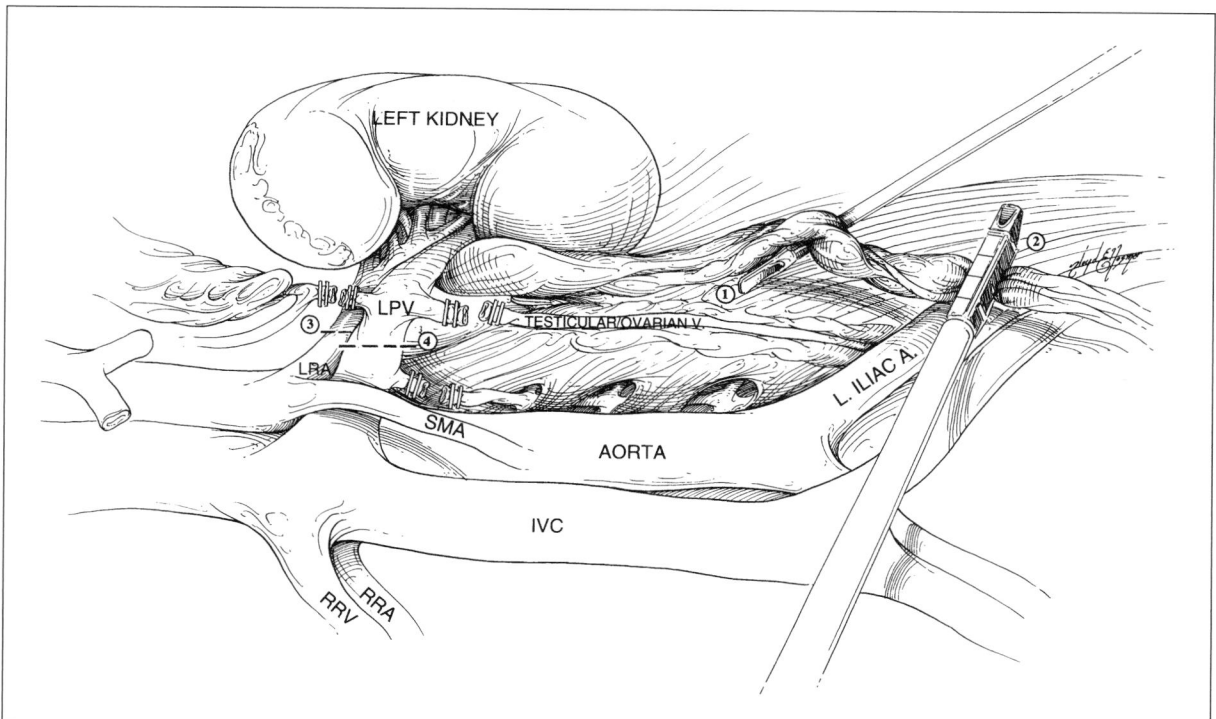

Figure 7.12-3. Anatomy for laparoscopic live-donor nephrectomy. (Reproduced with permission from Cho ES, Flowers JL: Laparoscopic live-donor nephrectomy. In *Surgical Laparoscopy*, 2nd edition. Zuker KA, ed. Lippincott Williams & Wilkins, 2001.)

The **hand-assisted laparoscopic donor nephrectomy** is similar to the pure laparoscopic approach described above; however, a midline 8-10 cm incision is made at the level of the umbilicus to position a device (e.g., Lapdisc) that will allow the surgeon to put one hand inside the abdomen without losing the pneumoperitoneum. The hand is used to help with retraction and exposure to the kidney. The warm ischemia time (clamping of the renal artery to perfusion) is reduced 50%. Operative time also may be reduced. This approach requires a longer abdominal incision and is associated with more wound complications than the pure laparoscopic approach.

In **open nephrectomy**, the **donor/patient** is placed in a lateral decubitus position on a flexible OR table with a kidney rest. A beanbag or sandbags are also helpful for positioning. An incision is made from the rectus muscle, angling slightly cephalic to cross into the flank just below the tip of the 12th rib. The retroperitoneum is exposed using a Thompson retractor. The kidney is then mobilized and the ureter is transected. A clamp is placed across the renal artery at the aorta and the renal vein at the IVC. Just before clamping the renal artery, furosemide and/or mannitol may be given to stimulate diuresis. It is important to keep the vascular volume expanded in these patients before kidney removal. The kidney is removed and taken to the back table where it is flushed with a cold preservation solution. It is then transported into the recipient room for reimplantation. Some surgeons use a full dose of heparin (75 U/kg) before clamping and use protamine afterwards. Smaller incisions and muscle-sparing incisions are now used to improve postop recovery.

Usual preop diagnosis: Donor nephrectomy

SUMMARY OF PROCEDURES

	Laparoscopic Nephrectomy	**Open Nephrectomy**
Position	Lateral decubitus	⇐
Incision	3-4 ports; retrieval incision, Pfannenstiel's or vertical suprapubic	Flank; may require 12th rib resection
Special instrumentation	Foley catheter; flexible OR table with kidney rest; beanbag; SCDs for DVT prophylaxis; harmonic scalpel	Foley catheter; Thompson retractor; flexible OR table with kidney rest; beanbag or sandbags; SCDs for DVT prophylaxis
Unique considerations	Avoid ETT dislodgement when turning patient from supine to flank position; vigorous hydration.	Possible pneumothorax; avoid ETT dislodgement when turning patient from supine to flank position. Vigorous hydration to encourage urine production.
Antibiotics	Cefazolin 1 g	Cefazolin 1 g, 1 h preop
Surgical time	2.5-4.5 h	2-2.5 h
Closing considerations	–	Delfex table to facilitate closure
EBL	Minimal	100 ml
Postop care	PACU → room; PCA for pain management	CXR to r/o pneumothorax. Epidural or PCA (morphine) is helpful for pain management. PACU → room.
Mortality	< 0.1%	⇐
Morbidity	Ileus: 2-5%	5-10%
	Urinary retention: 2-5%	5-10%
	Wound infection: 1-2%	1-3%
	Bleeding: 0.1-0.5%	⇐
		Pneumothorax: 1%
Pain score	3-5	7

PATIENT POPULATION CHARACTERISTICS

Age range	18-70 yr
Male:Female	1:1
Incidence	Up to 50% of all kidney transplants at some centers
Etiology	N/A
Associated conditions	Good health is mandatory for renal donation.

ANESTHETIC CONSIDERATIONS

See Anesthetic Considerations following Kidney Transplant Nephrectomy, p. 546.

KIDNEY TRANSPLANT NEPHRECTOMY

SURGICAL CONSIDERATIONS

Description: With improvements in graft survival and immunosuppressive therapy, the necessity of removing a kidney transplant graft for uncontrolled rejection has decreased significantly. This operation is divided into categories: **early nephrectomy,** performed during the first month posttransplant, and **late nephrectomy,** thereafter. **Early transplant nephrectomy** may be required for primary nonfunction, vascular thrombosis, and, rarely, refractory rejection. In these cases, an **extracapsular approach,** through the original transplant incision, is used. The kidney is freed up from the surrounding adhesion to obtain vascular control of the renal artery and renal vein. These structures are clamped and oversewn individually. The ureter is ligated as close as possible to the bladder and excised completely, with primary repair of the bladder. A suction drain is used if minimal oozing or lymph drainage is present. **Late transplant nephrectomy** is performed most commonly for acute, irreversible rejection with failure of the renal allograft. Most of these patients have returned to dialysis and the immunosuppressive medications have been stopped. Chronic infection and HTN associated with nonfunctional grafts are also an indication for surgical removal of the kidney allograft. It may be a difficult operation, as intense inflammatory adhesions are present between the renal capsule and the surrounding tissue. In the setting of acute late rejection, the graft is usually swollen and enlarged. Hematuria may be present, and the graft is friable. Spontaneous rupture and hemorrhage have been reported. The surgical approach is through the same incision as the implantation. In contrast to early transplant nephrectomy, extracapsular dissection may not be possible with late nephrectomy. To avoid injury to extrarenal structures, such as the iliac vessels, an **intracapsular approach** may be preferred. The kidney is mobilized gently from within the capsule toward the hilum. The capsule is reopened on the medial side to have access to the renal vessel high in the hilum. When the hilum is sufficiently mobilized, a strong vascular clamp is applied high in the hilum of the kidney away from the iliac vessels. After clamping the hilum en bloc, confirmation of distal pulses is obtained; then the kidney is excised over the vascular clamp. A running suture is used over the clamp, which is then released, and hemostasis is obtained. The ureter is identified and excised as close as possible to the bladder. The intracapsular dissection of the kidney may be associated with significant bleeding, as the kidney may fracture. This step should thus be done expeditiously to avoid excessive bleeding. The patient must have good vascular access for fluid resuscitation. Blood must be available for transfusion. After hemostasis is obtained, a low-pressure suction drain may be placed before closing.

Usual preop diagnosis: Transplant rejection

SUMMARY OF PROCEDURE

Position	Supine
Incision	Previous incision used for kidney transplant
Instrumentation	Self-retaining retractor; vascular instruments
Unique considerations	Large-bore vascular access; PRBCs available; stress dose of steroids, if chronic usage; protection of shunt or fistula
Antibiotics	Cefazolin 1 g
Surgical time	1-2.5 hr
EBL	200-2,000 ml
Postop care	PCA for pain management → PACU → room
Mortality	1-3%
Morbidity	Overall: 3-5%
	Wound infection: 3-5%
	Abscess formation: 1-2%
	Exsanguinating hemorrhage: < 1%
Pain score	5

PATIENT POPULATION CHARACTERISTICS

Age range	3-75 yr
Male:Female	1:1
Incidence	60/1,000,000
Etiology	Failed kidney transplant
Associated conditions	CAD (40%); HTN (25%); uremic and/or diabetic neuropathy (25%); hyperparathyroidism (15-20%)

ANESTHETIC CONSIDERATIONS FOR LIVE-DONOR AND POSTTRANSPLANTATION NEPHRECTOMY

PREOPERATIVE

In order to be a live donor, one must be in good health with bilaterally functional kidneys. Diabetes, HIV infection, liver disease, and malignancy are all contraindications to kidney donations.

Cardiovascular	R/O HTN, CAD.
Renal	Normal bilateral renal function is required. **Tests:** IVP; Cr, creatinine clearance
Fluid status	Adequate hydration is important and UO should be >1.5 ml/kg/h. Various regimes are used to ensure adequate hydration, usually with iv fluid starting the night before.
Premedication	Adequate anxiolysis is beneficial. These patients are making a great sacrifice and should be treated with special care. Standard premedication (see p. B-2).

INTRAOPERATIVE

Anesthetic technique: GETA ± epidural for postop pain management

Induction	Standard induction (see p. B-2).	
Maintenance	Standard maintenance (see p. B-3). Avoid long-acting, renally excreted drugs. Ventilate to maintain eucapnia to avoid possible renal artery vasoconstriction. Use of an epidural with local anesthetic and/or narcotic may aid both intraop and postop pain relief, but ↓BP should be avoided.	
Emergence	Routine extubation in OR	
Blood and fluid requirements	IV: 14 ga × 2 NS/LR @ 6-8 ml/h Warm all fluids. Humidify gases. UO 1.5 ml/kg/h	Aim for a minimum of 1.5 ml/kg/h UO. Mannitol (0.25-1 g/kg) given iv once kidney is being manipulated, and if UO decreases. Consider dopamine infusion to ↑BP as needed . Limit use of direct vasoconstrictors.
Monitoring	Standard monitors (see p. B-1).	CVP or invasive arterial monitoring are rarely required.
Positioning	✓ and pad pressure points. ✓ eyes.	Positioning may impair venous return → ↓BP. Ensure that the head is properly padded and that the C-spine is in line with thoracic spine.
Complications	Hemorrhage	Because the vessels are tied close to the aorta and IVC, the possibility of severe hemorrhage exists.
	Pneumothorax	Pneumothorax is always possible, especially when the 12th rib is resected.

POSTOPERATIVE

Complications	Pneumothorax Hemorrhage Infection Pulmonary problems Hypokalemia (diuretics) Ileus	
Pain management	Epidural narcotics (see p. C-2). PCA (see p. C-3).	Epidural analgesia is recommended.
Tests	CXR Hct	

References for Kidney Transplantation

1. Flye MW, ed: *Atlas of Organ Transplantation.* WB Saunders, Philedelphia: 1995.
2. Kahan BD, Ponticelli C: *Principles and Practice of Renal Transplantation.* Martin Dunitz, Ltd. London: 2000.
3. Morris PJ: *Kidney Transplantion.* WB Saunders, Philadelphia: 2001.

4. Odorico JS, Sollinger HW: Technical immunosuppressive advances in transplantation for insulin-dependent diabetes mellitus. *World J Surg* 2002; 26:194-211.

5. Simmons RL, Finch ME, Ascher NL, Najarian JS, eds: *Manual of Vascular Access, Organ Donation and Transplantation.* Springer-Verlag, New York: 1984.

6. Sprung J, Kapural L, Bourke DL, O'Hara JF Jr: Anesthesia for kidney transplant surgery. *Anesth Clin North Am* 2000; 18(4): 919-51.

LIVER TRANSPLANTATION

SURGICAL CONSIDERATIONS

Description: Liver transplantation is the treatment of choice for patients with acute and chronic end-stage liver disease (ESLD). Patients with ESLD, besides intrinsic liver dysfunction, also may have other organ system dysfunction, including hepatorenal and hepatopulmonary syndrome → oliguria and hypoxia, respectively. Patients with alcohol-mediated cirrhosis and Wilson's disease are at risk for significant cardiomyopathy, while those with fulminant hepatic failure may have significantly elevated intracranial pressures. These additional comorbidities present an added level of complexity to the anesthetic and surgical management of the liver transplant recipient. The liver transplant operation can be divided into three stages: (1) hepatectomy; (2) anhepatic phase, which involves the implantation of the liver; and (3) postrevascularization, which includes hemostasis and reconstruction of the hepatic artery and common bile duct.[16] There are many variations in the technical aspects of the liver transplant operation that may result in physiologic changes during anesthesia. The anesthesiologist must be aware of these technical variations to optimize the intraop management of the liver transplant recipient. Examples of these variations include: cross-clamping of the vena cava during the implantation of the liver, which results in impairment of the systemic venous return, with subsequent profound hypotension; utilization of the venovenous bypass, which may be associated with thrombus, air embolism, and/or fibrinolysis; and the use of a 'cutdown liver,' which may → significant bleeding from the raw surface following revascularization.

The **hepatectomy** may be a formidable task in patients with severe portal HTN, coagulopathy, and previous surgery in the upper abdomen. In such circumstances, blood loss is significant and may be minimized by placing the patient on venovenous bypass or by creating a temporary portocaval shunt to relieve the portal HTN. Table 7.12-1 lists factors that may be associated with significant blood loss during the transplant operation. The hepatectomy is usually much easier in patients with acute fulminant hepatitis or primary biliary cirrhosis than in patients with shrunken cirrhotic livers, such as in postnecrotic cirrhosis from hepatitis B or C, alpha-1 antitrypsin deficiency, or Wilson's disease, among others. The incision usually extends from the left midclavicular line across the midline to just medial of the right 12th floating rib, along with a vertical midline extension from the xiphoid process to the transverse incision. This provides wide exposure to the upper abdomen.

Table 7.12-1. Contributing Factors Associated with Increased Blood Loss in Liver Transplantation
1. Severe coagulopathy
2. Severe portal HTN
3. Portal or splenic vein thrombosis
4. Previous surgery in the RUQ
5. Renal failure
6. Uncontrolled sepsis
7. Retransplantation
8. Transfusion reaction
9. Venous bypass-induced fibrinolysis
10. Primary graft nonfunction
11. Intraop vascular complications

The hepatectomy usually begins with manual exploration of the abdomen to ensure that there are no occult malignancies, abscesses, or other abdominal processes that may be a contraindication to proceeding with the transplant. The liver is then mobilized by freeing the falciform and left cardinal ligaments, followed by entering the lesser sac through the division of the gastrohepatic ligament. The mobilization of the liver and the subsequent dissection of the portahepatis may be significantly complicated and a tedious process due to large, thin-walled varices that require careful dissection and ligation. The dissection of the portahepatis begins with identification and ligation of the hepatic artery, followed by the common bile duct. The portal vein is carefully dissected from its bifurcation into left and right branches, proximally to its emergence from behind the pancreas. If the degree of portal HTN is severe—such that mobilization of the liver may result in significant blood loss—or the patient is hemodynamically unstable—then portal vein mobilization may be performed early so that a temporary portocaval shunt or venous bypass may be instituted to allow decompression of the varices and enhance venous return to the heart.

Once the portal dissection has been completed, the right lobe of the liver is mobilized. The infrahepatic vena cava is carefully dissected to prevent injury to the right renal and adrenal veins, followed by mobilization of the suprahepatic vena cava. The liver can be removed easily by cross-clamping and dividing the supra- or infrahepatic vena cava, with or without the use of venous bypass. Alternatively, the recipient vena cava may be left in situ by further mobilization of the liver with division of the short hepatic veins that run from the anterior surface of the vena cava into the posterior aspect of the liver. To gain access to the short hepatic veins, the liver must be lifted and rotated to the left. This maneuver may result in partial occlusion of the inferior vena cava, which may impair venous return → temporary ↓BP. The piggyback technique, where the recipient vena cava is left in situ, has the advantage that venous return is not compromised during the anhepatic phase and thus precludes the need for venous bypass.

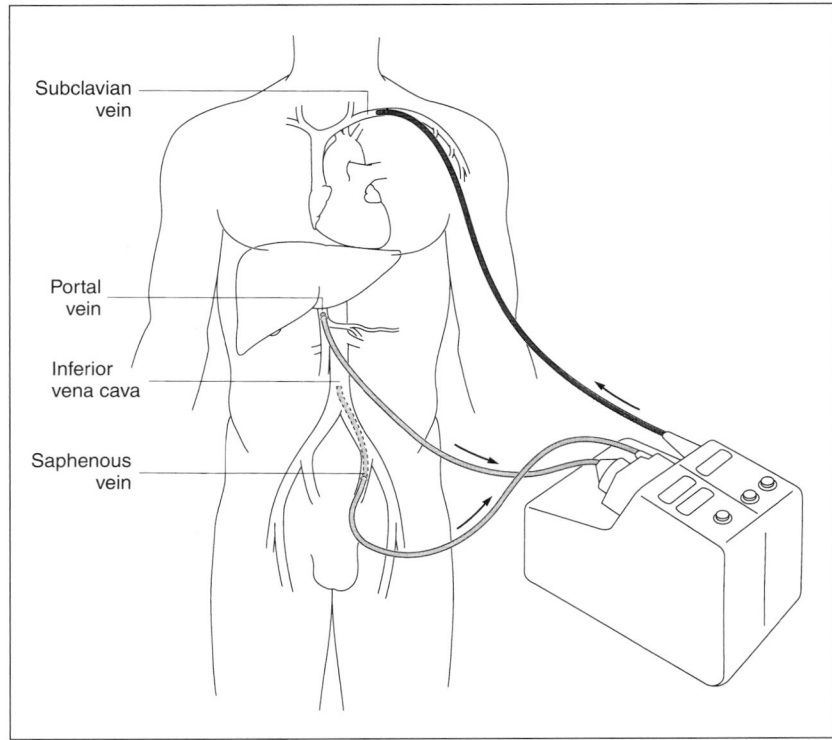

Figure 7.12-4. Setup for venovenous bypass during hepatic transplantation. Cannulas are placed into the portal vein to decompress the splanchnic bed and inferior vena cava (through the greater saphenous vein) to decompress the lower extremities and kidneys during the anhepatic phase of the transplant. A centrifugal pump is used to deliver bypassed blood to the central circulation by means of a cannula passed into the axillary vein. Cannulas also may be placed percutaneously directly into the femoral and subclavian veins. (Reproduced with permission from Greenfield LJ, et al, eds: *Surgery: Scientific Principles and Practice*, 3rd edition. Lippincott Williams & Wilkins, 2001.)

The **anhepatic phase** may be associated with significant hemodynamic changes, depending on the technique used for vascular control. This stage of the operation consists of implantation of the liver allograft, with or without venous bypass. The use of venous bypass is particularly helpful in coagulopathic patients with severe portal HTN. In these high-risk patients, the goal of the venous bypass system is to relieve the portal HTN by 'bypassing' the liver.[13] Cannulas, placed in the femoral and portal veins, draw the blood out of the systemic and splanchnic venous systems into a Biomedicus pump that delivers the blood into the axillary vein, maintaining the venous return (Fig 7.12-4). This system allows the interruption of the vena cava with mild-to-moderate hemodynamic changes, depending on the blood flow rate through the system. The benefits and potential complications of the venous bypass system are listed in Table 7.12-2.[13]

Table 7.12-2. Benefits and Potential Complications of the Venovenous Bypass System

Benefits	Complications
Improved hemodynamics during anhepatic phase	PE
↓blood loss	Air embolism
May improve perioperative renal function.*	Brachial plexus injury
	Wound seroma/infection
	Vascular injury

* In a prospective randomized trial comparing venovenous bypass with no bypass, no difference was found in the periop renal function between the two groups.[5]

Wound complications and nerve injuries may be prevented by introducing the bypass cannulas percutaneously, rather than approaching the vessels through a surgical incision. A subclavian or IJ line may be placed preop, and can be easily and rapidly exchanged during the operation to bypass cannulas using the **Seldinger technique**. If lines are placed preop for the specific purpose of venous bypass, a confirmatory CXR should be performed to ensure that the 15 Fr or larger bypass cannula will lie in the appropriate vessel when placed later in the operation. This also obviates the need for a CXR when the bypass cannula is placed later, when the patient may be unstable. Because of the potential complications, several transplant teams have opted not to use the venous bypass. In those cases, vascular control is obtained by placing vascular clamps across the supra- and infrahepatic vena cava and the portal vein. The systemic and splanchnic venous return is interrupted during the anhepatic phase, leading to significant ↓BP unless preventive measures, as reviewed in Anesthetic Considerations (p. 554), are taken (Fig 7.12-5).

In a **standard orthotopic liver transplant**, with or without venous bypass, the recipient's vena cava is removed, leaving two cuffs—one just below the diaphragm and the other above the entry of the renal veins. A cadaveric donor liver comes with a segment of the vena cava that is used for restoring the continuity of the recipient's vena cava. The first vascular anastomosis consists of an end-to-end anastomosis of the allograft suprahepatic vena cava and the cuff of the recipient's infradiaphragmatic vena cava. This is followed by the reconstruction of the infrahepatic vena cava with an end-to-end anastomosis. Immediately prior to completion of the infrahepatic vena caval anastomosis, the liver is purged with chilled or room temperature albumin and/or crystalloid solution via the allograft portal vein to remove the University of Wisconsin (UW) preservative solution, which contains ~145 mEq/L K⁺. Additionally, flushing the liver also removes a significant amount of the air that gets introduced during the procurement and preparation of the allograft for transplantation. Finally, the portal vein reconstruction is completed with an end-to-end anastomosis. At this point, the clamps are removed, ending the anhepatic phase of the operation.

Venous bypass is not necessary in **piggyback liver transplantation,** since the diseased liver is separated from the vena cava (systemic venous return remains unimpaired), and vascular control is obtained by placing a clamp across the confluence of the hepatic veins as they join the vena cava (Fig 7.12-6). A temporary portocaval shunt may be created to minimize bleeding in cases with severe portal HTN. The first anastomosis is between the suprahepatic vena cava of the liver allograft and the cuff created from the hepatic veins. The infrahepatic vena cava of the liver allograft is ligated, and the portal vein reconstruction is completed. The clamps are then removed and the liver is revascularized.

The **postrevascularization stage** of the transplant begins with the removal of the vascular clamps. The reperfusion of the liver may be the most critical part of the operation. Despite flushing the liver to remove the high K⁺-containing organ preservation solution, hyperkalemia may be troublesome following liver reperfusion, particularly with livers that sustained significant injury during preservation and reperfusion. Additionally, massive air embolism is an immediate concern following revascularization, as it may quickly lead to cardiac arrest. It is also during this stage that the patient may experience pulmonary HTN → RV failure and ↓↓BP. This must be treated aggressively with inotropic agents; otherwise, the liver is subjected to high outflow resistance → congestion and worsening of the preservation injury. The cause of this phenomenon is not well understood; fortunately, it is seen in very few patients. Another reperfusion phenomenon is that of systemic ↓BP 2° ↓SVR. This may be due to the release of systemic inflammatory mediators, which include kinins, cytokines, and free radicals. Reperfusion of the liver also can have dramatic effects on coagulation, such as fibrinolysis or hypercoagulation that may → venous thrombosis and massive PE with cardiovascular collapse.

Following revascularization, the patient usually is given methylprednisolone (250-1000 mg) as part of the immunosuppression regimen, as well as an adjunct to counteract the systemic effects of ischemia-reperfusion injury of the liver. At this point, all of the vascular anastomoses, the retroperitoneum, and the liver (especially the cut surface in segmental or reduced-size grafts) are inspected for surgical bleeding.

The hepatic artery reconstruction is performed after stabilization of the patient following revascularization of the liver. Once the hepatic arterial anastomosis is completed, it is important to maintain adequate arterial BP (MAP > 65 mmHg) to prevent hepatic artery thrombosis. This is especially critical in pediatric transplant recipients, where the hepatic artery diameter ranges from 1-3 mm. The last part of the procedure involves hemostasis, removal of the gallbladder, and reconstruction of the bile duct (Fig 7.12-7). There are two basic methods for the **bile duct reconstruction:** an end-to-end anastomosis, with or without a T tube (in patients with normal common bile ducts), or a choledochojejunostomy to a Roux-en-Y (Fig 7.12-8) (in patients with biliary atresia, primary sclerosing cholangitis, or diseased common bile ducts, or when there is a size discrepancy between the donor and recipient common bile duct). In cadaveric or live-donor segmental transplantation, the technique for the recipient's hepatectomy and the implantation of the allograft is not different from that of full-size liver transplantation; however, the technique of piggyback liver transplantation must be used with live donors since the allograft segment does not include the vena cava. The anesthesiologist must be alert during the reperfusion of a segmental graft, since significant bleeding may ensue from the raw surface of the liver.

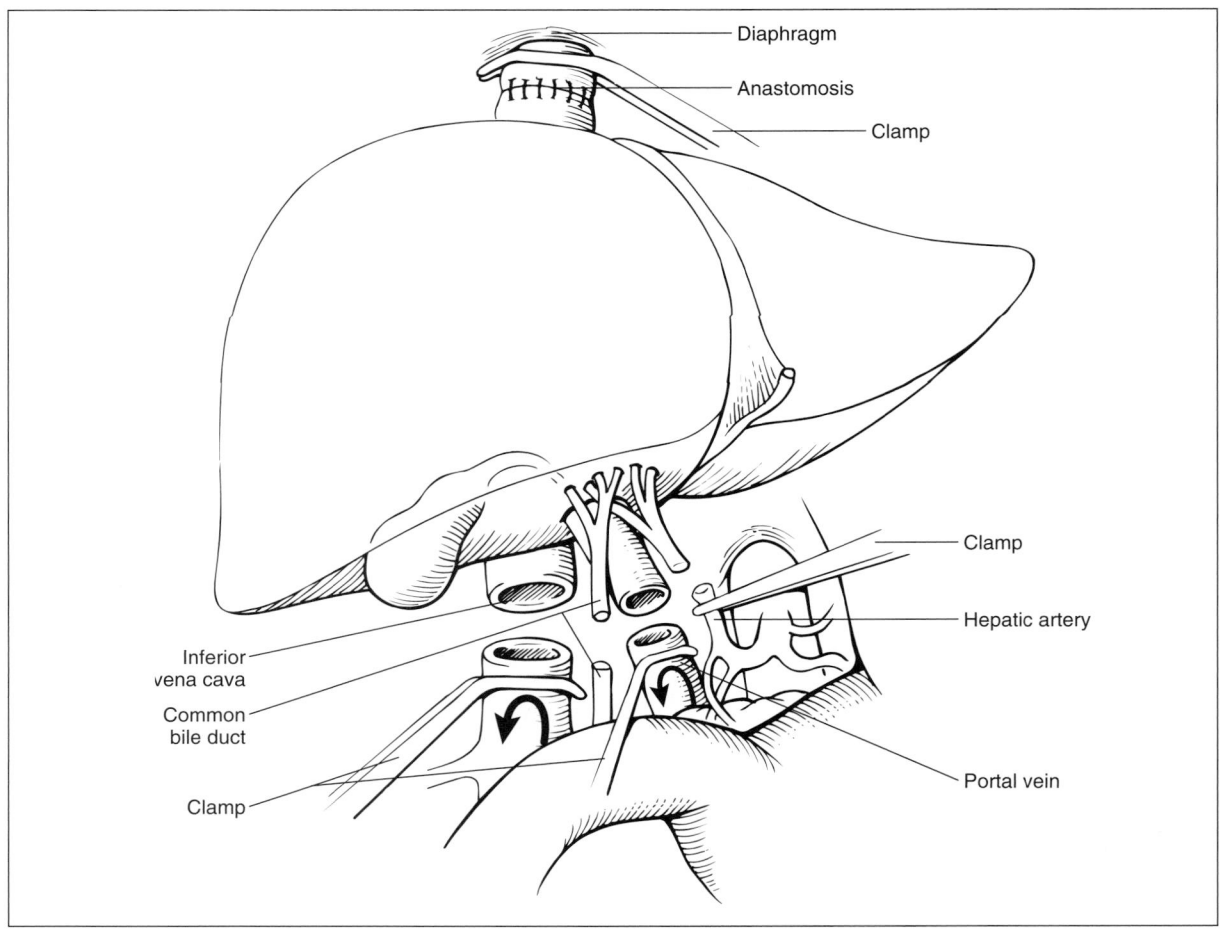

Figure 7.12-5. Standard liver transplantation without venovenous bypass. Venous return is significantly impaired.

Once the biliary reconstruction is completed and hemostasis has been achieved, a feeding jejunostomy tube and 2-3 closed-suction drains may be placed. The position of an OG or NG tube (placed at the beginning of the case) is confirmed and the abdomen is closed.

Usual preop diagnosis: ESLD

SUMMARY OF PROCEDURE

Position	Supine; arms tucked. Left arm and left groin area out for access to the axillary and femoral veins if venous bypass is used.
Incision	Bilateral subcostal, in children; in adults, incision must extend cephalad to the xiphoid process.
Special instrumentation	Upper hand retractor; venous bypass pump; rapid-infusion system; Cell Saver; argon beam coagulator
Unique considerations	Thrombus or air embolism may occur during removal of clamps from vena cava. RV failure, ↓BP, and ↓SVR may be observed after revascularization. Continuous AV hemofiltration may be required if renal failure is present. Head and extremities should be covered with plastic to maintain body T, particularly in children. OG tube required.
Antibiotics/drugs	Ampicillin (1 g q 8 h) and ceftriaxone (1 g q 24 h) prior to making incision. Methylprednisolone and antilymphocyte antibody preparations for immunosuppression. Aprotinin is used occasionally during the hepatectomy and anhepatic phase in patients with severe coagulopathy and fibrinolysis (venous thrombus formation and pulmonary embolism can be seen with aprotinin use).
Surgical time	4-12 h

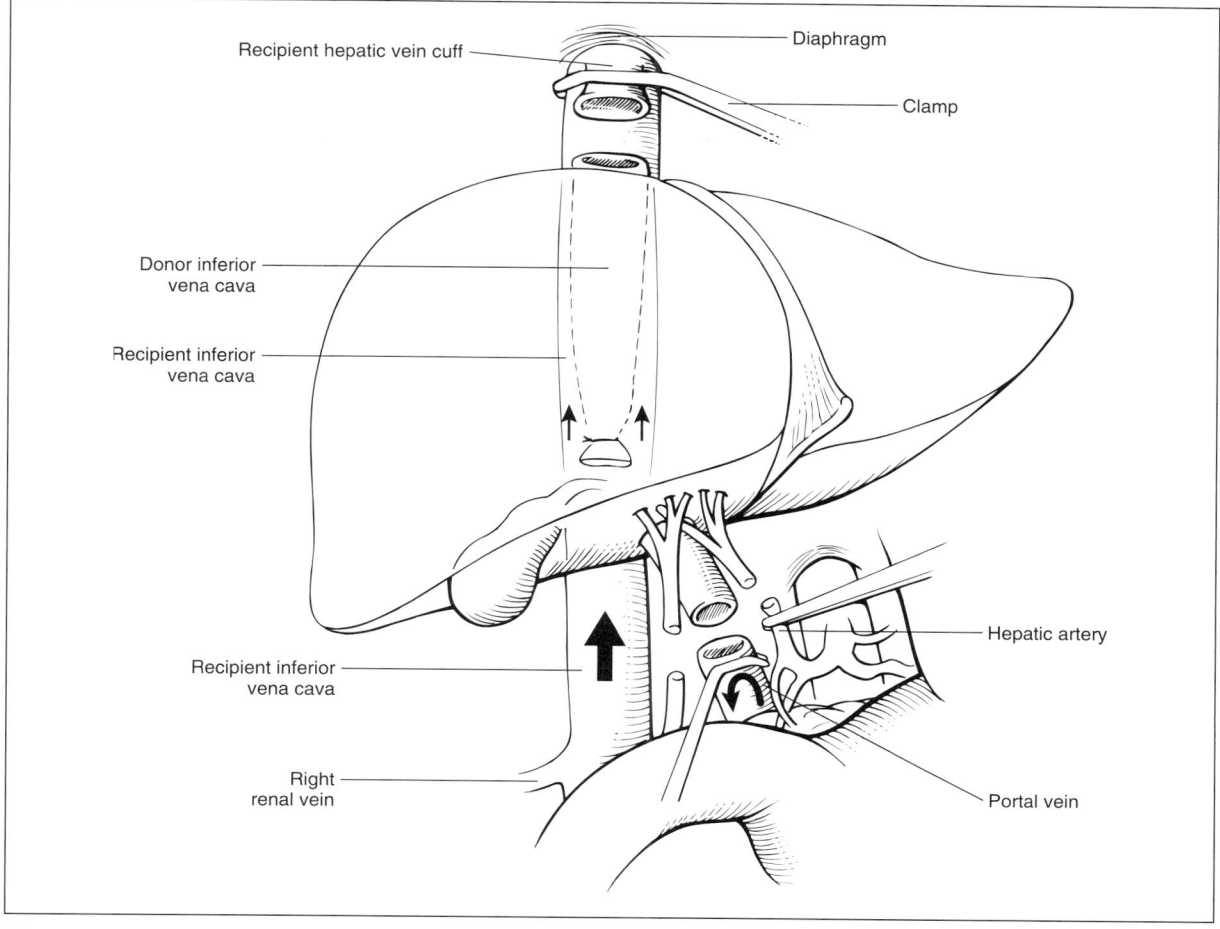

Figure 7.12-6. Piggyback liver transplantation. Note that the recipient's vena cava is left intact and systemic venous return is unimpaired.

EBL	6 U average blood loss (range 0-100 U)
Postop care	ICU: 1-2 d. HTN commonly seen.
Mortality	10% at 1 yr
Rejection	35-70% during first yr
Morbidity	Infectious complications: 20-50%
	Biliary stenosis or leaks: 6-15%
	Retransplantation: 6-14%
	Primary graft nonfunction: 2-6%
	Hepatic artery thrombosis: 0-6%
	Portal vein thrombosis: 1-4%
Pain score	7-8

PATIENT POPULATION CHARACTERISTICS

Age range	Neonate-70 yr
Male:Female	1:1
Incidence	10/million/yr (15% pediatrics)
Etiology	Adult: hepatitis C cirrhosis; alcoholic cirrhosis; primary biliary cirrhosis; primary sclerosing cholangitis; hepatitis B cirrhosis; hepatocellular carcinoma
	Pediatric: biliary atresia; inborn errors of metabolism
Associated conditions	Coagulopathy; hypoalbuminemia; ascites; cardiomyopathy (in alcoholic patients, hemochromatosis, and Wilson's disease); hepatorenal syndrome; hypoglycemia in acute fulminant hepatitis

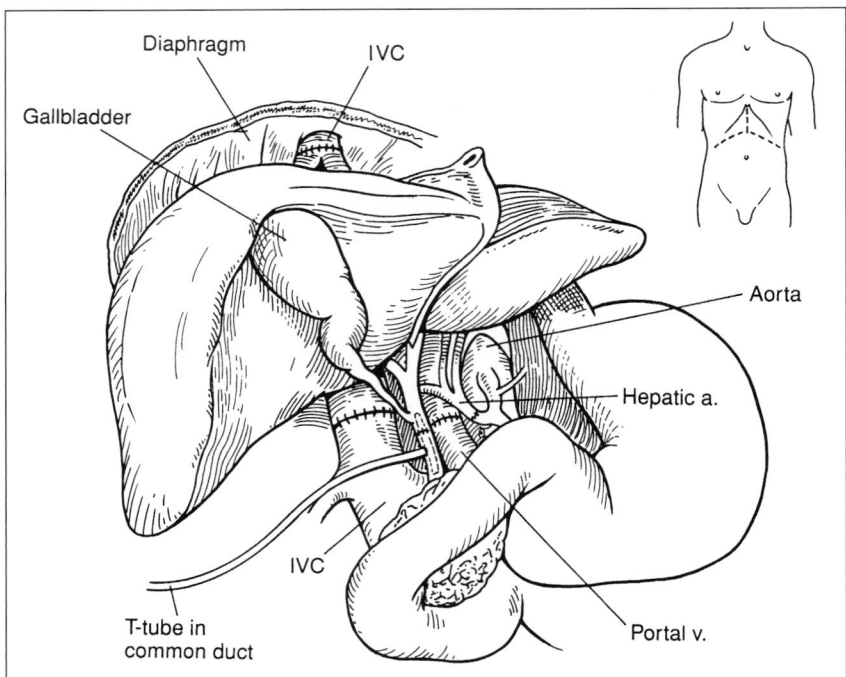

Figure 7.12-7. Liver transplantation. Anastomoses—including suprahepatic and infrahepatic IVC, portal vein, hepatic artery, and common bile duct—are complete as shown here. Roux-en-Y loop of small intestine is an alternative biliary drainage conduit. Inset shows a chevron incision with midline extension. (Reproduced with permission from Hardy JD: *Hardy's Textbook of Surgery*, 2nd edition. JB Lippincott, 1988.)

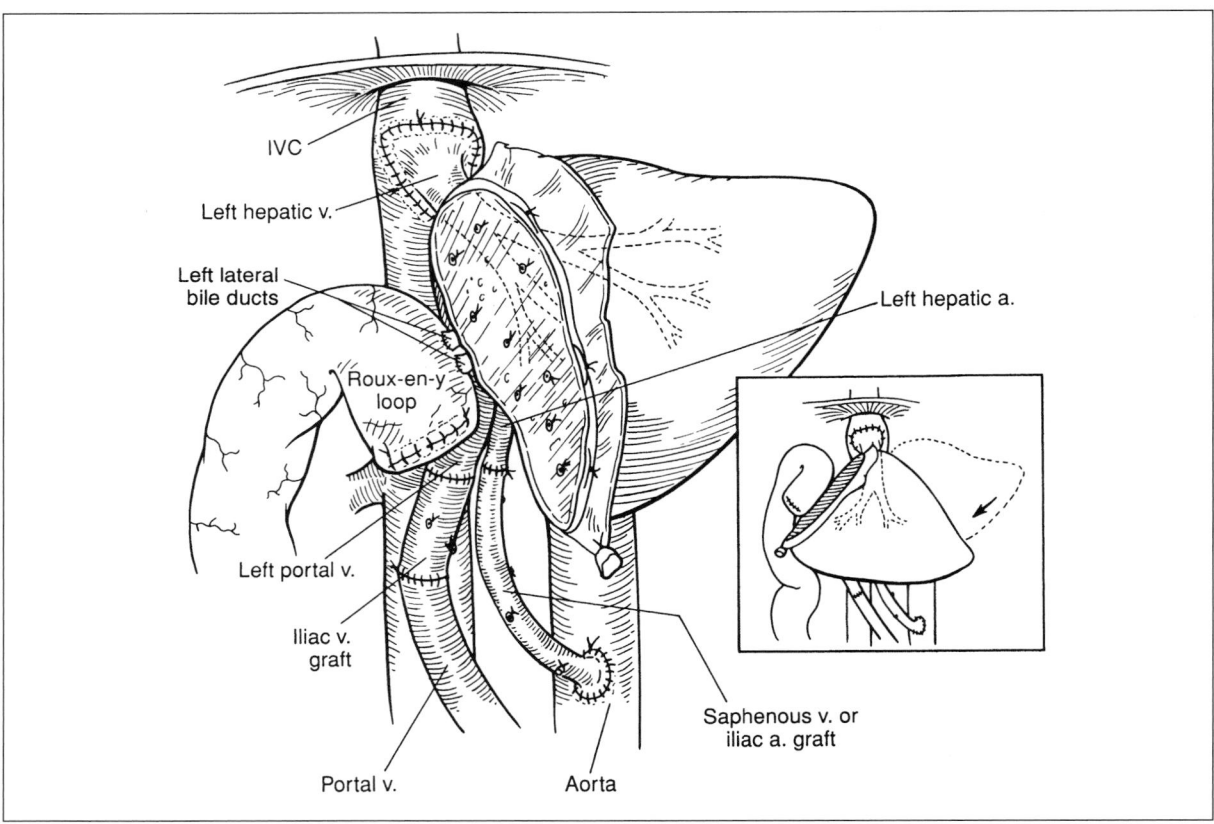

Figure 7.12-8. Liver transplantation (child) using left lateral segment from an adult liver. The hepatic artery and portal vein are extended with donor iliac artery and vein, respectively. The final position of the graft is shown (inset). A Roux-en-Y loop of small intestine is used to drain the bile duct(s). The IVC is left intact. The cut surface of the liver can bleed excessively if CVP is too high. (Reproduced with permission from Broelsch CE, et al: Liver transplantation in children from living related donors: surgical techniques and results. *Ann Surg* 1991; 214(4):432.)

ANESTHETIC CONSIDERATIONS

PREOPERATIVE

Patients presenting for liver transplantation represent a formidable challenge to the anesthesiologist. Frequently, these patients present for surgery with multiorgan system failure. Due to the emergent nature of the surgery, there may be insufficient time available for the customary evaluation and correction of abnormalities in this patient population.

Respiratory

These patients are often hypoxic because of ascites, pleural effusions, atelectasis, V/Q mismatch, pulmonary AV shunting, or hepatopulmonary syndrome. As a result, they are usually tachypneic and have a respiratory alkalosis. Evidence of pulmonary infection is usually a contraindication to surgery, but ARDS that may occur with hepatic failure is not.

Tests: ABG; PFT, as indicated. CXR: ✓ infection, effusions, atelectasis.

Cardiovascular

These patients demonstrate a hyperdynamic state with ↑plasma volume, ↑CO, and ↓SVR 2° arteriolar vasodilation in the splanchnic circulation, with intense vasoconstriction in other vascular territories (e.g., renal, brain, muscle, spleen). This inefficient circulatory state is manifested by a high SO_2. The SVR usually is not responsive to α-agents. AV fistulae may occur across the pulmonary circulation, so that precautions to prevent air embolism are important. Ejection fraction (EF) is usually high (> 60%), but some patients have cirrhotic cardiomyopathy → ↓contractility 2° ↓β-receptors, alterations in myocardial cell membrane properties, and ↑myocardial depressant substances. This cardiac dysfunction, however, usually is masked by a reduction in afterload. Pericardial effusions may be present, and should be drained at surgery. Many of these patients will have dysrhythmias, HTN, pulmonary HTN (very high risk), valvular disease, cardiomyopathy (alcoholic disease, hemochromatosis, Wilson's disease), and CAD. These patients will require appropriate preop consultation and workup.

Tests: ECG; ECHO: ✓ EF, contractility, pulmonary HTN, wall motion abnormalities, valve problems. If abnormal, consider a persantine thallium scan and/or right- and left-heart catheterization with coronary artery angiography.

Neurological

Patients are often encephalopathic and may be in hepatic coma; however, other organic causes of coma should be ruled out. In fulminant hepatic failure, ↑ICP is common, accounting for 40% of mortality (herniation), and may require prompt treatment (mannitol, hyperventilation, etc.).

Tests: Continuous ICP monitoring in fulminant hepatic failure

Hepatic

Hepatitis serology and the cause of hepatic failure should be determined. Vascular abnormalities, previous RUQ surgery or portal-vein decompressive surgery places the patient in a high-risk group. Albumin usually low, with consequent low plasma oncotic pressure → edema, ascites. The magnitude and duration of drug effects may be unpredictable, but, generally, these patients have ↑sensitivity to all drugs and their actions are prolonged.

Tests: Bilirubin; PT; ammonia level; SGOT; SGPT; albumin

Gastrointestinal

Portal HTN, esophageal varices, and coagulopathies ↑ risk of GI hemorrhage. Gastric emptying is often slow and, together with the emergent nature of this surgery, warrants rapid-sequence induction (see p. B-5). H_2-antagonists are indicated preop.

Renal

↓renal function, especially in fulminant hepatic failure (hepatorenal syndrome). The kidneys often recover after transplantation, but simultaneous kidney transplantation may be justified. These patients are often hypervolemic, hyponatremic, and possibly hypokalemic. Ca^{++} is usually normal. Metabolic alkalosis may be present. Consider preop dialysis and intraop continuous AV hemofiltration. Low-dose dopamine (2-4 μg/kg/min) and/or mannitol (0.5-1 g/kg) often are used intraop to maintain renal function.

Tests: BUN; Cr, creatinine clearance; electrolytes; ABG

Endocrine

Patients often glucose-intolerant or frankly diabetic, although acute hypoglycemia may be seen in acute hepatic failure. Hyperaldosteronism may be present.

Tests: Glucose; electrolytes

Hematologic

These patients are often anemic 2° either blood loss or malabsorption. Coagulation is impaired because of ↓hepatic synthetic function (all factors except VIII and fibrinogen are ↓), abnormal fibrinogen production, ↓/impaired Plt, fibrinolysis, and low-grade DIC.

Tests: PT; PTT; Plt count; bleeding time; fibrinogen; fibrin-split products (FSP); TEG

Premedication	Low doses of benzodiazepines may be used judiciously, but often nothing is given prior to surgery. Usually good preop evaluation and discussion suffice. Intramuscular injection should be avoided. Full-stomach precautions are justified. Metoclopramide 10 mg iv, ranitidine 50 mg iv and Na citrate 0.3 M 30 ml po should be given prior to surgery.

INTRAOPERATIVE

Anesthetic technique: GETA. These patients are extremely complex to manage because of the hemodynamic instability, massive blood loss, coagulopathy, and metabolic problems. It is convenient to divide the operation into three stages: preanhepatic, anhepatic and neohepatic (discussed below).

Induction	Often, a narcotic (e.g., fentanyl 2-5 μg/kg) is given just before induction; and rapid-sequence induction is preferred. STP (3-5 mg/kg) or etomidate (0.3 mg/kg) with succinylcholine (1-2 mg/kg), together with cricoid pressure.
Maintenance	Standard maintenance (see p. B-3) with fentanyl 10-50 μg/kg. A benzodiazepine (e.g., midazolam 0.1-0.3 μg/kg or scopalamine) often is given to ensure amnesia during periods of hemodynamic instability when the volatile agent may need to be off. N_2O is avoided because of bowel distention and possible air embolism. Ventilation with $FiO_2 > 0.5$ and $PaCO_2 = \sim 35$ mmHg. Occasionally, PEEP (5 cm H_2O) is added. Antibiotics and immunosuppressants should be given per surgeon's direction. Muscle relaxation usually is maintained with vecuronium.
Preanhepatic phase	The **preanhepatic phase** starts at skin incision and ends with removal of the recipient liver. Pleural and pericardial effusions are drained, which may improve oxygenation. Hyperglycemia is common during this period. A drop in filling pressures may be 2° hemorrhage or vascular compression. Hemorrhage can be severe 2° portal HTN. Coagulation problems usually increase during this stage, although fibrinolysis is not usually a problem. Blood loss replacement is accomplished with blood (PRBC) and FFP. Cryoprecipitate and Plts are given as needed, but a hypercoaguable state should be avoided, particularly if venovenous bypass is contemplated. Hemodynamic instability is not uncommon during the hepatic vascular dissection 2° manipulation of the liver and ↓venous return.
	Venovenous bypass relieves most of the complications of portal and IVC cross-clamping (↓venous return, low CO, tachycardia, acidosis, ↓renal function, intestinal swelling.) Blood is pumped from the femoral vein and the portal system (either portal vein or inferior mesenteric) via a centrifugal pump to the left axillary or subclavian vein. Generally, no heparin is used, but heparin-bonded cannulas and tubing are used. Bypass flows need to be at least 1 L/min to avoid possible thromboembolism. Bypass flow depends on venous inflow and is drawn into the pump by negative pressure. Low flows may be caused by hypovolemia or obstructed cannulae. Complications include unexpected decannulation, thromboembolism, and air embolism, all of which may need rapid termination of bypass and treatment of ↓BP; fibrinolysis is seen with prolonged venovenous bypass.
	Massive blood transfusion is associated with ↓Ca^{++}, and replacement is usually needed (± 500 mg/1000 ml of blood/FFP/plasmalyte mixture). If hyperkalemia occurs, it should be treated aggressively. Metabolic acidosis > 5 mEq/L should be treated with bicarbonate. Occasionally, inotropic support is needed, but α-adregenic agents should be avoided because of ↓renal and peripheral perfusion. UO needs to be maintained by ensuring adequate intravascular volume; occasionally, low-dose dopamine and/or mannitol may be needed.
Anhepatic phase	The **anhepatic phase** begins with clamping of the hepatic vessels and vena cava and removal of the liver; it ends with the reperfusion of the donor liver. Problems during this period include hemorrhage, increasing coagulopathy and fibrinolysis, acidosis, hypothermia, and ↓renal function. The hemodynamic instability associated with clamping of the hepatic vessels and the congestion of the bowel that occurs can be decreased by venovenous bypass (see above). Care should be taken to maintain intravascular volume, while avoiding volume overload, since this would worsen fluid overloading on reperfusion. At the completion of vena caval anastomoses, the liver is flushed via the portal vein to remove air, preservation fluid, and metabolites. Reperfusion may take place after completion of the portal vein anastomosis or after both portal vein and hepatic artery anastomoses are completed. As in the preanhepatic phase, acidosis, ↓Ca^{++}, glucose, coagulation, and other electrolyte abnormalities should be treated. Fibrinolysis usually starts in this period, but is not usually treated unless severe, because of the potential for embolism during venovenous bypass.
Neohepatic phase	The **neohepatic phase** begins with the unclamping of the portal vein, hepatic artery, and vena cava and reperfusion of the donor liver. Preparation for this phase is important because this may be a

Neohepatic phase, cont.	period of great hemodynamic instability. Before removal of the clamps, acidosis should be corrected, ionized Ca^{++} should be normal, and K^+ should be < 4.5 mEq/L. $CaCl_2$, $NaHCO_3$, and epinephrine should be readily available. Fluid overload prior to declamping should be avoided. High venous filling pressures decrease hepatic perfusion, especially prior to hepatic artery anastomosis. Declamping can be attended by ↓BP, ↓HR, dysrhythmias, hypothermia, lactic acidosis, coagulopathy, hyperglycemia, and thromboembolism.	
Reperfusion syndrome	**The 'reperfusion syndrome'** (which can occur in this phase) is characterized by ↓HR, ↓BP (30% of patients develop MAP < 70% of baseline), conduction defects, and ↓SVR in the face of acutely ↑RV filling pressures. Cause unknown. A rapid ↑K^+ can → cardiac arrest. (Rx: ensure normal pH and electrolytes prior to unclamping; rapid therapy when it occurs.) ↓BP and ↓HR are treated with epinephrine (10 μg increments), while $CaCl_2$ and $NaHCO_3$ are used to correct hyperkalemia and acidosis. Pulmonary edema may occur as a result of fluid overload and can be treated with diuretics, inotropes, and phlebotomy. A high venous pressure will cause graft congestion and should be avoided. Reperfusion is associated with severe coagulopathy due to fibrinolysis (usually primary), release of heparin, and hypothermia. As liver function returns, there should be an improvement in coagulation, acid-base status (metabolic alkalosis may occur), ↓lactic acidosis, return of glucose to normal, and bile production. Hypokalemia may occur 2° uptake by the liver. Graft failure is associated with coagulopathy, ↑lactic acid, citrate intoxication, hyperglycemia, and ↓bile formation.	
Emergence	Extubation is deferred to ICU, with patient intubated and ventilated. These patients generally are ventilated postop until they are stable and able to be weaned from ventilatory support. Apart from the usual tests, hepatic function needs to be monitored, immunosuppression provided, infection controlled, analgesia ensured (usually fentanyl), and peptic ulcer prophylaxis given (ranitidine preferred).	
Blood and fluid requirements	Massive blood loss IV: 10 Fr × 2 Plasmalyte A or Normasol UO >1 ml/kg/h Warm all fluids. Humidify gases. Rapid-infusion system Cell Saver 20 U PRBC 20 U FFP 20 U PLT	Generally, ivs are placed in the right antecubital fossa, left or right IJ or EJ. The left arm is avoided because the axillary or subclavian vein is used for venovenous bypass. Plasmalyte A or Normasol are preferred (absence of glucose, Ca^{++}, and lower Na^+ content) over NS/LR. Hypernatremia can be a problem due to administration of $NaHCO_3$. The ability to give up to 1.5 L/min of blood should be available. Usually a mixture of Normasol (250 ml), PRBC (1 U), and FFP (1 U) is used, yielding Hct = 26-30%. Actual blood loss estimation is extremely difficult, and usually replacement is judged by hemodynamic status, UO, and S_vO_2. Cell Savers are used to conserve blood. Anticoagulation is with a citrate solution to avoid heparin contamination, and cells are washed with Normasol/Plasmalyte A. D/C use before biliary reconstruction (infection) or in neoplasms, hepatitis B, or spontaneous bacterial peritonitis.
Monitoring	Standard monitors (see p. B-1). ECG (5-lead) Temp-bladder ETN_2 Arterial line(s) PA catheter/S_vO_2/CO	Include 5-lead ECG and bladder T. (These patients sustain significant heat loss.) A full-time anesthesia technologist and lab/blood bank runner are useful. Lab and blood bank should be notified of the expected transplant. An automated data acquisition system also is useful, since there are times during the case when the record may be neglected in favor of working with the patient. One or two arterial lines are placed at the outset—one in the right radial, for ongoing lab and blood gas sampling, with 1 port being designated as heparin-free; another line, in the right femoral artery is utilized for continuous pressure measurement. All flush solutions contain citrate for anticoagulation to avoid heparin contamination. A PA catheter is essential for management of hemodynamics in these patients because of the rapid changes in VS. A catheter capable of measuring mixed-venous O_2

Monitoring, cont.		sat is very useful, as it gives early clues to impending decompensation. Coagulopathy complicates the placement of central lines, and the use of ultrasound-guidance is recommended.
	TEE	TEE is useful to monitor cardiac filling and function and to diagnose problems such as PE or air embolism. Care needs to be taken in placing the TEE, since many of these patients have esophageal varices.
	ICP	ICP should be measured in patients with fulminant hepatic failure if ↑ICP is a concern.
		ABG, acid base status, electrolyte, lactate, osmolality, Ca^{++}, PT, PTT, Plt, Hct—all should be monitored on a regular basis (hourly or half-hourly; occasionally, more frequently).
	Thromboelastograph (TEG)	TEG is useful for monitoring coagulation (see discussion of coagulation management, below).
Coagulation management	PT PTT Plt counts Fibrinogen FSP	Patients are prone to a variety of coagulopathies (↓Plt, ↓coagulation factors, DIC, fibrinolysis, etc.) because of preop factors, massive hemorrhage, anhepatic period, and reperfusion of the new liver; therefore, monitoring and treatment are necessary. Also, states of hypercoagulopathy need to be avoided because of unheparinized venovenous bypass.
	TEG	While PT, PTT, Plt counts, fibrinogen, and FSP may provide relevant information, they may not reflect the true coagulability of patient's blood, and tend to take considerable time to perform. Thus, in some centers, TEG has gained in popularity. It measures whole blood coagulability, not specific factors. TEG works by measuring viscoelastic properties of blood as it forms clot (fibrin connections) between a rotating cuvette and a spindle. Characteristic patterns are formed by the various coagulopathies with the common types shown in Fig 7.12-9.
		Evaluation of the TEG leads to more rational transfusion therapy, reducing the number of U of blood/blood products used. Comparing specimens of native whole blood vs blood mixed with EACA or protamine can guide pharmacologic therapy of coagulopathies. Table 7.12-3 gives specific recommendations.
Positioning	✓ and pad pressure points. ✓ eyes.	Table and arm boards should be very well padded. Head should be placed on a foam rest. Particular care should be taken to pad the retractor supports where they may impinge on the arms and on the radial nerve as it curls around the humerus.
Temperature control	Warming blanket Humidifier	Patient's arms, head, and legs should be wrapped in plastic to protect against heat loss. Plastic drapes and the use of a cesarian section-type drape to protect the ECG electrodes and direct fluid flow off the table are useful to prevent the patient from lying in a pool of fluid. A warming blanket under the patient and over the lower legs is very useful.
Complications	Coagulopathy Hemorrhage Air embolism RV failure Metabolic acidosis	

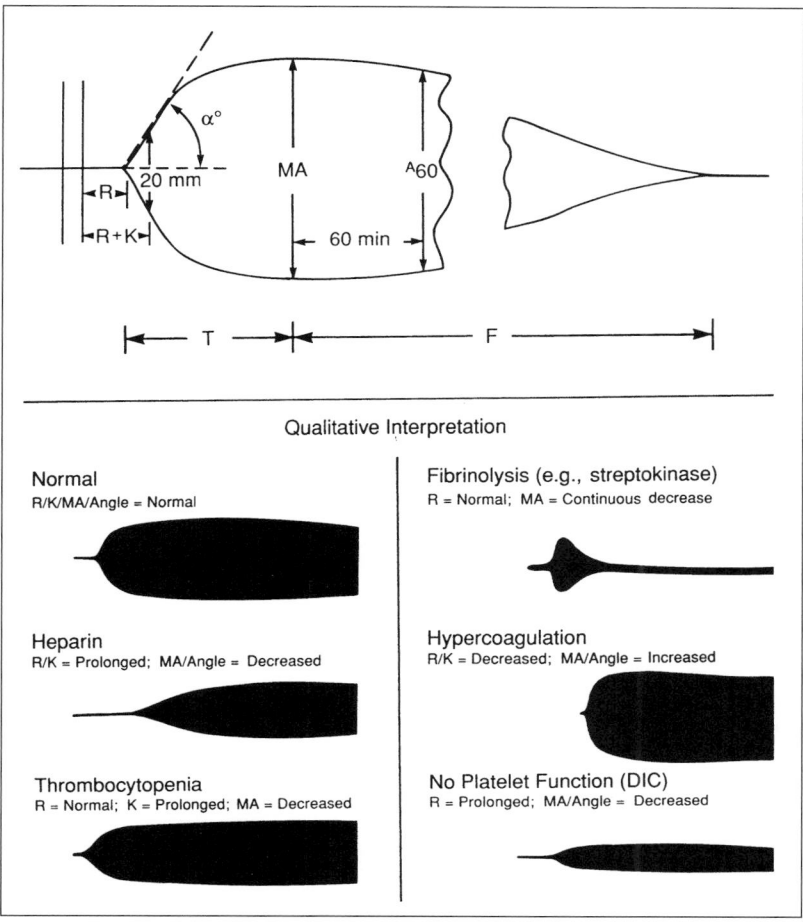

Qualitative Interpretation

Normal
R/K/MA/Angle = Normal

Heparin
R/K = Prolonged; MA/Angle = Decreased

Thrombocytopenia
R = Normal; K = Prolonged; MA = Decreased

Fibrinolysis (e.g., streptokinase)
R = Normal; MA = Continuous decrease

Hypercoagulation
R/K = Decreased; MA/Angle = Increased

No Platelet Function (DIC)
R = Prolonged; MA/Angle = Decreased

Figure 7.12-9. Variables and normal values measured by TEG:

R = reaction time, 6-8 min

R + k = coagulation time, 10-12 min

α = clot formation rate, > 50°

MA = maximum amplitude, 50-70 mm

A_{60} = amplitude 60 min after MA

A_{60}/MA-100 = whole blood clot lysis index, > 85%

F = whole blood clot lysis time, > 300 min

(Reproduced with permission from Kang YG, et al: Intraoperative changes in blood coagulation and thromboelastographic monitoring in liver transplantation. *Anesth Analg* 1985; 64:891.)

POSTOPERATIVE

Monitoring of hepatic function	Serial LFTs PT, PTT Ammonia level Lactate TEG Bile output	Initial LFTs often show very high liver enzymes, which subside over a period of days. PT generally improves to normal levels, while lactic acidosis usually corrects quickly. Often a metabolic alkalosis follows and may need HCl treatment.
Complications	Bleeding Partial vein thrombosis Hepatic artery thrombosis Biliary tract leaks Primary nonfunction Rejection Infection Pulmonary complication HTN Electrolyte abnormalities (hypokalemia, $\downarrow Ca^{++}$, $\uparrow Na$) Alkalosis Renal failure Peptic ulceration Neurologic	This is not a complete list. Feared complications that may → graft loss include portal vein thrombosis, hepatic artery thrombosis, bile leaks, and rejection. These are attended by ↑LFTs, lactic acidosis, coagulopathy, hypoglycemia, ↓renal function, and poor bile formation.

Table 7.12-3. Coagulation Therapy Guided by TEG Monitoring[6]

1. Maintenance fluid
   RBC: FFP: Plasmalyte A = 300:200:250 ml
2. Replacement therapy
   a. FFP (2 U) for prolonged reaction time (R > 15 min)
   b. Plt (10 U) for small MA (MA < 40 mm)
   c. Cryoprecipitate (6-12 U) for persistent slow-clot formation rate ($\alpha < 40°$) with normal MA
3. Pharmacologic therapy
   a. Compare coagulability of whole blood, blood treated with protamine sulfate, and blood treated with epsilon aminocaproic acid.
   b. Epsilon aminocaproic acid (1 g) for severe fibrinolysis (F < 60 min)
   c. Protamine sulfate (50 mg) for severe heparin effect
   d. Heparin (1000-2000 U) for hypercoagulable state

References for Liver Transplantation

1. Carmicheal FJ, Lindop MJ, Farman JV: Anesthesia for hepatic transplantation: cardiovascular and metabolic alterations and their management. *Anesth Analg* 1985; 64(2):108-16.
2. Carton EG, Rettke SR, Plevak, et al: Perioperative care of the liver transplant patient. Parts I & II. *Anesth Analg* 1994; 78: 120-33, 382-99.
3. Casavilla A, Gordon RD, Starzl TE: Techniques of liver transplantation. In *Surgery of the Liver and Biliary Tract*. Blumgart LH, Fong Y, eds. Churchill Livingstone, New York: 2000, 2155-80.
4. Gelman S, Kang YG, Pearson JD: Anesthetic consideration in liver transplantation. In *Anesthesia for Organ Transplantation*. Fabian JA, ed. JB Lippincott, Philadelphia: 1992, 115-39.
5. Grande L, Rimola A, Cugat E, Alvarez L, Garcia-Valdecasas JC, Taura P, et al: Effect of venovenous bypass on perioperative renal function in liver transplantation: results of a randomized controlled trial. *Hepatology* 1996; 23:1418-28.
6. Kang YG: Anesthesia for liver transplantation. *Anes Clin North Am* 1989; 7(3):507.
7. Kang YG, Lewis JH, Navalgund A, Russell MW, Bontempo FA, Niren LS, Starzl TE: Epsilon-aminocaproic acid for treatment of fibrinolysis during liver transplantation. *Anesthesiology* 1987; 66(6):766-73.
8. Kang YG, Martin DJ, Marguez J, Lewis JH, Bontempo FA, Shaw BW Jr, Starzl TE, Winter PM: Intraoperative changes in blood coagulation and thromboelastic monitoring in liver transplantation. *Anesth Analg* 1985; 64(9):888-96.
9. Kutt JL, Mezon BR: Anesthesia and liver transplantation. *Anesth Clin North Am* 1994; 12(4):717-28.
10. Jawan B, Cheung HK, Lee JH: Anesthesia for living related donor liver transplantation. *Transplant Proc* 1996; 28(4):2409-11.
11. Nakazato PZ, Concepcion W, Bry W, Limm W, Tokunaga Y, Itasaka H, et al: Total abdominal evisceration: an en bloc technique for abdominal organ harvesting. *Surgery* 1992; 111:37-47.
12. Ozaki CF, Katz SM, Monsour HP, et al: Surgical complications of liver transplantation. *Surg Clin North Am* 1994; 74(5): 1155-67.
13. Paulsen AW, Whitten CW, Ramsay MA, Klintmalm GB: Considerations for anesthetic management during veno-venous bypass in adult hepatic transplantation. *Anesth Analg* 1989; 68(4):489-96.
14. Ramsey MAE: Anesthesia for liver transplantation. In *Transplantation of the Liver*. Busuttil RW, Klintmalm GB, eds. WB Saunders, Philadelphia: 1996, 419-33.
15. Shaw BW, Martin DJ, Marquez JM, Kang YG, Bugbee AC, Iwatsuki S, et al: Venous bypass in clinical liver transplantation. *Ann Surg* 1984; 200:524-34.
16. Starzl TE, Demetris AJ: Liver transplantation: a 31-year perspective, Part III. *Curr Probl Surg* 1990; 27:181-240.
17. Starzl TE, Iwatsuki S, Esquivel CO, Todo S, Kam I, Lynch S, et al: Refinements in the surgical technique of liver transplantation. *Semin Liver Dis* 1985; 5:349-59.
18. Washburn WK, Lewis WD, Jenkins RL: Percutaneous venovenous bypass in orthotopic liver transplantation. *Live Transpl Surg* 1995; 1(6):377-82.

LIVING-DONOR LIVER TRANSPLANTATION

SURGICAL CONSIDERATIONS

Description: The success of cadaveric liver transplantation has resulted in an ever-increasing number of patients with end stage liver disease (ESLD) waiting for transplantation; however, the number of cadaveric donors has remained relatively constant. Consequently, the waiting time to receive an organ has increased significantly, and ~1/4 patients will die while waiting. The success of **living-donor renal transplantation,** coupled with the experience in adult-to-pediatric living-donor liver transplantation, as well as advances in surgical and postsurgical care of patients undergoing major liver resections, has lead to the implementation of adult-to-adult living-donor liver transplantation.[1,5] This provides a potentially larger source of healthy livers for transplantation.

Potential liver donors undergo extensive medical and psychosocial evaluation to ensure psychological as well as physical fitness to undergo a major surgical procedure with no medical benefits to the donor. Donors must have full blood typing to ensure compatibility with the recipient, and then fill out an extensive medical questionnaire, followed by a complete physical exam and screening lab tests. Any evidence of diabetes, HTN, or renal, pulmonary, cardiovascular, or hepatic abnormalities usually is a contraindication to donation. Once the potential donor is medically and psychosocially cleared, they undergo a detailed imaging study of the liver; and, if there are no anatomical contraindications, then an elective living-donor transplant is scheduled.[3]

The donor and recipient operations usually are conducted simultaneously to minimize the ischemic injury to the donor liver segment. The donor operation, however, is initiated first, with the recipient operation started only after the donor liver has been inspected intraop and no barriers to proceeding are found. The donor operation is similar to either a right or left hepatic lobectomy, although there are some differences that can have a significant impact on anesthetic management, as detailed below.

The donor may elect to have an epidural catheter for postop analgesia, and this usually is placed before surgery. A vertical midline incision is made from the xiphoid to just above the umbilicus and extended transversely to the right anterior axillary line. Occasionally, bisubcostal incisions are required. Following exploration of the abdomen, intraop ultrasound may be performed to map the hepatic venous anatomy so the plane of dissection can be delineated. Additionally, an intraop cholangiogram is performed via the cystic duct (a cholecystecomy is performed in a right or left hepatic lobectomy) or the common bile duct, to define the biliary anatomy. Once this is performed, the corresponding portal vein and hepatic artery are isolated. Unlike in a hepatic lobectomy for tumor, the venous and arterial inflow to the liver segment are not ligated; thus, the transaction of the liver parenchyma may → significant hemorrhage. Next, the respective lobe of the liver is mobilized from its attachments, and the liver is dissected from the retrohepatic vena cava, with the short-hepatic veins being ligated. This maneuver can → ↓BP 2° torque and compression of the IVC and hepatic veins, as well as potential bleeding from the vena cava itself. Next, the hepatic vein is isolated, and the liver can be divided, which may be a slow and tedious process. Once the parenchyma is divided, the liver segment is ready to be removed. Heparin (80-100 U/kg) is given to prevent intrahepatic clot formation. Following heparinization, the hepatic artery and portal vein are ligated and divided, followed by the hepatic vein. The donated hepatic lobe is immediately placed in ice and flushed with Viaspan preservation solution. Once the donated liver segment is flushed, the recipient's hepatic vein stump is oversewn and the abdomen and cut surface of the remaining liver are inspected for hemostasis and bile leak. Closed drains are placed, after which the abdomen is closed. Essentially, the same procedure is followed for a left lateral segmentectomy (adult-to-child), except that the extent of liver resection is about 25%, compared with 40% or 60% for a left or right lobectomy, respecively.

Usual preop diagnosis: Healthy, living liver donor

SUMMARY OF PROCEDURE

Position	Supine; arms tucked
Incision	Vertical midline with a right and/or left subcostal extension, depending on liver segment being utilized
Special instrumentation	Retractor; ultrasonic aspirator; irrigating bipolar cautery; argon beam coagulator; Cell Saver; rapid-infusion system
Unique considerations	Intraop cholangiogram and/or ultrasound. Hemodilution immediately before surgery, with removal of 1 U whole blood if Hct ≥ 40. Patients also may have donated 1-2 U of autologous blood. Heparin (80-100 U/kg).
Antibiotics	Ampicillin 1 g and ceftriaxone 1 g before skin incision
Surgical time	3-5 hr
EBL	250-500 ml
Postop care	ICU overnight or surgical floor. Hospital stay 5-7 d.

Mortality	7 deaths reported world-wide (as of December 2002) following ~1000 donor operations.
Morbidity	Infectious complications: 3%
	Biliary leak: 1%
	Reoperation: 3-5%
	Acute hepatic failure: < 0.1%
Pain score	7-9

PATIENT POPULATION CHARACTERISTICS

Age range	8-55 yr
Male:Female	1:1
Incidence	Uncommon

ANESTHETIC CONSIDERATIONS

See Anesthesia for Hepatic Resection, p. 442.

References

1. Broelsch CE, Emond JC, Whitington F, et al: Application of reduced size liver transplants as split grafts, auxiliary orthotopic grafts and living related segmental transplants. *Ann Surg* 1990; 212:368-75.
2. Everhart JE, Lombardero M, Detre KM, et al: Increased waiting time for liver transplantation results in higher mortality. *Transplantation* 1997; 64(9):1300-06.
3. Singer PA, Siegler M, Whitington PF, et al: Ethics of liver transplantation with living donors. *N Eng J Med* 1989; 321:620-2.
4. Strong RW, Lynch SV: Live related donors in liver transplantation. In *Surgery of the Liver and Biliary Tract*. Blumgart LH, Fong Y, eds. Churchill Livingstone, New York: 2000, 2129-40.
5. Strong RW, Lynch SV, Ong TH, Matsunami H, Koido Y, Balderson GA: Successful liver transplantation from a living donor to her son. *N Eng J Med* 1990; 322:1505-07.

MULTIORGAN PROCUREMENT

SURGICAL CONSIDERATIONS

Description: The families of brain-dead patients may allow donation of the patient's functioning organs—which may include, but is not limited to, heart, lungs, liver, kidneys, pancreas, and small intestine. The process of organ procurement can be chaotic, with multiple operative teams and technicians working simultaneously. Moreover, brain-dead patients tend to be hemodynamically unstable, sometimes requiring multiple pressors, and the possibility of acute decompensation is ever present.

The donor patient's chest and abdomen are opened in the midline from sternal notch to pubis (Fig 7.12-10). The chest is opened with a sternal saw and generally an extra-large Balfour retractor is used to widely retract the abdomen. The aorta and IVC are dissected first to allow rapid placement of a flush line in the event that the patient experiences a cardiovascular collapse. Following this, the liver vasculature is identified in the hepatoduodenal ligament and is dissected out. This part of the procedure generally takes about 1.5 h. In cases where the pancreas is procured, an additional 45-60 min is required for mobilization of the pancreas. During pancreas procurement, a Betadine/amphotericin B solution is administered through an NG tube into the stomach and duodenum. A total of about 300-500 ml of the Betadine solution is passed in two divided aliquots. Once the heart, liver, pancreas, and kidneys have been mobilized, the supraceliac aorta just below the diaphragm is dissected for placement of the aortic cross-clamp. Immediately before cross-clamping, 30,000 U of heparin (300 U/kg) is given systemically, with the α-antagonist phentolamine in some cases. The supraceliac aorta is then clamped and the organs are perfused with Viaspan, a hyperosmotic and hyperkalemic solution containing insulin, glucose, and reducing agents. At this point, the ventilator can be turned off, except in cases where the lungs are being procured. In this case, the lungs must be inflated with 100% O_2 just before removal. The heart is the first organ to be removed, followed by the lungs.

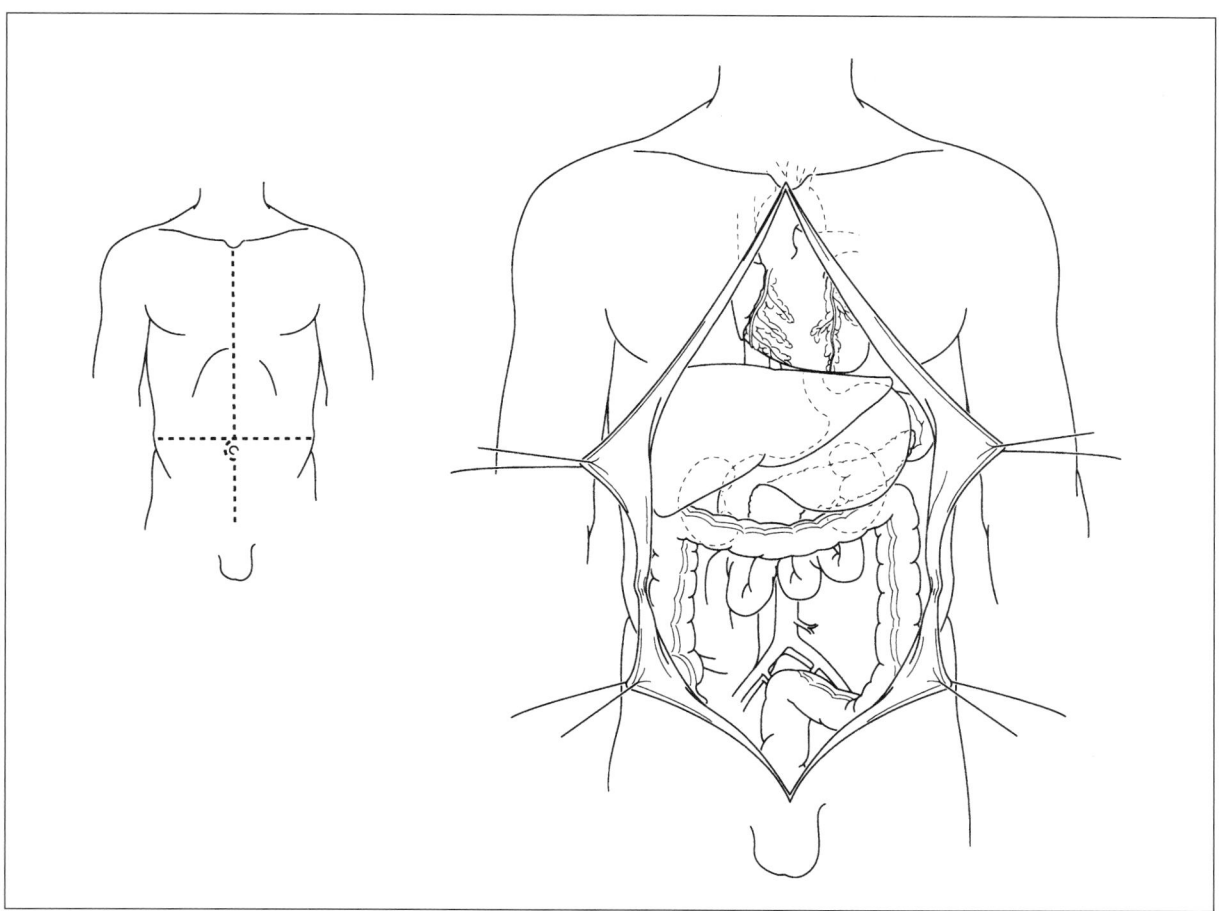

Figure 7.12-10. A complete midline incision, from suprasternal notch to pubis, is made for multiple organ procurement; and the sternum is split. If necessary, cruciate abdominal incisions are added to facilitate exposure of the intraabdominal organs. (Reproduced with permission from Greenfield LJ, et al, eds: *Surgery: Scientific Principles and Practice*, 3rd edition. Lippincott Williams & Wilkins, 2001.)

If the lungs are procured, an extra 20-30 min of perfusion time is required. After removal of the heart and/or lungs, the liver can be removed, followed by the pancreas, small intestines, and kidneys. After the organs are removed, spleen and lymph nodes for tissue typing are obtained from the abdominal and thoracic cavities; and, because of the possible need for vascular reconstruction in the recipients, bilateral iliac veins and arteries are removed. The total time for multiorgan procurement is ~4 h, although the anesthesia time typically ends with aortic cross-clamping.

Variant procedures: During the **'rapid-flush' technique** used by some procurement teams, the dissection of individual abdominal organs is minimized and an en bloc resection is done after clamping the aorta below the diaphragm and flushing preservation solution through the distal aorta. The en bloc organs are then dissected ex vivo, often at the transplant center, in preparation for transplantation. This technique is more rapid, requiring only about 1.5 h.

A second variant procedure, developed in response to the chronic shortage of transplantable organs, is the use of non-heart-beating donors. Patients, who are not brain-dead, but who have no hope of recovery (due to irreversible brain injury or pulmonary or cardiac failure), may be suitable donors. In this case, the patient is taken to the OR and, under the supervision of a physician who is not part of the transplant team, the life-sustaining treatment (e.g., pressors, ventilator) is D/C'd. When it has been determined that the donor has suffered cardiac death, the body is rapidly cooled with Viaspan through a cannula that is located in the aorta at the level of the renal arteries. Depending on the regional regulations, this cannula may be placed before cardiac death, or immediately following the declaration of cardiac death. Once the preservative flush is initiated, the abdomen is entered as rapidly as possible and the peritoneal cavity is packed with ice and the organs are removed expeditiously. The anesthesiologist's role is ended when cardiac death has been declared. The disadvantage of this approach is that there can be significant warm ischemia from the time the life-sustaining treatment is stopped to the time that cardiac death is reached.

Usual preop diagnosis: Brain death

SUMMARY OF PROCEDURE

Position	Supine
Incision	Midline only, neck to pubis, ± bilateral transverse extensions
Special instrumentation	Chest and abdominal retractors
Unique considerations	Maintain oxygenation and BP as if live patient. May require pressors and/or blood transfusion. Temporarily deflate lungs for sternal sawing.
Antibiotics	Ampicillin (1 g iv), ceftriaxone (1 g iv); Betadine via NG tube for pancreas (with duodenal segment) procurement. Heparin, relative. (Betadine/Amphotericin in B solution)
Surgical time	4 h; rapid-flush technique: 1.5 h
EBL	200 ml

PATIENT POPULATION CHARACTERISTICS

Age range	Neonate–70 yr
Male:Female	N/A
Incidence	Approximately 5000/yr in U.S.
Etiology	Usually head trauma (e.g., motor vehicle accidents, gunshot wounds to the head) or intracranial bleeding
Associated conditions	Vasomotor instability; diabetes insipidus (DI); intracranial HTN

ANESTHETIC CONSIDERATIONS

PREOPERATIVE

In general, organ donors are previously healthy individuals who have suffered catastrophic, irreversible brain injury of known etiology, most commonly due to blunt head trauma, penetrating head injury, or intracranial hemorrhage. A declaration of brain death by physicians not participating in the organ procurement must be documented. This documentation, together with certification of death and familial consent, should be verified by the anesthesiologist before organ procurement. The United Network for Organ Sharing (UNOS) has produced *The Critical Pathway for the Organ Donor* to facilitate the administrative aspects of organ procurement (http://www.unos.org/resources/donorManagement.asp). There should be no evidence of disease or trauma involving the organs targeted for donation and, in general, the patient should be hemodynamically stable with minimal inotropic requirements. Once brain death has been declared, it is important to shift the emphasis away from cerebral resuscitation efforts and to focus instead on the maintenance of adequate tissue perfusion and oxygenation. Brain death is frequently followed by a series of pathophysiological events that may complicate the management of these patients.

Respiratory Pulmonary dysfunction following brain death has many possible etiologies: aspiration, atelectasis, pneumonia, and pulmonary edema. In addition, trauma may cause pulmonary dysfunction related to contusion, pneumothorax, or hemothorax. Meticulous pulmonary toilet is essential to prevent atelectasis and pneumonia. Maintenance of adequate oxygenation is requisite to ensure preservation of other organs for transplantation. Use mechanical ventilation with TVs of 10-12 ml/kg and a minute ventilation that maintains $PaCO_2$ 30-35 mmHg and pH 7.35-7.45. The FiO_2 should ensure a PaO_2 75-150 mmHg and arterial saturation > 95%. PEEP usually is applied at 3-5 cmH_2O and should not exceed 7.5 cmH_2O because of the deleterious effects on CO and regional blood flow, and possible barotrauma. The FiO_2 generally should be increased to 100% before transport to the OR. An important exception is in the case of heart-lung or lung retrieval, where it is important to maintain FiO_2 < 40% to minimize possible effects of O_2 toxicity. Ideally, PIP should be < 30 cmH_2O to minimize possible barotrauma to the lungs.

Tests: Frequent ABGs, including immediate preop period. Proper position of the ETT should be confirmed preop.

Cardiovascular Hypotension should be anticipated in all organ donors. This results most commonly from neurogenic shock (derangement of descending vasomotor control → progressive ↓SVR and venous pooling) and hypovolemia. Hypovolemia is usually the result of dehydration therapy for cerebral edema, hemorrhage, DI, or osmotic diuresis 2° hyperglycemia. Hypothermia, LV dysfunction, and endocrine abnormalities also can contribute to ↓BP. Fluid resuscitation with crystalloid, colloid, and PRBCs to maintain Hct > 30% should be initiated preop. Hemodynamic goals are: (1) CVP 10-12 cmH_2O

Cardiovascular, cont.	(6-8 cmH$_2$O if lungs are to be procured); (2) MAP between 60-100 mmHg; (3) SBP > 100 mmHg; (4) PCWP ≤ 12 mmHg; (5) SVR 800-1200 dyne/section; and (6) UO > 1 ml/kg/h. Donors are often placed on inotropic therapy to maintain these parameters; however, following adequate volume resuscitation, preop inotropic therapy often may be gradually decreased or D/C'd. If inotropic therapy remains necessary, typically it would consist of dopamine (2-10 μg/kg/min), followed by dobutamine (3-15 μg/kg/min) or epinephrine (0.1-1.0 μg/kg/min), then norepinephrine. The latter 3 agents may be combined with dopamine (2-3 μg/kg/min) in an attempt to augment or preserve renal, mesenteric, and coronary arterial blood flow. It should be noted that brain death may be accompanied initially by a transient hypertensive crisis that may require short-term treatment with SNP and/or esmolol. ECG abnormalities are common in patients with intracranial injury and are of no pathologic consequence. Atrial and ventricular dysrhythmias and various degrees of conduction block occur frequently in organ donors; the etiology may be electrolyte imbalance, ABG disturbance, ↑ICP, loss of the vagal motor nucleus, inotropic therapy, hypothermia, or myocardial contusions or ischemia. Antidysrhythmic therapy should follow the usual guidelines except for ↓HR, which is resistant to atropine in this setting. Bradycardia, if accompanied by ↓BP, should be treated with isoproterenol, dopamine, epinephrine, or temporary cardiac pacing. **Tests:** ECG; ECHO (to assess wall motion abnormalities) and possibly coronary angiography (if CAD is suspected).
Neurological	Diabetes insipidus (DI) frequently occurs in brain-dead donors; it is likely the result of destruction of the hypothalamic-pituitary axis. Untreated, it may cause marked hypovolemia and electrolyte disturbances (↑Na, ↑Mg, ↓K, ↓PO$_4$, ↓Ca). Therapy with iv vasopressin (titrated from 2 μg/kg/min) or DDAVP (titrated from 0.3 μg/kg/min) often is initiated to maintain UO < 1.5-3 ml/kg/h. Many believe that the benefits of minimizing electrolyte imbalance, fluid shifts, and reduction of core T outweigh the risks of vasopressin or desmopressin therapy, including coronary and renal vasoconstriction and possible organ ischemia or uneven distribution of the preservation solutions during flushing. It may be prudent, however, to D/C vasopressin or DDAVP infusions for at least 1 h prior to aortic cross-clamping and infusion of preservation solutions. Thermoregulation is abnormal in brain-dead donors due to hypothalamic dysfunction; and core T should be monitored (bladder, esophageal, or rectal). Aggressive warming techniques may have to be employed early to maintain a core T > 34-35°C, as there are numerous undesirable consequences of significant hypothermia (< 32°C) in the organ donor (e.g., cardiac dysrhythmia, cardiac instability, ↓GFR and cold diuresis, a left shift in the oxyhemoglobin dissociation curve, and pancreatitis). While other endocrine or metabolic disturbances may exist as a result of destruction of the hypothalamic-pituitary axis, currently there is no consistent recommendation for any other hormonal replacement therapy. **Tests:** Serum electrolytes and osmolality every 4 h
Hematologic	Donors may be anemic from hemodilution and/or hemorrhage. To ensure adequate tissue O$_2$ delivery, PRBCs are transfused to maintain Hct > 30. Some donors may exhibit a coagulopathy; clinically significant bleeding should be treated with clotting factors and Plts. Persistent or severe primary fibrinolysis or DIC may require rapid transfer of the donor to the OR for organ retrieval. Administration of epsilon-aminocaproic acid to treat fibrinolysis is avoided for fear of microvascular thrombosis in the donor organs. **Tests:** Hb/Hct; PT; PTT; Plt count; DIC screen as clinically indicated.
Other	The role of oxygen-free radicals, with regard to reperfusion injury, has prompted the suggested use of mannitol and steroids (and other compounds) as scavengers.

INTRAOPERATIVE

Anesthetic technique: Although anesthesia is unnecessary in brain-dead organ donors, both visceral and somatic reflexes can lead to physiologic responses during the procedure. The goals of intraop management with regard to respiratory, cardiovascular, hematologic, and neurologic status are identical to those discussed under preop considerations, above.

Induction	Settings for mechanical ventilation parallel those of the ICU, although it may be advisable to begin with an FiO$_2$ of 100% until the first ABG result is obtained. The exception is when procurement of the lungs or heart-lungs is anticipated; then FiO$_2$ should not exceed 40%. To eliminate reflex neuromuscular activity and to facilitate surgical retraction, a long-acting neuromuscular blocking agent, such as pancuronium or pipecuronium (0.15 mg/kg), should be given at the beginning of the procedure and supplemented as necessary.

Maintenance	Reflex hypertensive responses to surgical stimulation occur frequently and may → excessive intraop blood loss and damage to donor kidneys; management should include the weaning of vasopressors and the initiation of vasodilator therapy with isoflurane, SNP, or NTG. Anesthetic care continues until the proximal aortic cross-clamp is applied. D/C all monitoring and supportive therapy at this point. The notable exception is the case of heart-lung or lung procurement; in this situation, all monitoring except FiO_2 should cease with proximal aortic cross-clamping. All supportive care is terminated, with the exception of mechanical ventilation of the lungs at 4 breaths/min or as directed by the transplant team, and suctioning of the ETT after cessation of mechanical ventilation just prior to removal of the tube. Extubation marks the termination of anesthetic care of the heart-lung or lung donor.	
Blood and fluid requirements	IV: 14-16 ga × 1-2 NS/LR @ 2-4 ml/kg/h	Significant 3rd-space losses; may need to administer large volumes of crystalloid, colloid (up to 1 L) and PRBCs (not uncommon to transfuse 2 or more U to maintain Hct >30). Central venous access is necessary for monitoring and for vasoactive drug delivery.
Monitoring	Standard monitors (see p. B-1). Intraarterial BP CVP line UO	If a PA catheter is in place, it may be used or removed based on concerns of catheter-related, right-side endocardial lesions. Rarely is insertion of a PA catheter warranted in these operations. ABG, Hb/Hct, serum electrolytes, and glucose should be monitored hourly; for operations involving procurement of lungs or heart-lungs, ABGs should be obtained at least every 30 min.
Complications	↓BP	Most commonly 2° hypovolemia and neurogenic shock (loss of descending vasomotor control). Ensure adequate volume repletion as described above, then institute or increase inotropic/vasopressor therapy as previously outlined.
	Dysrhythmias	Multiple possible etiologies as described above. Standard treatment and diagnosis should be employed, with the exception of bradycardia, which is atropine-resistant and should be treated with isoproterenol, dopamine, epinephrine, or transvenous pacing.
	Cardiac arrest	CPR should be instituted in an effort to maintain the viability of the liver, kidneys, and other abdominal viscera intended for transplantation. Procurement of the liver and kidneys should proceed rapidly to aortic cross-clamping at the diaphragm and administration of cold preservation fluid into the aorta and portal vein. This series of events will undoubtedly preclude use of the heart and lungs for transplantation.
	Oliguria	Ensure adequate volume replacement and BP as outlined, then add dopamine (2-3 µg/kg/min), if not previously instituted to promote renal vasodilation and to increase renal blood flow, glomerular filtration rate, and UO. If these measures are ineffective at restoring adequate UO (> 1 ml/kg/h), then furosemide or mannitol may be used, after consultation with the transplant team.
	Diabetes insipidus (DI)	Fluid and electrolyte therapy as determined by filling pressures and hourly serum electrolyte values. Adjustment of vasopressin or DDAVP infusion to maintain UO < 1.5-3.0 ml/kg/h; initiation of this infusion should be done in consultation with the transplant team. As previously discussed, it may be advisable to D/C vasopressin or DDAVP at least 1 h before aortic cross-clamping.
	Coagulopathy	Transfuse Plt, FFP, and cryoprecipitate as necessary for clinical bleeding in the setting of abnormal coagulation studies. Avoid EACA due to risk of microvascular thrombosis in the donor organs.

Complications, cont.	Hyperglycemia	Avoid dextrose-containing solutions, which may aggravate existing hyperglycemia and contribute to osmotic diuresis and electrolyte abnormalities.
	Hypothermia	Early aggressive attempts to minimize intraop heat loss are essential and include warming the OR, use of a warming blanket, insulating exposed areas (head, neck, shoulders), warming all fluids, and using heated, humidified inspired gases.
Special considerations	Heart-lung procurement	Division of the mediastinal pleura and tracheal dissection with manipulation of each lung outside the mediastinum may result in ↓↓BP and may cause problems with oxygenation and ventilation. Adequate intravascular volume is essential, and inotropic therapy may be required during this period. Problems with ventilation and oxygenation must be communicated immediately to the transplant team. Following aortic cross-clamping and infusion of cardioplegia solution, the lung preservation fluid will be infused via the right and left PAs. During this period, the lungs should be ventilated manually with 4 bpm, or as otherwise directed by the transplant team. It is prudent early on in the procurement procedure to verify the position of the ETT with the transplant surgeon to ensure that the tube does not contribute to mucosal injury at the site of the anticipated suture line.
	Organ preservation	Therapy aimed at improving organ preservation may require several pharmacologic manipulations, as directed by the transplant team. Agents commonly used during organ procurement include dopamine (2-3 μg/kg/min), furosemide, mannitol, allopurinol (free-radical scavenger), chlorpromazine and phentolamine (vasodilators), heparin (prevents microvascular thrombosis and promotes reperfusion), and PGE_1 (vasodilator, membrane stabilizer, antiplatelet effect). Systemic infusion of PGE_1 prior to aortic cross-clamping (commonly used in heart-lung or lung procurement) will lead to predictable and profound ↓BP; efforts at volume resuscitation toward optimal CVP should continue until the aortic cross-clamp is applied. If heparin is to be administered iv, a catheter should be used after verifying the ability to freely aspirate blood. Methylprednisolone (30 mg/kg) is commonly administered at least 2 h before organ retrieval in an effort to protect the heart and kidneys from ischemic injury.

References for Multiorgan Procurement

1. Gelb AW, Robertson KM: Anaesthetic management for the brain dead for organ donation. *Can J Anaesth* 1990; 37(7):806-12.
2. Phillips MG, ed: *Organ Procurement, Preservation and Distribution in Transplantation.* William Byrd Press, Richmond, VA: 1991.
3. Powner DJ, Kellum JA, Darby JM: Abnormalities in fluids, electrolytes, and metabolism of organ donors. *Prog in Transplantation* 2000; 10(2):88-94.
4. Robertson KM, Cook DR: Perioperative management of the multiorgan donor. *Anesth Analg* 1990; 70(5):546-56.
5. Salter DR, Dyke CM: Cardiopulmonary dysfunction after brain death. In *Anesthesia for Organ Transplantation.* Fabian JA, ed. JB Lippincott, Philadelphia: 1992, 81-94.

Surgeons

David A. Spain, MD
J. Augusto Bastidas, MD

7.13   TRAUMA SURGERY

Anesthesiologist

Linda E. Foppiano, MD

INITIAL ASSESSMENT AND AIRWAY MANAGEMENT FOR TRAUMA SURGERY

The Advanced Trauma Life-Support System (ATLS), developed by the American College of Surgeons' Committee on Trauma, represents the best current approach to the severely injured patient. The sequence of management includes: 1) primary survey and initial resuscitation, 2) evaluation of initial treatment and continued resuscitation, and 3) secondary survey with definitive management.

The primary survey attempts to identify and treat immediate life-threatening conditions. This is accomplished by following the ABCs: **airway control,** with cervical spine precautions; assisted **breathing** or mechanical ventilation; and support of the **circulation** via volume resuscitation and tamponade of external bleeding. Once alveolar ventilation is ensured, the next priority is to optimize O_2 delivery by maximizing cardiovascular performance. Hypovolemia is the most likely etiology of postinjury shock; therefore, fluid resuscitation should be initiated via two large-bore iv cannulas placed in the antecubital veins. Any external source of bleeding should be controlled with manual compression. When vascular collapse precludes peripheral percutaneous access, femoral vein cannulation in the groin or saphenous vein cutdown at the ankle are preferred alternatives. ECG monitoring, serial vital signs, rapid physical examination, rectal temperature reading, and initiation of flow sheet complete the primary survey. Response of the patient to fluid resuscitation is then evaluated and, if crystalloid volume exceeds 50 ml/kg, type-specific or O(-) blood should be given. If shock persists despite fluid resuscitation, ongoing hemorrhage, cardiac tamponade, or tension pneumothorax should be considered. Ongoing hemorrhage should be treated operatively without delay to attempt correction of vital signs. Tension pneumothorax should be vented immediately through a needle inserted into the second interspace in the midclavicular line, followed by chest tube placement. Cardiac tamponade will require operative decompression.

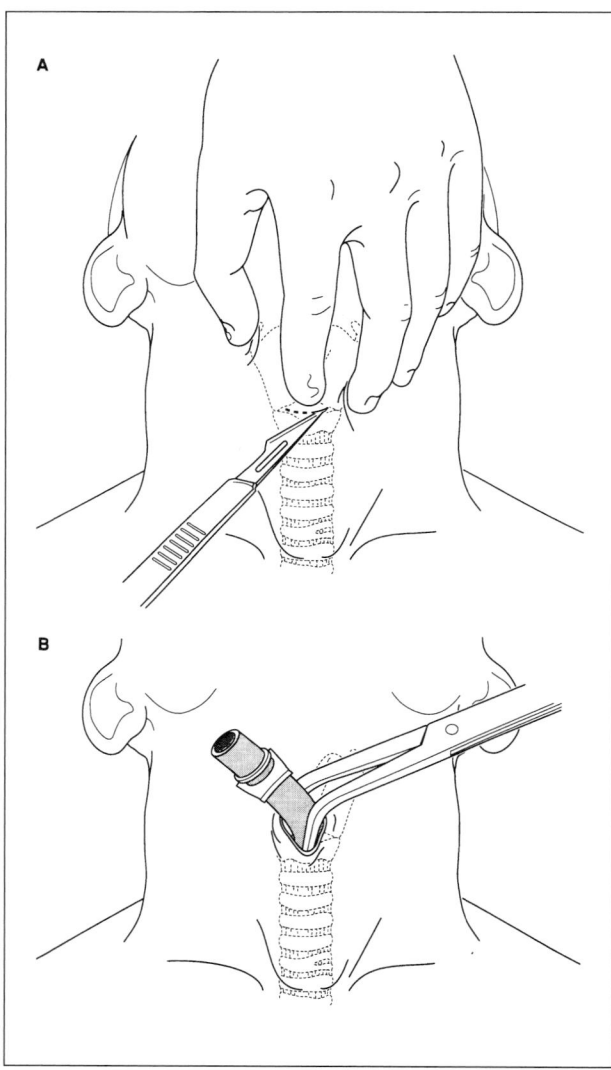

Figure 7.13-1. Cricothyroidotomy (vertical skin incision not shown). **(A)** Identification of the cricothyroid membrane by palpation and incising the membrane transversely. **(B)** Insertion of a tracheostomy tube or ETT through the cricothyroid membrane, which is spread with a tracheal dilator. (Redrawn with permission from Greenfield LJ, et al, eds: *Surgery: Scientific Principles and Practice, 2nd edition.* Lippincott-Raven, Philadelphia: 1997.)

MANAGEMENT OF AIRWAY

Airway obstruction, inadequate ventilation, hypoxemia, abnormal mental status, and cardiovascular instability are the usual indications for airway intervention. The three commonly accepted methods of airway control are: **blind nasotracheal intubation, orotracheal intubation,** and **cricothyroidotomy.**

Nasotracheal intubation, recommended for spontaneously breathing trauma patients, can be performed without the use of pharmacologic agents or special equipment. It is, however, associated with higher incidence of vomiting and aspiration and, in the intoxicated patient with a depressed level of consciousness, the success rate may be as low as 65%. Blind nasal intubation is contraindicated in patients with unstable midface fractures, penetrating neck trauma, or significant neck hematomas.

Oral intubation, with the use of appropriate neuromuscular blockade and the Sellick maneuver, is the preferred choice in many trauma centers. The approach is rapid, but at least three people are required to perform it safely in the patient with suspected C-spine injury.

In-line stabilization of the neck has replaced in-line traction as the protective measure. Because a failed intubation may force operative airway intubation, equipment for cricothyrotomy should be immediately accessible. Patients in respiratory distress with severe facial or neck trauma or unstable cervical spine injury require a surgical airway.

Cricothyrotomy (Fig 7.13-1) is the preferred method in adults who require a surgical airway. The important anatomic landmarks of the superior and inferior borders of the thyroid and cricoid cartilages are palpated. The thyroid cartilage is then stabilized, a vertical skin incision is made and rapidly advanced through subcutaneous tissue. The cricothyroid membrane lies very superficially, being covered by only the skin and platysma muscle. The cricothyroid membrane is incised transversely with the scalpel. In emergency situations, a standard ETT is generally easier to insert than a tracheostomy tube (Fig 7.13-1B). Cricothyrotomies should be converted to tracheotomies within 72 h after the initial injury, provided the patient's condition permits.

Tracheostomy is indicated for patients requiring surgical airway in less dramatic situations or if cricothyroidotomy cannot be performed due to direct laryngeal injury. It can be accomplished through the same incision, extended caudally, if laryngeal injury is found (see p. 568). On rare occasion, the injury is in the distal cervical or proximal intrathoracic trachea. In such cases, it may be necessary to intubate the distal end of the airway through the wound. A subsequent median sternotomy may be required to expose the injury. Right thoracotomy provides access to the more distal intrathoracic trachea (see Chest Trauma, p. 576).

Usual preop diagnosis: Airway compromise

SUMMARY OF PROCEDURE

Position	Supine
Incision	Midline longitudinal incision in the neck
Unique considerations	The large number of legal claims involving failed intubation suggests that surgical cricothyroidotomy remains an underutilized technique.
Antibiotics	Usually not given until clear indications related to the primary injury are apparent.
Surgical time	2 min
EBL	Minimal
Postop care	Mechanical ventilation
Mortality	Related to the primary injury
Morbidity	Cricothyrotomy is more likely to result in airway stricture or damage to more proximal structures in the larynx. On this basis, cricothyrotomies are converted to tracheostomies within 48-72 h of admission if patient's general condition permits.
Pain score	3

EMERGENCY TUBE THORACOSTOMY

SURGICAL CONSIDERATIONS

Description: In the United States, trauma is the most common cause of death in young people; 25% of these deaths (approximately 16,000 per year) are the result of thoracic trauma. Most of these are due to lethal injuries at the scene (e.g., cardiac rupture, free aortic transection). For patients who reach the hospital, proper management is crucial, as many deaths can be prevented. Early deaths are due to airway obstruction, tension pneumothorax, massive hemothorax, flail chest, cardiac tamponade, and open pneumothorax. Later deaths are due to respiratory failure, sepsis, and unrecognized injuries.

Eighty percent of blunt thoracic injuries are caused by motor vehicle collisions (MVCs). Penetrating injuries to the chest are almost as common as blunt trauma. The death rate in hospitalized patients with isolated chest injury is 4-8%; this increases to 10-15% when one other organ system is involved and to 35% if multiple additional organs are injured. Eighty-five percent of chest injuries do not require thoracotomy, and the patient can be managed with relatively simple measures, such as airway control and tube thoracostomy. Blunt trauma can induce injury by three distinctive mechanisms: direct blow, deceleration injury and compression injury. Rib fracture is the most common sign of blunt thoracic trauma. Fracture of the upper ribs (1st-3rd), clavicle, or scapula implies high-energy impact and is associated with a higher likelihood of major vascular injury.

Life-threatening injuries caused by penetrating trauma are distinctly different from those caused by blunt trauma. In penetrating chest injuries, pneumothorax is almost always present and hemothorax is present in 80% of cases. Hypovolemia from intrathoracic hemorrhage is second only to rib fractures as a sequela of thoracic trauma.

Tension pneumothorax may be caused by blunt or penetrating trauma. Venous return to the heart is impaired by the increased intrathoracic pressure and compression of the vena cava, → ↓BP and distended neck veins. Loss of lung volume on the ipsilateral side and subsequent compression of the contralateral side leads to impaired ventilation and hypoxia. The diagnosis of tension pneumothorax is made clinically. The presence of respiratory distress and absent or diminished breath sounds warrant immediate needle decompression (14-16 ga catheter through the 2nd intercostal space, midclavicular line), followed by subsequent tube thoracostomy. Treatment should not be delayed for radiographic confirmation. Since sequelae of thoracic injuries interfere with air exchange, treatment must take high priority, just after securing the airway, obtaining iv access, and beginning fluid resuscitation. In the hemodynamically stable patient, however, suspicion of a pneumothorax should be confirmed by x-ray. On the CXR, a 20% loss of lung dimension corresponds to ~50% loss of lung volume. A small, simple pneumothorax (<10%) with no respiratory compromise may be observed in patients with isolated injuries who do not require mechanical ventilation. These patients require close observation in the hospital and a repeat CXR in 4-6 h. Tube thoracostomy should be performed for a large pneumothorax (>10%), for patients with respiratory compromise or multiple injuries, or when it is not possible to adequately monitor the patient (e.g., during extended transport).

As much as 40% of the circulating blood volume can accumulate in a **hemothorax**. The most frequent sources of bleeding are the intercostal and internal mammary vessels. Some degree of hemothorax is present in almost every patient with chest injury. A supine CXR may miss up to 1 L of blood. Although an upright CXR is more sensitive, this is generally impractical in a multiple-trauma patient (whose spine often has not been fully evaluated). Following chest tube placement, blood loss > 1200-1500 ml or an ongoing loss of 250 ml/h for 4 h suggests the need for surgical intervention.

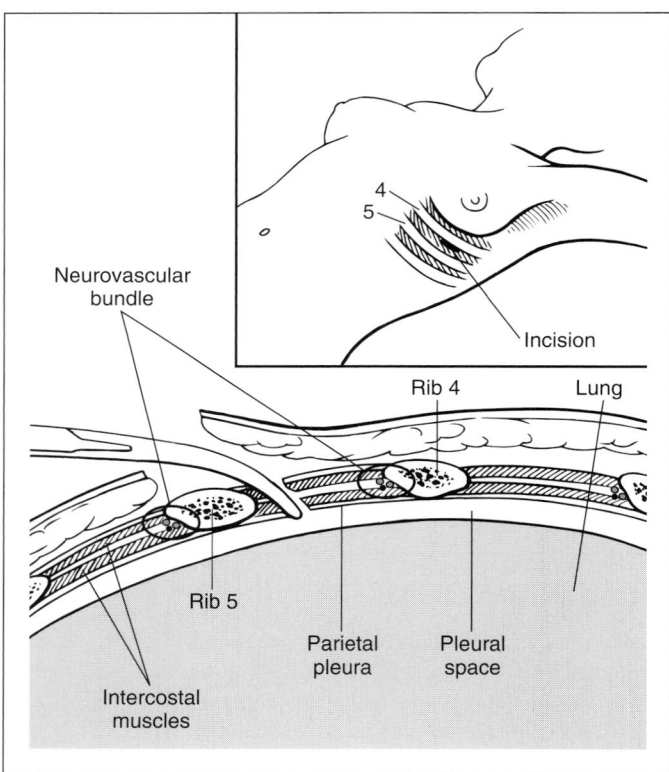

Figure 7.13-2. Tube thoracostomy. Incision through 4th or 5th interspace at anterior axillary line. Forceps are used to tunnel over the superior edge of the rib and to bluntly enter the pleural space.

Simple pneumothorax without associated hemothorax can be treated with a 20-22 Fr chest tube placed in the 4th intercostal space in the midaxillary line or in the 5th intercostal space in the anterior axillary line. Hemothorax and tension pneumothorax require a large-bore, 38-40 Fr chest tube placed in the midaxillary line through the 5th intercostal space (Fig 7.13-2). A 20 ml syringe with 1% lidocaine can be used not only to provide local anesthesia, but also to locate the upper edge of the rib in the obese patient. A generous, 3 cm incision should be made one interspace below the targeted level. The subcutaneous tissues are dissected bluntly, creating a tunnel that is directed upwards. The pleural space should be entered just above the upper edge of the rib to avoid injury to the intercostal neurovascular bundle, located just below the lower edge of the rib. After the pleural space has been entered bluntly, it should be explored with the operator's finger swept around to ensure proper location and to free potential adhesions. The chest tube should be inserted and advanced in the posterior and superior direction. The tube then should be connected to a suction/collection system under 20 cm of water-negative pressure, preferably through an autotransfusion device. CXR should immediately follow chest tube placement to evaluate decompression and assess for other injuries. If the pleural space still contains blood, another chest tube could be inserted or video-assisted thoracoscopy (VAT) could be considered if major vascular injury is not suspected.

Usual preop diagnosis: Tension pneumothorax; pneumothorax; hemothorax

SUMMARY OF PROCEDURE

Position	Supine, with arm abducted 90°
Incision	3 cm in interspace below 5th intercostal space in midaxillary line
Special instrumentation	38-40 Fr chest tube should be used in most patients. Small, 20-22 Fr tube reserved for simple pneumothorax in stable patients. Autotransfusion device should be available in ER.
Unique considerations	In tension pneumothorax, a large-bore needle inserted either in the 2nd intercostal space on the midclavicular line, can relieve tension and save a patient's life.
Antibiotics	Cefazolin 1 g iv.
Surgical time	5 min
EBL	Minimal, from tube placement. Variable amounts drained out, depending on extent of hemothorax and associated injuries.
Postop care	Chest tube may be removed after at least 48 h, when there is no air leak from lung and < 100-150 ml of fluid drainage per 24 h.
Mortality	If multiple additional organs injured: 35%
	In isolated chest injury: 4-8%
	When one other organ system is involved: 0-15%
Morbidity	Clotted hemothorax
	Empyema
	Lung abscess
	Lung contusion
Pain score	5

EMERGENCY DEPARTMENT THORACOTOMY

SURGICAL CONSIDERATIONS

Description: Rarely, emergency department thoracotomy may offer the only chance of survival in highly selected trauma patients. Its use should be restricted largely to patients who show signs of life in the emergency department (ED) but lose such signs shortly thereafter. The usual indications are: 1) massive exsanguination in the left chest, usually due to cardiac, vascular, or pulmonary injuries; and 2) pericardial tamponade. For patients with penetrating cardiac injuries who show signs of life in the ED, survival may be as high as 50%. For blunt trauma in this setting, survival is < 2%, regardless of presentation. With either mechanism, functional survival is almost unprecedented if the patient arrives without vital signs and unreactive pupils.

A **left anterolateral thoracotomy** is the preferred approach, since pericardiotomy, open cardiac massage, and aortic occlusion are best achieved by this means. This incision can be extended easily across the sternum and into the right chest to improve exposure and to control massive blood loss and/or air embolism from the right lung. The entire chest is prepped liberally, and left anterolateral thoracotomy is performed rapidly in the 5th intercostal space using a large-blade scalpel. Heavy scissors can be used to quickly divide the intercostal muscles and to cut across the sternum. If pericardial tamponade is encountered, the pericardium is opened longitudinally, anterior to the phrenic nerve. Blood and clot are evacuated and bleeding sites controlled with gentle digital pressure. Large, full-thickness lacerations that extend into the chambers may be controlled by inserting a Foley catheter, inflating the balloon, and pulling it snug against the myocardium. The open end of the Foley can be clamped or used as an infusion line for resuscitation. During ED thoracotomy, placement of clamps on the atria or ventricles should be avoided as they may extend the laceration. Attempts to repair cardiac lacerations should be delayed until resuscitative measures have been completed. In the nonbeating heart, suturing is performed prior to defibrillation. If coronary or systemic air embolism is present, the appropriate hilum is cross-clamped and air is aspirated from the left ventricle through the elevated apex. Cardiac arrest is an indication for immediate internal massage. The two-hand method is preferred, and internal defibrillation should be instituted. If internal defibrillation does not restore proper cardiac activity, cross-clamping of the aorta will improve coronary perfusion. To cross-clamp the aorta, the left lung is retracted anteriorly and superiorly and the posterior pleura is dissected under direct vision. Despite proper exposure and an NG tube in the esophagus, cross-clamping the aorta in the ED is difficult.

Usual preop diagnosis: Penetrating chest trauma with cardiac arrest and recent recorded signs of life

SUMMARY OF PROCEDURE

Position	Supine
Incision	Left anterolateral thoracotomy. Extension of incision across sternum could be considered for improved exposure.
Special instrumentation	ED thoracotomy tray; internal defibrillator paddles; suction device; Foley catheter; rapid-infusion device; O(-) blood
Unique considerations	Airway should be secured first. NG tube should be placed if possible. Typically, patients are not anesthetized for this procedure.
Antibiotics	Cefazolin, 1 g iv
Surgical time	10 min
EBL	1-2 L
Postop care	ICU
Mortality	Blunt trauma: 98%
	All penetrating chest injuries requiring ED thoracotomy: 85%
	Penetrating cardiac injury: 50%
Morbidity	Arrhythmias
	Acute MI
Pain score	10

EXPLORATORY SURGERY FOR NECK TRAUMA

SURGICAL CONSIDERATIONS

Description: The cervical region contains a greater variety of vital structures than any other region of the body (Fig 7.13-3). The cardiovascular, respiratory, digestive, endocrine, and CNS systems are all represented in the neck; injury to any of these can be fatal.

Injuries to the neck may result from blunt or penetrating trauma. In blunt trauma, < 5% of cases will have C-spine injuries. Since the consequences are so grave, however, all patients should be evaluated for C-spine injuries (H&P, x-rays, CT), and full spinal precautions should be maintained until the C-spine is cleared. Blunt airway injuries can be devastating and present significant management difficulties; however, the majority of blunt neck trauma consists of minor soft-tissue injuries that can be managed nonoperatively.

Penetrating trauma is defined as penetration of the platysma muscle. For these injuries, the neck is usually divided into three horizontal zones (Fig 7.13-3, inset). Zone I extends from the sternal notch to the cricoid cartilage. Penetrating injuries in this area are associated with a high mortality. Zone II extends from the cricoid cartilage to the angle of the mandible. Because this is the most exposed region of the neck, injuries can be evaluated and explored relatively easily. Zone III extends from the angle of the mandible to the base of the skull. Because of anatomic constraints, injuries to Zones I and III can be difficult to identify and repair. In patients with a Zone I injury, iv access should be established in the contralateral upper extremity because of possible injury to ipsilateral IJ vein or subclavian vein.

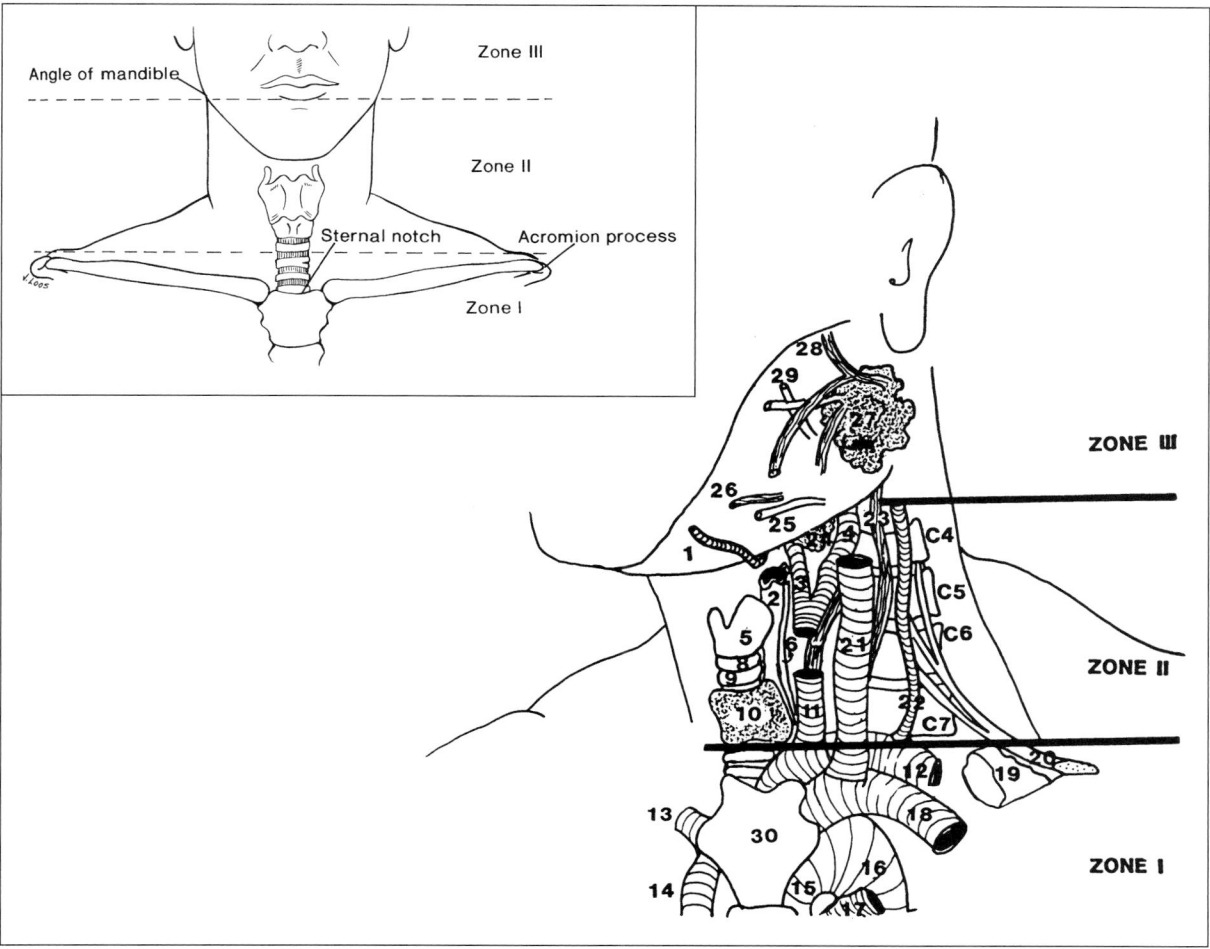

Figure 7.13-3. Cervical structures contained in Zones I, II and III: (1) facial artery; (2) esophagus; (3) internal carotid artery; (4) external carotid artery; (5) thyroid cartilage; (6) sympathetic trunk; (7) vagus nerve; (8) cricothyroid membrane; (9) cricoid cartilage; (10) thyroid cartilage; (11) common carotid artery; (12) subclavian artery; (13) right innominate vein; (14) SVC; (15) ascending aorta; (16) descending aorta; (17) PA; (18) subclavian vein; (19) clavicle; (20) brachial plexus; (21) IJ vein; (22) vertebral artery; (23) phrenic nerve; (24) submandibular gland; (25) lingual artery; (26) hypoglossal nerve; (27) parotid gland and duct; (28) facial nerve and its branches; (29) maxillary artery; (30) sternal manubrium. The thoracic duct is not shown in this figure. (Adapted with permission from Ordog GJ, et al. *J Trauma* 1985; 25:238). (Inset reproduced with permission from Baker RJ, Fischer JE: *Mastery of Surgery*. Lippincott Williams & Wilkins, Philadelphia, 2001.)

Until recently, evaluation and management of stable patients with neck injuries that penetrated the platysma depended on location of injury. Injuries to Zones I and III were evaluated radiographically, whereas injuries to Zone II were indications for mandatory exploration. With the increased availability of CT and arteriography, however, a selective exploration strategy is now favored. Evaluation of the larynx, pharynx, trachea, and esophagus should be performed if Sx are present; however, a penetrating neck wound should never be probed or explored locally, as this may dislodge a clot and precipitate a significant hemorrhage or air embolus.

Management of hemodynamically unstable or symptomatic patients with penetrating neck injuries should be limited to applying direct pressure, protecting the airway, establishing iv access, and obtaining CXR. Exploration and definitive management of the injury in the OR should follow as soon as possible. In stable patients with penetrating injuries and no indications for exploration, CT is generally the first diagnostic test.

Possible **median sternotomy incision** is used for patients with right-neck Zone I injuries or if injuries to mediastinum involving innominate artery or right subclavian artery are suspected. Exposure of injuries to the proximal left subclavian artery is extremely difficult via median sternotomy. In this case, a left anterior thoracotomy is necessary. The chest and left arm should be prepped and draped so as to allow arm manipulation.

Usual preop diagnosis: Penetrating neck injury

SUMMARY OF PROCEDURE

Position	Supine with head turned away from side of exploration and neck extended. If both sides of neck require exploration, head should be in midposition. It is helpful to clear the C-spine before exploration.
Incision	Sternocleidomastoid
Unique considerations	Monitor BP and HR carefully during carotid sinus manipulation.
Antibiotics	Cefazolin 1 g iv. If pharyngoesophageal injury: ampicillin 1 g + gentamicin 80 mg iv.
Surgical time	1 h
Closing considerations	Wound requires drainage, especially in Zone I exploration and if esophagus or airway was violated.
EBL	Variable
Postop care	ICU 12-24 h for neurologic and airway monitoring. After carotid injury repair, angiography should be considered.
Mortality	1%
Morbidity	Hemorrhage: acute from injuries; delayed from pseudoanuerysms
	Airway injury: acute loss of airway; delayed tracheal stenosis
	Damage to neural or vascular structures
	Esophageal fistula
Pain score	4

PATIENT POPULATION CHARACTERISTICS

Age range	Typically young adult
Etiology	Typically male
Incidence	5-10% of all trauma involves neck structures.
Associated conditions	Intrathoracic injuries; spinal cord injuries; recurrent laryngeal nerve injury; phrenic nerve injuries; thoracic duct injury

ANESTHETIC CONSIDERATIONS FOR NECK TRAUMA SURGERY

PREOPERATIVE

Patients with neck injuries often present unique challenges for ET intubation. Extensive internal damage may be present despite minimal external signs. High-velocity deceleration events, or 'clothesline' injuries, are often associated with airway compromise. Vascular injuries, particularly involving the carotid artery, can markedly distort internal anatomy and prevent visualization of laryngeal structures or passage of an ETT. Known or suspected C-spine injuries will restrict optimal positioning of the head and neck for laryngoscopy. Facial or dental injuries may impede access for laryngoscopy because of limited mouth opening or the presence of blood in the oropharynx. The use of alternative methods to secure the airway (e.g., fiber optic bronchoscopy) or a surgical approach may be the safest option.

Airway	Preop assessment of the airway and nature and extent of the cervical injury is crucial. Stridor and hoarseness may be present with laryngeal injury or compression of the trachea. Assess patient's ability to talk as a part of the airway evaluation. C-spine injury (though not common with penetrating neck injuries) should be evaluated by x-ray or CT scan. Airway injury can be associated with subcutaneous emphysema or pneumothorax. The extent of mouth opening, dental injuries, and any distortion of internal and external structures due to tissue swelling or hematoma should be determined before induction. The CXR should be examined carefully for evidence of tracheal deviation compression or pneumothorax.
	Tests: X-ray; CT scan; ABG
Cardiovascular	The patient should be evaluated for the extent of blood loss (BP, HR, capillary refill, peripheral pulse, skin condition). In addition to vascular injuries, associated facial and dental injuries may result in significant occult blood loss accumulated in the stomach. Venous lacerations possibly can allow VAE.
Neurological	Deficits associated with acute compromise of cerebral arterial blood flow should be evaluated on physical exam. Damage to the recurrent laryngeal nerve can occur, resulting in changes in voice and ↑aspiration risk. C-spine injuries should be assessed by physical exam (neck pain, neurologic examination) and radiologic studies (lateral C-spine x-rays [including C-7], CT scan, MRI).
Premedication	Full-stomach precautions (see p. B-5).

INTRAOPERATIVE

Anesthetic technique: GETA

Induction	The induction technique will depend on the associated injuries and physical exam. In the hypovolemic patient, induction doses of STP or propofol should be reduced by 50-75% to minimize ⬇⬇BP. Consider etomidate (0.2-0.3 mg/kg) or ketamine (0.5-1 mg/kg iv) as alternative induction agents. A rapid-sequence iv induction with cricoid pressure is usually required. In the presence of a vascular injury, the cough reflex and the BP response to intubation should be suppressed (e.g., remifentanil 1 μg/kg iv), in addition to induction agents, to prevent expansion of the hematoma. A wide range of ETT sizes (5.0-8.0 mm) should be available. If C-spine injury is suspected, in-line stabilization of the patient's head and neck should be provided by an assistant. In the presence of an unstable C-spine, cricoid pressure should be avoided to prevent further injury. If a difficult intubation is anticipated, fiber optic intubation (see p. B-6) or an awake surgical airway (cricothyrotomy or tracheotomy) should be considered. In patients with penetrating neck injuries, 'blind' intubation techniques (nasal inhalation, light-wand) should be avoided.
Maintenance	Standard maintenance (p. B-3) is usually appropriate for the normotensive neck-trauma patient. In cases of vascular injury, careful control of BP in the low normal range is advantageous. When nerve testing is anticipated, either no muscle relaxation or a short-acting agent (e.g., mivacurium) should be used.
Emergence	Awake extubation is the goal in patients with minimal distortion of the airway at the conclusion of the procedure. Postop intubation and mechanical ventilation is prudent in patients with residual neurological deficits or oropharyngeal swelling. BP control at low normal levels and slight elevation of the head of the bed (10-20°) will help to resolve tissue edema.
Blood and fluid requirements	IV: 14-16 ga × 2 NS/LR @ 4-6 ml/kg/h	Blood transfusion may be necessary with vascular injuries.
Monitoring	Standard monitors (see p. B-1). ± Arterial line	Invasive monitoring may be indicated for patients with major vascular injuries; however, the placement should not delay the start of emergency surgery.
Positioning	✓ and pad pressure points. ✓ eyes.	With suspected or known C-spine injuries, stabilization of the head and neck in the neutral position is required.
Complications	Awareness Hypothermia	

POSTOPERATIVE

Complications	Hemorrhage Hematoma Airway compromise	BP control at low normal levels (SNP infusion, labetalol, NTG) and elevation of the head of the bed (10-20°) will help minimize tissue edema and hematoma formation, which could lead to airway compromise.
Pain management	See Appendix C.	
Tests	As indicated.	

References:

1. Kendall JL, Anglin D, Demetriades D: Penetrating neck trauma. In *Emerg Med Clin North Am: Contemporary Issues in Trauma*. Eckstein M, Chan D, eds. WB Saunders, Philadelphia: 1998, 16(1), 85-106.
2. Wisner D, Blaisdell FW: Neck injuries. In *Scientific American Surgery*, Vol 1. Scientific American, New York: 1998.

CHEST TRAUMA: PERICARDIAL WINDOW, RELEASE OF TAMPONADE, REPAIR OF CARDIAC LACERATION

SURGICAL CONSIDERATIONS

Description: Cardiac contusions may occur in patients with blunt chest trauma. The degree of injury varies from localized contusion to cardiac rupture, but most are clinically insignificant if the patient survives to the hospital. Autopsy studies of victims of immediately fatal accidents show that as many as 65% have rupture of one or more cardiac chambers and 45% have pericardial lacerations. Most of the patients with cardiac rupture die at the scene; however, survivors are reported if vital signs are present during transport. Early clinical findings in cardiac contusion are most commonly dysrhythmias, but occasionally patients can develop cardiac failure. The initial ECG in the ED is the most sensitive diagnostic test. The most common abnormalities are atrial arrhythmias and right bundle branch block. Serial cardiac monitoring is indicated only if the initial ECG is abnormal. Serum enzymes are not helpful. Management is symptomatic. Arrhythmias should be treated in the standard fashion and are not a contraindication to surgery. Pericardial lacerations from stab wounds tend to seal and cause tamponade, present in 80-90% of patients with stab wounds to the heart. Accumulation of 150 ml of blood in the pericardium may impair preload and cause shock. **Beck's triad** of distended neck veins, muffled heart sounds, and ↓BP is present in only 30% of patients with tamponade. Pulsus paradoxus is even less reliable. The diagnostic test of choice is ultrasound, performed in the ED (the so-called **FAST scan**—focused assessment by sonography for trauma).

Treatment of penetrating cardiac injuries has gradually changed from initial management by **pericardiocentesis** to prompt **thoracotomy** and **pericardial decompression**. Pericardiocentesis, with ultrasound guidance, may be used to stabilize a patient until sternotomy or thoracotomy can be performed. A subxiphoid pericardial window is an option, but is best performed in the OR.

Gunshot wounds (GSWs) produce more extensive myocardial damage, multiple perforations, and massive bleeding into the pleural space. Hemothorax, shock, and exsanguination occur in nearly all cases of cardiac GSWs. Pericardial tamponade is often absent. Hemodynamically stable patients with penetrating injuries close to the heart should have ECG evaluation in the ED only if equipment is immediately available. The presence of pericardial fluid should be evaluated with a FAST scan. If a hemopericardium is confirmed, blood should be evacuated and injury treated in the OR.

Patients who are stable enough to be transported to the OR have excellent prognosis, with reported survival of 97% for stab wounds and 71% for GSWs. In contrast, patients who require ED thoracotomy have only a 25% survival rate for penetrating injuries.

Subxiphoid pericardial window under local or GA: The entire chest is prepped for potential sternotomy. A vertical midline incision is made over the xiphoid process and upper epigastrium. The xiphoid is elevated or excised, allowing access to the pericardiophrenic membrane and anterior mediastinum. Pericardium is opened between two stay sutures and inspected for the presence of blood. If blood is found, definitive repair should follow without delay. With the use of FAST scanning, this operation is rarely indicated as a diagnostic procedure.

Median sternotomy provides excellent exposure to the heart, great vessels, and pulmonary hila. This approach is ideal for anterior injuries and for the unstable patient, but is less well suited for posterior injuries and left subclavian injuries.

Left anterior/anterolateral thoracotomy in the 5th intercostal space can be used in a stable patient. The pericardium is opened anterior to the phrenic nerve and tamponade is relieved. The bleeding heart is controlled with digital occlusion and the laceration is closed with mattress sutures, with care being taken not to occlude coronary flow. Small coronary branches can be ligated, while others should be repaired and may even require CPB.

Usual preop diagnosis: Cardiac laceration

SUMMARY OF PROCEDURE

Position	Supine, L arm abducted 90°
Incision	Median sternotomy or left anterior or anterolateral thoracotomy in 5th intercostal space. (See Fig 7.13-4.) Further exposure may be obtained by transsternal extension into the R chest.
Special instrumentation	Rapid-infusion device; active rewarming system; internal defibrillator
Unique considerations	Massive blood loss is expected upon opening pericardium and during repair of laceration. Large-bore peripheral lower extremity iv and central venous access recommended for monitoring of volume replacement. A Foley catheter can be used to occlude laceration and as access for infusion. Arrhythmias are common.
Antibiotics	Cefazolin 1 g iv
Surgical time	45 min
Closing considerations	Hypothermia and coagulopathy contribute to mortality.

EBL	1-2 L
Postop care	ICU
Mortality	Without tamponade: ~90%
	With tamponade: ~30%
Morbidity	Overall: 50%
	Pulmonary complications
	Acute MI
	Arrhythmias
	Intracardiac shunts
	Ventricular aneurysms
	Valvular lesions
	Retained foreign bodies
Pain score	8

PATIENT POPULATION CHARACTERISTICS

Age range	Usually young adult
Etiology	GSWs, stab wounds, blunt trauma
Associated conditions	Hemothorax; pneumothorax; great-vessel injury; lung contusion

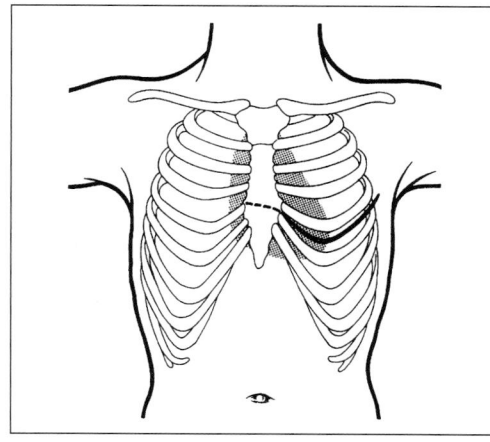

Figure 7.13-4. Incision (dashed/solid line) for ED thoracotomy: made immediately below the nipple, extending from sternum as far laterally as possible. (Reproduced with permission from Baker RJ, Fischer JE: *Mastery of Surgery.* Lippincott Williams & Wilkins, Philadelphia: 2001.)

ANESTHETIC CONSIDERATIONS

See Anesthetic Considerations for Chest Trauma, p. 580.

CHEST TRAUMA: REPAIR OF GREAT VESSELS

SURGICAL CONSIDERATIONS

Description: Thoracic great vessel injury accounts for 8-9% of all vascular injuries seen in the trauma center. The subclavian artery and descending thoracic aorta are the vessels injured most often (21% of cases), followed by PA (16%), subclavian vein (13%), vena cava (11%), innominate artery and pulmonary veins (9%).

Rupture of the thoracic aorta is the most lethal injury following blunt chest trauma and causes up to 50% of fatalities in MVCs. Proposed mechanism of injury is a deceleration force causing flexion or torsion of the aortic arch and subsequent disruption of the aortic wall at the ligamentum arteriosum immediately distal to the left subclavian artery. Survival of the patient depends on retention of the hematoma by the adventitial layer of the aorta. Although this protective mechanism is temporary, in patients with severe head injury or pulmonary contusion, repair may be delayed, provided that BP is adequately controlled. The mechanism of injury and the mediastinal silhouette on CXR are the two most sensitive markers for an injured thoracic aorta. Depressed left mainstem bronchus, apical capping, and a deviated trachea or esophagus (NG tube) seen on CXR may be suggestive of aortic injury. Arteriography is the standard for evaluating aortic injuries and may reveal pseudoaneurysms, AV fistulas, or intimal flaps. CT angiogram of the chest also may be used and is preferred in some trauma centers as a screening test.

Ascending aorta: Rupture requires median sternotomy, CPB and repair with a Dacron graft. Penetrating injury to the anterior aspect of the aorta can be repaired primarily; if there is additional posterior injury, CPB is required for successful repair.

Aortic arch: Complete exposure of the great vessels is required; median sternotomy with extension to the neck and division of the innominate vein may be utilized. Complex injuries may require CPB.

Innominate artery, right carotid artery: Approach is via a median sternotomy with right cervical extension and division of the innominate vein, if necessary. Blunt trauma typically involves the proximal innominate artery, in contrast to penetrating trauma, which usually involves the distal portion of the artery near the carotid or subclavian bifurcation. Injuries are repaired using an interposition graft of Dacron or Gore-Tex. Since cerebral perfusion is maintained through the L carotid and subclavian arteries, shunting is not necessary.

Descending thoracic aorta: 97% of patients with great-vessel injury who arrive alive at the hospital will have an injury at the isthmus. Clamping and direct reconstruction are required under temporary bypass shunt or pump-assisted shunt. Posterolateral thoracotomy via the 4th intercostal space is the preferred access. Distal control of the descending aorta is obtained first; then the transverse aortic arch is exposed and umbilical tape is applied between L carotid and L subclavian arteries. Vascular clamps are applied at the proximal aorta, distal aorta, and subclavian artery. Graft interposition is utilized in 85% of cases. An aortic cross-clamp time of < 30 min minimizes the incidence of paraplegia.

Subclavian artery or vein: Approach is via a cervical extension of the median sternotomy for right-sided injuries. Exposure of injuries to the proximal, left, subclavian artery via median sternotomy is usually inadequate. In patients with such injuries, a high left thoracotomy, often with either a supraclavicular or trap-door incision, is needed. Graft interposition is often necessary.

Pulmonary artery and veins: In major hilar injury, a pneumonectomy may be necessary, despite high mortality. Cross-clamping of the hilum prevents air embolus and hemorrhage. Simultaneous cross-clamping of the vessels and bronchus may reduce mortality. Fluid administration should be kept to a minimum to prevent right heart failure.

Thoracic vena cava: Intrathoracic IVC injury may cause hemopericardium and tamponade. Repair often is performed through the R atrium. SVC repair often is performed via a lateral venorrhaphy.

Usual preop diagnosis: Thoracic great vessel injury

SUMMARY OF PROCEDURE

Position	Supine
Incision	Anterolateral thoracotomy is preferred as it provides access to the descending aorta for cross-clamping, good access to heart, and may be extended across sternum into right chest.
Special instrumentation	Intraop blood recovery device; rapid-infusion device; graft materials for any vessels larger than 5 mm. CPB may be necessary.
Unique considerations	Use of vasodilators (SNP) prevents cardiac strain during cross-clamping of the aorta. Large amount of fluid is required to prevent hypotension after clamp removal.
Antibiotics	Cefazolin 1 g iv
Surgical time	1-3 h
EBL	$\geq$ 1-2 L
Postop care	ICU. Careful hemodynamic monitoring is critical since underlying pulmonary contusion may be worsened by inappropriate fluid administration. PA catheter may be necessary to optimize hemodynamic parameters, particularly in older patients. Coagulation studies must be carefully monitored and corrected with appropriate blood products.
Mortality	In general, mortality is associated with multisystem trauma and usually 2° concomitant head injury, infection, respiratory insufficiency, and renal insufficiency. Pulmonary artery or vein, suprahepatic IVC or SVC: > 70% Ascending thoracic aorta, aortic arch (in patients with stable vital signs on arrival): 50% Blunt injury to the descending thoracic aorta: 5-25% Subclavian artery injury: 5%
Morbidity	Paraplegia: ~8% (with descending aortic injuries)
Pain score	10

PATIENT POPULATION CHARACTERISTICS

Age range	Typically young adult
Incidence	Thoracic great vessel injury accounts for 8-9% of all vascular injuries seen in the trauma center.
Etiology	Blunt trauma from MVC; penetrating trauma from stab wounds or GSWs
Associated conditions	Pneumothorax; hemothorax; head injury

ANESTHETIC CONSIDERATIONS

See Anesthetic Considerations for Chest Trauma, p. 580.

CHEST TRAUMA: PNEUMONECTOMY, LOBECTOMY, REPAIR OF TRACHEOBRONCHIAL INJURY

SURGICAL CONSIDERATIONS

Description: Penetrating injuries to the chest can be divided into high- and low-velocity injuries. All stab wounds are classified as low-velocity injuries. GSWs may be considered low- or high-velocity injuries, depending on energy of the bullet. The majority of GSWs seen in the ED are low velocity; however, higher velocity injuries are being seen with increased frequency. The extent of tissue destruction in high-velocity; injuries is related to blast effect, tumbling and fragmentation of the missile, and secondary missiles such as bone fragments. Patients with such injuries are more likely to require thoracotomy and pulmonary resection. In general, pulmonary resection is required in 1% of stab wounds and 2% of GSWs. The indications for early operation are continued shock, prolonged bleeding, a larger air leak with inability to oxygenate or ventilate the patient, and suspected concomitant injuries to the vital intrathoracic structures. In most patients with stab wounds or low-velocity GSWs, bleeding from the lung tissue stops spontaneously after evacuation of the hemothorax and reexpansion of the lung. Only 5-10% of such patients will require thoracotomy to control bleeding, compared to a thoracotomy rate of 70% for high-velocity injuries. Pulmonary contusion is a frequent sequela of GSWs or blunt trauma to the chest. Pulmonary contusion occurs in 75% of patients with flail chest but also can occur following blunt trauma without rib fracture. Alveolar rupture with fluid transudation and extravasation of blood are early findings.

The incidence of tracheobronchial injuries reported in the autopsy series from MVC is 1%. Mechanisms of injury include rapid deceleration, direct blow, or sudden increase of intratracheal pressure against a closed glottis. The most common injury is transverse rupture, occurring in 74%, followed by longitudinal rupture in 18%, and complex in the remaining 8%. Approximately 80% of cases with tracheal rupture occur within 2.5 cm of the carina. Patients with injury to the airway may present in severe dyspnea and with massive subcutaneous emphysema. About 90% of these patients will have an abnormal CXR, showing pneumothorax, pneumomediastinum, subcutaneous emphysema, or pleural effusion.

Tracheobronchoscopy should be performed in all patients with suspected tracheobronchial injuries to establish the diagnosis and plan operative treatment.

Parenchymal lacerations are repaired by the simplest method available to stop bleeding or air leak. If pulmonary resection is required, formal segmental resection is not necessary. A stapling device should be used to preserve as much lung tissue as possible.

Anatomic pulmonary resections are indicated when bronchial injury repair is not feasible or may lead to complete lobar collapse. **Pneumonectomy** may be required for major hilar injuries but is associated with a mortality rate of 75%. **Primary repair of tracheobronchial injuries** should be performed as soon as possible. Transverse rupture may require the placement of a sterile tracheal tube into the distal trachea through the operative field. After posterior sutures are placed, an orotracheal tube is advanced beyond the area of injury. **Main-stem bronchial repair** is performed under OLV. High-frequency jet ventilation may be required to maintain oxygenation. Occasionally, total CPB is necessary for repair of complex airway injuries. Before closing, the suture line is pressure-tested and evaluated by fiber optic bronchoscopy.

Usual preop diagnosis: Tracheobronchial injury; penetrating/blunt chest trauma

SUMMARY OF PROCEDURE

Position	Supine, with neck extended for proximal tracheal injury, or lateral decubitus
Incision	Transverse cervical for almost all proximal tracheal injuries
	Right posterolateral thoracotomy in 5th intercostal space for thoracic trachea and right bronchial wounds
	Left posterolateral thoracotomy for L bronchial injury
Special instrumentation	Fiber optic bronchoscope, intrabronchial tube, jet ventilator/oscillator
Unique considerations	In patients with lobar resection or after pneumonectomy, PEEP may result in bronchopleural fistula
Antibiotics	Cefazolin 1 g iv
Surgical time	2-3 h
EBL	Variable
Postop care	ICU (typically)
Mortality	Pneumonectomy for trauma: 75%
	Penetrating tracheobronchial injuries: ~15%

Morbidity	Bronchopleural fistula: 10%
	Empyemia: 5%
	Hemothorax: 2-5%
	Pneumothorax
	ARDS (depends on extent of injuries)
Pain score	Cervical approach: 5-7
	Thoracic approach: 8-10

ANESTHETIC CONSIDERATIONS FOR CHEST TRAUMA SURGERY

Hemopericardium may rapidly progress to pericardial tamponade, requiring immediate pericardiocentesis or pericardial window, followed by surgical exploration and repair of the cardiac or vascular laceration. These patients typically present in shock ($\downarrow\downarrow$BP) with distended neck veins ($\uparrow\uparrow$venous pressure) and distant heart sounds (Beck's triad) without evidence of tension pneumothorax. Preop, and particularly during the induction of GA, the patient's intravascular volume must be expanded and myocardial contractility, HR, and SVR maintained. Inotropes and antiarrhythmic drugs may be required if hemodynamic instability occurs and does not respond to iv fluid administration. CPB is usually not required.

PREOPERATIVE

Respiratory   Associated injuries, such as hemothorax and/or pneumothorax, may be present, requiring thoracostomy tube placement. A widened mediastinum, apical pleural capping, or fracture of the first or second rib often occurs with injury to the great vessels. Multiple rib fractures are often associated with pulmonary contusions, which may not be apparent on the initial CXR, but can progressively impair oxygenation. With tamponade, spontaneous respiration is preferred over PPV ($\rightarrow\downarrow$venous return + $\downarrow$CO).

Tests: CXR (PA + lateral views). Upright inspiratory films best delineate chest structures; expiratory films enhance visualization of pneumothorax, but are difficult to obtain in multiple-trauma patients; ABG.

Cardiovascular   BP and HR should be followed and responses to fluid resuscitation noted. With adequate resuscitation, the EJ veins should appear full. CO can be significantly reduced despite normal BP measurements. Pulsus paradoxus may be present, with decreases in SBP of 10-12 mmHg during inspiration. Preop, intravascular volume should be restored and myocardial contractility supported with inotropes (e.g., dopamine 5-10 μg/kg/min) as necessary. Correction of metabolic acidosis with iv bicarbonate is indicated (e.g., 1 mEq/kg, then ✓ ABG). Myocardial contusion also can occur and can be associated with atrial or ventricular arrhythmias, RBBB, and RV failure, since the right heart is substernal and most directly involved in blunt trauma to the sternum. Supportive therapy with antiarrhythmics (e.g., lidocaine 1-2 mg/min) and inotropes (dopamine or epinephrine) may be required.

Tests: ABG, serial ECGs with myocardial contusion. FAST-scan is the test of choice for detection of pericardial effusions.

Neurological $\downarrow$BP and $\downarrow$CO may compromise cerebral perfusion. Associated head injury also can contribute to alterations in mental status. Pupil size and reactivity should be noted. Glasgow Coma Scale score ≤ 8 indicates significant brain injury.

Musculoskeletal   Known or suspected C-spine fractures require intubation precautions, with laryngoscopy performed while an assistant provides in-line stabilization of the patient's head in the neutral position.

Tests: Lateral C-spine x-rays, including C-7; CT; MRI

INTRAOPERATIVE

★ **Anesthetic technique:** GETA with full-stomach precautions (see p. B-5). **NB:** In the patient with an unstable C-spine, cricoid pressure (~10 lbs) may cause spinal cord injury, and consideration should be given to the establishment of a surgical airway under local anesthesia.

Induction   GETA is required for exploration through a median sternotomy or left thoracotomy. In the latter case, a DLT or BB is desirable. Rapid-sequence induction with ketamine (0.5-2.0 mg/kg) and succinylcholine is attractive since higher doses of ketamine are usually associated with $\uparrow$HR, $\uparrow$BP and $\uparrow$CO. Etomidate (0.2-0.6 mg/kg) is a useful alternative for patients with head injuries. Inotropic

Induction, cont.	agents (ephedrine, dopamine, epinephrine) should be immediately available to treat ↓BP. Agents which tend to decrease SVR, such as inhalational anesthetics and narcotics, should be introduced with caution. The potential for sudden and substantial blood loss exists and PRBCs (cross-matched, type-specific or O[-]) should be available in the OR prior to induction.	
Maintenance	Initially, low-dose inhalational agents and low-dose narcotics may be used, as tolerated. ↓BP may require dopamine infusion (1-10 μg/kg/min). Muscle relaxation and PPV are used. N_2O should be avoided if laceration of the heart or great vessel is suspected. If the patient is hypotensive and acidotic, scopolamine (0.2-0.4 mg iv) will provide amnesia. As cardiac and vascular injuries are repaired, BP and CO often will improve, permitting increased depth of anesthesia and decreased inotropic support.	
Emergence	Trauma patients often require prolonged intubation; however, hemodynamically stable patients with limited injuries may be extubated awake. Patients who received significant blood replacement (> 50% of blood volume), those requiring inotropic support, and those with head injuries should remain intubated and mechanically ventilated postop.	
Blood and fluid requirements	Be prepared for large blood loss. IV: 14 ga × 2 Fluid warmer Rapid-infusion device Airway humidifier T&C PRBCs.	Large blood losses occur occasionally, depending on the severity of the injury. Crystalloid and/or blood products should be infused to maintain BP and CVP (full jugular veins).
Monitoring	Standard monitors (see p. B-1). Arterial line CVP ± PA catheter ± TEE	ECG should be observed for changes associated with myocardial contusion (atrial/ventricular dysrhythmias, RBBB, ST-T wave changes). CVP monitoring can be useful in guiding fluid management. With release of tamponade, CVP rapidly drops toward normal.
Positioning	✓ and pad pressure points. ✓ eyes. ± C-spine: neutral position	Axillary roll, if lateral decubitus position; chest roll if median sternotomy.
Complications	Hypothermia Awareness Renal failure Coagulopathy	Hypothermia → dysrhythmias + ↓CO → acidosis. Rx: warm OR, warm iv fluids, humidify gases, and use patient warming devices. May be unavoidable in unstable patients. Rx: Consider scopolamine 0.2-0.4 mg iv. Usually 2° ↓renal perfusion (prerenal). Rx: Restore CO with volume and isotopes. Most commonly 2° dilutional thrombocytopenia. DIC may require replacement therapy with Plts, FFP and cryoprecipitate. Maintain nl Ca^{++} (1.05-1.3 mM/L).

POSTOPERATIVE

Complications	↓BP Arrhythmias Hypothermia ARDS Coagulopathy Renal failure	Cardiogenic shock may be 2° prolonged ↓BP or cardiac contusion. Hemodynamic instability with atrial/ventricular disrhythmias may occur. Treatment with inotropic infusions (dopamine 5-10 μg/kg/min or epinephrine 50-200 ng/kg/min) and antiarrhythmics. Active warming of iv fluids and warming blankets should be continued in ICU or PACU if hypothermia persists. Interstitial and alveolar edema → progressively worsening pulmonary function requiring prolonged mechanical ventilation. Based on clinical assessment and laboratory data (PT, Plt count, fibrinogen); transfusion of Plts, FFP, and/or cryoprecipitate may be indicated.

| Pain management | PCA (p. C-3) or parenteral narcotics
Epidural (p. C-2) | Epidural infusions of narcotic and/or low-dose local anesthetics can be effective in patients without coagulopathy. |

ABDOMINAL TRAUMA: DAMAGE CONTROL

SURGICAL CONSIDERATIONS

Description: The incidence of abdominal injuries requiring laparotomy approaches 25% for penetrating and 5% for blunt abdominal trauma. In blunt trauma, liver and spleen injuries occur with an incidence of ~50%. In penetrating trauma, the most common injuries are small bowel (29%), liver (28%), colon (23%), and stomach (13%). Many preventable deaths in trauma patients are related to shock from unrecognized intraabdominal hemorrhage caused by solid viscus injury.

Victims of severe multisystem trauma are particularly susceptible to development of a fatal coagulopathic state 2° hypothermia, acidosis, dilution, and consumption. Replacement of two or more blood volumes with NS or PRBCs will decrease the level of coagulation factors to 15%. Because of delays in obtaining coagulation profile results, coagulation factors should be replaced empirically in the setting of a large transfusion requirement (e.g., 1 U FFP/4 U PRBC). Metabolic acidosis affects both the circulatory system and coagulation, →↓CO and triggering DIC. Chances of salvaging a patient with pH < 7.0 are close to zero. To stop this self-perpetuating downward cycle, the concept of 'Damage Control' has evolved. This involves rapid laparotomy to control hemorrhage and GI spillage, followed by temporary closure of the abdomen and subsequent exploration after the patient has been rewarmed and stabilized. With the use of this technique, ~40% of critically injured patients can be saved from otherwise fatal injuries.

With the patient on a heated operating table, the abdomen and chest are prepped from the thighs to the neck and draped, and the abdomen is entered through a midline incision. This critical moment can be associated with significant blood loss and may require rapid blood transfusion. Four-quadrant packing with laparotomy pads is performed in the abdominal cavity, and manual compression of the subdiaphragmatic aorta may be instituted if packing alone does not control the hemorrhage. If necessary, the operation is stopped and blood/fluid resuscitation is performed. After consultation with the anesthesiologist, the surgeon proceeds with the sequential unpacking of each of the four quadrants and identifying injuries. Vascular injuries are controlled with clamping and ligation, bowel injuries are stapled across, but no attempt is made for primary repair. Liver and retroperitoneal injuries are controlled with packing alone. When damage control is performed, the abdomen is closed with a running skin suture, if possible; otherwise, a temporary vacuum dressing is used. PIP should be monitored during closure, as patients may develop abdominal compartment syndrome (↑↑intraabdominal pressure →↑PIP, ↓UO, nl filling pressures). The patient is then transported to ICU and actively rewarmed and resuscitated. Reoperation should be performed at 24-48 h and definitive repair of the injured organs should be completed.

Usual preop diagnosis: Intraabdominal trauma and hemorrhage

SUMMARY OF PROCEDURE

Position	Supine
Incision	Midline abdominal
Special instrumentation	Fluid-warming, rapid-infusion device
Unique considerations	Autotransfusion device (e.g., Cell Saver) may be of use if no contamination of abdominal cavity.
Antibiotics	Cefotetan 1 g iv
Surgical time	45 min
Closing considerations	Even temporary closure may not be possible because of severe bowel edema. A silo made from a plastic iv bag may be used to cover the bowel. Monitor PIP and UO during abdominal wall closure, as abdominal compartment syndrome may develop.
EBL	Average transfusion requirement: 12 L crystalloids, 20 U PRBCs, 5 U FFP, 6 U Plts
Postop care	ICU; patient remains intubated. Active rewarming is of primary importance.
Mortality	70%

Morbidity	Intraabdominal abscesses: 30%
	Fistulas: 10%
Pain score	10

PATIENT POPULATION CHARACTERISTICS

Age range	Typically young adult
Male:Female	9:1
Incidence	25% for penetrating and 5% for blunt abdominal trauma
Etiology	MVC; penetrating injury (e.g., GSW or stab wound)
Associated conditions	Chest trauma; closed head trauma; pelvic fracture

ANESTHETIC CONSIDERATIONS

See Anesthetic Considerations for Abdominal Trauma Surgery, p. 586.

ABDOMINAL TRAUMA: HEPATIC AND SPLENIC INJURIES

SURGICAL CONSIDERATIONS

Description: The liver is the most commonly injured organ in patients with penetrating trauma, while the spleen is the most commonly injured organ with blunt trauma. Approximately 30% of all patients requiring laparotomy for trauma will have hepatic injuries. Minor injuries (grades I and II) are managed nonoperatively unless other injuries mandate laparotomy. Thus, most liver injuries that require operation are complex (grades IV-V), with large blood loss and high mortality (up to 30%).

Several maneuvers can be used to facilitate **repair of liver injuries: Manual compression** temporarily controls bleeding and allows time for volume resuscitation. **Portal triad occlusion (Pringle maneuver)** (Fig 7.13-5) decreases blood loss and identifies the patient who might benefit from selective hepatic artery ligation. Perihepatic packing and planned reexploration is a life-saving maneuver and should be used early for patients with severe injuries, before they become hypothermic, coagulopathic, and acidotic. Extensive liver mobilization, parenchymal disruption (i.e., finger fracturing), and atriocaval shunts are rarely indicated. Hepatic angiogram and embolization in the immediate or early postop phase may be very useful for patients with severe injuries. At reexploration, intrahepatic omental packing is good for obliterating dead space. Closed suction drains should be used in all patients.

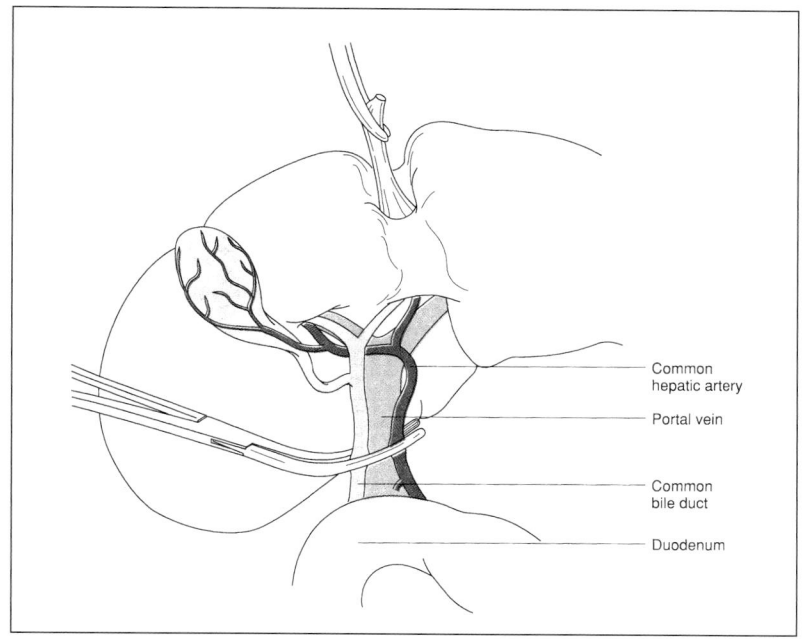

Common hepatic artery
Portal vein
Common bile duct
Duodenum

Figure 7.13-5. Pringle maneuver compression of the portal triad structures with a noncrushing vascular clamp for hepatic inflow control. (Reproduced with permission from Greenfield LJ, et al, eds: *Surgery: Scientific Principles and Practice*, 3rd edition. Lippincott Williams & Wilkins, Philadelphia: 2001.)

Portal triad (portal vein, hepatic artery, common bile duct) injuries, although rare, are associated with extremely high mortality. Isolated portal vein injuries are associated with a 70% mortality. The portal vein should be repaired if possible; however, ligation can be tolerated. Careful volume resuscitation should follow portal vein ligation to avoid ↓BP 2° fluid sequestration in the splanchnic bed. Simple ligation of the hepatic artery, preferably proximal to the gastroduodenal artery, is recommended for most major hepatic artery injuries. Shock and transfusion-related coagulopathy occurring in the immediate postop period are responsible for 80% of the deaths in liver injury patients. Control of hemorrhage remains the critical component in the successful management of liver injuries.

More than 90% of splenic injuries are caused by blunt trauma. Approximately 75-85% of these patients can be managed nonoperatively. Of the remaining patients, most will require splenectomy since usually only grade IV (active intraperitoneal bleeding) or V (shattered/avulsed injuries) require operation. Massive bleeding from the LUQ is probably caused by splenic injury. For severe injuries, the spleen is delivered into the wound by blunt dissection. The spleen is removed by cross-clamping the hilum and dividing the short gastric vessels. The LUQ is packed and reinspected for hemostasis once better resuscitation is provided. The splenic salvage rate in the pediatric population approaches 90%.

In a patient with massive **intraabdominal hemorrhage**, sudden cardiovascular collapse is predictable when the abdomen is opened. Laparotomy with manual compression of the aorta at the aortic hiatus is recommended. Access for subsequent aortic clamping is rapidly obtained by blunt finger dissection of the lesser sac. After removing all clots and free blood, four-quadrant packing is used to control bleeding. Significant liver bleeding should be controlled with manual compression, the Pringle maneuver, and perihepatic packing.

Usual preop diagnosis: Hepatic injury; splenic injury

SUMMARY OF PROCEDURE

Position	Supine
Incision	Midline abdominal
Special instrumentation	Active rewarming device; Cell Saver
Unique considerations	Most emergency laparotomies require close cooperation between anesthesiologist and surgeon. The procedure may need to be interrupted for fluid or blood resuscitation if patient becomes hypotensive. The entire chest and abdomen, including both groins, need to be accessible to the surgeon; ECG electrodes are placed preferably on the patient's back.
Antibiotics	Cefazolin 1 g iv
Surgical time	1-2 h
Closing considerations	After massive fluid resuscitation, interstitial edema may preclude primary fascial closure. Absorbable mesh or nonabsorbable synthetics may be necessary to close the abdomen.
EBL	2-10 L (transfusion requirement 6-20 U)
Postop care	ICU—shock and coagulopathy management. Monitoring for possible rebleeding and abdominal compartment syndrome.
Mortality	Liver: 10%
	Spleen: 10% (usually due to associated injuries)
Morbidity	Liver – perihepatic abscess: 10%
	Spleen – septic complications: 7%
Pain score	8-10

PATIENT POPULATION CHARACTERISTICS

Age range	Any age
Male:Female	3:1
Incidence	Liver: 30% of patients requiring laparotomy for trauma
	Spleen: 10% of patients requiring laparotomy for trauma
Etiology	Liver: penetrating wound (80%) with gunshot wounds responsible for 60% and stab wounds for 40%
	Spleen: blunt trauma (90%), mostly due to MVC
Associated conditions	Liver: isolated hepatic injury (30%); injury to one or two other organs (50%), with diaphragm, major vascular structures, stomach, lung, and colon being most common.

ANESTHETIC CONSIDERATIONS

See Anesthetic Conditions for Abdominal Trauma Surgery, p. 586.

ABDOMINAL TRAUMA: VASCULAR INJURIES

SURGICAL CONSIDERATIONS

Description: Penetrating trauma is the most common cause of abdominal vascular injuries — IVC/hepatic veins, 36%; celiac/mesenteric vessels, 30%; iliac vessels, 11%; and aorta, portal/splenic, and renal vessels, each 5%. Patients with gunshot wounds to the abdomen have ~25% incidence of major vascular injury; however, only ~10% of patients with penetrating stab wounds will have vascular injuries. Patients sustaining blunt abdominal trauma who require laparotomy have a 5-10% incidence of vascular injury.

Initial resuscitation of the patient with abdominal vascular injuries depends on the patient's condition. Multiple large-bore catheters should be inserted in the upper extremities or, if necessary, central venous access should be obtained. Because of the probable intraabdominal venous injury, lower-extremity venous access is not indicated. Blood replacement during resuscitation is done preferably with type-specific blood. It is a good practice to have two U of O(-) blood available immediately in the ED in case there is no time for a limited cross-match. Efforts to limit hypothermia should start as soon as patient arrives (use of prewarmed fluids and high-flow blood warmers and covering the patient with prewarmed blankets).

Injuries to the abdominal vessels can be grouped into four regions, which require different surgical approaches:

Midline supramesocolic hemorrhage or hematoma (superior to the transverse mesocolon) is usually 2° injury to the suprarenal aorta, celiac axis, proximal superior mesenteric artery, or proximal renal artery. Proximal aortic control should be obtained at the hiatus by either aortic compression or manually by entering the lesser sac and digitally splitting the muscle fibers of the crura. Once this is done, direct access to the vessels is achieved through medial visceral rotation of all left-sided viscera. Injuries to the aorta are then repaired directly or with the appropriate graft. An injured celiac axis probably can be ligated safely if the remaining visceral vessels are intact. Superior mesenteric artery injuries must be repaired, usually with a jump graft. Repair of the superior mesenteric vein is preferred, but the vein may be ligated if complex injuries are present. These patients require substantial fluid resuscitation postop and are at high risk for abdominal compartment syndrome. Injuries to the IVC or right side of the aorta can be exposed by **duodenal mobilization (Kocher maneuver)**.

Midline inframesocolic hemorrhage or hematoma results from infrarenal aorta or IVC injury. Exposure is obtained by incising posterior peritoneum in the midline after displacement of the small bowel and cephalic retraction of the transverse mesocolon. A proximal aortic clamp is then placed just below the left renal vein, with a distal clamp near the aortic bifurcation. The defect is repaired primarily, using patch aortoplasty, end-to-end anastomosis, or a graft. If the aorta is intact and an inframesocolic hematoma seems to be more extensive on the right side, or if there is active bleeding coming through the base of the mesentery, then injury to the IVC should be suspected. Access to the infrahepatic IVC is preferably obtained by mobilization of the R colon and duodenum. Proximal and distal control are best obtained by either digital compression or two sponge sticks. The injury is then repaired directly. Blind clamping should be avoided, but occasionally, with good exposure, a **Satinsky clamp** can be placed. In young patients with exsanguinating hemorrhage, the infrarenal IVC can be ligated, providing time for appropriate fluid management. These patients require significant fluid postop and will likely have chronic venous insufficiency.

Lateral perirenal hematoma or hemorrhage suggests injury to the renal vessels or kidney. In patients with blunt abdominal trauma who have a negative abdominal CT, IVP, or arteriogram, surgery is not required. A penetrating injury usually requires surgical exploration. Vascular control of the ipsilateral renal artery is obtained before the hematoma is entered. If there is active bleeding from the kidney or overlying retroperitoneum, then the kidney is exposed via a lateral incision, and a vascular clamp is applied to the renal vessel. This usually is followed by nephrectomy (after palpation and a one-shot IVP to verify function of a normal contralateral kidney). If the contralateral kidney is missing or nonfunctional, then back-table salvage surgery and autotransplantation of the injured kidney should be attempted. Only 30-40% of kidneys with arterial injuries can be salvaged.

Lateral pelvic hematoma or hemorrhage indicates injury to the iliac vessels. Pelvic hematoma 2° blunt trauma and pelvic fracture should not be explored. Primary control of bleeding is by external fixation of the pelvis and angiography/embolization. For penetrating injuries, vascular control is obtained at the aortic bifurcation proximally and close to the inguinal ligament distally. The internal iliac artery is best visualized by elevating common and external iliac arteries on vascular tapes. Unilateral internal iliac artery injuries can be ligated. Common or external iliac artery injuries can be repaired or a graft can be inserted. Grafts may be used even in the presence of GI contamination, provided the abdomen is thoroughly irrigated and the retroperitoneum is closed over the graft. Injuries to the iliac veins are treated with lateral venorrhaphy or ligation.

Usual preop diagnosis: Abdominal vascular injury

SUMMARY OF PROCEDURE

Position	Supine, with left arm abducted 90°
Incision	Midline abdominal
Special instrumentation	Autotransfusion device (e.g., Cell Saver); thoracotomy tray; aortic compressor
Unique considerations	Prevent heat loss and warm all infusions and irrigation solutions. For the patient requiring massive transfusion, 1 U FFP/4 U PRBCs. After prolonged aortic cross-clamp, prophylactic administration of $NaHCO_2$ (1-2 mEq/kg) may be indicated to prevent 'washout' acidosis.
Antibiotics	Cefazolin 1 g iv
Surgical time	Variable
Closing considerations	Once vascular injuries are repaired, hepatic injuries are controlled with packing, bowel injuries are closed with staplers, and the abdominal wall is closed temporarily.
EBL	5-10 L
Postop care	ICU; Patients after infrarenal vena cava ligation require volume expansion and prevention of lower extremity venous pooling. Elastic wraps and lower-extremity elevation should be maintained for at least 1 wk. Similarly, after superior mesenteric vein ligation, splanchnic hypervolemia requires vigorous fluid resuscitation and lasts approximately 3 d.
Mortality	Combined injury to the suprarenal aorta and IVC: 100%
	Aorta: 60%
	Infrarenal abdominal aorta: 50%
	Superior mesenteric artery: 40-80%
	Iliac artery: 40%
	Iliac vein: 30%
	Infrarenal vena cava: 30%
	Superior mesenteric vein: 20%
	Renal artery: 15%
Morbidity	Abdominal compartment syndrome ($\uparrow\uparrow$abdominal pressure $\rightarrow$$\uparrow$PIP + $\downarrow$UO)
	Acute renal failure
	Intraabdominal infection
	Fistula
Pain score	8-10

PATIENT POPULATION CHARACTERISTICS

Age range	Typically young adult
Male:Female	Male > female
Incidence	15% of patients with abdominal trauma
Etiology	10% of penetrating stab wounds and 25% of gunshot wounds to the abdomen will cause a major vascular injury.
Associated conditions	Multiple vascular injuries; hollow viscus perforation; fecal contamination

ANESTHETIC CONSIDERATIONS FOR ABDOMINAL TRAUMA SURGERY

Abdominal injuries range from relatively simple penetrating injuries (e.g., a stab wound) to severe blunt trauma (e.g., liver lacerations and pelvic fractures) and are often associated with massive hemorrhage. Head injuries and spinal fractures may complicate management plans. The ability to provide rapid, aggressive volume replacement is often the key to survival. Coagulopathy (DIC) and hypothermia present additional challenges.

PREOPERATIVE

Respiratory	Associated injuries, such as hemothorax and/or pneumothorax, may be present, requiring thoracostomy tube placement. A widened mediastinum, apical pleural capping, or fracture of the 1st or 2nd rib often occur with serious vascular injuries. Multiple rib fractures suggest possible pulmonary contusions, which may not be evident on initial CXR, but can progressively impair oxygenation and ventilation.
	Tests: CXR (PA + lateral views); ABG
Cardiovascular	BP and HR should be followed and responses to fluid resuscitation noted. Tachycardia can maintain an adequate BP with reduced pulse pressure, despite 25-30% loss of blood volume. Attempt to quantify overt blood loss (e.g., scalp lacerations, open fracture sites). Blunt chest trauma (e.g.,

Cardiovascular, cont.	steering wheel contact) may result in myocardial contusion with various dysrhythmias, most often premature ventricular or atrial complexes. **Tests:** Serial Hct; ECG in patients > 50 yrs of age or with blunt chest trauma
Neurological	Seek physical evidence of open or closed head injuries, such as palpable depressions of the skull or scalp lacerations, abrasions, or contusions. Pupil size and reactivity should be noted. Intubation in the ER is necessary for patients who are unable to protect their airway, require hyperventilation, or are combative and unable to cooperate with medical staff for exam and treatment. In general, any patient with a Glasgow Coma Scale (GCS) ≤ 8 (no spontaneous eye opening, inappropriate or incomprehensible speech and only reflexive motor responses) requires intubation. Motor and/or sensory deficits may reflect spinal cord injury and may be associated with neurogenic ('spinal') shock, particularly with upper thoracic or cervical cord injuries. **Tests:** C-spine x-rays (lateral view, including C7), is a good screening exam: ✓ for altered vertical alignment and unequal disk interspaces. CT scan or MRI of head: ✓ for gross asymmetry, hemorrhage, or midline shift.
Musculoskeletal	Known or suspected C-spine injuries require intubation precautions. In urgent cases, intubation without neck extension is achieved with an assistant providing in-line stabilization of the head in the neutral position. If time permits, awake, blind, or fiber optic intubation may be attempted. Basilar skull fractures contraindicate nasal ET or NG tubes. Pelvic and femur fractures may represent sources of significant (>1000 ml) occult blood loss. **Tests:** Radiographs of C-spine (see above), skull, extremities
Hematologic	Depending on estimations of prior, ongoing, and anticipated surgical blood losses, preop blood T&C may be desired. O(-) or type-specific blood should be available until the T&C is complete. **Tests:** Serial Hct; T&C; ✓ Ca^{++} following massive transfusions.
Laboratory	Other tests, as indicated from H&P or suspected injuries, including electrolytes, liver panel, toxicology screen, blood alcohol level.
Premedication	Premedication is rarely useful due to the urgency of the procedures and the need to have an alert, responsive patient for serial evaluations of mental status or abdominal pain. Sedative premedication should be avoided in patients who are hemodynamically unstable and those with probable head injuries. Virtually all patients are considered to have full stomachs, and any compromise of the ability to protect the airway is inappropriate. Na citrate (30 ml po) may be administered to patients at risk for aspiration; however, ranitidine and metoclopramide may not reach effective levels in the short interval before induction.

INTRAOPERATIVE

Anesthetic technique: GETA with full-stomach precautions (p. B-5)

Induction	Before induction, a variety of laryngoscope blades (e.g., Miller 1 and 2, Mac 3 and 4) and ETTs with stylets (6.0, 7.0, and 8.0 mm) should be ready. LMA may be useful for providing temporary airway control without C-spine manipulation if direct laryngoscopy is difficult. LMA may be used as a conduit for ET intubation (fiber optic or fast-track LMA). A size 7.0 mm ETT will pass through a #4 LMA. Equipment for emergent cricothyrotomy (a 14 ga iv catheter + adapter) and jet ventilation should be in OR. Most often, preoxygenation is followed by a rapid-sequence iv induction with cricoid pressure (Sellick's maneuver) using STP (3-5 mg/kg) and succinylcholine (1.0-1.5 mg/kg). If hypotension is present or a concern, alternate induction agents (e.g., ketamine 0.5-2.0 mg/kg iv or etomidate 0.1-0.3 mg/kg iv) may be used. Axial head and neck stabilization is necessary if C-spine injury is present or suspected. Some trauma patients will have been intubated in the ED. Induction consists of verifying ETT placement by auscultation and $ETCO_2$ monitoring. Very low $ETCO_2$ values may be obtained in patients with markedly reduced CO. Ventilation with 100% O_2 and muscle relaxation with pancuronium or vecuronium (0.1 mg/kg iv) is appropriate. Ongoing fluid resuscitation should be continued during this time.
Maintenance	O_2/air, muscle relaxants, narcotics, and volatile agents are titrated as tolerated. Avoid N_2O in the presence of pneumothorax, pneumocephalus, bowel distention, or prolonged procedures. Shorter-acting agents (e.g., volatile agents, remifentanil, rocuronium), carefully titrated, may be preferred

Maintenance, cont.	in patients with head injuries to facilitate early postop assessment of neurologic status. If ↓BP precludes use of volatile agents, low-dose scopolamine (0.1-0.2 mg iv) or ketamine (0.25 mg/kg/15-30 min) can provide amnesia. Heated or passive humidifiers should be used, particularly in prolonged cases. Forced-air warming blankets, elevated OR temperatures, and warmed irrigation fluids (surgical field, bladder) also may be necessary if hypothermia becomes problematic.	
Emergence	Prior to extubation, patient should be awake and able to protect his/her airway, and should be hemodynamically stable and spontaneously ventilating with ease through the ETT. Patients who should not be extubated at the end of the case include those with inadequate preop evualations, elderly patients with rib fractures, hemodynamically unstable patients, those who have received massive fluid and blood product transfusion (e.g., with evidence of intestinal edema), or those with coagulopathy.	
Blood and fluid requirements	Anticipate large blood loss. IV: 14-16 ga × 2 or 7-9 Fr × 2 NS/LR @ 8-10 ml/kg/h Fluid warmers Rapid-infusion device Airway humidifier/warmer ± T&C PRBCs.	Large blood losses may be anticipated, depending on the mechanism of injury (e.g., liver lacerations, major vascular injury, pelvic fractures). Crystalloid, colloid and PRBCs should be given to preserve blood volume as estimated by blood losses, systemic BP, CVP/PCWP and Hct. With massive transfusion, Plts and FFP will also be needed. In general, 2 U FFP and 6 U of Plts should be transfused after ~10 U of PRBCs (1 blood volume in a 70-kg person) have been given. Postop hypothermia is best minimized by warming all iv and irrigating fluids, maintaining OR temperature @ 78-80°F, warming and humidifying inspired gases, and using warming blankets.
Monitoring	Standard monitors (see **B-1**). Urinary catheter ± Arterial line ± CVP line ± PA catheter ± TEE	Standard monitoring should be applied as soon as the patient enters the OR. Arterial lines may be useful in unstable patients or those in whom frequent blood samples are anticipated. CVP line or PA catheter may be useful if vasoactive drips are needed or if ventricular dysfunction is apparent. In truly emergent cases, the placement of additional monitoring should be accomplished without delaying the surgical control of hemorrhage or without interrupting aggressive volume resuscitation.
Positioning	✓ and pad pressure points. ✓ eyes.	If C-spine has not been cleared by radiographs, the neck should remain immobilized intraop and postop.
Complications	Hypothermia Awareness Coagulopathy Renal failure	Hypothermia→dysrhythmias+↓CO→acidosis. Rx: warm OR, warm iv fluids, humidify gases, and use patient warming devices. May be unavoidable in unstable patients. Rx: Consider scopolamine 0.2-0.4 mg iv. Usually 2° dilutional thrombocytopenia. DIC may require replacement therapy with Plts, FFP, and cryoprecipitate.

POSTOPERATIVE

Complications	Hypothermia Atelectasis, V/Q mismatch Coagulopathy	Active warming of blood products and forced-air warming blankets (Bair-Hugger) and warm room temperatures should be continued in PACU if hypothermia persists. Pulmonary compliance is often increased with large volumes of fluid replacement. Pulmonary contusions may aggravate this problem and severely compromise oxygenation and ventilation, requiring high inspired O_2 concentration, high PIP and PEEP. Coagulation products may be necessary, based on Plt counts, PT/PTT, and ongoing RBC transfusion requirements.

Pain management	PCA or parenteral narcotics (see p. C-3, C-2), epidural narcotic	Patients with rib fractures benefit from epidural narcotic and/or low-dose local anesthetic infusions.
Tests	Hb/Hct CXR, if postop intubation or intraop central line or thoracostomy tubes were placed.	PT/PTT, Plt counts, if unexplained bleeding postop Fibrinogen, fibrin split products, if DIC is suspected.

PEDIATRIC TRAUMA: AIRWAY AND VASCULAR ACCESS

SURGICAL CONSIDERATIONS

Description: Children younger than 15 yr are victims in about 25% of all trauma occurring in the U.S. This incidence translates to approximately 200,000 hospitalizations and 10,000 deaths annually. Another 10,000-12,000 children sustain permanent impairment as a result of their injuries. According to the National Pediatric Trauma Registry, 40% of all pediatric injuries occur as a result of MVC and 35% are injuries sustained at home. Falls remain the most common cause of severe injury in infants and toddlers, while bicycle accidents cause most of the injuries in older pediatric groups. The majority of pediatric injuries occur 2° blunt trauma, and infants < 2 yr of age are known to have higher mortality rates for the same level of injury compared to older children.

The same sequence of primary survey, resuscitation, secondary survey, and definitive care should be followed as in adults. Confirmation of a patent airway is the essential first step. The best method for restoring airway patency is the **jaw thrust maneuver** and removal of any debris from the mouth. The most common reason for intubation in the pediatric trauma patient is loss of consciousness or as part of resuscitation from shock. Only 2% of children sustaining trauma will present with complete mechanical obstruction to the airway. In the rare child who presents with acute airway obstruction, **needle cricothyroidostomy** is the preferred method of securing the airway until definitive airway control can be achieved. This technique of ventilation uses the principle of jet insufflation as defined in the adult. **Surgical cricothyrotomy** in children results in a high incidence of subglottic stenosis, but it is still a viable option if needle cricothyroidostomy fails to be effective.

Because infants are obligatory nasal and diaphragmatic breathers, fractures and soft-tissue injuries that occlude the nostrils may actually obstruct the airway. Since air swallowed by the infant or insufflated into the stomach may cause acute gastric distention and restrict diaphragmatic excursion, the stomach should be decompressed with an OG tube.

Once the airway is secured and breathing is assured, attention should be given to the circulation. In the noncrying child, the SBP should be approximately 80+ their age in years × 2. Children may compensate for as much as 25% of circulating volume blood loss without a change in BP. Poor peripheral perfusion, decreased level of consciousness and ↓UO are suggestive of hypovolemia. IV access must be obtained rapidly to begin crystalloid resuscitation in any child with impending signs of shock. If the peripheral iv access is difficult to obtain, as is often the case, saphenous vein cutdown at the saphenofemoral junction should be performed. In infants, if iv access cannot be obtained within 2 min, intraosseous access should be attempted (Fig 7.13-6). Once iv access has been obtained, as many as 3 boluses of crystalloid, using a volume of 20 ml/kg, can be given. If the hypovolemic shock state has not been reversed after the second bolus, and other causes of shock—such as spinal injury, cardiac tamponade, or pneumothorax—were excluded, blood (10 ml/kg) should be administered without delay.

Another important problem in the management of pediatric trauma is related to high ratio of body surface area to body mass and lack of substantial subcutaneous tissue. A small infant who is hypothermic may be refractory to therapy; therefore, every attempt should be made to prevent heat loss, and all iv fluids should be warmed.

Needle cricothyrostomy: With the head in neutral position (which may require placement of towels under the shoulders), the neck should be prepped from the jaw to the chest. The neck is protected by in-line immobilization. The cricothyroid membrane should be identified, and the thyroid cartilage immobilized with the surgeon's left hand. The cricothyroid membrane is punctured perpendicularly with a 14-16 ga iv catheter over a needle. The needle is then redirected caudally, the catheter slid off into the trachea, and jet insufflation initiated. Placement of a permanent airway should follow.

Saphenous cutdown: The groin should be prepped and draped and a curvilinear incision made 1-2 cm below and parallel to the inguinal ligament. The saphenous vein is identified at the saphenofemoral junction medially to the femoral artery, and two ligatures are passed underneath if the distal ligature is tied and used to apply tension to the vein. The vein is punctured with a scalpel blade (No. 11) and cut, creating a small flap. Tension applied to the proximal ligature reduces backbleeding during cannulation. A catheter is then introduced, the proximal ligature is tied, and the distal ligature is used to secure the catheter in place.

Intraosseous infusion: After skin preparation, an incision is made 2 cm distal to the tibial tuberosity on the flattened medial aspect of the tibia. An 18-20 ga spinal needle (with obturator) can be used in children < 18 mo of age. Older patients may require use of a 13-16 bone marrow biopsy needle. Pressure and rotatory motion are applied

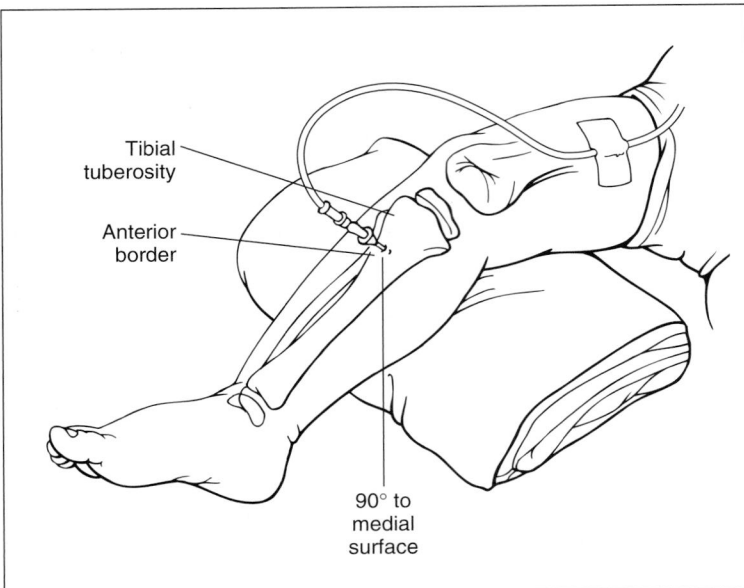

Figure 7.13-6. Intraosseous infusion. (Reproduced with permission from *Textbook of Pediatric Life Support*. American Heart Association, 1994.)

in a direction perpendicular to the bone until a decrease in resistance is felt. Position of the needle can be confirmed by bone marrow or blood aspiration. This route can be used for rapid fluid infusion and most resuscitation medications can be given this way. Interosseus infusion, however, is only an emergency maneuver and should be used to restore circulating volume to the level that enables more permanent iv access.

Usual preop diagnosis: Airway obstruction; hypovolemic shock; hypovolemic shock with difficult iv access

General Trauma Surgery References

1. Capan LM, Miller SM: Trauma and Burns. In *Clinical Anesthesia*, Barash PG, Cullen BF, Stoelting RK, eds. Lippincott Williams & Wilkins, Philadelphia: 2001, 1255-96.
2. Dutton RP, Sharar SR, eds: Trauma. *International Anesthesiology Clinics,* 40(3). Lippincott Williams & Wilkins, Philadelphia: 2002.
3. Hirshberg A, Mattox KL: Damage control surgery. *Surg Clin North Am* 1997; 77(4):909-20.
4. Karlin A: Anesthesia for Trauma. In *Reference Courses in Anesthesiology*. American Society of Anesthesiologists, Lippincott-Raven Publishers, Philadelphia: 1997; Vol 25, 107-16.

8.0 OBSTETRIC/GYNECOLOGIC SURGERY

Surgeons

O.W. Stephanie Yap, MD
Amreen Husain, MD
Daniel S. Kapp, MD, PhD
Nelson N. Teng, MD, PhD

8.1 GYNECOLOGIC ONCOLOGY

Anesthesiologists

Ian Carroll, MD
Myer H. Rosenthal, MD, FACCP

STAGING LAPAROTOMY FOR OVARIAN, FALLOPIAN TUBE, AND PRIMARY PERITONEAL CANCER

SURGICAL CONSIDERATIONS

Description: Ovarian carcinoma has the highest mortality rate of all gynecologic malignancies because it is usually discovered in advanced stages, with pelvic mass, omental caking, and ascites being common findings at presentation. Surgery is used for staging as well as therapy. Studies have demonstrated an inverse relationship between postop residual tumor mass and survival; therefore, the goals of surgery are: accurate staging and optimal tumor debulking (< 1 cm residual disease). The standard procedure consists of a meticulous exploration of the abdominopelvic cavity, abdominopelvic cytology, multiple random and targeted biopsies, **total abdominal hysterectomy (TAH)**, **bilateral salpingo-oophorectomy (BSO)**, **pelvic** and **paraaortic lymph node dissection**, **infracolic omentectomy**, and **appendectomy**. After access to the abdomen is obtained through a midline abdominal incision, cytologic washings of the pelvis, pericolic gutters, lesser sac, and hemidiaphragms are done. The peritoneal cavity is carefully explored. A TAH/BSO is performed by ligating and transecting the round, infundibulopelvic, broad, cardinal, and uterosacral ligaments on both sides. The specimen is cut away from the vagina and the cuff closed. The pelvic and paraaortic lymph nodes are dissected in a manner similar to that described under Radical Hysterectomy, p. 621. All residual tumor is removed,

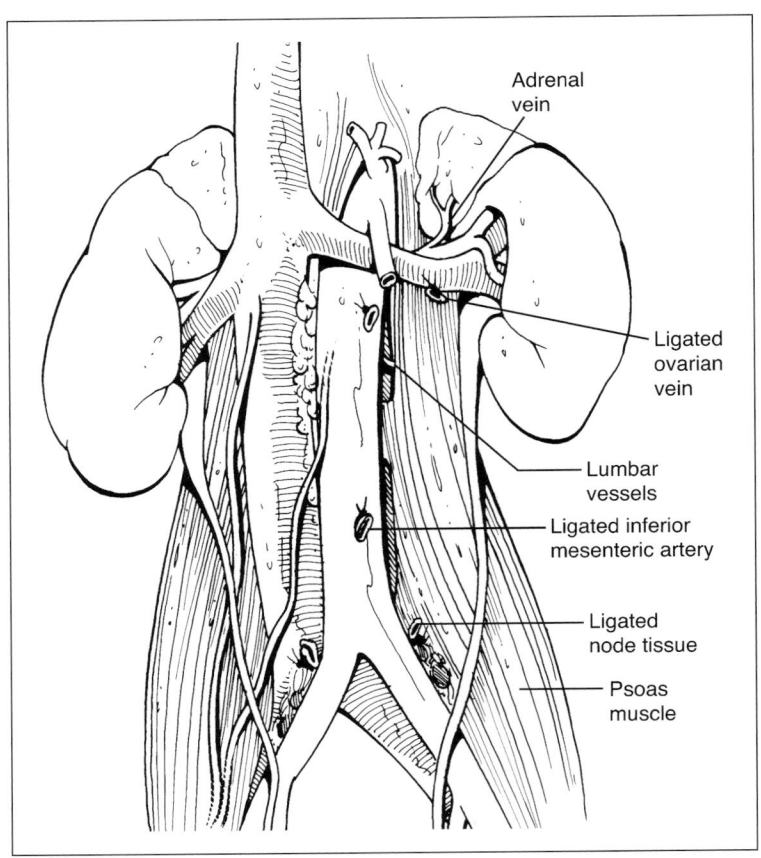

Figure 8.1-1. Aortic node dissection in staging laparotomy for ovarian cancer. In this case, both right and left node dissections have occurred, leaving the kidney, renal hilum, and psoas muscle exposed. Because the dissection is infrarenal and anterior to the lumbar vessels, there is residual fatty and nodal tissue at the posterior limit of the dissection.

using sharp dissection and/or CUSA and/or argon beam coagulator (ABC), and then an appendectomy usually is performed. The omentum is clamped, transected and ligated along its attachment to the transverse colon. A bowel resection with possible colostomy formation may be necessary to achieve optimal cytoreductive surgery (see Pelvic Exenteration, p. 613). Next, the peritoneal cavity is irrigated copiously with warm water. Targeted and random biopsies of bladder, cul-de-sac of Douglas, pericolic gutters, hemidiaphragms, small bowel, large bowel, and anterior abdominal wall are performed. A permanent peritoneal port may be placed subcutaneously for use in future dose-intensive intraperitoneal chemotherapy. A less extensive surgical procedure may be appropriate if a large volume of unresectable tumor is discovered. Surgery in these cases must be individualized.

In some Stage I lesions, a **unilateral salpingo-oophorectomy** is sufficient therapy. The decision to use this approach depends on cell type, age, reproductive status, and extent of disease. Generally, a retroperitoneal **lymph node dissection**, **omentectomy**, and **appendectomy** also are performed. Approximately 25% of patients undergoing **cytoreductive surgery** for advanced stages of ovarian carcinoma require bowel resection with either primary reanastomosis or colostomy. A splenectomy is not routinely done unless the spleen is involved with tumor. A permanent central venous infusion port may be placed for convenient venous access. This usually is done at the completion of the abdominal surgery following skin closure. Some patients with unresectable disease and bowel obstruction will require a gastrostomy tube placement at this time.

Usual preop diagnosis: Ovarian cancer/pelvic mass

SUMMARY OF PROCEDURE

Position	Supine
Incision	Midline or paramedian abdominal
Special instrumentation	CUSA, Vital View (suction-irrigation device combined with light source) helpful; laparoscopic biopsy forceps (laparoscope, laparoscopic instruments for evaluation of upper abdomen through lower vertical abdominal incision); ABC; TA, GIA, EEA stapling devices.
Unique considerations	Removal of large amounts of ascites may → fluid shifts and intravascular volume depletion intraop and postop.
Antibiotics	Cefotetan 2 g iv on call to OR; then q 12 h × 2 doses
Surgical time	1-4 h; 4-5 h, including splenectomy and bowel surgery for more advanced stages
Closing considerations	NG tube placement by anesthesiologist; permanent peritoneal or central venous access for subsequent chemotherapy
EBL	500-1000 ml; 250-500 ml for Stage I lesions; 1300 ml for more advanced stages
Postop care	Extensive peritoneal raw surfaces → intraperitoneal fluid 3rd-spacing. Patients require good hydration to maintain intravascular volume. Central hemodynamic monitoring and ICU admission are useful in selected patients. Use SCDs and mini-dose heparin for DVT prophylaxis.
Mortality	1-2/1000
Morbidity	Postop fever: 14-19%
	Wound infection: < 5%
	Wound dehiscence: 0.3-3%
	PE: 1-2%
	Ureteral injury: < 1%
	Vaginal vault prolapse: Rare
Pain score	7-8

PATIENT POPULATION CHARACTERISTICS

Age range	All age groups; most common, 50-59 yr.
Incidence	15/100,000 (26,700+ new cases/yr); 1.4% lifetime risk of ovarian cancer
Etiology	Unknown
Predisposing factors	Family Hx of ovarian carcinoma; personal or family Hx of breast cancer (BRCA gene mutations); ↑age at first pregnancy; gonadal dysgenesis; exposure to radiation; environmental factors
Associated conditions	Familial cancer syndromes (e.g., endometrial, colon, breast); Peutz-Jeghers syndrome—5% of cases develop gonadal stromal tumor; XY gonadal dysgenesis—gonadoblastomas; multiple nevoid basal cell carcinoma (Gorlin's syndrome); ataxia telangiectasia (hereditary, progressive cerebellar lack of muscular coordination associated with recurrent pulmonary infections and ocular and cutaneous telangiectasias)

ANESTHETIC CONSIDERATIONS

PREOPERATIVE

Ovarian carcinoma is usually diagnosed at a relatively late stage and, therefore, the patient may have significant ascites and a fairly large tumor mass. Surgery is indicated for cure of localized tumor and for staging of distant and local metastases. Additional procedures, such as bowel resection or lymph node dissection, occasionally are performed at the same time.

Respiratory	Significant ascites may distend the abdomen and produce respiratory compromise. The presence of orthopnea, tachypnea, or other signs of impaired ventilation need to be investigated. Underlying lung diseases, such as asthma, also may be exacerbated by the abdominal distension. **Tests:** Consider CXR; others as indicated from H&P.
Cardiovascular	An ECHO, MUGA scan, or other studies may be requested to evaluate cardiac function. Exercise tolerance should be evaluated in every patient and any preexisting cardiac disease explored in the preop visit. Irreversible, dose-dependent cardiotoxicity may result from doxorubicin chemotherapy. **Tests:** Consider ECG, as indicated from H&P.
Gastrointestinal	Patient should have adequate preop iv hydration if given a bowel prep overnight.
Neurological	Not usually significant. Taxol and cisplatin can → peripheral neuropathy.

Hematologic	Bone marrow suppression common following chemotherapy. Carboplatin, commonly used for ovarian cancer, often induces thrombocytopenia. **Tests:** Hct; WBC; Plt
Laboratory	LFT; CT scan of abdomen and pelvis
Premedication	Anxiolytic, such as midazolam 1-2 mg iv, on the morning of surgery

INTRAOPERATIVE

Anesthetic technique: GETA ± epidural analgesia. Typically, a balanced anesthetic with inhalational agents or propofol infusion (100-200 μg/kg/min) and narcotics. An epidural catheter may be placed for postop pain management and also may be used intraop to ↓ anesthetic requirements.

Induction	Standard induction (see p. B-2).	
Maintenance	Standard maintenance (p. B-3). Continue muscle relaxant, based on nerve stimulator response. Epidural 2% lidocaine with epinephrine 1:200,000 (~10 ml/h) if catheter is placed preop. A NG tube should be placed after induction and kept on low suction to help prevent postop N/V. Patients with combined regional/GA may require increased fluids due to vasodilation.	
Emergence	The patient may be extubated at the conclusion of surgery, unless hemodynamically unstable or requiring continued vigorous fluid resuscitation. Reverse muscle relaxant with neostigmine 0.07 mg/kg and glycopyrrolate 0.01 mg/kg, and give supplemental O_2 after extubation. It is reasonable to schedule a postop ICU bed for unstable patients or those who require invasive monitoring for fluid management. Consider PONV prophylaxis (e.g., ondansetron 4 mg iv).	
Blood and fluid requirements	± Significant blood loss IV: 16 ga × 2 NS/LR @ 4-6 ml/kg/h 5% albumin 6% hetastarch	Blood loss may be 1-2 L. Give PRBCs to keep Hct ~27%. 5% albumin or 6% hetastarch are useful for rapid volume replacement if Hct is acceptable. If large volumes of ascites are removed, significant ↓BP can develop from fluid shifts. Third-space losses, therefore, may be 10-15 ml/kg/h. Alternating NS and LR is recommended to avoid development of a nonanion gap hyperchloremic acidosis 2° excessive NS.
Monitoring	Standard monitors (p. B-1) ± Arterial catheter ± CVP/PA catheter Foley catheter NG tube	Arterial and PA catheters are indicated for extensive surgery and/or patients with underlying medical conditions (e.g., CAD, COPD). The measurements of cardiac filling pressures and CO help to guide fluid replacement when surgery is extensive.
Positioning	✓ and pad pressure points. ✓ eyes. Antiembolism stockings and SCD	
Complications	Hypothermia	These patients tend to become hypothermic, so it is important to warm all iv fluids and humidify inspired gases. A heating blanket on the bed and a forced-air warmer are helpful, as is wrapping the head with toweling or plastic. Keep OR as warm as practical. Central T should be monitored in the bladder or esophagus during surgery. Periop hypothermia may ↑ the incidence of wound infections, prolong hospital stays, and ↑ blood loss.
	Renal failure	Renal dose dopamine (1-3 μg/kg/min) with adequate preload may be indicated to maintain UO > 0.5 ml/kg/h in patients with borderline renal function; however, adequate levels of preload are essential to maintain renal perfusion.

POSTOPERATIVE

Complications	Excess fluid requirement	If patient required large volumes of fluid, extubation may need to be delayed until a diuresis can be started. IPPV

Complications,		with PEEP may be beneficial in maintaining lung volumes
cont.		and decreasing lung-water accumulation. Measurement of
		cardiac filling pressures is helpful in guiding therapy. Pul-
		monary edema may develop 3-5 d postop.
Pain management	PCA	See PCA and epidural narcotic recommendations on
	Epidural spinal narcotics	pages C-2 and C-3. Epidural may ↓ pain, PONV, and risk
		of DVT.
	PONV	Incidence of PONV ranges from 18-25% Rx: granisetron
		100 μg.

References

1. Burghardt E, et al: Pelvic lymphadenectomy in operative treatment of ovarian cancer. *Am J Obstet Gynecol* 1986; 155(2): 315-19.
2. Cruikshank DP, Buchsbaum HJ: Effects of rapid paracentesis. Cardiovascular dynamics and body fluid composition. *JAMA* 1973; 225(11):1361-2.
3. Curtin JP, Malik R, Venkataraman ES, et al: Stage IV ovarian cancer: impact of surgical debulking. *Gynecol Oncol* 1997; 64:9.
4. DiSaia PJ, Creasman WT: Epithelial ovarian cancer. In *Clinical Gynecologic Oncology*. DiSaia PJ, Creasman WT, eds. CV Mosby, St Louis: 2002; 289-350.
5. Halpin TF, McCann TO: Dynamics of body fluids following the rapid removal of large volumes of ascites. *Am J Obstet Gynecol* 1971; 110(1):103-6.
6. Morrow CP, Curtin JP: Surgery for ovarian neoplasia. In *Gynecologic Cancer Surgery*. Churchill Livingstone, New York: 1996, 627-716.
7. Ozols RF, Rubin SC, Thomas G, Robboy S: Epithelial ovarian cancer. In *Principles and Practice of Gynecologic Oncology, 3rd edition*. Hoskins WJ, Perez CA, Young RC, eds: Lippincott Williams & Wilkins, Philadelphia: 2000, 981-1073.
8. Sessler D: Mild perioperative hypothermia. *N Engl J Med* 1997; 336:1730-7.
9. Wheeless CR Jr: Staging of gynecologic oncology patients with exploratory laparotomy. In *Atlas of Pelvic Surgery*, 3rd edition. Williams & Wilkins, Baltimore: 1997, 380-1.
10. Wiklund RA, Rosenbaum S: Anesthesiology: Second of two parts. *N Engl J Med* 1997; 337(17):1215-19.
11. Wu PC, Lang JH, Huang RL, et al: Lymph node metastasis and retroperitoneal lymphadenectomy in ovarian cancer. *Bailliere's Clin Obstet Gynaecol* 1989; 3:143.
12. Young RC, Decker DG, Wharton JT, et al: Staging laparotomy in early ovarian cancer. *JAMA* 1983; 230:3072.

SECOND-LOOK/REASSESSMENT LAPAROTOMY FOR OVARIAN CANCER

SURGICAL CONSIDERATIONS

Description: The clinical evaluation of an ovarian cancer patient's response to chemotherapy may be unreliable because tumor that may defy detection by noninvasive methods can be present in the abdominopelvic cavity. Surgery in the form of **'second-look' laparotomy** is the only reliable method of evaluation of disease status in ovarian cancer patients after chemotherapy. It usually is undertaken to determine whether the patient is surgically and pathologically free of disease, after an appropriate number of treatment cycles with platinum-based (CDDP or carboplatin) chemotherapy. The recent advent of tumor markers (CA-125) and imaging techniques (CT, MRI, PET), however, have significantly reduced the incidence of 'second look' surgery. In addition, in cases where optimal debulking could not be performed, a second-look debulking laparotomy is done to achieve optimal cytoreduction. The surgery involves methodical and meticulous exploration of all of the abdomen and pelvis, multiple cytologies and biopsies, lysis of adhesions, resection of the residual tumor, as well as the pelvic and periaortic lymph nodes (if not done at time of first surgery). This procedure also may be done laparoscopically (see p. 496).

Usual preop diagnosis: Ovarian carcinoma

SUMMARY OF PROCEDURE

Position	Supine
Incision	Midline or paramedian vertical abdominal
Antibiotics	Cefotetan 2 g preop; then q 12 h × 2 doses
Surgical time	2-3 h
Closing considerations	Placement of permanent central venous or intraperitoneal access
EBL	350-700 ml
Postop care	PACU → room
Mortality	1-2/1000
Morbidity	Postop fever: 14-19%
	Wound infection: < 5%
	Wound dehiscence: 0.3-3%
	PE: 1-2%
	Incisional hernia: 0.5-1%
	Ureteral injury: 0.5-1%
	Necrotizing fasciitis: Rare
	Posthysterectomy prolapse of vaginal vault: Rare
Pain score	7-8

PATIENT POPULATION CHARACTERISTICS

Age range	All ages; most common, 50-59 yr
Incidence	15/100,000; 26,700+ new cases/yr; 1.4% lifetime risk of ovarian cancer
Etiology	Risk factors include: positive family Hx; nulliparity; ↑age at first pregnancy; gonadal dysgenesis; exposure to radiation; environmental factors
Associated conditions	Familial cancer syndromes (e.g., endometrial, colon, breast); Peutz-Jeghers syndrome (5% of cases develop gonadal stromal tumor); XY gonadal dysgenesis (gonadoblastomas); multiple, nevoid basal-cell carcinoma (Gorlin's syndrome); ataxia telangiectasia

Table 8.1-1. Toxicities of Selected Antineoplastic Chemotherapeutic Agents

Agent	Toxic Effects
Vincristine, vinblastine	Neuropathies, SIADH, myelosuppression
Cyclophosphamide	Prolonged neuromuscular block
Mechlorethamine	Prolonged neuromuscular block
Bleomycin	Pulmonary fibrosis
Doxorubicin, daunorubicin	Cardiotoxicity, GI upset, myelosuppression
Methotrexate	Myelosuppression, GI upset, stomatitis, pulmonary infiltrates
Fluorouracil	Myelosuppression, hepatic and GI alterations, nervous system dysfunction
Mercaptopurine	Myelosuppression
Thioguanine	Myelosuppression
Actinomycin D	Myelosuppression, GI upset, stomatitis
Mitomycin	Myelosuppression, GI upset
Cisplatin, carboplatin	Peripheral neuropathy, GI upset, electrolyte disturbances, nephrotoxicity, myelosuppression
Paclitaxel	Myelosuppression, peripheral neuropathy, GI upset, arthralgia/myalgias, mucositis
Docetaxel	Myelosuppression, peripheral neuropathy, malaise, maculopapular rash, GI upset

ANESTHETIC CONSIDERATIONS

PREOPERATIVE

Patients having a second-look laparotomy have undergone surgical resection of a tumor with lymph node biopsy, usually followed by chemotherapy and/or radiation therapy. Depending on the type of adjunctive treatment given, the patient may come to surgery in poor physical condition from malnutrition or toxicity from chemotherapy (see Table 8.1-1). Vascular access may be difficult to obtain due to sclerosis or thrombosis of peripheral veins.

Respiratory	Pulmonary function may be impaired by several chemotherapeutic drugs, most commonly bleomycin. Patients often have a Hickman catheter or other central line already in place, which can be used for induction of anesthesia. A preop CXR is mandatory to assess the presence of lung injury. Patients who have dyspnea at rest or with mild exertion, or who have known pulmonary fibrosis, should be evaluated by PFTs, including FVC, FEV_1, $MMEF_{25-75}$, and ABGs. Patients who have received bleomycin should not receive $O_2 > 39\%$ intraop, but arterial O_2 saturation ideally should be kept $\geq 93\%$. The pulmonary toxicity of bleomycin is dose-related, with a much higher incidence occurring if over 200 mg/m². Combination chemotherapy with vincristine or cisplatin also increases pulmonary toxicity. Severe lung disease is an indication for the use of spinal or epidural anesthesia whenever possible; otherwise, postop mechanical ventilation may be necessary. **Tests:** Consider CXR; others as indicated from H&P.
Cardiovascular	Cardiotoxicity is seen with several antineoplastic agents, especially daunorubicin and doxorubicin. The cardiomyopathy produced by these drugs occurs in two forms: (1) acute—ST-T wave changes and dysrhythmias, which are transient and usually not a serious problem; and (2) chronic—a dose-related toxicity manifested by CHF. Total doses of doxorubicin as low as 250 U can cause myocardial damage, but is more common at doses > 400 U. Cardiac irradiation, or combination chemotherapy with cyclophosphamide, increases the risk of cardiac toxicity. Patients who have received cardiotoxic drugs are usually followed by serial ECHOs or MUGA scans, and the results of these tests should be reviewed preop. Patients with CHF or ECG changes should have a cardiology consultation preop to optimize their medical condition. **Tests:** ECG; others as indicated from H&P.
Neurological	Peripheral neuropathies are produced by vincristine, cyclophosphamide, Taxol (paclitaxel), 5-fluorouracil and several other drugs. Vincristine can also → SIADH. Other CNS effects include N/V, Sz, and cerebellar dysfunction. A preop neurologic exam is required for patients with evidence of neurotoxicity. It is important to document the presence of neurologic deficits preop for subsequent comparisons.
Endocrine	Steroids such as prednisone are commonly used with chemotherapeutic agents, as treatment for pulmonary fibrosis and other complications of chemotherapy. The use of steroids for several wk suppresses the endogenous secretion of the adrenal cortex, which may take up to 6 mo to recover fully. Hydrocortisone 100 mg iv, therefore, is given periop q 8 h to cover the stress associated with surgery. The dose is tapered rapidly over 2 or 3 d postop. If the patient is receiving hormone replacement for hypothyroidism, it may be continued as scheduled periop. Diabetics should be managed to keep blood sugar at 150-250 mg/dL. A glucose and insulin infusion (100 U regular insulin/L D5W) is useful for maintaining proper blood glucose levels intraop. Infuse at 10-20 ml/h, based on the results of hourly blood glucose determinations during surgery; 20 mEq KCl/L may be added in patients with normal renal function to prevent hypokalemia. Oral hypoglycemic agents should be withheld on the day of surgery. **Tests:** Fasting blood sugar (if diabetic)
Renal	Many chemotherapeutic drugs have renal toxicity; therefore, a preop set of renal function tests is mandatory. Patients with impaired renal function should be given appropriate dosages of medications (e.g., antibiotics), which depend on renal excretion. **Tests:** Renal function tests
Musculoskeletal	Vincristine produces a neurotoxicity manifested by numbness and tingling in the extremities, weakness, foot drop, loss of reflexes, ataxia, and muscle pains. Muscle weakness in the arms and legs indicates that the drug should be D/C'd. Muscle weakness also may involve the larynx and extraocular eye muscles. Reduced amounts of NMBs should be used intraop and a nerve stimulator used to follow twitches.
Gastrointestinal	Consider hydration overnight if given a bowel prep or if there is significant N/V. **Tests:** Consider serum electrolytes, if indicated from H&P.
Hematologic	Bone marrow suppression is a very common side effect of antineoplastic drugs. The toxicity usually produces a reversible drop in leukocytes, erythrocytes, and Plt, with a nadir 10-14 d posttreatment.

Hematologic, cont.	Patients with a total neutrophil count of < 1,000 should be kept in isolation until counts improve. A low Plt count (< 75,000) is an indication for Plt transfusion preop. Regional anesthesia in patients with thrombocytopenia needs to be considered carefully due to ↑risk of bleeding complications. It is useful to ✓ PT/PTT preop when in doubt about the coag status of a patient. A preop transfusion of Plts and/or RBCs is recommended if lab values are below acceptable limits (Plt < 75,000, Hct < 25).
	Tests: Hb/Hct; WBC; Plt; PT; PTT
Laboratory	LFTs if indicated by H&P.
Premedication	Anxiolytic such as midazolam 1-5 mg im or iv. Stress-dose hydrocortisone (100 mg) if indicated.

INTRAOPERATIVE

Anesthetic technique: GETA usually indicated. Combined GETA/epidural or spinal are also excellent choices; however, surgery should be done under regional anesthesia in patients with severe bleomycin pulmonary toxicity.

General anesthesia:

Induction	Standard induction (see p. B-2). Consider renal function and surgery duration when deciding on agent.
Maintenance	Standard maintenance: see Anesthetic Considerations for Staging Laparotomy, p. 596. An epidural may be used to reduce GA requirements (p. B-3).
Emergence	Extubate when patient is responsive and neuromuscular block is fully reversed. In patients with borderline pulmonary function, extubation may be delayed until patient is in the PACU or ICU, and after ABG is checked while the patient breathes spontaneously. Consider PONV prophylaxis (e.g., ondansetron 4 mg iv).

Regional anesthesia:

Epidural	2% lidocaine ± epinephrine 1:200,000 (10-15 ml) or 0.5% bupivacaine (10-15 ml) are used; then at ~10 ml/h. Narcotics, such as morphine (2-4 mg) or hydromorphone (0.3-0.5 mg), may be given in the epidural for postop pain control.	
Blood and fluid requirements	IV: 16-18 ga × 1-2 NS/LR @ 7-10 ml/kg/h Keep UO > 0.5 ml/kg/h. PRBC for Hct < 30% 5% albumin 6% hetastarch	Excessive use of NS can lead to hyperchloremic metabolic acidosis; therefore, alternating NS and LR solutions makes sense when giving large volumes of iv fluids. 5% albumin or 6% hetastarch may be used as volume replacement when Hct > 30%, although they have no proven advantages over crystalloid solutions.
	FFP/Plt	FFP and Plts are used if there is evidence of coagulopathy (↑PT, ↑PTT, ↓Plt).
Monitoring	Standard monitors (see p. B-1). ± Arterial line ± CVP/PA catheter Foley catheter NG tube	Arterial and CVP catheters are indicated for patients with compromised cardiac or pulmonary function or patients having extensive surgical procedures.
Positioning	✓ and pad pressure points. ✓ eyes. Anti-embolism stockings and SCD	It is useful to maintain access to at least one arm for blood drawing and additional iv access.
Complications	Hypothermia	Warm all fluids; keep heating pad on bed; wrap patient's head in plastic or towels; use forced-air warmer. Avoidance of hypothermia may ↓ wound infections, hospital stay, and blood loss.
	Bleeding	✓ PT; PTT, Plts periodically for large blood loss.

POSTOPERATIVE

Complications	Bleeding PONV Infection Respiratory insufficiency	Antiemetics should be given for nausea. Supplemental O_2 should be given in PACU. PONV = 18-25% or more.

Pain management	PCA (see p. C-3). Epidural/spinal narcotics (see p. C-2).	Surgeons may infiltrate wound edges with 0.25% bupivacaine in those patients without epidurals. Consider iv ketorolac (30 mg).
Tests	CXR ABG	As indicated by postop clinical findings.

References

1. Chabner BA, Ryan DP, Paz-Ares S, et al: Antineoplastic agents. In *Goodman and Gilman's: The Pharmacologic Basis of Therapeutics*, 10th edition. Hardman JG, Limbird LE, Gilman AG, eds. McGraw Hill, New York: 2001, 1389-1459.
2. Copeland LJ, Gershenson DM, Wharton JT, Atkinson EN, Sneige N, Edwards CL, Rutledge FN: Microscopic disease at second-look laparotomy in advanced ovarian cancer. *Cancer* 1985; 55(2):472-8.
3. Creasman WT: Second look laparotomy in ovarian cancer. *Gynecol Oncol* 1994; 55:S122-S127.
4. DiSaia PJ, Creasman WT: Epithelial ovarian cancer. In *Clinical Gynecologic Oncology*. DiSaia PJ, Creasman WT, eds. CV Mosby, St. Louis: 2002, 289-350.
5. Ozols RF, Rubin SC, Thomas G, Robboy S: Epithelial ovarian cancer. In *Principles and Practice of Gynecologic Oncology*, 3rd edition. Hoskins WJ, Perez CA, Young RC, eds. Lippincott Williams & Wilkens, Philadelphia: 2000, 981-1073.
6. Podratz KC, Cliby WA: Second look surgery in the management of epithelial ovarian carcinoma. *Gynecol Oncol* 1994; 55: S128-S133.
7. Podratz KC, Kinney WK: Second-look operation in ovarian cancer. *Cancer* 1993; 71:1551.
8. Rubin SC, Lewis JL Jr: Second-look surgery in ovarian carcinoma. *Crit Rev Oncol Hematol* 1988; 8(75):91.
9. Sessler D: Mild perioperative hypothermia. *N Engl J Med* 1997; 336:1730-7.
10. Williams L: The role of secondary cytoreductive surgery in epithelial ovarian malignancies. *Oncology* 1992; 6:25.

RADICAL VULVECTOMY

SURGICAL CONSIDERATIONS

Description: En bloc dissection of the inguinal-femoral region and the vulva is the time-honored treatment for invasive vulvar carcinoma. The surgery involves bilateral excision of lymphatic and areolar tissue in the inguinal and femoral regions, combined with removal of the entire vulva between the labia-crural folds, from the perineal body to the upper margin of mons pubis (Fig 8.1-2). A large surgical wound is created and, if 1° closure without tension is not possible, a skin or myocutaneous graft may be necessary. Deep pelvic nodes are almost never involved with metastases when the superficial and deep groin nodes are free of disease; therefore, a **pelvic lymphadenectomy** is no longer routinely performed. If presence of tumor is documented in the groin nodes, particularly in Cloquet's sentinel nodes (the most cephalad, deep inguinal nodes), a **deep pelvic lymphadenectomy** may be performed. **Postop radiation therapy**, however, is widely used instead of a pelvic lymph node dissection to minimize operative morbidity and confer a survival advantage.

A skin incision in the shape of a bull's head (Fig 8.1-2) allows access to the inguinal-femoral region. (The incision ideally should extend 2+ cm beyond the tumor margin.) The inguinal ligament and rectus fascia should be cleared bilaterally of all nodal tissues,

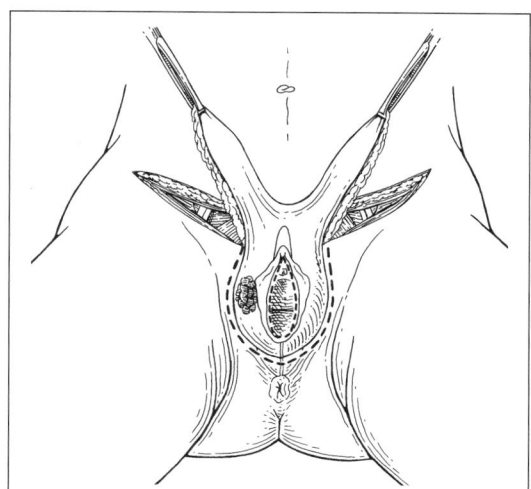

Figure 8.1-2. En bloc radical vulvectomy incisions shown; bilateral inguinal lymphadenectomy is complete. (Reproduced with permission from Rock JA, Thompson JD: *TeLinde's Operative Gynecology*, 8th edition. Lippincott Williams & Wilkins, 1997.)

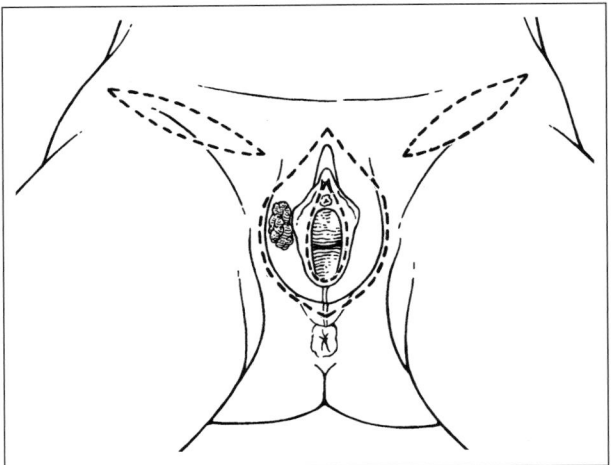

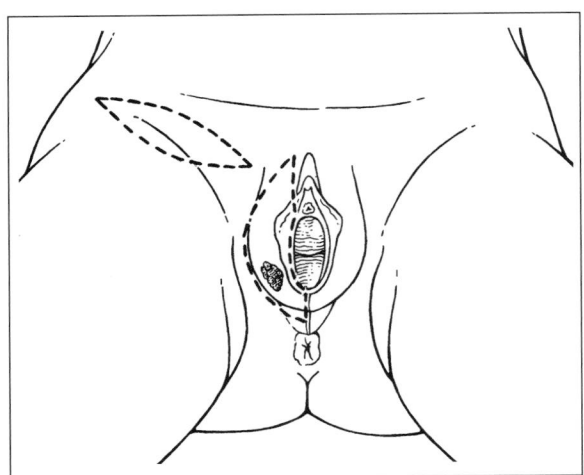

Figure 8.1-3. 3-incision radical vulvectomy and bilateral inguino-femeral lymphadenectomy. (Produced with permission from Rock JA, Thompson JD: *TeLinde's Operative Gynecology*, 8th edition. Lippincott Williams & Wilkins, 1997.)

Figure 8.1-4. Unilateral lymphadenectomy for a well lateralized lesion. (Produced with permission from Rock JA, Thompson JD: *TeLinde's Operative Gynecology*, 8th edition. Lippincott Williams & Wilkins, 1997.)

and the fossae ovalis on both sides identified. The lateral aspect of the femoral sheath is incised along the sartorius muscle, with care being taken not to injure the femoral nerve or vessels, and the cribriform fascia is cleaned off the femoral artery. The external pudendal artery, which marks the entrance of the saphenous vein into the fossa ovalis, should be identified and ligated. The proximal and distal segments of the saphenous vein should be ligated and excised as the fibrofatty, lymph-bearing tissue of the femoral sheath is resected. Cloquet's nodes at the femoral ring beneath the inguinal ligaments on both sides should be resected and submitted for frozen-section pathology evaluation. The deep inguinal lymphatic chain is removed on both sides by opening the inguinal canal from the external inguinal ring. The vulvar incision is carried down through the labia-crural folds. The internal pudendal vessels at the posterior lateral margin of the vulvar incision are identified as they emerge from Alcock's canal, then are ligated and incised.

Use of electrocautery in this portion of the procedure usually tends to decrease operative blood loss. The dissection is continued along the periosteum of the symphysis at the level of the fascia of the deep muscles of the urogenital diaphragm. The bulbocavernosus, ischiocavernosus, and superficial transverse perinei muscles are removed. A circumferential vaginal incision, excluding the urethral meatus, is then performed and the vulva is removed. The incisions overlying the groin node dissections should be closed with minimal tension after placement of closed-suction Jackson-Pratt drains. The vulvar surgical wound is closed by slightly undermining the skin of the edges of the incision and suturing them to the vaginal mucosa. A **vulvar reconstruction**, using myocutaneous flaps, also can be performed at this time (see Pelvic Exenteration, p. 613).

Variant procedure or approaches: In 1962, Byran and associates popularized a **3-incision technique** first described by Kehrer in 1918. This 3-incision technique, with separate vulva and groin incisions, is the most common approach (Fig 8.1-3). This operative approach has led to a significant decrease in wound infection and breakdown, apparently without increasing tumor recurrence in the inguinal dermal bridge above the symphysis pubis. Another variant is the **hemivulvectomy** (Fig 8.1-4), in which unilateral radical hemivulvectomy and groin node dissection are performed in selected stage I, nonmidline, unifocal vulvar cancer patients. This procedure will minimize morbidity, disfigurement, and sexual dysfunction. The observation that almost no contralateral groin metastases occur in the absence of positive ipsilateral groin nodes allows the surgeon to perform only a **unilateral groin node dissection**. **Lymphatic mapping** and **sentinel lymph node identification** techniques are under development for the management of patients with vulvar cancer.

Usual preop diagnosis: Invasive vulvar cancer

SUMMARY OF PROCEDURES

	En Bloc Dissection	**3-Incision**	**Hemivulvectomy**
Position	Modified dorsolithotomy in Allen universal stirrups	⇐	⇐
Incision	Bull's head, from iliac crest to iliac crest and along labia-crural folds (Fig 8.1-2)	2 separate groin incisions from iliac crest to pubic tubercle; 1 vulvar incision (Fig 8.1-3)	1 or 2 separate groin incisions from iliac crest to pubic tubercle; vulvar incision (Fig 8.1-4)

	En Bloc Dissection	3-Incision	Hemivulvectomy
Special instrumentation	ABC	⇐	⇐
Unique considerations	Two-team approach to minimize surgical time. Preop bowel prep and constipating medications (e.g., Lomotil) to ↓ postop bowel movements.	⇐	⇐
Antibiotics	Cefotetan 2 g iv on call to OR; then 2 g iv q 12 h × 72 h.	⇐	⇐
Surgical time	3-4 h	⇐	2-3 h
Closing considerations	Possible skin graft; vulvar and groin suction drains	⇐	⇐
EBL	500-1000 ml	⇐	250-1000 ml
Postop care	PACU or ICU, if necessary; SCDs and mini-dose heparin ★ for DVT prophylaxis. (**NB:** trauma to femoral vessels at time of groin lymph node dissection increases risk of thrombophlebitis and PE. Aggressive local wound care.)	⇐	⇐
Mortality	1-2%	⇐	⇐
Morbidity	Wound infection and breakdown: 40-80%	15%	< 15%
	Introital stenosis and dyspareunia: 50%	⇐	⇐
	Lymphedema of lower extremities: 25-30%	⇐	< 25% (if deep groin nodes not dissected)
	Lymphocysts: 10%	⇐	⇐
	Genital prolapse: 7%	⇐	1-2%
	Stress incontinence: 5%	⇐	1-2%
	Thrombophlebitis: 3-5%	⇐	1-2%
	Hernia: 1-2%	⇐	⇐
	PE: 1-2%	⇐	⇐
Pain score	8	8	7

PATIENT POPULATION CHARACTERISTICS

Age range	Median = 70 yr
Incidence	2.5/100,000; 3-5% of female genital malignancies
Etiology	Exact etiology unknown; risk factors include vulvar dystrophies; granulomatous disease of vulva; Bowen's disease; condyloma acuminata
Associated conditions	Diabetes; obesity; HTN; arteriosclerosis; nulliparity; positive serology for syphilis; cervical malignancy; human papilloma virus infection

---

ANESTHETIC CONSIDERATIONS

PREOPERATIVE

Patients with vulvar carcinoma are typically in the 6th or 7th decade of life and, hence, have a high incidence of concurrent medical problems, such as HTN, CAD, and diabetes. Radical vulvectomy is performed for invasive tumor that has not metastasized to distant sites. An ICU bed should be reserved for patients with a significant medical Hx.

Respiratory	The presence of lung disease and smoking Hx should be discussed with the patient preop. CXR or PFTs are indicated for patients with significant respiratory disease. The response to bronchodilators should be tested in patients with bronchospastic disease or COPD. **Tests:** Consider CXR; others as indicated from H&P.

Cardiovascular	There is an increased incidence of HTN and atherosclerosis in these patients. A cardiology consultation is indicated for angina, recent MI, CHF, or heart murmurs. An ECG should be ordered for all patients > 50 yr old. **Tests:** ECG; others as indicated from H&P.
Renal	In old age, creatinine clearance is decreased 2° ↓renal mass, but serum creatinine remains unchanged because of decreased muscle mass. Consider ✓ing creatinine clearance in patients > 70 yr old, or with known renal dysfunction. **Tests:** Serum creatine; others as indicated from H&P.
Gastrointestinal	Patients should have iv hydration preop if given bowel prep overnight.
Neurological	Document a neurological exam if Hx of stroke, Sz, or other neurologic disease. Hx of peripheral neuropathy or autonomic dysfunction should be assessed in diabetic patients. **Tests:** As indicated from H&P.
Endocrine	Diabetes, obesity, and hypothyroidism are common in this patient population. **Tests:** Fasting blood sugar; thyroid function; others as indicated from H&P.
Hematologic	Chronic anemia may be present. Encourage autologous blood donation if Hct is adequate. **Tests:** Hb/Hct; Plt count
Laboratory	LFTs, if indicated.
Premedication	Usually no premedication is needed, but occasionally small doses of midazolam (1-3 mg iv) are useful for anxiety.

INTRAOPERATIVE

Anesthetic technique: GETA or regional anesthesia, alone or in combination. Regional techniques may be supplemented by the use of a propofol infusion (25-100 μg/kg/h).

General anesthesia:

Induction	Standard induction (see p. B-2). Elderly patients usually require reduced dosages of medications. Titration to effect is advised when using any induction agent.
Maintenance	Standard maintenance (see p. B-3).
Emergence	No special considerations

Regional anesthesia:

Epidural	2% lidocaine ± epinephrine 1:200,000 (10-20 ml) or 0.5% bupivacaine (10-20 ml) are used; then @ ~10 ml/h. Narcotics such as morphine (2-4 mg) in the epidural for postop pain control.
Spinal	Tetracaine (12 mg) or bupivacaine (13-15 mg), preservative-free morphine (0.3-0.5 mg) → T8 sensory level.

Blood and fluid requirements	IV: 16 ga × 2 NS/LR @ 6-8 ml/kg/h Warm iv fluids. UO > 0.5 ml/kg/h PRBCs for Hct < 25% in healthy patients and < 30% in patients with cardiac or pulmonary disease	Occasionally, femoral vessels may be injured, requiring rapid blood replacement. Use forced-air warming. Hypothermia may ↑ wound infections, bleeding, and hospital stay.
Monitoring	Standard monitors (p. B-1) ± Arterial line ± CVP line Foley catheter	Invasive monitors indicated for patients in poor condition or with cardiovascular or respiratory disease. An arterial catheter is useful for drawing labs in surgery to check Hct, glucose, or ABGs.
Positioning	✓ and pad pressure points. ✓ eyes. Antiembolism stockings and SCD	

POSTOPERATIVE

Complications	Hypothermia	
	Nerve injury	Dx of nerve injury may be delayed by epidural anesthesia.
	Bleeding	
	Atelectasis	Give supplemental O_2 postop.
Pain management	PCA (p. C-3)	Incisions may be left open to granulate in, or be covered with skin grafts. Epidural analgesia allows earlier ambulation with less sedation in elderly patients. Multimodal analgesia with local anesthetics, opioids, NSAIDs, and even low-dose ketamine, may ↓ pain and PONV.
	Epidural or spinal narcotics (p. C-2)	
Tests	Tests as indicated.	From postop clinical findings

References

1. Burke TW, Eifel P, McGuire W, Wilkinson EJ: Vulva. In *Principles and Practice of Gynecologic Oncology,* 3rd edition. Hoskins WJ, Perez CA, Young RC, eds. Lippincott Williams & Wilkins, Philadelphia: 2000, 775-810.
2. Burke TW, Levenback C, Coleman RC, et al: Surgical therapy of T1 and T2 vulvar carcinoma: further experience with radical wide excision and selective inguinal lymphadenectomy. *Gynecol Oncol* 1995; 57:215-20.
3. DiSaia PJ, Creasman WT: Invasive cancer of the vulva. In *Clinical Gynecologic Oncology.* DiSaia PJ, Creasman WT, eds. CV Mosby, St. Louis: 2002, 211-39.
4. DiSaia PJ, Creasman WT, Rich WM: An alternate approach to early cancer of the vulva. *Am J Obstet Gynecol* 1979; 133(7):825-32.
5. Eifel P, Levenback C: Surgery for vulvar cancer. In *American Cancer Society Atlas of Clinical Oncology, Cancer of the Female Lower Genital Tract.* BC Decker, Hamilton: 2001, 203-16.
6. Hoffman MS, Cavanagh LD: Malignancies of the vulva. In *TeLinde's Operative Gynecology.* Rock JA, Thompson JD, eds. Lippincott Williams & Wilkins, Philadelphia: 1997, 1331-83.
7. Morrow CP, Curtin JP: Surgery for vulvar neoplasia. In *Gynecologic Cancer Surgery.* Churchill Livingstone, New York: 1996, 381-450.
8. Siller BS, et al: T2/3 vulva cancer: A case-controlled study of triple incision versus en bloc radical vulvectomy and inguinal lymphadenectomy. *Gynecol Oncol* 1995; 57:335.
9. Stehman FB, Bundy BN, Dvoretsky PM, Creasman WT: Early stage I carcinoma of the vulva treated with ipsilateral superficial inguinal lymphadenectomy and modified radical hemivulvectomy: a prospective study of the Gynecologic Oncology Group. *Obstet Gynecol* 1992; 79:490-7.
10. Wheeless CR Jr: Radical vulvectomy with bilateral inguinal lymph node dissection. In *Atlas of Pelvic Surgery.* Williams & Wilkins, Baltimore: 1997, 405-11.
11. White PF: The role of non-opioid analgesic techniques in the management of pain after ambulatory surgery. *Anesth Analg* 2002; 94(3):577-85.

CONIZATION OF THE CERVIX

SURGICAL CONSIDERATIONS

Description: Conization of the cervix can be used for both diagnostic and therapeutic purposes. It is performed in cases of biopsy-proven dysplasia with unsatisfactory colposcopy (inadequate visualization of the endocervical canal) or following endocervical curettage showing dysplasia or atypical glandular epithelial cells (Fig 8.1-5). Persistent abnormal cytology associated with normal colposcopy, colposcopic suspicion of invasion, and/or cervical biopsy showing microinvasive cancer are also indications for this procedure. The surgery consists of the annular removal of a cone-shaped wedge of tissue from the cervix with a scalpel. With the advent of the LEEP (loop electrosurgical excision procedure), most cone biopsies are done under local paracervical/intracervical block in an office setting and do not require the services of an anesthesiologist.

Variant procedure or approaches: In selected patients, a **laser** is used in place of the scalpel. This procedure can be performed under local anesthesia with less blood loss, but operative time is usually longer. The thermal effect of the laser at the cone margins, although usually minimal, may interfere with pathologic interpretation. In pregnant patients, a **shallower cone** is done to minimize complications. Approximately 1% of women with cervical carcinoma are pregnant at the time of diagnosis, and 1/1240 pregnancies is complicated by cervical cancer. Recognition and therapy of preinvasive cervical lesions during pregnancy, therefore, are of paramount importance. Because of the increased vascularity of the pregnant uterus and cervix, conization is usually associated with increased blood loss and morbidity.

Usual preop diagnosis: Cervical dysplasia

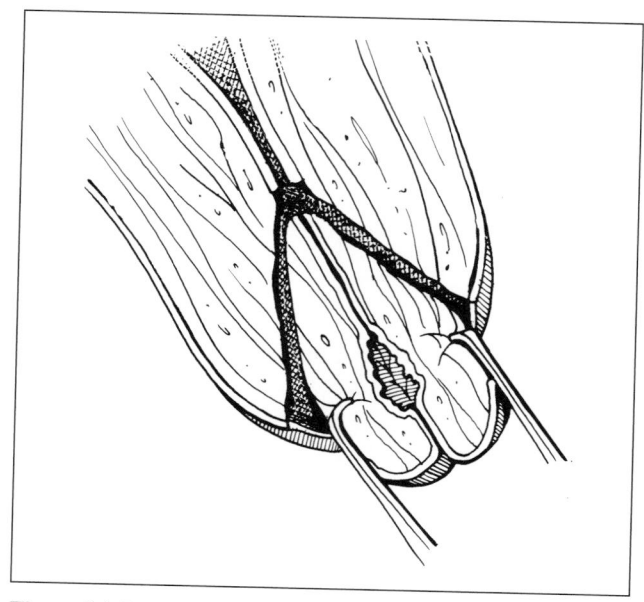

Figure 8.1-5. Cut across endocervix to complete cone excision.

SUMMARY OF PROCEDURES

	Conization	Laser Conization	Shallow Cone In Pregnancy
Position	Lithotomy	⇐	Lithotomy; with left lateral tilt in 3rd trimester
Incision	Cervical	⇐	⇐
Special instrumentation	Colposcope	CO_2 laser; protective eye wear; colposcope	Colposcope
Unique considerations	Infiltration of cervix with dilute vasopressin or phenylephrine solution. A 1:200,000 epinephrine solution also can be used. Vaginal pack necessary in selected patients.	⇐	Phenylephrine, vasopressin, or epinephrine should not be used during pregnancy. Liberal use of hemostatic sutures should be made.
Antibiotics	None	⇐	⇐
Surgical time	30-60 min	30-90 min	⇐
EBL	50-200 ml	50 ml	100-350 ml
Postop care	Be aware of postop bleeding.	⇐	⇐
Mortality	< 0.01%	⇐	⇐
Morbidity	Hemorrhage: 5-10%	⇐	10-15%
	Cervical incompetence: 2-3%	⇐	⇐
	Cervical stenosis: 2-3%	⇐	⇐
	Dysmenorrhea: Rare	⇐	⇐
	Infertility: Rare	⇐	⇐
	Injury to rectum and bladder: Rare	⇐	⇐
	Pelvic cellulitis: Rare	⇐	–
	Uterine perforation: Rare	⇐	–
			Fetal loss: 10-15% (up to 30% in 1st trimester)*
			Premature labor: 5-10% (controversial)
			Rupture of membrane: 2-5%
Pain score	3	3	3

* The naturally higher incidence of spontaneous miscarriages in the 1st trimester contributes to this figure.

PATIENT POPULATION CHARACTERISTICS

Age range	Reproductive and postreproductive years
Incidence	~5% of Pap smears (+ for dysplasia); 10-17% of patients who undergo colposcopic exams
Etiology and predisposing factors	Smoking; human papilloma virus (HPV); herpes simplex virus (HSV); multiple sexual partners; early age of onset of coitus; multiparity; lower socioeconomic status; HIV; immunocompromised hosts

ANESTHETIC CONSIDERATIONS

PREOPERATIVE

Conization is done for diagnosis and treatment of cervical lesions. Occasionally it is necessary to perform the procedure during pregnancy, which increases the risk of bleeding complications. The effect of anesthetic agents on the fetus (especially 1st trimester) also needs to be considered when choosing anesthetic technique (see p. 675).

Respiratory   Not usually a problem, unless there is Hx of lung disease or smoking.

Cardiovascular   These patients are generally young and, therefore, less likely to have significant heart disease.

Neurological   Usually not significant, unless there is Hx of seizure disorder or other neurologic illness.

Hematologic   **Tests**: Hct

Laboratory   Consider pregnancy test.

Premedication   Usually none, although an anxiolytic may be given if not pregnant. Na citrate (0.3 M) 30 ml po should be given 30 min prior to induction in all pregnant patients.

INTRAOPERATIVE

Anesthetic technique: Usually a local or MAC anesthetic; occasionally, GETA or spinal. Pregnancy makes it desirable to perform the procedure under local or regional anesthesia, if possible. The minimalist approach to pharmacologic intervention is appropriate in a pregnant patient.

General anesthesia:

Induction   Standard induction (p. B-2). In pregnant patients, rapid-sequence induction (p. B-5) with cricoid pressure is appropriate. If patient is to be intubated, use either succinylcholine 1 mg/kg iv or vecuronium 0.1 mg/kg iv for muscle relaxation; otherwise, in nonpregnant patients, mask or LMA ventilation may suffice.

Maintenance   Standard maintenance (p. B-3). It is not necessary to maintain muscle relaxation throughout the case; and either controlled or spontaneous ventilation can be used.

Emergence   Reverse muscle relaxants with neostigmine or edrophonium and ensure that the patient is awake and able to protect her airway prior to extubation. It may be prudent to give an antiemetic, such as metoclopramide 10 mg iv or 30 min prior to emergence in nonpregnant patients.

Regional anesthesia: Both spinal and epidural techniques are acceptable, and may be preferred for pregnant patients who cannot tolerate local anesthesia. Prehydration with 1000 ml LR before block is recommended. Treat ↓BP with ephedrine 5-10 mg iv, titrated to effect.

Blood and fluid requirements
Minimal blood loss
IV: 18 ga × 1
NS/LR @ 2-4 ml/kg/h

Monitoring
Standard monitors (see p. B-1).
Fetal monitoring may be indicated for pregnancies > 16 wk.

A labor and delivery nurse should accompany patient. Monitor for Sx of fetal distress or onset of labor. Mg++ or terbutaline may be necessary to suppress a sudden onset of premature labor. Consult with obstetrician on the need for these tocolytic agents. Any evidence of fetal distress should be communicated to the surgeon immediately.

Positioning	✓ and pad pressure points. ✓ eyes. Left uterine displacement	★ **NB**: peroneal nerve compression at lateral fibular head → foot drop. Left uterine displacement with a wedge under mattress should be used for pregnant patients (after ~20 wk).
Complications	Laser eye damage Fire Premature labor	If a laser is used, eye protection is required for the patient and all OR personnel; be alert for fire hazards when using a laser.

POSTOPERATIVE

Complications	Peroneal nerve injury (2° lithotomy position) PONV Premature labor Bleeding PDPH	Nerve injury manifested as foot drop and loss of sensation over dorsum of foot. Rx: metoclopramide 10 mg iv Tocolytic agents (e.g., terbutaline, magnesium) may be needed, administered in consultation with obstetrician. May require epidural blood patch.
Pain management	Oral analgesic	Acetaminophen (325-360 mg po) or ketorolac (30 mg iv)

References

1. Averette HE, Nasser N, Yankow SL, Little WA: Cervical conization in pregnancy. Analysis of 180 operations. *Am J Obstet Gynecol* 1970; 106(4):543-9.
2. Copeland LJ, Landon MB: Malignant disease in pregnancy. In *Obstetrics. Normal and Problem Pregnancies*. Gabbe SG, Niebyl JR, Simpson JL, eds. Churchill Livingstone, New York: 2002, 1255-81.
3. Delmore J, Horbelt DV, Kallail KJ: Cervical conization: cold knife and laser excision in residency training. *Obstet Gynecol* 1992; 79(6):1016-19.
4. DiSaia PJ, Creasman WT: Cancer in pregnancy. In *Clinical Gynecologic Oncology*. DiSaia PJ, Creasman WT, eds. CV Mosby, St. Louis: 2000, 439-72.
5. Duggan BD, Felix JC, Muderspach LI, et al: Cold-knife conization versus conization by the loop electrosurgical excision procedure: a randomized, prospective study. *Am J Obstet Gynecol* 1999; 180:276-82.
6. Hannigan EV, Whitehouse HH, Atkinson WD, et al: Cone biopsy during pregnancy. *Obstet Gynecol* 1982; 60:450.
7. Hoffman MS: Cervical conization. In *Gynecologic Surgery*. Mann WJ, Stovall TG, eds. Churchill Livingstone, New York: 1996, 265-83.
8. Kristensen GB: The outcome of pregnancy and preterm delivery after conization of the cervix. *Arch Gynecol* 1985; 236: 127.
9. Matseoane S, Williams SB, Navarro C, et al: Diagnostic value in the conization of the uterine cervix. Management of cervical neoplasia: a review of 756 consecutive patients. *Gynecol Oncol* 1992; 47:287.
10. Mazze RI, Kallen B. Reproductive outcome after anesthesia and operation during pregnancy: a registry study of 5405 cases. *Am J Obstet Gynecol* 1989; 161(5):1178-85.
11. Tabor A, Berget A: Cold knife and laser conization for cervical intra-epithelial neoplasia. *Obstet Gynecol* 1990; 76(4):633-5.

ANESTHETIC CONSIDERATIONS FOR LASER THERAPY TO VULVA, VAGINA, CERVIX

PREOPERATIVE

Laser therapy is indicated for preinvasive lesions of the vulva, vagina, or cervix. It destroys tissues by the selective application of light energy focused into a beam. Vaporized tissues tend to heal without scarring, and blood loss is minimal due to the cauterizing effect of the laser.[1] Most gynecological laser procedures are done with local anesthesia in the clinical setting and do not require the services of an anesthesiologist.

Respiratory	Not significant, unless there is underlying lung disease.
Cardiovascular	In elderly patients, exercise tolerance should be assessed. **Tests:** ECG if > 50 yr
Hematologic	**Tests:** Hct
Laboratory	Consider pregnancy test in young women.
Premedication	Anxiolytic, such as midazolam 1-2 mg iv, if needed

INTRAOPERATIVE

Anesthetic technique: Usually MAC; occasionally, GETA/LMA or regional technique may be used. Sedation with propofol, midazolam, and fentanyl in small doses usually is adequate.

General anesthesia:

Induction	Standard induction (p. B-2)
Maintenance	Standard maintenance (see p. B-3). Muscle relaxation not necessary. A technique with relatively rapid emergence (e.g., propofol or sevoflurane/desflurane) is useful for outpatient surgery.
Emergence	No special considerations

Regional anesthesia: Spinal or epidural anesthesia may be used with a sensory level to T10. Either lidocaine, tetracaine, or bupivacaine is acceptable, depending on anticipated length of surgery. Provide supplemental O_2 if sedation given.

Spinal	A T10 sensory level is desirable; and lidocaine 75 mg, tetracaine 10 mg or bupivacaine 12 mg can be used. Small-diameter spinal needles (e.g., 26 ga Quincke or 25 ga Sprotte needles) minimize chance of postdural puncture headache (PDPH).
Epidural	2% lidocaine, ± epinephrine 1:200,000 (10-15 ml), or 0.5% bupivacaine (10-15 ml) is used; then @ ~10 ml/h. Narcotics, such as morphine (4 mg) or hydromorphone (0.5 mg), may be given in the epidural for postop pain control.

Blood and fluid requirements	Minimal blood loss IV: 18 ga × 1 NS/LR @ 2-4 ml/kg/h	Give 1000 ml LR prior to regional block to compensate for vasodilatation.
Monitoring	Standard monitors (see p. B-1).	
Positioning	✓ and pad pressure points. ✓ eyes.	
Complications	Eye injury OR fires Aerosolization of viral particles	Goggles should be worn by both patient and all OR personnel during laser use to prevent injury to eyes from light. If the patient is asleep, cover eyes with saline-soaked gauze. Whenever laser is in use, be prepared for fires: know where fire extinguisher is located, and watch for improper handling of lasers. Vaporization of condyloma may produce aerosolization of viral particles; therefore, appropriate ventilation is suggested to disperse smoke.

POSTOPERATIVE

Complications	PONV PDPH	N/V may respond well to 10 mg iv metoclopramide. PDPH may require epidural blood patch for treatment.
Pain management	Oral analgesics	E.g., acetaminophen 325-650 mg po

Reference

1. McKenzie AL, Carruth JA: Lasers in surgery and medicine. *Phys Med Biol* 1984; 29(6):619-41.

SUCTION CURETTAGE
FOR GESTATIONAL TROPHOBLASTIC DISEASE

SURGICAL CONSIDERATIONS

Description: Suction curettage is the most efficient method of evacuating a gestational trophoblastic neoplasm (mole). The procedure involves dilation of the cervix by instruments or by laminaria tents, followed by insertion of suction cannula of appropriate diameter into the uterine cavity. Standard negative pressures used are in the range of 30-70 mmHg. IV oxytocin—to maintain uterine contraction and minimize blood loss—is started after a moderate amount of tissue has been removed. Suction curettage is followed by gentle, sharp curettage of the uterus to ensure adequate evacuation. Paracervical injection of dilute vasopressin solution or 1% xylocaine with 1:200,000 epinephrine may ↓ operative blood loss (in cases not complicated by thyrotoxicosis or HTN).

Variant procedure or approaches: Evacuation of a mole > 16 wk gestation size is associated with a significant risk of trophoblastic embolization and cardiorespiratory embarrassment (2° pulmonary HTN/edema, cyanosis, ↓CO, ↓BP, right heart failure). Central hemodynamic monitoring using a PA catheter is useful in the management of cardiovascular changes associated with trophoblastic embolization and to prevent inadvertent fluid overload.

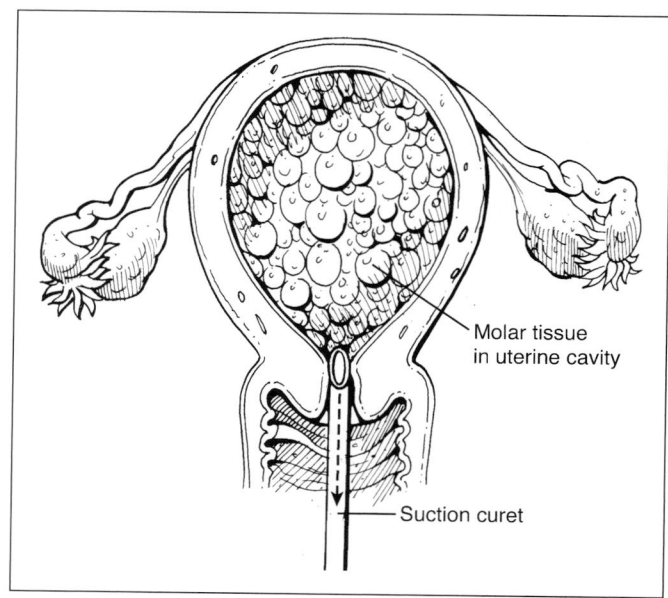

Figure 8.1-6. Suction curettage of a molar pregnancy.

Usual preop diagnosis: Gestational trophoblastic disease (GTD)

SUMMARY OF PROCEDURES

	Small Mole < 16 Weeks' Size	Large Mole > 16 Weeks' Size
Position	Lithotomy	⇐
Incision	None	⇐
Special instrumentation	Suction evacuation kit	⇐
Unique considerations	If mole > 12 wk size, laparotomy setup should be readily available. Oxytocin drip. In some cases, thyrotoxicosis may be present, requiring control with β-blockers.	⇐ + Central hemodynamic monitoring with PA catheter; avoid overzealous use of crystalloids and blood transfusions. Preop ABG.
Antibiotics	Cefotetan 2 g iv on call to OR	⇐
Surgical time	30-60 min	⇐
EBL	200-400 ml	⇐
Postop care	Outpatient (usually)	ICU admission in selected cases
Mortality	Rare	⇐
Morbidity	Trophoblastic embolization: 2.6%	11-27%
	Excessive bleeding: 2%	10%
	Infection: < 2%	⇐
	Uterine perforation: < 1%	1-2%
		Acute pulmonary edema: 2-11%
Pain score	3	3

PATIENT POPULATION CHARACTERISTICS

Age range	Reproductive age group
Incidence	1/1200 deliveries in U.S.

Etiology	Genetics: androgenous (all chromosomes in true moles are paternal in origin); nutritional deficiency: protein, folic acid, carotene (vitamin A)
Associated conditions	Lower socioeconomic status; Asian, Hispanic populations; hyperemesis gravidarum ($2°$ ↑levels of HCG); preeclampsia in 1st trimester; thyrotoxicosis (because of its analogy to TSH molecule, ↑levels of HCG can bind TSH receptors and cause thyrotoxicosis); prior GTD (incidence ↑ to 0.6-2.0%)

ANESTHETIC CONSIDERATIONS

PREOPERATIVE

Some 80% of cases are diagnosed at 12-18 wk of development.[6] Most patients have an unusually large uterus for the length of the pregnancy and vaginal bleeding is common. Trophoblastic disease is classified by the degree of invasiveness; **retained mole** is the most common type, and the least invasive; **invasive mole** involves the wall of the uterus; and **metastatic mole** involves more distant sites. Chemotherapy with methotrexate and actinomycin D usually is given postop for invasive or metastatic disease.[8] (See Table 8.1-1 for toxicities of chemotherapeutic agents.)

Respiratory	Pulmonary edema may complicate preeclampsia, which occurs in 25% of patients with GTD. If respiratory distress is present, it also may be $2°$ embolization of tumor to lungs. Avoid overhydration → pulmonary complications in patients with large moles. **Tests:** ABGs should be obtained preop if there is a question about the patient's pulmonary function and in patients at high risk of developing trophoblastic embolization. Others as indicated by H&P.
Cardiovascular	Blood volume is often depleted $2°$ hyperemesis and vaginal bleeding. Patients may be dehydrated $2°$ hyperemesis gravidarum preop, and adequate hydration should be given preop if patient shows Sx of hypovolemia (e.g., tachycardia, orthostatic ↓BP, low UO). Preeclampsia also may complicate this disease and can be diagnosed by HTN, proteinuria, and edema. If the patient has preeclampsia, invasive monitoring of BP may be advisable. Also, if patient is receiving Mg^{++} therapy, a serum level should be ✓'d preop. Mg^{++} therapy may inhibit myocardial contractility in high doses. Ca^{++} is the preferred antidote for myocardial depression. $MgSO_4$ → uterine atony → ↑blood loss.
Neurological	Sz prophylaxis with Mg^{++} is indicated for women with severe preeclampsia. If Sz occur, a small dose of STP (50-100 mg) or diazepam (2.5-5 mg) should be given iv and respiration assisted with supplemental O_2 by mask. The trachea should be intubated for airway protection in patients with full stomachs and in those who are difficult to ventilate by mask.
Musculoskeletal	✓ reflexes if patient has received Mg^{++}. Reduce amount of NMR to compensate for the effects of Mg^{++} on muscle strength.
Hematologic	Anemia may be masked by hypovolemia. Rh– patients with Rh+ partners should receive 300 μg of Rh immune globulin (RhoGAM) within 72 h postop to ↓ possibility of Rh isoimmunization in future pregnancies. **Tests:** CBC; ✓ Plt in preeclamptics. If patient has received chemotherapy recently, ✓ HCT; complete blood count (WBC, Plt). Plt count also should be ✓'d in women who have preeclampsia.
Endocrine	Hyperthyroidism occurs in 5% of women with hydatidiform moles[2] and is $2°$ the thyroid-stimulating effects of HCG. **Tests:** Thyroid function tests should be ✓'d preop in women with Sx of hyperthyroidism, and corrected before surgery.
Laboratory	Serum HCG level; consider thyroid function tests; LFTs; PT; PTT; Plt count; Mg^{++} level; UA—as indicated from H&P.
Premedication	Usually an anxiolytic such as midazolam 1-2 mg iv. A nonparticulate antacid (Na citrate 30 ml 0.3 M) should be given po just before induction.

INTRAOPERATIVE

Anesthetic technique: Usually GETA, although may be carried out under spinal or epidural anesthesia. Chemical sympathectomy in regional anesthesia may ↓ blood loss.

General anesthesia:

Induction	A rapid-sequence induction (p. B-5) with cricoid pressure should be used; STP 5 mg/kg iv or propofol 2-3 mg/kg iv usually is recommended. Analgesia is provided by fentanyl 1-3 μg/kg iv or sufentanil 0.1-0.3 μg/kg iv. Succinylcholine (1 mg/kg iv) or rocuronium (0.5 mg/kg iv) provides muscle relaxation for intubation.
Maintenance	Standard maintenance (p. B-3). Prophylaxis for N/V (e.g., metoclopramide 10 mg iv or ondansetron 4 mg is recommended. Control BP, if preeclamptic, with labetalol, hydralazine, or SNP. Try to keep DBP at 90-100 mmHg.
Emergence	Extubate when fully awake and protective airway reflexes have returned. Watch for emesis after extubation. Give supplemental O_2.

Regional anesthesia:

Spinal	A T8 sensory level is desirable; and lidocaine (75 mg), tetracaine (10-12 mg), or bupivacaine (10-12 mg) can be used. Small-diameter spinal needles (e.g., 26-ga Quincke or 25-ga Sprotte needles) will minimize the chances of postdural puncture headache (PDPH).
Epidural	Use 2% lidocaine ± epinephrine 1:200,000 (10-15 ml) or 0.5% bupivacaine (10-15 ml).

Blood and fluid requirements	Possible large blood loss IV: 18-16 ga × 1 NS/LR @ 2-4 ml/kg/h	One large-volume iv line should be placed and blood readily available. The usual causes of bleeding are uterine perforation, cervical laceration, or uterine atony.
Control of bleeding	Oxytocin (30 U/L) infusion Isoflurane < 1%	Oxytocin is begun about halfway through procedure at 30-60 drops/min (consult obstetrician). Try to keep isoflurane < 1% to prevent uterine relaxation. Large oxytocin boluses may → ↓↓BP.
	Ergonovine maleate 0.2 mg im	Ergonovine may be given for severe bleeding. Since this drug can cause HTN, it is contraindicated in cases of preeclampsia with elevated BP.
Monitoring	Standard monitors (p. B-1). ± Arterial catheter ± CVP/PA catheter Foley catheter	An arterial catheter and CVP are indicated in cases of thyrotoxicosis, preeclampsia, or significant hemorrhage. The use of vasodilators, such as SNP, is also an indication for invasive monitors.
Positioning	✓ and pad pressure points. ✓ eyes.	★ **NB**: peroneal nerve compression at lateral fibular head → foot drop. Lifting the legs may cause the level of spinal or epidural anesthesia to move cranially if performed too quickly after the block.
Complications	Embolization of trophoblastic material	Embolization may occur, especially if > 16 wk gestation. Significant respiratory compromise can occur, requiring postop ventilation and PEEP.

POSTOPERATIVE

Complications	Bleeding PONV HTN ↓BP	Continue oxytocin infusion. Significant hemorrhage should be evaluated by surgeons for possible perforation, laceration, or atony. Antiemetics such as Compazine (5-10 mg) or metoclopramide (10 mg) may be useful. BP should be monitored closely in preeclamptics. Consider ICU admission if unstable.
	Peroneal nerve injury (2° to lithotomy position)	Nerve injury manifested as foot drop and loss of sensation over dorsum of foot.
Pain management	Oral analgesics	Acetaminophen (325-650 mg po) or ketorolac (30 mg iv). Patients receiving Mg^{++} for preeclampsia may requie less opioid for pain control. This may be 2° NMDA receptor antagonism.

References

1. Amir SM, Osathanondh R, Berkowitz RS, et al: Human chorionic gonadotropin and thyroid function in patients with hydatidiform mole. *Am J Obstet Gynecol* 1984; 150:723.
2. Bagshawe KD, Noble MIM: Cardio-respiratory aspects of trophoblastic tumors. *QJM* 1966; 137:39.
3. Bakri YN, Berkowitz RS, Khan J, et al: Pulmonary metastases of gestational trophoblastic tumor: risk factors for early respiratory failure. *J Reprod Med* 1994; 39:175.
4. Berkowitz R, Goldstein DP: Gestational trophoblastic disease. In *Principles and Practice of Gynecologic Oncology,* 3rd edition. Hoskins WJ, Perez CA, Young RC, eds. Lippincott Williams & Wilkins, Philadelphia: 2000, 1117-37.
5. Berkowitz RS, Goldstein DP: Presentation and management of molar pregnancy. In *Gestational Trophoblastic Disease.* Hancock BW, Newlands ES, Berkowitz RS, eds. Chapman and Hall, London: 1997, 127.
6. Bruun T, Kristoffersen K: Thyroid function during pregnancy with special reference to hydatidiform mole and hyperemesis. *Acta Endocrinol* 1978; 88(2):383-9.
7. Burger RA, Creasman WT: Gestational trophoblastic neoplasia. In *Clinical Gynecologic Oncology.* DiSaia PJ, Creasman WT, eds. CV Mosby, St. Louis: 2000, 185-210.
8. Curry SL, Hammond CB, Tyrey L, Creasman WT, Parker RT: Hydatiform mole: Diagnosis, management and long-term followup of 347 patients. *Obstet Gynecol* 1975; 45(1):1-8.
9. Guido RS, Stovall DW: Dilation and curettage and hysteroscopy. In Mann WJ, Stovall TG, eds *Gynecologic Surgery.* Churchill Livingstone, New York: 1996; 225-63.
10. Hammond CB, Weed JC Jr, Currie JL: The role of operation in the current therapy of gestational trophoblastic disease. *Am J Obstet Gynecol* 1980; 136(7):844-58.
11. Tramier MR, Schneider J, Marti RA, Rifat K: Role of magnesium in postoperative analgesia. *Anesthesiology* 1996; 84(2):340-7.
12. Twiggs LB, Morrow CP, Schlaerth JB: Acute pulmonary complications of molar pregnancy. *Am J Obstet Gynecol* 1979; 135:189.
13. Wheeless CR Jr: Suction curettage for abortion. In *Atlas of Pelvic Surgery.* Williams & Wilkins, Baltimore: 1997, 205-7.

PELVIC EXENTERATION

SURGICAL CONSIDERATIONS

Description: Pelvic exenteration was introduced by Brunschwig as an ultraradical surgical approach for advanced and radioresistant cervical cancer. Although advanced vaginal and vulvar carcinoma occasionally have been treated with this procedure, its most important role is in the management of centrally recurrent, surgically resectable, radioresistant cervical carcinoma. **Total pelvic exenteration** involves **en bloc resection** of all pelvic tissues, including uterus, cervix, vagina, bladder, and rectum. Involvement of the distal vagina may require resection of vulva and groin nodes. The goal of this procedure is curative, with removal of all cancer tissue and reconstruction of appropriate diversions for the urine and stool if the colon cannot be reanastomosed to the rectum. It is rare for cervical and vaginal cancer to involve the lower 5 cm of the rectum and anus. It is, therefore, possible to mobilize the descending colon and anastomose it primarily to the distal rectum. A continent or incontinent urinary diversion, **omental pelvic carpet** or **sling** and **gracilis myocutaneous flaps** for vaginal and perineal reconstruction are performed. A **rectus abdominis muscle flap** also can be used

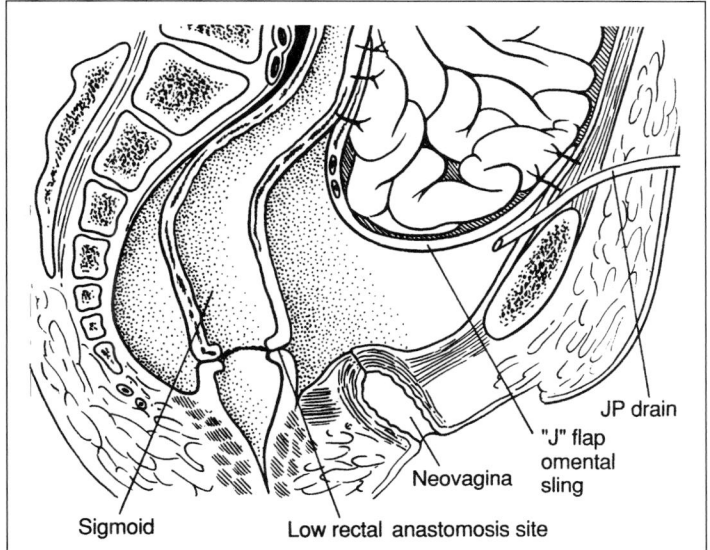

Figure 8.1-7. Sagittal section of the pelvis after a total pelvic exenteration. Note that all the reproductive organs, along with their supporting structures, the rectum and the bladder, have been resected. Drains can be placed through separate stab incisions in the abdomen. The small bowel is kept away from the operative site by a pelvic lid. The urinary and fecal diversions are not diagrammed. (Reproduced with permission from Wheeless CR: *Atlas of Pelvic Surgery.* Lea & Febiger: 1988.)

for vaginal reconstruction. This type of flap yields excellent aesthetic and functional results. In cases where an omental sling (shown in Fig 8.1-7) cannot be developed, an absorbable synthetic mesh is sutured to the pelvic peritoneum to create a pelvic lid (like a hammock) to keep the small bowel off the denuded pelvic peritoneum, thus decreasing the possibility of small-bowel obstruction. In general, an additional 2-3 h of surgical time and an additional 300 ml of EBL are expected when a vaginal reconstruction is undertaken. An exploratory laparotomy is needed prior to initiation of the exenterative procedure to r/o spread of disease outside the pelvis and/or extension to pelvic sidewalls and pelvic lymph nodes, all of which are absolute contraindications to this procedure.

Resectability is evaluated by examination of pelvic and paraaortic lymph nodes, liver, hemidiaphragms, and peritoneal surfaces of the upper abdomen and pelvic wall. Washings are obtained for cytology. A thorough lymph node dissection is then performed and all suspicious nodes are submitted for frozen-section pathologic examination. The pararectal, paravesical, and presacral spaces are then developed. If the patient is found to be inoperable, CUSA can be used to decrease the tumor burden. Consideration also should be given to IORT, which may provide an adjunctive treatment to radical surgery in the setting of: 1) recurrent disease close to the pelvic sidewalls; and 2) microscopically positive surgical margins or 'close' resection margins. If the patient is deemed operable, the space of Retzius is developed. The round ligaments are then transected close to the pelvic sidewall bilaterally; and the infundibulopelvic ligaments also are ligated and transected. The ureters are divided as close to the bladder as possible. The superior hemorrhoidal vessel is ligated and transected; and the colon is transected at the appropriate level. The anterior divisions of the internal iliac artery on both sides are ligated and divided; and the web of tissue is clamped close to the pelvic sidewall, transected, and suture-ligated. Following this, sharp dissection can be done to free up the specimen from the low attachments to the levator muscles. In larger tumors, the levator muscle is partially removed with the specimen to provide adequate margins. From a combined perineal and abdominal approach, the distal vagina, urethra, and perineum (± rectum) can be resected. The specimen is handed off the field, hemostasis is achieved, and the bladder is reconstructed with a continent urinary diversion using an ileocolonic segment, ileal loop, or transverse colon conduit. A low rectal anastomosis is performed, vaginal reconstruction is undertaken, and the pelvic floor is covered. An ileal loop or other urinary conduit is performed, a low rectal anastomosis is done, vaginal reconstruction is undertaken, and the pelvic floor is covered. (Figs 8.1-7 and 8.1-8 show the completed exenteration.)

Variant procedure or approaches: Anterior pelvic exenteration is technically similar to a total pelvic exenteration, except the rectum is left intact. **Posterior pelvic exenteration** involves preservation of bladder. Posterior exenteration has proved more useful in cancer of vulva or vagina than in cervical cancer. Anterior and posterior exenterations are used in selective cases because of the increased risk of an incomplete tumor resection and multiple complications and malfunctioning of the preserved organ.

Usual preop diagnosis: Recurrent cervical carcinoma following radiotherapy

SUMMARY OF PROCEDURE

Position	Modified dorsolithotomy with Allen stirrups
Incision	Midline longitudinal, perineal
Special instrumentation	Vital View, ABC may be helpful; EEA, GIA, TA staplers; Robo-retractor or similar devices
Unique considerations	Full and thorough mechanical and antibiotic intestinal prep. NG tube placement intraop. SCD and minidose heparin intraop for DVT prophylaxis. Preop PFTs. Consider preop Greenfield IVC filter placement to avoid PE for high-risk patients. Consider intraop radiation of tumor bed and/or of resection margins. Abort case if extrapelvic metastases and/or tumor extension to pelvic sidewalls noted.
Antibiotics	Cefotetan 2 g iv q 12 h to begin, 12 h preop, and continue 72 h postop. Alternatively, a combination of ampicillin (1 g), gentamicin (80 mg), and metronidazole (500 mg).
Surgical time	8-12 h (2-team approach); 5-10 h (for anterior and posterior exenteration)
Closing considerations	Abdominal drains; colostomy; ureteral stents; urostomy; intraop radiation therapy. Triple-lumen central line placement. Copious irrigation of the operative sites.
EBL	1200-4000 ml
Postop care	ICU: 2-3 d. Correction of electrolyte imbalance. Extensive peritoneal raw surfaces → intraperitoneal fluid 3rd-spacing. Patients require good hydration to maintain intravascular volume. SCDs and minidose heparin for DVT prophylaxis. Consider concentrated albumin infusion to maintain intravascular volume. Early and aggressive use of TPN is important. Maintain Hct in the low 30s, as concentrated blood may → sludging and contribute to flap necrosis and wound breakdown. Remove ureteral stents 1-2 wk postop, when the edema at the ureterointestinal site has subsided.
Mortality	5-11%

Morbidity	Intraop hemorrhage requiring a median of 5 U PRBC transfusion

Infectious:
 Nonspecific: 25%
 Flap necrosis: 20%
 Pelvic cellulitis: 19%
 Pyelonephritis: 17%
 Wound infection: 6%
 Sepsis: 3%
Psychiatric:
 Confusion: 24%
Intestinal:
 Ileus: 18%
 GI fistula: 13%
 Stoma breakdown: 3%
 Small bowel obstruction: 5%
Renal:
 Ureteral fistulae: 14%
 Failure: 5%
Cardiovascular:
 CHF: 8%
 Venous thrombosis: 3-7%
 DIC: 3%
 Dysrhythmia: 3%
 MI: 3%
Pulmonary:
 Pneumonia: 3%
 PE: 2%
Neurologic:
 CVA: 2%
 Spinal cord infarction: < 2%

Pain score 7-8

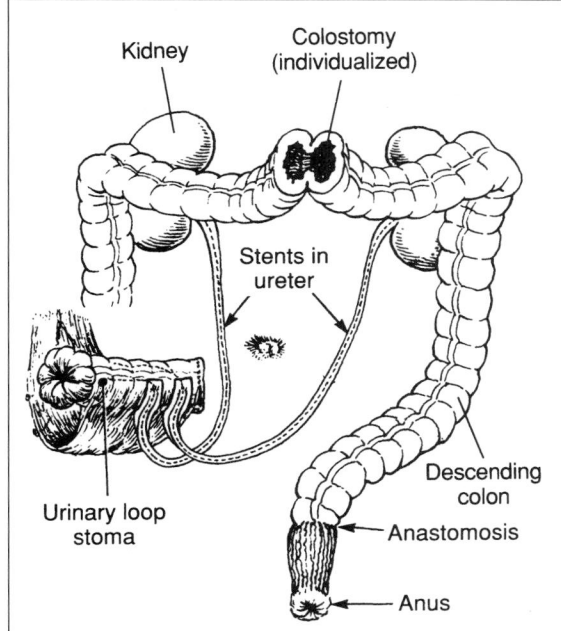

Figure 8.1-8. Conceptual drawing shows the urinary and fecal diversions after a total pelvic exenteration. (Reproduced with permission from Wheeless CR: *Atlas of Pelvic Surgery*. Williams & Wilkins: 1997.)

PATIENT POPULATION CHARACTERISTICS

Age range	All age groups
Incidence	1.5-17% of cervical cancers treated with radiation therapy (depending on stage and cell type)
Associated conditions	Advanced or recurrent gynecologic malignancies; radiation injury

ANESTHETIC CONSIDERATIONS

PREOPERATIVE

This procedure is performed for recurrent rectal, cervical, or other gynecologic carcinomas and involves removal of all pelvic tissues. Occasionally, the bladder or rectum is preserved, if not involved with tumor. Most patients have undergone preop radiation or chemotherapy.

Respiratory Usually not significant unless there is Hx of smoking or lung disease. Ask about prior chemotherapy. (See Anesthetic Considerations for Second-Look/Reassessment Laparotomy for Ovarian Cancer, p. 598.)
Tests: Consider CXR; others as indicated from H&P.

Cardiovascular Exercise tolerance should be assessed. Underlying CAD or CHF should be medically optimized preop in consultation with a cardiologist. Any exposure to cardiotoxic chemotherapy should be investigated and may require further tests, such as an ECHO.
Tests: Consider ECG; others as indicated from H&P.

Neurological Any Hx of stroke, Sz, carotid artery disease, or other neurologic disease should be evaluated and documented.

Endocrine	Any endocrine disease, such as diabetes, should be optimized in consultation with the patient's primary care physician or endocrinologist. Ask about recent corticosteroid use. **Tests:** Fasting blood sugar in the diabetic; others as indicated from H&P.
Gastrointestinal	Patients should have iv hydration if given a bowel prep. A long intestinal tube (Miller-Abbot or Cantor tube) should be placed preop for bowel decompression.
Hematologic	Many patients will be anemic from chronic disease and malnutrition. Preop transfusion of packed cells to ↑ Hct > 30% is indicated. Ask about recent NSAID usage. **Tests:** CBC, PT, PTT, if indicated.
Laboratory	LFTs; CT scan of pelvis and abdomen
Premedication	Anxiolytic such as midazolam (1-2 mg iv) or diazepam (10 mg po). Careful explanation about the procedure and the potential for postop intubation and mechanical ventilation is beneficial.

INTRAOPERATIVE

Anesthetic technique: GETA ± supplemental epidural anesthesia. Inhalation anesthetics or propofol infusion may be used in relatively healthy patients. A high-dose narcotic technique should be used for patients with significant CAD or in poor overall physical condition.

General anesthesia:

Induction	Standard induction (p. B-2), unless otherwise indicated by patient condition. Long-acting muscle relaxants (e.g., pancuronium [0.1 mg/kg]) should be used unless patient has significant renal dysfunction, in which case, cisatracurium (0.2 mg/kg) should be used.
Maintenance	Isoflurane, propofol (100-200 μg/kg/min) or high-dose fentanyl (50-75 μg/kg) combined with midazolam (0.1-0.5 mg/kg). Epidural anesthetic or epidural narcotic (morphine or hydromorphone) can be given to reduce anesthetic requirements when using inhalation agents. Cisatracurium infusion (1-2 mg/kg/min) should be used to maintain muscle relaxation in patients with renal dysfunction. High FiO$_2$ (0.8), avoiding hypothermia, and preop adminstration of cefotetan (2 g) may significantly ↓ risk of postop infection.
Emergence	If patient is hemodynamically stable, warm, and responsive at the end of surgery, extubation may be appropriate. Any patient who is unstable, hypothermic, has had a high-dose narcotic, has significant edema of the face or airway, or who has ongoing excessive fluid requirements should be ventilated overnight in the ICU before attempting extubation. Due to the large fluid shifts that can occur, all patients need to be monitored in ICU postop.

Regional anesthesia:

Epidural	2% lidocaine (10-15 ml), with or without epinephrine 1:200,000, or 0.5% bupivacaine (10-15 ml) are used; then, at ~10 ml/h. Narcotics, such as morphine (2-4 mg) or hydromorphone (0.3-0.5 mg), may be given in the epidural for postop pain control.

Ventilation	5 cm H$_2$O PEEP may help prevent atelectasis.	✓ ABGs during surgery. Adjust ventilation to keep normocarbic. HCO$_3$ is given for metabolic acidosis when pH < 7.20.
Blood and fluid requirements	Possible large blood loss IV: 14-16 ga × 2 NS/LR @ 10-15 ml/kg/h Colloid solutions Hetastarch PRBCs when Hct < 30% Keep PAWP < 20 mmHg.[12] Maintain UO of 0.5-1 ml/kg/h. Ionized Ca^{++}	Renal ultrafiltration improved by NS/LR, but bowel edema ↑'d. LR useful when acidosis occurs. NS is better when giving blood products or when metabolic alkalosis is present. Rapid-infuser should be available. Colloid solutions superior in restoring hemodynamic stability when large fluid volumes required. Use of 6% hetastarch should be limited to 1,000 ml due to potential coagulopathy with larger volumes. UO should guide fluid therapy, PA pressures, and CO. Dopamine 2-3 μg/kg/min may be used to maintain UO. Control ↓BP to MAP 60-70 mmHg in healthy patients to ↓ blood loss. Measure ionized Ca^{++} and K$^+$ after rapid administration of blood products; replace Ca^{++} as necessary.

Blood and fluid requirements, cont.	FFP/PLT	Plt or FFP may be given for coagulation abnormalities studies as necessary to treat significant bleeding.
Monitoring	Standard monitors (see p. B-1). ± Arterial line Foley catheter ± PA catheters ± TEE	Invasive hemodynamic monitoring with arterial and PA catheters usually is required. TEE allows intraop assessment of myocardial function and may be appropriate in selected patients.
Positioning	✓ and pad pressure points. ✓ eyes. Antiembolism stockings and SCD	★ **NB:** peroneal nerve compression at lateral fibular head → foot drop.
Complications	Hypothermia Bleeding Coagulopathy Trauma to kidney	Warm OR; use forced-air warmer; wrap head in towels; use warm saline lavage of abdomen. Rapid-infuser device is helpful for giving large volumes of iv fluids. Watch for hematuria or ↓UO.

POSTOPERATIVE

Complications	Bleeding Fluid overload Peroneal nerve injury 2° lithotomy position	✓ Hct and coags periodically. Be prepared for continued increased fluid requirements for 24 h postop. It is essential to maintain optimal cardiac filling pressures. After 24 h, fluid mobilization will begin, usually requiring diuretic therapy. Nerve injury manifested as foot drop and loss of sensation over dorsum of foot.
Pain management	Epidural or iv opiates	See p. C-2.
Tests	Hct	Others as indicated from H&P.

References

1. Craig RL, Poole GV: Resuscitation in uncontrolled hemorrhage. *Am Surg* 1994: 60:59.
2. DiSaia PJ, Creasman WT: Invasive cervical cancer. In *Clinical Gynecologic Oncology.* DiSaia PJ, Creasman WT, eds. CV Mosby, St. Louis: 2002, 53-111.
3. Eisenkop SM, Nalick RH, Teng NH: Modified posterior exenteration for ovarian cancer. *Obstet Gynecol* 1991; 78(5P+1): 879-85.
4. Fiorica JV, Roberts WS, Hoffman MS, Barton DP, Finan MA, Lyman G, Cavanagh D: Concentrated albumin infusion as an aid to postoperative recovery after pelvic exenteration. *Gynecol Oncol* 1991; 43(3):265-9.
5. Gemignani M, Alektiar KM, Leitao M, et al: Radical surgical resection and high-dose intraoperative radiation therapy (HDR-IORT) in patients with recurrent gynecologic cancers. *Int J Radiat Oncol Biol Phys* 2001; 50:687-94.
6. Greif R, Akca O, Horn EP, Kurz A, Sessler DI: Supplemental perioperative oxygen to reduce the incidence of surgical wound infection: *N Engl J Med* 2000; 342:161-7.
7. Hatch KD, Gelder MS, Soong SJ, Baker VV, Shingleton HM: Pelvic exenteration with low rectal anastomosis: survival, complications, and prognostic factors. *Gynecol Oncol* 1990; 38(3):462-7.
8. Hatch KD, Mann WJ: Exenterative surgery of the female pelvis. In *Gynecologic Surgery.* Mann WJ, Stovall TG, eds. Churchill Livingstone, New York: 1996, 535-54.
9. Hatch KD, Shingleton HM, Soong SJ, et al: Anterior pelvic exenteration. Gynecol Oncol 1988; 31:205.
10. Husain A, Curtin J, Brown C, et al: Continent urinary diversion and low-rectal anastomosis in patients undergoing exenterative procedures for recurrent gynecologic malignancies. *Gynecol Oncol* 2000; 78:208-11.
11. Martino M, Houvenaeghel G, Hardwigsen J, Moutardier V, et al: Pelvic recurrence of cancers of the uterine cervix. A study of a series of 49 cases. *Ann Chir* 1997; 51:36-45.
12. Matthews CM, Morris M, Burke TW, Gershenson DM, Wharton TJ, Rutledge FN: Pelvic exenteration in the elderly patient. *Obstet Gynecol* 1992; 79(5):773-7.
13. Morley GW, Hopkins MP, Lindenauer SM, et al: Pelvic exenteration, University of Michigan: 100 patients at 5 years. *Obstet Gynecol* 1989; 44:934.
14. Numa F, Ogata H, Suminami Y, Tsunaga N, et al: Pelvic exenteration for the treatment of gynecological malignances. *Arch Gynecol Obstet* 1997; 259:133-8.
15. Penalver MA, Benjany DE, Averette HE, et al: Continent urinary diversion in gynecologic oncology. *Gynecol Oncol* 1989; 34:274.
16. Ramirez PT, Modesitt SC, Morris M, et al: Functional outcomes and complications of continent urinary diversions in patients with gynecologic malignancies. *Gynecol Oncol* 2002; 85:285-91.

17. Rutledge FN, Smith JP, Wharton JT, O'Quinn AG: Pelvic exenteration: Analysis of 296 patients. *Am J Obstet Gynecol* 1977; 129(8):881-92.
18. Sessler D: Mild perioperative hypothermia. *N Engl J Med* 1997; 336:1730-7.
19. Soper JT: Grafts and flaps in gynecologic surgery. In *Gynecologic Surgery*. Mann WJ, Stovall TG, eds. Churchill Livingstone, New York: 1996, 555-86.
20. Soper JT, et al: Pelvic exenteration: Factors associated with major surgical morbidity. *Gynecol Oncol* 1989; 35:93.
21. Stanhope CR, Webb MJ, Podratz KC: Pelvic exenteration for recurrent cervical cancer. *Clin Obstet Gynecol* 1990; 33(4): 897-909.
22. Stehman FB, Perez CA, Kurman RJ, Thigpen JT: Uterine cervix. In *Principles and Practice of Gynecologic Oncology,* 3rd edition. Hoskins WJ, Perez CA, Young RC, eds. Lippincott Williams & Wilkins, Philadelphia: 2000, 841-918.
23. Symmonds RE, Pratt JH, Webb MJ: Exenterative operations: experience with 198 patients. *Am J Obstet Gynecol* 1975; 121(7):907-18.
24. Wheeless CR Jr: Total pelvic exenteration. In *Atlas of Pelvic Surgery*. Williams & Wilkins, Baltimore: 1997, 447-57.

EXPLORATORY LAPAROTOMY, HYSTERECTOMY/BSO FOR UTERINE CANCER

SURGICAL CONSIDERATIONS

Description: Currently, endometrial cancer is the most common gynecologic malignancy in the U.S. The first step in the management of this cancer is an **exploratory laparotomy**, concurrent with a **hysterectomy**. The objective, aside from 1° therapy, is to obtain as much surgical and pathological staging data as feasible for determination of adjuvant postop therapy. Careful exploration is carried out for evidence of omental, liver, peritoneal, and adnexal metastases. Aortic and pelvic areas are palpated for metastases, and suspicious nodes are removed. If no suspicious nodes are present, some pelvic and periaortic lymph nodes are sampled. Note that this is less extensive than the more complete lymph node dissection of a radical hysterectomy. The lymph node sampling may be omitted in the treatment of some uterine sarcomas. A **total hysterectomy** with **BSO** is then performed in the usual manner (see discussion of TAH/BSO in Staging Laparotomy for Ovarian Cancer, p. 594).

Variant procedure or approaches: A combined **laparoscopically assisted vaginal hysterectomy and BSO**, as well as laparoscopic pelvic and paraaortic node sampling, is appropriate in selected patients and is being performed with increasing frequency. The benefits of this approach are shorter hospital stay and convalescence and decreased postop pain. Adhesions of variable severity may be present from prior surgery or radiation. Care should be taken to avoid possible bowel injury at time of trocar insertion. Patient needs to be in steep Trendelenburg position for duration of the procedure; and both arms should be tucked in at the patient's sides. Since argon is a heavy gas, prolonged use of the endoscopic ABC in a patient in steep Trendelenburg can → significant facial and neck subcutaneous emphysema. As with the open technique, the lymph nodes being removed are in the immediate proximity of the great pelvic vessels. The surgeon and anesthesiologist should be mindful of the potential for severe hemorrhage if these vessels are injured.

Usual preop diagnosis: Endometrial carcinoma

SUMMARY OF PROCEDURES

	Open Technique	Laparoscopic Technique
Position	Supine	Modified dorsolithotomy in Allen stirrups
Incision	Midline longitudinal abdominal/transverse	Vertical infraumbilical and multiple small transverse incisions
Special instrumentation	None	Videolaparoscopy equipment. Endoscopic GIA staplers, endoscopic ABC, endoscopic vascular clips, and CO_2 laser.
Unique considerations	None	Mechanical bowel preop; steep Trendelenburg
Antibiotics	Cefotetan 2 g iv on call to OR; then 2 g iv q 12 h × 2 doses	⇐

	Open Technique	Laparoscopic Technique
Surgical time	2-4 h	2-3 h
Closing considerations	NG tube placement	Release the pneumoperitoneum completely. Closure of fascia at trocar sites ≥ 10 mm diameter
EBL	400-750 ml	100-500 ml
Postop care	Consider using SCDs and minidose heparin for DVT prophylaxis.	Begin early ambulation and feeding. Patients generally can be discharged on POD 1 or 2.
Mortality	0.1%	⇐
Morbidity	Hemorrhage requiring transfusion: 15%	0.3-3%
	Thrombophlebitis: 7%	⇐
	UTI: 7%	⇐
	Paralytic ileus: 2-5%	1-2%
	Wound infection: 3%	Rare
	PE: 1-2%	⇐
	Pelvic infection: 1.5%	⇐
	Wound dehiscence: 1%	N/A
	Bowel injuries: < 1%	1.1%
	Urinary tract injuries: < 1%	0.3-3%
		Trocar site herniation: 0.5-2%
		Trocar site tumor: 1.6% (estimated)
Pain score	7	2-3

PATIENT POPULATION CHARACTERISTICS

Age range	Reproductive and postreproductive ages (average = 61 yr)
Incidence	70-80/100,000
Etiology	Exposure to unopposed endogenous or exogenous estrogen; ↑extraglandular conversion of androstenedione to estrone; sequential oral contraceptive pills; exposure to radiation (sarcomas)
Associated conditions	Obesity; diabetes; HTN; nulliparity; late menopause; early menarche; family Hx; Stein-Leventhal syndrome; chronic anovulation; ovarian and colon cancer; granulosa cell ovarian tumors; arthritis; hypothyroidism

ANESTHETIC CONSIDERATIONS

PREOPERATIVE

Endometrial cancer usually is diagnosed in postmenopausal women who present with vaginal bleeding. Exploratory laparotomy and TAH/BSO are commonly performed for removal of the primary tumor as well as staging of metastatic disease. Occasionally, preop radiation therapy may be in progress, with consequent systemic effects.

Respiratory	✓ for Hx of lung disease or smoking. **Tests:** Others as indicated from H&P.
Cardiovascular	Hx of CAD, HTN, or CHF Sx (e.g., angina, dyspnea, or peripheral edema) should be investigated. Assess patient's exercise tolerance and current medications. Tests such as an exercise treadmill or ECHO may be indicated if patient has significant angina or CHF. **Tests:** All patients > 50 yr should have a preop ECG.
Neurological	Seldom a significant problem unless there is Hx of cerebrovascular disease, Sz, or other neurologic disease.
Endocrine	Inquire about the presence of endocrine diseases, such as diabetes and hypothyroidism, which have been associated with this tumor. If the patient has received corticosteroids within the previous 6 mo, a supplemental dose of hydrocortisone (100 mg iv q 12 h × 2 d) should be given for surgery. **Tests:** Consider tests if indicated from H&P.
Neuromuscular	Osteoarthritis and osteoporosis common in this patient population. Ask about NSAID usage. **Tests:** Bleeding time is indicated if considering regional anesthesia.
Hematologic	If vaginal bleeding has been profuse or of long duration, significant anemia may occur. Consider preop iron supplements if there are several days until surgery. **Tests:** CBC

Laboratory	LFTs; CT scan of abdomen and pelvis
Premedication	Anxiolytic, such as midazolam 1-5 mg iv, if necessary. Discuss anesthetic plan and options for postop pain management with patient.

INTRAOPERATIVE

Anesthetic technique: GETA ± epidural or spinal analgesia/anesthesia. In unusual circumstances (e.g., severe lung disease), surgery may be done under spinal or epidural anesthesia only.

General anesthesia:

Induction	Standard induction (p. B-2)
Maintenance	Standard maintenance (p. B-3). Continued muscle relaxation is usually required to facilitate surgery. Epidural 2% lidocaine with epinephrine 1:200,000 at 10 ml/h may be given to reduce anesthetic requirements.
Emergence	Reverse muscle relaxant with neostigmine (0.07 mg/kg with glycopyrrolate 0.01 mg/kg). Patient should awaken at the end of surgery and be extubated in the OR; provide supplemental O_2 until patient is fully recovered from anesthesia. Consider PONV prophylaxis (e.g., ondansetron 4 mg iv).

Regional anesthesia:

Epidural	2% lidocaine (10-20 ml), ± epinephrine 1:200,000, or 0.5% bupivacaine (10-20 ml) is used; then @ ~10 ml/h. Narcotics, such as morphine (2-4 mg) or hydromorphone (0.3-0.5 mg), may be given in the epidural for postop pain control.	
Spinal	Tetracaine (12-14 mg) ± preservative-free morphine (0.3-0.5 mg). Sensory level ~T5.	
Blood and fluid requirements	IV: 18-16 ga × 1 NS/LR @ 4-6 ml/kg/h PRBC for Hct < 25%	Crystalloid is used for volume replacement. If anemia is present preop, it may be necessary to give PRBCs to keep Hct > 25%.
Monitoring	Standard monitors (p. B-1) Foley catheter ± Arterial line, CVP NG tube	Direct monitoring of arterial pressure is indicated in patients with CAD, severe HTN, or lung disease. CVP or PA catheters may be appropriate in selected patients.
Positioning	✓ and pad pressure points. ✓ eyes. Antiembolism stockings and SCD	
Complications	Hypothermia (mild) Trauma or obstruction of ureter	Warm iv fluids; humidify inspired gases; use forced-air warmer. Heating pad on OR table. Wrap head in towels or plastic. Watch for hematuria or ↓UO.

POSTOPERATIVE

Complications	PONV	Consider PONV prophylaxis for this high-risk group.
Pain management	PCA (p. C-3) Epidural/spinal narcotics (p. C-2)	Ketorolac (30 mg im/iv) is useful for breakthrough pain. A multimodal approach—including local anesthetics, NSAIDs or acetaminophen, or even low-dose (0.1-0.2 mg/kg/h) ketamine—in the OR may provide analgesia and ↓ PONV.

References

1. Barakat RR, Grigsby PW, Sabbatini P, Zaino RJ: Corpus: epithelial tumors. In *Principles and Practice of Gynecologic Oncology,* 3rd edition. Hoskins WJ, Perez CA, Young RC, eds. Lippincott Williams & Wilkins, Philadelphia: 2000, 919-59.
2. Chuang L, Burke TW, Tomos C, et al: Staging laparotomy for endometrial carcinoma: assessment of retroperitoneal lymph nodes. *Gynecol Oncol* 1995; 58:189.
3. Dicker RC, Greenspan JR, Straus LT, et al: Complications of abdominal and vaginal hysterectomy among women of reproductive age in the United States. The Collaborative Review of Sterilization. *Am J Obstet Gynecol* 1982; 144(7):841-8.
4. DiSaia PJ, Creasman WT: Adenocarcinoma of the uterus. In *Clinical Gynecologic Oncology*. DiSaia PJ, Creasman WT, eds. CV Mosby, St. Louis: 2002, 137-71.

5. Edraki B, Schwartz PE. Operative laparoscopy and the gynecologic oncologist. Commentary and review. *Cancer* 1995; 76: 1987-91.
6. Foley K, Lee RB: Surgical complications of obese patients with endometrial carcinoma. *Gynecol Oncol* 1990; 39:171.
7. Liu CY: Complications of laparoscopic hysterectomy: prevention, recognition and management. In *Laparoscopic Hysterectomy and Pelvic Floor Reconstruction.* Liu CY, ed. Blackwell Science, Cambridge: 1996; 277-96.
8. Mohan DS, Samuels MA, Selim MA, et al: Long-term outcomes of therapeutic pelvic lymphadenectomy for Stage I endometrial adenocarcinomas. *Gynecol Oncol* 1998; 70:165.
9. Orr JW, Holloway RW, Orr PF, et al: Surgical staging of uterine cancer: An analysis of perioperative morbidity. *Gynecol Oncol* 1991; 42:209.
10. Stovall TG: Vaginal, abdominal, and laparoscopic-assisted hysterectomy. In *Gynecologic Surgery.* Mann WJ, Stovall TG, eds. Churchill Livingstone, New York: 1996, 403-44.

RADICAL HYSTERECTOMY

SURGICAL CONSIDERATIONS

Description: **Radical hysterectomy** is the preferred mode of therapy for young women with Stage IA, IB, or nonbulky IIA cervical carcinoma, who want to preserve ovarian function. It is also appropriate with Stage II endometrial and Stage I vaginal carcinoma. The operation involves the removal of the uterus, along with the upper vagina and all the parametrial tissues to the pelvic sidewall. A pelvic and paraaortic **lymph node dissection** usually is performed at the beginning of the procedure. Suspicious nodes are submitted for pathological frozen-section evaluation. The paravesical and pararectal spaces are then developed, with the 'web' of tissue between these two spaces being palpated carefully (Fig 8.1-9). If parametrial tumor extension is noted and/or the lymph nodes are positive on frozen section, the hysterectomy may be aborted. The radical hysterectomy is performed after the pararectal and paravesical spaces have been developed. The uterine arteries are divided at their origin from the anterior division of the internal iliac artery. The ureters are dissected free of the parametrial tissues, which are then transected close to the pelvic sidewall. Next, the rectovaginal space is developed (Fig 8.1-10). The uterosacral ligaments are transected between their uterine and sacral attachments. The upper third of the vagina is cross-clamped and divided in such a manner as to provide a 3 cm margin, and the specimen is delivered en bloc. Note that, during this procedure, the ureters and bladder are dissected free and left intact.

In reproductive-age women, who may require postop radiotherapy, ovarian function is preserved by performing an **oophoropexy**. This is accomplished by severing the uteroovarian ligament and mobilizing the ovarian vessels as they course through the infundibulopelvic ligament. The ovaries are then sutured outside the radiation therapy field and marked with metal clips for future identification.

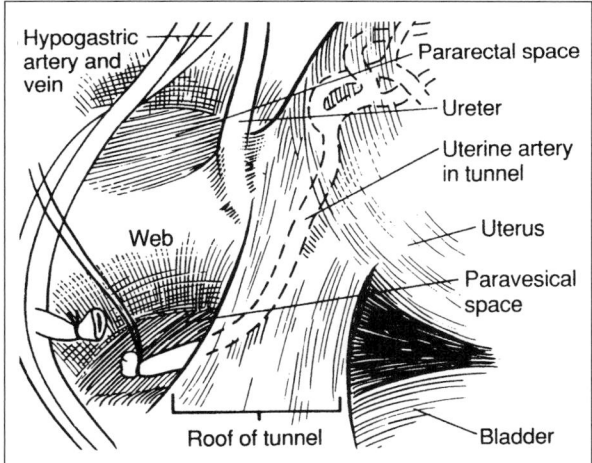

Figure 8.1-9. View of parametrial area, showing positions of ureter and uterine artery to web, hypergastric vessels, paravesical, and pararectal spaces. (Reproduced with permission from Wheeless CR: *Atlas of Pelvic Surgery.* Williams & Wilkins: 1997.)

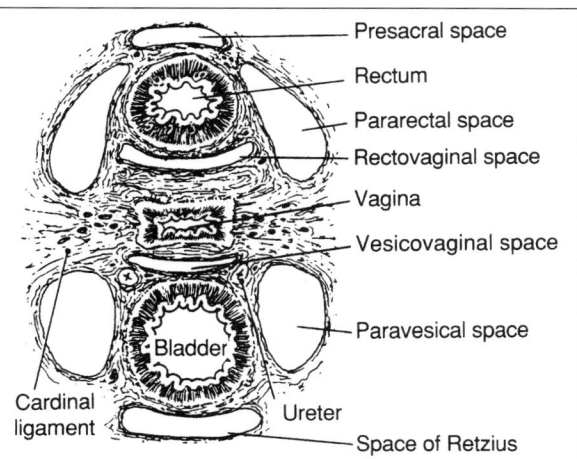

Figure 8.1-10. Schematic diagram of a cut in the anteroposterior plane with positions of all spaces in relation to pelvic organs. (Reproduced with permission from Wheeless CR: *Atlas of Pelvic Surgery.* Williams & Wilkins, 1997.)

Variant procedure or approaches: **Stallworthy, Dolstad, Novak, Rutledge, Wertheim,** and other surgeons have proposed several modifications in an effort to reduce the incidence of ureteral and bladder fistulae. These approaches include preservation of blood supply to the terminal 2 cm of the pelvic ureter by widely displacing ureters (not dissecting them from their fascial beds) and limiting parametrial dissection to the proximal 1/3 or 1/2.

Usual preop diagnosis: Stage IA, IB, or nonbulky IIA cervical carcinoma; Stage II endometrial or Stage I vaginal carcinoma (less common)

SUMMARY OF PROCEDURE

Position	Supine/modified lithotomy
Incision	Midline longitudinal or low transverse abdominal (Maylard/Cherney)
Special instrumentation	ABC, Vital View (suction, irrigation, and light source combined in 1 instrument) helpful
Unique considerations	Abort case if positive paraaortic lymph nodes found on frozen section, or if obvious parametrial involvement noted. Consider intraop radiation therapy (investigational), if patient is inoperable.
Antibiotics	Cefotetan 2 g iv on call to OR; then q 12 h × 2 doses
Surgical time	3-6 h
Closing considerations	Vaginal and abdominal drains; NG tube placement; suprapubic bladder catheter placement; oophoropexy; copious irrigation
EBL	500-1500 ml
Postop care	Transient ileus very common. Advance diet slowly. Transient bladder dysfunction very common; therefore, continued bladder drainage for 1+ wk may be necessary. Consider using SCDs and minidose heparin for DVT prophylaxis.
Mortality	0.3-2.0%
Morbidity	Paralytic ileus: 3-11%
	Pelvic lymphocyst: 6.4%
	Intraop hemorrhage: 5.6%
	Thrombophlebitis: 5%
	Pneumonia: 1.5-4%
	Wound infection: 3.5%
	Vesical injury: 2-3.5%
	Pelvic infection: 2.2%
	PE: 2.2%
	Vesical fistulae: 1.8%
	Small bowel obstruction: 1.5%
	Ureteral fistulae: 1.1%
	Ureteral injury: 1.1%
	Wound dehiscence: 1%
	Postop lymphedema: < 1%
	Rectal injury: < 1%
	Pelvic urinoma: Rare
Pain score	8

PATIENT POPULATION CHARACTERISTICS

Age range	Reproductive and postreproductive yr
Incidence	10/100,000
Etiology	Human papilloma virus (HPV), subtypes 16, 18 (most common), and others
Associated conditions	Smoking; venereal warts; genital herpes; multiple sexual partners; early-age onset of coitus; multiparity; lower socioeconomic status; HIV infection

ANESTHETIC CONSIDERATIONS

PREOPERATIVE

This surgery usually is performed for cervical carcinoma in young women who wish to preserve ovarian function, and whose tumor has not spread beyond local invasion. Lymph nodes are removed to confer a therapeutic advantage and to plan postop adjuvant therapy, if any.

Respiratory	These tumors have been associated with cigarette smoking. ✓ for preexisting lung disease. **Tests:** As indicated from H&P.
Cardiovascular	Patients > 50 yr need a preop ECG. **Tests:** As indicated from H&P.
Neurological	Not usually significant unless Hx of neurologic disease.
Musculoskeletal	Question patient about any joint or muscle disease and their exercise tolerance.
Gastrointestinal	Consider supplemental iv hydration in patients given a bowel prep.
Endocrine	Not usually important unless preexisting disease. ✓ for corticosteroid use in the previous 6 mo.
Hematologic	✓ NSAID usage in the previous wk. Encourage autologous blood donation. **Tests:** Consider coags if regional anesthetic planned; Hb/Hct; Plt count.
Laboratory	Electrolytes; renal panel; UA; CT scan of pelvis and abdomen (helpful but not necessary)
Premedication	Anxiolytic such as midazolam (1-2 mg iv)

INTRAOPERATIVE

Anesthetic technique: GETA ± epidural or spinal analgesia for postop pain control. (Surgery may be performed in patients with respiratory compromise under epidural or spinal anesthesia).

Induction	Standard induction (p. B-2)	
Maintenance	Standard maintenance (p. B-3). Muscle relaxation usually required to assist with surgical exposure. Prophylactic antiemetic (e.g., metoclopramide 10 mg iv) should be given before the end of surgery.	
Emergence	No special considerations	
Blood and fluid requirements	Occasional blood loss >1500 ml IV: 16-18 ga × 1-2 NS/LR @ 6-8 ml/kg/h Maintain UO > 0.5 ml/kg/h. Warm iv fluids. Humidify inspired gases.	Good iv access is necessary to deal with potential for bleeding. Controlled ↓BP to MAP = 60-70 mmHg may help ↓ blood loss. A lymph node dissection will ↑3rd-space losses and should be accounted for in fluid management. Fluid requirements generally are increased by a functioning epidural catheter 2° vasodilation. Controversy exists with regard to recurrence of cancer in patients who have received nonautologous blood transfusions.
Monitoring	Standard monitors (p. B-1) Foley catheter CVP catheter ± Arterial catheter	Invasive monitoring is indicated for patients with underlying cardiopulmonary disease or advanced age, or where controlled ↓BP is planned.
Positioning	✓ and pad pressure points. ✓ eyes. Antiembolism stockings and SCD	Heating pad on table
Complications	Injury to ureters Hypothermia	Watch for hematuria or ↓UO. Warm iv fluids; humidify gases; and use forced-air warmer, as hypothermia may ↑ risk of wound infections and prolong PACU and hospital stays.

POSTOPERATIVE

Complications	Atelectasis Hypothermia Bleeding	Give supplemental O$_2$ postop. Encourage use of incentive spirometer.
Pain management	PCA (p. C-3) Epidural or spinal narcotics (p. C-2)	Add ketorolac 30 mg im/iv q 8 h for breakthrough pain. Encourage surgeons to infiltrate local anesthetic (e.g., 0.5% ropivacaine or bupivacaine) into wound at end of case.

References

1. Anderson B, LaPolla J, Turner D, et al: Ovarian transposition in cervical cancer. *Gynecol Oncol* 1993; 49:206.

2. Averette HE, Nguyan HN, Donato DM, et al: Radical hysterectomy for invasive cervical cancer: a 25-year prospective experience with the Miami technique. *Cancer* 1993; 71:1422.

3. Ayhan A, Tuncer ZS: Radical hysterectomy with lymphadenectomy for treatment of early stage cervical cancer: clinical experience of 278 cases. *J Surg Oncol* 1991; 47(3):175-7.

4. Ayhan A, Tuncer ZS, Yarali H: Complications of radical hysterectomy in women with early stage cervical cancer: clinical analysis of 270 cases. *Eur J Surg Oncol* 1991; 17(5):492-4.

5. DiSaia PJ, Creasman WT: Invasive cervical cancer. In *Clinical Gynecologic Oncology.* DiSaia PJ, Creasman WT, eds. CV Mosby, St. Louis: 2002, 53-111.

6. Hoskins WJ, Ford JH Jr, Lutz MH, Averette HE: Radical hysterectomy and pelvic lymphadenectomy for the management of early invasive cancer of the cervix. *Gynecol Oncol* 1976; 4(3):278-90.

7. Lee YN, Wang KL, Lin MH, Liu CH, Wang KG, Lan CC, Chuang JT, Chen AC, Wu CC: Radical hysterectomy with pelvic lymph node dissection for treatment of cervical cancer: a clinical review of 954 cases. *Gynecol Oncol* 1989; 32:135-42.

8. Mann WJ: Radical hysterectomy. In *Gynecologic Surgery.* Mann WJ, Stovall TG, eds. Churchill Livingstone, New York: 1996, 481-512.

9. Meigs JV: Radical hysterectomy with bilateral pelvic lymph node dissections. A report of 100 patients operated on five or more years ago. *Am J Obstet Gynecol* 1951; 62:854-70.

10. Morrow CP, Curtin JP: Urological complications of radical pelvic surgery and radiation therapy. In *Gynecologic Oncology.* Coppleson M, ed. Churchill Livingstone, London: 1992, 1383.

11. Stehman FB, Perez CA, Kurman RJ, Thigpen JT: Uterine cervix. In *Principles and Practice of Gynecologic Oncology,* 3rd edition. Hoskins WJ, Perez CA, Young RC, eds. Lippincott Williams & Wilkins, Philadelphia: 2000, 841-918.

12. Symmonds RE, Pratt JH: Prevention of fistulas and lymphocysts in radical hysterectomy. *Obstet Gynecol* 1961; 17:57-64.

13. Webb MJ: Radical hysterectomy. *Baillieres Clin Obstet Gynaecol* 1997; 11(1):149-66.

INTERSTITIAL PERINEAL IMPLANTS

SURGICAL CONSIDERATIONS

Description: Radiotherapy is the treatment of choice for International Federation of Gynecology and Obstetrics (FIGO) Stage IIB-IVA carcinoma of the cervix; Stage I, II, III, and IVA vaginal cancers; selected vulvar cancers; and pelvic recurrences of gynecologic cancers. Often, **external-beam therapy** is combined with **brachytherapy**, either in the form of **intracavitary insertion** or as an **interstitial perineal template implant.** Intracavitary radiotherapy utilizes devices such as Fletcher-Suit tandem and ovoid applicators (Fig 8.1-11) or cylinders that are fitted into the vagina and provide a therapeutic boost to the vaginal apex region after external beam irradiation. In general, these devices do not require a laparotomy or

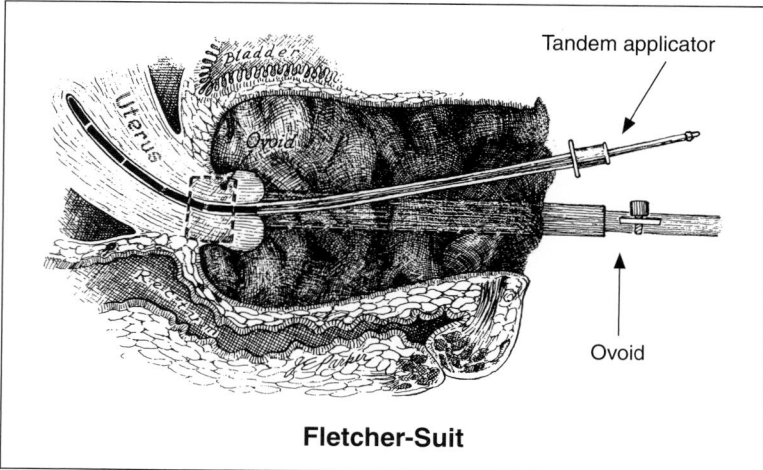

Fletcher-Suit

laparoscopy for guidance. For selected patients with distorted anatomy and/or bulky tumors, interstitial implants provide superior dose distribution and better local tumor control. The two most widely used systems are the **Martinez Universal Perineal Interstitial Template (MUPIT)** and the **Syed-Neblett applicator.** These systems have similar efficacy and both are performed in the OR with the patient under local or GA. A **laparotomy** is frequently performed at the time of interstitial implant placement to accurately guide the needles into their target tissues and to avoid radiation injury to bowel and/or other pelvic organs not involved with tumor. To minimize postop patient discomfort, some centers use **laparoscopy** instead of laparotomy for needle guidance. A two-team approach is used: a gynecologic

Figure 8.1-11. 'Fletcher-Suit.' The tandem and ovoid applicators are packed into the vagina, leaving the maxium distance between the bladder and radium sources. (Reproduced with permission from Wheeless CR: *Atlas of Pelvic Surgery.* Williams & Wilkins, 1997.)

oncology team performs the laparotomy or laparoscopy and guides the needles from above; a radiation oncology team inserts the implants from below. The implants are afterloaded with the appropriate radiation sources when the patient has returned to her shielded room. If a hysterectomy has been done previously, an omental pelvic carpet, or a pelvic lid made of delayed, absorbable mesh, is performed to provide additional space between the radiation source and bowel.

Usual preop diagnosis: Cervical, vaginal, vulvar carcinomas; pelvic recurrence of gynecologic malignancies

SUMMARY OF PROCEDURES

	Laparotomy-Guided	**Laparoscopy-Guided**
Position	Modified dorsolithotomy; Allen stirrups	⇐
Incision	Midline longitudinal abdominal	Vertical infraumbilical and multiple small transverse incisions at the pubic hairline
Special instrumentation	Syed-Neblett or MUPIT systems, or modifications thereof	⇐ + videolaparoscopy equipment, preferably with a 3-chip camera
Unique considerations	MRI and/or CT scans + information from physical exam are used to preplan implant with a computer dosimetry program. Patients require thorough preop mechanical and antibiotic bowel prep. Preop epidural placement or postop PCA (see pp. C-2–3) may prove helpful for pain control. Foley catheter needs to be inserted through an opening at the top of the clear plastic template prior to implant positioning.	⇐ + Adhesions of variable severity may be present from prior surgery or radiation. Care should be taken to avoid possible bowel injury at time of trocar insertion. Patient needs to be in steep Trendelenburg position for duration of procedure.
Antibiotics	Cefotetan 2 g iv on call to OR; then q 12 h × 3 doses	⇐
Surgical time	1.5-3 h	⇐
EBL	150-350 ml	Minimal
Closing considerations	Suture template to perineum. Perform rectal exam and adjust any needles that are too close to, or have protruded through, the rectal mucosa. Pack any space between template and perineum with Vaseline gauze. Obtain A-P and lateral orthogonal localization films with the patient in the supine bed-rest position. Insert Hypaque dye into Foley catheter balloon before localization films. Consider insertion of a large Foley into the rectum, and attach to a drainage bag. Consider NG tube placement.	⇐ + Release the pneumoperitoneum completely. Consider insertion of 1 L heparinized LR to cause the bowel to float and remain mobile, thus minimizing the risk of radiation injury.
Postop care	Patient is confined to bed while interstitial implants are in place. SCDs and minidose heparin for DVT prophylaxis. Vigorous use of incentive spirometry. Consider constipating medications (e.g., Lomotil). Patient must be placed in a shielded room. Visitors and medical personnel should interact with patient from behind a lead shield until radiation sources have been removed.	⇐
Mortality	0.1-0.3%	⇐
Morbidity	Hemorrhagic proctitis with diarrhea and tenesmus: 7-18%	⇐
	Radiation cystitis: 7-10%	⇐
	Cervical necrosis: 5-6%	⇐
	Rectovaginal fistula: < 5%	⇐
	Vesicovaginal fistula: < 5%	⇐
	Vaginal vault necrosis: 3-5%	⇐
	Rectal fibrosis: 2-5%	⇐
	Pelvic infection: 2-3%	⇐
Pain score	8-9	8-9

PATIENT POPULATION CHARACTERISTICS

Age range	Reproductive and postreproductive yr; childhood—rare
Etiology	Cervical, vaginal, or vulvar carcinomas; pelvic recurrence of gynecologic malignancies

ANESTHETIC CONSIDERATIONS

PREOPERATIVE

Radiation implants are used for palliation or cure in cervical, endometrial, and ovarian carcinoma. The implants concentrate the radiation close to the site of the tumor and may be supplemented by external beam radiation. The unusual tolerance of the uterus and vagina to radiation permit large doses to be given, and accounts for the success in treating cervical lesions. The sigmoid, rectum, and large bowel are much more sensitive to radiation injury, limiting the dose of radiation that may be given to the pelvis.

Respiratory	Usually not significant unless underlying lung disease is present.
Cardiovascular	Many patients with pelvic tumors are elderly and prone to cardiovascular disease. There are no specific recommendations except to ✓ a preop ECG in all patients > 50 yr who are otherwise asymptomatic. **Tests:** ECG; others as indicated from H&P.
Neurological	Usually not significant unless there is Hx of neurologic disease.
Musculoskeletal	Inquire about Hx of arthritis or osteoporosis. ✓ NSAID usage.
Hematologic	**Tests:** CBC; PT; PTT
Laboratory	UA; electrolytes; renal panel
Premedication	An anxiolytic, such as midazolam (1-3 mg iv), may be used if necessary.

INTRAOPERATIVE

Anesthetic technique: Regional or GA, depending on site involved. A postop epidural is useful for pain management.

Induction	Standard induction (see p. B-2).
Maintenance	Standard maintenance (see p. B-3). It is not necessary to maintain neuromuscular blockade after intubation.
Emergence	Metoclopramide (10 mg iv) can be given for prophylaxis against nausea 30 min before emergence.
Blood and fluid requirements	Small blood loss IV: 18-20 ga × 1 NS/LR @ 2-4 ml/kg/h
Monitoring	Standard monitors (see p. B-1).
Positioning	✓ and pad pressure points. ✓ eyes. Antiembolism stockings and SCD

POSTOPERATIVE

Pain management	Epidural narcotics (see p. C-2). PCA (see p. C-3).	Ketorolac 30-60 mg im/iv q 6 h is useful for breakthrough pain, unless the patient has PUD or renal insufficiency.

References

1. Ampuero F, Doss LL, Khan M, Skipper B, Hilgers RD: The Syed-Neblett interstitial template in locally advanced gynecological malignancies. *Int J Radiat Oncol Biol Phys* 1983; 9(12):1897-1903.
2. Aristizabal SA, Surwit EA, Hevezi JM, Heusinkveld RS: Treatment of advanced cancer of the cervix with transperineal interstitial irradiation. *Int J Radiat Oncol Biol Phys* 1983; 9(7):1013-17.
3. DiSaia PJ: Radiation therapy in gynecology. In *Obstetrics and Gynecology*, 8th edition. Scott JR, DiSaia PJ, Hammond CB, Spellacy WN, eds. Lippincott-Raven, Philadelphia: 1999, 909-26.

4. Edraki B, Teng NN, Kapp DS, O'Hanlan KA: Laparoscopically assisted interstitial perineal implantation and pelvic lid construction: description of an effective and minimally invasive method (abstract). *Gynecol Oncol* 1995; 56:133.

5. Fu KK, Snead PK, Leibel SA, Nori D, Peschel RE: Carcinoma of the cervix. In *Interstitial Brachytherapy: Physical, Biological, and Clinical Considerations*. Anderson LL, Nath R, Weaver KA, Nori D, Phillips TL, Son YU, Chin-Tsao ST, Meigooni AS, Meli JA, Smith V, eds. Interstitial Collaborative Working Group. Raven Press, New York: 1990, 179-88.

6. Hughes-Davies L, Silver B, Kapp DS: Parametrial interstitial brachytherapy for advanced or recurrent pelvic malignancy: the Harvard/Stanford experience. *Gynecol Oncol* 1995; 58:24-7.

7. Martinez A, Edmundson GK, Cox RS, Gunderson LL, Howes AE: Combination of external beam irradiation and multiple-site perineal application (MUPIT) for treatment of locally advanced or recurrent prostatic, anorectal, and gynecologic malignancies. *Int J Radiat Oncol Biol Phys* 1985; 11(2):391-8.

8. Monk BJ, Walker JL, Tewari K, Ramsinghani NS, Syed AM, DiSaia PJ: Open interstitial brachytherapy for the treatment of local-regional recurrences of uterine corpus and cervix cancer after primary surgery. *Gynecol Oncol* 1994; 52:222-8.

9. Paley PJ, Koh WJ, Stelzer KS, et al: A new technique for performing Syed template interstitial implants for anterior vaginal tumors using an open retropubic approach. *Gynecol Oncol* 1999; 73:121-5.

10. Perez CA, Hall EJ, Purdy JA, Williamson J: Biologic and physical aspects of radiation oncology. In *Principles and Practice of Gynecologic Oncology,* 3rd edition. Hoskins WJ, Perez CA, Young RC, eds. Lippincott-Raven Publishers, Philadelphia: 2000, 327-402.

11. Phillips TL, Nori D, Peschel RE: Carcinoma of the vagina and vulva. In *Interstitial Brachytherapy: Physical, Biological, and Clinical Considerations*. Anderson LL, Nath R, Weaver KA, Nori D, Phillips TL, Son YU, Chin-Tsao ST, Meigooni AS, Meli JA, Smith V, eds. Interstitial Collaborative Working Group. Raven Press, New York: 1990, 189-97.

12. Syed AM, Puthawala AA, Abdelaziz NN, et al: Long-term results of low-dose-rate interstitial-intracavitary brachytherapy in the treatment of carcinoma of the cervix. *Int J Radiat Oncol Biol Phys* 2002; 54(1):67-78.

13. Tewari K, Cappuccini F, Syed AM, et al: Interstitial brachytherapy in the treatment of advanced and recurrent vulvar cancer. *Am J Obstet Gynecol* 1999; 181(1):91-8.

LAPAROSCOPIC SURGERY IN GYNECOLOGIC ONCOLOGY

SURGICAL CONSIDERATIONS

Description: With the advent of minimally invasive laparoscopic techniques and instrumentation, the role of laparoscopic procedures in gynecologic cancer treatment continues to be actively defined. The potential advantages of a laparoscopic approach include a shorter hospital stay, better pain control, faster recovery time, ↓morbidity, and cosmetically appealing smaller incision. There is an acceptable complication rate; however, questions with regard to safety of use in malignant diseases, ↑operative time, and cost remain to be studied. The authors believe that there is a role for laparoscopy in select situations, such as:

- Second-look evaluation for ovarian cancer;
- Assessment of adnexal masses and diagnosis of ovarian cancer;
- Laparoscopic lymphadenectomy with laparoscopically assisted vaginal hysterectomy or laparoscopic hysterectomy in staging of endometrial cancer;
- Laparoscopically assisted radical vaginal hysterectomy or laparoscopic radical hysterectomy with lymphadenectomy in early-stage cervical cancer; and
- Laparoscopically assisted application of interstitial brachytherapy implants.

Details of each of these procedures are beyond the scope of this section; however, common principles of laparoscopic techniques (e.g., adhesiolysis, biopsies, oophorectomy, omentectomy) apply (see discussion in Laparoscopic Procedures for Gynecologic Surgery, p. 692). The patient is placed in the dorsal lithotomy position, with the buttocks extended over the edge of the table to allow for instrument manipulation, and may need to be placed in steep Trendelenburg position during surgery. Various techniques are used for entry into the abdominal cavity, but the open laparoscopic technique is favored by many and may ↓ risk of vascular or visceral injuries. Other incision-related complications include dehiscence and hernia.

Usual preop diagnosis: Ovarian tumor and other gynecological cancers/tumors

SUMMARY OF PROCEDURE

Position	Dorsal lithotomy; legs in Allen universal stirrups; steep Trendelenburg
Incisions	Intraumbilical; bilateral suprapubic; midline suprapubic
Special instrumentation	CO_2 laser; bipolar Kleppinger forceps; suction irrigator; may require Harmonic Scalpel; various laparoscopic stapling instruments.
Unique considerations	Extended operative time and period of abdominal insufflation for radical procedures. Possible rapid need for laparotomy. Extensive use of electrocautery, ABC, CO_2 laser.
Antibiotics	Cefazolin 1 g or cefotetan 2 g
Surgical time	1.5-5 h
Closing considerations	< laparotomy; but fascia of all 10- to 12-mm ports need to be closed. 5- mm trocar sites can be closed in a subcuticular fashion.
EBL	50-1400 ml, depending on extent of procedure
Postop care	Clear liquid diet; ambulate POD 1.
Mortality	4.4/100,000
Morbidity	Overall complication rate: 0.2-10.3%
	Conversion to laparotomy: 2.1-7%
	Port-site metastasis: < 1%
	Subcutaneous emphysema: 0.3-2%
	Pneumomediastinum: 0.26%
	Brachial plexus neuropathy: 0.16%
	Incisional hernia: 0.06-1%
	Visceral injury: 0.06-0.5%
	Major vascular injury: 0.04-0.08%
	Bladder/ureteral injury: 0.02-1.7%
	Gas embolism: 0.0014%
	Wound infection: Uncommon
Pain score	3-4

PATIENT POPULATION CHARACTERISTICS

Age range	Reproductive and postreproductive yr
Incidence	Depends on primary disease
Etiology	Numerous, depending on primary disease (see appropriate sections earlier in this chapter).
Associated conditions	See specific procedures in this chapter.

ANESTHETIC CONSIDERATIONS

See Anesthetic Considerations for Laparoscopic Procedures for Gynecologic Surgery, p. 692.

References

1. Canis M, Dauplat J, Pomel C, et al: Laparoscopic radical hysterectomy for cervical cancer. Results from about 41 cases (IGCS abstract). *Int J Gynecol Cancer* 1997; 7:3.
2. Canis M, Rabischong B, Houlle C, et al: Laparoscopic management of adnexal masses: a gold standard? *Curr Opin Obstet Gynecol* 2002; 14:423-8.
3. Childers JM, Brainard CM, Martel MK, et al: Laparoscopically assisted transperineal interstitial irradiation and surgical staging for advanced cervical carcinoma. *Endocuriether/Hypertherm Oncol* 1994; 10:83-6.
4. Childers JM, Brzechffa PR, Hatch KD, et al: Laparoscopically assisted surgical staging (LASS) of endometrial cancer. *Gynecol Oncol* 1993; 49:24-9.
5. Dargent DF: Laparoscopic surgery in gynecologic oncology. *Surg Clin North Am* 2001; 81:949-64.
6. Herd J, Fowler JM, Shenson D, et al: Para-aortic lymph node sampling: development of a technique. *Gynecol Oncol* 1992; 45:46-51.
7. Husain A, Chi DS, Prasad M, et al: The role of laparoscopy in second-look evaluations for ovarian cancer. *Gynecol Oncol* 2001; 80:44-7.
8. Joshi GP: Complications of laparoscopy. *Anesthesiol Clin North Am* 2001; 19:89-105.
9. Magrina JF: Complications of laparoscopic surgery. *Clin Obstet Gynecol* 2002; 45:469-80.

10. Magrina JF, Mutone NF, Weaver AL, et al: Laparoscopic lymphadenectomy and vaginal or laparoscopic hysterectomy with bilateral salpingo-oophorectomy for endometrial cancer: morbidity and survival. *Am J Obstet Gynecol* 1999; 181:376-81.
11. Morrow CP, Curtin JP: Minimal access surgery. In *Gynecologic Cancer Surgery*. Churchill Livingstone, New York: 1996, 745-67.
12. Munro MG: Laparoscopic access: complications, technologies, and techniques. *Curr Opin Obstet Gynecol* 2002; 14:365-74.
13. Pasic R, Hilgers R, Levine R: The role of laparoscopy in the management of gynecologic malignancies. *J Surg Oncol* 2000; 75:60-71.
14. Querleu D, Dargent D, Ansquer Y, et al: Extraperitoneal endosurgical aortic and common iliac dissection in the staging of bulky or advanced cervical carcinomas. *Cancer* 2000; 88:1883-91.

Surgeons

Bertha Chen, MD
Eva D. Littman, MD (*Infertility surgery*)
Amin A. Milki, MD (*Infertility surgery*)
Lynn M. Westphal, MD (*Infertility surgery*)

8.2 GYNECOLOGY/INFERTILITY SURGERY

Anesthesiologist

Karen A. Giarrusso, MD

DILATATION AND CURETTAGE (D&C)

SURGICAL CONSIDERATIONS

Description: During dilatation and curettage (D&C), the endometrial lining of the uterus and coexisting lesions (myoma, polyp) are removed. This procedure is performed to diagnose and treat bleeding from uterine and cervical lesions, to complete an incomplete or missed spontaneous abortion, or to treat cervical stenosis. It is used infrequently as a method for pregnancy termination. A D&C is performed less frequently with the advent of the office endometrial biopsy and medical management of bleeding problems.

With the patient in the dorsal lithotomy position, the surgeon initially performs a bimanual examination under anesthesia to obtain information about both the presence of adnexal pathology and anatomic detail of the uterus. A speculum is inserted into the vagina, and the cervix is grasped with a clamp. The cervix is pulled gently toward the operator, who then uses a uterine probe to delineate the length of the uterus and the angulation between the cervical canal and uterus. The uterine cavity is reached by dilating the cervical canal with progressively larger dilators (Hegar's or Pratt) to an 8-9 mm diameter. A ureteral stone forceps is often used at this stage to remove existing polyps; and a curette is used to systematically remove the endometrial lining (Fig 8.2-1).

Usual preop diagnosis: Uncontrolled uterine bleeding refractory to hormonal treatment in young women; abnormal uterine bleeding; incomplete, missed, or induced abortion; pregnancy termination; cervical stenosis causing dysmenorrhea or obstruction of menstral flow

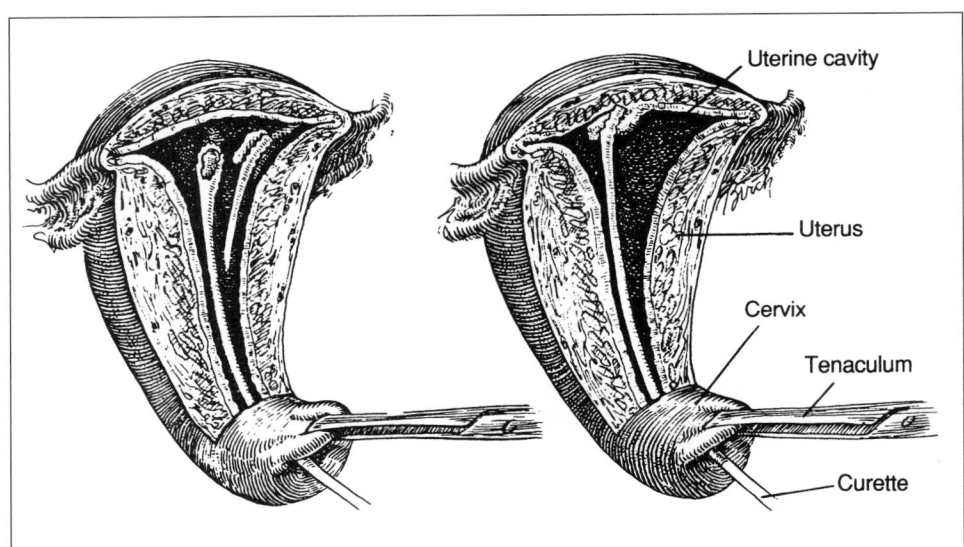

Figure 8.2-1. Curettage of endometrial lining. (Reproduced with permission from Rock JA, Thompson JD, eds: *Te-Linde's Operative Gynecology*, 8th edition. Lippincott Williams & Wilkins, 1997.)

SUMMARY OF PROCEDURE

Position	Dorsal lithotomy with stirrups
Incision	None
Special instrumentation	To prevent peroneal nerve injury, the area of the leg leaning against the stirrup should be well cushioned.
Unique considerations	Following induction, perineum is positioned at the very end of the table to ensure optimum exposure. During the cervical dilatation, a vasovagal response can occur, with subsequent bradycardia and ↓BP. Uterine perforations will often manifest as severe postop pain.
Antibiotics	None
Surgical time	5-15 min
EBL	50-100 ml
Mortality	Minimal
Morbidity	Postop fever: 1.7% Uterine perforation: 0.63% Severe immediate postop bleeding (caused by either uterine artery perforation or cervical injury): < 1%
Pain score	3-5

PATIENT POPULATION CHARACTERISTICS

Age range	20-80 yr
Incidence	> 1/50 females
Etiology	Dysfunctional uterine bleeding
Associated conditions	Obesity; HTN

ANESTHETIC CONSIDERATIONS

See Anesthetic Considerations following Therapeutic Abortion, Dilatation and Evacuation, p. 635.

References

1. Mackenzie IZ, Bibby JG: Critical assessment of dilatation and curettage in 1029 women. *Lancet* 1978; 2(8089):566-8.
2. Rock JA, Thompson JD, eds: *TeLinde's Operative Gynecology*, 8th edition. Lippincott Williams & Wilkins, Philadelphia: 1997, 465-75.

THERAPEUTIC ABORTION, DILATATION AND EVACUATION (D&E)

SURGICAL CONSIDERATIONS

Description: **Therapeutic abortion (TAB)** is the elective termination of a pregnancy prior to viability (usually considered to be 24 wk). In 1982, 1,574,000 legal abortions were performed in the U.S., a ratio of 426 abortions per 1,000 live births. **Suction curettage** is the most efficient method to terminate pregnancies during the first trimester (< 12 wk), and the great majority of abortions are performed this way. Few (< 5%) of first trimester abortions in the U.S. are performed with a sharp curette. Increased operative time and blood loss is seen with this method, resulting in its being practiced mainly in locations where a suction apparatus is not available. Suction curettage for a spontaneous abortion is performed in a manner identical to a regular TAB, except that a cervical dilatation might not be needed and the blood loss is usually 2-3 times greater. Very early termination (< 4 wk following LMP) can be performed without anesthesia via medical termination.

The **TAB procedure** consists of a standard cervical dilatation (required for gestations > 6 wk), followed by vacuum aspiration of the uterine contents, using a plastic suction curette (Fig 8.2-2). Alternatively, the cervical canal can be dilated > 6 hr prior to the operation with laminaria or synthetic osmotic dilators which, after insertion, swell to provide dilatation. A sharp curette often is used at the very end to gently verify the emptiness of the cavity, followed by reaspiration. Due to the risk of missing the pregnancy, most physicians wait until 7-8 wk following the LMP before performing the operation. Ergonovine maleate (0.2 mg im) and oxytocin (Pitocin) 20-30 U/1000 ml

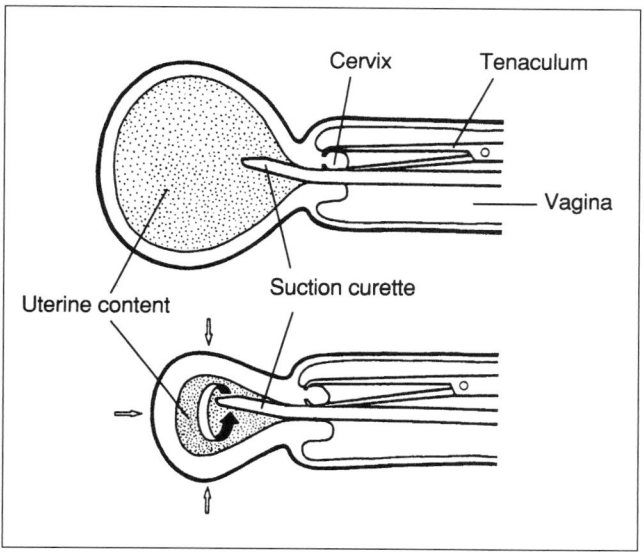

Figure 8.2-2. Uterine aspiration. Top—uterus at beginning of procedure; bottom—at conclusion of procedure. (Reproduced with permission from Rock JA, Thompson JD, eds: *TeLinde's Operative Gynecology*, 8th edition. Lippincott Williams & Wilkins, 1997.)

iv is often used during the procedure to reduce bleeding, although the efficacy of oxytocin has been questioned. The procedure is performed under either local or GA; it is generally felt that local is safer. Regardless of the method used, the obtained product of conception (POC) is sent for histological examination to exclude the presence of trophoblastic neoplasm or ectopic pregnancy.

Variant procedure: Dilatation and evacuation (D&E) remains the safest method for mid-trimester pregnancy termination.[2] It is performed similarly to first-trimester suction curettage, with the addition of using large-ring forceps to grasp and remove fetal parts intermittently. This procedure is often performed under GA.

Usual preop diagnosis: Pregnancy (viable or nonviable): 52% within 8 wk estimated gestational age; 90% within 12 wk estimated gestational age

SUMMARY OF PROCEDURES

	1st-Trimester Suction Curettage		**2nd-Trimester D&E**	
Position	Dorsal lithotomy with patient in Allen stirrups. Following induction, perineum positioned at end of table to ensure optimum exposure.		⇐	
Incision	None		⇐	
Special instrumentation	Suction		⇐ + Large-ring forceps	
Unique considerations	To prevent peroneal nerve injury, the area of the leg leaning against stirrup should be well cushioned. During cervical dilatation, a vasovagal reaction can occur → ↓HR + ↓BP. During injection of lidocaine for paracervical block, seizures may occur if > 12 ml of 1% solution are injected. Uterine perforations often will cause excessive postop pain.		⇐	
Antibiotics	Doxycycline 100 mg iv		⇐	
Surgical time	5-15 min		15-45 min	
EBL[6]	No. wk gestation: 1-4 – 10 ml 5-8 – 10-30 ml 9-10 – 30-80 ml 11-12 – 80-200 ml 13-14 – 200-400 ml		300-500 ml	
Postop care	PACU		⇐	
Mortality	0-3.1/100,000[3,4]		13/100,000[2]	
Morbidity	Mild infection	1/216	T > 38° for > 1 d	13.4/1,000
	Resuctioned day of surgery	1/553	Cervical injury	11.6/1,000
	Resuctioned subsequently	1/596	Cervical tear	10/1,000
	Cervical stenosis causing amenorrhea	1/6,071	Retained POC	9/1,000
	Cervical incompetence	1/9,444	Hemorrhage	7.1/1,000
	Underestimation of gestational age	1/15,454	UTI	1.8/1,000
	Convulsive Sz (after local anesthesia)	1/25,086		
	Total	1/118		
Complications requiring hospitalization	Incomplete abortion	1/3,617	Endometritis	8.5/1,000
	Sepsis	1/4,722	Uterine perforation	3.2/1,000
	Uterine perforation	1/10,625	Need for laparotomy	2.1/1,000
	Vaginal bleeding	1/14,166	Need for blood transfusion	1.9/1,000
	Inability to complete	1/28,333		
	Coexisting tubal pregnancy	1/42,500		
	Total	1/1,405		
Pain score	5		5	

PATIENT POPULATION CHARACTERISTICS

Age range	15-45 yr
Incidence	Abortions: 21.3/1000 women age 15-44 yr in the U.S. (2000)
Etiology	Desire for pregnancy termination

ANESTHETIC CONSIDERATIONS FOR D&C, TAB, D&E

PREOPERATIVE

These are among the most common procedures performed in gynecology. Patients presenting for these procedures are generally healthy; however, bleeding and sepsis may alter ASA status.

Cardiovascular	Hemodynamic status may be impaired 2° preop uterine bleeding, and patient may be septic from retained uterine products. ✓ BP, HR, orthostatic vital signs. **Tests:** As indicated from H&P.
Laboratory	Hb/Hct; other tests as indicated from H&P.
Premedication	Anxiolytic (e.g., midazolam 1-2 mg iv) as needed.

INTRAOPERATIVE

Anesthetic technique: Local, regional, or GA all may be appropriate. In the younger patient population, spinal anesthesia may be less desirable because of increased incidence of postdural puncture headache (PDPH).

Local anesthesia: Some obstetricians/gynecologists perform these procedures under local anesthesia. Paracervical block has the potential for inadvertent iv administration, with consequent toxic reaction.

Regional anesthesia: A T10 sensory level is sufficient to provide anesthesia for procedures on the uterus.

Spinal	5% lidocaine 75-100 mg (controversial); 0.75% bupivacaine 10-15 mg in 8.25% dextrose. (See Anesthetic Considerations for Cesarean Section, p. 664.) If spinal anesthesia is indicated, a pencil-point spinal needle (e.g., Whitacre or Sprotte) should be used to decrease the incidence of PDPH.[9]
Epidural	1.5-2.0% lidocaine with epinephrine 5 μg/ml, 15-25 ml; supplement with 5-10 ml as needed. Supplemental iv sedation. (See Anesthetic Considerations for Cesarean Section, p. 663.)
CSE	**Combined spinal/epidural (CSE):** An alternative technique combining the rapid onset and density of spinal anesthesia with the flexibility of continuous epidural anesthesia. Apply monitors, administer fluid, and position patient as for spinal or epidural. The most common technique is the needle-through-needle. After the epidural space is located with a standard 17 ga Tuohy needle, insert a 4″ 26-27 ga pencil-point spinal needle through it to administer 0.6 ml of spinal bupivacaine (0.75%) ± fentanyl 10 μg and morphine sulfate 0.1-0.2 mg. Secure the epidural catheter and use if needed (a test dose is advisable).

General anesthesia:

Induction	Standard induction (see p. B-2).
Maintenance	Standard maintenance (see p. B-3) used commonly, although frequently done by mask with O_2/N_2O + volatile anesthetic and spontaneous respiration. May also use propofol infusion (100-250 μg/kg/min), with N_2O, without volatile anesthetic. A small amount of opiate may be used. High incidence of postop N/V warrant prophylactic treatment with metoclopramide (5-10 mg iv) and/or a 5-HT_3-antagonist (e.g., ondansetron 4 mg iv, dolasetron 12.5 mg iv).
Emergence	Be ready with suction in the event of vomiting on emergence.

Blood and fluid requirements	Minimal blood loss IV: 18 ga × 1 (unless hypovolemic) NS/LR @ 2 ml/kg/h	Usual replacement of maintenance fluids and overnight deficit with crystalloid. Blood replacement rarely indicated.
Control of blood loss	Oxytocin (Pitocin) 20-30 U Ergonovine maleate (0.2 mg)	Oxytocin causes uterine contraction, with a consequent decrease in blood loss. Rapid iv bolus may lead to hypotension. Oxytocin is usually diluted in 1 L of crystalloid and then infused. Ergonovine maleate also causes uterine contraction and is usually given im. Side effects include HTN, myocardial ischemia and dysrhythmias, especially if given iv.[7]
Monitoring	Standard monitors (p. B-1)	
Positioning	✓ hip, leg, hand position. ✓ and pad pressure points. ✓ eyes. Shoulder abducted < 90°	Lithotomy position can be deleterious to pulmonary function, as it may impair respiratory mechanics. Rarely, hemodynamic changes can occur on elevation of the legs into the stirrups, as this increases venous return to the heart. Problems with hypotension on lowering legs postop are more common.

Vagal stimulation	Bradycardia	When cervix is grasped and dilated, patient may have excessive vagal stimulation, which can be treated by prompt cessation of stimulation and with atropine (0.4 mg iv), if indicated.
Complications	Nerve injury	Common peroneal nerve palsy (e.g., foot drop) is possible if pressure on the nerve over the fibula is not prevented by adequate padding or positioning. Hyperflexion of the hip joint can cause femoral and lateral femoral cutaneous nerve palsy. Obturator and saphenous nerve injury are also complications of the lithotomy position.[1]
	Finger trauma	Take care to ensure safety of patient's fingers when manipulating foot of the bed. Avoid finger injury by placing patient's arms on arm boards or by wrapping her hands.[6]

POSTOPERATIVE

Complications	High incidence of N/V Uterine perforation with severe abdominal pain (rare) Severe hemorrhage, necessitating blood transfusion (rare)	Antiemetics, including metoclopramide 10 mg iv and/or a 5-HT$_3$-antagonist (e.g., ondansetron 4 mg iv, dolasetron 12.5 mg iv), can be useful in this setting. Severe immediate postop bleeding caused by uterine atony, retained POCs, uterine perforation, or cervical injury.[2]
Pain management	IV opiate	Oral pain medications may be satisfactory. Extreme pain may be caused by uterine perforation.
Tests	Hb/Hct, if hemorrhage	

References

1. Courtney, MA: Neurologic sequelae of childbirth and regional anesthesia. In *Manual of Obstetric Anesthesia*. Churchill Livingstone, New York: 1992.
2. Grimes DA et al: Mid-trimester abortion by dilatation and evacuation. *N Engl J Med* 1977; 296(20):1141-5.
3. Grimes DA, Cates W Jr: Complications from legally-induced abortion: a review. *Obstet Gynecol Surg* 1979; 34(3):177-91.
4. Hakim-Elahi E: Complications of first-trimester abortion: a report of 170,000 cases. *Obstet Gynecol* 1990; 76(1):129-35.
5. Nakata DA, Stoelting RK: Positioning. *In Patient Safety in Anesthetic Practice*. Morell RC, Eichhorn JH, eds. Churchill Livingstone, New York: 1997, 293-318.
6. Pernoll ML, ed: *Current Obstetrics and Gynecologic Diagnosis and Treatment*. Appleton & Lange, Norwalk, CT: 1991, 686-91.
7. Rock JA, Thompson JD, eds: *TeLinde's Operative Gynecology*, 8th edition. Lippincott Williams & Wilkins, Philadelphia: 1997.
8. Ross BK, Chadwick HS, Mancuso JS, Benedetti C: Sprotte needle for obstetric anesthesia: Decreased incidence of post dural puncture headache. *Reg Anesth* 1992; 17:29-33.

HYSTEROSCOPY

SURGICAL CONSIDERATIONS

Description: Hysteroscopy is a procedure in which the endometrial cavity can be examined, allowing for direct visualization of lesions. The procedure is used primarily to investigate abnormal uterine bleeding, often caused by intrauterine submucous myoma and polyps. After the diagnosis, these lesions can be removed through the operative hysteroscope using a variety of techniques.

Variant procedure or approaches: Diagnostic hysteroscopies can be performed under both GA and local anesthesia, while **operative hysteroscopies** are usually performed under GA. An examination under anesthesia is performed, followed by the insertion of open speculum and the attachment of a tenaculum to the cervix. The cervical canal is dilated until the hysteroscope can be introduced with its sheath (Fig 8.2-3). A distention medium—usually a low-viscosity fluid—is then used to provide visualization of the uterine cavity. In the past, other media, such as CO_2 gas and Hyskon, were used frequently to distend the uterus; however, these have been replaced by low-viscosity fluids, due to the ease of its use and safety concerns about Hyskon. (Case reports of ARDS, pulmonary edema, DIC, anaphylactoid reactions, and platelet dysfunction have been reported when large volumes of Hyskon have been used.[5,6,12] It has been recommended that no more than 300 ml of this solution be infused, to avoid these potentially serious complications.) The most commonly used low-viscosity fluids are NS, sorbitol 3%/mannitol 0.5%, and mannitol 5% solutions. NS is most commonly used for diagnostic hysteroscopies, while the other nonconductive fluids are used for operative hysteroscopies. Certain bipolar operative hysteroscopies also allow the use of NS.

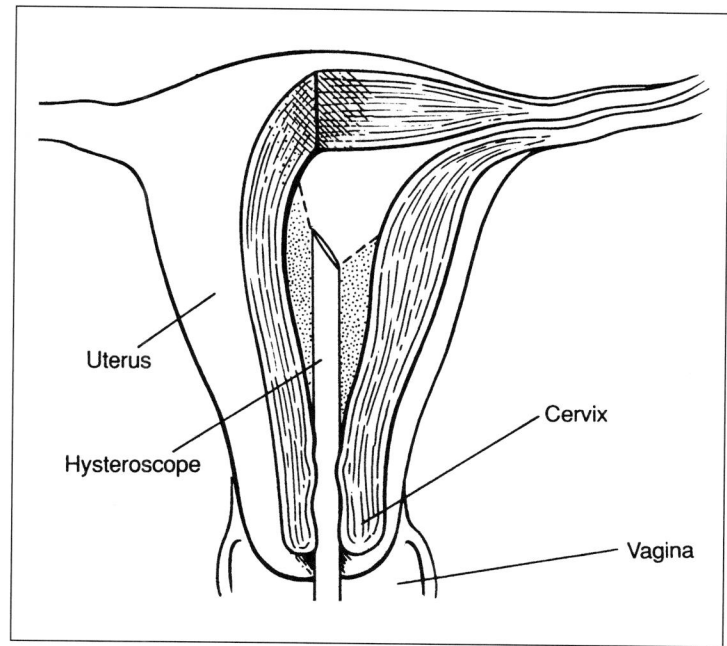

Figure 8.2-3. Hysteroscopy. (Reproduced with permission from Baggish MS, Barbot S, Valle RF: *Diagnostic & Operative Hysteroscopy.* Year Book Medical Pub, 1989.)

The distension medium is delivered to the hysteroscope by means of gravity or by a pump. Most systems use gravity, whereby the fluid is delivered via a wide-bore tubing and the maximum intrauterine pressure (IUP) is determined by the height of the fluid container above the uterus. The maximum IUP is thus limited by gravity, making this system relatively safe. The lowest IUP necessary to provide adequate visualization should be used to decrease the rate of absorption of the distention medium. A video camera can be attached to the hysteroscope to allow for easier visualization. During operative cases, an accompanying laparoscope is sometimes introduced from the abdomen to evaluate the progress of the hysteroscopy and to safeguard against uterine perforation and potential bowel injury.

Usual preop diagnosis: Abnormal uterine bleeding; infertility; recurrent pregnancy loss

SUMMARY OF PROCEDURE

Position	Dorsal lithotomy (Allen stirrups)
Incision	None
Special instrumentation	Fluid pump; laser; electrocautery equipment
Unique considerations	Accelerated fluid absorption with prolonged procedures or with resections may → pulmonary edema. Laparoscopy may accompany this procedure.
Surgical time	15 min-2 h
Antibiotics	Cefazolin 1 g iv
EBL	0-100 ml
Postop care	Excessive postop bleeding can be controlled by using a 5 ml Foley balloon catheter in the uterus for several h.[6]
Mortality	Minimal
Morbidity	Pleural effusion can be seen with use of low-viscosity medium.[1,3]
Pain score	3-5

PATIENT POPULATION CHARACTERISTICS

Age range	20-80 yr
Incidence	> 1/50
Etiology	Unexplained uterine bleeding; infertility
Associated conditions	Obesity

ANESTHETIC CONSIDERATIONS

PREOPERATIVE

Hysteroscopy may be performed for diagnostics or treatment of intrauterine pathology. Patients presenting for this procedure are generally healthy.

Cardiovascular	As patient may be undergoing hysteroscopy for uterine bleeding, BP, HR, and orthostatic vital signs should be noted. **Tests:** As indicated from H&P.
Laboratory	Hb/Hct if bleeding Hx. Other tests as indicated from H&P.
Premedication	Anxiolytic (e.g., midazolam 1-2 mg iv) as needed.

INTRAOPERATIVE

Anesthetic technique: Local, regional, or GA may be used. In the younger patient population, spinal anesthesia may be less desirable because of increased incidence of postdural puncture headache (PDPH). If spinal anesthesia is indicated, pencil point spinal needles (e.g., Sprotte or Whitacre) should be used to decrease the incidence of PDPH.[9]

Local anesthesia: Some procedures may be done under local, especially if they are diagnostic. Paracervical block has the potential for an inadvertent intravenous administration, with consequent toxic reaction.

Regional anesthesia: A T10 sensory level is sufficient to provide anesthesia for these procedures.

Spinal	5% lidocaine 75-100 mg (controversial); 0.75% bupivacaine 10-15 mg in 8.25% dextrose. (See Anesthetic Considerations for Cesarean Section, p. 664.)
Epidural	1.5-2.0% lidocaine with epinephrine 5 μg/ml, 15-25 ml; supplement with 5-10 ml as needed. Supplemental iv sedation. (See Anesthetic Considerations for Cesarean Section, p. 663.)
CSE	**Combined spinal/epidural (CSE):** An alternative technique combining the rapid onset and density of spinal anesthesia with the flexibility of continuous epidural anesthesia. Apply monitors, administer fluid, and position patient as for spinal or epidural. The most common technique is the needle-through-needle. After the epidural space is located with a standard 17 ga Tuohy needle, insert a 4″ 26-27 ga pencil-point spinal needle through it to administer 0.6 ml of spinal bupivacaine (0.75%) ± fentanyl 10 μg and morphine sulfate 0.1-0.2 mg. Secure the epidural catheter and use if needed (a test dose is advisable).

General anesthesia:

Induction	Standard induction (see p. B-2).
Maintenance	Standard maintenance (see p. B-3). Patients have a high incidence of vomiting, so prophylaxis (e.g., metoclopramide 10 mg iv), as in patients for D&C, is warranted.
Emergence	Be ready with suction in the event of vomiting on emergence.

Blood and fluid requirements	Minimal blood loss IV: 18 ga × 1 (unless hypovolemic) NS\LR @ 2 ml/kg/h	Usual replacement of maintenance fluids and overnight deficit in the form of crystalloid. Blood replacement is almost never indicated.
Positioning	✓ hip, leg, and hand positions. ✓ and pad pressure points. ✓ eyes. Shoulder abduction < 90°	Lithotomy position can be deleterious to pulmonary function, as it may impair respiratory mechanics. Rarely, hemodynamic changes occur on elevation of legs into the stirrups, as this increases venous return to the heart. Problems with hypotension on lowering legs postop are common. Common peroneal nerve palsy is possible if pressure on the nerve over the fibula is not prevented by adequate padding or positioning. Hyperflexion of hip joint can cause femoral and lateral femoral cutaneous nerve palsy. Obturator and saphenous nerve injury are also complications of the lithotomy position.[3]
Monitoring	Standard monitors (see p. B-1).	
Surgical stimulation	When cervix is grasped and dilated, patient may have excessive vagal nerve stimulation.	RX: prompt cessation of stimulation by surgeons and treatment with atropine, if indicated.

Complications	Pulmonary and cerebral edema (2° hypotonic fluid overload) Coagulopathy Air embolism Anaphylactoid reactions	Air embolism can occur with the use of gas distention media, thus, most institutions currently use low-viscosity fluids for distension. Low-viscosity media can be grouped, based on their tonicity and electrolyte content: 1) hypotonic, electrolyte-free media that may cause hypotonic fluid overload; and 2) isotonic, electrolyte-containing media that may cause isotonic fluid overload. It is important to monitor the volume of fluid used during the procedure. It is not uncommon to use 10–20 L of distention fluid during an operative hysteroscopy. If fluid overload is suspected, diuretic treatment should be considered.
	Finger injury (2° positioning)	When manipulating the foot of the bed, avoid finger injury by placing patient's arms on arm boards or by wrapping her hands.

POSTOPERATIVE

Complications	High incidence of PONV Respiratory compromise from excessive fluid absorption	Antiemetics, including metoclopramide 10 mg iv and/or a 5-HT_3-antagonist (e.g., ondansetron 4 mg iv, dolasetron 12.5 mg iv), can be useful in this setting.
Pain management	Small dose of titrated opiate	Patients usually tolerate oral pain medications.
Tests	Consider CXR and ABG. Serum electrolytes	If respiratory compromise

References

1. Adoni A, et al: Postoperative pleural effusion caused by dextran. *Int J Gynaecol Obstet* 1980; 18(4):243-4.
2. Borten M, Seibert CP, Taymor ML: Recurrent anaphylactic reaction to intraperitoneal dextran 75 used for prevention of postsurgical adhesions. *Obstet Gynecol* 1983; 61(6):755-7.
3. Cooper JM, Brady RM: Intraoperative and early postoperative complications of operative hysteroscopy. *Obstet Gynecol Clin North Am* 2000; 27(2):247-66.
4. Courtney MA: Neurologic sequelae of childbirth and regional anesthesia. In *Manual of Obstetric Anesthesia*. Churchill Livingstone, New York: 1992.
5. Jedeikin R, Olsfanger D, Kessler I: Disseminated intravascular coagulopathy and adult respiratory distress syndrome: life-threatening complications of hysteroscopy. *Am J Obstet Gynecol* 1990; 162(1):44-5.
6. Leake JF, Murphy AA, Zacur HA: Noncardiogenic pulmonary edema: a complication of operative hysteroscopy. *Fertil Steril* 1987; 48(3):497-9.
7. Nakata DA, Stoelting RK: Positioning. In *Patient Safety in Anesthetic Practice*. Morell RC, Eichhorn JH, eds. Churchill Livingstone, New York: 1997, 293-318.
8. Pellicer A, Diamond MP: Distending media for hysteroscopy. *Obstet Gynecol Clin North Am* 1988; 15:23-8.
9. Rock, JA, Thompson JD, eds: *TeLinde's Operative Gynecology*, 8th edition. Lippincott-Raven, Philadelphia: 1997.
10. Ross BK, Chaduck HS, Mancuso JJ, Benedelti C. Sprotte needle for obstetric anesthesia: Decreased incidence of post dural puncture headache. *Reg Anesth* 1992; 17:29-33.
11. Soderstrom RM, ed: *Operative Laparoscopy*, 2nd edition. Lippincott-Raven, Philadelphia: 1998.
12. Vercellini P, Rossi R, Pagnoni B, Fedele L: Hypervolemic pulmonary edema and severe coagulopathy after intrauterine dextran instillation. *Obstet Gynecol* 1992; 79(5[P + 2]):838-9.

PELVIC LAPAROTOMY

SURGICAL CONSIDERATIONS

Description: Laparotomy and its variants are all common gynecological procedures. Laparotomy is most frequently performed via a Pfannenstiel's incision, which permits good pelvic exposure. A vertical incision is used in oncological surgery or in the presence of a large uterus. A knife or Bovie is used to cut through the skin and underlying tissue until the rectus fascia is reached. The fascia is nicked, and then sharply incised bilaterally 2-4" with scissors or electrocautery (Bovie). The rectus muscle is separated sharply in the midline down to the pubis and the peritoneum is entered. The peritoneal incision is then extended vertically or transversely. The pelvis and entire abdominal cavity are explored first by palpation. Then the bowels usually are packed in a cephalad direction with surgical laparotomy sponges (laps) to prevent them from falling back into the pelvis. Good muscle relaxation is important during this stage to ensure optimal packing. A self-retaining retractor frequently is used to keep the laps in place and to enhance exposure. After the desired operation has been performed, the retractor and packs are removed. During the peritoneal closure, abdominal muscle relaxation is again critical to minimize tension on this layer and risk of bowel injury with the needle. The rectus fascia, the subcutaneous tissue, and the skin are closed in succession.

Variant procedures: Myomectomies are performed to remove myomata that are causing pain, abnormal bleeding, or infertility. Myomata are heavily vascularized at the base, and the surgeon has several ways to minimize this bleeding. A clamp can be placed across the uterine vasculature to minimize blood flow to the uterus. A common alternative is the use of a vasoconstrictor, such as diluted epinephrine (1:200,000) or vasopressin solution (1-5 U/10 ml NS). The solution (2-10 ml) is injected around the myoma prior to incising the uterus, which invariably → ↑HR and ↑BP. Gonadotropin releasing hormone (Gn-RH) agonists may be used for a few months prior to the operation to render the patient hypoestrogenic and, thus, decrease the vascularity of the myomata. After the myomata have been removed, the uterine defects are closed with several layers of suture, and the uterine serosa is closed.

Ovarian cystectomies are performed to alleviate related pain and to diagnose the identity of asymptomatic cysts. Small, single-functional ovarian cysts are found at different stages in a woman's menstrual cycle. At times, these cysts can increase in size and quantity, which may cause severe pain. The ovary also can contain various nonfunctional cysts (e.g., tumors) which have to be removed, even if asymptomatic, to r/o malignancy. After the pelvic structures are well visualized, the cystic ovary is stabilized with instruments or surgical laps. Sharp or blunt dissection is used to shell out the cyst intact. If there is any suspicion about the nature of the cyst, an intraop frozen section is obtained. The ovary is then reapproximated and the abdomen closed. If the cyst is large and little healthy ovarian stroma remains, an **oophorectomy** is performed.

Ectopic pregnancies are usually medical emergencies. Increasingly, **laparoscopy** is being used to treat this condition (see p. 687), although laparotomies for ectopic pregnancies are still widely performed. The abdomen is entered, and the pregnancy located quickly. An attempt is made to control the bleeding with the surgeon's hand, a clamp, or suture. Frequently, large amounts of blood in the pelvis are suctioned and the ectopic pregnancy is removed via a **partial tubal resection, salpingostomy**, or **salpingectomy**; then the abdomen is closed. A **D&C** is often performed at the end to prevent late bleeding from the pregnancy-induced endometrial proliferation (see p. 632).

In **abdominal colpopexy** (fixation of vagina), the patient is placed in the lithotomy position, usually with Allen stirrups, to perform an examination under anesthesia, as well as to insert a vaginal pack needed to identify the vaginal apex. A urethral catheter is inserted prior to staging the laparotomy. A rectus fascia graft is obtained during the opening of the abdomen (a synthetic graft can be used instead). The bowel is packed and the defect is examined from the abdominal perspective. Frequently there is an accompanying enterocele which must be closed initially (see **Moschowitz procedure,** below). The peritoneum over the vaginal apex is then entered and the neighboring rectum and bladder are dissected a distance away from the vaginal apex. The peritoneum over the sacrum is incised and the cephalad end of the graft is sutured to the anterior sacral ligament of the third vertebrae. Severe bleeding can occur if there is injury to the middle sacral artery. The caudal end of the graft is attached to the vaginal apex, with the surgeon frequently using a vaginal hand to place these last sutures. The peritoneum and abdomen are closed, and the patient's legs are elevated to the dorsal lithotomy position for a high posterior **colporrhaphy** (repair of vagina).

The **Moschowitz procedure** is used to reduce enteroceles via an abdominal approach. The abdomen is entered in the usual fashion, the uterus held up with a traction suture, the bowel packed, and the patient placed in the Trendelenburg position. Multiple concentric purse-string sutures are used to close the defect in the pouch of Douglas; and the abdomen is closed.

The **presacral neurectomy** is an operation performed for women with severe chronic midline pelvic pain. Usually the patient has a history of prior surgeries to diagnose and treat the problem. A laparotomy is initially performed with packing of the bowels. The rectosigmoid is brought over to the left to make a vertical, posterior, parietal, peritoneal incision over the sacral area. The anatomy is examined closely and the presacral nerves are obliterated or excised; then the peritoneum and abdomen are closed. Severe bleeding can be seen intraop from the hemorrhoidal and sacral veins, but usually can be controlled with pressure.

Usual preop diagnosis: Myomata (pelvic pain, hypermenorrhea, infertility); ovarian cysts and pelvic pain with undiagnosed ovarian mass; ectopic pregnancy; vaginal vault prolapse; enterocele; presacral neurectomy (chronic pelvic pain)

SUMMARY OF PROCEDURE

Position	Supine or lithotomy
Incision	Pfannenstiel's or low midline abdominal
Unique considerations	Muscle relaxation is important during bowel packing and abdominal closure. Vasoconstrictor substances for controlling myomata bleeding (1:200,000 epinephrine and 1-5 U vasopressin/10 ml NS) are often used and can alter BP and HR.
Antibiotics	1-2 g iv cefoxitin or cefotetan
Surgical time	45 min-4 h
	Abdominal colpopexy: 4-5 h
EBL	150-1000 ml (maximum related to procedure)
Postop care	PACU
Mortality	Minimal
Morbidity[2]	Gastric dilatation: 3%
	Thrombophlebitis: 3%
	PE: 2%
	Ureteral stenosis: 1%
Pain score	8

PATIENT POPULATION CHARACTERISTICS

	Myomectomy	Ovarian Cystectomy, Oophorectomy	Ectopic Pregnancy	Abdominal Colpopexy, Moschowitz	Presacral Neurectomy
Age range	20-45 yr	20-85 yr	15-45 yr	40-80 yr	20-50 yr
Incidence	> 1/5 females	⇐	1/100 females	1/500 females	⇐
Etiology	Congenital	Endometriosis Anovulation Adenoma	Preexisting tubal disease	Multiparous Obesity Chronic cough	Endometriosis
Associated conditions	Menorrhagia	Endometriosis	Pelvic adhesions	Pelvic relaxation	Endometriosis

ANESTHETIC CONSIDERATIONS

See Anesthetic Considerations following Infertility Operations, p. 644.

References

1. Rock JA, Thompson JD, eds: *TeLinde's Operative Gynecology*, 8th edition. Lippincott Williams & Wilkins, Philadelphia: 1997.
2. Uyttenbroeck F: *Gynecologic Surgery - Treatment of Complications and Prevention of Injuries*. Masson Publishing, New York: 1980.

TRANSVAGINAL OOCYTE RETRIEVAL (TVOR)

SURGICAL CONSIDERATIONS

Description: Transvaginal oocyte retrieval (TVOR) is performed on patients who have undergone ovarian stimulation using ovulation-inducing agents. This procedure is performed 35-36 h after the patient has been injected with human chorionic gonadotropin (HCG) to induce oocyte maturation. It is very important for the success of the procedure that retrieval be performed within this time period. If a retrieval is performed too late, ovulation will have occurred and oocyte retrieval will no longer be possible.

In the procedure room, the patient is placed in the dorsal lithotomy position, and conscious sedation is usually started at this time. A sterile speculum is inserted into the vagina and a vaginal prep is performed. After the prep, the speculum is removed and an ultrasound probe with a 16 ga needle on a needle guide is placed into the patient's vagina. One of the ovaries is identified and entered by inserting the needle through the vaginal fornix. Patients may experience a combination of pain and pressure at this point of the procedure. Once the needle is in the ovary, the surgeon will then proceed with sequential aspiration of the ovarian follicles. It is important that the patient remain relaxed and motionless during this part of the procedure, as movement may prevent aspiration of oocytes and increase the risk of injury to the surrounding organs and vessels. After retrieval is completed in the first ovary, the needle is withdrawn; the other ovary is identified, and a second puncture is made through the vaginal fornix. Depending on the number of follicles present, the entire procedure may last anywhere from 10-30 min. After all of the follicles have been aspirated, the needle and ultrasound probe are removed from the vagina. A sterile speculum is then reintroduced into the vagina and the vaginal wall and cervix are inspected for hemostasis. It is possible that a few minutes of applied pressure using sterile gauze are needed to obtain adequate hemostasis. Subsequently, the patient is taken to the recovery room and discharged after a recovery period of 30-90 min.

SUMMARY OF PROCEDURE

Position	Dorsal lithotomy
Incision	Vaginal punctures (usually 2)
Special instrumentation	Ultrasound probe with needle guide, 16-17 ga needle
Unique considerations	Requires complete relaxation/sedation to prevent injury and loss of oocyte during follicle aspiration.
Antibiotics	Cefotetan 1 g prior to procedure
Procedure time	Setup: 5-10 min
	Procedure: 10-30 min (depending on # of follicles)
Postop care	Recovery room→home
Morbidity	Bleeding: Rare
	Infection: Rare
Pain Score	1-3 (abdominal cramping)

PATIENT POPULATION CHARACTERISTICS

Age Range	18-50 yr (rare after age 43)
Incidence	It is estimated that at least 14% of American couples of reproductive age who desire pregnancy are unable to conceive within 1 yr.
Etiology	A male factor is responsible for 35%; pelvic factor, 25%; ovulatory factor, 20%; cervical factor, 10%; and 10% are unexplained.
Associated conditions	Thyroid disorders; polycystic ovarian syndrome; endometriosis; depression

ANESTHETIC CONSIDERATIONS

PREOPERATIVE

This is generally a fit, healthy patient population. Little is required beyond routine tests, unless otherwise indicated.

Laboratory	Tests as indicated from H&P
Premedication	Anxiolytic (e.g., midazolam 1-2 mg iv) as needed

INTRAOPERATIVE

Anesthetic technique: Conscious sedation or, rarely, local or regional anesthesia and GA have been used. Intravenous sedation (hypnotic agent, ± benzodiazepine, ± a narcotic analgesic), however, is the most commonly used and the safest technique for IVF.[2] The most stimulating parts of the procedure occur when the vaginal fornix is pierced on each side and when the ovarian follicles are entered for aspiration of the eggs.

MAC	Propofol infusion (25-100 μg/kg/min), with midazolam (2-4 mg iv) and fentanyl, alfentanil, or remifentanil titrated to achieve the desired combination of heavy sedation and analgesia (see p. B-4).
Blood and fluid requirements	Minimal blood loss
	IV: 18-20 ga × 1

Blood and fluid requirements, cont.	NS/LR @ 2 ml/kg/h	Usual replacement of overnight deficit in the form of crystalloid.
Monitoring	Standard monitors (p. B-1)	
Positioning	✓ hip, leg, and hand positions. ✓ and pad pressure points.	
Complications	Nerve injury	Common peroneal nerve palsy (e.g., foot drop) is possible if pressure on the nerve over the fibula is not prevented by adequate padding and positioning. Hyperflexion of the hip joint can cause femoral and lateral femoral cutaneous nerve palsy. Obturator and saphenous nerve injury are also complications of the lithotomy position.[1]
	Finger trauma	Ensure safety of patient's fingers when manipulating the foot of the bed by placing patient's arms on arm boards or by wrapping her hands.

POSTOPERATIVE

| **Complications** | PONV | Metoclopramide 10 mg iv and/or a 5-HT$_3$-antagonist (e.g., ondansetron 4 mg iv, dolasetron 12.5 mg iv) |
| **Pain management** | Minimal postop pain | Oral analgesics are usually sufficient. |

References

1. Courtney MA: Neurologic sequelae of childbirth and regional anesthesia. In *Manual of Obstetric Anesthesia.* Churchill Livingstone, New York: 1992.
2. Hadimioglu N, Titiz TA, Dosemeci L, Erman M: Comparison of various sedation regimens for transvaginal oocyte retrieval. *Fertility and Sterility* 2002; 78(3):648-9.
3. Meniru GI: *Cambridge Guide to Infertility Management and Assisted Reproduction.* Cambridge University Press, Cambridge: 2001, 130-1.
4. Mosher WD: Reproductive impairments in the United States, 1965-1982. *Demography* 1985; 22(3):415-30.

INFERTILITY OPERATIONS/IN VITRO FERTILIZATION

SURGICAL CONSIDERATIONS

Description: These operations all deal with reproductive problems. The general trend is to avoid laparotomies and to perform operations using outpatient laparoscopy and hysteroscopy techniques whenever possible.

Fimbrioplasty is used to repair distal fallopian tubal occlusion—a common cause for infertility—which is usually a consequence of pelvic inflammatory disease (PID). The operation may be performed by **pelvic laparotomy** or **laparoscopy** (see p. 639). If done by laparotomy, a urethral catheter is inserted to empty the bladder, followed by the insertion of a transcervical uterine catheter for chromopertubation (dye injection). The abdomen is opened and the pelvic structures are exposed. During the operation, microsurgical techniques are followed closely to minimize trauma. Meticulous hemostasis is important. A wound protector is often used instead of self-retaining retractors. The peritoneum and pelvic structures are kept moist with intermittent irrigation. Salpingolysis and ovariolysis may be performed microsurgically. Once the adnexae have been freed, they are elevated by loosely packing the pouch of Douglas with insulated pads (plastic sheathed covered laps). Chromopertubation is then performed and, if occlusion is present, a new stoma is created using microsurgical instruments and sutures. The abdomen is then closed.

Tubal reanastomosis, performed to restore fertility, is very similar to fimbrioplasty, with microsurgical techniques followed diligently. After the tubal segments have been freed slightly from their underlying mesosalpinx, the occluded ends are cut and chromopertubation is performed to ensure patency. After patency has been established, anastomosis is performed in two layers. The mesosalpinx is reapproximated to the tubal serosa and the abdomen closed.

The uterus is embryologically formed by the fusion of two paramesonephric tubes. At times, the fusion is incomplete and a septated uterus or bicornuate uterus is formed. The malformed uterus is associated with an increased risk for miscarriages and preterm labor. **Metroplasty** is used to correct this condition. The **Strassmann procedure** (extremely rare) for bicornuate uteri uses a standard pelvic laparotomy. Following uterine exposure, an incision is made on the medial side of each hemicorpus and carried down until the uterine cavity is entered. The edges are reapproximated to form a single uterus. Septated uteri are usually repaired via a hysteroscopic approach (see Hysteroscopy, p. 636) with scissors or laser.

Proximal tubal cannulation is a procedure in which proximal tubal occlusion can be repaired through either fluoroscopic or hysteroscopic approach. The hysteroscopic approach, usually performed under GA, allows the surgeon to insert a small cannula to restore tube patency. This procedure is often done with laparoscopy to follow the progress of the cannulization and to visualize the chromopertubation (see Hysteroscopy, p. 636, and Laparoscopy, p. 683).[2]

Gamete intrafallopian transfer[7] (GIFT) and **tubal embryo transfer** (TET) are methods of **advanced reproductive technology.** Couples who have undergone extensive infertility workups and treatment without success eventually become candidates for GIFT and TET procedures. Ovarian follicles are stimulated to grow with the help of gonadotropins. These follicles are then punctured with a needle transvaginally to 'harvest' the eggs. These eggs can be mixed with semen and placed directly into the distal end of the fallopian tube (GIFT) using laparoscopic techniques and a small tubal catheter (see Laparoscopy, p. 683). In the TET procedure, the semen and eggs are allowed to incubate a few days in vitro; embryos form and are transferred to the fallopian tubes in a manner similar to the GIFT procedure.

Usual preop diagnosis: Infertility; history of multiple spontaneous abortion and preterm labor

SUMMARY OF PROCEDURE

(For summaries of specific procedures, see Laparoscopy, p. 683; Hysteroscopy, p. 636; or Pelvic Laparotomy, p 639.)

PATIENT POPULATION CHARACTERISTICS

Age range	18-45 yr
Incidence	1/20 women
Etiology	PID; endometriosis; idiopathic
Associated conditions	Obesity

ANESTHETIC CONSIDERATIONS

(Procedures covered: pelvic laparotomy for myomectomy; ovarian cystectomy; oophorectomy; ectopic pregnancy removal; abdominal colpopexy; Moschowitz enterocele repair; presacral neurectomy; infertility operations)

PREOPERATIVE

This is generally a healthy patient population; however, this procedure can be performed for a wide variety of pathologic conditions.

Cardiovascular	Patients undergoing myomectomy and, especially, ectopic pregnancy removal, may have had a significant amount of preop bleeding; therefore, BP, HR and orthostatic vital signs should be noted. **Tests:** As indicated from H&P.
Laboratory	Hb/Hct. Patients with ectopic pregnancy may have urine/serum pregnancy tests, as well as pelvic ultrasound.
Premedication	Patients with ruptured ectopic pregnancies may come to the OR urgently, and should be treated as for full stomach. This includes premedication with a nonparticulate antacid, Na citrate 30 ml po, metoclopramide 10 mg iv, and ranitidine 50 mg iv.

INTRAOPERATIVE

Anesthetic technique: GETA is preferred in patients undergoing laparoscopic surgery and in patients presenting for emergency surgery. Regional anesthesia is best avoided in hemodynamically unstable patients (i.e., ectopic pregnancies), and for laparoscopy where breathing difficulty may develop 2° to pneumoperitoneum and Trendelenburg position. Regional anesthesia may be suitable for simple laparotomies. In the younger patient population, spinal anesthesia is less desirable because of an increased incidence of postdural puncture headache (PDPH). If spinal anesthesia is indicated, a pencil-point needle (e.g., Whitacre, Sprotte) should be used in order to decrease the incidence of PDPH.[7]

General anesthesia:

Induction	Standard induction (see p. B-2). A patient with an intact ectopic pregnancy undergoing laparoscopy should have an ETT placed and be mechanically ventilated to assure adequate oxygenation, ventilation and acid-base balance.[4] In a patient with a ruptured ectopic pregnancy, ketamine 1-2 mg/kg or etomidate 0.1-0.4 mg/kg may be preferable if a large blood loss has occurred. These patients may also have full stomachs; and, in this case, they require a rapid-sequence induction (p. B-5) with cricoid pressure and immediate ET intubation (succinylcholine 1.5 mg/kg).
Maintenance	Standard maintenance (see p. B-3). A high incidence of N/V warrants prophylaxis with metoclopramide 10 mg iv, and ondansetron 4 mg iv or granisetron 100 μg iv.
Emergence	Be ready with suction in the event of vomiting on emergence.

Regional anesthesia: A T4-6 sensory level is recommended for pelvic/lower abdominal surgery.

Spinal	5% lidocaine 75-100 mg (controversial); 0.75% bupivacaine 10-15 mg in 8.25% dextrose. (See Anesthetic Considerations for Cesarean Section, p. 664.)
Epidural	1.5-2.0% lidocaine with epinephrine 5 μg/ml, 15-25 ml; supplement with 5-10 ml as needed. Supplemental iv sedation. (See Anesthetic Considerations for Cesarean Section, p. 663.)
CSE	**Combined spinal/epidural (CSE):** An alternative technique combining the rapid onset and density of spinal anesthesia with the flexibility of continuous epidural anesthesia. Apply monitors, administer fluid, and position patient as for spinal or epidural. The most common technique is the needle-through-needle. After the epidural space is located with a standard 17 ga Tuohy needle, insert a 4″ 26-27 ga pencil-point spinal needle through it to administer 0.6 ml of spinal bupivacaine (0.75%) ± fentanyl 10 μg and morphine sulfate 0.1-0.2 mg. Secure the epidural catheter and use if needed (a test dose is advisable).

Blood and fluid requirements	Possible heavy blood loss IV: 16-18 ga × 1-2 NS/LR @ 5-7 ml/kg/h	Patients with ectopic pregnancies may have large blood loss both preop and intraop. Adequate iv access is imperative in these patients, as is the availability of blood.
Control of blood loss	Epinephrine Vasopressin	During myomectomies, surgeons may inject vasopressors into the area surrounding myomata prior to excision. This can cause HTN and cardiac dysrhythmias.
Monitoring	Standard monitors (p. B-1) ± Foley catheter Ectopic pregnancy: ± Arterial catheter	Patients with ectopic pregnancies may need intraarterial monitoring if major hemorrhage occurs.
Positioning	✓ and pad pressure points. ✓ eyes.	During abdominal colpopexy, patient is placed intermittently in both the lithotomy and supine positions. (See p. 635 for concerns regarding the lithotomy position.)
Complications	Respiratory: Pneumoperitoneum ↑$PaCO_2$, ↓PaO_2 ETT migration	Pneumoperitoneum with CO_2 and steep Trendelenburg position cause cephalad displacement of diaphragm with ↓FRC, ↓pulmonary compliance, and ↑airway closure/atelectasis. Hypercarbia and hypoxia, due to respiratory compromise, can result unless ventilation is controlled during GA. Check for endobronchial migration of ETT upon assumption of Trendelenburg position.
	Pneumothorax	Pneumothorax due to retroperitoneal dissection of insufflated gas into the mediastinum can cause hypoxemia, ↑airway pressure, subcutaneous emphysema, and ↓BP.
	Cardiovascular: ↓BP	↓BP can result from ↓venous return caused by pneumoperitoneum.

Complications, cont.	Hemorrhage Dysrhythmias	Hemorrhage can result from blood vessel injury or rapid reversal of head-down position. Unintended intravascular injection of CO_2 gas can → ↓BP and dysrhythmias.
	Neurological: Nerve injury Brachial plexus injury Nerve root compression	Use of Trendelenburg position incurs risk of nerve injury. Hyperextension of arm may result in brachial plexus injury and careful padding of vulnerable points is necessary. Shoulder brace can compress nerve roots in retroclavicular region.

POSTOPERATIVE

Complications	PONV Anemia Shoulder pain	Rx: metoclopramide 10 mg iv and/or a 5-HT_3-antagonist (e.g., ondansetron 4 mg iv, dolasetron 12.5 mg iv) Postop pain may be referred to the shoulder, due to irritation of diaphragm by residual pneumoperitoneum or bleeding.
Pain Management	PCA (p. C-3)	
Tests	Hb/Hct, if hemorrhage occurs.	

ANESTHETIC CONSIDERATIONS FOR IN VITRO FERTILIZATION

PREOPERATIVE

This is generally a fit, healthy patient population. Little is required beyond routine tests, unless otherwise indicated.

Laboratory	Tests as indicated from H&P.
Premedication	Standard premedication (see p. B-1).

INTRAOPERATIVE

Anesthetic technique: Conscious sedation, local anesthesia, regional (e.g., spinal and epidural) and GA all have been employed for in vitro fertilization. If the in vitro fertilization technique consists of transvaginal egg retrieval and embryo transfer (not laparoscopic technique), one study suggests higher pregnancy and delivery rates if conscious sedation or epidural anesthesia is used as opposed to GA.[2] Laparoscopy is only performed for GIFT, not for in vitro fertilization. For TVOR, use conscious sedation. Regional anesthesia provides adequate pain relief, but breathing difficulty can develop due to pneumoperitoneum and Trendelenburg position. Therefore, GETA with controlled ventilation is most commonly used. If GA is used, isoflurane-N_2O vs propofol-N_2O is controversial. A recent study suggests no difference in pregnancy rates with the use of isoflurane, propofol, N_2O, or midazolam.[1]

Induction	Standard induction (see p. B-2). Avoidance of succinylcholine may decrease postop myalgia.	
Maintenance	Standard maintenance (see p. B-3). N_2O does not appear to adversely affect success of fertilization.[5]	
Emergence	No special considerations	
Blood and fluid requirements	Minimal blood loss IV: 18 ga × 1 NS/LR @ 2 ml/kg/h	Blood loss minimal, unless trauma to vasculature. Rarely, trauma to blood vessels or organs following laparoscopy may necessitate laparotomy.
Monitoring	Standard monitors (p. B-1)	
Positioning	✓ and pad pressure points. ✓ eyes.	
Complications	Respiratory: Pneumoperitoneum: ↑$PaCO_2$, ↓PaO_2 ETT migration	Pneumoperitoneum with CO_2 and steep Trendelenburg position cause cephalad displacement of diaphragm with ↓FRC, ↓pulmonary compliance, and ↑airway closure/atelectasis. Hypercarbia and hypoxia, due to respiratory compromise, can result unless ventilation is controlled during GA. Check for endobronchial migration of ETT upon assumption of Trendelenburg position.

Complications, cont.	Pneumothorax	Pneumothorax due to retroperitoneal dissection of insufflated gas into the mediastinum can cause hypoxemia, ↑airway pressure, subcutaneous emphysema and ↓BP.
	Cardiovascular: ↓BP Hemorrhage VAE (CO_2) Dysrhythmias	↓BP can result from ↓venous return caused by pneumoperitoneum. Hemorrhage can result from blood vessel injury or rapid reversal of head-down position. Unintended intravascular injection of CO_2 gas (VAE) can lead to ↓BP and dysrhythmias.
	Neurological: Nerve injury Brachial plexus injury Nerve root compression Bowel injury	Use of Trendelenburg position incurs risk of nerve injury. Hyperextension of arm may result in brachial plexus injury and careful padding of vulnerable points is necessary. Shoulder brace can compress nerve roots in retroclavicular region.

POSTOPERATIVE

| Complications | Shoulder pain | Postop pain may be referred to the shoulder, due to irritation of diaphragm by residual pneumoperitoneum or bleeding. |
| Pain management | Oral analgesics are usually sufficient. | |

References

1. Beilin Y, Bodian C, Eisenkraft J, et al: The use of propofol, nitrous oxide, or isoflurane does not affect the reproductive success rate following gamete intrafallopian transfer (GIFT). *Anesthesiology* 1999; 90:36-41.
2. Confino ET: Transcervical balloon tuboplasty: a multicenter study. *JAMA* 1990; 264:2079-82.
3. Gonen O, Shulman A, Ghetler Y, Shapiro A, Judekin R, Beyth Y, Ben-Nun I. The impact of different types of anesthesia or *in vitro* fertilization-embryo transfer treatment outcome. *J Assist Reprod Genet* 1995; 12(10): 678-82.
4. Resiner, LS. The pregnant patient and the disorders of pregnancy. In *Anesthesia and Uncommon Diseases*. WB Saunders, Philadelphia: 1990, 165-6.
5. Rosen MA, Roizen MF, Eger EI II, Glass RH, Martin M, Dandekar PV, Dailey PA, Litt L: The effect of nitrous oxide on *in vitro* fertilization success rate. *Anesthesiology* 1987; 67(1):42-4.
6. Rock JA, Thompson JD, eds: *TeLinde's Operative Gynecology*, 8th edition. Lippincott-Raven, Philadelphia: 1997.
7. Ross BK, Chaduck HS, Mancuso JJ, Benedelti C. Sprotte needle for obstetric anesthesia: Decreased incidence of post dural puncture headache. *Reg Anesth* 1992; 17:29-33.
8. Tanbo T: Assisted fertilization in infertile women with patent tubes: a comparison of *in vitro* fertilization, gamete intra-fallopian transfer and tubal embryo stage transfer. *Hum Reprod* 1990; 5:266-70.

HYSTERECTOMY—VAGINAL OR TOTAL ABDOMINAL

SURGICAL CONSIDERATIONS

Description: After cesarean section (C-section), **hysterectomy** is the most commonly performed operation in the U.S. (650,000/year). Two approaches are possible: vaginal and abdominal. The **vaginal approach**, performed with the patient in a dorsal lithotomy position, is preferred since it offers significantly less morbidity and mortality. Its use is limited by situations in which pelvic bony architecture, uterine size, pelvic adhesions, or the presence of gynecological cancers require an **abdominal approach**. The approach may be changed in the OR, where a pelvic examination under anesthesia will determine the true uterine size, degree of prolapse, and the presence of pelvic pathology. A laparoscopy may be performed at the outset of surgery to evaluate the pelvis and free up adhesions that would have made a vaginal approach initially unsafe. In patients

≥ 45 years, **bilateral sal-pingo-oophorectomy** (BSO) is often performed in addition to the hysterectomy to provide ovarian cancer prophylaxis. Pelvic relaxation syndrome is the most frequent preop diagnosis in patients having a vaginal hysterectomy. Pelvic relaxation includes one or more of the following: prolapse of the uterus; intestine into the pouch of Douglas (enterocele); bladder into the anterior vaginal wall (cystocele); urethra into the anterior vaginal wall (urethrocele); and rectum into the posterior vaginal wall (rectocele). In these cases, the hysterectomy is often accompanied by an anterior/posterior colporrhaphy, bladder neck suspension, and perineoplasty.

Variant approaches: Abdominal hysterectomy is performed through a Pfannenstiel's or midline incision, depending on the uterine size and the need to perform a lymph node dissection for cancer. A Pfannenstiel's incision often can be improved

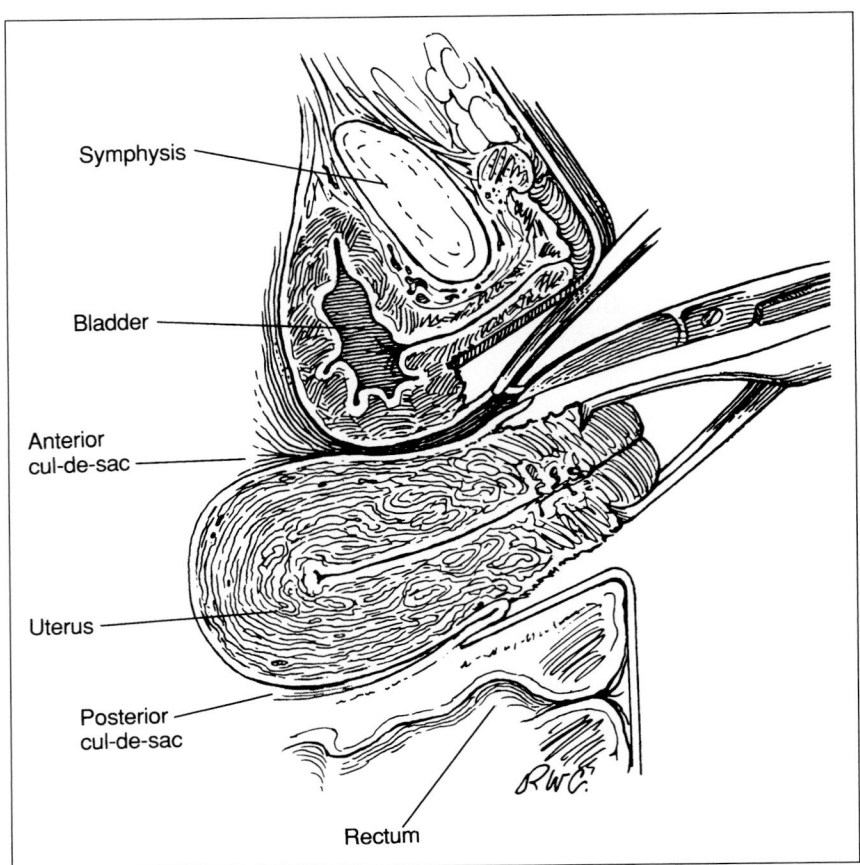

Figure 8.2-4. Surgical anatomy for vaginal hysterectomy. (Reproduced with permission from Rock JA, Thompson JD, eds: *TeLinde's Operative Gynecology*, 8th edition. Lippincott Williams & Wilkins, 1997.)

with two types of muscle-splitting steps: the **Maylard**, in which the rectus muscles are cut, or a **Cherney rectus muscle detachment** performed at the pubic insertion. After entering the abdomen, a self-retaining retractor is placed and the round, ovarian, and broad ligaments are clamped, cut, and tied, in that order. The uterine vessels are identified and ligated, followed by the creation of a bladder flap and, finally, the cutting and ligation of the uterosacral and cardinal ligaments. The vagina is entered and the cervix removed. Then the vaginal cuff is closed in a way to incorporate the uterosacral ligaments for support. The visceral peritoneum is reapproximated, the retractor removed, and the abdominal layers closed.

In a **vaginal hysterectomy**, the cervix is retracted, a paracervical incision is made, and the anterior and posterior cul de sacs are entered (Fig 8.2-4). The uterosacral and cardinal ligaments and the uterine vessels are cut and ligated. With steady downward traction, the broad ligament is ligated in a step-wise manner until either the ovarian or infundibulopelvic ligament is reached, and one of the two is ligated, depending on whether the ovaries are to be removed or not. After the uterus has been removed, the peritoneum is reapproximated, followed by the closing of the vaginal cuff, which often includes the uterosacral and cardinal ligaments for support. A vaginal pack often is left in place. Frequently, laparoscopy is being combined with vaginal hysterectomy to evaluate the pelvis for unrecognized disease and to ensure prophylactic adnexectomy in women ages ≥ 40-45 yr.

Usual preop diagnosis: Uterine myoma; pelvic relaxation syndrome; pelvic pain 2° endometriosis or adhesions; uncontrolled uterine bleeding/dysmenorrhea; endometrial hyperplasia; gynecological cancers

SUMMARY OF PROCEDURES

	Abdominal Approach	Vaginal Approach
Position	Supine	Lithotomy. Following induction, position patient so that the perineum is at the end of operating table to ensure optimum surgical exposure.

	Abdominal Approach	**Vaginal Approach**
Incision	Pfannenstiel's or low midline. The Pfannenstiel's incision can be extended with a Maylard muscle-splitting procedure or a Cherney rectus muscle detachment at pubic insertion.	Pericervical vaginal
Special instrumentation	None	Stirrups
Unique considerations	None	To prevent peroneal nerve injury, the area of leg leaning against stirrup should be well cushioned. Often, vasoconstriction agents (1:200,000 epinephrine and vasopressin) are used to cut down perioperative vaginal cuff bleeding.[3]
Antibiotics	1-2 g cefoxitin or cefotetan + clindamycin 600 mg iv	⇐
Surgical time	1-2 h	45 min-1.5 h
EBL	200-300 ml	100-200 ml
Postop care	PACU	⇐
Mortality[2,4,10]	Overall (10,000 patients): 14.6	20
	< 25 yr: 8.9	0
	25-34 yr: 4.7	0.9
	35-44 yr: 3.8	0.5
	45-54 yr: 6.5	2.7
	55-64 yr: 41.3	1.9
	65-74 yr: 93.0	18.3
	> 75 yr: 255.8	56.8
Morbidity[1,2,3,4,6,10]	Infection:	⇐
	Unexplained fever: 10-20%	5-8%
	Pelvic infection: 3.2-10%	3.9-10%
	Wound infection: 4-8%	–
	Urinary tract: 1.1-5%	1.7-5%
	Femoral nerve injury: 11.6%	–
	Hemorrhage:	⇐
	Intraop: 1-2%	0.7-2-5%
	Requiring transfusion: 2-12%	2-8.3%
	Unintended major procedures: 1.7%	5.1%
	Injury:	⇐
	Bladder: 1-2%	0.5-1.5%
	Bowel: 0.1-0.5%	0.1-0.8%
	Ureter: 0.1-0.5%	0.05-0.1%
	Vesicovaginal fistula: 0.1-0.2%	⇐
	Thromboembolic events: 0.4-1.3%	0.62-1.7%
Pain score	5-8	4-6

PATIENT POPULATION CHARACTERISTICS

Age range	30-80 yr
Incidence	> 1/5 females; 650,000/yr in U.S.
Etiology	Uterine myomata; endometriosis; uterine prolapse; uterine cancer
Associated conditions	Stress urinary incontinence; obesity

ANESTHETIC CONSIDERATIONS

PREOPERATIVE

Although many patients presenting for this procedure are otherwise healthy, others may have metastatic cancer.

Respiratory   CXR may be indicated to r/o pleural effusion or other lung pathology in cancer patients. Additionally, ABGs, ± PFTs, may be indicated preop in patients with significant pulmonary involvement.
Tests: As indicated from H&P.

Cardiovascular	Patient may have blood loss from the primary problem. Additionally, she may have undergone bowel prep, which can cause dehydration and electrolyte abnormalities. Assessment of volume status, using BP and orthostatic vital signs, is important. **Tests**: As indicated from H&P.
Hematologic	Hb/Hct. Patients with Hx of easy bruising or bleeding should have coagulation parameters evaluated (PT, PTT, Plt).
Laboratory	Other tests as indicated from H&P.
Premedication	Anxiolytic (e.g., midazolam 1-2 mg iv) as needed.

INTRAOPERATIVE

Anesthetic technique: GA is commonly used; however, either spinal, epidural, or combined spinal-edpidural (CSE) anesthesia is appropriate for adequately hydrated patients who are undergoing simple hysterectomy through a Pfannenstiel's incision, or vaginal hysterectomy. In the younger patient population, spinal anesthesia may be less desirable because of the increased incidence of post-dural puncture headache (PDPH) in using this technique. If spinal anesthetic is indicated, a pencil-point needle (e.g., Sprotte or Whitacre) should be used to decrease the incidence of PDPH.[8] Patients with extensive cancer who undergo exploratory laparotomy with lymph node dissection may benefit from combined epidural/GA with decreased postop pulmonary complications and early ambulation. Some studies advocate the use of epidural anesthesia to decrease intraop blood loss.[6]

General anesthesia:

Induction	Standard induction (see p. B-2).
Maintenance	Standard maintenance (see p. B-3). Muscle relaxation is necessary if the procedure is performed abdominally. These patients have a high incidence of N/V, and prophylaxis with metoclopramide 10 mg iv and ondansetron 4 mg iv, or, often, $5HT_3$-antagonist is indicated.
Emergence	Be ready with suction in the event the patient vomits on emergence.

Regional anesthesia: A T4-6 sensory level is sufficient to provide anesthesia for procedures on the uterus.

Spinal	5% lidocaine 75-100 mg (controversial); 0.75% bupivacaine 10-15 mg in 8.25% dextrose. (See Anesthetic Considerations for Cesarean Section, p. 664)
Epidural	1.5-2.0% lidocaine with epinephrine 5 µg/ml, 15-25 ml; supplement with 5-10 ml as needed. Supplemental iv sedation. (See Anesthetic Considerations for Cesarean Section, p. 663.)
CSE	**Combined spinal/epidural (CSE):** An alternative technique combining the rapid onset and density of spinal anesthesia with the flexibility of continuous epidural anesthesia. Apply monitors, administer fluid, and position patient as for spinal or epidural. The most common technique is the needle-through-needle. After the epidural space is located with a standard 17 ga Tuohy needle, insert a 4″ 26-27 ga pencil-point spinal needle through it to administer 0.6 ml of spinal bupivacaine (0.75%) ± fentanyl 10 µg and morphine sulfate 0.1-0.2 mg. Secure the epidural catheter and use if needed (a test dose is advisable).

Blood and fluid requirements	Possible heavy blood loss IV: 16-18 ga × 2 Warm all fluids. Heat, humidify gases. Autologous blood donation	Preop autologous blood transfusion may not be possible in patients who are already anemic. Blood and evaporative losses are usually greater in patients undergoing abdominal, rather than vaginal, hysterectomy. Patients having a Pfannenstiel's incision should also have smaller fluid requirements than those having a larger midline incision.
Control of blood loss	**Vaginal hysterectomy:** Moderate blood loss NS/LR @ 4-5 ml/kg/h. **Abdominal hysterectomy:** Moderate-to-heavy blood loss NS/LR @ 6-10 ml/kg/h	To avoid blood transfusion, consider colloid infusion in patients who have good cardiac function and can tolerate a low Hct. May need blood transfusion.
Monitoring	**Vaginal hysterectomy:** Standard monitors (p. B-1) ± Foley catheter	A Foley catheter may be helpful (to monitor fluid status) during vaginal hysterectomy if the procedure is expected to be longer than usual. Trendelenburg position may make drainage diffuclt.

Monitoring, cont.	**Abdominal hysterectomy:** Standard monitors (p. B-1) Foley catheter	During abdominal hysterectomy, a Foley catheter is useful, since this procedure is longer and involves more fluid shifts than the vaginal approach, and may involve a significant blood loss.
	± Arterial line ± CVP line	Intraarterial and CVP monitoring are useful in patients undergoing large tumor resections and in whom large blood losses are anticipated.
Positioning	✓ and pad pressure points. Shoulder abduction < 90°	The lithotomy position has several considerations for safety. (See p. 635 for details.)
Complications	**Vaginal hysterectomy:** Cervical stimulation Epinephrine/vasopressin injection → HTN or cardiac dysrhythmias	Vagal stimulation may occur when the surgeons grasp the cervix, and subsequent bradycardia may ensue. This can be treated by cessation of the surgical stimulus and treatment with atropine if indicated. The surgeons may use epinephrine or vasopressin to decrease local bleeding; however, either of these agents may cause HTN or cardiac dysrhythmias.[7]
	Abdominal hysterectomy: Blood loss Cervical stimulation Epinephrine/vasopressin injection	Hemorrhage is possible with large tumor resections, and must be treated with adequate fluid and blood replacement. Attention must be given to possible associated problems, such as hypothermia, hypocalcemia, and dilutional coagulopathy.

POSTOPERATIVE

Complications	PONV Anemia	Rx: metoclopramide 10 mg iv and/or a 5-HT_3-antagonist (e.g., ondansetron 4 mg iv, dolasetron 12.5 mg iv)
Pain management	Epidural opiates (p. C-2) PCA (p. C-3)	If catheter to be used postop.
Tests	Hct CXR (if CVP catheter placed intraop)	CXR to evaluate central line placement and rule out pneumothorax.

References

1. Carley ME, McIntire D, Carley JM, Schaffer J: Incidence, risk factors and morbidity of unintended bladder or ureter injury during hysterectomy. *Int Urogynecol J Pelvic Floor Dysfunct* 2002; 13(1):18-21.
2. Clough TF: Perioperative morbidity of hysterectomy for benign gynaecological disease. *J Obstet Gynaecol* 2001; 21(5):504-6.
3. Davies A, Hart R, Magos A, Hadad E, Morris R: Hysterectomy: surgical route and complications. *Eur J Obstet Gynecol Reprod Biol* 2002; 104(2):148-51.
4. Dicker RC, Greenspan JR, Strauss LT et al: Complications of abdominal and vaginal hysterectomy among women of reproductive age in the United States. The Collaborative Review of Sterilization. *Am J Obstet Gynecol* 1982; 144(7):841-8.
5. Guaschino S, De Santo D, De Seta F: New perspectives in antibiotic prophylaxis for obstetric and gynaecological surgery. *J Hosp Infect* 2002; 50(Suppl A):S13-6.
6. Harris WJ: Early complications of abdominal and vaginal hysterectomy. *Obstet Gynecol Surv* 1995; 50(11):795-805.
7. Modig, J: Regional anaesthesia and blood loss. *Acta Anaesthesiol Scand Suppl*: 1988, 89; 44-8.
8. Rock JA, Thompson JD, eds: *TeLinde's Operative Gynecology*, 8th edition. Lippincott Williams & Wilkins, Philadelphia: 1997.
9. Ross BK, Chaduck HS, Mancuso JS, Benedetti C: Sprotte needle for obstetric anesthesia: Decreased incidence of post dural puncture headache. *Reg Anesth* 1992; 17:29-33.
10. Varol N, Healey M, Tang P, Sheehan P, Maher P, Hill D: Ten-year review of hysterectomy morbidity and mortality: can we change direction? *Aust NZ J Obstet Gynaecol* 2001; 41(3)295-302.
11. Wingo PA, et al: The mortality risk associated with hysterectomy. *Am J Obstet Gynecol* 1984; 152(7):803-8.

ANTERIOR AND POSTERIOR COLPORRHAPHY, ENTEROCELE REPAIR, VAGINAL SACROSPINOUS SUSPENSION

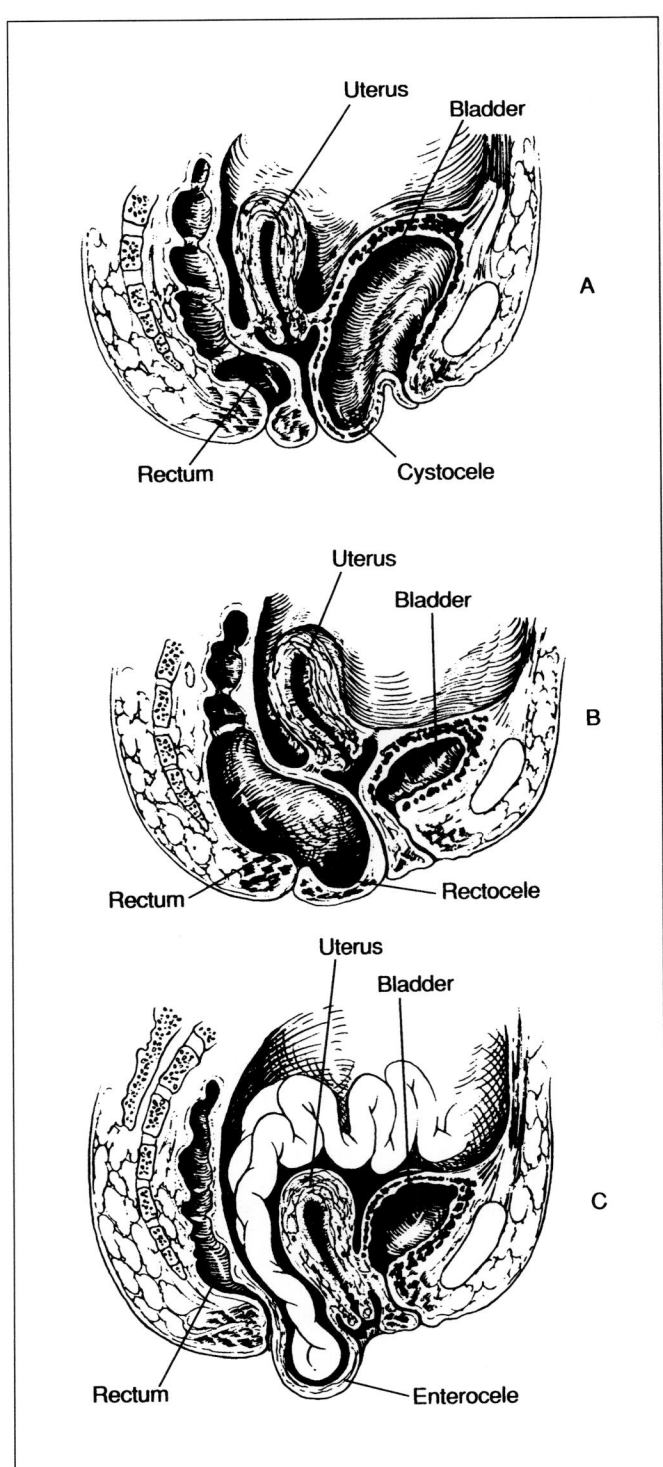

Figure 8.2-5. (A) Anatomy of cystocele. (B) Anatomy of rectocele. (C) Anatomy of enterocele. (Reproduced with permission from Pernoll ML, ed: *Current Obstetrics and Gynecological Diagnosis and Treatment*. Appleton & Lange: 1991.)

SURGICAL CONSIDERATIONS

Description: Cystocele (Fig 8.2-5A) and rectocele (Fig 8.2-5B) are prolapses (relaxations) of the anterior and posterior vaginal wall, respectively. They occur 2° multiparity and congenital weakening of pelvic tissue. The term 'pelvic relaxation syndrome' includes the often coexisting anatomical 'relaxations' (e.g., enterocele [Fig 8.2-5C] and uterine prolapse). Cystoceles are often symptomatic due to bladder protrusion past the introitus during straining. Often this relaxation will allow the bladder neck to lose its important anatomical relationship to the urethra and the rest of the bladder. The result can be bothersome stress urinary incontinence for the patient (see Operations for Stress Urinary Incontinence, p. 654). The rectocele often is experienced as a vaginal bulge during straining, and tends to cause incomplete evacuation of stool. The goal of the colporrhaphy is to restore the original anatomy. Due to the frequent coexisting relaxations, a posterior colporrhaphy (vaginal repair), enterocele repair, and vaginal hysterectomy are frequently performed at the same time.

In an **anterior colporrhaphy**, the patient is placed in a high dorsal lithotomy position with the perineum at the end of the operating table for surgical access. The bladder is emptied and a weighted speculum is inserted into the vagina. A **vaginal hysterectomy** is performed at this point, if indicated (see Vaginal Hysterectomy, p. 647). The extent of the urethrocystocele is determined manually and the vaginal mucosa is grasped at its cephalic border with two clamps. From this point to the external urethral meatus, the mucosa is undermined with a vasoconstrictive solution (epinephrine 5-10 ml, 1:200,000), phenylephrine (1:200,000), or vasopressin (1-5 U/10 ml NS). This decreases blood loss significantly and helps to determine the depth of the vaginal mucosa. The mucosa is cut over this undermined area and, with the help of sharp and blunt dissection, the mucosa is dissected laterally from its underlying fascia. A series of fascial plication sutures are placed to reduce the cystourethrocele. The redundant mucosa is excised and the edges are reapproximated. A suprapubic catheter is most often inserted at the end to prevent bladder overdistention.

Paravaginal repair is another procedure for repair of cystocele, and can be performed via the abdomen or the vagina. The space between the bladder and pubic bone is entered, and the bladder is dissected off the pelvic sidewall, taking care to avoid injury to the obturator nerve and vessels. The arcus tendineus fascia pelvis is visualized, running from the inferior margin of the pubic symphysis posteriorly to the ischial spine. The surgeon places a hand in the vagina to elevate the lateral vaginal sulcus to the arcus tendineus fascia. Multiple fine sutures are placed to secure the paravaginal tissues to the arcus tendineus fascia pelvis. The same is done for the opposite pelvic sidewall if bilateral defects are present.

If necessary, a **posterior colporrhaphy** may be performed. A small portion of perineum posterior to the introitus is removed initially. The vaginal mucosa over the rectocele is undermined with vasoconstrictor fluid prior to incision, followed by dissection of the overlying mucosa in a manner nearly identical to anterior colporrhaphy. One or several layers of stitches are placed to plicate the pararectal fascia, allowing for reduction of the rectocele. Redundant mucosa is excised and the edges are reapproximated. A vaginal pack is usually placed to minimize bleeding.

An **enterocele** often is first noticed during a posterior colporrhaphy procedure, and is repaired prior to finishing the posterior repair. The enterocele is well identified and dissected away from the surrounding tissue. Two or more parallel purse-string stitches are used to close the enterocele. The enterocele tissue distal to the purse-string closure is excised. To reduce the enterocele in an optimal fashion, intraabdominal pressure has to be at a minimum.

Variant procedure or approaches: Vaginal sacrospinous suspension with the Miya hook is an elegant alternative to the abdominal colpopexy procedure for women with severe uterine and/or vaginal vault prolapse. The patient is placed in a dorsal lithotomy position and an examination under anesthesia is performed. A vasoconstrictive solution is injected (usually 1:200,000 epinephrine 3-5 ml) in the posterior vaginal wall. A vertical incision is made and the mucosa is bluntly dissected off the rectum in an anterolateral direction. An enterocele, if found, is repaired at this time. The pararectal tissue is then bluntly pierced to enter the pararectal space. The anatomy surrounding the sacrospinous ligament is well palpated and, with the help of the special Miya hook, a large suture is placed into the sacrospinous ligament. The other end of the suture is placed at the apex of the vagina, which, after tying, is pulled in a lateral cephalad direction. The mucosa is finally closed.

Uterosacral ligament suspension, or **high McCall's culdoplasty**, is an alternate procedure for vaginal apex support. After the uterus is removed by a vaginal hysterectomy, the uterosacral ligaments are identified. Two separate permanent sutures are placed along the uterosacral ligament as far cephalad (toward the sacrum) as possible. The same is done on the opposite side. A cystoscopy is then carried out, with all four stitches placed on tension in order to r/o ureteral obstruction due to ligation or kinking of the ureters. The stitches are replaced if obstruction is observed. Once ureteral patency has been confirmed, these stitches are sutured to the fibromuscular layer of the vaginal cuff and tied, to bring the apex as cephalad as possible. The vaginal cuff is closed with absorbable sutures.

The **Le Fort procedure** is now a rare operation and is performed in very elderly women with complete prolapse of the uterus and/or vagina who do not desire to remain sexually active. With the patient in a dorsal lithotomy position, a rectangular strip from the anterior and posterior vaginal wall is removed initially, followed by closure of the margins each to the other. The result is a near-complete closure of the vagina.

Usual preop diagnosis: Symptomatic cystocele; symptomatic uterine prolapse; enterocele; rectocele causing severe constipation; dyspareunia

SUMMARY OF PROCEDURE

Position	Dorsal lithotomy
Incision	Vaginal mucosal; peritoneum for enterocele repair
Unique considerations	To prevent peroneal nerve injury, the area of the leg leaning against the stirrup should be well cushioned. Putting the legs in a high position increases venous return to the heart. Infiltration with epinephrine and vasopressin often are used to reduce intraop bleeding. This causes changes in CO, HR, and BP. Low intraabdominal pressure (good muscle relaxation) is needed during the enterocele reduction.
Antibiotics	1-2 g iv cefoxitin/cefotetan
Surgical time	45 min (anterior colporrhaphy)
	30 min (posterior colporrhaphy/enterocele repair)
	45 min (uterosacral ligament suspension)
	1 h (paravaginal repair)
Closing considerations	Suprapubic catheter (anterior colporrhaphy); vaginal pack (enterocele repair)
EBL	20-500 ml
Postop care	PACU
Mortality	1%

Morbidity	**Anterior colporrhaphy[1]**	**Vaginal sacrospinous suspension (Miya hook)**
	Delayed voiding 1-7 d: 30%	Bleeding in gluteal and pudendal vessels
	Foul vaginal discharge: 14%	Pararectal burning pain $\geq$ 2 mo
	Bacteriuria: 13%	Sciatic pain (indicating misplaced sutures, which must
	Pyrexia (>100.4F): 11%	be removed)
	Atelectasis: 3%	Peritoneal tear (during Miya hook insertion)
	Delayed voiding > 7 d: 0.6%	
	Need for blood transfusion: 0.6%	**Paravaginal repair**
	Urethrovaginal fistula: 0.4%	Obturator vessel laceration
	Acute gastric dilatation: 0.2%	Obturator nerve injury
		Ureteral obstruction
	Uterosacral ligament suspension	Bladder laceration
	Ureteral obstruction	
	Perirectral abscess due to stitch in rectum	
Pain score	5-8	

PATIENT POPULATION CHARACTERISTICS

Age range	40-80 yr
Incidence	> 1/5 women
Etiology	Multiparous state; obesity; chronic cough; previous pelvic surgery
Associated conditions	Pelvic relaxation syndrome

ANESTHETIC CONSIDERATIONS

See Anesthetic Considerations following Operations for Stress Urinary Incontinence, p. 656.

References

1. Beck RP, et al: A 25-year experience with 519 anterior colporrhaphy procedures. *Obstet Gynecol* 1991; 78(6):1011-18.
2. DeCherney AH, Pernoll ML, eds: *Current Obstetrics and Gynecologic Diagnosis and Treatment.* Appleton & Lange, Norwalk, CT: 1994.
3. Miyazaki F: Miya hook ligature carrier for sacrospinous ligament suspension. *Obstet Gynecol* 1987; 70(2):286-8.
4. Rock JA, Thompson JD, eds: *TeLinde's Operative Gynecology,* 8th edition. Lippincott Williams & Wilkins, Philadelphia: 1997, 951-1086.

OPERATIONS FOR STRESS URINARY INCONTINENCE

SURGICAL CONSIDERATIONS

Description: Stress urinary incontinence is a common condition affecting mostly older and multiparous women. It is a disorder of the musculofascial support to the bladder neck and pelvic floor. These patients usually have extensive preop workup to exclude urge incontinence and many have been treated with pelvic floor exercises (Kegel) prior to surgery. Two surgical approaches exist: **abdominal suspension** procedures and **suspension by the vaginal route**. Ongoing controversy exists concerning which approach is best. Patient position is crucial for all vaginal surgery.

Vaginal approaches: The **Kelly urethral plication** often has been used as the primary surgical treatment, especially when other vaginal surgery is needed to be performed. The patient initially is placed in a high dorsal lithotomy position with the perineum at the end of the operating table for surgical exposure. The bladder is emptied and a weighted speculum is inserted into the vagina. The extent of the cystourethrocele is determined and the vaginal mucosa is grasped at its cephalic border with two clamps. From this point to the external urethral meatus, the mucosa usually is undermined with 5-10 ml of a vasoconstrictive solution (epinephrine 1:200,000, phenylephrine 1:200,000, or vasopressin 1-5 U/10 ml NS). This decreases blood loss significantly and helps to determine the depth of the mucosa. With the help of sharp and blunt dissection, the mucosa is freed laterally from its underlying adherent fascia. A series of vertical mattress sutures are placed in the mobilized paraurethral and paravesicle fascia to reduce the cystourethrocele and elevate the posterior urethra to a high retropubic position. The redundant mucosa is excised and the edges are reapproximated. A suprapubic catheter is often inserted at the end of the surgery to prevent bladder overdistention.

Two anterior vesicle neck suspension techniques—Stamey and modified **Pereyra**—are very similar procedures wherein the vaginal mucosa is incised and dissected off the underlying paraurethral fascia, much the same way as in the Kelly plication. Instead of using a layer of mattress sutures, both suspension methods use two lateral sutures that suspend the vesicle neck on each side (see Fig 9-21, p. 728). The ends of the sutures are tied over the rectus fascia to provide support. The Stamey method uses a small Dacron cuff to prevent the suture from tearing through the paravesicle fascia, while in the modified Pereyra method, the posterior loop is attached firmly to the pubourethral ligament. One or two small suprapubic abdominal incisions must be made to allow for the tying of the sutures. Specialized long needles are used to help the placement of these sutures, and a cystoscope often is used to verify their placement. Perforation of the bladder is a common complication found upon cystoscopy. Finally, a suprapubic catheter is placed at the end of the operation. (See Urology, p. 728.)

Abdominal approaches: The **Marshall-Marchetti-Krantz (M-M-K)** and **Burch** (urethropexy) are probably the most common abdominal suspension procedures. The patient is placed in the frog-leg position with a urethral catheter in place. A Pfannenstiel's incision is used to enter the space of Retzius, which lies between the parietal peritoneum and the rectus fascia under the pubic bone. Blunt dissection is used to open and extend this space. The surgeon then inserts two fingers into the vagina to raise the anterior vagina and bladder neck. This enables the surgeon to place two or more sutures in the tissue just lateral to the urethra and attach them to Cooper's ligament (Burch) or to the periosteum of the posterior pelvic bone (M-M-K).

The **urethral sling procedure** was once reserved for women with low urethral pressure and/or for whom other incontinence operations had failed. It is now also used as primary treatment for stress urinary incontinence. The goal of the sling procedure is to produce extrinsic compression of the urethrovesical junction with the help of a strip anchored to the rectus fascia or pubic bone (see Fig 9-21, p. 728). With the patient in the dorsal lithotomy position, a urethral catheter is placed and the vaginal mucosa incised and dissected off the underlying paravesicle and paraurethral fascia, similar to the Kelly plication. The retropubic space is entered through a Pfannenstiel's incision and a strip of rectus fascia, is obtained. The strip is then brought through the vagina, around the urethra, and back to the abdomen, where it is fastened to the rectus fascia, creating a sling under the urethra at the junction of the bladder neck. The vaginal and abdominal incisions are closed, and a suprapubic catheter is placed. If donor fascia lata or synthetic material is used, a small (~2″) horizontal incision is made above the pubic bone for attachment of the sling.

Tension-free vaginal tape (TVT) is a new 'sling' type procedure for treatment of stress urinary incontinence. A Prolene mesh sling is used to support the urethra, although it is not attached to the fascia. The Prolene is woven in such a way that the sling cannot slide out over time. Fibroblasts grow into the sling to anchor it throughout the endopelvic fascia and around the dependent surface of the urethra. Placement of the sling material is through a vaginal incision similar to that of the Kelly plication. The TVT curved needle is introduced from the vagina through the space of Retzius on each side of the urethra, and is brought out to the abdomen above the pubic bone. The sling mesh is attached to the ends of each needle; thus, when both needles are pulled through the abdominal sites, the mesh will rest under the urethra. A cystoscopy is done before pulling the mesh through to verify that neither needle is in the bladder or the urethra. The mesh is then adjusted so that the urethra is resting on the sling, under no tension.

Usual preop diagnosis: Stress urinary incontinence; intrinsic sphincter deficiency

SUMMARY OF PROCEDURES

	Kelly Plication	**M-M-K/Burch**	**Urethral Sling**
Position	Dorsal lithotomy	Frog-leg	⇐
Incision	Vaginal mucosa	Pfannenstiel's	Vaginal
Unique considerations	Cushion area of leg against stirup to prevent peroneal injury. Epinephrine (1:200,000) or vasopressin are often infiltrated to reduce intraop bleeding for vaginal approaches. This causes changes in CO, bleeding, HR, and rhythm. The urethral catheter is frequently removed and reinserted during surgery.	⇐	⇐
Antibiotics	Cefoxitin 1-2 g iv	⇐	⇐
Surgical time	1 h	⇐	⇐
Closing considerations	Suprapubic catheter	⇐	⇐

	Kelly Plication	**M-M-K/Burch**	**Urethral Sling**
EBL	50 ml	100-200 ml	50-100 ml
Postop care	Inpatient	⇐	± outpatient
Mortality	Minimal	⇐	⇐
Morbidity	Detrusor instability: Rare (due to vaginal approach)	14%	–
	Enterocele: Rare	15%	N/A
	Incisional hernia: Rare	0.09%	Rare
	Osteitis pubis: Rare	⇐	⇐
	Voiding difficulties: Rare	2%	~40%
	Wound infection: Rare	8.7%	Rare
			Prolonged catheter time: > 50%
			Outlet obstruction: 10-20%
			Urethral perforation: 7%
			Bladder perforation: 1%
Pain score	4-6	6-8	4-6

PATIENT POPULATION CHARACTERISTICS

Age range	40-80 yr
Incidence	>1/5 women
Etiology	Multiparous state; obesity; chronic cough
Associated conditions	Other components of pelvic relaxation syndrome (rectocele, uterine prolapse, enterocele)

ANESTHETIC CONSIDERATIONS

(Procedures covered: anterior and posterior colporrhaphy; enterocele repair; vaginal sacrospinous suspension; operations for stress urinary incontinence)

PREOPERATIVE

This is usually an older patient population, past child-bearing age. Patient may be relatively healthy otherwise. ✓ for concurrent disease.

Laboratory	Hb/Hct, as indicated from H&P.
Premedication	Anxiolytic (e.g., midazolam 1-2 mg iv) as needed.

INTRAOPERATIVE

Anesthetic technique: Regional or GA may be used. In the younger patient population, spinal anesthesia may be less desirable because of increased incidence of postdural puncture headache (PDPH). If spinal anesthesia is indicated, a pencil-point needle (e.g., Sprotte or Whitacre) should be used to decrease the incidence of PDPH.[5]

Regional anesthesia: A T10 sensory level is sufficient to provide anesthesia for procedures on the uterus and bladder, but a T4 level is recommended if the peritoneum is opened.

Spinal	5% lidocaine 75-100 mg (controversial); 0.75% bupivacaine 10-15 mg in 8.25% dextrose. (See Anesthetic Considerations for Cesarean Section, p. 664.)
Epidural	1.5-2.0% lidocaine with epinephrine 5 μg/ml, 15-25 ml; supplement with 5-10 ml as needed. Supplemental iv sedation. (See Anesthetic Considerations for Cesarean Section, p. 663.)
CSE	**Combined spinal/epidural (CSE):** An alternative technique combining the rapid onset and density of spinal anesthesia with the flexibility of continuous epidural anesthesia. Apply monitors, administer fluid, and position patient as for spinal or epidural. The most common technique is the needle-through-needle. After the epidural space is located with a standard 17 ga Tuohy needle, insert a 4″ 26-27 ga pencil-point spinal needle through it to administer 0.6 ml of spinal bupivacaine (0.75%) ± fentanyl 10 μg and morphine sulfate 0.1-0.2 mg. Secure the epidural catheter and use if needed (a test dose is advisable).

General anesthesia:

Induction	Standard induction (see p. B-2).

Maintenance	Standard maintenance (see p. B-3).	
Emergence	No special considerations	
Blood and fluid requirements	Normally minimal blood loss IV: 16-18 ga × 1 NS/LR @ 2-4 ml/kg/h	Only 1 iv is normally necessary for adequate intraop hydration.
Control of blood loss	Epinephrine, vasopressin, phenyl-ephrine used by surgeons.	Surgeons may inject vasopressors into the submucosa to minimize blood loss. This may cause intraop and cardiac dysrhythmias.
Monitoring	Standard monitors (p. B-1)	Although bladder catheterization prior to incision is normal, the catheter is not left in place throughout surgery in those patients undergoing anterior and posterior colporrhaphy, enterocele repair, and Kelly urethral plication. Suprapubic bladder catheters are placed toward the end of surgery in these procedures, as well as in the Stamey, Pereyra, and urethral sling procedures.
Positioning	✓ and pad pressure points. ✓ eyes.	See p. 635 for concerns regarding the lithotomy position.

POSTOPERATIVE

Complications	PONV	Rx: metoclopramide 10 mg iv and/or a 5-HT$_3$-antagonist (e.g., ondansetron 4 mg iv, dolasetron 12.5 mg iv)
Pain management	IV opiates Usually rapid conversion to po pain medications	
Tests	None indicated.	

References

1. Blaivas JG, et al: Pubovaginal fascial sling for the treatment of complicated stress urinary incontinence. *J Urol* 1991; 145(6): 1214-18.
2. Galloway NT, et al: The complications of colposuspension. *Br J Urol* 1987; 60(2):122-4.
3. Lee RA, et al: Surgical complications and results of modified Marshall-Marchetti-Krantz procedure for urinary incontinence. *Obstet Gynecol* 1979; 53(4):447-50.
4. Pereyra AJ, et al: Pubourethral supports in perspective: modified Pereyra procedure for urinary incontinence. *Obstet Gynecol* 1982; 59(5):643-8.
5. Ross BK, Chaduck HS, Mancuso JS, Benedetti C: Sprotte needle for obstetric anesthesia: Decreased incidence of post dural puncture headache. *Reg Anesth* 1992; 17:29-33.
6. Stamey TA: Endoscopic suspension of the vesical neck for urinary incontinence in females. *Ann Surg* 1980; 192(4):465-71.
7. Varner RE, Sparks JM: Surgery for stress urinary incontinence. *Surg Clin North Am* 1991; 71(5):1111-34.
8. Wall LL: Urinary stress incontinence. In Rock JA, Thompson JD, eds: *TeLinde's Operative Gynecology*, 8th edition. Lippincott Williams & Wilkins, Philadelphia: 1997, 1087-1134.

Surgeons

M. Mark Taslimi, MD
Yasser El-Sayed, MD

8.3 OBSTETRIC SURGERY

Anesthesiologists

Brendan Carvalho, MBBCh, FRCA
Sheila E. Cohen, MB, ChB, FRCA

CESAREAN SECTION—LOWER SEGMENT AND CLASSIC

SURGICAL CONSIDERATIONS

Description: Cesarean section (C-section) is the delivery of the fetus through a horizontal or, more commonly, through a vertical incision in the **lower uterine segment**. The skin incision is made either as a Pfannenstiel's (transverse in the crease above the pubis), a **Maylard** (in extremely obese patients), or vertical midline from umbilicus to pubis. The peritoneal cavity is entered as in any laparotomy. A retractor is placed inferiorly and the reflection of visceral peritoneum from the bladder dome to the anterior lower segment of the uterus (bladder flap) is incised and displaced inferiorly, along with the bladder. The uterus is entered sharply and the incision extended with digital pressure and/or bandage scissors. The fetal head is elevated out of the pelvis and delivered through the uterine incision. In cases of nonvertex lie, the infant's breech or foot is grasped and brought out of the incision. After the delivery of the fetus, the cord is double-clamped and cut, and cord blood is obtained for analysis. The placenta is removed manually and the uterine cavity cleared of all

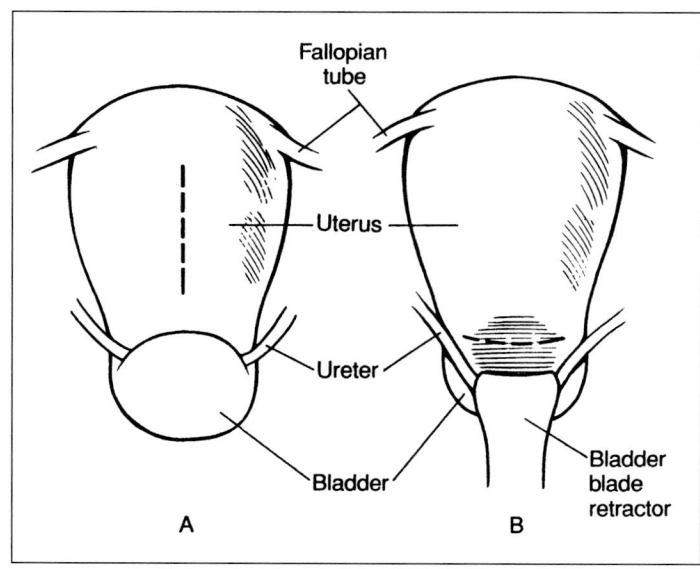

Figure 8.3-1. Typical C-section incisions. (A) Classic incision, in upper uterine segment. (B) Low transverse incision.

debris and clots. The uterine incision is closed with a running, interlocking stitch, followed by a 2nd imbricating layer. The bladder flap and parietal peritoneum do not require closure. Finally, the fascia is closed and the skin reapproximated with staples. **Classic C-section** usually involves a vertical skin incision and fundal vertical uterine incision (Fig 8.3-1). Patients with a history of prior classical C-section should be delivered abdominally via a repeat C-section, since the risk of uterine rupture with labor of vaginal delivery is 2%.

Usual preop diagnosis: Failure to progress in labor; elective repeat C-section; fetal distress; malpresentation

SUMMARY OF PROCEDURES

	Lower-Segment C-Section	Classic C-Section
Position	Supine with left lateral tilt. (In obese patients, the pannus may be lifted superiorly by tape or towel clips.)	⇐
Incision	Skin: transverse low abdominal (Pfannenstiel's) or repeat vertical. Uterus: transverse (Kerr) or low vertical (for premature infants or nonvertex lie)	Skin: Pfannenstiel's or, more commonly, vertical midline. Uterus: vertical fundal
Special instrumentation	Bladder blade retractor; small ring forceps; bandage scissors; suction bulb; DeLee suction trap (if meconium)	⇐
Unique considerations	✓ fetal heart tones before procedure. If for CPD: cervical exam within last 15 min before procedure. If for fetal distress: continuous monitoring until skin incision.	⇐
Antibiotics	If in labor or membranes ruptured: cefazolin 2 g iv, immediately after cord clamping.	⇐
Surgical time	20-90 min	40-90 min
Closing considerations	Low transverse: closed in 2 layers. Low vertical: 2 layers; may require additional operative time for repair of incision if extension into cervix or fundus.	3-layer closure requires additional time.

	Lower-Segment C-Section	**Classic C-Section**
EBL	750-1000 ml	1000-2000 ml
Postop care	Observation for bleeding and ↓BP	Special attention to VS needed due to additional blood loss.
Mortality	< 0.1%	⇐
Morbidity	Infection:	
	Not in labor: < 5%	⇐
	In labor/ruptured membranes: ≤ 50% (antibiotics reduce to 15%)	⇐
	Small-bowel obstruction (SBO): Rare	⇐
Pain Score	4	7

PATIENT POPULATION CHARACTERISTICS

Age range	14-40+ yr
Incidence	10-25%
Etiology[6]	Failure to progress (30%); repeat C-section (30%); fetal anomaly/other (20%); abnormal presentation (10%); fetal distress (10%)
Associated conditions	Preeclampsia/eclampsia; DIC; hemolysis, elevated liver enzyme, low Plt count (HELLP) syndrome; obstetrical hemorrhage/shock; chorioamnionitis

ANESTHETIC CONSIDERATIONS

(Procedures covered: C-section; emergent obstetrical hysterectomy; repair of uterine rupture)

PREOPERATIVE

In general, these patients are young and healthy, although the pregnant patient has undergone profound physiologic changes that affect the conduct of anesthesia. Patients present for emergency C-section for fetal distress and hemorrhage (placenta previa, abruptio placenta, and, rarely, uterine rupture).

Respiratory	The pregnant patient has a compensated respiratory alkalosis (PCO_2 = 32-34), ↑minute ventilation (MV) (↑50%), and ↓FRC (↓20%). ↑O_2 consumption (↑20%) with ↓FRC results in rapid onset of hypoxemia if ventilation is compromised. Small airway closure due to elevation of diaphragm (exaggerated by obesity and supine position) can → shunting and ↓PaO_2. ↑MV and ↓FRC enhance uptake of inhalational anesthetics. Mucosal capillary engorgement in upper airways may necessitate a smaller ETT and mandates careful airway suctioning to avoid bleeding. **Tests:** As indicated from H&P.
Cardiovascular	Typically, there is a ↓SVR (↓15%), ↓diastolic pressure and ↓MAP (↓15%) with ↑HR (↑30%) and ↑CO (↑30%). To minimize aortocaval compression and ↓BP, the supine position should be avoided by the use of left lateral tilt. Immediately postpartum, 600-800 ml blood enters the central circulation, due to placental transfusion, with further ↑ in CO. **Tests:** As indicated from H&P.
Hematologic	These patients have ↑blood volume (↑35%), ↑plasma volume (↑45%), ↑red cell mass (↑20%). WBC count may ↑ to 15,000/mm². Iron deficiency anemia often is superimposed on the dilutional anemia of pregnancy (Hct 33%). The typical blood loss of 500-800 ml is usually well tolerated. Excessive blood loss is possible with multiple gestation, previous C-section, PIH, placenta previa, abruptio placenta, and uterine atony. Repeat C-section associated with placenta previa poses high risk for hemorrhage because of placenta accreta. **Tests:** Hb/Hct
Gastrointestinal	Abnormalities, including ↓gastric motility (after onset of labor), gastroesophageal reflux, raised intragastric pressure, and gastric hyperacidity, predisposes to aspiration pneumonitis. All parturients should be considered to have full stomachs and should receive clear antacid (e.g., 0.3 M Na citrate 30 ml) immediately prior to GA or regional anesthesia. Administer iv metoclopramide 10 mg and ranitidine 50 mg before emergent C-section. Before elective C-section, parturients at high risk for aspiration (e.g., planned or potential GA, difficult airway, or any patient with esophageal reflux or obesity) should receive an H_2-blocker (e.g., ranitidine 150 mg po) the night before and the morning of surgery.

Hepatic	Liver enzymes can be mildly elevated and plasma protein concentration is diminished (↑unbound drug levels); however, liver function is usually normal. **Tests:** As indicated from H&P.
Renal	These patients have ↑renal blood flow (↑50%), ↑GFR, and ↑creatinine clearance, and ↓serum creatinine and ↓blood urea N_2. Dependent edema results from increased water and Na^+ retention 2° resetting of the osmotic threshold for thirst and vasopressin secretions. **Tests:** As indicated from H&P.
Laboratory	T&S maternal blood if risk factors for blood loss are present (e.g., third C-section). Cross-match unnecessary unless significant blood loss is anticipated. Routine autologous blood donation is not recommended. Coagulation studies and Plt count recommended with PIH, abruptio placenta, heavy maternal bleeding. BUN; Cr; UA; fasting blood glucose; others as indicated from H&P.
Premedication	Agents to decrease risk of aspiration pneumonitis are discussed on p. B-5. Sedatives are not routinely administered. In extremely anxious patients, however, 0.5-1.0 mg midazolam iv is an excellent anxiolytic, without apparent affect on maternal memory or alertness or neonatal condition.

SPECIAL CONSIDERATIONS

Pregnancy-induced hypertension (PIH)	PIH is characterized by generalized vasoconstriction with relative intravascular volume depletion and, occasionally, diffuse capillary leak. There may be ↑ risk of hypotension with regional anesthesia. Cautious hydration prior to regional anesthesia is necessary to prevent hypotension or pulmonary edema. Hepatic dysfunction may be present (HELLP syndrome). Epidural, spinal, and combined spinal-epidural (CSE) are all considered safe techniques in PIH. Cardiovascular stability is better with regional than GA, provided intravascular volume is adequate. Abnormal coagulation (↓Plt count or dysfunctional Plt) contraindicates regional anesthesia. If GA is necessary, control BP with small doses of labetalol (5-20 mg iv over 3-5 min) and/or low doses of a short-acting opioid (e.g., fentanyl 50-100 μg) prior to induction to blunt hypertensive response to laryngoscopy. There is a potential for difficult intubation in PIH due to airway edema; therefore, a small ETT (6.0 mm) should be available. $MgSO_4$ potentiates neuromuscular blocking agents; avoid defasiculating dose of muscle relaxant before induction, use smaller than normal doses of nondepolarizing agents, and monitor neuromuscular function. **Tests:** PT; PTT; Plt; TEG or bleeding time; LFTs
Eclampsia	Treat eclamptic Sz with adequate oxygenation and a small dose of STP (50-100 mg) or diazepam (5 mg). Intubate if necessary to protect airway. Initiate $MgSO_4$ therapy (loading dose: 4-6 g iv over 20-30 min; then infuse @ 1-2 g/h).
Massive maternal hemorrhage: • **Placenta previa** • **Abruptio placenta** • **Ruptured uterus**	Insert 2 large-bore iv catheters (14-16 ga). Assure immediate availability of cross-matched blood. Rapidly restore intravascular volume with crystalloid, colloid, or both. Induction of GA with ketamine (1-1.5 mg/kg) is preferred in hypovolemic patients. DIC can follow abruptio placenta or amniotic fluid embolism. Dilutional thrombocytopenia following massive blood loss might require Plt transfusion. Uterine atony is treated with oxytocin 20-40 U/L; NS @ rate sufficient to control atony (risk of ↓BP with boluses); methylergonovine, 0.2 mg im (risk of HTN); or 15-methylprostaglandin F_2-alpha, 0.25 mg im or intramyometrially (risk of pulmonary HTN, bronchospasm). Uterine artery embolization is often effective in controlling continued postpartum bleeding and may be considered before surgical artery ligation or hysterectomy.[10] Emergency hysterectomy, however, may be the only solution to continued bleeding. Induction of GA may be necessary if massive bleeding occurs during regional anesthesia.
Diabetes	Diabetic patients have an increased propensity to ↓BP following regional anesthesia, with the fetus becoming more acidotic than normal as a result. Determine blood glucose hourly and maintain at 80-100 mg/dL. Insulin requirements decrease drastically after delivery, and insulin dosage must be reduced to prevent maternal hypoglycemia. **Tests:** Fasting blood glucose; UA
Response to anesthetic drugs	In pregnant patients, MAC is ↓ ≤ 40% for inhaled agents; combined with more rapid uptake, this predisposes to anesthetic overdose. Sensitivity to local anesthetics also is increased. Epidural space capacity is decreased 2° engorgement of epidural veins; this decreases requirements for local anesthetics and increases possibility of intravascular injection of drugs. Increased sensitivity to nondepolarizing muscle relaxants (especially in patients receiving $MgSO_4$) mandates careful

Response to anesthetic drugs, cont. monitoring and use of reduced doses. Decreased protein binding may increase toxicity of highly protein-bound drugs such as bupivacaine.

INTRAOPERATIVE

Anesthetic technique: General considerations involve primarily the choice of anesthetic. Compared with regional anesthesia, the risks of aspiration and difficult intubation with GA significantly increase maternal morbidity and mortality.[2, 5] Anesthetic choice in specific circumstances depends on maternal and fetal conditions and degree of urgency. Properly conducted GA or regional anesthesia probably are equally safe for the fetus.

Spinal anesthesia is preferred for elective or semielective C-section (unless patient has an existing epidural) when no contraindications to regional anesthesia exist (e.g., patient refusal, coagulopathy, active neurological disease, hypovolemia, sepsis). With the use of pencil-point needles (e.g., Sprotte, Whitacre), the risk of headache is low (1-2%). Advantages of spinal over epidural anesthesia include: technical ease, more rapid onset of block, more solid anesthesia, and less shivering. ↓BP, however, is more common with spinal anesthesia. Fluid loading (1-1.5 L crystalloid/500 ml colloid), leg wrapping (e.g., compression stockings), and vasopressors reduce the incidence and severity of ↓BP[7,8] but do not eliminate it. Pressors (e.g., ephedrine [5-10 mg], phenylephrine [50-100 μg], and atropine [0.4 mg iv]) should be used as appropriate to treat ↓BP ± ↓HR. Ephedrine, even in large doses, may not reverse severe ↓BP, and may ↑fetal acidosis. Consider using epinephrine (50-100 μg iv) if other pressors/fluids are unsuccessful.

General anesthesia normally is used when regional anesthesia is contraindicated or when there is inadequate time to institute regional blockade. Obstetric emergencies for which rapid induction of GA may be indicated include: severe maternal hemorrhage, prolapsed umbilical cord, severe fetal bradycardia, severe persistent fetal decelerations, or the need for intrauterine manipulation. Less dire situations often permit the performance of a 'quick spinal' or extension of a functioning epidural block with an agent having a rapid onset (e.g., 15-20 ml 3% 2-chloroprocaine or 2% lidocaine with epinephrine). Continuous monitoring of the fetal heart rate (FHR) in the OR may allow use of regional anesthesia if the FHR tracing is reassuring. Constant communication with the obstetrician regarding maternal and fetal condition is essential. Although situations exist in which a GA is preferable to regional, the risks must be weighed against the benefits for patients with greater potential for complications. If difficult intubation is anticipated, rapid-sequence induction of GA should not be undertaken. Alternative approaches include awake intubation, spinal anesthesia, or local infiltration by the obstetrician. Sometimes, a nonreassuring FHR pattern is diagnosed as 'fetal distress' and the fetus is delivered immediately. Fetal distress is an imprecise and nonspecific term with little positive predictive value. The severity of any FHR abnormality should be considered when the urgency of delivery and type of anesthesia are determined. C-section performed for a nonreassuring FHR pattern does not necessarily preclude the use of regional anesthesia.

Regional anesthesia:

Epidural Apply monitors, fluid load, and place the patient in the sitting or lateral decubitus position. A 3 ml test dose of 1.5-2% lidocaine (45-60 mg) with 1:200,000 epinephrine (15-20 μg) is given through the epidural needle or catheter to exclude intravascular injection (Sx: tachycardia, palpitations, dizziness, tinnitus, new taste in mouth) or subarachnoid placement (motor/sensory block in lower extremities). After 3-5 min, inject 15-20 ml 2% (300-400 mg) lidocaine with 1:200,000 epinephrine (75-100 μg) incrementally over 5 min. Sodium bicarbonate, 1 mEq/10 ml lidocaine, hastens onset of block, but increases risk of ↓BP. Bupivacaine, levobupivacaine, or ropivacaine 0.5%, 15-20 ml (75-100 mg), with or without epinephrine 1:200,000 and/or fentanyl (50-75 μg), or 3% 2-chloroprocaine, 15-20 ml (450-600 mg) also can be used. To ensure a T4 level of anesthesia throughout surgery, additional local anesthetic often is needed. If a functioning epidural catheter is in place and an urgent C-section becomes necessary, 15-20 ml 3% 2-chloroprocaine (450-600 mg) or 2% lidocaine with epinephrine should produce adequate surgical anesthesia within 5-10 min.

Tilt table or use left hip elevation. Administer O_2 by mask or nasal cannula, and check FHR prior to abdominal prep. Monitor BP every min until stable, then every 3-5 min. Treat ↓20% in BP or SBP < 95-100 mmHg with further uterine displacement, additional fluids, and ephedrine 5-10 mg or phenylephrine 50-100 μg iv. For inadequate anesthesia, give additional epidural local anesthetic, 50-100 μg fentanyl iv or epidurally, 50% N_2O/O_2, ketamine 5-10 mg iv and/or infiltrate with local anesthetic. The patient must remain conscious to avoid risk of aspiration. If anesthesia is still inadequate, induce GA (see below).

After delivery of infant and placenta, rapidly infuse oxytocin 20-30 U/L. Antibiotics given at surgeon's request. Observe for excessive blood loss. Chest pain, mild oxyhemoglobin desaturation and SOB after delivery may be due to irritation of diaphragm by blood or packs, too high or inadequate level of anesthesia, or venous air or amniotic fluid embolization. S-T segment changes on ECG occur, but do not usually signify myocardial ischemia.[6]

Spinal	Apply monitors, administer fluid, and position as for epidural anesthesia. Metoclopramide 10 mg iv, 5-10 min prior to block decreases intraop N/V. Insert 24-25 ga pencil-point needle and verify free flow of CSF. In urgent situations, a larger pencil-point needle (e.g., 22 ga Sprotte) is easier and faster to place with minimal increase in headache. Inject hyperbaric 0.75% spinal bupivacaine 11.25-12.0 mg (1.5-1.6 ml) ± fentanyl 10-15 μg or preservative-free morphine 0.1-0.2 mg, and position the patient with left uterine displacement. Monitor and treat ↓BP as for epidural. Adjust operating table position to insure a T4 level of anesthesia. If anesthesia is inadequate and time permits, consider repeating block with CSE, repeat spinal (caution with dosing), or placement of an epidural catheter. Treat persistent inadequate anesthesia as for epidural. Induce GA if other measures fail.
Combined spinal-epidural (CSE)	An alternative technique combining the rapid onset and density of spinal anesthesia with the flexibility of continuous epidural anesthesia (e.g., if necessary to extend the duration or intensity of the block). Apply monitors, administer fluid, and position as for spinal/epidural. The most common technique is the needle-through-needle. When the epidural space is located with a 17 ga Tuohy needle, insert a 26-27 ga pencil-point spinal needle through it and administer 11.25-12 mg of spinal bupivacaine. Secure the epidural catheter and use if needed. (A test dose is advisable.)

General anesthesia:

Induction	Tilt table or use left hip displacement and administer 500-750 ml dextrose-free crystalloid before induction. Preoxygenation for 3 min is optimal; however, 4 maximal inspiratory breaths in 30 sec is a satisfactory substitute in an emergency. Place patient in maximal 'sniff' position with elevation of shoulders, if necessary, to optimize position for intubation. After patient is prepped and draped and obstetric team is ready to begin, perform rapid-sequence induction with cricoid pressure (p. B-5). Administer STP 4-5 mg/kg (or ketamine 1-1.5 mg/kg in hypovolemic patients) and succinylcholine 1-1.5 mg/kg to induce GA and facilitate intubation. Inflate cuff of ETT and verify tracheal placement by ETCO$_2$ waveform and auscultation of bilateral breath sounds.
Failed intubation[1, 4]	If tracheal intubation is unsuccessful, monitor O$_2$ sat and mask ventilate, maintaining cricoid pressure. Summon experienced help and quickly decide whether surgery must proceed. The risks of continuing with mask GA and cricoid pressure must be weighed against the risk of allowing the mother to awaken. If mask ventilation is impossible, quickly attempt ventilation with an LMA. If this succeeds, either continue to use throughout the case or place an ETT (6 mm ID) through LMA blindly, or with FOL; alternatively, use an intubating LMA. If LMA fails to allow ventilation, attempt emergency transtracheal ventilation using a 12-14-ga iv catheter and appropriate tubing to connect to a high-pressure O$_2$ source (e.g. jet ventilator). If these measures are unsuccessful, an emergency cricothyrotomy or tracheostomy should be performed by experienced personnel. **Planning for a failed intubation must occur before it actually happens.** A difficult-intubation tray, including equipment for emergency jet ventilation, must be immediately accessible in the delivery room.
Maintenance	50% N$_2$O/O$_2$ with 0.7-1.0% isoflurane or sevoflurane, or 0.5% halothane. Control ventilation, avoiding extreme hypocapnia (PCO$_2$ < 30 mmHg), which decreases umbilical blood flow. After delivery, substitute an opioid (e.g., fentanyl 50-100 μg) for volatile agent and increase concentration of N$_2$O to 70%. Administer small doses of muscle relaxants (e.g., vecuronium 2-3 mg) as needed. Reverse with neostigmine 0.05 mg/kg and glycopyrrolate 0.01 mg/kg or atropine 0.02 mg/kg. Midazolam (1-2 mg), given after delivery, helps avoid maternal awareness, which occasionally occurs with this anesthetic technique.
Emergence	Delay extubation until patient is fully awake and muscle strength has returned to normal.
Blood and fluid requirements	Moderate blood loss IV: 16-18 ga × 1 NS/LR 1-3 L typical replacement	Infuse 1-2 L dextrose-free crystalloid immediately prior to regional anesthesia. Typical blood loss = 500-800 ml. A rapid-fluid infuser and blood warmer should be available in the event that large-volume blood transfusion is required.
Monitoring	Standard monitors (p. B-1) FHR monitor ± CVP or PA catheter ± arterial line	Arterial BP monitoring via automated BP device or arterial line for severe or labile HTN. CVP useful in PIH for oliguric patients unresponsive to fluid challenges. Occasionally, a PA catheter is indicated (e.g., for pulmonary edema, unresponsive oliguria).

Positioning	Left uterine displacement (blanket under right hip and/or table tilt)	Minimizes aortocaval compression.
Complications	Amniotic fluid embolism	Rare cause of hemodynamic instability, hypoxemia, and DIC. Often fatal. Rx: supportive – 100% O_2, PEEP, and vasopressors. Correct Plt, clotting factors, and metabolic disturbances. CPB has been used successfully.

POSTOPERATIVE

Complications	PE	DX: pleuritic chest pain, hypoxemia, ↑RR, ↑HR, ↑A-a gradient. Rx: supportive – 100% O_2, volume expansion, and vasopressors.
	Postpartum hemorrhage	See Anesthetic Considerations for Removal of Retained Placenta, p. 666.
Pain management	**Epidural:** 4-5 mg preservative-free morphine in 10 ml after delivery. **Intrathecal:** morphine 0.1-0.2 mg given with spinal local anesthetic. Chloroprocaine interferes with analgesia from epidural opioids.	Common side effects include: pruritus 70%, nausea 30-40% and, rarely, respiratory depression. Nalbuphine (5-10 mg) and naloxone (0.1-0.4 mg) are used for reversal of these side effects. Metoclopramide (10 mg iv) and/or ondansetron (4 mg iv) may be needed for persistent nausea. Risk of delayed respiratory depression in healthy patients is small; however, adequately trained nursing staff and a protocol for treatment of complications are mandatory if intraspinal opioids are used. These patients should not routinely receive sedatives or other systemic opioids for 12 h, and close monitoring of RR and level of consciousness is necessary. Pulse oximetry is recommended in high-risk patients.
	Parenteral opioids: iv or im opioids or PCA instituted in recovery room. **Oral analgesics:** NSAIDs (e.g., ibuprofen), acetaminophen ± codeine (or equivalent oral narcotics), once patient can tolerate oral medication.	
Tests	As indicated.	

References

1. Caplan RA, et al: ASA Task Force on Difficult Airway Management. *Practice Guidelines for Management of the Difficult Airway.* (Approved Oct 1992, Amended Oct 2002). American Society of Anesthesiologists, Illinois.
2. Chadwick HS: An analysis of obstetric anesthesia cases from the American Society of Anesthesiologists closed claims project database. *Int J Obstet Anesth* 1996; 5:258-63.
3. Cunningham FG, MacDonald PC, Gant NF, Leveno KJ, Gilstrap LC, Hankins GDV, Clark SL, eds: Cesarean delivery and postpartum hysterectomy. In *Williams Obstetrics,* 21st edition. Appleton & Lange, Stamford, CT: 2001.
4. Ezri T, Szmuk P, Evron S, Geva D, Hagay Z, Katz J: Difficult airway in obstetric anesthesia: a review. *Obstet Gynecol Surv* 2001; 56(10):631-41.
5. Hawkins JL, Koonin LM, Palmer SK, Gibbs CP: Anesthesia-related deaths during obstetric delivery in the United States, 1979-1990. *Anesthesiology* 1997; 86:277-84.
6. McLintic AJ, Pringle SD, Lilley S, Houston AB, Thorburn J: Electrocardiographic changes during cesarean section under regional anesthesia. *Anesth Analg* 1992; 74(1):51-6.
7. Mercier FJ, Riley ET, Frederickson WL, Roger-Christoph S, Benhamou D, Cohen SE: Phenylephrine added to prophylactic infusion during spinal anesthesia for elective cesarean section. *Anesthesiology* 2001; 95(3):668-74.
8. Morgan PJ, Halpern SH, Tarshis J: The effects of an increase of central blood volume before spinal anesthesia for cesarean delivery: a qualitative review. *Anesth Analg* 2001; 92(4):997-1005.
9. Richardson MG: Regional anesthesia for obstetrics. *Anesthesiol Clin North America* 2000;18(2):383-406.
10. Vedantham S, Goodwin SC, McLucas B, Mohr G: Uterine artery embolization: an underused method of controlling pelvic hemorrhage. *Am J Obstet Gynecol* 1997; 176(4):938-48.

MEDICAL AND SURGICAL MANAGEMENT
OF POSTPARTUM HEMORRHAGE

SURGICAL CONSIDERATIONS

Description: The most common indication for postpartum uterine devascularization and hysterectomy is **intractable postpartum hemorrhage (PPH)**. PPH is clinically defined as any uncompensated postpartum blood loss → tissue hypoperfusion. There are four major causes of PPH: retained products of conception (POC), laceration of the genital tract, uterine atony, and coagulopathies. Inherited coagulopathies include von Willebrand's disease, hemophilia, and factor XI deficiency. Acquired coagulopathies are most often related to thrombocytopenia 2° preeclampsia/eclampsia, hypofibrinogenemia 2° long-standing fetal demise, placental abruption, and DIC related to massive blood loss.

Postpartum blood loss can be reduced by prophylactic use of oxytocin, methylergonovine, or prostaglandins, and these same agents are used as the first line of treatment for PPH. A concentrated oxytocin infusion (e.g., 80-100 U in 500 ml over 30 min) is most effective. Methylergonovine should be given im only (0.2 mg q 2-4 h up to 1 mg), since iv infusion has been reported to cause acute HTN, stroke, and Sz. Ergot derivatives are contraindicated in patients with Hx of HTN, asthma, Raynaud's syndrome, or migraine. $PGF_2\alpha$ (Hemabate) may be injected im (intramyometrial) at a dose of 0.25, up to a total of 2 mg.[2] Misoprostol, an inexpensive PGE, may be given rectally (up to 800 μg).

Simultaneously, the surgeon should explore the cause of PPH and apply a specific treatment. Surgical management of intractable PPH includes **uterine artery embolization, uterine devascularization**, and **hysterectomy**. If PPH is not controlled with treatment of uterine atony, and after volume replacement and correction of any coagulopathy, the patient is transferred to Radiology. Under fluoroscopic control, uterine arteries are selected, and pledgets of absorbable gelatin sponge are introduced. Treatment may be repeated until bleeding is stopped. In anticipation of PPH, catheters have been placed in uterine arteries before C-section in known cases of placenta accreta.[4]

The decision for surgical intervention is made when other options (i.e., medical, interventional radiology) have not been successful in decreasing the hemorrhage. Volume and coagulation factor replacement should continue while proceeding with surgery. Operative management includes use of hemostatic uterine sutures to compress the uteral cavity, vascular ligation, and hysterectomy.

Causes of **uterine rupture** include breakdown of a previous uterine scar, obstructed labor, or uterine trauma. The emergent nature of these conditions requires rapid intervention by the anesthesiologist, including iv fluid resuscitation and blood and blood product administration, if necessary. The patient's oxygenation and coagulation parameters must be monitored closely, given the risk of hypoxia and DIC 2° massive blood loss, and she should be transferred promptly to an OR that is well equipped for obstetric emergencies.

The technique for an **emergent obstetrical hysterectomy** is largely similar to a hysterectomy for other indications. Of note is the engorged and prominent nature of the vessels supplying the gravid uterus. The edematous tissues surrounding the uterus are very friable and may bleed profusely if improperly manipulated. A **supracervical** or **total hysterectomy** may be performed. Through a midline or Pfannenstiel's incision, the uterus is elevated out of the abdominal cavity. The round ligaments are clamped, transected, and ligated; and the anterior leaf of the broad ligament is incised bilaterally from the transected round ligaments to the vesicouterine reflection. The posterior leaf of the broad ligament adjacent to the uterus is entered at a level just below that of the fallopian tubes and uteroovarian ligaments. These are then clamped, transected, and ligated. Next, incision of the posterior leaf of the broad ligament toward the cardinal ligaments is performed. With gentle blunt dissection, the bladder and attached vesicouterine peritoneal flap are dissected off the lower uterine segment. The ascending uterine arteries and veins are identified bilaterally, then clamped, transected, and ligated. If a **subtotal hysterectomy** is planned, the body of the uterus is amputated at this level, and the cervical stump is closed with interrupted sutures. If a total hysterectomy is planned, dissection of the bladder off the cervix is continued until the cervicovaginal margin is identified. The cardinal and uterosacral ligaments are clamped, transected, and ligated, with clamps placed as close to the cervix as possible without including cervical tissue. Once the level of the lateral vaginal fornix is reached, a clamp is swung below the cervix, across the lateral vaginal fornix. The cervix is then amputated off the vaginal cuff. Throughout the procedure, it is vital to clamp and ligate any bleeding vessels and to take extra care to avoid damage to the ureter or bladder. Following removal of the uterus and cervix, the vaginal cuff angles are sutured to the ipsilateral cardinal ligament stumps, and the vaginal cuff is closed with a running locked stitch. The abdominal wall is closed in layers.

Usual preop diagnosis: Intractable postpartum bleeding; rupture of gravid uterus

SUMMARY OF PROCEDURE

Position	Supine, with left lateral tilt
Incision	Pfannenstiel's or midline longitudinal
Unique considerations	Monitoring of coagulation parameters and correction of DIC. Consider central venous hemo-dynamic monitoring. Pediatrics team present, if indicated.
Antibiotics	Cefotetan 2 g iv q 12 h; total 3 doses
Surgical time	2-3 h
Closing considerations	Subcutaneous intraperitoneal drains, if indicated.
EBL	3000-4000 ml
Postop care	ICU if blood loss severe; patient may require continued intubation and mechanical ventilatory support. Monitor for infectious morbidity and acute renal failure.
Mortality	< 1%
Morbidity	Hemorrhage
	Postop febrile morbidity
	DIC
	Wound infection
	Sheehan's syndrome
	Bladder injury
	Intraperitoneal bleeding requiring reoperation
	Vesicovaginal fistula
	Ureterovaginal fistula
	Transfusion-related complications
Pain score	7

PATIENT POPULATION CHARACTERISTICS

Age range	Reproductive age
Incidence	0.11% of obstetric patients
Etiology	Unknown
Associated conditions	Placenta accreta; uterine atony nonresponsive to medical or other surgical intervention; extension of cervical tear to lower uterine segment; placenta previa; uterine rupture; uterine inversion

ANESTHETIC CONSIDERATIONS

See Anesthetic Considerations following Cesarean Section, p. 661.

References

1. Al-Sibai MH, Rahman J, Rahman MS, Butalack F: Emergency hysterectomy in obstetrics—a review of 117 cases. *Aust NZ J Obstet Gynaecol* 1987; 27(3):180-84.
2. Bukowski R, Hankins GDV: Managing postpartum hemorrhage. *Contemporary OB/GYN* 2001; 9:92-105.
3. Chestnut DH, Dewan DM, Redick LF, Caton D, Spielman FJ: Anesthetic management for obstetric hysterectomy: a multi-institutional study. *Anesthesiology* 1989; 70(4):607-10.
4. Chitkara U: Personal communications, 2002.
5. Cho JH, Jun HS, Lee CN: Hemostatic suturing technique for uterine bleeding during cesarean delivery. *Obstet Gynecol* 2000; 96(1):129-31.
6. Cunningham FG, MacDonald PC, Gant NF, Leveno KJ, Gilstrap LC, Hankins GDV, Clark SL: Cesarean delivery and cesarean hysterectomy. In *Williams Obstetrics*, 20th edition. Appleton & Lange, Stamford, CT: 1997, 509-32.
7. Gilstrap LC III, Ramin SM: Postpartum hemorrhage. *Clin Obstet Gynecol* 1994; 37(4)824-30.
8. Mousa H, Walkinshaw S: Major postpartum hemorrhage. *Curr Opin Obstet Gynecol* 2001; 13(6):595-603.
9. O'Grady JP, Gimovsky ML, McIlhargie, eds: *Operative Obstetrics*. Williams & Wilkins, Baltimore: 1995, 264-67.
10. Plauche WC: Peripartum hysterectomy. *Obstet Gynecol Clin North Am* 1988; 15(4):783-95.
11. Tamizian O, Arulkumaraqn S: The surgical management of postpartum hemorrhage. *Curr Opin Obstet Gynecol* 2001; 13(2):127-31.

REPAIR OF UTERINE RUPTURE

SURGICAL CONSIDERATIONS

Description: Rupture of the gravid uterus is considered a true obstetric emergency and can be catastrophic, with significant maternal and fetal mortality. The classic symptoms are 'shearing' pain, cessation of uterine contractions, loss of fetal heart tones, and the onset of vaginal bleeding. Unfortunately, these warning symptoms occur only in a minority of uterine rupture cases. Extrusion of the placenta through the uterine rupture may result in late decelerations due to uteroplacental insufficiency. Extrusion of the umbilical cord may be manifested by recurrent variable decelerations. Suprapubic pain as the only symptom has not been associated with uterine rupture. In cases where the uterine rupture occurs at the site of a prior uterine scar, the clinical course is usually less severe and the blood loss less than in cases of primary rupture of an intact uterus. The incidence of uterine rupture at the site of the old scar is 0.5% for lower-uterine transverse C-sections, and 2% for classic C-sections. Uterine rupture mimics abruptio placenta in its presentations; however, once the diagnosis is made, prompt surgical intervention is mandated. **Total abdominal hysterectomy** (see p. 647), or **supracervical hysterectomy** (p. 666), is the definitive therapy; however, depending on the clinical situation and patient's wishes for future fertility, a **uterine repair** may be undertaken. This consists of a 2- to 3-layered closure of the defect, using synthetic absorbable sutures. A transverse abdominal incision is made ~3 cm above the symphysis pubis and carried to the anterior rectus fascia. The fascia is incised and the muscles of the anterior abdominal wall separated sharply and bluntly from the midline. The peritoneum is elevated and entered sharply. Because of the emergent nature of this condition and the possible massive blood loss associated with rupture of a gravid uterus, the anesthesiologist must act quickly. Prompt O_2 administration, together with aggressive iv fluid resuscitation, is indicated. Serious consideration should be given to the use of unmatched O(-) or type-specific blood until cross-matched blood becomes available. Intraop hypogastric or uterine artery ligation may help minimize blood loss. Patient's coagulation parameters must be monitored, since hypoxia and massive blood loss are associated with DIC.

Usual preop diagnosis: Uterine rupture

SUMMARY OF PROCEDURE

Position	Supine with left-lateral tilt
Incision	Pfannenstiel's (low, transverse abdominal) or midline longitudinal
Unique considerations	Pediatrics team present for infant resuscitation, if necessary. Thorough surgical exploration of the urinary tract (bladder and ureters) since ~10% of cases are associated with bladder lacerations. Cell Saver may be helpful.
Antibiotics	Cefotetan 2 g iv q 12 h × 3 doses
Surgical time	1-2 h
EBL	500-3000 ml
Postop care	ICU if blood loss severe; continued intubation and mechanical ventilatory support if aggressive fluid resuscitation results in pulmonary edema. Acute renal failure may occur 2° hypoxic and hypovolemic renal injury at time of acute uterine rupture with massive bleeding; monitor UO and serial renal function tests.
Mortality	Fetal: 35-45%
	Maternal: 5%
Morbidity	Blood transfusion > 5 U: 58.3%
	Postop wound infection: 33%
	Pelvic abscess: 8.3%
	Repeat uterine rupture with subsequent pregnancies: 5%
Pain score	6

PATIENT POPULATION CHARACTERISTICS

Age range	Reproductive age
Incidence	1/1400 deliveries
Etiology	Prior uterine surgery; grand multiparity; obesity; manual removal of placenta; injury from tools of abortion; direct or indirect violence; oxytocin use; intraamniotic or vaginal prostaglandins; breech extractions; internal or external version; forceps rotation; shoulder dystocia; fundal pressure; neglect (cephalopelvic disproportion, etc.); congenital uterine anomaly; cornual pregnancy; gestational trophoblastic neoplasia; placenta percreta; abruptio placenta

ANESTHETIC CONSIDERATIONS

See Anesthetic Considerations following Cesarean Section. p. 661.

References

1. Akasheh F: Rupture of the uterus. Analysis of 104 cases of rupture. *Am J Obstet Gynecol* 1968; 101(3):406-8.
2. Chazotte C, Cohen WR: Catastrophic complications of previous cesarean section. *Am J Obstet Gynecol* 1990; 163(3):738-42.
3. Claman P, Carpenter RJ, Reiter A: Uterine rupture with the use of vaginal prostaglandin E_2 for induction of labor. *Am J Obstet Gynecol* 1984; 150(7):889-90.
4. Cunningham FG, MacDonald PC, Gant NF, Leveno KJ, Gilstrap LC, Hankins GDV, Clark SL: Surgical sterilization. In *Williams Obstetrics*, 21st edition. Appleton & Lange, Stamford, CT: 2001, 1555-62.
5. Eden RD, Parker RT, Gall SA: Rupture of the pregnant uterus: a 53-year review. *Obstet Gynecol* 1986; 68(5):671-74.
6. Golan A, Sandbank O, Rubin A: Rupture of the pregnant uterus. *Obstet Gynecol* 1980; 56(5):549-54.
7. Plauche WC, VonAlmen W, Muller R: Catastrophic uterine rupture. *Obstet Gynecol* 1984; 64(6):792-97.
8. Reyes-Ceja L, Cabrera R, Insfran E, Herrera-Lasso F: Pregnancy following previous uterine rupture. Study of 19 patients. *Obstet Gynecol* 1969; 34(3):387-89.
9. Sawyer MM, Lipshitz J, Anderson GD, Dilts PV Jr: Third-trimester uterine rupture associated with vaginal prostaglandin E_2. *Am J Obstet Gynecol* 1981; 140(6):710-11.
10. Yussman MA, Haynes DM: Rupture of the gravid uterus. A 12-year study. *Obstet Gynecol* 1970; 36(1):115-20.

POSTPARTUM TUBAL LIGATION

SURGICAL CONSIDERATIONS

Description: **Postpartum tubal ligation (PPTL)** is female surgical sterilization performed at the time of cesarean section (C-section) after delivery of the infant and repair of the uterine incision or within the first several days after a vaginal delivery. Although PPTL can be performed immediately postpartum, problems in the neonate may not be immediately evident, and a delay in surgery may be appropriate. If performed after a vaginal delivery, a small infraumbilical incision is made in the skin and carried down through the parietal peritoneum. The fallopian tubes are identified and brought out of the incision. It is important to identify the fimbriated end of the tube to ensure that the structure ligated is not the round ligament. A midsegment portion of the tube over an avascular portion of mesosalpinx is selected and tubal patency is disrupted by a variety of methods (**Pomeroy, Parkland, Irving, Uchida,** etc.). The Pomeroy, or a modification of it, is the most common technique used. The segment of tube grasped is ligated with absorbable suture and the knuckle of tube formed is excised. The cut ends of the tubes should be hemostatic before replacing the tubes into the abdomen. The wound is closed in layers in the usual fashion.

The consent for sterilization requires special consideration. The procedure is strictly elective and voluntary and must be considered permanent, even though reversal may be possible. Some patients will eventually regret the decision to undergo permanent sterilization. The risk of sterilization failure and an increased risk of ectopic pregnancy in case of failure must be reviewed. The full range of alternatives to PPTL, including an interval sterilization procedure (sterilization performed remote from pregnancy) must also be considered.

Usual preop diagnosis: Desire for permanent sterilization

SUMMARY OF PROCEDURE

Position	Supine; steep Trendelenburg often required to allow bowel to fall away for exposure.
Incision	Infraumbilical
Special instrumentation	Small Richardson and Army/Navy retractors; Babcock clamps; vein retractor
Unique considerations	A special consent form for sterilization must be signed by the patient in advance of the surgery. The bladder must be drained prior to the procedure.
Antibiotics	None recommended
Surgical time	15-25 min (Uchida technique may ↑ operative time)

EBL	10 ml
Postop care	Routine postpartum care after recovery from anesthesia
Mortality	3/100,000
Morbidity	Hemorrhage
	Infection
	Incidental damage to bowel or bladder
Pain score	3

PATIENT POPULATION CHARACTERISTICS

Age range	Reproductive age
Incidence	The most common contraceptive procedure in the U.S.

ANESTHETIC CONSIDERATIONS

PREOPERATIVE

Optimal timing of tubal ligation is controversial. The patient with a functioning epidural catheter may benefit from having surgery immediately after delivery. Many surgeons, however, favor waiting 8-24 h, when adequate assessment of the neonate should be complete and risk of maternal hemorrhage lessened. Alternatively, the epidural catheter can be left in place and reinjected later (successful epidural reactivation within 24 h is possible in 92% of patients[7]). Because pulmonary aspiration remains a theoretical risk, initiation of GA or spinal anesthesia often is delayed 8-24 h until the acute GI changes of pregnancy have regressed. There is no benefit to delaying surgery beyond this time. Shorter hospital stays after vaginal delivery are encouraging more tubal ligations during the first 12 h after delivery. It is unknown whether this will affect morbidity or mortality.

Respiratory	FRC returns to normal almost immediately after delivery. Laryngeal edema may persist in preeclamptic and postpartum patients after protracted expulsive efforts during labor → requirement for a small ETT. **Tests:** As indicated from H&P.
Cardiovascular	The physiologic changes of pregnancy return to normal at varying intervals after delivery. For example, risk of aortocaval compression disappears immediately. Blood volume returns to prepregnant values over several days. Postpartum hemorrhage can occur without warning. **Tests:** As indicated from H&P.
Gastrointestinal	Postpartum patients continue to be at risk for acid aspiration, although it is not known exactly when normal GI function returns. If elective PPTL is planned within 8 h of delivery, patient should have no oral intake of solid foods during labor and the postpartum period. Precautions for prevention of acid aspiration should be followed as discussed in Cesarean Section, p. 661.
Neurological	Local anesthetic requirements for spinal anesthesia remain decreased after delivery but are greater than for pregnant patients.[1]
Laboratory	Hct; other tests as indicated from H&P.
Premedication	Precautions should be taken to ↓ risk of aspiration pneumonitis, as discussed in Cesarean Section, p. 662.

INTRAOPERATIVE

Anesthetic technique: Spinal anesthesia is preferred, if a functioning epidural catheter is not in place. Epidural catheters frequently become dislodged after patient becomes ambulatory. GA is acceptable if patient has a strong preference or if contraindications to regional anesthesia exist. These patients may be at risk for aspiration of gastric contents at least 8-24 h postdelivery.

Regional anesthesia:

Spinal	For technique and monitoring for spinal anesthesia, see Cesarean Section, p. 664. Hyperbaric 5% lidocaine was the drug of choice for this procedure, but concerns about transient radicular irritation after spinal lidocaine have led some to abandon its use.[8] Most procedures for PPTL last 20-40 min, but some (e.g., Uchida, Irving) may last ~1 h. If more prolonged surgery is likely (e.g., obese patient, or patient with adhesions) or for routine use, bupivacaine (7.5-12 mg) ± fentanyl (10-25 μg) may be preferable. With the patient supine, adjust position of the operating table to obtain a T6 level of anesthesia. Sedate patient as necessary with small doses of iv midazolam 0.5-1.0 mg or opioid.

Epidural	A 3 ml epidural test dose, followed after 3-5 min by 15-20 ml 3% 2-chloroprocaine or 1.5-2% lidocaine with 1:200,000 epinephrine injected incrementally. Additional local anesthetic as needed to ensure adequate level of anesthesia.	
General anesthesia:		
Induction	Rapid-sequence induction (p. B-5) with STP (4-5 mg/kg) or propofol (1-2 mg/kg) and succinylcholine (1 mg/kg) for ET intubation.	
Maintenance	Standard maintenance (p. B-3)	
Emergence	Extubation should be delayed until patient is fully awake and protective airway reflexes have returned.	
Blood and fluid requirements	Minimal blood loss IV: 18 ga × 1 NS/LR @ 2-4 ml/kg/h	1-1.5 L dextrose-free crystalloid immediately prior to regional anesthesia
Monitoring	Standard monitors (p. B-1)	
Positioning	✓ and pad pressure points. ✓ eyes.	
Complications	None specific	

POSTOPERATIVE

Complications	Minimal bleeding	
Pain management	**Intraspinal opioids**: 10-25 μg fentanyl **Parenteral opioids**: IV or im opioids (e.g., morphine 2-4 mg iv (up to 20 mg) or meperidine 10-20 mg iv q 10-15 min, titrated to RR and patient's level of pain) instituted in recovery room.	Intrathecal fentanyl 10-25 μg, given with spinal local anesthetic, enhances intraop anesthesia, particularly with low doses of bupivacaine, and provides several h postop analgesia.
Tests	None routinely indicated.	

References

1. Abouleish EI: Postpartum tubal ligation requires more bupivacaine for spinal anesthesia than does cesarean section. *Anesth Analg* 1986; 65(8):897-900.
2. American College of Obstetricians and Gynecologists: ACOG Committee Opinion, Committee on Ethics: Sterilization of women, including those with mental disabilities. No 216, 1999 (replaces No 63, 1988, and No 73, 1989). *Int J Gynaecol Obstet* 1999; 65(3):317-20.
3. American College of Obstetricians and Gynecologists: ACOG Committee Opinion, Committee on Obstetrics, Maternal and Fetal Sterilization: Postpartum tubal sterilization. No 105, 1992. *Int J Gynaecol Obstet* 1992; 39(3):244.
4. American College of Obstetricians and Gynecologists: ACOG technical bulletin. Sterilization. No 222, 1996 (replaces No 113, 1988). *Int J Gynaecol Obstet* 1996;53(3):281-8.
5. Bucklin BA, Smith CV: Postpartum Tubal Ligation: Safety, Timing, and Other Implications for Anesthesia. *Anesth Analg* 1999; 89(5):1269-75.
6. Cunningham FG, MacDonald PC, Grant NF, et al, eds: Surgical sterilization. In *Williams Obstetrics*, 21st edition. Appleton & Lange, Stamford, CT: 2001.
7. Goodman EJ, Dumas SD: The Rate of Successful Reactivation of Labor Epidural Catheters for Postpartum Tubal Ligation Surgery. *Reg Anesth Pain Med* 1998; 23(3):258-61.
8. Hampl KF, Schneider MC, Pargger H, Gut J, Drewe J, Drasner K: A similar incidence of transient neurologic symptoms after spinal anesthesia with 2 percent and 5 percent lidocaine. *Anesth Analg* 1996; 83:1051-54.
9. Hatcher RA, Stewart F, Trussell J, et al: *Contraceptive Technology*, 15th revised edition. Irvinton Publishers, New York: 1990, 387-421.
10. Hughes SC, Levinson G, Rosen MA, Shnider SM, eds: *Shnider and Levinson's Anesthesia for Obstetrics*, 4th edition. Lippincott Williams & Wilkins, Philadelphia: 2002.
11. Practice Guidelines for Obstetrical Anesthesia: a report by the American Society of Anesthesiologists' Task Force on Obstetrical Anesthesia. *Anesthesiology* 1999; 90:600-11.
12. Viscomi CM, Rathmell JP: Labor epidural reactivation or spinal anesthesia for delayed postpartum tubal ligation: a cost comparison. *Anesthesiology* 1994; 81:A1160.
13. Wheeless CR Jr: *Atlas of Pelvic Surgery*, 2nd edition. Lea & Febiger, Philadelphia: 1988, 282-88.

REPAIR OF VAGINAL/CERVICAL LACERATIONS

SURGICAL CONSIDERATIONS

Description: Vaginal and cervical lacerations may occur 2° trauma of spontaneous and operative vaginal delivery. Adequate repair requires optimal surgical assistance, exposure, and patient comfort. Repair may be performed in a birthing bed, or may require patient positioning, lighting, anesthesia, or monitoring capabilities available only in an OR. Vaginal and cervical lacerations can extend into the perineum, rectum, urethra, bladder, lower uterine segment, broad ligament, or peritoneal cavity.

Lacerations of the lower vagina generally are easy to identify and repair. Small, superficial lacerations that do not bleed often do not need repair, while larger ones should be approximated. Deep lacerations may cause profuse bleeding; if it persists despite placement of multiple stitches, brief tamponade may be adequate to achieve hemostasis, or vaginal packing may be required. Lacerations involving the perineum are classified as follows: First degree—involves break in mucosa and skin. Second degree—involves deeper tissue (bulbocavernosus and levator ani fascia and muscle). Third degree—involves anal sphincter. Fourth degree—extends into rectal mucosa. First- and second-degree lacerations are repaired in layers with continuous or interrupted stitches. The skin usually is closed with a subcuticular stitch. When the anal sphincter is lacerated, it often retracts. The ends are grasped with Allis clamps and approximated with multiple stitches. When the laceration extends into the rectum, the rectal mucosa usually is closed in two layers, with the second layer imbricating the first. With periurethral lacerations, a catheter may need to be placed in the urethra to prevent passing a stitch through it. A laceration involving the urethra or bladder should be closed in multiple layers, followed by bladder drainage for several days.

Lacerations of the upper vagina are often difficult to visualize. Uterine bleeding and the umbilical cord of an undelivered placenta can obscure the field, and it can be difficult to determine if bleeding is vaginal or uterine. It is helpful to deliver the placenta and control uterine bleeding before proceeding. Once visualization is adequate, it is important to place the first stitch above the apex of the laceration to control bleeding from vessels that may have retracted. Again, vaginal packing may be required if oozing of blood persists.

Superficial **lacerations of the cervix** occur with most deliveries but usually do not require treatment. Deep lacerations can cause significant blood loss, especially when they involve larger branches from the uterine artery or extend into the lower uterine segment. Again, the first stitch must be placed above the apex of the laceration to control bleeding from vessels that may have retracted. A **laparotomy** may be necessary if a laceration extends into the lower uterine segment or broad ligament and is causing significant bleeding that cannot be controlled otherwise. Alternatively, uterine artery embolization may be considered.

Usual preop diagnosis: Vaginal or cervical laceration

SUMMARY OF PROCEDURE

Position	Dorsal lithotomy
Incision	None (unless exploratory laparotomy is performed)
Special instrumentation	Right-angle retractors; ring forceps; Allis clamps; Gelpi retractor; vaginal packing
Antibiotics	May be used for lacerations involving entry into the peritoneal cavity or the rectal mucosa.
Surgical time	10-45 min (possibly longer if exploratory laparotomy is performed)
EBL	Variable. Possible need for transfusion. Areas that persistently ooze after repeated placement of suture may be managed with vaginal packing.
Postop care	PACU → ward
Mortality	Rare
Morbidity	Hemorrhage
	Hematoma
	Infection
	Rectovaginal fistula
	Vesicovaginal fistula
Pain score	3

PATIENT POPULATION CHARACTERISTICS

Age range	Reproductive age
Incidence	Not uncommon
Etiology	Trauma 2° spontaneous or operative vaginal delivery (98%); other vaginal/pelvic trauma (2%)
Associated conditions	Major blood loss possible; with nonobstetric etiology, the possibility of sexual assault needs to be explored.

ANESTHETIC CONSIDERATIONS

PREOPERATIVE

Vaginal and cervical lacerations may go undetected until considerable blood loss has occurred. Patients should be examined carefully for Sx of hypovolemia with appropriate volume resuscitation prior to anesthesia.

Respiratory	FRC returns to normal almost immediately after delivery. **Tests:** As indicated from H&P.
Cardiovascular	The physiologic changes of pregnancy return to normal at varying intervals after delivery. For example, risk of aortocaval compression disappears immediately. Blood volume returns to prepregnant values over several days. Postpartum hemorrhage can occur without warning. Ensure adequate fluid resuscitation prior to induction of GA or regional anesthesia. **Tests:** As indicated from H&P.
Gastrointestinal	Postpartum patients continue to be at risk for acid aspiration, although it is not known exactly when normal GI function returns. Precautions for prevention of acid aspiration should be followed as discussed in Cesarean Section, p. 661.
Neurological	Local anesthetic requirements for spinal anesthesia remain decreased after delivery.
Laboratory	Hct; other tests as indicated from H&P.
Premedication	Precautions should be taken to ↓ risk of aspiration pneumonitis, as discussed in Cesarean Section, p. 661.

INTRAOPERATIVE

Anesthetic technique: In many patients, a functioning epidural catheter will be in place, and supplemental doses of anesthetic may be given to provide adequate analgesia for the surgery. If no epidural is placed and the patient is hemodynamically stable, a spinal anesthetic may be satisfactory. Occasionally, GA may be required.

Regional anesthesia:

Epidural	Supplemental doses of local anesthetic (2-chloroprocaine or 1.5-2% lidocaine 10-15 ml) injected incrementally with patient in sitting position (if tolerated) to promote perineal anesthesia.
Spinal	Hyperbaric lidocaine 5% 50-70 mg (see comments regarding transient radicular irritation on p. 664) or hyperbaric bupivacaine 0.75% 7.5-10 mg with patient in sitting position, if tolerated. 24-25 ga pencil-point needle (Sprotte or Whitacre) to ↓ incidence of spinal headache. Anesthesia to T10 is usually adequate. Repair of more extensive lacerations may require a higher level and, consequently, a higher dose of anesthetic.
Combined spinal-epidural (CSE)	An alternative technique combining the rapid onset and density of spinal anesthesia with the flexibility of continuous epidural anesthesia (e.g., if necessary to extend the duration or intensity of the block). Apply monitors, administer fluid, and position as for spinal/epidural. The most common technique is the needle-through-needle. When the epidural space is located with a 17 ga Tuohy needle, insert a 26-27 ga pencil-point spinal needle through it and administer 7.5-10 mg of spinal bupivacaine. Secure the epidural catheter and use if needed. (A test dose is advisable.)

General anesthesia:

Induction	Rapid-sequence induction (p. B-5) with STP (4-5 mg/kg) and succinylcholine (1 mg/kg) for ET intubation. If significant blood loss, ketamine 1.5 mg/kg is preferred for induction.
Maintenance	Standard maintenance (p. B-3). If significant blood loss, ketamine 1.5 mg/kg is preferred for induction.
Emergence	Extubation should be delayed until patient is fully awake and protective airway reflexes have returned.
Blood and fluid requirements	IV: 16-18 ga × 1 NS/LR @ 2-4 ml/kg/h	1-1.5 L dextrose-free crystalloid immediately prior to regional anesthesia. Blood loss may be extensive until laceration is repaired.
Monitoring	Standard monitors (p. B-1)
Complications	Bleeding

| Positioning | ✓ and pad pressure points. ✓ eyes. | ★ **NB:** peroneal nerve compression at lateral fibular head → foot drop. |

POSTOPERATIVE

Complications	Bleeding Peroneal nerve injury (2° lithotomy position)	Nerve injury manifests as foot drop and loss of sensation over dorsum of foot.
Pain management	**Intraspinal opioids**: 10 μg fentanyl **Parenteral opioids**: iv or im opioids (e.g., morphine 2-4 mg iv (up to 20 mg) or meperidine 10-20 mg iv q 10-15 min (up to 100 mg) instituted in recovery room.	Intrathecal fentanyl 10 μg given with spinal local anesthetic – enhances intraop anesthesia and provides several h postop analgesia.
Tests	Hct	

References

1. American College of Obstetricians and Gynecologists: ACOG Educational Bulletin: Postpartum hemorrhage. No 243, 1998 (replaces No 143, 1990). *Int J Gynaecol Obstet* 1998; 61(1):79-86.
2. Cunningham FG, MacDonald PC, Grant NF, eds: Obstetrical hemorrhage. In *Williams Obstetrics*, 21st edition. Appleton & Lange, Stamford, CT: 2001, 619-69.
3. Golan A, David MP: Repair of birth injuries. In *Operative Perinatology: Invasive Obstetric Techniques*. Iffy L, Charles D, eds. MacMillan, New York: 1984, 730-50.
4. Zuspan P, Quilligan EJ, eds: *Douglas-Stromme: Operative Obstetrics*, 5th edition. Appleton & Lange, New York: 1988.

CERVICAL CERCLAGE—ELECTIVE AND EMERGENT

SURGICAL CONSIDERATIONS

Description: Cervical cerclage is the reinforcement of the cervix to prevent premature cervical dilation in a patient with an incompetent cervix. With cervical incompetence, there is painless dilation of the cervix in the midtrimester of pregnancy. The membranes bulge through the cervix and rupture, followed by delivery of a severely premature infant.

An **elective cerclage** is performed prophylactically before pregnancy or usually after the first trimester of pregnancy on a patient with a Hx of cervical incompetence. If cerclage is performed before pregnancy, it may need to be removed because of spontaneous abortion or fetal anomalies. It generally is performed between 14-16 wk gestation, but may be performed as early as 10 wk gestation. An **emergent cerclage** is performed in a patient who presents in the second trimester with painless cervical dilation and/or effacement. Ultrasound is performed before the procedure to confirm viability and to r/o major congenital anomalies. An emergent cerclage should not be performed if there is advanced cervical dilation or any evidence of infection, contractions, or uterine bleeding.

There are two types of cerclage procedures generally performed: the McDonald and the Shirodkar. The **McDonald cerclage** is technically easier, and the one most commonly performed. A purse-string stitch with nonabsorbable monofilament suture is placed high around the cervix near the level of the internal os and tied at the twelve o'clock position. The end of the suture is cut long to facilitate removal. The cerclage is removed electively at term or earlier if there is rupture of membranes, persistent contractions, bleeding, or evidence of infection. The **Shirodkar cerclage** involves incising the cervix transversely, anteriorly, and posteriorly, and advancing the bladder off the cervix. A nonabsorbable monofilament suture is placed submucosally between the incisions, and the mucosa is closed, burying the stitch. A Shirodkar cerclage may be left for future pregnancies if abdominal delivery is performed.

Usual preop diagnosis: Cervical incompetence

SUMMARY OF PROCEDURE

Position	Dorsal lithotomy, with use of cane stirrups. Left lateral pelvic tilt (if performed during pregnancy); Trendelenburg
Incision	None with McDonald cerclage; transverse cervical with Shirodkar cerclage
Special instrumentation	Right-angle retractors; monofilament, nonabsorbable stitch
Unique considerations	For emergent cerclage, when prolapsing membranes are present, they may be reduced by filling the bladder and/or possibly removing amniotic fluid transabdominally.
Antibiotics	None recommended.
Surgical time	30 min-1 h (may be longer for Shirodkar cerclage)
EBL	25-50 ml (may be higher with the Shirodkar cerclage)
Postop care	PACU → ward; tocolysis with indomethacin or other agent can be considered.
Mortality	Rare
Morbidity	Morbidity is increased for emergent cerclage, especially when performed later in 2nd trimester. The McDonald cerclage is associated with less trauma and bleeding than the Shirodkar cerclage.
	Cervical trauma
	Rupture of membranes
	Chorioamnionitis
	Preterm labor
	Spontaneous abortion
Pain score	McDonald—2; Shirodkar—3

PATIENT POPULATION CHARACTERISTICS

Age range	Reproductive age
Incidence	Not uncommon
Etiology	Cervical trauma from previous vaginal delivery; cervical trauma at time of previous D&C; previous treatment for cervical dysplasia (laser therapy, cryotherapy, loop electrosurgical excision procedure [LEEP]/large loop excision of transitional zone [LLETZ], cone biopsy); congenital anomalies; idiopathic

ANESTHETIC CONSIDERATIONS

PREOPERATIVE

This is a generally fit and healthy patient population. Little will need to be done other than routine tests, unless otherwise indicated. Cerclage is usually performed between 14-24 wk of pregnancy. When performed after 20 wk, relevant physiologic changes are as discussed under Cesarean Section, p. 661. Patient may receive drugs such as ß-sympathomimetics (e.g., terbutaline), nifedipine, or indomethacin to decrease uterine irritability.

Laboratory	Hct; other tests as indicated from H&P.
Premedication	None usually. If > 18 wk gestation, precautions should be taken to decrease risk of aspiration pneumonitis, as discussed in Cesarean Section, p. 661.

INTRAOPERATIVE

Anesthetic technique: Drug exposure during the critical period of organogenesis (15-56 d) should be minimized, although no particular anesthetic techniques or agents have proven teratogenic in humans. Through an action on vitamin B_{12}, N_2O inhibits methionine syntase, which is involved in thymidine and methionine synthesis. This may explain why N_2O is teratogenic in rodents. There is no evidence, however, that N_2O is teratogenic when used for cervical cerclage or other operations in humans. Large, retrospective analysis has shown no increase in congenital abnormalities following surgery under anesthesia.[5,7] Avoid diazepam during the period of organogenesis (may → cleft lip). Ensure adequate uteroplacental perfusion and fetal oxygenation by maintaining normal maternal BP and oxyhemoglobin saturation. Use left uterine displacement after 20 wk gestation. Maternal hyperventilation and IPPV may diminish uteroplacental and umbilical blood flow. Monitoring FHR may permit optimization of fetal well-being by adjustment of anesthetic technique or patient position. Spinal anesthesia is ideal as it minimizes fetal drug exposure and provides good operating conditions. Risk of headache is low with the use of pencil-point needles (e.g., Sprotte, Whitacre). Epidural anesthesia is an appropriate alternative for this procedure. GA may be used if regional anesthesia is contraindicated.

Regional anesthesia:

Spinal	Hyperbaric 5% spinal lidocaine 70-80 mg (see comments regarding transient radicular irritation, p. 664) or bupivacaine 7-10 mg ± fentanyl 10-15 μg. Position patient to obtain T8 block. Monitor BP every min until stable, then every 3-5 min. Treat > 20% ↓ in BP or SBP < 95-100 mmHg with additional fluids and ephedrine 5-10 mg iv.

General anesthesia:

Induction	Standard induction (p. B-2). If > 18 wk gestation, rapid-sequence induction is indicated (p. B-5).
Maintenance	Standard maintenance (p. B-3). If < 15-18 wk gestation, use of LMA or mask anesthesia with O_2/N_2O/volatile agent/opioid is appropriate. If > 18 wk gestation, ET intubation will be necessary.
Emergence	If > 18 wk gestation, extubate patient when fully awake and protective airway reflexes have returned.

Blood and fluid requirements	Minimal blood loss IV: 18 ga × 1 NS/LR @ 4 mg/kg/h	1-1.5 L dextrose-free crystalloid immediately prior to regional anesthesia
Monitoring	Standard monitors (p. B-1) ± FHR monitor	Consider FHR monitoring for viable fetuses and in earlier gestation, as the FHR may indicate inadequate placental perfusion and can guide BP management.
Positioning	Left uterine displacement, if > 20 wk gestation ✓ and pad pressure points. ✓ eyes.	Left uterine displacement with a wedge under mattress should be used for pregnant patients. ★ **NB:** peroneal nerve compression at lateral fibular head → foot drop.

POSTOPERATIVE

Complications	Preterm labor Maternal dysrhythmias Hypotension Peroneal nerve injury	Observe for preterm labor in recovery area. Tocolytic agents (β-adrenergic agents) given to inhibit uterine contractions can cause maternal dysrhythmias or ↓BP. Nerve injury manifests as foot drop and loss of sensation over dorsum of foot.
Pain management	**Intraspinal opioids**: 10-15 μg fentanyl **Parenteral opioids**: iv or im opioids (e.g., morphine 2-4 mg iv (up to 20 mg) or meperidine 10-20 mg q 15 min (up to 100 mg) instituted in recovery room.	Intrathecal fentanyl given with spinal improves intraop analgesia and provides short-period postop analgesia. Risk of delayed respiration depression minimal in healthy patients.

References

1. Aldridge LM, Tunstall ME: Nitrous oxide and the fetus. A review and the results of a retrospective study of 175 cases of anaesthesia for insertion of a Shirodkar suture. *Br J Anaesth* 1986; 58(12):1348-56.
2. American College of Obstetricians and Gynecologists: Cervical cerclage, prophylactic. ACOG Criteria, Set 17. Washington, DC: ACOG, 1996.
3. American College of Obstetricians and Gynecologists: Cervical cerclage, therapeutic. ACOG Criteria, Set 18. Washington, DC: ACOG, 1996.
4. Crawford JS, Lewis M: Nitrous oxide in early human pregnancy. *Anaesthesia* 1986; 41(9):900-5.
5. Czeizel AE, Pataki T, Rockenbauer M: Reproductive outcome after exposure to surgery under anesthesia during pregnancy. *Arch Gynecol Obstet* 1998; 261(4):193-9.
6. Goodman S: Anesthesia for nonobstetric surgery in the pregnant patient. *Semin Perinatol* 2002; 26(2):136-45.
7. Mazze RI, Kallen B: Reproductive outcome after anesthesia and operation during pregnancy: a registry study of 5405 cases. *Am J Obstet Gynecol* 1989; 161(5):1178-85.
8. O'Grady JP, Gimovsky ML, McIlhargie, eds: *Operative Obstetrics*. Williams & Wilkins, Baltimore: 1995, 44-51.
9. Safra MJ, Oakley GP Jr: Association between cleft lip with or without cleft palate and prenatal exposure to diazepam. *Lancet* 1975; 2(7933):478-84.

REMOVAL OF RETAINED PLACENTA

SURGICAL CONSIDERATIONS

Description: In most deliveries, the placenta is easily removed with gentle cord traction and uterine massage. If, after 30 min, the placenta remains undelivered, **manual removal**, following either parenteral analgesia or GA, must be initiated. NTG (100-200 μg iv or 0.4 mg sublingually) may induce uterine relaxation during manual removal. A possible alternative to manual removal involves injection of 10 ml of oxytocin (10 U/ml) into the umbilical vein; however, the success of this procedure is unpredictable. A retained placental fragment may cause immediate or late postpartum hemorrhage. An ultrasound evaluation of the uterus may help in the detection of a retained fragment. If retained products are found, **curettage** is recommended. Frequently, the retained product will already have been flushed out of the uterus by brisk bleeding. In such cases, iv oxytocin, im prostaglandins or methylergonovine may be administered to contract the uterus prior to curettage.

Bleeding from a retained placenta or fragment is frequently brisk, so the anesthesiologist must be ready to administer iv fluids and O_2, and to correct any coagulopathy. Cross-matched blood must be available. Placenta accreta, if extensive, can cause profuse bleeding at delivery, and a hysterectomy is often necessary.

Oxytocin 20-40 U in 1000 ml of LR should be administered at a rate sufficient to maintain uterine tone after manual removal of the placenta or after sharp/suction curettage of a retained placental fragment.

Usual preop diagnosis: Retained placenta

SUMMARY OF PROCEDURE

Position	Dorsal lithotomy
Incision	None
Special instrumentation	Banjo curette/suction cannula
Unique considerations	IV fluids; use of blood and blood products, as needed; monitoring of VS
Antibiotics	Cefotetan 2 g iv q 12 h; 3 total doses
Surgical time	30 min
EBL	Variable—300-900 ml
Postop care	PACU → ward. Monitor for infection and further bleeding.
Mortality	Rare
Morbidity	Hemorrhage
	Endometritis
	Uterine perforation 2° curettage
	Asherman's syndrome
	Transfusion-related morbidity (hepatitis, HIV, transfusion reactions)
Pain score	5

PATIENT POPULATION CHARACTERISTICS

Age range	Reproductive age
Incidence	0.25-0.8% of vaginal deliveries
Etiology	Unknown
Associated conditions	Placenta accreta; avulsed cotyledon; succenturiate lobe

ANESTHETIC CONSIDERATIONS

PREOPERATIVE

The degree of urgency associated with these patients may vary dramatically. Some patients may be hemodynamically unstable as a result of continued bleeding in the postpartum period; others may have a retained placenta with minimal bleeding. Patient's volume status should be carefully assessed.

Respiratory	FRC returns to normal almost immediately after delivery.
	Tests: As indicated from H&P.
Cardiovascular	Restore intravascular volume prior to institution of analgesia or anesthesia. Extension of existing lumbar epidural blockade may aggravate hypovolemia and should proceed with caution. Consider possibility of placenta accreta (placental villi are attached to myometrium).

Gastrointestinal	Postpartum patients continue to be at risk for acid aspiration, although it is not known exactly when normal GI function returns. Precautions for prevention of acid aspiration should be followed as discussed in Cesarean Section, p. 661.
Neurological	Local anesthetic requirements for spinal anesthesia remain decreased after delivery.
Hematologic	Coagulopathy can develop with retained placenta if bleeding is severe and persistent. **Tests:** Hct, PT, PTT, Plt, FSP, as indicated.
Laboratory	Other tests as indicated from H&P. T&C for 2 U+ if time permits. Emergency transfusion with Type O(-) or type-specific blood may be necessary.
Premedication	Precaution should be taken to decrease risk of aspiration, as discussed in Cesarean Section, p. 661.

INTRAOPERATIVE

Anesthetic technique: Anesthesia for the removal of a retained placenta may vary from MAC to GA performed as an emergency. In the multiparous patient, MAC may be sufficient to enable the obstetrician to empty the uterus. If better analgesia and additional uterine relaxation are needed, however, then GA may be required. The incidence of retained placenta is about 1%. If intravascular volume has been restored and an existing epidural catheter is in place, the block can be extended to provide adequate anesthesia. Initiating spinal anesthesia is also an option if intravascular volume status is adequate, there is no active bleeding, and uterine relaxation is not required. Small doses of opioids and midazolam sometimes provide sufficient analgesia and sedation to allow removal of a retained placenta without compromising maternal safety. If this proves inadequate or hemorrhage is severe, however, GA with ET intubation is required. Anecdotal experience indicates that NTG in 100-200 μg iv boluses or sublingual NTG 400 μg provides uterine relaxation and delivery of retained placenta in normovolemic patients receiving iv analgesia.[4,8]

Regional anesthesia:

Spinal	For technique and monitoring of spinal anesthesia, see Cesarean Section, p. 664. Hyperbaric 5% spinal lidocaine 50-75 mg (controversial, see comments on p. 670) or bupivacaine 8-10 mg; adjust the position of operating table to obtain T8 level of anesthesia.
Epidural	For technique and monitoring, see Cesarean Section, p. 663. Administer increments of 3% 2-chloroprocaine or 2% lidocaine with 1:200,000 epinephrine until block level adequate. Additional local anesthetic as needed to ensure adequate level of anesthesia.
MAC	Titrate small doses opioid (e.g., fentanyl 25-50 μg) and midazolam 0.5-1.0 mg or ketamine 0.1 mg/kg. Sedation ± analgesia should be titrated carefully, due to the potential risk of pulmonary aspiration in the parturient with an unprotected airway. Ensure patient is awake and responsive throughout. Consider NTG 100-200 μg iv for uterine relaxation, repeated as necessary to obtain the desired effect. Transient ↓BP may follow vasodilation due to NTG, and should be treated with volume and pressors if necessary.

General anesthesia:

Induction	Preoxygenation, rapid-sequence induction with cricoid pressure (p. B-5), and hydration, as discussed in Cesarean Section (p. 662). Ketamine (1 mg/kg) is preferred for induction of hypotensive patient; but, in larger doses (> 1.5 mg/kg), it theoretically may increase uterine tone and make removal of placenta more difficult. Anesthesia with N_2O/O_2 + opioid (but no volatile agent) often permits delivery of the placenta.	
Maintenance	If uterine relaxation is necessary, administer volatile agent (> 1 MAC) or NTG (see above) until uterine tone decreases.	
Emergence	Extubation should be delayed until patient is fully awake and protective airway reflexes have returned.	
Blood and fluid requirements	Anticipate large blood loss IV: 16-18 ga × 1-2 NS/LR @ 6-8 ml/kg/h	Infuse crystalloid solution to maintain BP (1-1.5 L iv) prior to regional anesthesia. Treat ↓BP with fluids and ephedrine, and by decreasing concentration of volatile agent. Surgery is usually brief; additional muscle relaxation not usually necessary.
Monitoring	Standard monitors (p. B-1)	

| **Complications** | Bleeding | Uterine atony: Oxytocin infusion (30 U in 1 L crystalloid), uterine massage, ± methylergonovine 0.2 mg im (may → ↑BP), ± $PGF_2\alpha$ (Hemabate) 250 μg iv/im/intrauterine (may → cardiovascular collapse/bronchospasm). |
| **Positioning** | ✓ and pad pressure points.
✓ eyes. | ★ **NB:** peroneal nerve compression at lateral fibular head → foot drop. |

POSTOPERATIVE

Complications	Peroneal nerve injury (2° lithotomy position) Bleeding	Nerve injury manifested as foot drop and loss of sensation over dorsum of foot. See uterine atony, above.
Pain management	IV or im opioids, titrated to effect, as usual, instituted in recovery room.	
Tests	Hct	

References

1. Clark SL: Placenta previa and abruptio placentae. In *Maternal-Fetal Medicine: Principles and Practice*, 4th edition. Creasy RK, Resnik R, eds. WB Saunders, Philadelphia: 1999, 616-31.
2. Cunningham FG, MacDonald PC, Gant NF, eds: Obstetrical hemorrhage. In *Williams Obstetrics*, 21st edition. Appleton & Lange, Stamford CT: 2001, 619-69.
3. Decherney AH, Pernoll ML, ed: *Current Obstetric and Gynecologic Diagnosis and Treatment,* 8th edition. Appleton & Lange, Stamford CT: 1994, 575-9.
4. Desimone CA, Norris MC, Leighton BL: Intravenous nitroglycerin aids manual extraction of a retained placenta. [Letter] *Anesthesiology* 1990; 73(4):787.
5. Hughes SC, Levinson G, Rosen MA, Shnider SM, eds: *Shnider and Levinson's Anesthesia for Obstetrics,* 4th edition. Lippincott Williams & Wilkins, Philadelphia: 2002.
6. O'Grady JP, Gimovsky ML, McIlhargie, eds: *Operative Obstetrics.* Williams & Wilkins, Baltimore: 1995, 503-4.
7. Practice Guidelines for Obstetrical Anesthesia: a report by the American Society of Anesthesiologists' Task Force on Obstetrical Anesthesia. *Anesthesiology* 1999; 90:600-11.
8. Riley ET, Flanagan B, Cohen SE, Chitkara U: Intravenous nitroglycerin: a potent uterine relaxant for emergency obstetrical procedures. Report of 3 cases and review of literature. *Int J Obstet Anesth* 1996; 5:264-8.

MANAGEMENT OF UTERINE INVERSION

SURGICAL CONSIDERATIONS

Description: Uterine inversion is associated with fundal implantation of the placenta whereby a thinning of the uterine wall, together with placental separation, causes an invagination of the myometrium, resulting in inversion. Vigorous fundal pressure or cord traction also can contribute to uterine inversion, which can be complete or incomplete. **Complete inversion** results in the inverted fundus extending beyond the cervix and appearing at the vaginal introitus, whereas in an **incompletely inverted uterus**, the fundus does not extend beyond the external cervical os. Uterine inversion can cause hemorrhage and shock out of proportion to observed bleeding, and must be managed as an obstetrical emergency. An anesthesiologist must be called to the delivery room as soon as a diagnosis of uterine inversion is made. The ready availability of GA is paramount. IV access with two infusion systems and appropriate fluid resuscitation must be initiated emergently. Blood and blood products should be available for administration as indicated.

Frequently, **reinversion** can be accomplished with iv tocolytics, such as terbutaline, $MgSO_4$, and, more recently, NTG; however, GA with a volatile agent may be necessary. Three primary methods for uterine reinversion are the Johnson, Huntington and Haultain procedures. Normally, the **Johnson method** is attempted first. Persistent pressure applied to the fundus is used to elevate the uterus into the vagina. The placenta, if attached, is not removed until iv resuscitation has been initiated, and iv tocolytics (or anesthesia) have been administered. Oxytocin is given when the uterus has been reinverted. Laparotomy must be performed if reinversion with the Johnson method is unsuccessful. The **Huntington procedure** involves grasping the round ligaments and applying upward traction on them, while an assistant exerts upward pressure on the uterus via a hand in the vagina. If the inverted uterus is trapped below the cervical ring, the **Haultain procedure** is used. This procedure involves making a longitudinal fundal incision posteriorly to allow easier reinversion of the fundus.

Usual preop diagnosis: Uterine inversion

SUMMARY OF PROCEDURES

	Manual Reinversion	Huntington/Haultain
Position	Dorsal lithotomy	Supine
Incision	None	Pfannenstiel's or midline longitudinal
Unique considerations	Prompt O_2 and iv fluid resuscitation; use of blood and blood products as necessary.	⇐
Antibiotics	Cefotetan 2 g iv q 12 h; total 3 doses	⇐
Surgical time	30 min	1-2 h
EBL	150-4000 ml	⇐
Postop care	± ICU. ARDS may necessitate mechanical ventilation. Monitor for acute renal failure 2° hypoxia and hypovolemia.	⇐
Mortality	Rare	⇐
Morbidity	Febrile morbidity	⇐
	Clinical shock	⇐
	Infectious morbidity from blood transfusion	⇐
Pain score	5	7

PATIENT POPULATION CHARACTERISTICS

Age range	Reproductive age
Incidence	1/2000-6000 deliveries
Etiology	Unknown
Associated conditions	Fundal implantation of the placenta; primiparity; intrapartum oxytocin; placenta accreta; therapy of preeclampsia with $MgSO_4$; macrosomic fetus

---

ANESTHETIC CONSIDERATIONS

PREOPERATIVE

These patients often present in shock out of proportion to blood loss; and immediate resuscitation may be necessary. Since patient condition will improve as soon as the uterus is replaced, however, surgical treatment should not be delayed.

Respiratory	FRC returns to normal almost immediately after delivery. **Tests:** As indicated from H&P.
Cardiovascular	Massive hemorrhage and pain usual with complete inversion. Prior to induction, insert large-bore iv and rapidly infuse fluids, including colloid, to treat ↓BP. Blood transfusion may be necessary, although is seldom available until after surgery.
Gastrointestinal	Postpartum patients continue to be at risk for acid aspiration, although it is not known exactly when normal GI function returns. Precautions for prevention of acid aspiration should be followed as discussed in Cesarean Section, p. 661.
Neurological	Local anesthetic requirements for spinal anesthesia remain decreased after delivery.
Laboratory	Hct; Plt; other tests as indicated from H&P. T&C for 2 U; keep 2 U ahead.
Premedication	Na citrate 30 ml po within 30 min of induction. If time permits, other agents to decrease risk of aspiration pneumonitis, as discussed in Cesarean Section, p. 661.

INTRAOPERATIVE

Anesthetic technique: Attempted uterine replacement and induction of anesthesia should not await intravascular volume replacement. Bleeding usually stops when uterus is replaced. IV NTG is very effective in providing uterine relaxation to facilitate replacement, and can be given immediately in the patient's room. (See p. 618 for dosages.) Other tocolytics, such as terbutaline or Mg^{++}, also may help. **Do not give oxytocin before uterine replacement.** Sometimes, however, GETA is required, often with increasing concentrations of volatile agents to facilitate uterine replacement. If regional anesthesia (e.g., epidural or spinal) was used for delivery, replacement of uterus may be accomplished with little further anesthetic intervention, with or without NTG. If regional anesthesia was not used for delivery, iv analgesia with small doses of fentanyl (25-50 μg iv) occasionally allows reduction.

Induction	Rapid-sequence induction (p. B-5) with ketamine (1.0 mg/kg) preferred. Higher dose may adversely increase uterine tone.	
Maintenance	Halothane, isoflurane, and sevoflurane are all effective uterine relaxants, but sevoflurane is most rapidly eliminated. ↓BP should be treated with fluids + vasopressors.	
Emergence	Extubation should be delayed until patient is fully awake and protective airway reflexes have returned.	
Blood and fluid requirements	Significant blood loss IV: 16-18 ga × 1 or 2	Possible continued blood loss after reduction of uterus, due to uterine atony.
Monitoring	Standard monitors (p. B-1)	Arterial line may be useful, if time allows.
Positioning	✓ and pad pressure points. ✓ eyes.	
Complications	Uterine atony Massive blood loss	Rx: ↓volatile anesthetic concentrations. Oxytocin infusion, uterine massage, ± methylergonovine 0.2 mg im (may →↑BP) ± PGF$_2\alpha$ (Hemabate) 250 μg iv/im/intrauterine (may → cardiovascular collapse/bronchospasm).

POSTOPERATIVE

Complications	Bleeding
Pain management	Parenteral opiates
Tests	Hct

References

1. American College of Obstetricians and Gynecologists: ACOG Educational Bulletin: Postpartum hemorrhage. No 243, 1998 (replaces No 143, 1990). *Int J Gynaecol Obstet* 1998; 61(1):79-86.
2. Bowes W: Clinical aspects of normal and abnormal labor. In *Maternal-Fetal Medicine: Principles and Practice,* 4th edition. Creasy RK, Resnik R, Bralow L, eds. WB Saunders, Philadelphia: 1999, 548-49.
3. Cunningham FG, MacDonald PC, Gant NF, eds: *Williams Obstetrics,* 21st edition. Appleton & Lange, Stamford CT: 2001.
4. Hostetler DR, Bosworth MF: Uterine inversion: a life threatening obstetric emergency. *J Am Board Fam Pract* 2000; 13(2): 120-3.
5. Hughes SC, Levinson G, Rosen MA, Shnider SM, eds: *Shnider and Levinson's Anesthesia for Obstetrics,* 4th edition. Lippincott Williams & Wilkins, Philadelphia: 2002.
6. Riley ET, Flanagan B, Cohen SE, Chitkara J: Intravenous nitroglycerin: a potent relaxant for emergency obstetrical procedures. Review of literature and reports of 3 cases. *Int J Obstet Anesth* 1996; 5:264-8.

Surgeon

Camran R. Nezhat, MD

8.4 LAPAROSCOPIC PROCEDURES FOR GYNECOLOGIC SURGERY

Anesthesiologist

Lindsey Vokach-Brodsky, MBChB, FFARCSI

LAPAROSCOPIC SURGERY FOR ENDOMETRIOSIS

SURGICAL CONSIDERATIONS

Description: There are numerous theories about the etiology of endometriosis, including: (1) The peritoneal cavity is seeded with endometrial cells via the fallopian tubes during menses.[7] (2) Totipotential cells in the peritoneal cavity are transformed by hormonal exposure into endometrial cells. (3) Endometrial cells are transported intravascularly or via lymphatics to ectopic sites, where they respond to hormonal stimuli (this theory has been used to explain the presence of endometriosis in the brain and pleura). (4) Decreased cytotoxic response of the immune system suggests that it is a failure of natural killer-cell activity to eliminate ectopic endometrial cells. (5) It is an inherited disorder, since the incidence of endometriosis is higher in first-degree relatives. Intervention usually is indicated for intractable pain, infertility, or impaired function of the gastrointestinal (GI) or genitourinary (GU) tracts. GU endometriosis may range from superficial involvement of peritoneum overlying the ureters and bladder to frankly invasive endometriosis penetrating through to bladder mucosa. Scarring and fibrosis can → ureteral obstruction and hydronephrosis with renal insufficiency. Patients with GI endometriosis may have thickening of the rectovaginal septum, suggesting obliteration of the posterior cul-de-sac or rectosigmoid involvement. Adhesions may make rectovaginal examination difficult or painful. Pelvic structures may be immobile, suggesting adhesions are fixing bowel or bladder to the uterus. Sigmoidoscopy should be performed to r/o malignancy and to determine whether endometriosis has penetrated through to the bowel mucosa.

Two treatment approaches can be taken. **Hysterectomy** and **bilateral salpingo-oophorectomy (BSO)** may be indicated for patients with severe symptoms who have not responded to medical or conservative surgical treatment and who do not desire fertility (see Laparoscopic Hysterectomy, p. 690). **Bilateral oophorectomy** might be necessary to eliminate the estrogen that sustains and stimulates the ectopic endometrium.[3] Conservative surgery is indicated for women who desire pregnancy and whose disease is responsible for their symptoms of pain or infertility. Though seldom curative, surgery improves fertility and offers at least temporary pain relief. **Laparoscopy** (Fig 8.4-1) is the most appropriate surgical technique for the diagnosis and treatment of endometriosis. Data from animal and clinical studies suggest that laparoscopic surgery is more effective for adhesiolysis, causes fewer de novo adhesions than laparotomy and reduces impairment of tuboovarian function.[8] Special consideration must be given to the patient's past Hx of abdominal or pelvic surgery, pelvic inflammatory disease (PID) and endometriosis, as this will affect the choice of surgical approach. Ovarian endometriosis is common and can be challenging to diagnose and treat. It can be divided into Type I (primary endometriomas or small cysts measuring > 3 cm on the ovarian surface) or Type II (secondary endometriomas, usually functional [e.g., follicular] in origin, which become enlarged to > 3 cm). Regardless of classification, it is critical to remove all endometriotic lesions to prevent exacerbation and recurrence.

Bladder endometriosis: If the lesions are superficial, **hydrodissection** and **vaporization** are adequate for removal. Using hydrodissection, the areolar tissue between the serosa and muscularis beneath the implants is dissected. The lesion is circumscribed with a laser and fluid is injected into the resulting defect. The lesion is grasped with forceps and dissected with the laser. Traction allows the small blood vessels supplying the surrounding tissue to be coagulated as the lesion is resected. Frequent irrigation is necessary to remove char, ascertain the depth of vaporization, and ensure that the lesion does not involve the muscularis and mucosa. Endometriosis extending to the muscularis but without mucosal involvement can be treated laparoscopically, and any residual or deeper lesions may be treated successfully with hormonal therapy. When endometriosis involves **full bladder-wall thickness**, the lesion is excised and the bladder reconstructed in one layer.[2] Simultaneous cystoscopy is performed and bilateral ureteral catheters are inserted. The bladder dome is held near the midline with the grasping forceps and the endometriotic nodule is excised 5 mm beyond the lesions. An incision is made with the CO_2 laser, using the suction-irrigating probe as a backstop. The specimen is removed from the abdominal cavity with a long grasping forceps. The lesion is regrasped and removed with the laparoscope as one unit. CO_2 distends the bladder cavity, allowing excellent observation of its interior. After again identifying the ureters and examining the bladder mucosa, the bladder is closed. Cystoscopy is performed to identify possible leaks. The duration of laparoscopic segmental cystectomy is ~35 min. Patients are discharged the following day and instructed to take trimethoprim and sulfamethoxazole for 2 wk. The Foley catheter is removed 7-14 d later, and cystograms are made.

GI/GU endometriosis: In a patient with no Hx of pelvic surgery, the **direct-trocar insertion method** may be used with an intraumbilical incision. The incision is made within the umbilicus because this is the anatomical area closest to the fascia and peritoneum and involves the least risk of injury to retroperitoneal structures.[5] Once the incision is made, the trocar is placed through the skin incision. Using an intraumbilical incision and inserting the trocar at 90° facilitates access to the abdominal cavity and decreases the risk of aortocaval injury. This technique of direct-trocar insertion may not be recommended for patients who have had prior laparotomy or laparoscopy that revealed adhesive disease. After insufflation of the abdomen with CO_2, assessment of intraabdominal and pelvic structures is made. A second skin incision is made 2-3 cm above the symphysis. A Foley catheter should be in place throughout the procedure to allow continuous drainage of the bladder, thereby

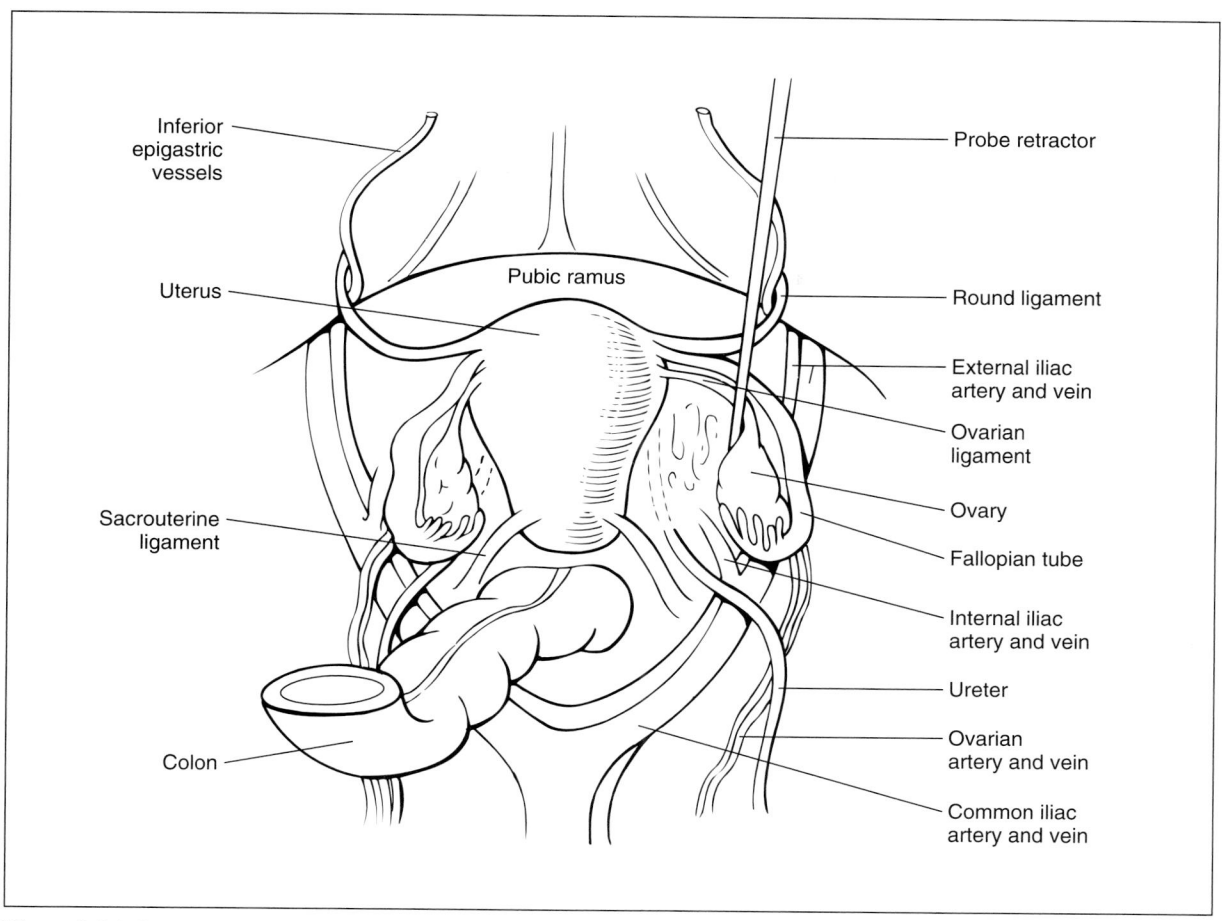

Figure 8.4-1. Laparoscopic view of the female pelvis.

reducing the likelihood of trocar injury to the bladder. A 5 mm trocar is placed under direct visualization, with attention to peritoneal vessels and bladder. Two lateral ports are placed in a similar fashion, taking care to avoid the inferior epigastric vessels. The suction irrigator, a blunt grasper, and the bipolar cautery are placed into the trocars. Filmy adhesions of the bowel or omentum to the anterior abdominal wall or uterus are lysed using CO_2 laser, bipolar cautery, monopolar scissors, or hydrodissection. Treatment of peritoneal endometriosis ranges from laser ablation of superficial peritoneal implants to excision and dissection of deeply embedded, fibrotic areas. Scarring from endometriosis that has penetrated the peritoneum to involve deeper structures destroys normal surgical planes and distorts anatomical relationships. Identification of structures and landmarks is critical before attempting to treat the peritoneal disease. At laparoscopy, normal anatomic relationships along the pelvic sidewall may appear distorted. Because scarring from endometriosis may change these relationships, patients are at risk for accidental ureteral or vascular injury at the time of surgery. Identification of ureters and blood vessels is critical prior to treatment of pelvic sidewall disease. Although different modalities have been used, hydrodissection and high-power superpulse or ultrapulse CO_2 lasers are the best options for endometriosis treatment.[2] Because the CO_2 laser does not penetrate water, this fluid backstop allows the surgeon to work on selected tissue with a greater safety margin.

Ovarian endometriosis: A Type I endometrioma of < 2 cm is vaporized using laser or bipolar coagulation. Larger Type I lesions may require excision using scissors or biopsy forceps. For Type IIA endometriomas, the procedure begins with lysis of periovarian adhesions using laser or monopolar scissors. The ovarian cortex is evaluated, the endometrioma cyst is identified, the cyst wall is perforated (using laser or scissors), and an irrigation device is inserted to assess cyst contents and wall. Suspicious areas are biopsied and sent for frozen-section analysis. A plane is developed between the cyst wall and ovary by grasping the wall and separating it from ovarian stroma, using traction and countertraction. Difficult areas where endometriosis has embedded through the cyst wall, disrupting the planes, require hydrodissection and bipolar cautery to control bleeding vessels in the ovarian bed. In some cases, it is necessary to remove a portion of the ovary attached to the cyst wall until a plane can be found. Redundant ovarian tissue is approximated with low-power laser or electrosurgery to avoid adhesions. Suturing should be avoided; but, if necessary, 4-0 polydioxanone sutures can be placed to close the defect.

Usual preop diagnosis: Endometriosis

SUMMARY OF PROCEDURES

	Ovarian Endometriosis Procedure	GI/GU Endometriosis Procedure
Position	Dorsal lithotomy, legs in stirrups ± steep Trendelenburg	⇐
Incision	Intraumbilical; lateral suprapubic; or midline suprapubic	⇐
Special instrumentation	CO_2 laser or other cutting instrument; bipolar Kleppinger forceps; suction irrigator	⇐ ± Ureteral stenting, cystoscope, sigmoidoscope
Antibiotics	Cefotetan 1 g iv	⇐
Surgical time	45 min–3 h, depending on extent of disease	1-4 h
Closing considerations	Close fascia of all 10-12 mm ports; subcuticular closure for 5 mm trocar sites	⇐
EBL	Minimal	⇐
Postop care	Mild disease: PACU → home; otherwise, discharge on POD 1 (peritoneal disease).	Ambulate POD 0; Foley catheter.
Mortality	0.08-0.2/1000[5]	⇐
Morbidity	Overall complication rate: 2.5% Conversion to laparoscopy: 0.42% VAE (CO_2 embolism) Peroneal nerve damage Vascular damage Bowel injury: Rare Urinary tract injury: Rare	Urinary tract injury
Pain score	4-8	4-8

PATIENT POPULATION CHARACTERISTICS

Age range	Reproductive age	20s–40s
Incidence	10-15% of all reproductive age women/25% of all gynecologic laparotomies	1-11% of women with known endometriosis
Etiology	Numerous theories (see above).	Extensive disseminated endometriosis
Associated conditions	Infertility; pelvic pain; bladder or bowel symptoms; HTN (2° to urinary tract involvement); GI tract involvement (3-7%)	Pelvic pain; GI or GU symptoms

ANESTHETIC CONSIDERATIONS

See Anesthetic Considerations following Laparoscopic Hysterectomy, p. 692.

References

1. Chantigian RC, Chantigian PDM: Anesthesia for laparoscopy. In *Complications of Laparoscopy and Hysteroscopy.* Corfman RS, Diamond MP, DeCherney A, eds. Blackwell Scientific Publications, Cambridge: 1993, 11.

2. Nezhat C, et al: *Operative Gynecologic Laparoscopy: Principles and Techniques,* 2nd edition. McGraw Hill, New York: 2000.

3. Nezhat F, et al: Videolaseroscopy for oophorectomy. *Am J Obstet Gynecol* 1991; 165:1323-30.

4. Nezhat F, Kalir T: Comparative immunohistochemical studies of endometriosis lesions and endometriotic cysts. *Fertil Steril* 2002; 78:820-4.

5. Querleu D, Chapron C: Complications of gynecologic laparoscopic surgery. *Curr Opin Obstet Gynecol* 1995; 7:257-61.

6. Samper ER, et al: Colonic endometriosis, its clinical spectrum. *South Med J* 1984; 77:912.

7. Samson JA: Peritoneal endometriosis due to menstrual dissemination of endometrial tissue into the pelvic cavity. *Am J Obstet Gynecol* 1927; 14:422.

8. Schenken SR, et al: Reoperation after initial treatment of endometriosis with conservative surgery. *Am J Obstet Gynecol* 1978; 131:416.

LAPAROSCOPIC SURGERY FOR ECTOPIC PREGNANCY

SURGICAL CONSIDERATIONS

Description: Ectopic pregnancy is defined as a pregnancy occurring outside the uterus. The majority of ectopic pregnancies occur in the fallopian tubes (95-97%); the remainder occur in the cornua (2-4%), ovary (0.1%), cervix (0.1%), or abdomen (0.03%). Ectopic pregnancy remains a leading cause of maternal morbidity and mortality. Predisposing factors include Hx of tubal ligation or other tubal surgery, pelvic inflammatory disease (PID), IUD use, and Hx of in vitro fertilization (IVF) or other treatments for infertility. Other associations include developmental anomalies of the Müllerian system, intrauterine polyps, or myomas.

Patients present with lower quadrant pain, vaginal bleeding, and an ↑β-hCG. Shoulder pain from subdiaphragmatic intraperitoneal blood is a less frequent finding. Treatment options for an asymptomatic ectopic gestation include operative laparoscopy or a trial of medical management with intramuscular methotrexate. In cases where the size of the ectopic pregnancy is too large for conservative medical management (> 3.5 cm), and the patient is hemodynamically stable, operative management is essential.[3] Hypotension or an acute abdomen in the presence of a positive β-hCG value are strongly suggestive of rupture and require expeditious surgical intervention.

Access to the abdomen is obtained in the usual fashion (e.g., through a Veress needle or direct-trocar insertion, followed by insufflation and insertion of accessory trocars). Ruptured tubal pregnancies can be treated endoscopically if the bleeding has ceased or can be controlled. Actively bleeding vessels are identified and cauterized, and forced irrigation is used to dislodge clots and trophoblastic tissue. Depending on their size, the products of conception (POCs) are removed through either a 5 or 10 mm trocar sleeve or placed into an endoscopic bag for removal; or a minilaparotomy can be performed. Copious irrigation should follow to ensure hemostasis and identify and remove any remaining trophoblastic tissue. Trophoblast is invasive, and residual tissue may implant into bowel, bladder, peritoneum, or other abdominal structures and cause significant future morbidity.

For an unruptured ectopic pregnancy, the tube is identified and stabilized using laparoscopic forceps. To minimize bleeding, 5-7 ml of a solution of 50 U vasopressin in 100 ml NS is injected into the mesosalpinx just below the ectopic pregnancy and over the antimesenteric surface of the tubal segment containing the gestation. Intravascular injection of vasopressin solution can precipitate acute arterial HTN, bradycardia, or even death; therefore, care must be taken to avoid such injection. A linear incision is made over the thinnest portion of the tube. The pregnancy usually protrudes through the incision, and forceful irrigation will dislodge the gestation from its implantation site. Oozing from the tube is common, but usually ceases spontaneously.

In a ruptured tubal or isthmic pregnancy, resection of the tubal segment containing the gestation is preferable to salpingostomy. **Segmental tubal resection** is performed with bipolar electrosurgery, laser (KTP, argon, Nd:YAG, or CO_2), sutures, or stapling devices. Similarly, **total salpingectomy** can be performed by progressive coagulation and cutting the mesosalpinx, which is separated from the uterus using bipolar coagulation and scissors or laser. The isolated tube segment containing the ectopic pregnancy is removed intact or in sectioned parts through the 10 mm trocar sleeve. At the completion of the procedure, the abdomen is irrigated and inspected and incisions are closed in the usual fashion.

Usual preop diagnosis: Ectopic pregnancy

SUMMARY OF PROCEDURE

Position	Dorsal lithotomy, legs in Allen universal stirrups, steep Trendelenburg
Incision	Intraumbilical, lateral suprapubic, midline suprapubic
Special instrumentation	CO_2 laser; laparoscopic instrumentation
Unique considerations	Intraperitoneal hemorrhage and hemodynamic instability are potential risks. Patient should be cross-matched for 2 U PRBCs.
Antibiotics	Cefotetan 1 g iv
Surgical time	45 min-2 h
Closing considerations	Fascia of 10-12 mm trocar sites closed in layers. Smaller 5 mm ports closed in a subcuticular fashion.
EBL	100 ml – severe hemorrhage, if ruptured.
Postop care	The patient may be admitted overnight for observation. Quantitative β-hCG should be followed until undetectable, to r/o the possibility of retained trophoblastic tissue.
Mortality	5/1000. For any laparoscopy: 0.08-0.2/1000.
Morbidity	Overall complication rate: 2.5% Hemorrhage and need for transfusion

Morbidity, **cont.**	Conversion to laparotomy: 4.2/1000 Air embolism: Rare Unintended puncture of a viscus: Rare Puncture of a major vessel: Rare Insufflation of incorrect site: Rare
Pain score	3-5

PATIENT POPULATION CHARACTERISTICS

Age range	Reproductive-age females
Incidence	1/100 pregnancies
Etiology	Distorted tubal or uterine anatomy
Associated conditions	Hx of PID; endometriosis; tubal damage; IUD; IVF

ANESTHETIC CONSIDERATIONS

See Anesthetic Considerations following Laparoscopic Hysterectomy, p. 692.

References

1. Chantigian RC, Chantigian PDM: Anesthesia for laparoscopy. In *Complications of Laparoscopy and Hysteroscopy.* Corfman RS, Diamond MP, DeCherney A, eds. Blackwell Scientific Publications, Cambridge: 1993, 11.
2. Luciano AA: Ectopic pregnancy. In *Current Therapy in Obstetrics and Gynecology.* Quilligan EJ, Zuspan PP, eds. WB Saunders, Philadelphia: 1990, 226.
3. Nezhat C, Nezhat F, Luciano AA, et al: *Operative Gynecologic Laparoscopy.* McGraw Hill, New York: 2000.
4. Querleu D, Chapron C: Complications of gynecologic laparoscopic surgery. *Curr Opin Obstet Gynecol* 1995; 7:257-61.

LAPAROSCOPIC MYOMECTOMY

SURGICAL CONSIDERATIONS

Description: Uterine myomata or fibroids are the most common uterine neoplasm, affecting ~20-25% of women of reproductive age.[1,6] Their growth is influenced by many factors, such as estrogen acting alone or synergistically with growth hormone and human placental lactogen in pregnancy. The severity of symptoms depends on the number, size, and location of the tumors. Symptoms may include constipation, pelvic or abdominal pressure, urinary frequency and, most commonly, menorrhagia. While leiomyomata are seldom the cause of infertility, there is a link between fibroids, fetal wastage, and premature delivery.[1] Patients present with profound anemia from menorrhagia or menometrorrhagia, the usual indications for surgery. Other indications include rapidly changing size, ureteral compression, hydroureter, or hydronephrosis and size > 12 wk. Size, number, and location are the primary factors that will determine surgical approach to myomata.

The simplest approach is a combination of **laparoscopy** and **minilaparotomy** for removal of myomas. This approach limits operative time. Three major objectives of laparoscopic myomectomy are: minimizing blood loss, which can be severe; minimizing postop adhesion formation; and maintaining uterine-wall integrity. Preop treatment with GnRH analogues to shrink fibroids has been shown to decrease the size of the myoma and reduce the need for transfusion.[2,5] Although myomectomy is performed to preserve fertility, postop adhesion formation often jeopardizes this goal. This can be minimized by using a single, vertical, anterior midline uterine incision.[3]

The abdomen is entered in the usual fashion for laparoscopy (e.g., through Veress needle or direct trocar insertion, followed by insufflation and insertion of accessory trocars). To reduce blood loss in pedunculated myomas, diluted vasopressin (3-5 ml) is injected into the base of the stalk where it joins the uterine wall. IV vasopressin can cause ↑BP, myocardial ischemia, dysrhythmias, or cardiac arrest, and should be avoided. The pedicle is coagulated with the bipolar forceps and cut with CO_2 laser or scissors. For subserosal or intramural myomas, diluted vasopressin is injected between the myometrium and the myoma pseudocapsule. An incision is made on the serosa overlying the myoma using the CO_2 laser or monopolar needle. As the incision is made, the myometrium is retracted away from graspers to expose the tumor. Vessels are coagulated prior to cutting. After the myoma is removed, the myoma bed is irrigated with LR, and bleeding points are coagulated again. After closure, the serosa is irrigated with LR. An adhesion barrier may be placed over the incision site to prevent future adhesion formation. Uteroperitoneal fistulae may follow laparoscopic myomectomy, because meticulous laparoscopic approximation of all layers of the myometrium is impossible. The use of electrocoagulation for hemostasis inside the uterine defect also may increase this risk.

Removal of the specimen is frequently the most challenging aspect of the operation. The myoma can be removed either by **morcellation of the specimen** or by extending the suprapubic incision. Alternatively, **posterior culdotomy** may be performed and the myoma removed via the vagina. A retractor is placed in the vagina and the laser is used to cut along the tented vaginal mucosa. After the myoma is removed, the incision can be closed using laparoscopic suturing. Minilaparotomy or culdotomy facilitate removal but increase postop wound complication risks, such as infection or hernia formation. After myoma removal, the abdomen and pelvis are irrigated, the patient is taken out of the Trendelenburg position, and any fluid that might have tracked into the upper abdomen is suctioned. The ports are closed in the usual fashion.

Usual preop diagnosis: Uterine myoma, fibroids

SUMMARY OF PROCEDURE

Position	Dorsal lithotomy; steep Trendelenburg to move bowel out of operating field
Incisions	Infraumbilical, 5 mm lateral and 5-12 mm midline suprapubic; minilaparotomy via extension of suprapubic incision or posterior culdotomy for removal of large myomata
Special instrumentation	CO_2 laser; laparoscopic instrumentation
Unique considerations	For large myomata: pretreatment with GnRH analogues (3-6 mo). Intraop injection of dilute vasopressin (1 IU in 100 ml LR) into myometrium to ↓ bleeding.
Antibiotics	Cefotetan 1 g iv
Surgical time	1-3 h
Closing considerations	Close fascia of all 10-12 mm ports; 5 mm ports are closed in a subcuticular fashion. Fascial closure essential in minilaparotomy. Posterior culdotomy requires laparoscopic suturing or vaginal closure.
EBL	100-600 ml
Postop care	1-2 d hospital stay; early ambulation; clear liquids POD 0; gradually advance diet after discharge home.
Mortality	0.08-0.2/1000
Morbidity	Rates: 1.3-5.9/100
	Peroneal nerve damage from positioning
	Severe bleeding with possible need for transfusion
	Uteroperitoneal fistulae
	Infertility
	Hyponatremia from peritoneal absorption of irrigant
	Air embolism
	Puncture of a major vessel
	Insufflation in the wrong place
	Need for emergent laparotomy
	Uterine rupture in pregnancy: 2%
	Adhesion formation
Pain score	4-6

PATIENT POPULATION CHARACTERISTICS

Age range	Reproductive-age women; myomas shrink in postmenopausal women and are less symptomatic.
Incidence	20-25% of all women
Etiology	Benign transformation and proliferation of a single smooth-muscle cell
Associated conditions	Menorrhagia; anemia; ureteral obstruction; pelvic pain or pressure

ANESTHETIC CONSIDERATIONS

See Anesthetic Considerations following Laparoscopic Hysterectomy, p. 692.

References

1. Buttram VC, Reiter RC: Uterine leiomyomata: etiology, symptomatology and management. *Fertil Steril* 1981; 36:433.
2. Friedman AJ, Rein NS, Harrison-Atlas D, et al: A randomized, placebo-controlled, double blind study evaluating leuprolide acetate depot treatment before myomectomy. *Fertil Steril* 1989; 52:728.
3. Operative Laparoscopy Study Group: Postoperative adhesion development after operative laparoscopy: evaluation at early second-look procedures. *Fertil Steril* 1991; 55:700-4.
4. Querleu D, Chapron C: Complications of gynecologic laparoscopic surgery. *Curr Opin Obstet Gynecol* 1995; 7:257-61.
5. Shaw RW: Mechanism of LHRH analogue action in uterine fibroids. *Horm Res* 1989; 32:150.
6. Vollenhoven BJ, Lawrence AS, Healy DL: Uterine fibroids: a clinical review. *Br J Obstet Gynecol* 1990; 97:285.

LAPAROSCOPIC HYSTERECTOMY

SURGICAL CONSIDERATIONS

Description: Hysterectomy is the second most common gynecologic operation, after cesarean section. The indications for **hysterectomy ± salpingo-oophorectomy** include: leiomyomata (38%); malignancy (15%); ovarian tumors (10%); abnormal bleeding (13%); adenomyosis (9%); pelvic pain or adhesions (5%); endometriosis (3%); and uterine prolapse (1%).[3] Other less common indications include parametrial disease, pelvic infection, and complications of pregnancy and delivery. Selection of surgical approach to hysterectomy requires consideration of the patient's age, medical Hx, Hx of prior pelvic surgery, the presence or possibility of adhesions or endometriosis, uterine size, adnexal pathology, and the presence or amount of uterine prolapse.

Laparoscopic hysterectomy offers the advantages of excellent visibility and exposure. There is shorter recovery time, rapid return of bowel function, less pain, and a lower wound complication rate. The disadvantages are higher cost and the level of surgical expertise required.[2] The most commonly performed procedure is the **laparoscopically assisted vaginal hysterectomy** (LAVH), in which hysterectomy is begun by laparoscopy, but four or more steps are performed vaginally.[2] Variants include: **total laparoscopic hysterectomy** (TLH), in which all steps are performed laparoscopically; **subtotal laparoscopic hysterectomy** (SLH), a supracervical hysterectomy; and **vaginally assisted laparoscopic hysterectomy** (VALH), in which four steps are completed laparoscopically and the procedure is completed vaginally. Combinations are usually performed, depending on findings at surgery. A mechanical and antibiotic bowel preparation is advised. Consultation with a urologist, bowel surgeon, and oncologist are sought as necessary.

Access to the abdomen is obtained in the usual fashion (e.g., through a Veress needle or direct-trocar insertion, followed by insufflation and insertion of accessory trocars). Diagnostic laparoscopy is performed, adhesions lysed, and any endometriosis treated. The course of the ureters is noted through the peritoneum until they are no longer visible at the level of the cardinal ligaments. When ureters cannot be identified clearly because of severe scarring or endometriosis, they are dissected retroperitoneally, and the dissection proceeds as for a radical hysterectomy. At the cardinal ligaments, the peritoneum is opened above or below the ureter and hydrodissection is performed to lift the peritoneum off the ureter without damaging it. Routine hysterectomy using hydrodissection to identify tissue planes and limit blood loss can be performed following identification of the ureters.

If the ovaries are to be spared, the uteroovarian ligament, proximal tube and mesosalpinx are cauterized and cut progressively, and the posterior leaf of the broad ligament is opened with hydrodissection. The bladder is dissected free from the cervix and uterus; and, if bladder trauma is suspected, 5 ml of indigo carmine injected iv (possible ↑BP) may help identify the site of perforation. Next, the uterine vessels are identified, noted to be free of ureter, desiccated, and cut. At the level of the cardinal ligaments, the ureters and descending branches of the uterine artery are close to one another and the cervix; therefore, cardinal ligament dissection and cautery must be precise to prevent bleeding and ureteral injury. A small uterus can be removed easily through the vagina. In benign disease, a large uterus can be morcellated and then removed segmentally through the vagina. Pneumoperitoneum will be lost during this procedure, and care must be taken to keep instruments free of bowel or other abdominal structures as this occurs.

If the procedure is to be completed entirely laparoscopically, pneumoperitoneum can be maintained by placing a glove containing two 4" × 4" sponges in the vagina. The vaginal wall is cut circumferentially, and the uterus is pulled to mid vagina, but not removed, to preserve the pneumoperitoneum. Alternatively, the uterus may be morcellated and removed through a 10 mm suprapubic port, or placed in a laparoscopic specimen bag. The suprapubic incision also may be extended into a minilaparotomy incision for specimen removal. The vaginal cuff is closed transversely using laparoscopic sutures, and any coexisting cystocele or enterocele is repaired. Once the uterus is removed and the vaginal cuff closed, the pelvic and abdominal cavities are reevaluated, irrigated, and cleared of blood and debris. The skin and fascia are closed in the usual fashion.

Variant procedure: In patients with severe rectovaginal and vesical endometriosis, the retroperitoneal space is entered using hydrodissection, and the external iliac vessels, hypogastric artery, and ureter are identified. In cases where extensive dissection and resultant blood loss is anticipated, coagulation or ligation of the hypogastric artery with laparoscopic clips may be performed. Endometriosis of the rectum, rectovaginal septum, and uterosacral ligaments is treated by vaporization, excision, or a combination of these. Sigmoidoscopy with concurrent laparoscopic visualization of the pelvis may be necessary to r/o the presence of incidental enterotomy. Cystoscopy with ureteral stenting also may be indicated to identify anatomy. (Treatment of bladder and bowel endometriosis have been described in Laparoscopic Surgery for Endometriosis, p. 684.) Once the ureter is identified along its course and entry into the bladder, the uterine vessels are retracted medially and separated from the ureter using a CO_2 laser. The uterus is retracted medially and the ureter laterally as the cardinal and uterosacral ligaments are cauterized and cut with the ureter under direct visualization. After these vascular pedicles have been ligated and all endometriosis treated, the hysterectomy and specimen removal proceed as described above.

Usual preop diagnosis: leiomyomata; malignancy; ovarian tumors; abnormal bleeding; adenomyosis; pelvic pain or adhesions; endometriosis; uterine prolapse; parametrial disease; pelvic infection; complications of pregnancy and delivery

SUMMARY OF PROCEDURE

Position	Dorsal lithotomy; legs in Allen universal stirrups; steep Trendelenburg
Incisions	Intraumbilical; bilateral suprapubic; midline suprapubic (5 or 10 mm)
Special instrumentation	CO_2 laser; laparoscopic instruments
Unique considerations	Extensive ureterolysis and treatment of endometriosis may require addition of cystoscopy, ureteral stent placement, and/or sigmoidoscopy.
Antibiotics	Cefotetan 1 g iv
Surgical time	2-6 h. Operative time is increased in cases of extensive adhesiolysis or endometriosis.
Closing considerations	Close fascia of all 10-12 mm ports; 5 mm trocar sites closed in a subcuticular fashion. Minilaparotomy closure if needed.
EBL	100-800 ml, depending on anatomy and difficulty of dissection
Postop care	Clear liquid diet; ambulate POD 1.
Mortality	0.08-0.2/1000
Morbidity	Overall complication rate: 2.5%
	Conversion to laparotomy: 4.2/1000
	Air embolism: Rare
	Peroneal nerve damage from positioning: Rare
	Unintended puncture of a viscous: Rare
	Puncture of a major vessel: Rare
	Insufflation of incorrect site: Rare
	Urinary and ureteral trauma, including fistulae: 1.6%
Pain score	6-9

PATIENT POPULATION CHARACTERISTICS

Age range	30s–70s
Incidence	20% of women < 40 yr; 37% of women < age 65[6]
Etiology	See Associated Conditions.
Associated conditions	Myomata; abnormal uterine bleeding; adenomyosis; malignancy; pelvic pain; endometriosis

References

1. Chantigian RC, Chantigian PDM: Anesthesia for laparoscopy. In *Complications of Laparoscopy and Hysteroscopy.* Corfman RS, Diamond MP, DeCherney A, eds. Blackwell Scientific Publications, Cambridge: 1993, 11.
2. Nezhat C, Nezhat F, Luciano AA, et al: *Operative Gynecologic Laparoscopy.* McGraw Hill, New York: 2000.
3. Nezhat C, Nezhat F: Operative laparoscopy (minimally invasive surgery) state of the art. *J Gynecol Surg* 1992; 8:111-41.
4. Querleu D, Chapron C: Complications of gynecologic laparoscopic surgery. *Curr Opin Obstet Gynecol* 1995; 7:257-61.
5. Saidi MH, Sadler RK, Vancaillie TG, Akright BD, Farhart SA, White AJ: Diagnosis and management of serious urinary complications after major operative laparoscopy. *Obstet Gynecol* 1996; 87:272-6.
6. Thompson JD, Warshaw J: Hysterectomy. In *TeLinde's Operative Gynecology.* Rock JA, Thompson JD, eds. Lippincott-Raven Publishers, Philadelphia: 1997, 771-854.

ANESTHETIC CONSIDERATIONS

(Procedures covered: laparoscopic surgery for endometriosis, ectopic pregnancy, myomectomy, hysterectomy)

PREOPERATIVE

With the exception of tubal pregnancies, most of these cases are done electively in an otherwise healthy patient population.

Respiratory	There can be intraop respiratory compromise from ↑intraabdominal pressure 2° CO_2 insufflation; however, patients without significant respiratory disease tolerate the insufflation quite well. **Tests:** As indicated from H&P.
Cardiovascular	Insufflation of the abdomen (typically with pressures of 14-22 mmHg) → ↑SVR and ↓venous return. ↑$PaCO_2$ → ↑dysrhythmias. These are usually well tolerated in the otherwise healthy patient. **Tests:** As indicated from H&P.
Gastrointestinal	Patients often have a bowel prep the night before. Check for Sx of dehydration (↓skin turgor, orthostatic ↓BP, ↑HR, etc.) and hypokalemia (e.g., weakness, flattened T waves, dysrhythmias, etc.). The combination of ↑intraabdominal pressure + Trendelenburg position → ↑aspiration risk. **Test:** Electrolytes
Hematologic	These patients often are having surgery for abnormal uterine bleeding → anemia. **Test:** Hct
Laboratory	Other tests as indicated from H&P.
Premedication	Many of these patients suffer chronic pelvic pain. They can be quite anxious and on chronic anxiolytic medication. Large doses of preop sedatives are often needed 2° extreme anxiety and drug tolerance. For the anxious patient, diazepam 10 mg po 1-2 h before surgery is often useful. In addition, midazolam can be titrated to effect (e.g., 2-4 mg) in the immediate preop period. Patients with risk factors for regurgitation (e.g., obesity, DM, hiatus hernia) may benefit from Na citrate 15-30 ml po and other full-stomach precautions preinduction (see p. B-5).

INTRAOPERATIVE

Anesthetic technique: GETA—a balanced technique with inhalational agents and narcotics. Neuromuscular blockade allows maximal insufflation of the abdomen with lower intraabdominal pressures.

Induction	To give the surgeons optimal operating conditions, care must be taken not to inflate the stomach and bowel with gas during positive-pressure mask ventilation. Preoxygenate 3 min and induce with propofol (1.5-2.5 mg/kg iv) and muscle relaxants (e.g., vecuronium 0.1 mg/kg). Following intubation, pass an OG tube to empty the stomach. Rapid-sequence induction (see B-5) usually is indicated for patients with an ectopic pregnancy.
Maintenance	Narcotics and inhalational agents: If the estimated time for the case is > 1 h, do not use N_2O, to avoid bowel distention. Continue neuromuscular blockade, since relaxation improves surgical access.
Emergence	Extubation at conclusion of surgery, following reversal of iv neuromuscular blockade. Give prophylactic antiemetic (e.g., metoclopramide 10 mg iv and ondansetron 4 mg iv or dolasetron 12.5 mg).
Blood and fluid requirements	Usually minimal blood loss IV: 18 ga × 1	Before induction, these patients may need extra fluid 2° dehydration caused by the bowel prep. During surgery, large

Blood and fluid requirements, cont.	NS/LR @ 2-4 ml/kg/h	volumes of fluid are sometimes given intraabdominally for irrigation and hydrodissection → fluid overload; therefore, maintenance iv fluid should be kept to a minimum.
Monitoring	Standard monitors (see p. B-1). Foley catheter	
Positioning	✓ and pad pressure points. ✓ eyes.	See Neuropathies, below.
Complications	Bradyarrhythmias	Attributed to peritoneal or fallopian-tube stimulation. Rx: stop surgery; deflate pneumoperitoneum; administer atropine 0.5 mg or glycopyrrolate 0.4-0.6 mg.
	Hypothermia	2° the large volume of fluid and CO_2 infused into the abdomen. All fluids should be warmed + use a heated forced-air device to warm the patient.
	Extraabdominal insufflation	Occasionally, large volumes of the insufflating gas can enter a vein, hollow viscera, subcutaneous tissue, thorax, mediastinum, or pericardium. Fortunately, since the gas is usually CO_2, small volumes are absorbed quickly and usually do not cause major physiologic compromise; however, large volumes may → cardiopulmonary collapse (e.g., 2° pneumothorax, VAE). Subcutaneous air can compromise the airway in some cases. ✓ airway before extubation.
	Neuropathies	These can be long cases, with the patient in lithotomy position. Make sure that the pressure points are padded well and, if the arms are out, relieve stress on the brachial plexus.
	Fluid overload	✓ fluid volume entering and exiting the abdomen. Fluid absorption → fluid overload → CHF, edema.

POSTOPERATIVE

Complications	PONV	↑↑N/V associated with laparoscopic cases. Use prophylactic antiemetics and treat PONV aggressively.
Pain management	Pain control is usually not a major problem.	Patients may complain of shoulder pain due to diaphragmatic irritation.

References

1. Healzer JM, Nezhat C, Brodsky JB, Brock-Utne JG, Seidman DS: Pulmonary edema after absorbing crystalloid irrigating fluid during laparoscopy [letter]. *Anesth Anal* 1994; 78(6):1207.
2. Moore SS, Green CR, Wang FL, Pandit SK, Hurd WW: The role of irrigation in the development of hypothermia during laparoscopic surgery. *Am J Obstet Gyn* 1997; 176(3):598-602.
3. Polati E, Verlato G, Finco G, Mosaner W, Grosso S, Gottin L, Pinaroli AM, Ischia S: Ondansetron versus metoclopramide in the treatment of postoperative nausea and vomiting. *Anesth Analg* 1997; 85(2):395-99.
4. Schwartz RO: Complications of laparoscopic hysterectomy. *Obstet Gyn* 1993; 81(6):1022-4.

Surgeons

Harcharan S. Gill, MD
Fuad S. Freiha, MD, FACS

9.0 UROLOGY

Anesthesiologists

Steven A. Deem, MD
Ronald G. Pearl, MD, PhD

DIAGNOSTIC TRANSURETHRAL (ENDOSCOPIC) PROCEDURES

SURGICAL CONSIDERATIONS

Description: Many urologic diseases are diagnosed and evaluated endoscopically through the urethra with the use of specialized instruments, such as cystoscopes and resectoscopes. With the patient in a lithotomy position, the cystoscope is introduced into the urethra and advanced under direct vision all the way into the bladder (Figs 9-1, 2), allowing inspection of the urethra (**urethroscopy**) and bladder (**cystoscopy**). If pathology is noted, a biopsy can be obtained easily through the cystoscope. It is also possible to introduce a small catheter into the ureteral orifice and advance it up to the kidney for radiologic evaluation (**retrograde pyelography**), to collect a urine specimen, or to bypass areas of obstruction. If the upper urinary tract needs to be visualized, a ureteroscope is introduced through the urethra into the bladder and through the ureteral orifice into the ureter and advanced up to the kidney, allowing inspection of the ureter (**ureteroscopy**) and intrarenal collecting system (**nephroscopy**). These procedures often precede a major surgical operation.

Usual preop diagnosis: Hematuria; hydronephrosis; benign prostatic hypertrophy; cancer of the urethra, prostate, bladder, ureter, and renal pelvis; urinary tract stones; strictures; ureteropelvic junction obstruction; hemorrhagic or interstitial cystitis

SUMMARY OF PROCEDURES

	Urethroscopy/ Cystoscopy	Ureteroscopy/ Nephroscopy
Position	Lithotomy	⇐
Incision	None	⇐
Special instrumentation	Cystoscope	Ureteroscope
Unique considerations	Use of x-ray and fluoroscopy	⇐
Antibiotics	Gentamicin 80 mg iv, slowly	⇐
Surgical time	15 min	45 min
EBL	None	⇐
Postop care	PACU → home	⇐
Mortality	Minimal	⇐
Morbidity	Infection: 5%	⇐
		Ureteral perforation: < 5%
Pain score	1	1

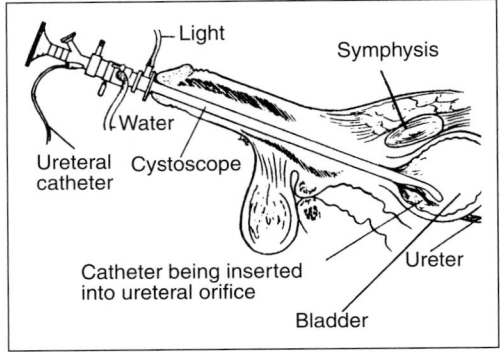

Figure 9-1. Cystoscope introduced into bladder via urethra (male anatomy). (Reproduced with permission from Hardy JD: *Textbook of Surgery*. JB Lippincott, 1988.)

PATIENT POPULATION CHARACTERISTICS

Age range	All ages	⇐
Male:Female	1:1	⇐
Incidence	30% of all urologic procedures	⇐
Etiology	Hematuria	⇐
	Urethral and bladder tumors	⇐
	Stones	⇐
	Urethral strictures	⇐
		Ureteropelvic junction obstruction
Associated conditions	Prostatic hypertrophy	Hydronephrosis
	Cystitis	⇐

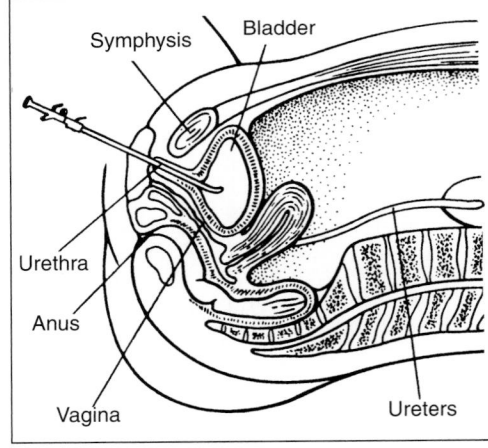

Figure 9-2. Cystoscope introduced into bladder (female anatomy). (Reproduced with permission from Govan DE: *Roche Manual of Urologic Procedures*. Hoffmann-LaRoche, 1976.)

ANESTHETIC CONSIDERATIONS

See Anesthetic Considerations following Therapeutic Transurethral Procedures (Except TURP), p. 698.

References

1. Bagley, DH: Ureteroscoy. In *Smith's Textbook of Endourology,* Vol 1, 1st edition. Smith AD, et al, eds. Quality Medical Publications, Inc. St. Louis: 2000, 369-513.
2. Carter HB: The urologic examination and diagnostic techniques. In *Campbell's Urology*, Vol 1, 7th edition. Walsh PC, et al, eds. WB Saunders, Philadelphia: 1998, 331-41.
3. Huffman JL: Ureteroscopy. In *Campbell's Urology*, Vol 3, 6th edition. WB Saunders, Philadelphia: 1992, 2195-2230.

THERAPEUTIC TRANSURETHRAL PROCEDURES (EXCEPT TURP)

SURGICAL CONSIDERATIONS

Description: Therapeutic transurethral procedures, the most common urologic operations, require the use of specialized instruments, such as cystoscopes and resectoscopes. Because of continuously improving instrumentation and fiber optics, the range and complexity of these operations are widening, and more operations are being done transurethrally now than ever before. These operations are: **transurethral resection (TUR)** of any urethral, prostatic, or bladder pathology; **fulguration** of bleeding vessels; **instillation of chemicals,** such as oxychlorosene (chloropactin) and formalin, into the bladder; **extraction** of stones; and **incision and dilation** of strictures.

With the patient in the lithotomy position, the cystoscope or resectoscope is introduced into the urethra and advanced under direct vision into the bladder, allowing inspection of the urethra and bladder (Figs 9-1, 2). The pathology is identified. If it is a tumor, it is resected piecemeal with the electrode of the resectoscope, using the cutting current and cauterizing the base of the tumor with the coagulating current. If the pathology is a stone, it is extracted with special forceps or a stone basket. Large stones have to be fragmented, prior to extraction, with a mechanical lithotrite, electrohydraulic probe, ultrasound lithotrite or laser (Holmium or pulsed-dye). Chemicals can be instilled through the cystoscope to control interstitial and hemorrhagic cystitis. Bleeding vessels can be coagulated with the electrode. Strictures of the urethra can be dilated or incised with an endoscopic knife. Strictures of the ureter also can be treated endoscopically by dilatation with a balloon catheter or by incision with electrocautery. Balloon catheters with attached cutting electro-wires (Accucise) often are used. A temporary ureteral stent is placed at the end of most endoscopic ureteral surgeries.

Variant procedure or approaches: Occasionally, access to the intrarenal collecting system (renal pelvis and calyces) and upper ureter is easier and more appropriately done by a **percutaneous nephrostomy** than a transurethral procedure. The patient is placed in a prone or flank position, a percutaneous stab wound is made at the costovertebral angle, and a tube is introduced into the kidney under fluoroscopic control.

Usual preop diagnosis: Tumors of the urinary tract; stones; interstitial or hemorrhagic cystitis; strictures

SUMMARY OF PROCEDURES

	Transurethral	Percutaneous
Position	Lithotomy	Flank or prone
Incision	None	Stab wound
Special instrumentation	Cystoscope; resectoscope; catheters; stents	Percutaneous nephrostomy kit; nephroscope; urethroscope; catheters; stents
Unique considerations	Use of x-rays, fluoroscopy, and electrocautery	⇐
Antibiotics	Gentamicin 80 mg iv, slowly	⇐
Surgical time	1 h	2-3 h
EBL	100 ml	500 ml
Postop care	Irrigation of tubes and catheters to clear clots and prevent obstruction	⇐
Mortality	< 1%	⇐

	Transurethral	**Percutaneous**
Morbidity	Bleeding: 10%	⇐
	Infection: 5%	⇐
	Perforation: 2%	⇐
	Retained stones: 2%	⇐
Pain score	1	3

PATIENT POPULATION CHARACTERISTICS

	Transurethral	**Percutaneous**
Age range	All ages	⇐
Male:Female	1:1	⇐
Incidence	10% of urologic diseases involve these procedures	⇐
Etiology	Urethral and bladder tumors; bladder and ureteral stones; interstitial cystitis; hemorrhagic cystitis; urethral stricture	Kidney stones; upper ureteral stones; ureteropelvic junction obstruction

ANESTHETIC CONSIDERATIONS FOR TRANSURETHRAL PROCEDURES (EXCEPT TURP)

PREOPERATIVE

Patients of all ages may present for ureteral stone extraction. Paraplegics and quadriplegics have a predilection for nephrolithiasis and may present for repeated cystoscopies. Bladder tumors usually are seen in older patients, who may present for cystoscopy or TUR. These patients may have preexisting medical problems, including CAD, CHF, PVD, cerebrovascular diseases, COPD, and/or renal impairment. Preop evaluation should be directed toward the detection and treatment of these conditions prior to anesthesia.

Neurological	Paraplegics and quadriplegics may present for repeated cystoscopies and stone extractions. Note Hx of autonomic hyperreflexia (AH); Sx may include flushing, headache, and nasal stuffiness, associated with voiding or noxious stimuli below the level of spinal cord injury (see below).
Musculoskeletal	Contractures and pressure sores may make positioning difficult in paraplegics or quadriplegics.
Laboratory	Tests as indicated from H&P.
Premedication	Sedation prn anxiety (e.g., lorazepam 1-2 mg po 1-2 h before surgery; midazolam 1-2 mg iv in preop area).

INTRAOPERATIVE

Anesthetic technique: Spinal, continuous lumbar epidural, and GA are acceptable, with the choice dependent on type and length of procedure, age, coexisting disease, and patient preference. Simpler transurethral procedures (e.g., cystoscopy) are amenable to topical anesthesia, while longer and more complex procedures (e.g., ureteral stone extraction) will require regional or GA (see discussion below regarding AH). Note that many of these procedures are done on an outpatient basis and the anesthetic should be planned accordingly. For regional anesthesia, a sacral block is required for urethral procedures, T9-T10 level for procedures involving the bladder, and as high as T8 for procedures involving the ureters.

Regional anesthesia:

Topical	2% lidocaine jelly
Spinal	0.75% bupivacaine 10-12 mg. For shorter procedures (< 1 h), consider low-dose bupivicaine (0.75%, 7.5 mg); mepivicaine (1.5%, 45 mg); or procaine (10%, 100-150 mg). Lidocaine may be used, but the incidence of transient neurologic symptoms may be as high as 30% for procedures performed in the lithotomy position.
Lumbar	1.5-2.0% lidocaine with epinephrine 5 μg/ml, 15-25 ml; supplement with 5-10 ml boluses as needed.
epidural	Supplemental iv sedation

General anesthesia:

Induction	Standard induction (see p. B-2). ET intubation may not be necessary for shorter procedures; consider LMA. Succinylcholine should be avoided in paralyzed (e.g., paraplegic, quadriplegic) patients 2° $\uparrow K^+ \rightarrow$ VF or asystole.

Maintenance	Pure inhalation anesthetic (e.g., N_2O, sevoflurane/desflurane) for short cases. IV technique (e.g., propofol 100-200 μg/kg/min; supplement with N_2O ± volatile anesthetic ± narcotic). Muscle relaxation not essential. Narcotics unnecessary since postop pain is usually minimal.	
Emergence	No specific considerations	
Blood and fluid requirements	Usually minimal blood loss IV: 18 ga × 1 NS/LR @ 2-4 ml/kg/h	
Monitoring	Standard monitors (see p. B-1).	
Positioning	✓ and pad pressure points. ✓ eyes.	★ **NB**: In lithotomy position, peroneal nerve compression at lateral fibular head → foot drop.
Complications	Anticipate ↓BP upon returning from lithotomy position. Autonomic hyperreflexia (**AH**): • Severe HTN • Bradycardia • Dysrhythmias • Cardiac arrest	Rx: volume (200-500 ml NS/LR) or ephedrine (5 mg iv) may be necessary. Patients with spinal cord injury level above T10 are at risk for **AH** associated with stimulation below the level of transection. Transection levels below T5 may be associated with less severe manifestations. AH can be prevented by GA, spinal, or epidural anesthesia. If AH occurs intraop, it should be treated by deepening the level of anesthesia, and iv antihypertensive agents (e.g., SNP 0.5-5 μg/kg/min; labetalol 5-10 mg iv; phentolamine 2-5 mg iv), if necessary.

POSTOPERATIVE

Complications	Peroneal nerve injury 2° lithotomy position Fever/bacteremia Bladder perforation	Peroneal nerve injury manifested as foot drop with loss of sensation over dorsum of foot. Seek neurology consultation. Bladder perforation may present as shoulder pain in the awake patient, but may go unnoticed in a patient under GA. Sx include unexplained HTN, tachycardia, ↓BP (rare).
Pain management	Pain usually mild	Rx: morphine 2-4 mg iv q 10-15 min prn, fentanyl 25-50 μg iv, ketorolac 30 mg im or iv

References

1. Amzallog M: Autonomic hyperreflexia. *Int Clin Anesth* 1993; 31:87-102.
2. Hambly PR, Martin, B: Anesthesia for chronic spinal cord lesions. *Anesthesia* 1998; 53:273-89.
3. Mebust WK: Transurethral Surgery. In *Campbell's Urology*, Vol 2, 7th edition. Walsh PC, Retite AB, Stamey TA, Vaughn ED Jr, eds. WB Saunders, Philadelphia: 1998, 1511-28.

TRANSURETHRAL RESECTION OF THE PROSTATE (TURP)

SURGICAL CONSIDERATIONS

Description: **TURP** is one of the most common urologic operations, performed to relieve bladder outlet obstruction by an enlarging prostate gland. It is often preceded by **cystoscopy**, which is used to evaluate the size of the prostate gland and to rule out any other pathology, such as bladder tumor or stone. The operation is performed with the resectoscope, a specialized instrument having an electrode capable of transmitting both cutting and coagulating currents.

The resectoscope is introduced into the bladder (Fig 9-3) and the tissue protruding into the prostatic urethra is resected in small pieces called 'chips.' Bleeding vessels are coagulated with the coagulating current. The resection is performed with continuous irrigation using an isotonic solution, such as sorbitol 2.7% with mannitol 0.54%. Once the obstructing prostatic tissues are completely resected and bleeding vessels coagulated, the chips are irrigated from the bladder and the resectoscope is removed. An indwelling Foley catheter is introduced into the bladder. The time of transurethral resection should not exceed 2 h because excessive absorption of the irrigating fluid may → dilutional hyponatremia, confusion, seizures, and heart failure. The size of the enlarged prostate or adenoma, therefore, needs to be carefully assessed preop to determine if it is possible to complete the resection within 2 h. If not, an **open prostatectomy** is performed. This variant approach is discussed under Open Prostate Operations, p. 703.

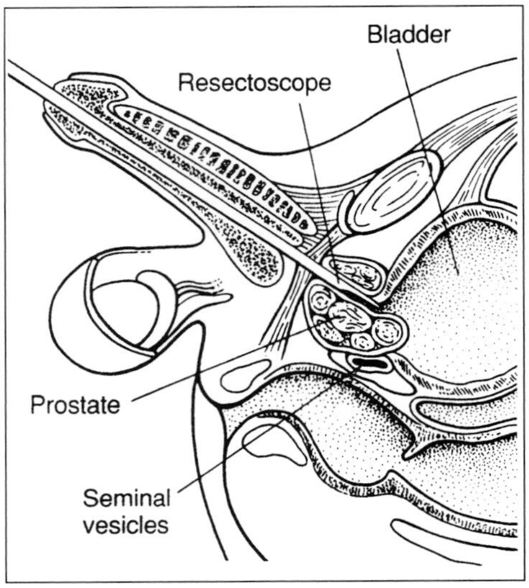

Variant procedure or approaches: A number of techniques have been developed to avoid the morbidity of TURP. These are either **vaporization** (electrocautery or laser) or **thermocoagulation** of the prostate (laser, microwave, radiofrequency). The following techniques are available and approved:

Figure 9-3. Transurethral resection of prostate using a resectoscope. (Reproduced with permission from Govan DE: *Roche Manual of Urologic Procedures.* Hoffmann-LaRoche, 1976.)

Bipolar TURP: To avoid fluid absorption and reduce blood loss, the traditional monopolar loop TURP is slowly being replaced by a bipolar technique, although at present there are few manufacturers of the bipolar devices. NS is used as the irrigant fluid and, thus, hyponatremia should be avoidable.

TUVP: Transurethral vaporization of the prostate with a standard resectoscope using a roller ball electrode at 275-300 watts setting.

VLAP: Visual laser ablation of the prostate is done with Nd:YAG or Ho:YAG laser through a standard cystoscope. All personnel in the OR, including the patient, must wear protective glasses to protect the eyes from inadvertent exposure from a break in the laser fiber.

TUNA: Transurethral needle ablation of the prostate is done with a special disposable device connected to a radiofrequency generator.

TUMT: Transurethral microwave thermotherapy is done with a catheter that has a microwave antenna attached to it. A microwave generator is needed for this procedure.

All of the above have several advantages over TURP, including shorter surgical time, no blood loss, reduced risk of fluid absorption, and all can be done as outpatient procedures.

Usual preop diagnosis: Benign prostatic hypertrophy; prostate cancer

SUMMARY OF PROCEDURES

	TURP	Thermotherapy
Position	Lithotomy	⇐
Incision	None	⇐
Special instrumentation	Cystoscope; resectoscope; catheters; electrocautery	Cystoscope; resectoscope; catheters; electrocautery (standby); laser equipment
Unique considerations	During resection, the patient should be absolutely still, because any movement may lead to perforation or injury to the external sphincter, → postop incontinence.	During resection, the patient and all personnel should wear protective eyeglasses.
Antibiotics	Gentamicin 80 mg iv, slowly	⇐
Surgical time	1-2 h (not to exceed 2 h)	1 h
EBL	500 ml	None
Postop care	Irrigation of the Foley catheter to clear it of clots and keep it from being blocked. Determination of serum Na$^+$	⇐
Mortality	< 1%	⇐

	TURP	Thermotherapy
Morbidity	Significant intraop bleeding: 10%	Prolonged catheterization: 10%
	Intraop perforation, which may require laparotomy: 1%	Postop bleeding: 1%
	Postop bleeding, which may necessitate a return to OR for fulguration of bleeding vessels: 5%	
	Absorption of irrigating fluid, which may → dilutional hyponatremia, mental confusion, and heart failure: 2%	
Pain score	1	1

PATIENT POPULATION CHARACTERISTICS

Age range	49-90 yr; typically, 70s and 80s
Incidence	Very common; 90% of men will develop benign hypertrophy; 20% may need surgical intervention.
Etiology	Aging; benign prostatic hypertrophy; prostate cancer
Associated conditions	COPD (10%); heart disease (10%); HTN (10%); diabetes mellitus (DM) (5%); DIC (1-2% of patients with prostate cancer may also have a low-grade, subclinical DIC, which becomes clinically manifest postop).

ANESTHETIC CONSIDERATIONS

PREOPERATIVE

Patients presenting for prostate surgery are generally elderly and may have preexisting medical problems, including CAD, CHF, PVD, cerebrovascular disease, COPD, and renal impairment. Preop evaluation should be directed toward the detection and treatment of these conditions before anesthesia.

Respiratory	COPD common in this age group. Patients with > 50 pack/year smoking Hx, or with any respiratory Sx, may need PFTs. For dyspnea with moderate exercise, ✓ VC, FEV_1, MMEF. If VC < 80%, FEV_1 < 60%, or MMEF < 40% predicted, ✓ ABG. If ABG and PFT markedly abnormal, consider postponing surgery until patient's respiratory condition has been optimized. **Tests**: PFT; CXR; ABG, as indicated from H&P.
Cardiovascular	HTN, CAD common in this age group. Assess exercise tolerance by H&P (e.g., should be able to climb a flight of stairs without difficulty or SOB). **Tests**: ECG; others as indicated from H&P.
Neurological	Cerebrovascular disease, Alzheimer's, and other neurologic problems may be present in this age group. Assess mental status to guide evaluation of any intraop or postop changes.
Renal	Anticipate renal impairment 2° chronic obstruction. **Tests**: BUN; Cr; electrolytes. If ↑BUN and ↑Cr, ✓ creatinine clearance (nl = 95-140 ml/min).
Musculoskeletal	Various arthritides in this age group may cause problems with positioning for regional anesthesia and surgery.
Endocrine	Increased incidence of DM.
Hematologic	Moderate blood loss expected with larger glands. If gland < 80 g, no T&C necessary; gland ≥ 80 g, T&C 2 U PRBCs. **Test:** Hct
Laboratory	Other tests as indicated from H&P.
Premedication	Continue commonly used drugs (e.g., digitalis, β-blockers, NTG) to prevent cardiovascular problems. Sedation prn anxiety (e.g., lorazepam 1-2 mg po 1-2 h before surgery).

INTRAOPERATIVE

Anesthetic technique: Regional or GA. Choice of technique depends on coexisting disease and patient preference. Regional anesthesia may hold some advantage over GA for TURP in that it allows evaluation of mental status and, thus, earlier detection of TURP syndrome. The incidence of postdural puncture headache is very low in this age group (< 1%). A T9 level is optimal. Continuous lumbar epidural anesthesia has no advantage over spinal anesthesia for TURP, since sacral block may be less reliable, the procedure is relatively short, and supplemental doses are usually not necessary.

Regional anesthesia:

Spinal	0.75% bupivacaine, 12 mg in 7.5% dextrose solution (1.6 ml)

General anesthesia:

Induction	Standard induction (see p. B-2).	
Maintenance	Standard maintenance (see p. B-3). Muscle relaxation is not mandatory, although patient movement during the procedure must be avoided.	
Emergence	Postop pain is usually not significant. Anticipate ↓BP when legs are repositioned from lithotomy. Avoid stress on lumbar spine by slowly and simultaneously bringing legs together and returning to supine position.	
Blood and fluid requirements	Moderate blood loss (TURP) Minimal blood loss (thermotherapy) IV: 16-18 ga × 1 NS/LR @ 2-4 ml/kg/h	Blood loss can be large (TURP) if venous sinuses are entered; it also can be difficult to quantify because of irrigant. To flush away blood and tissue and to promote visibility during TURP (or thermotherapy), continuous irrigation is used. For monopolar procedures, irrigating fluid must be nonelectrolytic to prevent dispersion of current, but near iso-osmotic to prevent hemolysis. For these reasons, sorbitol (2.7%) with mannitol (0.54%) or glycine (1.5%) are added to distilled water to produce solutions that are nearly isotonic.
Monitoring	Standard monitors (see p. B-1).	Regional anesthesia allows monitoring of mental status. Invasive monitoring, if indicated from H&P.
TURP syndrome	Intravascular volume overload Hyponatremia Hypotonicity 2° absorption of irrigant Symptoms include: • N/V • Visual disturbances • Mental status changes • Coma • Sz • HTN • Angina • Cardiovascular collapse	Factors which influence the absorption of irrigant include: surgical technique (TURP or thermotherapy); hydrostatic pressure of irrigant (height of bag); number of venous sinuses opened; peripheral venous pressure; duration of surgery; and experience of the surgeon. Resections should optimally be limited to 1 h or less. Some CNS manifestations are 2° glycine and its metabolites. Rx may include observation, diuresis (e.g., furosemide 5-20 mg iv), and administration of hypertonic saline (e.g., 100 ml 3% saline over 1-2 h). Serum sodium < 120 is associated with more severe symptoms, and the goal of therapy is to restore sodium to > 120. In milder cases, observation and water restriction may be sufficient.
Positioning	✓ and pad pressure points. ✓ eyes.	★ **NB**: In lithotomy position, peroneal nerve compression at lateral fibular head → foot drop.
Complications	Bladder perforation TURP syndrome	Bladder perforation may produce shoulder pain in the awake patient. Bladder perforation (and TURP syndrome) may go unnoticed under GA; Sx: ↑BP, ↑HR (occasionally ↓BP).

POSTOPERATIVE

Complications	TURP syndrome Bladder perforation Fever/bacteremia/sepsis Hypothermia	See discussion of TURP syndrome, above.
Pain management	Minimal postop pain	Rx: Morphine 1-4 mg iv prn until comfortable.
Tests	Hct; electrolytes Blood cultures if febrile	Consider serum osmolarity, CXR, ECG in TURP syndrome

References

1. Abrams PH, Shah PJ, Bryning K, et al: Blood loss during transurethral resection of the prostate. *Anaesthesia* 1982; 37(1): 71-3.
2. Jensen V: The TURP syndrome. *Can J Anaesth* 1991; 38(1):90-6.
3. Malhotra V: Transurethral resection of the prostate. *Anesthesiol Clin North Am* 2000; 18(4):883-97.
4. Mebust WK: Transurethral surgery. In *Campbell's Urology*, Vol 2, 7th edition. Walsh PC, Retite AB, Stamey TA, Vaughn ED Jr, eds. WB Saunders, Philadelphia: 1998, 1511-29.

OPEN PROSTATE OPERATIONS

SURGICAL CONSIDERATIONS

Description: Open (in contrast to transurethral or endoscopic) operations on the prostate gland are common. They include: **simple prostatectomy**; **radical prostatectomy**; and **retropubic exposure of the prostate for brachytherapy** through either a midline extraperitoneal incision, which extends from the umbilicus to the symphysis pubis, or through a Pfannenstiel's incision (Fig 9-4, inset).

Simple prostatectomy: When the benign prostatic hypertrophy or adenoma is too large to be resected transurethrally, it is removed by a simple prostatectomy. The prostate gland is exposed through a retropubic approach (Fig 9-4A) and the anterior capsule is incised, exposing the adenoma—the central part of the prostate which is excised, 'shelled' out by blunt dissection (Fig 9-4B), leaving behind the peripheral prostate and all the associated structures. A Foley catheter is left indwelling in the urethra, and the incision in the prostate capsule is closed. In a **suprapubic prostatectomy**, the incision is made in the bladder and the adenoma shelled from within the bladder.

Radical prostatectomy: The term 'radical prostatectomy' may be misleading. It is used to differentiate this cancer operation from a simple prostatectomy (used for benign prostatic hypertrophy). Radical prostatectomy can be achieved through either a **retropubic** or **perineal approach**, the choice being a matter of training, expertise, and surgeon's preference. In radical prostatectomy, all of the prostate gland is removed, together with the bladder neck, the seminal vesicles, and the ampullae of the vas deferens. A **limited pelvic lymphadenectomy** (Fig 9-5) also is performed. After the prostate gland and its associated structures are removed, the bladder neck is reduced to 1 cm diameter and anastomosed to the membranous urethra over an indwelling Foley catheter. Most of the blood loss occurs during control of the dorsal vein complex. In the past 10 yr, attempts have been made to preserve potency by preserving the nerves to the corpora cavernosa.

Usual preop diagnosis: Benign prostatic hypertrophy; prostate cancer

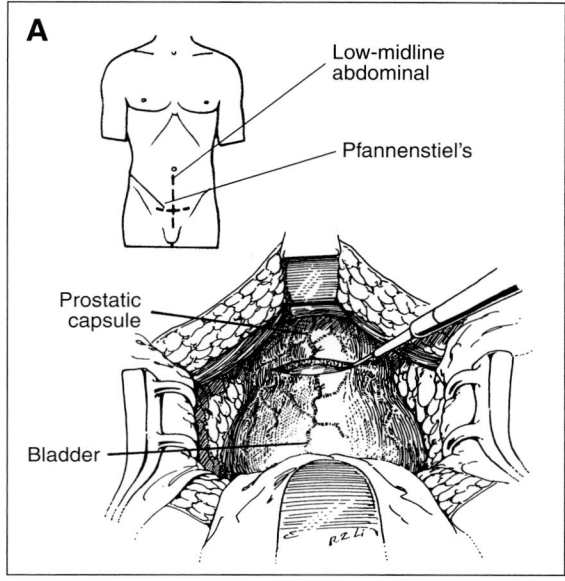

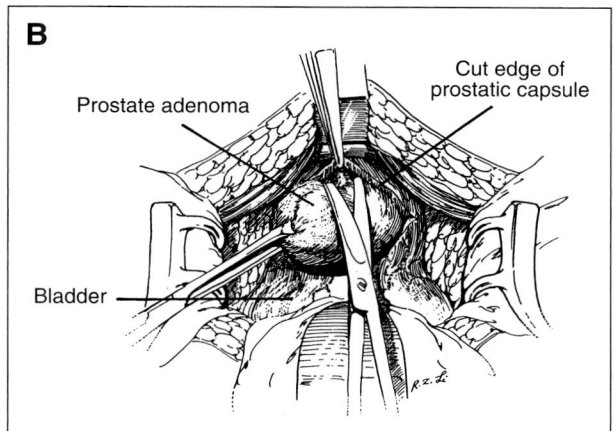

Figure 9.4. Retropubic prostatectomy: (A) A transverse capsulotomy is made between heavy hemostatic stay sutures, and (B) the cleavage plane between the adenoma and the surgical capsule is developed with scissors. (Reproduced with permission from Fowler JE: *Urologic Surgery*. Little, Brown, 1990.)

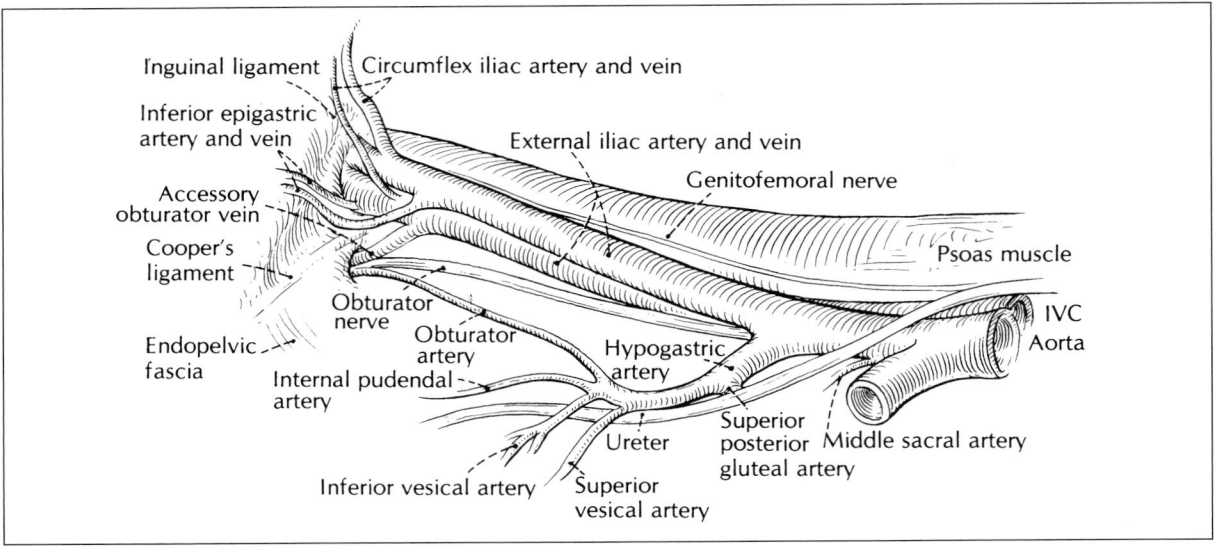

Figure 9-5. Right lateral pelvic wall. Anatomy of pelvic blood vessels and nerves encountered in a pelvic lymph node dissection. (Reproduced with permission from Graham SD Jr: *Glenn's Urologic Surgery*. Lippincott Williams & Wilkins, 1998.)

SUMMARY OF PROCEDURES

	Simple Prostatectomy	Radical–Retropubic	Radical–Perineal
Position	Supine	⇐	Lithotomy
Incision	Extraperitoneal, low midline, or Pfannenstiel's (Fig 9-4A, inset)	⇐	Perineal (Fig 9-6)
Unique considerations	None	⇐	Extreme hip flexion
Antibiotics	Gentamicin 80 mg iv, slowly	⇐	⇐
Surgical time	1 h	3 h	⇐
EBL	500 ml	1500 ml	500 ml
Postop care	Irrigate catheter to clear blood clots and prevent obstruction; frequently, if urine is bloody.	⇐	⇐
Mortality	< 1%	⇐	⇐
Morbidity	Bleeding: 2%	⇐	⇐
	DVT: 2%	⇐	⇐
	Infection: 2%	⇐	⇐
	PE: 1%	⇐	⇐
		Impotence: Non nerve-sparing: 100% Nerve-sparing: 50% Lymphocele: 4%	
Pain score	8	8	6

PATIENT POPULAT2ION CHARACTERISTICS

Age range	40-80 yr
Incidence	20% of men will develop symptomatic benign prostatic hypertrophy; 9% will develop clinically evident prostate cancer.
Etiology	Aging
Associated conditions	COPD (10%); CAD (10%); HTN (10%); diabetes mellitus (5%); renal failure (1%)

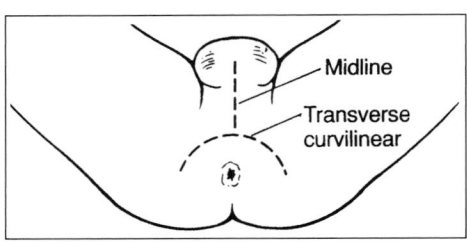

Figure 9-6. Perineal incisions.

ANESTHETIC CONSIDERATIONS

PREOPERATIVE

Patients presenting for prostate surgery are generally elderly and may have preexisting medical problems, including CAD, CHF, PVD, cerebrovascular disease, COPD, and renal impairment. Preop evaluation should be directed toward the detection and treatment of these conditions prior to anesthesia.

Respiratory COPD common in this age group. Patients with Hx of >50 pack-year smoking, or with respiratory Sx, may require PFTs. For dyspnea with moderate exercise, check VC, FEV_1, MMEF. If VC < 80%, FEV_1 < 60%, or MMEF < 40% predicted, ✓ABG. If ABG and PFT are markedly abnormal, consider postponing surgery until patient's respiratory condition has been optimized.
Tests: PFT; CXR; ABG, as indicated from H&P.

Cardiovascular HTN, CAD common in this age group. Assess exercise tolerance by H&P (e.g., should be able to climb a flight of stairs without difficulty or SOB).
Tests: ECG; others as indicated from H&P.

Neurological Cerebrovascular disease, Alzheimer's, and other neurologic problems may be present in this age group. Assess mental status to guide evaluation of any intraop or postop changes.

Renal Anticipate renal impairment 2° chronic obstruction.
Tests: Cr

Musculoskeletal Various arthritides may cause problems with positioning for regional anesthesia and surgery.

Endocrine Increased incidence of diabetes mellitus.

Hematologic Moderate blood loss expected with larger glands. For glands < 30 g, no T&C necessary; for glands 30-80 g, T&C 2 U PRBCs; for glands > 80 g, T&C 4 U PRBCs.
Tests: Hct

Laboratory Other tests as indicated from H&P.

Premedication Continue commonly used drugs (e.g., digitalis, β-blockers, diuretics, NTG) to prevent cardiovascular complications. Sedation prn anxiety (e.g., lorazepam 1-2 mg po on call to OR).

INTRAOPERATIVE

Anesthetic technique: Regional (spinal, continuous spinal, continuous lumbar epidural), GA, or combined techniques are acceptable. If regional anesthesia used, optimal block level is T8-T10 (depending on incision site). Advantages of regional anesthesia include potential for lower intraop blood loss, possible lower incidence of DVT postop, and faster return of bowel function. Disadvantages include positioning considerations (see below).

Regional anesthesia:

Spinal Bupivacaine (0.75%) 12 mg in 7.5% dextrose solution (1.6 ml) or hyperbaric tetracaine 10-15 mg with epinephrine 200 μg (0.2 ml of 1:1000 solution).

Epidural 1.5-2% lidocaine with epinephrine 5 μg/ml, 15-25 ml, supplemental iv sedation as necessary. Additional epidural lidocaine (5-10 ml boluses) may be needed, depending on length of procedure. Alternatively, smaller volumes of bupivacaine (0.25-0.5%), levobupivacaine (0.25-0.5%), or ropivacaine (0.5-1%) may be used. The addition of opiates has been associated with ↑urinary retention in noncatheterized patients.

General anesthesia:

Induction Standard induction (see p. B-2).

Maintenance Standard maintenance (see p. B-3).

Emergence No special considerations

Blood and fluid requirements Moderate-to-large blood loss
IV: 14-16 ga × 1-2
NS/LR @ 4-6 ml/kg/h

Additional requirements dependent on type of anesthesia. Regional techniques are associated with higher fluid requirement because of sympathectomy and systemic vasodilation; it also may be associated with lower blood loss than GA.[2]

Monitoring	Standard monitors (see p. B-1). Depending on underlying disease: ± CVP ± Arterial line	Some patients require CVP to aid in assessment of volume status. Arterial line is often useful for continuous BP monitoring and frequent blood draws. Patients at particularly high risk (e.g., Hx of preexisting cardiopulmonary disease) should probably have both.
Positioning	Anticipate ↓BP on return from lithotomy position. ✓ and pad pressure points. ✓ eyes.	Rx: volume (200-500 ml NS/LR) or ephedrine (5 mg iv) may be necessary. Elderly patients with arthritis or respiratory impairment may not tolerate the extreme positioning associated with perineal prostatectomy for extended periods of time, thus precluding the use of regional anesthesia. ★ (A combined technique with GA may be considered.) **NB:** In lithotomy position, peroneal nerve compression at lateral fibular head → foot drop.
Complications	Indigo carmine reaction Hemorrhage Hypothermia VAE	Indigo carmine → false ↓O_2 sat ± ↑BP; rare allergic reaction → rash + bronchoconstriction + ↓BP.

POSTOPERATIVE

Complications	Peroneal nerve injury 2° lithotomy position DVT	Manifested by foot drop with loss of sensation on dorsum of foot. Seek neurology consultation. Incidence of DVT less with regional than GA. Sx: variable, with pain and tenderness over involved area.
Pain management	Significant postop pain. Rx: morphine 0.1-0.3 mg/kg iv in incremental doses (e.g., 2-4 mg q 10-15 min prn).	Consider epidural infusion of dilute local anesthestics/opiates or PCA (see p. C-3).
Tests	Hct	

References

1. Donald JR: The effect of anaesthesia, hypotension, and epidural analgesia on blood loss in surgery for pelvic floor repair. *Br J Anaesth* 1969; 41(2):155-66.
2. Eastham JA, Scardino PT: Radical prostatectomy. In *Campbell's Urology*, 7th edition. WB Saunders, Philadelphia: 1998, 2547-64.
3. Gibbons RP: Radical perineal prostatectomy. In *Campbell's Urology*, Vol 3, 7th edition. WB Saunders, Philadelphia: 1998, 2589-2604.
4. Hendolin H, Mattila MA, Poikolainen E: The effect of lumbar epidural analgesia on the development of deep vein thrombosis of the legs after open prostatectomy. *Acta Chir Scand* 1981; 147(6):425-9.
5. Oesterling JE: Retropubic and suprapubic prostatectomy. In *Campbell's Urology*, Vol 2, 7th edition. Walsh PC, et al, eds. WB Saunders, Philadelphia: 1998, 1529-42.
6. Whalley DG, Berrigan MJ: Anesthesia for radical prostatectomy, cystectomy, nephrectomy, pheochromocytoma, and laparoscopic procedures. *Anesthesiol Clin North Am* 2000; 18(4):899-917.

NEPHRECTOMY

SURGICAL CONSIDERATIONS

Description: Nephrectomies fall into three basic groups: simple, partial, and radical. (Surgical anatomy is shown in Fig 9-7.)

Simple nephrectomy, performed for benign conditions, is the surgical excision of the kidney and a small segment of proximal ureter. The dorsal approach is well suited for this operation, and begins with an incision extending from the 12th rib to the iliac crest along the lateral edge of the sacrospinalis muscle and quadratus lumborum muscle. The dorsolumbar fascia is opened, exposing Gerota's fascia and the perinephric fat (Fig 9-8). The kidney is mobilized until the hilum is exposed. The artery and vein are tied, suture-ligated, and transected. The ureter is followed distally as far as possible, tied, and transected. The kidney is delivered out of the incision, which is then closed by approximating the dorsolumbar fascia and the fascia of the sacrospinalis muscle.

Usual preop diagnosis: Chronic hydronephrosis; hypoplastic kidney; renovascular HTN; double collecting system

Partial nephrectomy is the surgical excision of the segment of the kidney harboring the pathology. It is performed for small renal-cell carcinomas and benign tumors of the kidney, such as angiomyolipomas, and for duplicated collecting systems with a diseased moiety. If the partial nephrectomy is being done for

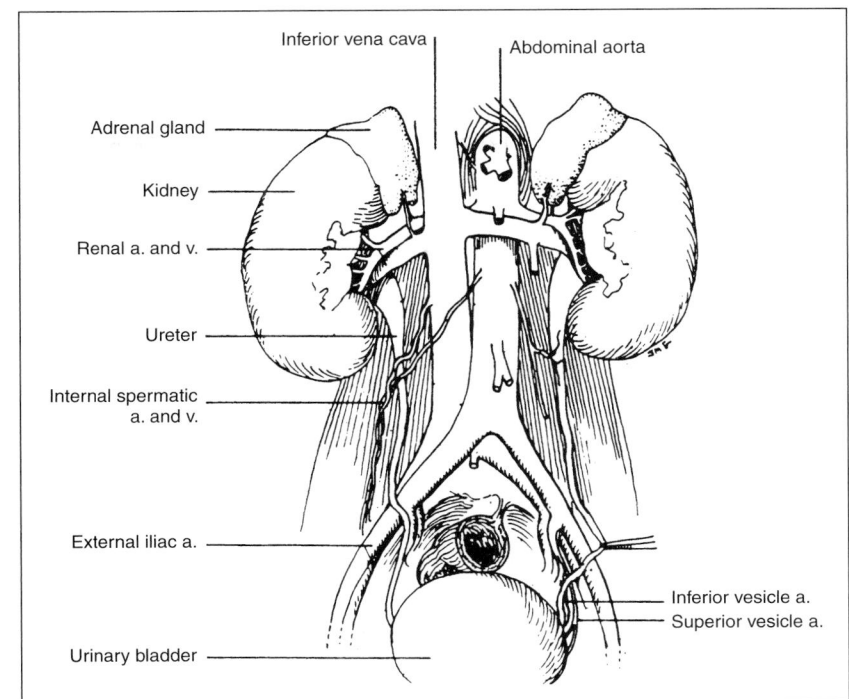

Figure 9-7. Surgical anatomy of the urinary tract. (Reproduced with permission from Hardy JD: *Textbook of Surgery.* Lippincott, 1988.)

renal-cell carcinoma, it may be accompanied with a **regional lymphadenectomy**. The flank approach (Fig 9-9A) is well suited for this operation and begins with an incision over the 12th or 11th rib, or in between, and extends anteriorly over the external and internal oblique muscles, which are transected. The transversalis muscle and fascia are opened, exposing Gerota's fascia. The renal capsule is exposed at the planned site of resection. Control of the renal vessels is advised for control of bleeding, if excessive. Incision in the renal parenchyma is made by sharp and blunt dissection, suture-ligating all bleeders. If the collecting system is opened, it should be closed with absorbable sutures. After complete hemostasis, Gelfoam or perinephric fat is used to cover the raw surface of the kidney.

Usual preop diagnosis: Renal-cell carcinoma; double collecting system

Radical nephrectomy is the surgical excision of the kidney, with its surrounding perinephric fat and Gerota's fascia, and the proximal 2/3rds of the ureter, accompanied by paracaval or paraaortic **lymphadenectomy**. It is performed for renal-cell carcinoma. Early control of renal vessels is advised before excessive manipulation of the tumor, to minimize blood loss and hematogenous spread. Transabdominal or flank approaches (Fig 9-9A, B) are best suited for this operation.

Laparoscopic nephrectomy: A pneumoperitoneum is created by insufflating CO_2 to a pressure of 14-16 mmHG. Three to four trochars are inserted as necessary (Fig 9-10). Typically, the patient is placed in a flank position as in an open radical

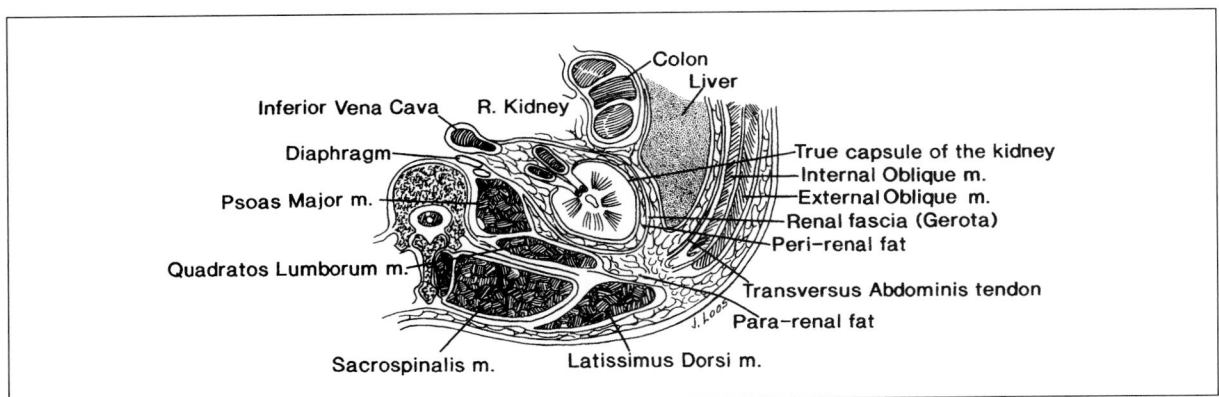

Figure 9-8. Transverse section showing the relation of the renal fascias to the right kidney. (Reproduced with permission from Baker RJ, Fischer JE: *Mastery of Surgery*, 4th edition. Lippincott Williams & Wilkins, 2001.)

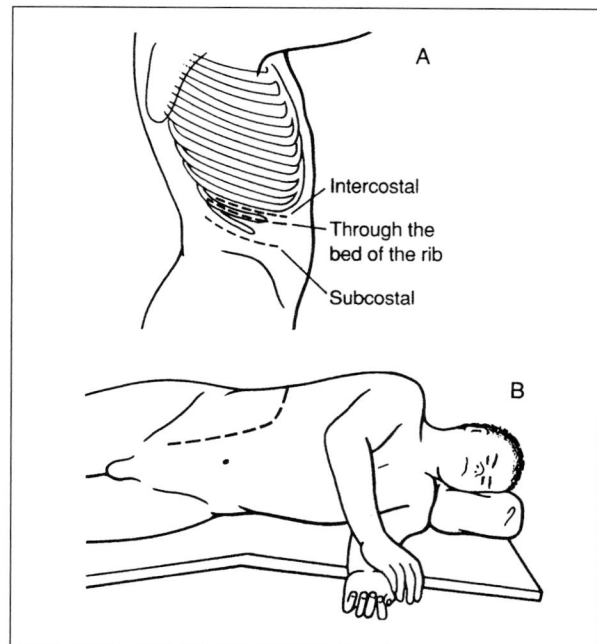

Figure 9-9. (A) Flank incisions. (B) Subcostal transabdominal incision.

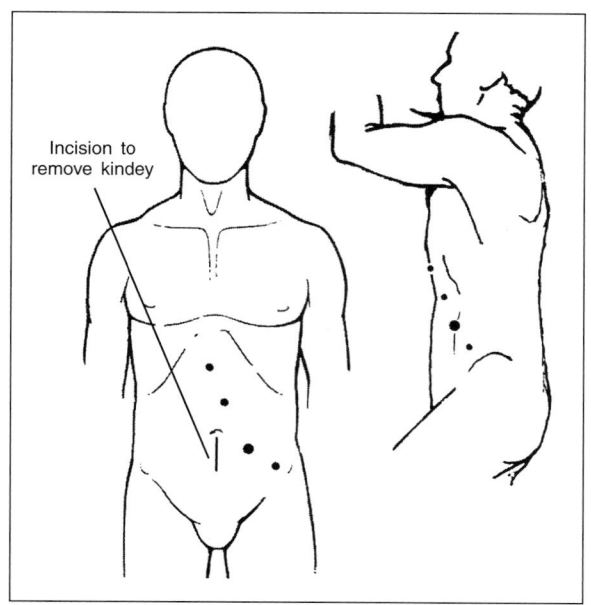

Figure 9-10. Incision and placement of trocars in laparoscopic nephrectomy. (Reproduced with permission from Scott-Conner CEH, Dawson DL: *Operative Anatamy*, 2nd edition. Lippincott Williams & Wilkins, 2003.)

nephrectomy. This procedure can be either **transperitoneal** or **retroperitoneal**, depending on the surgeon's preference or experience. The transperitoneal approach may be modified by using a hand assistance device through one of the ports (**hand-assisted laparoscopic nephrectomy**).

Usual preop diagnosis: Renal-cell carcinoma, nofunctioning kidney 2° infection or obstruction; kidney donation

Nephroureterectomy is a radical nephrectomy with ureter resection, including the ureteral orifice and a cuff of bladder wall around it. It is accompanied by a regional lymphadenectomy, since it is performed for a cancerous condition. The approach is either **transabdominal** or **extraperitoneal** through an extended flank incision, starting at the tip of the 11th rib and curving caudally along the lateral edge of the rectus abdominis muscle down to the pubic bone (Fig 9-9B). Some surgeons prefer two separate incisions: a flank incision for the radical nephrectomy part and a lower abdominal incision for the ureterectomy.

Usual preop diagnosis: Renal-cell carcinoma; Wilms' tumor; transitional-cell carcinoma of the renal collecting system or ureter

SUMMARY OF PROCEDURES

	Simple Nephrectomy	Partial Nephrectomy	Radical Nephrectomy	Laparoscopic Nephrectomy
Position	Flank or prone	Flank	Supine or flank	Flank
Incision	Flank (Fig 9-9A) or dorsal along paraspinous muscles	Flank (Fig 9-9A)	Midline or subcostal transabdominal (Fig 9-9B) or flank; subcostal or intercostal or through bed of 11th or 12th rib (Fig 9-9A)	3-4 ports (Fig 9-10)
Unique considerations	None	⇐	If tumor involves renal vein and/or IVC, clamp IVC.	Risk of emergent conversion to open case
Antibiotics	None	⇐	⇐	⇐
Surgical time	2-3 h	3-4 h	⇐	⇐
Closing considerations	Chest tube may be required if pleura opened with flank incision.	⇐	⇐	A small incision is made at the end of the case to remove the specimen.

	Simple Nephrectomy	Partial Nephrectomy	Radical Nephrectomy	Laparoscopic Nephrectomy
EBL	500 ml	1200 ml	500 ml	300 ml
Mortality	< 1%	⇐	1%	⇐
Morbidity	Prolonged ileus: 5% Pneumothorax 2° unrecognized pleural perforation: 2%	⇐	⇐	Vascular injury requiring conversion to open case
Pain score	10	10	10	4

PATIENT POPULATION CHARACTERISTICS

	Simple Nephrectomy	Partial Nephrectomy	Radical Nephrectomy	Laparoscopic Nephrectomy
Age range	All ages	⇐	⇐	⇐
Male:Female	1:1	⇐	⇐	⇐
Incidence	< 1%	⇐	⇐	⇐
Etiology	Double collecting system; chronic hydronephrosis; hypoplastic kidney; renovascular HTN	Localized renal-cell carcinoma	Wilms' tumor (8% of all childhood malignancies); transitional cell carcinoma (7% of all kidney tumors); renal-cell carcinoma (3% of adult malignancies)	⇐
Associated conditions	HTN if nephrectomy is used for renovascular HTN.			

ANESTHETIC CONSIDERATIONS

See Anesthetic Considerations following Operations on the Renal Pelvis and Upper Ureter, p. 710.

References

1. Cadeddu JA, Ono Y, Clayman RV: Laparoscopic nephrectomy for renal cell cancer. Evalution of efficacy and safety: a multicenter experience. *Urology* 1998; 52:773-7
2. Coleman DL: Control of postoperative pain: non-narcotic and narcotic alternatives and their effect on pulmonary function. *Chest* 1987; 92(3):520-8.
3. Novic AC, Streem SB: Surgery of the Kidney. In *Campbell's Urology*, Vol 3, 7th edition. WB Saunders, Philadelphia: 1998, 2973-3061.

OPERATIONS ON THE RENAL PELVIS AND UPPER URETER

SURGICAL CONSIDERATIONS

Description: Operations on the renal pelvis and upper ureter are becoming less common because of the increasing use of endoscopic and percutaneous procedures. The basic surgical approach is the same as that for nephrectomy (see p. 706). Specific procedures include:

Pyeloplasty is the surgical correction of congenital ureteropelvic junction stenosis to relieve obstruction. The most commonly used is the **dismembered pyeloplasty**, or **Anderson-Heinz pyeloplasty**, wherein the diseased ureteropelvic junction is excised, the redundant renal pelvis is reduced, and an anastomosis is established between the renal pelvis and ureter (Fig 9-11).

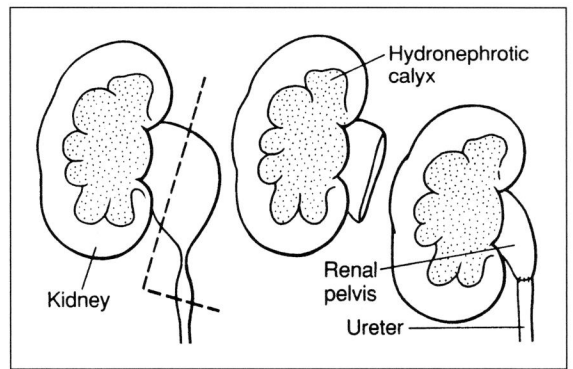

Figure 9-11. Dismembered pyeloplasty

Usual preop diagnosis: Ureteropelvic junction obstruction

Pyelolithotomy and ureterolithotomy are used to remove calculi from the renal pelvis or ureter. The upper ureter and renal pelvis are exposed, usually through a flank approach, the calculus is palpated and an incision is made in the ureter or renal pelvis over the calculus, which is then delivered. The incision is closed with fine, absorbable sutures.

Usual preop diagnosis: Renal pelvic or ureteral stone

Transureteroureterostomy is the transposition of one ureter across the midline and anastomosing it to the other ureter (Fig 9-12). This operation is performed whenever the distal ureter is traumatized or diseased, and the proximal ureter is not long enough to reimplant into the bladder. The recipient ureter should be normal.

Usual preop diagnosis: Traumatic loss of distal ureter; distal ureteral tumor requiring distal ureterectomy

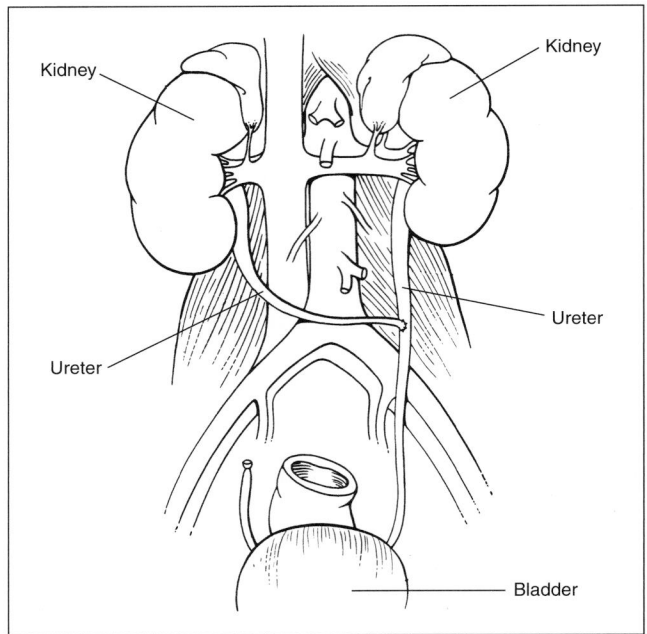

Figure 9-12. Transureteroureterostomy

SUMMARY OF PROCEDURES

	Pyeloplasty	Pyelolithotomy/Ureterolithotomy	Transureteroureterostomy
Position	Flank or prone	⇐	Supine
Incision	Flank (Fig 9-9A) or dorsal	⇐	Midline abdominal (Fig 9-4A, inset)
Antibiotics	None	⇐	⇐
Surgical time	3 h	1-2 h	3 h
EBL	Minimal	⇐	⇐
Mortality	< 1%	⇐	⇐
Morbidity	Urinary leakage: 5%	⇐	⇐
	Infection: 2%	⇐	⇐
Pain score	10	10	10

PATIENT POPULATION CHARACTERISTICS

Age range	All ages	⇐	⇐
Male:Female	1:1	⇐	⇐
Incidence	Rare	Extremely rare	⇐
Etiology	Ureteropelvic junction obstruction: 80% (of causes of dilated collecting system in the newborn)	Renal pelvic and upper ureteral stone	Traumatic loss of lower ureter; lower ureteral tumor
Associated conditions	Renal failure: 1%		

ANESTHETIC CONSIDERATIONS

(Procedures covered: nephrectomy and operations on the renal pelvis and upper ureter)

PREOPERATIVE

Patients presenting for nephrectomy and operations on the renal pelvis and upper ureter may be of any age, depending upon the etiology of the abnormality. Many patients may have renal insufficiency 2° the underlying problem or from renovascular HTN. Elderly patients frequently have preexisting medical problems, including CAD, CHF, PVD, cerebrovascular disease, COPD, and renal impairment. Preop evaluation should be directed toward the detection and treatment of these conditions prior to anesthesia.

Respiratory	Increased postop pulmonary complications because of location of incision (nonlaparoscopic). If Hx of pulmonary disease (e.g., asthma, COPD), consider postop respiratory therapy. **Tests:** As indicated from H&P.
Cardiovascular	Consider possibility of renal HTN.
Hematologic	Polycythemia may be seen in association with polycystic kidney disease, renal-cell carcinoma. Consider preop blood donation for autologous transfusion. **Tests**: Hct
Laboratory	Electrolytes; BUN; Cr; other tests as indicated from H&P.
Premedication	Standard premedication (see p. B-2).

INTRAOPERATIVE

Anesthetic technique: GA is recommended for these procedures; technique depends on underlying disease. Regional techniques (spinal or epidural) may be alternatives for some open procedures, but are less than optimal because of awkward positioning that may → patient discomfort and pain resulting from diaphragmatic stimulation. Consider combined technique with regional opiates.

Induction	Standard induction (see p. B-2).	
Maintenance	Standard maintenance (see p. B-3). If intraperitoneal or laparoscopic approach is used, consider limiting N_2O to avoid distention of bowel and interference with operative field.	
Emergence	No specific considerations	
Blood and fluid requirements	Mild-to-moderate blood loss IV: 14-16 ga × 1 NS/LR @ 6-8 ml/kg/h Warm all fluids.	Intraperitoneal approach associated with higher fluid requirements (8-10 ml/kg/h). When renal vessels are to be cross-clamped, mannitol (0.5 g/kg) is often given prior to occlusion (20 min maximum).
Monitoring	Standard monitors (see p. B-1). Urinary catheter Arterial line (partial nephrectomy) ± CVP line	Invasive monitoring if indicated from H&P. CVP line useful for partial nephrectomy in patients with solitary kidneys (↑↑blood loss).
Positioning	Use axillary roll if lateral. Avoid stretching brachial plexus – limit abduction to 90°. If prone, repeatedly ✓ eyes and pressure points. Assure free excursion of abdomen.	The lateral position with kidney rest and table flexion may →↓BP, possibly 2° vena cava obstruction. Moderate iv volume administration and gradual assumption of the position are recommended to avoid this complication.
Complications	Pneumothorax ↓BP with positioning (see above). Indigo carmine →↑BP, ↑SVR Methylene blue →↓BP	Sx of pneumothorax include: ↑RR, ↑PIP, hypoxemia, hypercarbia. If in doubt, ✓ CXR.

POSTOPERATIVE

Complications	Postnephrectomy syndrome Eye injury (if prone) Brachial plexus injury (if lateral) Pneumothorax Atelectasis Pneumonia	Postnephrectomy syndrome 2° retractor injury. L1 nerve root damage with resulting pain, dysesthesia, and sensory loss in L1 dermatome distribution.
Pain management	Morphine 0.1-0.3 mg/kg iv in incremental doses Consider epidural narcotic	Postop analgesia critical to minimize pulmonary complications. PCA. See pp. C-2 – C-3.
Tests	Hct CXR	Others dependent on operative course, coexisting disease.

Reference

1. Franke JJ, Smith JA: Surgery of the ureter. In *Campbell's Urology*, Vol 3, 7th edition. Walsh PC, et al, eds. WB Saunders, Philadelphia: 1998, 3062-84.

CYSTECTOMY

SURGICAL CONSIDERATIONS

Description: Open (in contrast to transurethral or endoscopic) bladder operations (cystectomies) account for 15-20% of all urological procedures. They are grouped as simple, partial, and radical procedures.

Simple cystectomy is performed for benign conditions of the bladder, such as severe hemorrhagic cystitis, radiation cystitis, and contracted bladder. It involves the removal of the bladder only. The operation is performed through a lower abdominal incision. The peritoneal reflections are incised down to the pouch of Douglas; the vasa deferentia and superior vesical arteries are identified, cross-clamped, transected, and tied. The ureters are identified, separated from the surrounding tissues, cross-clamped near the bladder, transected, and tied. The bladder is bluntly separated from the anterior rectal wall all the way to the apex of the prostate. The lateral pedicles of the bladder are cross-clamped, cut, and tied. The endopelvic fascia is incised, separating the prostate from the lateral pelvic wall. The puboprostatic ligaments are transected and the dorsal vein of the penis is suture-ligated. The tied dorsal vein and urethra are incised just distal to the apex of the prostate. The specimen is delivered out of the incision and hemostasis secured with electrocautery. An ileal conduit is then performed (see below).

Partial cystectomy is the excision of only the part of the bladder containing the pathology. This is not a commonly performed operation and is reserved for tumors located in the dome of the bladder of older patients who are poor surgical risks for major operations, such as radical cystectomy. The operation is preceded by a cystoscopy to identify the site of pathology. Beginning with a lower abdominal incision, the dome and lateral walls of the bladder are separated from the surrounding tissues, which are covered by wet packs to minimize contamination. An incision is made in the dome of the bladder at least 2 cm away from the pathology. The inside of the bladder is inspected and the pathology identified. The incision in the bladder is continued around, and at least 2 cm away from, the pathology, until the latter is completely excised. Bleeders in the wall of the bladder are electrocoagulated. The bladder wall is then closed in two layers—a through-and-through layer and an inverting layer—using absorbable material. Wet packs are removed, a drain is left in the region, and the abdominal incision is closed.

Radical cystectomy (or **radical cystoprostatectomy**) is performed for treatment of invasive bladder cancer. It encompasses the removal of the bladder and the lower ureters, the prostate gland, and seminal vesicles in men (Fig 9-13A), and the uterus, ovaries, and anterior vaginal wall in women (Fig 9-13B). Accompanied by a **pelvic lymphadenectomy**, it is performed in the supine position, except when a concomitant **urethrectomy** is required, wherein a lithotomy position is used.

Following cystectomy, whether radical or simple, some form of **urinary diversion** is required. This can be accomplished with either a standard ileal conduit or a bladder substitution. The **ileal conduit** is constructed from 6-8 inches of terminal ileum isolated, with its blood supply, from the small intestine. The continuity of the small intestine is accomplished by a simple anastomosis. The ureters are implanted into the proximal end of the conduit and the distal end is brought through the abdominal wall as a stoma (Fig 9-14). **Bladder substitution** is a more complex operation wherein a longer segment of bowel is isolated, with its blood supply, and fashioned into a pouch. The ureters are implanted in the pouch and the most dependent part of the pouch is connected to the membranous urethra, avoiding a stoma (Fig 9-15). Not all patients undergoing cystectomies are candidates for bladder substitution. For example, patients who require a urethrectomy are not candidates because of the need to remove the urethra.

Usual preop diagnosis: Bladder cancer; contracted bladder; hemorrhagic cystitis; radiation cystitis; bladder diverticulum

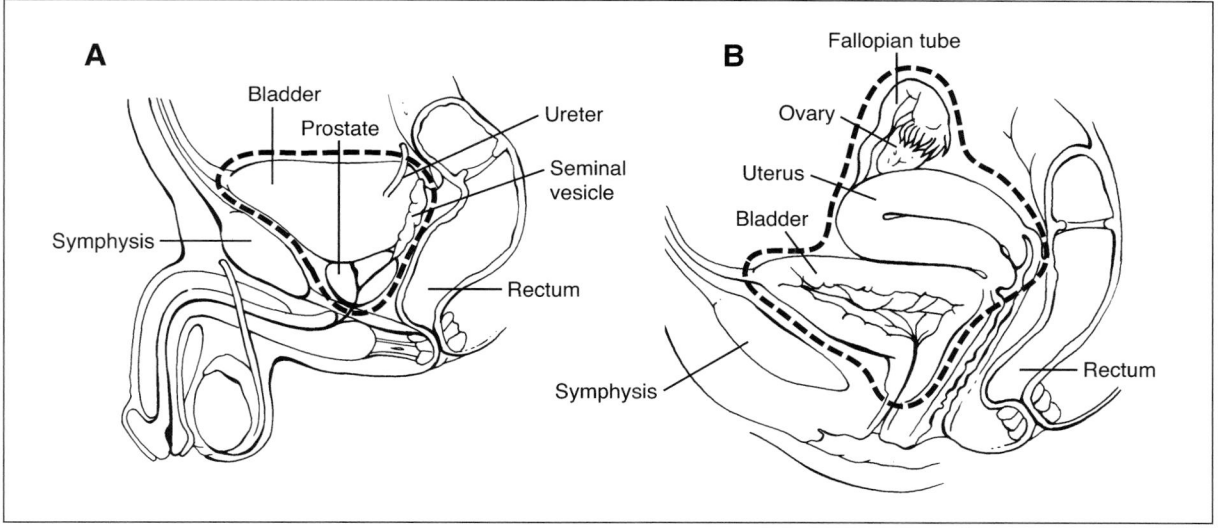

Figure 9-13. Anatomy of the pelvis with tissue to be excised outlined by dashed line: (A) male; (B) female.

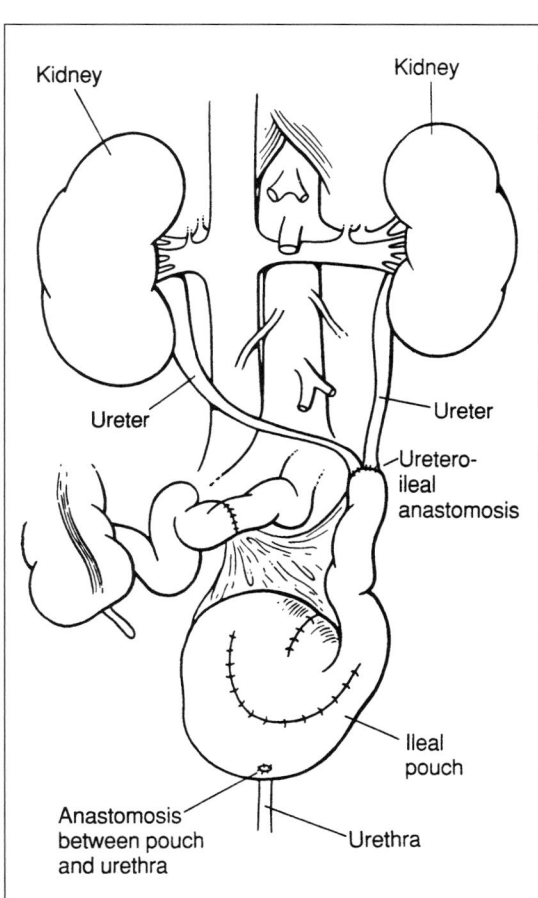

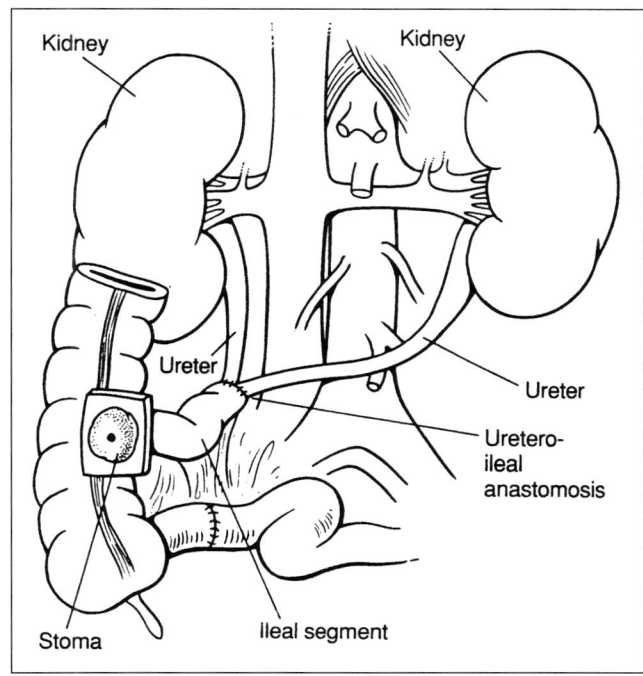

↑**Figure 9-14.** Ileal conduit: A segment of ileum is isolated from terminal ileum and continuity of the bowel is reestablished with an end-to-end anastomosis. Ureters are joined to the proximal end of the ileal segment and the distal end is brought out to the skin as a stoma.

← **Figure 9-15.** Bladder substitution: A segment of ileum is fashioned into a pouch and anastomosed to the urethra. The ureters are joined to the proximal, nondetubularized segment.

SUMMARY OF PROCEDURES

	Simple Cystectomy	Partial Cystectomy	Radical Cystectomy
Position	Supine	⇐	Supine or lithotomy
Incision	Transperitoneal, midline	⇐	⇐
Antibiotics	Cefotetan or ceftriaxone 1 g	⇐	⇐
Surgical time	4 h	2 h	6 h

	Simple Cystectomy	Partial Cystectomy	Radical Cystectomy
EBL	1000 ml	Minimal	1500 ml
Postop care	Care of the stoma	Catheter care	Care of the stoma
Mortality	1%	< 1%	2%
Morbidity	Prolonged ileus: 5%	–	5%
	Infection: 2%	–	2%
		Hematuria: 5%	
Pain score	10	10	10

PATIENT POPULATION CHARACTERISTICS

Age range	40-80 yr	⇐	⇐
Male:Female	3:1	⇐	⇐
Incidence	40,000 new cases of bladder cancer diagnosed/yr; 20% treated with cystectomy.	⇐	⇐
Etiology	Contracted bladder; hemorrhagic and radiation cystitis	Bladder cancer; bladder diverticulum	⇐
Associated conditions	Heart disease (10%); HTN (10%); COPD (5%); diabetes mellitus (5%)	Heart disease (10%)	⇐

ANESTHETIC CONSIDERATIONS

PREOPERATIVE

Patients presenting for cystectomy are frequently elderly and may have preexisting medical problems, including CAD, CHF, PVD, cerebrovascular disease, COPD, and renal impairment. Preop evalution should be directed toward the detection and treatment of these conditions prior to anesthesia.

Respiratory	✓ for pulmonary disease in older patients. **Tests:** As indicated from H&P.
Cardiovascular	✓ for cardiac disease, HTN in older patients. **Tests:** Consider ECG; others as indicated from H&P.
Gastrointestinal	Bowel prep likely and may cause dehydration and electrolyte disturbances. **Tests:** Electrolytes, if indicated.
Hematologic	T&C for 2-4 U PRBC. **Tests:** Hct
Laboratory	Other tests as indicated from H&P.
Premedication	Sedation prn anxiety in adults (e.g., lorazepam 1-2 mg po 1-2 h preop; midazolam 1-2 mg iv in preop area).

INTRAOPERATIVE

Anesthetic technique: Spinal, continuous lumbar epidural, or GA are acceptable, with choice dependent on length of procedure, coexisting disease, and patient preference. A combined technique using GA and regional anesthesia may be preferable. A T4 sensory level is recommended since peritoneal stimulation is likely during this procedure.

Regional anesthesia:

Spinal	0.75% bupivacaine 12-15 mg in 7.5% dextrose; hyperbaric tetracaine 10-15 mg with 200 μg epinephrine for procedures > 3 h.
Epidural	1.5-2% lidocaine with epinephrine 5 μg/ml, 15-25 ml; supplement with 5-10 ml as needed. Supplemental iv sedation (e.g., midazolam 1 mg iv prn; fentanyl 50 μg iv prn). Bupivacaine (0.25-0.5%), levobupivacaine (0.25-0.5%), or ropivacaine (0.5-0.75%), with or without sufentanil or fentanyl, may also be used. The addition of opiates has been associated with ↑urinary retention in noncatheterized patients.

General anesthesia:

Induction	Standard induction (see p. B-2). These patients may be significantly dehydrated and require volume replacement before induction.	
Maintenance	Standard maintenance (see p. B-3).	
Emergence	No specific considerations	
Blood and fluid requirements	Significant blood loss possible IV: 16 ga × 1 NS/LR @ 6-10 ml/kg/h Warm fluids. Humidify gases.	Blood loss may be less with regional than GA.
Monitoring	Standard monitors (see p. B-1). Arterial line CVP line	Consider PA catheter in patients with cardiopulmonary disease. UO as measure of volume status may be lost during procedure.
Complications	Major blood loss 3rd-space losses Hypothermia	

POSTOPERATIVE

Complications	Hypothermia	
Pain management	Morphine 0.1-0.3 mg/kg iv in incremental doses Consider epidural narcotics or PCA.	See pp. C2 – C-3.
Tests	Hct	Others as indicated by intraop course.

Reference

1. Marshall FF: Surgery of the bladder. In *Campbell's Urology*, Vol 3, 7th edition. Walsh PC, et al, eds. WB Saunders, Philadelphia: 1998, 3274-98.
2. Whalley DG, Berrigan MJ: Anesthesia for radical prostatectomy, cystectomy, nephrectomy, pheochromocytoma, and laparoscopic procedures. *Anesthesiol Clin North Am* 2000; 18(4):899-917.

OPEN BLADDER OPERATIONS (OTHER THAN CYSTECTOMY)

SURGICAL CONSIDERATIONS

Description: Open bladder operations include:

Augmentation cystoplasty (or **enterocystoplasty**): Small, contracted bladders can be enlarged and their size and capacity augmented with a segment of intestine. The bladder is opened widely, anteroposteriorly, or from side-to-side, or with a cruciate incision. A segment of intestine—either small bowel, cecum, or colon—is isolated from the intestinal tract, detubularized, and added on to the bladder.

Variant procedure: The antrum of the stomach can also be used (**gastrocystoplasty**).

Usual preop diagnosis: Contracted bladder from chronic cystitis

Repair of vesicovaginal or enterovesical fistulas: The communication between the vagina and bladder or bladder and bowel is identified and excised, and the edges freshened until normal, noninflamed tissues are exposed. The openings in the bladder and in the vagina or bowel are closed, and omentum is interposed in between to promote healing and prevent recurrence. With enterovesical fistulas, often the diseased segment of the intestine is excised and an **end-to-end anastomosis** of the intestine is performed.

Variant procedure: Transvaginal repair of vesicovaginal fistula (see Vaginal Operations, p. 728).

Usual preop diagnosis: Vesicovaginal or enterovesical fistula

Ureteral reimplantation, performed to correct vesicoureteral reflux, is more commonly used in the pediatric group than in adults. In adults, it is performed mainly for lower ureteral injuries, iatrogenic or traumatic. The lower ureter is identified and dissected proximally until adequate length is obtained. The bladder is opened and a 2-3 cm submucosal tunnel is created in or near the trigone, and the ureter is brought into the tunnel and fixed with sutures. If there is a large gap between the ureter and the bladder, a **psoas hitch procedure** is necessary. The bladder is mobilized and stitched to the psoas muscle in order to reach the ureter. In children, if the ureter is dilated, its diameter is reduced by imbrication before reimplantation. In adults, a nonrefluxing implantation is usually not necessary if the operation is being performed for ureteral injury.

Usual preop diagnosis: Vesicoureteral reflux; lower ureteral injuries

SUMMARY OF PROCEDURES

	Augmentation Cystoplasty	Repair of Fistulas	Ureteral Reimplantation
Position	Supine	Supine or lithotomy	Supine
Incision	Low abdominal	⇐	⇐
Antibiotics	Gentamicin 80 mg iv, slowly	⇐	⇐
Surgical time	4 h	3 h	⇐
EBL	Minimal	⇐	⇐
Postop care	Care of catheters and stents	⇐	⇐
Mortality	< 1%	⇐	⇐
Morbidity	Infections: 5%	⇐	⇐
	Urinary leakage: 1%	⇐	⇐
Pain score	10	10	10

PATIENT POPULATION CHARACTERISTICS

Age range	All ages	⇐	⇐
Male:Female	1:4	⇐	⇐
Incidence	Rare	⇐	⇐
Etiology	Contracted bladders from chronic cystitis	Traumatic fistulas; vesicovaginal; regional enteritis; diverticulitis; colon cancer	Vesicoureteral reflux; injury to lower ureters

ANESTHETIC CONSIDERATIONS

PREOPERATIVE

Patients presenting for open bladder operations may be of any age, depending on the etiology of the abnormality. Elderly patients frequently have preexisting medical problems, including CAD, CHF, PVD, cerebrovascular disease, COPD, and renal impairment. Preop evaluation should be directed toward the detection and treatment of these conditions prior to anesthesia.

Respiratory	✓ for pulmonary disease in elderly patients. **Tests:** As indicated from H&P.
Cardiovascular	✓ for of cardiac disease in elderly patients. **Tests:** Consider ECG; others, if indicated from H&P.
Neurological	Paraplegics and quadriplegics may present for operations on the bladder and urinary tract. Obtain Hx of autonomic hyperreflexia (AH). Sx are: flushing, HA, nasal stuffiness, and HTN associated with voiding or noxious stimuli below level of transection.

Laboratory	Other tests as indicated from H&P.
Premedication	Sedation prn anxiety (e.g., lorazepam 1-2 mg po 1-2 h before surgery; midazolam 1-2 mg iv in preop area).

INTRAOPERATIVE

Anesthetic technique: Spinal, continuous lumbar epidural, or GA are acceptable, with choice dependent on length of procedure, coexisting disease, and patient preference. A combined technique using light GA with regional anesthesia is also acceptable. A T10 sensory level is sufficient to provide anesthesia for procedures on the bladder, but a T4 level is recommended if the peritoneum is opened. (See Anesthetic Considerations for Transurethral Procedures [except TURP] p. 698, for patients with AH.)

Regional anesthesia:

Spinal	0.75% bupivacaine 10-12 mg. For shorter procedures (< 1 hr), consider low-dose bupivacaine (0.75%, 7.5 mg); mepivicaine (1.5%, 45 mg); or procaine (10%, 100-150 mg). Lidocaine may be used, but the incidence of transient neurologic symptoms is significant (30%).
Epidural	1.5-2% lidocaine with epinephrine 5 μg/ml, 15-25 ml; supplement with 5-10 ml as needed. Supplemental iv sedation. Bupivacaine (0.25-0.5%), levobupivacaine (0.25-0.5%), or ropivacaine (0.5-0.75%), with or without sufentanil or fentanyl, may also be used. The addition of opiates has been associated with ↑urinary retention in noncatheterized patients.

General anesthesia:

Induction	Standard induction (see p. B-2).	
Maintenance	Standard maintenance (see p. B-3). Consider limiting N_2O for long intraperitoneal procedures to minimize bowel distention.	
Emergence	No specific considerations	
Blood and fluid requirements	Minimal-to-moderate blood loss IV: 16-18 ga × 1 NS/LR @ 2-4 ml/kg/h Warm fluids. Humidify gases for lengthy procedures.	Intraperitoneal procedures have considerably higher requirements (e.g., NS/LR @ 6-10 ml/kg/h).
Monitoring	Standard monitors (see p. B-1) for simpler procedures. ± Arterial/CVP lines	UO as a measure of volume status may be lost during the procedure. Consider arterial line, CVP for longer, more complex procedures.
Positioning	✓ and pad pressure points. ✓ eyes.	★ **NB**: In lithotomy position, peroneal nerve compression at lateral fibular head → foot drop.
Complications	AH in spinal cord injured patients	See discussion in Anesthetic Considerations for Transurethral Procedures, p. 702.

POSTOPERATIVE

Complications	Hypothermia Fever, bacteremia	
Pain management	Morphine 0.1-0.3 mg/kg in incremental doses. Consider epidural narcotics or PCA.	See pp. C-2, C-3.
Tests	Hct Blood cultures if febrile	Others as indicated by intraop course.

Reference

1. Marshall FF: Surgery of the bladder. In *Campbell's Urology*, Vol 3, 7th edition. Walsh PC, et al, eds. WB Saunders, Philadelphia: 1998, 3274-98.

INGUINAL OPERATIONS

SURGICAL CONSIDERATIONS

Description: Inguinal operations are very common, and are usually performed on an outpatient basis. Groin dissection, however, may necessitate inpatient care.

Inguinal herniorrhaphy: A 3" inguinal incision is made, starting 1" medial to the anterior-superior iliac spine, and ending at the pubic tubercle. The external oblique aponeurosis is excised, opening the external inguinal ring. The spermatic cord and the hernial sac are freed off the inguinal canal; then the hernial sac is dissected off the spermatic cord and followed proximally into the internal inguinal ring, where it is suture-ligated and excised. The floor of the inguinal canal is strengthened by approximating the conjoined tendon to the reflected part of the inguinal ligament.

Usual preop diagnosis: Inguinal hernia (See Figs 9-16, 17 for details of anatomic relationships.)

Orchiopexy is performed through the same incision as used in herniorrhaphy. Once the inguinal canal is exposed, a search for the undescended testis begins. The testis and cord are dissected free from all surrounding tissue until adequate length is obtained to bring the testis down to the scrotum. Next, a pouch is created in the wall of the scrotum by incising the scrotal skin and dissecting it off dartos fascia. The testis is brought down into the pouch and fixed to the dartos fascia with sutures, and the incisions are closed. Often a **herniorrhaphy** is performed at the same time.

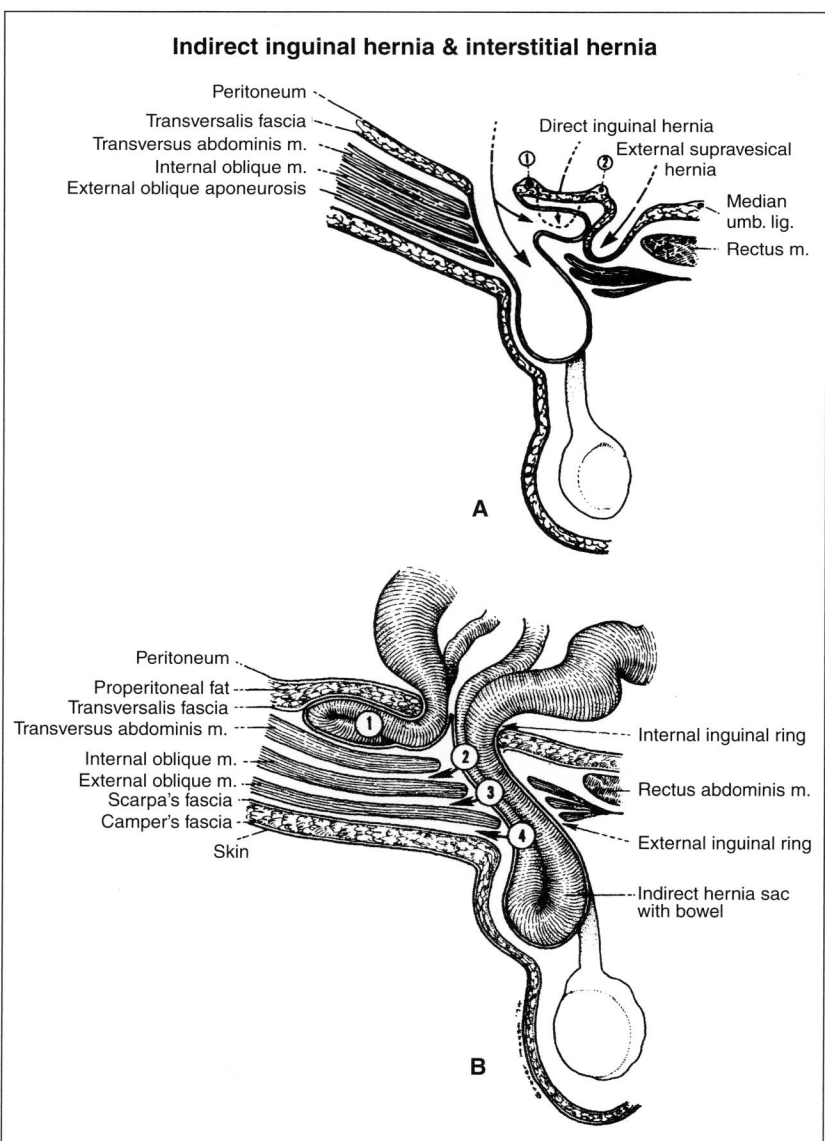

Usual preop diagnosis: Undescended testis

Figure 9-16. (A) Relationships of four groin hernias in one patient. Indirect inguinal hernia with intraparietal diverticulum, direct hernia, and external supravesical hernia. 1= lateral umbilical ligament; 2 = medial umbilical ligament. Arrows indicate different sites of origin of each hernia. (Reproduced with permission from Skandalakis JE, Gray SW, Burns WB, et al: Internal and external supravesical hernia. *Am Surg* 1976; 42:142.) (B) Diagram of intraparietal hernia. The sac, entering at the internal ring, may pass into any one or more spaces between layers of the abdominal wall. 1, properitoneal; 2 and 3, interstitial; 4, superficial. An indirect hernia also may be present. (Reproduced with permission form Skandalakis JE, Gray SW, Akin JT Jr: The surgical anatomy of hernial rings. *Surg Clin North Am* 1974; 54:1227.)

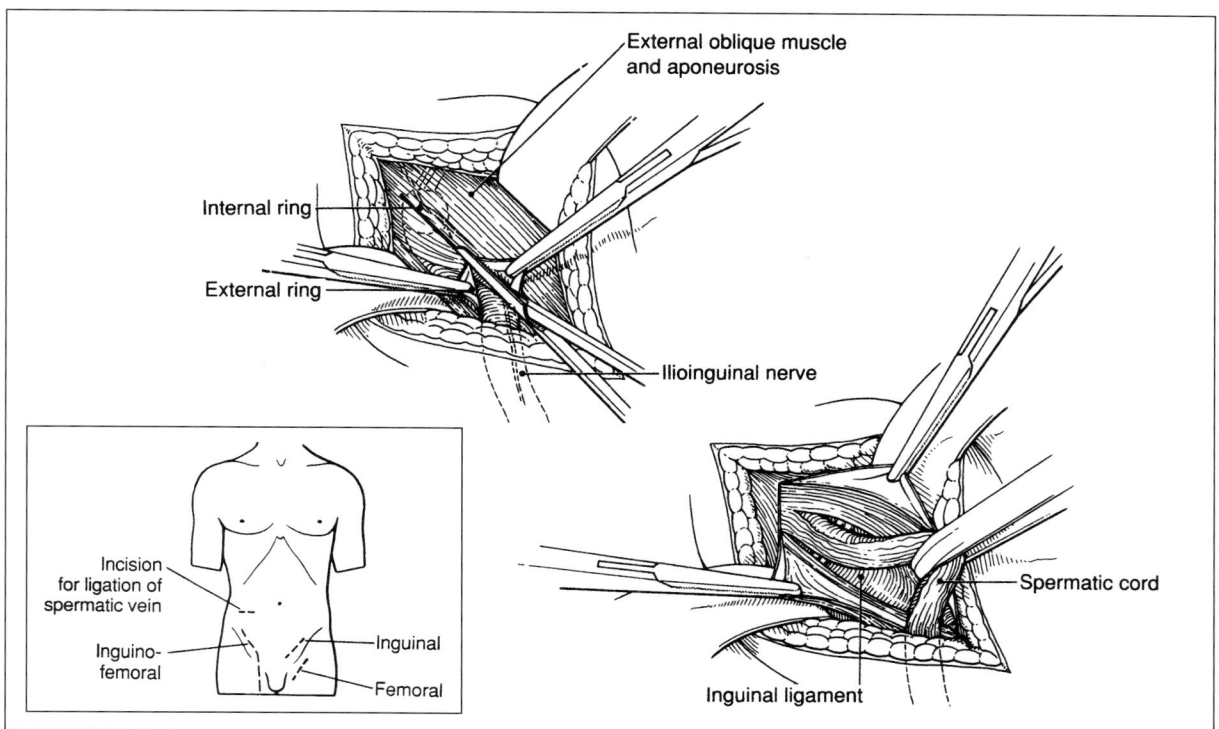

Figure 9-17. Incisions, and exposure of the spermatic cord for inguinal hernia repair. (Reproduced with permission from Scott-Conner CEH, Dawson DL: *Operative Anatomy*, 2nd edition. Lippincott Williams & Wilkins, 2003.)

Radical orchiectomy is performed through a herniorrhaphy incision (described above). The spermatic cord is freed and cross-clamped at the internal inguinal ring, transected, and suture-ligated. The testis, with its tunica vaginalis, is then delivered through the incision by blunt and sharp dissection and the inguinal incision is closed. Sometimes, a testicular prosthesis is inserted and fixed in the scrotum before the inguinal incision is closed.

Usual preop diagnosis: Testicular cancer

Ligation of spermatic vein is performed through a small, transverse incision 1-2" above the internal inguinal ring. Muscles are split and peritoneum reflected medially to expose the spermatic vessels; the vein is identified and ligated.

Usual preop diagnosis: Varicocele causing infertility

Groin dissection, or **inguinofemoral lymphadenectomy** (lymph node dissection), is the most critical of the inguinal operations. It is performed through either an inguinal incision (Fig 9-17, inset) curved distally over the femoral vessels or through 2 incisions, inguinal and upper-thigh (Fig 9-17, inset), over the femoral triangle. A complete inguinal and femoral lymphadenectomy is performed.

Usual preop diagnosis: Penile cancer

SUMMARY OF PROCEDURES

	Herniorrhaphy, Orchiopexy, Orchiectomy	Ligation of Spermatic Vein	Groin Dissection
Position	Supine	⇐	⇐
Incision	Inguinal (Fig 9-17, inset)	Transverse groin (Fig 9-17, inset)	Inguinal and upper thigh (Fig 9-17, inset)
Antibiotics	None	⇐	⇐
Surgical time	1 h	⇐	3 h
EBL	Minimal	⇐	200 ml
Postop care	PACU → home	⇐	PACU → ward; leg elevation
Mortality	< 1%	⇐	⇐
Morbidity	Wound infection: 2%	⇐	⇐
Pain score	7	5	7

PATIENT POPULATION CHARACTERISTICS

	Herniorrhaphy, Orchiopexy, Orchiectomy	Ligation of Spermatic Vein	Groin Dissection
Age range	All ages	Young adults	Middle age
Incidence	Hernia: 5% of population Undescended testis: 0.8% of male children Testis cancer: 6/100,000	1% of young men	Extremely rare, < 1% of all males
Etiology	Unknown; congenital	Varicocele	Penile cancer (very rare)

ANESTHETIC CONSIDERATIONS

PREOPERATIVE

Typically, patients presenting for inguinal operations are healthy, with most returning home on the day of surgery. The most common inguinal operation is herniorrhaphy. In these patients, consider causes of increased intraabdominal pressure during H&P. (Pediatric inguinal operations are discussed in Pediatric General Surgery, p. 1058+.) A hernia may strangulate → acute abdomen.

Respiratory   Chronic cough is a common precipitating factor.

Gastrointestinal   Constipation may be a precipitating factor.

Laboratory   Tests as indicated from H&P.

Premedication   Sedation for adults prn anxiety (e.g., lorazepam 1-2 mg po 1-2 h before surgery; midazolam 1-2 mg iv in preop area).

INTRAOPERATIVE

Anesthetic technique: Local anesthesia (with sedation), spinal, epidural, or GA are acceptable techniques, with choice dependent on patient age and coexisting disease, type and length of procedure, and patient preference. Local anesthesia is acceptable for simple herniorrhaphy, although discomfort may be elicited if the peritoneum is manipulated. If a spinal or epidural anesthetic is chosen, a T6 level should be sought. Most inguinal procedures are done on an outpatient basis, and the anesthetic should be planned appropriately.

Regional anesthesia:

  Spinal   0.75% bupivacaine 10-12 mg. For shorter procedures (< 1 h), consider low-dose bupivacaine (0.75%, 7.5 mg); mepivicaine (1.5%, 45 mg); or procaine (10%, 100-150 mg). Lidocaine may be used, but the incidence of transient neurologic symptoms is significant.

  Epidural   1.5-2.0% lidocaine with epinephrine 5 μg/ml, 15-25 ml; supplement with 5-10 ml as needed. Supplemental iv sedation with local or regional technique in adults; e.g., midazolam (1-2 mg iv), fentanyl (25-50 μg iv prn anxiety or discomfort); or propofol infusion (25-50 μg/kg/min).

General anesthesia:

  Induction   Standard induction (see p. B-2). ET intubation and/or controlled ventilation may not be needed for shorter cases; consider LMA.

  Maintenance   Standard maintenance (see p. B-3); consider propofol infusion (100-200 μg/kg/min). Muscle relaxation usually not required.

  Emergence   No specific considerations

Blood and fluid requirements   Usually minimal blood loss
IV: 18 ga × 1
NS/LR @ 1-2 ml/kg/h   Minimize NS/LR to avoid postop urinary retention after herniorrhaphy.

Monitoring   Standard monitors (see p. B-1).

POSTOPERATIVE

Complications   PONV
Failure to void   May delay discharge from PACU → home.

Pain management Local anesthesia
Ketorolac 30 mg im or iv in adults
± morphine 2-4 mg iv or fentanyl 25-
50 μg iv

Instillation (2 min) or infiltration of wound with 0.25% bupivacaine or ilioinguinal nerve block provides prolonged postop analgesia and decreases need for narcotics in outpatients. This can be used in both adult and pediatric patients.

References

1. Casey WF, Rice LJ, Hannallah RS, et al: A comparison between bupivacaine instillation versus ilioinguinal/iliohypogastric nerve block for postoperative analgesia following inguinal herniorrhaphy in children. *Anesthesiology* 1990; 72(4):637-9.
2. Goldstein M: Surgical management of male infertility and other scrotal disorders. In *Campbell's Urology*, Vol 2, 7th edition. WB Saunders, Philadelphia: 1998, 1331-78.
3. Herr HW: Surgery of penile and urethral carcinoma. In *Campbell's Urology*, Vol 3, 7th edition. WB Saunders, Philadelphia: 1998, 3395-409.
4. Rozanski T, Bloom DA, Colodny A: Surgery of the scrotum and testis in childhood. In *Campbell's Urology*, Vol 2, 7th edition. WB Saunders, Philadelphia: 1998, 2193-209.

PENILE OPERATIONS

SURGICAL CONSIDERATIONS

Penectomy is the total or partial resection of the penis for squamous-cell carcinoma of the penile skin. If the tumor can be resected with a safe margin of at least 2 cm, partial penectomy is usually enough. A tourniquet is placed at the base of the penis, which is amputated at least 2 cm proximal to the tumor. The corpora cavernosa are sutured and the tourniquet is released, followed by inspection for bleeding. The edges of the urethra are sutured to the ventral skin and the lateral and dorsal skin edges are approximated over the ends of the corpora cavernosa. Often, an **inguinal lymph node biopsy** follows the penectomy.

Usual preop diagnosis: Squamous-cell carcinoma of the penile skin

Insertion of penile prosthesis is performed for impotence. The prosthesis is inserted into the corpora cavernosa (Fig 9-18) through a penile or suprapubic incision. Penile prostheses are either malleable or inflatable. The latter have a reservoir in the retropubic space and a pump in the scrotum.

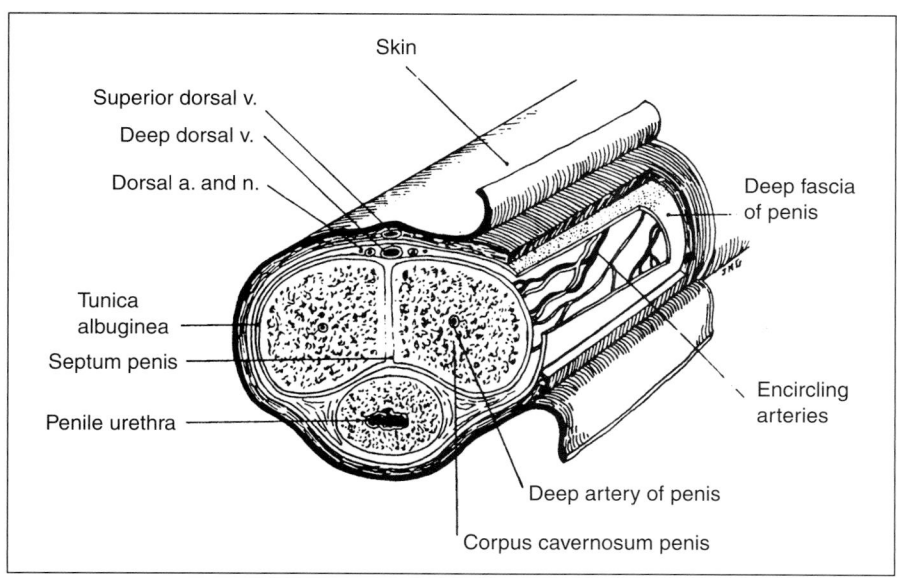

Figure 9-18. Anatomy of the penis. (Reproduced with permission from Hardy JD: *Textbook of Surgery.* JB Lippincott, 1988.)

Usual preop diagnosis: Impotence

Hypospadias repair is performed primarily on children < 5 yr. (See Pediatric Urology, p. 1075.)

SUMMARY OF PROCEDURES

	Penectomy	Insertion of Penile Prosthesis
Position	Supine	⇐
Incision	Circumferential penile	Bilateral incisions at base of penis
Special instrumentation	None	⇐
Unique considerations	None	⇐
Antibiotics	None	Gentamicin 80 mg iv, slowly; ampicillin 2 g iv
Surgical time	2 h	⇐
Closing considerations	None	⇐
EBL	200 ml	⇐
Postop care	PACU → home	⇐
Mortality	< 1%	⇐
Morbidity	Penile hematoma: 5%	Malfunction: 10%
		Edema: 5%
		Infection: 2%
		Extrusion of the prosthesis: 1%
Pain score	5	5

PATIENT POPULATION CHARACTERISTICS

Age range	Adults	⇐
Incidence	< 1% of all males	1-2% of all males
Etiology	Poor hygiene	Organic impotence

ANESTHETIC CONSIDERATIONS

PREOPERATIVE

Patients presenting for insertion of a penile prosthesis are frequently elderly and often have preexisting medical problems, including CAD, CHF, PVD, cerebrovascular disease, COPD, and renal impairment. Preop evaluation should be directed toward the detection and treatment of these conditions prior to anesthesia.

Neurological   Patients presenting for insertion of a penile prosthesis often have Hx of diabetes or spinal cord injury. Note presence of neuropathy or Hx of autonomic hyperreflexia (AH) (see Anesthetic Considerations for Transurethral Procedures [except TURP], p. 698). Sx suggestive of AH include HA, flushing, nasal stuffiness, and HTN associated with voiding or noxious stimuli below the level of transection. It is important to document neurological deficits prior to regional anesthesia.

Hematologic   Coagulation defects may be present in patients with priapism. There is a high incidence of priapism in patients with sickle-cell anemia.
Tests: Hct, if indicated from H&P.

Laboratory   Other tests as indicated from H&P.

Premedication   Sedation prn anxiety in adults (e.g., lorazepam 1-2 mg po 1-2 h prior to surgery; midazolam 1-2 mg iv in preop area).

INTRAOPERATIVE

Anesthetic technique: Spinal, caudal, or lumbar epidural and GA are acceptable, with choice dependent on length of procedure, patient age, coexisting disease, and patient preference. Sacral anesthesia (saddle block) is sufficient; lumbar epidural anesthesia may be less reliable than spinal or caudal at blocking sacral fibers.

Regional anesthesia:

Spinal   5% lidocaine 50 mg (controversial); 0.75% bupivacaine 10 mg in 7.5% dextrose; hyperbaric tetracaine 10 mg with epinephrine for longer procedures

Caudal	0.5% bupivacaine with epinephrine 5 μg/ml 15-20 ml
Epidural	1.5% lidocaine with epinephrine 5 μg/ml 15-25 ml; supplement with 5-10 ml as needed. Supplemental iv sedation
General anesthesia:	
Induction	Standard induction (see p. B-2). ET intubation may not be necessary for shorter procedures; consider LMA.
Maintenance	Standard maintenance (see p. B-3). Deeper levels of anesthesia usually are required to obtund autonomic reflexes (e.g., HTN, laryngospasm) resulting from intense surgical stimulation that may occur during these procedures.
Emergence	No specific considerations
Blood and fluid requirements	Minimal blood loss IV: 18 ga × 1 NS/LR at 2 ml/kg/h
Monitoring	Standard monitors (see p. B-1).
Complications	AH See Anesthetic Considerations for Transurethral Procedures, p. 702.

POSTOPERATIVE

Complications	Urinary retention
Pain management	Morphine 0.05-0.1 mg/kg iv or fentanyl 25-50 μg iv prn; ketorolac 30 mg im or iv

References

1. Herr HW: Surgery of penile and urethral carcinoma. In *Campbell's Urology*, Vol 3, 7th edition. WB Saunders, Philadelphia: 1998, 3395-3409.
2. Lewis R: Penile prosthesis. In *Campbell's Urology*, Vol 2, 7th edition. WB Saunders, Philadelphia: 1998, 1216-26.
3. Lewis R: Surgery for erectile dysfunction. In *Campbell's Urology*, Vol 2, 7th edition. WB Saunders, Philadelphia: 1998, 1215-36.
4. Lynch DF, Schellhammer PF: Tumors of the penis. In *Campbell's Urology*, Vol 3, 7th edition. WB Saunders, Philadelphia: 1998, 2453-86.

SCROTAL OPERATIONS

SURGICAL CONSIDERATIONS

Description: Scrotal operations are minor, common urologic procedures, performed on an outpatient basis.

Simple orchiectomy is performed as an alternative to medical castration, using either estrogens or LH-RH agonists on men with metastatic prostate cancer for androgen ablation. It is always bilateral. A small scrotal incision is made and the testis delivered. The spermatic cord is cross-clamped, transected, and suture-ligated.

Usual preop diagnosis: Metastatic prostate cancer

Vasovasostomy is the reestablishment of the continuity of the vas deferens and fertility following a previously performed vasectomy. Through a small scrotal incision, the testis and spermatic cord are delivered. The site of previous vasectomy is identified and excised and the two ends of the vas deferens anastomosed. It is bilateral and requires the use of either the operating microscope or magnifying loupes.

Usual preop diagnosis: Infertility 2° vasectomy

Hydrocelectomy: The testis, with the surrounding hydrocele (Fig 9-19), is delivered through a scrotal incision. The wall of the hydrocele is excised and the edges sutured around the epididymis to prevent recurrence.

Variant procedure or approach: Aspiration used as a temporizing approach since recurrence is almost 100%.

Usual preop diagnosis: Hydrocele

Spermatocelectomy: A spermatocele is a cyst of the epididymis, usually excised with the part of the epididymis from which it arises.

Variant procedure: Aspiration as a temporizing maneuver until the operation can be performed.

Usual preop diagnosis: Spermatocele or epididymal cyst

Insertion of testicular prosthesis: A small incision is made in the scrotal skin and a pouch is created by blunt dissection in dartos fascia. The prosthesis is placed in the pouch and fixed to the dartos fascia to prevent prosthesis migration.

Usual preop diagnosis: Absent testis, either congenital or following orchiectomy

Reduction of testicular torsion is an emer-

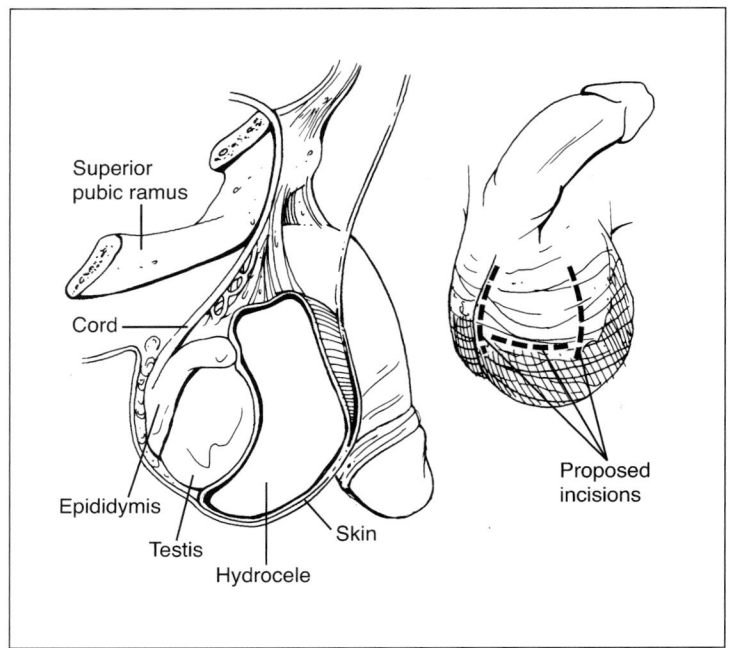

Figure 9-19. Scrotal hydrocele; scrotal incision.

gency operation which must be performed within 6 h of occurrence to prevent irreversible ischemic damage to the testis. Through a small scrotal incision, the testis is reduced and fixed to the dartos fascia to prevent retorsion.

Usual preop diagnosis: Acute testicular torsion

SUMMARY OF PROCEDURE

Position	Supine
Incision	Scrotal (Fig 9-19, inset)
Special instrumentation	Operating microscope; magnifying loupe for vasovasostomy
Antibiotics	None
Surgical time	1 h
EBL	Negligible
Postop care	PACU → home
Mortality	< 1%
Morbidity	Scrotal hematoma: 2%
	Wound infection: 2%
Pain score	4

PATIENT POPULATION CHARACTERISTICS

Age range	All ages
Incidence	Common
Etiology	See preop diagnosis for each procedure, above.

ANESTHETIC CONSIDERATIONS

PREOPERATIVE

Patients presenting for scrotal operations typically fall into two groups: young, otherwise healthy patients and an older population who may present with metastatic prostate cancer accompanied by other medical conditions. The latter group is the focus of the preop evaluation.

Respiratory   Pulmonary disease may be present in elderly patients requiring orchiectomy.
                              Tests: As indicated from H&P.

Cardiovascular	Cardiac disease may be present in elderly patients requiring orchiectomy. **Tests:** Consider ECG; others, if indicated from H&P.
Neurological	Document neurologic exam before regional anesthesia in patients with metastatic prostate carcinoma (spinal-cord or nerve-root compression may be present preop).
Musculoskeletal	✓ for presence of spinal metastases if orchiectomy is done for palliation of prostate carcinoma. Extensive lumbar metastases may preclude the use of spinal or epidural anesthesia (relative contraindication). **Tests**: L-spine films if Hx suggestive of spinal metastases.
Laboratory	Other tests as indicated from H&P.
Premedication	Sedation prn anxiety (e.g., lorazepam 1-2 mg po 1-2 h prior to surgery; midazolam 1-2 mg iv in preop area).

INTRAOPERATIVE

Anesthetic technique: Local anesthesia (with sedation) is acceptable for simpler operations (vasectomy, orchiectomy). Procedures that are longer or more complex may require spinal, epidural, or GA. A sensory level of T10 is required to block pain 2° testicular manipulation. Many of these procedures are done on an outpatient basis, and the anesthetic should be appropriately planned.

Regional anesthesia:

Spinal	0.75% bupivacaine 10-12 mg. For shorter procedures (< 1 h), consider low-dose bupivacaine (0.75%, 7.5 mg); mepivicaine (1.5%, 45 mg); or procaine (10%, 100-150 mg). Lidocaine may be used, but the incidence of transient neurologic symptoms is significant.
Epidural	1.5-2% lidocaine with epinephrine 5 μg/ml, 15-20 ml; supplement with 5-10 ml as needed. Supplemental iv sedation with local or regional techniques (e.g., midazolam 1-2 mg, fentanyl 25-50 μg iv prn anxiety or discomfort).

General anesthesia:

Induction	Standard induction (see p. B-2). Consider use of LMA.
Maintenance	Standard maintenance (see p. B-3). Muscle relaxation usually not imperative. Deeper levels of anesthesia are usually required to obtund autonomic reflexes (e.g., HTN, laryngospasm) resulting from intense surgical stimulation that may occur during these procedures.
Emergence	No specific considerations
Blood and fluid requirements	Minimal blood loss IV: 18 ga × 1 NS/LR @ 2 ml/kg/h
Monitoring	Standard monitors (see p. B-1).
Positioning	✓ and pad pressure points. ✓ eyes.	★ **NB**: peroneal nerve compression at lateral fibular head → foot drop.

POSTOPERATIVE

Complications	Peroneal nerve injury 2° lithotomy position	Peroneal nerve injury manifested by foot drop and loss of sensation on dorsum of foot. Seek neurology consultation.
Pain management	Ketorolac 30 mg im or iv in adults ± morphine 2-4 mg iv or fentanyl 25-50 μg iv prn	Following orchiopexy, high incidence of postop pain, N/V, which may be reduced by ilioinguinal/iliohypogastric nerve blocks.

References

1. Hannallah RS, Broadman LM, Belman AB, et al: Comparison of caudal and ilioinguinal/iliohypogastric nerve blocks for control of post-orchiopexy pain in pediatric ambulatory surgery. *Anesthesiology* 1987; 66(6):832-4.
2. Rozanski T, Bloom DA, Colodny A: Surgery of the scrotum and testis in childhood. In *Campbell's Urology*, Vol 2, 7th edition. WB Saunders, Philadelphia: 1998, 2193-209.

PERINEAL OPERATIONS

SURGICAL CONSIDERATIONS

Urethroplasty: Urethral strictures that do not respond to transurethral dilation and incision are corrected with urethroplasty. A transverse or longitudinal perineal incision is made and carried down to the urethra, which is dissected free from surrounding tissues. The strictured area is excised and end-to-end anastomosis is performed over a catheter. Repair of a long urethral stricture may require placement of a patch from the scrotum, foreskin, or buccal mucosa.

Variant procedure: Transurethral incision and dilation, which is associated with a 30-50% recurrence rate.

Usual preop diagnosis: Urethral stricture, usually posttraumatic

Urethrectomy: Partial or total urethrectomy is done through a longitudinal perineal incision.

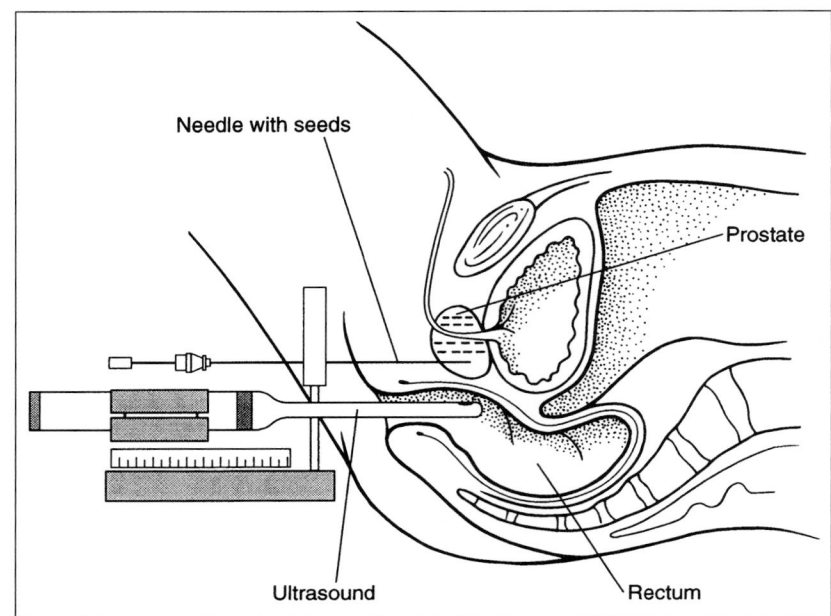

Figure 9-20. Transperineal brachytherapy of prostate gland.

The urethra is dissected free of surrounding tissues and followed proximally and distally from the membranous urethra to the external urethral meatus. In total urethrectomy, a tubularized skin graft is interposed between membranous urethra and perineal skin.

Usual preop diagnosis: Urethral carcinoma

Insertion of artificial urinary sphincter, performed for incontinence, consists of a perineal incision, through which a cuff is inserted around the bulbar urethra. A suprapubic incision is made to place the reservoir and pump, which inflates and deflates the cuff.

Usual preop diagnosis: Urinary incontinence

Transperineal prostate seed implantation (brachytherapy): High doses of radiation can be delivered to the prostate by implanting radioactive seeds directly into the prostate gland. Using a transrectal ultrasound probe, radioactive seeds (iodine 125 or palladium 103) are implanted into the prostate (Fig 9-20). The patient is placed in lithotomy position, and a rectal ultrasound probe, with a perineal grid attached, is introduced to image the prostate. Radioactive seeds are then placed transperineally using preloaded needles. Preop dosing calculations determine the number and location of the seeds. This procedure is done by a combined team of radiation oncologists and urologists. No special radiation precautions are necessary for the OR team.

Usual preop diagnosis: Prostate cancer

SUMMARY OF PROCEDURES

	Urethroplasty	Urethrectomy	Insertion of Sphincter	Brachytherapy
Position	Lithotomy	⇐	⇐	⇐
Incision	Perineal (Fig 9-6)	⇐	⇐ and scrotal (Fig. 9-19, inset)	None
Antibiotics	Gentamicin 80 mg im/iv	⇐	⇐	⇐
Surgical time	3 h	2 h	3 h	2 h
EBL	100 ml	300 ml	Minimal	⇐
Postop care	PACU → room	⇐	⇐	PACU, outpatient
Mortality	< 1%	⇐	⇐	⇐

	Urethroplasty	Urethrectomy	Insertion of Sphincter	Brachytherapy
Morbidity	Wound infection: 2%	⟸	⟸ Erosion of the urethra: 10% Extrusion of sphincter: 2%	Urinary retention
Pain score	3	3	4	3

PATIENT POPULATION CHARACTERISTICS

	Urethroplasty	Urethrectomy	Insertion of Sphincter	Brachytherapy
Age range	All ages	Adults	Older adults	50-80 yr
Incidence	< 1% of urologic procedures	⟸	2% of radical prostatectomy	10% of prostate cancer
Etiology	Traumatic strictures	Unknown	Radical prostatectomy (2%); incontinence	Aging

ANESTHETIC CONSIDERATIONS

PREOPERATIVE

This is a generally healthy patient population; preop considerations should be based on H&P.

Laboratory	Tests as indicated from H&P.
Premedication	Sedation prn anxiety in adults (e.g., lorazepam 1-2 mg po 1-2 h prior to surgery; midazolam 1-2 mg iv in preop area).

INTRAOPERATIVE

Anesthetic technique: Spinal or GA are acceptable, with choice dependent on length of procedure, position, patient age, coexisting disease, and patient preference. A sacral sensory level (saddle block) is usually sufficient. Lumbar epidural anesthesia may be less reliable at providing sacral anesthesia, and offers no advantages over the above techniques for shorter procedures, although caudal anesthesia may be an acceptable alternative.

Regional anesthesia:

Spinal	0.75% bupivacaine 10 mg in 7.5% dextrose; hyperbaric tetracaine 10 mg (with epinephrine [200 μg] for longer procedures)
Caudal	0.5% bupivacaine with epinephrine 5 μg/ml 15-20 ml. Supplemental iv sedation.

General anesthesia:

Induction	Standard induction (see p. B-2). Consider use of LMA.
Maintenance	Standard maintenance (see p. B-3); muscle relaxation usually not required. Deeper levels of anesthesia are usually required to obtund autonomic reflexes (e.g., HTN, laryngospasm) resulting from intense surgical stimulation that may occur during these procedures.
Emergence	No specific considerations
Blood and fluid requirements	Minimal blood loss IV: 18 ga × 1 NS/LR at 2 ml/kg/h
Monitoring	Standard monitors (see p. B-1).
Positioning	✓ and pad pressure points. ✓ eyes.	Patients with arthritis or other musculoskeletal disorders may not tolerate the exaggerated lithotomy position, ★ thus precluding the use of a regional technique. **NB**: In lithotomy position, peroneal nerve compression at lateral fibular head → foot drop.
Complications	Anticipate ↓BP on return from lithotomy position.	Rx: volume (200-500 ml NS/LR) or ephedrine (5 mg iv) may be necessary.

POSTOPERATIVE

Complications	Peroneal nerve injury 2° lithotomy position	Peroneal nerve injury manifests as foot drop with loss of sensation over dorsum of foot. Seek neurology consultation.
Pain management	Mild-to-moderate pain	Rx: morphine 0.05-0.1 mg/kg iv prn

VAGINAL OPERATIONS

SURGICAL CONSIDERATIONS

Description: Vaginal operations are performed by both urologists and gynecologists. They include the following:

Repair of vesicovaginal fistulas: The vaginal approach is usually recommended for small and distally located vesicovaginal fistulas; otherwise, a transabdominal repair is performed (see Open Bladder Operations, p. 715). An incision is made in the anterior vaginal wall around the fistula, which is excised. Bladder and vaginal walls are separated and closed with interposition of tissues or flaps to separate the incisions and prevent recurrence. A Foley catheter is left indwelling. **Variant approach:** Transabdominal repair of vesicovaginal fistula (see Open Bladder Operations, p. 715).

Usual preop diagnosis: Vesicovaginal fistula

Operations to correct stress urinary incontinence: Many procedures have been designed to correct female urinary incontinence. They fall into two basic groups: (1) operations to correct hypermobility of the urethra, and (2) operations to correct nonfunctioning urethra. The operation most commonly used by urologists to correct hypermobility is the **Stamey procedure** (Fig 9-21), or endoscopic **vesical neck suspension.** The operation is performed through two small suprapubic incisions, one on each side of the midline, and an anterior vaginal incision. A nylon suture is placed in a loop from either side of the bladder neck and not around it. Cystoscopy is used to ensure proper placement and to prevent the suture from transversing the bladder. When the sutures are pulled up and tied over the anterior rectus sheath, they pull the bladder neck up to its original position behind the symphysis pubis and restore the acute posterior ureterovesical angle. A variant of this procedure is the **Raz bladder neck suspension,** where bolsters are not used.

Operations to correct a nonfunctioning urethra include **submucosal collagen injection** at the bladder neck or construction of a **sling.** Rectus fascia, fascia lata of the thigh or the vaginal wall can be used to construct a sling around the urethra. All these techniques involve a combined suprapubic and vaginal approach.

Sling operations are the most common procedures done for correction of stress incontinence. These procedures can be done vaginally or open via a suprapubic incision. A variety of materials, both natural and synthetic, have been used. Many modifications have been made with reference to the placement of anchorage of the sling; therefore, there are a large number of procedures with different names utilizing the same principle. Most slings are placed midurethra.

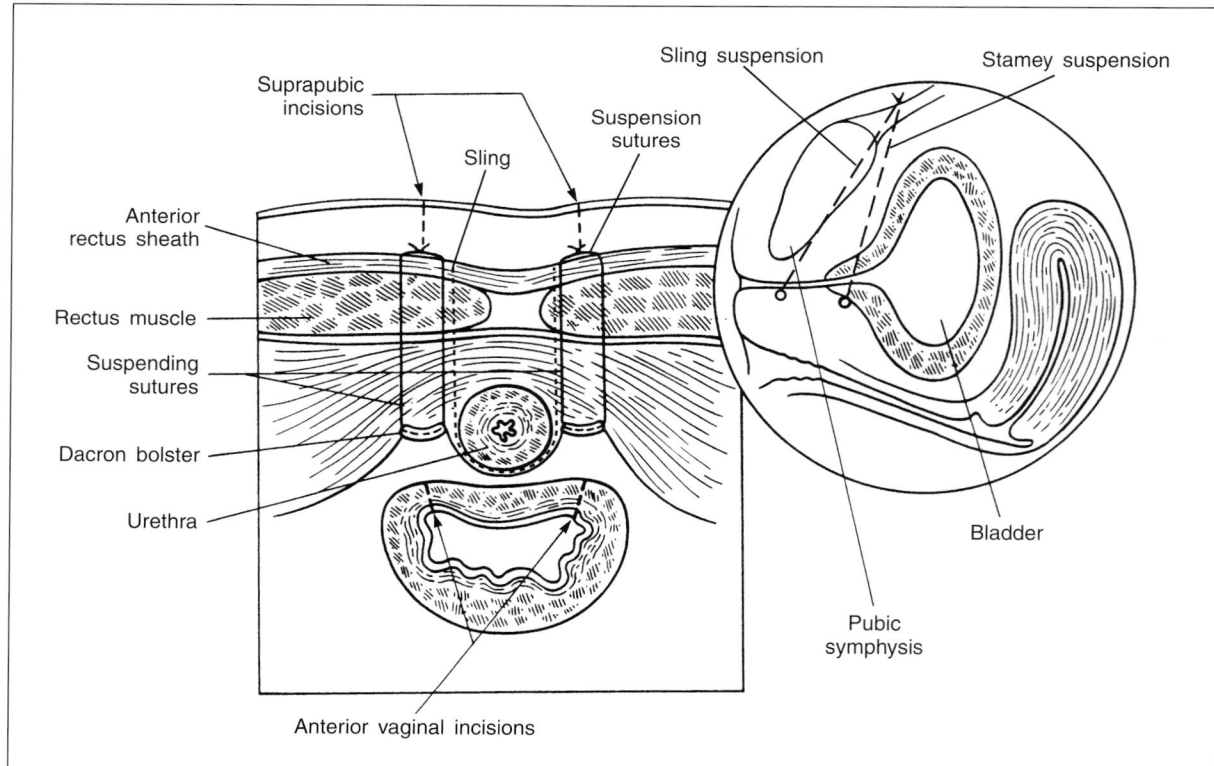

Figure 9-21. Stamey and sling procedures, sectional view; inset shows lateral view.

728

Variant approach: The **Marshall-Marchetti-Krantz operation**, which is performed retropubically, sutures the anterior portion of the urethra, bladder neck, and bladder to the pubic bone.

Usual preop diagnosis: Stress urinary incontinence

Excision of urethral diverticulum: Urethral diverticula are extremely rare and need excision only if they are the cause of recurrent UTIs. An incision is made in the anterior vaginal wall over the urethral diverticulum, which is dissected all around until it is attached only by its neck. It is excised and the neck closed. A Foley catheter is left indwelling, and the vaginal incision is closed.

Usual preop diagnosis: Recurrent UTI 2° infected urethral diverticulum

Repair of cystocele and rectocele: Some patients with urinary incontinence also present with prolapse of the bladder or rectum into the vagina. These can be repaired at the same time as incontinence surgery. A vaginal incision (anterior for cystocele, posterior for rectocele) is made and dissected laterally to free the bladder or rectum from the vagina. The defect is repaired and the redundant vaginal wall excised.

Usual preop diagnosis: Incontinence with pelvic prolapse, cystocele, or rectocele

SUMMARY OF PROCEDURES

	Repair of Vesicovaginal Fistula	Correction of Stress Incontinence	Excision of Urethral Diverticulum
Position	Lithotomy	⇐	⇐
Incision	Anterior vaginal	Anterior vaginal; suprapubic	Anterior vaginal
Special instrumentation	None	Cystoscope	None
Antibiotics	Gentamicin 80 mg iv, slowly	⇐	⇐
Surgical time	2 h	1 h	⇐
EBL	200 ml	500 ml	200 ml
Postop care	PACU → room	⇐	⇐
Mortality	< 1%	⇐	⇐
Morbidity	Infection: 2%	⇐	⇐
	Recurrence: 2%	10%	⇐
		Urinary retention: 20%	
Pain score	3	5	3

PATIENT POPULATION CHARACTERISTICS

Age range	20-80 yr	⇐	⇐
Incidence	< 1% of urologic procedures	5% of urologic procedures	< 1% of urologic procedures
Etiology	Traumatic delivery; iatrogenic following hysterectomy (< 1%)	Childbirth	Congenital (extremely rare)

ANESTHETIC CONSIDERATIONS

PREOPERATIVE

This is a generally healthy patient population. Preop considerations should be based on H&P.

Laboratory	Tests as indicated from H&P.
Premedication	Standard premedication (see p. B-2).

INTRAOPERATIVE

Anesthetic technique: Spinal, continuous lumbar epidural, or GA are acceptable, with choice dependent on age, coexisting disease, and patient preference. A block level of T9-T10 is recommended for operations involving the bladder, whereas somewhat higher levels of anesthesia may be necessary if a suprapubic incision is made. Epidural anesthesia may be less reliable than spinal in providing sacral anesthesia.

Regional anesthesia:

Spinal	0.75% bupivacaine 10-12 mg (1.6 ml)

Epidural	2% lidocaine with epinephrine 5 µg/ml, 15-20 ml. Supplemental iv sedation.
General anesthesia:	
Induction	Standard induction (see p. B-2).
Maintenance	Standard maintenance (see p. B-3). Muscle relaxation not imperative.
Emergence	No specific considerations
Blood and fluid requirements	Minimal blood loss IV: 18 ga × 1 NS/LR @ 2-4 ml/kg/h
Monitoring	Standard monitors (see p. B-1).
Positioning	✓ and pad pressure points. ✓ eyes.	★ **NB**: In lithotomy position, peroneal nerve compression at lateral fibular head → foot drop.
Complications	Anticipate ↓BP when returning from lithotomy. Bladder perforation	Rx: volume (200-500 ml NS/LR) or ephedrine (5 mg iv) may be necessary. Bladder perforation may present as shoulder pain in the awake patient, but may go unnoticed in the patient under GA. Sx include unexplained HTN, tachycardia, ↓BP (rare).

POSTOPERATIVE

Complications	Peroneal nerve injury 2° lithotomy position Bladder perforation (see above).	Peroneal nerve injury is manifested as foot drop with loss of sensation on dorsum of foot. Seek neurology consultation.
Pain management	Consider ketorolac 30 mg iv/im in adults; supplement with morphine 0.05-0.1 mg/kg iv prn.	

References

1. Leach GE, Trockman BA: Surgery for vesicovaginal and urethrovaginal fistula and urethral diverticulum. In *Campbell's Urology*, Vol 1, 7th edition. WB Saunders, Philadelphia: 1998, 1135-54.
2. Raz S, Stothers L, Chopra A: Vaginal reconstructive surgery for incontinence and prolapse. In *Campbell's Urology*, Vol 1, 7th edition. WB Saunders, Philadelphia: 1998, 1059-94.

10.0 ORTHOPEDIC SURGERY

Surgeons

Vincent R. Hentz, MD
Gordon A. Brody, MD

10.1 HAND SURGERY

Anesthesiologist

Eric Rey Amador, MD

DARRACH PROCEDURE

SURGICAL CONSIDERATIONS

Description: The **Darrach procedure** (Fig 10.1-1) is a resection of the distal ulna. The distal 2 cm of the ulna is resected subperiosteally, and local soft tissues are used to stabilize and cover the remaining ulna. It is commonly performed in patients who have had a disruption of the distal radioulnar joint with subluxation of the ulna. It also is indicated for patients who have had a malunion of a distal radius fracture such that the radius has shortened relative to the ulna or is abnormally angulated, resulting in dorsal subluxation of the ulna and impingement of the ulnar head upon the carpus. This causes painful motion of the wrist and forearm and posttraumatic degenerative arthritis of the ulnar head, carpus, and sigmoid notch of the distal radius. Disorders of the distal radioulnar joint and degeneration of the ulnar head, which may lead to attrition rupture of the overlying extensor tendons, are common in rheumatoid arthritis. This dorsal prominence of the ulnar head is treated by **Darrach resection**, combined with a soft-tissue procedure to stabilize the remaining ulna. Osteoarthritic degeneration of the distal radioulnar joint, either 2° trauma (see above) or due to idiopathic osteoarthritis, responds well to this procedure.

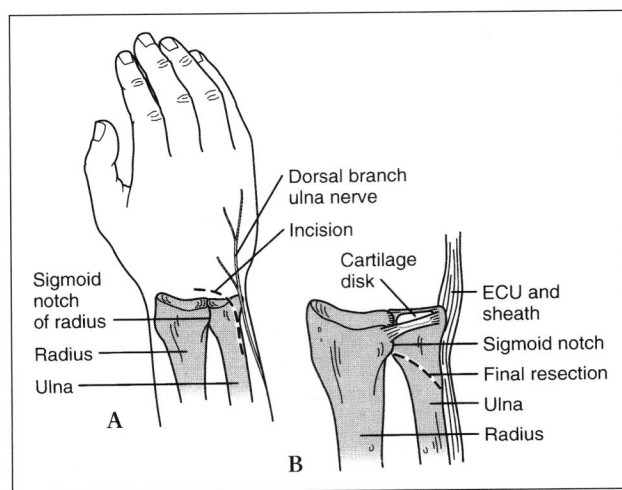

Figure 10.1-1. The Darrach procedure. (A) Skin incision. Avoid dorsal cutaneous branch of the ulnar nerve. (B) The distal ulna is resected at the radioulnar articulation just proximal to the sigmoid notch. (ECU=extensor carpi ulnaris) (Reproduced with permission from Chapman MW: *Chapman's Orthopaedic Surgery*, 3rd edition. Lippincott Williams & Wilkins, 2001.)

Variant procedure or approaches: Modifications of the Darrach procedure, such as the **hemiresection interposition technique of Bowers** and the **Soavé-Kapandji procedure**, are performed for the same indications as above.

Usual preop diagnosis: Arthritis or derangement of the distal radioulnar joint; rheumatoid arthritis; ulnar impingement syndrome; malunion of Colles' fracture or other fracture of the distal radius

SUMMARY OF PROCEDURE

Position	Supine, with arm extended on hand-surgery table
Incision	Dorsal-ulnar, over distal ulna
Special instrumentation	Pneumatic tourniquet
Antibiotics	Cefazolin 1 g iv
Surgical time	1-2.5 h, depending on associated procedures
Tourniquet	150 mmHg above systolic; max time = 120 min
Closing considerations	Routine skin closure; postop splint placed at conclusion of procedure.
EBL	Minimal; performed under tourniquet control.
Postop care	Elevation to minimize swelling. PACU → home, or overnight stay in observation bed.
Mortality	None associated with procedure
Morbidity	Ulnar nerve injury: Rare
	Postop swelling (rarely requires specific treatment)
Pain score	5-7

PATIENT POPULATION CHARACTERISTICS

Age range	Late teens–elderly
Male:Female	Slight predominance of females, due to incidence of malunion of Colles' fractures in women with senile osteoporosis
Incidence	Not uncommon
Etiology	See Usual Preop Diagnosis, above.
Associated conditions	Rheumatoid arthritis

ANESTHETIC CONSIDERATIONS

See Anesthetic Considerations for Wrist Procedures, p. 740.

Reference

1. Nolan WB, Eaton RG: Darrach procedure for distal ulnar pathology derangements. *Clin Orthop* 1992; 275:85-9.

DORSAL STABILIZATION AND EXTENSOR SYNOVECTOMY OF THE RHEUMATOID WRIST

SURGICAL CONSIDERATIONS

Description: This procedure is indicated for patients with rheumatoid arthritis and extensor tenosynovitis refractory to medical treatment, as well as extensor tendon ruptures and/or intercarpal synovitis. The procedure is performed under tourniquet control through a straight dorsal incision over the wrist. A **radical tenosynovectomy** of the extensor tendons in all six extensor compartments is carried out. Tendon ruptures or impending ruptures are repaired with tendon grafts or side-to-side anastomoses. Bone spurs are removed and a synovectomy of the distal radioulnar joint is carried out. A **modified Darrach procedure**, with resection or osteoplasty of the distal ulna, is usually performed. If there is evidence of synovitis within the wrist joint, a synovectomy is performed through a dorsal arthrotomy. A flap of the extensor retinaculum is transposed beneath the extensor tendons to reinforce the dorsal wrist ligaments

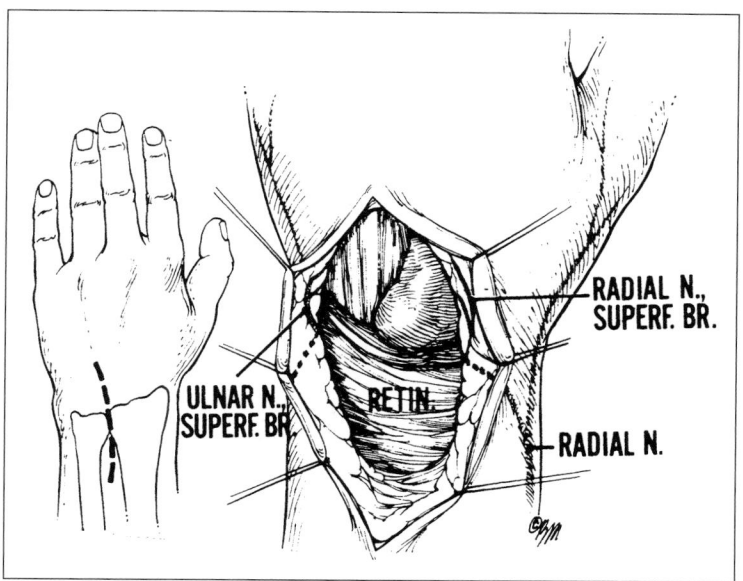

Figure 10.1-2. Incision and exposure for dorsal tenosynovectomy. Note superficial branches of radial and ulnar nerves protected in skin flaps. (Illustration by Elizabeth Roselius, © 1988. Reproduced with permission from Green DP: *Operative Hand Surgery*, 2nd edition. Churchill Livingstone: 1988.)

and, thus, stabilize the wrist to prevent volar subluxation of the carpus. A posterior interosseous neurectomy is carried out at the same time. The remaining extensor retinaculum is divided into two transverse strips and one is used to stabilize the distal ulna. The second strip is placed dorsal to the extensor tendons so they will not bowstring during wrist extension.

Usual preop diagnosis: Rheumatoid arthritis with extensor tendon tenosynovitis; extensor tendon rupture; distal radioulnar joint synovitis and/or subluxation

SUMMARY OF PROCEDURE

Position	Supine, with arm extended on hand-surgery table
Incision	Dorsal wrist (Fig 10.1-2)
Special instrumentation	Pneumatic tourniquet
Antibiotics	Cefazolin 1 g iv
Surgical time	2 h
Tourniquet	150 mmHg above systolic; max time = 120 min
Closing considerations	Postop splint
EBL	Minimal; tourniquet used until dressing in place.
Postop care	Admitted overnight for pain control and limb elevation.

Mortality	None associated with procedure
Morbidity	Extremity swelling (typically does not require treatment)
	Delayed healing 2° immunosuppression and steroid use
	Wound infection: Rare (unless patient is immunosupressed)
Pain score	3-5

PATIENT POPULATION CHARACTERISTICS

Age range	Procedure uncommon before 4th decade
Male:Female	As in all patients with rheumatoid arthritis, females more common.
Incidence	Not uncommon
Etiology	Connective tissue disorder; rheumatoid arthritis or variant
Associated conditions	All conditions associated with connective tissue disorders, including active rheumatoid arthritis, steroid dependency, immunosuppressive therapy, and/or skin fragility

ANESTHETIC CONSIDERATIONS

See Anesthetic Considerations for Wrist Procedures, p. 740.

Reference

1. Millender LH, Terrono AL: Synovectomy and tendon reconstruction. In *The Wrist*. Gelberman RH, ed. Raven Press, New York: 1994, 221-37.

METACARPOPHALANGEAL AND INTERPHALANGEAL JOINT ARTHROPLASTY

SURGICAL CONSIDERATIONS

Description: Joint replacement in the hand is most commonly indicated in patients with rheumatoid arthritis with severe joint destruction → pain and dysfunction. It is rarely indicated in patients with osteoarthritis. The most common prostheses, made of silicone rubber and popularized by Swanson, differ from total joint replacement in the hip or knee in that they do not function as true joints, but rather as spacers in a **resection arthroplasty**. Most of the stability and motion of these joints depend on meticulous soft-tissue reconstructions involving tendon and ligament transfers, as well as intensive postop physical therapy. To obtain good results, patients must be well motivated and understand their disease process and what will be asked of them during the recovery period. The results for **metacarpophalangeal (MP) arthroplasty** are far better than those obtained in the proximal interphalangeal joints. **Proximal interphalangeal joint arthroplasty** is now indicated only for the central middle and ring digits in patients with good ligamentous and tendinous structures. **Distal interphalangeal (DIP) arthroplasty** is rarely performed, since these patients do well with fusions. The procedure for the MP joints is performed through a dorsal transverse incision under tourniquet control. The metacarpal heads are removed with an oscillating saw and the intramedullary canals reamed to accept the stems of the prostheses. Once they have been placed with a no-touch technique, the capsule is closed and the supporting ligaments are reconstructed with centralization of extensor tendons. A splint with support for each finger is placed at the conclusion of surgery. Reconstructive procedures of the wrist and fingers can be combined with arthroplasty.

Variant procedure or approaches: Some surgeons favor longitudinal incisions rather than a transverse incision for the approach to the MP joints.

Usual preop diagnosis: Rheumatoid arthritis or other connective-tissue disorder

SUMMARY OF PROCEDURE

Position	Supine, with arm extended on hand-surgery table
Incision	Dorsal hand, transverse, or longitudinal
Special instrumentation	MP or PIP joint prostheses and associated instruments for preparing the medullary canal; pneumatic tourniquet
Antibiotics	Cefazolin 1 g iv
Surgical time	2.5 h
Tourniquet	150 mm above systolic; max time = 120 min
Closing considerations	Critical postop splinting
EBL	Minimal; tourniquet used throughout procedure.
Postop care	Admitted to hospital for pain control and limb elevation.
Mortality	None associated with procedure
Morbidity	Swelling (may require early splitting of dressing)
	Wound infection: Rare (if it occurs, requires removal of prosthesis)
	Prosthesis infection: Rare
Pain score	3-6

PATIENT POPULATION CHARACTERISTICS

Age range	> 50 yr
Male:Female	As in rheumatoid arthritis, females predominate.
Incidence	Uncommon
Etiology	Rheumatoid arthritis or other connective-tissue disorder
Associated conditions	As in rheumatoid arthritis (e.g., skin fragility, steroid dependency, immunosuppression)

ANESTHETIC CONSIDERATIONS

See Anesthetic Considerations for Wrist Procedures, p. 740.

ARTHRODESIS OF THE WRIST

SURGICAL CONSIDERATIONS

Description: A variety of arthrodeses can be performed about the wrist. These include **radiopancarpal arthrodesis** (**total wrist fusion**), and radiolunate, radioscapholunate, and intercarpal arthrodeses (**partial wrist fusions**). Radiopancarpal arthrodesis is generally performed as a salvage procedure for wrist pathology that cannot be treated with a procedure that preserves wrist motion. These indications include posttraumatic degenerative arthritis following fractures and dislocations, idiopathic osteoarthritis and/or rheumatoid arthritis. In the nonrheumatoid patient, an effective procedure is an arthrodesis using an iliac crest bone graft fixed with plate and screws. More recent techniques with improved plate designs rarely require iliac crest bone graft. Local bone from the distal radius is commonly utilized. Alternative techniques with other forms of fixation also are used. It has been shown that a position of fusion in 10-15° of dorsiflexion provides the greatest grip strength. In the rheumatoid patient, a technique using intramedullary fixation with a large-diameter Steinmann pin is preferred. Rheumatoid bone is osteoporotic, 2° disuse and chronic steroid administration. Screw fixation is not ideal in this soft bone. Bone graft is obtained locally in these patients, usually from the resected ulnar head. **Radiolunate fusion** also is indicated in rheumatoid patients who have progressive ulnar translation of the carpus. The lunate acts to block this translation of the carpus. **Radioscapholunate fusion** is indicated in patients with radiocarpal arthritis. This procedure preserves about 50% of wrist motion that occurs at the midcarpal joint. Bone graft is necessary and is easily obtained from the distal radius through the same incision. There are a variety of **intercarpal arthrodeses**, including **triscaphe** (scaphotrapezialtrapezoid), **scaphocapitate**, **lunotriquetrel** and **four-corner** (capitate-hamate-triquetral-lunate). These procedures are indicated for the treatment of intercarpal arthritis, carpal instabilities due to intercarpal ligament tears and Kienbock's disease (aseptic necrosis of the lunate). Each procedure requires bone graft, which may be obtained from the distal radius or the iliac crest. The **Cloward cervical spine fusion instrumentation** is useful for obtaining a bicortical plug of bone from the iliac crest with minimal dissection.

Usual preop diagnosis: Posttraumatic arthritis; osteoarthritis or rheumatoid arthritis; Kienbock's disease; carpal instability

SUMMARY OF PROCEDURE

Position	Supine, with arm extended on hand-surgery table. The iliac crest may be prepped and elevated with a sandbag beneath the ipsilateral buttock.
Incision	Dorsal wrist, transverse (for intercarpal fusion), or longitudinal
Special instrumentation	Pneumatic tourniquet
Unique considerations	Bone-graft donor site
Antibiotics	Cefazolin 1 g iv
Surgical time	2 h
Tourniquet	150 mmHg above systolic; max time = 120 min
Closing considerations	Immobilization with splints
EBL	Minimal; procedure is performed under tourniquet control. If iliac crest bone graft is used, there may be up to 500 ml of blood loss.
Postop care	PACU → room for pain and edema control
Mortality	None associated with procedure
Morbidity	Nonunion of fusion: ≤ 20%
Pain score	5-7, if no iliac graft; 6-9, if iliac graft used

PATIENT POPULATION CHARACTERISTICS

Age range	> 40 yr
Male:Female	Females predominate in rheumatoid arthritis; males in posttraumatic arthritis.
Incidence	Common
Etiology	Trauma (common); rheumatoid arthritis (common)
Associated conditions	Typical for rheumatoid arthritis (e.g., skin fragility, steroid dependency, immunosuppression)

ANESTHETIC CONSIDERATIONS

See Anesthetic Considerations for Wrist Procedures, p. 740.

Reference

1. Green DP: *Operative Hand Surgery*, 4th edition. Churchill Livingstone, New York: 1999.

TOTAL WRIST REPLACEMENT

SURGICAL CONSIDERATIONS

Description: The major indication for this procedure is rheumatoid arthritis of the wrist. **Total wrist replacement (TWR)** is often recommended in patients with bilateral wrist disease. An arthrodesis will be carried out on the nondominant helping hand and a TWR on the dominant hand to preserve dexterity. Many surgeons prefer to avoid **bilateral wrist arthrodesis**, although some patients with bilateral fusions have been able to function relatively well. Currently available protheses are suitable only for low-demand patients, and are not indicated for high-demand patients with posttraumatic arthritis. These patients will do better with wrist arthrodesis. Silastic wrist prostheses are associated with a high failure rate and silicone synovitis, and their use has been abandoned by many surgeons. The most commonly used prostheses today are metal on ultra-high-molecular-weight polyethylene articulations that are fixed with methylmethacrylate cement or bone ingrowth into porous stems. All of these prostheses depend on intact, normally functioning wrist extensor tendons, especially the extensor carpi radialis brevis, for balance and function. Absence of this tendon is felt by many to be an absolute contraindication to this procedure. Because these tendons are so commonly affected by rheumatoid arthritis, the patient population for this procedure is limited. In addition to functioning tendons, meticulously accurate placement of the components in relation to the centers of rotation of the wrist is critical for success. If the centers of rotation of the prosthesis do not duplicate those of the normal wrist, early component loosening and failure is likely. Intraop radiographs are useful in verifying component position. These patients frequently have other upper extremity deformities that will require reconstruction. Because of the complexity of TWR, other reconstructive procedures are not carried out at the same time.

Usual preop diagnosis: Rheumatoid arthritis

SUMMARY OF PROCEDURE

Position	Supine, with arm extended on hand-surgery table
Incision	Dorsal wrist
Special instrumentation	TWR instrumentation; pneumatic tourniquet
Antibiotics	Cefazolin 1 g iv
Surgical time	2 h
Tourniquet	150 mmHg above systolic; max time = 120 min
Closing considerations	Postop splint
EBL	Minimal; procedure performed under tourniquet control.
Postop care	PACU → room
Mortality	None associated with procedure
Morbidity	Infection: Rare (but requires removal of prosthesis and methylmethocrylate cement, if used)
	Poor wound healing
Pain score	4-8

PATIENT POPULATION CHARACTERISTICS

Age range	Rare before 4th decade; most in 6th and 7th decades
Male:Female	Females outnumber males, as in rheumatoid arthritis.
Incidence	Rare
Etiology	Rheumatoid arthritis
Associated conditions	Rheumatoid arthritis

ANESTHETIC CONSIDERATIONS

See Anesthetic Considerations for Wrist Procedures, p. 740.

Reference

1. Green DP: *Operative Hand Surgery*, 4th edition. Churchill Livingstone, New York: 1999.

THUMB CARPOMETACARPAL JOINT FUSION/ ARTHROPLASTY/STABILIZATION

SURGICAL CONSIDERATIONS

Description: Patients with degenerative arthritis of the carpometacarpal (CMC) joint of the thumb present with subluxation, pain, and synovitis of the joint. A **synovectomy and ligament reconstruction** to restore stability will treat pain and prevent further degeneration. This procedure is performed through a curvilinear incision over the joint. A distally attached graft of the radial 1/2 of the flexor carpi radialis tendon is passed through a drill hole in the base of the metacarpal and woven into the joint capsule. In the later stages of degeneration, patients must be treated with either an arthroplasty or an arthrodesis. A variety of **arthroplasty techniques** are available to the surgeon. The most successful methods involve resection of all or part of the trapezium and replacement with a biological spacer—usually a rolled up tendon graft commonly referred to as an 'anchovy.' These procedures also stabilize the first metacarpal with a tendon transfer through a drill hole in the bone. **Arthrodesis** (fusion) is another alternative. Fixation may be obtained with Kirschner wires and intraosseous compression wires. The time to fusion with this technique is 6 wk. These patients have very few limitations and perform almost all normal activities of daily living. This procedure requires very little postop hand therapy, compared with arthroplasty techniques. It also is well suited to active patients. In some patients with extensive bone loss and cyst formation, bone graft is necessary and can be obtained from the distal radius.

Variant procedure or approaches: Newer techniques, such as the tension-band intraosseous wire and sliding cortical graft, have much lower failure rates (although silicone rubber prostheses are associated with particulate synovitis).

Usual preop diagnosis: Osteoarthritis of CMC joint; basal joint arthritis; synovitis of CMC joint; CMC joint dislocation; trauma

SUMMARY OF PROCEDURE

Position	Supine, with arm extended on hand-surgery table
Incision	Curvilinear over joint at base of thumb. Tendon graft for interposition can be obtained through multiple small transverse incisions.
Special instrumentation	Pneumatic tourniquet
Antibiotics	Cefazolin 1 g iv
Surgical time	1.5-2 h
Tourniquet	150 mmHg above systolic; max time = 120 min
EBL	Minimal; procedures performed under tourniquet control.
Postop care	Postop splintage; overnight hospital stay for pain control
Mortality	None associated with procedure
Morbidity	Nonunion of arthrodesis: ≤ 20%
	Particulate synovitis (silicone rubber prostheses)
Pain score	8-9

PATIENT POPULATION CHARACTERISTICS

Age range	Joint stabilization in 3rd-5th decades; arthroplasty and arthrodesis in 5th-8th decades
Male:Female	Basal joint instability and arthritis much more prevalent in women
Incidence	Common
Etiology	Trauma may play a role in producing instability. Intraarticular fracture of the base of the first metacarpal with a nonanatomic reduction → incongruence of the joint → posttraumatic arthritis. Rheumatoid arthritis → instability and degeneration of the joint. Congenital ligamentous laxity → unstable basal joints and arthritis in many patients.
Associated conditions	Rheumatoid arthritis; osteoarthritis; carpal tunnel syndrome (CTS)

ANESTHETIC CONSIDERATIONS FOR WRIST PROCEDURES

(Procedures covered: Darrach procedure; dorsal stabilization and extensor synovectomy of the rheumatoid wrist; metacarpophalangeal and interphalangeal joint arthroplasty; arthrodesis of the wrist; total wrist replacement; thumb carpometacarpal joint fusion/arthroscopy/stabilization)

PREOPERATIVE

Airway	Rheumatoid involvement of the C-spine, TMJ, and cricoarytenoid joint (CAJ) are common in this patient population. Erosion of cervical vertebrae → unstable C-spine (e.g., atlantoaxial subluxation) necessitates extreme care in head and neck manipulation. C-spine fusion (↓neck ROM), TMJ arthritis (↓mouth opening) and CAJ arthritis (laryngeal narrowing, hoarseness, DOE, stridor) portend difficult intubation and may necessitate awake fiber optic intubation (p. B-6). In the case of CAJ arthritis, use of a smaller ETT may be required.
Respiratory	Rheumatoid patients may exhibit Sx of pleural effusion (✓ CXR) or pulmonary fibrosis (dyspnea, diffuse rales, ↓diffusing capacity, honeycomb appearance in CXR).
	Tests: Consider CXR, PFTs, ABGs in affected patients.

Cardiovascular	Rheumatoid patients may suffer from pericarditis, myocarditis, valvular disease, and cardiac conduction defects. Because of the physical limitations imposed by the disease process, it may prove difficult to evaluate these patients' cardiovascular status; hence, cardiology consultation, ECG, and ECHO may be useful in preparing for surgery. **Tests:** Consider ECG and ECHO, especially in patients with severe rheumatoid arthritis.
Neurological	Rheumatoid patients may have cervical or lumbar radiculopathies that should be documented carefully preop. In addition, peripheral neuropathy with consequent sensory/motor defects may be present. **Tests:** Consider C-spine radiographs to r/o occult subluxations in rheumatoid patients with neck pain or upper extremity radiculopathy.
Musculoskeletal	Bony deformities or muscle contractures may necessitate special attention to positioning.
Hematologic	Anemia, eosinophilia, and thrombocytosis may be present. Venous access may be difficult 2° vasculitis and ↑skin fragility (steroid-induced). Virtually all of these patients will be on some type of anti-inflammatory medication that may result in anemia or Plt inhibition. Ideally, patients should discontinue NSAIDs at least 5 d preop; aspirin, 7 d preop.
Endocrine	Rheumatoid patients are likely to be on oral corticosteroids and require supplemental periop steroids (e.g., 100 mg hydrocortisone q 8 h iv) to treat adrenal suppression, although the routine use of 'stress-dose steroids' has been questioned.
Laboratory	Hb/Hct serves as a minimum in otherwise healthy rheumatoid patients. Severe rheumatoid patients may require more extensive testing to screen for drug effects, etc. (e.g., serum electrolytes; glucose; kidney function tests; LFTs).
Premedication	Mild-to-moderate premedication (e.g., in adults, midazolam 1-2 mg iv, fentanyl 50-100 µg iv, titrated to effect) is often desirable before placement of a regional block.

INTRAOPERATIVE

Anesthetic technique: Regional anesthesia, GA, or a combination of the two are commonly used. A brachial plexus block via the axillary or infraclavicular approach is excellent for this procedure; it is a means of avoiding tracheal intubation for GA if airway difficulty is anticipated. Furthermore, it decreases admission rate, speeds discharge from PACU in day surgery setting, and increases patient satisfaction. Intravenous regional anesthesia (Bier block) is most useful for short procedures (< 1 h). If regional anesthesia is contraindicated, rheumatoid patients may require awake fiber optic intubation (see p. B-6).

Regional anesthesia: 1.5% mepivacaine 30-40 ml with alkalization for routine, superficial cases; 0.5% bupivacaine or 0.5% levobupivacaine/0.5% ropivacaine, if available, 30-40 ml for procedures > 2.5 h or if extended analgesia is desired. Epinephrine (2.5-5µg/ml) should be added whenever possible to decrease peak plasma concentrations of local anesthetics.

Infraclavicular block	The coracoid approach makes this a safe and effective regional technique. A single injection will provide anesthesia distal to the mid humerus. No additional injections are necessary, and the patient's arm does not need to be abducted for block placement. If intraop sedation is necessary, propofol (50-100 µg/kg/min) by continuous infusion or intermittent bolus injection of opioid/benzodiazepine are good choices.
Axillary block	The medial aspect of the upper arm is innervated by the intercostobrachial nerve (T2) and requires a separate subcutaneous field block in the axilla, especially when a tourniquet is used. The lateral cutaneous nerve of the forearm, a sensory branch of the musculocutaneous nerve supplying sensation to the lateral forearm, is frequently missed by the axillary approach to the brachial plexus. Thus, a block of this nerve at the elbow or within the proximal coracobrachialis muscle is sometimes necessary. If intraop sedation is necessary, propofol (50-150 µg/kg/min) by continuous infusion or intermittent bolus injection of opioid/benzodiazepine are good choices.
Bier block	The Bier block (intravenous regional anesthesia) is an excellent technique for short (< 60 min), superficial wrist and hand surgeries. 40-50 ml of 0.5% lidocaine is commonly used. A very brief operative procedure may be an indication to reduce the dose of iv anesthetic agent by, for example, having the surgeon use a forearm tourniquet instead of an upper arm tourniquet. The OR staff should be alerted that iv regional anesthesia is being used, so that all are ready to proceed once the tourniquet is inflated (i.e., surgical prep ready to be performed; surgeons scrubbed, gowned, and gloved). Tourniquet pain and postop pain is reduced by adding ketorolac (20 mg) or clonidine (1 µg/kg) to the lidocaine solution.

General anesthesia:

Induction	Standard induction (p. B-2) in patients with normal airways
Maintenance	Standard maintenance (p. B-3)
Emergence	Skin closure frequently is followed by application of a splint, and the patient should remain anesthetized during the splinting procedure. Cases with difficult airways require awake extubation.

Blood and fluid requirements	Minimal blood loss IV: 18 ga × 1 NS/LR @ 1.5-3 ml/kg/h	IV placed in the contralateral upper extremity.
Monitoring	Standard monitors (p. B-1)	
Positioning	Special handling required. ✓ and pad pressure points. ✓ eyes. ✓ C-spine instability.	As with nearly all orthopedic cases, positioning is a subtle, yet crucial aspect of anesthetic management. Rheumatoid patients may have contractures that require special attention. Steroid-dependent patients require special handling because of fragile skin.
Infraclavicular block complications	Local anesthetic toxicity Inadequate block Intravascular injection Pneumothorax Persistent paresthesia	Less frequent occurrence, compared with axillary block. Pneumothorax is very rare with the lateral coracoid approach.
Axillary block complications	Local anesthetic toxicity Inadequate block Intravascular injection Persistent paresthesia Axillary hematoma Axillary artery thrombosis	Very minimal doses of local anesthetic can cause CNS toxicity if reverse flow occurs during an intraarterial injection. Axillary thrombosis is extremely rare.
Bier block complications	Local anesthetic toxicity Inadequate block Thrombophlebitis	Proper exsanguination and tourniquet function is critical. Tourniquet should remain inflated a minimum of 25 min. Systemic toxic reaction to the local anesthetic may occur as a result of tourniquet leak or inadvertent premature (< 20 min) tourniquet release. Treatment is supportive. Sz are controlled with STP or midazolam, with appropriate airway protection. Even with a functioning tourniquet, it is possible to overcome tourniquet pressure by injecting too vigorously. Care must be taken when switching from proximal to distal tourniquet; never deflate proximal tourniquet until verifying that distal tourniquet is working.

POSTOPERATIVE

Pain management	PCA (p. C-3), in combination with regional block	Regional or combined regional-general anesthetic techniques are excellent for wrist procedures, especially with respect to postop pain management.
Tests	None routinely indicated.	

References

1. Brockway MS, Wildsmith JA: Axillary brachial plexus block: method of choice? *Br J Anaesth* 1990; 64(2):224-31.
2. Gerancher JC: Upper extremity nerve blocks. *Anes Clin North Am* 2000; 18(2):1-16.
3. Green DP: *Operative Hand Surgery*, 4th edition. Churchill Livingstone, New York: 1999.
4. Keenan MA, Stiles CM, Kaufman RL: Acquired laryngeal deviation associated with cervical spine disease in erosive polyarticular arthritis. *Anesthesiology* 1983; 58(5):441-9.
5. Ramamurthy S, Hickey R: Anesthesia. In *Operative Hand Surgery*, 4th edition. Green DP, ed. Churchill Livingstone, New York: 1999, 22-48.
6. Sia, S: Axillary brachial plexus block using peripheral nerve stimulator: A comparison between double- and triple-injection techniques. *Reg Anesth Pain Med* 2001; 26(6):499-503.

7.   Salazar CH: Infraclavicular brachial plexus block. *Reg Anesth Pain Med* 1999; 24(5):411-6.

8.   Steinberg, RB: The dose-response relationship of ketorolac as a component of intravenous regional anesthesia with lidocaine. *Anesth Analg* 1998; 86(4):791-3.

9.   Vandam LD: Anesthesia for hand surgery. In *Flynn's Hand Surgery*, 4th edition. Jupiter JB, ed. Williams and Wilkins, Baltimore: 1991, 46-54.

10. White RH: Preoperative evaluation of patients with rheumatoid arthritis. *Semin Arthritis Rheum* 1985; 14(4):287-99.

11. Wilson JL: Infraclavicular brachial plexus block: parasagittal anatomy important to the coracoid technique. *Anesth Analg* 1998; 87(4):870-3.

EXCISION OF GANGLION OF THE WRIST

SURGICAL CONSIDERATIONS

Description: Ganglion cysts about the wrist most commonly occur dorsally, originating from the scapholunate joint. The second most common site is volar to the scaphotrapezial joint. To prevent recurrence, these synovial fluid-filled outpouchings of the joint capsule must be excised completely. This requires isolating the stalk of the cyst to its origin, and excising a small cuff of normal joint capsule with the cyst. The joint, therefore, must be entered for a complete excision. Older studies found that the recurrence rate was decreased by the use of GA, as opposed to local or regional anesthetics. This was due to the fact that a more complete excision was performed when the patient was under GA. Hand specialists today feel that regional anesthetics are quite acceptable for this procedure, as long as the surgeon performs a meticulous excision. Volar wrist ganglions commonly involve the radial artery, which is at risk during excision. A preop Allen test should be performed to ensure that, if the radial artery is interrupted, there will not be ischemia in the hand.

Usual preop diagnosis: Ganglion cyst, primary or recurrent

SUMMARY OF PROCEDURE

Position	Supine, with arm extended on hand-surgery table
Incision	Longitudinal or transverse directly over cyst
Special instrumentation	Pneumatic tourniquet
Antibiotics	Cefazolin 1 g iv
Surgical time	0.5-1.5 h
Tourniquet	150 mmHg above systolic; max time = 120 min
Closing considerations	Routine skin closure. Large recurrent cysts may require a repair of the wrist capsule. Splint applied in OR.
EBL	Minimal; performed under tourniquet control.
Postop care	Elevation to prevent swelling
Mortality	None associated with procedure
Morbidity	Injury to radial artery: Rare (Because of the vascular interconnections between radial and ulnar arteries, loss of radial artery flow rarely → complications.)
Pain score	2-4

PATIENT POPULATION CHARACTERISTICS

Age range	Infants–elderly
Male:Female	1:1
Incidence	Very common
Etiology	Unknown. Trauma has been associated with ~50% of ganglion cysts. Underlying carpal instabilities, such as scapholunate instability, have been implicated.
Associated conditions	Carpal instability; trauma (wrist sprains and strains)

ANESTHETIC CONSIDERATIONS

See Anesthetic Considerations following Repair of Flexor Tendon Laceration, p. 746.

PALMAR AND DIGITAL FASCIECTOMY

SURGICAL CONSIDERATIONS

Description: This procedure is indicated for the treatment of Dupuytren's contractures of the digits, which produces a neoplastic thickening of the palmar and digital fascia. These pathologic cords (whose active cell is the myofibroblast) contract and, through their connections with the skin, tendon sheath, and phalangeal bone, cause flexion contractures of the metacarpophalangeal, proximal interphalangeal, and distal interphalangeal joints. The disease is progressive, and the only treatment is surgical excision of the fascia. In addition to the pathologic changes in the fascia of the hands, many patients also have thickening of the plantar fascia of the foot (Ledderhose's disease) and the dorsal fascia of the penis (Peyronie's disease). Patients with severe contractures that have been neglected may require amputation. Because the pathologic fascia is so intimately connected to the skin, it is sometimes necessary to excise the skin and replace it with full-thickness skin grafts. The groin is an excellent donor site for these grafts.

There are many different surgical approaches, most requiring the creation of Z-plasties for a tension-free closure. The **McCash technique** has been quite successful for the excision of palmar disease. This method consists of excising the palmar fascia through transverse incisions that are not sutured closed, but rather are left open to granulate and contract over a 3 wk postop period. These patients have a very low complication rate.

Usual preop diagnosis: Dupuytren's contracture

SUMMARY OF PROCEDURE

Position	Supine, with arm extended on hand-surgery table
Incision	Transverse or longitudinal palmar. Groin may be used as a full-thickness skin graft donor site.
Antibiotics	None
Surgical time	1-3 h
Tourniquet	150 mmHg above systolic; max time = 120 min. Because of the need to deflate tourniquet so that hemostasis can be obtained, Bier block is not suitable.
Closing considerations	Must obtain meticulous hemostasis. Z-plasties and skin grafts used frequently.
EBL	Minimal; dissection done under tourniquet control. A small amount of blood loss occurs when tourniquet is released and hemostasis is obtained.
Postop care	Pain control is essential. Patient may be admitted for initial postop period. Limb elevation to minimize swelling. Regional techniques that provide postop pain relief are very useful.
Mortality	None associated with procedure
Morbidity	Hematoma (usually requires operative intervention)
	Skin necrosis (may require secondary skin grafting)
	Digital nerve and artery injury (Nerve injuries typically recognized immediately. An operating microscope may be needed, and the procedure will be prolonged.)
	Reflex-sympathetic dystrophy (so-called sympathetic 'flare' reaction; requires prompt treatment, including stellate ganglion blockade)
Pain score	7-8

PATIENT POPULATION CHARACTERISTICS

Age range	Typically, 40-60 yr; can occur in teens.
Male:Female	More common in males
Incidence	Common
Etiology	Definite heritance—associated with strong family Hx. Ethnic diathesis for northern Europeans with fair hair and skin, blue eyes. Almost never seen in Blacks. Experimental studies suggest that microhematomas 2° repetitive trauma may be important in the disease process.
Associated conditions	Cigarette smoking; alcoholism; antiseizure medications

ANESTHETIC CONSIDERATIONS

See Anesthetic Considerations following Repair of Flexor Tendon Laceration, p. 746.

REPAIR OF FLEXOR TENDON LACERATION

SURGICAL CONSIDERATIONS

Description: The prognosis and difficulty of a flexor tendon repair depends on the anatomic site of the laceration. There are five zones of injury in the upper extremity (Fig 10.1-3). Zone I is distal to the flexor digitorum superficialis (FDS) tendon insertion and involves only the flexor digitorum profundus (FDP) tendon. Zone II extends from the entrance to the fibroosseous sheath at the metacarpal head to the FDS insertion. Lacerations usually involve both the FDS and FDP. These are the most difficult to repair and have the worst prognosis, as the tendons are apt to become scarred to each other and limit gliding. Zone III is the palm; Zone IV is within the carpal canal; and Zone 5 is in the forearm. Lacerations in these areas are easier to repair and have good prognoses for restoration of tendon gliding and, thus, digit motion. Associated injuries to the neural structures are common. Digital nerve lacerations are seen in Zone II; median nerve injuries, in Zone IV. Occasionally, nerve injuries occur in Zone V.

In general, nerve injuries are repaired at the time of the tendon repair. Tendons lacerated in the finger are often pulled back into the palm by muscular contraction. A palmar incision is required to retrieve the tendon, which must then be threaded carefully through the pulleys in the digit. Suture techniques for tendon repair create a juncture that is far weaker than an intact tendon. For this reason, the juncture must be protected from mechanical stress for a period of 8 wk or more. This is done by splinting the hand with the wrist and digits flexed so that the pull on the tendon by its muscle is limited. It is important that the patient emerges gently from anesthesia to limit the stress on the tendon. The best results are obtained when repair is carried out within 7 d of the injury, although primary repair can be performed up to 3 wk. After 7 d, the muscle begins to undergo irreversible contracture. If the flexor tendon is advanced after this has occurred, a flexion contracture

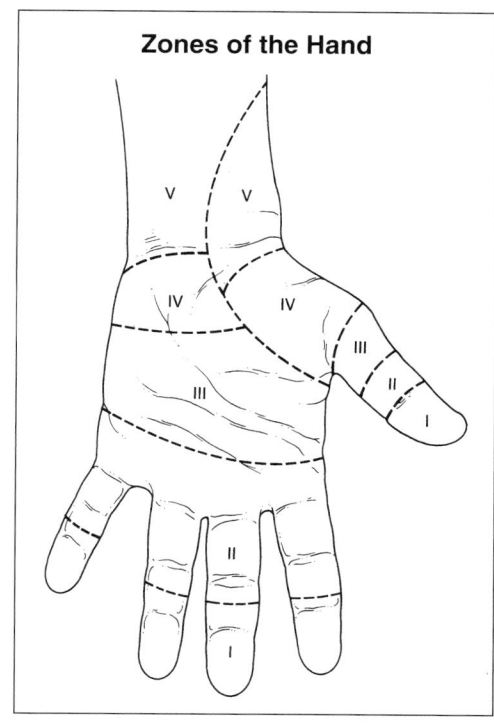

Figure 10.1-3. Zone classification of flexor tendon injuries. (Reproduced with permission from Scott-Conner CEH, Dawson DL: *Operative Anatomy*, 2nd edition. Lippincott Williams & Wilkins, 2003.)

results. If a flexor tendon laceration is neglected, a palm-to-fingertip tendon graft, using a different flexor tendon, should be performed. If the tendon bed is suitable for gliding, the graft can be accomplished in one stage. If not, a Silastic tendon spacer (rubber rod) must be placed at the first stage; 6-8 wk later, a palm-to-fingertip graft is placed in the bed prepared with the Silastic rod. Tendon graft donor sites include the palmaris longus tendon and toe extensors.

A variant of the sharp flexor tendon laceration is the FDP avulsion from its insertion in Zone 1. This is the so-called 'jersey finger.' This injury occurs during forceful grasp, and most commonly affects the ring finger. A common mechanism is the football or rugby player who is grasping the jersey of a ball carrier. The FDP tendon retracts and should be repaired within 7 d. If neglected, these patients should be treated with a **distal interphalangeal (DIP) arthrodesis**. A flexor tendon graft through an intact FDS tendon usually is not indicated, as tendon adhesions will commonly interfere with the function of the FDS, leading to decreased overall active motion of the digit. The most common complication is the development of tendon adhesions, which limit tendon gliding and digit motion. If these patients fail to improve within a 3- to 6-mo course of physical therapy, they require an operative tendolysis to lyse the adhesions.

Usual preop diagnosis: Flexor tendon laceration; FDP avulsion ('jersey finger'); digital nerve laceration; median nerve laceration

SUMMARY OF PROCEDURE

Position	Supine, with arm extended on hand-surgery table. The foot may be prepped for a tendon graft.
Incision	Zig-zag hand or wrist
Special instrumentation	Pneumatic tourniquet
Antibiotics	Cefazolin 1 g iv
Surgical time	1-2 h; may be extended for nerve repair and treatment of associated injuries.
Closing considerations	Tendon and nerve repairs must be protected with splints before emergence from GA. Smooth extubation (see Emergence, below).

EBL	Minimal; procedure performed under tourniquet control.
Postop care	PACU → home
Mortality	None associated with procedure.
Morbidity	Tendon adhesions: 25%
	Rupture of tendon repair:
	< 5%
	Infection: Rare
Pain score	2-4

PATIENT POPULATION CHARACTERISTICS

Age range	Infant–elderly
Male:Female	Slight male predominance, due to occupational injuries
Incidence	Not uncommon
Etiology	Trauma

ANESTHETIC CONSIDERATIONS

(Procedures covered: excision of ganglion of the wrist; palmar and digital fasciectomy; repair of flexor tendon laceration)

PREOPERATIVE

The majority of patients presenting for these procedures are usually otherwise healthy. Many of them present for elective surgery as a result of progressive functional impairment and pain, and preop workup is routine.

Neurological	If regional anesthesia is contemplated, preexisting sensory or motor defects should be documented carefully.
Laboratory	Hb/Hct (healthy patients); otherwise, as indicated from H&P.
Premedication	Mild-to-moderate premedication (e.g., in adults, midazolam 1-2 mg iv, fentanyl 50-100 μg iv, titrated to effect) is often desirable before placement of a regional block.

INTRAOPERATIVE

Anesthetic technique: Regional anesthesia (most common), GA, or a combination of the two may be used. Intravenous regional anesthesia (Bier block) is most useful for short procedures which last for < 1 h (see Anesthetic Considerations, p. 751). A brachial plexus block via the axillary or infraclavicular approach is excellent for this procedure. Because most of these procedures are done on an outpatient basis, brachial plexus block without GA is usually preferred to promote early 'street-readiness.'

Regional anesthesia: 1.5% mepivacaine 30-40 ml with alkalization for routine, superfical cases; 0.5% bupivacaine or 0.5% levobupivacaine/0.5% ropivacaine, if available, 30-40 ml for procedures > 2.5 h or if extended analgesia is desired. Epinephrine (2.5-5 μg/ml) should be added whenever possible to decrease peak plasma concentrations of local anesthetics.

Infraclavicular block	The coracoid approach makes this a safe and effective regional technique. A single injection will provide anesthesia distal to the mid humerus. No additional injections are necessary, and the patient's arm does not need to be abducted for block placement. If intraop sedation is necessary, propofol (50-100 μg/kg/min) by continuous infusion or intermittent bolus injection of opioid/benzodiazepine are good choices.
Axillary block	The medial aspect of the upper arm is innervated by the intercostobrachial nerve (T2) and requires a separate subcutaneous field block in the axilla, especially when a tourniquet is used. The lateral cutaneous nerve of the forearm, a sensory branch of the musculocutaneous nerve supplying sensation to the lateral forearm, is frequently missed by the axillary approach to the brachial plexus. Thus, a block of this nerve at the elbow or within the proximal coracobrachialis muscle is sometimes necessary. If intraop sedation is necessary, propofol (50-100 μg/kg/min) by continuous infusion or intermittent bolus injection of opioid/benzodiazepine are good choices.
Bier block	The Bier block (intravenous regional anesthesia) is an excellent technique for short (< 60 min), superficial wrist and hand surgeries. 40-50 ml of 0.5% lidocaine is commonly used. A very brief operative procedure may be an indication to reduce the dose of iv anesthetic agent by, for example,

Bier block, cont.	having the surgeon use a forearm tourniquet instead of an upper arm tourniquet. The OR staff should be alerted that iv regional anesthesia is being used, so that all are ready to proceed once the tourniquet is inflated (i.e., surgical prep ready to be performed; surgeons scrubbed, gowned, and gloved). Tourniquet pain and postop pain is reduced by adding ketorolac (20 mg) or clonidine ($1\mu g/kg$) to the lidocaine solution.	
General anesthesia:		
Induction	Standard induction (p. B-2)	
Maintenance	Standard maintenance (p. B-3)	
Emergence	Standard emergence (p. B-4). Skin closure is frequently followed by application of a splint; patient should remain anesthetized during splinting procedure.	
Blood and fluid requirements	Minimal blood loss IV: 18 ga × 1 NS/LR @ 1.5-3 ml/kg/h	An 18 ga iv catheter placed in the contralateral upper extremity should be adequate.
Monitoring	Standard monitors (p. B-1)	
Positioning	✓ and pad pressure points. ✓ eyes.	
Infraclavicular block complications	Inadequate block Intravascular injection Pneumothorax Persistent paresthesia Local anesthetic toxicity	Less frequent occurrence, compared with axillary block. Pneumothorax is very rare with the lateral coracoid approach.
Axillary block complications	Local anesthetic toxicity Intravascular injection Inadequate block Persistent paresthesia Axillary hematoma Axillary artery thrombosis	Minimal doses of local anesthetic can cause CNS toxicity during an accidental intravascular injection. Sz should be treated with STP or midazolam titrated to effect, accompanied by airway control. If there is any question of a full stomach, intubation should be accomplished rapidly. Axillary thrombosis is very rare.
Bier block complications	Local anesthetic toxicity Inadequate block Thrombophlebitis	Proper exsanguination and tourniquet function is critical. Tourniquet should remain inflated a minimum of 25 min. Systemic toxic reaction to the local anesthetic may occur as a result of tourniquet leak or inadvertent premature (< 20 min) tourniquet release. Treatment is supportive. Sz are controlled with STP or midazolam, with appropriate airway protection. Even with a functioning tourniquet, it is possible to overcome tourniquet pressure by injecting too vigorously. Care must be taken when switching from proximal to distal tourniquet; never deflate proximal tourniquet until verifying that distal tourniquet is working.

POSTOPERATIVE

Pain management	Oral analgesics are usually sufficient.	The lingering analgesia of the brachial plexus block is often sufficient for pain relief in the recovery room; oral analgesic therapy can be instituted prior to discharging patient to home.
Tests	None routinely indicated.	

References

1. Brockway MS, Wildsmith JA: Axillary brachial plexus block: method of choice? *Br J Anaesth* 1990; 64(2):224-31.
2. Gerancher JC: Upper extremity nerve blocks. *Anes Clin North Am* 2000; 18(2):1-16.
3. Goldberg ME, et al: A comparison of three methods of axillary approach to brachial plexus blockade for upper extremity surgery. *Anesthesiology* 1987; 66(6):814-16.
4. Green DP: *Operative Hand Surgery*, 4th edition. Churchill Livingstone, New York: 1999.

5. Ramamurthy S, Hickey R: Anesthesia. In *Operative Hand Surgery*, 4th edition. Green DP, ed. Churchill Livingstone, New York: 1999, 22-48.
6. Sia, S: Axillary brachial plexus block using peripheral nerve stimulator: A comparison between double- and triple-injection techniques. *Reg Anesth Pain Med* 2001; 26(6):499-503.
7. Salazar CH: Infraclavicular brachial plexus block. *Reg Anesth Pain Med* 1999; 24(5):411-6.
8. Steinberg, RB: The dose-response relationship of ketorolac as a component of intravenous regional anesthesia with lidocaine. *Anesth Analg* 1998; 86(4):791-3.
9. Vandam LD: Anesthesia for Hand Surgery. In *Flynn's Hand Surgery*, 4th edition. Jupiter JB, ed. Williams and Wilkins, Baltimore: 1991, 46-54.
10. Wilson JL: Infraclavicular brachial plexus block: parasagittal anatomy important to the coracoid technique. *Anesth Analg* 1998; 87(4):870-3.

TENDOLYSIS OF FLEXOR OR EXTENSOR TENDON
(WITH CAPSULOTOMY OF JOINTS)

SURGICAL CONSIDERATIONS

Description: Tendolysis refers to the surgical division of fibrous adhesions between tendons and surrounding tissues. These adhesions, or scar, form as a sequelae of injury either to the tendons themselves (e.g., tendon lacerations) or to the surrounding tissues (e.g., fractures). The adhesions bind the tendons to surrounding tissues and restrict their normal gliding movement, resulting in ↓ joint mobility, with loss of strength and function. Commonly, joint contracture is the result of tendons becoming solidly bound by scar to surrounding structures. For this reason, tendolysis procedures frequently are combined with an operative procedure, called **capsulotomy**, to restore better passive motion of the joint. A tourniquet is used frequently for the initial parts of the procedure, which can be combined with intravenous (**Bier**) regional anesthesia.

The operative steps include a number of skin incisions adequate for exposure. Tendolysis of the flexor tendons within the fingers may require exposure of the entire tendon sheath, from palm to fingertip. Adhesions are identified and sharply divided. If the associated joint(s) require(s) capsulotomy, this is performed in conjunction with tendolysis. Depending on whether the joint is stiff in extension or flexion, all periarticular tissues—including dorsal and volar capsules and collateral ligaments—potentially may need to be assessed. The involved tendons are grasped and pulled to determine whether adequate tendolysis has been performed. Once full passive motion has been restored, if circumstances permit and an iv regional block has been given, the tourniquet is released, the arm and hand allowed sufficient time to reperfuse, and the patient is asked to attempt to flex and extend the operative digit. In this way, the surgeon and patient can be assured that the procedure was successful.

Usual preop diagnosis: Laceration and primary repair of flexor or extensor tendons; replantation of amputated digits; joint dislocations; fractures; burns; crush injuries; frequently, diagnosis of 'joint contracture'

SUMMARY OF PROCEDURE

Position	Supine, arm extended on a hand table
Incision(s)	Varies according to location of pathology
Special instrumentation	Pneumatic tourniquet
Antibiotics	Cefazolin 1 g
Surgical time	30-90 min
Tourniquet	100-150 mmHg above SBP
Closing considerations	Local infiltration anesthesia, following iv regional
EBL	Minimal
Postop care	Elevation; PACU → home or overnight observation
Mortality	None associated with procedure.
Morbidity	Delayed wound healing
	Nerve injury
	Tendon rupture
Pain score	2-6

PATIENT POPULATION CHARACTERISTICS

Age range	Teens – elderly
Male:Female	Males predominate
Incidence	Very common hand surgery procedure
Etiology	See Usual preop diagnosis, above.
Associated conditions	See Usual preop diagnosis, above.

ANESTHETIC CONSIDERATIONS

See Anesthetic Considerations following Carpal Tunnel Release, p. 751.

WRIST ARTHROSCOPY

SURGICAL CONSIDERATIONS

Description: Wrist arthroscopy may be performed for either diagnostic or therapeutic indications. A smaller diameter version of the standard arthroscope is used for visualizing the wrist joint. All of the entry portals are on the dorsum of the wrist and course between the extensor compartments. Irrigation is used during the procedure and a cannula is routinely placed ulnar to the extensor carpi ulnaris tendon. Unlike the knee joint, where visualization is obtained by distention of the joint, in-the-wrist visualization is obtained by distraction. The digits are placed in finger traps and up to 10 lbs of traction can be placed on the wrist. Specialized instrumentation is available to resect and debride intraarticular structures and to place sutures to repair torn ligaments. The use of the Ho:YAG laser and radiofrequency energy generator for debridement, synovectomy, and excision of tears of the triangular fibrocartilage has led to shorter operative times. Arthroscopic techniques also can be used to irrigate and debride the infected wrist joint. If an open procedure, such as repair of an intercarpal ligament, is contemplated following diagnostic arthroscopy, either GA or regional block is preferred.

Variant procedure or approaches: The standard approach is to suspend the forearm vertically in traction. The forearm also can be placed horizontally on the hand table in traction.

Usual preop diagnosis: Internal derangement of the wrist of unknown etiology; tears of the triangular fibrocartilage complex; intercarpal instability due to intercarpal ligament tears; rotatory subluxation of the scaphoid; scapholunate dissociation; luno-triquetral dissociation; fracture of distal radius; ulnar impingement syndrome; rheumatoid synovitis; intraarticular infection

SUMMARY OF PROCEDURE

Position	Supine, with arm extended on hand-surgery table
Incision	Small incisions are made on the dorsum of the wrist for instrument insertion.
Special instrumentation	2.7 mm diameter arthroscope, 0 or 30° field of view; light source and video camera; television monitor; surgical power shaver; joint irrigation system; traction device for forearm; pneumatic tourniquet
Unique considerations	Patient is often awake and observes surgery on monitor.
Antibiotics	Cefazolin 1 g iv
Surgical time	30 min-2 h
Tourniquet	150 mmHg above SBP; max time = 120 min
Closing considerations	Arthroscopic portals are each closed with a single skin suture.
EBL	Minimal; procedure performed with tourniquet control.
Postop care	PACU → home
Mortality	None associated with procedure.
Morbidity	Infection: < 1%
	Swelling (2° to irrigation fluid): Common
	Nerve and artery damage: Uncommon
Pain score	1-3

PATIENT POPULATION CHARACTERISTICS

Age range	Adolescent–elderly. This procedure is not indicated in children.
Male:Female	1:1
Incidence	Least common form of arthroscopy
Etiology	See Usual preop diagnosis, above.
Associated conditions	Degenerative arthritis (posttraumatic and osteo-); rheumatoid arthritis

ANESTHETIC CONSIDERATIONS

See Anesthetic Considerations following Carpal Tunnel Release, p. 751.

Reference

1. Green DP: *Operative Hand Surgery*, 4th edition. Churchill Livingstone, New York: 1999.

CARPAL TUNNEL RELEASE

SURGICAL CONSIDERATIONS

Description: This is the most commonly performed procedure in hand surgery. It consists of the transection of the transverse carpal ligament through either an open-palmar or an endoscopic approach (Fig 10.1-4). The procedure may include synovectomy of the flexor tendons, tendon transfers to restore thumb opposition and the excision of masses from within the carpal canal. In patients with severe synovitis, as in rheumatoid arthritis, a synovectomy should be performed at the same time. If there is advanced thenar atrophy and weakness of thumb opposition, a tendon transfer also should be done at that time. The most common transfer is the **Camitz opponensplasty**, in which the palmaris longis tendon is prolonged with palmar fascia and transferred to the thumb. Transfers of the extensor indicis proprius and superficial flexor tendons also can be performed. Because of the great danger of lacerating a nerve during endoscopic carpal tunnel release, it is recommended that the procedure be performed under a local anesthetic with infiltration only into the skin. Thus, the nerves remain sensate and can be probed and identified by the awake patient. Short-acting sedation can be used during the insertion of the trocar and sheath into the carpal canal.

Usual preop diagnosis: Carpal tunnel syndrome (CTS); median nerve compression at the wrist

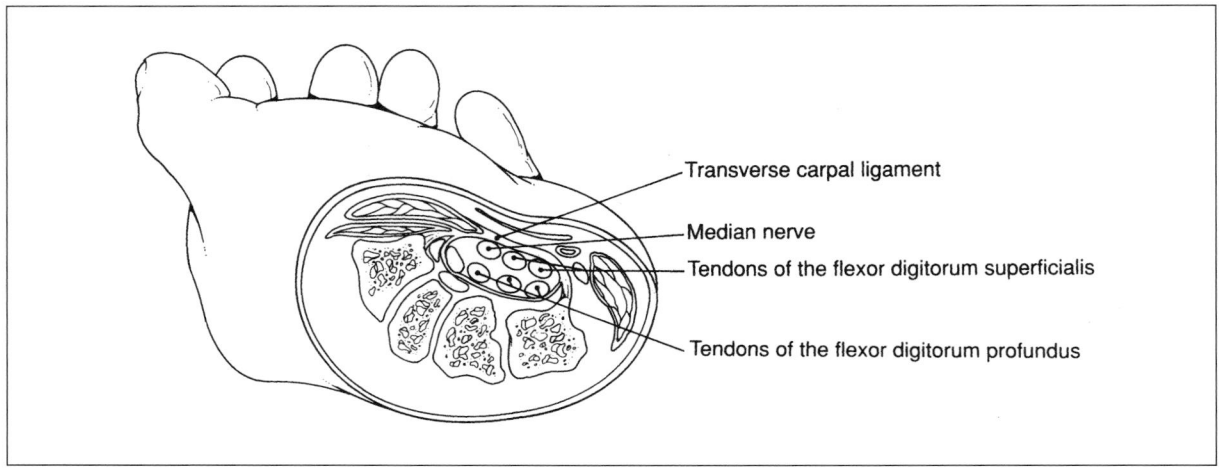

Figure 10.1-4. Exposure of the carpal tunnel. (Reproduced with permission from Scott-Conner CEH, Dawson DL: *Operative Anatomy*, 2nd edition. Lippincott Williams & Wilkins, 2003.)

SUMMARY OF PROCEDURES

	Open Carpal Tunnel Release	Endoscopic Carpal Tunnel Release
Position	Supine	⇐
Incision	Longitudinal incision in palm; may extend to forearm.	2 cm transverse at proximal flexion crease of wrist; 1 cm, mid-palm
Special instrumentation	Pneumatic tourniquet	Endoscopic carpal tunnel release system: endoscope, sheath and trocar, special cutting tools
Unique considerations	None	Danger of intraop injury to digital nerves, median nerve, tendons, superficial vascular arch
Antibiotics	Cefazolin 1 g iv	⇐
Surgical time	30-90 min	30 min
Tourniquet	150 mmHg above SBP; max time = 120 min	⇐
Closing considerations	Simple skin closure	⇐
EBL	Minimal; performed under tourniquet control.	Minimal
Postop care	Splint; elevation	No splint, early motion, elevation
Mortality	None associated with procedure	⇐
Morbidity	Overall complication rate: 4%	⇐
	Reflex sympathetic dystrophy (RSD): < 5%	Rare
	Hematoma: Rare	Complications of ulnar nerve palsy
	Infection: Uncommon	Tendon and nerve laceration: Rare (< 1%)
		Vascular injury: Less common than nerve injury
Pain score	1-2	1-2

PATIENT POPULATION CHARACTERISTICS

Age range	20-80 yr; 50% are 40-60 yr
Male:Female	1:2
Incidence	Common
Etiology	Compression of the median nerve within the carpal tunnel by synovitis; mass effect 2° tumor or fracture fragments, peripheral neuropathy, gout, anomalous structures, thrombosis of a persistent median artery, and idiopathic; repetitive trauma (e.g., computer use)
Associated conditions	Rheumatoid arthritis; thyroid imbalance; diabetes; amyloidosis; multiple myeloma; alcoholism; hemophilia; pregnancy; menopause; gout; fractures of the distal radius; Kienbock's disease

ANESTHETIC CONSIDERATIONS

(Procedures covered: tendolysis of flexor or extensor tendon; wrist arthroscopy; carpal tunnel release)

PREOPERATIVE

In general, there are two patient populations involved: (1) healthy patients with Hx of wrist trauma, and (2) rheumatoid patients. (See Anesthetic Considerations for Wrist Procedures, p. 740, for discussion of preop concerns in the rheumatoid patient.)

Laboratory	Hb/Hct (healthy patients); otherwise, as indicated from H&P.
Premedication	Mild-to-moderate premedication (e.g., in adults, midazolam 1-2 mg iv, fentanyl 50-100 μg iv, titrated to effect) is often desirable before placement of a regional block.

INTRAOPERATIVE

Anesthetic technique: Intravenous regional anesthesia is an excellent technique for procedures that are < 1 h. For longer procedures, an axillary or infraclavicular brachial plexus block are good alternatives. Both of these techniques are especially appropriate for outpatients.

Intravenous regional block	The Bier block (intravenous regional anesthesia) is an excellent technique for short (< 60 min), superficial wrist and hand surgeries. 40-50 ml of 0.5% lidocaine is commonly used. A very brief

Intravenous regional block, cont.	operative procedure may be an indication to reduce the dose of iv anesthetic agent by, for example, having the surgeon use a forearm tourniquet instead of an upper arm tourniquet. The OR staff should be alerted that iv regional anesthesia is being used, so that all are ready to proceed once the tourniquet is inflated (i.e., surgical prep ready to be performed; surgeons scrubbed, gowned, and gloved). Tourniquet pain and postop pain is reduced by adding ketorolac (20 mg) or clonidine (1µg/kg) to the lidocaine solution.	
Blood and fluid requirements	Minimal blood loss IV: 18 ga × 1 NS/LR @ 1.5-2 ml/kg/h	An 18 ga iv catheter placed in the nonoperative upper extremity should be adequate.
Monitoring	Standard monitors (p. B-1)	
Positioning	✓ and pad pressure points. ✓ eyes.	
Intravenous regional block complications	Local anesthetic toxicity Inadequate block Thrombophlebitis	Proper exsanguination and tourniquet function are critical. A tourniquet should remain inflated a minimum of 25 min. Systemic toxic reaction to the local anesthetic may occur as a result of tourniquet leak or inadvertent premature (< 20 min) tourniquet release. Treatment is supportive. Sz are controlled with STP or midazolam, with appropriate airway protection. Even with a functioning tourniquet, it is possible to overcome tourniquet pressure by injecting too vigorously. Care must be taken when switching from proximal to distal tourniquet; never deflate proximal tourniquet until verifying that distal tourniquet is working.

POSTOPERATIVE

Pain management	Oral analgesics usually sufficient	Residual analgesia with iv regional anesthesia is minimal unless ketorolac or clonidine are used. Some iv opioid may be necessary until the patient is tolerating fluids in the recovery room.
Tests	None routinely indicated.	

References

1. Davies JA, Wilkey AD, Hall ID: Bupivacaine leak past inflated tourniquets during intravenous regional analgesia. *Anaesthesia* 1984; 39(10):996-9.
2. Gorgias NK: Clonidine versus ketamine to prevent tourniquet pain during intravenous regional anesthesia with lidocaine. *Reg Anesth Pain Med* 2001; 26(6):512-17.
3. Grice SC, Morell RC, Balestrieri FJ, et al: Intravenous regional anesthesia: evaluation and prevention of leakage under the tourniquet. *Anesthesiology* 1986; 65(3):316-20.
4. Ramamurthy S, Hickey R: Anesthesia. In *Operative Hand Surgery*, 4th edition. Green DP, ed. Churchill Livingstone, New York: 1999, 22-48.
5. Steinberg, RB: The dose-response relationship of ketorolac as a component of intravenous regional anesthesia with lidocaine. *Anesth Analg* 1998; 86(4):791-3.
6. Sukhani R, Garcia CJ, Munhall RJ, et al: Lidocaine disposition following intravenous regional anesthesia with different tourniquet deflation technics. *Anesth Analg* 1989; 68(5):633-7.
7. Vandam LD: Anesthesia for hand surgery. In *Flynn's Hand Surgery*, 4th edition. Jupiter JB, ed. Williams and Wilkins, Baltimore: 1991, 46-54.

REPAIR OF FRACTURES AND DISLOCATIONS
OF THE DISTAL RADIUS, CARPUS, AND METACARPALS

SURGICAL CONSIDERATIONS

Description: Patients with fractures of the distal radius, carpus, and/or metacarpals that cannot be treated adequately with closed methods, require **open reduction and internal fixation** (ORIF). The criteria for adequate treatment include anatomic reduction of the fracture fragments and stable maintenance of this reduction. Closed, unstable, distal radius fractures often are treated by traction and application of an external fixator in the OR to maintain the reduction by ligamentotaxis. Patients with wrist dislocation and distal radius fractures frequently have signs of neurologic compromise, such as carpal tunnel syndrome (CTS). Vascular compromise of the hand associated with these injuries is rare, usually occurring in patients with severe crush or high-energy injuries. The devascularized hand is a surgical emergency, and revascularization must be carried out as soon as possible. Fractures of these structures are associated with blast and crush injuries, as well as low-velocity gunshot wounds (GSW). These injuries have significant soft-tissue components that must be treated. The possibility of a coexisting compartment syndrome should be considered; and a fasciotomy may be needed at the time of surgery. Treatment of these fractures often involves a bone graft from the iliac crest to augment the reduction. A variety of fixation devices, including screws and plates and Kirschner wires, are used. Open fractures are, by definition, contaminated and should be irrigated and debrided within 8 h of the injury. Surgical approaches are direct through longitudinal or transverse incisions. Some fractures of the articular surface of the distal radius are amenable to arthroscopically guided percutaneous pin fixation. Screw fixation of the scaphoid also can be accomplished by arthroscopy. Fluoroscopy often is utilized, as are standard portable radiographs to monitor and assess the quality of the reduction of the fracture.

Soft-tissue coverage of these injuries may be problematic, and **local flaps** or **free microvascular tissue transfers** may be indicated. Free transfers can come from the same limb (radial forearm flap, based on the radial artery; lateral upper arm flap, based on the posterior radial collateral artery) or a remote site (latissimus dorsi muscle, based on the thoracodorsal artery; or scapular skin flap, based on the circumflex scapular artery). Remote flaps require special patient positioning and draping. Microsurgical tissue transfers also may need special pharmacological considerations, such as the administration of heparin or dextran to prevent thrombosis of the anastomosis.

Usual preop diagnosis: Fractures of the distal radius (Colles', Barton's, Smith's are common eponyms); wrist dislocations (perilunate, lunate); fractures of the metacarpals; GSW; crush injuries; blast injuries

SUMMARY OF PROCEDURE

Position	Supine, with arm extended on hand-surgery table. Iliac crest bone graft may be indicated and should be prepped with a sandbag beneath the ipsilateral buttock.
Incision	Longitudinal or transverse
Special instrumentation	Fluoroscopy; wrist arthroscopy instrumentation; internal and external fixation devices and power tools; operating microscope; pneumatic tourniquet
Unique considerations	Associated injuries and soft-tissue problems in high-energy fractures
Antibiotics	Indicated during the treatment of infected fractures. Treatment of both open and closed fractures requires broad spectrum cephalosporin prophylaxis. Special cases of contamination, such as soil and human bite injuries, require specific extended coverage.
Surgical time	30 min-3 h. Microsurgical tissue transfers can have surgical times of 8 h or more.
Tourniquet	150 mmHg above SBP; max time = 120 min
Closing considerations	Some injuries require local flaps or free microsurgical tissue transfers for closure. Fasciotomy wounds usually are left open. Splint applied at surgery.
EBL	Minimal for fracture treatment, as tourniquet control is used. Iliac crest or free-tissue donor sites can result in blood loss of 500-2000 ml.
Postop care	Monitor free-tissue transfers with temperature monitoring and visual inspection.
Mortality	Usually 2° associated injuries
Morbidity	Loss of reduction, requiring repair
	Nonunion (requires additional surgical procedure)
	Infection
Pain score	3-9 (Great variation, probably depending on degree of median, ulnar, or dorsal radial sensory nerve involvement. Postop pain management is often problematic. Early use of stellate ganglion blocks may be beneficial in preventing the development of sympathetic mediated pain syndromes.)

PATIENT POPULATION CHARACTERISTICS

Age range	All ages. More conservative approaches are used with elderly patients.
Male:Female	1:1
Incidence	Very common
Etiology	Trauma
Associated conditions	Traumatic injuries

ANESTHETIC CONSIDERATIONS

PREOPERATIVE

The majority of patients presenting for these procedures are relatively young and healthy. Most present for elective repair of a traumatic injury, and preop workup is routine. Replantation and some wrist procedures, such as repair of a compound fracture, require immediate attention and necessitate emergency surgery and full-stomach considerations (see p. B-5).

Neurologic	If regional anesthesia is contemplated, preexisting sensory or motor defects should be documented carefully preop.
Laboratory	Hb/Hct (healthy patients); otherwise, as indicated from H&P.
Premedication	Mild-to-moderate premedication (e.g., in adults, midazolam 1-2 mg iv, fentanyl 50-100 μg iv, titrated to effect) is often desirable before placement of a regional block.

INTRAOPERATIVE

Anesthetic technique: GETA, regional anesthesia, or a combination are commonly used. A brachial plexus block via the axillary or infraclavicular approach are excellent for short (1-2 h) procedures on the wrist and hand. Regional anesthesia alone is a means of avoiding the risk of aspiration pneumonitis associated with GA in the patient with a full stomach whose operation must be done emergently (see Rapid-Sequence Induction of Anesthesia, p. B-5). Unfortunately, because these cases often require the use of bone grafts harvested from the iliac crest, regional anesthesia alone usually is not feasible. For similar reasons, regional anesthesia also is not appropriate for cases that require a free-tissue transfer.

General anesthesia:

Induction	Standard induction (p. B-2)
Maintenance	Standard maintenance (p. B-3)
Emergence	Skin closure is frequently followed by application of a splint; patient should remain anesthetized during splinting procedure.

Regional anesthesia: 1.5% mepivacaine 40 ml with alkalization for routine superficial cases; 0.5% bupivacaine or 0.5% levobupivacaine/0.5% ropivacaine, if available, 40 ml for procedures > 2.5 h or if extended analgesia is desired. Epinephrine (2.5-5μg/ml) should be added whenever possible to decrease peak plasma concentrations of local anesthetics.

Infraclavicular block	The coracoid approach makes this a safe and effective regional technique. A single injection will provide anesthesia distal to the mid humerus. No additional injections are necessary, and the patient's arm does not need to be abducted for block placement. If intraop sedation is necessary, propofol (50-100 μg/kg/min) by continuous infusion or intermittent bolus injection of opioid/benzodiazepine are good choices.
Axillary block	The medial aspect of the upper arm is innervated by the intercostobrachial nerve (T2) and requires a separate subcutaneous field block in the axilla, especially when a tourniquet is used. The lateral cutaneous nerve of the forearm, a sensory branch of the musculocutaneous nerve supplying sensation to the lateral forearm, is frequently missed by the axillary approach to the brachial plexus. Thus, a block of this nerve at the elbow or within the proximal body of the coracobrachialis muscle is sometimes necessary. If intraop sedation is needed, propofol (50 μg/kg/min) by continuous infusion or intermittent bolus injection of opioid/benzodiazepine (e.g., midazolam 0.5-1.0 mg iv q 5 min and alfentanil 5-10 μg/kg iv q min titrated to effect) are good choices.
Blood and fluid requirements	Minimal-to-moderate blood loss IV: 18 ga $\times$ 1 NS/LR @ 1.5-3 ml/kg/h	An 18 ga iv catheter placed in the nonoperative upper extremity should be adequate.

Monitoring	Standard monitors (p. B-1)	
Positioning	✓ and pad pressure points. ✓ eyes.	
Infraclavicular block complications	Local anesthetic toxicity Inadequate block Intravascular injection Pneumothorax Persistent paresthesia	Less frequent occurrence, compared with axillary block. Pneumothorax is very rare with the lateral coracoid approach.
Axillary block complications	Inadequate block Intravascular injection Persistent paresthesia Axillary hematoma Axillary artery thrombosis	Minimal doses of local anesthetic can cause CNS toxicity during an accidental intravascular injection. Sz should be treated with STP or midazolam titrated to effect, accompanied by airway control. If there is any question of a full stomach, then intubation should be accomplished rapidly. Axillary thrombosis is extremely rare.

POSTOPERATIVE

Pain management	PCA (p. C-3), in combination with regional block	Regional or combined regional-general anesthetic techniques are excellent for wrist procedures, especially with respect to postop pain management.
Tests	None routinely indicated.	

References

1. Brockway MS, Wildsmith JA: Axillary brachial plexus block: method of choice? *Br J Anaesth* 1990; 64(2):224-31.
2. Gerancher JC: Upper extremity nerve blocks. *Anes Clin North Am* 2000; 18(2):1-16.
3. Goldberg ME, et al: A comparison of three methods of axillary approach to brachial plexus blockade for upper extremity surgery. *Anesthesiology* 1987; 66(6):814-16.
4. Green DP: *Operative Hand Surgery*, 4th edition. Churchill Livingstone, New York: 1999.
5. Ramamurthy S, Hickey R: Anesthesia. In *Operative Hand Surgery*, 4th edition. Green DP, ed. Churchill Livingstone, New York: 1999, 22-48.
6. Sia, S: Axillary brachial plexus block using peripheral nerve stimulator: A comparison between double- and triple-injection techniques. *Reg Anesth Pain Med* 2001; 26(6):499-503.
7. Salazar CH: Infraclavicular brachial plexus block. *Reg Anesth Pain Med* 1999; 24(5):411-6.
8. Vandam LD: Anesthesia for hand surgery. In *Flynn's Hand Surgery*, 4th edition. Jupiter JB, ed. Williams and Wilkins, Baltimore: 1991, 46-54.
9. Wilson JL: Infraclavicular brachial plexus block: parasagittal anatomy important to the coracoid technique. *Anesth Analg* 1998; 87(4):870-3.

DIGIT AND HAND REPLANTATION

SURGICAL CONSIDERATIONS

Description: Patients with traumatic amputations of digits and the hand are candidates for emergency microsurgical replantation of these parts. In children, replantation is attempted for essentially all amputations. In the adult, replantation is carried out for amputations of the thumb, multiple digits, and amputations through the palm. In general, amputations of a single digit are not candidates for replantation because of the minimal loss of function in relation to the long rehabilitation period and expected outcome. Certainly, a single digit amputated proximal to the insertion of the flexor digitorum superficialis (FDS) tendon (Zone II) (Fig 10.1-3) should not be replanted. The condition of the amputated part plays an important role in the decision to proceed with replantation. A severely crushed, contaminated, or burned part cannot be expected to survive and function. The patients also may have associated traumatic injuries (i.e., intraabdominal bleeding with a positive peritoneal lavage, chest injuries), which will take preference over replantation. The patient's overall health status must be assessed. A patient with unstable angina probably should not be subjected to a lengthy microsurgical procedure.

There are a variety of reasons that people suffer amputations. Many of these patients are substance abusers or intoxicated at the time of injury. Studies of these patients also have shown a high incidence of psychopathology, along with substance abuse. Because these procedures are emergent, patients often arrive at the hospital with full stomachs. While regional anesthesia techniques provide peripheral vasodilation through their sympatholytic effect, many surgeons prefer GA because of the unpredictable length of the procedures. While the patient is being readied for induction, the surgeon prepares the amputated part in the OR. At this time, the structures to be repaired are tagged, which saves a great deal of anesthetic time. When the patient is prepped and draped, the hand is irrigated and debrided, and the corresponding structures are tagged in similar manner. The amputated part is brought to the field and the actual replantation is performed. Once arterial blood flow is reestablished, the patient must be kept warm to prevent vasospasm. As with other microsurgical procedures, pharmacologic intervention is indicated to prevent thrombosis; iv heparin and dextran are normally administered. Skin grafts for soft-tissue coverage and vein grafts to replace segmental vascular defects are commonly used. Vein grafts can be obtained from the ipsilateral upper extremity or from the lower extremity, especially the dorsum of the foot. The lateral thigh or abdomen are excellent donor sites for split-thickness skin grafts. Rarely is an immediate microsurgical free-tissue transfer indicated for soft-tissue coverage.

Usual preop diagnosis: Traumatic amputation of the digits or hand

SUMMARY OF PROCEDURE

Position	Supine, with arm extended on hand-surgery table
Incision	Extensile exposures of neurovascular structures. Lower extremity prepped and draped as donor site for vein grafts from dorsum of foot, split-thickness skin graft from the thigh.
Special instrumentation	Operating microscope; microsurgical instrumentation
Unique considerations	Emergency procedure
Antibiotics	Cefazolin 1 g iv
Surgical time	3-12 h
Tourniquet	150 mmHg above systolic; max time = 120 min
Closing considerations	Routine volar hand splint
EBL	< 500 ml
Postop care	ICU → requires monitoring in intensive nursing environment. Should be kept pain-free for extended period postop to minimize vessel spasm. Patients will benefit from postop sedation.
Mortality	Minimal for digit and hand. Mortality becomes an important issue when large amounts of muscle are part of the reattachment.
Morbidity	Loss of replanted part (vessel thrombosis): 10%
	Infection: Rare
Pain score	3-5

PATIENT POPULATION CHARACTERISTICS

Age range	All ages, infant–8th decade
Male:Female	1:1
Incidence	Uncommon
Etiology	Trauma
Associated conditions	Substance abuse; alcoholism

ANESTHETIC CONSIDERATIONS

PREOPERATIVE

In general, there are two patient populations for hand replantation: (1) isolated hand injury patients (common), and (2) multiple trauma victims (rare).

Respiratory	As suggested by coexisting disease or acute trauma injuries. Evidence of occult chest injury, including pneumothorax and pulmonary contusion, should be sought.
	Tests: Consider CXR, ABGs in victims of significant trauma.
Cardiovascular	As suggested by coexisting disease or acute trauma injuries. ✓ for evidence of occult cardiac or mediastinal injuries, such as myocardial contusion or great vessel rupture.
	Tests: Consider CXR (with NG tube in place to assess mediastinal widening), and ECG in victims of significant trauma.

Neurological	As suggested by coexisting disease or acute trauma injuries. The possibility of closed head injury should be addressed in multiple-trauma victims. Verify integrity of C-spine. **Tests:** Consider head CT prior to beginning a long procedure under GA in a patient with evidence of head trauma; C-spine x-ray.
Gastrointestinal	All patients should be considered to have full stomachs and, therefore, at increased risk for aspiration pneumonitis. In general, they should receive preop medication to reduce stomach volume and acidity (e.g., metoclopramide 10 mg iv and ranitidine 50 mg iv).
Hematologic	Multiple-trauma victims are likely to suffer from acute blood loss. Although blood loss from these procedures is generally modest, a preop T&C for several U PRBCs is wise for trauma patients. **Tests:** CBC
Metabolic	~50% of trauma victims are intoxicated. Anesthesia-related implications of ethanol intoxication include decreased anesthetic requirements, diuresis, vasodilation, and hypothermia.
Laboratory	As suggested by coexisting disease or acute trauma injuries. In general, most victims of significant trauma are best served by obtaining a wide variety of baseline lab studies to screen for unrecognized injury. These studies normally include: ABGs; UA; renal function tests; LFTs; serum amylase; tox screen.
Premedication	Full-stomach precautions: Na citrate 0.3 M 30 ml, metoclopramide 10 mg iv; H$_2$-blocker

INTRAOPERATIVE

Anesthetic technique: GETA, after rapid-sequence induction (see p. B-5). Because of the unpredictable length of these procedures and the possible need for bone and/or vessel grafts, regional anesthesia is not feasible as the primary technique. A concurrent, continuing brachial plexus block, however, will provide sympathetic blockade, as well as postop analgesia, and catheter placement should be considered before inducing GA. The hand injury repair may be done concurrently with other procedures in multiple-trauma victims.

Induction	Rapid-sequence induction (p. B-5) is mandatory in emergency cases, unless awake intubation is performed. C-spine fracture patients and those with facial injuries may require awake fiber optic intubation (p. B-6). Hemodynamically unstable, acute-trauma patients may be induced more safely with etomidate or ketamine.	
Maintenance	Standard maintenance (p. B-3) for stable patients. Hemodynamically unstable, acute-trauma victims undergoing emergency surgery may be better served by using a combination of medications designed to have minimal hemodynamic consequences (e.g., fentanyl for analgesia, vecuronium for muscle relaxation, and scopolamine or midazolam for amnesia). N$_2$O is best avoided in the trauma patient.	
Emergence	Difficult airway or full-stomach cases require awake extubation. Trauma victims who have undergone a prolonged procedure or who have significant associated cardiopulmonary injuries usually are left intubated for postop mechanical ventilation.	
Blood and fluid requirements	Significant blood loss IV: 16 ga × 1 NS/LR @ 1.5-3 ml/kg/h + replacement of blood loss Fluid/blood warmers, heating blanket, warmed circuit humidifier	A 16 ga iv catheter in nonoperative upper extremity should be adequate in hemodynamically stable patients. Acute-trauma victims who are unstable require a minimum of 2 large-bore iv catheters or large-bore central lines.
Monitoring	Standard monitors (p. B-1)	Invasive hemodynamic monitoring and TEE should be considered in acute, multiple-trauma victims.
Positioning	✓ and pad pressure points. ✓ eyes.	
Complications	Hemodynamic instability	Previously unrecognized injuries (e.g., pneumothorax, cardiac tamponade, intracranial bleeding) should be considered as a cause of unexplained intraop hemodynamic instability in all acute-trauma victims.

POSTOPERATIVE

Complications	Sepsis ARDS	Many trauma victims survive the initial insult only to die later of sepsis or ARDS.

Pain management   PCA (p. C-3)

Tests   None routinely indicated.

References

1. Carr DB, Kwon J: Anesthesia techniques and their indications for upper limb surgery. In *Surgery of the Hand and Upper Extremity.* McGraw-Hill, New York: 1996, 199-239.
2. Cullings HM, Hendee WR: Radiation risks in the orthopaedic operating room. *Contemp Orthop* 1984; 8:48-52.
3. Green DP: *Operative Hand Surgery*, 4th edition. Churchill Livingstone, New York: 1999.
4. Johnstone RE: Acute trauma with multiple injuries. *Current Opin in Anesthesiol* 2000; 13(2):175-9.
5. Nicholls BJ, Cullen BF: Anesthesia for trauma. *J Clin Anesth* 1988; 1(2):115-29.
6. Ramamurthy S, Hickey R: Anesthesia. In *Operative Hand Surgery*, 4th edition. Green DP, ed. Churchill Livingstone, New York: 1999, 22-48.
7. Soderstrom CA, Cowley RA: A national alcohol and trauma center survey. Missed opportunities, failures of responsibility. *Arch Surg* 1987; 122(9):1067-71.

Surgeons

Amy L. Ladd, MD
Andrew C. Karich, MD

10.2 SHOULDER/ARM SURGERY

Anesthesiologist

Eric Rey Amador, MD

ARTHROSCOPIC SHOULDER SURGERY

SURGICAL CONSIDERATIONS

Description: The role of arthroscopy in shoulder surgery has advanced tremendously in the past 5-10 yr. In the past, arthroscopy was used primarily for diagnostic purposes, followed by a definitive open procedure. Advances in arthroscopy and instrumentation now permit many procedures to be done 'all inside.' Arthroscopic procedures include **subacromial decompression (SAD); distal clavicle resection (Mumford procedure); debridement** for labral tear, infection, or synovitis; and, more recently, **rotator cuff (RC) repair, anterior capsule-labral repair** for recurrent dislocation (**Bankart repair**), and **repair of SLAP lesions** (superior labral anterior-posterior tears). Less common procedures include **capsular plication** for multidirectional instability (MDI), **capsular release for frozen shoulder**, and the **OATS** procedure (osteochondral autograft transfer system) for focal cartilage lesions or Hill-Sachs lesions. **Arthroscopic capsular shrinkage (thermal capsulorrhaphy)** is a controversial technique used for MDI or as an adjunct to arthroscopic Bankart repair in traumatic instability.

Procedures done arthroscopically are less painful postop than their respective open counterparts, produce less trauma to normal tissues, and may accelerate rehabilitation. The surgeon may insert an intraarticular catheter (local anesthetic infusion for analgesia that lasts from 2-3 d); alternatively, interscalene block has been shown to provide excellent postop analgesia of shorter duration.

Arthroscopic shoulder surgery may be performed in the beach-chair or lateral decubitus position. Numerous commercial beach-chair positioners are available with a trough for the head and a breakaway shoulder pad to provide access to the posterior shoulder. The lateral decubitus position utilizes distal traction of 5-10 lbs, with the arm abducted 30-45°. Both are safe positions for the brachial plexus, as the shoulder is not excessively abducted.

Initially, an 18 ga spinal needle is inserted into the glenohumeral joint, passing through the posterior deltoid and infraspinatus muscle and the posterior capsule of the joint (see shoulder anatomy, Fig 10.2-1). Placement is verified by injecting saline to inflate the joint capsule. A stab incision is made using a No. 11 blade in the direction previously defined by the finder needle. Sharp, then blunt trocars are used to gain access to the joint and permit insertion of the arthroscopic device. Improper insertion of the instruments can injure the axillary or suprascapular nerves and the cartilage of the glenohumeral joint. Initial diagnostic arthroscopy is carried out through the posterior portal. Bupivacaine 0.5% with epinephrine 1:200,000 often is infiltrated into portals and the joint or subacromial space at the onset of surgery to help with hemostasis. An anterior portal is used for instrumentation within the glenohumeral joint. After joint arthroscopy, the scope is placed into the subacromial space, where a direct lateral portal is used for instrumentation. Accessory portals are established as needed, depending on the procedure performed. Joint debridement, anterior stabilization, and bone grafting procedures are performed within the joint. SAD, RC repair, and distal clavicle resection are done within the subacromial space (deep to the deltoid and superficial to the RC). Epinephrine (1 mg/3 L) in the irrigation fluid and maintaining MAP < 80 mmHg help control bleeding, thus enhancing visualization during surgery.

Usual preop diagnosis: Rotator cuff tear; subacromial impingement; glenohumeral instability; AC arthritis; labral tear

SUMMARY OF PROCEDURE

Position	Lateral decubitus or beach-chair
Incision	Posterior arthroscopic portal, anterior instrumentation portal, lateral instrumentation portal for visualizing subacromial bursa; superior portal for semisitting position
Special instrumentation	Arthroscope; power burrs; arthroscopic shavers; suture-passing instruments; bone anchors; radiofrequency cautery
Unique considerations	Rigid eye patch over ipsilateral eye, to prevent corneal abrasion, suggested. Positioning of the head with appropriate support, removing upper section of operating table, if possible, for better access with semisitting position. ETT taped to opposite side of face. MAP ≤ 80.
Antibiotics	Cefazolin 1 g iv preop, particularly if bone work performed.
Surgical time	Positioning the patient is time-intensive; can add as much as 45 min. Diagnostic: < 1-1.5 h Reconstructive: 1-4 h
EBL	Minimal: < 200 ml (less with use of epinephrine, electrocautery, and laser)
Postop care	Frequently outpatient; may be overnight if interscalene or supraclavicular block is given or reconstructive procedure performed. Intraarticular pain catheter commonly used.
Mortality	Rare
Morbidity	VAE possible Extravasation of fluid (NS or LR): > 50% Brachial plexus injury (lateral decubitus position): Rare

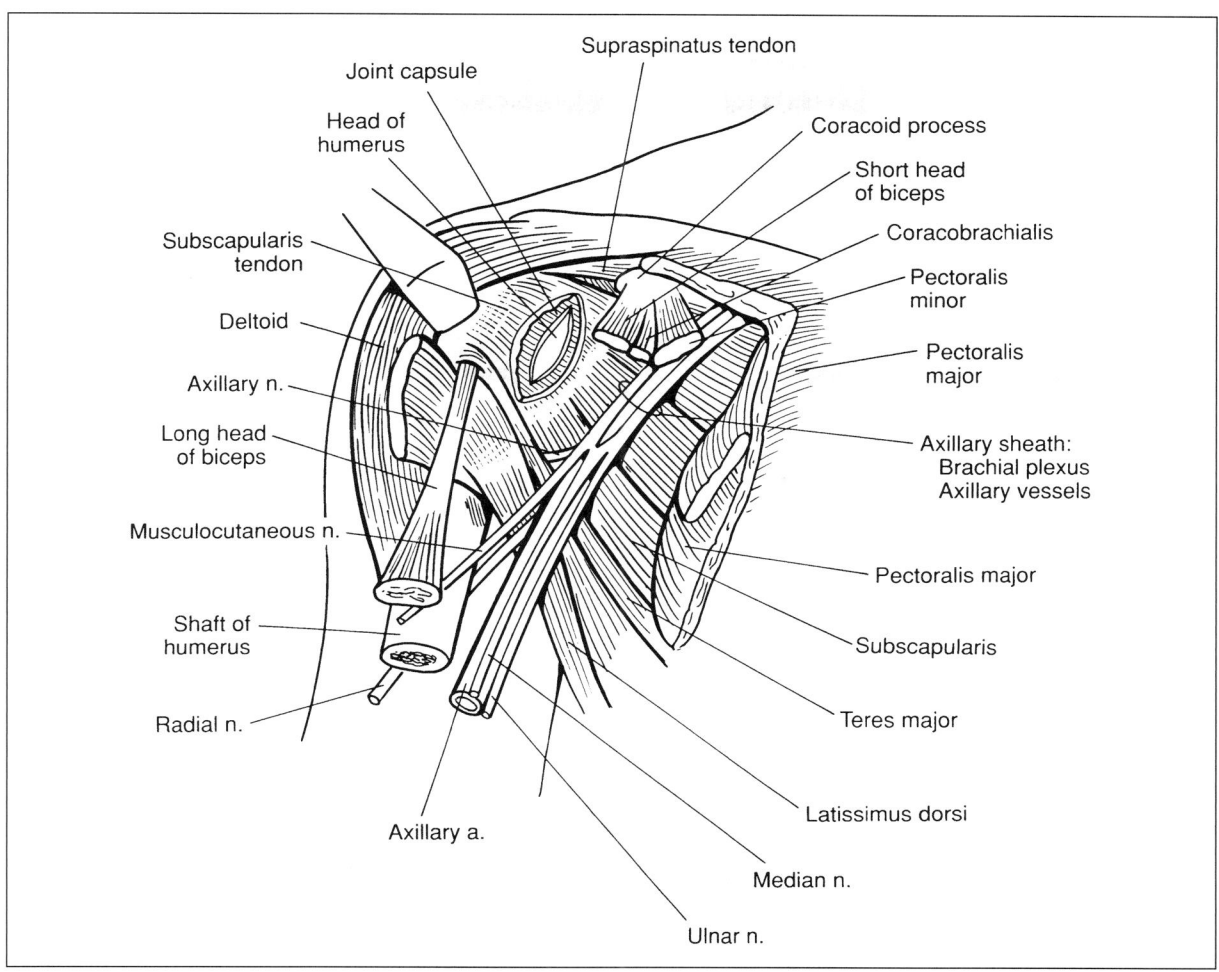

Figure 10.2-1. Anatomy of the shoulder joint, anterior. (Reproduced with permission from Hoppenfeld S, deBoer P, *Surgical Exposures in Orthopaedics: The Anatomic Approach*, 2nd edition. Lippincott Williams & Wilkins, 1994.)

Morbidity, cont.	Breakage of instruments: < 1%
	Infection: 0-3%
Pain score	4 (diagnostic); 5-7 (reconstruction)

PATIENT POPULATION CHARACTERISTICS

Age range	15-40 yr (instability); 35-75 yr (rotator cuff and acromial pathology)
Male:Female	2:1-4:1
Incidence	Very common: > 50,000/yr
Etiology	Young patients: usually sports-related
	Older patients: cuff and acromial pathology; age-wear phenomenon
	Rotator cuff pathology and acromial impingement (frequently coexist)
Associated conditions	Cervical arthritis and radiculopathy with rotator cuff pathology

ANESTHETIC CONSIDERATIONS

See Anesthetic Considerations following Surgery for Shoulder Dislocations or Instability, p. 766.

References

1. Al-Kaisy A, McGuire G, Chan VW, Bruin G, Peng P, Miniaci A, Perlas A: Analgesic effect of interscalene block using low-dose bupivacaine for outpatient arthroscopic shoulder surgery. *Reg Anesth Pain Med* 1998; 23(5):469-73.

2. Altchek DW, Carson EW: Arthroscopic acromioplasty. Current status. *Orthop Clin Am* 1997; 20(2):157-68.
3. Altchek DW, Warren RF, Skyhar MJ: Shoulder arthroscopy. In *The Shoulder*. Rockwood CA Jr, Matsen FA III, eds. WB Saunders, Philadelphia: 1990, 258-77.
4. Baechler MF, Kim DH: Patient positioning for shoulder arthroscopy based on variability in lateral acromion morphology. *Arthroscopy* 2002; 18(5):547-9.
5. Bigliani LU, Flatow EL, Deliz ED: Complications of shoulder arthroscopy. *Orthop Rev* 1991; 20(9):743-51.
6. Burkhart SS, Danaceau SM, Athanasiou KA: Turbulence control as a factor in improving visualization during subacromial arthroscopy. *Arthroscopy* 2001; 17(2):209-12.
7. Matthews LS, Fadale PD: *Technique and Instrumentation for Shoulder Arthroscopy: Instructional Course Lectures.* American Academy of Orthopedic Surgeons, Park Ridge, IL: 1989, Vol 38.
8. Mileski RA, Snyder SJ: Superior labral lesions in the shoulder: pathoanatomy and surgical management. *J Am Acad Orthop Surg* 1998; 6(2):121-31.
9. Pearsall AW IV, Osbahr DC, Speer KP: An arthroscopic technique for treating patients with frozen shoulder. *Arthroscopy* 1999; 15(1):2-11.
10. Ruotolo C, Nottage WM, Flatow EL, Gross RM, Fanon GS: Controversial topics in shoulder arthroscopy. *Arthroscopy* 2002; 18(2Supp 1):65-75.
11. Segmuller HE, Hays MG, Saies MD: Arthroscopic repair of glenolabral injuries with an absorbable fixation device. *J Shoulder Elbow Surg* 1997; 6(4):383-92.

SURGERY FOR ACROMIAL IMPINGEMENT, ROTATOR CUFF TEARS, AND ACROMIOCLAVICULAR JOINT ARTHRITIS

SURGICAL CONSIDERATIONS

Description: **Subacromial impingement** is a common degenerative condition of middle age. It may be related to anatomic factors (e.g., hooked acromion) or may be brought on by acute or chronic trauma. The subacromial space (space between the acromion and humeral head) is occupied by the supraspinatus (superior rotator cuff [RC]) muscle and tendon and the bursa, which allows for smooth gliding of the cuff tendon under the acromion. Trauma produces hemorrhage and inflammation in the bursa; swelling of the bursa decreases the space available under the acromion. These tissues may then, with abduction of the shoulder, be 'pinched' between the greater tuberosity of the humerus and the lateral aspect of the acromion (Fig 10.2-2). This further increases the inflammation, producing a vicious cycle.

Impingement of the lateral acromion on the insertion of the supraspinatus (along with poor vascularity of this part of the cuff) is a leading hypothesis for the etiology of degenerative **RC tears**. **AC joint arthritis** is a common x-ray finding in adults, but it is often asymptomatic. While undersurface spurs of the AC joint are removed during **subacromial decompression (SAD)**, distal clavicle excision is done for clinically symptomatic AC joint arthritis.

Subacromial impingement: Surgical treatment of subacromial impingement is indicated when nonoperative treatment (e.g., cortisone injection, physical therapy) fails. Surgery involves resection of the anterolateral aspect of the undersurface of the acromion (creating more room in the subacromial space). This may be accomplished

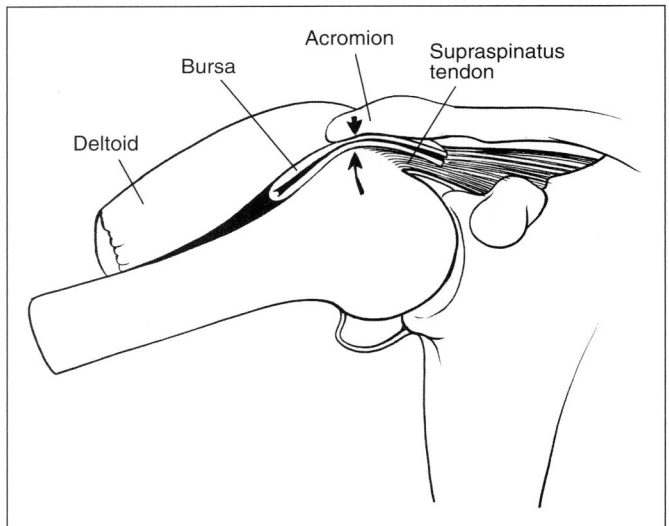

Figure 10.2-2. Abduction of the arm can impinge the subacromial bursa between the greater tuberosity and the undersurface of the acromion and coracoacromial ligament. (Reproduced with permission from Hoppenfeld S, deBoer P: *Surgical Exposures in Orthopaedics: the Anatomic Approach,* 2nd edition. Lippincott Williams & Wilkins, 1994.)

with open techniques in combination with open RC repair, but it is more commonly done arthroscopically. The bursa is usually inflamed and quite vascular. Bleeding may obscure arthroscopic visualization and is controlled with electrocautery, epinephrine in the irrigant, and by maintaining relative ↓BP (MAP < 80 mmHg).

Rotator cuff tears: RC (Fig 10.2-3) repair may be performed using the **direct lateral open approach, the mini-open (deltoid-splitting) approach** in conjunction with arthroscopy, or, more recently, all arthroscopically. If a deltoid-splitting incision is used, care is taken not to extend the split more than 5 cm distal to the acromion because of possible injury to the axillary nerve, which innervates the deltoid 5 cm or more from the lateral aspect of the acromion. If the beach-chair position is used for open RC surgery or arthroscopy, the upper limb is draped free. The arm is manipulated, and traction is frequently applied. It is important that the head is secured (the head may be taped to the table or special beach-chair positioner), the eyes are protected, and that the anesthesiologist frequently checks to see that the surgeon is not pulling the patient off the table (not always apparent from the surgeon's side of the drape). Traction on the brachial plexus is more likely in the lateral decubitus position 2° arm traction.

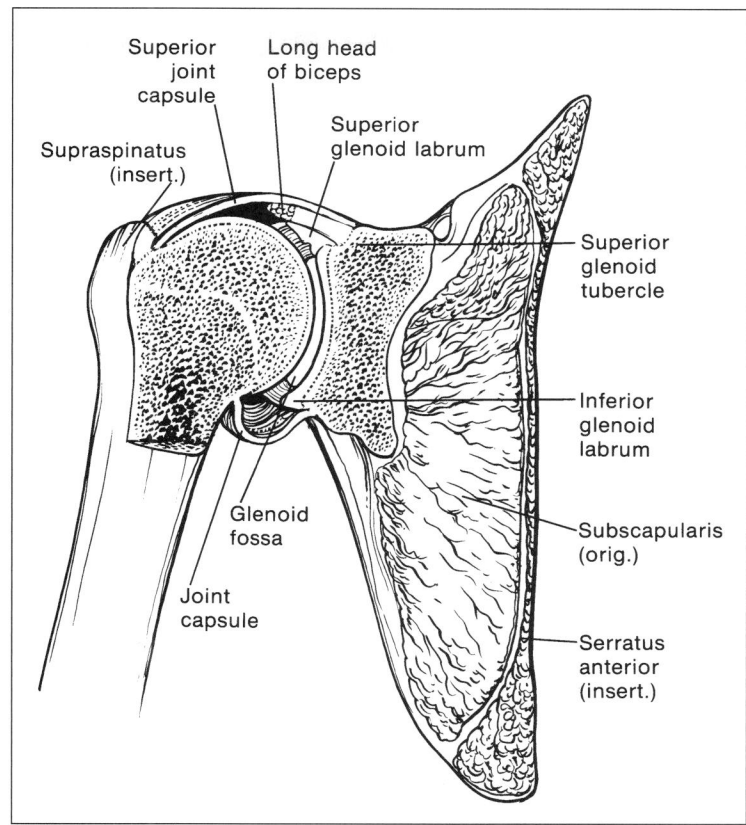

Figure 10.2-3. Cross section of the joint: The joint capsule is redundant inferiorly to allow abduction. The long head of the biceps tendon traverses the joint. The tendon is surrounded by synovium and, therefore, is anatomically intracapsular but extrasynovial. (Reproduced with permission from Hoppenfeld S, deBoer P: *Surgical Exposures in Orthopaedics: the Anatomic Approach*, 2nd edition. Lippincott Williams & Wilkins, 1994.)

Open RC repair involves suturing the cuff insertion back to the greater tuberosity through drill holes or with suture anchors. Arthroscopic repair requires percutaneous anchor placement and arthroscopic suture-passing and knot-tying. Bleeding is minimal with the arthroscopic technique, but may approach 400 ml with an open procedure. Both require that the patient remain relaxed until all dressings are applied and he/she is fitted with an abduction sling. Patients typically are admitted for 24 h for pain control or if a drain is used.

AC joint disease: Surgery for **AC joint arthritis** is usually performed in conjunction with SAD and/or RC repair and may be done open or arthroscopically. It involves simple resection of the distal 5 mm of the clavicle through an incision directly over the joint or through an accessory anterior portal. Again, relative ↓BP is required for the arthroscopic procedure.

Repair of AC joint dislocation ('shoulder separation') is uncommon. Most AC separations are treated nonoperatively, because long-term functional results are the same or better than those treated surgically. Severe AC separations occasionally require surgery, when the dislocated clavicle is buttonholed posteriorly through the trapezius, the deltoid origin has been avulsed from the clavicle, or the clavicle is displaced inferiorly below the cricoid process. Repair is performed in the beach-chair position with the incision carried out over the AC joint and distal third of the clavicle. The clavicle is reduced and held in place with a large screw into the base of the coracoid, a large suture wrapped around the coracoid, or with K-wires across the AC joint. The coracoclavicular ligament often is repaired or reconstructed with tendon graft, or the coracoacromial ligament is transferred from the edge of the acromion to the clavicle. Following reduction and fixation, the deltoid is reattached to the clavicle if it has been avulsed, and the patient is placed in an immobilizer after skin closure. The operation is technically challenging and there is a high failure rate. The brachial plexus and subclavian vessels are at risk with screw placement and with inferior dislocations.

Usual preop diagnosis: RC tears (partial or complete); AC arthritis; impingement; bursitis; bicipital tendinitis; AC separation

SUMMARY OF PROCEDURE

Position	Beach-chair; semisitting, ~ 40-70°; or lateral decubitus
Incision	Oblique, saber-type incision anteriorly over distal acromion; lateral or deltopectoral incision for wider exposure; deltoid-splitting incision for RC tears
Special instrumentation	Power equipment for bone work; self-retaining retractors for cuff repairs; suture anchors
Unique considerations	Rigid eye protection for ipsilateral eye and careful head positioning
Antibiotics	Cefazolin 1 g iv preop
Surgical time	1-3 h
Closing considerations	Muscle relaxation when mobilizing cuff and during closure. Arm in sling and swathe, or abduction pillow for large tears. Immobilizer should be positioned prior to awakening patient to minimize potential for rupture of repair.
EBL	200-400 ml
Postop care	Maintenance of position in sling and swathe; no active motion of shoulder girdle for 2 d - 6 wk, depending on procedure.
Mortality	Rare
Morbidity	Infection: 1-5%
	Axillary nerve damage: < 2%
	Musculocutaneous nerve damage: < 2%
	Breakage of instruments: < 1%
	Brachial plexus damage (position-dependent)
	Suprascapular nerve at risk for RC mobilization
Pain score	5-8

PATIENT POPULATION CHARACTERISTICS

Age range	Rotator cuff tears > 40 yr (younger for athletes)
Male:Female	3:1
Incidence[3,4]	5-30% of general population affected by RC and acromial conditions, depending on age, thickness of tear, associated conditions
Etiology	Age-related; trauma (70% involved in light work)
Associated conditions	Bursitis; tendinitis; impingement; RC disease (especially in first-time glenohumeral dislocations > 40 yr); diabetes and renal failure; hypermobility

ANESTHETIC CONSIDERATIONS

See Anesthetic Considerations following Surgery for Shoulder Dislocations or Instability, p. 766.

References

1. Altchek DW, Carson EW: Arthroscopic acromioplasty. Current status. *Orthop Clin Am* 1997; 20(2):157-68.
2. Chelly JE, Greger J, Al-Samsam T, Gebhard R, Masson M, Matuszczak M, Sciard D: Reduction of operating and recovery room times and overnight hospital stay with interscalene blocks as sole anesthetic technique for rotator cuff surgery. *Minerva Anestesiol* 2001; 67(9):613-19.
3. Cofield RH, Parvizi J, Hoffmeyer PJ, Lanzer WL, Ilstrup DM, Rowland CM: Surgical repair of chronic rotator cuff tears. A prospective long-term study. *J Bone Joint Surg Am* 2001; 83-A(1):71-7.
4. Flatow EL, Altchek DW, Gartsman GM, Ionnotti JP, et al: The rotator cuff. Commentary. *Orthop Clin North Am* 1997; 28(2): 177-94.
5. Hata Y, Saitoh S, Murakami N, Seki H, Nakatsuchi Y, Takaoka K: A less invasive surgery for rotator cuff tear: mini-open repair. *J Shoulder Elbow Surg* 2001; 10(1):11-16.
6. Martin SD, Baumgarten TE, Andrews JR: Arthroscopic resection of the distal aspect of the clavicle with concomitant subacromial decompression. *J Bone Joint Surg Am* 2001; 83-A:328-35.
7. Neer CS II: Impingement lesions. *Clin Orthop* 1983; 173:70-7.
8. Peterson CA II, Altchek DW: Arthroscopic treatment of rotator cuff disorders. *Clin Sports Med* 1996; 15(4):715-36.
9. Schlegel TF, Burks RT, Marcus RL, Dunn HK: A prospective evaluation of untreated acute grade III acromioclavicular separations. *Am J Sports Med* 2001; 29(6):699-703.
10. Tubiana R, McCullough CJ, Masquelet AC: *An Atlas of Surgical Exposures of the Upper Extremity.* JB Lippincott, Philadelphia: 1990.
11. Yamaguchi K, Ball CM, Galatz LM: Arthroscopic rotator cuff repair: transition from mini-open to all-arthroscopic. *Clin Orthop* 2001; 390:89-94.

SURGERY FOR SHOULDER DISLOCATIONS OR INSTABILITY

SURGICAL CONSIDERATIONS

Description: **Shoulder instability** is classified as multidirectional (MDI) or traumatic. MDI is associated with generalized ligamentous laxity (e.g., Ehlers Danlos or Marfan syndromes, or idiopathic), and is treated primarily nonoperatively with physical therapy. Occasionally, open or arthroscopic **capsular shift** or arthroscopic **thermal capsulorrhaphy** is performed for recalcitrant cases. This involves 'plication' of the capsule (taking up the slack) or actual shrinkage of the capsular tissue with a radiofrequency probe. A subset of patients with MDI, known as 'voluntary dislocators,' frequently have psychiatric disorders and are very poor candidates for surgery.

Traumatic instability is usually anterior and is quite common in the young, active population. Recurrent dislocation is common (80-90%) in these patients and is associated with avulsion of the capsule/labrum from the anterior-inferior glenoid rim (Bankart lesion). The population undergoing a **Bankart repair** is almost invariably young and healthy. First-time dislocators age >50 yr more commonly sustain rotator cuff (RC) tears or fractures, which do not result in chronic instability, but may require operative reduction and RC repair or fracture fixation. Posterior traumatic dislocation is much less common and is associated with high-energy trauma and grand mal Sz.

Instability surgery is classically performed as an open procedure in the beach-chair position. This often is preceded by exam under anesthesia and arthroscopic examination; however, more surgeons are now performing anterior stabilization arthroscopically, using either suture anchors or bioabsorbable tacks. The essential feature of instability surgery, whether arthroscopic or open, is the reattachment of the anterior capsule and inferior glenohumeral ligament to the rim of the glenoid, thus reestablishing the normal anatomy. Nonanatomic procedures (reconstructive) are much less common but are still performed occasionally. These include advancement of the subscapularis insertion (**Magnuson-Stack operation, Putti-Platt operation**), transfer of the coracoid process to the anterior glenoid rim (**Bristow procedure**), and rotational osteotomy of the proximal humerus for instability associated with large-impression fractures of the humeral head.

The **open Bankart repair** is performed in the beach-chair position using the deltopectoral approach, with the interval between the deltoid and pectoralis major. The subscapularis (anterior RC muscle) lies just anterior to the joint capsule (Fig 10.2-3), and this is either detached from its insertion or split. The capsule may then be opened to visualize the joint and rim of the glenoid. The glenoid rim is decorticated, providing bleeding bone to promote healing, and the anterior capsule is reattached through drill holes in the glenoid or with suture anchors. The capsule often is imbricated (overlapping folds) if it is redundant.

The shoulder and deltoid are highly vascular; however, bleeding is usually slight, with careful surgical technique. Major nerves are close but out of the plane of the operative field. The **musculocutaneous nerve** may be stretched by excessive medial retraction of the coracobrachialis (especially if a coracoid osteotomy is used) and the **axillary nerve** may be injured if the surgeon strays too far inferiorly.

If the **subscapularis-releasing technique** is used, the muscle is reattached and must be protected postop. External rotation of the shoulder is prevented for several wk while the repair heals, and the surgeon may want the patient to remain anesthetized until a shoulder immobilizer is applied.

The **arthroscopic Bankart repair** is similar to the open procedure but is performed through two anterior portals with the scope coming in posteriorly. This procedure is less painful postop and allows for more rapid rehabilitation, as the subscapularis is not detached. The use of absorbable pegs is technically easier, since fixation with suture anchors requires advanced arthroscopic techniques, including arthroscopic knot-typing, and typically adds 1 h to the total operative time.

Open surgery for posterior dislocation is similar to the open Bankart repair, but it is done in the lateral position and utilizes the interval between the infraspinatus and teres minor. The RC attachment is preserved, but the posterior deltoid is detached and must be protected postop.

Usual preop diagnosis: Recurrent traumatic anterior or posterior instability; MDI; fracture dislocation

SUMMARY OF PROCEDURES

	Open	Arthroscopic
Position	Beach-chair for anterior; lateral decubitus for posterior	Lateral decubitus or beach-chair
Incision[7, 11]	Deltopectoral (anterior); posterior approach (posterior)	Multiple small portals
Special instrumentation	High-speed laser; suture anchors; glenoid and humeral instrumentation	⇐ + arthroscopic instruments for suture-passing and knot-tying
Antibiotics	Cefazolin 1 g iv preop if bone work performed.	⇐

	Open	Arthroscopic
Surgical time	2-4 h	⇐
Closing considerations	Continuous anesthesia until application of sling and swathe or abduction pillow	⇐
EBL	200-400 ml	Minimal
Postop care	No active motion for 6 wk	⇐
Mortality	Minimal	⇐
Morbidity	Axillary nerve palsy: 15% (may be preexisting) Suprascapular nerve injury	
Pain score	8	5

PATIENT POPULATION CHARACTERISTICS

Age range	15-35 yr
Male:Female	2:1
Incidence	Common
Etiology	Trauma; hypermobility; Sz
Associated conditions	RC tears (> 50 yr); hypermobility syndrome; Sz disorder; Hill-Sachs lesion (humeral head defect) may require bone grafting; superior labral tears; in most axillary nerve palsies from the injury; iatrogenic (rare)

ANESTHETIC CONSIDERATIONS

(Procedures covered: shoulder arthroscopy; surgery for acromial impingement, RC tears, and AC disease; surgery for shoulder dislocations or instability)

PREOPERATIVE

Typically, three patient populations present for repair of RC tears or shoulder arthroscopy: (1) healthy posttrauma, (2) nonrheumatoid arthritic, and (3) rheumatoid arthritic. Individuals presenting for repair of shoulder dislocations also may include those with a joint hypermobility syndrome (e.g., Marfan or Ehlers-Danlos) or Sz disorder patients.

Respiratory	Arthritic patients may exhibit Sx of pleural effusion or pulmonary fibrosis. Hoarseness may indicate cricoarytenoid joint (CAJ) involvement → difficult intubation. (See Anesthetic Considerations for Wrist Procedures, p. 740.) Seizure disorder patients who suffer from recurrent shoulder dislocation as a result of frequent grand mal Sz also may suffer from occult aspiration pneumonia or pneumonitis. **Tests:** Consider CXR; PFTs; ABGs in debilitated rheumatoid patients
Cardiovascular	Arthritic patients may suffer from chronic pericardial effusions, valvular disease, and cardiac conduction defects. Patients presenting for shoulder stabilization because of joint hypermobility syndromes are likely to have valvular dysfunction and are vulnerable to aortic dissection 2° HTN. These patients may require antibiotic prophylaxis for bacterial endocarditis. **Tests:** Consider ECG, ECHO in patients with severe rheumatoid arthritis. Recent ECHO to assess valve function and aortic root size indicated in most patients with Marfan syndrome.
Neurological	Arthritic patients may have cervical or lumbar radiculopathies that should be documented carefully preop. For example, head flexion may cause cervical cord compression. Patients with severe Sz disorders can suffer from recurrent shoulder dislocations 2° frequent violent grand mal Sz. Such patients should be treated maximally for Sz disorder prior to elective surgery. Be aware that as many as 15% of shoulder dislocations can be accompanied by axillary nerve palsy, which should be documented carefully preop. **Tests:** Consider C-spine radiographs to r/o occult subluxations in arthritic patients with neck complaints or upper extremity radiculopathy. Verify therapeutic levels of antiepileptic medication in Sz disorder patients.
Musculoskeletal	Arthritic patients may have limited neck and jaw ROM and may require fiber optic intubation techniques. Bony deformities or muscle contractures may necessitate special attention to positioning. Patients with joint hypermobility syndromes presenting for shoulder surgery also may suffer other joint dislocations 2° positioning problems.

Hematologic	Virtually all patients will be on some type of anti-inflammatory medication that may result in anemia or Plt inhibition. Ideally, patients should D/C NSAIDs at least 5 d preop; aspirin, 7 d. In addition, selected patients with Ehlers-Danlos are known to have severe coagulation defects that may preclude the use of regional anesthesia. **Tests:** A coag profile is mandatory in Ehlers-Danlos patients.
Endocrine	Rheumatoid patients are likely to be on oral corticosteroids and may require supplemental peri-operative steroids (e.g., 100 mg hydrocortisone q 8 h iv) to treat adrenal suppression, although the routine use of 'stress-dose steroids' has been questioned.
Laboratory	Hb/Hct (in healthy patients); other tests as indicated from H&P. Patients with Ehlers-Danlos syndrome should always have banked blood available for surgery, except for the most trivial of procedures.
Premedication	Mid-to-moderate premedication (e.g., in adults, midazolam 1-2 mg iv, fentanyl 50-100 μg iv, titrated to effect) is often desirable before placement of a regional block.

INTRAOPERATIVE

Anesthetic technique: GETA or regional anesthesia (interscalene block), or a combination of the two techniques, can be used. A suprascapular block (less technically demanding and invasive than an interscalene block) can be used for intraop → postop pain control in arthroscopic shoulder procedures. When logistically feasible, a combined technique is ideal. Unless contraindicated, a long-acting local anesthetic should be used in regional anesthesia for shoulder surgery to ameliorate postop pain.

General anesthesia:

Induction	Standard induction (see p. B-2). Arthritic patients may require awake fiber optic intubation (see p. B-6).
Maintenance	Standard maintenance (see p. B-3).
Emergence	Management of emergence and extubation should be routine, except in difficult airway cases which require awake extubation.

Regional anesthesia:

Local anesthetics	2% lidocaine or 1.5% mepivacaine ± alkalization have similar onset times (10 min vs 15 min), with mepivacaine providing significantly longer postop pain control (8-10 h vs 4-6 h). If extended postop pain control is desired, 0.5% bupivacaine, levobupivacaine, or ropivacaine (each with epinephrine 1:400,000) can be used. Onset is usually within 30 min, with duration up to 18-20 h. Levobupivacaine or ropivacaine may be preferred for peripheral nerve block due to their decreased cardiotoxicity.
Interscalene block	Anesthetics and doses (epinephrine [2.5-5 μg/ml]) should be added to local anesthetic whenever possible to decrease peak plasma concentrations: • 2% lidocaine or 1.5% mepivacaine 30 ml for procedures ≤ 2.5 h. • 0.5% bupivacaine, levobupivacaine, or ropivacaine 30 ml for procedures lasting > 2.5 h. The skin on the top of the shoulder (C3-C4) and the medial aspect of the upper arm (T2) often require separate subcutaneous field blocks. Phrenic nerve block → hemidiaphragmatic paralysis is an inevitable consequence of the interscalene block, which may not be tolerated by patients with significant preexisting respiratory compromise. Major complications, such as total spinal or pneumothorax resulting from interscalene block, are extremely rare; therefore, this technique is suitable for use in outpatients. Interscalene block is contraindicated in patients with contralateral recurrent laryngeal nerve or phrenic nerve palsy (e.g., post CABG). If sedation is needed, midazolam (0.5-1.0 mg boluses), alfentanil (0.125-0.25 μg/kg/min by infusion) or propofol (50-100 μg/kg/min by infusion), given initially in subanesthetic doses and thereafter titrated to effect, are good choices.

Blood and fluid requirements	Minimal-to-moderate blood loss IV: 18 ga × 1 NS/LR @ 1.5-3 ml/kg/h	IV catheter placed in contralateral upper extremity.
Monitoring	Standard monitors (see p. B-1). ± Precordial Doppler ± Arterial line	To help detect VAE, consider precordial Doppler monitoring when semisitting position used. Consider intraarterial BP monitoring for patients with hypermobility disorders because of risk for aortic dissection 2° HTN.
Positioning	✓ and pad pressure points. ✓ eyes.	Postural ↓BP is the most common complication of the semisitting position. Changing to this position gradually

Positioning, cont.	↑VAE risk in semisitting position	can help prevent ↓BP, as can the use of antiembolism stockings, plus fluid-loading the patient. Marfan and Ehlers-Danlos patients require very gentle positioning to prevent joint dislocations.
Interscalene block complications	Total spinal Accidental epidural injection Local anesthetic toxicity (Sz/dysrhythmias) Stellate ganglion block (Horner's syndrome) Laryngeal nerve block Phrenic nerve block Pneumothorax Persistent paresthesia	Resuscitative equipment, including airway management tools, should be immediately available. When possible, nerve blocks should be performed in responsive patients to minimize complications. May last ≤ 6 wk.
Other complications	↓BP during surgical prep and positioning	↓BP during long surgical preps normally can be avoided by using light inhalation anesthesia (e.g., isoflurane 0.3-0.5%) to ensure amnesia, with moderate muscle relaxation to prevent bucking on the ETT, and maintaining adequate hydration. Antiembolism stockings will help prevent venous pooling in lower limbs.
	Cardiac dysrhythmia VAE	Dysrhythmias may be 2° to irrigation fluids containing epinephrine.

POSTOPERATIVE

Pain management	PCA (see p. C-3) or regional block techniques.	Combined regional-general anesthetic techniques are excellent for shoulder procedures, especially with respect to postop pain management.
Tests	None indicated routinely.	

References

1. Bak H, Spring BJ, Henderson JP: Inferior capsular shift procedure in athletes with multidirectional instability based on isolated capsular and ligamentous redundancy. *Am J Sports Med* 2000; 28(4):466-71.
2. Borgeat A: Acute and nonacute complications associated with interscalene block and shoulder surgery. *Anesthesiology* 2001; 95(4):875-80.
3. Bottoni CR, Wilckens JH, DeBerardino TM, D'Alleyrand JC, Rooney RC, Harpstrite JK, Arciero RA: A prospective, randomized evaluation of arthroscopic stabilization vs nonoperative treatment in patients with acute, traumatic, first-time shoulder dislocations. *Am J Sports Med* 2002; 30(4):576-80.
4. Dolan P, Sisko F, Riley E: Anesthetic considerations for Ehlers-Danlos syndrome. *Anesthesiology* 1980; 52(3):266-9.
5. Gerancher JC: Upper extremity nerve blocks. *Anes Clin N Am* 2000; 18(2):1-16.
6. Gill TJ, Micheli LJ, Gebhard F, Binder C: Bankart repair for anterior instability of the shoulder. Longterm outcome. *J Bone Joint Surg Am* 1997; 79(6):850-7.
7. Hoppenfeld S: *Surgical Exposures in Orthopaedics: The Anatomic Approach*, 2nd edition. Hoppenfeld S, deBoer P, eds. JB Lippincott, Philadelphia: 1994.
8. Keenan MA, Stiles CM, Kaufman RL: Acquired laryngeal deviation associated with cervical spine disease in erosive polyarticular arthritis. *Anesthesiology* 1983; 58(5):441-9.
9. Kim SH, Ha KI, Kim SH: Bankart repair in traumatic anterior shoulder instability: open vs arthroscopic technique. *Arthroscopy* 2002; 18(7):755-63.
10. Murphy DB: Upper extremity blocks for day surgery. *Tech in Reg Anes Pain Manag* 2000; 4(1):19-29.
11. Reginster JY, Damas P, Franchimont P: Anaesthetic risks in osteoarticular disorders. *Clin Rheum* 1985; 4:30-8.
12. Ritchie ED: Suprascapular nerve block for postoperative pain relief in arthroscopic shoulder surgery. *Anesth Analg* 1997; 84:1306-12.
13. Salathe M, Johr M: Unsuspected cervical fractures: a common problem in ankylosing spondylitis. *Anesthesiology* 1989; 70(5):869-70.
14. Sperber A, Hamberg P, Karlsson J, Sward L, Wredmark T: Comparison of an arthroscopic and open procedure for posttraumatic instability of the shoulder: a prospective, randomized multicenter study. *J Shoulder Elbow Surg* 2001; 10(2):105-8.
15. Urmey WF, Talts KH, Sharrock NE: One hundred percent incidence of hemidiaphragmatic paresis associated with interscalene brachial plexus anesthesia as diagnosed by ultrasonography. *Anesth Analg* 1991; 72(4):498-503.
16. Verghese C: Anaesthesia in Marfan's syndrome. *Anaesthesia* 1984; 39(9):917-22.

17. Weiss KS, Savoie FH III: Recent advances in arthroscopic repair of traumatic anterior instability. *Clin Orthop* 2002; 400: 117-22.
18. Wells DG, Podolakin W: Anaesthesia and Marfan's syndrome: case report. *Can J Anaesth* 1987; 34(3+Pt 1):311-14.
19. White RH: Preoperative evaluation of patients with rheumatoid arthritis. *Semin Arthritis Rheum* 1985; 14(4):287-99.

GLENOHUMERAL SHOULDER ARTHROPLASTY

SURGICAL CONSIDERATIONS

Description: Shoulder replacement is performed for pain associated with end-stage arthritis. Primary osteoarthritis (wear-and-tear arthritis) is much less common in the shoulder than in the weight-bearing joints, such as the hip and knee. The most common causes of shoulder arthritis requiring **total shoulder arthroplasty (TSA)** are rheumatoid arthritis; avascular necrosis (AVN); and osteoarthritis 2° trauma, such as fractures, massive rotator cuff (RC) tear (RC arthropathy), and chronic instability. Most patients are elderly and may have systemic autoimmune disorders, such as rheumatoid arthritis or systemic lupus erythematosus (SLE). AVN is associated with chronic alcoholism and systemic steroid use.

TSA involves replacement of the humeral head with a stemmed prosthesis and resurfacing the glenoid with a polyethylene component. Both components may be cemented or uncemented, depending on the surgeon's preference. **Hemiarthroplasty** involves only replacement of the humeral side. This is indicated when the humeral head is involved primarily and the glenoid is in good condition, as in severe proximal humerus fractures, AVN of the humeral head, and some chronic dislocators. Resurfacing the glenoid, however, is contraindicated in the presence of an unreconstructable massive RC tear. Some posttraumatic situations require glenoid osteotomy or grafting, which increases the complexity of the case and blood loss.

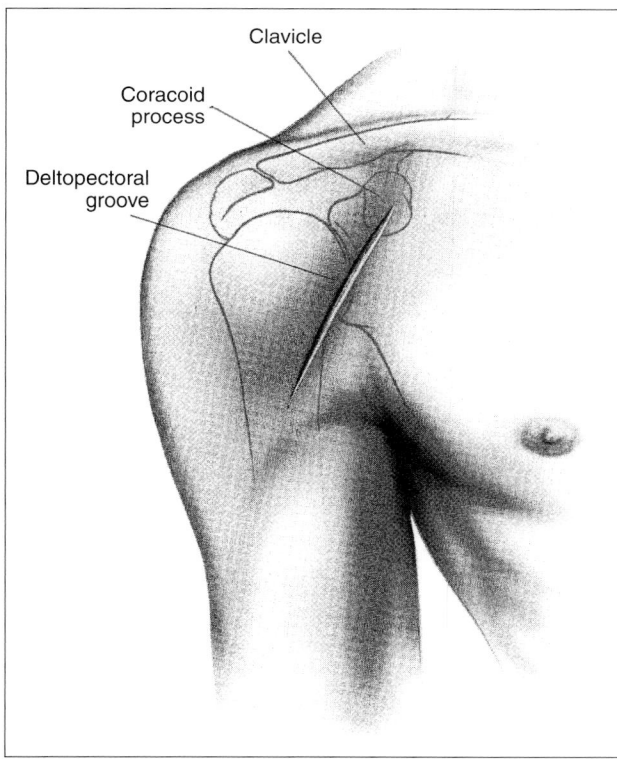

Figure 10.2-4. Incision in the deltopectoral groove. (Reproduced with permission from Hoppenfeld S, deBoer P: *Surgical Exposures in Orthopaedics: the Anatomic Approach*, 2nd edition. Lippincott Williams & Wilkins, 1994.)

Shoulder arthroplasty utilizes the beach-chair position and the deltopectoral incision (Fig 10.2-4), the 'workhorse' incision of shoulder surgery. The deltopectoral interval is developed; often a portion of the deltoid origin or insertion is incised to aid in exposure. The subscapularis insertion is incised and the muscle is reflected medially. The capsule is incised and the joint exposed. The humeral head is dislocated anteriorly and the head is removed with an oscillating saw. Reamers and broaches are used to prepare the proximal humerus for the prosthesis. If the glenoid is to be resurfaced, it is done before implantation of the final humeral component. The labrum is excised and a motorized reamer is used to remove the cartilage of the glenoid; 'peg holes' are made to conform to the back of the prosthesis. The glenoid prosthesis is cemented into place, with the component held in position manually until the cement hardens (~15 min). The humeral component is 'trialed' to determine the appropriate size, and the final humeral component is inserted with or without cement. The joint is reduced, and the subscapularis is repaired. Skin closure is followed by placement of a sling or shoulder immobilizer. Postop management includes early passive ROM, limiting active internal rotation, and passive external rotation until the subscapularis has healed. Additional limitations may be instituted in revision situations or if RC repair is performed. Some surgeons use epinephrine-soaked gauze in the canal prior to implanting the final prosthesis. Rarely, pressurization of the canal with cement is associated with hemodynamic changes.

Usual preop diagnosis: Rheumatoid arthritis; posttraumatic arthritis; AVN; RC arthropathy; 4-part proximal humerus fracture

SUMMARY OF PROCEDURE

Position	Semisitting, beach-chair
Incision	Deltopectoral incision (Fig 10.2-4) or extended incision for complex revision
Special instrumentation	Glenoid and humeral instrumentation, in addition to usual shoulder instruments; mixing and introduction of cement
Unique considerations	Systemic illnesses of the patient; systemic complications of use of cement in the patient; precautions in pregnant staff working with methylmethacrylate; usage of laminar flow or UV lighting for total joint precautions, depending on the surgeon's preference and capabilities of the OR.
Antibiotics	Cefazolin 1 g iv preop, and 48 h postop
Surgical time	2-5 h
Closing considerations	Drain; sling and swathe
EBL	200-1000 ml
Postop care	Immediate passive motion. No active internal rotation for 6 wk.
Mortality	< 1%
Morbidity	Blood loss
	Nerve injury: Rare
	↓BP 2° cement: Rare
	Infection
Pain score	8

PATIENT POPULATION CHARACTERISTICS

Age range[3]	45-80 yr
Male:Female	1:1
Incidence	Uncommon
Etiology	Osteoarthritis; inflammatory arthritis; trauma; avascular necrosis; systemic disease
Associated conditions	Inflammatory disease; systemic disease; alcoholism; RC pathology; arthritis and radiculopathy; cervical arthritis

ANESTHETIC CONSIDERATIONS

PREOPERATIVE

Typically, three patient populations present for shoulder arthroplasty: (1) healthy posttrauma, (2) nonrheumatoid arthritic, and (3) rheumatoid arthritic.

Respiratory	Rheumatoid arthritic patients may exhibit Sx of pleural effusion or pulmonary fibrosis. Hoarseness may indicate cricoarytenoid joint (CAJ) involvement → difficult intubation. (See Anesthetic Considerations for Wrist Procedures, p. 740.) **Tests:** Consider CXR; PFTs; ABGs in debilitated rheumatoid patients.
Cardiovascular	Rheumatoid arthritic patients may suffer from chronic pericardial effusions, valvular disease, and cardiac conduction defects. **Tests:** Consider ECG and ECHO in patients with severe rheumatoid arthritis.
Neurological	Arthritic patients may have cervical or lumbar radiculopathies that should be documented carefully preop. For example, head flexion may cause cervical cord compression.

Neurological, cont.	**Tests:** C-spine radiographs to r/o occult subluxations in rheumatoid patients with neck complaints or upper extremity radiculopathy
Musculoskeletal	Arthritic patients may have limited neck and jaw ROM that may require special intubation techniques. Bony deformities or muscle contracture may necessitate special attention to positioning.
Hematologic	Virtually all nontrauma patients will be on some type of anti-inflammatory medication that may result in anemia or Plt inhibition. Ideally, patients should D/C NSAIDs at least 5 d preop.
Endocrine	Rheumatoid patients are likely to be on oral corticosteroids and may require supplemental perioperative steroids (e.g., 100 mg hydrocortisone q 8 h iv) to treat adrenal suppression, although the routine use of 'stress-dose steroids' has been questioned.
Laboratory	Hb/Hct (healthy patients); other tests as indicated from H&P.
Premedication	Mild-to-moderate premedication (e.g., in adults, midazolam 1-2 mg iv, fentanyl 50-100 mg iv, titrated to effect) is often desirable before placement of a regional block.

INTRAOPERATIVE

Anesthetic technique: GETA or a combination of GETA and regional anesthesia can be used. An interscalene brachial plexus block in combination with GA is excellent for surgical procedures on the shoulder. Unless contraindicated, a long-acting local anesthetic should be used in regional anesthesia for shoulder surgery to ameliorate postop pain.

General anesthesia:

Induction	Standard induction (see p. B-2). Rheumatoid patients may require awake fiber optic intubation (see p. B-6).
Maintenance	Standard maintenance (see p. B-3). Because of the typically long duration of these cases, the opioid selected as part of the balanced anesthetic technique may be given by continuous infusion (e.g., iv sufentanil [0.25-1.0 μg/kg/h]). Some surgeons prefer muscle relaxation beyond that provided by volatile anesthetic.
Emergence	Management of emergence and extubation should be routine except in difficult airway cases that require awake extubation. Emergence from anesthesia should be delayed until patient's shoulder is securely immobilized in the sling and swathe to prevent undesired movement of the newly placed prosthesis.

Regional anesthesia:

Local anesthetics	Significant discomfort may be associated with this procedure; therefore, extended postop pain control is desirable. When a single-shot technique is used, 0.5% bupivacaine, levobupivacaine, or ropivacaine (each with epinephrine 1:400,000) can be used. Onset is usually within 30 min, with duration up to 18-20 h. Levobupivacaine or ropivacaine may be preferred for peripheral nerve block, due to their decreased cardiotoxicity. For continuous catheter techniques, a postop infusion of 8-12 ml/h of 0.2% of any of these agents is appropriate.
Interscalene block	Typical anesthetics and doses. Note that epinephrine [2.5-5 μg/ml] should be added to the local anesthetic whenever possible to decrease peak plasma concentrations: • 0.5% bupivacaine, levobupivacaine, or ropivacaine, 30 ml for the procedures The skin on the top of the shoulder (C3-C4) and the medial aspect of the upper arm (T2) often require separate subcutaneous field blocks. Phrenic nerve block → hemidiaphragmatic paralysis is an inevitable consequence of the interscalene block, which may not be tolerated by patients with significant preexisting respiratory compromise. A continuous interscalene catheter may be placed for postop pain management. Major complications, such as total spinal or pneumothorax resulting from interscalene block, are extremely rare. Interscalene block is contraindicated in patients with contralateral recurrent laryngeal nerve or phrenic nerve palsy. If sedation is needed, midazolam (0.5-1.0 mg boluses), or propofol (25-100 μg/kg/min by infusion), titrated to effect, are good choices.
Blood and fluid requirements	Moderate-to-significant blood loss IV: 16 ga × 1 NS/LR @ 1.5-3.0 ml/kg/h	RBC recovery and reinfusion techniques (e.g., Cell Saver) are advisable because blood loss can be considerable. IV in nonoperative upper extremity.
Monitoring	Standard monitors (see p. B-1).	Consider invasive, hemodynamic monitoring in the debilitated or elderly patient.

Monitoring, cont.	Precordial Doppler	Since VAE is a possible complication of the semisitting position, consider using precordial Doppler for cases done in this position.
Positioning	✓ and pad pressure points. ✓ eyes. ↑VAE risk	Postural ↓BP is the most common complication of the semisitting position. Changing patient to this position gradually can help prevent ↓BP, as can the use of antiembolism stockings and fluid-loading the patient.
Interscalene block complications	Total spinal Epidural anesthesia Local anesthetic toxicity (Sz/dysrhythmias) Stellate ganglion block (Horner's syndrome) Laryngeal nerve block Phrenic nerve block Pneumothorax Persistent paresthesia	Resuscitative equipment, including airway management tools, should be immediately available. May last ≤ 6 wk.
Other complications	Potential for embolic event ↓BP during prep and positioning	Because of the increased risk of VAE during shoulder arthroplasty, N_2O may be D/C'd during placement of humeral component. Use of methylmethacrylate cement has been associated with the sudden onset of ↓BP and even cardiac arrest, presumably due to profound vasodilation ± associated VAE. ↓BP during long surgical prep usually can be avoided by using light inhalation anesthesia (isoflurane 0.3-0.5%) to ensure amnesia, with moderate muscle relaxation to prevent bucking on ETT, and maintaining adequate hydration.

POSTOPERATIVE

| Pain management | PCA (see p. C-3) or regional block/catheter | Combined regional-general anesthetic techniques are excellent for shoulder procedures, especially for postop pain management. |
| Tests | None indicated routinely. | |

References

1. Andersen KH: Air aspirated from the venous system during total hip replacement. *Anaesthesia* 1983; 38(12):1175-8.
2. Borgeat A: Acute and nonacute complications associated with interscalene block and shoulder surgery. *Anesthesiology* 2001; 95(4):875-80.
3. Cofield RH: Degenerative and arthritic problems of the glenohumeral joint. In *The Shoulder*. Rockwood CA Jr, Matsen FA III, eds. WB Saunders, Philadelphia: 1990, 678-749.
4. Cushner MA, Friedman RJ: Osteonecrosis of the humeral head. *J Am Acad Orthop Surg* 1997; 5(6):339-46.
5. Gartsman GM, Roddey TS, Hammerman SM: Shoulder arthroplasty with or without resurfacing of the glenoid in patients who have osteoarthritis. *J Bone Joint Surg Am* 2000; 82(1):26-34.
6. Goldberg BA, Smith K, Jackins S, Campbell B, Matsen FA III: The magnitude and durability of functional improvement after total shoulder arthroplasty for degenerative joint disease. *J Shoulder Elbow Surg* 2001; 10(5):464-9.
7. Green A, Norris TR: Shoulder arthroplasty for advanced glenohumeral arthritis after anterior instability repair. *J Shoulder Elbow Surg* 2001; 10(6):539-45.
8. Keenan MA, Stiles CM, Kaufman RL: Acquired laryngeal deviation associated with cervical spine disease in erosive polyarticular arthritis. *Anesthesiology* 1983; 58(5):441-9.
9. Klein SM: Interscalene brachial plexus block with continuous catheter insertion system and a disposable infusion pump. *Anesth Analg* 2000; 91(6):1473-8.
10. Murphy DB: Upper extremity blocks for day surgery. *Tech in Reg Anes Pain Manag* 2000; 4(1):19-29.
11. Newens AF, Volz RG: Severe hypotension during prosthetic hip surgery with acrylic bone cement. *Anesthesiology* 1972; 36(3):298-300.
12. Reginster JY, Damas P, Franchimont P: Anaesthetic risks in osteoarticular disorders. *Clin Rheum* 1985; 4:30-8.
13. Salathe M, Johr M: Unsuspected cervical fractures: a common problem in ankylosing spondylitis. *Anesthesiology* 1989; 70(5):869-70.

14. Sanchez-Sotelo J, Cofield RH, Rowland CM: Shoulder hemiarthroplasty for glenohumeral arthritis associated with severe rotator cuff deficiency. *J Bone Joint Surg Am* 2001; 83-A(12):1814-22.
15. Shapiro J, Zuckerman JD: Glenohumeral arthroplasty: indications and preoperative considerations. *Instr Course Lect* 2002; 51:3-10.
16. White RH: Preoperative evaluation of patients with rheumatoid arthritis. *Semin Arthritis Rheum* 1985; 14(4):287-99.
17. Zuckerman JD, Scott AJ, Gallagher MA: Hemiarthroplasty for cuff tear arthropathy. *J Shoulder Elbow Surg* 2000; 9(3): 169-72.

SHOULDER GIRDLE PROCEDURES

SURGICAL CONSIDERATIONS

Description: Trauma about the shoulder girdle in young patients ranges from athletic injuries to life-threatening trauma. Some of these injuries include common athletic injuries, such as **acromioclavicular joint separations**, which rarely require surgery unless there are associated **acromial** or **clavicular fractures. Posterior sternoclavicular dislocations** may warrant surgical stabilization if the trachea is compressed. **Clavicle fractures**, frequently associated with **scapular fractures**, occasionally require open reduction.

Scapular fractures involving the glenoid also may require surgical stabilization. Extreme fractures involving the shoulder girdle (**scapulothoracic dissociations**) include scapular fracture, clavicle fracture, subclavian or axillary artery disruption, and brachial plexus injury. These may coexist with **proximal humerus fractures**, rib fractures, and pneumothorax. In the older, debilitated patient, the most common injury is proximal humeral fracture, which may be amenable to surgical stabilization, or may be so comminuted as to warrant hemi- or total arthroplasty.

For each of these fractures, the incision is made over the appropriate site, the fracture or dislocation is identified and reduced under manual or manipulative traction, and appropriate fixation proceeds. For instance, a displaced proximal humerus fracture in a young person may require fixation with a plate and screws through a deltopectoral approach (see Surgery for Shoulder Dislocations or Instability, p. 765, and Glenohumeral Shoulder Arthroplasty, p. 769). A scapular fracture in a scapulothoracic dissociation would be stabilized with a plate and screws via a posterior approach (see Surgery for Shoulder Dislocations or Instability, p. 765) after vascular repair of the subclavian artery and fixation of the clavicle, if necessary. Typically, a sling or sling-and-swathe-type immobilization is required. As with other shoulder procedures, relaxation is necessary upon awakening the patient.

Usual preop diagnosis: Trauma about the shoulder girdle

SUMMARY OF PROCEDURES

	Anterior	Posterior
Position	Semisitting or prone	Lateral decubitus (scapula)
Incision	Anterior, superior, or oblique for acromio-clavicular; supraclavicular for clavicle; delto-pectoral for proximal humerus and glenoid	Posterior lateral border or medial border of scapula, spinous scapula, depending on location
Special instrumentation	Plates and screws; tension band wiring; proximal humerus replacement for comminuted fractures	⇐
Unique considerations	Multiple trauma warrants early stabilization; may require vascular repair and brachial plexus exploration.	⇐
Antibiotics	Cefazolin 1 g iv	⇐
Surgical time	2-10 h	⇐
Closing considerations	Fracture-dependent; most commonly requires application of sling and swathe.	⇐
EBL	200-1200 ml or greater, depending on trauma	⇐

	Anterior	**Posterior**
Postop care	May require ICU for multiple-trauma patients; otherwise, early mobilization with physical therapy	⇐
Mortality	Mortality dependent on associated conditions: Infection Neurologic injury Respiratory failure Massive blood loss Unrecognized pneumothorax Cardiac tamponade	⇐
Morbidity	Nerve injury (axillary, brachial plexus) Stiffness Poor healing	Axillary and suprascapular ⇐ ⇐
Pain score	6-10	6 (clavicle and AC joint) 8 (scapula and proximal humerus)

PATIENT POPULATION CHARACTERISTICS

Age range	15-80 yr, depending on nature of trauma
Male:Female	5:1
Incidence	Common
Etiology	Trauma
Associated conditions	Axillary nerve palsy; musculocutaneous nerve palsy; brachial plexus injury; arterial disruption in high-energy trauma; brachial and great vessel injuries and posterior sternoclavicular dislocation pneumothorax

ANESTHETIC CONSIDERATIONS

See Anesthetic Considerations following Brachial Plexus Surgery, p. 776.

References

1. Butters KP: Fractures and dislocations of the scapula. In *Fractures in Adults*, Vol II, 4th edition. Rockwood CA Jr, Green DP, Bucholz RW, Heckman JD, eds. Lippincott-Raven, Philadelphia: 1996, 1163-92.
2. Craig EV: Fractures of the clavicle. In *Fractures in Adults*, Vol II, 4th edition. Rockwood CA Jr, Green DP, Bucholz RW, Heckman JD, eds. Lippincott-Raven, Philadelphia: 1996, 1109-62.
3. Collins DN, Harryman DT II: Arthroplasty for arthritis and rotator cuff deficiency. *Orthop Clin North Am* 1997; 20(2):225-39.
4. Imatani RJ: Fractures of the scapula: a review of 53 fractures. *J Trauma* 1975; 15(6):473-8.
5. Neviaser RJ: Injuries to the clavicle and acromioclavicular joint. *Orthop Clin North Am* 1987; 18(3):433-8.
6. Richards RR, Sherman RM, Hudson AR, Waddell JP: Shoulder arthrodesis using a pelvic-reconstruction plate. A report of eleven cases. *J Bone Joint Surg* [Am] 1988; 70(3):416-21.
7. Rockwood CA Jr, Matsen FA III, eds: *The Shoulder*. WB Saunders, Philadelphia, 1990.
8. Rockwood CA Jr, Williams GR, Young CD: Injuries to the acromioclavicular joint. In *Fractures in Adults*, Vol II, 4th edition. Rockwood CA Jr, Green DP, Bucholz RW, Heckman JD, eds. Lippincott-Raven, Philadelphia: 1996, 1341-1414.
9. Rockwood CA Jr, Wirth MA: Injuries to the sternoclavicular joint. In *Fractures in Adults*, Vol II, 4th edition. Rockwood CA Jr, Green DP, Bucholz RW, Heckman JD, eds. Lippincott-Raven, Philadelphia: 1996, 1415-78.

BRACHIAL PLEXUS SURGERY

SURGICAL CONSIDERATIONS

Description: Brachial plexus injuries occur most commonly in two groups: traumatic birth injuries and high-energy trauma. Surgery ranges from exploration with neurolysis, to repairs, to cable nerve grafting. Typically, the latter requires grafting with the sural nerve, and nerve pedicle transfer, such as transfer of the spinal accessory nerve to denervated paralyzed muscle, combined with muscle transfers. C5-C6 is most commonly injured in obstetrical (Erb's) palsy. Injuries in adults are more commonly closed-traction. Similar to obstetrical palsy, they occur with an outstretched, abducted arm with the neck rotated in the opposite direction. The most severe form includes complete avulsion at the preganglionic level, presenting with a Horner's syndrome, winging of the scapula, and a flail arm. These are typically 'supraclavicular' injuries, and have a poorer prognosis. Surgical exposure may proceed above the clavicle similar to an anterior neck dissection, or may require an extension below the clavicle. Occasionally, an osteotomy of the clavicle for extensive dissection is required. For axillary nerve dissection, a posterior approach also is used. Open injuries, such as gunshot or knife wounds, are typically 'infraclavicular' and have a better prognosis. (See diagram of brachial plexus, Fig 10.2-5.)

Usual preop diagnosis: Obstetrical palsy; adult trauma – most commonly motorcycle accident

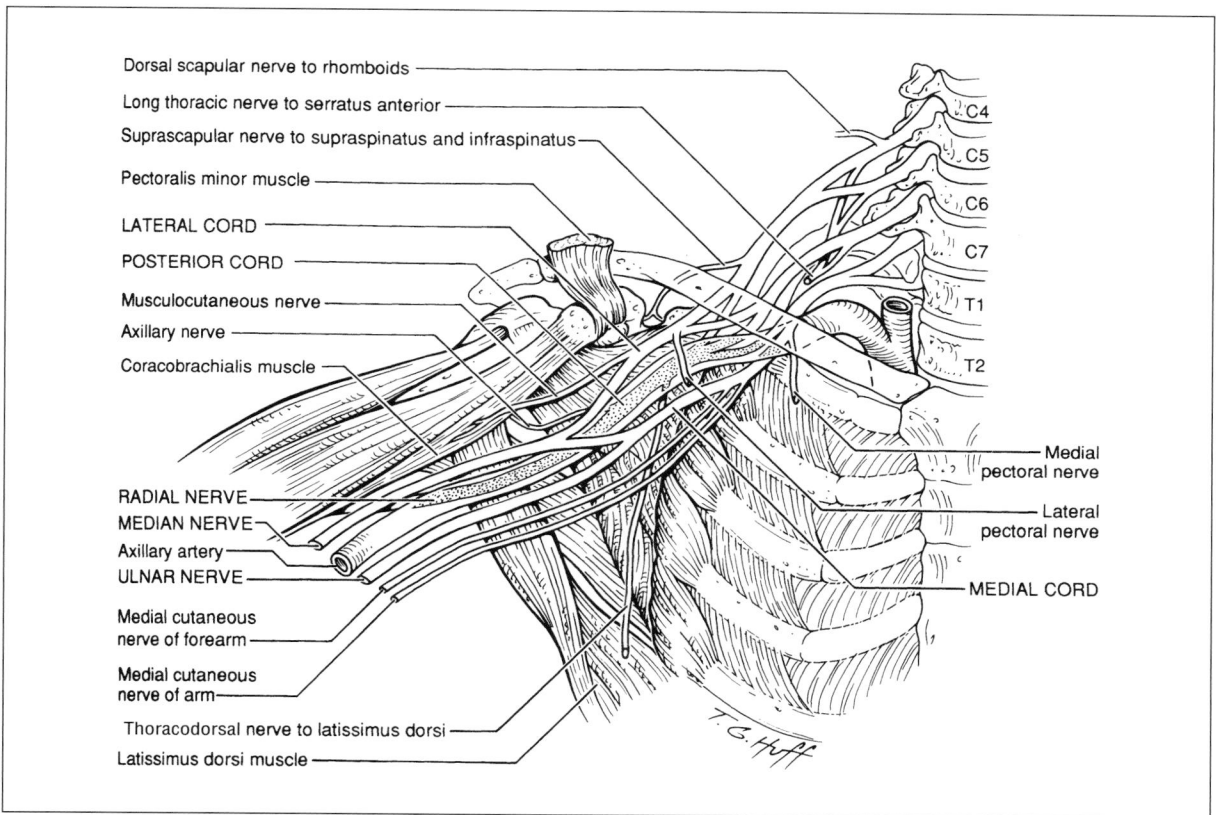

Figure 10.2-5. Brachial plexus: Its division into supraclavicular and infraclavicular portions is apparent. The proximal origin of the dorsal scapular nerve and the long thoracic nerve are demonstrated. The T1 spinal nerve arises below the head of the 1st rib. The relation of the cords of the plexus to the axillary artery at the level of the coracoid process (origin of the pectoralis minor and coracobrachialis muscles) is illustrated. The posterior cord and the radial nerve behind the axillary artery are stippled for clarity. (Reproduced with permission from Tindall GT, Cooper PR, Barrow DL: *The Practice of Neurosurgery*, Vol III. Williams & Wilkins, Baltimore, 1996.)

SUMMARY OF PROCEDURE

Position	Lateral decubitus or semisitting
Incision	Supra- or infraclavicular, extensile to include deltopectoral incision. Clavicle osteotomy incision will provide for improved exposure. Supraclavicular incision used for supraclavicular brachial plexus.

Special instrumentation	Nerve stimulator
Unique considerations	Associated trauma
Antibiotics	Cefazolin 1 g iv preop
Surgical time	4-10 h
Closing considerations	Other incisions if nerve grafts obtained.
EBL	400-2000 ml
Mortality	Minimal
Morbidity	Bleeding
	Hematoma
	Pneumothorax
	Clavicular nonunion
Pain score	8

PATIENT POPULATION CHARACTERISTICS

Age range	Infants and children: 3 mo-8 yr; adults: 20-40 yr
Male:Female	Adult: 5:1
Incidence	Infants: 0.3-8/1000 births; adults: commonly associated with motorcycle accidents
Etiology	Obstetrical palsy; trauma
Associated conditions	None known

ANESTHETIC CONSIDERATIONS

(Procedures covered: shoulder girdle procedures; brachial plexus surgery)

PREOPERATIVE

With the exception of traumatic birth injuries, most of these patients are healthy males who have suffered major blunt or penetrating trauma. For the acute and subacute trauma victim, the major anesthesia-related concerns center around associated traumatic injuries. Many adult trauma victims with brachial plexus injuries will be operated on in the first few days after their injury. For infants (usually operated on at 6-12 mo), the major anesthesia-related concerns are those routinely associated with pediatric anesthesia (See Pediatric Orthopedic Surgery, p. 1091.). Approximately half of all trauma victims are intoxicated. The anesthesia-related implications of ethanol intoxication include: decreased anesthetic requirements, diuresis, vasodilation, and hypothermia.

Respiratory	As suggested by coexisting disease or acute trauma injuries. Look for evidence of occult chest injury, including pneumothorax (tachypnea, wheezing, ↓BP, ↓PaO_2, CXR changes) and pulmonary contusion (multiple rib fracture, ↓PaO_2).
	Tests: Consider CXR and ABGs in victims of significant trauma; other tests as indicated from H&P.
Cardiovascular	As suggested by coexisting disease or acute trauma injuries. Look for evidence of occult cardiac or mediastinal injuries, such as myocardial contusion (e.g., ECG abnormalities typically consistent with ischemia) or great vessel rupture (e.g., widened mediastinum).
	Tests: Consider CXR (with NG tube in place to access mediastinal widening) and ECG in victims of significant trauma; others as indicated from H&P.
Neurological	Victims of shoulder trauma are vulnerable to brachial plexus damage. Look for evidence of upper extremity nerve dysfunction and document any injuries preop. The possibility of closed-head injury also should be considered.
	Tests: Head CT prior to beginning a procedure under GA in a patient with evidence of head trauma.
Musculoskeletal	As suggested by coexisting disease or acute trauma injuries. The amount of force necessary to produce a brachial plexus injury mandates a C-spine series to r/o C-spine fracture in all victims of brachial plexus trauma.
Laboratory	In general, most victims of significant trauma are best served by obtaining a wide variety of baseline lab studies to screen for unrecognized injury. These studies generally should include: Hct; CBC; ABGs; UA; renal function tests; LFTs; serum amylase.
Premedication	None

INTRAOPERATIVE

Anesthetic technique: GETA is preferred over regional techniques because of the unpredictable and prolonged length of these procedures and the need to evaluate brachial plexus function postop.

Induction	Rapid-sequence induction (see p. B-5) is mandatory in unscheduled cases, unless awake fiber optic intubation is performed (see Anesthetic Considerations for Thoracolumbar Neurosurgical Procedures, p. 97). C-spine fracture patients or those with facial injuries may require awake fiber optic intubation (see p. B-6) or other special airway techniques, as indicated from H&P. Hemodynamically unstable, acute-trauma patients can be induced more safely with etomidate (0.3-0.4 mg/kg iv) or ketamine (1-3 mg/kg iv).	
Maintenance	Balanced anesthesia with low-dose isoflurane (0.4-0.6%), iv sufentanil (0.25-1.0 μg/kg/h), and N_2O in O_2 is suitable for stable patients. Hemodynamically unstable, acute-trauma victims undergoing emergency surgery are not likely to tolerate this regimen and are better served by using a combination of medications designed to have minimal hemodynamic consequences (e.g., fentanyl for analgesia, vecuronium for muscle relaxation, and scopolamine or midazolam for amnesia). N_2O is best avoided in the trauma patient. For brachial plexus surgery, some surgeons prefer minimal muscle relaxation after tracheal intubation so that a nerve stimulator can be used to help identify surgical anatomy.	
Emergence	Management of emergence and extubation should be routine except in difficult airway or full-stomach cases, which require that extubation be delayed until the patient's airway reflexes have returned and the patient is fully awake.	
Blood and fluid requirements	Significant blood loss IV: 14-16 ga × 1-2 NS/LR @ 1.5-3 ml/kg/h + replacement of blood loss @ 3 × volume Fluid warmer Airway humidifier	IV catheter placed in the nonoperative upper extremity is usually adequate in hemodynamically stable patients. Unstable, acute-trauma victims require a minimum of 2 large-bore iv catheters or large-bore central lines.
Monitoring	Standard monitors (see p. B-1). ± SSEP ± TEE	Invasive hemodynamic monitoring and TEE should be considered in acute, multiple-trauma victims. Some surgeons request SSEP to make continuous assessment of preop intact brachial plexus possible. When using SSEP monitoring, high doses of volatile anesthetic agents should be avoided because they adversely affect SSEP readings.
Positioning	✓ and pad pressure points. ✓ eyes. VAE risk	Postural ↓BP is the most common complication of the semisitting position, particularly during the surgical prep period. SCD or antiembolism stockings may be beneficial. VAE is a potential complication of this position.
Complications	Hemodynamic instability Possible VAE	Previously unrecognized injuries (e.g., pneumothorax, cardiac tamponade, intracranial bleeding) should be considered as a cause of unexplained intraop hemodynamic instability in all acute-trauma victims. VAE risk is increased with patient in semisitting position.

POSTOPERATIVE

Complications	Sepsis ARDS	Many trauma victims survive the initial insult only to die later of sepsis or ARDS.
Pain management	PCA (see p. C-3).	
Tests	Based on concurrent injuries.	

References

1. Grundy BL: Intraoperative monitoring of sensory-evoked potentials. *Anesthesiology* 1983; 58(1):72-87.
2. Johnstone RE: Acute trauma with multiple injuries. *Curr Opin Anesthesiol* 2000; 13(2):175-9.
3. Leifert RD: Neurological problems. In *The Shoulder*. Rockwood CA Jr, Matsen FA III, eds. WB Saunders, Philadelphia: 1990, 750-8.

4. Nanakas AO: Injuries to the brachial plexus. In *The Pediatric Upper Extremity: Diagnosis and Treatment.* Bora FW Jr, ed. WB Saunders, Philadelphia: 1986, 247-58.
5. Thompson RW, Petrinec D, Toursarkissian B: I. Surgical treatment of thoracic outlet compression syndromes. II. Supraclavicular exploration and vascular reconstruction. *Ann Vasc Surg* 1997; 11(4):442-51.

ARM SURGERY

SURGICAL CONSIDERATIONS

Description: Surgical procedures on the arm are primarily for trauma or tumor surgery. Other procedures include extended approaches from the shoulder for significant trauma or tendon transfer. Exploration of peripheral nerves, most commonly of the radial nerve, are also included in this category, as are distal extensile approaches from the elbow for trauma or for lateral epicondylitis ('tennis elbow'). Depending on the lesion or fracture, the incision is developed through an internervous or intramuscular compartment. Procedures include **excisional biopsy** for soft tissue or bone tumors of the arm; **tumor excision**, which may be marginal, wide, or radical, depending on the tumor encountered; **tendon transfers**, such as pectoralis transfer to replace biceps function, used primarily for brachial plexus injuries; and **fractures and nonunion fractures of the humerus**. Positioning and location of incision is dependent on the level of the pathology. For example, for fractures involving the proximal half of the humerus, the standard **deltopectoral incision** may be extended distally along the interval between the biceps and triceps on the lateral aspect of the arm. This approach requires a beach-chair or, occasionally, supine position. Distal-third fractures are best approached posteriorly with the **triceps-splitting approach**. Distal fractures that extend into the elbow joint often require an olecranon osteotomy to visualize the fractured joint surface. Posterior approaches to the distal humerus are performed in either the lateral or prone position. Distal (intercondylar) humerus fractures are among the most difficult fractures to treat, with operative time ranging from 2-6 h, depending on the degree of comminution.

Usual preop diagnosis: Trauma; tumor

SUMMARY OF PROCEDURE

Position	Supine; semisitting position for extended deltopectoral; lateral decubitus or prone for distal humerus fractures
Incision	Anterolateral approach; posterior approach in the lateral decubitus or prone position
Special instrumentation	Plate and screws; external fixators; intramedullary rods; occasionally, methylmethacrylate cement for tumor surgery; sterile tourniquet for distal humerus; I.I. for fracture surgery
Unique considerations	CT-guided sclerotherapy preop for vascular tumors; longitudinal incisions for biopsy and tumor excisions (not violating fascial planes)
Antibiotics	Cefazolin 1 g iv preop
Surgical time	45 min-6 h
Closing considerations	Drain frequently required.
EBL	Minimal—500+ ml, depending on pathology
Mortality	Varies with pathology
Morbidity	Bleeding
	Shoulder stiffness
	Nerve injury
Pain score	4-9

PATIENT POPULATION CHARACTERISTICS

Age range	Varies with procedure
Male:Female	Varies with procedure
Incidence	Procedure-dependent
Etiology	Fractures; nerve entrapment (radial) following trauma; tumors
Associated conditions	Radial or ulnar nerve injury with humeral fractures

ANESTHETIC CONSIDERATIONS

PREOPERATIVE

With the exception of tumor patients, the majority of patients presenting for arm procedures are relatively young and healthy. Most of these patients present for elective repair of a traumatic injury; thus, the preop workup is routine. Some arm procedures, such as repair of a compound fracture, require immediate attention and necessitate emergency surgery and full-stomach considerations (p. B-5).

Laboratory   Hb/Hct (healthy patients); other tests as indicated from H&P.

Premedication Mild-to-moderate premedication (e.g., in adults, midazolam 1-2 mg iv, fentanyl 50-100 μg iv, titrated to effect) is often desirable before placement of a regional block.

INTRAOPERATIVE

Anesthetic technique: GETA or regional anesthesia, or a combination of the two, can be used for surgical procedures on the arm. A brachial plexus block via the supraclavicular or infraclavicular approaches are excellent for procedures on the distal arm. The interscalene approach to the brachial plexus is perhaps best for more proximal procedures near the shoulder. Regional anesthesia alone is a means of avoiding the risk of aspiration pneumonitis associated with GA in the patient with a full stomach.

General anesthesia:

Induction   Standard induction (see p. B-2) except in acute-trauma patients, where rapid-sequence induction is appropriate (see p. B-5).

Maintenance Standard maintenance (see p. B-3).

Emergence   Management of emergence and extubation should be routine, except in difficult airway cases, which require awake extubation. Skin closure is frequently followed by application of a splint; patient should remain anesthetized during splinting procedure.

Regional anesthesia:

Local anesthetics 2% lidocaine or 1.5% mepivacaine ± alkalization have similar onset times (10 min vs 15 min), with mepivacaine providing significantly longer postop pain control (8-10 h vs 4-6 h). If extended postop pain control is desired, 0.5% bupivacaine, levobupivacaine, or ropivacaine (each with epinephrine 1:400,000) can be used. Onset is usually within 30 min, with duration up to 18-20 h. Levobupivacaine or ropivacaine may be preferred for peripheral nerve block due to their decreased cardiotoxicity.

Interscalene block Typical anesthetics and doses. Note that the addition of epinephrine (2.5-5 μg/ml) will reduce peak plasma anesthetic concentrations:
• 2% lidocaine or 1.5% mepivacaine 30 ml for procedures lasting ≤ 2.5 h.
• 0.5% bupivacaine, levobupivacaine, or ropivacaine 30 ml for procedures lasting > 2.5 h.
Skin on the top of the shoulder (C3-C4) and the medial aspect of the upper arm (T2) often require separate subcutaneous field blocks. Phrenic nerve block → hemidiaphragmatic paralysis is an inevitable consequence of the interscalene block, which may not be tolerated by patients with significant preexisting respiratory compromise. Major complications (e.g., total spinal or pneumothorax) resulting from interscalene block, are very rare; therefore, this technique is suitable for outpatients. Interscalene block is contraindicated in patients with contralateral recurrent laryngeal nerve or phrenic nerve palsy. If sedation is needed, midazolam (0.5-1.0 mg boluses), alfentanil (0.125-0.25 μg/kg/min by infusion), or propofol (25-100 μg/kg/min by infusion), titrated to effect, are good choices.

Infraclavicular block Excellent for surgical procedures distal to the mid humerus. Fewer associated complications, compared with a supraclavicular block, and well tolerated by patients. 1.5% mepivacaine or 2% lidocaine 30-40 ml for routine cases; 0.5% bupivacaine, levobupivacaine, or ropivacaine 30-40 ml for procedures estimated to last > 2.5 h.

Supraclavicular block 1.5% mepivacaine or 2% lidocaine 30-40 ml for routine cases. 0.5% bupivacaine, levobupivacaine, ropivacaine 30-40 ml for procedures estimated to last > 2.5 h. The upper arm medial aspect is innervated by the intercostobrachial nerve (T2) and requires a separate subcutaneous field block in the axilla, especially with tourniquet use.

Supplemental sedation	Supplemental sedation may be accomplished with propofol by continuous infusion (50-150 μg/kg/min or intermittent bolus injection of opioid/benzodiazepine, titrated to effect.	
Blood and fluid requirements	Minimal blood loss IV: 18 ga × 1 NS/LR @ 1.5-3 ml/kg/hr	IV catheter should be placed in the contralateral upper extremity.
Monitoring	Standard monitors (see p. B-1).	
Positioning	✓ and pad pressure points. ✓ eyes.	
Complications: **Interscalene block**	Total spinal Epidural anesthesia Local anesthetic toxicity (Sz/dysrhythmias) Stellate ganglion block (Horner's syndrome) Laryngeal nerve block Phrenic nerve block Persistent paresthesia Pneumothorax	Resuscitative equipment, including airway management tools, should be immediately available. May last up to 6 wk.
Infraclavicular block	Inadequate block Intravascular injection Local anesthetic toxicity Persistent paresthesia Pneumothorax	↓risk of pneumothorax compared with supraclavicular approach
Supraclavicular block	Inadequate block Intravascular injection Hematoma Pneumothorax Horner's syndrome Phrenic nerve paralysis Local anesthetic toxicity Persistent paresthesia Recurrent laryngeal nerve paralysis	If accidental intraarterial injection occurs, minimal doses of local anesthetic can cause CNS toxicity. Pneumothorax is an important concern when the supraclavicular approach is used. A large pneumothorax may become symptomatic quickly; most take many hours to develop and may be without Sx. The possibility of pneumothorax associated with the supraclavicular block makes this approach less suitable for use with outpatient procedures. May last up to 6 wk.

POSTOPERATIVE

Pain management	PCA (see p. C-3). ± Regional block	Regional or combined regional-general anesthesia is excellent for arm procedures, especially with respect to postop pain management.
Tests	None routinely indicated.	

References

1. Gerancher JC: Upper extremity nerve blocks. *Anes Clin N Am* 2000; 18(2):1-16.
2. Henry AK: *Extensile Exposure*, 2nd edition, Churchill Livingstone, Edinburgh: 1973.
3. Hoppenfeld S, deBoer, eds: *Surgical Exposures in Orthopaedics: The Anatomic Approach*, 2nd edition. Lippincott Williams & Wilkins, Philadelphia: 1994, 51-146.
4. Moorthy SS, Schmidt SI, Dierdorf SF, Rosenfeld SH, Anagnostou JM: A supraclavicular lateral paravascular approach for brachial plexus regional anesthesia [see comments]. *Anesth Analg* 1991; 72(2):241-4.
5. Moran MC: Modified lateral approach to the distal humerus for internal fixation. *Clin Orthop* 1997; 340:190-7.
6. Safran O, Mosheiff R, Segal D, Liebergall M: Surgical treatment of intercondylar fractures of the humerus in adults. *Am J Orthop* 1999; 28(11):659-62.
7. Salazar CH: Infraclavicular brachial plexus block. *Reg Anesth Pain Med* 1999; 24(5):411-16.
8. Wilson JL: Infraclavicular brachial plexus block: parasagittal anatomy important to the coracoid technique. *Anesth Analg* 1998; 87(4):870-3.

Surgeon

Eugene J. Carragee, MD

10.3   SPINE SURGERY

Anesthesioloists

C. Philip Larson, Jr., MD, CM
Stanley I. Samuels, MB, BCh, FFARCS
Richard A. Jaffe, MD, PhD

MINIMALLY INVASIVE POSTERIOR LUMBAR DISCECTOMY (MICRODISCECTOMY)

SURGICAL CONSIDERATIONS

Description: Since the mid-1990s, a number of techniques have been developed to allow the decompression of lumbar roots (removal of disc material) with as little trauma to the nerves and surrounding tissues as possible. In most instances, little or no bone is removed and, therefore, this is not technically a laminectomy or laminotomy. These minimally invasive procedures typically are carried out in healthy young or middle-aged adults with sciatica and are not done for more involved pathology such as deformity, tumor, or infection. **Transpedicular fixation** and **short-segment fusions** may be attempted using modifications of these techniques.

Microdiscectomy approach: This can be done under GA, regional (epidural or spinal), or local anesthesia. The patient is placed in a prone or kneeling position and the posterior landmarks are palpated to identify the approximate level (e.g., L4/5); then the overlying skin is infiltrated with local anesthetic. A spinal needle is placed to the level of the lamina and an x-ray or fluoroscopic image is taken to confirm the level. A 1" incision is made over the proposed interspace and, using either traditional or specialized retractors, the soft tissue is displaced to expose the ligamentum flavum. With the use of an operating microscope, the ligamentum flavum is removed, the nerve retracted, and the extruded disc excised. For a single level, this should take between 30-90 min, depending on the size of the patient and whether there is any scarring or adhesions from previous surgery.

Variant approach: Percutaneous discectomy through a posterolateral approach is usually reserved for 'contained discs'—protrusions into, but not through, the outer annulus of the disc. These are usually done under MAC with local anesthetic. The percutaneous instruments may be positioned using fluoroscopic guidance with or without a fiber optic light source and camera/monitor setup. The disc space is entered posterolaterally. The surgeon usually avoids anesthetizing the area around the nerve root so that the patient can alert the team if the root is struck by an instrument (quite painful). Once the disc space is entered, fluoroscopic or camera images are used to guide the surgeon in the removal of herniated disc. The disc material can be removed with specialized grabbers or automatic power-driven shavers.

Usual preop diagnosis: Chronic back pain 2° herniated lumbar disc; lumbar radiculopathy

SUMMARY OF PROCEDURES

	Microdiscectomy	Percutaneous Discectomy
Position	Prone or kneeling, with bolster or frame support. The abdomen must hang free to decompress the epidural veins.	Prone or lateral decubitus
Incision	Posterior midline or slightly off midline, at the appropriate vertebral level	About 8-12 cm lateral to the midline at the appropriate vertebral level
Special instrumentation	Microscope; light source; specialized retraction and dissection instruments for working in a small, deep incision	Percutaneous instruments, including trocars, sounds, and arthroscopic-type grabbers and shavers; fluoroscopy; and, sometimes, camera/monitor and fiber optic light setup
Unique considerations	Often outpatient procedure. Need to make room for microscope at head of bed.	Patient must be alert enough to respond to pain if nerve roots are encountered.
Antibiotics	Cefazolin 1 g iv	⇐
Surgical time	0.5-1.5 h	1-2 h
Closing considerations	Minimal suturing	Usually no closure (Bandaids)
EBL	25-100 ml	Minimal
Postop care	PACU. Mobilization as soon as tolerated. Usually discharged within 24 h.	PACU → home. Mobilization as tolerated.
Mortality	Very rare	⇐
Morbidity	Nerve injury	Failure to decompress the nerve adequately
	Dural laceration	–
	Infection	⇐
Pain score	4	2

PATIENT POPULATION CHARACTERISTICS

Age range	16-60 yr
Male:Female	3:2
Incidence	Common
Etiology	Degenerative; trauma (rare)

ANESTHETIC CONSIDERATIONS

PREOPERATIVE

Young and middle-aged adults are usually healthy; the elderly may have cardiovascular and/or pulmonary disease.

Musculoskeletal Since these patients may have chronic back pain with radiculopathy, they may not be suitable candidates for regional anesthetic techniques. Postop exacerbation of symptoms may be incorrectly ascribed to the anesthetic technique. A careful motor and sensory evaluation of the lower extremities should be documented. Patients commonly taking centrally acting analgesics (e.g., Ultram); narcotics (e.g., Darvon, Darvocet, OxyContin, Percocet, Vicodin); NSAIDs (e.g., Feldene, Naprosyn, Relafen, Voltaren); or COX-2 inhibitors (e.g., Bextra, Celebrex, Vioxx) often require higher doses of sedative-hypnotics and analgesics in the periop period.

Hematologic Patients should stop taking aspirin or NSAIDs at least 2 wk before surgery. In addition, an INR or PT and PTT should be checked preop.
Tests: Hct; Plt; INR

Laboratory Other tests as indicated from H&P.

Premedication Standard premedication (see p. B-2).

INTRAOPERATIVE

Anesthetic technique: Microdiscectomies are commonly done under GA; however, local or regional anesthetic techniques are suitable in selected patients. Care must be taken to avoid encroaching on the surgical site. Percutaneous discectomies typically require only MAC with sedation. These patients must be awake in order to alert the surgeon to inadvertent nerve root contact. In some centers, regional anesthesia (spinal or epidural) is the anesthetic of choice.

General Anesthesia:

Induction Standard induction (see p. B-2). Consider using wire-reinforced ETT to prevent kinking, with patient in prone position.

Maintenance Standard maintenance (see p. B-3). Usually 1-2 h operation. Once exposure obtained, further relaxant use is unnecessary.

Emergence No special considerations

MAC See p. B-4.

Regional anesthesia:

Spinal Patient in sitting, lateral decubitus, or prone position for placement of subarachnoid block. Doses of local anesthetics should be adequate to provide a high lumbar level of sensory anesthesia (e.g., bupivacaine 6-10 mg with fentanyl 10 μg).

Epidural Patient in sitting or lateral decubitus position for placement of epidural catheter. A test dose (e.g., 3 ml of 1.5% lidocaine with 1:200,000 epinephrine [5 μg/ml]) is administered and the patient is observed for development of subarachnoid block or Sx of an intravascular injection. Titrate 2% lidocaine with epinephrine (3-5 ml at a time) until desired surgical level is obtained.

Blood and fluid requirements IV: 18-20 ga × 1   Blood not likely to be required.
NS/LR @ 5 ml/kg/h

Monitoring Standard monitors (see p. B-1).

| Positioning | ✓ and pad pressure points.
✓ eyes. | Prone position: Wilson frame or bolsters to support shoulders/hips and optimize ventilation.
Knee-chest position: Andrews table
Place head in cushioned holder with cutout for eyes, nose, chin (e.g., Andrews Gentle-Rest pillow). Make certain nose and chin do not touch table. Pad elbows, knees, other pressure points. |

POSTOPERATIVE

Complications	Urinary retention in the older patient Transient numbness/paresthesias, weakness	Rx: Consider catheterization. Due to nerve-root irritation from operation. Rx with analgesics and/or muscle relaxants (e.g., Flexeril, Robaxin, Soma).
Pain management	PCA (p. C-3) Ketorolac 30 mg iv Epidural analgesia (p. C-2)	PO analgesics may be suitable: acetaminophen and codeine (Tylenol #3 1-2 tab q 4-6 h) or oxycodone and acetaminophen (Percocet 1 tab q 6 h)
Tests	As indicated by patient status	Patient usually discharged from hospital within 24-48 h.

References

1. Bookwalter J III, Busch M, Nicely D: Ambulatory surgery is safe and effective in radicular disc disease. *Spine* 1994; 19: 526-30.
2. Carragee E, Helms E, O'Sullivan G: Are post-operative activity restrictions necessary after posterior lumbar discectomy? A prospective study of outcomes in 50 consecutive cases. *Spine* 1996; 21:1893-7.
3. Javedan S, Sonntag VK: Lumbar disc herniation: microsurgical approach. *Neurosurgery* 2003; 52(1):160-4.
4. Maroon JC: Current concepts in minimally invasive discectomy. *Neurosurgery* 2002; 51(5Suppl):137-45.
5. Rodriguez HE, Connolly MM, Dracopoulos H, Geisler FH, Podbielski FJ: Anterior access to the lumbar spine: laparoscopic versus open. *Am Surg* 2002; 68(11):978-83.
6. Schick U, Dohnert J: Technique of microendoscopy in medial lumbar disc herniation. *Minim Invasive Neurosurg* 2002; 45(3):139-41.
7. Spengler DM: Lumbar disc herniation. In *Chapman's Orthopaedic Surgery*, 3rd edition. Chapman MW, ed. Lippincott Williams & Wilkins, Philadelphia: 2001, 3765-74.
8. Zahrawi F: Microlumbar discectomy: Is it safe as an outpatient procedure? *Spine* 1994; 19:1070-3.

ANTERIOR SPINAL RECONSTRUCTION AND FUSION— THORACIC AND THORACOLUMBAR SPINE

SURGICAL CONSIDERATIONS

Description: Traditionally, most spinal procedures have been approached posteriorly. The advent of surgical treatment for vertebral TB and postpolio spinal deformities during the 1960s saw the development of surgical approaches to the anterior spine. These procedures initially were reserved for patients with significant deformities, especially kyphosis. More recently, the treatment of traumatic, neoplastic, and degenerative conditions have been included in the anterior approach. Regardless of the condition under treatment, the approach is similar for a given level. There are several more or less distinct types of surgical exposures, depending on the level.

Cervicothoracic approach: Most cephalad and difficult is the approach to the upper thoracic spine (T1-T3). This generally includes a modified anterior cervical exposure with a caudal extension, including a resection of the clavicle, part of the manubrium, and sometimes the rib at the thoracic outlet. Dangers in this exposure are to the great vessels at the thoracic outlet, trachea (rare) and esophagus (more common), lung parenchyma, sympathetic ganglia, lymphatic duct (on the left), and brachial plexus. Once the spine is exposed and the discs and/or vertebrae are removed, the spinal cord is at risk. This procedure occasionally involves entering the thoracic cavity, in which case it is usually done intrapleurally—that is, through the parietal pleura. The lung needs to be collapsed at least partially. Spinal cord monitoring is usually performed; wake-up tests are not. Manipulation of the carotid artery and aortic arch may cause wide HR and BP fluctuations.

Transthoracic approach:
Further down the spine, the levels from T5-T10 are more easily reached via a transthoracic approach (Fig 10.3-1). This involves a typical thoracotomy with the resection

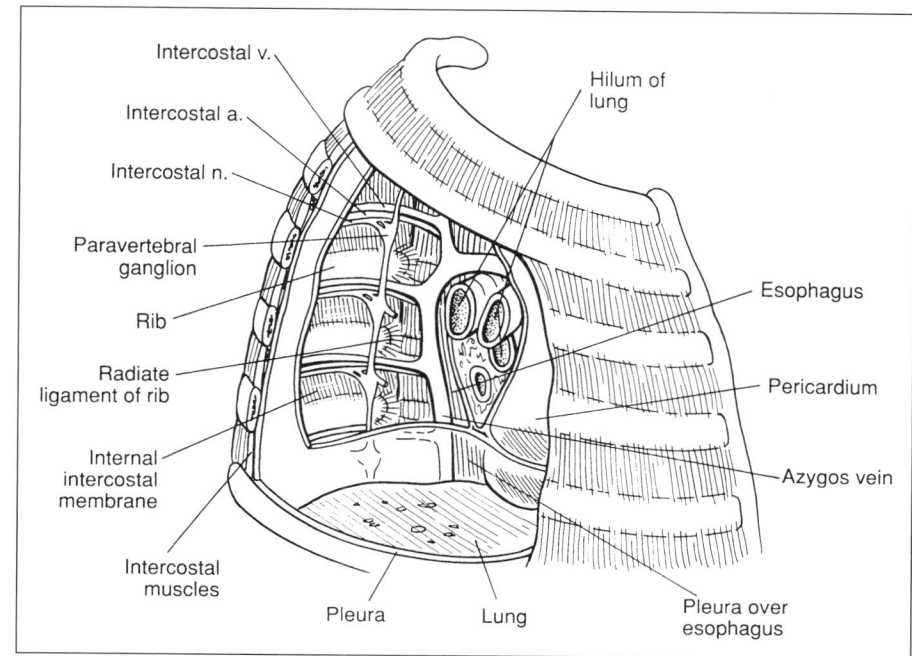

Figure 10.3-1. Surgical anatomy of the transthoracic approach. (Reproduced with permission from Hoppenfeld S, deBoer P: *Surgical Exposures in Orthopaedics*. JB Lippincott: 1984.)

of a rib. The level of the rib resection is usually 1-2 levels above the highest vertebral level being approached. The great vessels and lung parenchyma are at risk, as is the thoracic duct (on the left). The patient is in the lateral decubitus position and the mediastinum and heart usually fall to the opposite side, out of harm's way. Risk to the spinal cord depends on the difficulty and extent of the vertebral disease and the reconstruction. Spinal cord monitoring usually is performed intraop. The need for the lung to be deflated varies with the extent of the exposure. In centers where this procedure is frequently performed and the surgeons are accustomed to the respiratory motion during operation, DLTs are not routinely used. Since there is no (intended) violation of the lung parenchyma, air leaks and parenchymal repairs are not common.

Transdiaphragmatic approach: When the exposure must transverse the diaphragm, a combined retroperitoneal and transthoracic approach is used. This requires the diaphragm to be sectioned circumferentially from the chest wall and spine. If only the very low segments of the thoracic spine (T10-T12) are exposed, the required deflation of the involved lung is minimal. The risks are the same as those encountered with the transthoracic or retroperitoneal approaches alone. Regardless of the level of exposure, the operating table may be used during the procedure to manipulate the spine for better exposure and to 'lock in' implants, bone grafts, etc. Usually, the area of the spine to be exposed is centered above the 'breaking' joint and kidney rests of the table (Fig 10.3-2). After the initial exposure, the table is angled in the center with the head and legs pointing down and kidney rests elevated to 'open up' the section of spine facing the surgeon. After

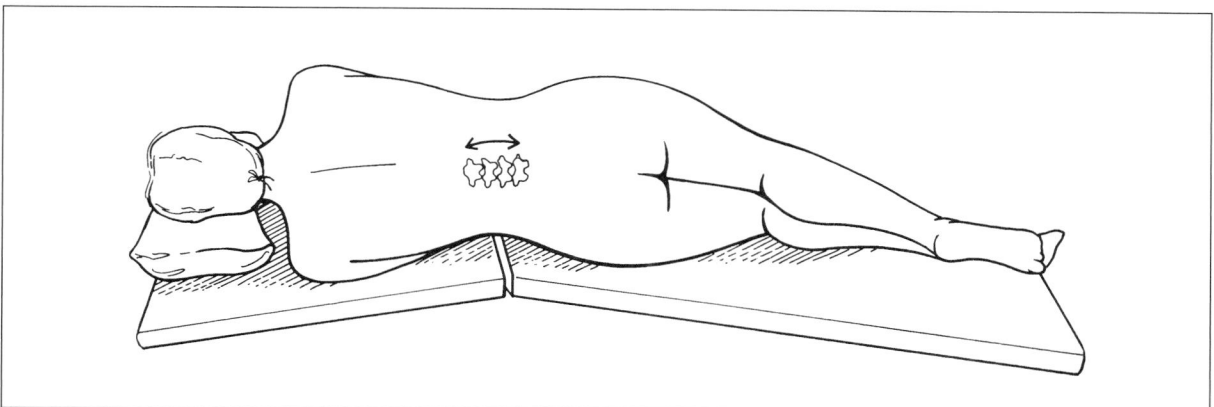

Figure 10.3-2. Patient position for transdiaphragmatic or retroperitoneal approach. (Reproduced with permission from Hoppenfeld S, deBoer P: *Surgical Exposures in Orthopaedics*. JB Lippincott, Philadelphia, 1984.)

removal of the disk, abscess, or tumor, a reconstruction—using bone graft, metal implants, bone cement, or a combination of these—is performed. The operating table is straightened and, with the spine in neutral alignment, the stability of the reconstruction is tested. This maneuver may need to be repeated several times.

The **morbidity** of these procedures depends primarily on the nature of the underlying disease. Obviously, bleeding and visceral injury are more likely when debriding a grapefruit-sized Potts abscess with several destroyed vertebrae than in removing a degenerated lumbar disk for fusion.

In some instances, the anterior procedure may be followed with a posterior fusion, either immediately or after 5-7 d of convalescence. If done immediately after, the patient needs to be repositioned prone, and the second procedure done through a midline exposure. Sometimes anterior and posterior surgery are performed simultaneously by two surgical teams. The most common reason for a staged anterior/posterior procedure (in the U.S.) is scoliosis; however, fractures at the thoracolumbar junction, after anterior decompression and reconstruction, are often instrumented and fused posteriorly.

Usual preop diagnosis: Fractures (usually at thoracic lumbar junction); idiopathic scoliosis; primary neoplasm or metastatic disease to the spine; pyogenic or TB osteomyelitis of the spine; Scheuermann's kyphosis

SUMMARY OF PROCEDURES

	Cervicothoracic Approach	Transthoracic Approach	Transdiaphragmatic Approach
Position	Supine; towel roll placed between shoulder blades, head slightly extended and turned away from operated side	Lateral decubitus (Fig 10.3-2); intended segments over the table break and kidney rests; axillary roll	⇐
Incision	Inverted 'L' longitudinally along manubrium to sternal notch, then transversely above clavicle	Along a rib, 2 levels above the highest segment to be exposed	⇐
Special instrumentation	Instrumentation rarely used. Strut grafts—using rib, fibula, clavicle or cement—may be used to replace excised vertebrae. ± DLT	For thoracolumbar scoliosis, a Zielke-type rod and screws may be used; more rigid instrumentation sometimes used in fractures. ± DLT	⇐ (More common to use instrumentation at the affected level than above.)
Unique considerations	Aortic arch and carotid manipulation may cause BP/HR changes. Postop respiratory distress well described.	During spinal reconstruction, manipulation of operating table may be essential to 'lock in' graft or implant (see above).	⇐
Antibiotics	Cefazolin 1 g iv (+ gentamicin 80 mg iv, if indwelling bladder catheter)	⇐	⇐
Surgical time	2-6 h	⇐	⇐
Closing considerations	Patient usually transferred to bed prior to emergence; sudden jerking motions may dislodge graft or implant.	⇐	⇐
EBL	200-5000 ml. Blood loss is extremely variable; when bleeding occurs, it may be torrential from the aorta, vena cava, or iliac vessels and branches. In nontumor or infection cases, 200-400 ml is usual.	⇐	⇐
Postop care	Chest drain; NG suction usually needed; short period of ICU observation is usual.	⇐	⇐
Mortality	< 0.1%, except in cases of malignancy or sepsis	⇐	⇐
Morbidity	For elective degenerative cases: 5-10% overall	⇐	⇐

	Cervicothoracic Approach	Transthoracic Approach	Transdiaphragmatic Approach
Morbidity, cont.	DVT: 6%	⇐	⇐
	Neurological: 3%	⇐	⇐
	Infection: 1%	⇐	⇐
	Sexual dysfunction	⇐	⇐
	For sepsis or tumor: 50-80% (overall)	⇐	⇐
	Cardiorespiratory failure	⇐	⇐
	Sepsis	⇐	⇐
Pain score	7-8 (if patient sensate at level of surgery)	7-8 (if patient sensate at level of surgery)	7-8 (if patient sensate at level of surgery)

PATIENT POPULATION CHARACTERISTICS

Age range	12-30 yr (scoliosis surgery); > 40 (tumor and infection surgery); 15-35 yr (fractures)
Male:Female	1:1, except more scoliosis surgery in females (1:4) and more fractures in males
Incidence	20,000/yr
Etiology	Scoliosis: idiopathic (50%), neuromuscular (15%), congenital (5%); trauma (20%); infections, tumors (10%)
Associated conditions	Pulmonary HTN and impaired pulmonary function; neuromuscular scoliosis (poliomyelitis, CP, muscular dystrophy, Friedreich's ataxia); aspiration; cardiomyopathy

ANESTHETIC CONSIDERATIONS

See Anesthetic Considerations for Spinal Reconstruction and Fusion, p. 789.

References

1. Butler J, Schafer MF: Anterior approach to scoliosis. In *Chapman's Orthopaedic Surgery*, 3rd edition. Chapman MW, ed. Lippincott Williams & Wilkins, Philadelphia: 2001, 4011-30.
2. Hoppenfeld S, deBoer P: *Surgical Exposures in Orthopaedics: An Anatomic Approach*, 2nd edition. Lippincott Williams & Wilkins, Philadelphia: 1994, 215-302.
3. Jain AK: Treatment of tuberculosis of the spine with neurologic complications. *Clin Orthop* 2002; 398:75-84.
4. McLain RF, Benson DR: Operative treatment of thoracic and thoracolumbar fractures. In *Chapman's Orthopaedic Surgery*, 3rd edition. Chapman MW, ed. Lippincott Williams & Wilkins, Philadelphia: 2001, 3725-45.
5. McLain RF, Lieberman I: Surgical treatment of adult scoliosis. In *Chapman's Orthopaedic Surgery*, 3rd edition. Chapman MW, ed. Lippincott Williams & Wilkins, Philadelphia: 2001, 4101-14.
6. Taft E, Francis R: Evaluation and management of scoliosis. *J Pediatr Health Care* 2003; 17(1):42-4.
7. Tay BK, Deckey J, Hu SS: Spinal infections. *J Am Acad Orthop Surg* 2002; 10(3):188-97.

ANTERIOR SPINAL RECONSTRUCTION AND FUSION— LUMBOSACRAL SPINE

SURGICAL CONSIDERATIONS

Description: The same general considerations apply here as in thoracolumbar reconstruction segments. The thoracic cavity is not entered, nor is the diaphragm sectioned. Careful preop assessment is needed, as these patients may have a wide range of coexisting diseases. The same operative procedure is performed for removal of a degenerative disk in a healthy patient as is carried out to decompress the cauda equina in a debilitated patient with metastatic breast carcinoma.

Retroperitoneal approach: Below the diaphragm, exposure of the lumbar spine (L2-S1) can be performed through a retroperitoneal approach (Fig 10.3-3). This often involves a flank incision, often with resection of the 11th or 12th rib. The patient lies in a decubitus or partial decubitus position. At risk here are the great vessels above and below the bifurcation of the aorta (L4-L5). The ureter crosses the operative field and must be identified and protected. The sympathetic chain may be damaged along the vertebrae, but the consequences of this are minimal. The presacral plexus further down may be injured and result in persistent retrograde ejaculation.

A Pfannenstiel's incision may be used to approach L5/S1 or L4/5. Regardless of the level of exposure, the operating table is used during the procedure to manipulate the spine for better exposure and to 'lock in' implants, bone grafts, etc. Usually the area of the spine to be exposed is centered above the 'breaking' joint and kidney rests of the table (Fig 10.3-2). After

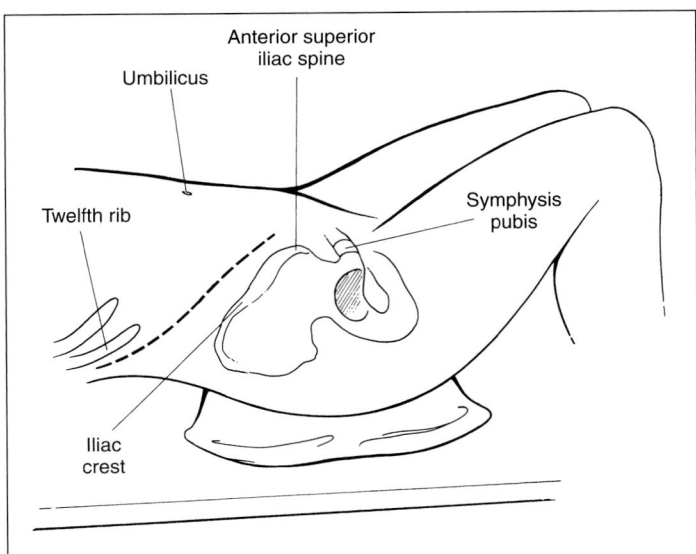

Figure 10.3-3. Retroperitoneal approach to lumbar spine. (Reproduced with permission from Hoppenfeld S, deBoer P: *Surgical Exposures in Orthopaedics.* JB Lippincott, 1984.)

initial exposure, the table is angled in the center with the head and legs pointing down and the kidney rests elevated to open up the section of spine facing the surgeon. After the removal of the disc, abscess, or tumor, a reconstruction—using bone graft, metal implants, bone cement, or a combination of these—is performed. The table is then straightened; with the spine in neutral alignment, the stability of the reconstruction is tested by this maneuver, which may need to be repeated several times.

In some instances, the anterior reconstruction and fusion is followed with a **posterior fusion**, either immediately or after 5-7 d of convalescence. If done immediately after, the patient needs to be positioned prone on the operating table, and the second procedure done through a midline exposure. Sometimes anterior and posterior surgeries can be performed simultaneously by two surgical teams. The most common reason for a staged anterior/posterior procedure (in the U.S.) was scoliosis. Recent trends in degenerative lumbar disk surgery indicate that anterior and posterior fusion has become more common, with some evidence suggesting better results in fusion and pain relief.

Variant procedure or approaches: When the L5 vertebra and sacrum need to be exposed widely, a **transperitoneal approach** may be needed. This involves a laparotomy or Pfannenstiel's incision, displacement of the bowels out of the pelvis, and exposure of the lumbosacral junction (Fig 10.3-4). The patient is supine for this procedure and the surgical risks are similar, as with other intraabdominal approaches.[10]

In a recent modification to the retroperitoneal approach, the patient is placed in the supine position. In this **supine retroperitoneal approach,** an incision is made in either a longitudinal or transverse fashion between the umbilicus and the pubis. The rectus abduminus fascia is incised and the rectus abduminus is retracted medially or laterally, allowing access to the retroperitoneal space without violating the peritoneal cavity. The advantage of this approach over the transperitoneal approach includes decreased need for bowel manipulation, →↓3rd-space loss of fluid and ↓heat loss.

Usual preop diagnosis: Degenerative disc disease; segmental instability; vertebral fractures requiring decompression; vertebral osteomyelitis or tuberculosis; neoplastic disease of the lumbar spine[10]

SUMMARY OF PROCEDURES

	Retroperitoneal Approach (Lateral)	**Transperitoneal Approach**
Position	Lateral decubitus, affected side up. The up hip and knee are flexed to relax psoas muscle and allow its reflection to expose the lumbar vertebral bodies.	Supine
Incision	Flank incision curving anteriorly to the lateral margin of the rectus abdominus (Fig 10.3-3)	Pfannenstiel's above the pubis
Special instrumentation	Occasional use of anterior instrumentation to stabilize fractures or to reconstruct the spine when entire vertebrae are removed	⇐

	Retroperitoneal Approach (Lateral)	Transperitoneal Approach
Unique considerations	In performing spinal reconstruction, manipulation of operating table is essential to 'lock in' graft or implant (see above).	⇐ + A general bowel prep usually is performed preop.
Antibiotics	Cefazolin 1 g iv (+ gentamicin 80 mg iv, if indwelling bladder catheter already in place); exception is when infection is suspected and specific cultures are obtained intraop.	⇐
Surgical time	3-6 h	⇐
Closing considerations	The spine may be more or less stable after reconstruction, and patient usually transferred to bed prior to being awakened. Sudden jerking motions, etc., may dislodge graft or implant.	⇐
EBL	200-5000 ml. Blood loss extremely variable. When bleeding occurs, it may be torrential from the aorta, vena cava, or iliac vessels and branches. In nontumor/infection cases, 200-400 ml is usual.	⇐
Postop care	Patients with degenerative conditions and elective surgeries normally recover in PACU and return to ward. Patients with infections, fractures, and tumors are usually observed in ICU for 24 h postop. Ileus for 24-72 h is usual; NG suction usually continues until bowel sounds and passing flatus are present. Generally, mobilization depends on final stability.	⇐
Mortality	Malignancy or sepsis: 1-2%	⇐
	Elective: < 0.1%	⇐
Morbidity	In patients with malignancy, sepsis or fractures with cauda equina compression, overall serious complications: 25-50%	⇐
	Cardiopulmonary failure	⇐
	Neurologic deficit	–
	Pneumothorax	–
	Sepsis	⇐
Pain score	6	6

PATIENT POPULATION CHARACTERISTICS

Age range	Variable (infant–adult)
Male:Female	1:1, except more scoliosis surgery in females (1:4)
Incidence	Uncommon
Etiology	Infection (osteomyelitis, TB); trauma; congenital; neoplasia; idiopathic

---

ANESTHETIC CONSIDERATIONS FOR SPINAL RECONSTRUCTION AND FUSION

(Procedures covered: anterior reconstruction and fusion of thoracic, thoracolumbar, and lumbosacral spine

PREOPERATIVE

Patients presenting for spinal reconstruction commonly have either idiopathic or acquired scoliosis, a complex deformity involving both lateral curvature and rotation of the spine, as well as an associated deformity of the rib cage. Types of scoliosis include: idiopathic, congenital, neuromuscular, myopathic, traumatic, tumor-related, and mesenchymal disorders. The majority of cases are idiopathic, with a male:female ratio of 1:4. Normally, the cervical spine and lumbar spine are lordotic, while the thoracic spine is kyphotic. Surgery is indicated when the curvature is severe (angulation beyond 40° in the thoracic or lumbar spine[7]) or progressing rapidly. The primary purpose of the operative correction of scoliosis is not to straighten the spine, but to prevent further curvature from developing. The instrumentation is intended to stabilize the spine until bony fusion of the spine has occurred. Once the fusion is solid (6-12 mo), the instrumentation may be removed if it is broken, causes protrusions or lumps in the back, or the patient is having residual back pain. Nonscoliotic patients presenting for this surgery may have spinal instability as a result of trauma, metastatic carcinoma or infection (e.g., TB). These patients are usually healthy, apart from their underlying pathology. The patients with disseminated lung or breast cancer may need a careful workup with regard to respiratory, nutritional, and chemotherapeutic status. (See Anesthetic Considerations for Lobectomy, Pneumonectomy, p. 210, or Mastectomy, p. 517.)

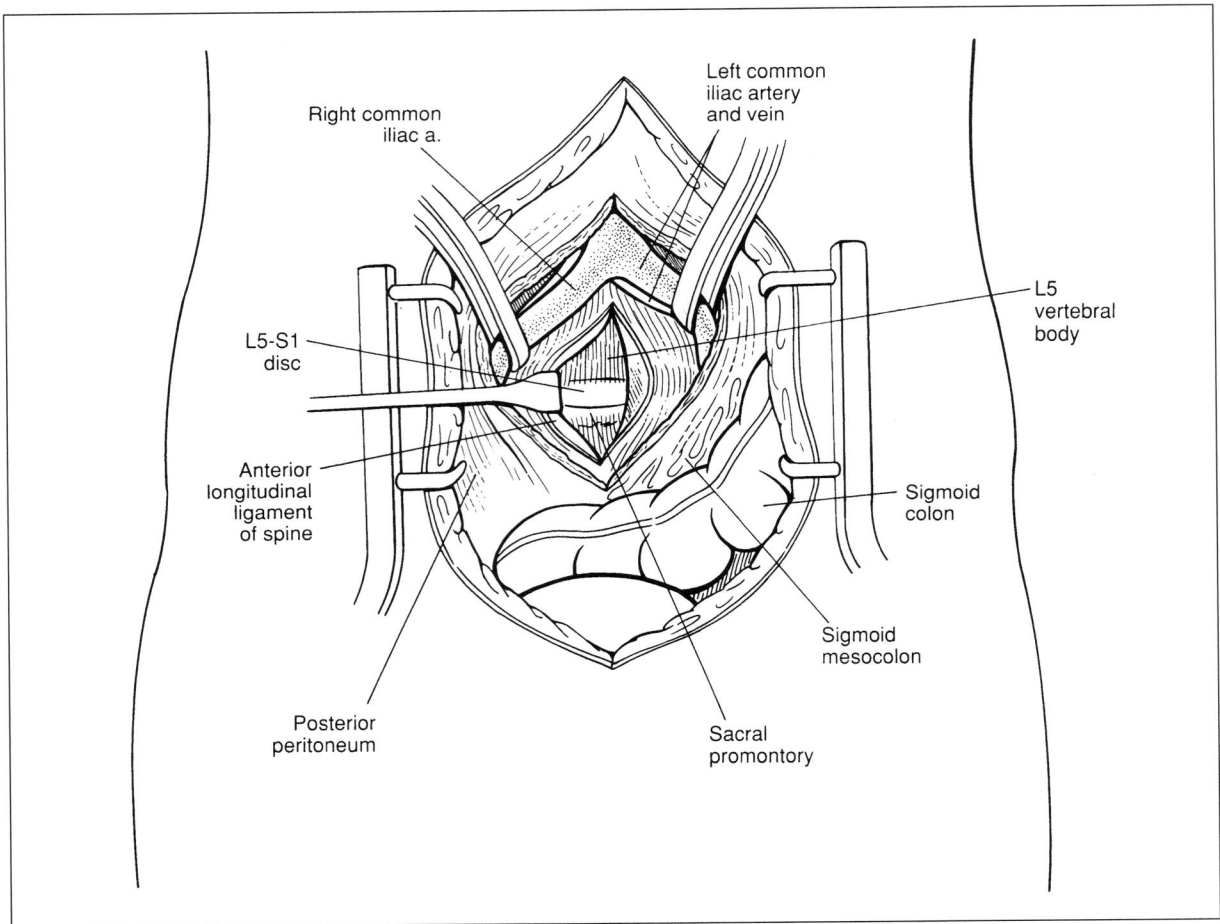

Figure 10.3-4. Transperitoneal approach to lumbosacral junction. (Reproduced with permission from Hoppenfeld S, deBoer P: *Surgical Exposures in Orthopaedics*. JB Lippincott: 1984.)

Respiratory	Respiratory impairment proportional to angle of lateral curvature (Cobb angle) (Fig 10.3-5)[22]		

Cobb Angle	30°-60°	60°- 90°	>90°
VC	↓25%	↓50%	↓70%
TLC	↓27%	↓37%	↓50%

Restrictive pattern: ↓TLC + ↓↓VC
- If VC >70% predicted, respiratory reserve is adequate.
- If VC < 40% predicted, postop ventilation usually is required.

Expect further significant (~40%) ↓VC immediately postop, requiring 7-10 d to resolve.

↑RR + ↓TV → ↑dead space + ↓alveolar ventilation → V/Q mismatch → hypoxemia.[12]

Patients with scoliosis of neuromuscular origin are more susceptible to aspiration and respiratory failure.

Tests: CXR; ABG; PFT; assess exercise tolerance by Hx.

Cardiovascular   ★ ↑PVR (**NB**: independent of severity of scoliosis). High incidence of CHD and mitral valve prolapse.

Tests: ECG; ECHO—consult cardiologist if apical systolic murmur or other evidence of cardiovascular impairment is present.[12]

Neurological   SSEPs (posterior cord) and MEPs (anterior cord) will be monitored in most patients who are undergoing spinal reconstruction. Some surgeons, however, may request that the patient be awakened

Neurological, cont.	intraop, after completion of the instrumentation, but before closure of the wound, to ensure that no motor deficits have developed as a result of the correction. Movement of the toes or feet bilaterally is sufficient to verify intact motor function. Inform the patient preop that this test will be performed, that it will only take a few minutes, that the patient will not be in severe pain while doing the test, and that full anesthesia will be reinstituted upon completion of the test. If focal neurological lesions exist preop as a result of disease (e.g., tuberculous spondylitis), their documentation is important to distinguish them from changes associated with correction.
Musculoskeletal	When the Cobb angle is > 25°, the degree of respiratory impairment will be significant and the need for postop ventilatory support becomes more likely. Patients with muscular dystrophy may be more sensitive to myocardial depression from anesthetic agents and also may require postop ventilation 2° muscle weakness. Succinylcholine may cause severe rhabdomyolysis with hyperkalemia. These patients also may be at risk for MH.

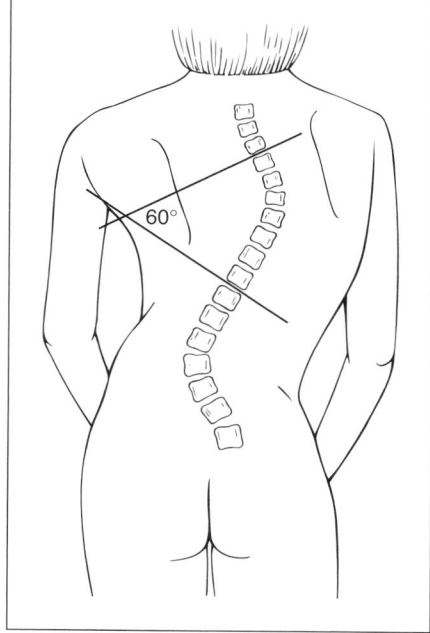

Figure 10.3-5. Cobb angle.

Hematologic	Avoid use of Plt inhibitors 2 wk before surgery. Encourage autologous or directed-donor blood

donations. Have at least 2 U PRBCs available at start of operation. Consider use of low-volume Cell Savers (e.g., OrthoPat, Medtronic Autolog). Discuss use of controlled ↓BP with surgeon. If anticipated blood loss is substantial, some institutions use isovolemic hemodilution by collecting 1-2 U blood at the start of anesthesia and replacing them with crystalloid or colloid solutions. Be aware that patients with previously placed spinal support (e.g., Milwaukee brace) for correction of scoliosis may have more blood loss than usual.

Laboratory	✓ INR, PT, PTT, and Plt count preop. ✓ Hct the morning of operation or after induction of anesthesia if autologous donations have been made since, with modest blood loss and fluid therapy, the Hct may rapidly ↓ to < 26%.
Premedication	Standard premedication (see p. B-2), if appropriate.

INTRAOPERATIVE

Anesthetic technique: GETA. For pediatric cases, preheat room to 78° F. For operations in the prone position, use a wire-reinforced tube to prevent kinking and airway obstruction. If a transthoracic approach is used, a DLT usually is necessary.

Induction	Standard induction (p. B-2). A DLT may facilitate surgical access in the patient undergoing an anterior correction. The smallest available DLT is size 28 Fr (OD = 8.9 mm), typically suitable for a child aged 12-14 yr.
Maintenance	Standard maintenance (p. B-3). It is important to minimize changes of potent inhalational agents during measurement of SSEPs. Optimal SSEP and MEP recordings are obtained using sevoflurane or isoflurane at MAC concentrations, supplemented by opiates and NMB drugs to prevent extraneous muscle movements while surgeon is dissecting muscle from bony spine. Avoid N_2O as it diminishes EP tracings and is inappropriate when OLV is used.
Emergence	The patient's trachea usually is extubated at the conclusion of the operation, unless there is a question of lung function following a transthoracic approach and OLV. Some surgeons may place an epidural catheter before closure for postop pain management or perform intercostal injections for the transthoracic approach. Prior to emergence, scoliosis patients usually are fitted with a plaster mold to be used as a permanent brace that will be worn for several mo postop. Transfer from the operating table to bed must be smooth and gentle.

Blood and fluid requirements	IV: 14-16 ga × 2 NS/LR @ 6-8 ml/kg/h	Anticipate substantial blood loss with scoliosis surgery from extensive dissection of muscles from bony spine; less so with isolated thoracic fusion. It may vary from 25%->100% of the patient's blood volume, although blood loss is usually less with the anterior approach (Dwyer's). Colloid is preferred since it will remain intravascular until metabolized.
	Hetastarch 6% ≤ 20 ml/kg or albumin prn Warm all fluids. Humidify gases. T&C 2-4 U PRBCs. ± Cell Saver	Low-volume units (e.g., OrthoPat, Autolog) are best.
Control of blood loss	Position to prevent venous engorgement. ↓MAP to 60-70 mmHg. ± ↓Hct to 25-28%.	Consider maintaining BP ≤ 20% below the lowest preop values to minimize blood loss during dissection. Generally maintain MAP > 60 mmHg in young, healthy patients, and > 80 mmHg in older patients, for spinal cord perfusion. Once dissection is complete, higher BP values acceptable. Maintain UO at 0.5-1 ml/kg/h during controlled hypotension.
Monitoring	Standard monitors (p. B-1) Arterial line CVP line Urinary catheter ± SSEP	CVP monitor helpful in selected, older patients to assess fluid Rx. Trends in CVP may be more reliable than measurement of UO to assess changes in volume status in patients in the prone and lateral positions.
Positioning	✓ and pad pressure points. ✓ eyes, neck.	Prone: Place head on cushioned head holder with cutout for eyes, nose, chin (e.g., Andrews Gentle-Rest pillow). Make certain that none of the face rests on bed. ✓ elbows, knees, feet. Lateral: Place head on donut in neutral position. Pad both arms in neutral position.
Wakeup test	30 min advance warning from surgeons is needed (sevoflurane). • Decrease inhalational agents. • Reverse muscle relaxants (and narcotics, if necessary). • Monitor train of four. • Request hand squeeze; if present, elicit bilateral foot movement. • Reinduce anesthesia with STP (2-3 mg/kg) or propofol (0.5-1 mg/kg). **Dangers:** Air embolus Dislodgement of spinal instrumentation Accidental extubation[25]	The wakeup test assesses integrity of motor pathways in the ventral cord. Uncontrolled patient movement during wakeup test can result in accidental extubation or dislodgement of the spinal instrumentation. Unrestrained inspiratory efforts may provoke venous air embolism. The anesthesiologist must be prepared to rapidly reanesthetize the patient.
SSEP and MEPs	SSEP: Dorsal cord function only MEPs: Ventral cord function	SSEP and, more recently, MEP are being used routinely. The technician needs to know when there are substantive changes in doses of inhalation anesthetics or ventilation. Optimal EP recordings are obtained with sevoflurane or isoflurane at MAC, supplemented with opiates and NMB drugs. N_2O added to sevoflurane and isoflurane worsens EPs.
Complications	Spinal cord ischemia Massive blood loss Fat embolism	SSEP indications of spinal cord ischemia should be treated by restoring normal BP and by ↓ cord traction. Prompt transfusion may be necessary and blood should be available in the room (2-4 U PRBC).

POSTOPERATIVE

Complications	Pulmonary insufficiency Hypothermia Pneumothorax Dislodgement of internal fixation	Postop ventilation may be required in patients with severe respiratory impairment (see Preoperative Considerations, above). In addition, thoracotomy, surgical trauma to the diaphragm and fat embolism may further ↑ the risk of post-op pulmonary insufficiency. Careful handling of patient in transfer is mandatory.
	Neurologic sequelae	Neurologic sequelae probably remain the most feared complication, and it is important to document postop neurologic exam.
Pain management	PCA (p. C-3) Intrathecal morphine 0.1-0.25 mg by surgeon intraop, dependent on age of patient Thoracic/lumbar epidural opiates	Pain is a significant problem for postop scoliosis patients. Most need analgesia × 3-4 d. Preop consultation with patient (and parents) about different pain management techniques is important. See p. C-2.
Tests	CXR; ABG; Hct	✓ for pneumothorax and line placement.

References

1. Chapman MW: *Operative Orthopaedics*, 3rd edition. Lippincott Williams & Wilkins, Philadelphia: 1993, 4011-73.
2. Colovic V, Walker RW, Patel D, Rushman S: Reduction of blood loss using aprotonin during spinal surgery in children for non-idiopathic scoliosis. *Paediatr Anaesth* 2002; 12(9):835.
3. Dwyer AF, Schafer MF: Anterior approach to scoliosis. Results of treatment in fifty-one cases. *J Bone Joint Surg* [Br] 1974; 56(2):218-24.
4. Fabregas N, Craen RA: Anaesthesia for minimally invasive neurosurgery. *Best Pract Res Clin Anaesthesiol* 2002; 16(1):81-93.
5. Floman Y, Penny JN, Micheli LJ, Riseborough EJ, Hall JE: Combined anterior and posterior fusion in seventy-three spinally deformed patients: indications, results and complications. *Clin Orthop* 1982; 164:110-22.
6. Fritzell P, Hagg O, Wessberg P, Nordwall A: Chronic low back pain and fusion: a comparison of three surgical techniques: a prospective multicenter randomized study from the Swedish Lumbar Spine Study Group. *Spine* 2002; 27(11):1131-41.
7. Goldstein LA, Waugh TR: Classification and terminology of scoliosis. *Clin Orthop* 1973; 93:10-22.
8. Goodarzi M, Shier N, Ogden J: Epidural versus patient-controlled analgesia with morphine for postoperative pain after orthopedic procedures in children. *J Pediatr Orthop* 1993; 13:663-67.
9. Hagberg CA, Welch WC, Bowman-Howard ML: Anesthesia and surgery for spine and spinal cord procedures. In *Textbook of Neuroanesthesia with Neurosurgical and Neuroscience Perspectives*. Albin MS, ed. McGraw-Hill, New York: 1997, 1039-82.
10. Hoppenfeld S, deBoer P: *Surgical Exposures in Orthopaedics: the anatomic approach,* 2nd edition. Lippincott Williams & Wilkins, Philadelphia: 1994, 215-302.
11. Horlocker TT, Wedel DJ: Anesthesia for orthopaedic surgery. In *Clinical Anesthesia*, 4th edition. Barash PG, Cullen BF, Stoelting RK, eds. Lippincott Williams & Wilkins, Philadelphia: 2001, 1103-18.
12. Kafer ER: Respiratory and cardiovascular functions in scoliosis and the principles of anesthetic management. *Anesthesiology* 1980; 52(4):339-51.
13. Kostuik JP, Carl A, Ferron S: Anterior Zielke instrumentation for spinal deformity in adults. *J Bone Joint Surg* [Am] 1989; 71(6):898-906.
14. McMaster MJ: Anterior and posterior instrumentation and fusion of thoracolumbar scoliosis due to myelomeningocele. *J Bone Joint Surg* [Br] 1987; 69(1):20-5.
15. Morrissy RT: *Atlas of Pediatric Orthopaedic Surgery*. JB Lippincott, Philadelphia: 1992, 75-97.
16. O'Brien T, Akmakjian J, Ogin G, Eilert R: Comparison of one-stage versus two-stage anterior/posterior spinal fusion for neuromuscular scoliosis. *J Pediatr Orthop* 1992; 12(5):610-15.
17. Perez-Cruet MJ, Fessler RG, Perin NI: Review: complications of minimally invasive spinal surgery. *Neurosurgery* 2002; 51(5Suppl):26-36.
18. Phillips WA, Hensinger RN: Control of blood loss during scoliosis surgery. *Clin Orthop* 1988; 229:88-93.
19. Sinatra RS, Torres J, Bustos AM: Pain management after major orthopaedic surgery: current strategies and new concept. *J Am Acad Orthop Surg* 2002; 10(2):117-29.
20. Sloan TB, Heyer EJ: Anesthesia for intraoperative neurophysiologic monitoring of the spinal cord. *J Clin Neurophysiol* 2002; 19(5):430-43.
21. Slosar PJ: Indications and outcomes of reconstructive surgery in chronic pain of spinal origin. *Spine* 2002; 27(22):2555-63.
22. Smyth RJ, Chapman KR, Wright TA, Crawford JS, Rebuck AS: Pulmonary function in adolescents with mild idiopathic scoliosis. *Thorax* 1984; 39(12):901-4.

23. Smyth RJ, Chapman KR, Wright TA, Crawford JS, Rebuck AS: Ventilatory patterns during hypoxia, hypercapnia, and exercise in adolescents with mild scoliosis. *Pediatrics* 1986; 77(5):692-97.

24. Soriano SG, McCann ME, Laussen PC: Neuroanesthesia. Innovative techniques and monitoring. *Anesthesiol Clin North Am* 2002; 20(1):137-51.

25. Sudhir KG, Smith RM, Hall J, Hall JE, Hansen DD: Intraoperative awakening for early recognition of possible neurologic sequelae during Harrington-rod spinal fusion. *Anesth Analg* 1976; 55(4):526-8.

26. Tay BK, Deckey J, Hu SS: Spinal infections. *J Am Acad Orthop Surg* 2002; 10(3):188-97.

Surgeons

Michael J. Bellino, MD
Stuart B. Goodman, MD, PhD, FRCSC, FACS

10.4 HIP, PELVIS, UPPER LEG SURGERY

Anesthesiologist

Frederick G. Mihm, MD

OPEN REDUCTION AND INTERNAL FIXATION (ORIF)
OF PELVIS OR ACETABULUM

SURGICAL CONSIDERATIONS

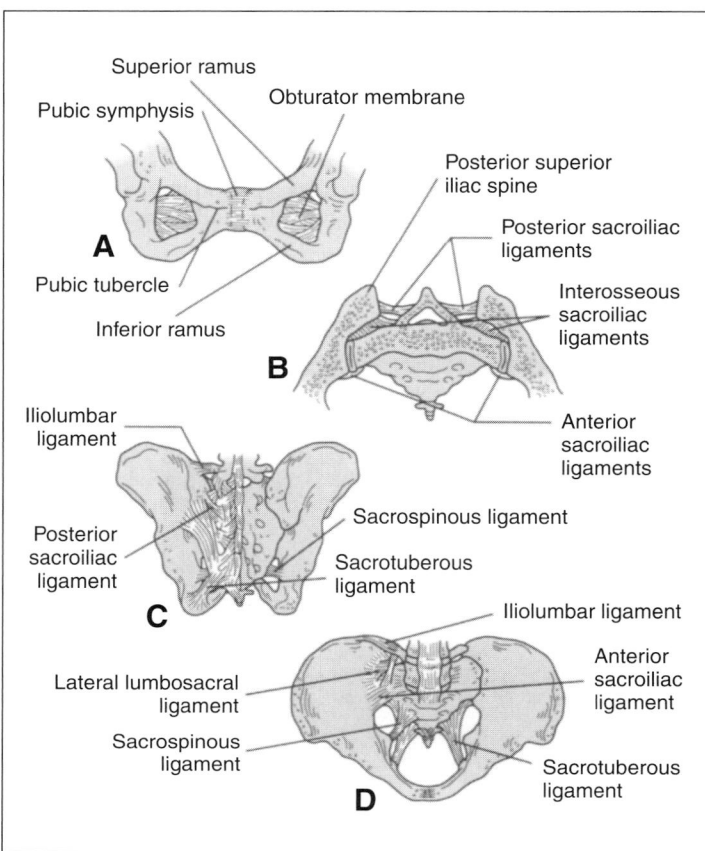

Figure 10.4-1. Schematic views of the pelvis with the principal ligamentous supports. (A) Symphysis pubis fibrocartilage. (B) Posterior SI ligaments. (C) Posterior view. (D) Anterior view. (Reproduced with permission from Chapman MW: *Chapman's Orthopaedic Surgery*, Vol 1, 3rd edition. Lippincott Williams & Wilkins, 2001.)

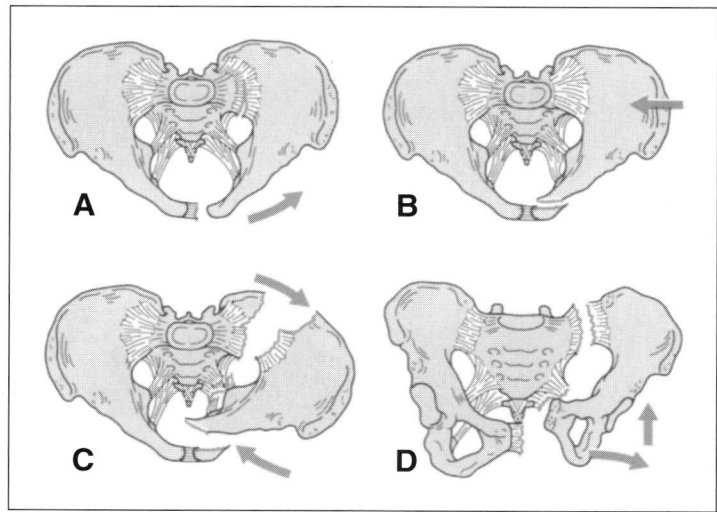

Description: Pelvic fractures present several challenging treatment problems. Surgical management is complex and often difficult in nature. Specialized training and equipment are required for a successful outcome. Major trauma mechanisms produce pelvic-ring injuries, and patients with pelvic-ring disruptions frequently have associated systemic injuries, which may be life-threatening (e.g., hemorrhagic shock). Pelvic stabilization and surgical control of hemorrhage may be performed acutely in the polytrauma patient who is hemodynamically unstable. This is in conjunction with an exploratory laparotomy performed by a trauma surgeon. The majority of patients with pelvic fractures who are treated operatively are taken to the OR on a delayed basis, after they have been stabilized. Pelvic fractures that do not heal are 'nonunions,' while those that heal in an unsatisfactory position are 'malunions.'

Anterior approaches to the pelvis include Pfannenstiel's and ilioinguinal incisions, which are utilized for reduction and fixation of dislocations and fracture/dislocations of the symphysis pubis, fractures of the pubic rami, and access to the anterior aspect of the sacroiliac (SI) joint. **Posterior approaches** to the pelvis involve either vertical or curved incisions along the iliac crest and are used for reduction and fixation of SI joint dislocations, fracture/dislocations of the SI joint, and fractures of the iliac wing and of the sacrum. These procedures are often lengthy and are staged, requiring changes in patient position. Reductions are facilitated by neuromuscular paralysis. The posterior approach requires a large operative field, which may prevent the use of an epidural catheter. In addition, postop anticoagulation for DVT prophylaxis is used uniformly, and may contraindicate the use of epidural catheters.

Figure 10.4-2. Schematic view of the principal pelvis injury patterns, as determined by the vector of the provocative blow. (A) Anteroposterior compression or external rotation injury. (B) Stable lateral compression or internal rotation injury. (C) Unstable lateral compression or internal rotation injury. (D) Unstable vertical shear disruption. (Reproduced with permission from Chapman MW: *Chapman's Orthopaedic Surgery*, Vol 1, 3rd edition. Lippincott Williams & Wilkins, 2001.)

The goal of pelvic reconstruction is to restore the anatomy and stability of the pelvis, which will decrease hemorrhage in the hemodynamically unstable patient, aid in mobilization of the multiply injured patient; and improve long-term function.

Usual preop diagnosis: Fractures of pelvis/acetabulum; nonunion/malunion of the pelvis/acetabulum

SUMMARY OF PROCEDURE

Position	Supine (anterior); prone (posterior)
Incision	Pfannensteil's, ilioinguinal (anterior); posterior, curving along iliac crest (posterior)
Special instrumentation	Radiolucent table; pelvic instruments and implants; Cell Saver; I.I.
Antibiotics	Cefazolin 1 g iv
Surgical time	1-6 h (anterior); 3-6 h (posterior)
Closing considerations	May require neuromuscular relaxation to aid reduction and closure; postop radiograph
EBL	≥ 1000 ml
Postop care	Multiple-trauma patient → ICU; others → PACU
Mortality	10%+, dependent on extent of multiple trauma
Morbidity	Ileus: Common
	Neurologic injury: Common
	Genitourinary injuries: Not uncommon
	Failure of fixation: Rare
	Infection: Rare
	Malunion: Rare
	Nonunion: Rare
Pain score	9

PATIENT POPULATION CHARACTERISTICS

Age range	Any age, but predominance of males < 30 yr
Male:Female	5:1
Incidence	1-2%
Etiology	Motorcycle and motor vehicle accidents (60-80%); falls (10-15%); crush injuries (5%); other (5%)
Associated conditions	Frequently associated with trauma to other organ systems, including head and neck, chest, abdomen, and extremities. These often will be addressed concurrently with pelvic or acetabular fracture.

ANESTHETIC CONSIDERATIONS

See Anesthetic Considerations for Procedures About the Pelvis and Hip, p. 806.

References

1. Burgess AR, Jones AL: Fractures of the pelvic ring. In *Fractures in Adults*, 4th edition. Rockwood CA Jr, Green DP, Bucholz RW, Heckman JD, eds. Lippincott-Raven, Philadelphia: 1996, 1575-1616.
2. Fishmann AJ, Greeno RA, Brooks LR, Matta JM: Prevention of deep vein thrombosis and pulmonary embolism in acetabular and pelvic fracture surgery. *Clin Orthop* 1994; 305:133-7.
3. Guyton JL: Fractures of hip, acetabulum, and pelvis. In *Campbell's Operative Orthopaedics*, Vol 3, 9th edition. Canale ST, ed. Mosby-Year Book, St. Louis: 1998, 2181-2280.
4. Jones A, Reinert C, Bucholz R: Complications of fractures of the pelvic ring and acetabulum. In *Complications in Orthopaedic Surgery*, 3rd edition. Epps CH Jr, ed. JB Lippincott, Philadelphia: 1994, 749-62.
5. Kane WJ: Complications of pelvic fractures and their treatment. In *Complications in Orthopaedic Surgery*. Epps CH Jr, ed. JB Lippincott, Philadelphia: 1986, 795-814.
6. LaVelle DG: Delayed union and nonunion of fractures. In *Campbell's Operative Orthopaedics*, 10th edition. Canale ST, ed. CV Mosby, St. Louis: 2003, 3125-67.
7. LaVelle DG: Delayed union and nonunion of fractures. In *Campbell's Operative Orthopaedics*, Vol 3, 9th edition. Canale ST, ed. Mosby-Year Book, St. Louis: 1998, 2537-78.
8. Leighton RK: Nonunions and malunions of the pelvis. In *Chapman's Orthopaedic Surgery*, Vol I, 3rd edition. Chapman MW, ed. Lippincott Williams & Wilkins, Philadelphia: 2001, 921-34.

9.   Mears DC, Durbhakula SM: Fractures and dislocations of the pelvic ring. In *Chapman's Orthopaedic Surgery*, Vol I, 3rd edition. Chapman MW, ed. Lippincott Williams & Wilkins, Philadelphia: 2001, 531-86.

10.   Mears DC, Rubash HE: *Pelvic and Acetabular Injuries*. Slack Inc., Thorofare NJ: 1986.

11.   Tile M: Fractures of the acetabulum. In *Fractures in Adults*, 4th edition. Rockwood CA Jr, Green DP, Bucholz RW, Heckman JD, eds. Lippincott-Raven, Philadelphia 1996, 1617-58.

12.   Tile M: *Fractures of the Pelvis and Acetabulum*, 2nd edition. Williams & Wilkins, Baltimore: 1995, 549-54.

CLOSED REDUCTION AND EXTERNAL FIXATION OF THE PELVIS

SURGICAL CONSIDERATIONS

Description: This procedure entails manipulating the pelvis to obtain an acceptable reduction by closed means under GA, and then applying an anterior external fixation device to maintain the reduction. The pins for the external fixator are inserted into the iliac crest either percutaneously or through small incisions. During this procedure, either radiographs or the I.I. is used to confirm that an acceptable reduction has been obtained. In some centers, this procedure is done in the emergency department as a life-saving procedure.

Usual preop diagnosis: Displaced fracture of the pelvis; unstable fracture of the pelvis

SUMMARY OF PROCEDURE

Position	Supine
Incision	Percutaneously or through small incisions along the iliac crest.
Special instrumentation	External fixation; often performed on a radiolucent table using I.I.
Antibiotics	Cefamandole 1 g iv. Combination antibiotics, if multiple severe, open fractures or other significant injuries are present.
Surgical time	1-1.5 h
EBL	Negligible from surgical procedure; however, anticipate large blood losses (4+ U) from the pelvic fracture alone.
Postop care	Multiple-trauma victim → ICU; others → PACU
Mortality	10% or more, depending on extent of multiple trauma; 50% in open fractures
Morbidity	Ileus: Virtually 100%
	Sacroiliac (SI) pain: 15-30%+
	Genitourinary problems, including bladder or urethral rupture: 13%
	Neurological deficit to lumbosacral plexus: 1-10%
	Malunion/severe deformity: 5%
	Leg-length discrepancy: 3-5%
	Impotence: 1-5%
	Residual instability: 1-3%
	Vascular complications: 1%
	Hypotension 2° to retroperitoneal hematoma: Common
	Respiratory distress: Common
	Gynecological and colorectal injuries: More common with open fractures/dislocations
	Delayed union, nonunion: Not uncommon
	Osteomyelitis: Rare
	Rupture of diaphragm: Rare
Pain score	7-10

PATIENT POPULATION CHARACTERISTICS

Age range	Any age, but predominance of males < 30 yr
Male:Female	5:1
Incidence	Common
Etiology	Motorcycle and motor vehicle accidents (60-80%); falls (10-15%); crush injuries (5%); other (5%)
Associated conditions	Frequently associated with trauma to other organ systems, including head and neck, chest, abdomen, and extremities. Patient sustaining a pelvic fracture also has a probability of having other injuries, including: musculoskeletal (85%); respiratory (60%); CNS (40%); GI (30%); urologic (12%); CVS (6%). These often will be addressed concurrently with the pelvic fracture.

ANESTHETIC CONSIDERATIONS

See Anesthetic Considerations for Procedures About the Pelvis and Hip, p. 806.

References

1. Bucholz RW, Brumback RJ: Fractures of the shaft of the femur. In *Fractures in Adults*, 4th edition. Rockwood CA Jr, Green DP, Bucholz RW, Heckman JD, eds. JB Lippincott, Philadelphia: 1996, 1827-1918.
2. Guyton JL: Fractures of hip, acetabulum, and pelvis. In *Campbell's Operative Orthopaedics*, Vol 3, 9th edition. Crenshaw AH, ed. Mosby-Year Book, St. Louis: 1998, 2042-80.
3. Jones A, Reinert C, Bucholtz R: Complications of fractures of the pelvic ring and acetabulum. In *Complications in Orthopaedic Surgery*, 3rd edition. Epps CH Jr, ed. JB Lippincott, Philadelphia: 1994, 749-62.
4. Kane WJ: Complications of pelvic fractures and their treatment. In *Complications in Orthopaedic Surgery*. Epps CH Jr, ed. JB Lippincott, Philadelphia: 1986, 795-814.
5. Mears DC, Durbhakula: Fractures and dislocations of the pelvic ring. In *Chapman's Orthopaedic Surgery*, Vol I, 3rd edition. Chapman MW, ed. Lippincott Williams & Wilkins, Philadelphia: 2001, 531-86.
6. Mears DC, Rubash HE: *Pelvic and Acetabular Injuries*. Slack Inc, Thorofare NJ: 1986.
7. Tile M: *Fractures of the Pelvis and Acetabulum*, 2nd edition. Williams & Wilkins, Baltimore: 1995, 549-54.

OPEN REDUCTION AND INTERNAL FIXATION (ORIF) OF ACETABULUM FRACTURES

SURGICAL CONSIDERATIONS

Description: Although the acetabulum is contained within the bony architecture of the pelvis, surgical management of acetabulum fractures are approached separately from pelvic fractures. The goal of surgical treatment of acetabulum fractures is to preserve the hip joint by accurately reconstructing the supporting bony anatomy. Surgical treatment of these challenging injuries are performed by surgeons who have undergone specialized training in orthopedic pelvic surgery. The mechanism of injury is usually high-energy trauma (e.g., motor vehicle, motorcycle accidents), industrial accidents, or a fall from a height that drives the femur into the acetabulum. Associated injuries to the pelvis are common, as are associated systemic injuries.

Optimal results are achieved when surgery is performed within 7 d. The approach is dictated mainly by the unique characteristics of the fractures. Essentially, three approaches are commonly used: the **ilioinguinal** (anterior, Fig 10.4-3), the **extended iliofemoral** (lateral, Fig 10.4-4), and the **Kocher-Langenbeck** (posterior, Fig 10.4-5). The most difficult portion of the procedure is the reduction; it may be facilitated by neuromuscular relaxation, pelvic reduction instruments, and traction. The I.I. is used frequently throughout the procedure to assess the reduction and position of implants, which necessitates the use of lead aprons. A radiograph also is obtained at the end of the case to verify a satisfactory reduction and position of the implants. Patients are anticoagulated in the postop period to prevent thromboembolic complications. Weight-bearing restrictions are maintained until enough healing has occurred to permit functional ambulation.

Usual preop diagnosis: Fracture of the acetabulum; nonunion/malunion of the acetabulum

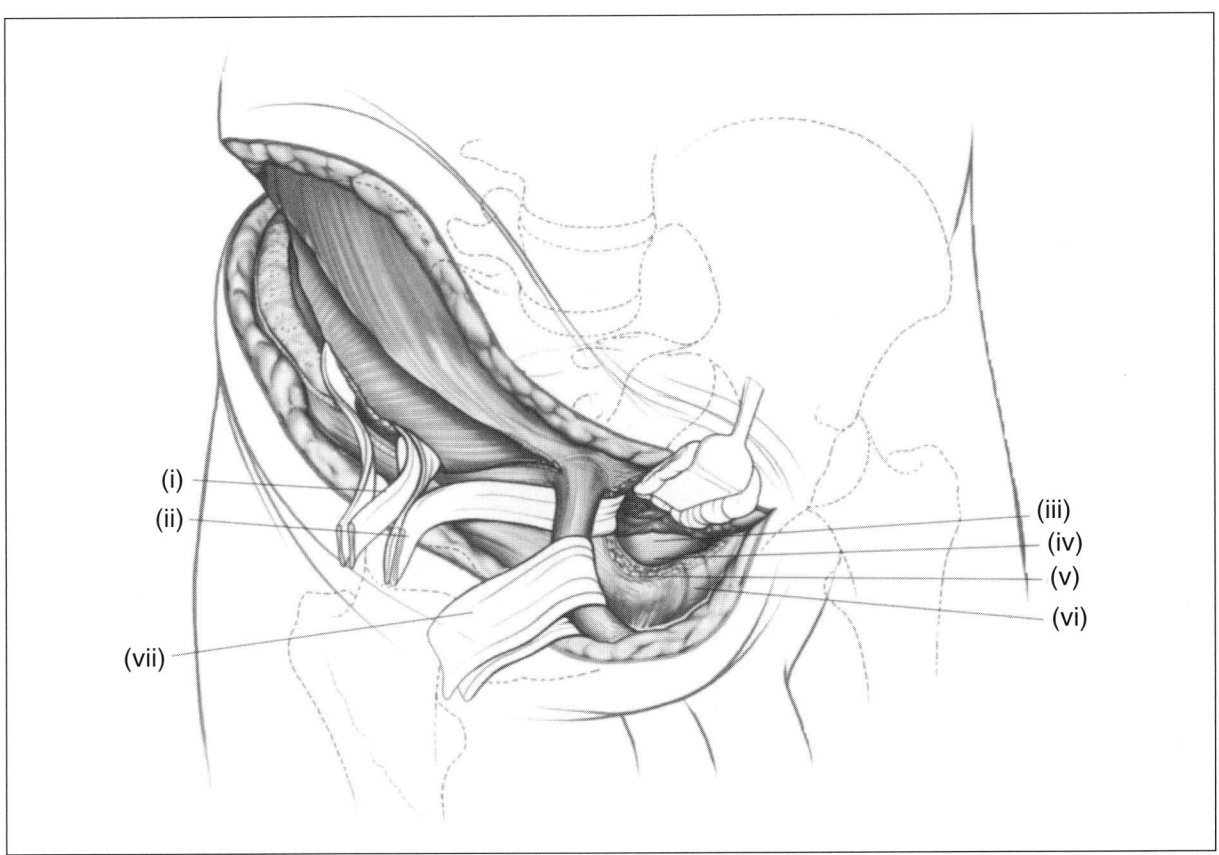

Figure 10.4-3. Ilioinguinal approach, right side: (i) Penrose drain around iliopsoas, femoral nerve, and lateral femoral cutaneous nerve; (ii) Penrose drain around femoral vessels; (iii) bladder and space of Retzius; (iv) pubis; (v) pubic tubercle; (vi) symphysis pubis; (vii) Penrose drain around spermatic cord. (Reproduced with permission from Sledge CB, ed: *The Hip.* Lippincott-Raven, 1998.)

SUMMARY OF PROCEDURE

Position	Supine (anterior); lateral decubitus (lateral); prone (posterior)
Incision	Ilioinguinal (anterior, Fig 10.4-3); extended iliofemoral (lateral, Fig 10.4-4), Kocher-Langenbeck (posterior, Fig 10.4-5)
Special instrumentation	Pelvic table; pelvic instruments and implants; I.I.; Cell Saver
Antibiotics	Cefazolin 1 g iv
Surgical time	2-5 h
EBL	100-2000 ml
Postop care	Multiple-trauma: ICU; others: PACU
Mortality	2.28%
Morbidity	Ectopic ossification: 24.4%
	Osteoarthritis after perfect reduction: 10.2%; after imperfect reduction: 35.7%
	Lateral cutaneous nerve of the thigh: 12%
	Sciatic nerve damage: 6.3%
	Infection: 4.2%
	Avascular bone necrosis: 4.1%
	DVT: 3%
	Wound hematoma: 1.5%
	Secondary displacement of fracture site: 1.5%
	PE: 1%
	Pseudoarthrosis: 0.7%
	Ileus after ilioinguinal approach: Common
Pain score	7-8

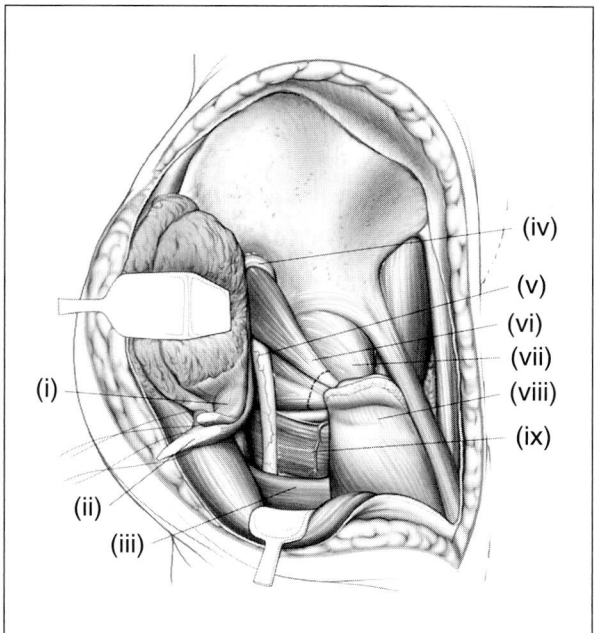

Figure 10.4-4. Extended iliofemoral approach: (i) Gluteus minimus tendon; (ii) gluteus medius tendon; (iii) gluteus maximus tendon; (iv) superior gluteal neurovascular bundle; (v) sciatic nerve; (vi) piriformis and conjoint tendons; (vii) hip joint capsule; (viii) greater trochanter; (ix) medial femoral circumflex artery overlying quadratus femoris. (Reproduced with permission from Sledge CB, ed: *The Hip*. Lippincott-Raven, 1998.)

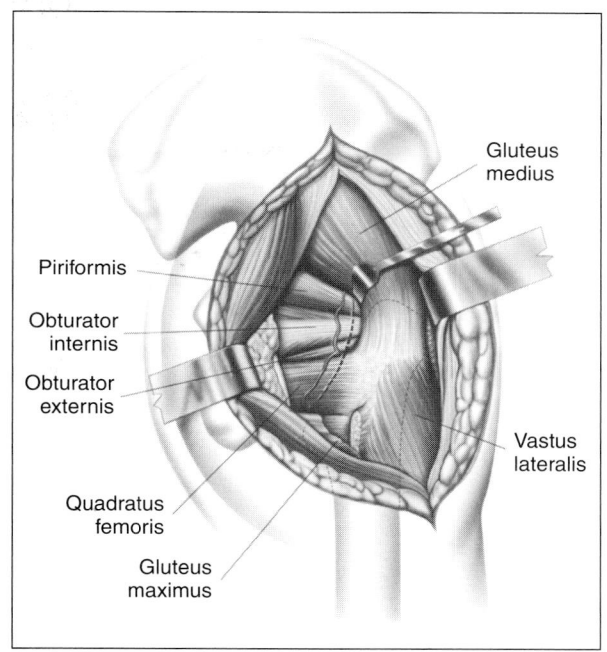

Figure 10.4-5. Kocher-Langenbeck approach. (Reproduced with permission from Sledge CB, ed: *The Hip*. Lippincott-Raven, 1998.)

PATIENT POPULATION CHARACTERISTICS

Age range	12-85 yr
Male:Female	65.6% (M); 34.6% (F)
Etiology	Motor vehicle accidents (70%); motor vehicle/pedestrian accidents (13%); falls (14%); other (3%)

ANESTHETIC CONSIDERATIONS

See Anesthetic Considerations for Procedures About the Pelvis and Hip, p. 806.

References

1. Fishmann AJ, Greeno RA, Brooks LR, Matta JM: Prevention of deep vein thrombosis and pulmonary embolism in acetabular and pelvic fracture surgery. *Clin Orthop* 1994; 305:133-7.
2. Johnson EE, Matta JM, Mast JW, Letournel E: Delayed reconstruction of acetabular fractures 21-120 days following injury. *Clin Orthop* 1994; 305:20-30.
3. Letournel E, Judet R: *Fractures of the Acetabulum*, Spring, New York: 1993.
4. Matta JM: Fractures of the acetabulum: reduction accuracy and clinical results of fractures operated within three weeks of injury. *J Bone Joint Surg* 1996; 78A:1632-45.
5. Olson SA, Matta JM: Fractures of the acetabulum, hip dislocations, and femoral head fractures. In *Chapman's Orthopaedic Surgery*, Vol I, 3rd edition. Chapman MW, ed. Lippincott Williams & Wilkins, Philadelphia: 2001, 587-616.

OSTEOTOMY AND
BONE GRAFT AUGMENTATION OF THE PELVIS

SURGICAL CONSIDERATIONS

Description: Acetabular insufficiency (acetabular dysplasia) is characterized by deficient anterior and lateral coverage of the acetabulum on the femoral head. This condition of the hip produces joint incongruity and instability, eventually leading to arthrosis and a dysfunctional hip joint. Treatment is aimed at reorienting the dysplastic acetabulum (Fig 10.4-6). In children, bone grafting alone may be sufficient; in adults, however, pelvic osteotomy, to reorient or broaden the weight-bearing surface, is necessary. A supplemental bone graft to expand the weight-bearing surface may be added. In certain instances following pelvic osteotomy, incongruity of the hip may persist. In this situation, the pelvic osteotomy is combined with a proximal femoral osteotomy to restore congruence. Pelvic and proximal femoral osteotomies usually are fixed internally with screws and plates to allow early mobilization without displacement. Weight-bearing is permitted after healing of the osteotomy at ~8 wk.

Usual preop diagnosis: Acetabular dysplasia; developmental dysplasia of the hip

SUMMARY OF PROCEDURE

Position	Supine
Incision	Anterior: ilioinguinal or iliofemoral and Smith-Peterson
Special instrumentation	Pelvic instruments and implants; special osteotomes and saws; I.I., Cell Saver
Unique considerations	Intraop radiographs and use of I.I.
Antibiotics	Cefazolin 1 g iv
Surgical time	3 h
EBL	500+ ml
Postop care	PACU → room; usually on protected, weight-bearing walker or crutches × 8 wk
Mortality	Minimal
Morbidity	Ileus: 100%
	Leg-length discrepancy: Uniformly present after pelvic osteotomy
	Neurological deficit:
	Injury to lateral cutaneous nerve: Common (50%)
	Sciatic nerve: Uncommon (1%)
	Thromboembolism: 5-10%
	Wound infection:
	Septic arthritis, osteomyelitis: 1-7%
	Delayed union, nonunion, malunion: 1-2%
	Genitourinary problems—urinary retention requiring catheterization: Common
	Hematoma: Common
	Hypotension 2° to retroperitoneal hematoma: Rare
	Vascular complications: Rare
Pain score	8

PATIENT POPULATION CHARACTERISTICS

Age range	20-50 yr
Male:Female	3-4 × higher incidence in females for congenital hip dysplasia; equal incidence for other causes
Etiology	Congenital hip dysplasia; neuromuscular disorders (cerebral palsy, meningomyelocele); pediatric trauma to acetabular growth plate
Associated conditions	Depends on Dx

ANESTHETIC CONSIDERATIONS

See Anesthetic Considerations for Procedures About the Pelvis and Hip, p. 806.

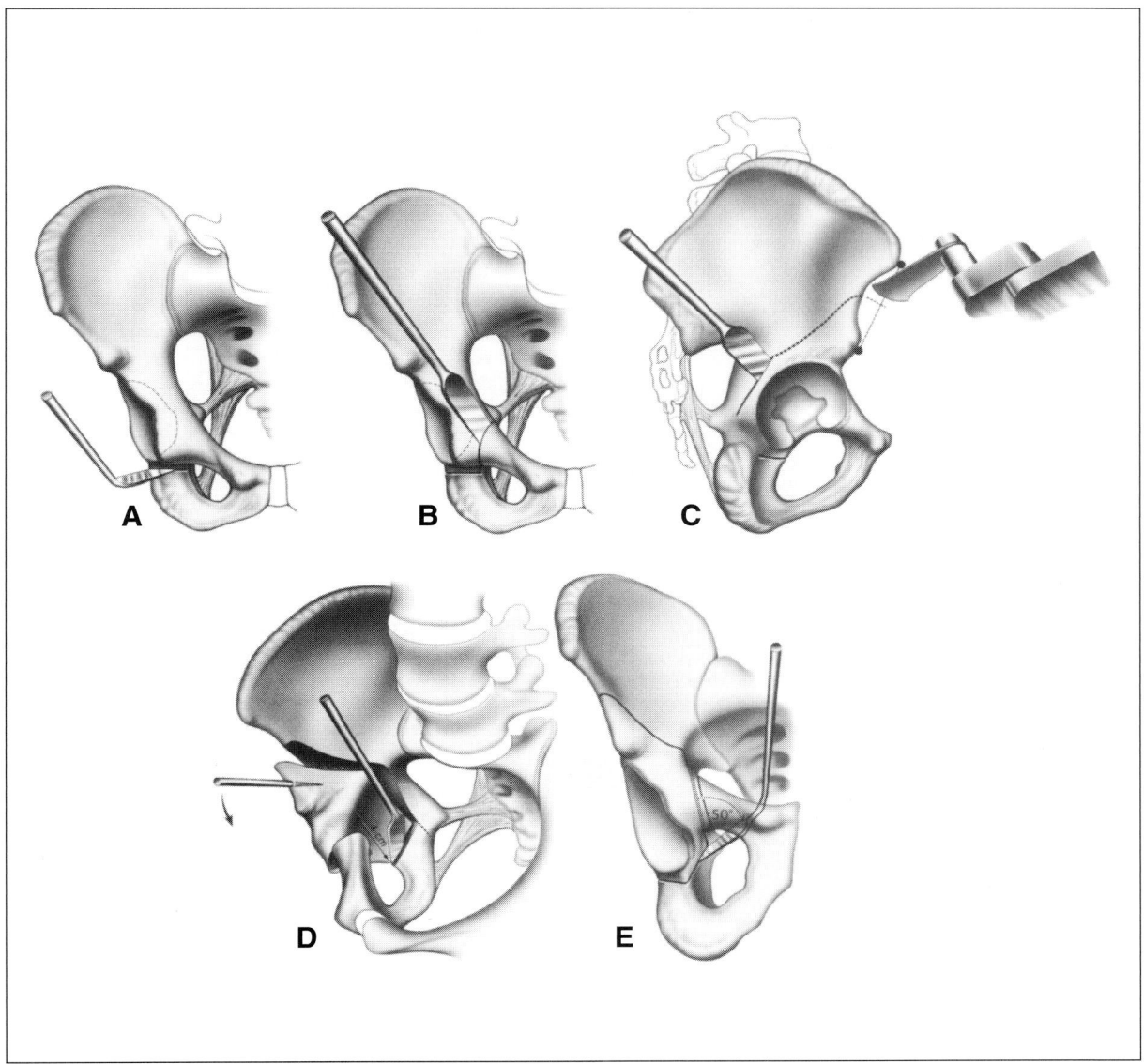

Figure 10.4-6. The Bernese periacetabular osteotomy. (Reproduced with permission from Ganz R, et al: A new periacetabular osteotomy for the treatment of hip dysplasias: Technique and preliminary results. *Clin Orthop* 1988; 232:26-36.)

References

1. Chiari K: Iliac osteotomy in young adults. In *The Hip: Proceedings of the 7th Open Meeting of the Hip Society*. CV Mosby, St. Louis: 1979, 260-77.
2. Ganz R, Klaue, K, Vihn TS, Mast JW: A new periacetabular osteotomy for the treatment of hip dysplasias. *Clin Orthop* 1988; 232:26-36.
3. Hersch O, Casillas M, Ganz R: Indications for intertrochanteric osteotomy after periacetabular osteotomy for adult hip dysplasia. *Clin Orthop* 1998; 347:19-26.
4. Salter RB, Thompson GH: The role of innominate osteotomy in young adults. In *The Hip: Proceedings of the 7th Open Meeting of the Hip Society*. CV Mosby, St. Louis: 1979, 278-312.
5. Sutherland DH, Greenfield R: Double innominate osteotomy. *J Bone Joint Surg* [Am] 1977; 59(8):1082-91.

ARTHRODESIS OF THE SACROILIAC JOINT

SURGICAL CONSIDERATIONS

Description: In this procedure, a painful and/or unstable sacroiliac (SI) joint is fused, usually by excising the joint through an **anterior** or **posterior approach** and employing an iliac crest bone graft. Supplemental screw fixation of the joint is used. The incision follows the iliac crest from the anterior superior iliac spine past the convexity of the iliac tubercle; the aponeurosis of the external abdominal musculature is elevated from the iliac crest. The internal iliac fossa is exposed subperiosteally, posterior to the SI joint; then the joint cartilage is excised and packed with cancellous bone strips. The SI joint is fixed with plates and screws. Alternatively, a posterior approach to the SI Joint may be used. A straight vertical incision is made just lateral to the posterior superior iliac spine. The origin of the gluteus maximus is elevated from its origin off the posterior ilium and sacrum and reattached laterally. The SI joint is identified, debrided of cartilage, and packed with strips of cancellous bone. It is then fixed with screws.

Variant procedure or approaches: Anterior or posterior approach

Usual preop diagnosis: Arthritis or arthrosis of the SI joint; pelvic instability

SUMMARY OF PROCEDURE

Position	Supine (anterior) or prone (posterior)
Incision	Lateral portion of ilioinguinal (anterior); posterior approach to SI joint (posterior)
Special instrumentation	Radiolucent table; pelvic instruments and implants; I.I.; Cell Saver
Unique considerations	Intraop radiographs or use of I.I.
Antibiotics	Cefazolin 1 g iv
Surgical time	2-3 h
EBL	250-500 ml
Postop care	Usually on protected, weight-bearing walker or crutches × 6-8 wk; anticoagulation for DVT prophylaxis
Mortality	Extremely low
Morbidity	Ileus: Virtually always
	Osteomyelitis: < 1%
	Wound infection: < 1%
	Genitourinary problems; urinary retention requiring catheterization: Common
	Delayed union, nonunion, malunion, leg-length discrepancy: Not uncommon
	Neurological deficit; injury to lumbosacral plexus: Rare, unless present preop; L5 nerve root susceptible in anterior approaches
	Hypotension 2° to retroperitoneal hematoma: Rare
	Injury to bowel: Rare
	Vascular complications; injury to iliac arteries: Rare
	Thromboembolism
Pain score	7

PATIENT POPULATION CHARACTERISTICS

Age range	20-50 yr
Male:Female	Increased incidence in males (trauma)
Incidence	Rare
Etiology	Trauma—postpelvic fracture dislocation; painful septic arthritis

ANESTHETIC CONSIDERATIONS

See Anesthetic Considerations for Procedures About the Pelvis and Hip, p. 806.

References

1. Christian CA, Donley BG: Arthrodesis of the ankle, knee and hip. In *Campbell's Operative Orthopaedics*, Vol 1, 9th edition. Crenshaw AH, ed. Mosby-Year Book, St. Louis: 1998, 145-88.
2. Guyton JL: Fractures of hip, acetabulum, and pelvis. In *Campbell's Operative Orthopaedics*, Vol 3, 9th edition. Crenshaw AH, ed. Mosby-Year Book, St. Louis: 1998, 2042-80.

3. Jones A, Reinert C, Bucholtz R: Complications of fractures of the pelvic ring and acetabulum. In *Complications in Orthopaedic Surgery*, 3rd edition. Epps CH Jr, ed. JB Lippincott, Philadelphia: 1994, 749-62.
4. Kane WJ: Complications of pelvic fractures and their treatment. In *Complications in Orthopaedic Surgery.* Epps CH Jr, ed. JB Lippincott, Philadelphia: 1986, 795-814.
5. LaVelle DG: Fractures of hip and pelvis. In *Campbell's Operative Orthopaedics*, 10th edition. Canale ST, ed. CV Mosby, St. Louis: 1998.
6. Russell TA: Arthrodesis of the lower extremity and hip. In *Campbell's Operative Orthopaedics*, Vol 2, 9th edition. Crenshaw AH, ed. CV Mosby, St. Louis: 1998.

AMPUTATIONS ABOUT THE HIP AND PELVIS: DISARTICULATION OF THE HIP AND HINDQUARTER AMPUTATION

SURGICAL CONSIDERATIONS

Description: These surgical procedures accomplish an excision of the entire lower extremity. In a **hip disarticulation**, the amputation is performed through the hip joint. An anterior, racquet-shaped incision is made and all muscles crossing the hip joint are incised or detached. The femoral artery, vein, and nerve; obturator vessels; sciatic nerve; and deep vessels are isolated and ligated. The gluteal flap is brought anteriorly and sewn to the anterior portion of the incision. In a **hindquarter amputation**, excision of the lower extremity, hip joint and a portion of the pelvis is performed. Anterior and posterior incisions are used; and the iliac wing is divided posteriorly and the symphysis pubis is disarticulated anteriorly. Either the common iliac or external iliac vessels are ligated, as are all nerves to the lower extremity. Usually the gluteal flap is drawn anteriorly for closure. These procedures are performed very rarely—for severe trauma, tumor, or infection—and are often life-saving surgeries. They often are performed in conjunction with a general surgeon, and standard bowel prep is done. The operations are long and tedious, with extensive blood loss, in patients who are usually systemically ill.

Usual preop diagnosis: Malignant tumor of femur, hip or pelvis; traumatic amputation to femur, hip, or pelvis; uncontrollable infection to leg, hip, or pelvis (e.g., clostridia)

SUMMARY OF PROCEDURES

	Hip Disarticulation	**Hindquarter Amputation**
Position	Supine	Lateral decubitus; stabilized by bean bag and/or kidney rests.
Incision	Anterior racquet type (rare)	Anterior and posterior
Unique considerations	Urinary catheter should be placed.	Urinary catheter; NG tube; scrotum strapped to opposite thigh; anus stitched closed/sealed.
Antibiotics	Cefazolin or cefamandole 1 g iv q 6-8 h	⇐
Surgical time	3-4 h	4-5 h
EBL	1000-2000 ml (intraop blood salvage system recommended, except for tumors)	2000-3000 ml
Postop care	ICU	⇐
Mortality	Rare in patients undergoing elective amputation for trauma or localized tumor; higher for patients with debilitated trauma, chronic infection or extensive invasive malignant tumor; highest in clostridial infections: ~50%+	⇐
Morbidity	Anemia: Common	⇐
	Electrolyte abnormalities: Common	⇐
	Hematoma: Common	⇐
	Neurological injury to lumbosacral plexus or peripheral nerves: Common	⇐
	Paralytic ileus: Common	⇐
	Psychosocial problems: Common	⇐
	UTI: Common	⇐
	Flap necrosis: Not uncommon	⇐

	Hip Disarticulation	Hindquarter Amputation
Morbidity, cont.	Incomplete excision with recurrence of tumor or infection: Not uncommon	⇐
	Injury to peritoneal or retroperitoneal contents, including bowel and bladder: Not uncommon	⇐
	Vascular injury—iliac, other vessels: Not uncommon	⇐
Pain Score	10	10

PATIENT POPULATION CHARACTERISTICS

Age range	Any age
Male:Female	Similar, except higher incidence in males for traumatic etiologies
Incidence	Uncommon
Etiology	Malignant tumor; trauma; infection—clostridial myonecrosis, chronic osteomyelitis, etc.

ANESTHETIC CONSIDERATIONS FOR PROCEDURES ABOUT THE PELVIS AND HIP

(Procedures covered: ORIF, pelvis, acetabulum; closed reduction, external fixation, pelvis; osteotomy and bone graft of pelvis; arthrodesis of SI joint; amputations about hip and pelvis: disarticulation of hip and hindquarter amputation)

PREOPERATIVE

Patients presenting for pelvic surgery generally fall into two categories: 1) Major trauma—pelvic fracture requires substantial force and seldom occurs alone. These patients require aggressive fluid therapy with large-bore iv's and invasive monitors (arterial line and CVP). If the patient can be made hemodynamically stable with volume resuscitation, a thorough evaluation for coexisting neurological, thoracic, or abdominal trauma should be undertaken before anesthesia. 2) Tumor resection and amputation of thigh, hip, and pelvis. Because of large intraop blood loss and 3rd-spacing of fluids, invasive hemodynamic monitoring is necessary. Although epidural anesthesia is seldom adequate for surgery, postop epidural analgesia is an effective means of controlling the tremendous pain caused by this type of surgery. Other patient populations covered in this section include otherwise healthy patients with congenital or acquired hip dysplasia presenting for augmentation procedures.

Respiratory	Trauma patients are at risk for hemothorax, pneumothorax, pulmonary contusion, fat embolism (preop and postop), and aspiration. A chest tube will be needed before surgery if either a hemothorax or pneumothorax is present. Pulmonary fat embolus occurs in 10-15% of patients with long-bone fractures, and can occur after isolated pelvic fractures. Sx include hypoxemia, tachycardia, tachypnea, respiratory alkalosis, mental status changes, conjunctival petechiae, fat bodies in the urine, and diffuse pulmonary infiltrates. Sx of pulmonary aspiration are similar to those of fat embolism. Preop therapy for either should include supplemental O_2 to correct hypoxemia (may necessitate mechanical ventilation) and meticulous fluid management to prevent worsening of pulmonary capillary leak. **Tests:** CXR, or others as indicated from H&P.
Cardiovascular	Blunt chest trauma can produce both cardiac contusion and aortic tear. Preop ECG and CPK isoenzymes will help evaluate the presence of myocardial injury. A wide mediastinal silhouette suggests aortic tear, which requires evaluation with TEE or angiography. **Tests:** Consider ECG; CPK isoenzymes; others as indicated from H&P.
Neurological	The possibility of coexistent neurologic trauma necessitates a thorough preop mental status review and peripheral sensory exam. A CT scan of the head is indicated for any patient with loss of consciousness prior to anesthesia.
Musculoskeletal	For trauma patients, C-spine films will evaluate the stability of the C-spine before neck manipulation during ET intubation. Thoracic and lumbar x-rays also should be evaluated for the presence of traumatic spinal deformity or instability that would require special stabilization in the anesthetized patient. **Tests:** C-spine x-rays or others as indicated from H&P.

Hematologic   Restore Hct to 25% prior to inducing anesthesia. Have available 1 blood volume (70 ml/kg) or 1 total erythrocyte mass (20 ml/kg) for intraop transfusion. Transfusions of more than 1 blood volume will require monitoring and possible replacement of Plts and coag factors. The incidence of DVT is very high in these patients, and prophylaxis with SCDs or low-dose sc heparin is indicated whenever feasible.

Renal   Renal injury commonly results from trauma to the collecting system, myoglobinuria from rhabdomyolysis and ischemic, acute, tubular necrosis from hypovolemia or aortic dissection. Foley catheters should be placed only after urologic consultation for possible urethral tear. Suprapubic catheters are often necessary. Monitoring of UO is mandatory to detect intraop compromise of the collecting system, and to monitor adequacy of renal perfusion.
Tests: Consider UA; BUN; Cr; others as indicated from H&P.

Laboratory   Hct; electrolytes; other tests as indicated from H&P.

Premedication   In hemodynamically stable patients, pain can be treated with morphine (1-2 mg iv q 10 min titrated to pain relief) prior to anesthesia.

INTRAOPERATIVE

Anesthetic technique: GETA is indicated due to the duration and extent of the surgery, as well as the varied positions that are necessary to accomplish pelvic fixation. Regional anesthesia is generally inadequate for major pelvic surgery; however, in elective surgeries, serious consideration should be given to postop epidural analgesia.

Induction   A rapid-sequence induction (see p. B-5) is necessary for trauma patients to minimize aspiration risk. Elective cases can undergo a standard induction (see p. B-2).

Maintenance   Standard maintenance (see p. B-3).

Emergence   Extubate trauma patients when fully awake and protective airway reflexes have returned. Do not extubate patients with evolving pulmonary injuries (fat embolism, aspiration, or contusion). Monitoring in an ICU usually is indicated for trauma and cancer patients. Prolonged stays can be anticipated for patients with severe coexistent trauma.

Blood and fluid requirements	Large blood loss IV: 14-16 ga × 2 NS/LR @ 8-12 ml/kg/h 2-4 U PRBC in OR Warm fluids. Humidify gases.	Expect large blood losses (from 0.5-2 or more blood volumes) with all but augmentation procedures. Cell-scavenging techniques are useful to reduce the requirement for blood. Care should be taken to ensure that cells have been adequately washed to minimize ↓BP on reinfusion.
Control of blood loss	Deliberate hypotension Hemodilution	Patients with severe cardiovascular disease or carotid artery stenosis are not candidates for ↓BP. Full replacement of any volume deficit is mandatory before inducing ↓BP. Commonly used agents are isoflurane (1-3%) or esmolol (50-200 μg/kg/min) ± SNP (0.25-3 μg/kg/min). These agents are titrated to produce a 30% ↓ in preop MAP (but not < 60 mmHg).
Monitoring	Standard monitors (see p. B-1). Arterial line CVP line ± PA catheter ± TEE UO	Patients for shelf procedures may require only standard monitoring. Patients with myocardial dysfunction should have fluid and inotropic/pressor therapy, guided by a PA catheter and/or TEE.
Positioning	✓ and pad pressure points. ✓ eyes.	Meticulous padding of the chest, pelvis, and extremities is imperative to prevent nerve injury and ischemia of the extremities. ↓BP → risk of neurovascular injury.
Complications	Hypothermia Damage to urinary collecting system Major blood loss Coagulopathy	Warming of hypothermic patient may unmask severe volume depletion that will increase fluid requirement to well above apparent losses.

POSTOPERATIVE

Complications	Nerve root damage Peripheral nerve damage	Preop or intraop damage to L4-S5 nerve roots and cauda equina, resulting in hemiplegia and bladder and bowel dysfunction. Neuropathy of the femoral, genitofemoral, and lateral femoral cutaneous nerves can result from pressure on the ilioinguinal ligament during surgery.
Pain management	IV morphine Spinal opiates	Morphine 1-2 mg iv q 10 min prn Epidural hydromorphone 50 μg/ml infused at 100-250 μg/hr, ± bupivacaine 0.125-0.25% at 4-8 ml/h, provides excellent analgesia.
Tests	Hct CXR Coag profile, as indicated.	

References

1. Fung DL: Anesthesia and pain management. In *Chapman's Orthopaedic Surgery,* 3rd edition, Vol I. Chapman MW, ed. Lippincott Williams & Wilkins, Philadelphia: 2001, 133-56.
2. McCollough NC III: Complications of amputation surgery. In *Complications in Orthopaedic Surgery,* 3rd edition. Epps CH Jr, ed. JB Lippincott, Philadelphia: 1994.
3. Tooms RE: Amputations of lower extremity. In *Campbell's Operative Orthopaedics*, Vol 1, 9th edition. Crenshaw AH, ed. CV Mosby, St. Louis: 1998, 532-47.

ARTHROPLASTY OF THE HIP

SURGICAL CONSIDERATIONS

Description: **Total hip arthroplasty** is one of the most successful procedures in orthopedic surgery. In this procedure, the hip joint (Fig 10.4-7) is approached through one of several standard incisions. The femoral head is dislocated from the acetabulum, and the arthritic femoral head and a portion of the neck are excised. The acetabulum is reamed to accept a cemented or cementless cup made of metal and plastic. The femoral stem and head are usually modular, allowing for numerous shapes, sizes, lengths, etc. The metallic femoral component may be cemented or cementless. A hybrid total hip combines a cemented femoral stem and a cementless acetabular cup. After relocation of the new prosthetic hip joint and closure of the tissues, the patient usually is placed in traction or positioning devices to prevent dislocation. Mobilization takes place over the ensuing days.

Variant procedure or approaches: **Unipolar** (only the femoral side is replaced); **bipolar** (both the femoral side and the acetabular side are replaced; the acetabular cup is not fixed to the pelvis). **Revision procedures** are more arduous and time-consuming, as the 'failed' or loose component(s) must be removed and the bone prepared to accept new cemented or cementless components. These procedures require more specialized equipment for extracting prostheses and cement, and rebuilding the femoral or acetabular bone stock (allografts, autografts, etc.). Often, special components are needed for implantation of a new prosthesis. In the **Girdlestone procedure** (**resection arthroplasty**), the components are removed, but not replaced. This procedure is usually performed for infection.

Usual preop diagnosis: Fracture of femoral neck; arthritis of hip; arthrosis of hip; loose (or malpositioned) hip prosthesis; chronic dislocation of hip arthroplasty; infected hip arthroplasty

SUMMARY OF PROCEDURES

	Unipolar, Bipolar, Total Hip Replacement	Revision, Total Hip Replacement	Girdlestone Resection Arthroplasty
Position	Supine (for anterior or antero-lateral approaches); lateral decubitus position (for lateral or posterior approaches)	⇐	⇐

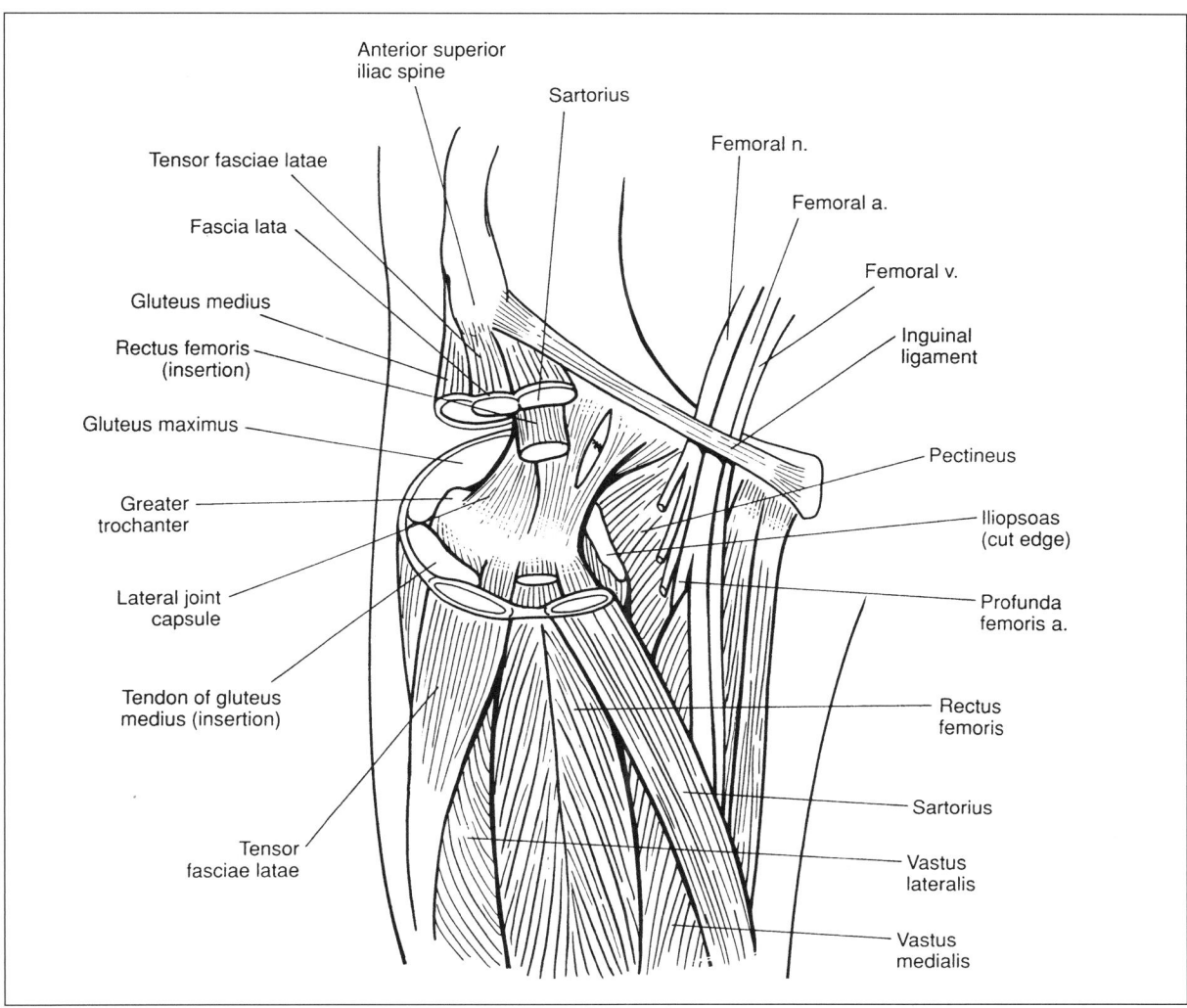

Figure 10.4-7. Surgical exposure of the hip joint: The hip joint may be exposed through a number of approaches. The relevant anatomical landmarks are shown here. (Reproduced with permission from Hoppenfeld S, deBoer P: *Surgical Exposures in Orthopaedics*. JB Lippincott: 1984.)

	Unipolar, Bipolar, Total Hip Replacement	Revision, Total Hip Replacement	Girdlestone Resection Arthroplasty
Incision	Anterolateral, lateral or postero-lateral over hip joint	⇐	⇐
Special instrumentation	Appropriate prostheses and instrumentation	Special instruments for excising cement	⇐
Unique considerations	In lateral decubitus position, patient is usually stabilized by bean bag and/or kidney rests. SCDs used.	A trochanteric osteotomy is frequently performed.	⇐
Antibiotics	Cefazolin or cefamandole 1 g iv q 6 h × 48 h	⇐	⇐ after intraop cultures
Surgical time	2-3 h	3-6 h or more	3 h or more
EBL	500-750 ml (intraop blood retrieval system may be useful).	≥ 1000 ml; intraop blood retrieval recommended.	⇐
Postop care	Patient's legs immobilized between abduction wedge; or operated leg suspended in a splint or placed in traction.	⇐	⇐

	Unipolar, Bipolar, Total Hip Replacement	Revision, Total Hip Replacement	Girdlestone Resection Arthroplasty
Mortality	1-2% (increasing with age)	⇐	⇐
Morbidity	DVT:	⇐	⇐
	Without prophylaxis: ≥ 50%	⇐	⇐
	With low-molecular-weight heparin, coumadin, SCDs, or antiembolism stockings: 10-20%	⇐	⇐
	Heterotopic ossification: 3-50% (average, 13%; significant, 4-5%)	> 3-50%	⇐
	Intraop cementless fracture: 5-20%	⇐	⇐
	UTI: 7-14%	⇐	⇐
	Late aseptic loosening requiring revision: 5-10% (after 10 yr)	> 5-10%	⇐
	Wound infection: 1% Primary psoriatic and diabetic patients: 5-10% Primary OA: 1%	3-10%	⇐
	Hematoma (major): < 5%	⇐	5-10%
	Femoral/sciatic nerve injury: 0.7-3.5%	⇐	⇐
	PE: 1.8-3.4% (if no prophylaxis)	⇐	⇐
	Intraop cemented fracture: 1-3%	2-3%	1-3%
	Postopsubluxation/dislocation: 0.5-3%	⇐	–
	Vascular injury to iliac vessels: < 0.5%	> 0.5%	⇐
	Urinary retention requiring catheterization: Common	⇐	⇐
	GI bleed, MI, cholecystitis: Rare	⇐	–
			Neurological injury: 3-10%
Pain score	7	8	8

PATIENT POPULATION CHARACTERISTICS

Age range	Hip fracture and cases of arthrosis of the hip joint: generally > 60 yr
	Arthritis of the hip (e.g., rheumatoid arthritis or juvenile rheumatoid arthritis, traumatic arthritis): all ages
Male:Female	Dependent on disease etiology
Incidence	Common: approximately 200,000/yr in U.S.
Etiology	Osteoarthritis; seropositive or seronegative arthritis; avascular necrosis; traumatic arthritis; congenital dislocation of the hip
Associated conditions	Dependent on primary conditions (e.g., rheumatoid arthritis patients may have numerous deformities, cardiorespiratory disease, etc.)

ANESTHETIC CONSIDERATIONS

See Anesthetic Considerations for Hip Procedures, p. 813.

References

1. Berry DJ: Primary total hip arthroplasty. In *Chapman's Orthopaedic Surgery,* 3rd edition, Vol III. Chapman MW, ed. Lippincott Williams & Wilkins, Philadelphia: 2001, 2769-94.

2. Bierbaum BE, Pomeroy DL, Berklacich FM: Late complications of total hip replacement. In *The Hip and its Disorders*. Steinberg ME, ed. WB Saunders, Philadelphia: 1991, 1061-96.
3. Harkey JW: Arthroplasty of hip. In *Campbell's Operative Orthopaedics*, Vol I, 9th edition. Crenshaw AH, ed. Mosby-Year Book, St. Louis: 1998, 473-520.
4. Ranawat CS, Figgie MP: Early complications of total hip replacement. In *The Hip and its Disorders*. Steinberg ME, ed. WB Saunders, Philadelphia: 1991, 1042-60.
5. Shaw JA, Greer RB III: Complications of total hip replacement. In *Complications in Orthopaedic Surgery*, 3rd edition. Epps CH Jr, ed. JB Lippincott, Philadelphia: 1994, 1013-1106.

ARTHRODESIS OF THE HIP

SURGICAL CONSIDERATIONS

Description: In adults, this procedure is accomplished by fusing the femur to the acetabulum. Some form of internal fixation is usually employed; a spica cast is sometimes placed immediately postop or a few days later. The patient is usually not a good candidate for total hip arthroplasty (e.g., a young, healthy male with unilateral traumatic arthritis). The hip usually is fused in 30° of flexion, 10-30° of external rotation, and neutral-to-slight adduction. The surgical procedure may be performed through anterior, lateral, or posterior incisions, with the lateral being most common. A **trochanteric osteotomy** facilitates exposure. After excising the cartilage surfaces, internal fixation, using screws ± a plate, is performed (Fig 10.4-8).

Usual preop diagnosis: Arthritis or arthrosis of the hip; previous septic arthritis of the hip; recurrent subluxation or dislocation of the hip

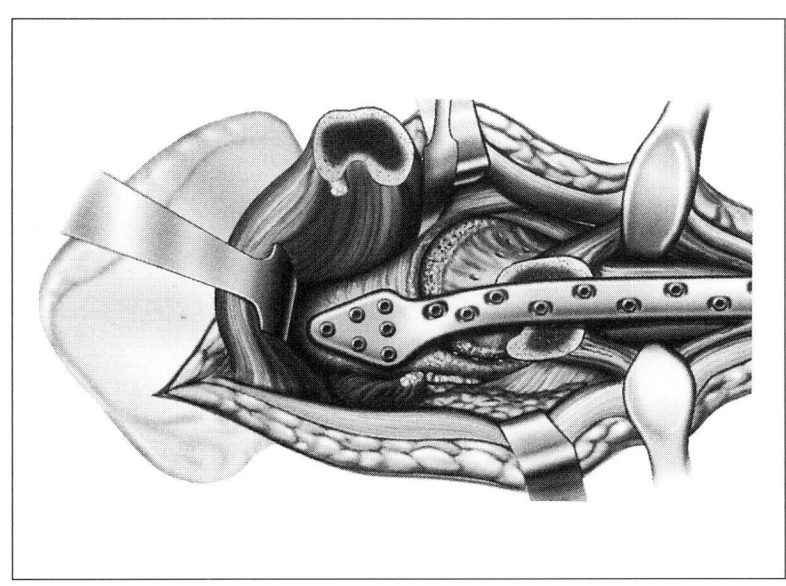

Figure 10.4-8. Application of cobra plate after it has molded to the shape of the acetabulum and femur, and initial fixation with one proximal + distal outrigger compression screws. (Reproduced with permission from Sledge CB, ed: *The Hip*. Lippincott-Raven, 1998.)

SUMMARY OF PROCEDURE

Position	Usually supine; occasionally lateral decubitus
Incision	Anterior or lateral thigh
Special instrumentation	Plates and screws or other internal fixation; reamers from surface replacement arthroplasty set also may be useful; intraop x-ray; fracture table
Unique considerations	Intraop radiographs or I.I. used with patient on fracture table
Antibiotics	Broad-spectrum cephalosporin (e.g., cefazolin 1 g iv q 6 h × 48 h)
Surgical time	3-4 h
EBL	500-1000 ml; Cell Saver recommended.
Postop care	Spica cast
Mortality	Extremely low

Morbidity	Limb shortening: Some shortening is always present
	Delayed union, nonunion, malunion: 10-15%
	Femoral shaft fracture: 5-10%
	Wound infection: < 1%
	Genitourinary problems: urinary retention requiring catheterization: Common
	Ileus: Common
	Late degenerative arthritis of other lower extremity joints or back: Common, many yr later
	Injury to iliac or femoral vessels: Rare
	Neurological deficit; injury to lateral cutaneous nerve, sciatic, or femoral nerves: Not uncommon
	Osteomyelitis: Rare
	Vascular complications: Rare
	Superior mesenteric artery syndrome causing duodenal obstruction: Extremely rare
	Thromboembolism: See Arthroplasty of the Hip, p. 810.
Pain score	9

PATIENT POPULATION CHARACTERISTICS

Age range	18-50 yr
Male:Female	Usually males > females
Incidence	Rare
Etiology	Trauma, general; neuromuscular disorders (cerebral palsy, meningomyelocele); trauma to acetabular growth plate; congenital hip dysplasia
Associated conditions	Depends on etiology.

ANESTHETIC CONSIDERATIONS

See Anesthetic Considerations for Hip Procedures, p. 813.

References

1. Carnesale PG, Stewart MJ: Complications of arthrodesis surgery. In *Complications in Orthopaedic Surgery*. Epps CH Jr, ed. JB Lippincott, Philadelphia: 1986, 1289-1306.
2. Gill PS, Paprosky WG: Failed hip arthroplasty: revision and arthrodesis. In *Chapman's Orthopaedic Surgery,* 3rd edition, Vol III. Chapman MW, ed. Lippincott Williams & Wilkins, Philadelphia: 2001, 2795-2858.
3. Matta JM, Siebenrock KA, Gautier E, Mehne D, Ganz: Hip fusion through an anterior approach with the use of a ventral plate. *Clin Orthop* 1997; 337:129-39.
4. Russell TA: Arthrodesis of the lower extremity and hip. In *Campbell's Operative Orthopaedics,* Vol 2. Crenshaw AH, ed. CV Mosby, St. Louis: 1987, 1091-1130.

SYNOVECTOMY OF THE HIP

SURGICAL CONSIDERATIONS

Description: An **arthrotomy** of the hip joint is performed through one of several standard approaches (anterior, anterolateral, lateral, posterior). A **capsulotomy** is performed, and is closed with reabsorbable sutures later in the case. Generally, the hip is not dislocated, but the cartilage surfaces are inspected and documented. The synovium, as well as any loose bodies, cartilage flaps, and osteophytes, are excised. Although weight-bearing is usually protected, ROM and strengthening exercises are begun early.

Usual preop diagnosis: Chronic synovitis of hip; loose bodies in hip; juvenile and adult rheumatoid arthritis; pigmented villonodular synovitis

SUMMARY OF PROCEDURE

Position	Supine for anterior or anterolateral surgical approaches; lateral decubitus for posterior approaches
Incision	Overlying hip joint, depending on specific surgical approach
Unique considerations	Patient may have systemic disease (e.g., rheumatoid arthritis); careful positioning of limbs is necessary to avoid fracture or skin slough.
Antibiotics	Cefazolin or cefamandole 1 g iv q 6-8 h
Surgical time	2 h
EBL	< 500 ml
Mortality	Rare
Morbidity	Thromboembolism: 10-50%
	Neurovascular injury—femoral or sciatic nerve, or iliac vessels: < 3%
	Wound infection or dehiscence: < 3%
	Septic arthritis and osteomyelitis: < 1% (unless synovectomy is performed for infection).
	Avascular necrosis of femoral head: Rare (if hip is not dislocated).
	Hematoma: Rare (if drainage tubes used).
	Inability to void, requiring urinary catheterization: Common
Pain score	7-8

PATIENT POPULATION CHARACTERISTICS

Age range	< 60 yr
Male:Female	Dependent on disease etiology (e.g., preponderance of females in rheumatoid arthritis)
Incidence	Rare
Etiology	Septic arthritis (very common); rheumatoid arthritis, juvenile/adult (rare); pigmented villonodular synovitis (rare); trauma (rare)
Associated conditions	See Etiology, above.

ANESTHETIC CONSIDERATIONS FOR HIP PROCEDURES

(Procedures covered: hip arthroplasty, arthrodesis, synovectomy)

PREOPERATIVE

Osteoarthritis is the most common indication for hip arthroplasty. These patients are usually elderly and their anesthetic management is tailored to any concurrent disease. Rheumatoid and other inflammatory arthritides form another group of candidates for these procedures and the special anesthetic considerations for these patients are outlined below. Avascular necrosis of the hip is seen in patients with sickle-cell disease and in heart transplant patients.

Respiratory	Patients with rheumatoid arthritis frequently have associated pulmonary complications. SOB on performing activities of daily living or exercise (e.g., climbing a flight of stairs) warrants further evaluation with PFTs. Pulmonary effusions are common. Pulmonary fibrosis (rare) often manifests as cough and dyspnea. Rheumatoid arthritis involvement of the cricoarytenoid joints may produce glottic narrowing (requiring small ETT) and manifest as hoarseness. Arthritic involvement of the TMJ limits mouth opening and may necessitate special techniques (e.g., fiber optic or light wand) for ET intubation.
	Tests: As indicated from H&P.
Cardiovascular	The severity of the arthritis often limits exercise; thus, a dobutamine stress ECHO and/or dipyridamole/thallium imaging may be necessary for adequate cardiac evaluation in patients with poor exercise tolerance. HTN and cardiovascular disease are common in elderly patients (dysrhythmias/TIAs → fall → hip fracture). Rheumatoid arthritis is associated with pericardial effusion, cardiac valve fibrosis, cardiac conduction abnormalities and aortic regurgitation (AR). An ECG is indicated in all rheumatoid arthritis patients, and ECHO is indicated for patients with physical Sx suggestive of tamponade or cardiovascular disease.
	Tests: As indicated from H&P.
Neurological	In patients with rheumatoid arthritis, a thorough neurological exam preop often yields evidence of cervical nerve-root compression. Patients with arthritis involving the cervical spine should have

Neurological, cont.	lateral neck films preop to determine the stability of the atlanto-occipital joint. After the stability of the spine has been established, full ROM of the neck should be evaluated for evidence of further nerve-root compression or cerebral ischemia (suggesting vertebral artery compression). Evidence of cerebral ischemia mandates a neurovascular evaluation to plan intraop BP management. **Tests:** As indicated from H&P.
Musculoskeletal	Pain and ↓joint mobility make positioning and regional anesthesia difficult in patients with arthritis.
Hematologic	Rheumatoid arthritis patients often have anemia. Also, anemia may be 2° NSAID gastritis. Patients with Hb > 12 g/dL are candidates for preop autologous blood donation. Hip fracture → potential large-volume blood loss at fracture site. DVT is common after hip surgery, and prophylaxis for its occurrence reduces mortality. Effective preventive measures include SCDs and sc heparin. NSAID-induced coagulopathy may preclude the use of regional anesthesia. **Tests:** As indicated from H&P.
Renal	Estimation of renal function may be useful to predict drug clearance and the need for invasive monitoring in this elderly population. **Tests:** As indicated from H&P.
Laboratory	Other tests as indicated from H&P.
Premedication	In the absence of limited pulmonary reserve or severe cardiac disease, a standard premedication (see p. B-2) is appropriate. Full-stomach precautions (p. B-5) may be necessary for patients in acute pain.

INTRAOPERATIVE

Anesthetic technique: GETA or regional anesthesia (may be difficult 2° pain on positioning).

General anesthesia:

Induction	The lateral position may mandate ET intubation for patients undergoing GA. A careful preop airway evaluation will determine the need for special airway techniques (e.g., fiber optic intubation or light wand). Aggravation of cricoarytenoid arthritis that is common in rheumatoid arthritis patients can be minimized if a small ETT (6-7 mm cuffed) is used. For otherwise healthy patients, standard induction (p. B-2) is appropriate.
Maintenance	Standard maintenance (p. B-3). Neuromuscular blockade facilitates the placement and testing of the prosthesis. In otherwise healthy patients, induced hypotension (e.g., ↓20%) → ↓blood loss.
Emergence	No special considerations

Regional anesthesia: Induction of regional anesthesia, with its attendant positioning requirements, can be uncomfortable in patients with limited joint mobility. Rheumatoid arthritis patients, however, rarely have involvement of the lumbar spine, and regional anesthesia offers the advantages of decreased periop DVT, decreased intraop blood loss and no need for airway manipulation. Anesthesia to T10 is adequate. Full motor blockade is essential for placement of the prosthesis and assessment of the passive ROM. Lumbar epidural block (15-20 ml 2% lidocaine with epinephrine 1:200,000, administered over 15 min) has the advantage of slow onset, allowing time to treat the induced cardiovascular changes. Postop epidural opiates can provide excellent analgesia. Spinal anesthesia, with 15 mg of bupivacaine 0.5% and morphine 0.2 mg placed at L3-L4, has a more rapid onset than epidural anesthesia and yields analgesia for up to 24 h postop.

Blood and fluid requirements	Major blood loss IV: 14-16 ga × 2 NS/LR @ 4-8 ml/kg/h	Cell scavenging helps reduce total transfusion requirement. Care should be taken to ensure that cells have been adequately washed to minimize ↓BP on reinfusion.
Control of blood loss	Regional anesthesia Controlled hypotension	These techniques may be appropriate in selected patient populations.
Monitoring	Standard monitors (see p. B-1). ± CVP line ± Arterial line	Invasive monitoring is indicated in the presence of exercise-limiting cardiac or pulmonary disease.
Positioning	Axillary roll, bean bag ✓ and pad pressure points. ✓ eyes.	Meticulous padding of extremities and maintaining a neutral neck position are mandatory. A bean bag and axillary roll also are necessary to stabilize patient in the lateral position and to protect dependent arm from neurovascular compression injuries.

| **Complications** | Methylmethacrylate: | Embolization of air, fat, bone fragments, and cement may occur during insertion of the femoral prosthesis. Systemic ↓BP and pulmonary HTN may occur. Care should be taken to ensure that patient is adequately hydrated before procedure, and pressors may be necessary to maintain BP (ephedrine 5-20 mg iv or epinephrine 10-100 μg iv and increasing the dose as necessary). |

Complications   Methylmethacrylate:
      ↓BP 2° vasodilation
      ↓PaO$_2$ 2° embolization
      Cardiovascular collapse
      VAE
      Major blood loss
      DVT (femoral vein: 80%)
      Nerve damage
      Femur fracture

Embolization of air, fat, bone fragments, and cement may occur during insertion of the femoral prosthesis. Systemic ↓BP and pulmonary HTN may occur. Care should be taken to ensure that patient is adequately hydrated before procedure, and pressors may be necessary to maintain BP (ephedrine 5-20 mg iv or epinephrine 10-100 μg iv and increasing the dose as necessary).

POSTOPERATIVE

Complications   Nerve damage
      DVT
      Continued blood loss

Sciatic nerve injury is evidenced by foot drop and an inability to flex the knee.

Pain management   Spinal opiates
      Epidural analgesia

Epidural hydromorphone 50 μg/ml infused at 100-250 μg/hr provides excellent analgesia.

Tests   Hct
      CXR, if CVP was placed.
      Monitor UO

References

1. Dutkowsky JP: Miscellaneous nontraumatic disorders. In *Campbell's Operative Orthopaedics*, Vol 1, 9th edition. Crenshaw AH, ed. Mosby-Year Book, St. Louis: 1998, 787-856.
2. Fung DL: Anesthesia and pain management. In *Chapman's Orthopaedic Surgery*, 3rd edition, Vol I. Chapman MW, ed. Lippincott Williams & Wilkins, Philadelphia: 2001, 133-56.

OPEN REDUCTION AND INTERNAL FIXATION (ORIF) OF PROXIMAL FEMORAL FRACTURES

(FEMORAL NECK, INTERTROCHANTERIC, SUBTROCHANTERIC FRACTURES)

SURGICAL CONSIDERATIONS

Description: Fractures of the proximal femur are seen in two distinct populations: most commonly in elderly patients as the result of falls, and in younger patients following trauma. In elderly patients, the fracture occurs through osteoporotic bone in the femoral neck, intertrochanteric or subtrochanteric area (Fig 10.4-9). Displaced femoral neck fractures are usually treated by **prosthetic replacement**. Nondisplaced or minimally displaced femoral neck fractures are usually treated by **closed reduction and percutaneous pinning** of the fracture. Intertrochanteric and subtrochanteric fractures, whether displaced or nondisplaced, are usually treated by **ORIF with a nail/plate or nail/rod device** (Fig 10.4-10). Prosthetic replacement

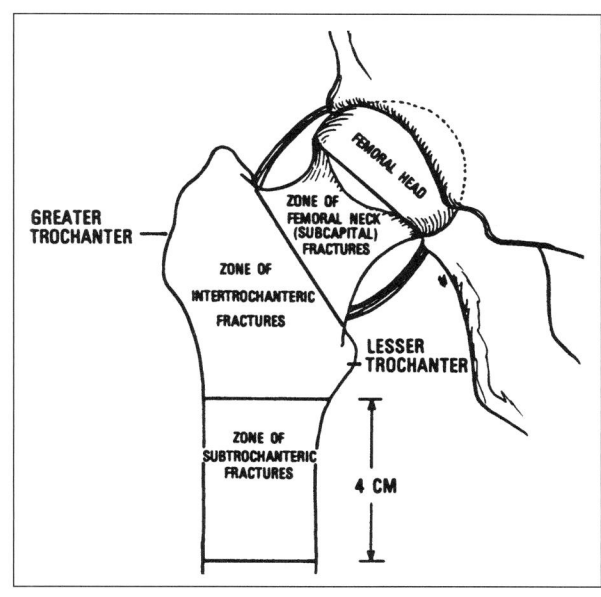

Figure 10.4-9. Anatomical classification of fractures of the proximal femur. (Reproduced with permission from Hardy JD: *Hardy's Textbook of Surgery*, 2nd edition. JB Lippincott, 1988.)

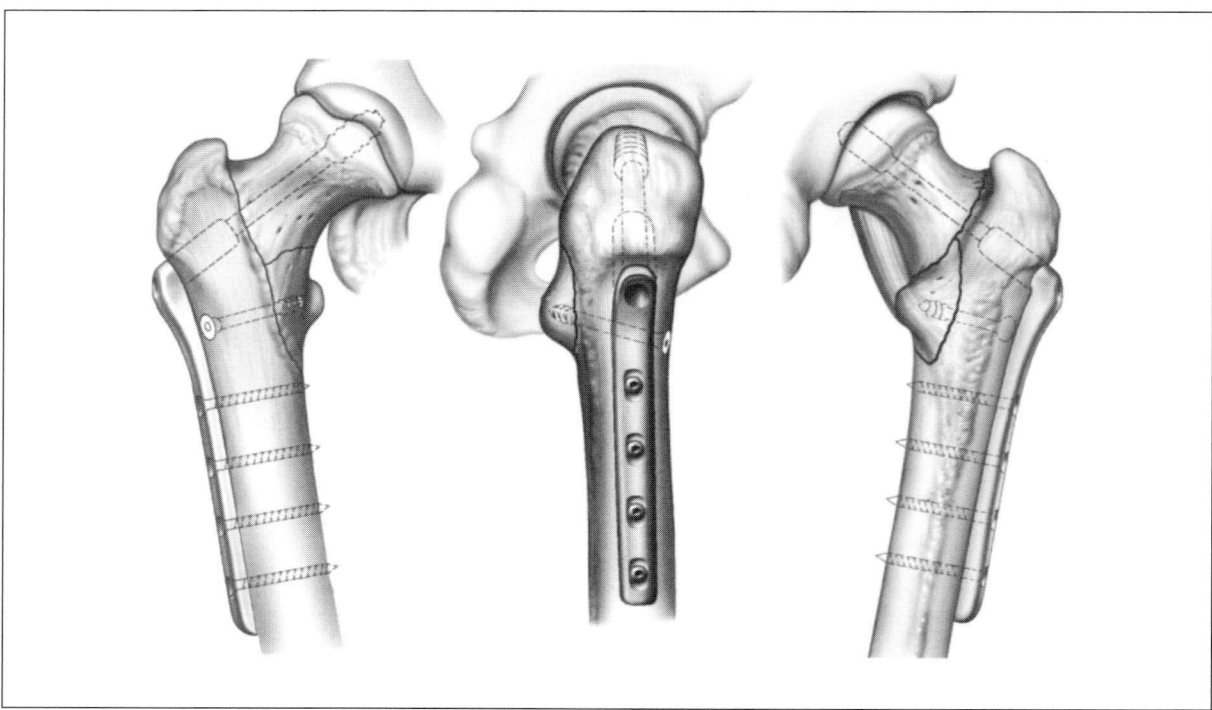

Figure 10.4-10. Intertrochanteric hip fracture treated with dynamic hip screw. (Reproduced with permission from Sledge CB, ed: *The Hip*. Lippincott-Raven, 1998.)

is performed only rarely. Elderly patients frequently have numerous medical problems, which means that the fractures require prompt internal fixation/prosthetic replacement to facilitate early mobilization. In younger patients (16-40 yr), proximal femoral fractures are almost always treated by ORIF with screws, plates and screws, or intramedullary devices. These are normally much higher energy fractures, often associated with multiple trauma.

Variant procedure or approaches: Variants include: **percutaneous pinning** of nondisplaced femoral neck fracture; **ORIF of displaced femoral neck fracture** (also see Arthroplasty of the Hip, p. 808); **ORIF of intertrochanteric or subtrochanteric fracture.**

Usual preop diagnosis: Nondisplaced femoral neck fracture; displaced femoral neck fracture (those not requiring prosthetic replacement); intertrochanteric ± subtrochanteric fracture

SUMMARY OF PROCEDURES

	Nondisplaced Femoral Neck Fracture	**Displaced Femoral Neck Fracture**	**Intertrochanteric ± Subtrochanteric Fracture**
Position	Supine, on fracture table	⇐	⇐
Incision	Proximal lateral thigh	⇐	⇐
Special instrumentation	Usually multiple percutaneous pins	Multiple screws or other devices	Screw-plate device or intramedullary device
Unique considerations	Fracture table and I.I. used. Percutaneous pinning may be accomplished with local anesthesia only.	⇐	⇐
Antibiotics	Broad-spectrum cephalosporin (e.g., cefazolin or cefamandole 1 g iv q 6-8 h × 48 h)	⇐	⇐
Surgical time	1 h	1.5-2 h, including placing patient on fracture table and obtaining adequate reduction of fracture	1.5-3 h
EBL	< 100 ml	250-500 ml	500+ ml

	Nondisplaced Femoral Neck Fracture	Displaced Femoral Neck Fracture	Intertrochanteric ± Subtrochanteric Fracture
Postop care	Generally PACU → room; if medically unstable, → ICU	⇐	⇐
Mortality	10-30% in first 12 mo postop in elderly; in younger patients, depends on other involved trauma.	⇐	⇐
Morbidity	Dysrhythmias: ~50%	⇐	⇐
	MI: ~50%	⇐	⇐
	Respiratory failure: ~50%	⇐	⇐
	Urinary retention requiring catheterization: ~50%	⇐	⇐
	UTI: ~50%	⇐	⇐
	Thromboembolism: 40%+	⇐	⇐
	Avascular necrosis and late segmental collapse: 10-20%	≥15-35%	1%
	Infection, deep: 2-17%	⇐	⇐
	Infection, superficial: 2-17%	⇐	⇐
	Septic arthritis: 2-17%	⇐	⇐
	Nonunion: 5-15%	20-30%	2%
	Malunion: < 10%	> 10%	10-20%
	Loss of reduction: < %5	> 10%	10%
	Hematoma	–	–
	Intraop comminution of the fracture	–	–
	Neurological injury: Rare	⇐	⇐
	Vascular injury: Rare	⇐	⇐
Pain score	5-6	7	8

PATIENT POPULATION CHARACTERISTICS

Age range	Usually > 60 yr (patients with an intertrochanteric fracture average 65-70 yr); occasionally, younger patients, 16-35 yr (as part of multiple-trauma situation)
Male:Female	Elderly 1:4-5
Incidence	Extremely common—about 5-100/100,000; femoral neck fractures are about twice as common as intertrochanteric fractures.
Etiology	Accidents and falls (may be 2° TIA, stroke, MI, dysrhythmia); pathological fracture; multiple trauma (younger patients); stress fracture
Associated conditions	Numerous serious medical conditions often present in elderly; senile dementia; multiple trauma often

ANESTHETIC CONSIDERATIONS

See Anesthetic Considerations for Lower-Extremity Procedures, p. 863.

References

1. Chapman MW: Fractures of the hip and proximal femur. In *Chapman's Orthopaedic Surgery,* Vol I, 3rd edition. Chapman MW, ed. Lippincott Williams & Wilkins, Philadelphia: 2001, 617-70.
2. Guyton JL: Fractures of the hip, acetabulum, and pelvis. In *Campbell's Operative Orthopaedics*, Vol 3, 9th edition. Crenshaw AH, ed. CV Mosby, St. Louis: 1998, 2181-2280.
3. Kyle RF, Schmidt AH, Campbell SJ: Complications of the treatment of fractures and dislocations of the hip. In *Complications in Orthopaedic Surgery*, 3rd edition. Epps CH Jr, ed. JB Lippincott, Philadelphia: 1994, 443-86.
4. LaVelle DG: Delayed union and nonunion of fractures. In *Campbell's Operative Orthopaedics*, Vol 3, 9th edition. Crenshaw AH, ed. CV Mosby, St. Louis: 1998, 2579-2630.

OPEN REDUCTION AND INTERNAL FIXATION (ORIF) OF DISTAL FEMUR FRACTURES

SURGICAL CONSIDERATIONS

Description: ORIF of the distal femur fracture involves a longitudinal incision along the femoral shaft, obtaining reduction by direct visualization of the fracture fragments, and applying plates and screws along the femur for rigid internal fixation. An iliac crest bone graft may be necessary. Some intramedullary devices are also available for fixation of these fractures.

Usual preop diagnosis: Fracture of the distal femur; nonunion/malunion of the distal femur; degenerative arthritis of knee, with deformity

SUMMARY OF PROCEDURE

Position	Supine. Patient usually arrives at OR in balanced traction if fracture is acute.
Incision	Anterior knee, lateral or medial thigh along the femoral shaft
Special instrumentation	Special plates, screws, rods, reduction clamps; radiolucent table; intraop blood salvage
Unique considerations	Usually requires intraop radiographs; tourniquet.
Antibiotics	Broad-spectrum cephalosporin (e.g., cefazolin or cefamandole 1 g iv q 6-8 h × 48 h)
Surgical time	3 h (or more, depending on difficulty)
EBL	750 ml or more
Postop care	Multiple-trauma victim → ICU; others → PACU
Mortality	~3-4%, depending on the extent of multiple trauma
Morbidity	Nonunion: 4-33%
	Malunion: 4-31%
	Infection, osteomyelitis, septic arthritis; closed/open:
	Grade I: 1-5%
	Grade II: 5-20%
	Grade III: > 20%
	Delayed union: 0-17%
	Vascular complications: 2-3%
	Neurological deficit to peripheral nerves, peroneal nerve: ~3%
	Compartment syndrome: Rare
	Hypotension: Rare
	Leg-length discrepancy: Rare
	Respiratory distress and fat embolism: Rare
Pain score	8

PATIENT POPULATION CHARACTERISTICS

Age range	Any age; predominance of males < 40 yr (trauma); degenerative arthritis of knee < 60 yr. Special rare case is elderly patient with a supracondylar fracture above a total knee replacement.
Male:Female	5:1
Incidence	Common in trauma center patients; rare in cases of degenerative arthritis of knee (osteotomy) or elderly patient with a supracondylar fracture above a total knee replacement.
Etiology	Motorcycle and motor vehicle accidents; falls; industrial injury; degenerative arthritis of knee
Associated conditions	Frequently associated with trauma to other organ systems.

ANESTHETIC CONSIDERATIONS

See Anesthetic Considerations for Lower-Extremity Procedures, p. 863.

References

1. LaVelle DG: Delayed union and nonunion of fractures. In *Campbell's Operative Orthopaedics*, Vol 3, 9th edition. Crenshaw AH, ed. CV Mosby, St. Louis: 1998, 2579-2630.
2. Mize R: Supracondylar and articular fractures of the distal femur. In *Chapman's Orthopaedic Surgery,* 3rd edition, Vol I. Chapman MW, ed. Lippincott Williams & Wilkins, Philadelphia: 2001, 709-23.

3. Mize R, Johnson EE, Hohl M: Complications of fractures and dislocations of the knee. In *Complications in Orthopaedic Surgery*, 3rd edition. Epps CH Jr, ed. JB Lippincott, Philadelphia: 1994, 525-56.
4. Whittle AP: Fractures of lower extremity. In *Campbell's Operative Orthopaedics*, Vol 3, 9th edition. Crenshaw AH, ed. CV Mosby, St. Louis: 1998, 2042-2180.
5. Whittle AP: Malunited fractures. In *Campbell's Operative Orthopaedics*, 9th edition. Crenshaw AH, ed. Mosby, St. Louis: 1998, 2579-2630.
6. Wiss DA, Watson JT, Johnson EE: Fractures of the knee. In *Rockwood and Green's Fractures in Adults*, 4th edition. Rockwood CA Jr, Green DP, Bucholz RW, Hickman JD, eds. Lippincott-Raven, Philadelphia: 1996, 1919-2000.

OPEN REDUCTION AND INTERNAL FIXATION (ORIF) OF THE FEMORAL SHAFT WITH PLATE

SURGICAL CONSIDERATIONS

Description: ORIF of the femoral shaft involves obtaining a reduction by open means, usually through a longitudinal lateral incision along the length of the femur, and applying plates and screws along the femur to maintain the reduction. An iliac crest bone graft may be necessary.

Usual preop diagnosis: Fracture of femur

SUMMARY OF PROCEDURE

Position	Supine or lateral decubitus
Incision	Lateral thigh along length of femur ± iliac crest incision
Special instrumentation	Special plates, screws; reduction clamps; blood salvage device
Unique considerations	Fracture or radiolucent table; I.I. Patient usually arrives at OR in balanced traction.
Antibiotics	Broad-spectrum cephalosporin (e.g., cefazolin or cefamandole 1 g iv q 6-8 h)
Surgical time	3 h or more, depending on difficulty
EBL	750 ml; Cell Saver recommended.
Postop care	Multiple-trauma victims: ICU
	Others: PACU
Mortality	Dependent on extent of multiple trauma
Morbidity	Knee stiffness: 20-30%
	Delayed union, nonunion, malunion: 5-21%
	Leg-length discrepancy: 0-11%
	Failure of fixation: 5-10%
	Infection, osteomyelitis: < 5%
	Hypotension: Not uncommon
	Respiratory distress and fat embolism: Not uncommon, often subclinical
	Compartment syndrome: Rare
	Neurological deficit to peripheral nerves: Rare
	Vascular complications: Rare
Pain score	9

PATIENT POPULATION CHARACTERISTICS

Age range	Any age, but predominance of males < 30 yr
Male:Female	5:1
Incidence	Unknown
Etiology	Motorcycle and motor vehicle accidents; falls; industrial injuries
Associated conditions	Frequently associated with trauma to other organ systems

ANESTHETIC CONSIDERATIONS

See Anesthetic Considerations for Lower-Extremity Procedures, p. 863.

References

1. Azer R, Rankin EA: Complications of femoral shaft fractures. In *Complications in Orthopaedic Surgery*, 3rd edition. Epps CH Jr, ed. JB Lippincott, Philadelphia: 1986, 487-524.
2. Bucholz RW, Brumback RJ: Fractures of the shaft of the femur. In *Rockwood and Green's Fractures in Adults*, 4th edition. Rockwood CA Jr, Green DP, Bucholz RW, Heckman JD, eds. JB Lippincott, Philadelphia: 1996, 1827-1918.
3. LaVelle DG: Delayed union and nonunion of fractures. In *Campbell's Operative Orthopaedics*, Vol 3, 9th edition. Crenshaw AH, ed. CV Mosby, St. Louis: 1998, 2579-2630.
4. Matta JM, Siebenrock KA, Gautier E, Mehne D, Ganz R: Hip fusion through an anterior approach with the use of a ventral plate. *Clin Orthop* 1997; 337-129-39.
5. Whittle AP: Malunited fractures. In *Campbell's Operative Orthopaedics*, 9th edition. Crenshaw AH, ed. Mosby, St. Louis: 1998, 2579-2630.

INTRAMEDULLARY NAILING OF FEMORAL SHAFT

SURGICAL CONSIDERATIONS

Description: Intramedullary nailing of the femur is the standard procedure for fractures of the femoral shaft. It is indicated for virtually any fracture, from the lesser trochanter to the distal femur, within 7 cm of the articular surface. The procedure also is used for the treatment of nonunions and malunions of the femoral shaft. Typically, the nail is placed in an antero-grade fashion from proximal to distal. There are, however, indications in which the nail is inserted in a retrograde fashion from distal to proximal (e.g., bilateral femur fractures; ipsilateral femur and tibia fractures; distal femur fractures; and multiple-trauma, obese, and pregnant patients). Early fixation of femoral shaft fractures in severe polytrauma has several benefits. The advantages of early fixation of long bones include improved pain control, early mobilization, improved pulmonary function, and decreased morbidity and mortality.

Femoral nails are inserted after reaming the intramedullary canal, which allows a larger diameter implant and improves the mechanical properties of the bone implant interface. Reaming may produce systemic effects by embolic showering of medullary contents to the pulmonary vasculature, a phenomenon that has been documented by TEE. This situation may be exacerbated in the polytrauma patient with pulmonary injury, and may produce posttraumatic pulmonary failure. Patients with femur fractures may have associated injuries.

Patients may arrive from the ICU in skeletal traction or from the emergency department, especially in the case of an open fracture. Hemorrhage up to 1 L may be contained in the thigh following a femur fracture; therefore, patients may be hypovolemic at the start of the procedure. Since the procedure is essentially percutaneous, apparent blood loss may be underestimated because of the hemorrhaged blood contained in the thigh.

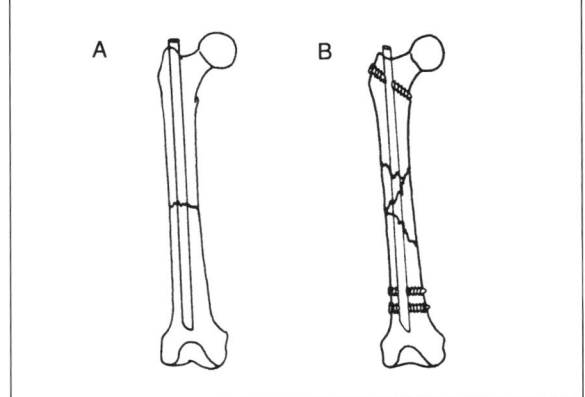

Figure 10.4-11. (A) Simple and (B) locked intramedullary fixation of femoral shaft. (Reproduced with permission from Hardy JD: *Hardy's Textbook of Surgery*, 2nd edition. JB Lippincott, 1988.)

The patient is placed in the supine or lateral decubitus position on either a radiolucent table or a fracture table. Ante-grade insertion of the nail requires a lateral incision several cm in length proximal to the greater trochanter. The hip abductors are split, and portal into the femoral canal is created in the piriformis fossa. The femoral canal is reamed over a guide wire. The intramedullary nail is then inserted into the intramedullary canal with gentle taps, using a hammer.

Retrograde insertion of the nail is performed through an incision several cm long over the anterior aspect of the knee. The knee joint is entered and the portal to the intramedullary canal is made in the nonweight-bearing portion of the inter-condylar notch. The nail is inserted in the same fashion as the anterior nail. Cross-locking screws are commonly used, and they are inserted through the rod.

Variant procedure or approaches: The application of femoral nailing has been expanded to treat nonunions, malunions, posttraumatic deformities of the femur, and leg-length differences. Specialized additional equipment, such as an intramedullary saw or an external fixator, may be required for these procedures.

Usual preop diagnosis: Femur fracture; nonunion/malunion of the femur; leg-length discrepancy

SUMMARY OF PROCEDURE

Position	Supine or lateral decubitus
Incision	Proximal lateral thigh or anterior knee
Special instrumentation	Intramedullary nails; intramedullary saw for closed femoral shortening of femur; fracture or radiolucent table; I.I.
Unique considerations	Patient may have multiple trauma with other associated injuries. Procedure is heavily dependent on I.I.
Antibiotics	Broad-spectrum cephalosporin (e.g., cefazolin 1 g iv q 6-8)
Surgical time	2-3 h; 3+ h for nonunion/malunion of femur or closed femoral shortening of femur
EBL	250-500 ml; ≥ 750 ml for nonunion/malunion of femur or closed femoral shortening of femur (Cell Saver recommended).
Postop care	If surgery performed acutely, patient is usually a multiple-trauma victim with numerous injuries and extensive blood loss; usually goes to ICU.
Mortality	Dependent on extent of trauma

Morbidity	Respiratory distress and fat embolism: 10%
	Malunion: 5-10%
	Infection, osteomyelitis:
	  Open technique: 1-10%
	  Closed technique: 0-1%
	Neurological deficit to peripheral nerves: 2%
	Vascular complications: ~2% (up to 15% have occult vascular abnormalities)
	Delayed union: 1%
	Nonunion: 1%
	Hypotension: Common in multiple-trauma situations
	Knee stiffness: Common
	Leg-length discrepancies: Not uncommon
	Compartment syndrome: Rare
	Failure of fixation: Rare

Pain score	6

PATIENT POPULATION CHARACTERISTICS

Age range	Any age, but predominance of males < 30 yr
Male:Female	5:1
Incidence	Very common
Etiology	Motorcycle and motor vehicle accidents (60-80%); falls (5-10%); industrial injuries (5-10%); previous trauma (rare)
Associated conditions	Frequently associated with trauma to other organ systems.

ANESTHETIC CONSIDERATIONS

See Anesthetic Considerations for Lower-Extremity Procedures, p. 863.

References

1. Azer R, Rankin EA: Complications of femoral shaft fractures. In *Complications in Orthopaedic Surgery*, 3rd edition. Epps CH Jr, ed. JB Lippincott, Philadelphia: 1986, 487-524.
2. Bone LB, Johnson KD, Weigelt J: Early versus delayed stabilization of femoral fractures: a prospective randomized study. *J Bone Joint Surg* (Am) 1989; 71(3):336-40.
3. Bucholz RW, Brumback RJ: Fractures of the shaft of the femur. In *Rockwood and Green's Fractures in Adults*, 4th edition. Rockwood CA Jr, Green DP, Bucholz RW, Heckman JD, eds. Lippincott-Raven, Philadelphia: 1996, 1827-1918.
4. Chapman MW: Diaphyseal fractures of the femur. In *Chapman's Orthopaedic Surgery,* 3rd edition, Vol I. Chapman MW, ed. Lippincott Williams & Wilkins, Philadelphia: 2001, 671-708.
5. Chapman MW: Fractures of the hip and proximal femur. In *Chapman's Orthopaedic Surgery,* 3rd edition, Vol I. Chapman MW, ed. Lippincott Williams & Wilkins, Philadelphia: 2001, 617-70.

6. LaVelle DG: Delayed union and nonunion of fractures. In *Campbell's Operative Orthopaedics*, Vol 3, 9th edition. Crenshaw AH, ed. CV Mosby, St. Louis: 1998, 2579-2630.

7. Mize RD: Supracondylar and articular fractures of the distal femur. In *Chapman's Orthopaedic Surgery*, 3rd edition, Vol I. Chapman MW, ed. Lippincott Williams & Wilkins, Philadelphia: 2001, 709-23.

8. Pape HC, Regel G, Dwenger A: Influences of different methods of intramedullary femoral nailing on lung function in patients with multiple trauma. *J Trauma* 1993; 35(5):709-16.

9. Wenda K, Runkel M, Degeif J: Pathogenesis and clinical relevance of bone marrow embolism in medullary nailing—demonstrated by intraoperative echocardiography injury. *Injury* 1993; 24(Suppl 3):73-81.

10. Whittle AP: Malunited fractures. In *Campbell's Operative Orthopaedics*, 9th edition. Crenshaw AH, ed. Mosby, St. Louis: 1998, 2579-2630.

REPAIR OF NONUNION/MALUNION OF PROXIMAL THIRD OF FEMUR, PROXIMAL FEMORAL OSTEOTOMY FOR OSTEOARTHRITIS

SURGICAL CONSIDERATIONS

Description: Operations for nonunion/malunion of the proximal femur entail realigning the bones with a femoral osteotomy (as necessary); stabilizing the reduction with internal fixation (using a nail/plate-nail/rod device); and supplementing this with a bone graft. In young patients (< 50 yr) in whom early osteoarthritis of the hip spares some of the cartilage, the hip may be realigned with **proximal femoral osteotomy**. This entails cutting the bone at the level of the lesser trochanter, realigning the hip and stabilizing the osteotomy with internal fixation.

Variant procedure or approaches: Osteotomy of proximal 1/3 of femur for degenerative arthritis of hip

Usual preop diagnosis: Nonunion/malunion of proximal 1/3 of femur; early degenerative arthritis of hip

SUMMARY OF PROCEDURES

	Repair Nonunion/Malunion	Proximal Femoral Osteotomy
Position	Supine or lateral decubitus	⇐
Incision	Proximal lateral thigh	⇐
Special instrumentation	Plates, screws; reduction clamps; occasionally, an intramedullary device. Cell Saver recommended. Some surgeons use fracture or radiolucent table with I.I.	⇐
Antibiotics	Broad-spectrum cephalosporin (e.g., cefazolin or cefamandole 1 g iv q 6-8 h)	⇐
Surgical time	2 h for bone grafting alone; 3 h or more if difficult malunion	3 h
EBL	500-750 ml or more	500 ml +
Mortality	Rare: < 1%	⇐
Morbidity	Leg-length discrepancy: Common	–
	Technical complications/fixation failure: 1-5%	⇐
	Superficial, deep infection/osteomyelitis: 1%	⇐
	Malunion: Not uncommon	–
	Compartment syndrome: Rare	⇐
	Neurological deficit to peripheral nerves: Rare	⇐
	Vascular complications: Rare	⇐
		Progressive pain/arthritis (by 5-10 yr): 40-50%
		Delayed union: 5-10%
		Nonunion: 1-5%
Pain score	8	8

PATIENT POPULATION CHARACTERISTICS

	Repair Nonunion/Malunion	Proximal Femoral Osteotomy
Age range	Any age	⇐
Male:Female	1:1	⇐
Incidence	Rare	⇐
Etiology	Previous surgery (rare); previous trauma (rare)	Early degenerative arthritis of the hip (not uncommon)
Associated conditions	May accompany multiple traumas	⇐

ANESTHETIC CONSIDERATIONS

See Anesthetic Considerations for Lower-Extremity Procedures, p. 863.

References

1. Barr RJ, Santore RF: Osteotomies about the hip. In *Chapman's Orthopaedic Surgery,* 3rd edition, Vol 3. Chapman MW, ed. Lippincott Williams & Wilkins, Philadelphia: 2001, 2723-68.
2. Kyle RF, Schmidt AH, Campbell SJ: Complications of the treatment of fractures and dislocations of the hip. In *Complications in Orthopaedic Surgery*, 3rd edition. Epps CH Jr, ed. JB Lippincott, Philadelphia: 1994, 443-86.
3. LaVelle DG: Delayed union and nonunion of fractures. In *Campbell's Operative Orthopaedics*, Vol 3, 9th edition. Crenshaw AH, ed. CV Mosby, St. Louis: 1998, 2579-2630.
4. Whittle AP: Malunited fractures. In *Campbell's Operative Orthopaedics*, Vol 3, 9th edition. Crenshaw AH, ed. CV Mosby, St. Louis: 1994, 2537-78.

CLOSED REDUCTION AND EXTERNAL FIXATION OF FEMUR

SURGICAL CONSIDERATIONS

Description: This procedure entails manipulating the femur to obtain an acceptable reduction by closed or limited-open means, then applying an external fixation device to maintain the reduction. The pins for the external fixator are inserted percutaneously or through small incisions. This method of treatment may be used for severe open fractures (e.g., Grade III) with extensive bone and soft-tissue injury.

Usual preop diagnosis: Displaced, open fracture of the femur

SUMMARY OF PROCEDURE

Position	Supine or lateral
Incision	Done percutaneously or through small incisions
Special instrumentation	External fixation device of surgeon's choice; radiolucent table with I.I.
Unique considerations	Fracture is usually an open, extremely comminuted fracture in a multiple-trauma patient.
Antibiotics	Broad-spectrum cephalosporin (e. g., cefazolin or cefamandole 1 g iv q 6-8 h) + gentamicin (80 mg iv q 8 h until wound closed); adjust for renal status for Grade III open fractures.
Surgical time	1 h
EBL	Operative blood loss usually 100-200 ml; however, blood loss may be extensive before surgery.
Postop care	Multiple-trauma victims → ICU; others → PACU
Mortality	Dependent on extent of trauma

Morbidity	Refracture: 2-12%
	Hypotension 2° blood loss and other injuries: Common
	Stiffness of knee: Common
	Delayed union, nonunion, malunion: More common in comminuted, open fractures
	Leg-length discrepancy: More common in severely comminuted fractures
	Osteomyelitis: More common in open fractures
	Respiratory distress: More common in multiple-trauma situations
	Amputation: Rare
	Compartment syndrome: Rare
	Neurological deficit to peripheral nerves: Rare
	Vascular complications: Rare
Pain score	9-10 (due to extensive open fracture)

PATIENT POPULATION CHARACTERISTICS

Age range	Any age, but predominance of males < 30 yr
Male:Female	5:1
Incidence	Common
Etiology	Motorcycle and motor vehicle accidents; falls; industrial injury
Associated conditions	Frequently associated with trauma to other organ systems, including head and neck, chest, abdomen, and extremities; these will often be treated simultaneously with the femur fracture.

ANESTHETIC CONSIDERATIONS

See Anesthetic Considerations for Lower-Extremity Procedures, p. 863.

References

1. Azer SN, Rankin EA: Complications of femoral shaft fractures. In *Complications in Orthopaedic Surgery*, 3rd edition. Epps CH Jr, ed. JB Lippincott, Philadelphia: 1986, 487-524.
2. Bucholz RW, Brumback RJ: Fractures of the shaft of the femur. In *Rockwood and Green's Fractures in Adults*, 4th edition. Rockwood CA Jr, Green DP, Bucholz RW, Heckman JD, eds. JB Lippincott, Philadelphia: 1996, 1827-1918.
3. Chapman MW: Diaphyseal fractures of the femur. In *Chapman's Orthopaedic Surgery,* Vol I, 3rd edition. Chapman MW, ed. Lippincott Williams & Wilkins, Philadelphia: 2001, 671-708.
4. LaVelle DG: Delayed union and nonunion of fractures. In *Campbell's Operative Orthopaedics*, Vol 3, 9th edition. Crenshaw AH, ed. CV Mosby, St. Louis: 1998, 2579-2630.
5. Whittle AP: Malunited fractures. In *Campbell's Operative Orthopaedics*, Vol 3, 9th edition. Crenshaw AH, ed. CV Mosby, St. Louis: 1994, 2537-78.

Surgeons

John J. Csongradi, MD
Stuart B. Goodman, MD, Phd, FRCSC, FACS

10.5   KNEE SURGERY

Anesthesiologist

Frederick G. Mihm, MD

ARTHROPLASTY OF THE KNEE

SURGICAL CONSIDERATIONS

Description: In this procedure, an arthrotomy of the knee joint is performed, and metallic and plastic components are used for replacement of the knee joint surfaces (**total knee replacement**). The femur, patella, and tibia are exposed; cartilage and minimal bone are excised with a saw. The new components may be cemented or uncemented. Alternatively, arthroplasty may be performed on only one compartment of the knee (i.e., medial/lateral **unicompartmental knee replacement**). In **revision procedures**, one or more components of the old joint are removed and new components are placed. In **resection or excision arthroplasty** of the knee, usually for infection of the prosthesis, the components are removed but not replaced.

Usual preop diagnosis: Arthritis of knee; arthrosis of knee; loose (or malpositioned) knee prosthesis; infected knee

SUMMARY OF PROCEDURES

	Knee Replacement	Revision	Resection/Excision
Position	Supine	⇐	⇐
Incision	Anterior or anteromedial over patella	⇐	⇐
Special instrumentation	Appropriate prostheses and instrumentation	Special instruments for excising cement	⇐
Unique considerations	± Tourniquet; ± SCD	⇐	⇐
Antibiotics	Broad-spectrum cephalosporin (e.g., cefazolin or cefamandole 1 g iv q 6-8 h × 48 h)	Broad spectrum cephalosporin, after cultures taken	⇐
Surgical time	2 h	3-4 h or more	3 h
Closing considerations	In infected or complex revision cases (rare), a local or free flap is required.	⇐	⇐
EBL	300-500 ml	500-1000 ml	⇐
Postop care	Bulky dressing or splint; or continuous passive motion (CPM) is begun, using a machine.	⇐	Splint/cast
Mortality	Rare	⇐	⇐
Morbidity	DVT, without prophylaxis: 50-75%	⇐	⇐
	DVT, with prophylaxis (e.g., low molecular weight heparin, coumadin, SCD, antiembolism stockings): 10-20%	⇐	⇐
	Postop subluxation/dislocation of patella: ≤ 35%	> 35%	–
	Superficial wound necrosis: 10-15%	> 10-15%	≥ 10-15%
	Wound infection:	> 5-10%	Rare
	Primary rheumatoid or psoriatic arthritis, diabetes: 5-10%		
	Primary osteoarthritis (OA): 1%		
	PE: 1-7%	⇐	⇐
	Postop subluxation/dislocation of knee joint: 1-6%	≥ 1-6%	–
	Late aseptic loosening requiring revision after ~10 yr: 5%	–	–
	Peroneal nerve injury: 1-5%	> 1-5% (more common in difficult revisions)	1-5%
	Urinary retention requiring catheterization: Common	–	–

	Knee Replacement	Revision	Resection/Excision
Morbidity, cont.	Hematoma: Rare (1%)	–	
	Hypotension	–	–
	Knee stiffness	–	–
	Intraop fracture: Rare	⇐	–
	Wound dehiscence: Rare	–	⇐
	Fat embolism: Extremely rare	–	–
	Vascular injury to popliteal vessels: Extremely rare	–	–
Pain score	7	8	
			9

PATIENT POPULATION CHARACTERISTICS

Age range	Generally, > 60 yr. Arthritis of the knee (e.g., rheumatoid arthritis or juvenile rheumatoid arthritis); hemophilia, ≥18 yr
Male:Female	1:1
Incidence	Common (~150,000/yr in U.S.)
Etiology	Arthrosis of the knee (degenerative joint disease [DJD] or OA); seropositive or seronegative arthritis; traumatic arthritis; hemophiliac arthropathy of the knee
Associated conditions	Dependent on primary condition

ANESTHETIC CONSIDERATIONS

See Anesthetic Considerations For Knee Procedures, p. 835.

References

1. Blaster RB, Matthews LS: Complications of prosthetic knee arthroplasty. In *Complications in Orthopaedic Surgery*, 3rd edition. Epps CH Jr, ed. JB Lippincott, Philadelphia: 1994, 1057-86.
2. Burke DW, O'Flynn H: Primary total knee arthroplasty. In *Chapman's Orthopaedic Surgery*, 3rd edition. Chapman MW, ed. Lippincott Williams & Wilkins, Philadelphia: 2001, 2869-96.
3. Guyton JL: Arthroplasty of the ankle and knee. In *Campbell's Operative Orthopaedics*, 9th edition. Crenshaw AH, ed. Mosby-Year Book, St. Louis: 1998, Vol 1, 232-94.
4. Insall JN: Total knee replacement. In *Surgery of the Knee*. Insall JN, ed. Churchill Livingstone, New York: 1984, 587-695.
5. Vince KG: Revision knee arthroplasty and arthrodesis of the knee. In *Chapman's Orthopaedic Surgery*, 3rd edition. Chapman MW, ed. Lippincott Williams & Wilkins, Philadelphia: 2001, 2897-2952.

ARTHRODESIS OF THE KNEE

SURGICAL CONSIDERATIONS

Description: In this procedure, the femur is fused to the tibia, obliterating the knee joint. Through a midline incision and anterior arthrotomy, the cartilage surface and a small amount of bone are excised. The cut ends are opposed and aligned in 0-20° of flexion and 5-10% of valgus. The bones are stabilized with plates, screws, an intramedullary rod, or an external fixator.

Usual preop diagnosis: Arthritis or other arthrosis of the knee; previous septic arthritis of the knee; failed or infected knee arthroplasty

SUMMARY OF PROCEDURE

Position	Usually supine
Incision	Anterior midline over knee
Special instrumentation	External fixator; internal fixation with plates and screws or intramedullary nail
Unique considerations	Intraop radiographs or I.I.; tourniquet
Antibiotics	Cefazolin or cefamandole 1 g iv q 6-8 h × 48 h
Surgical time	3 h (+ 1 h, if necessary, to excise total knee arthroplasty)
Closing considerations	Cast or splint while anesthetized
EBL	< 100 ml, if tourniquet and local fixation used. 500-1000 ml, if no tourniquet used, or if intramedullary procedures are used.
Mortality	Rare, but depends primarily on age and medical condition of patient.
Morbidity	Thromboembolism – ≥ incidence following total knee replacement:
	DVT (without prophylaxis): 50-75%
	DVT (if prophylaxis used): 10-20%
	PE (if no prophylaxis; reduced if anticoagulation or SCDs used): 1-7%
	Failure of fusion (nonunion), malunion: 10%
	After failed knee replacement: 19-44%
	With Charcot joint: as high as 50%
	Pin tract infection: ≥ 1-10%
	Wound infection: 5%
	Deep infection and osteomyelitis
	Urinary retention requiring catheterization, UTI: Common
	Breakage or failure of internal or external fixation: Rare
	Fat embolism: Rare
	GI bleed, MI: Rare
	Hematoma: Rare
	Hypotension: Rare
	Intraop femoral or tibial fracture: Rare
	Neurological injury, usually popliteal nerve or peroneal nerve: Rare
	Superficial wound necrosis and wound dehiscence: Rare
	Vascular injury to popliteal vessels: Rare
	Amputation: Extremely rare (usually 2° acute arterial occlusion or uncontrollable local sepsis)
Pain score	9

PATIENT POPULATION CHARACTERISTICS

Age range	Any age
Male:Female	1:1
Incidence	Rare
Etiology	Failed or infected total knee replacement (probably most common etiology); trauma to knee—unreconstructable, intraarticular fractures; total unstable knee or failed ligament repairs with severe DJD in a young patient

ANESTHETIC CONSIDERATIONS

See Anesthetic Considerations For Knee Procedures, p. 835.

References

1. Blaster RB, Matthews LS: Complications of prosthetic knee arthroplasty. In *Complications in Orthopaedic* Surgery, 3rd edition. Epps CH Jr, ed. JB Lippincott, Philadelphia: 1994, 1057-86.
2. Carnesale PG, Stewart MJ: Complications of arthrodesis surgery. In *Complications in Orthopaedic Surgery*, 3rd edition. Epps CH Jr, ed. JB Lippincott, Philadelphia: 1994, 1279-1308.
3. Christian CA, Donley BG: Arthrodesis of the ankle, knee, hip. In *Campbell's Operative Orthopaedics*, 9th edition. Canale ST, ed. Mosby-Year Book, St. Louis: 1998, Vol 1, 145-88.
4. Mize R, Johnson EE, Hohl M: Complications of fractures and dislocations of the knee. In *Complications in Orthopaedic Surgery*, 3rd edition. Epps CH Jr, ed. JB Lippincott, Philadelphia: 1994, 525-56.
5. Vince KG: Revision knee arthroplasty and arthrodesis of the knee. In *Chapman's Orthopaedic Surgery,* 3rd edition. Chapman MW, ed. Lippincott Williams & Wilkins, Philadelphia: 2001, 2897-2952.

OPEN REDUCTION AND INTERNAL FIXATION (ORIF) OF PATELLAR FRACTURES

SURGICAL CONSIDERATIONS

Description: In ORIF of patellar fractures, a short incision over the patella is used to perform a reduction by direct visualization of the fracture fragments of the patella. Since this is generally an intraarticular fracture, the fragments should be reduced precisely. The torn quadriceps retinaculum is also repaired. Part or all of the patella may be excised; pins, wires, and/or screws are normally used to fix the patellar fragments together internally. Thereafter, the knee is casted, or early motion of the knee is started.

Usual preop diagnosis: Fracture of patella; severe degenerative arthritis of patellofemoral joint

SUMMARY OF PROCEDURE

Position	Supine
Incision	Anterior over patella
Special instrumentation	Wire, pins, screws as necessary
Unique considerations	Intraop radiographs may be obtained; tourniquet
Antibiotics	Cefazolin or cefamandole 1 g iv q 6 h × 48 h
Surgical time	1.5-2 h
Closing considerations	Splint or cast usually applied.
EBL	< 100 ml
Mortality	< 1%
Morbidity	Late degenerative arthritis of patellofemoral joint: ~50-60%
	DVT: ~5%
	Wound infection, septic arthritis, osteomyelitis: ~5%
	Delayed union, nonunion, malunion: ~2-5%
	Knee stiffness: Common
	Weakness: Common
	Avascular necrosis: Rare
	Sympathetic dystrophy: Rare
	Following patellectomy—quadriceps strength: ~75% of normal
Pain score	7

PATIENT POPULATION CHARACTERISTICS

Age range	Any age; frequently seen in young, active, healthy adults.
Male:Female	1:1
Incidence	~1% of all skeletal injuries
Etiology	Trauma: falls (60%); motorcycle and motor vehicle accidents (25-35%); industrial injury (6%); degenerative arthritis of patellofemoral joint (rare)

ANESTHETIC CONSIDERATIONS

See Anesthetic Considerations for Knee Procedures, p. 835.

References

1. Mize R, Johnson EE, Hohl M: Complications of fractures and dislocations of the knee. In *Complications in Orthopaedic Surgery*, 3rd edition. Epps CH Jr, ed. JB Lippincott, Philadelphia: 1994, 525-56.
2. Whittle AP: Fractures of lower extremity. In *Campbell's Operative Orthopaedics*, Vol 3, 9th edition. Canale ST, ed. Mosby-Year Book, St. Louis: 1998, 2042-2180.
3. Whittle AP: Malunited fractures. In *Campbell's Operative Orthopaedics*, Vol 3, 9th edition. Canale ST, ed. Mosby-Year Book, St. Louis: 1998, 2537-78.
4. Wiss DA, Watson JT, Johnson EE: Fractures of the knee. In *Rockwood and Green's Fractures in Adults*, 5th edition. Rockwood CA Jr, Green DP, Bucholz RW, Heckman JD, eds. Lippincott-Raven, Philadelphia: 1996, 1919-71.

REPAIR OR RECONSTRUCTION OF KNEE LIGAMENTS

SURGICAL CONSIDERATIONS

Description: Collateral ligaments usually are repaired by direct suture or by stapling the torn ligaments to bone. Cruciate tears are generally repaired only if bone is avulsed at one end of the ligament, again with direct suture, staples, or screws. For collateral ligament repair, a longitudinal incision is made directly over the ligament medially or laterally. The ligament is exposed by deep dissection and elevation of skin flaps. The torn ligament is repaired by direct suture or by fixing it to bone with a screw or staple. Following closure, the knee is immobilized with a long leg splint or cast. Cruciate ligaments are repaired in similar fashion, except for the approaches: medial parapatellar (with anterior arthrotomy) for the anterior cruciate ligament (ACL) and posteromedial (with posterior arthrotomy) for the posterior cruciate ligament (PCL). Cruciate ligament reconstruction is performed for instability 2° intrasubstance tears of these ligaments. Homografts, such as a portion of the patellar tendon or semitendinosus tendon, normally are used, but allografts or synthetics also are available. (The ligaments of the knee are illustrated in Figs 10.5-1, 10.5-2.)

Usual preop diagnosis: Trauma

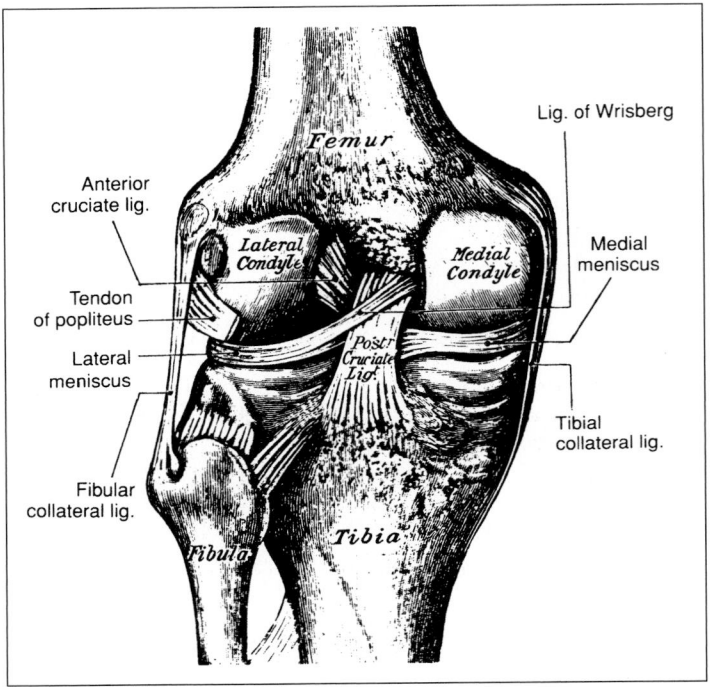

Figure 10.5-1. Left knee joint (from behind), showing interior ligaments. (Reproduced from Goss CM, ed: *Gray's Anatomy of the Human Body*, 27th edition. Lea & Febiger: 1959.)

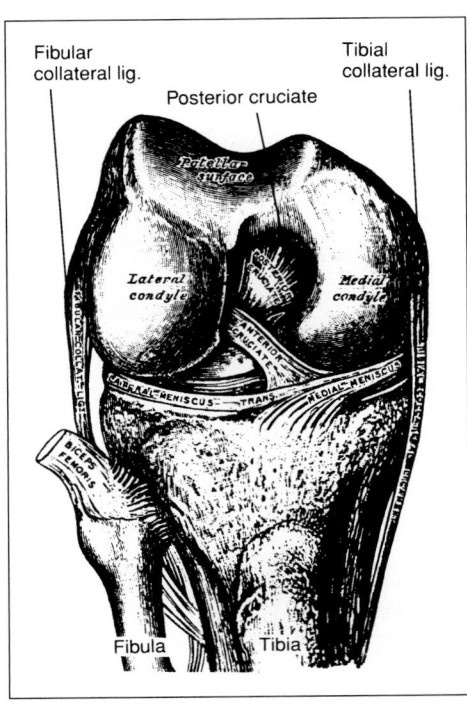

Figure 10.5-2. Right knee joint, dissected from the front. (Reproduced from Goss CM, ed: *Gray's Anatomy of the Human Body*, 27th edition. Lea & Febiger: 1959.)

SUMMARY OF PROCEDURES

	Repair or Collateral Reconstruction	Repair or Cruciate Reconstruction
Position	Supine	⇐
Incision	Over collateral ligament	Anterior and lateral ACL or medial PCL
Special instrumentation	Staples	Drill guides, staples, screws
Unique considerations	Often arthroscopically assisted; tourniquet	⇐
Antibiotics	Cefazolin 1 g iv preop	⇐
Surgical time	2 h	⇐
Closing considerations	Splint or cast while anesthetized	⇐
EBL	100 ml	⇐
Postop care	PACU → room or home	⇐
Mortality	Minimal	⇐

	Repair or Collateral Reconstruction	Repair or Cruciate Reconstruction
Morbidity	Infection: < 1%	⇐
	Thrombophlebitis: < 5%	⇐
Pain score	4	7

PATIENT POPULATION CHARACTERISTICS

Age range	Young adult
Male:Female	2:1
Incidence	Common
Etiology	Trauma: 100%

ANESTHETIC CONSIDERATIONS

See Anesthetic Considerations for Knee Procedures, p. 835.

References

1. Canale ST, ed: *Campbell's Operative Orthopaedics*, 10th edition. Mosby, St. Louis: 2003.
2. Marder RA, Ertl JP: Dislocations and multiple ligamatous injuries of the knee. In *Chapman's Orthopaedic Surgery,* 3rd edition. Chapman MW, ed. Lippincott Williams & Wilkins, Philadelphia: 2001, 2417-34.

PATELLAR REALIGNMENT

SURGICAL CONSIDERATIONS

Description: The goal of this procedure is prevention of chronic subluxation or dislocation of the patella. Soft tissue components of the surgery include incision (release) of the lateral patellar retinaculum and reefing or tightening of the medial retinaculum (Fig 10.5-3). In cases of severe malalignment of the extensor mechanism, the insertion of the patellar tendon may be moved to a new, more medial location (**tibial tubercle transfer**). In this procedure, the tibial tubercle generally is detached with a saw or osteotomes, leaving a bone pedicle attached distally. The tubercle is then rotated medially on the pedicle and fixed in its new position with a screw. Many surgeons routinely perform an **anterior compartment fasciotomy** to prevent postop compartment syndrome.

Usual preop diagnosis: Chronic patellar subluxation or dislocation

SUMMARY OF PROCEDURES

	Patellar Realignment	Tibial Tubercle Transfer
Position	Supine	⇐
Incision	Anteromedial or anterolateral to knee	⇐
Special instrumentation	None	Screws or staples
Unique considerations	Tourniquet	⇐
Antibiotics	None	Cefazolin 1 g iv preop
Surgical time	1 h	1.5 h
Closing considerations	None	Splint or cast while anesthetized
EBL	50 ml	100 ml
Postop care	PACU → room or home	⇐
Mortality	Minimal	⇐
Morbidity	Hemarthrosis: 100%	5%
	Redislocation: 20%	25%
	Thrombophlebitis: 10-20%	⇐

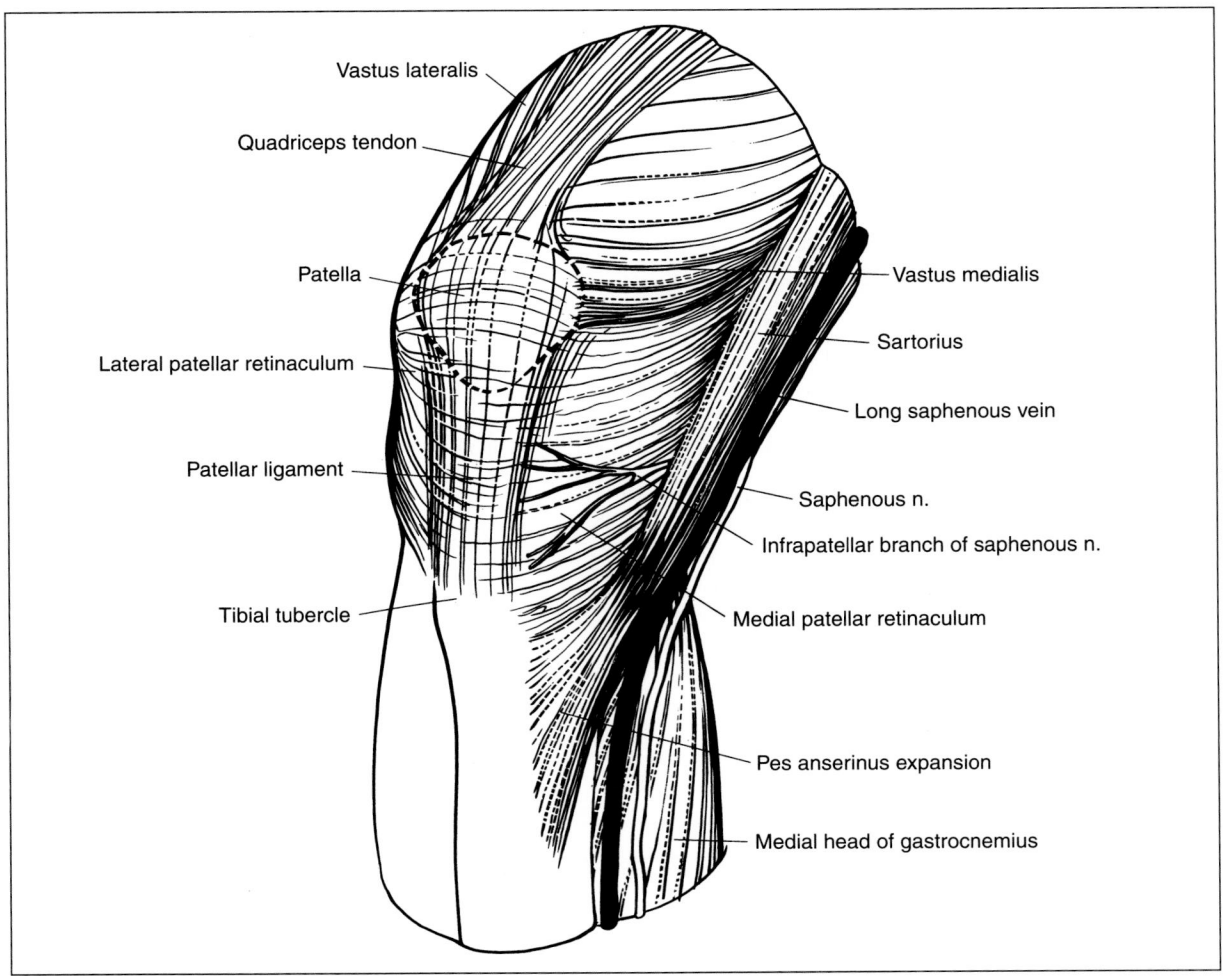

Figure 10.5-3. Outer layer of anteromedial aspect of the knee joint. Shows anatomy of the patellar retinaculum. (Reproduced with permission from Hoppenfeld S, deBoer P: *Surgical Exposures in Orthopaedics: The Anatomic Approach.* Lippincott Williams & Wilkins: 1994.)

	Patellar Realignment	**Tibial Tubercle Transfer**
Morbidity, cont.	Compartment syndrome: < 1%	⇐
	Infection: < 1%	⇐
Pain score	6	7

PATIENT POPULATION CHARACTERISTICS

Age range	Usually young adult
Male:Female	1:2
Etiology	Trauma (70%); congenital (30%)
Associated conditions	Patellofemoral dysphasia (60-70%)

ANESTHETIC CONSIDERATIONS

See Anesthetic Considerations for Knee Procedures, p. 835.

References

1. Epps CH Jr, ed: *Complications in Orthopaedic Surgery*, 3rd edition. JB Lippincott, Philadelphia: 1994.
2. Griffin LY, Duralde XA: Adolescent sports injuries. In *Chapman's Orthopaedic Surgery,* 3rd edition. Chapman MW, ed. Lippincott Williams & Wilkins, Philadelphia: 2001, 2493-2536.

ARTHROSCOPY OF THE KNEE

SURGICAL CONSIDERATIONS

Description: **Knee arthroscopy** is used to diagnose and treat intraarticular problems, most commonly torn meniscus, but the procedure is also used for ligament injuries (Fig 10.5-1, 10.5-2), osteochondral fractures, loose bodies, arthritis, and infections. In knee arthroscopy, multiple portals or entry points for the arthroscope and instruments generally are used. The most common portals are anteromedial and anterolateral adjacent to the patellar ligament. Other portals may be suprapatellar, parapatellar, and posterior. Portals are made by making a stab wound with a knife and then entering the joint with a combination of sharp and blunt trochars. A diagnostic inspection from one of the anterior portals is normally performed at the outset. A second portal is used with a nerve hook to manipulate intraarticular tissues. If resection or repair is performed, the appropriate instruments are inserted through one of the portals. Meniscus repair and cruciate reconstruction may require separate longitudinal incisions, which are usually posteromedial or posterolateral, for placement of sutures and/or drill holes.

Meniscectomy and/or **debridement** often are performed in conjunction with arthroscopy. **Cruciate ligament reconstruction** usually is performed with arthroscopic assistance. At the end of the procedure, the knee joint is copiously irrigated with NS or LR solution through one of the portals. Portals are closed with Steri-Strips or a single suture; compression bandages are applied; and often a knee immobilizer is used.

Usual preop diagnosis: Torn meniscus; cruciate ligament tear; arthritis

SUMMARY OF PROCEDURES

	Arthroscopy	Meniscectomy/Debridement	Cruciate Reconstruction
Position	Supine	⇐	⇐
Incision	3-4.5 cm portals	⇐	⇐ + anterior midline and lateral
Special instrumentation	Arthroscopic video system; small biters and graspers	⇐ + shaver	⇐ + drill guides and drills; fixation screws
Unique considerations	Thigh holder; foot of table 90°; ± tourniquet	⇐	⇐
Antibiotics	None	⇐	Cefazolin 1 g iv preop
Surgical time	0.5 h	1-2 h	2-3 h
Closing considerations	No splint; local anesthetic injected	⇐	⇐
EBL	Minimal	⇐	50 ml
Postop care	PACU → home	⇐	⇐ or overnight
Mortality	< 0.1%	⇐	⇐
Morbidity	Hemarthrosis: 5-20%	5%	⇐
	Thrombophlebitis: < 2%	⇐	⇐
	Infection: 0.1%	⇐	⇐
	Stiffness: < 0.1%	< 4%	⇐
Pain score	3	4	6

PATIENT POPULATION CHARACTERISTICS

Age range	10-70 yr (usually 20-40 yr)
Male:Female	2:1
Incidence	The most common arthroscopic procedure (85% of total)
Etiology	Trauma (~85%); arthritis (~10%); infection (~5%)
Associated conditions	Usually healthy; systemic arthritis (< 5%)

ANESTHETIC CONSIDERATIONS

See Anesthetic Considerations for Knee Procedures, p. 835.

References

1. Coward DB: Principles of arthroscopy of the knee. In *Chapman's Orthopaedic Surgery,* 3rd edition. Chapman MW, ed. Lippincott Williams & Wilkins, Philadelphia: 2001, 2269-98.
2. McGinty JB, ed: *Operative Arthroscopy.* 3rd edition. Lippincot Williams & Wilkins, Philadelphia: 2002.

KNEE ARTHROTOMY

SURGICAL CONSIDERATIONS

Description: **Arthrotomy** of the knee is the opening of the joint for drainage, excision of intraarticular tissue (synovium, meniscus, loose bodies), ligament repair/reconstruction, or fracture fixation. The knee generally is opened with a parapatellar incision, either medial or lateral, and the joint capsule is incised just adjacent to the patella. After the intraarticular pathology is addressed, a tight capsular closure is performed, followed by subcutaneous tissue and skin closure.

Variant procedure or approaches: **Arthrotomy with debridement** may be used for infection or arthropathy which produces debris. In both cases, **synovectomy** may be necessary.

Usual preop diagnosis: Infection; trauma (fracture, sprain, torn meniscus); arthritis

SUMMARY OF PROCEDURES

	Arthrotomy	Arthrotomy with Debridement	Arthrotomy with Synovectomy
Position	Supine	⇐	⇐
Incision	Medial or lateral parapatellar	⇐	⇐
Special instrumentation	Tourniquet	⇐	⇐
Antibiotics	Cefazolin 1 g iv preop	⇐	⇐
Surgical time	1 h	2 h	2-3 h
Closing considerations	Compressive dressing; may be splinted; suction drain	⇐	⇐
EBL	100 ml	⇐	⇐
Postop care	PACU → room	⇐	⇐
Mortality	Minimal	⇐	⇐
Morbidity	Hemarthrosis: 100%	⇐	⇐
	Degenerative arthritis: 5-20%	⇐	⇐
	Stiffness: 5%	⇐	⇐
	Thrombophlebitis: 5%	⇐	⇐
	Infection: 1%	10%	20%
Pain score	7	7	8

PATIENT POPULATION CHARACTERISTICS

Age range	Infant–elderly (usually young adult)
Male:Female	1:1
Incidence	Common
Etiology	Infection; trauma; arthritis
Associated conditions	Inflammatory arthritis (20%)

ANESTHETIC CONSIDERATIONS

See Anesthetic Considerations for Knee Procedures, p. 835.

Reference

1. Epps CH Jr, ed: *Complications in Orthopaedic Surgery*, 3rd edition. JB Lippincott, Philadelphia: 1994.

REPAIR OF TENDONS—KNEE AND LEG

SURGICAL CONSIDERATIONS

Description: Acute ruptures of tendons in the lower limb are repaired by **direct suture** and sometimes reinforced with part of another tendon. At the knee, patellar tendon ruptures are most common; at the ankle, Achilles tendon ruptures are most common. A longitudinal incision generally is made directly over the tendon. The tendon sheath is opened and tendon ends reapproximated with a nonabsorbable tendon stitch. If necessary, the repair may be augmented by synthetic tape or fascia or protected with a wire that takes tension off the repair. The tendon sheath is closed separately from the skin incision; and a cast or splint is applied. **Achilles tendon repair** and **posterior tibial tendon repair** require different positioning. For an Achilles tendon repair, the patient is placed prone, and a longitudinal incision is made just medial to the tendon, spanning the rupture. The tendon sheath is incised and carefully protected. Torn ends of the tendon are approximated with multiple tendon stitches and may be protected with a fascial flap developed from the gastrocnemius fascia. The tendon sheath is closed carefully, followed by skin wound closure. A splint or cast is applied with the foot in equinus.

Usual preop diagnosis: Tendon rupture

SUMMARY OF PROCEDURES

	Posterior Tendon Repair	Achilles Tendon Repair
Position	Supine	Prone
Incision	Over tendon	⇐
Special instrumentation	Wire or synthetic tape for augmentation	⇐
Unique considerations	Tourniquet	⇐
Antibiotics	If young, none; in elderly or infirm, cefazolin 1 g iv preop	⇐
Surgical time	1 h	⇐
Closing considerations	Splint or cast while anesthetized	⇐
EBL	Minimal	⇐
Postop care	PACU → room or home	⇐
Mortality	Minimal	⇐
Morbidity	Weakness: ~10%	⇐
	Wound slough: 5%	⇐
	Adhesions: < 1%	⇐
	Infection: < 1%	⇐
		Rerupture: 5-10%
Pain score	3	3

PATIENT POPULATION CHARACTERISTICS

Age range	Any age
Male:Female	1:1
Incidence	Uncommon
Etiology	Trauma (90%); chronic tendinitis (10%)
Associated conditions	Obesity; diabetes mellitus (DM); inflammatory arthritis

ANESTHETIC CONSIDERATIONS FOR KNEE PROCEDURES

(Procedures covered: arthroplasty; arthrodesis; ORIF of patellar fractures; repair/reconstruction of ligaments; patellar realignment; arthroscopy; arthrotomy; tendon repair—knee and leg)

PREOPERATIVE

Trauma and osteoarthritis (OA) are the most common indications for these procedures. Trauma patients (e.g., those with sports injuries) are often young and healthy, whereas arthritic patients are often elderly and anesthetic management must be tailored to any concurrent disease. Patients with rheumatoid and other inflammatory arthritides form another group of candidates for these procedures; the special anesthetic considerations for these patients are described in Anesthetic Considerations for Hip Procedures, p. 813. A final group of patients undergoing these procedures are hemophiliacs, who develop arthritis from recurrent bleeding into their joints. The hematologic management of these patients is discussed below.

Respiratory	These patients often have **rheumatoid arthritis** and associated pulmonary conditions. For example, pulmonary effusions are common. Limited respiratory reserve warrants further evaluation. Pulmonary fibrosis (rare) often manifests as a cough and dyspnea. Rheumatoid arthritis involving the cricoarytenoid joints may manifest as hoarseness, glottic narrowing, and difficult intubation. Arthritic involvement of the TMJ and cervical spine may further complicate airway management. **Tests:** As indicated from H&P.
Cardiovascular	The severity of the arthritis often limits exercise and makes assessment of cardiovascular status difficult. Dobutamine stress, ECHO, and dipyridamole thallium imaging may be necessary for an adequate cardiac evaluation. Rheumatoid arthritis is associated with pericardial effusion, cardiac valve fibrosis, cardiac conduction abnormalities and aortic regurgitation (AR). **Tests:** ECG and others as indicated from H&P.
Neurological	In arthritic patients, a thorough preop neurological exam often yields evidence of cervical nerve root compression. After the stability of the neck has been established, the full range of neck motion should be evaluated for evidence of nerve compression and cerebral ischemia (suggesting vertebral artery compression). Consider preop lateral neck films to determine stability of atlantooccipital joint and evidence of vertebral spurs that may interfere with intubation. **Tests:** As indicated from H&P.
Musculoskeletal	Pain and ↓joint mobility may make positioning and regional anesthesia difficult in this patient population.
Hematologic	**Hemophiliacs** require restoration of clotting factors preop. Administer 1 U of factor concentrate/kg body weight for each 2% increase necessary to achieve clotting factor activity of 40% normal. FFP contains 1 U/ml and cryoprecipitate 20 U/ml. Hemophilia B (Factor IX def), but not hemophilia A (Factor VIII def), can be treated with prothrombin complex concentrate; however, these products can activate clotting factors and → DIC. Approximately 10% of hemophiliacs develop antibodies to exogenous clotting factors, and the care of these patients should be guided by a hematologist. **Tests:** Hct; other tests as indicated from H&P.
Laboratory	Other tests as indicated from H&P.
Premedication	Standard premedication (see p. B-2). Preop patellar pain is treated effectively with a femoral nerve block at the inguinal ligament, using 10 ml of lidocaine 1.5% with epinephrine 1:200,000.

INTRAOPERATIVE

Anesthetic technique: For many of these patients, regional anesthesia may be the preferred technique, offering the advantages of ↓blood loss, ↓DVT, minimal respiratory impairment, and effective postop analgesia. Patients with rheumatoid arthritis rarely have involvement of the lumbar spine. Since rheumatoid arthritis frequently affects the C-spine, however, these patients may have limited range of neck motion, an unstable atlantooccipital joint, and cricoarytenoid and TMJ arthritis. Careful airway evaluation, therefore, is important to determine the appropriateness of special intubation techniques (e.g., fiber optic).

Regional anesthesia: Either subarachnoid or epidural blocks are useful techniques, depending on the patient population (e.g., younger patients may be at ↑risk of spinal headache following SAB). Anesthesia extending from S2 to T12 (T8, if tourniquet is used) is adequate for knee surgery. Full motor blockade is essential for fixation of the patella, or placement of the joint prosthesis and assessment of the passive ROM of the prosthesis. Typical drugs and doses include: subarachnoid—15 mg of 0.75% bupivacaine with morphine 0.2 mg; epidural—15-20 ml 2% lidocaine with epinephrine 1:200,000 in divided doses.

General anesthesia:

Induction	Standard induction (see p. B-2) is appropriate for patients with normal airways.
Maintenance	Standard maintenance (see p. B-3). Neuromuscular relaxation facilitates the placement of the prosthesis. Hemophiliacs will require infusion of clotting factors. For hemophilia A and von Willebrand's disease, 1.5 U/kg/h; for hemophilia B, 0.75 U/kg/h.
Emergence	The tourniquet is deflated around the time of emergence. In patients with moderate-to-severe lung disease, controlled ventilation should be continued until after the lactic acid that has accumulated in the leg has been metabolized (3-5 min), since these patients may be unable to increase ventilation to buffer this acid load.

Blood and fluid requirements	IV: 14-16 ga × 1 NS/LR @ maintenance during the case, and 5-10 ml/kg bolus prior to tourniquet deflation	A tourniquet blocks intraop blood loss. When it is deflated, prepare for a 1-2 U blood loss over the ensuing h; more, if the posterior tibial artery has been damaged in the dissection.
Control of blood loss	Tourniquet	Inflation pressure is typically 100 mmHg > systolic pressure. Maximum 'safe' tourniquet time is 1.5-2 hr, followed by a 5-to-(preferably) 15-min reperfusion interval, if further tourniquet time is necessary.
Monitoring	Standard monitors (see p. B-1). ± CVP line ± Arterial line	A CVP line is indicated in the presence of significant cardiac or pulmonary disease.
Positioning	✓ and pad pressure points. ✓ eyes.	In rheumatoid arthritic patients, meticulous padding of the extremities is mandatory.
Complications	Posterior tibial artery trauma Peroneal nerve palsy	A 20% fall in mean BP is common on tourniquet deflation. Additional crystalloid (5-10 ml/kg) may be necessary to replace edema fluid and blood loss to the leg.

POSTOPERATIVE

Complications	Hemorrhage from the posterior tibial artery	✓ surgical drain output.
	Peroneal nerve palsy → foot drop Tourniquet-related nerve injury Post-tourniquet syndrome (PTS)	Examine patient for evidence of neurologic dysfunction and notify surgeons as necessary. PTS is a self-limiting condition in which the affected limb is edematous, pale, and weak.
Pain management	Spinal opiates: • Epidural anesthesia • Spinal anesthesia	Epidural hydromorphone 50 μg/ml infused at 100-250 μg/h provides excellent analgesia. Intrathecal morphine 0.2-0.3 mg provides analgesia for up to 24 h after administration.
Tests	Hct; other studies as indicated.	Patients with coagulopathies require replacement therapy for 6-10 d.

References

1. Epps CH Jr, ed: *Complications in Orthopaedic Surgery*, 3rd edition. JB Lippincott, Philadelphia: 1994.
2. Heiden EA: Tendinopathies about the knee. In *Chapman's Orthopaedic Surgery*, 3rd edition. Chapman MW, ed. Lippincott Williams & Wilkins, Philadelphia: 2001, 2339-46.

Surgeon

John J. Csongradi, MD

10.6 LOWER LEG, ANKLE, FOOT, AND OTHER LOWER-EXTREMITY PROCEDURES

Anesthesiologist

Frederick G. Mihm, MD

OPEN REDUCTION AND INTERNAL FIXATION (ORIF) OF THE TIBIAL PLATEAU FRACTURE

SURGICAL CONSIDERATIONS

Description: **ORIF of the tibial plateau** or proximal tibia fracture involves making a longitudinal incision along the proximal leg, lateral to the knee, obtaining a reduction by direct visualization of the fracture fragments, and applying plates and screws along the tibia for rigid internal fixation. An iliac crest bone graft may be necessary. A **proximal tibial osteotomy** involves correcting malalignment (valgus and varus) of the lower extremity by excising a wedge of bone from the tibia and correcting the mechanical axis.

Usual preop diagnosis: Tibial plateau or proximal tibial fracture; nonunion/malunion of the tibial plateau or proximal tibia; degenerative arthritis of the knee, with varus or valgus deformity

SUMMARY OF PROCEDURES

	ORIF Tibial Plateau Fracture	Proximal Tibial Osteotomy
Position	Supine	⇐
Incision	Lateral to knee, usually; medial, rarely	Transverse or lateral incision
Special instrumentation	Special plates, screws; reduction clamps; radiolucent table	⇐
Unique considerations	Intraop radiographs or I.I.; tourniquet	⇐
Antibiotics	Cefazolin or cefamandole 1 g iv q 6-8 h × 48 h	⇐
Surgical time	~2.5-3 h; more, depending on difficulty	⇐
Closing considerations	Splint, cast while anesthetized	⇐
EBL	< 200 ml	⇐
Postop care	Multiple-trauma victim → ICU; others → PACU; ± CPM	PACU → ward
Mortality	Rare, except in severe multiple trauma	None
Morbidity	Compartment syndrome: 10-20%	< 25%
	Wound infection: 7-15%	~2%
	DVT (symptomatic): 3-5%	2%
	Delayed union, nonunion, malunion: < 5%	⇐
	Peripheral nerve damage: 3%	0.2%
	Intraarticular fracture: 2%	
	Hypotension (multiple trauma)	
	Leg-length discrepancy	
	Osteomyelitis, septic arthritis	
	Respiratory distress and fat embolism	
	Vascular complications	
Pain score	7	7

PATIENT POPULATION CHARACTERISTICS

Age range	Any age; fracture most common in younger trauma patients and elderly Degenerative arthritis of knee, < 60 yr
Male:Female	1:1
Incidence	Common
Etiology	Trauma: falls, motorcycle and motor vehicle accidents, industrial injuries Degenerative: arthritis of knee

ANESTHETIC CONSIDERATIONS

See Anesthetic Considerations for Lower-Extremity Procedures, p. 863.

References

1. Aglietti P, Chambat P: Fractures of the knee. In *Surgery of the Knee*. Insall JN, ed. Churchill Livingstone, New York: 1984, 395-490.
2. Egol KA, Koval KJ: Fractures of the tibial plateau. In *Chapman's Orthopaedic Surgery,* 3rd edition, Vol I. Chapman MW, ed. Lippincott Williams & Wilkins, Philadelphia: 2001, 737-54.

3. LaVelle DG: Delayed union and nonunion of fractures. In *Campbell's Operative Orthopaedics,* Vol 3. Canale ST, ed. CV Mosby, St. Louis: 1998, 2579-2630.
4. Mize R, Johnson EE, Hohl M: Complications of fractures and dislocations of the knee. In *Complications in Orthopaedic Surgery,* 3rd edition. Epps CH Jr, ed. JB Lippincott, Philadelphia: 1994, 525-56.
5. Whittle AP: Malunited fractures. In *Campbell's Operative Orthopaedics*. Canale ST, ed. Mosby, St. Louis: 1998, 2537-78.
6. Wiss DA, Watson JT, Johnson EE: Fractures of the knee. In *Rockwood and Green's Fractures in Adults*, 4th edition. Rockwood CA Jr, Green DP, Bucholz RW, Heckman JD, eds. Lippincott-Raven, Philadelphia: 1996.

INTRAMEDULLARY NAILING, TIBIA

SURGICAL CONSIDERATIONS

Description: In intramedullary nailing of the tibia, a metal nail is placed into the medullary canal of the tibia to stabilize (or prevent) a fracture. The affected leg generally is placed in traction, on a fracture table, via stirrup or calcaneal pin. Following the incision, an awl is used to make an entry hole in the proximal metaphysis of the tibia, through which a guide wire is introduced. The guide wire is placed across the aligned fracture, and the nail is introduced and driven over the guide wire. Before nail insertion, the medullary canal often is reamed to allow use of a larger nail. Most nails are interlocked both proximally and distally with screws that pass from the bone through holes in the nail.

Usual preop diagnosis: Fracture, nonunion or malunion of the tibia

SUMMARY OF PROCEDURE

Position	Supine, on fracture table. Consider inducing anesthesia before moving patient.
Incision	Proximal longitudinal incision over the patellar tendon; stab wound for screws
Special instrumentation	Nails, screws, and insertion instruments; intramedullary reamers; I.I.
Antibiotics	Cefazolin 1 g iv preop
Surgical time	2 h
Closing considerations	No splint or cast
EBL	200 ml
Postop care	PACU → room
Mortality	Minimal
Morbidity	Compartment syndrome: < 5%
	Infection: < 2%
	Neuropraxia: < 1%
Pain score	5

PATIENT POPULATION CHARACTERISTICS

Age range	> 16 yr
Male:Female	5:1
Etiology	Trauma (95%); tumor (5%)
Associated conditions	Multiple trauma (50%); compartment syndrome (5%)

ANESTHETIC CONSIDERATIONS

See Anesthetic Considerations for Lower-Extremity Procedures, p. 863.

Reference

1. Bucholz RW, Heckman JD, eds: *Rockwood and Green's Fractures in Adults*, 5th edition. Lippincott Williams & Wilkins, Philadelphia: 2001.

EXTERNAL FIXATION, TIBIA

SURGICAL CONSIDERATIONS

Description: Fractures of the tibia are fixed with percutaneous pins that are clamped to an external frame. Stainless steel pins are drilled into the proximal and distal fragments of the fracture through stab wounds in the skin and subcutaneous tissues. Usually 2-3 pins are placed on either side of the fracture. Pin clamps and an external frame are attached and the fracture aligned with the assistance of the I.I. or under direct vision. Following fracture alignment, the pin clamps and frames are tightened to hold fracture alignment. External fixation is often used with open fractures. **Small-pin fixators** (e.g., Ilizarov) are used for fracture fixation, leg lengthening, and treatment of bony defects. Wound irrigation and debridement often accompany application of the fixation frame.

Usual preop diagnosis: Tibial fracture; tibial nonunion or malunion; tibial shortening

SUMMARY OF PROCEDURE

Position	Supine
Incision	Stab wounds. Small-pin fixator may require metaphyseal incision for osteotomy.
Special instrumentation	Pins; fixation frame; I.I.
Antibiotics	Cefazolin 1 g iv preop
Surgical time	0.5-1 h
	Small-pin fixator: 3-5 h
Closing considerations	May be open fracture (usually left open)
EBL	50 ml; small-pin fixator, 100 ml
Postop care	PACU → room
Mortality	Minimal
Morbidity	Infection: 15%
	Compartment syndrome: < 2%
	Neuropraxia: < 1%
Pain score	2-3

PATIENT POPULATION CHARACTERISTICS

Age range	All ages
Male:Female	5:1
Incidence	Common
Etiology	Trauma (95%); shortened limb (< 2%); ununited or malunited fracture (< 2%)
Associated conditions	Open fracture (95%); compartment syndrome (< 2%); congenital anomaly (< 1%)

ANESTHETIC CONSIDERATIONS

See Anesthetic Considerations for Lower-Extremity Procedures, p. 863.

Reference

1. Bucholz RW, Heckman JD, eds: *Rockwood and Green's Fractures in Adults*, 5th edition. Lippincott Williams & Wilkins, Philadelphia: 2001.

OPEN REDUCTION AND INTERNAL FIXATION (ORIF) OF DISTAL TIBIA, ANKLE, AND FOOT FRACTURES

SURGICAL CONSIDERATIONS

Description: ORIF is nearly always required for displaced fractures involving the ankle or joints in the foot. A longitudinal incision is made over the fractured medial and/or lateral malleoli. Dissection is carried directly down to the bone and the fracture is identified and reduced under direct vision.

Open fractures may require **irrigation and debridement**. The fractures are realigned under direct vision and fixed and stabilized with pins, plates, and/or screws. An intraop radiograph is obtained to confirm reduction and placement of hardware. The incisions are closed and a splint or cast is applied.

Usual preop diagnosis: Fracture of the distal tibia, ankle, or foot

SUMMARY OF PROCEDURES

	ORIF Ankle	With Irrigation and Debridement
Position	Supine	⇐
Incision	Longitudinal over fracture site	⇐ + extension of existing wound
Special instrumentation	Pins, plates, and screws; tourniquet; x-ray or I.I.	⇐
Antibiotics	Cefazolin 1 g iv preop	⇐
Surgical time	2 h	2-3 h
Closing considerations	Splint or cast while anesthetized	Splint or cast; may leave wound open.
EBL	50 ml	100 ml
Postop care	PACU → room	⇐
Mortality	Minimal	⇐
Morbidity	Wound dehiscence: 10%	⇐
	Loss of reduction: 7%	⇐
	Infection: 3%	15%
Pain score	4	4

PATIENT POPULATION CHARACTERISTICS

Age range	Infant–elderly (usually > 60 yr)
Male:Female	1:1
Incidence	~ 250,000 cases/yr in U.S.
Etiology	Trauma: 100%
Associated conditions	Alcohol abuse; obesity; diabetes mellitus (DM)

ANESTHETIC CONSIDERATIONS

See Anesthetic Considerations for Lower-Extremity Procedures, p. 863.

References

1. Bucholz RW, Heckman JD, eds: *Rockwood and Green's Fractures in Adults*, 5th edition. Lippincott Williams & Wilkins, Philadelphia: 2001.
2. Carragee EJ, Csongradi JJ, Bleck EE: Early complications in the operative treatment of ankle fractures. Influence of delay before operation. *J Bone Joint Surg* [Br] 1991; 73(1):79-82.
3. Epps CH Jr, ed: *Complications in Orthopaedic Surgery*, 3rd edition. JB Lippincott, Philadelphia: 1994.

REPAIR NONUNION/MALUNION, TIBIA

SURGICAL CONSIDERATIONS

Description: This procedure is used to treat a fracture that has not healed or was misaligned upon healing. The fracture is mobilized, usually grafted with autogenous or allograft bone, and realigned. With an anterior approach, a longitudinal incision is made anteromedial or anterolateral to the shaft of the tibia. Dissection is carried directly down to the bone and the nonunion identified. If the tibia is approached with a posterolateral incision, the patient is turned prone and a longitudinal incision is made just posterior to the fibula. Dissection is carried down posteriorly to the interosseous membrane, to the tibia, and the procedure becomes identical to the anterior approach. Tissue interposed between the bone ends may or may not be debrided. The cortex of the bone adjacent to the nonunion is roughened with an osteotome. Autogenous or allograft bone is placed adjacent to or in the nonunion site. In the case of a malunion, the bone may be osteotomized with a saw or osteotomes to allow realignment. If skeletal fixation is used, a plate may be attached to the bone through the same incision. Alternatively, an intramedullary nail may be placed through an incision anterior to the tibial tubercle. If an intramedullary device is used, the canal may be reamed with intramedullary reamers prior to placement of the nail. A third type of **skeletal fixation** is the external fixator that stabilizes the nonunion via percutaneous pins placed into the proximal and distal tibia, which are then spanned by a device with pin clamps at both ends. An intraop x-ray is often used to confirm fixation and placement of devices; alternatively, an I.I. may be used.

Variant procedure or approaches: Autogenous **bone grafting from the iliac crest** is commonly used to stimulate healing. An incision is made directly over the iliac crest and muscles are stripped from the crest and table of the ilium. Osteotomes and gouges are used to remove either the inner or outer table of the ilium and cancellous bone between the two tables. The wound is closed over a suction drain.

Usual preop diagnosis: Ununited or malunited fracture

SUMMARY OF PROCEDURES

	Basic Repair	With Iliac Graft	With Skeletal Fixation
Position	Supine (prone with posterior lateral graft)	⇐	⇐
Incision	Anteromedial or posterolateral to shaft of tibia	Anteromedial, parallel to iliac crest	⇐
Special instrumentation	Tourniquet; x-ray or I.I.	⇐	Pins, plates, screws, rods, external fixator; tourniquet; x-ray or I.I.
Antibiotics	Cefazolin 1 g iv preop. (If infected nonunion anticipated, antibiotics are withheld until cultures are obtained.)	⇐	⇐
Surgical time	2 h	2.5 h	3 h
Closing considerations	Splint or cast applied while anesthetized.	⇐	No splint or cast
EBL	100 ml	200-300 ml	⇐
Postop care	PACU → room	⇐	⇐
Mortality	Minimal	⇐	⇐
Morbidity	Thrombophlebitis: 5%	⇐	⇐
	Compartment syndrome: 1%	⇐	⇐
	Infection: 1%	⇐	⇐
	Hematoma: < 1%	5%	1-3%
Pain score	5	8	5-8

PATIENT POPULATION CHARACTERISTICS

Age range	10-80 yr (usually 20-40 yr)
Male:Female	5:1
Incidence	5-10% of tibia fractures; 50-75% of open fractures
Etiology	Trauma: 100%
Associated conditions	Poor nutrition (50%); infection (10%); metabolic disease (10%)

ANESTHETIC CONSIDERATIONS

See Anesthetic Considerations for Lower-Extremity Procedures, p. 863.

References

1. Csongradi JJ, Maloney WJ: Ununited lower limb fractures. *West J Med* 1989; 150(6):675-80.
2. Epps CH Jr, ed: *Complications in Orthopaedic Surgery*, 3rd edition. JB Lippincott, Philadelphia: 1994.
3. Goulet JA, Hak DJ: Nonunions and malunions of the tibia. In *Chapman's Orthopaedic Surgery,* 3rd edition, Vol I. Chapman MW, ed. Lippincott Williams & Wilkins, Philadelphia: 2001, 977-1000.

ARTHROSCOPY OF THE ANKLE

SURGICAL CONSIDERATIONS

Description: **Ankle arthroscopy** is usually a diagnostic procedure, although it may be used for debridement or removal of loose bodies. The ankle joint generally is inspected through anterolateral and anteromedial portals (entry wounds). Postero-lateral and posteromedial portals also may be used. Each portal is made via a 5 mm stab wound in the skin (Fig 10.6-1); then instrumentation is placed, using trochars. If the ankle joint is tight, a mechanical distractor (external fixator distraction appa-ratus spanning the ankle joint) may be used. The distractor is attached to the bones via percutaneous pins, as in the case of the application of an external fixator. The portals are closed with sterile tape or a single suture. **Debridement** may be used to reduce local or generalized articular damage.

Usual preop diagnosis: Trauma; infection; arthritis

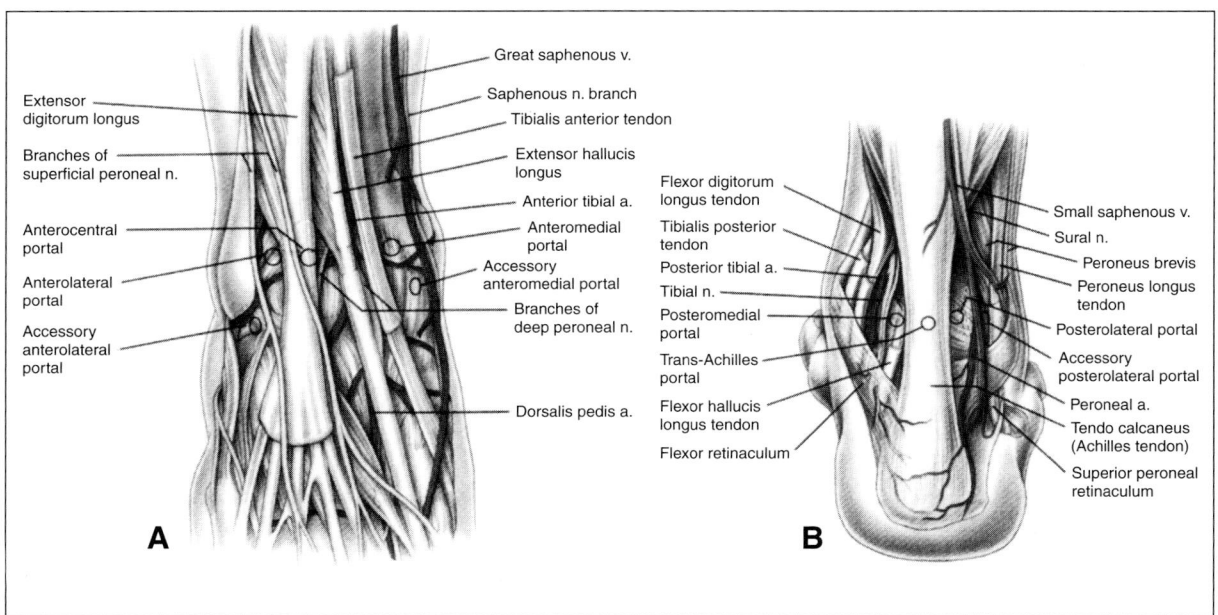

Figure 10.6-1. Portals for ankle arthroscopy. (A) Anterior anatomy and portals. The anterolateral and anteromedial portals are used routinely. (B) Posterior anatomy and portals. The posterolateral portal also is used routinely. (Reproduced with permission from Ferkel RD: *Arthroscopic Surgery: The Foot and Ankle*. Lippincott-Raven, 1996.)

SUMMARY OF PROCEDURES

	Arthroscopy	Arthroscopy + Debridement
Position	Supine	⟸
Incision	0.5 cm portals (incisions)	⟸
Special instrumentation	Arthroscopic video system; small biters and graspers	⟸ + shaver
Unique considerations	± Tourniquet. May use distractor with pins through tibia and calcaneus.	⟸
Antibiotics	Cefazolin 1 g iv preop (optional)	⟸
Surgical time	1 h	1-2 h
Closing considerations	No splint; incisions injected with local anesthetic.	⟸
EBL	Minimal	50 ml
Postop care	PACU → home	⟸
Mortality	< 0.01%	⟸
Morbidity	Hemarthrosis: 5%	⟸
	Thrombophlebitis < 2%	⟸
	Infection: < 1%	⟸
Pain score	2-3	3

PATIENT POPULATION CHARACTERISTICS

Age range	12-70 yr (usually 20-40 yr)
Male:Female	1:1
Incidence	Uncommon
Etiology	Trauma (70%); arthritis (20%); infection (5%)
Associated conditions	Usually healthy; may have systemic arthritis.

ANESTHETIC CONSIDERATIONS

See Anesthetic Considerations for Lower-Extremity Procedures, p. 863.

References

1. Ferkel RD, McGrath SJ: Arthroscopy of the ankle. In *Chapman's Orthopaedic Surgery,* 3rd edition, Vol 3. Chapman MW, ed. Lippincott Williams & Wilkins, Philadelphia: 2001, 2441-66.
2. McGinty JB, ed: *Operative Arthroscopy*, 3rd edition. Lippincott Williams & Wilkins, New York: 2002.

ANKLE ARTHROTOMY

SURGICAL CONSIDERATIONS

Description: Arthrotomy of the ankle is the opening of the joint for drainage, debridement, or fracture treatment. The joint usually is opened with an anterolateral midline or anteromedial longitudinal incision. Tendons and neurovascular structures are carefully retracted to expose the joint capsule, which is then opened in line with the skin incision. After intraarticular pathology is addressed, careful closure of the capsule is performed, taking care to obtain good hemostasis.

Usual preop diagnosis: Infection; trauma; arthritis

SUMMARY OF PROCEDURE

Position	Supine
Incision	Anterior midline or anteromedial longitudinal
Special instrumentation	Tourniquet

Antibiotics	Cefazolin 1 g iv preop
Surgical time	1 - 2 h
Closing considerations	± Splint while anesthetized; may have suction drain.
EBL	Minimal
Postop care	PACU → room
Mortality	Minimal
Morbidity	Hemarthrosis: 20%
	Thrombophlebitis: 5%
	Infection: 1%
Pain score	5

PATIENT POPULATION CHARACTERISTICS

Age range	Infant – elderly
Male:Female	1:1
Incidence	Rare
Etiology	Trauma (70%); arthritis (20%); infection (10%)
Associated conditions	Inflammatory arthritis; multiple trauma; immunosuppression

ANESTHETIC CONSIDERATIONS

See Anesthetic Considerations for Lower-Extremity Procedures, p. 863.

Reference

1. Crenshaw AH, ed: *Campbell's Operative Orthopaedics*, 10th edition. Mosby, St. Louis: 2003.

ANKLE ARTHRODESIS

SURGICAL CONSIDERATIONS

Description: An **ankle fusion** may need to be performed for severe pain 2° arthritis of the ankle. In most cases, an anterior approach is made to the ankle joint. An alternative approach is through the medial malleolus. The ankle joint is exposed and the surfaces of the joint are debrided either with osteotomes or a burr. Cancellous bone is exposed on the distal tibia and talus, and the joint is clamped together either with a simple external fixation device with pins going through the distal tibia and talus, or with bone screws that go from the distal tibia into the talus. The wound is closed over a drain, and a splint may be applied.

Usual preop diagnosis: Arthritis of the ankle

SUMMARY OF PROCEDURE

Position	Supine
Incision	Anterior midline over distal tibia
Special instrumentation	Tourniquet; external fixator or bone screws
Unique considerations	Intraop radiographs; tourniquet use
Antibiotics	Cefazolin 1 g iv preop
Surgical time	2 h
Closing considerations	May be splinted; suction drain.
EBL	100 ml
Postop care	PACU → room
Mortality	Minimal

Morbidity	Nonunion (late): 15%
	Thrombophlebitis: 10%
	Hematoma: 5%
	Wound dehiscence: 5%
	Infection: 1%
Pain score	8

PATIENT POPULATION CHARACTERISTICS

Age range	All adult
Male:Female	1:1
Etiology	Degenerative arthritis; trauma; avascular necrosis of talus; septic arthritis
Associated conditions	Inflammatory arthritis; any disease requiring steroids

ANESTHETIC CONSIDERATIONS

See Anesthetic Considerations for Lower-Extremity Procedures, p. 863.

References

1. Chapman MW, ed: *Operative Orthopaedics*. 3rd edition. Lippincott Williams & Wilkins, Philadelphia: 2000.
2. Crenshaw AH, ed: *Campbell's Operative Orthopaedics*, 10th edition. Mosby, St. Louis: 2003.

REPAIR/RECONSTRUCTION OF ANKLE LIGAMENTS

SURGICAL CONSIDERATIONS

Description: Lateral ankle ligaments may be repaired acutely, but generally are reconstructed at a later date, if necessary, with the peroneus brevis used in most reconstructions. An incision is made posterior to the distal fibula, curving around the lateral malleolus and ending in the anterolateral foot. The peroneus brevis tendon is identified and detached from its musculotendinous junction in the leg, and the peroneus brevis muscle is sutured to the peroneus longus tendon. A hole is drilled from anterior to posterior in the distal lateral malleolus; then the detached end of the peroneus brevis tendon is threaded through the hole. It is then attached to either the calcaneus or the talus, anterior to the lateral malleolus, with a staple or by suturing into a hole in the bone. The skin and subcutaneous tissues are closed and a splint or cast is applied.

Usual preop diagnosis: Lateral instability of the ankle

SUMMARY OF PROCEDURE

Position	Supine or lateral decubitus
Incision	Posterolateral aspect of ankle
Special instrumentation	Bone staples; tourniquet
Antibiotics	Cefazolin, 1 g iv preop
Surgical time	2 h
Closing considerations	Splint or cast while still anesthetized.
EBL	Minimal
Postop care	PACU → room or home
Mortality	Minimal
Morbidity	Infection: < 1%
	Reruption: < 1%
	Wound dehiscence: < 0.1%
Pain score	5

PATIENT POPULATION CHARACTERISTICS

Age range	Young adults
Male:Female	2:1
Etiology	Ankle sprain
Associated conditions	Alcohol abuse; obesity; diabetes mellitus (DM)

ANESTHETIC CONSIDERATIONS

See Anesthetic Considerations for Lower-Extremity Procedures, p. 863.

Reference

1. Epps CH Jr, ed: *Complications in Orthopaedic Surgery*, 3rd edition. JB Lippincott, Philadelphia: 1994.
2. Marder RA: Ankle ligament injuries. In *Chapman's Orthopaedic Surgery,* 3rd edition, Vol 3. Chapman MW, ed. Lippincott Williams & Wilkins, Philadelphia: 2001, 2473-84.

AMPUTATION THROUGH ANKLE (SYME)

SURGICAL CONSIDERATIONS

Description: **Syme's amputation** (Figs 10.6-2, 10.6-3) is ankle disarticulation with closure, using a posterior flap, including the heel pad. It is more functional than below-knee amputation because patients can bear weight on the end of the stump; however, success is poor in patients with vascular disease or peripheral neuropathy. The posterior flap is dissected directly from the calcaneus, carefully preserving the tough heel pad and its blood supply. The heel pad is sutured directly to the distal tibia to prevent migration and to cover the bone end. The posterior flap is then sutured to the anterior flap with interrupted sutures and a compression dressing applied.

Usual preop diagnosis: Trauma; infection

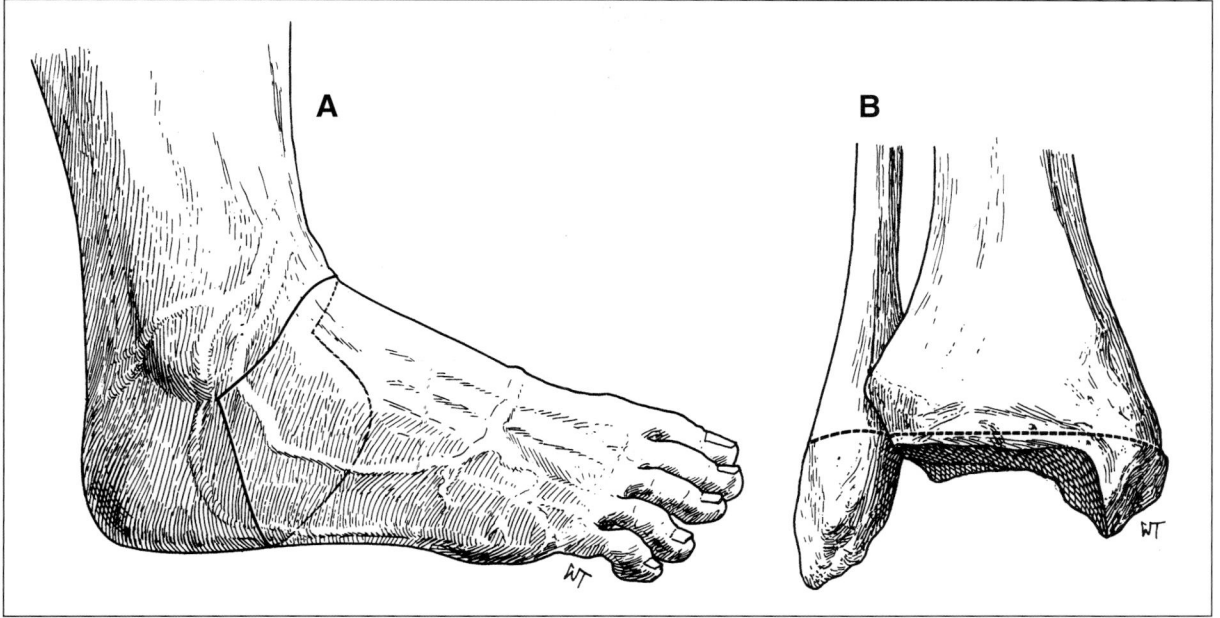

Figure 10.6-2. Syme's amputation. (A) Skin incisions. (B) Level of bone transection in adults. (Reproduced from Bohne WHO: *Atlas of Amputation Surgery*. Thieme Medical, 1987.)

SUMMARY OF PROCEDURE

Position	Supine
Incision	Anterior and posterior flaps
Special instrumentation	Tourniquet
Antibiotics	Cefazolin 1 g iv preop
Surgical time	1.5-2 h
Closing considerations	Bulky dressing; if infection present, wound may be left open.
EBL	100 ml
Postop care	PACU → room
Mortality	Minimal
Morbidity	Phantom pain: 90%
	Infection: 10-15%
	Wound breakdown: 10-15%
	Pneumonia: 12%
	MI: 7%
	PE: 6%
	Hematoma: 5%
	Stroke: 5%
Pain score	5

PATIENT POPULATION CHARACTERISTICS

Age range	Typically, > 60 yr
Male:Female	3:1
Incidence	20,000-30,000/yr
Etiology	Trauma (50%); infection (30%); congenital anomaly (5%)
Associated conditions	Peripheral vascular disease (30-40%); diabetes mellitus (DM) (< 20%)

ANESTHETIC CONSIDERATIONS

See Anesthetic Considerations for Lower-Extremity Procedures, p. 863.

References

1. Bohne WHO, Ertl JP: Amputations of the lower extremity. In *Chapman's Orthopaedic Surgery,* 3rd edition, Vol 3. Chapman MW, ed. Lippincott Williams & Wilkins, Philadelphia: 2001, 3157.
2. Epps CH Jr, ed: *Complications in Orthopaedic Surgery*, 3rd edition. JB Lippincott, Philadelphia: 1994.

AMPUTATION, TRANSMETATARSAL

SURGICAL CONSIDERATIONS

Description: This amputation, usually for infection or ischemic necrosis of the toes, is performed at the midmetatarsal level, leaving the patient able to walk without a prosthesis. A transverse dorsal incision is made at the transmetatarsal level, and a plantar incision is made beginning at the corners of the dorsal incision and extending distally to the metatarsal heads to create a long plantar flap. The plantar flap is reflected proximally to the midmetatarsal level and tapered distally. The metatarsals are sectioned with a saw, and nerves and tendons are sectioned proximal to the osteotomies. The plantar flap is then brought over the ends of the bones and sutured with interrupted sutures to the dorsal flap. A compression dressing is applied.

Variant procedure or approaches: Other partial-foot amputations, such as **midtarsal** and **ray amputation**, are much less common. They are managed in a fashion similar to that of the transmetatarsal amputation.

Usual preop diagnosis: Gangrene of the toes; infection

SUMMARY OF PROCEDURE

Position	Supine
Incision	Dorsal and plantar flaps
Special instrumentation	Tourniquet
Antibiotics	Cefazolin 1 g iv preop
Surgical time	1-2 h
Closing considerations	Bulky dressing
EBL	50 ml
Postop care	PACU → room
Mortality	Minimal
Morbidity	Phantom pain: 90%
	Infection: 10-15%
	Wound breakdown: 10-15%
	Hematoma: 5%
Pain score	5

PATIENT POPULATION CHARACTERISTICS

Age range	> 60 yr
Male:Female	3:1
Incidence	20,000-30,000 total amputations/yr
Etiology	Vascular disease (70%); infection (25%) trauma (< 5%); congenital anomalies (< 1%)
Associated conditions	Vascular disease (70%); diabetes mellitus (30%); pulmonary disease (30%)

ANESTHETIC CONSIDERATIONS

See Anesthetic Considerations for Lower-Extremity Procedures, p. 863.

References

1. Bohne WHO, Ertl JP: Ampuations of the lower extremity. In *Chapman's Orthopaedic Surgery,* 3rd edition, Vol 3. Chapman MW, ed. Lippincott Williams & Wilkins, Philadelphia: 2001, 3152-5.
2. Canale ST, ed: *Campbell's Operative Orthopaedics*, 10th edition. Mosby, St. Louis: 2003.
3. Epps CH Jr, ed: *Complications in Orthopaedic Surgery*, 3rd edition. JB Lippincott, Philadelphia: 1994.

LENGTHENING OR TRANSFER OF TENDONS, ANKLE, AND FOOT

SURGICAL CONSIDERATIONS

Description: In cases of motor imbalance from neuromuscular disease or trauma, tendons are lengthened or transferred to a new insertion to partially restore balance or normalize joint motion. For **tendon lengthening**, a longitudinal incision generally is made directly over the tendon. Subcutaneous tissues and tendon sheath are incised to expose the tendon, which is transected with a Z-type incision. The tendon is placed in its lengthened position and the ends of the Z are closed with absorbable suture. If present, the tendon sheath is closed separately from the skin closure. In a **tendon transfer**, the tendon usually is cut close to its insertion and transferred to a new bony insertion, which often requires a separate incision. The tendon is attached to the bone either with a metal staple or by suturing it into a drill hole in the bone.

Variant procedure or approaches: **Achilles tendon lengthening** is used to bring the ankle out of equinus. A **posterior tibial tendon lengthening** and/or **posterior ankle capsulotomy** may accompany the procedure.

Usual preop diagnosis: Contracture of muscle

SUMMARY OF PROCEDURES

	Tendon Lengthening	Achilles Tendon Lengthening
Position	Supine	Prone
Incision	Over tendon; sometimes multiple incisions	Over tendon
Special instrumentation	Tourniquet	⇐
Antibiotics	If young, none; in elderly or infirm, cefazolin 1 g iv preop	⇐
Surgical time	2 h	1 h
Closing considerations	Splint or cast while anesthetized	⇐
EBL	10 ml	⇐
Postop care	PACU → room	PACU → room or home
Mortality	Minimal	⇐
Morbidity	Infection: < 1%	⇐
Pain score	4	3

PATIENT POPULATION CHARACTERISTICS

Age range	Any age
Male:Female	1:1
Incidence	Rare
Etiology	Neuromuscular disease (80%); trauma (20%)
Associated conditions	Static encephalopathy/cerebral palsy (75%); other neuromuscular disease (25%)

ANESTHETIC CONSIDERATIONS

See Anesthetic Considerations for Lower-Extremity Procedures, p. 863.

Reference

1. Canale ST, ed: *Campbell's Operative Orthopaedics*, 10th edition. Mosby, St. Louis: 2003.

AMPUTATION ABOVE THE KNEE

SURGICAL CONSIDERATIONS

Description: In above-the-knee amputations, the distal part of the lower extremity is excised, starting just above the knee at the level of the distal third of the femur (Fig 10.6-3). A stump is fashioned, and will require prosthetic fitting at a later time. The most commonly performed stumps incorporate anterior and posterior flaps of equal length. The underlying muscles (hamstrings and quadriceps) are either sewn to each other (**myoplasty**) or to bone (**myodesis**). In a **guillotine**, or **open amputation**, the stump is not fashioned (tissues are not closed) until later. This is a multistage procedure used for dirty, traumatic amputations, infection, or above-knee amputations with questionable survival, and usually is done as a life-saving measure. Internal fixation of part of the remaining femur may be indicated in traumatic amputations. The patient returns to the OR every 1-3 d for redebridement until closure of the clean stump can be performed.

Usual preop diagnosis: PVD or gangrene of lower extremity; trauma to lower extremity; open-femur fracture with traumatic amputation; tumor of lower extremity

SUMMARY OF PROCEDURE

Position	Supine
Incision	Anterior and posterior on thigh
Special instrumentation	Amputation saw and rasp; drill for myodesis
Unique considerations	Patient often very ill from sepsis, chronic disease, or trauma
Antibiotics	Cefazolin or cefamandole 1 g iv q 6-8 h), ± gentamicin (80 mg iv q 8 h); adjust dosage for renal status, ± penicillin (1-2 million U iv q 4 h).
Surgical time	1-2 h
Closing considerations	Compressive dressing ± special stump sock
EBL	250 ml or more; higher for traumatic amputations
Postop care	Generally PACU → room (if medically unstable → ICU)
Mortality	Approximately 10-20%; higher in PVD (10-39%)
Morbidity	Phantom limb: 85-95%
	Phantom pain: 2-15%
	Wound infection ± deep infection: < 15% in PVD
	Respiratory failure or pneumonia: 10-15%
	MI: 7-10%
	Thromboembolism: 6-10%
	Cerebrovascular accident: 5-10%
	Contractures – flexion and abduction: Common
	Urinary retention requiring catheterization: Common
	Failure to heal ± wound dehiscence: Uncommon
	Hematoma: Rare
	Neuromas: Rare
	Reamputation: Rare
	UTI: Rare
	Contralateral amputation, especially in diabetics and those with PVD
	Postop depression
Pain score	7-10

PATIENT POPULATION CHARACTERISTICS

Age range	PVD, diabetic gangrene: 70-90% > 60 yr
	Multiple trauma with traumatic amputation, tumor of lower extremity: 18-35 yr
Male:Female	Overall, 3-9:1
	Elderly, predominance of males
	Multiple trauma, 4-5:1
	Tumor 1:1
Incidence	Common for PVD patients; rare for trauma or tumor
Etiology	PVD and diabetic gangrene (70-90%); multiple trauma (younger patients) (rare—usually with severe Grade IIIC injuries with neurovascular severance); tumor (rare); uncontrollable infection (e.g., gas gangrene) (rare)
Associated conditions	Diabetes (70-80% of patients presenting for this procedure); numerous other serious medical conditions; multiple trauma in younger patients

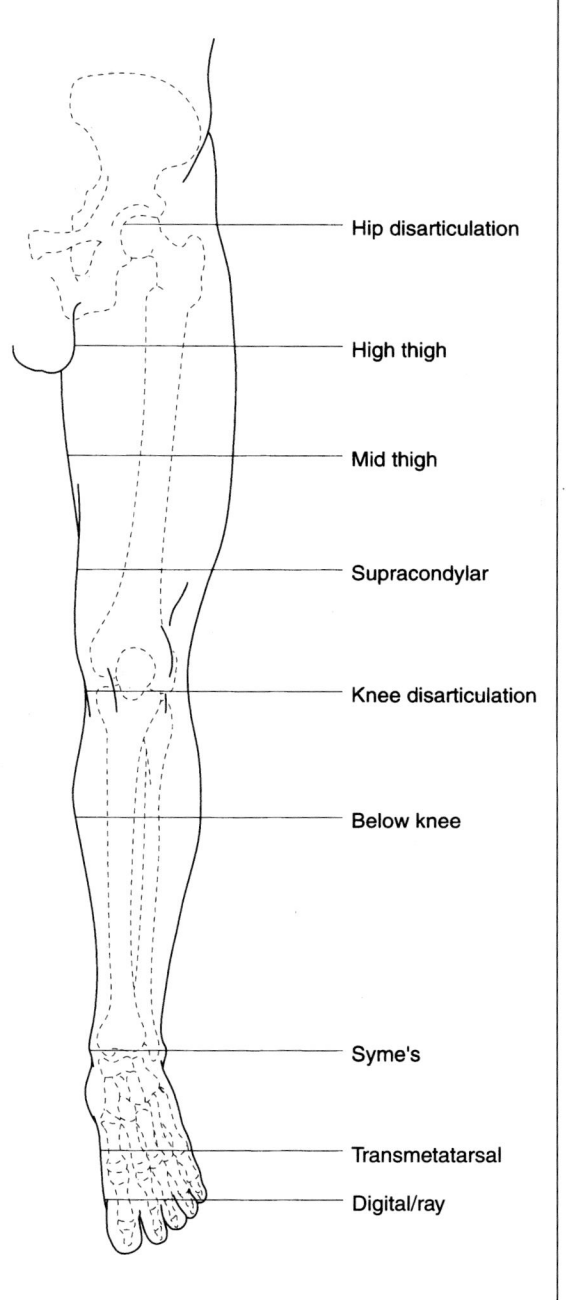

Figure 10.6-3. Common amputation levels for the lower extremity. (Reproduced with permission from Greenfield LJ, et al: *Surgery: Scientific Principles and Practices*, 3rd edition. Lippincott Williams & Wilkins, 2001.)

ANESTHETIC CONSIDERATIONS

See Anesthetic Considerations for Above- and Below-Knee Amputation, p. 855.

References

1. McCollough NC III, Epps CH Jr, Banks WJ Jr: Complications of amputation surgery. In *Complications in Orthopaedic Surgery*, 3rd edition. Epps CH Jr, ed. JB Lippincott, Philadelphia: 1994, 1279-1308.
2. Swiontkowski MF, Post PA: Surgical approaches to the lower extremity. In *Chapman's Orthopaedic Surgery,* 3rd edition, Vol I. Chapman MW, ed. Lippincott Williams & Wilkins, Philadelphia: 2001, 29-52.
3. Tooms RE: Amputations of lower extremity. In *Campbell's Operative Orthopaedics*, Vol 1, 9th edition. Canale ST, ed. Mosby-Year Book, St. Louis: 1998, 532-41.

AMPUTATION BELOW THE KNEE

SURGICAL CONSIDERATIONS

Description: **Below-the-knee amputation** is ablation of the lower limb, usually at the level of the midleg. A long, posterior flap normally is used to cover the stump. The condition of the soft tissues may dictate the level and/or type of flaps used. The procedure begins with an anterior transverse incision made over the midtibia. A long posterior flap, which is 2-3 times the diameter of the leg in length, is then made. The bone is exposed anteriorly and the anterolateral neurovascular structures and muscles are transected and ligated as appropriate (Fig 10.6-4A). The bone is then transected with a bone saw, and the posterior structures are transected and ligated as appropriate. The amputated leg and foot are then removed from the table and the posterior flap is tapered and shaped for closure (Fig 10.6-4B). Deep sutures are placed to secure the posterior muscles to the anterior tibia. The skin opening and subcutaneous tissues are closed with interrupted sutures. Finally, a drain is placed (sometimes), and either a compression dressing or an immediate postop cast is applied.

Variant procedure or approaches: **Guillotine amputation** may be used as the first of a two-stage procedure in infected or contaminated cases. With a guillotine amputation, the bone and soft tissues are transected very quickly in guillotine fashion at the midtibial level. Neurovascular structures are ligated as appropriate. These wounds are usually left open and a compression dressing applied.

Usual preop diagnosis: Dysvascular limb; infection; trauma

SUMMARY OF PROCEDURE

Position	Supine
Incision	Anterior and posterior flaps; for guillotine amputation, circumferential incision
Special instrumentation	Bone saw; tourniquet, if traumatic (tourniquet contraindicated if infected or avascular)
Antibiotics	Cefazolin 1 g iv preop
Surgical time	1.5 h; for guillotine amputation, 0.5 h
Closing considerations	May use cast; drain. Bulky dressing needed for guillotine amputation.
EBL	200 ml
Postop care	PACU → room
Mortality	10%
Morbidity	Phantom pain: 90%
	Infection: 10-15%
	Wound breakdown: 10-15%
	Pneumonia: 12%
	MI: 7%
	PE: 6%
	Hematoma: 5%
	Stroke: 5%
Pain score	5

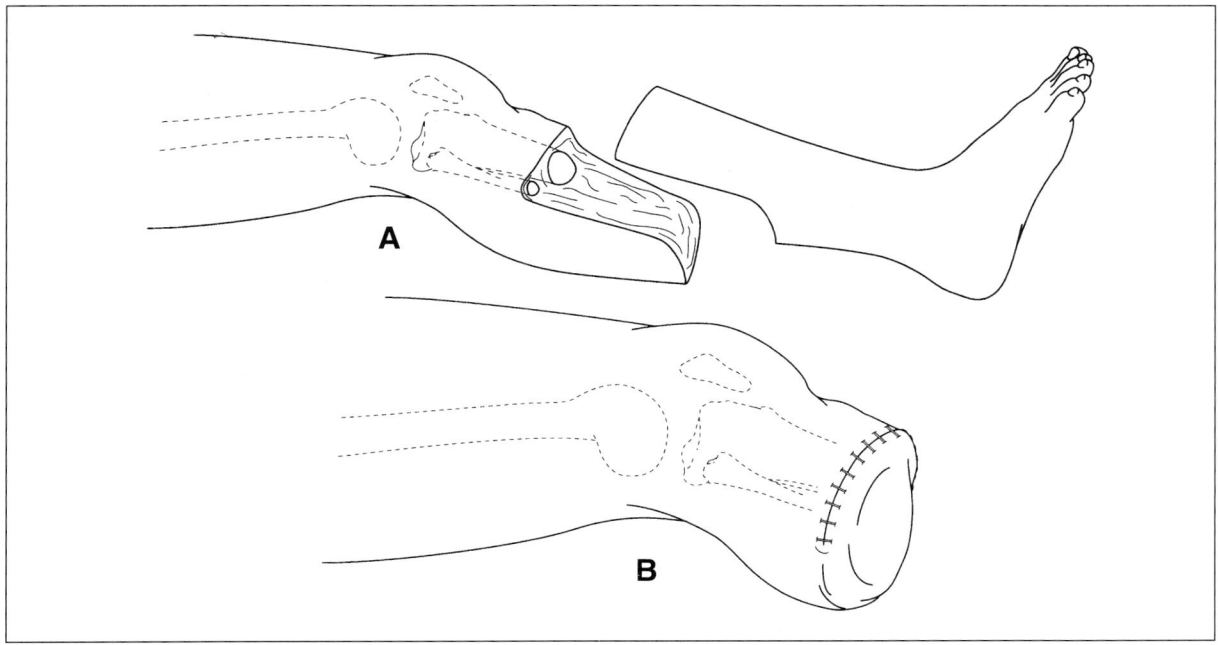

Figure 10.6-4. Below-knee amputation. (A) The tibia is transected 1 cm proximal to the skin incision, and the fibula is transected an additional 1 cm proximal to the level of the tibial transection. The posterior calf muscles are incised along the plane of the skin incision. (B) The posterior flap is rotated anteriorly and approximated. (Reproduced with permission from Greenfield LJ, et al, eds: *Surgery: Scientific Principles and Practice*, 3rd edition. Lippincott Williams & Wilkins, 2001.)

PATIENT POPULATION CHARACTERISTICS

Age range	Usually, > 60
Male:Female	3:1
Incidence	20,000-30,000 total amputations/yr
Etiology	Dysvascular limb (70%); trauma (20%); infection (5%); tumor (5%); congenital anomaly (< 1%)
Associated conditions	Vascular disease (70-80%); malnutrition (50%); diabetes mellitus (30%); pulmonary disease (30%)

ANESTHETIC CONSIDERATIONS FOR ABOVE- AND BELOW-KNEE AMPUTATION

PREOPERATIVE

Vascular disease and tumors are the two most common indications for these surgeries. Patients presenting for amputations often have severe systemic vascular disease. Their inability to perform exercise limits the usefulness of preop Hx in evaluating cardiopulmonary reserve, and often necessitates invasive studies for full evaluation.

Respiratory	Smoking is a risk factor common to both vascular and pulmonary diseases. Chronic bronchitis or COPD patients should have maximum medical therapy (e.g., inhaled bronchodilators, theophylline and steroids, when appropriate) prior to anesthesia. Regional anesthesia is an excellent choice for patients with severe pulmonary disease. **Tests:** As indicated from H&P.
Cardiovascular	Significant cardiovascular disease is present in 30% of patients presenting for vascular surgery. Particularly in diabetics, CAD is often silent. Dipyridamole thallium imaging of the heart can reveal the preop myocardium at risk of ischemia; however, therapy of stenotic coronary arteries usually can be undertaken only after the amputation. Medical management, to include ß-blockers when tolerated, will reduce perioperative MIs. **Tests:** ECG; others as indicated from H&P.

Neurological	Peripheral and autonomic neuropathies may be present in the diabetic patient. Hence, these patients may be more susceptible to injury from malpositioning and are less able to tolerate the hemodynamic changes associated with regional anesthesia. Preexisting neurological deficits should be carefully documented. Autonomic neuropathy is diagnosed by any of the following: postural ↓BP (in patient not bedridden); loss of sinus arrhythmia; resting ↑HR; miosis–abnormal response to darkness.
Musculoskeletal	Rhabdomyolysis can occur in the presence of partial ischemia. (See Renal, below.)
Hematologic	Often a trial of heparin, warfarin, or thrombolytic therapy will have been undertaken before amputation. Coag studies, including PT, PTT, and bleeding time are, therefore, often necessary to determine the appropriateness of epidural or intrathecal anesthesia. Warfarin-induced elevation of the PT can be reversed preop with FFP 5-10 ml/kg body weight. This therapy may induce fluid overload in patients with poor cardiac reserve. For these patients, diuretics should be administered to maintain normovolemia. **Tests:** As indicated from H&P.
Renal	Limb ischemia can result in myoglobinemia from rhabdomyolysis. Evidence of progressive renal failure or rising CPK-MM fractions should be treated with hydration, forced alkaline diuresis and prompt amputation. **Tests:** Consider Cr; BUN; CPK enzymes; urine myoglobin.
Laboratory	Diabetic patients require preop control of blood glucose and periop glucose monitoring.
Premedication	Standard premedication (see p. B-2).

INTRAOPERATIVE

Anesthetic technique: Either regional or GA may be appropriate.

Regional anesthesia: Both SAB and epidural blocks are useful techniques. Subarachnoid anesthesia has the advantage of limited spread of the block above the level of surgery, while obtaining adequate blockade of the sacral roots that are resistant to low-dose epidural techniques. Epidural anesthesia allows for extending the duration of anesthesia and for the administration of postop epidural analgesia. Anesthesia from T12 (T8 with tourniquet) is adequate. Full motor blockade is not necessary. Typical drugs and doses include: subarachnoid—75 mg of 5% lidocaine in 5% dextrose (controversial) with morphine 0.2 mg; epidural—12-15 ml 2% lidocaine with epinephrine 1:200,000 in divided doses.

General anesthesia:

Induction	Standard induction (see p. B-2) is appropriate for patients with normal airways. Intubation is indicated for diabetic patients with gastroparesis. Beware of difficult airway in long-standing insulin-dependent diabetics.	
Maintenance	Standard maintenance (see p. B-3).	
Emergence	No special considerations	
Blood and fluid requirements	Moderate blood loss IV: 16 ga × 1 NS/LR @ 4-6 ml/kg/h	Expect 100-200 ml blood loss, mostly during cleaning of the wound made while developing a flap.
Control of blood loss	Tourniquet may be used.	Inflation pressure is typically 100 mmHg > systolic pressure. Maximum 'safe' tourniquet time is 1.5-2 h, followed by a 5- to- (preferably) 15-min reperfusion interval, if further tourniquet is necessary.
Special considerations	Tourniquet deflation and limb reperfusion	Mild ↓BP is common. In patients with moderate-to-severe lung disease, continue controlled ventilation until after the lactic acid accumulated in the ischemic leg is metabolized (3-5 min), since these patients may be unable to increase ventilation adequately to buffer this acid load.
Monitoring	Standard monitors (see p. B-1). ± CVP line ± Arterial line	Invasive monitoring is indicated in the presence of severe cardiac or pulmonary disease. Serial blood glucose determination should be made in the diabetic patient.
Positioning	✓ and pad pressure points. ✓ eyes.	Meticulous padding of the extremities is necessary to prevent ischemic skin ulceration in patients with vascular insufficiency.

POSTOPERATIVE

Complications	Hematoma Bleeding	✓ drains.
Pain management	Spinal opiates Epidural analgesia	Epidural hydromorphone 50 μg/ml infused at 50-200 μg/h provides excellent analgesia.
Tests	CXR if CVP was placed.	Other studies as indicated.

References

1. Bohne WHO, Ertl JP: Ampuations of the lower extremity. In *Chapman's Orthopaedic Surgery,* Vol 3, 3rd edition. Chapman MW, ed. Lippincott Williams & Wilkins, Philadelphia: 2001, 3149-74.
2. Fung DL: Anesthesia and pain managment. In *Chapman's Orthopaedic Surgery,* Vol I, 3rd edition. Chapman MW, ed. Lippincott Williams & Wilkins, Philadelphia: 2001, 133-56.
3. McCollough NC III, Epps CH Jr, Banks WJ Jr: Complications of amputation surgery. In *Complications in Orthopaedic Surgery*, 3rd edition. Epps CH Jr, ed. JB Lippincott, Philadelphia: 1994, 1279-1308.

FASCIOTOMY OF THE THIGH

SURGICAL CONSIDERATIONS

Description: Increased intracompartmental pressure in the thigh requires surgical release of tight skin and fascial structures (Fig 10.6-5). This usually occurs after severe trauma to the thigh (e.g., crush injury, comminuted fracture, etc.), after prolonged vascular surgery (with ischemia to the thigh), or with infection. Compartment syndrome is a true emergency and must be treated within minutes of recognition. Failure to do so may result in loss of limb or death. Conventional devices may be used to measure intracompartmental pressure, which usually is abnormal if > 30-35 mmHg (normal = < 30 mmHg). **Fasciotomy of the thigh** involves incising the skin and fascia over the thigh and debriding any necrotic tissue. The wound is left open for later redebridement, delayed primary closure, or skin grafting. Thus, the fasciotomy begins a multistage procedure of incision and debridement, with subsequent reconstruction.

Usual preop diagnosis: Compartment syndrome of thigh; crush injury to thigh; necrotizing fasciitis

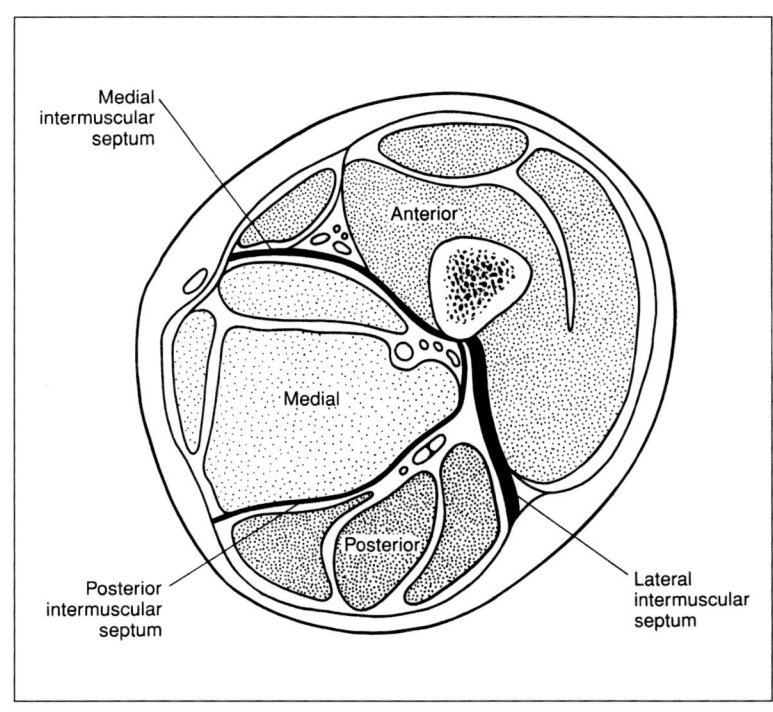

Figure 10.6-5. Cross-section of the thigh showing the 3 major compartments. (Reproduced with permission from Tarlow SD, Achterman C, Hayhurst J, Ovadin D: Acute compartment syndrome of the thigh. *J Bone Joint Surg* [Am] 1986; 68:1441.)

SUMMARY OF PROCEDURE

Position	Supine or lateral decubitus
Incision	Lateral thigh
Unique considerations	Patient may be very ill. If an ipsilateral femoral fracture is present with a compartment syndrome, the surgeon may want to perform ORIF, intramedullary nailing, or external fixation of the fracture.
Antibiotics	Cefazolin or cefamandole 1 g iv q 6 h
Surgical time	1.5-2 h for fasciotomy alone
Closing considerations	Wound left open and covered by sterile dressings.
EBL	250-500 ml
Postop care	If surgery is performed acutely, patient frequently will be a multiple-trauma victim with numerous injuries and extensive blood loss; usually goes to ICU.
Mortality	Dependent on extent of multiple trauma
Morbidity	Hypotension and fluid loss: Common
	Neurological deficit to peripheral nerves: Common, if decompression delayed
	Respiratory distress and fat embolism: Not uncommon, if concomitant femur fracture
	Vascular complications: Not uncommon
	Amputation: Rare, if decompression prompt
	Systemic sepsis: Rare
	Wound infection: Rare
	New compartment syndrome; insufficient fasciotomy: Rare
Pain score	7-8

PATIENT POPULATION CHARACTERISTICS

Age range	Any age, but predominance of males < 30 yr
Male:Female	5:1
Incidence	Extremely rare
Etiology	Trauma – motorcycle and motor vehicle accidents, falls, industrial injury, crush injuries; postsurgery – local hematoma and swelling; thrombosis or disruption of blood supply to thigh (e.g., failed proximal vascular bypass surgery, aortic dissection, etc.); massive infection of thigh compartment (e.g., gas gangrene)
Associated conditions	Burns; drug and alcohol overdose; frequently associated with trauma to other organ systems

ANESTHETIC CONSIDERATIONS

See Anesthetic Considerations following Fasciotomy of the Leg, p. 859.

References

1. Dutkowsky JP: Miscellaneous nontraumatic disorders. In *Campbell's Operative Orthopaedics*, Vol 1, 9th edition. Canale ST, ed. Mosby-Year Book, St. Louis: 1998, 787-856.
2. Meyer RS, Mubarak SJ: Compartment syndromes. In *Chapman's Orthopaedic Surgery*, 3rd edition. Chapman MW ed. Lippincott Williams & Wilkins, Philadelphia: 2001, 393-416.

FASCIOTOMY OF THE LEG

SURGICAL CONSIDERATIONS

Description: This procedure is the surgical decompression of fascial compartments for treatment or prevention of compartment syndrome. Patients are often very ill and unstable with other injuries or disease. Compartment syndrome is a true emergency and must be treated within minutes of recognition. Failure to do so may result in loss of limb or death. There are four compartments in the leg: anterior, lateral, deep posterior and superficial posterior (Fig 10.6-6). Generally, all four compartments are released during the procedure. A **four-compartment fascial decompression** can be performed through two incisions—medial and lateral. A medial longitudinal incision is made just posterior to the tibia; through this incision, the superficial and deep posterior compartments are identified and the fascia incised in longitudinal fashion. A straight, lateral, longitudinal incision is made and the deep fascia overlying the anterior and lateral compartments is identified. The fascia of each compartment is then incised longitudinally. Skin incisions are rarely closed because of the swelling. A compression dressing is applied and splints may be used.

Usual preop diagnosis: Compartment syndrome; vascular trauma

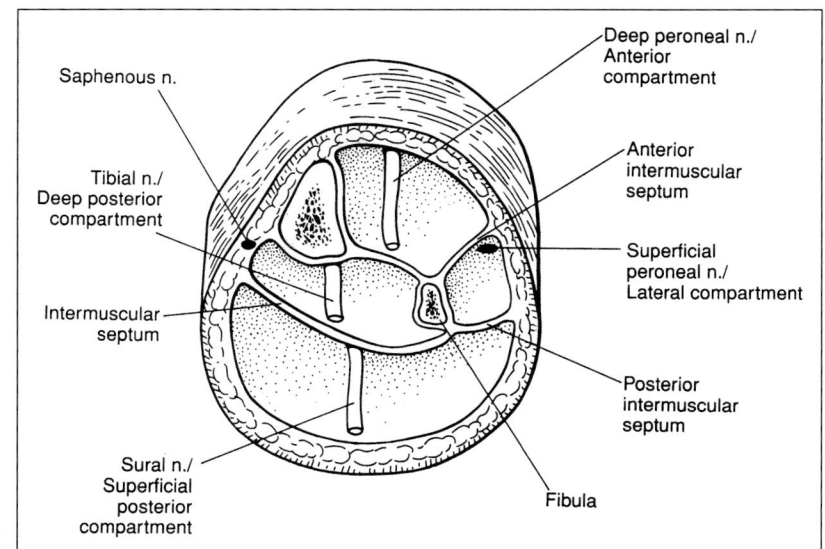

Figure 10.6-6. Cross-section of the left leg, middle lower third, showing the four compartments with associated peripheral nerves. (Reproduced with permission from Mubarak SJ, Owen CA: Double-incision fasciotomy of the leg for decompression in compartment syndromes. *J Bone Joint Surg* [Am] 1977; 59:184-7.)

SUMMARY OF PROCEDURE

Position	Supine
Incision	Medial and lateral parallel to tibia
Unique considerations	Often associated with fracture; may require fixation.
Antibiotics	Cefazolin 1 g iv preop
Surgical time	30 min +
Closing considerations	Wounds left open; splint may be required.
EBL	100 ml
Postop care	PACU → room; vascular monitoring is carried out clinically via a pulse oximeter on toes.
Mortality	Minimal
Morbidity	Myonecrosis: 50%
	Thrombophlebitis: 10-20%
	Infection: 10-15%
Pain score	3

PATIENT POPULATION CHARACTERISTICS

Age range	All ages
Male:Female	1:1
Incidence	~5% of tibia fractures
Etiology	Trauma – blunt fracture, vascular (90%); drug overdose (10%); burns (< 5%); revascularization (< 5%)
Associated conditions	Multiple trauma (60%); vascular disease (15%)

ANESTHETIC CONSIDERATIONS FOR FASCIOTOMY OF THIGH AND LEG

PREOPERATIVE

Compartment syndromes and necrotizing fasciitis are the indications for these procedures (necrotizing fasciitis also may cause compartment syndrome). Patients with compartment syndrome often have no systemic disease, while patients with necrotizing fasciitis have a rapidly life-threatening infection that requires prompt surgical debridement and often is complicated by rhabdomyolysis and DIC.

Respiratory   Usually no special considerations, unless massive sepsis.

Cardiovascular	Sepsis is uniformly present in patients with necrotizing fasciitis. Management includes antibiotics and hemodynamic support with dopamine (5-15 μg/kg/min) or epinephrine (0.02-0.25 μg/kg/min), with therapy guided by invasive hemodynamic monitoring, which may include PA catheter.
Neurological	If fasciotomy is for compartment syndrome, there may be compromise of distal nerves and blood flow. Perform a thorough neurologic exam of the involved extremity to document preop deficits.
Hematologic	If infection is the indication for the fasciotomy, DIC is likely. Evaluate for pathologic bleeding. Administer factors necessary to correct coagulopathy during the procedure. **Tests:** CBC; PT; PTT; fibrinogen; fibrin split products; Plt count
Renal	Both necrotizing fasciitis and compartment syndrome often cause myoglobinuria and rhabdomyolysis. Myoglobinuria can be inferred from urine that is dipstick-positive for occult blood but microscopically free of RBCs in the absence of hemolysis (therefore, no free Hb in the urine).
Laboratory	Hct; serial K^+ levels if there is an active diuresis; other studies as indicated from H&P.
Premedication	Standard premedication (see p. B-2).

INTRAOPERATIVE

Anesthetic technique: Regional techniques are appropriate for compartment syndrome decompression, unless there is evidence of DIC or systemic infection. These surgeries are usually of short duration (< 1 h). Sepsis and hemodynamic instability usually mandate GETA for fasciotomy in patients with necrotizing fasciitis.

Regional anesthesia: Either subarachnoid or epidural blocks are useful in the absence of systemic infection or severe coagulopathy. Subarachnoid anesthesia has the advantage of adequate blockade of the sacral roots that are resistant to low-dose epidural techniques. Anesthesia from T10-S2 is adequate. Typical drugs and dosages include: subarachnoid—15 mg of 0.5% bupivacaine; epidural—12-15 ml 2% lidocaine with epinephrine 1:200,000 in divided doses.

General anesthesia:

Induction	Standard induction (see p. B-2).	
Maintenance	Standard maintenance (see p. B-3).	
Emergence	Consider postop ventilation for patients with impaired oxygenation or ongoing hemodynamic instability; otherwise, no special considerations.	
Blood and fluid requirements	IV: 16 ga × 1 (compartment syndrome) 14-16 ga × 2 (necrotizing fasciitis) NS/LR @ 4-6 ml/kg/h	To prevent renal damage, insure adequate circulatory volume; induce osmotic diuresis with mannitol 0.25 g/kg iv. Furosemide 10-100 mg also may be necessary to maintain diuresis. Replace UO with 0.5 NS + 50 mEq bicarbonate/L, or as guided by invasive monitoring.
Monitoring	Standard monitors (see p. B-1). UO ± Arterial line ± CVP or PA catheter	Fluid losses (3rd-spacing, bleeding) may be significant. Patients with necrotizing fasciitis require an arterial line and either a CVP or PA catheter to guide fluid and inotropic/pressor therapy.
Positioning	✓ and pad pressure points. ✓ eyes.	

POSTOPERATIVE

Complications	DIC Renal failure 2° rhabdomyolysis Hypo/hyperkalemia Sepsis syndrome, including ARDS	
Pain management	PCA or epidural analgesia	See pp. C-3, C-2.
Tests	Hct Electrolytes UA (dipstick and microscopic)	For patients with sepsis: coag profile, including PT/PTT, fibrin split products, and Plt count

---

References

1. Bucholz RW, Heckman JD, eds: *Rockwood and Green's Fractures in Adults*, 5th edition. Lippincott Williams & Wilkins, Philadelphia: 2001.

2. Epps CH Jr, ed: *Complications in Orthopaedic Surgery*, 3rd edition. JB Lippincott, Philadelphia: 1994.
3. Meyer RS, Mubarak SJ: Compartment syndromes. In *Chapman's Orthopaedic Surgery*, 3rd edition. Chapman MW ed. Lippincott Williams & Wilkins, Philadelphia: 1993, 2001, 393-416.

BIOPSY, LEG AND FOOT

SURGICAL CONSIDERATIONS

Description: Biopsy is performed to excise tissues for pathologic evaluation, usually through a small, longitudinal wound. For **incisional biopsy**, a longitudinal incision is made over the mass. Overlying soft tissues are incised with minimal undermining. The area in question is incised and the biopsy removed, with care being taken to prevent spillage into the adjacent tissues. The pathologist often is asked to perform a frozen section to determine whether diagnostic tissue is present. The wound is closed with interrupted sutures and a compression dressing applied. A splint or cast may be used if a significant amount of bone has been removed. If the lesion is small, x-ray control or image intensification may be necessary for localization. **Needle biopsy** may be used for distinct osseous lesions to obtain small amounts of tissue for culture or histology. **Excisional biopsy** may be used for benign lesions like exostoses or lipomas.

Usual preop diagnosis: Tumor; infection

SUMMARY OF PROCEDURES

	Incisional Biopsy	Needle Biopsy	Excisional Biopsy
Position	Supine	⇐	⇐
Incision	Short longitudinal	Stab wound	Stab wound
Special instrumentation	Bone-cutting instruments; x-ray or I.I.	Trephine (e.g., Craig needle); x-ray or I.I.	X-ray or I.I.
Unique considerations	Tourniquet	⇐	⇐ (Bone graft may be necessary.)
Antibiotics	None (May be given postop.)	⇐	⇐
Surgical time	1 h	0.5 h	0.5-2 h
Closing considerations	May be splinted.	Usually no splint	May be splinted.
EBL	50 ml	Minimal	100-200 ml
Postop care	PACU → room or home	⇐	PACU → room
Mortality	Minimal	⇐	⇐
Morbidity	Hematoma: 5%	⇐	⇐
	Tumor spread: < 5%	⇐	⇐
	Infection: < 1%	⇐	⇐
Pain score	3	2	3

PATIENT POPULATION CHARACTERISTICS

Age range	All ages
Male:Female	1:1
Incidence	Rare
Etiology	Tumor (75%); infection (25%)
Associated conditions	Metastatic disease; immune compromise

ANESTHETIC CONSIDERATIONS

See Anesthetic Considerations for Lower-Extremity Procedures, p. 863.

Reference

1. Enneking WF: *Musculoskeletal Tumor Surgery*. Churchill Livingstone, New York: 1983.

BIOPSY OR DRAINAGE
OF ABSCESS/EXCISION OF TUMOR

SURGICAL CONSIDERATIONS

Description: This procedure involves obtaining a piece of tissue for histologic and/or bacteriologic Dx by closed, percutaneous means or by open biopsy. Subsequently, the area may be drained (abscess or infection) or an open excision of a tumor may follow (± internal fixation). For excision of tumors of the pelvis, acetabulum or femur, please consult the appropriate section describing fractures of the area. Each case must be individualized.

Variant procedure or approaches: Excision of infection or tumor of proximal or distal femur, femoral shaft, pelvis, or acetabulum.

Usual preop diagnosis: Femur: biopsy of mass; infection; osteomyelitis. Pelvis or acetabulum: biopsy of pelvis or acetabulum; drainage of abscess or infection of pelvis or acetabulum; osteomyelitis of pelvis or acetabulum; septic arthritis of acetabulum

SUMMARY OF PROCEDURE

Position	Supine or lateral decubitus
Incision	Percutaneous, short or long; location depends on surgical approach.
Special instrumentation	Biopsy needles and instruments to take core biopsy; bone cement may be used to plug biopsy site. Some surgeons use fracture table or radiolucent table with I.I.
Unique considerations	May require intraop frozen section and gram stain.
Antibiotics	After tissue has been obtained, cefazolin or cefamandole 1 g iv q 6 h × 48 h. A gram stain will help decide immediate antibiotic coverage, but cultures and sensitivities are ultimately necessary.
Surgical time	1 h for simple procedures; much longer (up to 12 h) for more extensive excisional procedures ± further reconstruction.
EBL	100-1000 ml or more
Postop care	If procedure is extensive with much blood loss, or the patient is unstable or ill from chronic sepsis or invasive tumor, it is prudent to send patient to ICU.
Mortality	Dependent on extent of procedure. Biopsy or drainage of a small, localized abscess in soft tissue or bone is rarely life-threatening. Wide/radical excision of a malignant tumor in the pelvis or extremities is frequently life/limb-threatening.
Morbidity	The following are dependent on site and procedure:
	Intraop fracture
	Nonunion
	Chronic osteomyelitis
	Compartment syndrome
	Residual instability of pelvis or hip joint
	Fracture of pelvis or acetabulum, nonunion
	Chronic osteomyelitis or septic arthritis
	Hypotension 2° to blood loss
	Respiratory distress
	Neurological injury to lumbosacral plexus, sciatic nerve, or other peripheral nerves
	Vascular injury to iliac or other vessels
	Injury to GI, genitourinary, or gynecological organs
Pain score	2-10

PATIENT POPULATION CHARACTERISTICS

Age range	Any age; predominance of elderly patients with tumors
Male:Female	1:1
Incidence	Rare
Etiology	Benign and malignant tumors (common); infection (rare); previous surgery (rare); previous trauma (rare)
Associated conditions	Metastatic disease or other foci of infection

ANESTHETIC CONSIDERATIONS FOR LOWER-EXTREMITY PROCEDURES

(Procedures covered: ORIF of femur, tibia, ankle, and foot; intramedullary nailing of femur and tibia; closed reduction and external fixation of femur and tibia; distal tibia, ankle and foot procedures; repair nonunion/malunion of femur and tibia; ankle arthroscopy, arthrotomy, arthrodesis; repair/reconstruction, ankle ligaments; Syme's amputation; transmetatarsal amputation; tendon (ankle, foot) lengthening; biopsy of leg and foot; biopsy or drainage of abscess/excision of tumor)

PREOPERATIVE

Trauma victims comprise the largest group of patients for these procedures. Minimizing the time between fracture and surgery for open wounds significantly reduces the incidence of wound infection. Evaluations for other injury, adequacy of fluid resuscitation and preexisting conditions need to be undertaken promptly and used as a guide for anesthetic management. Patients with bone cancer form another subset of patients and often have concurrent medical conditions and have undergone chemotherapy or radiation therapy preop.

Respiratory	Pulmonary fat embolus occurs in 10-15% of patients following bone fracture. Sx include hypoxemia, ↑HR, tachypnea, respiratory alkalosis, mental status changes, and conjunctival petechiae. Lab analysis may reveal fat in the urine. Preop therapy for this condition should include supplemental O_2 with mechanical ventilation, to correct hypoxemia, and meticulous fluid management to prevent worsening pulmonary capillary leak. **Tests:** Consider CXR; others as indicated from H&P.
Cardiovascular	Cardiac contusion or tamponade are possible if blunt chest trauma has occurred during the injury. A large volume of blood can be hidden around a long bone fracture site. ↑HR, orthostasis, or ↓BP indicate hypovolemia, and this should be corrected with crystalloid (10-40 ml/kg) or blood if Hct < 24%. In patients with a tibial or distal femur fracture, and who are presenting with hemodynamic instability and ongoing blood loss, consider applying a tourniquet to the thigh prior to induction. **Tests:** Consider ECG; CPK enzyme levels and ECHO will help evaluate the presence of cardiac injury.
Neurological	Perform a thorough neurological evaluation, including mental status and peripheral sensory exams. A CT scan of the head is indicated for any patient with prolonged loss of consciousness prior to anesthesia. Drug abuse is common in trauma patients and they should be asked specifically about any drug use. **Tests:** Patients with inappropriate behavior or a positive drug abuse Hx should undergo a urine and plasma drug screen.
Musculoskeletal	Consider cervical instability and obtain spine films if mechanism of injury included rapid deceleration or trauma to the head or neck. Myoglobinemia and ↑K^+ may result from crush injury.
Hematologic	Patients with cancer who have undergone chemotherapy and multiple transfusions often develop sensitivities to blood products and may require specialized blood products, such as leukocyte-poor PRBC or red cells negative for a particular antigen. The availability of these blood products should be confirmed before surgery. **Tests:** Hct and others as indicated from H&P.
Renal	**Tests:** UA
Laboratory	Other tests as indicated from H&P.
Premedication	Due to the risk of gastric aspiration, minimal or no premedication is given to trauma victims. For other patients, standard premedication (see p. B-2). Narcotic premedication (morphine 1-2 mg iv q 10 min titrated to effect) is appropriate for patients experiencing pain with movement.

INTRAOPERATIVE

Anesthetic technique: For trauma patients, regional anesthesia permits evaluation of mental status, provides intact airway reflexes, and ↓ blood loss. Combative patients and those requiring multiple concurrent surgical procedures or prolonged (> 2 h) procedures are often managed with GETA.

Regional anesthesia: Either subarachnoid or epidural blocks are useful techniques. Subarachnoid anesthesia has the advantage of adequate blockade of the sacral roots that are resistant to low-dose epidural techniques. Epidural anesthesia allows for the administration of postop epidural analgesia. Anesthesia from T12 (T8 with tourniquet) to S2 is adequate. Full motor blockade is desirable. Typical drugs and doses include: subarachnoid—15 mg of 0.5% bupivacaine with morphine 0.2 mg (omit if outpatient); epidural—12-15 ml 2% lidocaine with epinephrine 1:200,000 in divided doses (Na bicarbonate 0.1 mg/ml will speed onset of block).

General anesthesia:

Induction	Standard induction (see p. B-2) is appropriate for patients with normal airways. Trauma patients require a rapid-sequence induction (see p. B-5) and intubation with cricoid pressure to prevent gastric aspiration.	
Maintenance	Standard maintenance (see p. B-3). Trauma patients are often cold and require active warming if < 35°C (convection blanket and active humidifier). Warming the patient may unmask severe hypovolemia that should be corrected.	
Emergence	Trauma patients should have full return of protective airway reflexes and, given the possibility of fat embolus, evidence of adequate oxygenation on 50% O_2 prior to extubation.	
Blood and fluid requirements	IV: 14-16 ga × 2 NS/LR @ 4-8 ml/kg/h Warm fluids. Humidify gases.	Some fractures can involve large (30 ml/kg) blood losses that are hidden in the leg or thigh. Clinical signs of hypovolemia and serial Hct determination should guide fluid therapy.
Control of blood loss	Tourniquet	Inflation pressure is typically 100 mmHg > systolic pressure. Maximum 'safe' tourniquet time is 1.5-2 h, followed by a 5- to- (preferably) 15-min reperfusion interval, if further tourniquet time is necessary.
Monitoring	Standard monitors (see p. B-1). ± Arterial line ± CVP line	Arterial/CVP lines indicated for patients with ↓BP not readily correctable with crystalloid infusion, massive blood loss (> 1 blood volume), or the need for postop ventilation.
Positioning	✓ and pad pressure points. ✓ eyes.	
Special considerations	Release of tourniquet	A 20% fall in mean BP is common on tourniquet deflation. Additional crystalloid (5-10 ml/kg) may be necessary to replace edema fluid and blood loss to the leg.
Complications	Fat embolism Myoglobinemia	

POSTOPERATIVE

Complications	Hypoxemia	May be 2° fat embolism.

Pain management	Spinal opiates:
	  Epidural anesthesia
	  Spinal anesthesia
		Epidural hydromorphone 50 μg/ml infused at 100-250 μg/h provides excellent analgesia. Intrathecal morphine 0.2-0.3 mg provides analgesia for up to 24 h after administration. (Monitor for delayed respiratory depression.)

Tests	Hct CXR, if CVP placed or oxygenation is impaired.	Other studies as indicated.

References

1. Carnesale PG: General principles of tumors. In *Campbell's Operative Orthopaedics*, Vol 1, 9th edition. Canale ST, ed. Mosby-Year Book, St. Louis: 1998, 643-82.
2. Fung DL: Anesthesia and pain management. In *Chapman's Orthopaedic Surgery,* 3rd edition, Vol I. Chapman MW, ed. Lippincott Williams & Wilkins, Philadelphia: 2001, 133-56.
3. Warner WC Jr: General principles of infections. In *Campbell's Operative Orthopaedics*, Vol 1, 9th edition. Canale ST, ed. Mosby-Year Book, St. Louis: 1998, 563-77.

11.0 PLASTIC AND RECONSTRUCTIVE SURGERY

Surgeons

Lonny L. Ross, MD, FRCSC
David M. Kahn, MD

11.1 FACIAL COSMETIC SURGERY

Anesthesiologist

Tara Cornaby, MD

INTRODUCTION TO COSMETIC FACIAL SURGERY

The presenting Sx of the aging face are predictable, based on the effects of gravity, facial expression, sunlight (or other UV exposure), and connective tissue changes. Patients present with concerns of looking tired, angry, or older than they feel. They also may complain of functional difficulties, like loss of visual fields due to drooping brow or eyelids, or breathing difficulty due to previous nasal surgery. Other common complaints are creases or wrinkles around the eyes and mouth, and a sagging or fatty chin and neck.

Cosmetic facial surgery sets out to rejuvenate the facial form by surgical manipulation of the facial soft tissues. The techniques used involve any or all of the following: soft tissue release, resection, plication, and resuspension.

Facial aging takes place simultaneously in all areas of the face and neck; therefore, combined procedures are not uncommon. Generally, in combined procedures, facelift would precede necklift. If a browlift is added, it would be next. Blepharoplasty procedures are generally addressed after the 'lift' procedures, because they change the lid tissue posture. A rhinoplasty ideally comes last, as it can cause immediate bleeding and swelling, which can obscure other facial fields of surgery.

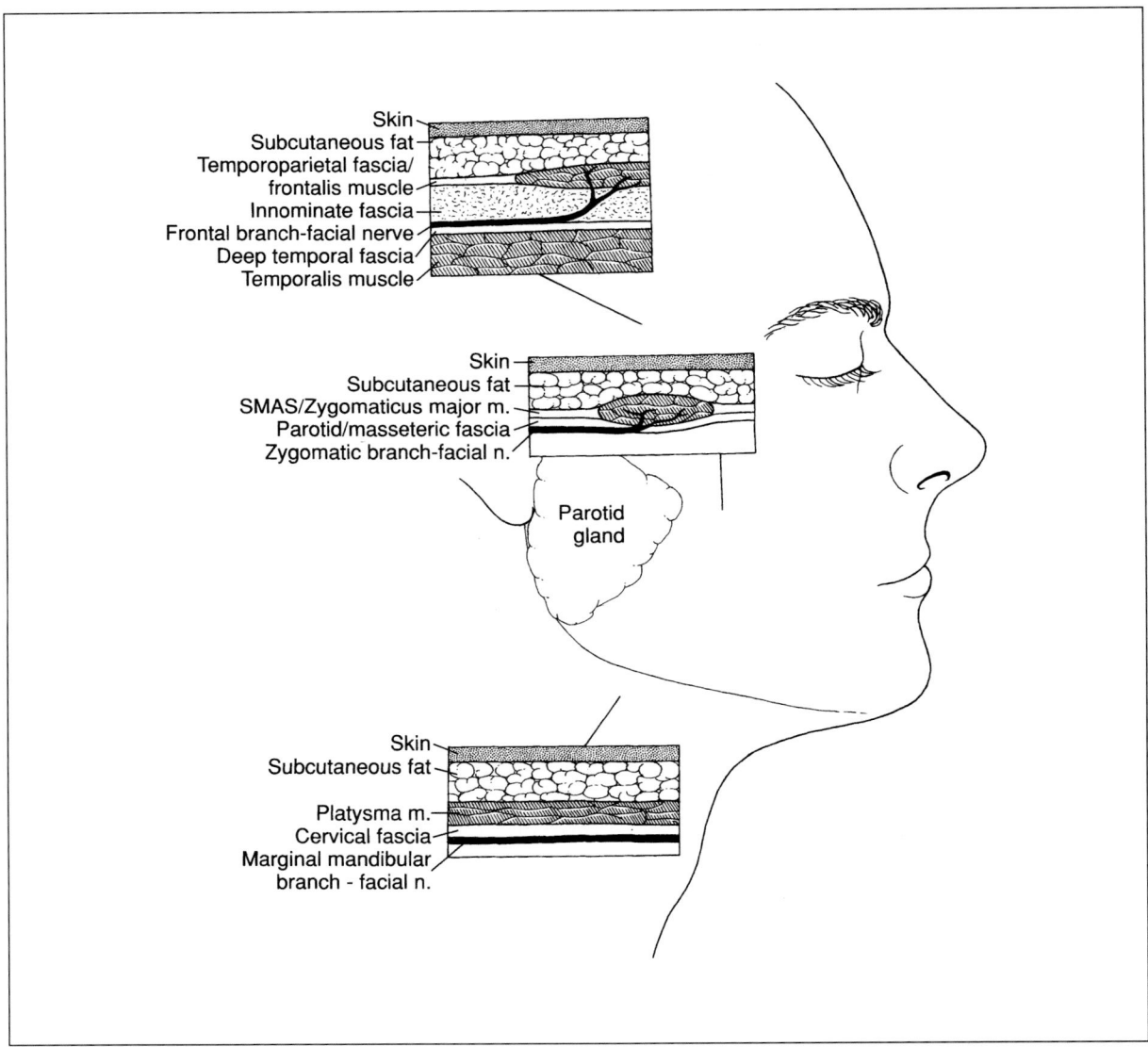

Figure 11.1-1. Anatomic layers of the face. Although the names vary, the arrangement persists, regardless of the area of the face. The facial nerve (CN VII) branches innervate their respective muscles of the SMAS layer via the deep surfaces. (Reproduced with permission from Thorne CHM, Aston SJ: Aesthetic surgery of the aging face. In *Grabb & Smith's Plastic Surgery*, 5th edition. Aston SJ, Beasley RW, Thorne CHM, eds. Lippincott-Raven, 1997.)

FACELIFT AND NECKLIFT

SURGICAL CONSIDERATIONS

Facelift (or Meloplasty or Rhytidectomy)

Description: Facelifts and **midfacial lifts** are procedures to rejuvenate the face by use of soft-tissue surgical manipulation, affecting the area between the inferior orbital rim and the inferior border of the mandible. The lips and nose are generally unaffected. Many types of 'facelift' procedures have been developed to solve the diversity of challenges of facial aging and rejuvenation.[12] Traditional facelift procedures took place in the subcutaneous plane, with some skin resection. Today, three planes of dissection are used (Fig 11.1-1). **Subcutaneous dissection** continues to be popular, traversing the adipose tissue below the skin and many of the vessels supplying the skin.[12,17] The next dissection plane is the subSMAS, which occurs between the superficial musculoaponeurotic system of the face (SMAS) and the parotid gland.[14,17] More recently, **subperiosteal dissections**[10,11,15] (midfacial lifts) have become popular, since they are much less likely to develop postop hematomas. (Recovery can be extended with subSMAS and subperiosteal techniques due to prolonged swelling.) Combinations of these dissection planes also have been described.

Local anesthetics with epinephrine are injected presurgically for the various procedures. A number of subcutaneous infiltration mixtures may be used, including one described by **Klein** that consists of NS 1000 ml with 1.0 ml epinephrine (1:1000) and 50 ml of 1%

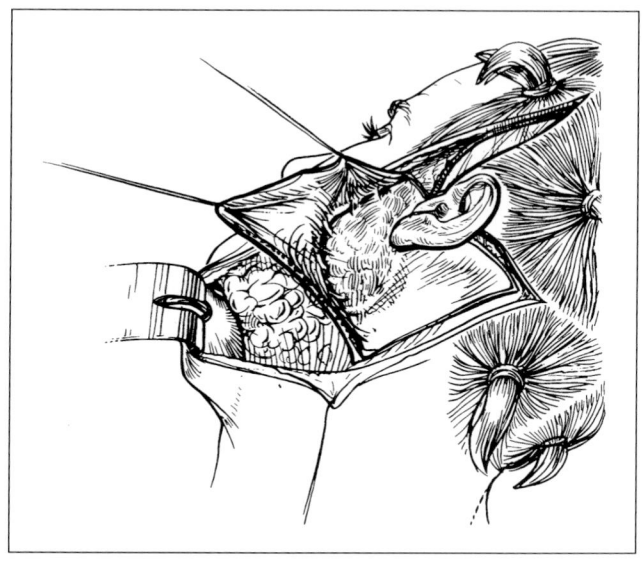

Figure 11.1-2. Dissection of SMAS/platysma flap. If a composite rhytidectomy is performed, the same plane of dissection is used. If SMAS dissection extends to the zygomaticus major muscle, it is termed 'extended.' (Reproduced with permission from Thorne CHM, Aston SJ: Aesthetic surgery of the aging face. In *Grabb & Smith's Plastic Surgery*, 5th edition. Aston SJ, Beasley RW, Thorne CHM, eds. Lippincott-Raven, 1997.)

lidocaine ± 12.5 ml of 8.5% sodium bicarbonate solution. It has been shown that 5-7 times the traditionally accepted maximum dose of lidocaine with epinephrine can be injected safely into the subcutaneous space.[20] This solution provides hemostasis and hydrodissection. Decreased OR time and excellent intraop and postop analgesia also have been attributed to its use.[5,16]

Traditional incisions typically are made in the preauricular region with temporal and inferior postauricular scalp extensions. The approaches for the subcutaneous and SMAS techniques resemble those used for bilateral facial palsy and parotid gland operations. The midfacial procedures may be carried out through intraoral and/or lower-lid incisions and may be combined with other facelift procedures.

A typical facelift may begin with subcutaneous dissection of the facial skin flap (Fig 11.1-2) on one side (± the neck on the same side), with meticulous hemostasis being accomplished with bipolar electrocautery. The SMAS layer can then be mobilized and resuspended. Some surgeons continue on the same side with skin resection and closure before starting the opposite side, while others temporarily pack the first side and perform an identical elevation and SMAS procedure on the opposite side. In this case, a second look for bleeding is made on each side after a waiting period.

Hematoma is the most common complication of facelift surgery, and HTN is the most common medical condition in the age group presenting for facelift;[13] thus, periop HTN is the facelift patient's worst enemy. It must be anticipated and treated preemptively. Commonly used salicylates and other NSAIDS are contraindicated in the immediate preop period (i.e., within 10 d of surgery; platelet life span=10 d).[7] Hematoma risk is highest in male patients, perhaps due to increased perfusion of the bearded region, hormonal gender differences, or increased sebaceous gland density.[13] Smoking also has been shown to be detrimental to facelift results, especially with regard to skin flap survival. Ideally, patients should not smoke for 2 wk before and after surgery.[13]

One of the least desirable long-term morbidities is injury to the facial nerve, which can produce a disastrous aesthetic result following a purely cosmetic surgery. Many surgeons prefer that no paralytics be used during the procedure to allow ongoing monitoring of facial nerve function.

Necklift

Description: Necklift is the rejuvenation of the area from the inferior mandibular margin to the clavicals. This procedure often is combined with facelift procedures to sharpen the chin and smooth the anterior neck (i.e., improve the cervicomental angle). It usually is achieved via extension of the facelift dissection inferiorly and a small submental incision ± skin excision, and may be combined with **submental liposuction** or **lipectomy** and **platysma muscle modifications** (plication, suspension, resection, or transection techniques).[8] The submental portion can be achieved before or after the facelift procedures. Some platysmal suspension techniques require the facelift incisions to remain open with continuity in the subcutaneous plane laterally.

Variant procedures or approaches: Laser resurfacing (see p. 881 and p. 1207), especially in the perioral and periorbital regions; **blepharoplasty** and **browlift** (see p. 872) are common adjunct procedures.

Usual preop diagnosis: Facelift: facial rhytids (wrinkles/creases); solar or senile elastosis; jowling; deep nasolabial folds; tear troughs; nasojugal folds; malar bags. Necklift: 'turkey gobbler' neck; platysmal bands; cervical laxity; cervical rhytids

SUMMARY OF PROCEDURES

	Facelift	Necklift	Midface lift
Position	Supine, reverse Trendelenburg	⇐	⇐
Incision	Preauricular, scalp	Extension of face-lift incision + sub-mental incision.	Intraoral ± subciliary or inferior lid
Special instrumentation	Infiltration equipment for super wet techniques; endoscopic equipment (more frequent with brow lifts)	⇐ ± liposuction in-strumentation.	–
Unique considerations	Oral intubation; ability to move ETT side-to-side. Watch for: occulocardiac reflex (OCR), retrobulbar hematoma with periorbital approaches.	⇐	⇐
	If laser is used: • Special fire-retardant ETT and drapes • Laser eye protection for all in room • Cannula-administered O_2 should be far away from laser (fire safety) • Smoke evacuation system (See Facial Laser Resurfacing, p. 882.)	⇐	⇐
	Infiltration of increased amounts of local and epinephrine in facelift and liposuction procedures	⇐	–
Antibiotics + other meds	Cefazolin 1 g iv, (± Solu-Medrol 125 mg iv). Antivirals periop if laser used (e.g., acyclovir 2400 mg × 2 d preop and 14 d postop)[1]	⇐	⇐
Surgical time	4-6 h	1-2 hr	2-4 h
Closing considerations	Trendelenburg for final hemostasis ± drains	⇐	⇐
	Some surgeons prefer gentle ↑ in BP during hemostasis.	⇐	⇐
	Tissue thrombin agents may be used between the elevated flaps.	⇐	–
	Sensory nerve blocks by surgeon	⇐	⇐
	± Full head/face wrap before patient awakens	⇐	⇐
	Gentle, nonagitated awakening to prevent sudden ↑BP.	⇐	⇐
EBL	100-200 ml	⇐	⇐
Postop care	Monitor for hematoma: most common complaint is pain; therefore, r/o hematoma before increased analgesia or sedation.[18]	⇐	⇐
	Lightly compressive dressing, ± drains: both removed at 24 h.	⇐	⇐
	2 wk no aspirin, moderate activity	⇐	⇐
Mortality	Rare	⇐	⇐

	Facelift	**Necklift**	**Midface lift**
Morbidity[3,4,9,11,13,14,17,18,19]	Early hematoma:	⇐	Very rare
	Large expanding: 1-15% (return to OR)	⇐	
	Small (< 30 ml): 10-15% (± aspiration in office)	⇐	
	Late hematoma (average = 9 d postop; 2° to exertion or aspirin use, from superficial temporal vessels)	⇐	–
	Infection: 0-0.33%	⇐	⇐
	Nerve injury:		
	Motor (temporal/marginal mandibular branches)	⇐	Very rare
	Temporary: 0.1-2.6%	⇐	
	Permanent: 0-0.66%	⇐	
	Motor (spinal accessory nerve): Rare	⇐	–
	Sensory injury:	⇐	–
	Great auricular nerve → ↓sensation in lower ½ of ear ± painful neuromas or paresthesias		
	Lesser occipital nerve painful → neuroma	⇐	–
	Alopecia: 0.4% (most temporary, along the incision)	⇐	–
	Skin slough: 14% (especially in retroauricular area) (12.5 × greater in smokers)	⇐	–
	Dehiscence: 0.1-0.35%	⇐	⇐
	Parotid cysts: Rare	⇐	–
	Poor cosmetic result:	⇐	⇐
	Hyperpigmentation		
	Telangiectasia (preexisting lesions may worsen)		
	Hypertrophic scarring		
	Keloids: Very rare		
	'Pixie' (pulled-down earlobe deformity (technique-dependant)		
	Hairline shifts		
	Ectropion (midface, approached via lid incisions only): Up to 3%		
Pain score	3	3	3

PATIENT POPULATION CHARACTERISTICS

Age range[2]	> 35 yr
Male:Female	1:9[2] to 1:5[17] (This has increased from 1:17 in the 1970s.[14,17])
Incidence[6]	124,531 facelift procedures in the U.S. (2001); 8% of total cosmetic procedures (5th most common cosmetic procedure)
Etiology	Facial rhytids 2° solar elastosis, senile elastosis, facial expression
Associated Conditions	Cancers of the skin (basal cell carcinoma, squamous cell carcinoma and precursors, and melanoma), in solar elastosis cases, especially fair-skinned patients

ANESTHETIC CONSIDERATIONS

See Anesthetic Considerations following Browlift and Blepharoplasty, p. 876.

References:

1. Alster TS, Apfelberg DB, eds: *Cosmetic Laser Surgery: A Practitioner's Guide*, 2nd edition. Wiley-Liss, New York: 1999.
2. American Society of Plastic Surgeons website: www.plasticsurgery.org. 444 East Algonquin Rd, Arlington Heights, IL 60005-4664.
3. Baker DC, Conley J: Avoiding facial nerve injuries in rhytidectomy. *Plast Reconstr Surg* 1979; 64(6):781-95.
4. Baker TJ, Gordon HL: Complications of rhytidectomy. *Plast Reconstr Surg* 1967; 40(1):31-9.
5. Brody GS: The tumescent technique for facelift. *Plast Reconstr* Surg 1994; 94:563.
6. Desnoyers Y, Custeau P, Berthiaume J, Dagenais G: Anaesthesia for facial rhytidectomy. *Can Anaesth Soc J* 1979; 26(3): 222-4.
7. Dumanian GA, Bontempo FA, Johnson PC: Evaluation and treatment of the plastic surgical patient having a potential to bleed. *Plast Reconstr Surg* 1995; 96(1):211-18.

8.   Feldman JJ: Corset platysmaplasty. *Plast Reconstr Surg* 1990; 85(3):333-43.
9.   Goldwyn RM: Late bleeding after rhytidectomy from injury to the superficial temporal vessels. *Plast Reconstr Surg* 1991; 88(3):443-5.
10. Heinrichs HL, Kaidi AA: Subperiosteal face lift: A 200-case, 4-year review. *Plast Reconst Surg* 1998; 102(3):843-55.
11. Hester TR Jr, Codner MA, McCord CD, Nahai F, Giannopoulos A: Evolution of technique of the direct transblepharoplasty approach for the correction of lower lid and midfacial aging: Maximizing results and minimizing complications in a 5-year experience. *Plast Reconstr Surg* 2000; 105(1):393-408.
12. Hoefflin SM: The extended supraplatysmal plane (ESP) face lift. *Plast Reconstr Surg* 1998; 101(2):494-503.
13. Kaye, BL: Complications of face-lift. *Adv Plast Reconstr Surg* 1990; 6:125-76.
14. Lemmon ML, Hamra ST: Skoog rhytidectomy: A five-year experience with 577 patients. *Plast Reconstr Surg* 1980; 65(3): 283-97.
15. Little JW: Three-dimensional rejuvenation of the midface: Volumetric resculpture by malar imbrication. *Plast Reconstr Surg* 2000; 105(1):267-85.
16. Mottura AA: The tumescent technique for face lifts? *Plast Reconstr Surg* 1995; 96(1):231.
17. Pitanguy I: Facial cosmetic surgery: A 30-year perspective. *Plast Reconstr Surg* 2000; 105(4):1517-27.
18. Rees TD, Lee YC, Coburn RJ: Expanding hematoma after rhytidectomy. *Plast Reconstr Surg* 1973; 51(2):149-53.
19. Schnur PL, Burkhardt BR, Tofield JJ: The second-look technique in face lifts—Does it work? *Plast Reconstr Surg* 1980; 65(3):298-301.
20. Schoen SA, Taylor CO, Owsley TG: Tumescent technique in cervicofacial rhytidectomy, *J Oral Maxillofac Surg* 1994; 52: 344-7.
21. Sullivan SA, Dailey RA: Endoscopic subperiosteal midface lift. *Opthal Plast Reconstr Surg* 2002; 18(5):319-30.

BROWLIFT AND BLEPHAROPLASTY

SURGICAL CONSIDERATIONS

Browlift (or Forehead Lift)

Description: Browlift is the resuspension of the brows and elimination of upper facial rhytids to help restore the youthful appearance of the upper face. This procedure has a large effect on the results of an upper blepharoplasty, with which it is frequently paired. Patients presenting for browlift usually have specific concerns about lateral brow hoods, forehead wrinkles, and glabellar creases that give them an angry appearance.

Like facelift procedures, browlifts have been performed in the relatively avascular subgaleal/subperiosteal[6] or subcutaneous[12] planes. The subgaleal/subperiosteal plane approach has become more popular with the incorporation of **endoscopic techniques.** Incisions may be complete bicoronal or interrupted elliptical incisions. They may be along the hair line or within the hair-bearing scalp (Fig 11.1-3). In the open technique, the bicoronal flap is peeled off of the upper face (Fig 11.1-4). The brows are elevated by **scalp resuspension ± resection** (Fig 11.1-5). The scalp suture closure helps hold the resuspension position; also, the soft tissues may be fixated directly to the cranium with plates and screws and to the temporal fascia with suture to maintain their new positions. Release of the periosteum along the superior orbital rims is generally a prerequisite to adequate resuspension when using a subperiosteal approach. Elimination of the upper facial rhytids (i.e., glabellar wrinkles) is achieved by resection of the medial brow musculature (corrugator and procerus muscles) from beneath the elevated flap. Muscular bleeding is controlled with bipolar electrocautery.

Variant procedures or approaches: The browlift has become the facial plastic surgery procedure most adaptable to the techniques of **endoscopy.** Multiple smaller (1-1.5″) incisions are used within the scalp for access, and small, elliptical excisions also may be used to achieve the desired effect. The muscle resection is accomplished endoscopically with very small biting forceps from beneath the flap.[7,11]

Usual preop diagnosis: Brow ptosis; brow droop; upper facial rhytids (wrinkles or creases)

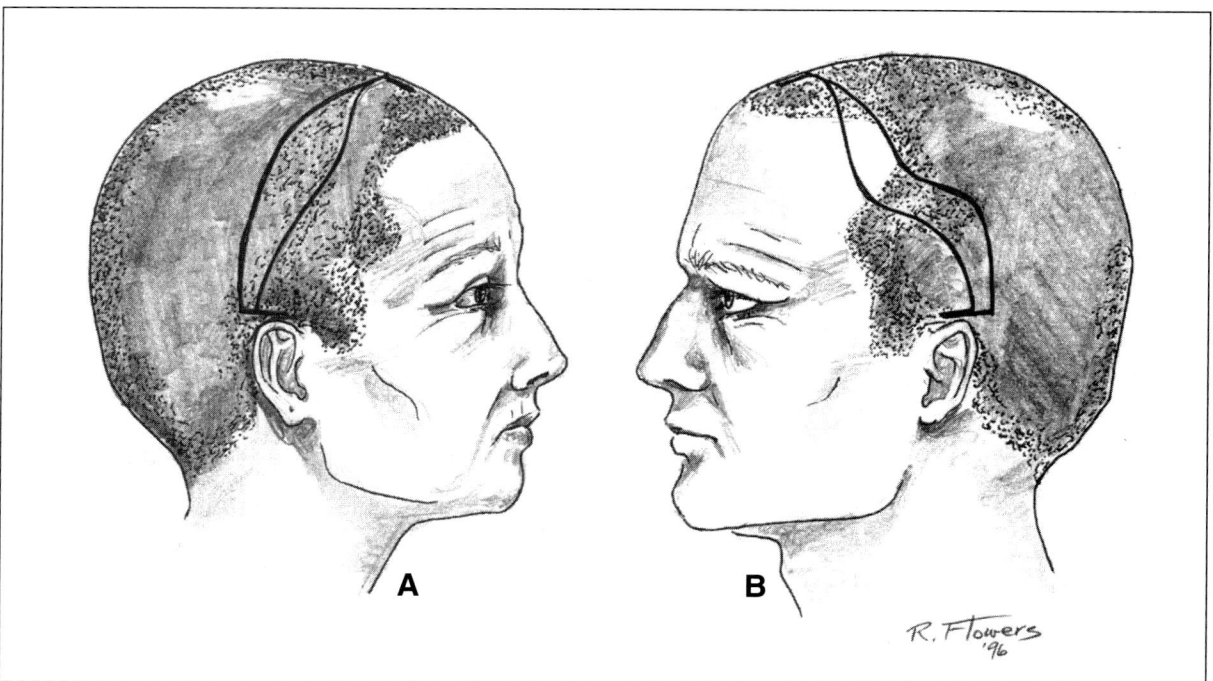

Figure 11.1-3. Incisions for forehead/brow lifting. Consistent blepharoplasty results demand appropriate frontal lifting technique. (A) Standard coronal incision and (B) male and female balding incision. Note the posterior displacement of the ascending incision for maximum camouflage. Hair perimeter incisions are rarely necessary. The central brow corrects nicely from only parietotemporal scalp excisions (after appropriate supraperiosteal release). (Reproduced with permission from Flowers RS, DuVal C: Blepharoplasty and periorbital aesthetic surgery. In *Grabb & Smith's Plastic Surgery*, 5th edition. Aston SJ, Beasley RW, Thorne CHM, eds. Lippincott-Raven, 1997.)

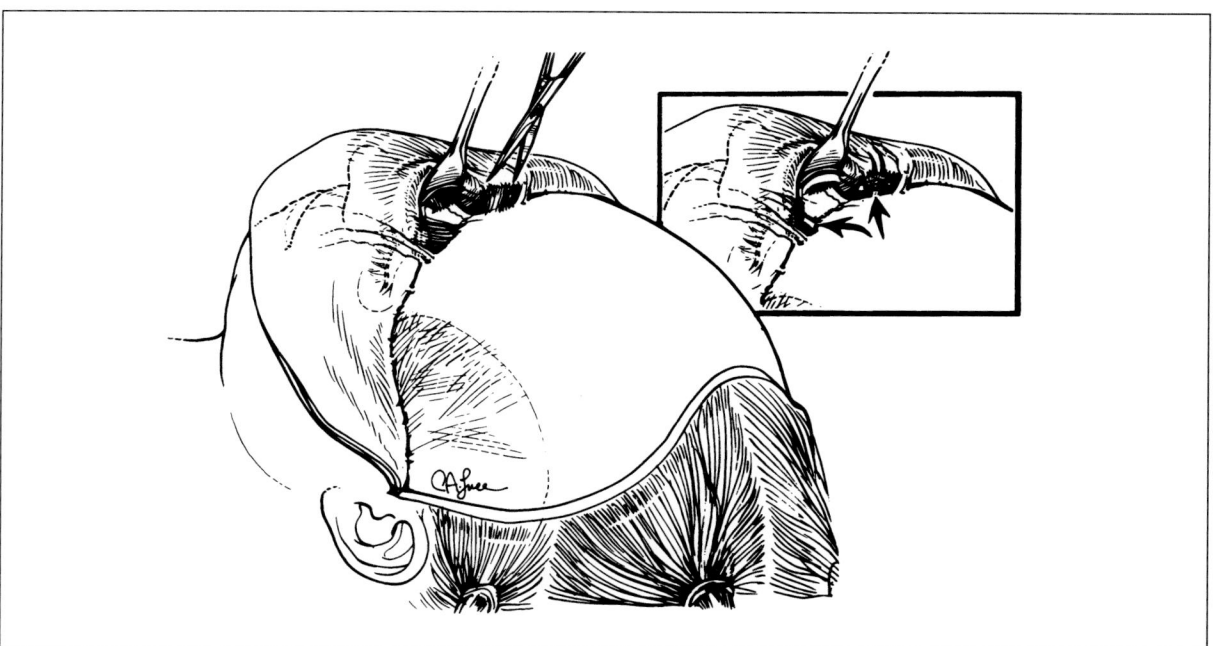

Figure 11.1-4. Exposure after subgaleal, supraperiosteal dissection of the forehead. The supraorbital nerves can be seen easily, but the supratrochlear nerves are more superficial and are hidden by the corrugator muscles. Scissors are used to tease through the corrugator muscles to locate the supratrochlear nerve branches. The muscle is then aggressively resected, preserving the sensory branches. (Reproduced with permission from Thorne CHM, Aston SJ: Aesthetic surgery of the aging face. In *Grabb & Smith's Plastic Surgery*, 5th edition. Aston SJ, Beasley RW, Thorne CHM, eds. Lippincott-Raven, 1997.)

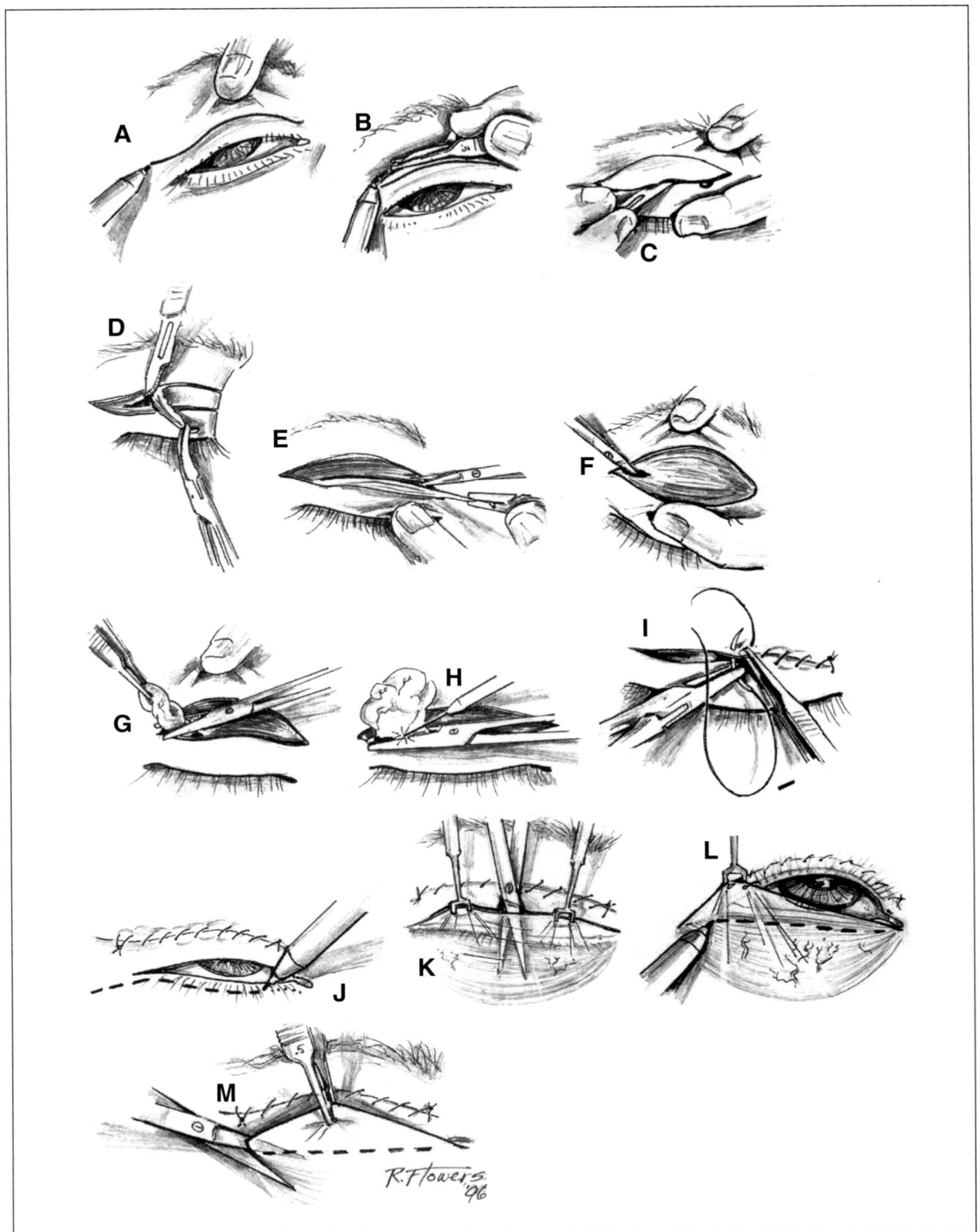

Figure 11.1-5. Traditional blepharoplasty technique. (A) The caudal margin of the excision is marked and (B) the upper eyelid skin is pinched. Skin and muscle are excised (C, D, E); excess or herniated fat is removed from medial and lateral compartments (F, G, H); and the wound is closed (I). On the lower lid, the traditional approach is flap elevation, consisting of skin or skin with attached muscle (J, K). The skin is draped upward and outward so the surgeon can assess and remove excess skin (L, M). (Reproduced with permission from Flowers RS, DuVal C: Blepharoplasty and periorbital aesthetic surgery. In *Grabb & Smith's Plastic Surgery*, 5th edition. Aston SJ, Beasley RW, Thorne CHM, eds. Lippincott-Raven, 1997.)

Blepharoplasty (or Lidlift)

Description: Blepharoplasty (Fig 11.1-5), or lidlift, is the surgical rejuvenation of the periorbital region to eliminate the tired and aged appearance of the eyes. Westernizing the Asian eyelid also has become quite common-place. Presenting complaints include excess lid skin, prominent periorbital fat, and absence of upper lid folds. Blepharoplasty can involve resection of skin, muscle (orbicularis occuli), and fat. Many patients presenting for this procedure will require a simultaneous browlift to establish the baseline position of the brows to reveal the true amount of upper-lid soft-tissue redundancy.[3] Eyelid ptosis repair also can be achieved in the same surgery.

Although a seemingly benign procedure, the manipulation of periorbital fat can have very serious consequences. Retrobulbar hematoma and blindness[9] can occur postop, and occulocardiac reflex (OCR) can complicate the intraop course with ↓HR and ↓BP. This generally resolves with elimination of the stimulus.[4]

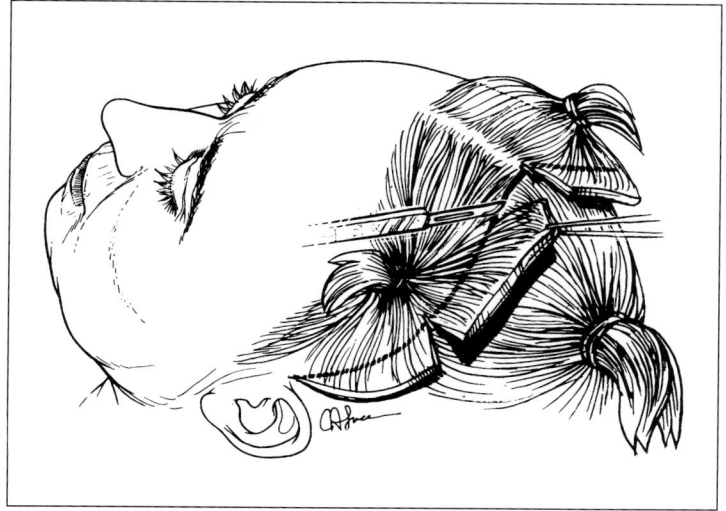

Figure 11.1-6. Redraping the forehead/brow using 'key' fixation sutures. Maximal tension is placed laterally to elevate the lateral brow to a greater extent than the medial brow. (Reproduced with permission from Thorne CHM, Aston SJ: Aesthetic surgery of the aging face. In *Grabb & Smith's Plastic Surgery*, 5th edition. Aston SJ, Beasley RW, Thorne CHM, eds. Lippincott-Raven, 1997.)

Blepharoplasty, as an isolated procedure, is often carried out with local anesthetics and iv sedation so that patients can open and close their eyes during the procedure. This ensures a good result without excess skin removal and lagophthalmos, and is especially important if a ptosis repair is also planned.[10]

Variant Procedures or Approaches: CO_2 **laser blepharoplasty** techniques have proven effective[5] but must be done under the safety parameters of eye protection and fire and burn prevention (see p. 882). With this technique, the fat and skin resections are achieved with a laser to replace use of a scalpel. Laser resurfacing techniques to gain some of the skin tightening of a blepharoplasty also have been described.

Usual preop diagnosis: Blepharochalasis; periorbital fat; blepharoptosis; supratarsal fold absence; Asian eyelid

SUMMARY OF PROCEDURES

	Browlift	Blepharoplasty
Position	Supine; table rotated 90 or 180°	⇐
Incision	Hairline, coronal; multiple scalp for endoscopic procedure	Upper: tarsal fold; lower: subciliary, transconjunctival
Special instrumentation	Fibrin glue, miniplates and screws for suspension; endoscopic equipment	Bipolar electrocautery
Unique considerations	Local anesthetic with epinephrine	Retrobulbar hematoma; OCR; local anesthetic with epinephrine
Antibiotics	Cefazolin 1 g iv ± Solu-Medrol 125 mg iv	⇐
Surgical time	1-2 h	⇐
Closing considerations	Place dressing before arousing patient. Gentle arousal from anesthesia (↑ in BP or emesis → risk of hematoma)	No dressing (ointment)
EBL	50 ml	Minimal
Postop care	PACU → room/home	⇐
	Lightly compressive dressing	Cool packs
	Head of bed elevated	⇐
		Ophthalmic lubricant
		Vision checks
Mortality	Rare	⇐

	Browlift	**Blepharoplasty**
Morbidity	Hematoma: Rare	⇐
	Alopecia: Rare (more common with bicoronal approach)	–
	Infection: < 1%	⇐
	Frontalis paralysis: Rare (usually transient)	–
	Poor cosmetic result	⇐
	Sensory nerve dysfunction	⇐
	Lagophthalmos	⇐
		Blindness: Extremely rare
		Ectropion
		Entropion
Pain score	3	2-3

PATIENT POPULATION CHARACTERISTICS

Age range[1]	Most ≥ 35 yr
Male:Female[1]	Blepharoplasties: 1:4
	Browlifts: 1:7.33
Incidence[1]	Blepharoplasties: 238,213, or 15% of all cosmetic procedures (3rd most common cosmetic procedure) in U.S. (2001) (137% increase from 1992-2001)
	Browlifts: 74,987, or 5% of all cosmetic procedures in U.S. (2001) (229% increase from 1992-2001)
Etiology	Facial rhytids 2° solar elastosis, senile elastosis, facial expression, and increased muscle resting tone; Asian eyelids
Associated conditions	Cancers of the skin (basal cell carcinoma, squamous cell carcinoma and precursors, and melanoma) in solar elastosis cases, especially fair-skinned patients

---

References:

1. American Society of Plastic Surgeons website: www.plasticsurgery.org, 444 East Algonquin Rd, Arlington Heights, IL 60005-4664.
2. Flowers RS: The art of eyelid and orbital aesthetics: multiracial surgical considerations. *Clin Plast Surg* 1987; 14(4):703-21.
3. Flowers RS, Caputy GC, Flowers SS: The biomechanics of brow and frontalis function and its effect on blepharoplasty. *Clin Plast Surg* 1993; 20(2):255-68.
4. Matarasso A: The oculocardiac reflex in blepharoplasty surgery. *Plast Reconstr Surg* 1989; 83(2):243-50.
5. Mittelman H, Apfelberg DB: Carbon dioxide laser blepharoplasty—advantages and disadvantages. *Ann Plast Surg* 1990; 24(1):1-6.
6. Ortiz-Monasterio F, Barrera G, Olmedo A: The coronal incision in rhytidectomy—the brow lift. *Clin Plast Surg* 1978; 5(1):167-79.
7. Ramirez OM: Endoscopically assisted biplanar forehead lift. *Plast Reconstr Surg* 1995; 96(2):323-33.
8. Ramirez OM: Endoscopic techniques in facial rejuvenation: an overview. Part 1. *Aesth Plast Surg* 1994; 18:141-7.
9. Sacks SH, Lawson W, Edelstein D, Green RP: Surgical treatment of blindness secondary to intraorbital hemorrhage. *Arch Otolaryngol Head Neck Surg* 1988; 114:801-3.
10. Stasior OG, Ballitch HA II: Ptosis repair in aesthetic blepharoplasty. *Clin Plast Surg* 1993; 20(2):269-73.
11. Steinsapir KD, Shorr N, Hoenig J, Goldberg RA, Baylis HI, Morrow D: The endoscopic forehead lift. *Opthal Plast Reconstr Surg* 1998; 14(2):107-18.
12. Wolfe SA, Baird WL: The subcutaneous forehead lift. *Plast Reconstr Surg* 1989; 83(2):251-6.

ANESTHETIC CONSIDERATIONS

(Procedures covered: facelift, necklift; browlift, blepharoplasty)

PREOPERATIVE

Cosmetic facial surgery is elective and should be performed preferably on ASA I or II patients. Often, several cosmetic procedures (including facial laser resurfacing) are performed during the same surgical session. A preop discussion with the surgical team is important to help define the anesthetic plan. The above procedures are predominantly done under GA in the hospital, but can also be done under MAC with local anesthesia. Several authors describe the use of a propofol/ketamine MAC or 'dissociative anesthetic' in the office-based setting (see p. 1208). There are varying descriptions of this technique, generally involving a propofol infusion with incremental ketamine boluses or infusion, resulting in elimination or significant reduction in the administration of iv opiates.

Airway	A careful inspection of the airway should be performed. Surgeon may request intraop manipulation of the oral ETT from side-to-side.
Cardiovascular	A thorough cardiovascular evaluation should be performed, since HTN is the most common medical condition in this patient population. Many procedures involve the use of significant amounts of local anesthetic with epinephrine, placing the patient at higher risk for HTN, dysrhythmias, and coronary artery spasm. Additionally, consider patient suitability for the use of controlled, mild controlled ↓BP (particularly the facelift patient). **Tests:** ECG, if indicated from H&P.
Hematologic	✓ for recent aspirin/NSAID use. **Tests:** CBC, if indicated from H&P.
Laboratory	Others tests as indicated from H&P.
Premedication	Preop sedation with clonidine (adjunctive hypnotic and antihypertensive agent) or midazolam usually is appropriate. Preop steroids (dexamethasone 4-8 mg) also may be used to reduce postop pain and PONV, as well as swelling.

INTRAOPERATIVE

Anesthetic technique: See above. Cases are predominantly done under GA, using an ETT or LMA, as appropriate. MAC with local anesthetic also is an option and may be advantageous for certain patients (e.g., with Hx of PONV) or for cases that benefit from a patient's intraop ability to follow commands (e.g., ptosis repair).

Induction	For those procedures done under GETA, a standard induction (p. B-2) is appropriate. An oral RAE ETT may be used to minimize intrusion into the surgical field. For cases involving a laser, a shielded ETT manufactured for laser surgery should be used and the cuff filled with NS and methylene blue, rather than air. (Note: no cuffed ETT is 100% laser-proof; always use standard precautions.)	
Maintenance	Standard maintenance (p. B-3) with volatile anesthetic ± propofol infusion is appropriate in most cases. Muscle relaxation should be avoided in cases with facial nerve monitoring. Mild, controlled ↓BP may be requested and used to facilitate hemostasis. HTN should be avoided and treated immediately if it occurs. Maintain anesthesia during application of head/face wrap.	
Emergence	Antiemetic prophylaxis (e.g., 5-HT$_3$-receptor antagonist) is recommended, as postop emesis greatly increases the likelihood of hematoma formation. Perform thorough oropharyngeal suctioning and ensure that all throat packing has been removed. A smooth emergence with no notable increase in BP is preferred.	
Blood and fluid requirements	Blood loss generally minimal IV: 18 ga × 1 NS/LR @ 2-4 ml/kg/h	
Monitoring	Standard monitors (p. B-1)	
Control of blood loss	Local infiltration with epinephrine Surgical hemostasis Mild degree of ↓BP	
Positioning	✓ and pad pressure points. Rotate OR table 90-180°.	Scleral shields ± ophthalmic ointment
Complications	OCR Local anesthetic toxicity Retrobulbar hematoma	Remove inciting stimulus. Consider atropine 0.5 μg and deepening anesthetic.

POSTOPERATIVE

Complications	PONV	Vigorous treatment of nausea is important.
Pain management	Local infiltration + iv/po narcotics, if needed	R/O expanding hematoma as cause of increasing pain.

Anesthesia References

1. Aasboe V, Raeder JC, Groegaard B: Betamethasone reduces postoperative pain and nausea after ambulatory surgery. *Anesth Analg* 1998; 87:319-23.
2. Barash PG, Cullen BF, Stoelting RK, eds: *Clinical Anesthesia*, 3rd edition. Lippincott Williams & Wilkins, Philadelphia: 1997.
3. Friedburg BL: Propofol-ketamine technique: dissociative anesthesia for office surgery; a review of 1,264 cases. *Aesth Plast Surg* 1999; 23:70.
4. Guit JB, Koning HM, Coster ML, et al: Ketamine as an analgesic for total intravenous anesthesia with propofol. *Anaesthesia* 1991; 46:24-7.
5. Richard MJ, Skues MA, Jarvis AP, Prys-Roberts C: Total iv anesthesia with propofol and alfentanil: dose requirements for propranolol and the effect of premedication with clonidine. *Br J Anaesth* 1990; 65:157-63.

RHINOPLASTY

SURGICAL CONSIDERATIONS

Description: Rhinoplasty, one of the greatest challenges of plastic surgery, is the surgical manipulation of the nasal form for aesthetic and/or functional improvement. In combination with nasal septal surgery, it is called **septorhinoplasty**. Common patient requests are for dorsal hump reduction and improved tip definition. Cosmetic surgery of the nose can be divided into four types: **tip rhinoplasty**,[5,6,7,13] **dorsal rhinoplasty**,[2,8] **alarplasty**, and **septoplasty**[3] and other ancillary procedures to enhance airway function.

Tip and **dorsal procedures** may be accomplished by either **reduction** or **augmentation**. Augmentation can be achieved with synthetic materials such as silicone, expanded fibrillated polytetrafluoroethylene polymer (Gore-Tex), porous polyethylene implants (Medpore), hydroxyapatite, etc.[4,11] Cadaveric tissue (cartilage, bone, fascia, or dermis) or autologous tissue also are utilized. Common donor sites for cartilage are the ear concha (via anterior or posterior approach), the nasal septum[7] (internal nasal approach), and the ribs. Bone harvest sites may include the outer table of cranium,[12] the iliac crest, and the ribs. Dermal graft is commonly harvested from the groin and fascial graft harvest is often taken from the temporoparietal region. (Table 11.1-1 shows the range of open and closed rhinoplasty techniques.)

A throat pack is useful to prevent aspiration or ingestion of blood, as significant blood pooling can occur in the naso/oropharynx area, especially with nasal osteotomies used to narrow or straighten the nasal dorsum. Cases where such pooling is expected are safer under GA with a throat pack. Often rhinoplasties are done with local or regional (nasociliary and infraorbital blocks) anesthesia with sedation. Vasoconstrictor-soaked nasal packs (cocaine vs epinephrine vs oxymetazoline) are placed before the first incision.[9,10]

Open versus closed technique is decided based on patient requirements and surgeon's preference. An **open approach** will utilize a transcolumellar incision to allow elevation of a nasal skin flap, degloving the lower alar cartilages for direct and wide exposure of the nasal framework. **Closed approaches** utilize intercartilaginous, intracartilaginous, infracartilaginous, rim, hemitransfixion, and transfixion incisions (all hidden within the nose).

A typical **closed rhinoplasty** (Figure 11.1-7) would begin with dorsal work through intercartilaginous incisions. The dorsum may be reduced using a scalpel and/or rasps beneath the undermined dorsal skin and periosteum. The septum is addressed as necessary through a hemitransfixion incision (± cartilage harvest). Tip reduction by scalpel or scissor resection of the lower alar cartilage ± tip suture is next. Nasal osteotomies with osteotome and mallet begin at the base of the nasal bones along the piriform aperture. Digital manipulation completes the fractures, and this is when most of the blood loss occurs. Dorsal and tip grafts are applied as necessary, with alar modifications made last. **Alar reduction** entails wedge resection of the lateral alar base and primary closure.

Open	**Closed/Open**	**Closed**
Incisions/skin flap elevation ↓ Tip analysis/cephalic crura excision ↓ Extramucosal tunnels ↓ Dorsal modification ↓ Caudal septum/anterior nasal spine ↓ Septoplasty/harvest ↓ Osteotomies ↓ Graft preparation ↓ Definitive dorsum/spreader grafts ↓ Tip: Columella strut/tip sutures ↓ Closure ↓ Alar base modification ↓ Dressing/postop management	Intercartilaginous/transfixion incisions ↓ Skin elevation/extramucosal tunnels ↓ Rasp bony hump/ excise cartilaginous hump ↓ Radix reduction ↓ Check profile line/septal angle ↓ Caudal septum/anterior nasal spine ↓ Infracartilaginous/ transcolumellar incisions ↓ Tip exposure and analysis ↓ Septal correction/harvest ↓ Osteotomies ↓ Definitive dorsum/spreader grafts ↓ Tip/columellar modification (excision/sutures/grafts) ↓ Closure ↓ Alar base modification ↓ Dressing	Transcartilaginous/ transfixion incision ↓ Skin elevation/extramucosal tunnels ↓ Rasp bony hump/ excise cartilage hump ↓ Radix reduction ↓ Check profile line/septal angle ↓ Caudal septum/anterior nasal spine ↓ Septoplasty/harvest ↓ Infracartilaginous incisions ↓ Alar cartilage delivery ↓ Excision/incision/sutures ↓ Osteotomies ↓ Grafts (spreader/dorsum/columella/tip) ↓ Closure ↓ Alar base modifications ↓ Dressing

Table 1. Rhinoplasty Techniques

Note: Only those steps appropriate for the individual case are performed.

Depending on the type of rhinoplasty performed, different dressings will be applied at the end of the procedure. When nasal bone osteotomies are used, the patient will require a dorsal nasal splint ± bilateral nasal packing. Nasal packing is generally removed at 24-72 h. When septal manipulation is needed, nasal packing or some sort of septal splint may be placed. The packs are removed within 3 d, but the splints (Silastic sheets, usually sutured in place) can be maintained much longer and the nasal airways kept patent with vasoconstrictor nasal sprays.

Variant procedures or approaches: Placement of a **columellar strut (cartilage graft)** and **release of the tip depressor muscle** often are achieved via intraoral vestibular incisions (behind the upper lip).

Usual preop diagnosis: Posttraumatic nasal deformity (including disordered breathing, 'saddle nose,' crooked nose, septal deviation); developmental nasal deformities (bulbous tip, flat tip, drooping tip, broad dorsum, dorsal hump, alar widening, 'Pinnochio nose'); congenital nasal malformation (cleft nasal deformities)

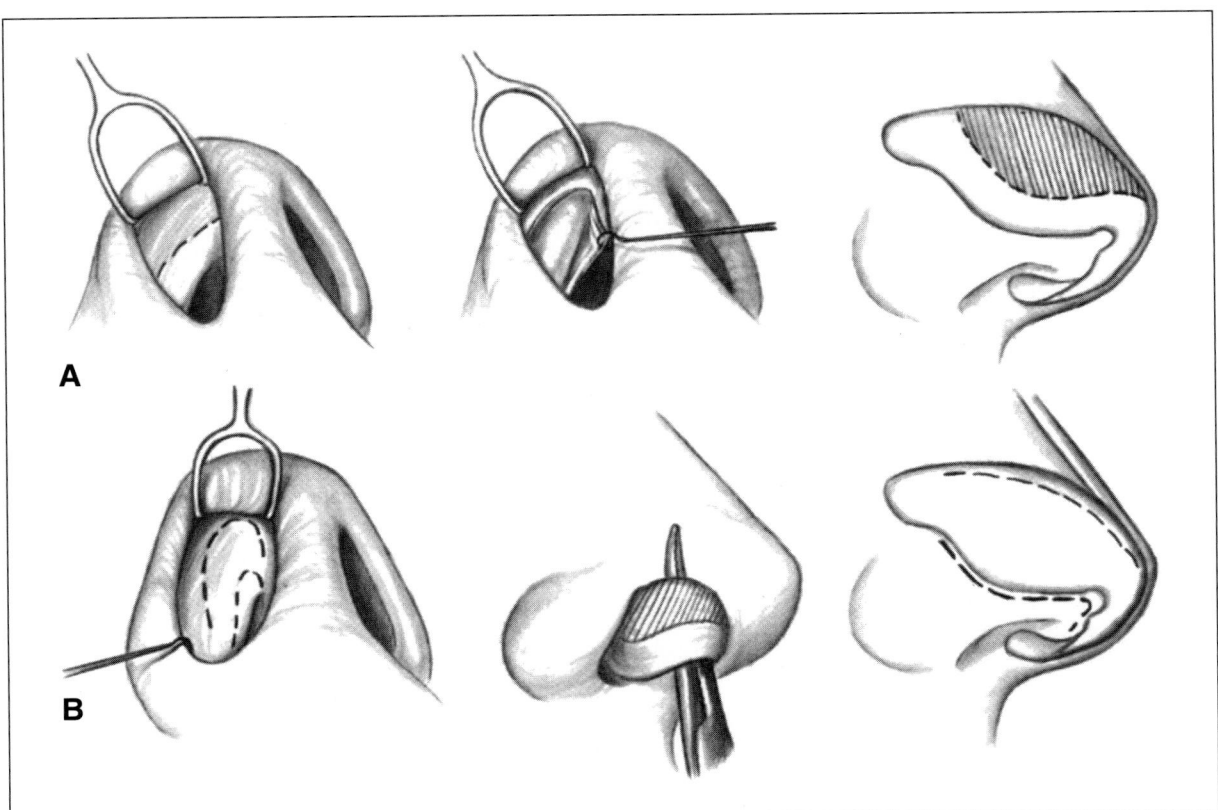

Figure 11.1-7. Closed rhinoplasty. (A) Transcartilaginous approach using an intracartilaginous incision. (B) Delivery approach, using a high intercartilaginous incision and a marginal incision to facilitate delivery of the lateral crura. (Reproduced with permission from Daniel RK: Rhinoplasty. In *Grabb & Smith's Plastic Surgery*, 5th edition. Aston SJ, Beasley RW, Thorne CHM, eds. Lippincott-Raven, 1997.)

SUMMARY OF PROCEDURE

Position	Supine, table may be rotated 180°. If GA: oral ETT toward foot of bed, shoulder roll, neck extended, scleral lubricant, shields
Incision	External vs internal nasal incisions
Special instrumentation	Headlight
Unique considerations	Throat pack for expected nasopharyngeal bleeding. Intranasal vasoconstrictors.
Antibiotics	Cefazolin 1 g iv
Surgical time	1-2.5 h
Closing considerations	Suction stomach via OG tube at the end of surgery. **Remove throat pack prior to extubation.**
EBL	Tip rhinoplasty: 20 ml
	Dorsum with osteotomies: 75-150 ml
	Septoplasty: + 50 ml
Postop care	PACU → room (most home the same day). Ensure minimal PONV; elevate head of bed; no pressure on nose (e.g., O_2 mask).
Mortality	Rare
Morbidity	Infection: < 1%
	Adverse cosmetic result:
	Alar notching
	Alar collapse
	Dorsal irregularity
	Asymmetry
	Tip droop
	Adverse functional result (i.e., poor airway)
	Septal perforation
Pain Score	3 (4 with osteotomies)

PATIENT POPULATION CHARACTERISTICS

Age Range	Most ≥ 15 yr
Male:Female[1]	1:1.7
Incidence[1]	370,968, or 23% of all cosmetic procedures in the U.S. (2001)
Etiology	Developmental; acquired (posttraumatic); congenital (see Secondary Cleft Lip and Nasal Surgery, p. 1145).
Associated conditions	Breathing difficulties; psychosocial issues (body dysmorphic disorder)

ANESTHETIC CONSIDERATIONS

See Anesthetic Considerations for Nasal and Sinus Surgery, pp. 154, 158.

References:

1. American Society of Plastic Surgeons website: www.plasticsurgery.org, 444 East Algonquin Rd, Arlington Heights, IL 60005-4664.
2. Becker DG, McLaughlin RB, Loevner LA, Mang A: The lateral osteotomy in rhinoplasty: clinical and radiographic rationale for osteotome selection. *Plast Reconstr Surg* 2000; 105(5):1806-19.
3. Byrd HS, Salomon J, Flood J: Correction of the crooked nose. *Plast Reconstr Surg* 1998; 102(6):2148-57.
4. Eppley BL: Alloplastic implantation. *Plast Reconstr Surg* 1999; 104(6):1761-83.
5. Gruber RP: Lengthening the short nose. *Plast Reconstr Surg* 1993; 91(7):1252-8.
6. Gruber RP, Friedman GD: Suture algorithm for broad or bulbous nasal tip. *Plast Reconstr Surg* 2002; 110(7):1752-68.
7. Gunter JP, Rohrich RJ: Correction of pinched nasal tip with alar spreader grafts. *Plast Reconstr Surg* 1992; 90(5):821-9.
8. Guyuron B: Nasal osteotomies and airway changes. *Plast Reconstr Surg* 1998; 102:856.
9. Molliex S, Navez M, Baylot D, Prades JM, Elkhoury Z, Auboyer C: Regional anaesthesia for outpatient nasal surgery. *Br J Anaesthesia* 1996; 76:151-3.
10. Niechajev I, Haraldsson PO: Two methods of anesthesia for rhinoplasty in outpatient setting. *Aesth Plast Surg* 1996; 20: 159-63.
11. Owsley TG, Taylor CO: The use of Gore-Tex for nasal augmentation: A retrospective analysis of 106 patients. *Plast Reconstr Surg* 1994; 94(2):241-50.
12. Sheen JH: Adjunctive techniques in rhinoplasty: harvesting cranial bone for nasal grafts. In *Video Perspectives in Plastic Surgery*. Quality Medical Publishing, St. Louis: 1989, 1-32.
13. Tebbetts JB: Shaping and positioning the nasal tip without structural disruption: A new, systematic approach. *Plast Reconstr Surg* 1994; 94(1):61-77.

Also see References for Secondary Cleft Lip/Nasal Surgery, p. 1149.

OTOPLASTY

See Chapter 12.8 Surgery for Craniofacial Malformations, Otoplasty, p. 1149.

FACIAL LASER RESURFACING

Description: Laser resurfacing is a technique by which a controlled burn is administered to the skin of the face with laser technology, creating a healing process which reduces the signs of aging or acne. **CO_2 laser resurfacing** is commonly used with facial cosmetic procedures. It is used widely for the periorbital and perioral creases and wrinkles not addressed by previously described facial cosmetic surgical techniques. Although complete facial resurfacing is sometimes done, it is not recommended in areas of undermined flaps. The laser is usually added at the end of another surgical procedure, and a large mobile laser machine is rolled into the OR for this purpose. Nerve blocks, local anesthesia, iv sedation, and GA are all possibilities for laser treatment and the choice depends more on the specific surgical procedures to be performed before the laser procedure is carried out. Laser resurfacing also is done frequently in an office-based setting (see Chapter 14.0 Office-Based Procedures, p. 1207). As laser resurfacing is usually an adjunct to another facial cosmetic procedure, the following discussion pertains primarily to the unique set of **safety issues** that must be addressed in the OR.

Ocular Hazards: These include direct and reflected injury to the eye. Everyone present, including the patient and all medical personnel, requires laser-specific (i.e., wavelength-specific) safety eyewear. (Scleral shields are available for the patient in cases where the patient's glasses would be in the operative field.) Protective eyewear must be undamaged and have:

- Permanent labels with wavelength and optical density tolerance
- Side shields
- Damage threshold of > 10 sec
- No surface reflection
- Good fit
- Approval from the laser safety officer

Fire and reflectivity hazards: Many items used in the OR (e.g., drapes, sponges, plastic cannulas, etc.) are made of materials that can be fire hazards if not kept from interaction with the high-intensity laser beam heat. Protection from fire and reflectivity is provided by:

- Having fire-retardant or moist draping
- Having water basin available
- Having fire extinguisher readily available
- Avoiding all alcohol-containing prep solutions
- Avoiding use of plastic and rubber instruments (may melt or ignite)
- Using special fire-resistant ETTs or wet sponge protection for plastic ETTs to decrease the possibility of tube breach or ignition
- Avoiding open sources of O_2 (nasal cannulas, etc.)
- Avoiding metal or other reflective materials

Airborne contaminants: The laser destruction of cells releases carbon particles, microbials, DNA, and toxic fumes. Protection for the patient and medical personnel is provided by:

- Utilizing a smoke evacuation system 2 cm from created plume
- Wearing high-filtration masks (recommended). (No masks exist that will filter all airborne contaminants.) Note that these masks generally become less effective when moistened from perspiration during a long case; therefore, a new mask may be required at the end of a case before the laser is to be used.

ANESTHETIC CONSIDERATIONS

See Anesthetic Considerations following Browlift and Blepharoplasty, p. 876, or Office-Based Laser Skin Resurfacing, p. 1208.

References

1. Alster TS, Apfelberg DB, eds: *Cosmetic Laser Surgery: a Practitioner's Guide*, 2nd edition. Wiley-Liss, New York: 1999.
2. Blakeley KR, Klein KW, White PF, et al: A total intravenous technique for outpatient facial laser resurfacing. *Anesth Analg* 1998; 87:827-9.

Surgeons

David M. Kahn, MD
Jeffrey D. Pardun, MD
George W. Commons, MD (*Liposuction*)

11.2   NONFACIAL AESTHETIC SURGERY

Anesthesiologists

Lindsey Vokach-Brodsky, MBChB, FFARCSI
Bruce D. Halperin, MD (*Liposuction*)

AUGMENTATION MAMMOPLASTY

SURGICAL CONSIDERATIONS

Description: Augmentation mammoplasty is accomplished through the use of a breast implant. The surgery itself may be performed under GA or local anesthesia with sedation. The patient is positioned either with the arms abducted at 90°, or with the hands on the abdomen. Local anesthetic (± epinephrine) is infiltrated into the skin at the incision site and under the glandular tissue. Implant insertion can be done through an inframammary, periareolar, or transaxillary incision. The implant is placed in a pocket that is created either under the mammary gland (subglandular) or under the pectoralis muscle (submuscular), depending on the surgeon's preference and the amount of tissue available. When the implant is placed in the submuscular position, the pectoralis muscle is divided from its insertion along the inframammary fold to allow the muscle to drape over the implant. If a saline implant or sizer is used, it is inflated with saline until the appropriate volume is reached. The patient may be placed in the seated position to assess the size, shape, and symmetry of the breasts. Once the desired result is achieved, the sizer is removed, the permanent prosthesis is placed and the wound is closed. A dressing is then applied (Fig 11.2-1). Augmentation mammoplasty usually is performed as an outpatient procedure, although some patients may want an overnight stay for initial pain management and antiemetics. PONV is not uncommon, and all efforts should be made to decrease its frequency.

Variant procedure or approaches: A transumbilical, endoscopic approach also has been described, but it is not commonly used.

Preop Diagnosis: Hypomastia

SUMMARY OF PROCEDURE

Position	Supine
Incision	Inframammary; periareolar; axillary; or umbilical
Antibiotics	Cefazolin 1 g iv
Unique considerations	May place patient in sitting position during procedure.
Surgical time	1 h
Closing considerations	May need patient in sitting position for application of dressings.
EBL	Minimal
Postop care	Outpatient procedure

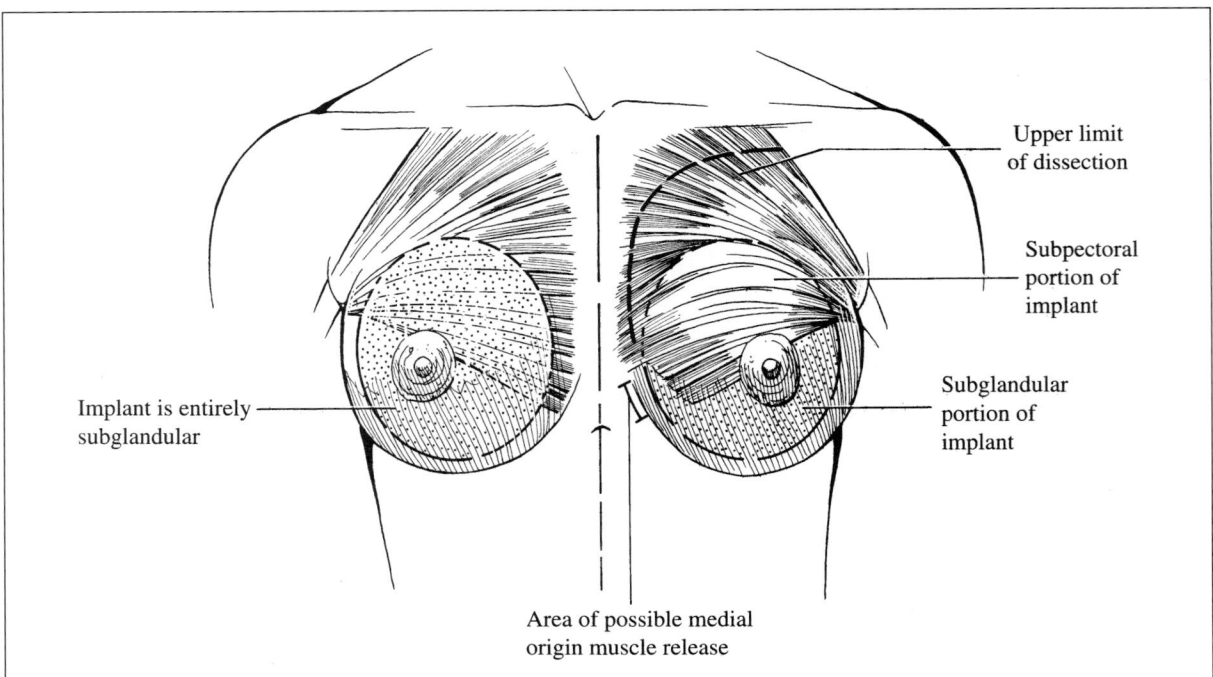

Figure 11.2-1. Breast augmentation. Implants may be placed in a subglandular or subpectoral position. (Reproduced with permission from Spear SL: *The Breast: Principles and Art.* Lippincott-Raven, 1998.)

884

Mortality	Rare
Morbidity	Prosthesis failure: 5%
	Capsular contracture: 5%
	Hematoma: 3%
	Infection: 2%
	Wound dehiscence: < 1%
	Cosmetic disappointments
Pain score	3-4

PATIENT POPULATION CHARACTERISTICS

Age range	17-45 yr, but also may be done on the contralateral breast in a patient undergoing breast reconstruction.
Incidence	219,883 performed in US in 2001[1]
Etiology	Developmental; age-related atrophy
Associated conditions	Not common, but can be seen with Poland's syndrome.

ANESTHETIC CONSIDERATIONS

See Anesthetic Considerations following Mastopexy/Breast Lift, p. 887.

References: See References following Mastopexy/Breast Lift, p. 888.

REDUCTION MAMMOPLASTY

SURGICAL CONSIDERATIONS

Description: Breast reduction surgery can be done as an outpatient procedure or with an overnight stay. One might choose to admit the patient overnight in a hospital setting to monitor for hematoma formation and evidence of ↓blood supply to the nipple-areola complex, or to aid in the management of PONV. In these patients, the pain from this procedure is relatively low; therefore, PONV tends to be more of a factor in the periop period.

The most common type of reduction performed in the U.S. is the **inferior pedicle technique** (Fig 11.2-2). The areola is marked circumferentially with an areola sizer and then incised. The remaining incision lines are scored with a scalpel. Next, the inferior pedicle, which contains the neurovascular supply to the nipple-areola complex, is deepithelialized. Excess skin and breast tissue are excised, preserving the pedicle of tissue that will make up the future breast mound. The resected tissue is weighed so that an appropriate amount of breast tissue can be excised from each breast to ensure symmetry. The amount of tissue removed from each breast can range from 200-1000 g. The skin envelope is closed temporarily with staples, while the procedure is carried out on the opposite breast. The patient is placed in a sitting position so that the breasts can be evaluated for symmetry. When the surgeon is satisfied with the appearance of the breasts, they are closed with sutures. Drains may be placed, depending on surgeon preference (Fig 11.2-2). Once the skin has been closed, the location of the nipple and areola are planned. Skin from this recipient site is excised and the nipple-areola complex is delivered into the wound and sutured into position. Soft, supportive dressings are placed.

Variant procedure or approaches: Liposuction may be used in combination with this procedure. Reduction mammoplasty using liposuction, alone, has recently increased in popularity.

Preop diagnosis: Macromastia/mammary hypertrophy

SUMMARY OF PROCEDURE

Position	Supine, arm abducted 90°
Incision	Marked preop. Most have circumareolar incision with an inferior anchor-shaped extension (Fig 11.2-2).

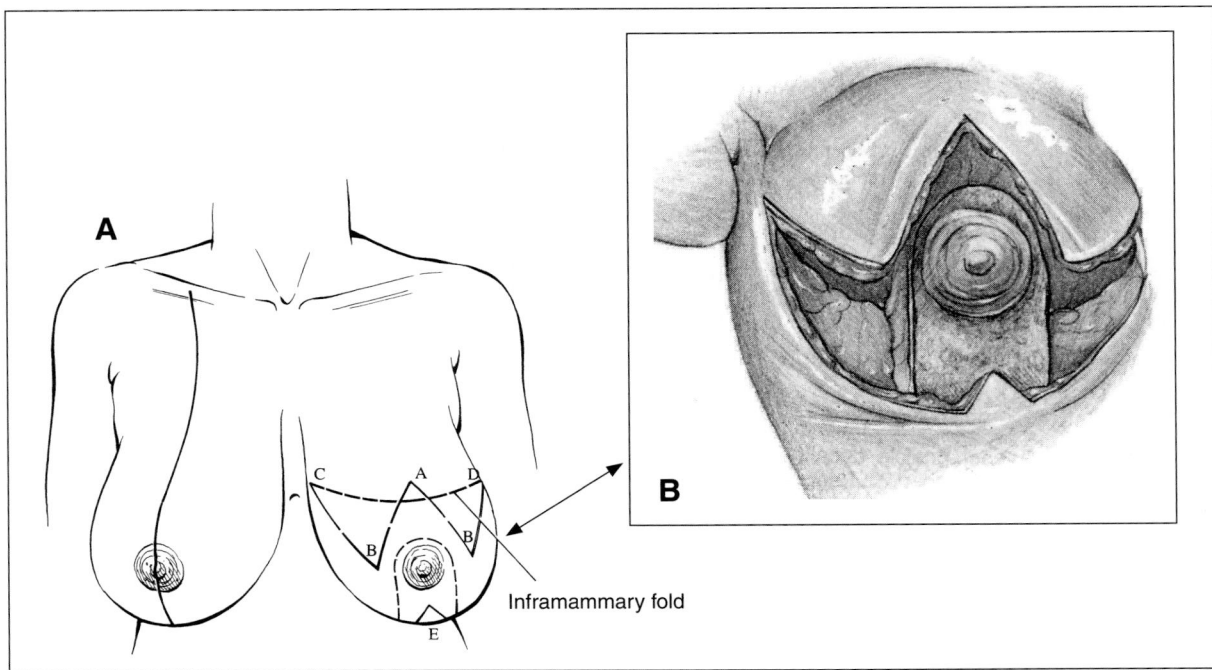

Figure 11.2-2. Reduction mammoplasty using an inferior pedicle technique. (A) The skin and breast tissue on the medial and lateral sides of the pedicle are resected, and (B) the medial and lateral skin envelopes are sutured at the midline, leaving an inverted-T shaped scar. (Reproduced with permission from Spear SL: *The Breast: Principles and Art*. Lippincott-Raven, 1998.)

Antibiotics	Cefazolin 1 g iv
Unique considerations	May place patient in sitting position during procedure to assess symmetry; Foley catheter; SCDs
Surgical time	3-5 h, depending on volume of reduction
Closing considerations	May place patient in sitting position for application of dressings.
EBL	100-200 ml
Postop care	Outpatient or 24-h stay for pain/nausea management. Avoid the use of toradol in the first 24 h because of the large, raw surface created between the skin flaps and breast tissue.
Mortality	Minimal
Morbidity	Dehiscence: 5%
	Infection: 1%
	Seroma/hematoma: < 1% (may require reexploration)
	Skin flap necrosis
	Loss of nipple-areola complex (may require urgent reexploration)
	Loss of nipple-areola sensation
	Hypertrophic scarring
	Cosmetic disappointments
Pain score	3-4

PATIENT POPULATION CHARACTERISTICS

Age range	25-65 yr
Incidence	99,428 performed in U.S. in 2001[1]
Etiology	Developmental; child-bearing; obesity
Associated conditions	None common

ANESTHETIC CONSIDERATIONS

See Anesthetic Considerations following Mastopexy/Breast Lift, p. 887.

References: See References following Mastopexy/Breast Lift, p. 888.

MASTOPEXY/BREAST LIFT

SURGICAL CONSIDERATIONS

Description: Mastopexy procedures to reduce the volume of the skin envelope are designed to treat ptosis ('droopy breasts'). Depending on the degree of ptosis, and the desire of the patient, the ptosis may be treated by augmentation alone to increase the volume of the breast to match the skin envelope, by removing excess skin from the breast, or a combination of a mastopexy and an augmentation.

The operation itself resembles a reduction mammoplasty, except that breast tissue generally is not removed, and an implant may be added. The patient is marked before surgery in the upright position. After the induction of anesthesia, the arms are positioned either on the abdomen or abducted 90°. The procedure begins with the areola being marked circumferentially with an areola sizer, and then incised. Next, the skin flaps are elevated. The breast tissue is moved to a higher position on the chest wall, and the skin is redraped and tailor-tacked closed. The patient is placed in a sitting position to assess for symmetry and nipple location. The nipple-areola complex is then brought out into its new position, and dressings are applied.

Preop diagnosis: Breast ptosis (droop)

SUMMARY OF PROCEDURE

Position	Supine
Incision	Circumareolar ± inferior extension or complete anchor
Antibiotics	Cefazolin 1 g iv
Unique considerations	May place patient in sitting position during procedure.
Surgical time	2-3 h
Closing considerations	May place patient in sitting position for application of dressings.
EBL	< 100 ml
Postop care	Outpatient or 24-h stay
Mortality	Minimal
Morbidity	Wound healing: 5%
	Infection: 1%
	Seroma/hematoma: < 1%
	Hypertrophic scarring
	Cosmetic disappointments
Pain score	3-4

PATIENT POPULATION CHARACTERISTICS

Age range	35-65 yr
Incidence	55,176 performed in U.S. in 2001[1]
Etiology	Age-related ptosis; child-bearing; weight loss
Associated conditions	None common

ANESTHETIC CONSIDERATIONS FOR MAMMOPLASTY/MASTOPEXY

PREOPERATIVE

Typically, three patient populations present for mammoplasty: 1) healthy individuals, for breast reduction/augmentation/lift or removal of an implant; 2) morbidly obese, for breast reduction; 3) breast cancer patients, for reconstruction after mastectomy. (For preop considerations in the morbidly obese patient, see Anesthetic Considerations for Abdominoplasty, p. 890.) Breast cancer patients undergoing mastectomy with immediate reconstruction will not have had either chemotherapy or radiation. The following considerations are for breast cancer patients undergoing delayed reconstruction postchemotherapy.

Respiratory	Pulmonary fibrosis may complicate chemotherapy. Alkylating agents (e.g., cyclophosphamide and melphalan), used to treat breast cancer, have some pulmonary toxicity. Consider pulmonary fibrosis in a patient reporting dyspnea, nonproductive cough, and fever. **Tests:** Consider CXR; ABG, PFTs as indicated from H&P.

Cardiovascular	Cardiomyopathy and CHF may result from chemotherapy, especially doxorubicin (Adriamycin) > 550 mg/m². **Tests:** Consider ECG; ECHO, if indicated from H&P.
Neurologic	Note any previous damage to long thoracic nerves, as evidenced by winged scapula deformity.
Musculoskeletal	Avoid iv and BP cuff on mastectomy side.
Hematologic	Leukopenia, thrombocytopenia, and anemia from chemotherapy may be present. **Tests:** CBC; Plt count
Renal/Hepatic	Methotrexate can produce some renal and hepatic dysfunction. **Tests:** Cr; LFTs
Laboratory	Other tests as indicated from H&P, prior chemotherapy, obesity.
Premedication	Midazolam 1-2 mg iv immediately preop. Surgeon may want to mark the patient's skin preop, with patient standing. Delay premedication until this has been done.

INTRAOPERATIVE

Anesthetic technique: GETA

Induction	Standard induction (p. B-2). ✓ with surgeons regarding use of a nerve stimulator during dissection (and the need to avoid muscle relaxants). Consider LTA to minimize coughing during position changes.
Maintenance	Standard maintenance (p. B-3). Surgeons may want patient sitting for part of the procedure. Pneumothorax should be considered with any change in lung inflation pressure, O₂ sat, or BP.
Emergence	During some of the procedure and for application of dressing, patient may be moved to sitting position, with consequent coughing, bucking, etc. (Rx: deeper anesthesia, e.g., propofol 0.5 mg/kg or lidocaine 1 mg/kg.) Watch BP carefully and treat orthostatic hypotension if it occurs, usually with a fluid bolus if the patient is not fluid sensitive (Hx of CHF or renal failure).
Blood and fluid requirements	IV 16-18 ga × 1 NS/LR @ 4-8 ml/kg/h	Minimal blood loss for simple reconstruction, augmentation, or reduction; larger blood losses anticipated for combined procedures (e.g., mastectomy with immediate reconstruction or flap reconstruction).
Monitoring	Standard monitors (p. B-1)	Arterial line in the morbidly obese
Positioning	Patient may need to be sitting for application of dressing.	Avoid HTN, bucking, and straining; these may cause or exacerbate bleeding at reconstruction site. Careful padding and unwrapping of arms to protect them during position change.

POSTOPERATIVE

Complications	Pneumothorax
Pain management	PCA (p. C-3)

References

1. American Society of Plastic Surgeons website: www.plasticsurgery.org.
2. Baker, JL: Augmentation Mammoplasty: General considerations. In *Surgery of the Breast: Principles and Art*. Spear SL, ed. Lippincott-Raven, Philadelphia: 1998, 845-54.
3. Desidero DP, Kross RA, Bedford RF: Evaluation of the patient with oncologic disease. In *Principles and Practice of Anesthesiology*, 2nd edition. Longnecker DE, Tinker JH, Morgan GE Jr, eds. Mosby-Year Book, St. Louis: 1998, 379-96.
4. Elliott LF: Circumareolar mastopexy with augmentation. *Clin Plast Surg* 2002; 29(3): 337-47.
5. Hoffman, S: Inferior pedicle technique in breast reduction. In *Surgery of the Breast: Principles and Art*. Spear SL, ed. Lippincott-Raven, Philadelphia: 1998, 761-72.
6. Matarasso A. Suction mammoplasty: the use of suction lipectomy alone to reduce large breasts. *Clin Plast Surg* 2002; 29(3): 433-43.
7. Shenkman Z, Shir Y, Brodsky JB: Perioperative management of the obese patient. *Br J Anaesth* 1993; 70(3):349-59.
8. Spear SL: Primary implant reconstruction. In *Surgery of the Breast: Principles and Art*. Lippincott-Raven, Philadelphia: 1998, 347-56.
9. Vasconez HC, Holley DT: Use of the TRAM and latissimus dorsi flaps in autogenous breast reconstruction. *Clin Plast Surg* 1995; 22(1):153-66.

ABDOMINOPLASTY

SURGICAL CONSIDERATIONS

Description: Patients who present for **abdominoplasty** have laxity in the abdominal wall musculature and excess skin and adipose tissue. This laxity may be associated with rectus muscle diastasis. Muscular laxity is treated by plicating the abdominal fascia with sutures; and the excess skin and adipose tissue are resected directly. **Liposuction** often is performed before abdominoplasty to remove additional adipose tissue and improve contour. Incision lines are marked on the patient preop (Fig 11.2-3). The umbilicus is circumscribed, with care taken to preserve its blood supply. An incision is made above the pubic hairline and extended bilaterally to each anterior superior iliac spine. Electrocautery is used to raise a flap of skin, subcutaneous tissue, and fat at the level of the abdominal wall fascia. The dissection extends cephalad to the costal margin. The operating table is flexed and the patient is placed in the semi-Fowler position. The elevated flap is pulled down to overlap the inferior incision, and the redundant soft tissue is excised in a tailor-tack fashion (Fig 11.2-4). The surgical area is inspected for hemostasis and irrigated. Sutures may be placed to plicate the abdominal wall musculature. Fibrin sealant may be sprayed to aid in hemostasis.

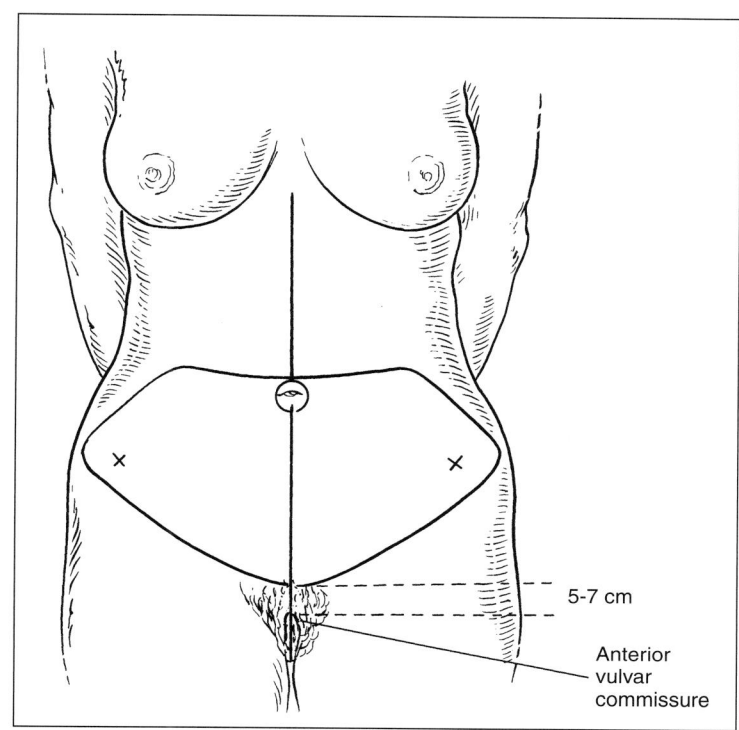

Figure 11.2-3. Abdominoplasty, markings for incisions. (Reproduced with permission from Aston SJ, Beasley RW, Thorne CHM: *Grabb & Smith's Plastic Surgery*, 5th edition. Lippincott-Raven, 1997.)

The wound is closed over drains, and the umbilicus is brought out through a new incision. Dressings, including an abdominal binder, are applied. The patient is maintained in the semi-Fowler position during transfer from the operating table. The patient may elect to have the procedure as an outpatient or with an overnight stay in a monitored facility.

Usual preop diagnosis: Abdominal wall laxity; rectus diastasis; lipodystrophy; redundant skin and soft tissue

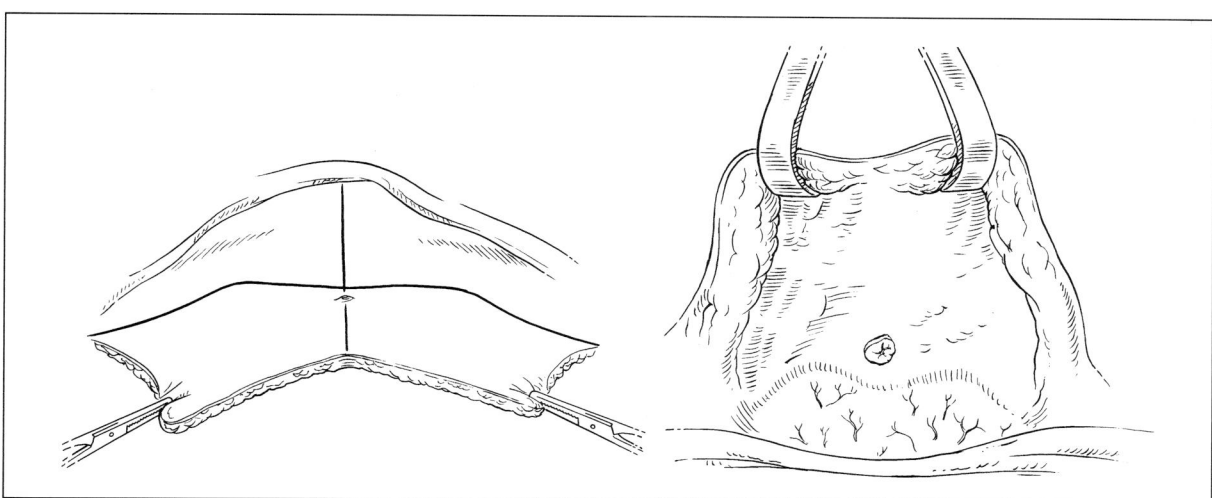

Figure 11.2-4. Once the lower incision has been made and the abdominal flap has been elevated, the flap is pulled down to overlap the inferior incision, and the redundant soft tissue is excised in a tailor-tack fashion. (Reproduced with permission from Aston SJ, Beasley RW, Thorne CHM: *Grabb & Smith's Plastic Surgery*, 5th edition. Lippincott-Raven, 1997.)

SUMMARY OF PROCEDURE

Position	Supine
Incision	Extended Pfannenstiel's; periumbilical
Unique considerations	Foley catheter; SCDs
Antibiotics	Cefazolin 1 g iv
Surgical time	2-4 h
Closing considerations	Flex table to facilitate closure.
EBL	~100 ml, not including blood contained in specimen.
Postop care	Maintain flexed position; avoid ketorolac 1st 24-48 h.
Mortality	0-1%
Morbidity	Ileus: 10%
	Infection: 2-3%
	Dehiscence: 1%
	Fat embolism: 1%
	DVT: 1%
	Hematoma
	Seroma
Pain score	4-6

PATIENT POPULATION CHARACTERISTICS

Age range	30-65 yr
Male:Female	1:5
Incidence	58,567 performed in U.S. in 2001.[1]
Etiology	Overeating; laxity of skin after pregnancy
Associated conditions	Obesity

ANESTHETIC CONSIDERATIONS

PREOPERATIVE

Typically, there are two patient populations for abdominoplasty: the generally healthy, and the morbidly obese. Some patients have Hx of amphetamine, cocaine, or thyroid hormone abuse,[2] and ↑incidence of hiatal hernia. The following considerations focus on the morbidly obese patient (body weight [kg] ≥ 2 × ideal weight. Ideal body weight [kg] is estimated by subtracting 100 [male] or 105 [female] from height in cm).

Respiratory	In the morbidly obese patient, findings include[1]: ↑O_2 consumption, ↑CO_2 production, restrictive lung disease, ↓FRC, ↓ERV, ↓VC, ↓IC, and ↓PaO_2. These changes are exacerbated by the supine position. Younger patients may show alveolar hyperventilation in response to hypoxemia; older patients may not, and may retain CO_2. Patients may have obesity hypoventilation syndrome (pickwickian syndrome) and sleep apnea; with intermittent airway obstruction, hypoxemia, and hypercarbia during sleep, which may → pulmonary HTN. Obese patients are at ↑risk of pulmonary aspiration due to ↑incidence of hiatal hernia, GERD, and ↑gastric volumes (typically > 25 ml with pH < 2.5). See Premedication, below, for aspiration prophylaxis.
	Tests: Consider CXR, room-air ABG, and PFT (helpful, but generally do not predict postop complications, e.g., atelectasis, pneumonia).
Cardiovascular	↑CO and ↑blood volume → LVH. Chronic hypoxia and pulmonary compromise may produce right heart failure, ↓↓exercise tolerance, ↑risk of CAD, and pulmonary systemic HTN. Patients with LVH may have ↑dysrhythmias. Some patients may have previously taken fenfluramine alone or in combination with phentermine for weight loss. Those patients should be evaluated for pulmonary HTN (e.g., dyspnea, central cyanosis, right axis deviation, and CXR changes) and valvular heart disease.
	Tests: ECG (↑HR, conduction abnormalities, LVH); CXR (cardiomegaly)
Metabolic	Increased incidence of diabetes, hypercholesterolemia, hypertriglyceridemia, liver abnormalities; ↓plasma folate, B_{12}; ↑incidence of cholelithiasis, nephrolithiasis. Determine whether electrolyte abnormalities are present in patient S/P ileojejunal bypass.
	Tests: As indicated from H&P.

Hematologic	Polycythemia suggests chronic hypoxemia (see Respiratory, above). **Tests:** Hb/Hct
Laboratory	Other tests as indicated from H&P.
Premedication	Sedative premedication is avoided in the morbidly obese due to their pulmonary compromise. Aspiration prophylaxis is essential: ranitidine 100 mg po or iv the evening before, and 60-90 min before surgery, plus nonparticulate antacid (Na citrate 0.3 M, 30 ml po) preinduction. Additionally, metoclopramide 10 mg iv may be given, although it has not been shown to be more effective in combination with an H_2-blocker than the H_2-blocker alone. For the healthy outpatient, midazolam 1-2 mg iv immediately preop may lessen anxiety.

INTRAOPERATIVE

Anesthetic technique: GETA. Morbidly obese patients may not tolerate the supine position for an extended period of time. Consider placement of thoracic epidural for postop pain control.

Induction	Standard induction (p. B-2) for healthy patients. Special considerations for the morbidly obese include prophylaxis for aspiration (see above), followed by rapid-sequence induction in an appropriately positioned patient (see Fig 7.2-6). If mandibular and cervical mobility are decreased by excessive soft tissue, plan awake fiber optic intubation (see p. B-6) with the patient sitting. Anticipate rapid O_2 desaturation during periods of hypoventilation, even with adequate preoxygenation.
Maintenance	Standard maintenance (p. B-3). Calculate drug dosage on basis of lean body mass. In the obese, increased plasma fluoride concentrations are found after anesthesia with halothane and enflurane; controlled ventilation with large TV and high inspired O_2 concentration is recommended. Since epinephrine infiltration generally is used to decrease blood loss, isoflurane is recommended as the ★ least dysrhythmogenic of the inhalation agents in the presence of epinephrine. **NB:** Midazolam has a prolonged half-life in obese patients, but awakening times from inhalational or narcotic-based anesthetics are comparable to those of nonobese patients.
Emergence	Smooth emergence with minimal bucking, coughing, or retching to minimize tension on the suture line; give antiemetics (metoclopramide 10 mg and dolasetron 12.5 μg or granisetron 1 mg) 20 min before conclusion of surgery. Maintenance of flexed position will minimize tension on suture line. Small additional doses of narcotic (e.g., meperidine 10 mg) may be titrated to RR if patient is allowed to resume spontaneous respiration before the end of the case.
Blood and fluid requirements	Moderate blood loss IV: 16-18 ga × 1 NS/LR @ 6-10 ml/kg/h	
Monitoring	Standard monitors (see p. B-1). ± Arterial line ± CVP line	Additional monitoring for the morbidly obese patient may include arterial and CVP lines.
Positioning	Flexed position Pillows under knees ✓ and pad pressure points. ✓ eyes.	Flexed position minimizes tension on suture line. Morbidly obese may require 2 OR tables side-by-side. Supine position may be poorly tolerated; monitor ventilation closely.
Complications	Fat emboli	More common during liposuction.

POSTOPERATIVE

Complications	Patients may have postop ileus of 1-2 d duration.	The morbidly obese should not be outpatients; they have an ↑incidence of wound infection, DVT, PE, and postop pulmonary complications. Provide supplemental O_2 for the first 2 d postop. Keep patient in semisitting or flexed position to avoid undue stress on wound.
Pain management	Epidural narcotics or PCA may be used (pp. C-2–C-3).	Monitor patient for postop respiration depression.
Tests	Pulse oximetry	Maximum reduction of arterial saturation may occur on postop day 2-3.[6]

References

1. Cooper JR, Brodsky JB: Anesthetic management of the morbidly obese patient. *Semin Anesth* 1987; Vol 6: 260-70.
2. Klein JA: Anesthesia for liposuction in dermatologic surgery. *J Dermatol Surg Oncol* 1988; 14(10):1124-32.
3. Lockwood T: High-lateral-tension abdominoplasty with superficial fascial system suspension. *Plast Reconstr Surg* 1995; 96(3):603-15.
4. Matarasso A: Liposuction as an adjunct to a full abdominoplasty. *Plast Reconstr Surg* 1995; 95(5):829-36.
5. Seung-Jun O, Taller SR: Refinements in abdominoplasty. *Clin Plast Surg* 2002; 29(1):95-109.
6. Shenkman ZZ, Shir Y, Brodsky JB: Perioperative management of the obese patient. *Br J Anaesth* 1993; 70(3):349-59.
7. Vaughan RW, Wise L: Postoperative arterial blood gas measurements in obese patients: effects of position on gas exchange. *Ann Surg* 1975; 182(6):705-9.
8. Vistnes, LM: *Procedures in Plastic and Reconstructive Surgery: How They Do It.* Little, Brown, Boston: 1991.

LIPOSUCTION

SURGICAL CONSIDERATIONS

Description: Liposuction remains the most commonly performed cosmetic surgical procedure in the U.S. The surgical technique has changed since the introduction of the procedure in the late 1970s. For example, the preaspiration injection of epinephrine-containing wetting solution into the adipose tissue has expanded the use of the surgical procedure. Patients who desire a more dramatic cosmetic surgical result may now have larger volumes of fat removed safely, without losing large quantities of blood during surgery. All members of the surgical team must function in a coordinated fashion to avoid the many pitfalls associated with liposuction. Complications such as PE, fat emboli, fluid overload, toxicity from local anesthetics, and body-cavity perforation from both the wetting solution cannula and the suctioning cannula have been reported.

The current standards for performance of liposuction involve the use of an epinephrine-containing wetting solution injected into the subcutaneous tissue prior to aspiration. Most wetting solutions contain 1 L of LR, to which 1 mg of epinephrine and 200-500 mg of lidocaine are added. Epinephrine in the 1/1,000,000 concentration will provide excellent vasoconstriction in the adipose tissue before suctioning. The concentration of lidocaine depends on the primary anesthetic modality. For patients having GA or regional anesthesia, the lower concentration of local anesthetic will provide satisfactory postop analgesia. Higher concentrations of local anesthetic are needed for patients having liposuction under local anesthesia/MAC. Following administration of the wetting solution to the surgical region, 10-20 min is allowed for vasoconstriction to take place before suctioning. The large volume of local anesthetic and epinephrine-containing solution represents substantial risk to the patient (local anesthetic toxicity, HTN, cardiac arrhythmia, coronary insufficiency), along with the risk of perforation with the cannula.

Ultrasonic liposuction may be used to liquefy fat in the surgical region prior to or simultaneously with its removal. Power-assisted liposuction utilizes pressurized gases or an electrical motor to power the tip of the lipo cannula to improve the efficiency of the procedure. Complications reported during the use of the new technologies include seroma formation, increased blood loss, and increased risk of body cavity perforation.

Following completion of the surgery, incision sites are closed and sterile dressings are applied. Compressive garments may be worn by the patient for several d or wk, depending on the extent of the surgery. Discomfort in the surgical regions varies greatly from patient to patient, but may last from several d to several wk.

Usual preop diagnosis: Obesity

SUMMARY OF PROCEDURE

Position	According to body region (repositioning often required).
Incision	Incisions may be hidden in skin folds. The use of long injection and lipo cannulas will reduce the number of incisions.
Special instrumentation	Cannulas, aspirating machine; ultrasonic or power-assist machinery
Antibiotics + other meds	Cefazolin 1 g. Dexamethasone 8 mg may be given during surgery.
Surgical time	2-7 h, depending on volume of resection and number of surgical sites
EBL	2-8% of total aspirate volume when using wetting solution before aspiration
Postop care	PACU for small-volume liposuction; hospitalization or postop monitoring for large-volume resection (> 5000 ml)
Mortality	19.1/100,000

Morbidity	Pulmonary emboli
	Fat emboli
	Fluid overload
	Local anesthetic toxicity
	Body cavity perforation
	Respiratory restriction from compressive garments has been noted in PACU.
Unique considerations	Wetting solution must be warmed before use to prevent hypothermia. Foley catheter monitoring is used for larger volume surgeries. TEDs, SCDs used on all cases.
Pain score	4-6

PATIENT POPULATION CHARACTERISTICS

Age range	Teens–70 yr
Male:Female	< 1:9
Etiology	Quest for eternal youth

ANESTHETIC CONSIDERATIONS
PREOPERATIVE

Patients considering liposuction should be in ASA category I or II. The ideal candidate for surgery should be physically active and have maintained a stable weight Hx for 6 mo-1 yr. Preop consultation with the surgical team is necessary for finalizing the anesthetic plan. Current techniques use the injection of wetting solution to reduce blood loss and to deliver local anesthetics for postop analgesia. Most wetting solutions contain lidocaine 200-500 mg/L combined with epinephrine 1 mg/L (1/1,000,000). Typically, 1 ml of wetting solution will be used for each 1 ml of anticipated fat resection. Because of the demand for more dramatic results, larger fat resections (large-volume liposuction > 5000 ml) are being performed. These large-volume procedures may require postop hospitalization for patient monitoring (fluid shifts, ↓Hct, pulmonary edema). Large volumes of wetting solution often are used in these procedures and require limiting iv fluids during surgery. In contrast, small-volume liposuction often requires larger volumes of iv fluid administration because of the small volumes of wetting solution that would be available for postop hydration.

Respiratory	Postop discomfort following chest, upper back, and upper abdomen liposuction may interfere with respiration. Restrictive compression garments applied to the chest or upper abdomen also may restrict breathing. Patients with respiratory impairment may not be candidates for this procedure.
Cardiovascular	Patients with Hx of CHF or those with MVP may not be candidates for high-volume liposuction. Fluid management is based on volume status and the quantity of tumescent fluid injected during surgery. Tumescent solution injected into the subcutaneous tissue is absorbed over 48 h. Postop pulmonary edema has been reported 2° fluid overload in patients receiving larger volumes of tumescent injection. Some patients may have previously taken fenfluramine alone or in combination with phentermine for weight loss. Those patients should be evaluated for pulmonary HTN (e.g., dyspnea, central cyanosis, right axis deviation and CXR changes) and valvular heart disease. All weight control drugs should be D/C'd at least 2 wk before surgery.
Neurologic	Preop neurologic exam should be normal. Local anesthetic administration during tumescent injection may cause areas of numbness postop.
Hematologic	Vasoconstriction from epinephrine-containing wetting solutions greatly reduces blood loss to 2-8% of the total aspirate volume. Blood transfusion is rarely needed, even in larger volume resections. **Tests:** Hct
Laboratory	Other tests as indicated from H&P.
Premedication	Midazolam 1-2 mg or oral benzodiazepine (e.g., lorazepam 1 mg po 1-2 h preop)

INTRAOPERATIVE

Anesthetic technique: Local anesthesia may be suitable for smaller volume liposuction. Regional anesthesia (spinal, epidural) may be used when the surgical regions are appropriate for this type of anesthetic. Concerns have been raised because of vasodilation → ↑blood loss + ↑fat embolization with regional anesthesia. GA ensures patient comfort and allows liposuction to be done on all body regions. Airway and ventilation control also provides safety during the surgery. SCDs or foot/ankle compression devices are used for all patients to reduce the risk of PE.

Induction	Standard induction (see p. B-2). Steroids (dexamethasone 8 mg) may be used to reduce postop swelling and may be of benefit in the event of fat embolism.

Maintenance	Standard maintenance (see p. B-3) with volatile anesthetics ± propofol infusion. Neuromuscular blockade as appropriate. GA is maintained during application of compression garments.	
Emergence	Antiemetic prophylaxis with metoclopramide (10 mg) and ondansetron (4 mg) or granisetron 100 μg is appropriate. Careful monitoring of respiratory function is necessary when surgery has been performed on the chest, back or upper abdomen, since compression garments may limit respiration.	
Blood and fluid requirements	IV: 18 or 20 ga × 1 NS/LR	NS/LR volume determined by the needs of the case. Transfusion rarely needed, diuretics may be needed for patients receiving large volumes of wetting solution (e.g., furosemide 5-10 mg).
Monitoring	Standard monitors (see p. B-1). ± Foley catheter	UO monitoring mandatory on all large-volume lipo cases. Careful T monitoring.
Positioning	✓ and pad pressure points. ✓ eyes. Repeat ✓s frequently.	Frequent intraop position checks are needed as patient position will change during surgery → potential for peripheral nerve injury.
Complications	Local anesthetic toxicity Excess blood loss Volume overload Abdominal cavity perforation Peripheral nerve injury Hypothermia Fat embolism	Lidocaine 35-55 mg/kg has been shown to produce safe serum levels when used in a highly dilute solution (0.05-0.1%) with epinephrine for tumescent injection during liposuction.[8,11] Peak plasma lidocaine level occurs 10-12 h after infusion. Vigorous efforts needed to maintain body temperature (e.g., fluid warmer, Bair-Hugger).

POSTOPERATIVE

Complications	Hypoxemia	Consider fluid overload, fat embolism, pneumothorax of pulmonary edema in differential diagnosis (DDx).
	HTN	Consider fluid overload and epinephrine effect in DDx.
	Respiratory compromise	May be 2° compression garments and pain.
Pain management	PO analgesics IV opiates	Patients often will be comfortable 2° residual local anesthesia, which may persist for 8-24 h. Oral analgesics are usually satisfactory for postop pain control.
Tests	Hct	✓ Hct following large-volume procedures.

References

1. Burk RW III, Guzman-Stein G, Vasconez LO: Lidocaine and epinephrine levels in tumescent technique liposuction. *Plast Reconstr Surg* 1996; 97:1379.
2. Commons GW, Chang CC, Vistnes D, Halperin BD: Role of liposuction in morbid obesity. In *Problems in General Surgery*. Lippincott Williams & Wilkins, Philadelphia: 2000.
3. Commons GW, Halperin BD: Considerations in large volume liposuction. *Sem Plast Surg* 2002; 16(2).
4. Commons GW, Halperin BD, Chang CC. Large volume liposuction: a review of 631 consecutive cases over 12 years. *Plast Reconstr Surg* 2001; 108:1753.
5. Gilliland M, Commons GW, Halperin BD: Safety issues in ultrasonic assisted large volume lipoplasty. *Clin Plast Surg* 1999.
6. Grazer FM, deJong RH: Fatal outcomes from liposuction: census survey of cosmetic surgeons. *Plast Reconstr Surg* 2000; 105(1):436-48.
7. Hunstad JP: Body contouring in the obese patient. *Clin Plast Surg* 1996; 23(4):647-70.
8. Klein JA: Tumescent technique for local anesthesia improves safety in large volume liposuction. *Plast Reconstr Surg* 1993; 92:1085-100.
9. Klein JA: Tumescent technique for regional anesthesia permits lidocaine doses of 35 mg/kg for liposuction. *J Dermatol Surg Oncol* 1990; 16:248-63.
10. Meister F: Possible association between tumescent technique and life-threatening pulmonary complications. *Clin Plast Surg* 1996; 23:642.
11. Ostad A, Kageymis N, Moy RL: Tumescent anesthesia with a lidocaine dose of 55 mg/kg is safe for liposuction. *Dermatol Surg* 1996; 22:921-7.
12. Pitman GH, Aker JS, Tripp ZD: Tumescent liposuction: a surgeon's perspective. *Clin Plast Surg* 1996; 23(4):633-41.
13. Samdal F, Amland PF, Bugge JF: Blood loss during liposuction using the tumescent technique. *Aesthetic Plast Surg* 1994; 18(2):157-60.

Surgeons

Lonny L. Ross, MD, FRCSC
Stephen A. Schendel, MD, DDS, FACS

11.3 CRANIOFACIAL SURGERY

Anesthesiologists

Tara Cornaby, MD
Stanley I. Samuels, MB, BCh, FFARCS
Richard A. Jaffe, MD, PhD

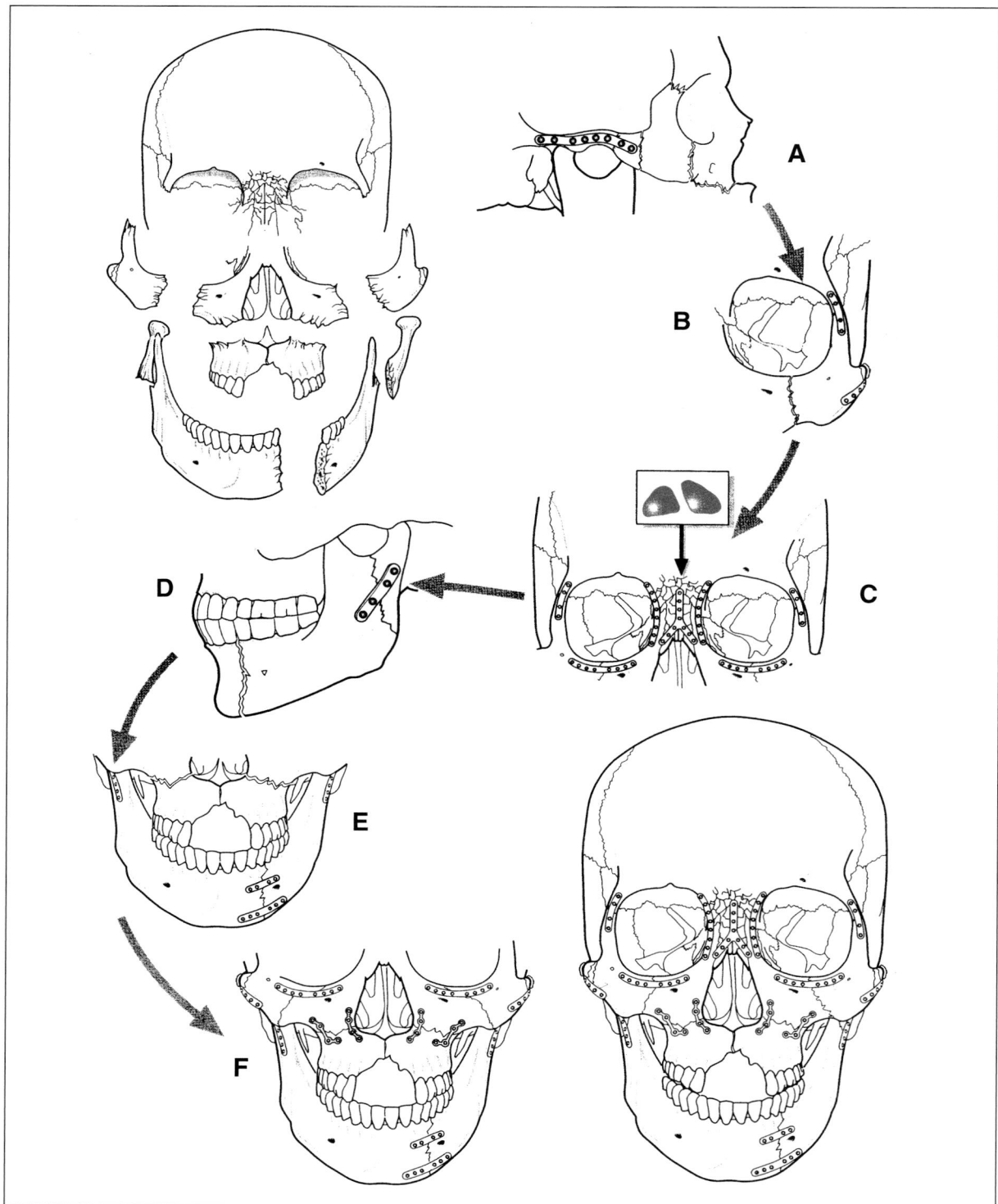

Figure 11.3-1. Panfacial fracture treatment protocol, based on reconstructing load-bearing structures of the facial skeleton. (A) Projection of the midface is created by reconstructing the zygomatic arches, starting from the stable part of the temporal bone. (B) The zygomas are fixed to the arches and to the frontal bone to create the final projection of the midface. (C) The width of the midface is reconstructed by repositioning the central midface (orbits and nose) to its correct position, in relation to the zygomas and frontal bone. Concomitantly, canthopexy is fixed and the frontal bone and sinus fractures are treated. (This procedure is independent of the occlusion.) (D) The posterior vertical height of the face is reconstructed by positioning and fixing the condylar fractures. (E) Intermaxillary fixation is applied and the mandible is reconstructed. (F) Finally, the LeFort I-level fractures are positioned to natural occlusion. (Reproduced with permission from Booth PW, Schendel SA, Hausamen J-E, eds: *Maxillofacial Surgery*. Churchill Livingstone, 1999.)

REPAIR OF FACIAL FRACTURES

SURGICAL CONSIDERATIONS

Description: Facial fractures are classified by location and the involved bones.

Upper and mid-face region: Frontal sinus fractures may involve the anterior wall alone, or also may involve the naso-frontal ducts and/or posterior wall. Nasofrontal duct disruption may require obliteration of the duct and sinus, which is done with an electric burr and loupe magnification to remove all mucosa before grafting the area with bone, fat, or peri-cranium. A posterior wall disruption is a fracture into the anterior cranial fossa that may require CSF leak repair ± cranialization of the sinus (complete removal of the posterior wall of the sinus). Each frontal bone forms a large component of the orbital roof and, as such, ocular injury or periorbital entrapment must be considered.

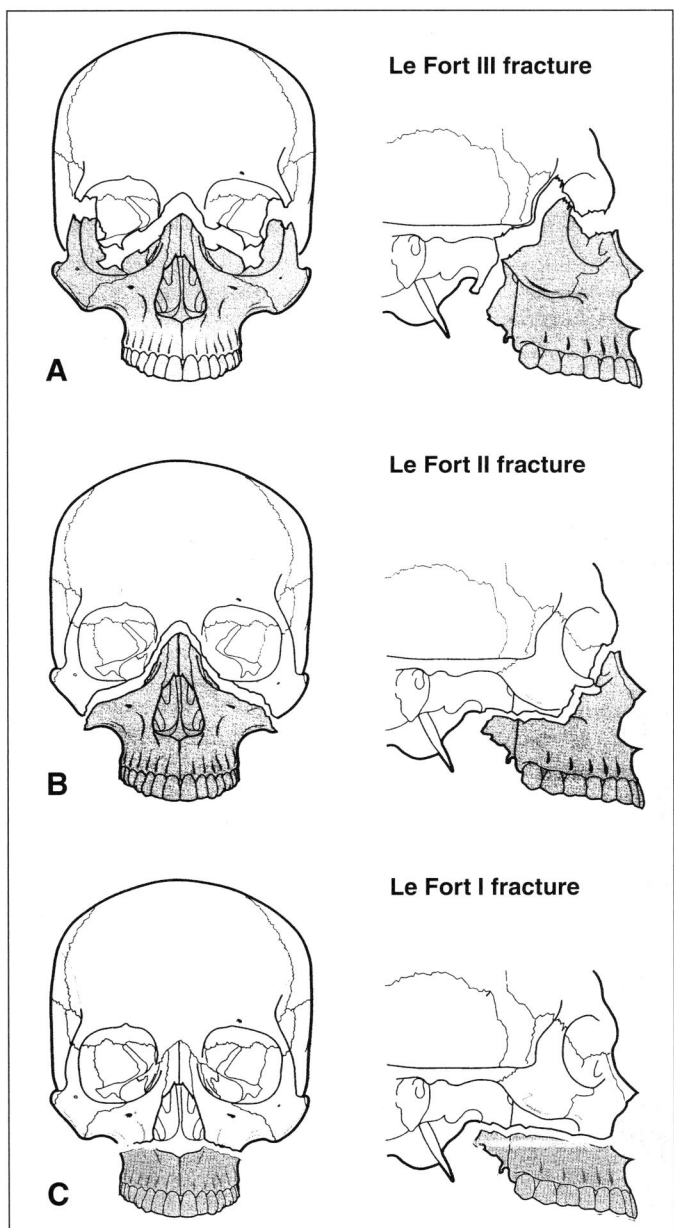

Fractures of the maxilla are classified as **LeFort I, II,** or **III,** depending on the level of the fracture (Fig 11.3-2). **LeFort I** is a horizontal fracture, separating the teeth and lower maxillary components from the upper facial structures. **LeFort II** is a triangular fracture with a fracture line across the nose, below the infraorbital rims, and extending through the entire lower maxillary structures. **LeFort III** is essentially a disassociation of the cranium and face. In these cases, the maxilla is usually mobile, or impacted posteriorly, occasionally closing off the posterior airway. Further mobility of the segments may be present with a sagittal split of the palate. Associated fractures in the maxillary region (Fig 11.3-2) include fractures of the zygoma; orbital fractures (most commonly orbital floor), isolated nasal fractures; naso-orbital-ethmoid (NOE) fractures (usually with severe comminution of the upper face); and cranial base fractures with the potential for dural tears and CSF rhinorrhea. Added procedures which may be required to complete the repair of these fractures include **local flap closure** of a CSF leak and **primary bone grafting,** usually from cranium or distant sites, such as the ilium, to highly comminuted areas (e.g., NOE, orbital floors).

Lower face: Fractures of the mandible are classified by the type of fracture and location (Fig 11.3-3), the most common being the subcondylar fracture. Fractures involving the mandibular body, such as a parasymphyseal fracture, may result in unstable mandibular segments. In cases of bilateral mandibular body fractures associated with symphyseal fractures, the mandible can be flail and fall posteriorly in the supine position, allowing the tongue to block off the airway. All of the fractures involving change in occlusion (LeFort maxillary and all mandibular fractures), require reestablishment of a normal occlusion by the application of arch bars and wires also called intermaxillary fixation (IMF). This may be

Figure 11.3-2. Schematic of the LeFort fracture lines. (A) LeFort III involves separation of cranium from facial bone structure. (B) LeFort II is a pyramid-shaped fracture, including the dentition and nasal structures. (C) LeFort I is a horizontal fracture involving mobilization of dentition and maxilla. (Reproduced with permission from Booth PW, Schendel SA, Hausamen J-E, eds: *Maxillofacial Surgery.* Churchill Livingstone, 1999.)

combined with rigid fixation, most commonly internal plates. In some cases, rigid fixation will allow removal of the IMF at the end of the case; in others, IMF may be required for postop healing. Removal of the throat pack prior to final IMF is of paramount importance.

Trismus may be associated with any of the above injuries 2° direct injury to the muscles of mastication, but is more commonly associated with fractures of these muscular attachments (e.g., mandible, zygoma). Associated **dentoalveolar fractures** of the maxilla or mandible may require preop wiring in the ER. The intent is to hold steady those segments with tenuous stability and blood supply. Intubation techniques should avoid displacing these segments. Fractures not involving change in occlusion (e.g., orbital zygomatic, nasal fracture) can be orally intubated. Most fractures with a change in occlusion should be nasally intubated with RAE or 60° curved connector. Exceptions include edentulous segments allowing tube to pass vs edentulous patient with splint fabricated for oral intubation. Another preop consideration is the amount of blood loss at the scene or in the ER. Facial and scalp vessels can bleed profusely (hypovolemia) and patients may arrive in the OR with both anterior and posterior nasal packs in place (difficult ventilation).

The **surgical approach** depends on the extent of fractures and associated lacerations. Periorbital incisions can be external, on or below the lower eyelid and over the brow, or internal, along the lower eyelid conjunctiva. Upper facial repair may include a bicoronal approach (Fig 11.3-4) designed to peel the face off the upper facial skeleton via an ear-to-ear scalp incision. Rainey clips are used to minimize scalp bleeding. Of note, periorbital dissection to explore and repair NOE or orbital floor fractures involves some retraction on the globe. This may cause ↓HR and ↓BP via the occulocardiac reflex. The mandible can be approached through external, preauricular or inferior border, or intraoral incisions.

Variant procedure or approaches: Endoscopic approaches are being developed for multiple fracture sites. **Resorbable plates and screws**, especially for pediatric cases, can be applied through the same surgical approaches.

Usual preop diagnosis: Facial trauma

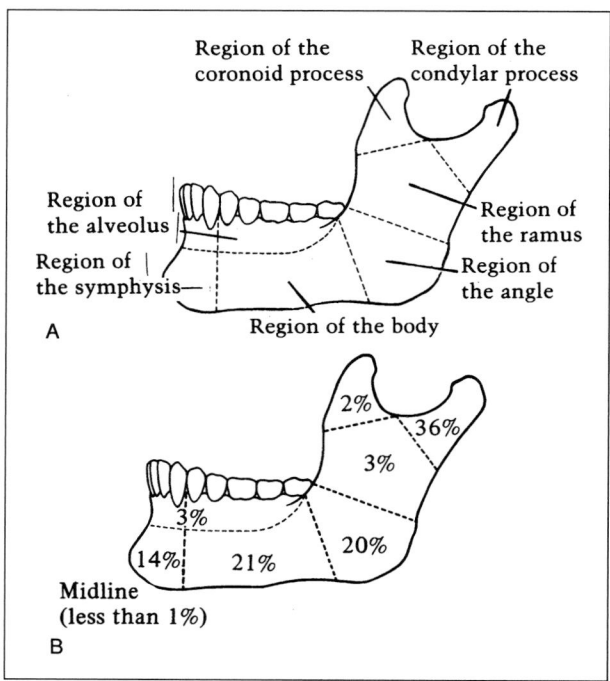

Figure 11.3-3. (A) Anatomic regions of the mandible and (B) frequency of fractures in those regions. (Reproduced with permission from Aston SJ, Beasley RW, Thorne CH, eds: *Grabb and Smith's Plastic Surgery*, 5th edition. Lippincott-Raven, 1997.)

SUMMARY OF PROCEDURES

	Mandibular	Maxillary Orbital/Zygomatic	Nasal
Position	Supine	⇐	⇐
Incision	Intraoral; lateral, submandibular	Intraoral, ± subciliary; possibly coronal	Closed reduction; possibly intranasal
Special instrumentation	Air power tools; plate fixation; headlight	⇐ + Periorbital malleable retractors; Rowe disimpaction forceps; acrylic dental split	⇐
Unique considerations	Nasal RAE (sutured to dentition or septum); throat pack; corticosteroids periop to ↓ edema.	Panfacial smash; airway swelling associated with head injury; burns or other system involvement. Consider preop tracheostomy. Close monitoring for and removal of stimulus until occulocardiac reflex recovery.	
Antibiotics + other meds	Cefazolin 1 g iv	Methylprednisolone 125 mg iv (adults or equivalent)	⇐
Surgical time	1-3 h	1-6 h (bicoronal approach adds 1.5 h)	1 h

	Mandibular	Maxillary Orbital/Zygomatic	Nasal
Closing considerations	NG at end of procedure, maintained for 24 h; IMF postop; ★ **NB:** throat pack removal.	⇐	–
EBL	100-800 ml, depending on extent of fractures, need for graft harvest, patient age	⇐	⇐
Postop care	Airway or respiratory status may be compromised (preop and postop swelling/aspiration/associated injuries), requiring maintenance of intubation → ICU.	⇐	⇐
Mortality	Minimal (↑ due to associated injuries and blood loss)	⇐	⇐
Morbidity	Trismus	⇐	–
	Poor occlusion	⇐	–
	Drooling	⇐	–
	Poor cosmetic result	⇐	⇐
	Chronic pain/sensation changes	⇐	⇐
	Loss of taste	Loss of smell	⇐
		Visual problems/epiphora	–
		Sinus problems	⇐
		Breathing difficulty	⇐
Pain score	4-8	4-8	4-8

PATIENT POPULATION CHARACTERISTICS

Age range	> 4 yr
Male:Female	1:1 (varies by age group)
Incidence	The most common are: nasal bones, zygoma and arch, mandible, and orbital floor (on the rise due to airbags in autos).
Etiology	**Adults:** Motor vehicle accidents (MVAs), mostly young males (43-67%); assaults (13-48.8%); sports-related (3.8%); falls (3.6%); gunshot wounds (3%) **Children:** Uncommon: only ~5% of all facial fractures occur in ages < 12 yr; falls (33%); MVA (28%); abuse (3%); dog bites (rare). 69% are periorbital or nasal.
Associated conditions	Airway compromise/closed head trauma (40%); extremity fractures (33%); thoracic injury (29%); open or radiographic brain injury (25%); intraabdominal (12%); globe injuries (11%); oral trauma (11%); pelvic fractures (10%); C-spine fractures (4%-10%); T-L spine injuries (4%); shock; multisystem trauma; burns; massive soft-tissue loss. Mandibular fractures during MVAs are associated with a 65% incidence of life-threatening injuries and mortality of up to 8%; up to 1/3 of LeFort fractures will require intubation, most often due to upper respiratory tract blood and secretions.

ANESTHETIC CONSIDERATIONS

PREOPERATIVE

The forces required to produce facial fractures are considerable and frequently result in other associated trauma (e.g., closed head trauma; spine injuries; thoracic injury, including pneumothorax and myocardial contusion; intraabdominal bleeding). Soft-tissue injury to the tongue or larynx can make airway management difficult. When in doubt, a tracheostomy under local anesthesia or awake intubation should be considered. In mandible or maxillary fractures, nasal intubation is usually best, because the patient will be placed in intermaxillary fixation (IMF) (teeth brought together via wires or rubber bands) at the conclusion of the procedure. In malar or nasal bone fractures, the fixation may be precarious, making it undesirable to use mask ventilation at the termination of the procedure and necessitating awake extubation. Facial nerve monitoring may be required, contraindicating the use of muscle relaxants.

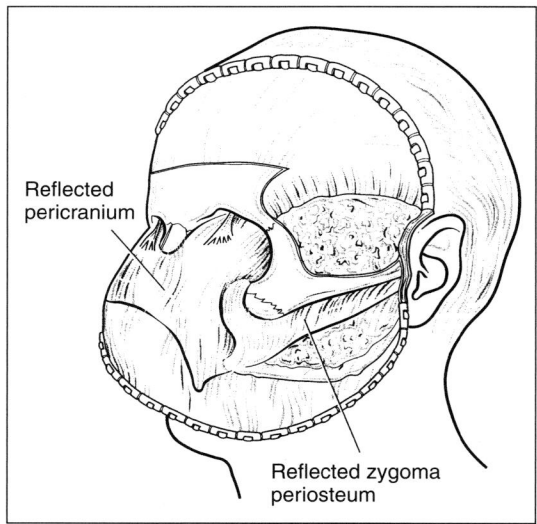

Figure 11.3-4. Bicoronal approach. (Reproduced with permission from Booth PW, Schendel SA, Hausamen J-E, eds: *Maxillofacial Surgery*. Churchill Livingstone, 1999.)

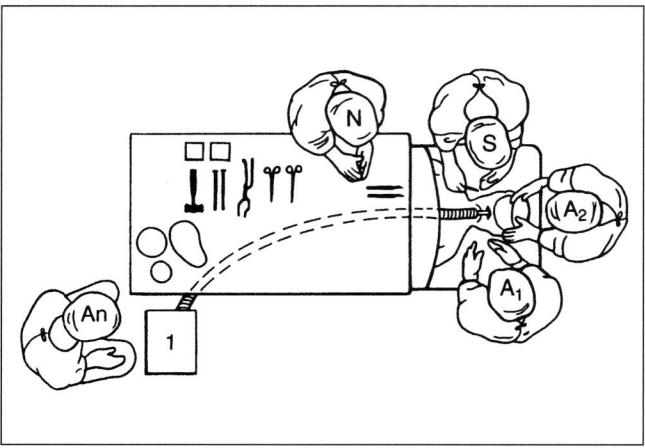

Figure 11.3-5. Standard anesthesia and surgical setup for a maxillofacial surgical procedure and certain craniofacial surgical procedures. The table may be rotated 90°-180° with anesthesia equipment and personnel at the foot or off to one side. (Reproduced with permission from Bell WH, ed: *Modern Practice of Orthognathic Surgery*, Vol I. WB Saunders, 1990.)

Frequently, the anesthesiologist's first encounter with these patients is in the ER, where prompt airway management decisions are essential—often before diagnostic imaging studies are complete. These patients should be treated with full-stomach precautions (see p. B-5) and may have already aspirated. Patients may be unable to open their mouths 2° pain or mechanical factors. The cause of limited mouth opening should be determined before induction of anesthesia. Several options exist. Often, the airway can be managed simply by inserting an oropharyngeal airway; failing this, an emergency intubation will be necessary. Blind nasal intubation should be avoided in patients with CSF rhinorrhea or other evidence of nasopharyngeal trauma, where the potential for creating false passages and additional trauma is significant. An awake oral intubation with topical anesthesia is often the safest approach. Emergency oral intubation may be complicated by an unstable C-spine and limited jaw opening, together with blood and debris in the oropharynx, making visualization difficult if not impossible. Often the only recourse is tracheostomy under local anesthesia. As with any trauma victim, attention is first directed toward maintaining the airway and restoration of fluid volume. The repair of the facial fracture may be carried out incidental to the primary trauma surgery or, more often, is deferred until the patient's condition is stabilized. This preop assessment will focus on the patient coming to the OR for semielective repair of a facial fracture.

Airway	**Semielective:** Usually, facial swelling and intraoral bleeding will have resolved, although mouth opening may be limited 2° pain or mechanical factors. Airway management requires knowledge of the fracture site(s). Patients with a maxillary fracture may benefit from an oral intubation to allow inspection of the nasopharynx before nasal intubation and definitive repair. The possibility of an awake fiber optic intubation (see p. B-6) should be discussed with the patient. Patients with an isolated orbital, zygomatic, or nasal fracture usually do not present airway management problems. The surgeon should be consulted regarding the preferred intubation route. **Trauma:** Airway and nasal obstruction following trauma can be extreme, as a result of soft-tissue swelling and accumulated blood and secretions. The extent of facial fractures, particularly in the midface, should be identified as they may preclude nasal intubation. Mandibular fractures may make access to the oropharynx difficult. Unstable dentoalveolar fractures may require preop wiring in the ER. In the case of massive trauma to the face, urgent tracheostomy should be considered. **Tests:** As indicated from H&P.
Respiratory	**Trauma:** Evaluate for associated trauma and respiratory insufficiency 2° aspiration. ✓ that chest tubes are functioning properly. **Tests:** CXR; others as indicated from H&P.
Cardiovascular	**Semielective:** Typically, several days will have elapsed since the initial trauma, and the patient should be hemodynamically stable. **Trauma:** Blunt chest trauma may be associated with myocardial contusion, pericardial effusion/tamponade, and aortic tear/dissection. **Tests:** ECG; others as indicated from H&P.

Neurological	**Semielective:** Document any neurological deficits and altered mental status. Meningitis may occur in patients with persistent CSF rhinorrhea or pneumocephalus.
	Trauma: Intracranial injury may be associated with facial fractures. Patients with head trauma may have ↑ICP; therefore, appropriate methods (e.g., CO_2 ↓, fluid ↓, smooth induction/intubation) are used to prevent further ↑ICP. Basilar skull fractures preclude passage of nasotracheal and NG tubes. In the presence of otorrhea or rhinorrhea, positive-pressure mask ventilation is inadvisable, due to the potential for causing pneumocephalus.
	Tests: Review skull and C-spine x-rays.
Musculoskeletal	**Semielective:** May be associated with other fractures and soft-tissue trauma that may affect patient positioning.
	Trauma: C-spine injuries are commonly associated with facial injuries. The C-spine should be cleared by clinical and x-ray exam before transport to OR. If C-spine cannot be cleared, intubation should be done with the head in a neutral position (splinted or with axial traction), using direct FOL (see p. B-6).
Hematologic	**Trauma:** Maxillary surgery may be associated with major blood loss and, for elective cases, autologous donation should be encouraged.
	Tests: Hct; others as indicated from H&P.
Laboratory	Other tests as indicated from H&P.
Premedication	Standard premedication (see p. B-2) is appropriate for nontrauma, neurologically intact patients with normal airways.
	Trauma: Trauma patients should be considered to have full stomachs, and sedative premedications are best avoided. Aspiration prophylaxis with 0.3 M Na citrate (30 ml po), ± metoclopramide 10 mg iv ± ranitidine 50 mg iv, should be considered.

INTRAOPERATIVE

Anesthetic technique: The majority of patients presenting for elective procedures are healthy and have normal airways. In the case of facial trauma, however, intubation of the trachea may be impossible. Hence, a tracheostomy under local anesthesia may be life-saving.

Induction	If there is any doubt regarding the ease of intubation, an awake FOL should be performed (see p. B-6). Nasal intubation is preferred for patients with mandibular and maxillary (LeFort) fractures involving a change in occlusion. Patients with orbital, zygomatic, or nasal fractures usually are intubated orally. In patients with normal airways, a standard induction (see p. B-2) is appropriate. Nasal or oral ETTs (RAE), or anode ETTs are commonly used to minimize intrusion into the surgical field.
Maintenance	Standard maintenance (see p. B-3); muscle relaxation usually is required except with facial nerve monitoring. Controlled ↓BP may be appropriate. Administration of an antiemetic (e.g., metoclopramide 10 mg iv or ondansetron 4 mg iv) is beneficial in patients who have their jaws wired or banded together.
Emergence	Patients with difficult airways or with jaws wired together should be extubated when fully awake. Extubation over a tube-changer may be appropriate. A wire cutter (or scissors for elastic bands) should be at the bedside at all times. Ensure that all throat packing has been removed before extubation. Thorough oropharyngeal suctioning is essential. NG tube may be used postop, so consider placement prior to extubation. Some patients with multiple trauma or extensive soft-tissue swelling may require continued postop intubation and mechanical ventilation.

Blood and fluid requirements	Moderate blood loss IV: 16-18 ga × 1 **Trauma:** NS/LR @ 6-8 ml/h **Other:** NS/LR @ 2-4 ml/h	Blood loss from facial fractures or orthognathic procedures can be extensive. T&C patient so blood is immediately available in OR.
Monitoring	Standard monitors (see p. B-1). ± Arterial line	Invasive monitoring may be required in patients with intracranial or other trauma, or for controlled ↓BP.
Control of blood loss	Surgical hemostasis Topical vasoconstrictors Posterior oropharyngeal packing	Surgical hemostasis should control most bleeding in these procedures. Topical vasoconstrictors, such as phenylephrine or cocaine, can be applied on the surgical field.

Control of blood loss, cont.	Controlled ↓BP	Posterior oropharyngeal packing can keep blood from passing undetected into the upper GI tract. Controlled ↓BP can be achieved simply by increasing volatile anesthetic levels.
Positioning	✓ and pad pressure points. ✓ eyes.	Some surgeons prefer that the OR table be rotated 90° or 180°. Be prepared with long hoses and appropriate connectors. Protect eyes with an ophthalmic ointment.
Complications	ETT damage	Nasal ETT may be wired inadvertently to the maxilla, making extubation difficult. In case of ETT damage, be prepared to reestablish the airway rapidly by reintubation, usually over an intubating stylet or gum elastic bougie.
	Oculocardiac reflex	Notify surgeon (stop surgical stimulus). Consider atropine and increasing depth of anesthesia.

POSTOPERATIVE

Complications	Airway obstruction	Wire cutters (or scissors) should be available at bedside to facilitate emergent reintubation or other form of airway management. Consider retained throat pack.
	PONV	Vigorous treatment of nausea is important.
Pain management	Parenteral narcotics (see p. C-2) or PCA with antiemetics (see p. C-3).	Local anesthetic infiltrated at end of procedure.

References

1. Booth PW, Schendel SA, Hausamen J-E, eds: *Maxillofacial Surgery*. Churchill Livingstone, New York: 1999, Chap 1-11.
2. Carlin CB, et al: Facial fractures and related injuries. *J Craniomaxillofac Trauma* 1998; 4(2):44-8.
3. Fischer K, et al: Injuries associated with mandible fractures sustained in motor vehicle collisions. *Plast Reconstr Surg* 2001; 108(2):328-31.
4. Fortunato MA, et al: Facial bone fractures in children. *Oral Surg Oral Med Oral Pathol* 1982; 53(3): 225-30.
5. Girotto JA: Long-term physical impairment and functional outcomes after complex facial fractures. *Plast Reconstr Surg* 2001; 108(2):312-27.
6. Hoffmann JF:, Naso-orbital-ethmoid complex fracture management. *Fac Plast Surg* 1998; 14(1):67-76.
7. Manson PN: Facial Injuries. In *Plastic Surgery*, Vol 2. McCarthy JG, ed. WB Saunders, Philadelphia: 1990, 867-1141.
8. Matarasso A: The oculocardiac reflex in blepharoplasty surgery. *Plast Reconstr Surg* 1989; 83(2):243-50.
9. Ng M, et al: Managing the emergency airway in LeFort fractures. *J Craniomaxillofac Trauma* 1998; 4(3):38-43.
10. Stanley RB Jr: Maxillofacial trauma. In *Otolaryngology—Head and Neck Surgery,* Vol I, 3rd edition. Cummings CW, Fredrickson JM, Harker LA, Krause CJ, eds. Mosby-Year Book, St. Louis: 1998, 453-85.
11. Strong EB, Sykes JM: Zygoma complex fractures. *Fac Plast Surg* 1998; 14(1):105-15.
12. Tu AH, Girotto JA, et al: Facial fractures from dog bite injuries. *Plast Reconstr Surg* 2002; 109(4):1259-65.

LEFORT OSTEOTOMIES

SURGICAL CONSIDERATIONS

Description: LeFort osteotomies are used to correct maxillary deformities. The most common is the **LeFort I**, a transverse osteotomy, above the apices of the teeth, used to correct maxillary retrusion or maxillary vertical excess or deficiency. One of the goals in achieving improved function is to improve the occlusion, as classified by Angle (Fig 11.3-6). One or both jaws may be moved to achieve normocclusion. An intraoral vestibular incision is used for this approach, followed by an osteotomy of the maxilla, with either a burr or a saw, and completed with osteotomes. The osteotomy extends through the maxillary sinus toward the ETT, within the piriform aperture. There is potential for nasal ETT damage with this maneuver. Of note, BP usually will increase at the start of the osteotomies, increasing bleeding if anesthesia/analgesia

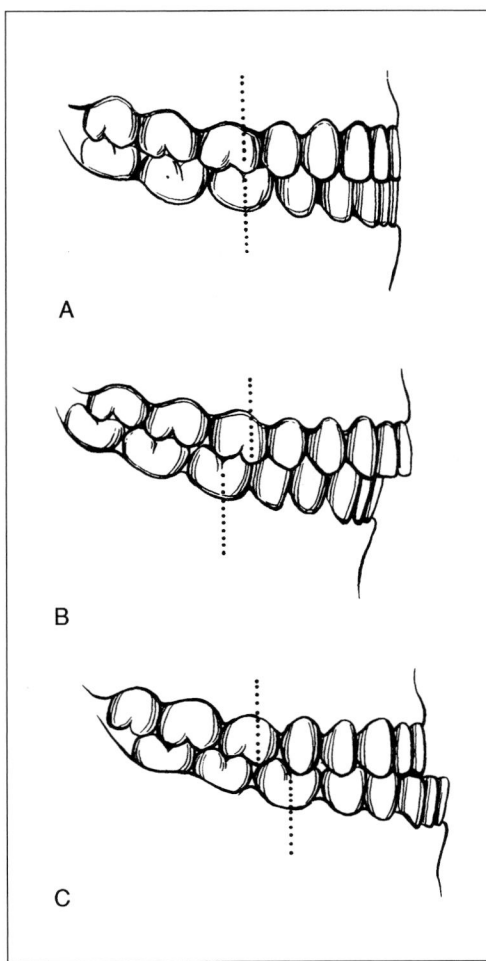

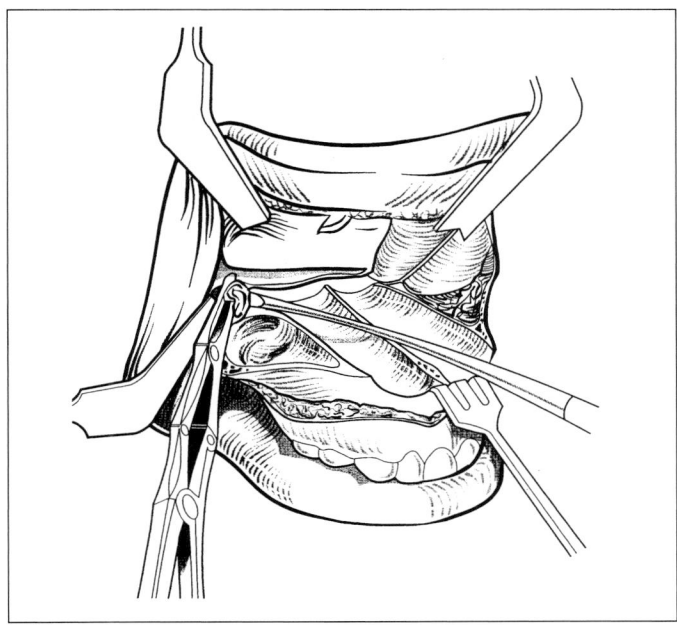

←**Figure 11.3-6.** The Angle classification of occlusion. (A) Class I, normal occlusion. (B) Class II, retroocclusion or mandibular deficiency. (C) Class III, prognathic occlusion (maxillary deficiency or mandibular excess). The key relationships to be discerned are those of the first molar teeth, cuspids, and incisors. (Reproduced with permission from Aston SJ, Beasley RW, Thorne CH, eds: *Grabb and Smith's Plastic Surgery*, 5th edition. Lippincott-Raven, 1997.)

↑**Figure 11.3-7.** Removal of bone around the perpendicular plate of the palatine bone. The descending palatine vessels may be ligated. (Reproduced with permission from Booth PW, Schendel SA, Hausamen J-E, eds: *Maxillofacial Surgery*. Churchill Livingstone, 1999.)

is inadequate. The maxilla is subsequently downfractured (Fig 11.3-7) and mobilized with Rowe disimpaction forceps. This is when most of the bleeding occurs. Further interdental osteotomies creating multiple maxillary segments may be required. LeFort II or LeFort III maxillary osteotomies may be used to correct severe midfacial retrusion. In these cases, infraorbital incisions are used with either brow or coronal (Fig 11.3-4) incisions. With maxillary advancements, iliac or cranial bone grafts are often necessary to close the bony gap created. Most of these patients have orthodontic appliances and will require intermaxillary fixation (IMF), with either wire or elastics at the end of the procedure, with or without a prefabricated splint. The maxilla is fixed rigidly in the new position with miniplates.

Variant procedure or approaches: Recently, **distraction osteogenesis** after LeFort osteotomy has been shown to be effective for correction of severe deformity that would be difficult to correct with single movements and internal fixation. This technique creates new bone as the osteotomized bones are slowly separated. No bone grafts are necessary. Distraction hardware is applied either internally or externally. External devices are stabilized via halo and compression bolts into the skull. IMF is not indicated, as the upper jaw must be free to be distracted in relation to the lower jaw. A second operation may be required for removal of distractor hardware. **Absorbable internal devices** also are available.

Usual preop diagnosis: Facial deformities; dentoskeletal dysplasia

SUMMARY OF PROCEDURES

	LeFort I	LeFort II	LeFort III	Distractor
Position	Supine; table may be rotated 90° or 180°	⇐	⇐	⇐
Incision	Intraoral	Intraoral and facial ± coronal	⇐	⇐
Special instrumentation	Miniplates and screws; burr or saws	⇐	⇐	Distractors

	LeFort I	LeFort II	LeFort III	Distractor
Unique considerations	Jaw frequently closed (wires or elastic); nasal RAE or armored tube. **NB: Keep SBP < 100 mmHg during osteotomy-closure.**	⇐	⇐	No IMF
	With cranial bone graft harvest, the nasal ETT goes opposite to the donor side and is repositioned later.	⇐	⇐	⇐
Antibiotics + other meds	Cefazolin 1 g iv; methylprednisolone 125 mg iv (or pediatric equivalent)	⇐	⇐	⇐
Surgical time	3-6 h	⇐	⇐	⇐
Closing considerations	★ **NB: Throat pack removal.** NG at end of case × 24 h. NSAIDs contraindicated.	⇐	⇐	⇐
EBL	400-800 ml	⇐	⇐	⇐
Postop care	PACU → room	ICU × 1 d	⇐	⇐
Mortality	Rare	⇐	⇐	⇐
Morbidity	Relapse	⇐	⇐	⇐
	Infection	⇐	⇐	⇐
	Bone/tooth loss: Uncommon	⇐	⇐	⇐
	Severe intraop bleeding: Uncommon	⇐	⇐	⇐
	Blindness: Very rare	⇐	⇐	⇐
	Temporomandibular joint dysfunction	⇐	⇐	⇐
	Nasal obstruction	⇐	⇐	⇐
	Nasolacrimal obstruction	⇐	⇐	⇐
	Oronasal fistulas (multi-piece osteotomies, uncommon)	⇐	⇐	⇐
	Poor cosmetic result	⇐	⇐	⇐
	Sensory nerve dysfunction	⇐	⇐	⇐
				Distractor malfunction
Pain score	4	5	5	5

PATIENT POPULATION CHARACTERISTICS

Age range	15 yr–adulthood, usually < 30 yr
Male:Female	1:1
Incidence	Up to 5% of population
Etiology	Usually developmental in nature; also cleft lip and palate patients Rarely syndromic: Apert (1/100,000); Crouzon (1/25,000)
Associated conditions	Usually none with developmental cases; sleep apnea; or part of a recognized condition associated with congenital anomalies (e.g., cleft lip and palate, proptotic eyes, severe mitten-hand syndactylies)

ANESTHETIC CONSIDERATIONS

See Anesthetic Considerations following Mandibular Osteotomies/Genioplasty, p. 906.

References

1. Frost DE: Orthognathic surgical techniques. In *Maxillofacial Surgery.* Booth PW, Schendel SA, Hausamen J-E, eds. Churchill Livingstone, Edinburgh: 1999, 1273-95.
2. Hilley MD, Ghali GE, Giesecke AU: Anesthesia for orthognathic surgery in modern practice. In *Orthognathic Reconstructive Surgery*, 2nd edition. Bell WH, ed. WB Saunders, Philadelphia: 1992, 128-53.
3. Lanigan DT, Hey JH, West RA: Major vascular complications of orthognathic surgery: hemorrhage associated with LeFort I osteotomies. *J Oral Maxillofac Surg* 1990; 48(6):561-73.
4. Lo LJ, Hung KF, Chen YR: Blindness as a complication of LeFort I osteotomy for maxillary distraction. *Plast Reconstr Surg* 2002; 109(2):688-700.
5. Richardson D, Pospisil OA: Avoiding surgical complications in orthognathic surgery. In *Maxillofacial Surgery.* Booth PW, Schendel SA, Hausamen J-E, eds. Churchill Livingstone, Edinburgh: 1999, 1307-20.
6. Schendel SA, Mason ME: Adverse outcomes in orthognathic surgery and management of residual problems. *Clin Plast Surg* 1997; 24(3):489-505.
7. Scully JR, Matheson JD: Emergency airway management in the traumatized patient. In *Oral and Maxillofacial Trauma,* 2nd edition. Fonseca RJ, Walker RV, eds. WB Saunders, Philadelphia: 1997, 105-37.

MANDIBULAR OSTEOTOMIES/GENIOPLASTY

SURGICAL CONSIDERATIONS

Description: Mandibular deformities include either a retruded mandible or a prognathic mandible involving a malocclusion (Class II or III), and may occur in combination with a small chin (microgenia). Surgical correction of the basic mandibular deformity involves either advancing or retruding the mandible. The most common procedure for this is the **sagittal ramus split osteotomy (Obwegesser)** (Fig 11.3-8). The mandible is split with the inferior alveolar nerve solely within the anterior segment, such that the tooth-bearing anterior segment can slide forward or backward to correct the original deformity. A variety of other techniques of mandibular osteotomies exist, often involving the ramus area of the mandible, and are performed via an intraoral approach.

In some very large deformities, an external incision (**Risdon** type) and bone graft placement may be necessary to complete the mandibular ramus reconstruction. Many patients will be treated for dentoskeletal deformities with a combination of LeFort movement and sagittal-split osteotomies of the mandible. When the mandible is set back, mandibular bone is resected and often can be used in combined procedures as bone graft for the LeFort osteotomy. This avoids cranial bone harvest and, therefore, avoids repositioning the ETT during the procedure for cranial bone access and avoids donor site morbidity. Occasionally, deformities may be corrected by mandibular body osteotomies.

Rigid fixation of mandibular osteotomies is often accomplished by the use of small miniplates and screws. Fixation also can be accomplished with elastic traction (rarely, wire fixation) between mandible and maxilla (IMF), placed either at the time of surgery, or several days following, and held in position for 1-2 wk. These procedures may be combined with a **genioplasty** to correct the chin deformity; or, genioplasty may be performed as an isolated procedure. The most common type is a horizontal osteotomy of the inferior mandible, with the chin segment repositioned with internal fixation (Fig 11.3-9A). Augmentation of the chin also is accomplished with alloplastic

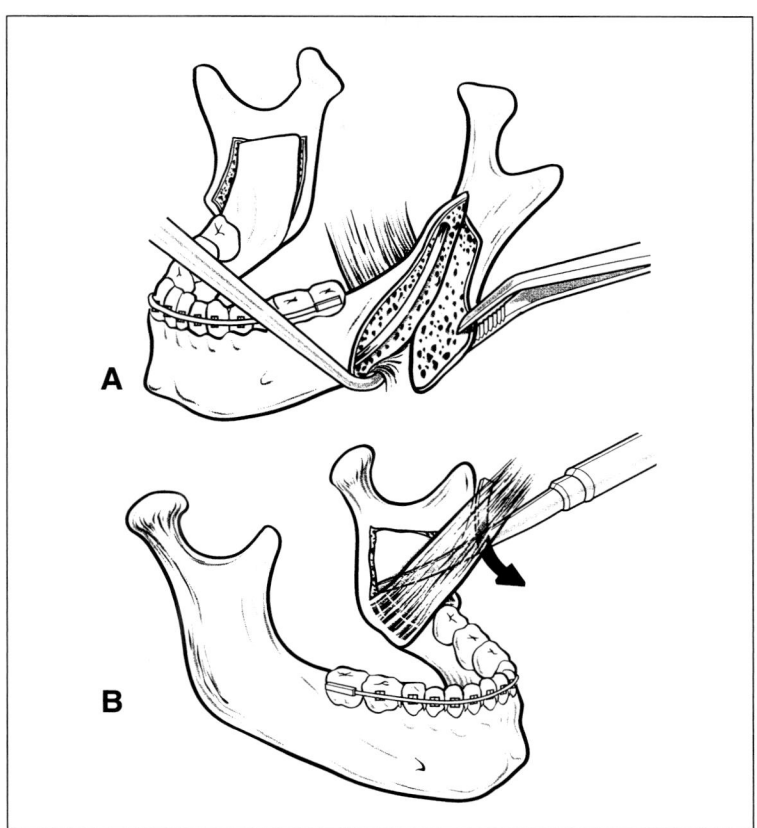

Figure 11.3-8. (A, B) "J" stripper used to remove muscle attachments from medial aspect of distal segment. Used through the osteotomy split. (Reproduced with permission from Booth PW, Schendel SA, Hausamen J-E, eds: *Maxillofacial Surgery.* Churchill Livingstone, 1999.)

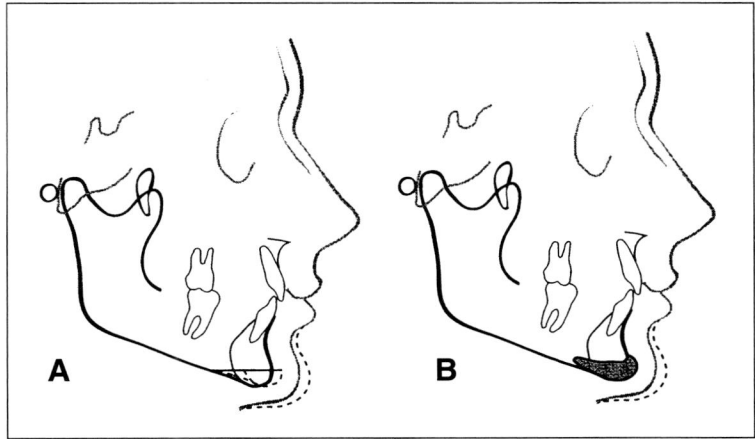

Figure 11.3-9. An osseous genioplasty (A) can be used to augment the chin, move it posteriorly, alter its vertical position or change the transverse position of the chin. Allopastic implants (B) can be used to augment the chin anteriorly. These are less effective for vertical augmentation. (Reproduced with permission from Booth PW, Schendel SA, Hausamen J-E, eds: *Maxillofacial Surgery.* Churchill Livingstone, 1999.)

onlay materials (Fig 11.3-9B) placed via either the oral route or the extraoral route through a small submental incision. As an isolated procedure, genioplasty is performed most frequently with local anesthesia and sedation.

Variant procedure or approaches: Distraction osteogenesis is being used more frequently in treating certain acquired and congenital jaw deformities. This involves a partial mandibular osteotomy and placement of a distraction device (Fig 11.3-10). Depending on the application, this may be an external or internal device. External devices are visible over the skin with percutaneous pins into the bone. Internal devices are placed beneath the oral soft tissues, with a single adjustment pin exposed.

Usual preop diagnosis: Mandibular deformity

SUMMARY OF PROCEDURE

Position	Supine; table may be rotated 90° or 180°. Nasal RAE tube toward head of bed (sutured through nasal septum), padded, and secured to forehead; shoulder roll; neck extended
Incision	Usually oral, but may be external in the submental or posterior mandibular area; preinjection with local anesthetic with epinephrine
Special instrumentation	Miniplates and screws; burrs/saws; osteotomes; distractor for distraction osteogenesis; throat pack
Unique considerations	Scleral lubricant and shields needed. Postop, patient may have IMF with inability to open the ★ mouth. (IMF not used with distractor cases. **NB: Remove throat pack** before extubation; thorough oro- and nasopharyngeal suction.
Antibiotics + other meds	Cefazolin 1 g iv; methylprednisolone 125 mg iv (adults)
Surgical time	Genioplasty: 0.5-1 h
	Mandibular osteotomy: 2-4 h
EBL	Genioplasty: 50 ml
	Mandibular osteotomy: 100-200 ml
Postop care	PACU → room. If sleep apnea present, ICU overnight + extubation.
Mortality	Rare
Morbidity	Mandibular relapse: ≤ 30%
	Mental nerve paresthesia: 5-20%
	Lingual nerve injury: 1-16%
	Infection/nonunion: < 1%
	Facial nerve injury: Rare (most reported cases resolve without treatment)
	Aseptic necrosis (buccal plate or genioplasty fragment)
	Worsening TMJ problems
	Adverse cosmetic result
Pain score	4

PATIENT POPULATION CHARACTERISTICS

Age range	Infant–adult
Male:Female	Unknown
Incidence	Unknown
Etiology	Developmental (90%); acquired (10%)
Associated conditions	Usually none with developmental cases; sleep apnea; congenitally small mandible may be associated with a large tongue and cleft palate (Pierre Robin syndrome), hemifacial microsomia (which may be associated with heart, vertebral, and other anomalies), Treacher Collins syndrome, or Nager's syndrome (many of the congenital cases may be tracheostomy- and gastrostomy-dependent, with associated TMJ ankylosis).

ANESTHETIC CONSIDERATIONS

(Procedures covered: LeFort osteotomies; mandibular osteotomies; genioplasty)

PREOPERATIVE

These surgeries are usually performed on patients with facial disproportion. In general, this patient population is young and healthy; however, many of them will present with challenging airway management problems. In addition, facial disproportion will often accompany congenital anomalies (e.g., Crouzon, Apert, Pierre Robin, and Treacher Collins

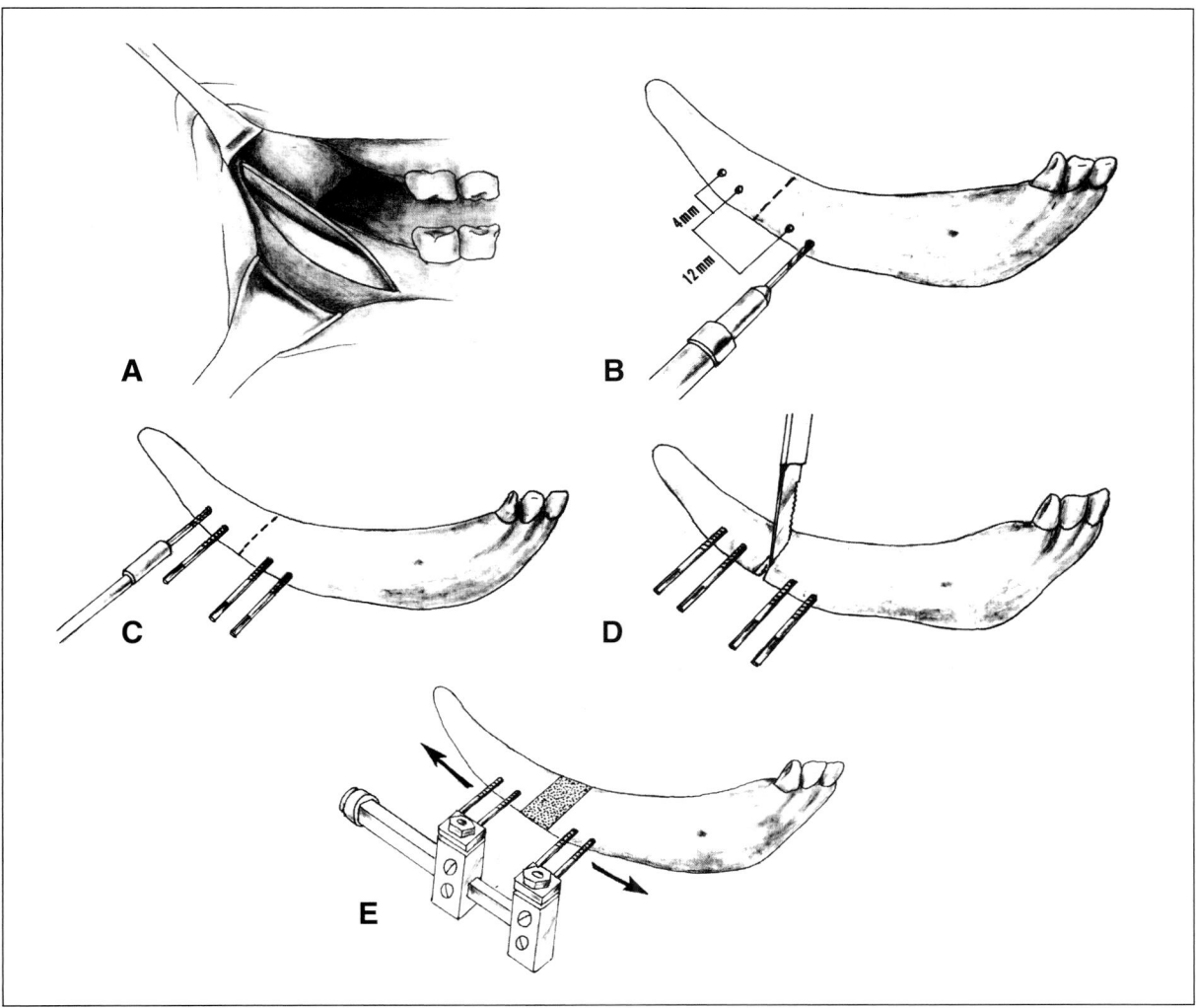

Figure 11.3-10. Mandibular distraction technique: (A) An intraoral incision is made along the oblique line of the mandibular remnant. (B) Sites of the pinholes and proposed osteotomy (interrupted line). (C) Pins have been inserted. (D) The osteotomy is performed. (E) Commencement of distraction with the appliance in position. The arrows designate the movement of the mandibular segments with formation of bony regenerate in the resulting gap. (Reproduced with permission from Aston SJ, Beasley RW, Thorne CH, eds: *Grabb and Smith's Plastic Surgery*, 5th edition. Lippincott-Raven, 1997.)

syndromes). (For discussion of specific syndromes, see Anesthetic Considerations for Pediatric Orthopedic Surgery of the Pelvis and Lower Limbs, p. 1121).

Airway	As usual, a careful airway evaluation is essential since many of these patients have abnormal airway anatomy and may be difficult to mask ventilate or intubate. Visual inspection often reveals the reasons for the surgery and allows the anesthesiologist to determine the safest approach to intubation. When a difficult intubation is anticipated, the need for awake fiber optic intubation (p. B-6) should be discussed with the patient.
Respiratory	Consider the anesthetic implications of associated congenital syndromes in this patient population. Obstructive sleep apnea (OSA, see p. 196) also may be associated with patients in need of mandibular surgery. **Tests:** As indicated from H&P.
Cardiovascular	As above, consider the implications of possible congenital syndromes. Assess whether patient is a suitable candidate for the use of controlled ↓BP, particularly those undergoing maxillary procedures. **Tests:** As indicated from H&P.
Hematologic	Encourage autologous blood donation for maxillary procedures. **Tests:** Hct

Laboratory	Other tests as indicated from H&P.
Premedication	Standard premedication (see p. B-2) is usually appropriate.

INTRAOPERATIVE

Anesthetic technique: GETA

Induction	If there is any doubt regarding the ease of intubation or ability to mask ventilate, an awake FOL should be performed (see p. B-6). Nasal intubation is preferred for patients undergoing mandibular or maxillary osteotomies, as well as genioplasty. In patients with normal airways, a standard induction (see p. B-2) is appropriate. Nasal or oral ETTs (RAE), or anode ETTs, are commonly used to minimize intrusion into the surgical field.
Maintenance	Standard maintenance (see p. B-3); muscle relaxation is usually required. Administration of an antiemetic (e.g., metoclopramide 10 mg iv or ondansetron 4 mg iv) is essential in patients who have their jaws wired or banded together.
Emergence	Patients with difficult airways or with their jaws wired (or banded) together should be extubated when fully awake. Perform thorough oropharyngeal suctioning. If not placed previously, an NG tube should be placed before extubation. A wire cutter (or scissors for elastic bands) should be at the bedside at all times. Ensure that all throat packing has been removed before extubation.

Blood and fluid requirements	Moderate blood loss IV: 16 ga × 1 NS/LR @ 5-8 ml/kg/h	Maxillary osteotomies may be associated with major blood loss (e.g., 1500-2000 ml). The majority of blood loss occurs when the maxilla is downfractured. Controlled ↓BP (SBP < 90 mmHg) may be particularly useful during this part of the case, and blood should be readily available for this and all maxillary procedures.
Monitoring	Standard monitors (see p. B-1). ± Arterial line ± CVP line or 2nd iv	Direct arterial pressure measurements are useful for deliberate ↓BP. Central venous access or a 2nd peripheral iv may be useful for vasodilator infusions.
Positioning	✓ and pad pressure points. ✓ eyes.	Eyes should be protected with an ophthalmic ointment and possible tarsorrhaphy by the surgeons. Some surgeons prefer to have the OR table rotated 90° or 180°. Be prepared with circuit-extension tubing.
Complications	ETT damage Hemorrhage	ETT may be cut during maxillary osteotomy, necessitating rapid reintubation.

POSTOPERATIVE

Complications	Airway obstruction PONV	Wire cutters (or scissors) should be available at bedside to facilitate emergent reinduction or other form of airway management. Consider retained throat pack. Vigorous treatment of nausea is important.
Pain management	Parenteral narcotics (see p. C-2) or PCA with antiemetics (see p. C-3).	

References:

1. Blanco G, Melman E, Cuairn V, Moyao D, Ortiz-Monasterio F: Fibreoptic nasal intubation in children with anticipated and unanticipated difficult intubation. *Paediatric Anaesthesia* 2001; 11(1):49-53.
2. Frost DE: Orthognathic surgical techniques. In *Maxillofacial Surgery*. Booth PW, Schendel SA, Hausamen J-E, eds. Churchill Livingstone, Edinburgh: 1999, 1273-95.
3. Hunt JA, Hobar PC: Common craniofacial anomalies: the facial dysostoses. *Plast Reconstr Surg* 2002; 110(7):1714-28.
4. Osses H, et al: Laryngeal mask for difficult intubation in children. *Paediatric Anaesthesia* 1999; 9(5):399-401.
5. Richardson D, Pospisil OA: Avoiding surgical complications in orthognathic surgery. In *Maxillofacial Surgery*. Booth PW, Schendel SA, Hausamen J-E, eds. Churchill Livingstone, Edinburgh: 1999, 1307-20.
6. Samchukov ML, Cope JB, Cherkashin AM, eds: *Craniofacial Distraction Osteogenesis*, Mosby-Year Book, St. Louis: 2001.
7. Schendel SA, Mason ME: Adverse outcomes in orthognathic surgery and management of residual problems. *Clin Plast Surg* 1997; 24(3):489-505.

Surgeons

Yvonne L. Karanas, MD
James Chang, MD
David M. Kahn, MD
Jeffrey D. Pardun, MD
William C. Lineaweaver, MD, FACS (*Scalp replantation*)
Kenneth C. W. Hui, MD, FACS (*Scalp replantation*)

11.4 FUNCTIONAL RESTORATION

Anesthesiologist

Tara Cornaby, MD

MICROSURGERY—FREE-FLAP RECONSTRUCTION

SURGICAL CONSIDERATIONS

Yvonne L. Karanas and James Chang

Description: Microsurgical recon-struction involves moving tissue from one site of the body to another (see Fig 11.4-1, Table 11.4-1). This may be muscle, skin, bone, or any combination of these tissues. An artery and vein that supply the tissues are connected to an artery and vein at the new recipient site, thereby reestablishing blood flow and ensuring tissue survival. Once transplanted, the tissue is molded and shaped to replace the missing part. Vascular anastomoses are performed on vessels as small as 1.5 mm in diameter. Complex reconstructions may require 12 h of GA with significant blood loss and fluid shifts. Patients with comorbid conditions may need additional medical tests before surgery to ensure that they are able to withstand this type of operation.

Peripheral, central, and arterial lines should be placed at the start of the case only after consultation with the reconstructive surgeon. For example, radial forearm flap may be injured by placement of a peripheral

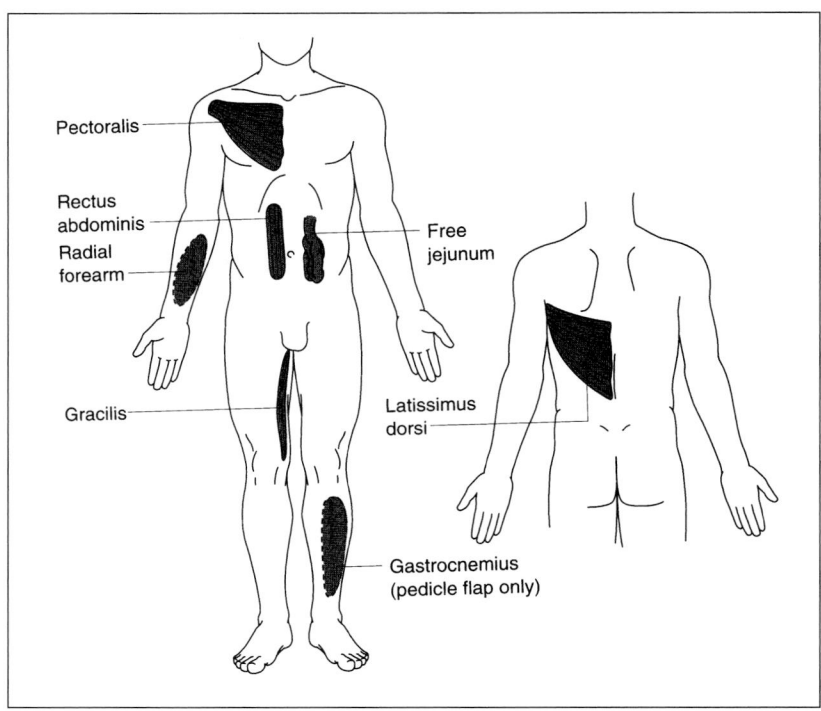

Figure 11.4-1. Locations of commonly used flaps. (Reproduced with permission from Greenfield, LJ, et al, eds: *Surgery: Principles and Practice*, 2nd edition. Lippincott-Raven, 1997.)

iv in the antecubital fossa or within the body of the flap. The neck is a common site for microvascular anastomoses in head and neck reconstruction. The placement of internal jugular lines should be discussed with the surgeon before surgery. The rectus muscle flap relies on the deep inferior epigastric vessels for its perfusion. Femoral arterial or venous line placement may injure these vessels and is, therefore, contraindicated. In bilateral breast reconstruction with free flaps, the iv lines should be placed in the lower extremities if possible. The reconstructive surgeon will try to operate in conjunction with the extirpative surgeon to minimize operating time. This often necessitates repositioning the patient as the case progresses.

Microsurgical reconstructions are often long operations, and large surface areas of the patient are exposed during the surgery. The patient's core temperature should be monitored closely with the use of a bladder or esophageal temperature probe. Body and fluid warmers should be used routinely to maintain the patient's body temperature. There is no standard practice for anticoagulation in microsurgery. No randomized prospective clinical trial has definitively documented the efficacy of a particular type of anticoagulation in routine reconstructive microsurgery. Aspirin, dextran, and heparin are the most commonly used agents. Close communication between the surgeon and anesthesiologist is critical so that the desired agent is administered at the appropriate time.

The survival of the flap relies on the patency of the anastomosis. Thrombosis requires reexploration and may → complete loss of the tissue. Anastomotic patency is diminished by vasospasm or vascular constriction. The common causes of vasoconstriction include dehydration, hypothermia, pain, and administration of vasoconstrictors; therefore, during microsurgery, vasoconstrictors are contraindicated and should be given only when absolutely necessary, after consultation with the reconstructive surgeon. The patient must be adequately hydrated so that there is good perfusion to the transplanted tissue. Diuretics should be avoided. Postop pain control is important to prevent vasoconstriction on emergence from anesthesia. After surgery, patients are transferred to an area of the hospital where the free flap can be monitored. In many hospitals, this is an ICU.

Usual preop diagnosis: Trauma, cancer, chronic wounds, congenital anomalies, and burns are some of the common diagnoses that result in the need for microsurgical reconstruction.

910

Table 11.4-1. Types of Flaps

Reconstruction	Commonly Used Flaps	Location	Positioning
Head and neck	Fibula	Leg	Supine
	Radial forearm	Arm	Supine
	Scapula	Back	Lateral decubitus
	Iliac crest	Hip	Supine
	Anterolateral thigh	Thigh	Supine
	Gracilis	Thigh	Supine
Breast	TRAM	Abdomen	Supine
	Gluteal	Buttocks	Lateral decubitus
	Rubens/iliac crest	Hip	Supine
	Tensor fascia lata	Lateral thigh	Supine
	Latissimus dorsi	Back	Lateral decubitus
Lower extremity	Rectus abdominis	Abdomen	Supine
	Latissimus dorsi	Back	Lateral decubitus
	Serratus anterior	Back	Lateral decubitus
	Gracilis	Thigh	Supine

SUMMARY OF PROCEDURE

Position — Requirements of the recipient site take precedence; optimal position for the donor site is then considered.

Incision — Each site will have specific incision.

Special instrumentation — Microscope; tourniquet for extremities

Unique considerations — Multiple surgical teams; avoid hypothermia; ± anticoagulation; if intraop nerve stimulation is planned, muscle relaxants should be avoided.

Antibiotics — Cefazolin (1 g iv) in uncomplicated cases; broader coverage in complicated circumstances

Surgical time — Simple flap: 4-6 h
Complex cases: 8-12 h

Closing considerations — Splints and dressings should be secured before emergence.

EBL — Skin flap: 200 ml
Muscle flap: 200-500 ml
Bone flap: 500-1000 ml

Postop care — ICU for flap perfusion monitoring

Mortality — < 2% (usually associated with coexisting disease)

Morbidity — Soft-tissue complications: 20-30%
Vascular complications requiring reexploration: 5-10%
Flap failure: 5%

Pain score — 3-5

PATIENT POPULATION CHARACTERISTICS

Age range — 2-90 yr
Male:Female — 1:1
Incidence — 50-200/yr/major center
Etiology — Malignancy; trauma; chronic infection

Associated conditions — Complications of underlying disease (e.g., anemia)

ANESTHETIC CONSIDERATIONS

PREOPERATIVE

These surgeries are carried out on patients who have sustained major soft-tissue losses and require flap procedures to cover the defects. There are four typical patient populations presenting for this surgery: (1) those presenting for reconstruction following cancer surgery (e.g., radical neck dissection and mastectomy); (2) patients following trauma, usually with upper or lower-limb defects; (3) patients with congenital defects; and (4) previous burn victims. In general, these patients should present few problems for the anesthesiologist. In a patient with a congenital lesion, however, it is prudent to look for evidence of CHD, musculoskeletal deformities, and airway problems.

Respiratory	Exposure of the thorax to radiation may produce pathologic changes in the lungs and related structures, including pneumonitis ($\to$ dyspnea, hypoxemia) that may progress to fibrosis ($\to$ $\downarrow$pulmonary compliance). Tracheal or bronchial fibrosis may $\to$ partial airway obstruction. Many burn patients have pulmonary pathology 2° smoke inhalation injury. The pathology usually include edema, inflammation, and loss of ciliary activity, but can vary depending on the length and amount of smoke exposure, as well as the composition of the material that burned. Patients with breast cancer may have been treated with chemotherapeutic agents (e.g., methotrexate, cyclophosphamide, bleomycin) that may cause pulmonary fibrosis, interstitial infiltrates, and pleural effusions. **Tests:** Consider CXR, PFT, and pulmonary consult.
Cardiovascular	Exposure of the heart to radiation may produce pathologic changes in the heart and related structures, including accelerated atherosclerotic changes, myocardial fibrosis, pericarditis, and valvular dysfunction. Patients with breast cancer may have been treated with doxorubicin (Adriamycin), which may produce cardiomyopathy (usually seen at total doses > 550 mg/m^2) $\to$ CHF. XRT increases the incidence of clinically significant cardiomyopathy.
Hematologic	Myelosuppression may be present in patients with Hx of chemotherapy. **Tests:** CBC, with differential and Plt count
Laboratory	Other tests as indicated from H&P.
Premedication	Standard premedication (see p. B-2).

INTRAOPERATIVE

Anesthetic technique: GETA. Coordinate iv and/or invasive monitoring sites with the surgical team. Adjunctive regional anesthesia is an option for the appropriate patient who will not be anticoagulated. Some authors propose that the resultant vasodilation causes $\uparrow$blood flow through the flap, but this has not been definitely shown in clinical trials.

Induction	Standard induction (see p. B-2) and intubation. Avoid succinylcholine in burn patients.	
Maintenance	Standard maintenance (see p. B-3). Muscle relaxation usually is required. The patient must be kept warm and well hydrated to minimize peripheral vasoconstriction, which might impair graft perfusion. Surgeon may request intraop anticoagulation, usually in the form of aspirin, dextran, or heparin.	
Emergence	Smooth emergence to avoid disrupting the surgical repair. Patients usually are transported to the ICU for continuous monitoring of flap perfusion.	
Blood and fluid requirements	Moderate blood loss IV: 16 ga × 1 NS/LR @ 4-5 ml/kg/h Warm fluids. Humidify gases.	Keep patient warm, and maintain a positive fluid balance. A Hct of 30-35% will provide adequate O$_2$ transport, while minimizing viscosity. Dextran 40 usually is used to further $\downarrow$ viscosity, thereby $\uparrow$ flap blood flow.
Monitoring	Standard monitors (see p. B-1). UO ± Arterial line	An arterial line may be useful for prolonged procedures where regular ABGs and blood chemistries will be needed.
Positioning	✓ and pad pressure points. ✓ eyes.	These can be very lengthy surgeries, and careful monitoring of pressure points is essential.
Complications	Hypothermia	Maintain normal body temperature with warming blankets, fluid, and airway warmers.
	Decubitus ulcer	Pressure necrosis can occur in as little as 2 h. Carefully pad and repeatedly ✓ pressure points.
	Dextran reaction	Prophylactic use of very low molecular weight dextran (Promit) usually prevents allergic reactions to higher-molecular-weight dextran. Adult dose = 20 ml 1-15 min before dextran infusion.

POSTOPERATIVE

Complications	Arterial thrombosis	May require reexploration.
	Hematoma	May require reexploration.
Pain management	Parenteral opiates (see p. C-2). PCA (see p. C-3).	Pain should be treated promptly to minimize reflex peripheral vasoconstriction and impaired graft perfusion.

References

1. Banic A, Krejei V, Erni D, Petersen-Felix S, Sigurdsson G: Effects of extradural anaesthesia on microcirculatory blood flow in free latissimus dorsi musculocutaneous flaps in pigs. *Plast Reconstr Surg* 1997; 100:945.
2. Buncke HJ, ed. *Microsurgery.* Lea & Febiger, Philadelphia: 1991.
3. Hynynen M, Eklund P, Rosenberg PH: Anaesthesia for patients undergoing prolonged reconstructive and microvascular plastic surgery. *Scand J Plast Surg* 1982; 16:201.
4. Jones NF: Resection and reconstruction of extensive and complex tumors of the head and neck. In *Excision and Reconstruction in Head and Neck Cancer.* Soutar D, Tiwari R, eds. Churchill Livingstone, Edinburgh: 1994, 405.
5. Khouris RK, Cooley BC, Kunselman AR, Landis JR, Yerarnian P, Ingram D, Natarajan N, Benes CO, Wallemark C: A prospective study of microvascular free-flap surgery and outcome. *Plast Reconstr Surg* 1998; 102:711-21.
6. Lineaweaver W: Microsurgery. In *Plastic Surgery.* Ruberg RL, Smith DJ, eds. CV Mosby, St. Louis: 1994, 65.
7. Lineaweaver W, Ching P, Siko P, Yim K, Alpert B, Buncke GM, Buncke H: Transfusion requirements for clinical elective muscle transplantation. In *Trans Third Vienna Muscle Symposium.* Frelinger G, Deutinger M, eds. Blackwell MZV, Vienna: 1992, 378.
8. Scott GR, Rothkopf DM, Walton RL: Efficacy of epidural anaesthesia in free flaps of the lower extremity. *Plast Reconstr Surg* 1993; 91:673.
9. Welch GW: Anesthesia for the patient with thermal injury. *Curr Rev Clin Anesth* 1992; 12:45.

MICROSURGERY—REPLANTATION

SURGICAL CONSIDERATIONS

Yvonne L. Karanas, James Chang, William C. Lineaweaver, and Kenneth C. W. Hui

Description: Patients who require replantation surgery are trauma victims and must be evaluated carefully preop, by both surgeons and anesthesiologists, to ensure that replantation is appropriate and that other injuries are not overlooked. In these cases, time is critical, as the amputated tissue is ischemic and may require immediate revascularization if it is to be salvaged. Coordination between the microsurgeon, anesthesiologist, and trauma team is important to minimize the time between injury and replantation.

As in any microsurgical procedure, it is critical to prevent vasoconstriction in these procedures. These patients may have experienced significant blood loss at the time of the trauma and require iv hydration and/or blood transfusion. The need for hemodynamic support often indicates another injury that may preclude transplantation. The patient may be hypothermic and require active rewarming. Vasoconstrictors and diuretics should be avoided unless absolutely necessary. During the replantation procedure, other tissues (e.g., skin, vein, bone) are required to aid in the reconstruction. These are routinely harvested from the leg, groin, or foot, which will be prepped into the surgical field.

The amputated stump is initially examined using loupe magnification. The arteries, veins, and nerves are dissected and tagged. The surgeon determines if the part is replantable. The amputated stump is prepared by dissecting the recipient arteries, veins, and nerves. The need for a vein graft may be determined at this time. The sequence of replantation varies; however, a general algorithm is:

Bone fixation → Extensor tendon repair → Flexor tendon repair → Arterial anastomosis → Skin closure

The replanted tissue must be monitored on an hourly basis to ensure continued viability. In many hospitals, this is performed in a microsurgical unit, while in others the ICU is used. Patients should be kept adequately hydrated, warm, and pain-free to prevent vasoconstriction and subsequent thrombosis. Vascular thrombosis requires immediate exploration and revision of the vascular anastomosis.

Specific variations of replantation procedures have unique features, as follows.

Replantation of fingers and hands: Generally, two surgeons work simultaneously. One surgeon at the back table explores the amputated parts, tagging significant nerves, vessels, and tendons. A second surgeon debrides the amputation sites and identifies the stumps of reparable structures. The surgeons then proceed with replantation. Generally, bone fixation and tendon repairs are performed first. Vessel and nerve repairs are performed next, using a microscope. The need for vein grafting and anticoagulation is determined intraop. Blood transfusions are rarely needed except when using anticoagulants.

Replantation of extremities: Replantation of arms or legs must be handled very efficiently since irreversible muscle damage occurs within 4 h of ischemia. Generally, the sequence of surgery is similar to finger replantation, with the exception being that a temporary arterial circulation (using a dialysis shunt) is established as soon as possible to minimize ischemia time in an amputated part. Ongoing venous blood loss occurs while skeletal repairs are done, and transfusion is frequently required. Definitive vessel repairs (often requiring vein grafts) and nerve repairs are done under the microscope.

Scalp replantation: Scalp avulsions are caused by entanglement of hair in machinery. These amputations are frequently replantable, sparing the patient a grotesque and unstable deformity. Initial evaluation should include careful assessment of the C-spine, since the patient transiently hangs by the neck until the scalp separates. Initial blood loss can be significant and should be replaced preop. Replantation proceeds by identifying matching vessels at the margin of the defect and the avulsed scalp. The superficial temporal vessels are most commonly repaired, and use of vein grafts should be anticipated. Following the first artery repair, brisk bleeding generally occurs at the scalp margin until vein repairs are completed. This blood loss should be anticipated.

Usual preop diagnosis: Trauma

SUMMARY OF PROCEDURES

	Fingers/Hands	Extremities	Scalp
Position	Supine, injured arm extended	Supine	Supine or side (depending on vessel position)
Incision	Conventional hand exposure	Extension of injury; fasciotomies may be done.	Preauricular
Special instrumentation	Microscope; hand table; tourniquet	Microscope; tourniquet	Microscope; neurosurgical headrest
Unique considerations	Anticoagulation	⇐	RAE or anode tube; table, turned 180°
Antibiotics	Cefazolin 1g iv	⇐	⇐
Surgical time	1st finger: 3-4 h; 2 h/subsequent finger Hand: 4 h	4-8 h	4 h
Closing considerations	Splint applied before emergence.	Cast or splint applied before emergence.	Elevate head as much as possible.
EBL	100-200 ml	2-6 U	2-8 U
Postop care	ICU for monitoring	⇐	⇐
Mortality	None	Rare	None
Morbidity	Replant failure: 5-15%	Failure: 10-20%	Vascular occlusion → reexploration
Pain score	5-6	5-6	3-5

PATIENT POPULATION CHARACTERISTICS

Age range	Childhood-old age	⇐	Young adult
Male:Female	> 10:1	⇐	1:2
Incidence	250/yr/major center	Rare	⇐
Etiology	Trauma	⇐	⇐
Associated conditions	Other injuries	Other injuries, blood loss	C-spine injuries, blood loss

ANESTHETIC CONSIDERATIONS FOR REPLANTATION

PREOPERATIVE

In general, there are two patient populations for replantation procedures: (1) isolated limb and scalp injury patients (common), and (2) multiple trauma victims (rare). Most patients are otherwise healthy and the preop workup is routine.

Gastrointestinal	All of these patients should be considered to have full stomachs and, therefore, are at increased risk for aspiration pneumonitis. In general, they should receive preop medication to reduce stomach volume and acidity (e.g., metoclopramide 10 mg iv and ranitidine 50 mg iv) 30-60 min before induction, time permitting.
Metabolic	~50% of trauma victims are intoxicated. Anesthesia-related implications of acute ethanol intoxication include: ↓ anesthetic requirements, diuresis, vasodilation, and hypothermia.
Neurologic	Assess for possible head or C-spine injury, particularly in the trauma patient presenting with facial or scalp injuries.
Laboratory	As suggested by coexisting disease.
Premedication	Standard premedication (see p. B-2). Full-stomach precautions: Na citrate 0.3 M 30 ml immediately before induction of anesthesia.

INTRAOPERATIVE

Anesthetic technique: GETA, after rapid-sequence induction. These procedures are often lengthy, and regional anesthesia is usually not appropriate as the primary technique but may be considered as an adjunct.

Induction	Rapid-sequence induction (see p. B-5) is mandatory in emergency cases, unless awake intubation is performed. C-spine fracture patients or those with facial injuries may require awake fiber optic intubation (see p. B-6).	
Maintenance	Standard maintenance (see p. B-2) for stable patients.	
Emergence	Difficult airway or full-stomach cases require awake extubation.	
Blood and fluid requirements	Significant blood loss possible IV: 16 ga × 1-2 (extremity/scalp) IV: 18 ga × 1 (digit) NS/LR @ 1.5-3 ml/kg/h + 3 × blood loss Fluid/blood warmers, heating blanket, warmed circuit humidifier	A 16 ga iv catheter in a nonoperated upper extremity should be adequate in hemodynamically stable patients. Keep patient warm and hydrated to maximize perfusion to the replanted site. Avoid vasoconstrictors if possible.
Monitoring	Standard monitors (see p. B-1). ± Arterial line, CVP	Invasive hemodynamic monitoring should be considered in cases where large blood loss is anticipated.
Positioning	✓ and pad pressure points. ✓ eyes.	
Control of blood loss	Tourniquet may be used.	Inflation pressure is typically 100 mmHg greater than systolic pressure. Maximum 'safe' tourniquet time is 1.5-2 h, followed by a 5- (preferably) 15 min reperfusion interval, if further tourniquet time is necessary.
Special considerations	Tourniquet deflation and limb reperfusion	Mild ↓BP is common. In patients with moderate-to-severe lung disease, continue controlled ventilation until after the lactic acid that has accumulated in the ischemic limb is metabolized (3-5 min), since these patients may be unable to increase ventilation adequately to buffer this acid load.
Complications	Hemodynamic instability	Previously unrecognized injuries (e.g., pneumothorax, cardiac tamponade, intracranial bleeding) should be considered as a cause of unexplained intraop hemodynamic instability in all acute-trauma victims.

POSTOPERATIVE

Complications	Reperfusion failure	May require immediate reexploration.
Pain management	PCA (p. C-3)	
Tests	None routinely indicated.	Reimplant perfusion must be monitored.

References

1. Alpert BS, Lineaweaver W, Buncke HJ: Surgical treatment of the avulsed scalp. In *Hair Transplantation,* 3rd edition. Unger WP, ed. Marcel Dekker, New York: 1995, 777.
2. Buncke HJ, Whitney TM, Valauri F, Alpert B: Replantation. In *Microsurgery.* Buncke HJ, ed. Lea & Febiger, Philadelphia: 1991, 594.
3. Carr DB, Kwon J: Anesthesia techniques and their indication for upper limb surgery. In *Surgery of the Hand and Upper Extremity.* Peimer CA, ed. McGraw-Hill, New York: 1996, 119-39.
4. Furnes H, Lineaweaver W, Buncke HJ: Blood loss associated with anticoagulation of patients with replanted digits. *J Hand Surg* 1992; 17A:226.
5. Gayle L, Lineaweaver W, Buncke GM, Oliva A, Alpert BS, Billys J, Buncke HJ: Lower extremity replantation. *Clin Plastic Surg* 1992; 18:437.
6. Goldner RD, Urbaniak JR: Replantation. In *Green's Operative Hand Surgery.* Green DP, Hotchkiss DP, Hotchkiss RN, Pederson WC, eds. Churchill Livingstone, San Francisco: 1999, 1139-58.
7. Khouri RK, Cooley BC, Kunselman AR, Landis JR, Yeramian P, Ingram D, Natarajan N, Benes CO, Wallemark C: A prospective study of microvascular free-flap surgery and outcome. *Plast Reconstr Surg* 1998; 102:7111-21.
8. Livingston KG: Safety of dextran in relation to other colloids—ten years' experience with hapten inhibition. *Infusionsther, Transfusionsmed* 1993; 20:206.
9. Partington M, Lineaweaver W, O'Hara M, Kitzmiller J, Valauri F, Buncke GM, Alpert BS, Buncke HJ: Unrecognized injuries in patients referred for emergency microsurgery. *J Trauma* 1993; 34:238.
10. Raggi RP: Balanced regional anesthesia for hand surgery. *Orthop Clin North Am* 1986; 17:473.
11. Sanders N, Anderson KR: Anesthesia for microsurgery. In *Microsurgery.* Buncke HJ, ed. Lea & Febiger, Philadelphia: 1991, 729.
12. Strauch B, Greenstein B, Goldstein R, Liebling RW: Problems and complications encountered in replantation surgery. *Hand Clin* 1986; 2:389.
13. Tamai S: Twenty years' experience of limb replantation: A review of 293 upper extremity replants. *J Hand Surg* 1982; 6: 549.

BREAST SURGERY—INTRODUCTION

David M. Kahn, Yvonne L. Karanas, Jeffrey Pardun

Patients presenting for plastic surgery of the breast can be grouped into four basic categories along a continuum ranging from amastia/hypomastia to hypertrophy. Plastic surgery procedures are designed to create or make adjustments in the amounts of skin and glandular tissue or to make adjustments in their relationship to each other to create an aesthetic breast. The first type of patient is one who has acquired amastia after undergoing a mastectomy; it is this patient who is featured in this section on functional restoration. In this patient, the goal is to replace the missing tissue, both skin and glandular, with like tissue or an implant. The second type is a person presenting for augmentation mammoplasty (see p. 884). In this situation, the breast is deficient of skin and glandular tissue. The third type is the patient who presents for a reduction mammoplasty (see p. 885). In this situation, there is an excess of glandular tissue and skin. The fourth type is the patient who presents for a mastopexy or breast lift (see p. 887). In this patient, there exists a discrepancy between the amount of glandular tissue present and the volume of the skin envelope, resulting in ptosis.

For all breast procedures, the patient's breasts are marked preop with the patient in either the sitting or standing position. This is a necessity, and its importance cannot be overstated. The appearance of the breasts in the supine position versus the upright position is significantly different due to the effects of gravity.

BREAST RECONSTRUCTION

SURGICAL CONSIDERATIONS

Description: The goal of breast reconstruction is to create an aesthetic breast that is symmetrical with the contralateral breast. Typically, this can be accomplished in three ways: expander/implant reconstruction; latissimus flap reconstruction, ± an implant; and TRAM flap reconstruction, performed using either a pedicled technique or a free-tissue transfer. Each type of reconstruction follows the principle of replacing glandular and cutaneous breast tissue. In patients undergoing mastectomy, reconstruction may be performed immediately after the mastectomy or it may be delayed and performed at a later date.

In **expander/implant reconstruction** (Fig 11.4-2), a tissue expander is placed underneath the pectoralis major muscle and a portion of the serratus anterior muscle, followed by skin closure. Thus, two layers exist above the implant—skin and muscle. The patient returns to the office for expansions, with saline being injected into the implant port. This is continued until the desired size is reached. Then, the patient returns to the OR for the exchange of the expander for a permanent implant that contains either saline or silicone gel as filler material. Except for the psychosocial aspects of patient management, much of the technique and perioperative concerns are similar to those for breast augmentation (see p. 884).

Autologous breast reconstructions: Two types of flaps are used for these procedures—latissimus myocutaneous flap and transverse rectus abdominus muscle (TRAM) flap. The **latissimus dorsi myocutaneous flap** consists of the muscle with overlying skin that is rotated from the back to the anterior chest for the creation of a breast. The flap does not supply sufficient bulk to be used in breast reconstruction unless the contralateral breast is very small. Usually a breast implant is placed between the latissimus and pectoralis muscles, thus increasing the volume of the reconstruction. The patient is placed in the lateral decubitus position for the latissimus flap harvest. The incision is designed to surround the skin paddle. The ellipse of skin is incised, and the dissection then proceeds along the superficial surface of the latissimus muscle towards its lateral, superior, and inferior borders. Dissection is performed underneath the latissimus muscle to separate it from the deep tissues of the back. The muscle is released from its insertions on the posterior superior iliac crest, medial fascial attachments, and surrounding muscle attachments (i.e., serratus anterior, teres major). The flap is tunneled through the axilla, and the back wound is closed (Fig 11.4-3). The patient is then returned to the supine position. The muscle is disinserted from the humerus, if necessary, and brought out onto the anterior chest wall. At this point, the muscle is inset into the mastectomy defect. An implant or tissue expander may be placed under the muscle if necessary for size and symmetry. Often, the patient is placed in the seated or semi-Fowler position for closure. The incisions are closed over a drain and dressings are applied. The skin flap is monitored postop for signs of flap ischemia and congestion, which may necessitate a return to the OR.

The **TRAM flap** procedure replaces the breast with an ellipse of abdominal skin and subcutaneous tissue based on the rectus abdominus muscle (Fig 11.4-4). In selecting patients for a TRAM flap reconstruction, the patient must have adequate lower abdominal tissue to make a breast; however, obese patients, smokers, diabetics, and those with a Hx of prior abdominal surgery may have a higher incidence of complications and flap loss. The benefit of this procedure is that it creates a natural appearing breast from the patient's own tissue without an implant. As a bonus, the abdominal donor site is closed

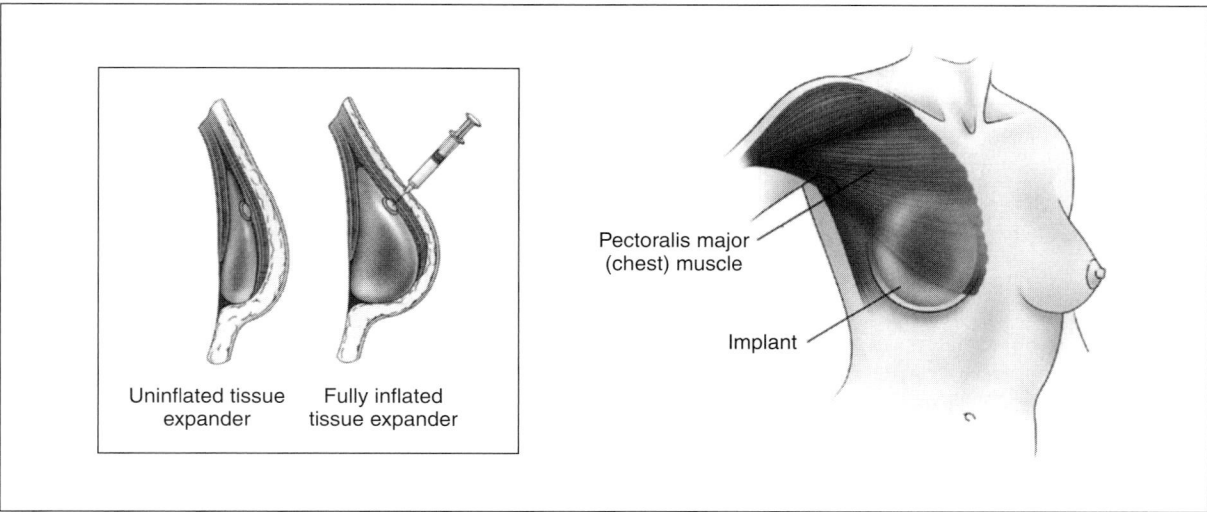

Figure 11.4-2. Expander–implant reconstruction. (Reproduced with permission from Greenfield LJ, et al, eds: *Surgery: Scientific Principles and Practices,* 3rd edition. Lippincott Williams & Wilkins, 2001.)

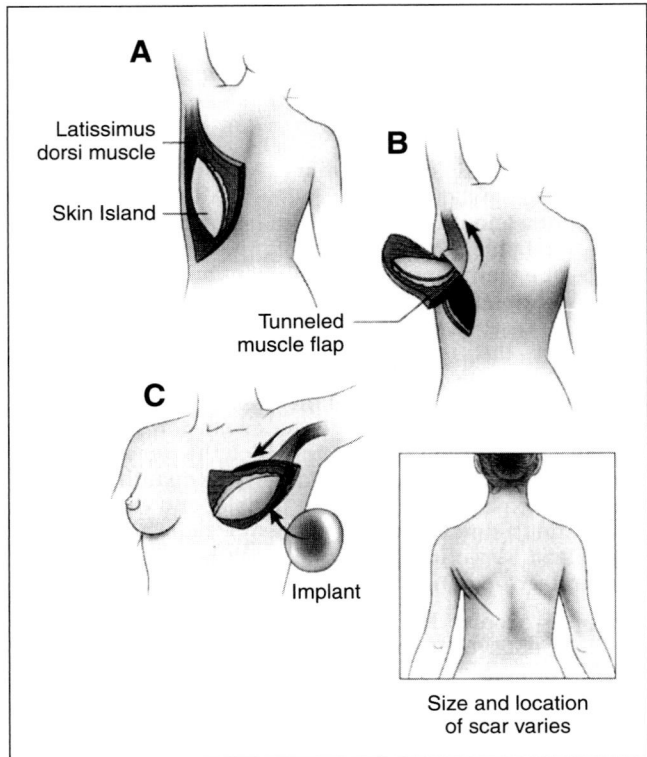

Figure 11.4-3. (A–C) Latissimus dorsi flap reconstruction. (Reproduced with permission from Greenfield LJ, et al, eds: *Surgery: Scientific Principles and Practices*, 3rd edition. Lippincott Williams & Wilkins, 2001.)

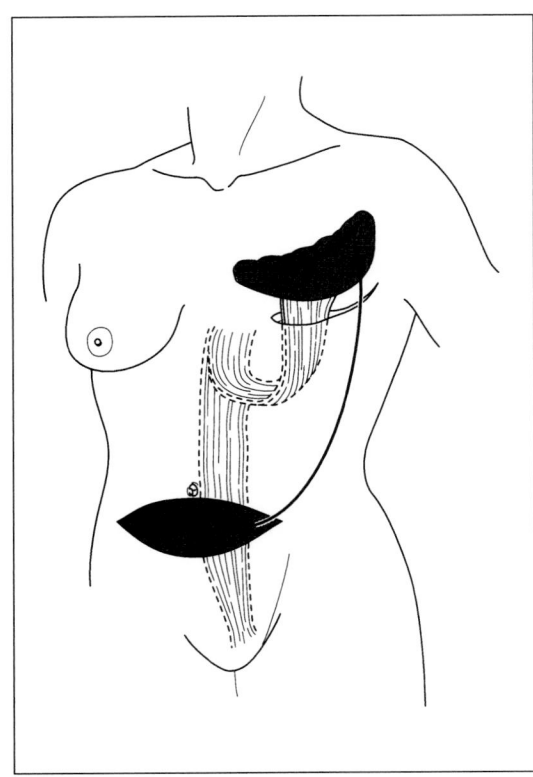

Figure 11.4.4. Breast reconstruction using free TRAM flap. (Reproduced with permission from Greenfield, LJ, et al, eds: *Surgery: Scientific Principles and Practice*, 2nd edition. Lippincott-Raven, 1997.)

as though the patient had undergone abdominoplasty ('tummy tuck'). The myocutaneous perforators that arise from the superior epigastric and inferior epigastric arteries provide blood supply to the flap. This flap can be harvested in either a pedicled fashion, based on the superior epigastric artery, or as a free flap, based on the inferior epigastric artery. The inset of the flap and closure of the donor site are the same in both cases. The basic difference between the two methods of flap transfer is that, in the free TRAM procedure, the flap is removed from the abdomen, brought into the mastectomy wound, and the operating microscope is used to suture the vascular pedicle of the flap to the recipient vessels, either the thoracodorsal or internal mammary arteries. In the case of the pedicled TRAM flap, the flap is passed through a tunnel, created under the skin, maintaining the blood supply via the superior epigastric artery. The flap is brought out into the mastectomy wound where it is sutured into position.

Pedicled TRAM flap: The patient is marked preop in the upright position. The midline and inframammary folds are marked, as is the abdominal ellipse. The arms are placed at 90° abduction. The breasts and abdomen are prepped and draped. A general surgeon performs the mastectomy and, if possible, the TRAM flap harvest is started at the same time. Incising the skin along the superior marking of the abdominal ellipse begins the harvest of the flap. The upper abdominal skin and subcutaneous fat are elevated off the abdominal wall fascia up to the level of the costochondral cartilage, as in an abdominoplasty. The table is then flexed, and the upper skin and subcutaneous tissue is brought to overlap the TRAM flap to ensure that the location of the marked incision at the lower border of the flap will allow for abdominal closure. The patient is returned to the supine position. The skin and subcutaneous tissue of the flap are raised from a lateral to medial direction off the abdominal wall fascia until the lateral border of the rectus muscle is identified. Care is taken to preserve the myocutaneous perforators supplying the flap. The anterior rectus sheath is incised and the rectus muscle is elevated away from the posterior rectus sheath. The inferior epigastric vascular pedicle is identified and divided, preserving as much length as possible. The portion of the rectus muscle below the flap is transected so that the muscle, along with the overlying ellipse of skin and subcutaneous tissue can be rotated into the mastectomy site. A tunnel is created under the skin to connect the abdominal wound and mastectomy site. The flap is passed through this tunnel and rotated into position on the chest wall (Fig 11.4-5).

In flap reconstructions, the harvested tissue receives its blood supply through a single artery and vein. It is important in these cases to maintain a stable BP that will allow for continued perfusion of the flap tissue. Vasopressors are to be avoided,

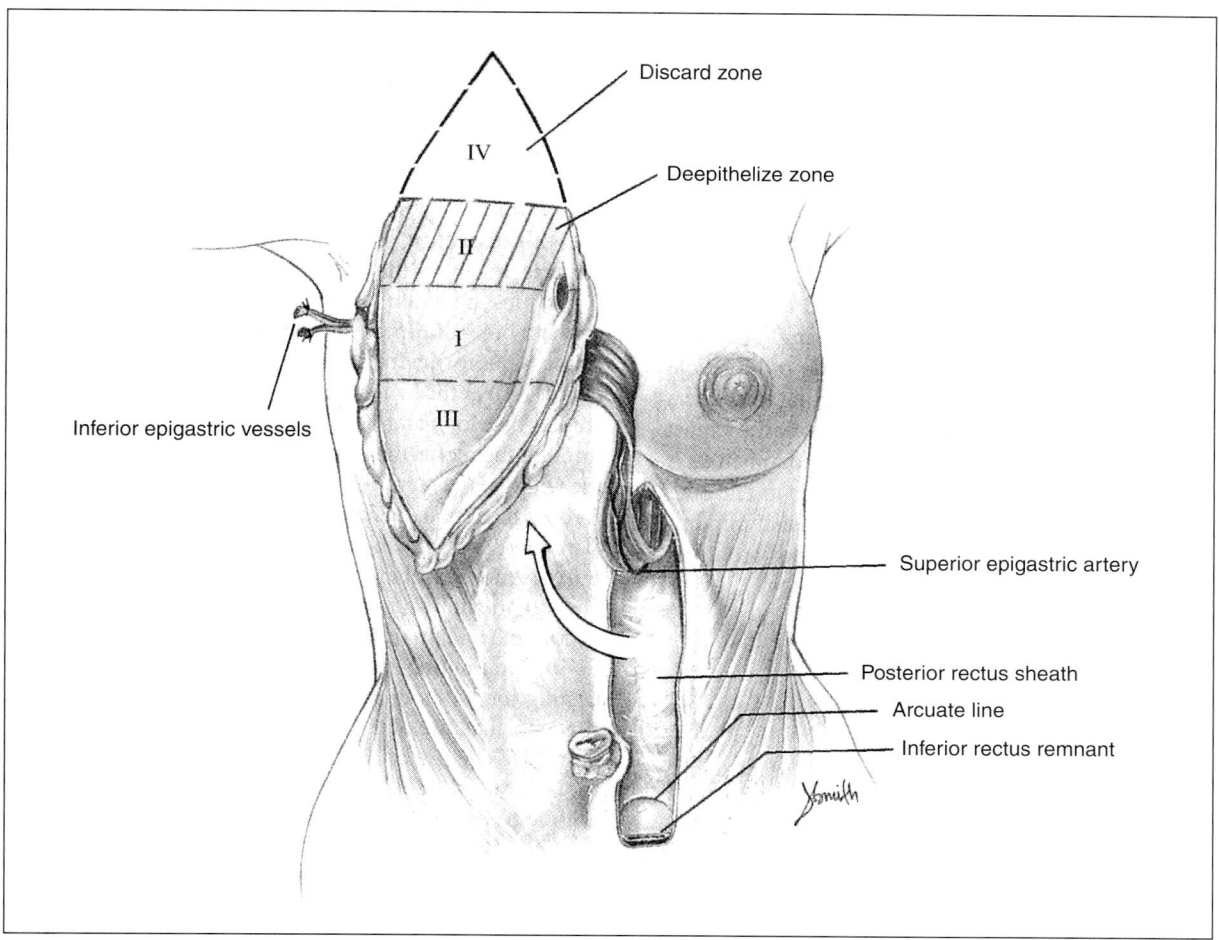

Figure 11.4-5. TRAM flap reconstruction of the breast. A contralateral pedicled TRAM flap has been elevated and will be tunneled under the skin to be inset at the mastectomy site. The zone of tissue furthest from the blood supply is discarded. A portion of the TRAM flap will be deepithelialized and placed under the mastectomy skin flaps. (Reproduced with permission from Spear SL: *Surgery of the Breast: Principles and Art.* Lippincott-Raven, 1998.

as they will constrict the artery and thus restrict the inflow into the flap. It is preferred, if possible, to maintain a stable BP with volume replacement. Once the flap is in place at the mastectomy site, the table is again flexed as much as 45-60° for closure. Drains are placed within both the chest and abdominal wound beds. The flap is trimmed and sutured into position to create symmetry with the contralateral breast. The abdomen is closed in a fashion similar to an abdominoplasty. Many surgeons prefer that N_2O (which can distend the abdomen) be avoided during the abdominal closure. The surgeon will evaluate the flap to monitor for signs of ischemia and congestion. This is done both by clinical evaluation (color, temperature, and turgor) and by Doppler. If inflow or outflow is inadequate for flap survival, blood flow may be supplemented by performing a microvascular anastomosis between the inferior epigastric pedicle and the thoracodorsal vessels. In some cases, the surgeon may choose to convert the pedicled flap to a free flap.

Usual preop diagnosis: Carcinoma of the breast; radiation therapy; cardiovascular surgery; Poland syndrome

SUMMARY OF PROCEDURES

	Tissue Expander/Implant	Latissimus Dorsi Flap	TRAM Flap
Position	Supine	Lateral decubitus → supine	Supine
Incision	Breast	Posterior (supine); lateral (thorax)	Abdominal
Unique considerations	May have to place patient in sitting position during procedure; SCDs; Foley catheter if case > 3-4 h.	⇐	⇐ + Avoid use of N_2O.

	Tissue Expander/Implant	Latissimus Dorsi Flap	TRAM Flap
Surgical time	1-2 h	4 h (+ mastectomy time)	6-8 h (free TRAM) 4 h (pedicled TRAM) (not including mastectomy time)
Closing considerations	Extensive dressing required	⇐	⇐ + Flex table for abdominal closure.
EBL	Minimal-100 ml	200-300 ml	200-400 ml
Postop care	PACU → room	⇐	⇐ (free TRAM flap → ICU)
Mortality	Rare	⇐	⇐
Morbidity	Capsular contraction: ± 30%	–	–
	Decreased sensation: 15%	⇐	⇐
	Hematoma: 2.2%	⇐	⇐
	Fat/skin necrosis: 1.7-1.9%	⇐	⇐
	Nipple areola necrosis: 1.4%	–	–
		Flap loss: Rare	⇐
			Abdominal hernia: Infrequent
Pain score	5	5	5

PATIENT POPULATION CHARACTERISTICS

Age range	30-70 yr
Male:Female	Mostly female
Incidence	Breast reconstruction is performed in 9% of female population
Etiology	Cancer; trauma; idiopathic; radiation or postcardiovascular surgery
Associated conditions	Breast cancer; cardiovascular disease; S/P chemotherapy; pulmonary disease

ANESTHETIC CONSIDERATIONS

See Anesthetic Considerations for Breast and Chest-wall Reconstruction, p. 921.

Reference

1. Abeloff MD, et al: Breast. In *Clinical Oncology.* Churchill Livingstone, New York: 1995.
2. American Society of Plastic Surgeons' Website: www.plasticsurgery.org.
3. Desidero DP, Kross RA, Bedford RF: Evaluation of the patient with oncologic disease. In *Principles and Practice of Anesthesiology*, 2nd edition. Longnecker DE, Tinker JH, Morgan GE Jr, eds. Mosby-Year Book, St. Louis: 1998, 379-96.
4. Spear SL, ed: Breast reconstruction. In *Surgery of the breast: Principles and art.* Lippincott-Raven, Philadelphia: 1998, 335-672.
5. Spear SL: Primary implant reconstruction. In *Surgery of the Breast: Principles and Art.* Lippincott-Raven, Philadelphia: 1998, 347-56.
6. Vasconez HC, Holley DT: Use of the TRAM and latissimus dorsi flaps in autogenous breast reconstruction. *Clin Plast Surg* 1995; 22(1):153-66.

CHEST-WALL RECONSTRUCTION

SURGICAL CONSIDERATIONS

Yvonne L. Karanas

Description: Chest-wall reconstruction is most commonly performed for infections, sternal dehiscence, tumor extirpation, and radiation injuries. Complications after median sternotomy make up a large number of these cases. The patients often have comorbidities and are at high risk for anesthetic and surgical complications. The goals of reconstruction are to provide a stable chest-wall for respiration, to eradicate infection, and to obtain a healed wound.

Sternal wound infections and dehiscences: Wound complications after median sternotomy include dehiscence of the sternum and mediastinitis. In these cases, radical debridement of all devitalized tissue is the cornerstone to a successful outcome. The initial debridement is, therefore, performed in conjunction with the cardiovascular surgeons. During this debridement, blood loss may be extensive, requiring transfusion. The resulting dead space around the heart and great vessels is obliterated, most commonly with **pectoralis major or rectus abdominis muscle (TRAM) flaps.** For patients who have failed the initial reconstruction or are not candidates for these flaps, a **latissimus dorsi muscle flap** may be used. In spite of radical excision of the sternum, the respiratory function of these patients remains adequate and no bony stabilization is required.

Tumor extirpation and radiation injury: Tumor resection or removal of osteoradionecrosis of the chest wall often involves the full-thickness removal of skin, muscle, and underlying rib cage. The rib cage may be reconstructed with prosthetic mesh or bone grafts. These structures are then covered with muscle flaps. The pectoralis major, rectus abdominis, and latissimus dorsi muscles are the muscle flaps most commonly used. After surgery, the patient's ventilatory capacity may be diminished by the rib resection, and this should be anticipated preop.

Usual preop diagnosis: Chest-wall infections; tumor; sternal dehiscence; radiation injuries

SUMMARY OF PROCEDURES

	Pectoralis Flap	**Latissimus Flap**	**Rectus (TRAM) Flap**
Position	Supine	Lateral decubitus → supine	Supine; table flexed
Incision	Chest	Posterolateral thorax	Abdominal
Antibiotics	Cefazolin 1 g	⇐	⇐
Surgical time	3 h	⇐	4-6 h
Closing considerations	✓ flap perfusion.	⇐	⇐
EBL	200-400 ml	⇐	300-500 ml
Postop care	PACU → room	⇐	⇐
Mortality	Rare	⇐	⇐
Morbidity	Thrombosis/flap failure	⇐	⇐
	Hematoma	⇐	⇐
	Fat/skin necrosis	⇐	⇐
			Abdominal hernia: Infrequent
Pain score	4-5	4-5	4-5

PATIENT POPULATION CHARACTERISTICS

Age range	30-80 yr
Male:Female	1:1
Incidence	Uncommon
Etiology	Cancer; trauma; radiation; postcardiovascular surgery
Associated conditions	Breast cancer; cardiovascular disease; S/P chemotherapy; pulmonary disease; mediastinitis

ANESTHETIC CONSIDERATIONS FOR BREAST AND CHEST-WALL RECONSTRUCTION

PREOPERATIVE

These surgeries are performed most commonly for reconstruction following cancer surgery, such as radical neck dissection and mastectomy (see Anesthetic Considerations for the primary procedure), as well as complications after median sternotomy. The following considerations focus on patients undergoing reconstruction postchemotherapy.

Respiratory   Pulmonary fibrosis may complicate chemotherapy. Bleomycin (> 200 mg/m^2) carries the greatest risk of pulmonary toxicity (10%), but alkylating agents (e.g., cyclophosphamide and melphalan) may cause a degree of pulmonary toxicity as well. Avoid $FiO_2 > 30\%$ in bleomycin patients (to prevent progressive pulmonary fibrosis and edema). Patients presenting with complications from a prior sternotomy may have ↓respiratory function/reserve and will require further work-up.
  Tests: CXR; ABG and PFTs as indicated from H&P.

Cardiovascular   Cardiomyopathy and CHF may result from chemotherapy, especially doxorubicin (Adriamycin) > 550 mg/m^2. Previous XRT increases risk of clinically significant cardiomyopathy. Patients with

Cardiovascular, cont.	median sternotomy-related complications who have undergone prior cardiac surgery will require careful evaluation of their current cardiovascular status. **Tests:** ECG; ECHO, if indicated from H&P.
Neurological	Note any previous damage to long thoracic nerves, as evidenced by winged scapula deformity.
Musculoskeletal	It is traditional to avoid iv and BP cuff on mastectomy side.
Hematologic	Myelosuppression/toxicity from chemotherapeutic agents may be present. **Tests:** CBC; Plt count; coag profile; Hb/Hct
Renal/Hepatic	Methotrexate can produce renal and hepatic dysfunction. Elevated alkaline phosphatase may suggest metastatic bone invasion. **Tests:** Electrolytes; BUN; Cr; LFTs
Gastrointestinal	Tamoxifen, used in hormonal chemotherapy, can cause preop N/V and dehydration.
Laboratory	Other tests as indicated from H&P, prior chemotherapy.
Premedication	Midazolam 1-2 mg iv immediately preop, or valium 5-10 mg po 1 h preop

INTRAOPERATIVE

Anesthetic technique: GETA

Induction	Standard induction (see p. B-2) and intubation. Avoid iv and NIBP monitoring on mastectomy side.
Maintenance	Standard maintenance (see p. B-3). Muscle relaxation is usually appropriate. These patients should be kept warm and well hydrated to minimize peripheral vasoconstriction, which might impair graft perfusion.
Emergence	During some of the procedure and for application of dressing, patient may be moved to sitting position, with consequent coughing, bucking, etc. (Rx: deeper anesthesia, e.g., propofol 0.5 mg/kg or lidocaine 1 mg/kg.) Watch BP carefully and treat orthostatic hypotension if it occurs, usually with a fluid bolus if the patient is not fluid-sensitive (e.g., Hx of CHF or renal failure).
Blood and fluid requirements	IV: 16 ga × 1 NS/LR @ 4-6 ml/kg/h Warm fluids. Humidify gases.	Extensive blood loss may occur with debridement of sternum in cases of infection or dehiscence. Keep patient warm and maintain a positive fluid balance. Hypothermia may impair flap perfusion.
Monitoring	Standard monitors (see p. B-1). UO	Use invasive monitoring in cardiovascular-challenged patients or in cases with significant expected blood loss, where regular ABGs and blood chemistries will be useful.
Positioning	✓ and pad pressure points. ✓ eyes.	
Complications	Pneumothorax	Pneumothorax should be considered with any ↑lung inflation pressure, ↓O_2 sat or ↓BP.
	Decubitus ulcer	Pressure necrosis can occur in as little as 2 h. Carefully pad and repeatedly ✓ pressure points.
	Dextran reaction	Prophylactic use of very low molecular weight dextran (Promit) usually prevents allergic reactions to higher molecular weight dextrans. Adult dose = 20 ml (pediatric dose = 0.3 ml/kg) iv 1-2 min (maximum 15 min) before dextran infusion.

POSTOPERATIVE

Complications	Pneumothorax ↓ Flap perfusion	
Pain management	Parenteral opiates (see p. C-2). PCA (see p. C-3).	Pain should be treated promptly to minimize reflex peripheral vasoconstriction and impaired graft perfusion.

References:

1. American Society of Plastic Surgeons' website: www.plasticsurgery.org.
2. Roth DA: Thoracic and abdominal wall reconstruction. In *Grabb and Smith's Plastic Surgery,* 5th edition. Aston SJ, Beasley RW, Thorne CHM, eds. Lippincott-Raven, Philadelphia: 1997, 1023-30.

PRESSURE-SORE RECONSTRUCTION

SURGICAL CONSIDERATIONS

Description: Pressure sores occur when constant pressure is placed on an area of the body. They tend to occur in debilitated, bedridden, paralyzed, and wheelchair-bound patients. Multiple factors—including altered sensory perception, poor nutrition, incontinence, moisture, and shear forces—also may contribute to the formation of the pressure sores. The most common locations are the sacrum, ischium, and greater trochanter regions, as well as the heel and scalp.

The management of pressure sores is multidisciplinary and involves more than just debridement and wound closure. Patient compliance is the most important factor of wound management, as recurrence rates after closure are high. All components that contributed to the formation of the ulcer must be addressed before wound closure. This is best done in a team setting, with the goal of preventing further sores. In this effort, nutrition must be optimized; infection, muscle spasm, and contractures controlled; pressure relief measures instituted; and the psychological issues addressed. Once these are in place, wound reconstruction may begin.

Reconstruction is based on adequate debridement, elimination of dead space and pressure points, and closure of the wound with healthy, durable tissue. Multiple flap designs have been described for the coverage of pressure sores, depending on their location (Fig 11.4-6). An important point in the design of a flap is the consideration for future reconstructions because of the high incidence of recurrent wounds. The choice of flap also needs to take into consideration the donor site morbidity. Skin-only flaps, fasciocutaneous flaps, and musculocutaneous flaps are commonly used.

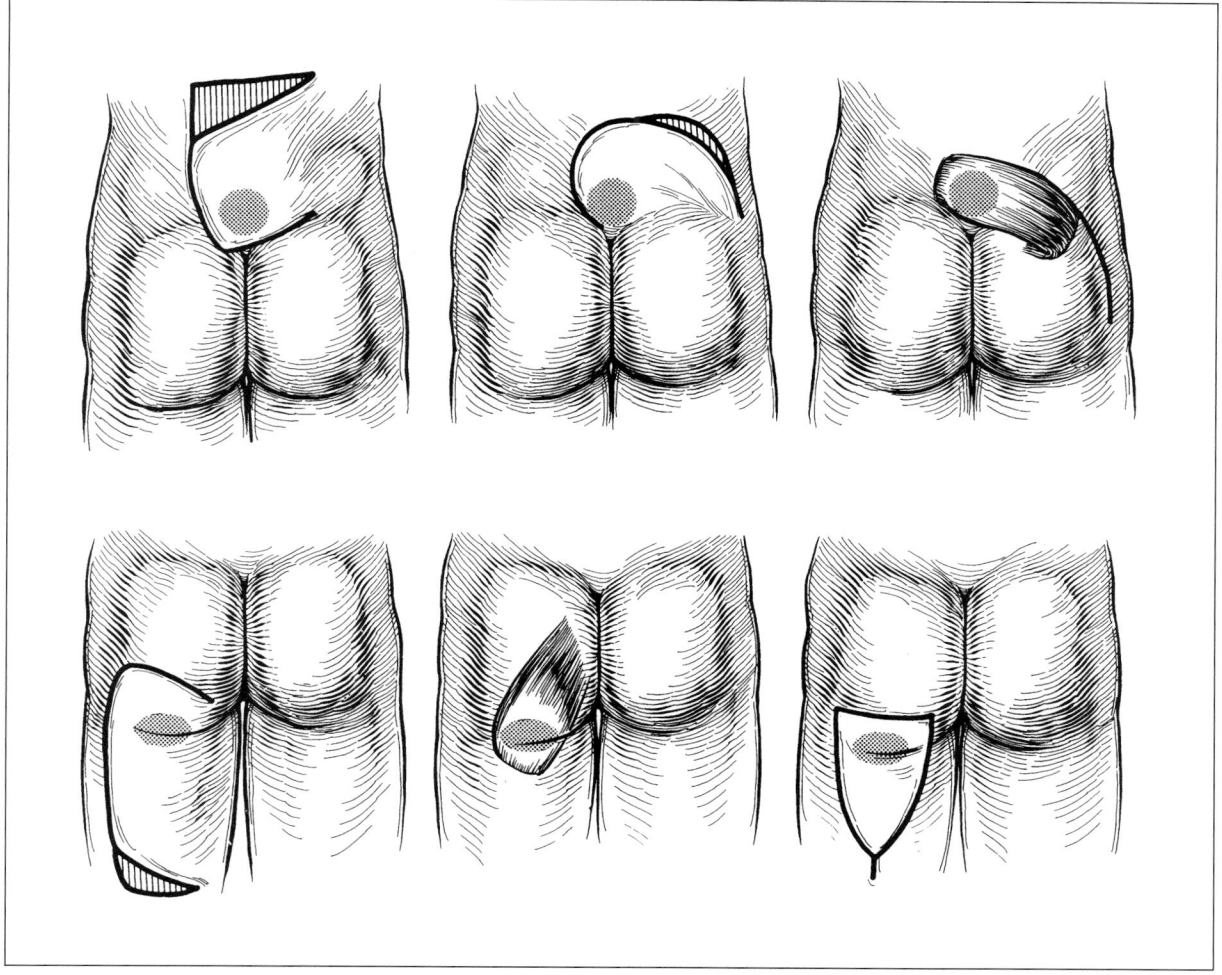

Figure 11.4-6. Commonly used flap designs for coverage of sacral and ischial pressure sores. (Reproduced with permission from Aston SJ, Beasley RW, Thorne CHM: *Grabb and Smith's Plastic Surgery*, 5th edition. Lippincott-Raven, 1997.)

The patient is placed in the prone position and may be jackknifed to facilitate exposure of the wound. Debridement of the wound is performed; and the bursa and underlying bony prominences may be removed. Hemostasis is obtained and the wound is irrigated with pulsed lavage. The flap to be used is designed over the vascular pedicle. The donor site for sacral, gluteal, and greater trochanteric wounds are typically the tissues of the buttocks and posterior thigh. The skin is incised and the flap is raised to include the appropriate layers of tissue, depending on whether a skin, fasciocutaneous, or musculocutaneous flap is to be used. The flap is then rotated into position in the wound. A portion of the flap may be deepithelialized and placed into the wound to eliminate dead space. Drains are placed into the wound and the flap is sutured into its new location. The donor site defect that occurs after rotation of the flap may be closed directly or may require a skin graft. Once the operation is complete, the patient is transferred to a pressure-relief bed (e.g., Clinitron or air-fluidized bed) and extubated.

Usual preop diagnosis: Pressure sores

SUMMARY OF PROCEDURE

Position	Prone or lateral decubitus
Incision	Gluteal or posterior thigh
Unique considerations	Foley catheter; SCDs
Antibiotics	Cefazolin 1 g iv. Some surgeons may prefer broader polymicrobial coverage.
Surgical time	3 h
Closing considerations	None
EBL	200-300 ml
Postop care	Strict bed rest on a pressure-relief bed for up to 3 wk. Care must be taken to ensure that the patient is turned every 2 h so that excessive pressure is not transferred to a new location. Antibiotics and the control of urine and stool are important to prevent soiling of the suture lines.
Mortality	0-1%
Morbidity	Infection: 2-3%
	Dehiscence: 1%
	DVT: 1%
	Recurrence
Pain score	4-6 (depends on spinal cord status)

PATIENT POPULATION CHARACTERISTICS

Age range	20-70 yr
Male:Female	Predominantly male
Etiology	Immobility; unrelieved pressure; altered sensation
Associated conditions	Paraplegia; debilitation; quadriplegia

ANESTHETIC CONSIDERATIONS

PREOPERATIVE

Typically, these surgeries are carried out on nonambulatory patients, with the spinal cord injury patient comprising a large subset. Anesthesia for plegic patients may well present several challenges, as discussed below.

Respiratory	Plegic patients may have intercostal muscle weakness → atelectasis and ↓clearance of secretions → recurrent URIs and V/Q mismatching → hypoxemia. **Tests:** PFT; ABG; others as indicated from H&P.
Cardiovascular	Autonomic hyperreflexia (AH) may present as acute episodes of uninhibited hyperactivity in the patient with an injury level of T10-T7 or above. The main clinical signs are paroxysmal HTN and bradycardia, in response to stimulation below the lesion. Severe HTN can result in pulmonary edema, myocardial ischemia and cerebral hemorrhage. Identify triggering stimuli (e.g., bowel or bladder distension, cutaneous stimulation). T4 or higher lesions may → ↓BP on induction of GA or regional anesthesia, initiation of IPPV, or postural changes. **Tests:** ECG; others as indicated from H&P.

Neurological	✓ level of cord injury. AH in patient with spinal cord injury (see Cardiovascular, above) may manifest as headaches, sweating, facial flushing or syncope. Hyperreflexia below injury level.
Musculoskeletal	Immobility → skeletal muscle atrophy, osteoporosis, and decubitus ulcer formation.
Gastrointestinal	Spinal cord injury → ↓GI function → constipation/full stomach.
Renal	Chronic spinal cord injury → recurrent UTIs and calculi → renal failure. Foley catheter placement may → AH. **Tests:** UA; BUN; Cr; others as indicated from H&P.
Laboratory	Immobility → ↑Ca⁺⁺ → dysrhythmia and nausea. **Tests:** Others as indicated from H&P.
Premedication	Standard premedication (see p. B-2) is usually appropriate. Patients with limited respiratory reserve should receive minimal sedation. Nifedipine (10 mg sublingually 5 min or po 20 min before induction) may be used to blunt AH.

INTRAOPERATIVE

Anesthetic technique: GETA. If flap donor and recipient sites are confined to the lower half of the body, regional anesthesia may be considered for short procedures. Spinal or epidural anesthesia will minimize AH; however, anesthetic level may be difficult to assess and regional anesthesia may not be tolerated for prolonged surgery. Lighter levels of GA will not prevent AH.

Induction	Standard induction (see p. B-2) and intubation. Although the risk of ↑K^+ 2° succinylcholine is reportedly decreased 6 mo after injury, NMRs are still preferred. AH may occur with Foley catheter placement.	
Maintenance	Standard maintenance (see p. B-3). Muscle relaxation is usually appropriate and may be necessary to reduce muscle spasticity. Avoid drugs that are primarily renally excreted in patients with CRI. Direct arterial vasodilators and alpha-adrenergic blocking agents should be readily available. Plegic patients are prone to hypothermia. These patients should be kept warm and well hydrated to minimize peripheral vasoconstriction, which might impair graft perfusion.	
Emergence	AH 2° distended bladder or rectum may occur on emergence from anesthesia.	
Blood and fluid requirements	IV: 16 ga × 1 NS/LR @ 4-6 ml/kg/h Warm fluids. Humidify gases.	Keep patient warm and maintain a positive fluid balance. Hypothermia may impair flap perfusion. Initial debridement of ulcer may be extensive and significant blood loss can occur. T&C as appropriate.
Monitoring	Standard monitors (see p. B-1). UO ± Arterial line	 An arterial line may be useful in patients susceptible to AH and for prolonged procedures where regular ABGs and blood chemistries will be useful.
Positioning	✓ and pad pressure points. ✓ eyes.	Many of these patients may be osteoporotic, so great care should be used in moving and positioning.
Complications	Hypothermia AH Decubitus ulcer	Patients with spinal cord injury often have impaired thermoregulation. Maintain normal body temperature with warming blankets, fluid, and airway warmers. AH should be promptly controlled with SNP bolus (5-50 μg) and infusion, while anesthesia is deepened. A continuous trimethaphan infusion (0.5-4 mg/min) is another option. Pressure necrosis can occur in as little as 2 h. Carefully pad and repeatedly ✓ pressure points.

POSTOPERATIVE

Complications	Respiratory insufficiency	Quadriplegic patients may have ↓VC and ↓ERV and be uniquely susceptible to residual respiratory depressant effects.

Complications, cont.	AH	AH may occur 2° distended bladder or rectum. Rx: phentolamine 1 mg iv q 1 min and/or SNP bolus/infusion; removal of stimulus.
Pain management	Parenteral opiates (see **C-2**). PCA (see **C-3**).	Pain should be treated promptly to minimize reflex peripheral vasoconstriction and impaired graft perfusion.

References:

1. Colen SR: Pressure Sores. In *Plastic Surgery.* McCarthy JG, ed. WB Saunders, Philadelphia: 1990, 3797-3838.
2. Niazi ZB, Salzberg CA: Surgical management of pressure ulcers. *Ostomy Wound Manage* 1997; 43(3):44-52.

Surgeon

Kenneth K.Yim, MD, FACS

11.5 BURN SURGERY

Anesthesiologist

Melissa T. Berhow, MD, PhD

FREE SKIN GRAFT FOR BURN WOUND
(WITH TANGENTIAL EXCISION, EXCISION TO FASCIA, OR DEBRIDEMENT)

SURGICAL CONSIDERATIONS

Description: Until the mid 1970s, management of burn wounds involved daily debridement, hydrotherapy, and spontaneous eschar separation, with subsequent skin grafts applied to the granulated tissue. Operative management has become much more aggressive with the description of **tangential excision** by **Janzekovic**.[5] There are two surgical approaches to burn wounds—tangential excision and fascial excision.

Tangential excision (TE) is the more frequently performed procedure. The concept of TE is extremely simple, but requires considerable experience and teamwork. Thin slices of burn eschar (burned, necrotic tissue), are shaved sequentially with manual or power dermatomes until a healthy wound bed is developed. Assessment of the wound bed is done with visualization of bleeding and/or the clinical appearance of the excised bed. Blood loss is generally diffuse and can be massive; therefore, communication between anesthesiologist and surgeon is essential. In large excision, PRBCs should be available in the OR before excision so that the anesthesiologist does not get behind in blood and fluid replacement.

Diffuse bleeding, especially dermal, is controlled by laparotomy pads soaked with warm 1:100,000 epinephrine solution. These pads are replaced every 3-5 min and, after ~10 min, are removed one at a time, with persistent bleeding points controlled by electrocautery. Although very high plasma epinephrine levels have been reported after major burn excision, systemic manifestations are very rare in acute burn patients[3] (probably 2° high-level endogenous catecholamine secretion).

TE in the extremities usually is accomplished with a pneumatic tourniquet to minimize blood loss. In some centers, subcutaneous injection of a diluted (1:1,000,000) epinephrine solution under the burn wound also is used to minimize blood loss; however, the resulting vasoconstriction makes the end-point of excision—i.e., bleeding—difficult to ascertain.

Fascial excision involves removing the burn eschar and all underlying fat en bloc to the level of muscle fascia, or beyond. Fascial excision can be performed more rapidly and with less blood loss than TE. Its disadvantages, however, are the marked cosmetic deformities and functional limitations that occur because of the loss of all soft tissue overlying the musculature. Because of its disadvantages, fascial excision is reserved for fourth-degree burns or for patients with very extensive, life-threatening, full-thickness (third-degree) burns.

In patients with serious burns (> 40% total body surface area [TBSA]), excision usually commences on postop day 2-5, after completion of fluid resuscitation, and is performed every 2-3 d, as the patient's condition permits. If eschar excision can be completed before secondary sepsis supervenes, management of the patient is easier and the complications and morbidity are lessened considerably.

The endpoints for surgical excision in large burns are: (1) operative time of 2-3 h; (2) core temperature of 35°C; or (3) blood loss of 10 U of PRBC. The violation of any of these parameters invites coagulopathy and increasing problems with hemostasis and VS stability. Adverse effects occurring after 3-4 h of operative time are usually the result of massive transfusion or hypothermia.

Due to loss of skin integrity and large exposed surfaces, these patients lose heat rapidly. Fluids, gases, and the OR should be warm, although there is no demonstrable benefit to warming the OR past the point of isothermic neutrality (~82°F [28°C]).[8] Many surgeons, however, will maintain the room at ~100°F (38°C). All areas not in the operative field should be covered, and a warming blanket (Bair Hugger) is used frequently.

Coverage: After excision of wounds and attainment of hemostasis, wounds are covered, using either an autograft or temporary coverage with an allograft, xenograft, or synthetic/biologic dressing. An autograft is used for coverage when the wound bed is deemed suitable, a donor site is available, and the patient is stable. A split-thickness skin graft (STSG) often is used for coverage of a burn wound. Since a STSG is harvested at the dermal level, bleeding also is controlled with topical epinephrine-soaked laparotomy pads before application of dressings. Depending on the location of donor sites, many surgeons use subcutaneous infiltration of diluted (1:1,000,000) epinephrine in saline solution to smooth out irregularities (e.g., underlying ribs) or to create a flat surface (e.g., scalp) to physically improve the ease of taking skin grafts. A substantial volume of saline may be infiltrated, and this should be added into the total fluids administered to the patient.

Intraop position change may be necessary between the burn excision and the STSG harvest. For example, donor skin may be harvested from the back for application to the chest or abdomen.

The STSG is held temporarily in place with staples or sutures. Uncontrolled patient movement may dislodge the graft. To protect against this eventuality, grafts are secured with circumferential dressings and splints. This procedure may be time-consuming, and any uncontrolled patient movement should be avoided.

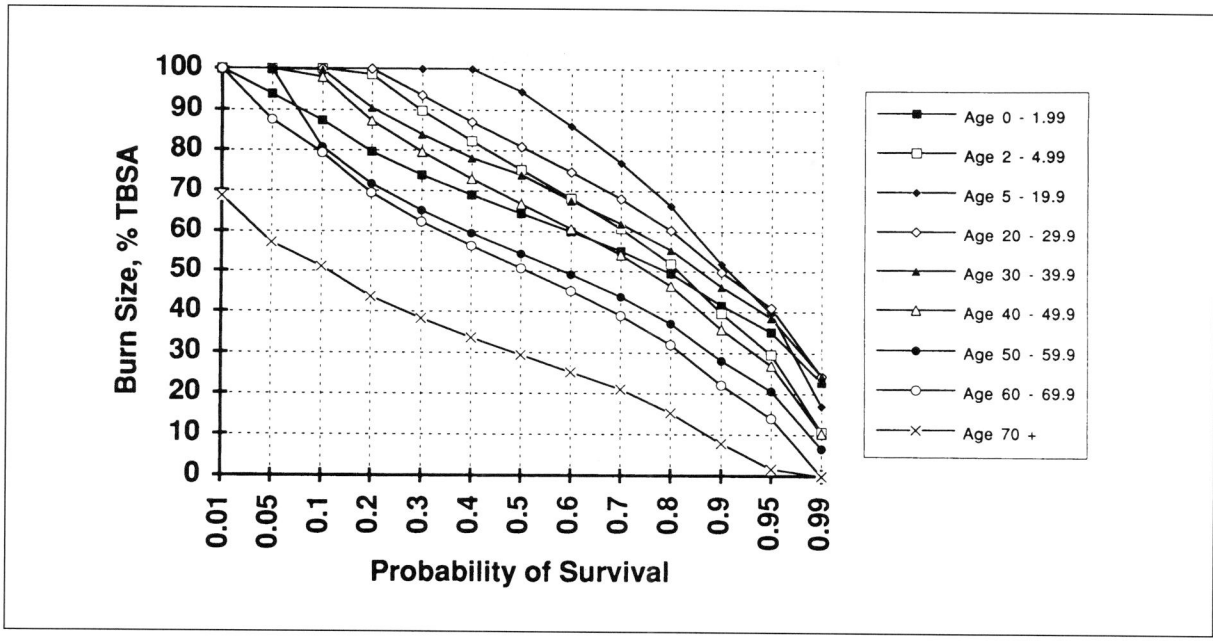

Figure 11.5-1. Probit Survival Curves for 6,417 patients by age groups. (Both Probit Survival figures reproduced with permission from Saffle JR, Davis B, Williams P, et al: Recent outcomes in the treatment of burn injury in the United States: A report from the American Burn Association Patient Registry. *J Burn Care Rehab* 1995; 16:219-32.)

It has become apparent that early eschar excision is advantageous even if wounds are so extensive they cannot be covered with autografts. In this situation, temporary coverage of the excised wound is accomplished with the application of an allograft, porcine xenograft, or synthetic/biologic dressing. The wound is maintained in this way, with further debridement and biologic dressing changes as necessary, until autograft becomes available.

Usual preop diagnosis: Thermal, electrical, or chemical burn

SUMMARY OF PROCEDURES

	TE	Fascial Excision
Position	Supine, prone, or lateral	⇐
Incision	Anywhere eschar is to be excised.	⇐
Special instrumentation	Dermatomes, as determined by the surgeon—manual or powered.	–
Temperature considerations	Keep room T at ~82°F (28°C).	⇐
Unique considerations	Possible subcutaneous infiltration of diluted epinephrine-saline solution.	None
Antibiotics	Cefazolin (adult = 1g; child = 15 mg/kg) iv on induction of anesthesia	⇐
Surgical time	2-3 h	⇐
EBL	Massive; limit to 10 U PRBC transfusion	250-500 ml
Postop care	Generally, patients can be extubated at the end of these procedures, recovered in the PACU, and returned to the burn center. If patient remains intubated, generally he/she is transported directly to the burn center, where body T can be maintained more easily.	⇐
Mortality	18-40% (Mortality is a function of burn size, plus other associated conditions, especially inhalation injury [Figs 11.5-1, 2].)	⇐
Morbidity	Massive blood loss	–
	Sepsis	⇐
	Infection 2° to catheters and lines	⇐
Pain score	2-5 (Most patients are maintained on sustained-release methadone or iv morphine, for periop pain control.)	⇐
		⇐

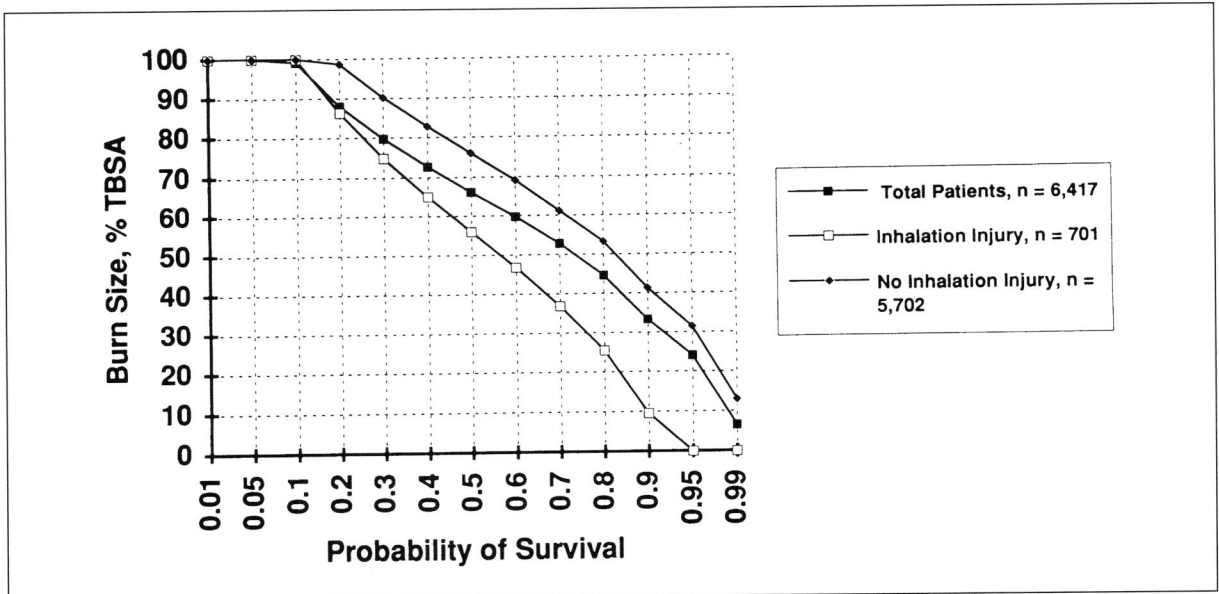

Figure 11.5-2. Probit Survival for patients with and without inhalation injury.

Table 11.5-1. Burn wounds—Classified According to Depth of Burn

Degree	Burn Depth	Tissue involved
First degree	Superficial	Epidermis only
Second degree	Partial thickness	Various thickness of dermis
Third degree	Full thickness	Entire thickness of dermis
Fourth degree	To underlying tissue	Beyond dermis (e.g., subcutaneous fat, fascia, or muscle)

PATIENT POPULATION CHARACTERISTICS

Age range	All
Male:Female	More commonly male
Incidence	45,000 burn center admissions/yr
Etiology	Scald; flame burns; chemicals; electric burns
Associated conditions	Generally few, except in elderly patients

ANESTHETIC CONSIDERATIONS

PREOPERATIVE

Burn injuries may result in a broad spectrum of physiologic impairments. These vary, depending on the percent of TBSA burned, location of burns, age of the patient, time elapsed since initial injury, and interim treatment. Ideally, burn patients are fluid-resuscitated and stabilized before being brought to the OR. Typically, skin grafts to cover the burn area start on post-injury day 3. Blood loss and hypothermia are the predominant considerations during surgery on burn patients. Blood loss can be rapid and massive, as much as 8 U in 15 min, and can be difficult to estimate as it generally is not collected into the suction.

Respiratory	**Upper airway:** A patient with burns around the airway (e.g., singed nose hairs) should be intubated as early as possible. Direct inhalational/thermal injury and fluid resuscitation may make delayed intubation more difficult 2° upper airway edema. **Lower airway:** Physiologic derangements may include pulmonary edema and ARDS. Additionally, burn patients can be severely hypermetabolic (e.g., a patient with 40% TBSA burns may have twice the normal metabolic rate), with corresponding increased CO_2 production. These patients may have

Respiratory, cont.	high PIPs and high minute ventilation requirements. Pressure control ventilation and high levels of PEEP may be useful. Other possible effects of severe burns include: ↓lung and chest-wall compliance, ↓FRC, ↑A-a gradient, ↑carboxyhemoglobinemia and ↑methemoglobinemia. **Tests:** ABG, depending on pulmonary status; CXR
Cardiovascular	The hypermetabolism associated with burns increases cardiac demand, and burn patients have greatly elevated circulating levels of catecholamines → ↑HR + ↑CO. **Tests:** As indicated from H&P.
Neurological	Evaluate for burn encephalopathy. Characterize baseline mental status before anesthesia to allow evaluation of recovery postop.
Musculoskeletal	Damaged muscle → ↑acetylcholine receptor density, resulting in ↓sensitivity to nondepolarizing muscle relaxants and potentially fatal elevations of K^+ in response to succinylcholine. In burns > 5% TBSA, avoid succinylcholine after 24 h postburn and for at least 1 yr thereafter for burns > 10% TBSA (↑↑K^+). Recovery of normal response to muscle relaxants does not occur until burns have healed completely.
Hematologic	Coagulopathies may result directly from the burn injury, as well as from rapid replacement of blood loss during operative procedures. **Tests:** Hb/Hct; electrolytes; coagulation profile
IV access	May be difficult; assess preop. Consider central line placement with a large-bore catheter, such as a Cordis.
Laboratory	Other tests as indicated from H&P.
Premedication	Patients are commonly placed on high-dose narcotics after the initial injury; additional narcotics are frequently required to provide adequate analgesia for transport and movement to the OR table.
Transport	For patients with severe ARDS, transportation from burn unit to OR may pose formidable challenges with regard to ventilation. Cardiopulmonary monitoring must be continued during transport; the ventilation system used in transport must be capable of delivering high minute-volumes, PEEP, and inspiratory pressures. These requirements may not be satisfied by standard bag-valve systems and may require a high-quality transport ventilator.

INTRAOPERATIVE

Anesthetic technique: GETA. Regional techniques are rarely feasible, given the multiple surgical sites for harvesting and grafting. LMAs are not recommended, given the potential for significant fluid resuscitation and subsequent airway edema, as well as the frequent repositioning of patient intraop.

Induction	If the patient is adequately volume-resuscitated, propofol (1.5-2.5 ml/kg iv) or thiopental (3-5 mg/kg) may be used. If the patient is intravascularly volume-depleted, etomidate (0.3 mg/kg) or ketamine (1-3 mg/kg) is recommended. Patients with extensive burns (> 30% TBSA) will develop a decreased sensitivity to nondepolarizing NMBs; therefore, 1.5 × the usual intubating dose of NMB is recommended: vecuronium (1.5 mg/kg), pancuronium (0.15 mg/kg), or rocuronium (1.5 mg/kg). If rapid-sequence induction is indicated, succinylcholine should not be used if the initial injury is > 24 h old. Under these circumstances, high-dose rocuronium (2 mg/kg) can be used. If the face is burned, awake FOI may necessary and securing the ETT may be difficult. Alternatives to taping the ETT include suturing the tube to the teeth or using umbilical tape.
Maintenance	Standard maintenance (see p. B-3). Physiologic derangements of the respiratory system (ARDS, pulmonary edema) and a hypermetabolic state may require minute-volumes > 30 L/min, and high inspiratory pressures and PEEP, for adequate ventilation. Depending on equipment availability, a Siemens or ICU ventilator (capable of PPV) may be necessary. Intraop, surgeons may use epinephrine-soaked sponges to ↓blood loss. Systemic absorption of epinephrine will cause tachycardia and increase the probability of dysrhythmias; therefore, it is best to avoid halothane or desflurane. Isoflurane and sevoflurane are acceptable.
Emergence	Estimation of an adequate dose of narcotic to provide postop analgesia may be difficult since these patients are often receiving high doses of narcotics preop. If large-volume resuscitation has occurred intraop, there is the possibility of clinically significant airway edema; use caution before extubating to ensure a patent airway.

Blood and fluid requirements	Extensive blood loss IV: 14-16 ga × 2 or a Cordis NS/LR @ 8-10 ml/kg/h Keep UO @ 0.5-1 ml/kg/h. Blood: ~200 ml/1% BSA excised and grafted.[5] Fluid warmer T&C 2-4 U PRBC (to keep ahead).	Blood must be in OR before induction. The major blood loss generally is associated with eschar excision, usually the first part of the procedure. For patients without contraindications to hemodilution (e.g., CAD, anemia), it is often better to delay PRBC transfusion until major blood loss is complete. IV hyperalimentation should be continued during surgery, or, replace with 10% dextrose infusion to avoid hypoglycemia. If sudden ↓BP occurs during very rapid infusion of blood (>150 ml/min), consider using Ca^{++} to counteract the chelating effect of citrate. Avoid fluid overload, especially if patient has ARDS, is a small child, or is elderly. As the surgical site is superficial, there is not much 3rd-space loss.
Thermal considerations	Room = 80-82°F Warm all fluids. Humidify gases. Warming blanket Reflective head cover	Temperature must be monitored throughout the case. The surgeon may be notified if patient's core T is dropping.
Monitoring	Standard monitors (see p. B-1). ± CVP line PA catheter	ECG may require needle electrodes or alligator clip electrodes to skin graft if there is no skin availability to apply adhesive electrodes. The hemodynamically unstable patient should be monitored with a PA catheter.
Positioning	✓ and pad pressure points. ✓ eyes.	The burn patient may be uniquely susceptible to laryngeal or upper airway edema in the prone position; therefore, examination of the upper airway before extubation is recommended to avoid emergent reintubation.
Complications	Massive blood loss	

POSTOPERATIVE

Complications	Hypothermia Coagulopathy	May occur as the result of massive blood loss and replacement.
Transport	Continue cardiopulmonary monitoring. High minute-ventilation requirements ↑PIP ↑PEEP	Verify adequacy of transport ventilation system before departing OR.
Pain management	Oral methadone or sustained-release morphine sulfate IV fentanyl or morphine sulfate	Titrate analgesia to effect.
Tests	Hct, ABG, electrolytes, PT, PTT, Plt, if massive transfusion given.	

References

1. Burke JF, Quinby WC Jr, Bondoc CC: Primary excision and prompt grafting as routine therapy for the treatment of thermal burns in children. *Surg Clin North Am* 1976; 56(2):477-94.
2. Capan LM, Miller SM: Trauma and burns. In *Clinical Anesthesia*. Barash PG, Cullen BF, Stoelting RK, eds. Lippincott Williams & Wilkins, Philadelphia: 2001, 1255-97.
3. Heimbach DM: Early burn excision and grafting. *Surg Clin North Am* 1987; 67(1):93-107.
4. Jurkovich GJ: Envenomation and environmental injuries. In *Surgery: Scientific Principles and Practice*. Greenfield LJ, et al, eds. Lippincott Williams & Wilkins, Philadelphia: 2001, 405-300.
5. Janzekovic Z: A new concept in the early excision and immediate grafting of burns. *J Trauma* 1970; 10(2):1103-8.
6. Moran KT, O'Reilly TJ, Furman W, Munster AM: A new algorithm for calculation of blood loss in excisional burn surgery. *Am Surg* 1988; 54(4):207-8.
7. Pavlin EG: *Surgical Management of the Burn Wound*. Heimbach DM, Engrav LH, eds. Raven Press. New York: 1985, 139-53.
8. Sheridan RL, Tompkins RG: Burns. In *Surgery: Scientific Principles and Practice*. Greenfield LJ, et al, eds. Lippincott Williams & Wilkins, Philadelphia: 2001, 431-49.

12.0   PEDIATRIC SURGERY

Surgeon

Stephen L. Huhn, MD

12.1 PEDIATRIC NEUROSURGERY

Anesthesiologists

William W. Feaster, MD
C. Philip Larson, Jr, MD

CRANIOFACIAL SURGERY

SURGICAL CONSIDERATIONS

Description: Craniofacial surgery is a broad term that refers to both cranial and/or facial reconstructive procedures for cranial dysostosis or craniofacial dysmorphism. Cranial dysostosis is the congenital maldevelopment of the cranial base and/or vault, 2° premature fusion of cranial sutures. More commonly referred to as **craniosynostosis**, the surgical correction of this disorder involves removal of the affected suture(s) and reconstruction of the cranial, orbital, or facial bones. The most common form of craniosynostosis—scaphocephaly—is caused by the fusion of the sagittal suture, which leads to a long and narrow calvarium. Other forms of craniosynostosis, in order of decreasing frequency, are coronal synostosis (brachycephaly), metopic synostosis (trigonocephaly), and lambdoidal synostosis. Deformational occipital plagiocephaly refers to flattening of the occiput 2° preferential sleep position and the resultant deformation of the skull. This condition is not a form of craniosynostosis and, despite the potential for significant flattening of the head, reconstructive surgery is not indicated. Crouzon and Apert syndromes are inherited craniofacial disorders associated with craniosynostosis and facial/orbital dysmorphism. The facial deformities common to Crouzon and Apert are shallow and misplaced orbits, exophthalmos, and midface hypoplasia. In each form of craniosynostosis, sporadic or predisposed, the abnormality is present at birth, but may not become recognizable until the rapid phase of brain growth, occurring in the first year of life, begins to accentuate the limitations on skull shape produced by the premature suture closure. In simple terms, the growth of the underlying brain drives the expansion of the skull, and closure of a suture produces abnormal skull growth in the opposite direction.

Early recognition and correction of craniosynostosis results in the best cosmetic outcome because, with release of the fused suture, the growing brain helps correct the abnormal cranial shape.[2,3] Most procedures are scheduled during the first 6 mo of life; thus, the issue of blood volume and replacement becomes a critical factor for surgical and anesthetic consideration. The main principles of surgical treatment of craniosynostosis involve removal of the abnormal suture through a craniectomy, followed by reconstruction of the calvarium and/or orbit to overcome the cranial deformity and optimize the chance for normal cranial development. The surgery may be done in conjunction with a pediatric neurosurgeon and a plastic surgeon. Patient positioning varies, depending on the approach to the craniectomy, and is generally prone for sagittal and lambdoidal synostosis, and supine for coronal and metopic synostosis. Another surgical principle important for synostosis surgery is to minimize intraop blood loss. The surgical team should make every effort to reduce blood loss during the procedure by infiltrating the scalp with 1:400,000 epinephrine, preserving the pericranium, and waxing the bone edges. The most common skin incision is a bicoronal opening that allows for access to the entire calvarium. The extent of the bone removal and reconstruction varies, depending on the type and number of sutures involved. Surgical correction of patients with Crouzon or Apert syndromes may often be staged with correction of the cranial component, followed by a later procedure for the face, as described by Tessier and colleagues.[7,8,9] Invariably, blood loss occurs from the scalp and bone, and the surgeon must remain mindful of the volume contained within the surgical field and readily communicate to the anesthesiologist when bleeding is felt to be either continuous or excessive. Injury to the underlying dural venous sinuses is rare, but the potential for catastrophic blood loss is great, if an opening in the dural sinus occurs. Recent advances in endoscopy have lead to the development of minimally invasive techniques for craniosynostosis in some centers, and reports suggest that use of the endoscope reduces blood loss.[4] Recombinant erythropoietin administered preop also has been studied in an attempt to reduce the need for intraop transfusion associated with repair of craniosynostosis.[1] Subgaleal and epidural drains are placed at the close of the procedure, and the patient is monitored closely in the ICU for postop bleeding that often requires additional transfusions in the first 24 h after surgery.

Usual preop diagnosis: Craniosynostosis (sagittal, coronal, metopic, lambdoidal); craniofacial dysmorphism; Apert syndrome; Crouzon syndrome

SUMMARY OF PROCEDURE

Position	Supine or prone (less common); or table 180°
Incision	Bicoronal, biparietal, Meisterschnitt, midsagittal
Special instrumentation	Midas Rex craniotome; absorbable plates and screws
Unique considerations	↑ICP and/or hydrocephalus may coexist. ↑ICP is usually seen with multiple-suture synostosis; it also occurs in single-suture craniosynostosis,[6] but is rare (< 5-10%). Hydrocephalus typically is seen in monogenic conditions (e.g., Apert, Crouzon). Most neurosurgeons shunt the hydrocephalus and treat the ↑ICP prior to craniosynostosis surgery.
Antibiotics	Vancomycin (13-15 mg/kg) or cloxacillin (25-50 mg/kg) for cranial surgery. Vancomycin or cloxacillin and cefotaxime (25-30 mg/kg) for craniofacial surgery involving nasal sinuses.
Closing considerations	Watch for ↑blood loss from the scalp after hemostatic skin clips are removed. To prevent excessive blood loss, reapproximate only one portion of the scalp at a time.

EBL	Highly variable; must be minimized. Amount depends on the number of sutures involved, age of the patient and magnitude of the repair. Operative injury to the superior sagittal sinus may be catastrophic if hemostasis cannot be achieved or volume loss is excessive.
Postop care	ICU. Postop Hct/Hb levels required. Blood transfusion often necessary in infants (< 10 kg).
Mortality	< 1-2%
Morbidity	Meningitis
	CSF rhinorrhea
	↑ICP (2° skull reshaping)
	Venous thrombosis
	Neurological injury: Rare
Pain score	1-3

PATIENT POPULATION CHARACTERISTICS

Age range	Newborn–young adult
Male:Female	1.2:1
Incidence	1/2,000/yr
Etiology	Sporadic; heritable (monogenic and chromosomal syndromes); environmentally induced (amniotic bands, iatrogenic)
Associated conditions	Congenital defects (limbs, heart, brain, kidneys); hydrocephalus; encephalocele (sincipital/basal); fibrous dysplasia; craniometaphyseal dysplasia; holoprosencephaly

ANESTHETIC CONSIDERATIONS

PREOPERATIVE

Craniofacial surgery encompasses a wide variety of procedures, with the two most common being linear craniectomy for craniosynostosis (or premature closure of the cranial sutures) and reconstructive (cosmetic surgery) for congenital deformities of the forehead, orbit ridges, and nose. Craniosynostosis usually manifests itself in the first yr of life, while surgery for other congenital deformities of the face and skull usually is performed from ages 1-6 yr.

Respiratory	As a result of craniofacial deformities, some children may present difficult intubations. Their airways should be carefully evaluated preop.
Neurological	Presenting Sx in infants with craniosynostosis include: progressive head deformation, progressively increasing irritability, crying, failure to eat, and failure to grow in head circumference. These Sx may be due in part to ↑ICP. On physical examination, one or more of the cranial sutures are fused. Infants with other types of craniofacial deformity usually have no Sx related to their abnormalities.
Laboratory	Tests as indicated from H&P.
Premedication	For children, midazolam 0.5 mg/kg po (see p. D-2) generally provides satisfactory preop sedation after ~30 min. For young children (< 5 yr) who refuse po meds, instillation of midazolam 0.3 mg/kg intranasally provides rapid amnesia, sedation, and easy separation from the parents.[5]

INTRAOPERATIVE

Anesthetic technique: GETA.

Induction	Standard pediatric induction (see p. D-2). Orotracheal tubes are preferred over nasotracheal tubes because the surgery may involve reflection of the scalp down over the eyes and nose, in which case a nasal tube would be in the way. Verify ETT placement (see p. D-3). Tape the tube firmly in place at one side of the mouth using benzoin adherent. When craniofacial surgery is performed, the surgeon usually places plastic corneal shields in the eyes and sutures the lids shut to protect eyes from injury.
Maintenance	Standard maintenance (see p. D-3). Muscle relaxation is usually provided. Maintain a near-normal BP. Maintain normal T by keeping the OR warm (78°F) and using warming lights as needed. Ventilation is controlled to PetCO$_2$ = 35-40 mmHg with a mechanical ventilator, from the start of anesthesia until the surgical wound is closed.
Emergence	No specific considerations. The ETT is removed at the conclusion of the anesthetic. Patient usually goes to PICU.

Blood and fluid requirements	Large blood loss IV: 18-20 ga × 1-2 NS/LR @ 4 ml/kg/h 5% albumin Fluid warmer	Administer crystalloid via a continuous infusion pump or Volutrel. Blood is often necessary. It is advisable to begin transfusion at the start of surgery, to avoid getting behind. In smaller children, it is better to administer warmed blood by syringe, in 10 ml increments. Serial Hct determinations are useful.
Monitoring	Standard monitors (see p. D-1). ± Foley catheter ± Doppler ± Arterial line ± CVP line	If operation is anticipated to last several h, a Foley catheter should be inserted. If patient is semi-sitting, a Doppler ultrasound probe may be placed on the chest to monitor for air embolism. Invasive monitoring is often appropriate. $\uparrow K^+$ and $\downarrow Ca^{++}$ are most common following transfusions with blood or FFP.
Positioning	OR table rotated 180° ✓ and pad pressure points. ✓ eyes.	
Complications	Major blood loss VAE	VAE may occur if dural sinus entered.

POSTOPERATIVE CONSIDERATIONS

Complications	Bleeding Hypovolemia	Major complications from these operations are uncommon.
Pain management	Parenteral opioids (see p. E-1). Avoid oversedation.	Fentanyl 1-2 μg/kg q 60 min, morphine 0.05-0.1 mg/kg q 2 h
Tests	Hct/Hb	Hct/Hb levels are necessary to determine adequacy of blood replacement.

References

1. Fearon JA, Weinthal J: The use of recombinant erythropoietin in the reduction of blood transfusion rated in craniosynostosis repair in infants and children. *Plast Reconstr Surg* 2002; 109(7):2190-6.
2. Hoffman HJ: Congenital malformations of the spine and skull. In *Practice of Surgery*. Goldsmith HS, ed. Harper & Row, New York; 1980.
3. Hoffman HJ, Hendrick EB: Early neurosurgical repair in craniofacial dysmorphism. *J Neurosurg* 1979; 51(6):796-803.
4. Jimenez DF, Barone CM, Cartwright CC, Baker L: Early management of craniosynostosis using endoscopic-assisted strip craniectomies and cranial orthotic molding therapy. *Pediatrics* 2002; 110:97-104.
5. Karl HW, Keifer AT, Rosenberger JL, Larach MG, Ruffle JM: Comparison of the safety and efficacy of intranasal midazolam or sufentanil for preinduction of anesthesia in pediatric patients. *Anesthesiology* 1992: 76(2):209-15.
6. Shillito J Jr, Matson DD: Craniosynostoses: a review of 519 surgical patients. *Pediatrics* 1968; 41(4):829-53.
7. Tessier P: Relationship of craniostenoses to craniofacial dysostoses and to faciostenoses: a study with therapeutic implications. *Plast Reconstr Surg* 1971; 48(3):224-37.
8. Tessier P: Total facial osteotomy. Crouzon's syndrome, Apert's syndrome: oxycephaly, scaphocephaly, turricephaly. *Ann Chir Plast* 1967; 12(4):273-86.
9. Tessier P, Guiot G, Rougerie J, Delbet JP, Pastoriza J: Cranio-naso-orbito-facial osteotomies. Hypertelorism. *Ann Chir Plast* 1967; 12(2):103-18.

CLOSURE OF MYELOMENINGOCELE

SURGICAL CONSIDERATIONS

Description: Myelomeningocele is a neural tube defect characterized by failure of the spinal cord to fuse posteriorly during primary neurulation. This results in an open neural placode joined to the incomplete epithelial defect, usually located in the thoracolumbar spine. Associated CNS conditions are hydrocephalus and Chiari II hindbrain malformation, both of which usually contribute more to long-term morbidity than the spinal cord defect itself. The presence of the myelomeningocele may be detected before birth by high-resolution ultrasound and/or elevated maternal serum alpha fetoprotein. The incidence of neural tube defects is declining in the U.S. due to maternal dietary folate supplementation and prenatal Dx and selective termination.[3]

The fundamental goals of surgery are preservation of neural tissue, reconstitution of a normal intrathecal environment, and complete skin closure to prevent a spinal fluid leak.[2,4] Despite a very thin parchment of dystrophic epithelium attached to the placode, most myelomeningoceles leak spinal fluid from the time of birth. Because of the risk of ventriculitis associated with the exposed subarachnoid space, closure of the myelomeningocele is recommended within 72 h after birth. Infants with neural tube defects have a higher incidence of other congenital anomalies, including hydronephrosis, malrotation of the gut, VSD or ASD, and craniofacial disorders. The neonate should be screened for these potential abnormalities before undergoing surgery and, in general, this can be accomplished within 24 h after birth. During the procedure, the child is in the prone position. The defect is dissected so that the various anatomic layers can be separated. The edges of the placode (spinal cord) are mobilized from the adjacent epithelium and imbricated to form a closed tube. The laterally displaced dura is dissected from the fascia and closed over the spinal cord, thus reconstituting the elements of the spine, except for the lamina defect that is not reconstructed. An attempt may be made to mobilize the lumbosacral fascia as a separate layer; however, in most cases, the subcutaneous and skin layers comprise the final layer. In cases of large defects, local skin or myocutaneous flaps may be necessary to cover the spinal defect adequately. Progressive hydrocephalus usually presents within days to weeks after closure of the myelomeningocele, but ~15% of patients will present at birth with significant hydrocephalus that requires early insertion of a VP shunt. Finally, in rare circumstances, prominent vertebral angulation, or kyphosis, at the defect could necessitate vertebrectomies to reestablish normal spinal alignment.

Variant procedure or approaches: The efficacy of **intrauterine myelomeningocele repair** is currently being explored through a randomized multicenter trial, and the results may alter future approaches in favor of intrauterine closure if the incidence of hydrocephalus is reduced in these patients.[1,4]

Usual preop diagnosis: Myelomeningocele; meningocele; myelodysplasia; spina bifida

SUMMARY OF PROCEDURE

Position	Prone
Incision	Surrounding the defect, preserving skin that can be utilized in the closure
Special instrumentation	Loupes or operating microscope (optional)
Unique considerations	Concomitant hydrocephalus, lower brain stem dysfunction. Need for blood replacement rare in straightforward cases.
Antibiotics	Cefotaxime (25-30 mg/kg iv), vancomycin (13-15 mg/kg iv, slowly)
Surgical time	1.5-3 h
Closing considerations	Skin closure may be complex and require rotation of flaps or aid of plastic surgeon.
EBL	Negligible–25 ml (in most cases)
Postop care	Neonatal nursery. Postop, child often nursed on stomach or side. Head size is monitored for development of hydrocephalus, which may require shunting at a later date.
Mortality	Approaching zero
Morbidity	Meningitis/ventriculitis
	Hind brain dysfunction
	Wound infection
	CSF leak
	Massive blood loss
Pain score	3-5

PATIENT POPULATION CHARACTERISTICS

Age range	Newborn (diagnosed at birth)
Male:Female	~1:1
Incidence	1/1000 live births
Etiology	Congenital
Associated conditions	Hydrocephalus; lower extremity weakness; bowel and/or bladder dysfunction (neurogenic bladder); scoliosis; Chiari II malformations; congenital cardiac anomalies

ANESTHETIC CONSIDERATIONS

PREOPERATIVE

Myelomeningoceles are congenital abnormalities of the spinal cord that result in a saccular protrusion near the base of the spine. The sac, containing neural elements and CSF, can vary in size from very small to a volume that occupies the whole lower spinal region. The Dx may be suspected from fetal ultrasound, and is confirmed at birth. It is generally believed that immediate removal of the sac and covering of the defect with skin is desirable to preserve neurological function and avoid infections. These newborns, therefore, usually are brought to surgery within 24 h after birth.

Cardiovascular	May have associated congenital anomalies. **Tests:** ECHO
Neurological	Although difficult to assess at this age, newborns may have motor and/or sensory deficits in the lower extremities, neurogenic bladder, and lower cranial nerve dysfunction. Most have an Arnold-Chiari malformation, which requires a ventriculoperitoneal shunt within days of the back repair.
Renal	May have associated congenital anomalies. **Tests:** Renal ultrasound
Laboratory	Routine preop studies
Premedication	None necessary

INTRAOPERATIVE

Anesthetic technique: GETA

Induction	Before induction, the patient is placed in the supine position, and the back defect is protected by a donut or rolls to prevent pressure or rupture. Patients usually will come to the OR with an iv in place, allowing for a standard iv induction (see p. D-2). If not, a standard inhalational induction (p. D-2), followed by establishment of iv access is indicated. Sevoflurane is preferred because of its low blood-gas partition coefficient and absence of airway irritability, which allows a smooth, rapid induction. Oral ETT intubation usually follows muscle relaxation with rocuronium (0.6-1 mg/kg) or vecuronium (0.1 mg/kg). Atropine (0.05-0.1 mg) may be administered before intubation to reduce secretions and to prevent reflex bradycardia. Verify ETT placement and tape tube securely in place at one side of the mouth with benzoin adherent to facilitate prone positioning.
Maintenance	Sevoflurane 2-3% or halothane 1% or less, with N_2O or air/O_2 mixture to maintain arterial O_2 sat at 95-96%. Depending on duration of operation, additional doses of vecuronium (0.1 mg/kg) or rocuronium (0.3 mg/kg) may be needed. Maintain a near-normal BP. Maintain normal T by keeping OR warm (78°F) and using warming lights as needed. Ventilation is controlled to maintain $PetCO_2$ = 35-40 mmHg with a mechanical ventilator or manually, from the start of anesthesia until surgical wound is closed.
Emergence	The ETT is removed at the conclusion of the anesthetic. The newborn is nursed in the prone or lateral positions for the first few d postop.
Blood and fluid requirements	IV: 22-24 ga × 1 D10 @ 2-4 ml/kg/h (newborn) D10 ¼ NS @ 4 ml/kg/h (> 24 h) Warm fluids.	Administer crystalloid, usually D10 ¼ NS, via a continuous infusion pump, etc. Blood is rarely, if ever, necessary.
Monitoring	Standard monitors (see p. D-1).
Positioning	✓ and pad pressure points. ✓ eyes.	Prone with shoulders and hips on bolsters to elevate abdomen off operating table. Head turned to the side, which results in the tube being furthest from the bed. ✓ tube placement by listening to breath sounds after positioning.

POSTOPERATIVE

Complications	CSF leak Infection Hydrocephalus
Pain management	Parenteral opiates (see p. E-3).

Reference

1. Cochrane D, Irwin B, Chambers K: Clinical outcomes that fetal surgery for myelomeningocele needs to achieve. *Eur J Pediatr Surg* 2001; 22(Suppl 1):S18-20.
2. Cohen AR, Robinson S: Early management of myelomeningocele. In *Pediatric Neurosurgery: Surgery of the Developing Nervous System*, 4th edition. McLone DG, ed. WB Saunders, Philadelphia: 2001, 241-60.
3. Cragen J, Roberts H, Edmonds L, et al: Surveillance for anencephaly and spina bifida and the impact of prenatal diagnosis-Unites States, 1985-1994. *Morbid Mortal Wkly Rep* 1995; 44(S-4):1-13.
4. Reigel DH: Myelomeningocele repair. In *Pediatric Neurosurgery: Surgery of the Developing Nervous System*, 4th edition. McLone DG, ed. WB Saunders, Philadelphia: 2001, 261-5.
5. Tulipan N, Sutton LN, Bruner JP, Cohen BM, Johnson M, Adzick NS: The effect of intrauterine myelomeningocele repair on the incidence of shunt-dependent hydrocephalus. *Pediatr Neurosurg* 2003; 38(1):27-33.

SURGICAL CORRECTION OF SPINAL DYSRAPHISM

SURGICAL CONSIDERATIONS

Description: **Occult spinal dysraphism** covers a spectrum of spinal anomalies generally related to defects in secondary neurulation, in contrast to a myelomeningocele, which occurs as a result of defective primary neurulation. These forms of congenital spinal defects are covered by intact skin and share the common pathophysiology of spinal cord tethering. Occult spinal dysraphism includes tight filum terminale, intramedullary lipoma, lipomyelomeningocele, split cord malformations (diastematomyelia), dermal sinus tracts, meningocele manqué, neuroenteric cyst, and myelocystocele. Each of these lesions can result in a tethering, or stretching, of the spinal cord as the vertebral axis elongates during normal growth. The fixed spinal cord is stretched by the growing spine, resulting in neurological dysfunction, most likely as a result of reduced pial blood flow.[3] Excision of the lesion and release of the tethering elements is recommended to prevent either the onset or worsening of cord dysfunction.

The surgical principles for correction of occult spinal dysraphism involve excision of the intradural lesion and release of the tissue element that is tethering the spinal cord, while preserving the normal neural structures.[1] In cases of tight filum terminale, this is easily accomplished with little threat to the spinal cord or nerve root function, whereas excision of lipomyelomeningoceles may be extremely challenging procedures. Any tethering lesion needs to be carefully separated from the spinal cord and adjacent nerve roots without disrupting neurological function.[4] Intraop neurophysiological monitoring may be a useful adjunct to monitor cord and nerve root function during the dissection and release of the tethering lesion.[2] Following the intradural procedure, closure of the dura is critical in prevention of postop spinal fluid leaks; and dural grafts may be necessary in some cases.

Usual preop diagnosis: Tethered spinal cord; fat filum terminale; lipomyelomeningocele; lipoma of the filum; diastematomyelia; spinal dysraphism; dermal sinus tract; caudal agenesis

SUMMARY OF PROCEDURE

Position	Prone
Incision	Posterior midline centered over abnormality
Special instrumentation	Operating microscope; laser
Unique considerations	Blood replacement with loss of significant amount of blood in the infant
Antibiotics	Cefotetan (25-30 mg/kg iv) and vancomycin (13-15 mg/kg iv slowly), appropriate for weight
Surgical time	1.5-5 h (longer for diastematomyelia and lipomyelomeningocele)
Closing considerations	Surgeon often wants to test integrity of dural closure with Valsalva maneuver: sustained (10-20 sec) inspiratory pressure at 20-40 cmH$_2$O.
EBL	5-100 ml
Postop care	Patient often kept flat postop to protect dural closure.
Mortality	Approaching zero

Morbidity	Infection
	Neurological deficit
	Aseptic meningitis
	CSF leak
	Massive blood loss
Pain score	3-5

PATIENT POPULATION CHARACTERISTICS

Age range	Newborn–adults
Male:Female	~1:1
Incidence	Uncommon
Etiology	Congenital
Associated conditions	Ankle/foot deformity (talipes); neurologic impairment; scoliosis; vertebral abnormalities; VACTERL/VATER association (vertebral, anal, cardiac, tracheoesophageal, renal, and limb anomalies); cutaneous anomaly over spine; syringomyelia; caudal agenesis; neurogenic bowel/bladder

ANESTHETIC CONSIDERATIONS

PREOPERATIVE

A variety of spinal abnormalities fall under the category of spinal dysraphism, the most common being a tethered cord or a lipoma of the spinal cord. In the case of the tethered cord, there may be a Hx of myelomeningocele repair at birth. Most patients range from 3-16 yr of age.

Neurological	Presenting Sx are usually pain in the lower back radiating into the legs and/or progressively worsening motor or sensory deficits in the anal region or involving the lower extremities (document carefully).
Musculoskeletal	Lower extremity sensory or motor deficits may be present and should be carefully documented.
Renal	Renal function may be impaired in patients with Hx of recurrent UTIs. **Tests:** UA; BUN; Cr; others as indicated from H&P.
Laboratory	Other tests as indicated from H&P.
Premedication	For children, midazolam 0.5 mg/kg po (see p. D-2) generally provides satisfactory preop sedation after ~30 min. For young children (< 5 yr) who refuse po meds, instillation of midazolam 0.3 mg/kg intranasally provides rapid amnesia, sedation, and easy separation from parents.
Latex allergy	Meningomyelocele patients may have developed a latex allergy (see Appendix G).

INTRAOPERATIVE

Anesthetic technique: GETA

Induction	Standard induction (see p. D-2) with sevoflurane or halothane, N_2O, and O_2. This is followed by establishment of iv access, then ETT intubation with the use of a muscle relaxant (e.g., vecuronium 0.15 mg/kg or rocuronium 1 mg/kg). Sevoflurane is preferred because of its rapid, smooth induction. Tape the tube firmly in place at one side of the mouth, using benzoin adherent, for prone positioning.	
Maintenance	Standard maintenance (see p. D-3). Upon completion of placement of the dural graft, and before closure of the wound, the surgeon will want to check the integrity of the graft to eliminate any CSF leaks. The surgeon will ask that positive pressure be applied to the airway to at least 20 cmH_2O for 10-20 sec. If graft leaks are detected, they will be repaired and the test repeated.	
Emergence	The ETT is removed at the conclusion of the anesthetic. The patient may be nursed flat in the prone or lateral position for the first few d postop to lessen the chance of a CSF leak developing.	
Blood and fluid requirements	IV: 18-20 ga × 1 NS/LR @ 4-6 ml/kg/h	In children, administer fluids via a volumetric infusion set. Blood is rarely, if ever, necessary.
Monitoring	Standard monitors (see p. D-1). ± Foley catheter ± UO	If the operation is anticipated to last several h, a Foley catheter should be inserted.

Positioning	✓ and pad pressure points. ✓ eyes.	Prone with the shoulders and hips on bolsters to elevate the abdomen off the operating table. Head turned to the side, resulting in the tube being furthest from bed. ✓ tube placement by listening to breath sounds after positioning.
Complications	Severe bradycardia Latex allergy	Manipulation of the spinal cord may produce ↓↓HR reflexly. See Appendix G for latex allergy considerations.

POSTOPERATIVE

Complications	Possible neurological deficits Infection CSF leak	Major complications from this operation are uncommon, but include new neurological deficits from irritation of the spinal cord during surgery, localized infection, and CSF leak from the wound site.
Pain management	Parental opiates or PCA (see p. E-3).	

References

1. Oakes WJ: Management of spinal cord lipomas and lipomyelomeningoceles. In *Neurosurgery Update II*. Wilkins RH, Rengachary S, eds. McGraw-Hill, New York: 1991, 345-52.
2. von Koch CS, Quinones-Hinojosa A, Gulati M, Lyon R, Peacock WJ, Yingling CD: Clinical outcome in children undergoing tethered cord release utilizing intraoperative neurophysiological monitoring. *Pediatr Neurosurg* 2002; 37(2):81-6.
3. Warf BC: Pathophysiology of tethered cord syndrome. In *Pediatric Neurosurgery: Surgery of the Developing Nervous System*, 4th edition. McLone DG, ed. WB Saunders, Philadelphia: 2001, 282-8.
4. Yamada S, Iacono RP: Tethered Cord Syndrome. In *Disorders of the Pediatric Spine*. Pang D, ed. Raven Press, New York: 1995, 159-74.

CRANIOTOMY FOR VEIN OF GALEN MALFORMATION

SURGICAL CONSIDERATIONS

Description: A vein of Galen aneurysm is a large, AV fistula between arteries, mainly of the posterior cerebral circulation, and a massively enlarged vein of Galen (deep venous drainage of the brain).[1] Patients can present with CHF (infants), progressive macrocephaly from hydrocephalus (infants, children, adults), or, rarely, IC hemorrhage in adult patients. Most cases present during the infant years, and immediate care is often directed toward stabilizing cardiac function related to CHF. Patients undergoing surgery without adequate stabilization of cardiac function carry the highest risk of periop mortality. Many patients will have some degree of accompanying hydrocephalus, but decisions regarding the placement of ventricular shunts are best postponed until the malformation has been treated, as hydrocephalus may improve with reduction in intracranial venous pressure. Once the issues of cardiac function and hydrocephalus have been addressed, the patient can be evaluated for treatment by cerebral angiography and endovascular techniques.

Treatment is directed at staged occlusion of the arterial feeders to the AV fistula and subsequent thrombosis of the fistula itself from the venous side.[2] Open microsurgical techniques, endovascular methods, or a combination of both may be used to reduce flow through the malformation. With reduction in the aneurysmal flow, CO will decrease, SVR will improve, and mixed venous PO_2 will decrease. Because of the high mortality associated with treatment by surgery alone and the advances in endovascular techniques, vein of Galen malformations currently are managed without direct primary surgical approaches. Surgery, as an option, is more likely to occur in the setting of staged or attempted embolizations.[3] Subtemporal, midline occipital, or bilateral occipital craniotomies can be used to isolate and occlude arterial feeders to the malformation.

Variant procedure or approaches: Alternative approaches may access the torcular (confluence) of venous sinuses through a burr hole to allow direct retrograde placement of thrombogenic coils in the AV fistula.

Usual preop diagnosis: Vein of Galen aneurysm; IC hemorrhage; hydrocephalus; progressive neurologic deficits

SUMMARY OF PROCEDURE

Position	Lateral decubitus, Concorde (modified prone), or semisitting; for burr hole, lateral
Incision	Temporal or occipital; for burr hole, occipital
Special instrumentation	Operating microscope, microscopic instruments; intraop angiography; for burr hole, endovascular catheters and equipment; intraop SSEP monitoring
Unique considerations	Careful attention to blood loss in infants
Antibiotics	Vancomycin (1 g iv slowly q 12 h for adults; 10-15 mg/kg iv slowly q 6 h for children); cefotaxime (1 g iv q 6 h for adults; 40 mg/kg iv q 6 h for children)
Surgical time	3-5 h
Closing considerations	Meticulous hemostasis; avoid ↓BP or HTN (MAP 80-90 adults; 70-80, children).
EBL	< 250 ml
Postop care	Monitor for ↑ICP (use of extraventricular drain) as a result of venous HTN 2° rapid occlusion of AV fistula. ICU × 1-3 d.
Mortality	Approaches 100% if in CHF
Morbidity	Deep venous infarct: 5-10%
	Hydrocephalus
	Stroke
	Subdural hygroma
	Infection: Rare
Pain score	3-4

PATIENT POPULATION CHARACTERISTICS

Age range	1 mo–3 yr (typically)
Male:Female	1:1
Incidence	Rare
Etiology	Congenital
Associated conditions	Other intracranial vascular malformations; high-output CHF

ANESTHETIC CONSIDERATIONS

PREOPERATIVE

Vein of Galen aneurysms are rare congenital abnormalities representing < 1% of all aneurysms.[1] They are usually diagnosed in infants because they cause an abnormal increase in head size due to the aneurysmal dilation and obstruction of the dural sinus. The abnormal vasculature constitutes a high-flow shunt, much like an AVM. If left untreated, the morbidity and mortality are high; however, treatment with radiologic embolization and/or surgical excision also is associated with high morbidity and mortality rates.

Cardiovascular	Because these lesions constitute high-flow shunts through the brain, the infants are prone to develop CHF, which is fatal in more than 40% of patients.
Neurological	Infants usually present with an abnormal head size, Sz disorder, or bizarre neurological signs, such as high-pitched crying, posturing, failure to eat or thrive, etc.
Laboratory	CT; MRI; cerebral angiography. The infant may need sedation and anesthetic management to obtain adequate diagnostic studies.
Premedication	None

INTRAOPERATIVE

Anesthetic technique: GETA, with the goals being the same as those for IC vascular malformations.

Induction	Whenever possible, an iv induction is preferred. STP 2-3 mg/kg, propofol 1-2 mg/kg, fentanyl 2-3 μg/kg, and vecuronium 0.1 mg/kg or rocuronium 1 mg/kg are satisfactory induction agents.
Maintenance	STP ≤ 5 mg/kg, fentanyl ≤ 5 μg/kg, isoflurane ≤ 1%, with N_2O or air 60-70% to keep O_2 sat = 95-98%. Additional doses or NMBs may be administered as needed to maintain a single-twitch response to nerve stimulation.
Emergence	Plan to leave ETT in place for at least 24 h postop; infant should receive controlled ventilation and sedation during that interval. If infant does not show evidence of serious neurological injury postop, the ETT may be removed within 1-2 d.

Blood and fluid requirements	IV: 20-22 ga × 1-2 20 ga CVP, either IJ or subclavian	Replace blood as it is lost. Limit crystalloid fluid therapy to no more than 10 ml/kg above UO.
Control of brain volume	Same as for AVMs (see p. 19).	
Monitoring	Same as for AVMs (see p. 19).	
Control of BP	Goal = normal range for age Neonate: 55-70/40 (HR = 180) 1 yr: 70-100/60 (HR = 140)	BP should be kept in the normal range for the infant with close monitoring from an arterial catheter. If HR becomes excessive, esmolol infusion is useful.
Positioning	Same as for AVMs (see p. 19).	
Complications	Coagulopathy	If large volumes of blood are needed, a coagulopathy may ensue. Monitoring of coagulation status during surgery may be necessary.
	Hypothermia	Once the aneurysm is surgically corrected, immediate efforts must be made to return infant to a normal body T by the conclusion of the operation.

POSTOPERATIVE

Complications	Neurological deficits IC hemorrhage Heart failure
Pain management	Codeine 1-1.5 mg/kg im
Tests	Same as for AVMs (see p. 20).

References

1. Lasjaunias P, Rodesch G, Pruvost P, Laroche FG, Landrieu P: Treatment of vein of Galen aneurysmal malformation. *J Neurosurg* 1989; 70(5):746-50.
2. Herman JM, Hamilton MG, Spetzler RF: Vein of Galen Malformations: surgical indications and techniques. In *Neurovascular Surgery*, Carter LP, Spetzler RF, eds. McGraw-Hill, New York: 1994, 1041-8.
3. Moriarity JL, Steinberg GK: Surgical obliteration for vein of Galen malformation: a case report. *Surg Neurol* 1995; 44:365-70.

VENTRICULOSCOPY AND THIRD VENTRICULOSTOMY

SURGICAL CONSIDERATIONS

Description: Ventriculoscopy is the technique of intraop visualization of the lateral, third, and, occasionally, fourth ventricles using fiber optic endoscopes inserted through standard cranial burr holes. The ventriculoscope permits direct inspection and limited navigation within the ventricle for both diagnostic and therapeutic purposes, and is most commonly applied in the setting of hydrocephalus. In addition to CT scans, preop MRI exam of the brain often is obtained to better depict the anatomy of the ventricular system, which is distorted frequently by congenital lesions. The enlarged ventricles produced by the hydrocephalus contribute to the safety and feasibility of most endoscopic approaches, enabling a variety of procedures.[1,2,7] The endoscope can be used to fenestrate multicompartmental periventricular or arachnoid cysts, position ventricular catheters during shunt insertion, biopsy or, in some cases, resect intraventricular tumors. Neuroendoscopy generally does not help in the initial cannulation of the ventricle (a common misconception).

Endoscopic ventriculoscopy may be performed through either frontal or parietal-occipital approaches, with the patient typically supine with the neck slightly flexed. Standard small incisions similar to shunt insertions are used. A twist drill or burr hole is created and the ventricle cannulated by insertion of the shunt catheter or an introducer with a peel-away sheath (for larger endoscopes). Endoscopes vary in size from 1.1 mm, for use inside a standard shunt catheter, to larger endoscopes (12-14 Fr), equipped with working channels, for more complex intraventricular procedures.[3] After the ventricle is 'tapped' through conventional methods, the endoscope can be inserted and the ventricular anatomy identified. Once the intraventricular anatomic landmarks—such as the choroid plexus—are recognized, the scope can be navigated to the site of interest. Smaller endoscopes are used to position the catheter in the optimal ventricular location during shunt placement or revision. Larger endoscopes equipped with channels for instrumentation are used for biopsy, tumor resection, cyst aspiration, or fenestration procedures. Most scope systems have a separate channel for fluid irrigation if minor bleeding or debris obscure visibility.

Intraop complications associated with neuro-endoscopic procedures include: minor or major intraventricular hemorrhage; air entrapment (pneumocephalus); injury to paraventricular structures (basal ganglia, hypothalamus, brain stem); cardiorespiratory depression; and de-layed arousal from anesthesia. Intraventricular hemorrhage is caused by direct or indirect in-jury to ependymal and extraependymal blood vessels. Fortunately, most bleeding encountered is minor, but may be sufficient to interfere with visualization and illumination of the ven-tricle. Cardiorespiratory depression and car-diac arrhythmia are due, at least in part, to phenomena attributed to ↑ICP from excessive irrigation without equal extracranial egress, rate of fluid installation, and/or nonisothermic irrigant irritating the hypothalamic nuclei adjacent to the third ventricle.[4]

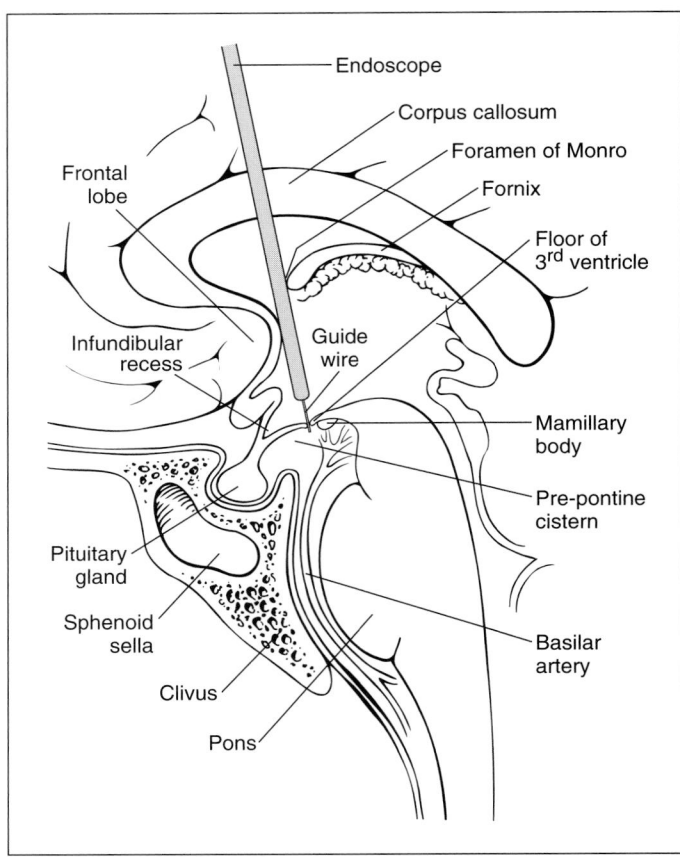

Figure 12.1-1. Endoscopic third ventriculostomy. The figure depicts fenestration of the floor of the third ventricle by a blunt probe inserted through the endoscope.

Third ventriculostomy is one of the more common endoscopic procedures and refers to fenestration of the floor of the third ventricle to create a communication between the third ventricle and the basilar cistern (Fig 12.1-1). The technique is most commonly applied to patients with obstructive, or noncommunicating, hydrocephalus, although broader indications are being explored.[5,6] This form of hydrocephalus results from impaired CSF flow through the Sylvian aqueduct or fourth ventricle outlets. For patients with noncommunicating hydrocephalus, successful third ventriculostomy allows CSF communication between the third ventricle and the interpeduncular subarachnoid space, thereby alleviating the hydrocephalus and avoiding shunt placement. The fenestration is conducted first by direct visualization of the floor of the third ventricle and then by perforation of the ependymal and arachnoid tissue between the mammillary bodies and the infundibular recess. The perforation can be dilated by inflation of a balloon catheter passed through the fenestration. Because of the proximity to the brain stem—in addition to the complications encountered with ventriculoscopy—third ventriculostomy carries the additional risk of mesencephalic injury, hypothalamic dysregulation, cranial nerve injury and hemorrhage from the basilar artery and adjacent perforating vessels. Minor bleeding can be controlled easily by steady irrigation. In the event of excessive bleeding, conversion to an open craniotomy is unlikely to improve control of the hemorrhage. Patients also may be prepped for shunt insertion in the event the ventriculostomy is aborted because of unfavorable third ventricular anatomy. A temporary extraventricular drain (EVD) may be left in place following some procedures to control CSF drainage postop and/or to allow assessment of ICP.

Usual preop diagnosis: Obstructive hydrocephalus; shunt malfunction; loculated multicompartmental hydrocephalus; intraventricular mass; arachnoid cyst; retained catheter

SUMMARY OF PROCEDURE

Position	Supine with head turned; table 90° or 180°
Incision	Small frontal or parietal-occipital
Special instrumentation	Endoscope (1.1-6 mm diameter); video system
Unique considerations	Hydrocephalus, ↑ICP; suspicion of latex allergy in patients with spina bifida (see p. G-1).

Antibiotics	Nafcillin (25 mg/kg q 4-6 h iv) or cefazolin (25 mg/kg q 8 h iv)
Closing considerations	Monitor for delayed intraventricular or subdural hemorrhage, ventricular collapse, acute hydrocephalus, CSF leak.
Postop care	Floor or ICU setting with cardiac and O_2 sat monitoring $\times$ 24 h. Measurement of serum sodium. Fluid intake/output recording. CT to r/o hemorrhage and to evaluate ventricular volume may be necessary. EVD used in cases of third ventriculostomy for draining CSF and testing ICP.
Mortality	0-7% (most series report 0%)
Morbidity	Intraventricular hemorrhage
	Acute hydrocephalus
	CSF leak/pneumocephalus
	Meningitis/ventriculitis
	Subdural effusions or hematoma
	Cranial nerve palsy
	Hemiparesis
	Diabetes insipidus
	SIADH
	Temperature dysregulation
Pain score	2-4

PATIENT POPULATION CHARACTERISTICS

Age range	Newborn–adult
Male:Female	1:1
Incidence	3/1000 live births (congenital only)
Etiology	Congenital and acquired
Associated conditions	Hydrocephalus; spinal dysraphism; Chiari malformation; posthemorrhagic hydrocephalus; arachnoid cyst

---

ANESTHETIC CONSIDERATIONS

PREOPERATIVE

Ventricular shunts are inserted to ameliorate hydrocephalus or cyst formations, which are either congenital or acquired.

Cardiovascular $\uparrow$ICP $\rightarrow$ $\uparrow$BP & $\downarrow\downarrow$HR (Cushing's response)
Tests: As indicated from H&P.

Neurological   The most common presenting Sx is HA. If hydrocephalus is severe, Sx of $\uparrow$ICP (>15 mmHg) (e.g., N/V, drowsiness, papilledema, Sz, and focal neurological defects) develop.

Laboratory   Tests as indicated by H&P.

Premedication   Usually not required; should be avoided in patients with $\uparrow$ICP.

INTRAOPERATIVE

Anesthetic technique: GETA

Induction   If $\uparrow$ICP, iv induction with STP (3-5 mg/kg) or propofol (0.15-0.3 mg/kg) is preferred, because of their ability to decrease cerebral blood volume and, hence, ICP. ETT intubation is accomplished with the use of a nondepolarizing NMB (e.g., vecuronium [0.1 mg/kg] or rocuronium [0.7-1 mg/kg]).

Maintenance   Isoflurane 1.5% or less or sevoflurane < 2% inspired with N_2O/O_2 mixture to maintain O_2 sat ~99%. Depending on duration of operation, additional doses of vecuronium (0.1 mg/kg) or rocuronium (0.2 mg/kg) may be needed. Maintain normal T in children by keeping OR warm (78°F) and using warming lights as needed. Ventilation is controlled mechanically (ventilator) or manually from the start of anesthesia until the surgical wound is closed. TV and frequency are adjusted so that $PetCO_2$ = 35-40 mmHg. Hyperventilation and hypocarbia are undesirable because they make cannulation of the ventricle(s) more difficult for the surgeon. Maintain normotension.

Emergence   ETT is removed at the conclusion of the anesthetic. Prophylactic antiemetic (e.g., metoclopramide 10 mg [0.1-0.2 mg/kg] or ondansetron 4 mg [0.1 mg/kg]) should be given 30-60 min before extubation.

Blood and fluid requirements	IV: 18-20 ga × 1 (22 ga for children) NS/LR @ 4-6 ml/kg/h	Administer crystalloid (via measured volume system in a child). Blood is rarely, if ever, necessary.
Monitoring	Standard monitors (see p. D-1).	
Positioning	Table turned 180° ✓ and pad pressure points. ✓ eyes.	Supine with a bolster under the shoulder on the operative side. The head, chest, and abdomen are prepped, so all anesthesia equipment and lines must be at the sides of the patient.
Complications	Infection Valve malfunction	Major complications from this operation are uncommon, but include infection at the valve site or in the tubing, and malfunction of the valve, either draining too little or too much CSF.

POSTOPERATIVE

Pain management	Children < 2 yr: Tylenol suppositories (up to 40 mg/kg intraop, then 10-15 mg/kg q 4 h). Other analgesics if required. (See Appendix E.)

References

1. Drake JM: Ventriculostomy for treatment of hydrocephalus. In *Neurosurgery Clinics of North America.* Butler AB, McLone DG, eds. 1993; 4(4):657-66.
2. Grant JA, McLone DG: Third ventriculostomy: A review. *Surg Neurol* 1997; 47:210-12.
3. Grotenhuis JA: *Manual of Endoscopic Procedures in Neurosurgery.* Uitgeverij Machaon, Nijmegen, The Netherlands: 1995.
4. Handler MH, Abbott R, Lee M: A near-fatal complication of endoscopic third ventriculostomy: case report. *Neurosurg* 1994; 35(3): 525-8.
5. Jones RFC, Kwok BCT, Stening WA, Vonau M: The current status of endoscopic third ventriculostomy in the management of non-communicating hydrocephalus. *Minim Invasive Neurosurg* 1994; 37:28-36.
6. Jones RFC, Kwok BCT, Stening WA, Vonau M: Third ventriculostomy for hydrocephalus associated with spinal dysraphism: indications and contraindications. *Eur J Pediatr Surg* 1996; 6(Suppl 1):5-6.
7. Kirolous RW, Javadpour M, May P, Mallucci C: Endoscopic treatment of suprasellar and third ventricle-related arachnoid cysts. *Childs Nsrv Syst* 2001; 17(12)713-8.
8. Walker ML, Petronio J, Carey CM: Ventriculoscopy. In *Pediatric Neurosurgery: Surgery of the Developing Nervous System.* Cheek WR, Marlin AE, McLone DG, Reigel DH, Walker ML, eds. WB Saunders, Philadelphia: 1994, 572-81.

Surgeon

D. M. Alcorn, MD

12.2   PEDIATRIC OPHTHALMIC SURGERY

Anesthesiologist

Alice A. Edler, MD

STRABISMUS SURGERY

SURGICAL CONSIDERATIONS

Description: Surgical correction of strabismus is a common procedure in ophthalmic practice, as strabismus occurs in 3-5% of the general population. Strabismus surgery is the most common pediatric eye surgery performed. The goal of this procedure is to correct the ocular misalignment caused by this condition. This can be achieved by several methods: (1) **weakening the muscles** (either by recession or marginal myotomy); (2) **strengthening the muscles**, by shortening their length (resection), moving the muscle's insertion toward the limbus (advancement), or tightening the muscle's fibers (plication or tuck); or (3) by **transposing the muscles**. Surgery can be performed on any of the four recti muscles (medial rectus, lateral rectus, superior rectus, and lateral rectus muscle) or the two oblique muscles (superior oblique and inferior oblique).

Often, **forced duction testing (FDT)** is performed during surgery to help differentiate a paretic muscle vs a restriction that may limit motility. The eyes should be immobile during FDT as well as during surgery. If succinylcholine has been used, at least 20 min should pass before performing duction testing, since succinylcholine causes contraction of extraocular muscles. Alternatively, a different muscle relaxant may be used.

Eye position under GA is well documented: the eyes will become more divergent and this tendency is increased in misaligned eyes; therefore, exotropic eyes appear more outwardly deviated and esotropic (inward deviation) eyes actually appear straighter (less esotropic).

The surgery usually is performed through one of two possible approaches. The **limbal incision** is made at the junction of the cornea and the conjunctiva, with radial relaxing incisions in the quadrants on either side of the muscle. The other is a **fornix** or **cul-de-sac incision**, which is made ~8 mm from the limbus in the quadrant beside the muscle. Comfort and cosmesis immediately postop are superior with the fornix incision.

Variant procedure or approaches: In very cooperative older children, an **adjustable suture** technique may be used. Unlike fixed sutures, an adjustable suture involves temporarily positioning the muscle, but not finally tying it down until the patient is awake. Once the patient is free of the effects of anesthesia, measurements are retaken, and the muscle is placed in its optimum position, to properly align the eyes, and then securely tied down. This adjustment may be performed the same day of surgery or the following day. **Adjustable strabismus surgery** ideally reduces the frequency of reoperations by eliminating undesirable early postop undercorrections or overcorrections and increases the rate of surgical success.

Although GA is most commonly used, strabismus surgery may be done using a **retrobulbar block**, or **peribulbar block** (sub-tenon's anesthesia), or even under topical anesthesia. Both topical and peribulbar anesthesia have the advantage of providing good akinesia and anesthesia but without the risks associated with a retrobulbar injection (e.g., hemorrhage, optic nerve damage, ocular perforation). When using topical anesthesia, this may be augmented by the use of minimal sedation and/or antianxiety medications.

Usual preop diagnosis: Strabismus

SUMMARY OF PROCEDURE

Position	Supine
Incision	Limbal or fornix
Antibiotics	Topical and/or subconjunctival antibiotics at completion of case
Unique considerations	Ask surgeons if they want neuromuscular blockade. If using succinylcholine, would need to wait 20 min before doing FDT. Keep patient under stable anesthesia, so the eyes are immobile and not drifting. Postop vomiting is common after strabismus surgery, with an incidence of 40-88%.
Surgical time	Dependent on type of surgery and number of muscles; usually 30-90 min.
EBL	Minimal
Mortality	Rare
Morbidity	Failure to achieve desired alignment
	Infection
	Hemorrhage
	Anterior segment ischemia
Postop care	PACU with discharge home within a few h. Typically no eye patches
Pain Score	2-4

PATIENT POPULATION CHARACTERISTICS

Age range	Children (most common)
Male:Female	1:1
Incidence	~5% of population
Etiology	Generally idiopathic; muscle palsies may be associated with trauma, inflammation, tumors, and/or ischemia; restrictive strabismus may occur with thyroid disease (Graves), fibrosis syndromes, or 2° to a scleral buckle or mass.
Associated conditions	↑incidence in premature infants, small-for-gestational-age infants, those with a positive family Hx of strabismus, craniosynostosis syndromes, or associated CNS disease

---

ANESTHETIC CONSIDERATIONS

PREOPERATIVE

In children, strabismus is the most frequent ophthalmic condition requiring surgical repair. Although most patients with this condition are otherwise healthy, there is an increased incidence of strabismus in children with cerebral palsy or meningomyelocele with hydrocephalus. Unlike many adult eye surgeries, which can be performed under regional anesthesia (retrobulbar or peribulbar block), in children, GA is almost always required to ensure good surgical conditions. The anesthesiologist should be aware of the potential problems that are associated with strabismus surgery, including: increased risk of malignant hyperthermia (MH); occurrence of the oculocardiac reflex (OCR); and increased incidence of postop N/V. It has been noted that individuals at risk for MH often have musculoskeletal abnormalities, such as strabismus or ptosis. It is, therefore, important to obtain a thorough family Hx of anesthetic problems. Avoid the use of succinylcholine since it can induce a tonic contracture of the extraocular muscles, which can interfere with the FDT. The surgeon performs the FDT by grasping the sclera of the operative eye and moving it into each field of gaze in order to determine if the strabismus is a result of paretic or restrictive extraocular muscles. This helps in forming the surgical plan.

Anesthetic technique: GETA, LMA

Induction	Following standard pediatric induction (p. D-2), a vagolytic dose of atropine (0.02 mg/kg) or glycopyrrolate (0.01 mg/kg) may be given to attenuate oculocardiac and oculorespiratory reflexes. The use of sevoflurane as an inhalation agent, however, significantly decreases the occurrence of these two vagally mediated responses.[2] FDT may be performed by the surgeon at this time, before the use of muscle relaxants. At completion, NMRs (e.g., rocuronium 0.6 mg/kg) can be used to assist ET intubation.
Maintenance	Techniques can include either inhalation agents or TIVA. The use of N_2O may ↑ risk for PONV, despite use of prophylactic antiemetics.[7] If a propofol drip is used, suggested dose ranges are 150-175 μg/kg/min. Postop analgesia should include fentanyl (1-2 μg/kg) and acetaminophen (30-40 mg/kg pr × 1). Preferred antiemetic medications include ondansetron (0.2-0.4 mg/kg up to 4 mg) and metoclopramide (0.15 mg/kg), ± dexamethasone (1 mg/kg up to 20 mg); used alone or in combination.
Emergence	In specific cases, the surgeon may request 'deep extubation.' Care should be taken to ensure control of airway.
Blood and fluid requirements	IV: 20-22 ga NS/LR to replace calculated deficit and maintain requirements.
Monitoring	Standard monitors (see p. B-1). Temperature
Positioning	Supine or supine with shoulder roll.
Complications	Oculocardiac reflex (OCR)/oculorespiratory reflex (ORR)	Traction on extraocular muscles can result in vagally mediated slowing of HR (> 20% of baseline), ± junctional, ventricular, or supraventricular arrhythmias. Additionally, decreases in spontaneous ventilation may occur.[1] Both of these complications are significantly decreased with use of sevoflurane anesthesia. OCR/ORR tend to fatigue with repeated manipulation. Treatment includes release of

Complications, cont.

	tension on extraocular muscles and administration of vagolytic agents (atropine or glycopyrrolate).
Malignant hyperthermia (MH)	Consider MH if the following are noted: unexplained tachycardia; ↑ETCO$_2$; muscular rigidity, masseter spasm; ↑temperature (a late sign). To evaluate, obtain ABGs. MH produces ↓PaO$_2$, ↑PaCO$_2$, ↑K$^+$, and acidosis. If MH is suspected, stop anesthetics and change anesthetic tubing and CO$_2$ absorbent. Stop surgery as soon as possible, hyperventilate patient with 100% O$_2$, treat acidosis with bicarbonate, and treat hyperkalemia (e.g., 15 U regular insulin/50 g glucose). Give dantrolene 2.5 mg/kg iv as soon as possible. Also cool the patient and maintain UO. Further doses of dantrolene may be necessary (can give up to 10 mg/kg).
Accidental extubation	Surgical repositioning or removal of surgical drapes may result in accidental extubation. ETT should be firmly secured and anesthesiologist should be attentive to changes in positioning or removal of drapes.

POSTOPERATIVE

Complications	PONV	See above for rescue doses of antiemetics.
	MH	See above.
Pain management	Continue po acetaminophen (10-12 mg/kg q 4) + antiemetics as needed.	Occasional need of opioid analgesics.

References

1. Alexander JP: Reflex disturbances of cardiac rhythm during ophthalmic surgery. *Brit J Ophthal* 1975; 59(9):518-23.
2. Alison CE, Delange JJ, Koole FD, Zuurmond WW, Ros HH, vanSchagen NT: A comparison of the incidence of the oculocardiac and oculorespiratory reflexes during sevoflurane and halothane anesthesia for strabismus surgery in children. *Anesth Analg* 2000; 90(2):306-10.
3. Braun U, Feise J, Muhlendyck H: Is there a cholinergic and adrenergic phase of the oculocardiac reflex during strabismus surgery? *Acta Anaesthesiol Scand* 1993; 37(4):390-5.
4. France NK, France TD, Woodburn JD, et al: Succinylcholine alteration of the forced duction test. *Ophthalmol* 1980; 87(2): 1282-7.
5. Hill R, et al: Cost effectiveness of prophylactic antiemetic therapy with ondansetron, droperidol or placebo. *Anesthesiology* 2000; 92(4):958-67.
6. Tramer M, Moore A, McQuay H: Prevention of vomiting after paediatric strabismus surgery: A systematic review using the numbers-needed-to-treat method. *Br J Anaesth* 1995; 75(5):556-61.
7. Watcha M, Simeon R, White PF, Stevens J: Effect of propofol on the incidence of postoperative vomiting after strabismus surgery in pediatric outpatients. *Anesthesiology* 1991; 75(2):204-9.

Surgeons

Anna H. Messner, MD
Kay W. Chang, MD

12.3 PEDIATRIC OTOLARYNGOLOGY

Anesthesiologists

Cathy R. Lammers, MD
Gregory B. Hammer, MD

PEDIATRIC OTOLARYNGOLOGY

INTRODUCTION—SURGEON'S PERSPECTIVE

ANESTHESIOLOGIST/SURGEON COOPERATION

Pediatric otolaryngology/head and neck surgery procedures frequently involve the oral cavity, pharynx, larynx, and tracheobronchial tree. This can result in competition for the airway between the anesthesiologist and the pediatric otolaryngologist. Preop, a ventilation plan should be discussed and agreed upon to avoid a poor outcome. Neither specialist should assume that the other intuitively knows which combination of anesthesia and ventilation is best for an individual case. Frequently, the table will be turned 90° during the procedure. Close communication must be maintained throughout the procedure.

TUBE POSITIONING

Many head and neck procedures require turning of the head during the procedure. This necessitates that the tube be securely fastened to the face, but not tightly anchored to the bed or chest. Delays can be avoided if the anesthesiologist and surgeon have discussed the positioning of the ETT (nasal or oral, taped to the left corner of mouth, etc.) preop.

SPONTANEOUS VENTILATION AND MUSCLE RELAXATION

If vocal cord function is to be visualized or the trachea examined for tracheomalacia, spontaneous ventilation of the patient is preferred. In some head and neck cases—such as parotidectomy and mastoidectomy—muscle relaxation is contraindicated to avoid interference with facial nerve monitoring, and so that facial movements can be seen. In other cases—such as esophagoscopy—muscle relaxation aids the surgeon in passing the esophagoscope through the cricopharyngeus. It is always best to discuss the use of muscle relaxants preop.

LASER CASES

If any foreign object, such as an ETT, is in the airway, the FiO_2 should not be raised above 0.3, to avoid an airway fire. All OR personnel need to be prepared to wear protective glasses during the case.

MYRINGOTOMY AND TYMPANOSTOMY TUBE PLACEMENT

SURGICAL CONSIDERATIONS

Description: Tympanostomy (PE or pressure equalizing) tubes are placed in the patient with chronic serous otitis media (fluid in the middle ear for > 3 mo) or recurrent acute otitis media (6 or more episodes of otitis media over the prior yr). Occasionally, PE tubes are placed in a child with meningitis of otitic origin or with acute otitis media that is unresponsive to antibiotics. The patient is supine and the OR table in the 0-degree position. The microscope is positioned over the bed and the head turned to expose the ear. An ear speculum is inserted into the ear canal, cerumen is removed, and an incision is made in the tympanic membrane. Fluid is sometimes suctioned from the middle ear; then, a tympanostomy tube is inserted into the ear, straddling the tympanic membrane. Antibiotic ear drops frequently are inserted into the external auditory canal. The surgeon changes to the other side of the table, the microscope is repositioned, the head is turned, and the procedure is repeated on the other ear.

Usual preop diagnosis: Chronic serous otitis media; acute otitis media

SUMMARY OF PROCEDURE

Position	Supine; head to anesthesia
Incision	Tympanic membrane
Special instrumentation	Operating microscope
Antibiotics	No parenteral antibiotics (except for SBE prophylaxis); topical antibiotic ear drops
Surgical time	10-20 min. Patients with small ear canals (e.g., Down syndrome) can take longer.
EBL	None

Postop care	PACU → home
Mortality	Rare
Morbidity	Bleeding from ear
	Purulent drainage from ear (otorrhea)
Pain score	1-3

PATIENT POPULATION CHARACTERISTICS

Age range	3 mo+ (most common, 1-3 yr)
Male:Female	1:1
Incidence	Most common surgical procedure requiring GA
Etiology	Chronic middle ear infections
Associated conditions	Cleft palate

ANESTHETIC CONSIDERATIONS

PREOPERATIVE

The majority of children presenting for PE tubes are < 3 yr and generally in good health. Many of these children, however, have recurrent URI, which contributes to edema of the eustachian tubes, predisposing to episodes of acute otitis media. Intervals between URI may be brief, and scheduling surgery during these interludes is often impractical. Children with mild URI generally can be anesthetized safely for PE tube placement if tracheal intubation is not performed. Surgery should be delayed for patients with acute, febrile illnesses, and in those with Sx referable to the lower airways (e.g., productive cough, wheezing). Surgery should not be delayed if fever is 2° acute otitis media.

Respiratory	Surgery in patients with URI Sx referable to the extrathoracic airway alone is generally not delayed. These Sx include nasal congestion and/or discharge and mild conjunctivitis. Fever, productive cough, and wheezing are Sx of lower respiratory tract involvement and should prompt rescheduling of the procedure 2-3 wk after these Sx have abated. In borderline cases (e.g., those with rales auscultated on chest exam but no other lower tract Sx), O_2 sat may be measured by pulse oximetry. Procedures in patients with SpO_2 < 95% should be deferred.
Laboratory	None
Premedication	Some practitioners advocate withholding premedication, as the duration of action of the premed may outlast the surgery. In general, however, we administer oral midazolam syrup to patients > 9-12 mo (see p. D-2) and have not found a significant, related delay in discharge from PACU. Alternatively, acetaminophen with codeine (1 mg/kg) may be given to provide mild sedation and postop analgesia.

INTRAOPERATIVE

Anesthetic technique: GA via face mask

Induction	A standard inhalation induction with sevoflurane or halothane, N_2O, and O_2 is performed with routine monitoring. An oral airway commonly is inserted, as soft tissue obstruction may occur when the head is turned fully to the side during surgery. CPAP 5-8 cmH_2O also may be useful in maintaining airway patency. Following induction, a one-time loading dose of rectal acetaminophen (30-40 mg/kg) may be given for postop analgesia. (↓ rectal dose if po acetaminophen is given at home or as premedication.)
Maintenance	If sevoflurane was used for induction, consider switching to isoflurane. Marked agitation has been noted following emergence from sevoflurane, unless fentanyl and/or midazolam have been used for premedication. An iv catheter is not placed routinely.
Emergence	For bilateral procedures, the inhalational anesthetic is D/C'd before or during the 2nd myringotomy to facilitate prompt emergence. N_2O is continued until the completion of surgery. As the patient is awakening, gentle oropharyngeal suctioning is performed.
Blood and fluid requirements	None
Monitoring	Standard monitors (see p. D-1).

Positioning	✓ and pad pressure points.	
	✓ eyes.	
Complications	Laryngospasm	Secretions → laryngospasm 2° irritation of the vocal cords, especially in children with URI. Rx: 100% O_2 and CPAP or manual ventilation with PEEP ≤ 20-25 cmH$_2$O. Rarely, succinylcholine (2-4 mg/kg im) may be needed if a significant decrease in SpO$_2$ occurs and ventilation is not possible. Atropine (0.01-0.02 mg/kg) should be given in the same syringe to mitigate the bradycardia associated with succinylcholine. Oropharyngeal suctioning and manual ventilation usually result in resolution of the laryngospasm. Rarely, tracheal intubation may be indicated for recurrent laryngospasm.

POSTOPERATIVE

Complications	Laryngospasm	Laryngospasm may occur, and should be treated as described above.
Pain management	Acetaminophen 10-15 mg/kg po ± Codeine 1 mg/kg or hydrocodone 0.15 mg/kg	Consider previously administered po and/or pr dosing.

References

1. Tait AR, Knight PR: The effects of general anesthesia on upper respiratory tract infections in children. *Anesthesiology* 1987; 67:930-5.
2. Tobias JD, Lowe S, Hersey S, et al: Analgesia after bilateral myringotomy and placement of pressure equalization tubes in children: acetaminophen vs acetaminophen with codeine. *Anesth Analg* 1995; 81:496-500.

TONSILLECTOMY AND ADENOIDECTOMY

SURGICAL CONSIDERATIONS

Description: The dissection is carried out with the patient supine, shoulders elevated by a shoulder roll (typically, a rolled towel), and head stabilized by a 'doughnut.' A mouth gag is inserted, and a small suction catheter is passed through the nose and brought out the mouth to elevate the soft palate and expose the nasopharynx. The adenoids are viewed with a mirror and/or palpated. A curette, adenotome, or suction Bovie is used to remove the adenoids; then, typically, the nasopharynx is packed. The tonsillectomy is performed by grasping the tonsil with Allis forceps and drawing it medially. A vertical incision is made in the anterior tonsillar pillar with a sickle knife, scissors, or electrocautery instruments; then, the tonsil is dissected from the surrounding tissue and removed. A snare may be used to amputate the inferior pole of the tonsil before removal. Hemostasis is obtained through use of packs and suction electrocautery. After hemostasis has been obtained in the tonsillar fossae, the pack is removed from the nasopharynx, and hemostasis is achieved in the nasopharynx using suction electrocautery.

Usual preop diagnosis: Obstructive sleep apnea (OSA); chronic tonsillitis and/or adenoiditis; tonsillar and adenoid hypertrophy; asymmetric enlargement of tonsils (to r/o cancer)

SUMMARY OF PROCEDURE

Position	Supine, shoulder roll, head extended; table turned 90°; surgeon at head of table
Incision	Intraoral mucosal
Special instrumentation	Mouth gag (McIvor, Crowe-Davis, Dingman)

Unique considerations	Observe for compression of ETT or accidental extubation when mouth gag is manipulated. Patients with Down syndrome must be evaluated preop for possible atlantoaxial subluxation, as the neck is typically extended. Steroids (e.g., dexamethasone 0.5-1 mg/kg) used routinely by some practitioners.
Antibiotics	Not used routinely.
Surgical time	30-60 min
EBL	10-200 ml. Monitor closely.
Postop care	Lateral position; suction in midline only. Most commonly, PACU → home. Overnight stay, if < 2 yr.
Mortality	Rare
Morbidity	Bleeding: 2-3%
	Aspiration: Rare
	Tooth damage: Rare
Pain score	Adenoidectomy, 3-5; tonsillectomy, 6-9

PATIENT POPULATION CHARACTERISTICS

Age range	1 yr+ (most common, 2-8 yr)
Male:Female	1:1
Incidence	500,000 cases/yr in U.S.
Etiology	OSA; chronic infection; peritonsillar abscess; snoring. (R/O lymphoma, carcinoma, lympho-proliferative disease.)
Associated conditions	Down syndrome

ANESTHETIC CONSIDERATIONS

PREOPERATIVE

While most children presenting for tonsillectomy and/or adenoidectomy are healthy, a variety of related medical problems may exist. Severe adenoidal hyperplasia may cause nasopharyngeal obstruction, obligate mouth breathing, failure to thrive 2° poor feeding, and disturbances of speech and sleep. Chronic nasal obstruction may result in narrowing of the upper airway and dental and facial changes (so-called 'adenoidal facies'). Tonsillar hyperplasia may cause airway obstruction, OSA, CO_2 retention and cor pulmonale, and failure to thrive. Most of these changes are reversible with removal of the adenoids and tonsils. Children presenting for adenoidectomy/tonsillectomy also frequently have URI (see Myringotomy and Tympanostomy Tube Placement, p. 955).

Respiratory	See discussion under Anesthetic Considerations for Myringotomy and Tympanostomy Tube Placement, p. 955.
Dental	Examination of the airway should include inspection of the teeth; and parents should be advised that loose teeth may be dislodged during placement of the mouth gag or laryngoscopy.
Cardiovascular	In children with severe OSA, CXR and ECG should be done to evaluate the presence of cor pulmonale. If significant RVH and/or cardiomegaly are present, consider ECHO and consultation by pediatric cardiologist.
Hematologic	A careful Hx is taken for Sx of easy bruising or bleeding. If present, a CBC with Plt count, as well as PT, PTT, and bleeding time are performed. In patients with a negative Hx, we order no preop lab tests.
Premedication	Children with severe OSA (airway obstruction) generally should not be premedicated. Patients who are very anxious may receive a reduced dose of oral midazolam (see p. D-2) in a well monitored environment (e.g., with an experienced RN or member of the anesthesia team present). SpO_2 should be monitored, if possible, following administration of premedication.

INTRAOPERATIVE

Anesthetic technique: GETA

Induction	A standard inhalational induction (see p. D-2); however, airway obstruction during induction is common in these patients, and usually is alleviated with placement of an oral airway and administration of CPAP 10-20 cmH$_2$O. An iv catheter should be placed as soon as possible to

Induction, cont.	facilitate administration of muscle relaxant ± glycopyrrolate (4-6 μg/kg) to reduce oral secretions. For patients with severe OSA, consider iv induction to facilitate prompt placement of the ETT. An oral RAE ETT is used and taped securely in the midline position to facilitate placement of the mouth gag. A cuffed ETT may be desirable because, in combination with a throat pack, it minimizes the risk of entry of blood and oral secretions into the trachea during surgery. Bilateral breath sounds and chest excursion should be confirmed after placement of the mouth gag, which may cause kinking and obstruction of the ETT. Acetaminophen (30-40 mg/kg) may be given pr after induction. (↓ dose if po acetaminophen given with premedications.)	
Maintenance	Standard maintenance (see p. D-3). An intermediate-acting NMR (e.g., vecuronium 0.1 mg/kg or rocuronium 0.6-1.0 mg/kg) is given to facilitate tracheal intubation. Opioids (e.g., fentanyl 2-3 μg/kg, morphine sulfate 0.1-0.15 mg/kg) are given for postop analgesia. The use of propofol, ± remifentanil, instead of anesthetic vapor, may ↓ the incidence of PONV, which is common following tonsillectomy/adenoidectomy. Administration of ondansetron (0.1 mg/kg, up to 4 mg) is controversial due to some evidence that it can mask postop bleeding, with retained blood in the stomach.	
Emergence	Blood and secretions should be suctioned from the oropharynx and stomach following the completion of surgery. The patient should be fully awake before tracheal extubation, which may be performed supine or in the lateral position with the head down. Verify removal of throat packs. Alternatively, extubating deep under anesthesia decreases coughing, but requires vigilance to avoid airway obstruction and aspiration at emergence and during transport to PACU.	
Blood and fluid requirements	IV: 22 or 20 ga × 1 NS/LR @ 5-10 ml/h	Blood loss is typically ~4 ml/kg and may accumulate in the stomach → N/V.
Monitoring	Standard monitors (see p. D-1).	
Positioning	✓ and pad pressure points. ✓ eyes.	
Complications	Airway obstruction ETT dislodgement/kinking	Usually caused by insertion/manipulation of mouth gag.

POSTOPERATIVE

Complications	Airway obstruction	Retention of throat pack → airway obstruction. Remove with Magill forceps. Recurrent airway obstruction may require application of positive pressure via face mask (CPAP vs manual ventilation with PEEP) ± placement of an oral airway. Severe postop airway obstruction is more common in patients < 2 yr. In these patients, admission to PICU may be necessary. CPAP via face mask or nasal mask may be helpful. On rare occasion, tracheal intubation and mechanical ventilation are required until swelling of the airway resolves.
	Hemorrhage	Bleeding may occur in the immediate postop period or several d later. Patients present with anemia and hypovolemia, as well as airway compromise and a full stomach 2° swallowed blood. IV fluid, including blood, should be given before induction. Rapid-sequence intubation (p. B-5) should be performed with cricoid pressure in preparation for surgical treatment.
Pain management	Morphine 0.025-0.05 mg/kg	May be given incrementally in PACU. Subsequently, acetaminophen with codeine 1 mg/kg or hydrocodone 0.15 mg/kg is given. Local anesthetic injection by the surgeon into the tonsillar and adenoidal beds ↓ postop opiod requirements.

References

1. Colclasure JB, Grahamm SS: Complications of outpatient tonsillectomy and adenoidectomy: a review of 3,340 cases. *Ear Nose Throat J* 1990; 69:155-60.

2. Linden BE, Gross CW, Long TE, et al: Morbidity in pediatric tonsillectomy. *Laryngoscope* 1990; 100:120-4.
3. Mather SJ, Peurtrell JM: Postoperative morphine requirements, nausea and vomiting following anaesthesia for tonsillectomy. Comparison of intravenous morphine and non-opioid analgesic techniques. *Paediatr Anaesth* 1995; 5:185-8.

BRONCHOSCOPY/ESOPHAGOSCOPY

SURGICAL CONSIDERATIONS

Description: Flexible bronchoscopy is performed when the dynamics of the larynx and trachea need to be visualized. The child is supine on the OR table, which is turned 90°-180°. With the child sedated or under GA, but breathing spontaneously, the bronchoscope is passed through the nose into the pharynx by way of an adapter attached to a standard anesthesia mask. The larynx is viewed with the patient breathing spontaneously so that vocal cord movement can be observed; then the anesthesia is deepened and the bronchoscope passed into the trachea. The trachea and bronchi are viewed and, when indicated, bronchoalveolar lavage or bronchial biopsy can be performed.

Rigid bronchoscopy is preferred when direct ventilation of the trachea is required and/or when foreign bodies (FBs) need to be removed. It also can be used for Dx of airway lesions. Direct laryngoscopy is performed; then the rigid bronchoscope is passed through the vocal cords into the trachea. The anesthesia tubing is connected to the bronchoscope and the patient is ventilated through the scope. If a FB is present, the telescope within the bronchoscope will be removed and optical forceps inserted through the bronchoscope to remove the FB. During the time when the telescope is being changed, a leak will be present in the ventilation system.

Usual preop diagnosis: Airway obstruction; bronchial FB; pneumonia (requiring bronchoalveolar lavage); tracheal or bronchial lesion

Flexible or rigid esophagoscopy can be performed for diagnostic or therapeutic (removal of FB) purposes. Flexible esophagoscopy can be performed under sedation; however, GETA is preferred for rigid esophagoscopy. The esophagoscope is inserted through the mouth into the esophagus, and the entire length of the esophagus is viewed. If a FB is to be removed with the rigid esophagoscope, the telescope and forceps are passed through the lumen of the esophagoscope. If a FB (especially food stuff) is to be removed with the flexible esophagoscope, the scope may need to be passed several times.

Esophageal dilation may be performed in one of several ways. Balloon dilation can be performed with the flexible esophagoscope. Alternatively, a guide wire can be passed through the esophagoscope, then Savary/Gilliard dilators, in successively larger sizes, are passed over the wire. Another option is to remove the esophagoscope after the stenosis has been visualized; then, Maloney or Hurst dilators are passed blindly through the mouth and into the esophagus. Care must be taken to avoid accidental extubation of the patient while the dilators are being inserted and removed.

Usual preop diagnosis: GERD; esophageal FB; esophageal stricture

SUMMARY OF PROCEDURES

	Bronchoscopy	Esophagoscopy
Position	Patient supine; table turned 90°	⇐
Unique considerations	Ventilate through rigid bronchoscope. Ventilate via mask with adapter for flexible bronchoscope. Dexamethasone (0.7-1 mg/kg) may be indicated, if glottic or subglottic edema is present.	Observe for accidental extubation. ETT taped to left side of mouth.
Antibiotics	None	⇐
Surgical time	10 min-1.5 h	15 min-1 h
EBL	None	< 10 ml
Postop care	Watch for airway compromise; PACU.	PACU
Mortality	Rare	⇐

	Bronchoscopy	**Esophagoscopy**
Morbidity	Laryngospasm	Esophageal perforation
	Laryngeal edema	Bleeding
	Dental trauma	⇐
Pain score	3-4	3-4

PATIENT POPULATION CHARACTERISTICS

Age range	Newborn+
Male:Female	1:1
Incidence	Common
Associated conditions	Bronchoscopy requiring bronchial alveolar lavage (BAL): immunocompromised patient
	Esophageal stricture: tracheoesophageal fistula (TEF)
	Esophageal FB: esophageal stricture

ANESTHETIC CONSIDERATIONS

See Anesthetic Considerations following Laryngoscopy, Supraglottoplasty, Excision of Laryngeal Lesions, p. 961.

LARYNGOSCOPY, SUPRAGLOTTOPLASTY, EXCISION OF LARYNGEAL LESIONS

SURGICAL CONSIDERATIONS

Description: Flexible laryngoscopy typically is performed in the clinic setting, but may be performed in the OR in an unstable or uncooperative child. The patient should be breathing spontaneously, and will be in a sitting (with support) or supine position. Topical anesthesia and vasoconstrictors are applied to the nose; then the scope is passed through the nose into the pharynx, and the larynx is viewed. Vocal cord function is best assessed with the child only mildly sedated.

Diagnostic direct laryngoscopy is performed with the child in a supine position, table turned 90°, with a small shoulder roll in place. The laryngoscope is introduced and, with a lifting motion, a thorough exam of the oropharynx, hypopharynx, and larynx is performed. If more than a brief exam is to take place, the vocal cords are anesthetized with topical lidocaine to help prevent laryngospasm. A telescope (often connected via camera to a video monitor) may be passed through the vocal cords to observe the trachea and major bronchi.

Microlaryngoscopy with removal/ablation of laryngeal lesions—most commonly papillomas, nodules, or polyps—is accomplished by suspending the laryngoscope from the Mayo stand or OR table, using a suspension apparatus. The patient continues to breath spontaneously or is paralyzed and jet ventilated. When the laser is used, the patient's eyes and face are covered with a damp cloth. OR personnel must wear protective glasses. A microscope with the laser attached is positioned so that the laser beam passes through the laryngoscope onto the vocal folds.

Young infants with severe laryngomalacia may undergo a **supraglottoplasty** for relief of airway obstruction. The laryngoscope is suspended and the laser or microlaryngeal instruments are used to remove redundant aryepiglottic fold tissue.

Usual preop diagnosis: Diagnostic laryngoscopy: hoarseness; airway obstruction; stridor. Operative laryngoscopy: laryngeal papillomas; laryngeal nodules; laryngeal web; laryngeal polyps; subglottic hemangioma or cysts; severe laryngomalacia

SUMMARY OF PROCEDURE

Position	Supine; table turned 90°; shoulder roll
Special instrumentation	± Jet ventilation; laryngoscope suspension apparatus; video equipment; operating microscope

Unique considerations	Potential laser precautions; patient usually not intubated; dexamethasone 0.7-1.0 mg/kg to prevent laryngeal edema; laryngeal topical lidocaine 0.4 mg/kg.
Antibiotics	None
Surgical time	15-90 min
EBL	< 5 ml
Postop care	Observe for airway obstruction in PACU.
Mortality	Rare
Morbidity	Laryngospasm
	Laryngeal edema
	Dental trauma
Pain score	3-5

PATIENT POPULATION CHARACTERISTICS

Age range	Newborn +
Male:Female	1:1
Incidence	Occasional
Etiology	Papillomas: Most commonly, viral infection contracted from mother during vaginal delivery)
	Nodules, polyps: Vocal abuse, gastropharyngeal reflux
	Subglottic hemangioma: Unknown
	Subglottic cyst: Prior intubation
	Laryngeal cysts, webs: Congenital malformation
	Laryngomalacia: Unknown
Associated conditions	Chronic hoarseness, stridor; GERD; FTT

ANESTHETIC CONSIDERATIONS

(Procedures covered: bronchoscopy; esophagoscopy; laryngoscopy; supraglottoplasty; excision of laryngeal lesions)

PREOPERATIVE

Direct laryngoscopy (DL) is performed most commonly for patients with stridor. In infants, stridor is most often 2° laryngomalacia, with vocal cord paralysis being less common. Patients with severe laryngomalacia and those with posttransplant lymphoproliferative disease involving the epiglottis may undergo supraglottoplasty. Older children may present with stridor 2° laryngeal masses or papillomatosis, for which laser excision may be performed. A careful H&P is contributory to Dx, after which flexible laryngoscopy in the ENT clinic can be confirmatory.

Laryngoscopy and **rigid bronchoscopy** also are performed for the removal of airway foreign bodies (FBs). A Hx of choking and/or coughing while eating is usually elicited. Children may present with agitation, wheezing, and cyanosis. This condition constitutes a true surgical emergency and the patient should be taken to the OR as soon as possible.

Airway/ Respiratory	Stridor usually is worsened with crying or agitation, and often less severe during sleep.
Dental	Any loose teeth may be dislodged.
Laboratory	No routine tests indicated. In stable patients with suspected FB aspiration, CXR may be obtained.
Premedication	Because stridor often is decreased during quiet breathing and sleep, premedication with oral midazolam is usually beneficial in patients > 9-12 mo. Children with FB aspiration generally should not be given po medications. They may benefit from small doses of iv midazolam. EMLA or ELA-max cream (4% lidocaine in a special base) may be applied 45 or 20 min (respectively) in advance to iv sites for topical anesthesia.

INTRAOPERATIVE

Anesthetic technique: GA. Primary and backup plans for airway management during the procedure should be discussed in detail with the ENT surgeon in advance of anesthetic induction.

Induction	Mask induction is followed by placement of an iv catheter, if not already in place. In cases where vocal cord function must be evaluated, spontaneous breathing is maintained under halothane or sevoflurane in 100% O_2. Alternatively, continuous infusion of propofol (50-100 μg/kg/min and remifentanil (0.05-1 μg/kg/min) may be used.

Maintenance	Prior to removal of the face mask for DL, a deep level of anesthesia is achieved. During DL, blow-by O_2 is administered.	

For patients in whom vocal cord function must be assessed, gradual offset of inhalational anesthesia should → ↑vocal cord excursion. Supraglottoplasty and laser excision of laryngeal lesions may be performed with intermittent mask anesthesia. Propofol with or without remifentanil may be used, thereby avoiding contamination of the OR with anesthetic vapor while providing continuous anesthesia. In general, the trachea is not intubated, as even a small ETT will interfere with the surgical procedure. Muscle relaxant may be given and jet ventilation maintained using a Sanders jet ventilator (see Fig 3-4, p. 151). Intermittent jets of 100% O_2 are delivered with a high-pressure (40-55 psi) gas source through a tube incorporated into the laryngoscope blade. As the jet is pointed toward the glottic opening, gas is entrained by the Venturi effect. Manual ventilation is performed while chest excursion is observed to ensure that excessive inflating pressures and volumes are avoided. During jet ventilation, anesthesia is maintained with iv agents. Propofol 150-200 μg/kg/min is infused with remifentanil 0.15-0.40 μg/kg/min. (Remifentanil 0.1 mg is added to each 10 ml of propofol in a single syringe; e.g., for a propofol infusion of 100 μg/kg/min, remifentanil 0.1 μg/kg/min is delivered.)

★ **NB:** fire hazard during laser surgery is minimal in the absence of a combustible material (e.g., plastic) in the field. An FiO_2 of 1.0 may, therefore, be used safely, unless a plastic ETT is in place. For selected laser procedures involving the tissues around the glottis, a metal or metal-wrapped ETT may be used. When a plastic ETT is in place, the lowest possible FiO_2 is used (O_2/air mixture) to maintain an acceptable SpO_2.

During rigid bronchoscopy, ventilation is performed through a side port of the bronchoscope. Assisted, spontaneous ventilation under deep inhalational anesthesia may be maintained. Alternatively, iv anesthesia and muscle relaxation may be preferred, as described above. For FB cases, maintenance of spontaneous ventilation generally is preferred to avoid distal displacement of the FB. Gentle, assisted ventilation may be required, however, to ensure adequate oxygenation and ventilation.

Emergence	A conventional ETT sometimes is placed after removal of the laryngoscope or bronchoscope, as laryngospasm following these procedures is common. Tracheal extubation is performed with the patient fully awake and following complete reversal of neuromuscular blockade, if applicable.	
Blood and fluid requirements	IV: 22 ga × 1 NS/LR @ 3-5 ml/kg/h	Blood loss is minimal.
Monitoring	Standard monitors (see p. D-1).	
Positioning	Table rotated 90° ✓ and pad pressure points. ✓ eyes.	Shoulder roll/neck extension for surgery Eyes covered with wet sponges or goggles when laser in use.
Complications	Hypoventilation Hypoxemia Airway injury Pneumothorax Laryngospasm Eye injury Airway fire	Adjust Sanders jet; mask ventilation prn. 2° jet ventilation, DL/bronchoscope Rx: 100% O_2, CPAP vs manual ventilation/PEEP Remove ETT; irrigate with NS; resume ventilation with 100% O_2 when fire extinguished.

POSTOPERATIVE

Complications	Dental trauma Bleeding Eye trauma Pneumothorax	
Pain management	Acetaminophen (10-15 mg/kg) ± Hydrocodone 0.15 mg/kg or codeine 1 mg/kg q 4 h	
Tests	CXR	If respiratory distress, ↓SpO_2 present.

References

1. Weeks DG: Laboratory and clinical description of the use of jet-Venturi ventilator during laser microsurgery of the glottis and subglottis. *Anesth Rev* 1985; 12:32-6.
2. Zalzal GH: Stridor and airway compromise. *Pediatr Clin North Am* 1989; 36:1389-1402.

REMOVAL OF BRANCHIAL CLEFT CYST OR THYROGLOSSAL DUCT CYST

SURGICAL CONSIDERATIONS

Description: Branchial cleft cysts and tracts typically present in the lateral neck; thyroglossal duct cysts, in the midline. Removal consists of making an incision in the neck around the opening of the tract (if present), or over the palpable cyst, and following the tract superiorly to its origin. A **Sistrunk procedure** is performed in the case of a thyroglossal duct cyst, and involves the removal of the middle section of the hyoid bone.

Usual preop diagnosis: Branchial cleft cyst; thyroglossal duct cyst

SUMMARY OF PROCEDURE

Position	Supine; head 180° from anesthesia; oral intubation
Incision	Horizontal neck
Antibiotics	Clindamycin 12 mg/kg or cefazolin 25 mg/kg
Surgical time	45-90 min
EBL	10-50 ml
Postop care	Routine
Mortality	Rare
Morbidity	Bleeding/neck hematoma
	Infection
	Recurrence of cyst
	Damage to CN XI, XII
Pain score	4-6

PATIENT POPULATION CHARACTERISTICS

Age range	Newborn-adult
Male:Female	1:1
Etiology	Congenital
Associated conditions	Branchio-oto-renal (BOR) syndrome

ANESTHETIC CONSIDERATIONS

See Anesthetic Considerations following Incision/Drainage of Deep Neck Abscess, p. 964.

INCISION/DRAINAGE OF DEEP NECK ABSCESS

SURGICAL CONSIDERATIONS

Description: Children with deep neck abscesses (retropharyngeal, parapharyngeal, peritonsillar) are at risk for acute airway obstruction; therefore, the abscesses are drained on an emergent basis. Retropharyngeal and peritonsillar abscesses typically are drained through an intraoral approach; parapharyngeal abscesses, through an external neck approach. In each case, the child must be intubated orally and placed in the supine position. The anesthesiologist or otolaryngologist who is intubating the child must be prepared for abnormal pharyngeal anatomy 2° the abscess. Care must be taken that the abscess is not ruptured in the intubation process. A tracheotomy tray should be in the OR at the time of intubation. In most cases, the child can be extubated immediately after the abscess is drained; however, in a small number of cases, the child may need to remain intubated until the pharyngeal edema subsides.

Usual preop diagnosis: Retropharyngeal, parapharyngeal, or peritonsillar abscess

SUMMARY OF PROCEDURE

Position	Supine; table turned 90°-180°; oral intubation
Incision	Intraoral (retropharyngeal or peritonsillar abscess); lateral neck (parapharyngeal abscess)
Unique considerations	Acute airway obstruction can occur with induction. Care must be taken to avoid rupture of abscess on intubation; ± dexamethasone 1 mg/kg.
Antibiotics	Clindamycin 12 mg/kg
Surgical time	30-90 min
EBL	< 30 ml
Postop care	May remain intubated postop.
Mortality	Rare
Morbidity	Aspiration (if abscess ruptures spontaneously)
	Airway obstruction 2° aspiration or edema
	Bleeding
Pain score	5

PATIENT POPULATION CHARACTERISTICS

Age range	Most common, 6 mo-3 yr; can occur at any age.
Male:Female	1:1
Incidence	Uncommon
Etiology	URI

ANESTHETIC CONSIDERATIONS

(Procedures covered: excision of branchial cleft and thyroglossal duct cyst; incision/drainage of neck abscess)

PREOPERATIVE

These patients generally are otherwise healthy children. A cystic hygroma (cystic lymphangioma), as with other neck masses, may cause airway obstruction and difficult intubation.

Respiratory	The size and extent of the neck mass should be defined carefully in an effort to detect the potential for airway compromise and to avoid soft-tissue trauma during intubation, with consequent acute airway obstruction. Inspiratory stridor suggests supraglottic obstruction, while expiratory stridor is associated with subglottic/intrathoracic obstruction. These patients should have had prior CT/MRI imaging; scans and anesthesia records for these studies should be reviewed. **Tests:** CXR; CT/MRI
Cardiovascular	Cervical masses may be adherent to and/or cause compression of the great vessels. **Tests:** CT/MRI
Hematologic	T&C for cystic hygroma, or if a cervical mass involves great vessels or extends into the mediastinum. **Tests:** Hct
Laboratory	Other tests as indicated from H&P.

964

Premedication	If > 9-12 mo and asymptomatic, midazolam (0.5-0.75 mg po) 30 min prior to arrival in OR. Avoid all premedication in patients with significant potential for airway compromise.

INTRAOPERATIVE

Anesthetic technique: GETA

Induction	Standard pediatric induction (see p. D-2) in patients without airway compromise. When airway obstruction is present, iv should be secured prior to mask induction, which may be done with halothane or sevoflurane in 100% O_2. As plane of anesthesia deepens, gently assist ventilation. Give atropine (0.01-0.02 mg/kg iv) prior to laryngoscopy. If partial airway obstruction exists, maintain spontaneous ventilation with CPAP and perform laryngoscopy at ~3 MAC of volatile agent. FOB should be available. Have full range of ETT sizes available, since airway narrowing may be present. Once airway is secured, proceed with neuromuscular blockade (e.g., vecuronium 0.1 mg/kg or rocuronium 1.0 mg/kg).
Maintenance	Standard pediatric maintenance (see p. D-3). Surgeon may infiltrate incision with local anesthetic. Limit lidocaine to 5 mg/kg when used without epinephrine, or 7 mg/kg when used with epinephrine, and bupivacaine to 2.5 mg/kg.
Emergence	Reverse neuromuscular blockade with neostigmine (0.07 mg/kg iv) and atropine (0.02 mg/kg iv). Extubate when fully awake.

Blood and fluid requirements	Minimal blood loss
	IV: 20-22 ga × 1
	Great vessel involvement:
	  IV: 20 ga × 1-2
	  NS/LR @ 3 ml/kg/h
		Minimal 3rd-space losses. Each ml blood loss can be replaced with 3 ml NS/LR. When great vessels involved, place at least 1 iv in lower extremity. Blood loss can be quite sudden; have blood available in OR.

Monitoring	Standard monitors (see p. D-1). ± Arterial line, 22 ga	An arterial line is used when there is risk of large blood loss or periop airway compromise.
Positioning	✓ and pad pressure points. ✓ eyes.	
Complications	ETT dislodged/loss of airway Laryngospasm Bronchospasm Hemorrhage	ETT must be secured carefully. Liberal use of benzoin adherent. Avoid tension on ETT by circuit hoses. Hold ETT during surgeon's intraoral examination to prevent accidental extubation.

POSTOPERATIVE

Complications	Subglottic edema Upper airway obstruction from edema related to tumor resection Recurrent laryngeal nerve injury	Dexamethasone (0.5-1 mg/kg iv) and nebulized racemic epinephrine (1.25%) with mist O_2 to treat subglottic edema.
Pain management	Morphine (0.025-0.1 mg/kg iv q 2-4 h) Acetaminophen (10-15 mg/kg po/pr q 4 h)	The majority of these procedures are performed on outpatient basis (except cystic hygroma).

References

1. Gregory GA, ed: *Pediatric Anesthesia*, 4th edition. Churchill Livingstone, New York: 2002.
2. Motoyama EK, Davis PC, eds: *Smith's Anesthesia for Infants and Children*, 5th edition. CV Mosby, St. Louis: 1990.
3. Tapper D: Head and neck-sinuses and masses. In *Pediatric Surgery*. Ashcraft KW, Holder TM, eds. WB Saunders, Philadelphia: 1993, 923-34.

CRICOID SPLIT, LARYNGOTRACHEOPLASTY

SURGICAL CONSIDERATIONS

Description: A **cricoid split** is most commonly performed in the NICU baby who fails extubation due to subglottic stenosis. **Diagnostic bronchoscopy** is performed; then the baby is reintubated or the bronchoscope is left in the airway and the procedure is performed over the bronchoscope. A horizontal neck incision is made over the cricoid cartilage. The strap muscles are separated in the midline; the laryngeal cartilage and trachea are exposed; and a vertical incision is made through the inferior portion of the thyroid cartilage, through the cricoid cartilage and first tracheal ring. Typically, an ETT 1/2 size larger than the previously placed ETT is inserted.

A **laryngotracheoplasty** is performed in the patient with moderate-to-severe subglottic stenosis. In most of these patients, a tracheotomy will already be present. During the procedure, the tracheotomy tube is switched for an anode tube, which is sutured or taped to the chest. After the airway is exposed, a costal cartilage, auricular cartilage, or thyroid cartilage graft will be harvested. The cartilage graft is then sutured into the anterior airway, keeping the cricoid split incision spaced open. Sometimes, a posterior cartilage graft is necessary in a severely stenotic airway, and this is placed after making an incision through the posterior cricoid.

In a single-stage procedure, the anode tube is removed from the tracheotomy, and the patient is intubated either orally or nasotracheally to maintain the airway. This ETT is kept in place for 2-7 d as a stent around which the airway heals. In a two-stage procedure, the tracheotomy tube is kept in place. In this circumstance, there is usually a stent attached to the superior aspect of the tracheotomy tube, which stents the airway open from the tracheostomy up through the subglottis.

Usual preop diagnosis: Subglottic stenosis

SUMMARY OF PROCEDURE

Position	Supine, shoulder roll
Incision	Horizontal neck
Unique considerations	After the cut is made into the airway, a leak may be present, depending on position of the cuff (if present).
Antibiotics	Clindamycin 12 mg/kg
Surgical time	Cricoid split: 45 min
	Laryngotracheoplasty: 1.5-4 h
EBL	5-30 ml
Mortality	Rare
Morbidity	Pneumothorax
	Bleeding
	Infection
	Stent dislodgement
	Residual/recurrent subglottic stenosis
Pain score	4-6; 6-8 if costal cartilege harvested.

PATIENT POPULATION CHARACTERISTICS

Age range	Newborn-adult
Male:Female	1:1
Incidence	Rare
Etiology	ETT intubation; congenital
Associated conditions	Prematurity with prolonged NICU course

ANESTHETIC CONSIDERATIONS

PREOPERATIVE

These procedures are performed in patients with subglottic stenosis with a lesion that is either congenital or acquired. Congenital subglottic stenosis varies with regard to the length of trachea involved and the degree of stenosis. Segmental stenosis may occur in the region of the cricoid cartilage, midtrachea, or just above the carina. Sx are severe retractions, especially with agitation or intercurrent URI, dyspnea, and stridor. If the stenotic segment is short and severe, excision with primary anastomosis may be performed. If the involved segment is long, tracheoplasty is usually performed.

966

Acquired subglottic stenosis occurs as a complication of prolonged tracheal intubation and mechanical ventilation, most commonly in neonates born prematurely with severe lung disease associated with prematurity (infant respiratory distress syndrome [IRDS]). The stenotic lesion usually is limited to the level of the cricoid cartilage, and is treated with the cricoid split procedure. In addition to tracheal stenosis, tracheomalacia may be present.

Respiratory	Patients may be intubated and mechanically ventilated in the PICU. A variable degree of lung disease may be present; some patients may be on minimal ventilatory support, while others may be receiving relatively high FiO_2 and/or inflating pressures. Some patients will have an indwelling tracheostomy tube that bypasses the stenotic lesion, and may be cared for at home. **Tests:** As indicated from H&P.
Cardiovascular	Although not common, cor pulmonale with RVH may be present 2° chronic lung disease.
Hematologic	Anemia is common, especially in infants with chronic lung disease. **Tests:** Hct
Premedication	Infants in PICU usually are receiving a regimen of sedative and analgesia drugs. These should be continued until the patient is transported to the OR, with supplemental doses given preop as needed. Tolerance may be present, and drug doses should be titrated to achieve an adequate level of sedation.

INTRAOPERATIVE

Anesthetic technique: GETA

Induction	In intubated or trached patients with iv access, an iv induction is performed; otherwise, induction is done with inhalation agents. In the absence of an ETT, a mask induction is performed, with care being taken to preserve upper airway patency, as even mild obstruction tends to exacerbate tracheal collapse. Following neuromuscular blockade, tracheal intubation is performed with an ETT smaller than normal for age. In patients with severe stenosis, an ETT as small as 2.5 mm may be required. If prolonged sedation and mechanical ventilation are planned postop, central venous access should be considered.
Maintenance	Plans for postop mechanical ventilation are discussed with the surgeon. In those patients for whom mechanical ventilation is planned for > 24 h, high-dose opioid anesthesia is appropriate (e.g., fentanyl 20-50 μg/kg), as well as a long-acting muscle relaxant (pancuronium). A mixture of air and O_2 is used to keep $SpO_2 \leq 95\%$ to minimize O_2 toxicity.
Emergence	The majority of patients are transported to the PICU with indwelling ETT and residual sedation, narcosis, and neuromuscular blockade. IV sedation may be achieved with midazolam, lorazepam, or diazepam before completion of surgery.
Blood and fluid requirements	IV: 24 or 22 ga × 1 NS/LR @ maintenance	Blood loss < 30 ml
Monitoring	Standard monitors (see p. D-1).
Positioning	✓ and pad pressure points. ✓ eyes.

Complications	Tracheal edema
	Injury to neck structures:
	  Trachea
	  Vascular structures
	  Recurrent laryngeal nerve injury
		Rx: dexamethasone (0.5-1 mg/kg)

POSTOPERATIVE

Complications	Tracheal disruption (leak)	Presents with subcutaneous emphysema of the neck, face and chest wall.
	Recurrent laryngeal nerve injury	May cause vocal cord dysfunction.
Sedation/ analgesia	Heavy sedation	To minimize head and neck movement and tracheal wound disruption while ETT is in place.

References

1. Allen TH, Stevens IM: Prolonged endotracheal intubation in infants and children. *Br J Anaesth* 1985; 37:566-73.
2. Cotton RT: Pediatric laryngotracheal stenosis. *J Pediatr Surg* 1984; 19:699.
3. Vinograd I, Klim B, Efrati Y: Airway obstruction in neonates and children: surgical treatment. *J Cardiovasc Surg* 1994; 35: 7-12.

CHOANAL ATRESIA REPAIR

SURGICAL CONSIDERATIONS

Description: Infants born with bilateral choanal atresia typically have severe airway distress shortly following birth because neonates are obligate nose breathers. The distress resolves after the child is intubated or a McGovern nipple (large nipple with cross-cuts in the end) or oral airway is positioned in the oral cavity. These infants undergo primary repair of the atresia within the first few d of life. Children with unilateral choanal atresia usually do not have any respiratory distress and, thus, surgery is often postponed until a later age.

Intranasal repair involves opening up the atretic area with nasal dilators or urethral sounds and placing an intranasal stent. If a transpalatal repair is performed, a Dingman mouth gag is placed in the mouth, a palatal flap is raised and the posterior portion of the hard palate and posterior septum is removed. A stent is positioned in the nose. The infant should be able to breathe spontaneously through the nose at completion of either procedure.

Usual preop diagnosis: Bilateral or unilateral choanal atresia

SUMMARY OF PROCEDURE

Position	Supine; head 90°-180° from anesthesia
Incision	Intranasal or intraoral
Special instrumentation	Nasal dilators; Dingman mouth gag
Antibiotics	Clindamycin 12 mg/kg
Surgical time	30 min-2 h
EBL	< 10 ml
Postop care	Observation in PICU for respiratory distress
Mortality	Rare
Morbidity	Bleeding
	Pressure necrosis to nasal ala from stent
	Infection
	Airway obstruction if stents become malpositioned
Pain score	3-6

PATIENT POPULATION CHARACTERISTICS

Age range	Newborn–young child
Male:Female	1:1
Incidence	Rare
Etiology	Congenital
Associated conditions	Coloboma, heart disease, atresia choanae, retarded growth, genital anomalies, and ear deformities (CHARGE) association (see Anesthetic Considerations, below).

ANESTHETIC CONSIDERATIONS

PREOPERATIVE

Because many neonates are nasal breathers, choanal atresia may present with cyanosis at rest, resolving with crying or placement of an oral airway. Unilateral atresia is usually asymptomatic; bilateral lesions usually → respiratory distress in the neonatal period, but occasionally are asymptomatic. Although choanal atresia is most commonly an isolated anomaly, it may present as part of the CHARGE association.

Respiratory	Classic findings include cyanosis at rest, resolving with crying.
Cardiovascular	When part of the CHARGE association, cardiac defects include tetralogy of Fallot, ASD, VSD, PDA, AV canal, or right-side aortic arch.
Neurologic	When part of the CHARGE association, a variety of CNS abnormalities may be present. Hypoxia 2° airway obstruction may cause CNS impairment and Sz.
Premedication	Repair of choanal atresia usually is performed in infancy, and premedication is not indicated.

INTRAOPERATIVE

Anesthetic technique: GETA

Induction	Standard pediatric induction (see p. D-2). Airway obstruction may develop during induction of anesthesia. Early placement of an oral airway, facilitated by topical anesthesia of the tongue with viscous lidocaine prior to induction, may prevent or relieve the obstruction. An oral RAE ETT is preferred, especially if a transpalatal repair is planned using a Dingman mouth retractor.
Maintenance	Inhalational or iv anesthesia is maintained during the procedure. During the first mo of life, opioids (other than remifentanil) should be avoided generally because of the risk of postop respiratory depression. For infants undergoing repair after the first mo of life, small doses of fentanyl (1-2 μg/kg) or morphine sulfate (0.05-0.1 mg/kg) may be given. Muscle relaxation does not need to be maintained following tracheal intubation.
Emergence	Nasal stents placed following the repair must be secure and free of secretions prior to tracheal extubation. Patients must be fully awake and capable of maintaining patency of their oropharynx in the event of postop swelling and transient obstruction of the nasopharynx.

Blood and fluid requirements	IV: 24 or 22 ga × 1 NS/LR @ maintenance	Blood loss is < 10 ml; may be greater in older infants.
Monitoring	Standard monitors (see p. D-1).	
Positioning	✓ and pad pressure points. ✓ eyes.	
Complications	Airway obstruction Bleeding	2° obstruction or displacement of nasal stents Especially in older infants

POSTOPERATIVE

Complications	See Intraop Complications, above.	
Pain management	Acetaminophen po/pr	Small doses of opioid may be given iv immediately post-op, with special attention to avoid respiratory depression/obstruction.

References

1. Harris J, Robert E, Kfallfen B: Epidemiology of choanal atresia with special reference to the CHARGE association. *Pediatrics* 1997; 99:363-7.
2. Menasse-Palmer L, Bogdanow A, Marion RW: Choanal atresia. *Pediatr Rev* 1995; 16:475-6.
3. Prescott CA: Nasal obstruction in infancy. *Arch Dis Child* 1995; 72:287-9.

PEDIATRIC TRACHEOSTOMY

SURGICAL CONSIDERATIONS

Description: A **tracheostomy** is performed in the infant or child with upper airway obstruction (subglottic stenosis, laryngeal web, etc.) or in the child in whom prolonged mechanical ventilation is anticipated. In most cases, the child will already be intubated and the procedure will be performed over the ETT. In selected infants, the tracheostomy can be performed with a rigid bronchoscope in the airway through which the patient is being ventilated. A midline horizontal neck incision is made just inferior to the cricoid cartilage. The dissection is carried out in the midline until the trachea is reached. In children, the tracheal incision is vertical; and the patient typically has a large air leak. As the ETT or bronchoscope is being removed, a tracheostomy tube is inserted in the neck. The ventilation tubing will be exchanged for new sterile tubing and the tracheostomy tube secured with neck sutures and/or ties around the neck. Stay sutures may be placed around the tracheal wall and taped to the right and left sides of the chest. In the case of accidental decannulation postop, these sutures can be used to pull open the tracheal incision to aid in replacement of the tracheostomy tube.

Usual preop diagnosis: Ventilator dependence; subglottic stenosis

SUMMARY OF PROCEDURE

Position	Supine; head to anesthesia; shoulder roll; neck extended
Incision	Horizontal neck
Special instrumentation	Tracheostomy hook
Unique considerations	Patient is draped to allow easy access to ETT. When trachea is opened, a large air leak may be present.
Antibiotics	Clindamycin 12 mg/kg or cefazolin 25 mg/kg
Surgical time	30 min-1 h
EBL	< 10 ml
Postop care	Close observation in PICU. CXR immediately following procedure to r/o pneumothorax.
Mortality	2-5%, usually 2° tracheostomy tube plugging or dislodgement
Morbidity	Pneumothorax
	Subcutaneous emphysema
	Bleeding
	Infection
	Plugging
	Skin abrasion around trach edges or trach ties in patient with short, chubby neck
Pain score	3-5

PATIENT POPULATION CHARACTERISTICS

Age range	Newborn-adult
Male:Female	1:1
Incidence	Uncommon
Etiology	Anatomical airway obstruction; ventilatory dependence; high, spinal-cord, or head injury
Associated conditions	Prematurity; trauma

ANESTHETIC CONSIDERATIONS

See Anesthetic Considerations following Tracheostomy, in Chapter 3.0 Otolaryngology, p. 183.

Surgeons

V. Mohan Reddy, MD
Frank L. Hanley, MD

12.4 PEDIATRIC CARDIOVASCULAR SURGERY

Anesthesiologists

M. Gail Boltz, MD
Chandra Ramamoorthy, MD

SURGERY FOR ATRIAL SEPTAL DEFECT (OSTIUM SECUNDUM)

SURGICAL CONSIDERATIONS

Description: Atrial septal defects (ASDs) are among the most common congenital cardiac defects. ASDs vary widely in size and location and are broadly classified as **ostium secundum, ostium primum, sinus venosus,** and **coronary sinus** types (Fig 12.4-1). Ostium secundum defects—the most common (80%)—result from an incompletely formed or fenestrated septum primum covering the fossa ovalis. A L→R shunt results in augmented pulmonary blood flow which, if left uncorrected, may → RV failure, atrial arrhythmias, pulmonary HTN, and rarely, pulmonary vascular occlusive disease (PVOD). In 1953, Gibbon successfully repaired an ASD using a pump-oxygenator and, in doing so, ushered in the era of open cardiac surgery.

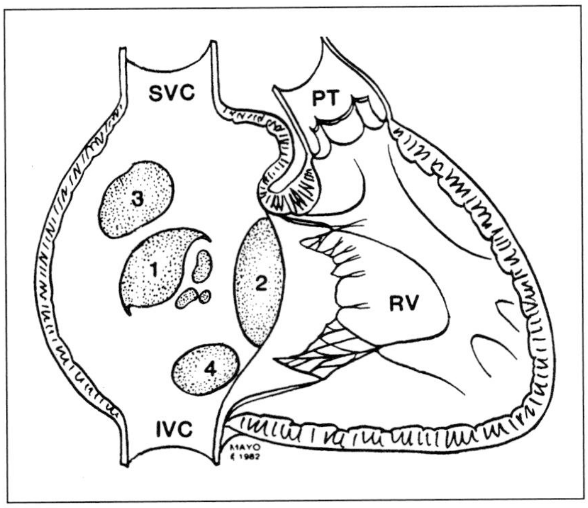

Secundum ASDs that fail to close spontaneously should be closed electively in early childhood to avoid long-term complications. Currently, ASD closure is performed through a minimally invasive approach on CPB. A right anterolateral thoracotomy through the 4th intercostal space also provides satisfactory exposure and provides female patients with better cosmesis. Once CPB and cardioplegic arrest have been instituted, a right atriotomy is created and the ASD is visualized.

Figure 12.4-1. Location of ASDs, numbered in decreasing order of frequency: 1 = secundum; 2 = primum; 3 = sinus venosus; 4 = coronary sinus type. IVC = inferior vena cava; PT = pulmonary trunk; RV = right ventricle; SVC = superior vena cava. (Reproduced with permission from the Mayo Foundation for Education and Research.)

Repair is effected by direct suture closure or patch closure, using autologous pericardium or prosthetic material (e.g., Gore-Tex, Dacron). After the repair is completed and the atriotomy is closed, standard deairing maneuvers are performed, the aortic cross-clamp is released, and CPB is D/C'd. The chest is then closed in the standard fashion.

Variant procedure or approaches: Currently, a **device closure** of ASD in the cathlab is a standard procedure. A **robotic approach** to ASD closure is undergoing clinical trials. Patent foramen ovale (PFO) in adults is becoming a common indication for device closure to avoid risk of paradoxical embolism and stroke during surgery.

Usual preop diagnosis: ASD; ostium secundum defect; other variants

SUMMARY OF PROCEDURE

Position	Supine or right lateral decubitus (thoracotomy)
Incision	Minimally invasive midline incision with limited right median sternotomy; right anterolateral thoracotomy (4th intercostal space)
Unique considerations	R→L shunt → systemic embolization
Antibiotics	Cefazolin 25 mg/kg q 8 h
Surgical time	Aortic cross-clamp: 20-30 min
	Total: 2 h
Closing considerations	Routine closure with chest tube in pericardial space; temporary atrial pacing wire (older patients); possible left atrial line for monitoring
EBL	Minimal
Postop care	Extubation in OR or within several h; 24 h monitoring in ICU
Mortality	Rare
Morbidity	Hemorrhage
	Postpericardiotomy syndrome
	Atrial arrhythmias
Pain score	6-8

PATIENT POPULATION CHARACTERISTICS

Age range	Neonate–adults
Male:Female	1:2

Incidence	10-15% of congenital heart defects
Etiology	Unknown; sometimes associated with such syndromes as Holt-Oram.
Associated conditions	ASD may coexist with nearly any of the other recognized congenital cardiac anomalies, but is more commonly associated with pulmonary stenosis (10%), partial anomalous pulmonary venous return (7%), VSD (5%), PDA (3%), and mitral stenosis (2%). ASDs are also part of other malformations, including tricuspid atresia, total anomalous pulmonary venous connection (TAPVC), and mitral atresia.

ANESTHETIC CONSIDERATIONS

PREOPERATIVE

Pathophysiology	Although the secundum ASD is the most common, periop management varies little among all types of ASDs (including ostium primum, sinus venosus, and coronary sinus types). One principle guideline in all L→R shunts is the estimation of shunt flow: Q_p:Q_s. This is determined by the amount of pulmonary blood flow (Q_p), size of the defect, and the PVR and SVR. Patients are generally asymptomatic until the Q_p:Q_s ratio exceeds 3.0. As the shunt flow increases, Sx of pulmonary overcirculation may develop (e.g., failure to thrive, tachypnea at rest, and feeding difficulties). L→R shunt → ↑pulmonary blood flow (Q_p) → ↑PA pressures → ↑PVR → RV overload → RV failure. The larger the area of the defect, the greater the shunt.
Cardiovascular and respiratory	Most infants with ASDs are asymptomatic and are detected on cardiac auscultation (fixed splitting of S2). Young children may have Hx of frequent URIs. Cyanosis is rare and indicates shunt reversal and development of pulmonary HTN. Surgical closure is advocated as these patients are at risk for paradoxical embolism, stroke, and bacterial endocarditis. Unlike ventricular septic defects (VSDs), ASDs rarely close spontaneously. Endovascular closure in the cath lab may be suitable for some patients, obviating the need for CPB. **Tests:** ECG: normal or RVH. CXR: cardiomegaly and ↑pulmonary vascular markings. ECHO. TEE: essential for locating and estimating size of defect, other valvular abnormalities, and identification of pulmonary vein anatomy.
Laboratory	Hb/Hct; T&C
Premedication	Generally not necessary for patients < 9 mo old. Midazolam 0.5-0.7 mg/kg po 20 min before induction.

INTRAOPERATIVE

Anesthetic technique: GETA + SAB (fast-tracking). Most of these patients are candidates for **fast-tracking**—the practice of extubation of cardiac patients in the OR within 4 h of completion of surgery. To achieve this goal, the anesthetic technique must be adjusted to permit early extubation. A combination of neuraxial (spinal) or iv anesthesia, combined with volatile anesthetic agents, is used at Stanford.

Criteria for fast-tracking include: patients > 4 mo of age, short CPB run, stable hemodynamic profile, minimal inotropic support, normal acid-base status, and adequate surgical hemostasis. Patients who are pacemaker-dependent are not suitable candidates for fast-tracking. Generally, patients selected for fast-tracking have undergone repair of either a secundum ASD, VSD (no evidence of postop pulmonary HTN), bidirectional Glenn and Fontan procedures, or a RV→PA conduit change. For patients with a single ventricle, resumption of spontaneous ventilation decreases intrathoracic pressure and improves the transthoracic (PA-LA) pressure gradient. This increases venous return and improves CO.

Induction	**Neuraxial fast-track:** Following inhalation induction using sevoflurane (NO/N_2O), an iv is placed and intubation facilitated with rocuronium (1 mg/kg). After ET intubation, an arterial line is placed for close BP monitoring. If neuraxial anesthesia is to be used, place the patient in the lateral decubitus position and 30° Trendelenburg tilt. Following usual sterile precautions, a 25 ga Quincke spinal needle is introduced at the L3-4 or L4-5 interspace. Following intrathecal injection of tetracaine, the patient is kept in Trendelenburg for a minimum of 15 mins. The spinal block should be completed in 1 h, before systemic heparinization. This high-spinal technique is not recommended in patients > 8 yr old, as these patients may manifest symptoms of a sympathetic blockade with ↓↓HR and ↓↓BP. **IV fast-track:** Intravenous techniques are used for fast-tracking patients who are not candidates for regional anesthesia (e.g., parent preference, spine abnormality, age). Inhalation induction (sevoflurane ± N_2O) is followed by placement of an iv arterial line. Fentanyl (2-5 μg/kg) and a muscle relaxant

Induction, cont.	(e.g., rocuronium 1 mg/kg) are administered and the airway is secured. Then, either an infusion of remifentanil (0.1-0.4 μg/kg) is started or single bolus iv methadone (0.2 mg/kg; max dose 20 mg) is administered.	
	Non fast-track: For patients who are not candidates for fast-tracking, the standard anesthetic is fentanyl 40-60 μg/kg in divided doses with supplemental isoflurane before and during CPB. Additional midazolam (0.1-0.3 mg/kg) may be administered to prevent recall and awareness. Smaller children generally tolerate an inhalation induction with sevoflurane in 50% $N_2O + O_2$. After induction, iv access is established and rocuronium (1 mg/kg), followed by remifentanil 1 μg/kg, is given. An iv induction should be used in patients with significant pulmonary HTN and/or RV failure. IV induction is accomplished with etomidate 0.1-0.3 mg/kg or ketamine 0.5-1 mg/kg, followed by a muscle relaxant (e.g., vecuronium 1 mg/kg).	
Maintenance	In the maintenance of anesthesia, isoflurane may be used with iv techniques before, during, and after CPB. In patients in whom immediate postop extubation is planned, anesthesia is maintained using a volatile agent in air + O_2, combined with remifentanil infusion. N_2O is turned off after induction to avoid expansion of any intraop VAE. In patients with pulmonary HTN, RV failure and/or other medical conditions requiring postop mechanical ventilation, a high-dose narcotic technique may be appropriate (e.g., fentanyl 50-150 μg/kg ± inhalation agent).	
Emergence	If the choice is made to extubate the patient receiving remifentanil in the OR, isoflurane is terminated during skin closure, muscle relaxant is reversed, and the remifentanil is turned off when the dressing is applied. When the patient meets standard extubation criteria (e.g., -25 cmH$_2$O NIF, spontaneous ventilation, adequate sat), remove the ETT and document spontaneous ventilation. If the patient is not extubated in the OR, transport the patient to the ICU sedated with remifentanil (0.1-0.4 μg/kg/min) or low-dose propofol (25-75 μg/kg/min), and extubate in the ICU. If the patient received methadone, standard criteria for extubation are used. Vasodilators are usually not required for BP control. O$_2$, bag, mask, airway equipment, and emergency drugs should be available during transport.	
Blood and fluid requirements	IV: appropriate for patient's size × 1-2 LR @ TKO Blood warmer ✓ for air bubbles. T&C 1 U PRBC.	★ **NB:** It is critical to avoid iv bubbles in all patients with intracardiac shunts. Meticulous attention must be paid to clearing the iv tubing and stopcocks of any bubbles to avoid paradoxical air embolism and possible stroke. Have blood available in the OR. Blood transfusion may be required in patients < 10 kg.
Monitoring	Standard monitors (see p. D-1). T (2 sites) Arterial line CVP line Urinary catheter ACT monitoring TEE	ABG, electrolytes, and Hct should be checked as needed during the procedure. Place at least two O$_2$ probes to ensure readings during critical times. Avoid dorsalis pedis and posterior tibial arterial lines (inaccurate 2° spasm post-CPB). Femoral arterial line may be used. Double lumen CVP in IJ preferable. TEE monitoring is used to assess anatomy and repair.
Positioning	✓ and pad pressure points. ✓ eyes.	
Pre-CPB	Heparinization (4 mg/kg) ✓ ACT > 400. ✓ NMB. ✓ UO.	
CPB	Hypothermia ✓ adequate flow and pressure during CPB. Ventilation stopped ✓ face for venous congestion. ✓ ABG and ACT. ✓ UO. Blood should be available.	The patient is not actively cooled for secundum ASD closure. The T is allowed to drift to 33-34° C. Secundum ASD may be repaired using ventricular fibrillation instead of cardioplegia with aortic cross-clamping.
Transition off CPB	Rewarming Vasoactive infusions started at 32°C.	Surgeon will deair heart, and this maneuver is monitored with TEE. Dopamine 3-5 μg/kg/min.

Transition off CPB, cont.	Flush lines. Zero transducers. Suction ETT. Resume ventilation. Observe inflation of both lungs.	
Post-CPB	Reversal of heparin with protamine ✓ UO. ± Modified ultrafiltration (MUF)	1 mg of protamine will reverse 100 U of residual heparin. MUF uses the CPB machine to remove excess water and inflammatory mediators. It has been shown to transiently ↓ postop edema and improve cardiopulmonary function.
Complications	Air embolism (VAE) Supraventricular dysrhythmias Heart block Ventricular dysfunction	Potential for paradoxical embolization Likely 2° atriotomy

POSTOPERATIVE

Complications	Bleeding Epidural or spinal hematoma	In regional anesthesia patients
Tests	ABG Electrolytes; Hct CXR	

References

1. Allen HD, Clark EB, Gutgesell HP, Driscoll DJ, eds. *Moss and Adams' Heart Disease in Infants, Children, and Adolescents*, 6th edition. Lippincott Williams & Wilkins, Philadelphia: 2001.
2. Castaneda AR, Jonas RA, Mayer JE Jr, Hanley FL: Atrial septal defect. In *Cardiac Surgery of the Neonate and Infant*. WB Saunders, Philadelphia: 1994, 143-55.
3. Cooper JR, Goldstein MT: Septal and endocardial cushion defects and double outlet right ventricle perioperative management. In *Pediatric Cardiac Anesthesia*, 3rd edition. Lake CL, ed. Appleton & Lange, Stamford, CT: 1998, 285-301.
4. Emmanouilides GC, Allen HD, Riemenschneider TA, Gutgesell HP: Atrial septal defects. In *Clinical Synopsis of Moss and Adams' Heart Disease in Infants, Children, and Adolescents*. Williams & Wilkins, Baltimore: 1998, 243-52.
5. Kopf GS, Laks H: Atrial septal defects and cor triatriatum. In *Glenn's Thoracic and Cardiovascular Surgery*, 6th edition. Baue AE, ed. Appleton & Lange, Stamford: 1996: 1115-25.
6. Mainwaring RD, Lamberti JJ: Atrial septal defects. In *Mastery of Cardiothoracic Surgery*. Kaiser LR, Kron IL, Spray TL, eds. Lippincott-Raven, Philadelphia: 1998, 677-86.
7. Reitz BA, Yuh DD, eds: *Congenital Cardiac Surgery*. McGraw-Hill, New York: 2002.

SURGERY FOR ATRIOVENTRICULAR CANAL DEFECT

SURGICAL CONSIDERATIONS

Description: Atrioventricular (A-V) canal defects comprise a spectrum of congenital cardiac anomalies stemming from the embryonic maldevelopment of endocardial cushions. This leads to the absence of septal tissue immediately above and below the level of the A-V valves and defects in the A-V valves in continuity with these septal defects. **Partial A-V canal defects** (or **ostium primum atrial septal defects**) involve the atrial septum, while **complete A-V canal defects** involve the atrial and ventricular septa. Pathophysiologically, these defects result in L → R shunting at the atrial and/or ventricular levels, leading to pulmonary HTN and CHF. A-V valvular insufficiency is also frequently observed with these defects, contributing to the early development of CHF.

Palliative repair of A-V canal defects consists of **pulmonary artery banding** (Fig 12.4-2) to reduce excessive pulmonary blood flow. Palliation is rare and is reserved for very small infants with complicating conditions, such as RSV and other pneumonias. **Total correction** is now performed routinely, even in neonates. Repair consists of the closure of atrial and ventricular septal defects (VSDs) with closure of the cleft in the anterior leaflet of the mitral valve, and repair of associated defects, such as a patent ductus arteriosus (PDA) or secundum atrial septal defect (ASD). The septal defects may be repaired with either a **'two-patch technique,'** consisting of a Dacron or pericardial patch on the ventricular septum and pericardial patch on the atrial septum, or a single patch (pericardium) covering both ASDs and VSDs. The ASD frequently is closed by placing the coronary sinus return on the left atrial side to avoid suturing in close proximity to the bundle of His.

Partial A-V canal defects: Exposure is obtained through a standard median sternotomy. CPB is instituted with aortic cross-clamping and cardioplegic arrest. Through a right atriotomy, the mitral valve cleft is sutured. A pericardial patch is placed across the top of the ventricular septum, around the coronary sinus orifice, and along the free edge of the superior portion of the ASD. The atriotomy is closed and the aorta unclamped after deairing. The patient is rewarmed and weaned from bypass.

Complete A-V canal defects: Following median sternotomy, CPB is instituted with aortic cross-clamping and cardioplegic arrest. In the **single-patch technique,** one

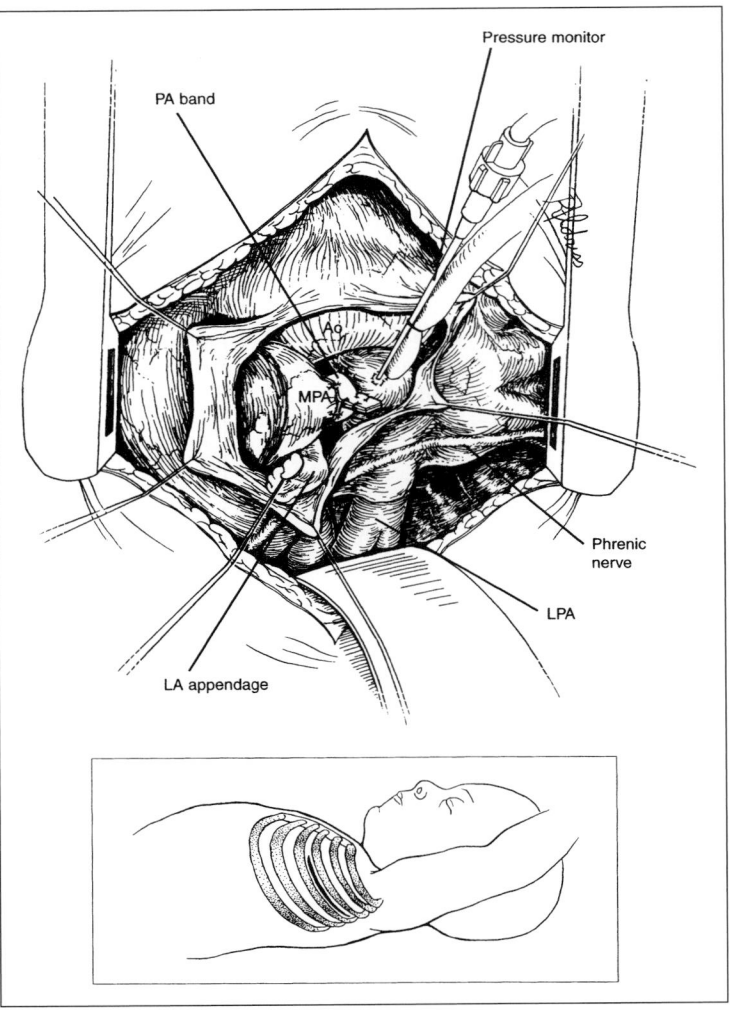

Figure 12.4-2. Placement of pulmonary artery band. PA = pulmonary artery; Ao = aorta; MPA = main pulmonary artery; LPA = left pulmonary artery; LA = left atrial. (Reproduced with permission from Kaiser LR, Kron IL, Spray TL, eds: *Mastery of Cardiothoracic Surgery*. Lippincott-Raven, Philadelphia, 1998.)

patch is used to close both the ASD and VSD components. The anterior and posterior bridging leaflets often are divided and resuspended to the patch, thereby creating two separate valves. The cleft in the left AV valve is usually closed. If AV valve regurgitation is present, repair is undertaken. In the two-patch technique, two separate patches are used to close the ASD and VSD, and the common AV valve is sandwiched in between the two patches. Repair of AV valve is the same in either technique. Closure of the right atrium, deairing, aortic unclamping, rewarming, and resuscitation of the heart are commenced, and CPB is D/C'd. Closure proceeds in the standard fashion. In ~5% of patients with complete A-V canal defects, tetralogy of Fallot (TOF) or left ventricular outflow tract obstruction (LVOTO) has to be addressed surgically.

Usual preop diagnosis: A-V canal defects (complete, intermediate, or partial); endocardial cushion defects

SUMMARY OF PROCEDURES

	Partial A-V Canal Defect	Complete A-V Canal Defect
Position	Supine	⇐
Incision	Standard median sternotomy/right anterolateral thoracotomy	Standard median sternotomy
Unique considerations	None	Repair performed through a right atriotomy; no ventriculotomies required.
Antibiotics	Cefazolin 25 mg/kg q 8 h	⇐

	Partial A-V Canal Defect	**Complete A-V Canal Defect**
Surgical time	Aortic cross-clamp: 30-40 min Total: 1.5-2 h	Aortic cross-clamp: 60-80 min Total: 2.5-3 h
Closing considerations	Chest tube in pericardial space; temporary ventricular pacing wire; possibly right or left atrial line for monitoring	⇐
EBL	Moderate	⇐
Postop care	ICU for 1-2 d, with 12-24 h assisted ventilation; minimal need for inotropes.	1-3 d assisted ventilation; pulmonary HTN protocol, including hyperventilation and sedation; need for pulmonary vasodilators (e.g., NO) is uncommon; use of inotropes for adequate CO. Avoid excessive volume to prevent distension and mitral valve regurgitation.
Mortality	0-1%	1-2%
Morbidity	Transient heart block Atrial dysrhythmias Hemorrhage Infection	Pulmonary vasospasm Right heart dysfunction Mitral valve regurgitation Low CO Heart block/atrial dysrhythmias Residual VSD Hemorrhage
Pain score	6-10	6-8

PATIENT POPULATION CHARACTERISTICS

Age range	1-20 yr (usually 2-3 yr)	2-6 mo (occasionally older; rarely, adults)
Male:Female	1:1	⇐
Incidence	0.5-1% of congenital heart defects	⇐
Etiology	Down syndrome: Rare, in patients with partial A-V canal defect	Commonly associated with Down syndrome (75% in patients with complete A-V canal defect)
Associated conditions	Left A-V valve insufficiency	Pulmonary HTN, left A-V valve insufficiency, minor associated cardiac anomalies (e.g., PDA or ASD); major associated anomalies (e.g., TOF, LVOTO)

ANESTHETIC CONSIDERATIONS

PREOPERATIVE

Pathophysiology	A-V canal defects may be either partial or complete. The partial A-V canal has no interventricular communication and has an ostium primum ASD. There is often a cleft in the anterior leaflet of the mitral valve → MR. The complete A-V canal has communication at both the arterial and ventricular levels with a single A-V valve that is regurgitant. Like all L→R shunt lesions, the degree of shunt depends on relative resistances in the systemic and pulmonary circuits. Patients with large L→R shunts are at risk of developing pulmonary HTN, requiring early surgical correction.
Respiratory	Look for pulmonary congestion or any infectious process. Pulmonary HTN can be present in patients with partial or complete A-V canal defects. **Tests:** CXR: enlarged heart + increased pulmonary markings
Cardiovascular	Complete A-V canal → CHF and biventricular failure. **Tests:** ECG: RAE, RVE; ECHO diagnostic; cardiac cath may be indicated to assess PVR.
Down syndrome	A-V canal defects account for 40% of cardiac defects in the Down syndrome patient. These patients are at risk of atlantoaxial instability (20%); therefore, avoid excessive flexion-extension of the head and neck. Additional airway considerations (subglottic stenosis, large tongue, hypotonia) make these patients unsuitable for fast-tracking and early extubation.
Laboratory	See ASD, p. 973.
Premedication	Midazolam 0.5-0.75 mg/kg po.

INTRAOPERATIVE

Anesthetic technique: GETA

Induction	Typically, mask sevoflurane in N_2O and O_2. If iv in place, fentanyl 10 μg/kg and rocuronium 1 mg/kg. Verify ETT position (see p. D-3). In children with Down syndrome, anticipate difficult airways and atlantoaxial instability. Avoid excessive neck flexion. In this population, candidates for early or immediate extubation have only partial A-V canals and small shunts.
Maintenance	Volatile anesthetic in O_2 is given. In patients requiring postop mechanical ventilation, fentanyl 50-100 μg/kg total, rocuronium prn, and midazolam (0.1-0.2 mg/kg) $\pm$ volatile agent ($FiO_2 = 1$) is used for anesthesia.
Emergence	Patients undergoing repair of A-V canal defects are seldom suitable for fast-tracking. On conclusion of procedure, the patient is taken to PICU, intubated, ventilated, sedated, and monitored. Transport to ICU.

Blood and fluid requirements	IV: 22-24 ga × 2 LR @ TKO Blood products	See Table 12.4-2, p. 992.
Monitoring	See ASD, p. 974. TEE	TEE is used to assess left A-V valve regurgitation, valvular function, residual shunt, and ventricular function.
CPB	Management of CPB is discussed in Intraoperative Considerations for TOF, p. 974.	In the immediate post-CPB period, TEE exam is valuable for evaluation of ventricular function and residual mitral valve regurgitation. Closure of VSD may → temporary or permanent heart block requiring use of a pacemaker.
Complications	Air embolism	Avoid air embolism in A-V canal patients (shunt reversal → paradoxical embolization).
	A-V block, ventricular dysfunction Persistent bleeding Hypothermia Pulmonary HTN	A-V block may be temporary 2° edema and/or cardioplegic arrest. Permanent injury can occur to the conduction system at the A-V node or bundle of His with repair of the VSD. Temporary atrial and ventricular pacing wires are placed. See treatment for pulmonary HTN, p. 343.

POSTOPERATIVE

Complications	Residual VSD/ASD AV valve regurgitation	
Tests	TEE	Analysis of post repair function is best done by TEE.

References

1. Allen HD, Clark EB, Gutgesell HP, Driscoll DJ, eds. *Moss and Adams' Heart Disease in Infants, Children, and Adolescents*, 6th edition. Lippincott Williams & Wilkins, Philadelphia: 2001.
2. Castaneda AR, Jonas RA, Mayer JE Jr, Hanley FL: Atrioventricular canal defect. In *Cardiac Surgery of the Neonate and Infant*. WB Saunders, Philadelphia: 1994, 167-86.
3. Lowe DA, Stayer SA, Rehman MA: Abnormalities of the atrioventricular valves. In *Pediatric Cardiac Anesthesia*, 3rd edition. Lake CL, ed. Appleton & Lange, Stamford, CT: 1998, 407-30.
4. Reitz BA, Yuh DD, eds: *Congenital Cardiac Surgery*. McGraw-Hill, New York: 2002.
5. Vick WG, Titus JL: Defects of the atrial septum including the atrioventricular canal. In *The Science and Practice of Pediatric Cardiology*. Garson A, Bricker JT, McNamara DG, eds. Lea & Febiger, Philadelphia: 1990.

SURGERY FOR VENTRICULAR SEPTAL DEFECT

SURGICAL CONSIDERATIONS

Description: Ventricular septal defect (VSD) is the most common congenital cardiac anomaly. VSDs can occur anywhere in the interventricular septum (Fig 12.4-3). One of the most common locations is the perimembranous (conoventricular) in the region of membranous septum near the tricuspid and aortic valves. Supracristal (subarterial) defects are common in the Pacific rim population. Muscular defects occur in the inlet, trabecular, or outlet muscular septum. A-V canal defects are present under the septal leaflet of the tricuspid valve. Physiologically, these defects result in L→R shunting in proportion to the defect size. Untreated, this defect can → RV volume overload and CHF in infancy and irreversible pulmonary HTN later in life. As PVR rises, shunt reversal to a R→L shunt can occur, producing hypoxemia and cyanosis; this is known as Eisenmenger's syndrome and occurs in ~10% of untreated, nonrestrictive VSDs (rare). Moderate-to-large VSDs that remain open > 6 mo of age should be closed. Severe, intractable CHF in infants refractory to medical therapy (e.g., diuretics, digoxin), or ↑PVR in infants > 6 mo are indications for earlier VSD repair.

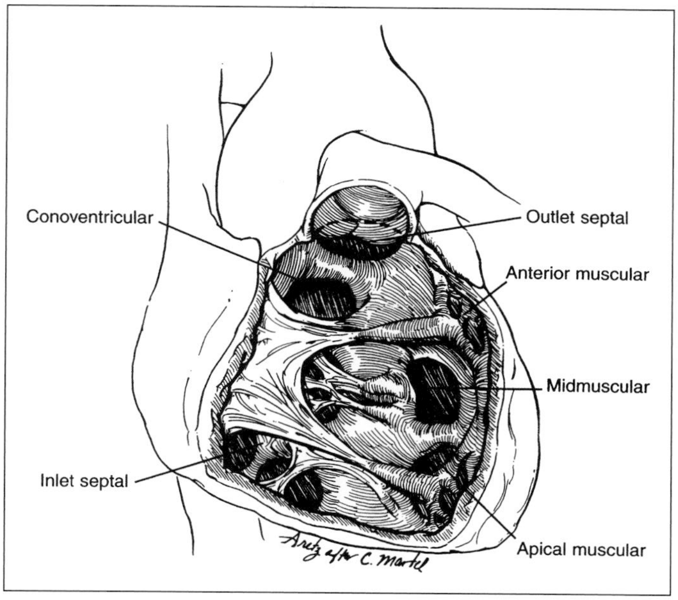

Lillehei, Varco, and colleagues performed the first successful VSD repairs using normothermic cross-circulation in 1955. Kirklin subsequently described successful VSD closure using extracorporeal circulation in 1957. VSD repair is performed now through a median sternotomy on CPB

Figure 12.4-3. The right ventricular free wall has been resected to show the VSDs: conoventricular = perimembranous; conal septal = outlet septal (subpulmonary); inlet septal = A-V canal type. Muscular (trabecular) defects may be midmuscular, anterior, or apical. The penetrating bundle is closely related to the inferior margin of the conoventricular defect and diverges away from this margin into the trabecular septomarginalis beneath the muscle of Lancisi. (Reproduced with permission from Kaiser LR, Kron IL, Spray TL, eds: *Mastery of Cardiothoracic Surgery.* Lippincott-Raven, Philadelphia, 1998.)

with bicaval cannulation. Deep hypothermia (18°C) with circulatory arrest is used in neonates < 1800 g to facilitate repair. Once CPB and cardioplegic arrest have been instituted, a right atriotomy is created and the VSD is visualized by retracting the tricuspid valve leaflets. The VSD is then closed with a patch (e.g., pericardium, Gore-Tex, Dacron), with care being taken not to place sutures through the nearby conduction fiber bundles or the aortic valve. After the repair is completed and the atriotomy is closed, standard deairing maneuvers are performed, the aortic cross-clamp is released, and CPB is D/C'd. The chest is then closed in the standard fashion.

Variant procedure or approaches: Supracristal defects may be more easily exposed through a pulmonary arteriotomy, while some inferiorly located muscular VSDs may be better accessed through a right ventriculotomy. Multiple VSDs or 'Swiss cheese' ventricular septum can be a challenging surgical problem. Many can be closed with approaches described above. Some may require a combined surgical and device closure. Palliative pulmonary artery banding may be required in Swiss cheese muscular VSD, with the hope that many of the VSDs may close spontaneously. At a second stage, the remaining VSDs are closed and the PA band is removed. Currently, device closure of muscular VSDs is experimental.

Usual preop diagnosis: VSD

SUMMARY OF PROCEDURE

Position	Supine
Incision	Standard median sternotomy
Antibiotics	Cefazolin 25 mg/kg q 8 h
Surgical time	Aortic cross-clamp: 15-45 min
	Total: 2-3 h
Closing considerations	Routine closure with chest tube in the pericardial space; temporary ventricular pacing wire; possibly right/left atrial and/or pulmonary arterial lines for monitoring

EBL	Minimal-to-moderate
Postop care	Extubation in OR or within several h; 24 h monitoring in ICU.
Mortality	≤ 1%
Morbidity	Hemorrhage
	Low CO
	Atrial dysrhythmias
	Complete A-V heart block
	Residual shunting; tricuspid regurgitation
Pain score	6-8

PATIENT POPULATION CHARACTERISTICS

Age range	Neonate – adult
Male:Female	1:1
Incidence	20% of congenital heart defects; 2/1000 births
Associated conditions	PDA (6%); coarctation of the aorta (5%); congenital AS (2%); congenital mitral valve disease (2%); also part of other malformations, including TOF, TGA, DORV, tricuspid atresia; truncus arteriosus; others

ANESTHETIC CONSIDERATIONS

PREOPERATIVE

Pathophysiology	VSDs are classified by their location and degree of shunt flow. Large VSDs offer little resistance to flow and are nonrestrictive (RV = LV pressure). Small VSDs (restrictive) may close spontaneously in early childhood. Patients with large VSDs present with CHF and other signs of pulmonary over-circulation (Q_p:Q_s > 3.0). Cyanosis indicates pulmonary HTN and shunt reversal (Eisenmenger's syndrome).
Cardiovascular and respiratory	Infants may present with feeding difficulty and failure to thrive (FTT). Children with small VSDs may be asymptomatic, while children with larger VSDs may have ↓exercise tolerance, fatigue, frequent URIs and Sx of CHF. A holosystolic murmur can be heard best at the left lower sternal border. Cyanosis is absent unless there is R→L shunting (suggesting pulmonary HTN). **Tests:** Obtain ECG, CXR, ECHO. If pulmonary HTN is suspected, cardiac catheterization is performed for measurement of PA pressures. If PA pressures are elevated, O_2 and NO responsiveness is tested. VSDs may be closed surgically or by a device in the cath lab if pulmonary HTN is not present.
Laboratory	Hct; electrolytes (children on diuretic Rx); others as indicated from H&P.
Premedication	See ASD, p. 973.

INTRAOPERATIVE

Anesthetic technique: The anesthetic management of a patient with VSD (without pulmonary HTN and CHF) is similar to the patient with ASD. These patients may be candidates for fast-tracking and early extubation. Refer to fast-tracking in ASD section (see p. 973). For patients with unrestrictive VSDs, avoid factors that ↓PVR and ↑shunt flow. This will compromise DBP and coronary perfusion. For patients who are not candidates for fast-tracking, the standard anesthetic is fentanyl 40-60 μg/kg in divided doses with supplemental isoflurane before and during CPB. Additional midazolam (0.1-0.3 mg/kg) may be administered to prevent recall and awareness.

Blood and fluid requirements	IV: appropriate for patient size × 1-2 LR @ TKO Blood warmer T&C	Minimize administration of iv fluids. Both ventricles are volume-overloaded in large VSDs.
Monitoring	Standard monitors (see p. D-1). Arterial line Surgical LA line Urinary catheter ACT monitoring	A transthoracic LA line may be placed by the surgeon if there is concern about postop mitral valve and LV dysfunction.

Monitoring, cont.	TEE	In the immediate post-CPB period, TEE exam is valuable for evaluation of residual VSD and ventricular function.
Pre-CPB	See ASD, p. 974.	
CPB	See ASD, p. 974.	Most VSDs are closed under mild/moderate hypothermic CPB (28-32°C).
Transition off CPB	See ASD, p. 974.	
Post-CPB	Maintenance of adequate filling pressure (LA = 5-10 mmHg)	
	Temporary pacemaker wires	Placed in patients with conduction disturbances; pacemaker wires are placed routinly, but may not be connected to a pacemaker.
	TEE	✓ for residual shunt and ventricular and valvular function.
	Pulmonary HTN	

POSTOPERATIVE

Complications	Persistent bleeding	
	Heart block: RBBB; bifascicular block	May appear early or later in postop course.
	Ventricular dysfunction/failure	Especially in patients with ventriculotomy Dx: TEE
Tests	ABGs	
	Electrolytes; Hct; coags prn	
	CXR	

References

1. Castaneda AR, Jonas RA, Mayer JE Jr, Hanley FL: Ventricular septal defect. In *Cardiac Surgery of the Neonate and Infant.* WB Saunders, Philadelphia: 1994, 187-201.
2. Emmanouilides GC, Allen HD, Riemenschneider TA, Gutgesell HP: Ventricular septal defects. In *Clinical Synopsis of Moss and Adams' Heart Disease in Infants, Children, and Adolescents.* Williams & Wilkins, Baltimore: 1998, 264-85.
3. Knott-Craig CJ: Ventricular septal defects. In *Mastery of Cardiothoracic Surgery.* Kaiser LR, Kron IL, Spray TL, eds. Lippincott-Raven, Philadelphia: 1998, 687-96.

SURGERY FOR PATENT DUCTUS ARTERIOSUS

SURGICAL CONSIDERATIONS

Description: Patent ductus arteriosus (PDA) usually is located between the proximal descending thoracic aorta and the main PA. Pathophysiologically, this results in L→R shunting and augmented pulmonary blood flow, which, if left untreated, may lead to pulmonary HTN and CHF. A relatively common congenital heart anomaly, comprising 12-15% of CHDs, PDA was first successfully ligated by Gross in 1938. Early administration of indomethacin may promote ductal closure in many premature infants, obviating surgical intervention; however, this mode of therapy generally is contraindicated in the setting of renal insufficiency or intracranial bleeding.

Surgical ductal closure is indicated for significant L→R shunting. The ductus usually can be exposed via a small, left, posterolateral thoracotomy in the 4th intercostal space, or via thorocoscopic approach. The ductus is identified and dissected, with special care taken to avoid injury to the phrenic and left recurrent laryngeal nerves (Fig 12.4-4). The ductus is interrupted with a surgical clip in neonates; in older children, the ductus is double- or triple-ligated or divided between vascular clamps, and the ends are oversewn. A small thoracostomy tube is placed, and the thoracotomy is closed. The thoracostomy tube is removed in the OR immediately after the chest is closed or a few h later.

Variant procedure or approaches: Percutaneous coil embolization and **thoracoscopic clip ligation** are standard alternative approaches. A **robotic approach** is experimental.

Usual preop diagnosis: PDA

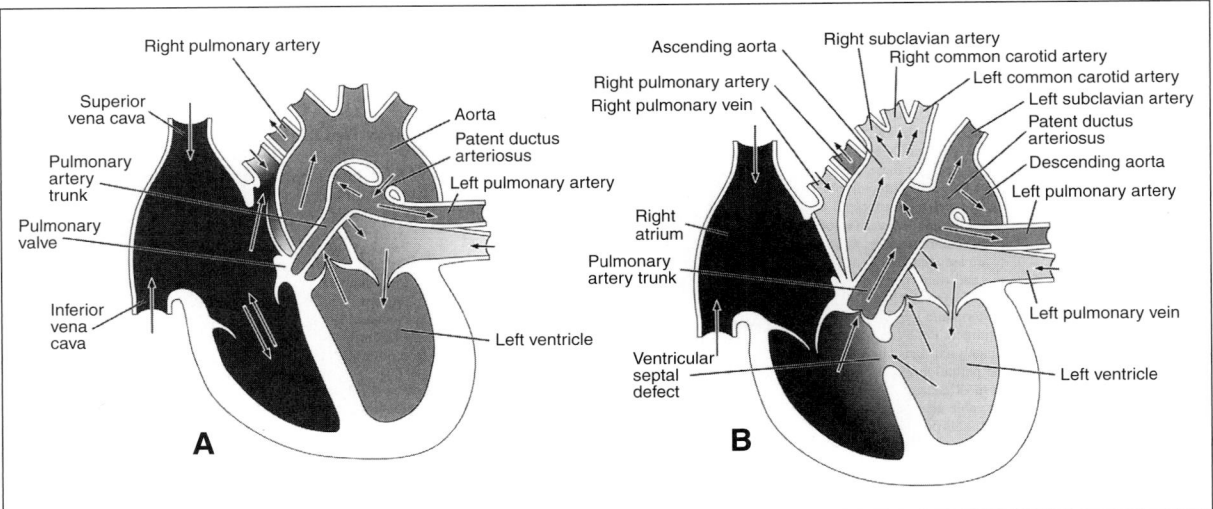

Figure 12.4-4. PDA. (A) Ductal dependency for pulmonary blood flow in pulmonary valvular atresia. The ductus arteriosus must be open for blood to enter the pulmonary arteries; as the ductus arteriosus closes, pulmonary blood flow is lost, and the patient becomes cyanotic. (B) Dependence on the ductus arteriosus for perfusion of the distal aorta is shown in a patient with interrupted aortic arch. Left ventricular blood (oxygenated) is able to cross the VSD and enter the PA, where it mixes with right ventricular blood. The flow is then distributed to the branch PAs and across the ductus arteriosus to the descending aorta. (Reproduced with permission from Ungerleider RM, Plunkett MD, Gaynor JW: Congenital heart disease. In *Surgery of Infants and Children.* Oldham KT, Colombani PM, Foglia RP, eds. Lippincott-Raven, 1997.)

SUMMARY OF PROCEDURE

Position	Right lateral decubitus
Incision	Small left posterolateral thoracotomy; 3rd or 4th intercostal space
Antibiotics	Cefazolin 25 mg q 8 h
Surgical time	30-60 min
Closing considerations	Routine closure ± left thoracostomy tube
EBL	Minimal
Postop care	24 h observation in ICU; extubation in the OR or within several h
Mortality	Rare
Morbidity	Hemorrhage
	Recurrent laryngeal nerve injury
	Chylothorax
Pain score	6-8

PATIENT POPULATION CHARACTERISTICS

Age range	1 mo–adulthood
Male:Female	1:2
Incidence	12-15% of congenital heart defects
Etiology	Failure of complete ductal closure

ANESTHETIC CONSIDERATIONS

PREOPERATIVE

Depends on surgical approach. Closure of PDA in the preterm infant is done at the bedside in the NICU. These patients are intubated, mechanically ventilated, hemodynamically unstable, and dependent on inotropic support. Older patients may be eligible for endovascular closure in the cath lab, leaving a small percentage for open surgical closure in the OR. Surgical closure may be performed with video-assisted thoracoscopy (VAT) or via thoracotomy. The following discussion for anesthetic management covers open thoracotomy only. The premature infant requiring surgical closure of PDA typically presents because indomethacin Rx has failed or is contraindicated. Premature infants often have primary pulmonary disease and multisystem organ problems. In the preterm infant, the symptoms of large L→R shunt and pulmonary overcirculation

→ cardiac and respiratory failure and ventilator dependence. The ductal runoff causes ↓DBP and compromises coronary blood flow and other organ perfusion. In older asymptomatic patients, risk of bacterial endocarditis necessitates closure. Permanent anatomic closure usually occurs within the first mo of life.

Cardiovascular	Clinical presentation depends on the size of the ductus. An infant with a large ductus can present in CHF with tachypnea, tachycardia, diaphoresis, failure to thrive (FTT), and hepatosplenomegaly. A continuous systolic murmur heard best at the left upper sternal border and widened pulse pressure with bounding pulses may be present. The older infant may have minimal shunt 2° ↑PVR. A small PDA may be detected by a murmur only. **Tests:** CXR: Normal or cardiomegaly with ↑PA size and ↑pulmonary vascular markings. ECG: Normal or LVH/RVH. ECHO diagnostic: documents patency, evaluates left-sided cardiac chamber sizes and aortic arch anatomy, and estimates size of shunt.
Laboratory	Hct; others as indicated from H&P.
Premedication	Not indicated in premature infants. Midazolam 0.5-0.7 mg orally 20 min prior to induction for children > 9 mo having routine PDA closure.

INTRAOPERATIVE

Anesthetic technique: Depends on the surgical approach. At the bedside of the preterm infant, anesthesia can be provided with ketamine (1-2 mg/kg) and muscle relaxant (e.g., rocuronium 1 mg/kg iv). Small doses of fentanyl (5-10 μg/kg) may be given for supplemental analgesia and BP control. During lateral decubitus positioning, careful attention to the airway and close monitoring of BP is necessary. Children presenting in the OR for elective operation generally tolerate an inhalation induction with sevoflurane in 50% N_2O + O_2. Once the patient is anesthetized, iv access is established, followed by oral intubation, with administration of a muscle relaxant (e.g., rocuronium 1 mg/kg). Most children presenting for elective closure of PDA via thoracotomy are candidates for thoracic epidural analgesia, while for those undergoing thoracoscopic closure, an epidural is not required. In patients > 25 kg, placement of a DLT for selective ventilation of the right lung will improve surgical access. With the exception of the preterm infant, all other patients are candidates for early extubation in the OR (see fast-track in ASD, p. 973). Avoid hyperoxia and hyperventilation → ↑SVR + ↓PVR → ↑ L→R shunt. In preterm neonates, because of lung disease and associated morbidity, it is important to avoid further ↑ PVR associated with positioning and light anesthesia (hypoventilation and hypoxemia can cause shunt reversal).

Induction	See above.	
Maintenance	In patients for whom immediate postop extubation is planned, anesthesia is maintained with isoflurane in air + O_2.	
Emergence	Patients may be extubated awake or in a deep plane of anesthesia. Postthoracotomy, an effective regional anesthetic is helpful for fast-tracking. For patients returning to the NICU intubated and ventilated, portable monitoring equipment, O_2, bag/mask airway equipment, and emergency drugs should be available during transport.	
Epidural	Thoracic level T8-10 preferred. Initial bolus of bupivacaine (0.25%, 0.3 ml/kg) with hydromorphone (5-10 μg/kg) ± clonidine (0.5-1 μg/kg). Infuse bupivacaine (1/8%) at 0.3-0.5 ml/h during surgery.	
Blood and fluid requirements	IV: 22-24 × 1-2 Continue iv dextrose. Blood warmer T&C ✓ for air bubbles.	Blood loss may become significant if the ductus is torn during ligation. Have blood available for rapid transfusion. Clear air bubbles from iv tubing and stopcocks (potential bidirectional shunt → paradoxical embolism).
Monitoring	Standard monitors (see p. D-1). ± Arterial line ± CVP line	Monitoring of the preductal BP (right arm) and a postductal saturation monitor (usually lower extremity) are required because of possible inadvertent ligation of the descending aorta. Place BP cuff on preductal (right arm) and pulse oximeter on the foot to monitor flow in the ascending and descending aorta. Inadvertent aortic occlusion → ↓LE pulses/pressure/perfusion. Inadvertent PA occlusion → ↓SpO₂ + ↓ETCO₂. Bradycardia may occur during manipulation of the ductus. The DBP will ↑ postligation.
Positioning	✓ and pad pressure points. ✓ eyes.	

Complications

Occlusion of aorta or PA
Torn ductus → hemorrhage
Residual PDA
Lung trauma ± pneumothorax

POSTOPERATIVE

Complications

Recurrent laryngeal nerve injury
Vagus nerve injury

Tests

Hct
CXR

Other tests as indicated.

References

1. Burke RP: Patent ductus arteriosus. In *Mastery of Cardiothoracic Surgery*. Kaiser LR, Kron IL, Spray TL, eds. Lippincott-Raven, Philadelphia: 1998, 657-62.
2. Castaneda AR, Jonas RA, Mayer JE Jr, Hanley FL: Patent ductus arteriosus. In *Cardiac Surgery of the Neonate and Infant*. WB Saunders, Philadelphia: 1994, 203-13.
3. Emmanouilides GC, Allen HD, Riemenschneider TA, Gutgesell HP: Patent ductus arteriosus. In *Clinical Synopsis of Moss and Adams' Heart Disease in Infants, Children, and Adolescents*. Williams & Wilkins, Baltimore: 1998, 286-308.
4. Haas G: Patent ductus arteriosus and aortopulmonary window. In *Glenn's Thoracic and Cardiovascular Surgery,* 6th edition. Baue AE, ed. Appleton & Lange, Stamford: 1996, 1137-61.

SURGERY FOR COARCTATION OF THE AORTA

SURGICAL CONSIDERATIONS

Description: Coarctation of the aorta is a congenital narrowing of the upper descending aorta, typically located at the juxtaductal region (Fig 12.4-5). Coexisting intracardiac defects are not uncommon. Surgical repair of aortic coarctation, first performed by **Crafoord** in 1944, consisted of resection of the narrowed aortic segment, followed by an **end-to-end repair.** The same year, **Blalock** and **Park** proposed an alternative technique in which the left subclavian artery was divided distally and sutured into the descending thoracic aorta, creating a bypass. Subsequently, the use of an onlay prosthetic graft to widen the area of coarctation and the use of a **subclavian artery flap** were described by **Waldhausen. Prosthetic interposition tube graft repairs** have been described in patients with diffuse aortic hypoplasia. Patients with an associated intracardiac L→R shunt (e.g., VSD) may require concomitant pulmonary artery banding following repair of the coarctation.

In infants, a left posterolateral thoracotomy approach is used. The lung is retracted anteriorly and the pleura is incised vertically over the aorta, along the left subclavian artery and the descending aorta. The aortic arch, all the arch branches, and the descending aorta are thoroughly mobilized. The PDA/ligamentum arteriosus is ligated and divided. Vascular clamps are placed across the aortic arch and the descending aorta. The aortic isthmus is ligated. The coarctated segment and all ductal tissue from the descending aorta are excised. An aortotomy is made in the aortic arch (may extend on to the distal ascending aorta) and the descending aorta is anastomosed to the aortic

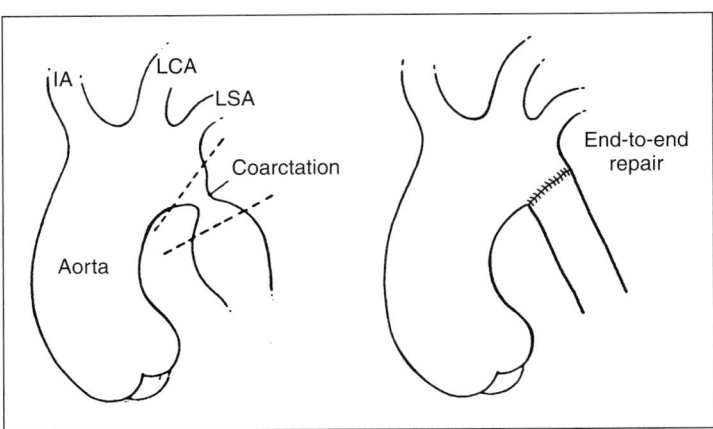

Figure 12.4-5. Coarctation of the aorta. (Redrawn with permission from Hardy JD: *Hardy's Textbook of Surgery*, 2nd edition. JB Lippincott, Philadelphia: 1988.)

arch. If a subclavian flap angioplasty is performed, the distal left subclavian artery is ligated and opened longitudinally down into the aorta, across the coarctation and into the descending aorta. The subclavian flap is then turned down and anastomosed to the descending aorta across the coarctated segment. Patch aortoplasty is performed by creating a longitudinal aortotomy above and below the coarctation and suturing a generously sized patch onto the defect. Following repair, the aortic cross-clamps are released, and hemostasis is secured. A pleural drainage tube is placed and the pleura is sutured over the aorta, followed by standard closure.

Variant procedure or approaches: In adults and older children (teens), **balloon dilatation with stent placement** is an acceptable alternative.

Usual preop diagnosis: Coarctation of the aorta

SUMMARY OF PROCEDURES

	Infant	Child or Adult
Position	Right lateral decubitus	⇐
Incision	Posterolateral left thoracotomy, 3rd-4th interspace	⇐
Unique considerations	Right upper limb arterial line. Avoid iv or arterial lines in left arm. Mild hypothermia and surface cooling (35°C).	Collateral circulation is adequate if distal aortic MAP > 50 mmHg. In rare cases of inadequate collateral circulation, left atrial-to-descending-aorta or femoral bypass should be considered. Mild hypothermia of 35° may be useful.
Antibiotics	Cefazolin 25 mg/kg q 8 h	⇐
Surgical time	Aortic cross-clamp: 12-20 min Total: 1-1.5 h	Aortic cross-clamp: 10-15 min Total: 2-2.5 h
Closing considerations	Thoracostomy tube	⇐
EBL	Minimal	1-2 ml/kg
Postop care	Early extubation in ICU; consider intercostal nerve block or epidural analgesia; careful control of MAP may require SNP or esmolol infusion.	⇐
Mortality	< 1%	⇐
Morbidity	Chylothorax	⇐
	Bleeding	⇐
	Infection	⇐
	Paraplegia: < 0.5%	⇐
Pain score	8-10	8-10

PATIENT POPULATION CHARACTERISTICS

	Infant	Child or Adult
Age range	1 wk–1 yr	1 yr–adult
Male:Female	2:1; 1:1 for coarctations with associated defects	⇐
Incidence	5-8% of congenital heart defects	5% of congenital heart defects
Etiology	Unknown. Ductal sling may be the single most contributory factor.	⇐
Associated conditions	PDA (50%); VSD (36%); congenital mitral stenosis (7%); single ventricle (7%); TGA/VSD (7%)	Usually an isolated defect. When repaired at a later age, bicuspid aortic valve.

ANESTHETIC CONSIDERATIONS

PREOPERATIVE

Pathophysiology Coarctation is a narrowing of the aortic arch, most commonly occurring at the junction of the ductus arteriosus. The clinical presentation of the neonate or infant with coarctation depends on: (1) location and degree of obstruction, (2) rate at which high-grade stenosis develops, (3) patency of the ductus,

Pathophysiology, cont. (4) PVR, and (5) associated cardiac anomalies. Patients with mild-to-moderate stenosis and no associated abnormalities will be asymptomatic with HTN and diminished lower extremity pulses. The ductus often will be closed. Neonates with critical stenosis will demonstrate ductal-dependent aortic flow. With the ductus open and ↑PVR, the neonate may be asymptomatic. R→L ductal flow, enhanced by ↑PVR, may → palpable lower extremity pulses, obscuring the Dx. As the ductus closes (after 4-10 d), lower torso hypoperfusion will become significant (acidemia, gut ischemia, cold lower extremities). In the absence of a VSD, rapid ductal closure will → an acute rise in LV afterload, without time for compensatory LVH, causing LV failure. If there is a significant VSD, ductal closure and a concomitant ↓PVR will result in a huge L→R shunt and LV failure from volume overload.

Respiratory **Tests:** CXR (cardiomegaly, characteristic aorta, PE)

Cardiovascular **Neonates:** Patients present with ↑BP, a pressure gradient between upper and lower extremities and a systolic murmur. Neonates present with 'critical' coarctation and are ductal-dependent. If the ductus is closing, PGE_1 may reopen the duct—or at least relax juxtaductal tissue—and improve perfusion. PGE_1 treatment may allow time for ECHO assessment of associated lesions.

Symptomatic infants: Young infants admitted with Sx of shock are medically managed until they have stabilized. Generally, small or moderate-size VSDs will not be addressed at first operation.

Asymptomatic infants: Surgery is indicated when ECHO or MRI scan demonstrates > 50% narrowing at the coarctation site, or > 20 mmHg resting gradient by cuff measurement.

Infants and older children: Often present with HTN, HA, and diminished or absent femoral pulses. The indication for operation is similar to that of asymptomatic infants. Systemic HTN and LVH may not resolve following repair.

Tests: ECHO; ECG; ABG; CXR—rib notching 2° collateral vessels. (This is a late finding.)

Renal **Tests:** BUN; Cr; electrolytes

CNS PGE_1 is associated with apnea in the newborn. Generally, the neonate is intubated once the prostaglandin infusion is started.

Laboratory Hct; T&C

Premedication Not appropriate in severely ill infants. Otherwise, midazolam 0.5-0.7 mg/kg po (maximum of 20 mg). For children > 25 kg, lorazepam 1-2 mg po 2 h before surgery.

INTRAOPERATIVE

Anesthetic technique: GETA. For the neonate, regional and fast-tracking are not appropriate.

Induction In sick neonates, an iv induction with fentanyl 2-5 μg/kg and rocuronium is appropriate. Avoid ↓SVR and myocardial depression, while maintaining a normal HR. Inhalation induction (sevoflurane and O_2) is well tolerated in the older patients. Regional anesthesia in coarctation of aorta patients is controversial because coincidental neurologic injury may occur when spinal cord blood flow is decreased from aortic cross-clamping. In most infants and children, single-lumen ETT is sufficient. In children > 10 kg, selective ventilation of the right lung with a DLT will facilitate surgery.

Maintenance When early postop extubation is planned, see fast-tracking, p. 973. A narcotic technique (10-20 μg/kg fentanyl ± volatile agent) is appropriate for critically ill neonates. Consider mild hypothermia (34-35°C) for CNS protection. The operation usually is done through a left thoracotomy. The aortic arch, isthmus, and descending aorta are mobilized. 100 U/kg of heparin may be given. The ductus arteriosus is ligated, then the aortic arch and descending aorta are occluded. The anesthesiologist should observe the arterial line trace closely during proximal occlusion and immediately inform the surgeon of any damping. Upper and lower extremity cuff pressures are measured.

Emergence Infants and children undergoing elective operation usually can be extubated in the OR. In neonates or infants with compromised cardiac function, extubation should be delayed until their clinical status has improved. Dopamine or milrinone are usually continued postop and the patient gradually weaned. In young infants, systolic pressure consistently > 120 mmHg should be treated. A chest tube is left in place to monitor blood loss, or the appearance of a chylous effusion.

Blood and fluid requirements

IV: appropriate for patient size × 1-2
LR @ TKO (D-5 LR in neonates)
Blood warmer
T&C 1-2 U.

As a rule, infants and children undergoing coarctation repair will not require transfusion. Infrequently, however, sudden and substantial blood loss can occur, necessitating rapid transfusion. Adequate iv access, and immediate availability of blood is essential in this operation.

Monitoring	Standard monitors (see p. D-1). RUE arterial line ± CVP	BP must be monitored above and below the level of coarctation. A right radial arterial line allows BP monitoring during occlusion of the aortic arch. If a percutaneous radial arterial line cannot be placed, a surgical cutdown should be performed or a right axillary arterial line should be placed.
	BP cuffs × 2 (UE + LE)	Both upper and lower extremity cuff pressures should be monitored. ✓ ABG, glucose, Hct at intervals.
Control of BP	Anesthetic depth	In neonates and infants, GA is usually sufficient to control BP during aortic cross-clamp; however, SNP may be necessary to control BP in some patients.
Aortic cross-clamping	± Heparin 100 U/kg Ductus arteriosus ligated Aorta cross-clamped × 2 ✓ arterial line for damping. Ischemia time = 10-20 min Maintain distal perfusion. Lactic acidosis → ↓SVR + ↓BP.	Aortic cross-clamping presents an acute afterload to the LV. In preparation for release of cross-clamp, decrease or eliminate volatile anesthetic. Have blood and other volume available. Sodium bicarbonate is frequently required (1-2 m Eq/kg). ✓ ABG and treat accordingly.
Complications	Spinal cord ischemia HTN Bleeding Hypothermia Residual coarctation	

POSTOPERATIVE

Complications	Paraplegia HTN Bleeding GI bleed Abdominal pain and ileus Recurrent laryngeal nerve injury Chylous effusion Residual or recurrent coarctation	Incidence = 0.14-0.4%. The cause is likely 2° spinal cord ischemia. If a regional anesthetic was placed preop, spinal or epidural hematoma must be r/o. Occurs infrequently. Attributable to mesenteric arteritis. Neonates are at risk for GI reperfusion injury following repair. These patients are kept npo for 12-24 h.
Tests	CXR Hct ABGs	

References

1. Allen HD, Clark EB, Gutgesell HP, Driscoll DJ, eds. *Moss and Adams' Heart Disease in Infants, Children, and Adolescents*, 6th edition. Lippincott Williams & Wilkins, Philadelphia: 2001.
2. Castaneda AR, Jonas RA, Mayer JE Jr., Hanley FL: Aortic coarctation. In *Cardiac Surgery of the Neonate and Infant.* WB Saunders, Philadelphia: 1994, 333-52.
3. Emmanouilides GC, Allen HD, Riemenschneider TA, Gutgesell HP: Left ventricular and pulmonary outflow abnormalities. In *Clinical Synopsis of Moss and Adams' Heart Disease in Infants, Children, and Adolescents.* Williams & Wilkins, 1998, 464-500.
4. Morriss MJH, McNamara DG: Coarctation of the aorta and interrupted aortic arch. In *Science and Practice of Pediatric Cardiology.* Garson A, Bricker JT, McNamara DG, eds. Lea & Febiger, Philadelphia: 1990.
5. Reitz BA, Yuh DD, eds: *Congenital Cardiac Surgery.* McGraw-Hill, New York: 2002.
6. Ungerleider RM: Coarctation of the aorta. In *Mastery of Cardiothoracic Surgery.* Kaiser LR, Kron IL, Spray TL, eds. Lippincott-Raven, Philadelphia: 1998, 704-15.

SURGERY FOR TETRALOGY OF FALLOT

SURGICAL CONSIDERATIONS

Description: In **tetralogy of Fallot (TOF)**, the RV infundibulum is maldeveloped, resulting in RV outflow tract obstruction (RVOTO), a large malalignment (overriding aorta) VSD, RVH (see Fig 12.4-6) and, occasionally, an ASD (**pentalogy of Fallot**). TOF is the most common cyanotic congenital cardiac defect. Pathophysiologically, RVOTO leads to significant R→L shunting across a nonrestrictive VSD, which, in turn, leads to inadequate pulmonary blood flow and varying degrees of cyanosis. The variation in presentation depends primarily on the severity and type of RVOTO.

Patients with TOF were first treated palliatively beginning in 1944, with the introduction of the **Blalock-Taussig (B-T) systemic-to-pulmonary artery shunt**. This procedure augments pulmonary blood flow and, hence, systemic oxygenation. Currently, however, most cases of TOF are treated routinely with early complete correction between 3-12 mo of age. Neonatal repair is performed in infants who are severely cyanotic ($SaO_2 < 80\%$, have ductal-dependent pulmonary blood flow, or have cyanotic spells. Initial palliation with the B-T procedure is now reserved for patients with severe pulmonary arterial hypoplasia and (by some surgeons) for an anomalous

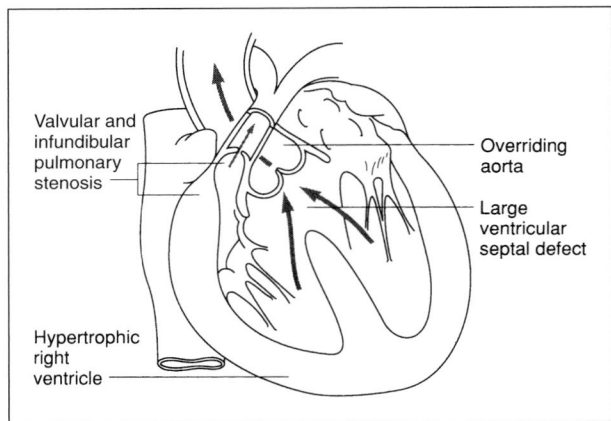

Figure 12.4-6. Anatomic features of tetralogy of Fallot. The primary morphologic abnormality, anterior and superior displacement of the infundibular septum, results in malalignment VSD, overriding the aortic valve and obstructing RV outflow. RV hypertrophy is a secondary occurrence. (Reproduced with permission from Greenfield LJ, et al, eds: *Surgery: Scientific Principles and Practice*, 2nd edition. Lippincott-Raven Publishers, 1997.)

left anterior descending coronary artery originating from the right coronary artery.

Surgical correction is performed through a standard median sternotomy on standard CPB with moderate hypothermia. During cooling, the modified B-T shunt, if present, is ligated and divided, followed by aortic cross-clamping, cardioplegic arrest, and topical cooling. The pulmonary valve and RVOT are accessed through a longitudinal pulmonary arteriotomy and the tricuspid valve (via a right atriotomy), respectively. RVOTO is treated as necessary by infundibular muscle resection, pulmonary valvotomy or valvectomy, and patch augmentation of the main PA or its branches. Autologous pericardium, Gore-Tex, or other type of synthetic/biologic material may be used for patch widening the RVOT at any level, from the RV to the PAs. The primary goal in relieving the RVOTO is to save the pulmonary valve, avoid a trans-cannular patch, and minimize pulmonary valve insufficiency. The VSD, accessed through the tricuspid valve, is closed with a patch (pericardial/Dacron) in the standard fashion, with care being taken to avoid injury to the bundle of His.

Variant procedure or approaches: In patients with severe hypoplasia or atresia of the RVOT, or in patients with an anomalous origin of the LAD coronary artery from the right coronary artery, a **Rastelli procedure** is performed. This operation consists of patch closure of the VSD and reconstruction of the RVOT in which a conduit, in the form of a cryopreserved homograft or valved prosthesis, is placed between the RV and the PA.

Usual preop diagnosis: TOF; cyanotic CHD; severe cyanotic spells; failure to thrive (FTT)

SUMMARY OF PROCEDURES

	Neonate Repair	Infant and Adult Repair With Standard CPB
Position	Supine	⇐
Incision	Standard median sternotomy	⇐
Unique considerations	R→L shunt → systemic embolization	⇐
Antibiotics	Cefazolin 25 mg/kg q 8 h	⇐
Surgical time	Aortic cross-clamp: 60 min	45-60 min
	CPB: 90-120 min	75-100 min
	Total: 3-4 h	3-4 h
Closing considerations	Chest tube in pericardial (and possibly pleural) space, if opened; temporary ventricular pacing wires; routine right- and left-atrial lines for monitoring.	⇐

	Neonate Repair	Infant and Adult Repair With Standard CPB
EBL	Moderate	⇐
Postop care	ICU × 2-3 d. 1-3 d assisted ventilation; inotropes for RV dysfunction	ICU for 1-2 d
Mortality	~2%	⇐
Morbidity	Junctional tachycardia	⇐
	Atrial dysrhythmias	⇐
	Hemorrhage	⇐
	Infection	⇐
	Low CO	⇐
	Stroke	⇐
	Heart block	⇐
	Residual VSD	⇐
	Transient, right-side CHF	⇐
Pain score	8-10	8-10

PATIENT POPULATION CHARACTERISTICS

Age range	Neonate-adult (usually < 6 mo)
Male:Female	3:2
Incidence	10% of congenital cardiac defects
Etiology	22 g microdeletion is seen in some patients, who also may have DiGeorge syndrome; higher than expected prevalence of older maternal age at time of conception of affected children.
Associated conditions	A-V canal; PDA; previous systemic-to-pulmonary arterial shunt; anomalous left coronary artery from pulmonary artery (ALCAPA); metabolic acidosis (profound hypoxia); right-sided aortic arch

ANESTHETIC CONSIDERATIONS

PREOPERATIVE

Pathophysiology   The clinical presentation of TOF is dependent on the wide anatomic variation of this tetrad. The critical factor is the degree of RVOTO, which determines the amount of R→L shunting across the VSD. This obstruction is dynamic and can be related to RV infundibular spasm, and variations in pH, $PaCO_2$ and PaO_2. The onset of hypercyanotic episodes is the indication for complete surgical repair.

'TET' spells   Hypercyanotic episodes, or 'TET' spells: These constitute medical and surgical emergencies; however, they are seen less frequently due to early surgical intervention. TET spells may present in early infancy and are related to infundibular spasm resulting in ↑R→L shunting. If untreated, these episodes can progress to unconsciousness, Sz, and death. For management of TET spells, see table 12.4-1.

Table 12.4-1. Treatment for TET Spells

Treatment Modalities	Effect
1. Knee-chest position	↑ SVR.
2. Abdominal compression	Simulates squatting, ↑ SVR.
3. Volume administration	↑ preload, opens RVOT.
4. O_2	Pulmonary vasodilator
5. Anesthesia and sedation	Negative inotropy → reduced RVOT spasm.
6. Alpha-agonist (phenylephrine)	↑ SVR. Dose: 10 μg/kg bolus.
7. Beta-blockers (esmolol)	Negative inotropy. Dose: 50 μg/kg bolus.

Respiratory	Infectious/asthmatic pulmonary processes will complicate preop and postop cardiopulmonary function. Optimize pulmonary function preop. **Tests:** CXR: ↓pulmonary vascular markings and characteristic heart shape.
Cardiovascular	CHF is rare in young patients, except in infants without a pulmonary valve, but more common in older children/adults 2° RV cardiomyopathy, chronic hypoxia, and functionally induced aortic insufficiency. An understanding of the patient's anatomic defects and their pathophysiology (e.g., is their RVOTO fixed or dynamic?) is essential for formulating the anesthetic plan. Avoid prolonged fasting to prevent profound decreases in preload on induction. **Tests:** ABG; ECG: ✓ for RVH, right axis deviation (RAD) ± complete or incomplete RBBB. CXR: ✓ heart size, 'coeur en sabot' (elevation of apex 2° RVH, RAE). Cardiac cath and ECHO: Locate site of pulmonary outflow obstruction, VSD, bronchopulmonary collaterals, PDA, abnormal patency of previous surgical shunts (e.g., B-T shunt). Define aortic arch anatomy, abnormal coronary or subclavian arteries, tricuspid regurgitation/aortic insufficiency (TR/AI), ventricular function.
Hematologic	Polycythemia (typical with chronic O_2 sat < 90%) → ↑blood viscosity → thromboembolic events. Polycythemia → ↓Plt + coagulopathy. Extreme polycythemia (> 70) may require isovolemic hemodilution intraop. **Tests:** CBC; Plt; bleeding time; coag profile
Laboratory	Electrolytes if on diuretics; otherwise, tests as indicated from H&P.
Premedication	As required to ↓ anxiety, avoid TET spells and facilitate separation from parents. Midazolam 0.5-0.75 mg po 20 min before induction in a monitored setting.

INTRAOPERATIVE

Anesthetic technique: GETA. Patients with TOF, pulmonary atresia, and MAPCAS (major aortopulmonary collaterals) requiring unifocalization, present a challenge for surgical and anesthetic management. Special periop requirements include: placement of cuffed ETTs and availability of inline bronchodilator therapy 2° an increased risk for severe bronchospasm. OLV also may be required to facilitate surgical exposure. Bronchial bleeding 2° extensive surgical dissection requires frequent ETT suctioning. A significant portion of the procedure is done off-CPB, and hemodynamic instability may occur during surgical dissection. Closely monitor blood loss and replace ml/ml with PRBCs. It is essential to monitor ECG for ST-segment changes during dissection. Avoid air bubbles in iv tubing/stopcocks.

Induction	Typically mask induction with sevoflurane, O_2 ± N_2O. If iv in place, ketamine (1-2 mg/kg) and/or fentanyl (10 µg/kg) with rocuronium (1 mg/kg) ± volatile agent. Avoid ↓↓SVR. Verify ETT position (see p. D-3).
Maintenance	For patients not undergoing unifocalization, anesthesia is maintained with isoflurane or sevoflurane. TET spells can occur 2° surgical manipulation. Hypercyanotic episodes can occur during surgical dissection for cannulation before CPB. The surgeon can provide direct aortic compression or urgently proceed to CPB. Refer to Table 12.4-1 for other treatment. For patients who are undergoing unifocalization, hypoxic pulmonary vasoconstriction is blunted by the use of volatile anesthetic agents, causing a further decrease in arterial saturation. As a result, we prefer to use total intravenous anesthesia with propofol/ketamine/midazolam infusion.
Emergence	Patients are transported to ICU monitored, intubated, and ventilated.

Blood and fluid requirements	IV: 22-24 ga × 2 LR @ TKO T&C PRBC	Blood in OR before incision. For all repeat sternotomy patients, have blood available for immediate administration.
Monitoring	Standard monitors Urinary catheter Arterial line (usually radial) CVP line TEE Transthoracic LA line: have transducer available.	 Double-lumen CVP placed in IJ or femoral vein.
Pre-CPB	Heparinization (4 mg/kg) ACT > 400 sec MAP ~70 mmHg	In the pre-CPB period, crystalloid and/or 5% albumin is administered as needed to compensate for bleeding and 3rd-space losses.

Pre-CPB, cont.	✓ muscle relaxation. ✓ pupils. ✓ UO.	
CPB	Ventilation stopped. Hypothermia: ~28°C Hct 30 typical during CPB ✓ adequate flow/pressure. ✓ anesthetic/NMB levels. ✓ pupils. ✓ face for venous congestion. ✓ ABG, electrolytes, UO, Hct, and ACT q 30 min.	Lasix (0.5-1 mg/kg) for ↓UO and hemoconcentration.
Transition off CPB	Rewarming Vasoactive infusions started at 32°C. Flush lines. TEE Zero transducers. Suction ETT. Resume ventilation. Observe lung inflation. Supplement NMB and deepen anesthesia. Rewarm to 36°C. ✓ bilateral breath sounds. ✓ ABGs, electrolytes, Hct (~30). ✓ ACT (> 400). ✓ ECG: pacing may be necessary.	Surgeons deair heart, which can be monitored by TEE. A measurement of the RV and LV pressure ratio helps to judge adequacy of repair of the RVOTO. TEE also is used to evaluate the anatomy, the repair, and pressures. These patients are at risk for development of junctional ectopic tachycardia (JET). Avoid excessive warming > 37°C. Have amiodarone (5-10mg/kg load) available.

Post-CPB	Inotropic support (dopamine, milnirone, epinephrine, and CaCl)
	Rx pulmonary HTN (↓PVR):
	   $FiO_2 = 1$
	   $PaCO_2$ ~30
	Minimize mean airway pressure.
	AV sequential pacemaker (heart block not uncommon).
	Transthoracic PA or LA line placed to monitor hemodynamics.
	Reverse anticoagulation.
	Rx coagulopathy
	Modified ultrafiltration (MUF)
		↓RV compliance is expected. RV afterload reduction is essential, initially through ventilatory efforts: clear unobstructed ventilation; do not allow wheezing (albuterol prn); use gentle hyperventilation on 100% O_2. Inotropic support of RV also typically is used—dopamine/dobutamine initially and epinephrine reserved for severe RV dysfunction.
		
		See Table 12.4-2 for blood product utilization (p. 992). MUF uses the CPB machine to remove excess H_2O and inflammatory medications (↓edema and improved cardiopulmonary function).

Positioning	✓ and pad pressure points. ✓ eyes.	
Complications	See Postoperative Complications, below.	

POSTOPERATIVE

Complications	Persistent bleeding Persistent RVOTO Dysrhythmias (JET)	For neonatal repairs, a PFO is left surgically open to allow RV decompression via a R→L intraatrial shunt. This often will result in ↓systemic O_2 sat. TEE will confirm the existence of intraatrial shunting.
Tests	ABGs + electrolytes Coag profile CXR: ✓ line, ETT placement.	

Table 12.4-2. Blood Product Utilization[8]

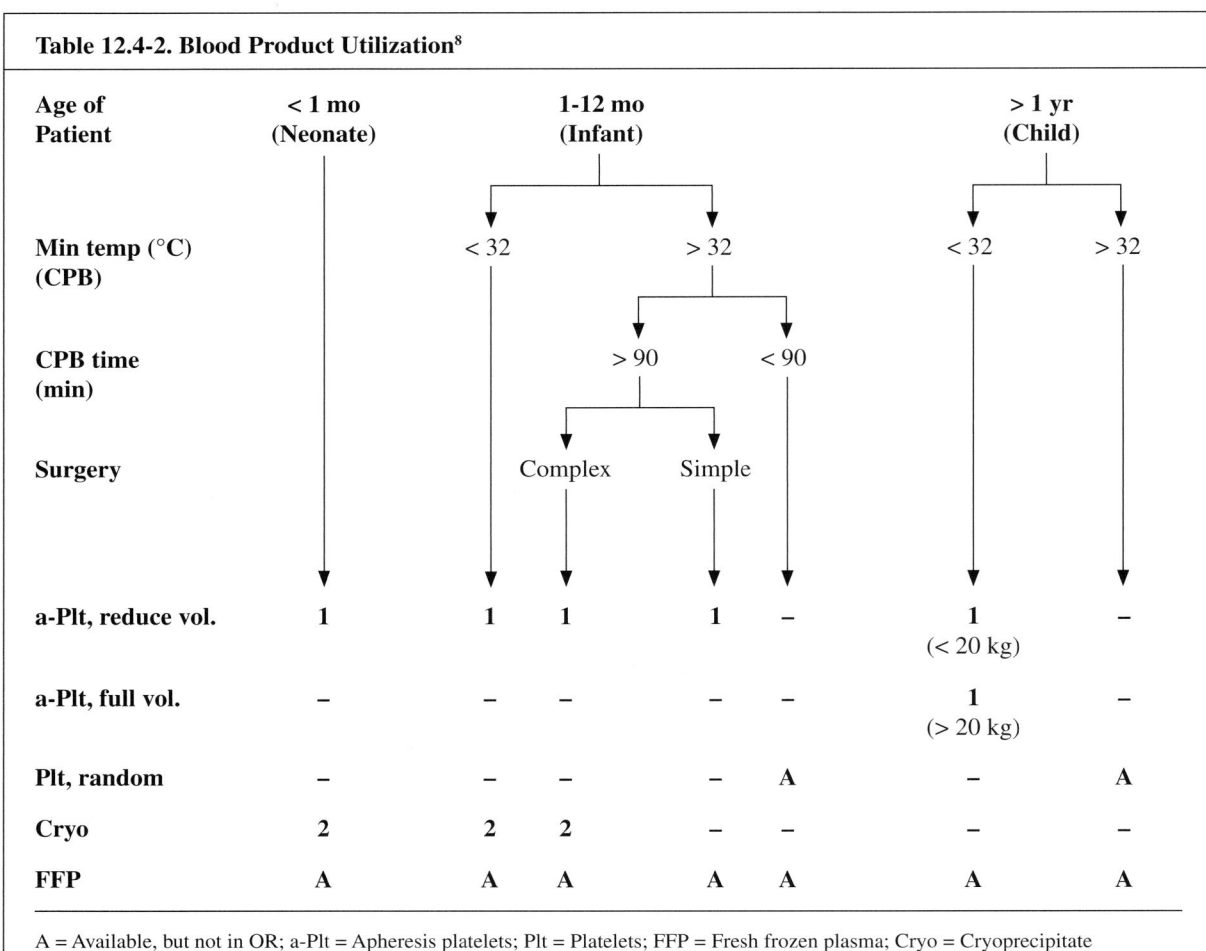

Age of Patient	< 1 mo (Neonate)	1-12 mo (Infant)				> 1 yr (Child)	
Min temp (°C) (CPB)		< 32	> 32			< 32	> 32
CPB time (min)			> 90		< 90		
Surgery			Complex	Simple			
a-Plt, reduce vol.	1	1	1	1	–	1 (< 20 kg)	–
a-Plt, full vol.	–	–	–	–	–	1 (> 20 kg)	–
Plt, random	–	–	–	–	A	–	A
Cryo	2	2	2	–	–	–	–
FFP	A	A	A	A	A	A	A

A = Available, but not in OR; a-Plt = Apheresis platelets; Plt = Platelets; FFP = Fresh frozen plasma; Cryo = Cryoprecipitate

References

1. Allen HD, Clark EB, Gutgesell HP, Driscoll DJ, eds. *Moss and Adams' Heart Disease in Infants, Children, and Adolescents,* 6th edition. Lippincott Williams & Wilkins, Philadelphia: 2001.
2. Castaneda AR, Jonas RA, Mayer JE Jr, Hanley FL: Tetralogy of Fallot. In *Cardiac Surgery of the Neonate and Infant.* WB Saunders, Philadelphia: 1994, 215-34.
3. Emmanouilides GC, Allen HD, Riemenschneider TA, Gutgesell HP: Tetralogy of Fallot. In *Clinical Synopsis of Moss and Adams' Heart Disease in Infants, Children, and Adolescents.* Williams & Wilkins, 1998, 409-33.
4. Karl TR: Tetralogy of Fallot. In *Glenn's Thoracic and Cardiovascular Surgery,* 6th edition. Baue AE, ed. Appleton & Lange, Stamford: 1996, 1211-19.
5. Perryman RA, Jaquiss DB: Tetralogy of Fallot. In *Mastery of Cardiothoracic Surgery.* Kaiser LR, Kron IL, Spray TL, eds. Lippincott-Raven, Philadelphia: 1998, 831-8.
6. Reitz BA, Yuh DD, eds: *Congenital Cardiac Surgery.* McGraw-Hill, New York: 2002.
7. Samuelson PN, Lell WA: Tetralogy of Fallot. In *Pediatric Cardiac Anesthesia,* 3rd edition. Lake CL, ed. Appleton & Lange, Stamford: 1998, 303-14.
8. Williams GD, Bratton SL, Riley EC, Ramamoorthy C: Association between age and blood loss in children undergoing open-heart surgery. *Ann Thorac Surg* 1998; 66:870-6.

SURGERY FOR TOTAL ANOMALOUS PULMONARY VENOUS CONNECTION

SURGICAL CONSIDERATIONS

Description: Total anomalous venous connection (TAPVC) is a rare congenital cardiac malformation in which the entire pulmonary venous return empties either directly into the systemic venous channels via anomalous veins or the right atrium (Fig 12.4-7). An interatrial R→L shunt, in the form of a PFO or an ASD, is required to maintain systemic output and, hence, survival in the postnatal period. The objective of surgical correction is to redirect the entire pulmonary venous return to the left atrium.

TAPVC was first successfully repaired in 1956 by Lewis and Varco at the University of Minnesota, by joining the pulmonary venous sinus to the left atrium and closure of the ASD. Although mortality for this lesion was initially quite high, particularly in infants with obstruction of the pulmonary veins, improvements in intraop and postop management have permitted successful correction in most neonates and infants. There are four TAPVC drainage patterns, as defined by Darling and associates. These include **supracardiac** (45%), **cardiac** (25%), **infracardiac** (25%), and **mixed** patterns (5%) of venous drainage. The anomalous drainage in supracardiac TAPVC is usually by a left vertical vein into the innominate vein. In cardiac TAPVC, drainage is usually into the coronary sinus and occasionally into the right atrium. In infracardiac TAPVC, drainage is usually into the portal vein. The mixed type consists of combinations of the other three varieties of TAPVC.

When pulmonary venous drainage is obstructed, patients present with cyanosis, severe pulmonary edema, pulmonary HTN, and ↓CO. Symptomatic TAPVC is repaired at any age. TAPVC with obstruction is a true

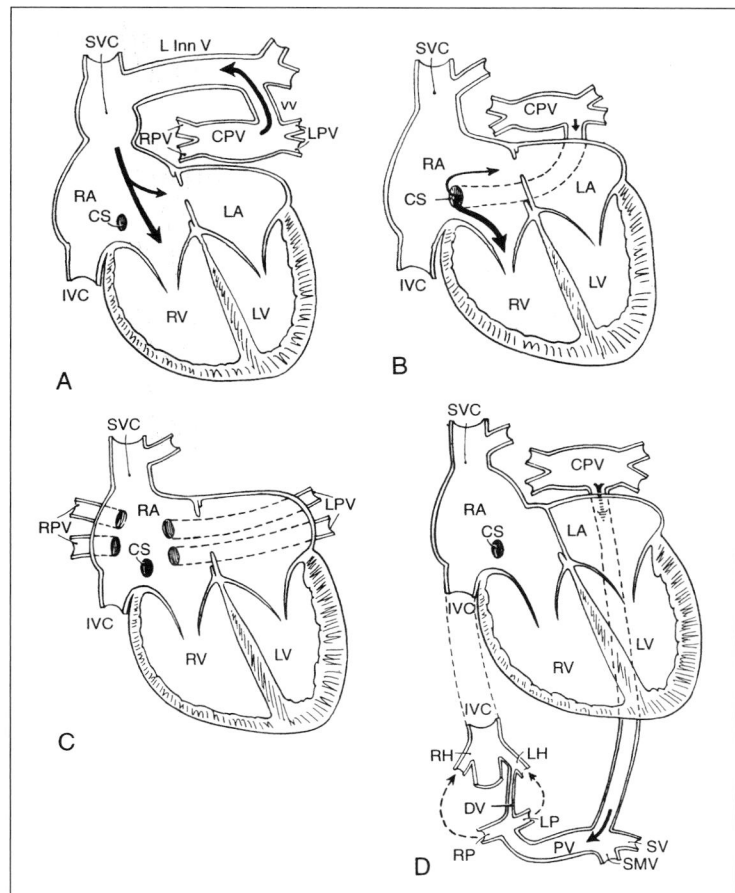

Figure 12.4-7. Common forms of TAPVC: (A) TAPVC to the left innominate vein (L inn V) by way of a vertical vein (VV). (B) TAPVC to coronary sinus (CS). The pulmonary veins join to form a confluence designated as the common pulmonary vein (CPV), which connects to the coronary sinus. (C) TAPVC to right atrium (RA) The left and right pulmonary veins (LPV and RPV) usually enter the RA separately. (D) TAPVC to the portal vein (PV). The PVs form a confluence, from which an anomalous channel arises. (Reproduced with permission from Emmanouilides GC, Allen HD, Riemenschneider TA, Gutgesell HP: *Clinical Synopsis of Moss and Adams' Heart Disease in Infants, Children, and Adolescents.* Williams & Wilkins, 1998.)

surgical emergency. Critically ill neonates with obstructed pulmonary venous return must undergo emergent correction after initial stabilization (i.e., intubation/ventilation, diuretics). Occasionally, preop ECMO may be required.

In most cases, the right and left pulmonary veins drain into a common pulmonary venous sinus, allowing for its anastomosis to the left atrium for a definitive repair. Through a standard median sternotomy, the aortic and venous cannulae are placed and CPB with cooling is initiated. The aorta is cross-clamped, immediately followed by cardioplegic arrest. The cardiac apex is lifted up, and the pulmonary veins are identified through the posterior pericardium. The left atrium is then opened transversely with extension onto the left atrial appendage, followed by the direct anastomosis of the pulmonary venous confluence to the left atrium. Finally, via a right atriotomy, the ASD or PFO is closed. The heart is deaired, aortic cross-clamp is released, and the patient is rewarmed and separated from bypass. Successful outcomes are dependent on early and immediate correction of TAPVC with obstruction, before lung damage ensues. Other important factors include repair without residual obstruction and postop control of pulmonary HTN.

Variant procedure or approaches: Alternatively, repair of TAPVC may be accomplished through a right atriotomy and across the atrial septum, constructing the anastomosis between the pulmonary venous confluence and left atrium from within the left atrium or through a transverse sinus approach.

Usual preop diagnosis: TAPVC; total anomalous venous return; total anomalous pulmonary venous drainage—all of these ± obstruction and either supracardiac, cardiac, or mixed types

SUMMARY OF PROCEDURE

Position	Supine
Incision	Standard median sternotomy
Unique considerations	Patients often require urgent or emergency surgery. Obligatory R→L shunting → risk of systemic embolization. Myocardial preservation using blood or crystalloid cardioplegia, in addition to topical myocardial hypothermia, is used.
Antibiotics	Cefazolin 25 mg/kg q 8 h
Surgical time	Aortic cross-clamp: 30-60 min Circulatory arrest: occasionally, 30-45 min Total: 2-3 h
Closing considerations	A fine polyvinyl catheter inserted through the free wall of the right ventricle and advanced into the pulmonary trunk will allow monitoring for pulmonary HTN. A chest tube is inserted into the pericardial space; temporary ventricular pacing wires are placed. Left atrial lines normally needed.
EBL	Moderate
Postop care	2-6 d of assisted ventilation, sedation and hyperventilation; pulmonary vasodilators, including isoproterenol, PGE_1, SNP; inotropes as needed for right heart dysfunction. Sometimes, if pulmonary injury is severe or pulmonary HTN is uncontrollable, ECMO may be indicated.
Mortality	2-10%, depending on presence of preop pulmonary venous obstruction and metabolic acidosis.
Morbidity	Pulmonary vasospasm: 25-40% Low CO: 10% Hemorrhage: 2-3%
Pain score	8-10

PATIENT POPULATION CHARACTERISTICS

Age range	1 d–20 yr (usually < 1 mo)
Male:Female	4:1 in infracardiac type; equal distribution in other types
Incidence	0.5%-2% of congenital heart defects
Etiology	Failure of fusion of the pulmonary vein evagination (from posterior left atrium) with the pulmonary venous plexus surrounding the lung buds.
Associated conditions	PDA present in nearly all infants within the first few wk of life and in about 15% of cases overall. VSD occasionally occurs (may be associated with TOF, DORV, interrupted aortic arch, and other lesions).

ANESTHETIC CONSIDERATIONS

PREOPERATIVE

Pathophysiology	In the supradiaphragmatic connection, all the pulmonary venous return drains into the right atrium via a common pulmonary vein. When this vein or confluence is stenotic or obstructed, severe pulmonary HTN, cyanosis, pulmonary edema, and shock ensue. This is a true surgical emergency, requiring immediate intervention. An ASD or PFO is essential for survival, and sometimes a balloon septostomy may be required for stabilization before surgery.
Respiratory	In patients with obstructed TAPVC, expect severe pulmonary edema and pulmonary HTN. **Tests:** ✓ CXR: ↑heart size, ↑pulmonary vascularity, 'figure-of-8,' or 'snowman' cardiac silhouette.
Cardiovascular	ECHO findings: large RV and small LA. Cardiac interventricular cath for balloon or blade septostomy in patients with restrictive ASD may be necessary to improve R→L shunting. **Tests:** ✓ ECG for right axis deviation (RAD), RAE and RVH.

Laboratory	ABG and Hct; other tests as indicated from H&P.
Premedication	Generally not indicated and not necessary in severely ill infants.
Transport of critically ill newborn	All critically ill neonates are intubated, ventilated, and often are on PGE$_1$ and/or dopamine for hemodynamic stability. This is in addition to TPN and sedative medication. Some neonates (with HLHS syndrome, truncus, TGA) may be on hypoxic mixtures to reduce pulmonary overcirculation and maintain systemic perfusion. Additionally, PEEP of 8-10 cmH$_2$O may be used to ↑PVR and ↓pulmonary blood flow. To facilitate transport of these patients, notify the nurse in advance and request all drips transferred to OR syringe pumps. D/C sedative and intralipid infusions. Maintain a dextrose-containing infusion during and after transport to ensure normoglycemia. An air-O$_2$ blender should be available so the inspired O$_2$ concentration can be adjusted as needed. Verify that the transport monitor has ECG, SaO$_2$ and invasive pressure transducers. Resuscitation medications and airway equipment must accompany the patient. Maintain the neonate's body T during transport with a warming pad and a head cover. Preop if an infant is on a hypoxic mixture in the NICU, nitrogen may be necessary for transport; however, patients can be transported on room air with gentle manual ventilation, taking care to avoid hyperventilation. Avoid oversedation and use of muscle relaxants before transport, as systemic blood flow is severely compromised if there is an acute ↑ in pulmonary blood flow.

INTRAOPERATIVE

Anesthetic technique: GETA. Profound hypothermic CPB (16°-18°C) with low flow may be required. Patients who weigh < 3.0 kg and are ventilator-dependent preop are at high risk to have continued decline in oxygenation and ventilation post-CPB. Frequently, the patient ventilator from the NICU is used in the OR, as this allows for maximum flexibility in ventilator support.

Induction	Infants are often severely ill and come to the OR intubated and ventilated, with invasive lines and inotropic support. Verify ETT placement. Patients are subject to rapid cardiovascular decompensation. Rocuronium (1 mg/kg) is given, as is fentanyl (10 μg/kg). Volatile agents are rarely tolerated in obstructed TAPVC.
Maintenance	Fentanyl (20-50 μg/kg) in divided doses. Rocuronium prn, midazolam 0.1-0.2 mg/kg. FiO$_2$ = 1.0. Ventilation maneuvers to ↓PVR. (See Post-CPB, p. 991.)
Emergence	Transport to ICU intubated and ventilated. If NO used in OR, must have delivery system ready for transport to ICU). There may be continued requirement for inotropic support.

Blood and fluid requirements	IV: 22-24 ga × 2, taped securely LR @ TKO Continue iv dextrose in neonates. 5% albumin PRBC Blood warmer	Avoid air bubbles with R→L shunt—can cause systemic embolization of air. ✓ blood glucose. Avoid hyperglycemia, especially during profound hypothermic CPB. See Table 12.4-2 for blood product utilization.
Monitoring	Standard monitors (see p. D-1). Transthoracic LA, PA, RA lines	Severely ill infants usually present with invasive monitoring and ETT. ✓ correct placement of UAC and UVC preop.
Complications	Bleeding Refractory pulmonary HTN	Pulmonary HTN may be difficult to control. Ventilation maneuvers (e.g., ↓PaCo$_2$; 100% O$_2$), vasodilators, and deep anesthesia to ↓ PVR. NO is started for refractory pulmonary HTN; if NO (20 ppm) is unsuccessful, ECMO may be instituted.
	Biventricular failure	Inotropic support (dopamine, milnirone, epinephrine, calcium chloride)
	Overdose of NO → methHb	✓ metHb while on NO therapy.

POSTOPERATIVE

Complications	See above.	
Tests	ABG Hct; electrolytes; coags Methemoglobin CXR	 Only if on NO

References

1. Allen HD, Clark EB, Gutgesell HP, Driscoll DJ, eds. *Moss and Adams' Heart Disease in Infants, Children, and Adolescents,* 6th edition. Lippincott Williams & Wilkins, Philadelphia: 2001.
2. Castaneda AR, Jonas RA, Mayer JE Jr, Hanley FL: Total anomalous pulmonary venous connection. In *Cardiac Surgery of the Neonate and Infant.* WB Saunders, Philadelphia: 1994, 157-66.
3. Cope JT, Kron IL: Anomalies of pulmonary venous return and cor triatriatum. In *Mastery of Cardiothoracic Surgery.* Kaiser LR, Kron IL, Spray TL, eds. Lippincott-Raven, Philadelphia: 1998, 867-79.
4. Emmanouilides GC, Allen HD, Riemenschneider TA, Gutgesell HP: Venous abnormalities. In *Clinical Synopsis of Moss and Adams' Heart Disease in Infants, Children, and Adolescents.* Williams & Wilkins, 1998, 349-68.
5. Lake CL: Anomalies of the systemic and pulmonary venous returns. In *Pediatric Cardiac Anesthesia,* 3rd edition. Appleton & Lange, Stamford: 1998, 353-71.
6. Lanier WL: Glucose management during cardiopulmonary bypass: cardiovascular and neurologic implications. *Anesth Analg* 1991; 72:423-7.
7. Reitz BA, Yuh DD, eds: *Congenital Cardiac Surgery.* McGraw-Hill, New York: 2002.

SURGERY FOR COMPLETE TRANSPOSITION OF THE GREAT ARTERIES

SURGICAL CONSIDERATIONS

Description: Complete **transposition of the great arteries (TGA)** is a congenital cardiac defect in which the aorta arises from the RV and the PA arises from the LV (Fig 12.4-8). TGA is associated with an intact ventricular septum (TGA/IVS) or a ventricular septal defect (TGA/VSD). Pathophysiologically, this discordant ventriculoarterial configuration results in systemic and pulmonary circulations placed in a parallel (normally in series) configuration. Thus, a L→R shunt in the form of an atrial septal defect (ASD), VSD, or patent ductus arteriosus (PDA) is required to permit oxygenated blood to enter the 'right-sided' systemic circulation. The earliest surgical treatment for TGA was described by **Blalock** and **Hanlon** in 1950, with a procedure in which an **atrial septectomy** was performed, improving the mixing of pulmonary and systemic blood at the atrial level. In the 1950s, a variety of partial physiologic corrections were developed in which the pulmonary veins or the vena cava were transposed to the alternate atria. Palliative treatment was advanced by **Rashkind's** description of a **balloon atrial septostomy** in 1966. More complete physiologic correction was obtained by **atrial switch** operations, described by **Senning** in 1959 and **Mustard** in 1963, in which systemic and pulmonary venous return were baffled to the appropriate ventricles. Postop complications with the atrial switch operations, however, led to the development of the more 'anatomic' **arterial switch** operations described by **Jatene, Yacoub,** and others beginning in the 1970s. By 1987, the arterial switch operation in neonates was widely accepted as the standard approach to TGA.

Total correction is now performed routinely in the first 2 wk of life. The heart is exposed through a standard median sternotomy and CPB is instituted. The aortic cross-clamp is applied, followed by cardioplegic arrest and induced hypothermia. The ascending aorta is transected at its midportion and the pulmonary trunk is transected just proximal to its bifurcation. Two buttons from the 'neopulmonary artery' (former aortic root) containing the origins of the left and right coronary arteries are transposed and anastomosed to the 'neoaorta' (former main pulmonary trunk). The distal aortic segment is swung beneath the PA bifurcation (**Lecompte maneuver**). Pericardial patches are used to repair the defects resulting from excision of the coronary artery buttons, and any associated ASDs and/or VSDs are repaired. The distal aortic segment is anastomosed to the neoaorta and the distal bifurcated pulmonary artery segment is anastomosed to the neopulmonary artery. If hypothermia has been induced, a brief period of circulatory arrest facilitates repair of the ASD and/or VSD, if present. The aortic cross-clamp is removed and rewarming is begun during the neopulmonary arterial anastomosis. CPB is then D/C'd and closure is routine.

Variant procedure or approaches: In children with TGA and VSD, additional cardiac anomalies are common. These include pulmonary stenosis, pulmonary atresia, straddling atrioventricular valves, hypoplasia of ventricular chambers, and coarctation or interruption of aorta. Dynamic or structural subpulmonic obstruction is also more common in TGA and VSD than in TGA/IVS.

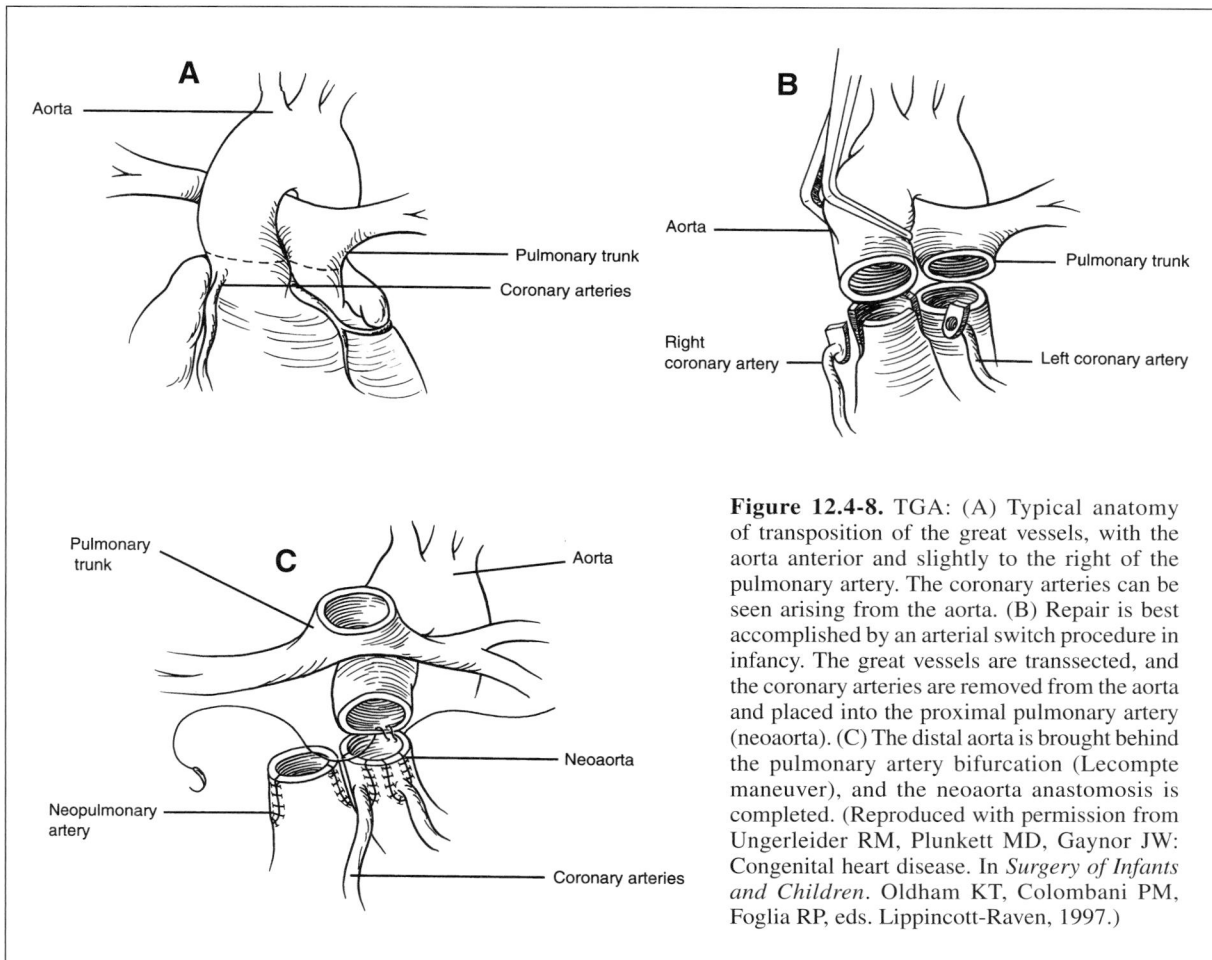

Figure 12.4-8. TGA: (A) Typical anatomy of transposition of the great vessels, with the aorta anterior and slightly to the right of the pulmonary artery. The coronary arteries can be seen arising from the aorta. (B) Repair is best accomplished by an arterial switch procedure in infancy. The great vessels are transsected, and the coronary arteries are removed from the aorta and placed into the proximal pulmonary artery (neoaorta). (C) The distal aorta is brought behind the pulmonary artery bifurcation (Lecompte maneuver), and the neoaorta anastomosis is completed. (Reproduced with permission from Ungerleider RM, Plunkett MD, Gaynor JW: Congenital heart disease. In *Surgery of Infants and Children.* Oldham KT, Colombani PM, Foglia RP, eds. Lippincott-Raven, 1997.)

Rastelli procedure: The VSD is baffled to the aorta with construction of a RV→PA valved conduit and is the procedure of choice for patients with TGA/VSD and pulmonary atresia or significant valvular pulmonary stenosis.

Coronary arteries in TGA: Abnormalities in the origin and course of coronary arteries are common in TGA and, in the past, influenced the success of surgery. A simple rule that accounts for virtually all variations is that the coronaries arise from the sinuses of Valsalva, which face the pulmonary artery, and follow the shortest route to their ultimate destination. Only a small number pose a problem in switching the great arteries.

Usual preop diagnosis: Complete TGA; transposition of the great vessels; transposition ± VSD; ASD; PDA

SUMMARY OF PROCEDURE

Position	Supine
Incision	Standard median sternotomy
Unique considerations	Operation to be performed before LV pressure falls substantially 2° ↓PVR.
Antibiotics	Cefazolin 25 mg/kg q 8 h
Surgical time	Aortic cross-clamp: 45-70 min
	Circulatory arrest: 10-15 min
	Total: 3 h
Closing considerations	Routine closure with chest tube in the pericardial space; temporary ventricular pacing wire; possible right or left atrial line for monitoring.
EBL	Moderate
Postop care	1-5 d of assisted ventilation; pulmonary HTN protocol consisting of hyperventilation and sedation and use of pulmonary vasodilators; inotropes for adequate CO.

Mortality	1-3%
Morbidity	Hemorrhage
	Atrial dysrhythmias
	↓CO
	Coronary artery kinking and myocardial ischemia
	Pulmonary HTN
Pain score	8-10

PATIENT POPULATION CHARACTERISTICS

Age range	1-21 d; ≤ 3-6 mo in TGA/VSD
Male:Female	2:1; for TGA/IVS, 3.3:1
Incidence	7-8% of congenital heart defects
Etiology	Usually no associated syndromes or other noncardiac abnormalities
Associated conditions	ASD; VSD; PDA; LVOTO; pulmonary atresia; coarctation of the aorta

---

ANESTHETIC CONSIDERATIONS

PREOPERATIVE

Pathophysiology In TGA, the pulmonary and systemic circulations flow in parallel, unlike the normal series circulation. Deoxygenated blood returns to the right heart and is pumped to the aorta and systemic circulation without passing through the lungs for gas exchange. The oxygenated blood returns via the pulmonary veins and recirculates through the LV back into the lungs. Survival depends on mixing of pulmonary and systemic blood at some level (ASD, VSD, PDA). In the absence of a septal defect, a balloon atrial septostomy (Rashkind) may be required before surgery to promote mixing.

Respiratory Some patients are maintained preop on PGE_1, to keep the ductus arteriosus open. PGE_1 can cause apnea; therefore, mechanical ventilation may be required.
Tests: CXR: ✓ enlarged heart and pulmonary edema.

Cardiovascular Patients with VSD have ↑pulmonary blood flow, ↑intercirculatory mixing → CHF. Marked cyanosis is seen in patients with TGA and intact ventricular septum, O_2 sat depends on degree of mixing (Q_P/Q_S ratio).
Tests: ECG: right axis deviation (RAD) and RVH. ECHO. Cardiac cath defines anatomy, coronary arteries, septal defects, PFO, PDA, bronchopulmonary collaterals, LVOT, pulmonic valve function and pressures, including PVR and LV:RV ratio. Balloon atrial septostomy (Rashkind-Miller) is required to improve mixing in some patients.

Laboratory Hct; coags; other tests as indicated from H&P.

Premedication Generally not necessary in children < 9 mo.

Transport of critically ill newborn All critically ill neonates are intubated, ventilated, and often are on PGE_1 and/or dopamine for hemodynamic stability. This is in addition to TPN and sedative medication. Some neonates (with HLHS syndrome, truncus, TGA) may be on hypoxic mixtures to reduce pulmonary overcirculation and maintain systemic perfusion. Additionally, PEEP of 8-10 cmH_2O may be used to ↑PVR and ↓pulmonary blood flow. To facilitate transport of these patients, notify the nurse in advance and request all drips transferred to OR syringe pumps. D/C sedative and intralipid infusions. Maintain a dextrose-containing infusion during and after transport to ensure normoglycemia. An air-O_2 blender should be available so the inspired O_2 concentration can be adjusted as needed. Verify that the transport monitor has ECG, SaO_2 and invasive pressure transducers. Resuscitation medications and airway equipment must accompany the patient. Maintain the neonate's body T during transport with a warming pad and a head cover. Preop if an infant is on a hypoxic mixture in the NICU, nitrogen may be necessary for transport; however, patients can be transported on room air with gentle manual ventilation, taking care to avoid hyperventilation. Avoid oversedation and use of muscle relaxants before transport, as systemic blood flow is severely compromised if there is an acute ↑ in pulmonary blood flow.

INTRAOPERATIVE

Anesthetic technique: GETA

Induction	Most neonates are placed on PGE$_1$ to maintain ductal patency and promote mixing of pulmonary and systemic blood. Anesthetic management is based on maintaining a balance between systemic and pulmonary blood flows. Excessive pulmonary blood flow → ↓systemic perfusion. Avoid factors that ↓ PVR (hyperoxia, hyperventilation, alkalosis). IV induction with fentanyl (e.g., 5-10 μg/kg slowly) and muscle relaxant (e.g., rocuronium 1 mg/kg) is the technique of choice. Inotropic infusion and PRBC transfusion may be required to support BP.	
Maintenance	For patients with inadequate intercirculatory mixing and ↓pulmonary blood flow, treatment should include ventilation maneuvers to ↓ PVR (see TOF, Post-CPB, p. 991) and improve mixing. Deep GA helps to blunt reactive pulmonary HTN. Avoid ↓HR → ↓CO in infants with limited myocardial reserve.	
Emergence	Control aortic BP and treat any coagulopathy. Monitor LA pressures closely. ✓ for myocardial ischemia, which can be 2° coronary air emboli or a problem with reimplantation of coronaries. Transport to ICU intubated and ventilated.	

Blood and fluid requirements	IV: 22-24 ga × 1-2 taped securely LR @ TKO Continue iv dextrose in neonates. 5% albumin	Avoid air bubbles in patients with R → L and L → R shunts. Maintain blood glucose ~50-200. See Table 2.4-2 for blood products utilization. Administer blood and products slowly, with close monitoring of LAP. Overtransfusion can cause systemic HTN, LA dilation, or pulmonary edema, producing additional suture line bleeding or mitral regurgitation.
Monitoring	Standard monitors (see **D-1**).	Severely ill infants often present with invasive monitoring and mechanical ventilation. Correct placement of UAC and UVC should be checked preop.
	Transthoracic monitoring lines (RA, LA, or PA)	Placed routinely on rewarming, before weaning from CPB. These are for monitoring and administration of inotropes and other medications. The LV is deconditioned and has not been exposed to systemic afterload; therefore, it may be dysfunctional and require inotropic support (dopamine, milrinone, epinephrine, and CaCl infusion). During weaning from CPB, it is critical to monitor LAP, as a reflection of left-sided filling, simultaneously with RA pressure monitoring.
	TEE	Abnormalities in coronary perfusion may manifest as changes in ECG rhythm and should be closely followed. TEE is useful both as a monitor of function and volume status. ECMO may be needed for severe ventricular dysfunction.
CPB	Management of CPB is discussed in Intraoperative Considerations for TOF, p. 990.	Low flow or moderate hypothermic CPB. Cool with pH stat management (T, corrected ABG). Warm on reperfusion with alpha stat.
Complications	Bleeding LV dysfunction and failure Myocardial ischemia Residual structural defects Dysrhythmias Pulmonary HTN	In patients with TGA and IVS, the LV may be inadequate to support the systemic circulation. The LV becomes deconditioned after the PVR drops in early infancy. The LV is then unable to function as the systemic ventricle. Inotropic support (dopamine and epinephrine) and afterload reduction (SNP or amrinone) may be necessary to separate from CPB. ECMO may be required for severe ventricular dysfunction.

POSTOPERATIVE

Complications	Hypothermia Bleeding Dysrhythmias Myocardial ischemia LV failure	Ischemia 2° coronary artery stenosis, stretching, spasm, compression. Spasm can be treated with NTG and ↑aortic pressure. If the now-anterior PA dilates (↓PaO$_2$, ↑PaCO$_2$, ↓T, ↓pH, excessive or too little PIP, or RV failure), the coronary arteries may be compressed. Measures to ↓ PA pressure are often essential.

Tests	ABGs; electrolytes; coag profile	
	CXR	✓ line, chest tube placement; ✓ for pneumothorax.
	TEE	

References

1. Castaneda AR, Jonas RA, Mayer JE Jr, Hanley FL: D-transposition of the great arteries. In *Cardiac Surgery of the Neonate and Infant.* WB Saunders, Philadelphia: 1994, 409-38.
2. Castaneda AR, Mayer JE: Neonatal repair of transposition of the great arteries. In *Fetal and Neonatal Cardiology.* Long WA, ed. WB Saunders, Philadelphia: 1990.
3. du Plessis AJ, Jonas RA, Wypij D, Hickey PR, Riviello J, Wessel DL, et al: Perioperative effects of alpha-stat versus pH-stat strategies for deep hypothermic cardiopulmonary bypass in infants. *J Thorac Cardiovasc Surg* 1997; 114:991-1001.
4. Emmanouilides GC, Allen HD, Riemenschneider TA, Gutgesell HP: Great artery anomalies. In *Clinical Synopsis of Moss and Adams' Heart Disease in Infants, Children, and Adolescents.* Williams & Wilkins, 1998, 501-14.
5. Lanier WL: Glucose management during cardiopulmonary bypass: cardiovascular and neurologic implications. *Anesth Analg* 1991; 72:423-7.
6. Quaegebeur JM, Auteri JS: Transposition of the great arteries. In *Glenn's Thoracic and Cardiovascular Surgery,* 6th edition. Baue AE, ed. Appleton & Lange, Stamford: 1996, 1393-1407.
7. Spray TL: Transposition of the great arteries. In *Mastery of Cardiothoracic Surgery.* Kaiser LR, Kron IL, Spray TL, eds. Lippincott-Raven, Philadelphia: 1998, 785-99.

SURGERY FOR TRUNCUS ARTERIOSUS

SURGICAL CONSIDERATIONS

Description: Truncus arteriosus is a rare cardiac anomaly in which there is a common aortopulmonary trunk originating from the base of the heart by way of a single, semilunar valve (truncal valve). This single great artery gives rise to the pulmonary, systemic, and coronary circulations. A nonrestrictive VSD is almost always found immediately below the truncal valve. An anatomic classification scheme proposed by **Collett** and **Edwards** in 1949 describes four types of truncus. In **type I** truncus (60%), a single arterial trunk gives rise to the aorta and main PA (Fig 12.4-9A). In **type II** truncus (20%), the right and left PAs arise separately from the posterolateral aspect of the truncus. **Type III** truncus (10%) designates cases in which the two PAs also originate from the posterior truncus, but with widely separated orifices. In **type IV** truncus (10%), the PA branches are absent, with pulmonary blood flow derived from aortopulmonary collaterals. Pathophysiologically, there is significant L→R shunting at the truncal and ventricular levels, leading to unrestricted pulmonary blood flow, CHF, and pulmonary HTN. Patients become symptomatic in infancy 2° CHF when the PVR ↓ and CO ↑. Untreated, 90% of infants die within 6 mo.

The first total repairs of this congenital anomaly were reported in the early 1960s and included the insertion of **nonvalved artificial conduits** and **aortic allograft and valve conduits.** In the early and mid-1970s, repair was performed at younger ages, with abandonment of palliative banding of the PA branches. Currently, early primary repair is carried out during the first few wk of life.

Through a median sternotomy, the truncus and PA branches are dissected and cannulation for CPB is performed. The PAs are snared to block pulmonary flow during perfusion. Hypothermia is induced and the aorta is cross-clamped. The PAs are separated from the main truncus, the resultant aortic defect is repaired with a patch, and a valved homograft (12-14 mm) is prepared. An end-to-end anastomosis of the distal homograft to the PA opening is performed, the VSD is closed through a right ventriculotomy, and the proximal end of the homograft is then anastomosed to the right ventriculotomy (Fig 12.4-9B). The heart is deaired, the aorta is unclamped, rewarming and resuscitation are performed, and CPB is D/C'd.

There are several **special considerations** associated with this repair that warrant mention. The truncal valve may exhibit insufficiency, necessitating valve repair or replacement using a cryopreserved aortic or pulmonary homograft. In older infants, the PVR may be elevated and pulmonary hypertensive crises should be anticipated. In some patients, an associated interruption of the aortic arch has to be addressed and increases the complexity of the procedure. Coronary artery abnormalities are common in patients with truncus arteriosus and may contribute to their mortality.

Usual preop diagnosis: Truncus arteriosus (types I, II, III, IV)

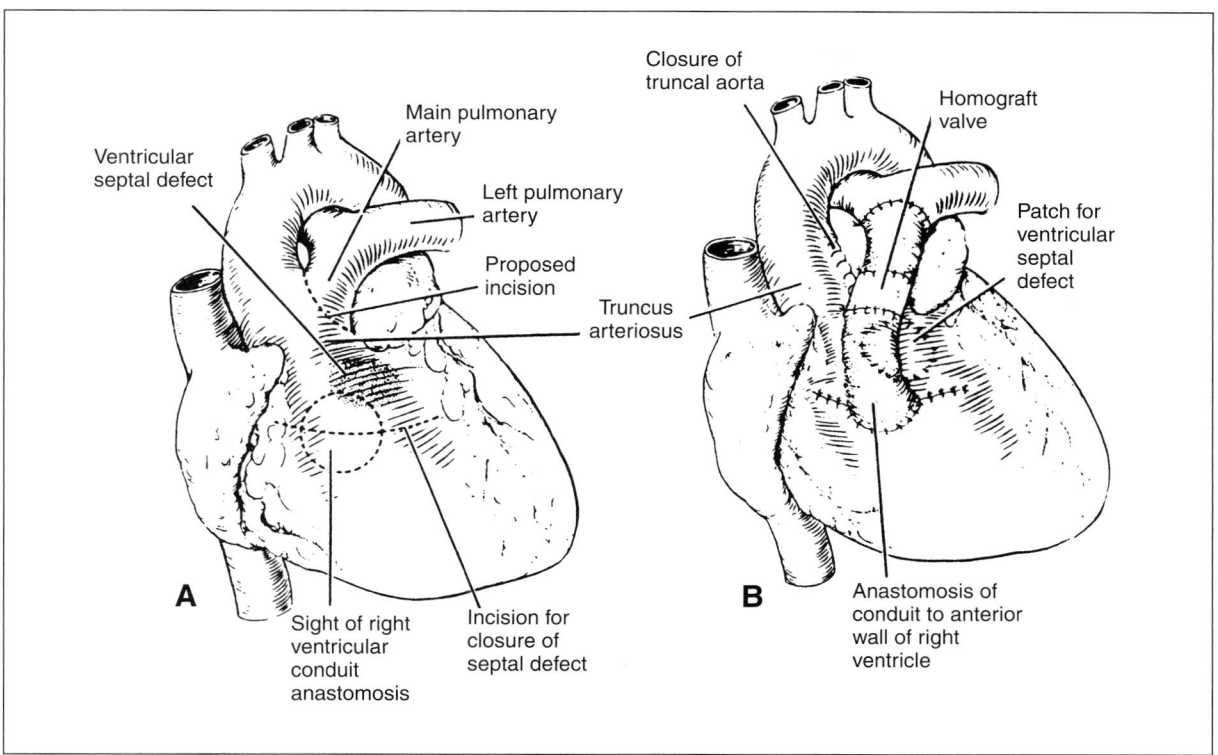

Figure 12.4-9. Truncus arteriosus. (**A**) Cohen-Edwards (Type I). (**B**) Surgical correction involves the separation of the main PA from the truncus, VSD patch closure and insertion of a conduit between the RV and the distal main PA. (Reproduced with permission from Way LW: *Current Surgical Diagnosis and Treatment*, 10th edition. Lange Medical Publications, 1973.)

SUMMARY OF PROCEDURE

Position	Supine
Incision	Standard median sternotomy
Antibiotics	Cefazolin 25 mg/kg q 8 h
Surgical time	Aortic cross-clamp: 30-90 min
	Circulatory arrest: 10-15 min
	Total: 2.5-3 h
Closing considerations	Routine closure with chest tube in the pericardial space; temporary ventricular pacing wire; possible right or left atrial line for monitoring
EBL	Moderate
Postop care	1-5 d of assisted ventilation; pulmonary HTN protocol consisting of hyperventilation and sedation and use of pulmonary vasodilators. Inotropes for adequate CO.
Mortality	< 3%
Morbidity	Hemorrhage
	Atrial dysrhythmias
	Pulmonary vasospasm
	Truncal valve insufficiency
	↓CO
Pain score	8-10

PATIENT POPULATION CHARACTERISTICS

Age range	3 wk–6 mo
Male:Female	1:1
Incidence	1.7-4.6% of congenital heart defects
Etiology	No known etiology
Associated conditions	Coexisting interrupted aortic arch or coarctation with PDA (10-20%); right aortic arch (16%); mitral valve anomalies (10%); moderate-size or large ASD (10%); DiGeorge syndrome

ANESTHETIC CONSIDERATIONS

PREOPERATIVE

Pathophysiology	A single, common aortopulmonary artery—the truncus—overlies the two ventricles and VSD. Depending on the configuration, the truncus gives rise to coronary and pulmonary arteries and ascending aorta. Complete mixing of systemic and pulmonary circulations occurs at the VSD and truncal valve, resulting initially in cyanosis. After birth, as PVR decreases, significant L→R shunting occurs at the level of the VSD. This → excessive pulmonary blood flow and CHF. Additionally, truncal valve insufficiency causes ventricular dilatation and low diastolic coronary perfusion, → myocardial ischemia. If untreated, 80% die of CHF in the first year. Early total correction is indicated.
Airway	The facial anomalies (e.g., micrognathia) in DiGeorge syndrome may make intubation difficult.
Respiratory	Typically, these infants present with the respiratory Sx of CHF (dyspnea, tachypnea, hypoxemia). **Tests:** CXR: ↑pulmonary markings and wide mediastinum.
Cardiovascular	Frequently, neonates are intubated and ventilated for hemodynamic support. Arterial saturation > 85% indicates excessive pulmonary blood flow. This may be controlled by the use of hypoxic gas mixtures (17-19% FiO_2), inspired CO_2 (3-5%), and PEEP. **Tests:** ECG. ECHO: Usually diagnostic. Identifies the origin of PA from the common trunk and the presence (subtype A) or absence (subtype B) of a VSD. Evaluates truncal valve competency.
Endocrine	In DiGeorge syndrome, thymic hypoplasia occurs with hypoparathyroidism and symptomatic hypocalcemia. **Tests:** ✓ Ca^{++} levels; parathyroid hormone
Premedication	Not indicated.
Transport to OR	See Transport of the Critically Ill Newborn, p. 995.

INTRAOPERATIVE

Anesthetic technique: GETA

Induction	The goal for induction is to maintain hemodynamic stability. If the patient is not intubated prior to induction, do not preoxygenate. IV induction (fentanyl 2-10 μg/kg) and muscle relaxant (e.g., rocuronium 1 mg/kg) is preferred. Once ETT is secured, avoid hyperventilation and maintain arterial saturation 75-85%. Keep DBP > 20 mmHg to maintain coronary perfusion. Treat ↓BP on induction with additional inotropes, transfusion of blood, or occlusion of a PA by the surgeon as soon as the chest is opened.	
Maintenance	Fentanyl (20-50 μg/kg). Rocuronium as needed ± midazolam 0.2 mg/kg ± volatile agent. FiO_2 = 0.21. Avoid hyperventilation (↓PVR → ↑shunt + CHF). PEEP may be useful to maintain PVR. The surgeon may leave a PFO to serve as a 'pop-off' to preserve systemic perfusion when ↑PVR and RV dysfunction occur. A surgical left atrial line is frequently placed for monitoring. In some cases, the sternum may be left open due to chest-wall and mediastinal edema and the presence of the anterior RV-PA conduit (Rastelli conduit).	
Emergence	Transport to ICU intubated and ventilated. Maintain narcotic infusion (e.g., fentanyl 1-10 μg/kg/h) for first few d postop to minimize pulmonary hypertensive crises.	
Blood and fluid requirements	See Tetralogy of Fallot (TOF), p. 990.	Continue dextrose infusion in neonates. Only irradiated blood and blood products should be used to prevent graft vs host disease. See Table 12.4-2 for blood product utilization.
Infusions	Inotropic support	These patients require inotropic support (dopamine, milrinone, epinephrine, and CaCl infusion).
Monitoring	Standard monitors + LA, RA, PA lines TEE	Transthoracic lines TEE is helpful to assess function, truncal valve compentency, RV function, and the direction of atrial shunt.
Positioning	See TOF, p. 991.	
CPB	See TOF, p. 991.	

Complications	Pulmonary HTN
	Truncal valve insufficiency
	Coronary artery insufficiency
	Residual lesion

POSTOPERATIVE

Complications	Bleeding	
	Pulmonary hypertensive crisis	Frequent in patients > 1 mo old. Rx: NO, sedation, PGE_1, hyperventilation.
	A-V block	Generally temporary, injury to conduction system unlikely because it is remote from VSD closure. Occasionally, a pacemaker may be required.
	Ventricular dysfunction	May require inotropic support.
	Residual lesions	Residual VSD, severe truncal valve incompetence or obstruction, obstruction of coronary flow, LVOTO.

References

1. Allen HD, Clark EB, Gutgesell HP, Driscoll DJ, eds. *Moss and Adams' Heart Disease in Infants, Children, and Adolescents*, 6th edition. Lippincott Williams & Wilkins, Philadelphia: 2001.
2. Castaneda AR, Jonas RA, Mayer JE Jr, Hanley FL: Truncus arteriosus. In *Cardiac Surgery of the Neonate and Infant*. WB Saunders, Philadelphia: 1994, 281-93.
3. Emmanouilides GC, Allen HD, Riemenschneider TA, Gutgesell HP: Truncus arteriosus. In *Clinical Synopsis of Moss and Adams' Heart Disease in Infants, Children, and Adolescents*. Williams & Wilkins, 1998, 434-41.
4. Ramamoorthy C, Tabbutt S, Kurth CD, Steven JM, Montenegro LM, Durning S, Wernovsky G, Gaynor JW, Spray TL, Nicolson SC: Effects of inspired hypoxic and hypercapnic gas mixtures on cerebral oxygen saturation in neonates with univentricular heart defects. *Anesthesiology* 2002; 96:283-8.
5. Reitz BA, Yuh DD, eds: *Congenital Cardiac Surgery*. McGraw-Hill, New York: 2002.
6. Spray TL: Truncus arteriosus. In *Mastery of Cardiothoracic Surgery*. Kaiser LR, Kron IL, Spray TL, eds. Lippincott-Raven, Philadelphia: 1998, 759-70.
7. Tabbutt S, Ramamoorthy C, Montenegro LM, Durning SM, Kurth CD, Steven, JM, Godinez RI, Spray TL, Wernovsky G, Nicolson SC: Impact of inspired gas mixtures on preoperative infants with hypoplastic left heart syndrome during controlled ventilation. *Circulation* 2001; 104(Supp I):I159-I164.

SURGERY FOR TRICUSPID ATRESIA

SURGICAL CONSIDERATIONS

Description: In tricuspid atresia, there is a developmental failure of the tricuspid valve, isolating the RA from the RV. There are three types of tricuspid atresia, based on the relationship of the great vessels to the ventricles, otherwise known as **ventriculoarterial concordance.** Type I, the most common (60-80%), consists of normal ventriculoarterial concordance. Type II (15-25%) consists of *d*-transposition, and Type III (3%) consists of *l*-transposition. In most cases of tricuspid atresia, the RV is hypoplastic, an ASD is present, and pulmonary blood flow is restricted 2° pulmonary stenosis or atresia. Together, these malformations lead to R→L shunting and varying degrees of cyanosis. Those patients with unobstructed pulmonary blood flow develop pulmonary overcirculation and CHF. Consequently, the initial palliative surgical management of this defect depends on the magnitude of pulmonary blood flow; the initial procedure may be either a modified **Blalock-Taussig systemic-to-PA shunt** or a **PA band.** The subsequent definitive surgical management consists of a bidirectional **Glenn shunt** and a modified **Fontan procedure.** Patients undergo these operations sequentially or, in rare cases, directly to the definitive Fontan operation.

The systemic-to-PA shunt, developed by **Blalock** and **Taussig** in 1944, was the first palliative treatment for this condition. Later, other shunts were introduced by **Potts** (descending aorta-to-left PA) and **Waterston** (ascending aorta-to-right PA). In 1958, Glenn described a shunt from the SVC to the right PA applied specifically to patients with tricuspid atresia. A modification of this shunt to a **bidirectional cavopulmonary anastomosis** was performed clinically by **Azzollina** in 1974 and has since gained widespread acceptance. In 1971, Fontan proposed a surgical repair for tricuspid atresia based on separation of the right and left circulations. Subsequent modifications to Fontan's original operation were designed

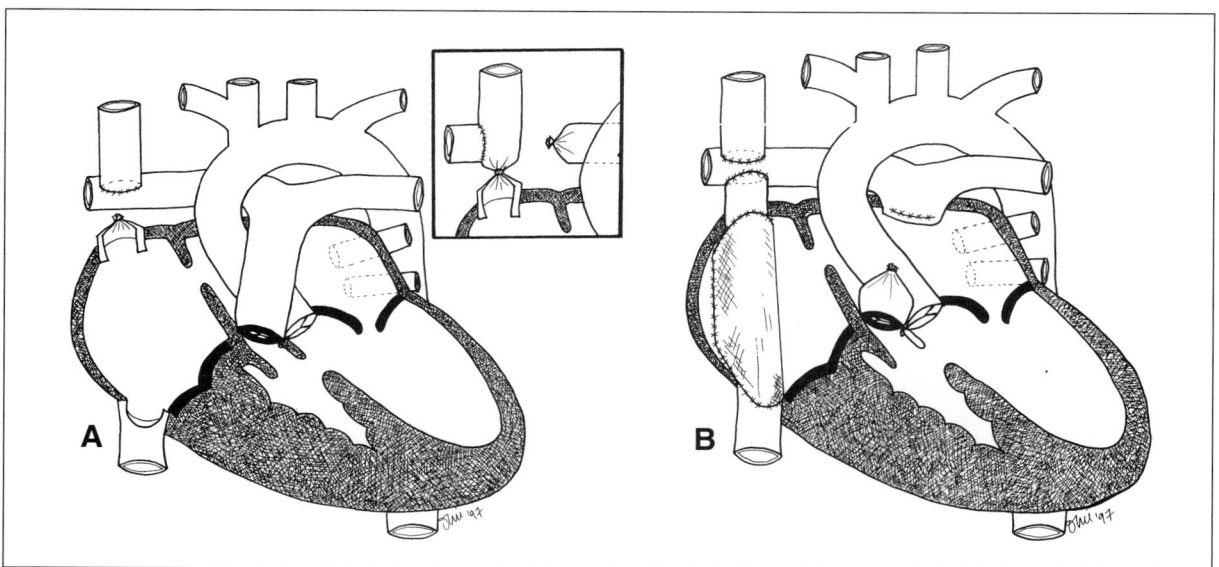

Figure 12.4-10. Surgery for tricuspid atresia. (A) Bidirectional Glenn shunt. Inset shows classic unidirectional Glenn shunt. (B) Lateral tunnel Fontan operation. (Reproduced with permission from Emmanouilides GC, Allen HD, Riemenschneider TA, Gutgesell HP: *Clinical Synopsis of Moss and Adams' Heart Disease in Infants, Children, and Adolescents*. Williams & Wilkins, 1998.)

to bypass the RV and direct systemic venous return to the pulmonary circulation. The most recent modifications divert vena caval blood directly to the PA—now referred to as a **total cavopulmonary connection** (modified Fontan). In 1988, **Laks** suggested leaving a small ASD between the right and left circulations, creating a R→L shunt for the purposes of augmenting systemic CO while still maintaining adequate oxygenation.

Modified Blalock-Taussig (B-T) shunt: In neonates with tricuspid atresia or other single ventricle variants with low pulmonary blood flow, a modified B-T shunt is the procedure of choice. The preferred approach is through a midsternotomy. The right PA and the right innominate and subclavian arteries are mobilized. The patient is heparinized and clamps are applied on the right PA and the innominate/subclavian arteries. Arteriotomies are performed and a Gore-Tex tube graft is interposed and anastomosed to the right PA and the subclavian/innominate arteries. The size of shunt (3-4 mm) is dictated by patient size and arterial anatomy. Alternatively, the procedure can be performed via right thoracotomy, or through a left thoracotomy if the morphology dictates a left-sided shunt. A midline approach can be used for any variation of the shunt and also gives the option of using CPB in case of patient instability.

Pulmonary artery banding: In patients with tricuspid atresia or other variants of single ventricle and increased pulmonary blood flow, PA banding is performed to protect the pulmonary vascular bed, prevent pulmonary HTN, and prevent CHF. A midline sternotomy is the preferred approach. The main PA is exposed and a 2-3 mm wide strip of Silastic band is placed around the main PA and tightened to adjust the pulmonary blood flow. The goal is a PaO_2 of ~80-85%.

Bidirectional Glenn shunt: A standard median sternotomy approach is used. If concomitant intracardiac repairs are not anticipated, the bidirectional Glenn shunt may be performed without CPB by placing a temporary shunt between the high SVC and the RA. If the patient has a preexisting Blalock-Taussig shunt on the right, it is divided after instituting CPB. A shunt on the left side may be left open, while the bidirectional Glenn shunt is created on the right. The SVC is divided and the cardiac end is oversewn. The remaining caval end is anastomosed end-to-side to the superior aspect of the right PA (Fig 12.4-10A).

Fontan procedure: The heart is accessed via a standard median sternotomy. Previously placed systemic-to-PA shunts are dissected and occluded prior to bypass. Bicaval cannulation and CPB with hypothermia are used. The IVC is transected at its PA junction and a Gore-Tex tube graft is interposed end-to-end between the IVC and the inferior surface of the right PA. This operation, in conjunction with the previously performed bidirectional Glenn shunt, establishes a total cavopulmonary connection (Fig 12.4-10B). After completing the anastomosis, the aortic cross-clamp is removed, the heart is rewarmed and the patient is weaned from CPB. Fenestration of the Fontan circuit may be desirable in high-risk patients, but is generally not required in patients with tricuspid atresia and good ventricular function.

Variant procedure or approaches: A **RA→RV connection** can be performed in patients with tricuspid atresia without pulmonary obstruction and an adequately functioning RV. This is accomplished with a direct anastomosis or a valved/ nonvalved conduit (e.g., aortic homograft, Dacron graft).

Usual preop diagnosis: Tricuspid atresia after B-T shunt or PA banding; univentricular heart or single ventricle after shunt or band; cyanotic congenital heart disease

SUMMARY OF PROCEDURES

	Bidirectional Glenn Shunt	Cavopulmonary Fontan Procedure
Position	Supine	⇐
Incision	Standard median sternotomy	⇐
Unique considerations	Particulate or gaseous emboli from iv lines can become systemic emboli.	Areas of PA stenosis need to be repaired concomitantly; subaortic obstruction needs to be considered if there is a restrictive VSD and the great vessels are transposed.
Antibiotics	Cefazolin 25 mg/kg q 8 h	⇐
Surgical time	If a simple anastomosis is constructed, the aorta is not cross-clamped. Total: 1.5-2 h	⇐ Total: 3-4 h
Closing considerations	Chest tube in the pericardial space; temporary ventricular pacing wire; possible atrial monitoring line to assess ventricular filling pressures	Chest tube in the pericardial space; possible pleural tubes; temporary ventricular and atrial pacing wires; possible atrial line to correlate with CVP to determine the transpulmonary gradient
EBL	Moderate	⇐
Postop care	Cardiac ICU; early extubation to minimize positive intrathoracic pressure	ICU or early extubation; inotropes for ventricular function, including low-dose dopamine, milrinone for afterload reduction. Maintain sinus rhythm, A-V pacing, if required.
Mortality	< 2%	2-4%
Morbidity	Bleeding	Pleural effusions
	Infection	–
	Atrial dysrhythmias	⇐
	↑SVC pressure	–
	Upper extremity edema (SVC syndrome)	–
	↓CO	⇐
	Cyanosis 2° ↓pulmonary blood flow	–
	Pulmonary arteriovenous fistula	Protein-losing enteropathy (late)
Pain score	8-10	8-10

PATIENT POPULATION CHARACTERISTICS

Age range	4 mo-1 yr	2-5 yr
Male:Female	1:1	⇐
Incidence	1-3% of congenital heart defects	⇐
Etiology	Unknown	⇐
Associated conditions	TGA; AV valve insufficiency requiring repair or replacement; residual PA obstruction from previous procedures; dextrocardia; asplenia or polysplenia syndromes	

ANESTHETIC CONSIDERATIONS

PREOPERATIVE

Pathophysiology	This is characterized by absence of the tricuspid valve and a hypoplastic RV with no communication between RA and RV. Survival in the neonatal period depends on interatrial communication. The degree of cyanosis reflects the size of the VSD and magnitude of RVOTO. 30% of patients have CHF from pulmonary overcirculation 2° a large VSD and unobstructed RVOT. These patients may require PA banding. Tricuspid atresia requires staged palliation, beginning with the establishment of adequate pulmonary blood flow. Patients undergo a balloon septostomy or a systemic-pulmonary artery shunt (B-T shunt) in the newborn period to augment pulmonary blood flow. At 3-4 mo of age, these infants undergo cardiac catheterization, and a palliative bidirectional Glenn shunt (SVC→PA)

Pathophysiology, cont.	is performed and the B-T shunt is ligated. The Glenn shunt reduces the volume overload of the systemic ventricle. The final palliative procedure—the Fontan operation—is done between 1.5-3 yr of age, where the IVC is connected to the PA via an extracardiac conduit. The pulmonary and systemic circulations are now in series.
Respiratory	Identify any infectious or asthma-related problems. Optimizing pulmonary function is very important because pulmonary blood flow will be supplied passively from the systemic venous return. **Tests:** CXR; O$_2$ sat
Cardiovascular	**Tests:** ECG, ECHO, cath
Laboratory	Hct; others as indicated by H&P.
Premedication	Midazolam 0.5-0.75 mg/kg po 20 min before induction in children > 1 yr old

INTRAOPERATIVE / POSTOPERATIVE

For intraop and postop considerations for tricuspid atresia, see Anesthetic Considerations for Surgery for HLHS, p. 1011.

References

1. Emmanouilides GC, Allen HD, Riemenschneider TA, Gutgesell HP: Tricuspid valve abnormalities. In *Clinical Synopsis of Moss and Adams' Heart Disease in Infants, Children, and Adolescents*. Williams & Wilkins, 1998, 369-84.
2. Mayer JE Jr: Tricuspid atresia/single ventricle and the Fontan operation. In *Mastery of Cardiothoracic Surgery*. Kaiser LR, Kron IL, Spray TL, eds. Lippincott-Raven, Philadelphia: 1998, 848-57.

SURGERY FOR DOUBLE-OUTLET RIGHT VENTRICLE

SURGICAL CONSIDERATIONS

Description: In double-outlet right ventricle (DORV), at least 50% of both of the great arteries arise from the RV. By necessity, there is a VSD that is usually large, but may in some cases be restrictive or, rarely, multiple and muscular. The VSD may be located primarily below the aorta (**DORV/subaortic VSD**) (Fig 12.4-11A), below the pulmonary valve (**DORV/subpulmonic VSD, or Taussig-Bing DORV**) (Fig 12.4-11B), below both great vessels (doubly committed, Fig 12.4-11C), or remote from both great vessels (noncommitted, Fig 12.4-11D). In DORV/subaortic VSD, oxygenated LV blood is directed to the aorta and deoxygenated systemic venous return from the RV is directed to the PA, resulting in minimal-to-no cyanosis. L→R shunting across the VSD, however, leads to pulmonary overcirculation, pulmonary HTN, and CHF. In DORV/subpulmonic VSD, oxygenated LV blood is directed to the PA and deoxygenated systemic venous return from the RV is directed to the aorta → pulmonary overcirculation and significant cyanosis. If early PA banding or primary correction is not performed in patients with pulmonary overcirculation, PVOD may result at an early age. In patients with some degree of pulmonary stenosis (usually infundibular), R→L shunting and cyanosis results; the natural history resembles that of patients with tetralogy of Fallot.

The first repairs of DORV were described by **Kirklin** in 1957. The Taussig-Bing DORV was first corrected in 1967. In recent years, management has been simplified for this variant by combining the **arterial switch operation** with an **intraventricular baffle to the pulmonary valve**. From a surgical standpoint, the anatomic variations and past attempts at correction may lead to unique intraop challenges. For example, if a previous Blalock-Taussig shunt has been performed, it needs to be controlled prior to initiating CPB. A previous pulmonary band may require removal and PA reconstruction.

DORV/subaortic VSD generally is repaired with an **intraventricular tunnel repair,** in which LV blood from the VSD is channeled through the RV to the aorta. Through a median sternotomy, CPB is instituted, and previous shunts are ligated. The aorta is cross-clamped and cardioplegia is administered. After performing a right atriotomy, the interior of the RV is inspected through the tricuspid valve; a right ventriculotomy may be necessary for adequate exposure. A tunnel constructed of pericardial or Dacron patch is then placed between the VSD and the subaortic infundibulum. Augmentation of the RVOT, in the form of an outflow patch or extracardiac RV→PA conduit, is often necessary if the outflow tract is obstructed or if the RVOT is encroached upon by the intraventricular tunnel. The heart is then rewarmed and resuscitated, CPB is D/C'd, and standard chest closure is begun.

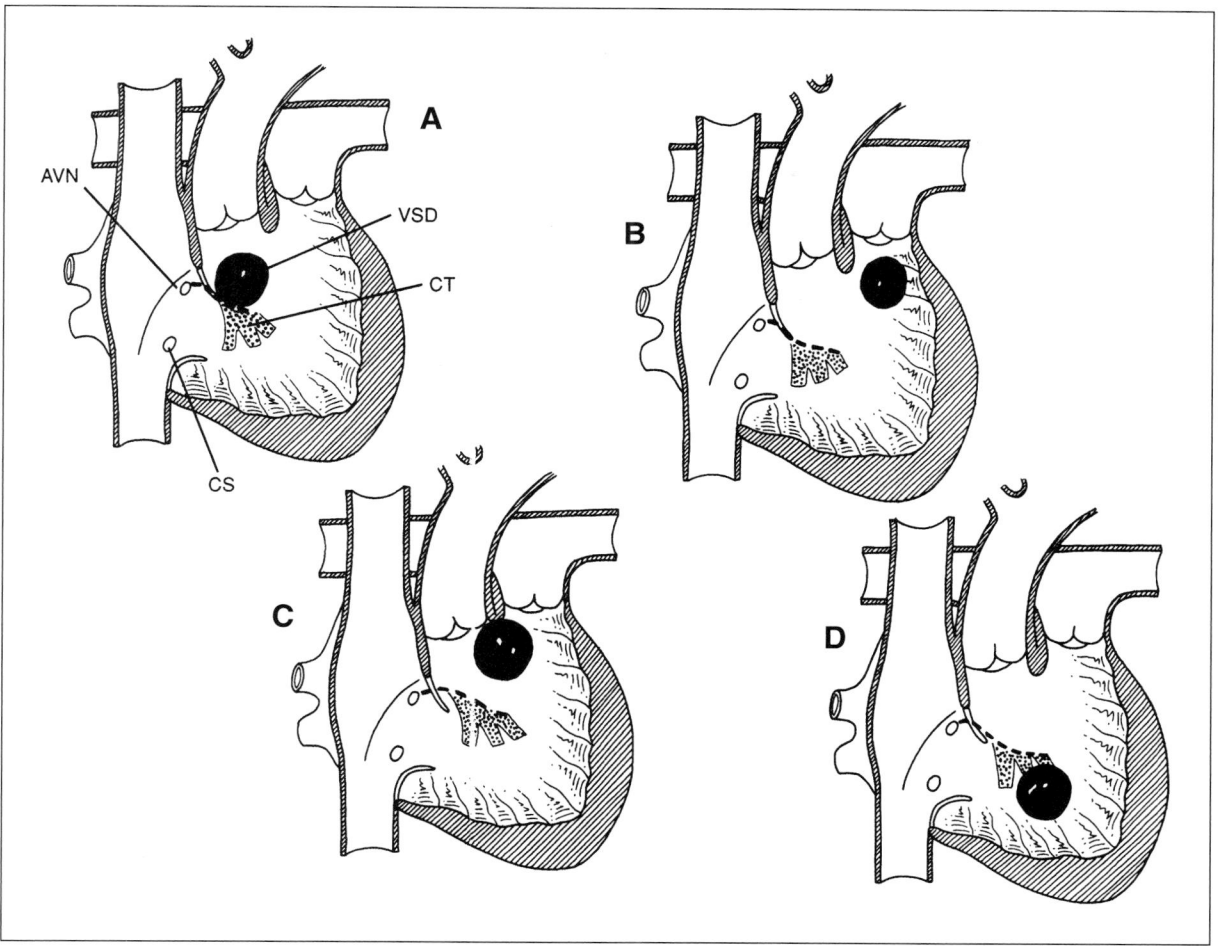

Figure 12.4-11. Types of double-outlet right ventricle classified by the relationship of the VSD to the great arteries. The location of the atrioventricular node and conduction tissue is depicted. (A) Subaortic VSD. (B) Subpulmonary VSD. (C) Doubly committed VSD. (D) Noncommitted VSD. AVN = atrioventricular node; CS = coronary sinus; CT = conduction tissue.(Reproduced with permission from Kaiser LR, Kron IL, Spray TL, eds: *Mastery of Cardiothoracic Surgery*. Lippincott-Raven, Philadelphia, 1998.)

DORV/subpulmonic VSD (Taussig-Bing DORV) can be corrected with an arterial switch operation and VSD closure under CPB (see Surgery for Complete Transposition of the Great Arteries, p. 996). DORV with significant pulmonary stenosis repair resembles that for the TOF (see p. 988). DORV with doubly committed VSD is similar to DORV/subaortic VSD. DORV with uncommitted VSD poses a surgical challenge. A two-ventricle repair requires intracardiac baffles. Alternatively, a single-ventricle approach is taken.

Usual preop diagnosis: DORV ± pulmonary stenosis; s/p PA band or modified Blalock-Taussig shunt; Taussig-Bing type of DORV; CHF

SUMMARY OF PROCEDURE

Position	Supine
Incision	Standard median sternotomy
Antibiotics	Cefazolin 25 mg/kg q 8 h
Surgical time	Aortic cross-clamp: 30-80 min
	Total: 2-3.5 h
Closing considerations	Routine closure with chest tube in the pericardial space; temporary ventricular pacing wire; possible LA line for monitoring
EBL	Minimal
Postop care	ICU for 1-4 d of controlled ventilation; possible pulmonary HTN protocol in cases of unrestricted pulmonary blood flow (see description of management for A-V canal defect, p. 975).

Mortality	~2%
Morbidity	Hemorrhage
	↓CO
	Atrial dysrhythmias
	RV dysrhythmias
	Intraventricular tunnel obstruction
	Baffle leakage; residual RVOTO
	Heart block
Pain score	8-10

PATIENT POPULATION CHARACTERISTICS

Age range	3-24 mo
Male:Female	1:1
Incidence	1-3% of congenital heart defects
Etiology	No specific correlations or associated conditions
Associated conditions	Pulmonary stenosis; complete A-V canal defect; coarctation of the aorta; interruption of the aortic arch; straddling tricuspid valve

ANESTHETIC CONSIDERATIONS

PREOPERATIVE

Pathophysiology   Both great vessels arise from the RV and there is a single, large VSD, whose location may vary (subaortic, subpulmonic). The pathophysiology varies according to the VSD location and other cardiac anomalies, such as aortic stenosis (AS) or pulmonary stenosis (PS). Those with subaortic VSD present with minimal or no cyanosis, but may have pulmonary overcirculation and CHF. In infants with PS in addition to subaortic VSD, the physiology is similar to TOF. In DORV with subpulmonic VSD, deoxygenated venous return from RV is directed to the aorta, leading to cyanosis. The oxygenated LV output is directed through the VSD into the PA, leading to pulmonary overcirculation. This physiology resembles TGA. The surgical approach may consist of VSD closure, or TOF or TGA repair.

Anesthetic management: Is dictated by specific surgical repair. See sections on VSD, p. 979, TOF, p. 988, and TGA, p. 996 for Anesthetic Considerations.

References

1. Emmanouilides GC, Allen HD, Riemenschneider TA, Gutgesell HP: Great artery anomalies. In *Clinical Synopsis of Moss and Adams' Heart Disease in Infants, Children, and Adolescents.* Williams & Wilkins, 1998, 501-14.
2. Kanter KR: Double-outlet ventricles. In *Mastery of Cardiothoracic Surgery.* Kaiser LR, Kron IL, Spray TL, eds. Lippincott-Raven, Philadelphia: 1998, 771-84.

SURGERY FOR HYPOPLASTIC LEFT HEART SYNDROME

SURGICAL CONSIDERATIONS

Description: Hypoplastic left heart syndrome (HLHS) represents a spectrum of left-sided cardiac malformations centered around a markedly hypoplastic LV, and an atretic or hypoplastic aortic valve and ascending aorta; the mitral valve is also usually hypoplastic or atretic (Fig 12.4-12). Consequently, the RV supports both the pulmonary and systemic circulations. The pulmonary venous return (PVR) enters the RA via an ASD, and the admixture of systemic and pulmonary venous return is delivered into the RV and main PA. Systemic flow is delivered into the aorta by way of a typically large PDA. Cyanosis, CHF, and systemic hypoperfusion result as PVR decreases and pulmonary blood flow increases at the expense of systemic blood flow.

Until the mid-to-late 1980s, patients born with this anomaly usually died within the first 2 wk of life, with survival beyond 6 wk being very rare. A palliative surgical treatment was reported by Norwood in 1983. This treatment of HLHS comprises staged operations, with the first stage designated as the '**Norwood operation.**' The procedure is directed toward establishing effective CO from the RV to the systemic circulation and to support the pulmonary circulation with a systemic-to-pulmonary arterial shunt. An adequate atrial septal communication is essential.

Norwood Stage I: A midline sternotomy approach is used. The innominate artery (alternatively, the main PA or ascending aorta, if it is of adequate size) and RA appendage are cannulated and CPB with cooling is instituted. The arch vessels and proximal descending thoracic aorta are dissected. Deep hypothermia with low-flow CPB technique is used. During arch reconstruction, cerebral blood flow is maintained, although many surgeons prefer total circulatory arrest. The ductus arteriosus is then divided and the pulmonary end is oversewn. Next, the main PA is divided and the distal PA is oversewn. An aortotomy is created, extending from the interior aspect of the aortic arch through the lateral aspect of the ascending aorta to the level of the transected pulmonary trunk. The entire aortic arch complex is then augmented, creating a 'neoaorta' from the proximal portion of

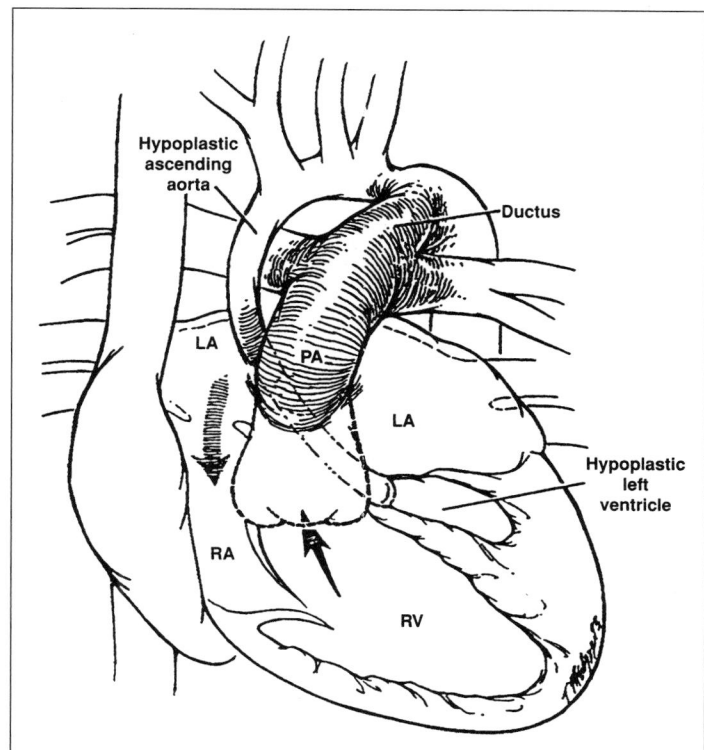

Figure 12.4-12. The anatomic features of hypoplastic left heart syndrome. The right atrium (RA), right ventricle (RV), and main pulmonary artery (PA) are larger than in neonates with normal circulation. LA = left atrium. (Reproduced with permission from Kaiser LR, Kron IL, Spray TL, eds: *Mastery of Cardiothoracic Surgery.* Lippincott-Raven, Philadelphia, 1998.)

the transected main PA, which is anastomosed to the ascending aorta and arch. A cryopreserved homograft patch is used to facilitate the repair. The RA is opened and the atrial septum is excised to maximize the size of the interatrial communication. The heart is deaired and rewarming is started with full CPB. If circulatory arrest was used, the cannulae are reinserted, and rewarming begins. Finally, a B-T systemic-to-PA shunt is created to provide pulmonary blood flow. The patient is weaned from CPB, a pericardial drainage tube is placed, and the chest is closed in standard fashion.

Recently, a modification of the Norwood procedure strongly advocated by Japanese surgeons is being adopted by many surgeons worldwide. This involves abandoning the modified B-T shunt in favor of RV-PA shunt ± valve. This modification eliminates the diastolic run-off and preserves coronary blood flow. The major advantage is a stable early postop course. The long-term implications of right ventriculotomy in a systemic RV are not known at the present time.

Stage II (bidirectional Glenn procedure): As the PVR normally falls in the weeks after the first-stage operation, excessive pulmonary blood flow from the B-T shunt may → RV volume overload and CHF. The second-stage procedure for HLHS is intended to reduce the volume load on the single ventricle, while maintaining adequate pulmonary blood flow. This operation consists of a bidirectional cavopulmonary (Glenn) shunt (see Surgery for Tricuspid Atresia, p. 1003), and usually is performed in children 4-6 mo old.

Stage III (Fontan procedure): The third, and final stage of the Norwood procedure usually is performed about 6-12 mo after the second stage and consists of the completion of the Fontan procedure (see Surgery for Tricuspid Atresia, p. 1003). It is designed to divide the systemic venous return from the pulmonary venous return by establishing continuity from the IVC to the confluence of the PA and SVC.

Variant procedure or approaches: Successful cardiac transplantation for this condition was performed by **Bailey** in 1985. Cardiac transplantation is associated with a lower operative mortality; however, a significant number of neonates on the waiting lists do not receive donor hearts. Moreover, cardiac transplantation is associated with lifelong immunosuppression and its associated risks.

Usual preop diagnosis: HLHS; mitral and aortic atresia

SUMMARY OF PROCEDURE

Position	Supine
Incision	Standard median sternotomy
Unique considerations	Hypothermia (< 18° C) ± circulatory arrest; manipulation of PVR and SVR, both preop and postop, is extremely important, with the FiO_2 and ventilation being crucial in regulating pulmonary blood flow. For very high pulmonary blood flows and O_2 sats > 85%, consider the addition of N_2 to lower the FiO_2 to < 20%; use of afterload reduction to manipulate SVR and ↓ ventricular work.
Antibiotics	Cefazolin 25 mg/kg q 8 h
Surgical time	Aortic cross-clamp: 30-60 min
	Circulatory arrest (if used): 30-45 min
	Total: 2.5-3.5 h
Closing considerations	Sternum often left open, with chest tube in the pericardial space, with closure delayed until POD 2-4; temporary ventricular pacing wire; possible left atrial line for monitoring
EBL	Minimal-to-moderate
Postop care	2-7 h of controlled ventilation; moderate need for inotropic drugs; balancing PVR and SVR to optimize pulmonary blood flow and systemic CO.
Mortality	10-20%
Morbidity	Hemorrhage
	Infection
	↓CO
	RV dysfunction
	Inadequate/excessive pulmonary blood flow
	Tricuspid regurgitation
Pain score	8-10

PATIENT POPULATION CHARACTERISTICS

Age range	5-30 d
Male:Female	2:1
Incidence	3-5% of congenital heart defects
Etiology	Often associated with genetic disorders, but no single associated defect
Associated conditions	CNS defects (29%); microencephaly (25-27%); VSD (5%); TGA

ANESTHETIC CONSIDERATIONS

PREOPERATIVE

Pathophysiology	HLHS is characterized by a hypoplastic or atretic aortic valve associated with hypoplasia of the LV, ascending aorta, and aortic arch. The mitral valve may be atretic or stenotic. Pulmonary venous return enters the LA and then passes into the RA via an ASD or the PFO. Rarely, pulmonary venous return is via TAPVC to the RA. The systemic circulation is supplied entirely through the ductus arteriosus. Perfusion of the ascending aorta, coronary arteries, and transverse arch is retrograde via the ductus. Maintenance of adequate systemic perfusion relies on ductal patency and is achieved with continuous administration of PGE_1. Maintaining ↑PVR by ↓ FiO_2 to 0.17-0.20, or by adding CO_2 to breathing gas mixture, may be necessary. As the ductus closes, the systemic perfusion is compromised, → ischemia, acidosis, and eventually death. Hence, survival depends on the patency of the ductus arteriosus, the adequacy of mixing at the atrial level, and maintaining a balance between PVR and SVR to ensure adequate pulmonary and systemic perfusion.
Cardiovascular	**Tests:** ECG; RAE/RVH; ECHO: assessment of tricuspid or common AV valve regurgitation. Severe TR is a contraindication for 1st stage repair.
Neurological	Preop head ultrasound to r/o intracranial anomaly (e.g., hemorrhage). Periop neurological monitoring, including cerebral oximeter can be useful.
Laboratory	BUN; Cr; Hb/Hct; Plt count
Premedication	Not indicated.

Transport to OR   See Transport of the Critically Ill Newborn, p. 995.

INTRAOPERATIVE

Anesthetic technique: GETA

Induction	On arrival in the OR, monitors are applied and ventilation should be adjusted to maintain arterial O_2 sat = 75-85%. Hypoxic gas mixtures may be necessary. Avoid hyperventilation ($\rightarrow \uparrow$pulmonary blood flow). Arterial sat > 85% will cause systemic hypoperfusion. See Truncus Arteriosus, p. 1002.
Maintenance	Fentanyl (20-50 μg/kg) with muscle relaxant in divided doses. Volatile anesthetic on CPB. Midazolam (0.1-0.2 mg/kg) as tolerated.
Emergence	Transport to ICU intubated, ventilated, and monitored.

Blood and fluid requirements	See Tetralogy of Fallot (TOF), p. 990. See Table 12.4-2 for blood product utilization.	Continue dextrose infusion in neonates. Blood loss can be due largely to dilutional coagulopathy and multiple suture lines.
Infusions	See Truncus Arteriosus, p. 1002.	
Monitoring	See Truncus Arteriosus, p. 1002.	
CPB	See TGA, p. 999.	
Transition off CPB and Post-CPB	See TOF, p. 991.	After Stage I (Norwood) surgical repair, the blood flow continues to be supplied in a parallel fashion from the single ventricle. At Stanford, a small homograft conduit is placed from the RV to PA (Sano modification) instead of the traditional modified B-T shunt. This prevents the diastolic run-off of the B-T shunt and improves coronary perfusion. Optimal PaO_2 30-50 mmHg with MAP 40-50 mmHg.

POSTOPERATIVE

Complications	Bleeding	
	Pulmonary overcirculation	
	Myocardial dysfunction and failure	A ventricular-assist device may be required.
	Aortic arch obstruction	
	Pulmonary HTN	
	CNS injury	

References

1. Allen HD, Clark EB, Gutgesell HP, Driscoll DJ, eds. *Moss and Adams' Heart Disease in Infants, Children, and Adolescents*, 6th edition. Lippincott Williams & Wilkins, Philadelphia: 2001.
2. Emmanouilides GC, Allen HD, Riemenschneider TA, Gutgesell HP: Left ventricular outflow abnormalities. In *Clinical Synopsis of Moss and Adams' Heart Disease in Infants, Children, and Adolescents*. Williams & Wilkins, 1998, 501-14.
3. Jacobs ML: Hypoplastic left heart syndrome. In *Mastery of Cardiothoracic Surgery*. Kaiser LR, Kron IL, Spray TL, eds. Lippincott-Raven, Philadelphia: 1998, 858-66.
4. Jacobs ML, Norwood WI: Hypoplastic left heart syndrome. In *Glenn's Thoracic and Cardiovascular Surgery,* 6th edition. Baue AE, ed. Appleton & Lange, Stamford: 1996, 1271-81.
5. Jacobs ML, Norwood WI: Hyperplastic left heart syndrome. In *Pediatric Cardiac Surgery: Current Issues*. Jacobs ML, Norwood WI, eds. Butterworth-Heinemann, Stoneham, UK: 1992, 182-92.
6. Kirkham FJ: Recognition and prevention of neurological complications in pediatric cardiac surgery. *Pediatr Cardiol* 1998; 19:331-45.
7. Nicolson SC, Steven JM, Jobes DR: Hypoplastic left heart syndrome. In *Pediatric Cardiac Anesthesia,* 3rd edition. Lake CL, ed. Appleton & Lange, Stamford: 1998, 337-52.
8. Ramamoorthy C, Tabbutt S, Kurth CD, Steven JM, Montenegro LM, Durning S, Wernovsky G, Gaynor JW, Spray TL, Nicolson SC: Effects of inspired hypoxic and hypercapnic gas mixtures on cerebral oxygen saturation in neonates with univentricular heart defects. *Anesthesiology* 2002; 96:283-8.
9. Reitz BA, Yuh DD, eds: *Congenital Cardiac Surgery*. McGraw-Hill, New York: 2002.
10. Tabbutt S, Ramamoorthy C, Montenegro LM, Durning SM, Kurth CD, Steven, JM, Godinez RI, Spray TL, Wernovsky G, Nicolson SC: Impact of inspired gas mixtures on preoperative infants with hypoplastic left heart syndrome during controlled ventilation. *Circulation* 2001; 104(Supp I):I159-64.

Surgeons

Baird M. Smith, MD
Christine Matthes-Kofidis, MD

12.5 PEDIATRIC GENERAL SURGERY

Anesthesiologists

Brenda Golianu, MD
Gregory B. Hammer, MD

RESECTION OF CYSTIC HYGROMA, BRANCHIAL CLEFT CYST, THYROGLOSSAL DUCT CYST, OR OTHER CERVICAL MASS

SURGICAL CONSIDERATIONS

Description: Common lesions requiring dissection in the neck and floor of the mouth include branchial cleft remnants; thyroglossal duct remnants; vascular malformations (hemangiomas); lymphatic malformations (cystic hygromas); and infected or enlarged lymph nodes refractory to antibiotic therapy.

Surgical approach: Ideally, an acutely inflamed node (*Staphylococcus aureus*) usually is incised and drained; a chronically infected node (cat-scratch disease, atypical TB) or an enlarged node (lymphoma) is excised. Remnants of the first and second (rarely third) branchial clefts are lateral masses found and excised from (respectively): the parotid region anterior to the ear sometimes extending to the external auditory canal, or the anterior border of the sternocleidomastoid muscle sometimes extending through the carotid bifurcation to the tonsillar fossa. Thyroglossal duct remnants are midline lesions that involve the central portion of the hyoid bone and may extend up to the base of the tongue. When acute infection is resistant to antibiotics, it is drained; when quiescent, thyroglossal duct remnants are excised. Occasionally, it is advantageous for the anesthesiologist to digitally depress the tongue near the foramen cecum to help the surgeon know when the dissection approaches this structure. Vascular and lymphatic malformations may overlap; they tend to be lateral and are sometimes extensive. Significant blood loss may result and resection may involve tedious dissection of neurovascular structures, including the carotid sheath, brachial plexus, sympathetic chain, phrenic nerve, and cranial nerves V, VII, X, XI, and XII.

Usual preop diagnosis: Cystic hygroma; branchial cleft cyst/fistula; thyroglossal duct cyst; atypical mycobacterial adenitis

SUMMARY OF PROCEDURES

	Lateral Lesions (Branchial Cleft Remnant Lymph Node, Vascular + Lymphatic Malformations)	Midline Lesions (Thyroglossal Duct Remnants)
Position	Neck extended, turned to contralateral side	Neck extended
Incision	Oblique	Transverse
Special instrumentation	Facial nerve monitor; nerve stimulator	None
Unique considerations	Nerve testing	None
Antibiotics	Cefazolin 25 mg/kg	⇐
Surgical time	1-6 h	1 h
EBL	5-20 ml/kg	< 5 ml/kg
Postop care	PICU; airway monitoring	None
Mortality	< 2%	< 1%
Morbidity	Airway compromise	⇐
	Fluid accumulation	⇐
	Infection	⇐
Pain score	3-4	3-4

PATIENT POPULATION CHARACTERISTICS

Age range	Newborn–school age
Male:Female	1:1
Incidence	Common
Etiology	Developmental anomaly; mycobacteria
Associated conditions	Hygroma-mediastinal airway involvement; branchial cleft – 10% (bilateral)

ANESTHETIC CONSIDERATIONS

PREOPERATIVE

These patients generally are otherwise healthy children. A cystic hygroma (cystic lymphangioma), as with other neck masses, may cause airway obstruction and difficult intubation.

Respiratory	The size and extent of the neck mass should be defined carefully in an effort to detect the potential for airway compromise and to avoid soft-tissue trauma during intubation, with consequent acute airway obstruction. Inspiratory stridor suggests supraglottic obstruction, while expiratory stridor is associated with subglottic/intrathoracic obstruction. These patients should have had prior CT/MRI imaging; anesthesia records for these studies should be reviewed. **Tests:** CXR ± CT/MRI scans
Cardiovascular	Cervical masses may be adherent to and/or cause compression of the great vessels. **Tests:** CT/MRI scans
Hematologic	T&C for cystic hygroma, or if a cervical mass involves great vessels or extends into the mediastinum (~3%). **Tests:** Hct
Laboratory	Other tests as indicated from H&P.
Premedication	If child is 1-10 yr old and asymptomatic, midazolam (0.5-0.75 mg/kg po) 30 min prior to arrival in OR. Avoid all premedication in patients with potential airway compromise.

INTRAOPERATIVE

Anesthetic technique: GETA with pediatric circle, and warm, humidified gases. OR temperature 75-80°; warming pad on OR table. Use air/O_2 mixture for ventilation. Maintain SpO_2 between 95-100% to minimize retinopathy in premature infants.

Induction	Standard pediatric induction (p. D-2) in patients without airway compromise. IV should be secured before induction when airway compromise is present or suspected. Mask induction with sevoflurane or halothane in 100% O_2. As plane of anesthesia deepens, gently assist ventilation. (Keep PIP < 20 cmH$_2$O). Give atropine (0.02 mg/kg iv), if < 9 mo, prior to laryngoscopy. If partial airway obstruction exists, maintain spontaneous ventilation and perform laryngoscopy under deep anesthesia (e.g., ~3 MAC of volatile agent). FOB should be available. Have full range of ETT sizes available, since airway narrowing may be present. Once airway is secured, proceed with NMB (e.g., vecuronium 0.1 mg/kg iv or pancuronium 0.1 mg/kg), unless monitoring facial nerve function.
Maintenance	Standard pediatric maintenance (p. D-3). Surgeon may infiltrate incision with local anesthetic. Limit bupivacaine to 2.5 mg/kg.
Emergence	Reverse neuromuscular blockade with neostigmine (0.07 mg/kg iv) and atropine (0.02 mg/kg iv). Confirm air leak around ETT and extubate when fully awake.

Blood and fluid requirements	Minimal blood loss IV: 20-22 ga × 1 Great vessel involvement – IV: 20 ga × 2 NS/LR @ 3 ml/kg/h	Minimal 3rd-space losses. Each ml blood loss can be replaced with 3 ml NS/LR. When great vessels involved, place at least one iv in lower extremity. Blood loss can be quite sudden; have blood available in OR.
Monitoring	Standard monitors (p. D-1) ± Arterial line – 22 ga	An arterial line is used when there is risk of large blood loss or periop airway compromise.
Positioning	✓ and pad pressure points. ✓ eyes.	
Complications	ETT dislodged/loss of airway Laryngospasm Bronchospasm Hemorrhage	ETT must be carefully secured. Liberal use of benzoin. Avoid tension on ETT by circuit hoses. Hold ETT during surgeon's intraoral examination.

POSTOPERATIVE

Complications	Subglottic edema Upper airway obstruction from edema related to tumor resection Recurrent laryngeal nerve injury	Dexamethasone (0.5-1 mg/kg iv) and nebulized racemic epinephrine (1.25%) with mist O_2 to treat subglottic edema.
Pain management	Morphine (0.05-0.1 mg/kg iv q 2-4 h) Acetaminophen (10-15 mg/kg po/pr q 4 h)	
Tests	As indicated.	

References

1. Fallat ME: Neck. In *Surgery of Infants and Children*. Oldham KT, Colombani PM, Foglia RP, eds. Lippincott-Raven, Philadelphia: 1997, 835-56.
2. Gregory GA, ed: *Pediatric Anesthesia*, 2nd ed. Churchill Livingstone, New York: 1989.
3. Motoyama EK, Davis PJ, eds: *Smith's Anesthesia for Infants and Children*, 6th edition. Mosby-Year Book, St. Louis: 1996.

ESOPHAGUS—FOREIGN BODY REMOVAL AND DILATION

SURGICAL CONSIDERATIONS

Description: Flexible, diagnostic **esophagogastroduodenoscopy**—a common procedure in pediatrics—usually is performed under GA or heavy sedation in an endoscopy suite or special procedure area. **Rigid esophagoscopy** usually is performed for therapeutic indications, such as removal of a foreign body (FB), dilation of an esophageal stricture, or injection of varices. The procedure is similar for each diagnosis and generally is performed with ET intubation. FB removal is normally a very short procedure, while dilation and variceal injection can be prolonged and may require multiple insertions/removals of the endoscope. Compression of the trachea, distal to the ETT by the rigid esophagoscope, is a common occurrence. **Radial balloon dilation**, which involves less shear stress than repeat bougienage, is becoming a popular method of dilation.

Usual preop diagnosis: Esophageal FB; stricture; esophageal varices

SUMMARY OF PROCEDURE

Position	Supine, head to the side for rigid esophagoscopy
Special instrumentation	Rigid esophagoscopes; forceps; dilators
Unique considerations	Esophagoscope may obstruct airway; dilation may perforate esophagus.
Surgical time	5 min-2 h
Closing considerations	Abrupt ending
EBL	< 5 ml/kg
Postop care	Airway support
Mortality	< 5%
Morbidity	Esophageal perforation: 2-5%
Pain score	2-3

PATIENT POPULATION CHARACTERISTICS

Age range	Newborn–school age
Male:Female	1:1
Incidence	1/1000
Etiology	Varices – portal HTN; FB – possible stricture
Associated conditions	Esophageal atresia – stricture; portal HTN – varices

ANESTHETIC CONSIDERATIONS

PREOPERATIVE

Esophagoscopy for FB removal is usually performed in healthy infants and children, although esophageal lodging of a FB can occur in any age group. All of these patients should be treated with full-stomach precautions (p. B-5). Esophageal dilation usually performed in three distinct patient populations: (1) those with prior tracheoesophageal fistula (TEF) repair; (2) those with prior ingestion of a caustic substance; and (3) those with skin and connective tissue diseases (e.g., epidermolysis bullosa [EB]).

Respiratory	Patients with prior caustic ingestion may have Hx of pulmonary aspiration, with resultant chemical pneumonitis and/or fibrosis. Prolonged intubation after TEF repair may → subglottic stenosis. ✓ any recent anesthesia records for ETT size required. Patients with EB may have limited mouth opening and require special care regarding placing and securing of ETT (see p. 1126). **Tests:** CXR, if clinically indicated.
Cardiovascular	There may be persistent congenital cardiac anomalies in the TEF patient. **Tests:** Cardiology consultation, as needed.
Laboratory	No routine lab analyses are required if patient has no underlying chronic illnesses.
Premedication	For esophageal dilation, patient preference is extremely important since some patients have undergone this procedure several times. For FB removal, iv access may be necessary before induction.

INTRAOPERATIVE

Anesthetic technique: GETA, using a pediatric circle or Bain circuit. Room temperature can be maintained at 65-70°F, as long as patient is covered.

Induction	If the patient is presenting for dilation alone and has no evidence to suggest reflux, a standard inhalation or iv induction may be performed. Rapid-sequence induction is usually appropriate for FB removal. Atropine (0.02 mg/kg if < 6-9 mo) is administered to attenuate bradycardia from succinylcholine and intubation. Preoxygenate for 2-3 min. Apply cricoid pressure. STP (4-6 mg/kg iv) or propofol (2-3 mg/kg), followed by succinylcholine (1-2 mg/kg). Confirm absence of train-of-four prior to laryngoscopy. Intubate trachea with age-appropriate ETT ([16 + age] ÷ 4). Once airway is secured, administer rocuronium (1 mg/kg) or vecuronium (0.1 mg/kg).	
Maintenance	Maintain anesthesia with volatile agent/N_2O/O_2 or propofol (100-200 μg/kg/min) + remifentanil (0.05-2 μg/kg/min). Supplement inhalation anesthetic with small doses of fentanyl (e.g., 1-2 μg/kg) or morphine (0.05-0.1 μg/kg). Maintain neuromuscular blockade. Movement must be avoided with rigid esophagoscopy.	
Emergence	Extubate when fully awake. Neostigmine (0.07 mg/kg) and atropine (0.02 mg/kg) to reverse neuromuscular blockade. Do not attempt reversal of neuromuscular blockade until first twitch of train-of-four has returned.	
Blood and fluid requirements	IV: 20-22 ga × 1 NS/LR @ 4-6 ml/kg/h	
Monitoring	Standard monitors (p. D-1) Peripheral nerve stimulator	Axillary roll as needed; avoid brachial plexus compression.
Positioning	✓ and pad pressure points. ✓ eyes. ✓ radial pulse of dependent arm.	Esophageal perforation, more common with rigid esophagoscopy, will → pneumothorax (R > L).
Complications	Pneumothorax Aspiration Accidental extubation Stridor 2° subglottic edema	

POSTOPERATIVE

Complications	Residual neuromuscular blockade Pneumothorax	
Pain management	Minimal postop pain	If patient reports marked substernal discomfort, suspect esophageal perforation.
Tests	None	

References

1. Gans SL, ed: Esophagoscopy. In *Pediatric Endoscopy*. Grune and Stratton, New York: 1983, 55-66.
2. Rodgers BM, McGahren ED III: Esophagus. In *Surgery of Infants and Children*. Oldham KT, Colombani PM, Foglia RP, eds. Lippincott-Raven, Philadelphia: 1997, 1005-20.

REPAIR OF TRACHEOESOPHAGEAL FISTULA AND ESOPHAGEAL ATRESIA

SURGICAL CONSIDERATIONS

Description: The majority of infants with tracheoesophageal fistulae (TEF) have an associated esophageal atresia (EA), as shown in Fig 12.5-1 (Type C). The Dx is made presumptively when a NG tube cannot be advanced past 8-13 cm and gas is present in the stomach. The complications of aspiration (gastric contents come up the fistula into the trachea) and GI distention compromising respiration (from passage of air down the fistula into the intestines) are diminished by repair within a few days of birth. Primary repair without gastrostomy is routine. A staged procedure—initial gastrostomy with deferred thoracotomy—may be used in babies < 1 kg, with pure EA, or with more critical associated anomalies.

Surgical approach: The operation is performed in left lateral decubitus position through a 4th interspace **right thoracotomy**. Preop ECG is advised to look for cardiac anomalies and confirm a normal left-sided aortic arch. In the case of a right-sided arch (10%), most surgeons approach the fistula through a **left thoracotomy**. Debate continues as to whether the best approach is retropleural or transpleural. The former is slower but may diminish the chances of empyema when the esophageal anastomosis leaks transiently.

Another approach is **thoracoscopy**. It is performed using three or four trocars in the modified (prone) left lateral decubitus position, causing the lung to drop forward as 5 mmHg capnothorax is achieved. Dividing the azygous vein is necessary to find the subjacent fistula, branching off the posterior aspect of the trachea (Type C). The right bronchus, aorta, and (rarely) left bronchus may be mistaken for this structure. Division of the fistula may dramatically improve ventilation; until this moment it is sometimes necessary to operate in short 3- to 5-min bursts, relaxing lung and mediastinal retraction for 1-2 min when saturations descend to critical levels. Afterwards, the proximal fistula is located (when the anesthesiologist pushes downward on the indwelling [Replogle] tube) and then is dissected upwards into the root of the neck to achieve sufficient length for anastomosis. After the posterior wall of the anastomosis is complete, some surgeons will ask for the NG tube to be replaced by a small (5 or 6 Fr) feeding tube, which is advanced into the stomach, separating the anterior from posterior esophageal wall during closure and permitting enteric feeds during the customary 1 wk before an esophagram is performed. This tube must be fixed in place since it has a tendency to become dislodged. If possible, spinal anesthesia is used and the patient is extubated on the table (otherwise, subsequently in the NICU). Because neck hyperextension places significant tension on the anastomosis, reintubation is to be avoided. When the length of native esophagus is too short, even after lengthening maneuvers, both ends can be tied to the prevertebral fascia or attached to monofilament sutures and brought tangentially out of the back skin (Foker). In the former case, one reoperates months later, after differential growth of the esophagus elongates it relative to the vertebral bodies—or if not, to replace it with stomach or bowel. In the latter case, stretching daily over 1-2 wk may provide sufficient length for secondary anastomosis. A chest tube usually is left in place.

Variant procedures or approaches: Pure EA without fistula (Type A) indicates a long gap—the initial operation is a feeding G-tube along the lesser gastric curve, followed by definitive operation months later or the **Foker procedure**. A pure fistula without EA (Type E) is usually diagnosed later in life and occurs in the neck; it is repaired through a cervical incision.

Usual preop diagnosis: EA; TEF

SUMMARY OF PROCEDURES

	Primary Repair	Gastrostomy
Position	Lateral	Supine
Incision	Posterolateral thoracotomy (side opposite aortic arch)	LUQ
Special instrumentation	NG tube in upper pouch	G-tube
Unique considerations	Loss of ventilation via fistula; lung compression	May be done under local anesthesia.
Antibiotics	Preop: ampicillin 25 mg/kg iv + gentamicin 2.5 mg/kg iv	⇐
Surgical time	2-4 h	1 h
Closing considerations	Extubation favored	Local anesthetic; wound infiltration
EBL	10 ml/kg	5 ml/kg
Postop care	NICU; humidified mist; avoid CPAP and neck hyperextension	⇐
Mortality	1-20%, depending on associated anomalies	5%
Morbidity	Stricture: 20-40%	–
	Leak: 10-20%	–

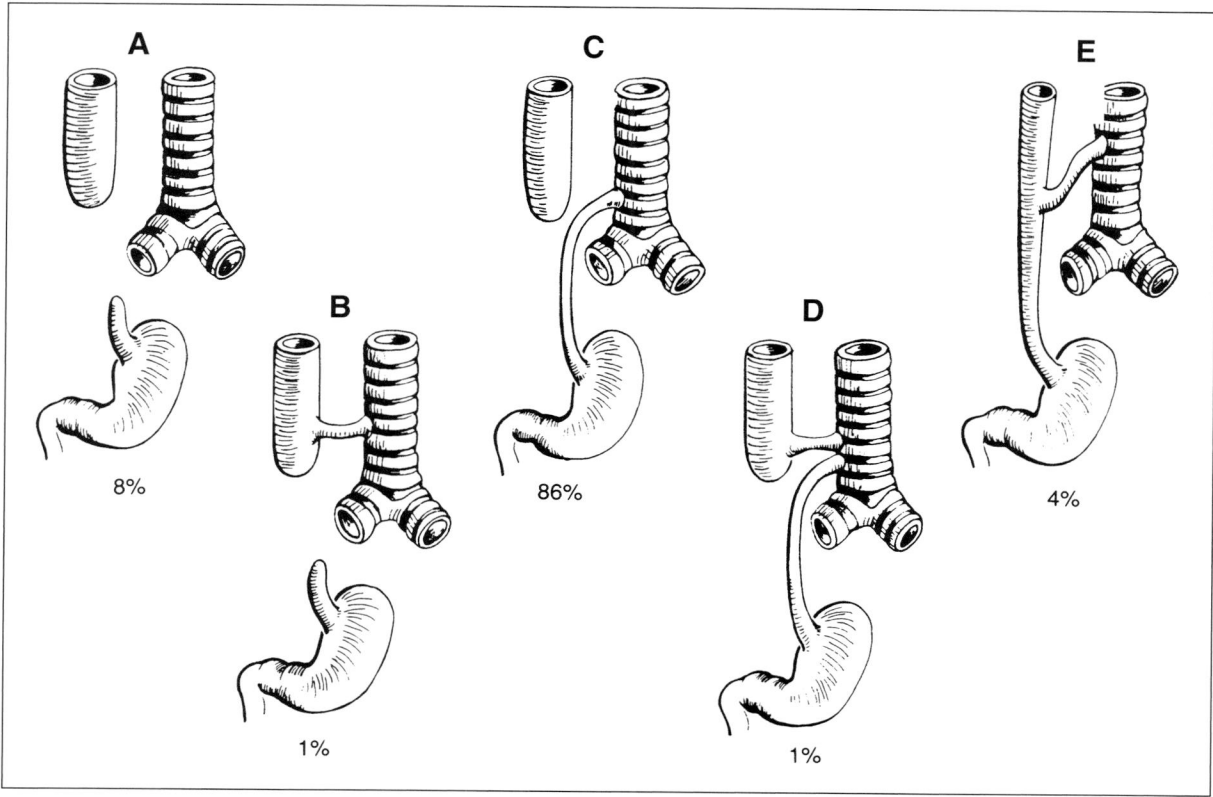

Figure 12.5-1. Types of esophageal atresia: (A) pure esophageal atresia; (B) proximal fistula; (C) esophageal atresia, distal fistula; (D) proximal and distal fistula; (E) pure tracheoesophageal fistula. (Redrawn from Ravitch MM, et al, eds: *Pediatric Surgery*, Vol 1, 3rd edition. Year Book Medical Pub: 1979.)

	Primary Repair	**Gastrostomy**
Morbidity, cont.	Aspiration	⇐
	Atelectasis	–
	Stridor	–
Pain score	7-8	3-4

PATIENT POPULATION CHARACTERISTICS

Age range	Days–weeks
Male:Female	1:1
Incidence	1/4000 births
Etiology	Unknown
Associated conditions	Vertebral, anal, TEF, renal (or radial) anomalies (VATER association); vertebral, anal, cardiac, TEF, renal, limb anomalies (VACTERL association); trisomy 13, 18; hydrocephalus

ANESTHETIC CONSIDERATIONS

PREOPERATIVE

EA and TEF usually are detected in the first day of life, although TEF without atresia may be difficult to diagnose until the patient experiences recurrent pneumonia, cyanosis associated with feeding, or abdominal distention. The fistula is usually at the distal trachea near the carina. Because of the risk of pulmonary aspiration, gastrostomy may be performed within hours of detection. Abnormalities frequently associated with TEF include prematurity (30-40%) and other congenital anomalies, particularly cardiac (20-35%). The VATER association includes the following defects: vertebral anomalies, anal atresia, TEF with EA, and radial (or renal) anomalies. Routine neonatal preop evaluation includes H&P, serum electrolytes, blood sugar, and Hct. Evidence of UO is needed before surgery.

Respiratory	The upper esophageal pouch is suctioned continuously to minimize aspiration. Premature infants are at risk for RDS. These patients frequently have respiratory insufficiency 2° meconium aspiration or RDS, and may be intubated and on mechanical ventilation with supplemental O_2 prior to surgery. **Tests:** CXR; ABG
Cardiovascular	Associated cardiac abnormalities include: VSD, PDA, tetralogy of Fallot, ASD, and coarctation of the aorta. At risk for pulmonary HTN with R→L shunt (e.g., PFO). **Tests:** ECG; ECHO; catheterization, as indicated from H&P in consultation with pediatric cardiologist.
Gastrointestinal	Multiple associated GI anomalies may occur (e.g., VATER association, pyloric stenosis, duodenal atresia).
Musculoskeletal	Musculoskeletal anomalies are usually of little anesthetic significance, except for C-spine involvement. **Tests:** C-spine flexion, extension
Hematologic	For the first 2-3 mo of life, the O_2-carrying capacity of blood is increased because of the presence of fetal Hb with its ↓sensitivity to 2,3-DPG. A shift to the right of the O_2 sat curve results in ↑O_2-Hb affinity. As a result, tissue oxygenation may be reduced, especially with anemia (Hb < 12 g/dl @ < 2-3 mo). Although TEF repair is not usually associated with significant blood loss, a T&C is indicated. **Tests:** Hct; T&C; others as indicated from H&P.
Laboratory	Serum electrolytes, UA, ABG, blood glucose, to determine metabolic state.
Premedication	Usually none

INTRAOPERATIVE

Anesthetic technique: Combined GETA/epidural, using a pediatric circle or Bain circuit with humidified and warmed gases. Maintain body temperature as close to 37°C as possible. Warm room to 78-80°F. If child is otherwise healthy and extubation is planned at end of the case, consider placing a caudal or lumbar epidural catheter (p. D-5) after airway is secured and the child is anesthetized. Patients with large fistulas may need awake gastrostomy or a Fogarty catheter placed via gastrostomy or trachea with FOB to occlude the fistula.

Induction	Atropine (0.02 mg/kg iv in children < 6-9 mo) is given before induction to ablate vagal response to laryngoscopy. IV induction, with care during ventilation to minimize PIP and potential inflation of stomach. Advance ETT to right mainstem and withdraw until bilateral breath sounds are present. Rotate ETT so the bevel faces posteriorly (to prevent intubation of the fistula). Have flexible pediatric bronchoscope available to verify placement of ETT and site of TEF. Keep air leak around ETT to a minimum (leak at 15-35 cmH₂O) to minimize alterations in ventilation 2° changes in chest and pulmonary compliance.
Maintenance	Avoid high FiO_2; use air/O_2 mixture for ventilation to maintain O_2 sat between 95-100%. Use low PIPs to avoid gastric distention by gases passing through fistula. Careful adjustment of ventilation will be necessary during surgical retraction of lung. Manual ventilation provides direct monitoring of pulmonary compliance. Air/O_2/opiate (e.g., fentanyl 5-10 μg/kg/h) and low-dose volatile technique preferred because of better hemodynamic stability. Muscle relaxation (pancuronium or vecuronium 0.1 mg/kg iv) is usually necessary. If combined epidural anesthetic is used, GA drug requirements will be reduced. Frequent tracheal suctioning may be needed.
Emergence	Extubation in OR is preferable, but not always possible. Supplemental O_2 is necessary to keep PaO_2 = 60-80 mmHg (SpO_2 = 95-100%). Cardiac or pulmonary complications, or any question regarding adequacy of ventilation, mandate continued intubation and ventilation. Reintubation may compromise new anastamosis.
Blood and fluid requirements	Blood loss usually minimal IV: 22-24 ga × 2 NS/LR (maintenance) @: 4 ml/kg/h – 0-10 kg 5% albumin	Continue dextrose-containing solution from NICU. Replace 3rd-space losses (6-8 ml/kg/h) with NS/LR. Replace blood loss with 5% albumin ml for ml blood loss; maintain Hct > 35%.
Monitoring	Standard monitors (p. D-1). Left axillary precordial stethoscope Arterial line (e.g., 24 ga)	ABG, Hct, and glucose q 60 min

Positioning	✓ and pad pressure points. ✓ eyes. Axillary roll Arms should be positioned to be visible and easily available to anesthesiologist.	The patient is turned to the left lateral decubitus position for a right thoracotomy. Monitor breath sounds in dependent lung.
Complications	Hypothermia Metabolic acidosis Hypo- or hyperventilation Aspiration Pneumothorax Atelectasis Mucus plug	ETT placement may interfere with TEF closure. Migration of ETT above fistula may lead to leak through gastrostomy and difficult ventilating. E.G., in ETT or bronchi

POSTOPERATIVE

Complications	Apnea Pneumothorax Hypoventilation Tracheal leak Inadequate NMB reversal Recurrent laryngeal nerve injury Pneumonia	Maintenance of normothermia lessens incidence of apnea, hypoventilation, and metabolic acidosis. Spontaneous hip flexion is the most reliable indication of adequate neuromuscular function.
Pain management	Acetaminophen: 10-20 mg/kg pr q 4 h prn Fentanyl 0.5-1.0 μg/kg iv q 60 min prn Epidural analgesia (p. E-5)[6]	
Tests	ABG; Hct	

References

1. Andropoulus DB, Row RW, Betts JM: Anesthetic and surgical airway management during tracheoesophageal fistula repair. *Paediatr Anesth* 1998; 8:313-19.
2. Beasley SW: Esophageal atresia and tracheoesophageal fistula. In *Surgery of Infants and Children.* Oldham KT, Colombani PM, Foglia RP, eds. Lippincott-Raven, Philadelphia: 1997, 1021-34.
3. Chittmittrapap S, Spitz L, Kiely EM, Brereton RJ: Anastomotic leakage following surgery for esophageal atresia. *J Pediatr Surg* 1992; 27(1):29-32.
4. Goh DW, Brereton RJ: Success and failure with neonatal tracheo-oesophageal anomalies. *Br J Surg* 1991; 78(7):834-7.
5. Holzki J: Bronchoscopic findings and treatment in congenital tracheo-oesophageal fistula. *Paediatric Anaesthesia* 1992; 2: 297-303.
6. Liu LM, Paug LM: Neonatal surgical emergencies in anesthesiology. *Clin North Am* 2001; 19(2):272-6.
7. Motoyama EK, Davis PJ, eds: *Smith's Anesthesia for Infants and Children*, 6th edition. Mosby-Year Book, St. Louis: 1996, 464-6.

MEDIASTINAL MASS—BIOPSY OR RESECTION

SURGICAL CONSIDERATIONS

Description: Mass lesions in the mediastinum are classified as anterior, middle, and posterior, based on their relationship to the heart, which occupies the middle mediastinum. **Anterior tumors** include lymphomas, thyroid tumors, teratomas, and thymomas. Large lymphomas and, less commonly, teratomas or metastatic germ cell tumors may cause **anterior mediastinal mass syndrome** and/or **SVC compression**. Patients will use accessory muscles, refuse to lie flat, may have a suffused face with venous distention, and are at great risk for distal airway obstruction during induction. As often as possible, operations are performed quickly, with the patient awake and semirecumbent. Steroids are very effective in shrinking lymphomas, causing massive cell death such that tumor histology may demonstrate only necrosis after 36 h. Preop preparation includes a rigid bronchoscope, plans to advance the ETT into a mainstem bronchus, and consideration of the need to rapidly roll the patient prone. These masses often are approached through a **3rd-rib anterior mediastinotomy (Chamberlain procedure)** or thoracoscopically. **Middle mediastinal tumors** include esophageal duplications, bronchogenic cysts, lymphangiomas and variants, pericardial cysts, and lymph nodes. They are typically approached through a 5th-intercostal space posterolateral thoracotomy or thoracoscopically. **Posterior mediastinal lesions** are usually neurogenic tumors; less commonly, neuroenteric cysts. The former may communicate with the spinal cord through the intervertebral foramina, giving them the appearance of central narrowing ('dumbbell tumor'). They usually arise from the sympathetic ganglia and, if high in the chest, when excised they may cause Horner's syndrome. They are approached thoracoscopically or via posterolateral thoracotomy.

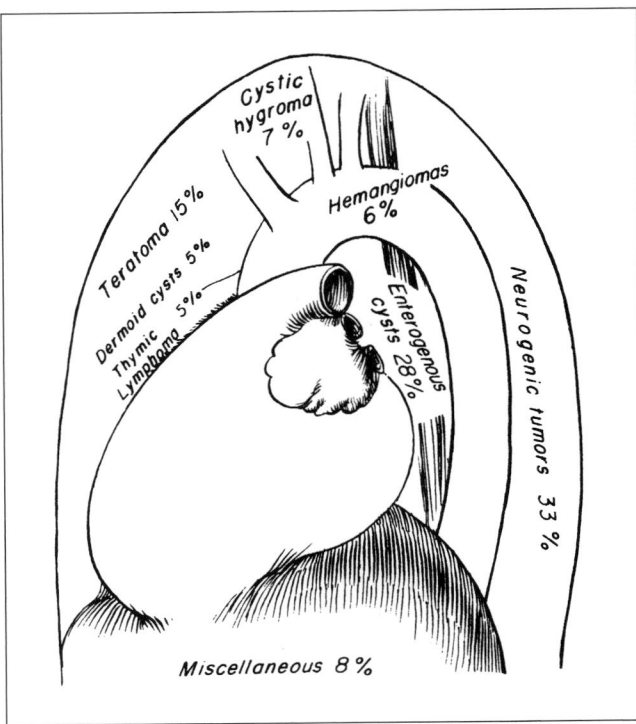

Figure 12.5-2. Distribution of mediastinal cysts and tumor. (Reprinted with permission from Ravitch MM, et al: *Pediatric Surgery*. Year Book Medical Publishers, Chicago: 1986.)

Surgical approach: The potential for blood loss and airway compromise must always be anticipated when operating on chest lesions adjacent to the great vessels and tracheobronchial tree. When SVC or anterior mediastinal mass syndromes are suspected, they may be confirmed clinically and should be discussed among surgeon, anesthesiologist, and oncologist. **Thoracotomy** remains the gold standard approach, although increasing expertise with **thoracoscopy** has benefited many patients.

Variant Procedure: In the past, it was a dictum that at least 1 cm^3 of tumor was needed for architecture to diagnose and classify lymphomas. In the age of histochemistry and chromosomal studies, this is less true. Sometimes the Dx can be made on bone marrow aspirate, pleural effusion aspirate, or a Tru-Cut needle biopsy. These alternatives should be considered when large anterior mediastinal masses are encountered.

Usual preop diagnosis: Neuroblastoma; teratoma; duplication cyst of foregut; mediastinal mass (lymphoma)

SUMMARY OF PROCEDURES

	Lateral Thoracotomy	**Median Sternotomy**
Position	Lateral	Supine or semirecumbent
Incision	Posterolateral	Median, parasternal
Special instrumentation	None	Bronchoscope; ± CPB
Unique considerations	Airway or cardiovascular collapse after induction in anterior mediastinal masses	⇐
Antibiotics	Preop: ampicillin 25 mg/kg iv + gentamicin 2.5 mg/kg iv; intraop: cephalosporin irrigation (1 g/500 ml NS)	⇐
Surgical time	2-4 h	1-4 h
Closing considerations	Lung inflation; intercostal block; epidural catheter	⇐
EBL	10-30 ml/kg	10-50 ml/kg
Postop care	Aggressive respiratory therapy; analgesia	⇐
Mortality	< 5%, except symptomatic anterior masses	⇐
Morbidity	Atelectasis/respiratory	⇐
	Cardiovascular collapse with anterior masses	⇐
Pain score	7-8	6-7

PATIENT POPULATION CHARACTERISTICS

Age range	Newborn–teens
Male:Female	1:1
Incidence	1/5000
Etiology	Unknown
Associated conditions	Cervical or axillary cystic hygroma; hemangioma; SVC syndrome

ANESTHETIC CONSIDERATIONS

PREOPERATIVE

The clinical presentation of a mediastinal mass is often nonspecific in an otherwise healthy child. Often, a routine CXR (for some incidental Sx) will show the presence of an anterior mediastinal mass. These patients may suffer acute cardiorespiratory compromise on induction of anesthesia. Hence, a careful preop workup is essential.

Respiratory	Respiratory Sx (e.g., dyspnea, cough, stridor, wheezing) are extremely important in guiding additional studies. Note that, when mild airway compromise is present in the awake patient, this can indicate that total obstruction may occur when the patient is anesthetized or after muscle relaxation. The ability to lie supine without respiratory embarrassment should be determined. Tracheal and bronchial compression from the tumor may be positional. Preop radiation therapy may ↓ tumor mass and relieve airway obstruction. **Tests:** CXR; supine-sitting flow/volume loops (useful for evaluating location and extent of airway obstruction); ABG (or pulse oximetry), if symptomatic; chest CT/MRI.
Cardiovascular	Sx of a mediastinal mass may include SVC syndrome (e.g., venous engorgement of head and neck, edema of upper body). Other Sx may include syncope and headaches (↑ICP) made worse in the supine position. Papilledema should be sought. **Tests:** ECHO; ECG, if symptomatic
Musculoskeletal	If thymoma present, ✓ for Sx of myasthenia gravis. **Tests:** Presence of acetylcholine-receptor antibodies
Laboratory	Electrolytes; CBC; T&C for 2-4 U, depending on body weight and tumor size; other tests as indicated from H&P.
Premedication	Avoid premedication in symptomatic patients.

INTRAOPERATIVE

Anesthetic technique: GETA, with warmed and humidified gases, OR temperature 70-75°; heating pad on OR table.

Induction	An iv is mandatory before induction. If SVC syndrome is present, it is important to have iv access in the lower extremity. Atropine (0.02 mg/kg iv) is given to dry secretions and prevent bradycardia from deep inhalation induction and laryngoscopy. An awake FOB and intubation in the sitting position may be necessary. Alternatively, a mask induction with sevoflurane or halothane/O$_2$ in the semi-Fowler's (reclining) position may be appropriate. Intubation should be performed with preservation of spontaneous ventilation. Have small ETTs available, in light of possible tracheal compression. FOB is useful to confirm ETT placement and to evaluate trachea/bronchi. Avoid muscle relaxants until the ETT is in place. Surgeon must be present with rigid bronchoscope immediately available ★ in the event of acute airway obstruction on induction. **NB:** A simple positional change (e.g., supine to lateral or sitting) may relieve cardiorespiratory collapse. Following induction, placement of a lumbar or thoracic epidural catheter is beneficial.
Maintenance	Spontaneous ventilation/assisted ventilation with volatile agent and 100% O$_2$ may be appropriate. Supplemental epidural analgesia may be administered (p. D-3). Have surgeon infiltrate wound with bupivacaine 0.25% to reduce volatile anesthetic and opiate requirements.
Emergence	Confirm air leak around ETT (with cuff deflated). Have all emergency airway equipment available and surgeon present. Patient should be fully awake before extubation.
Blood and fluid requirements	Usually minimal blood loss IV: 18-24 ga × 2, depending on age	If mediastinoscopy is performed, sudden blood loss from torn great vessel may occur. Volume-loading with NS/LR

Blood and fluid requirements, cont.	NS/LR @ 10-20 ml/kg iv	prior to induction may be appropriate because of myocardial depression and venodilation from deep inhalational induction.
Monitoring	Standard monitors (p. D-1) Arterial line	Pulse oximeter on ear lobe detects desaturation sooner than probes on extremities. Esophageal or precordial stethoscope earliest monitor of airway obstruction.
Positioning	✓ and pad pressure points. ✓ eyes.	If obstruction worsens acutely, be prepared to change to lateral decubitus position, which may alleviate tracheal, bronchial compression and cardiovascular collapse.
Complications	Respiratory failure Loss of airway Bronchospasm Laryngospasm Hypotension	Careful attention to ABCs (airway, breathing, circulation). Have all resuscitation drugs (e.g., epinephrine 10 μg/kg iv) drawn up.

POSTOPERATIVE

Complications	Respiratory failure Pneumothorax	Anesthesiologist must be readily available in the PACU to manage acute airway problems.
Pain management	Ketorolac 0.9 mg/kg (up to 30 mg) iv q 6 h × 24 h Epidural analgesia PCA (p. E-3)	Cervical biopsy/mediastinoscopy have minimal postop pain and can be effectively treated with NSAID and local anesthetic infiltration.
Tests	Hct, ABG, CXR, as clinically indicated.	

References

1. Ferrari LR, Bedford RF: General anesthesia prior to treatment of anterior mediastinal masses in pediatric cancer patients. *Anesthesiology* 1990; 72(6):991-5.
2. Hattmer SJ, Dodds TM: Use of laryngeal mask airway in managing a patient with a large anterior mediastinal mass: A case report. *AANAJ* 1996; 64(5):497-500.
3. Narang S, Harte BH, Body SC: Anesthesia for patients with a mediastinal mass. *Anesthesiol Clin North Am* 2001; 19(3):559-79.
4. Neuman GB, Weingarten AE, Abramowitz RM, Kushins LG, Abramson AL, Ladner W: The anesthetic management of the patient with an anterior mediastinal mass. *Anesthesiology* 1984; 60(2):144-7.
5. Rodgers BM, McGahren ED III: Mediastinum and pleura. In *Surgery of Infants and Children*. Oldham KT, Colombani PM, Foglia RP, eds. Lippincott-Raven, Philadelphia: 1997, 915-34.
6. Vas L, Naregal F, Nail V: Anaesthetic management of an infant with mediastinal mass. *Pediatr Anaesth* 1999; 9(5):439-43.
7. Watcha MF, et al: Comparison of ketorolac and morphine as adjuvants during pediatric surgery. *Anesthesiology* 1991; 76(3): 368-72.

NEONATAL LUNG RESECTION

SURGICAL CONSIDERATIONS

Description: Neonatal lung resection is performed for a few disorders relatively unique to children, including congenital cystic adenomatoid malformations (CCAM); sequestrations (intralobar 75%, extralobar 25%); congenital lobar overdistention (CLO, formerly called 'emphysema'); and congenital pulmonary cysts (Fig 12.5-3). Many lesions are asymptomatic; they are diagnosed by antenatal ultrasound or later when a CXR is performed for other reasons. CCAMs may compromise respiration and are at low risk for subsequent malignant degeneration. Sequestrations represent little danger, but are frequently fed by a large artery of near-aortic caliber (often from below the diaphragm) with independent venous drainage back into the vena cava, causing significant L→R shunting. CLO resection is performed when the volume of ineffective, dilated lung compresses adjacent functioning lobes, compromising their function. (This condition is worsened by artificial ventilation with high pressure.) The key therapy is surgical—opening the hemithorax enables an oversized lobe to herniate through the incision, decompressing the healthy lung beneath. Most resections are performed on a ventilated lung because it is difficult to selectively intubate small airways.

Surgical approach: Patients undergoing lateral thoracotomy through the 4th, 5th, or 6th intercostal space benefit from preop placement of an epidural catheter. In some institutions, throacoscopic resection may be performed. Significant blood loss is possible (infrequent). Often ventilation improves when aberrant lung segment is removed. A large CCAM, intralobar sequestration, or CLO usually requires formal **lobectomy**. Smaller CCAMs, pulmonary cysts, and extralobar sequestrations are treated with lesser resections. A chest tube usually is left in place at the end of the case.

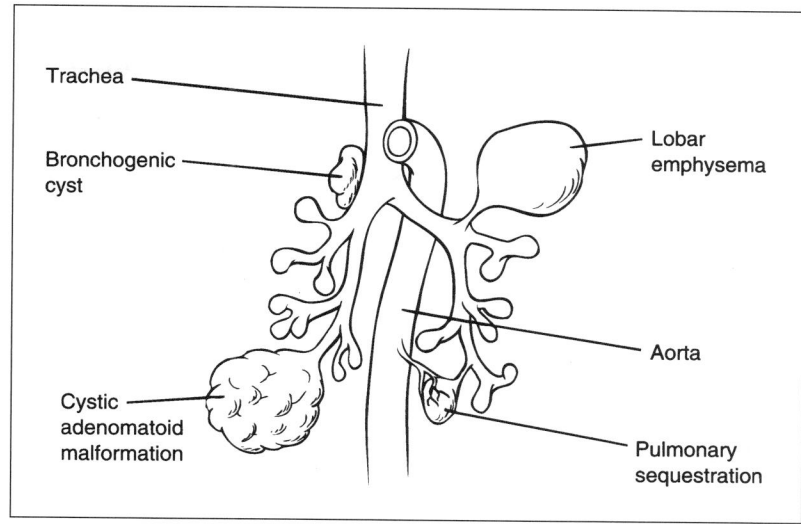

Figure 12.5-3. Classic developmental abnormalities of the tracheobronchial tree. (Reproduced with permission from Oldham KT, Colombani PM, Foglia RP: *Surgery of Infants and Children*. Lippincott-Raven, 1997. After Haller JA Jr, Golladay ES, Pickard LR, et al: Surgical management of lung bud anomalies: lobar emphysema, bronchogenic cyst, cystic adenomatoid malformation, and intralobar pulmonary sequestration. *Ann Thorac Surg* 1979; 28:34.)

Variant procedures or approaches: Thoracoscopic lobectomy has been described and is infrequently, but increasingly practiced. **Thoracoscopic segmentectomy** is easier and more widely performed. **Fetal surgery** for large CCAMs has been performed, when associated with hydrops fetalis, but without convincing benefit.

Usual preop diagnosis: CCAM; sequestration; CLO; pulmonary cysts; congenital diaphragmatic hernia; pneumothorax

SUMMARY OF PROCEDURE

Position	Lateral decubitus
Incision	Lateral thoracotomy
Special instrumentation	Pediatric rib retractor
Unique considerations	Rapid thoracotomy improves ventilation in CLO. Aggressive high-pressure ventilation should be avoided.
Antibiotics	Cefazolin 25 mg/kg
Surgical time	2 h
Closing considerations	Extubation preferable and aided by epidural catheter.
EBL	10 ml/kg
Postop care	NICU
Mortality	< 5%
Morbidity	Bleeding
	Air leak
	Atelectasis
Pain score	7-8

PATIENT POPULATION CHARACTERISTICS

Age range	Days-weeks
Male:Female	1:1
Incidence	1/5,000 live births
Etiology	Bronchopulmonary foregut maldifferentiation
Associated conditions	**Extralobar sequestration:** may occur below the diaphragm.
	Sequestrations: may be associated with high-output heart failure and diaphragmatic hernia.
	CCAM: may cause hydrops fetalis and fetal death. Intermediate forms of sequestration and CCAM exist.

ANESTHESIA FOR PEDIATRIC THORACIC SURGERY

PREOPERATIVE

In general, children have significantly decreased respiratory reserve compared with adults because:

1. FRC is closer to RV in children, thereby making airway closure more likely.

2. O_2 consumption is higher (6-8 ml/kg/min vs 3 ml/kg/min).

3. In adults, the decubitus position increases blood flow to the ventilated, dependent lung, while decreasing perfusion to the operated nondependent lung. In children, the nondependent lung may actually receive greater perfusion than the dependent lung, which may be due to a more compliant chest wall in infants and young children.

Premedication   Midazolam 0.5-0.7 mg/kg po or 0.05 mg/kg iv may be used (see p. D-2). If airway obstruction or severe pulmonary disease is present, avoid premedication, or use with extreme caution and continue pulse oximetry.

INTRAOPERATIVE

Anesthetic technique: Combined epidural/GETA, using a pediatric circle with humidified and warmed gases. For infants, warm OR to 75-80°F; use warming pad on OR table. Warming all iv fluids may help to maintain body temperature.

Induction   Either inhalation or iv induction may be performed. (For OLV, see below.) The trachea is intubated. An arterial line is indicated for children having a thoracotomy and for VATS in patients with significant lung disease. A CVP is generally not required if iv access is adequate.

One-lung ventilation (OLV) in pediatric patients   OLV is used to allow deflation of the operative lung, which is especially useful during VATS. Alternatively, the surgeon may insufflate CO_2 to compress the operative lung. OLV also isolates the lungs to help prevent contamination of the nonoperative lung with blood or purulent fluid from the operative lung.

The **three techniques for OLV** in infants and children include:

- Use of a **single-lumen tube**: a single-lumen tube is advanced into the mainstem bronchus of the nonoperative lung. FOB may be placed through ETT to confirm placement. Disadvantages: may obstruct upper lobe bronchus; cannot suction operative lung; may not have complete collapse of operative lung.

- Use of a **balloon-tipped catheter**: Operative lung intubated with ETT, guide wire passed through ETT, BB advanced over guide wire; second smaller ETT placed in trachea, alongside the BB. BB also can be advanced under direct visualization with FOB guidance via ETT. Multiport adapters allow oxygenation while positioning. Disadvantages: requires small ETT, FOB, or fluoroscopy.

- Use of a **double-lumen tube (DLT)**: Can be placed for older children (see table below for approximate sizes). (See Lobectomy, Pneumonectomy, p. 213, for details.)

Table 12.5-1. Tube Selection for OLV in Children

Age (yr)	ETT (Inner Diameter)	BB (Fr)	Univent Tube	DLT (Fr)
0.5-1	3.5-4.0	5		
1-2	4.0-4.5	5		
2-4	4.5-5.0	5		
4-6	5.0-5.5	5		
6-8	5.5-6	6	3.5	
8-10	6.0 cuffed	6	3.5	26
10-12	6.5 cuffed	6	4.5	26-28
12-14	6.5-7.0 cuffed	6	4.5	32
14-16	7.0 cuffed	7	6.0	35
16-18	7.0-8.0 cuffed	7	7.0	35

Maintenance   Standard maintenance (see p. D-3). Muscle relaxation is appropriate. Inhalation agent (e.g., sevoflurane) or TIVA (p. B-3) may be used; 100% O_2 or O_2/air mixture; N_2O is not used. Fentanyl 2-5 μg/kg or other iv opioid should be given when epidural opiates are not used.

Emergence	In most cases, the patient can be extubated at the end of surgery. An OG tube should be placed before, and suctioned prior to extubation. Ensure ability to oxygenate and ventilate adequately before extubation.	

Blood and fluid requirements	IV: 18-22 ga × 2
	NS/LR @ maintenance:
	  0-10 kg = 4 ml/kg/h
	  + 11-20 kg = 2 ml/kg/h
	  + > 20 kg = 1 ml/kg/h (e.g., 25 kg = 65 ml/h)
		Potential for moderate blood loss. Transfuse to maintain Hct > 23. If > 2 mo of age, dextrose-containing solutions are not required.

Monitoring	Standard monitors (see p. D-1). ± Arterial line (e.g., 22 ga) ± CVP Foley catheter ± TEE	Consider arterial line if patient has significant cardiac or respiratory compromise. For thoracotomy, ABG, Hct, and glucose should be evaluated as clinically indicated; UO monitored and kept at 1 ml/kg/h. CVP may be useful to evaluate fluid status if large fluid shifts or blood loss is anticipated.
Positioning	✓ and pad pressure points. ✓ eyes.	
Complications	Hypoxia Hypercarbia ↓BP	Movement of ETT or BB, compromising OLV; bronchospasm; obstruction of ETT by kinking or secretions; preexisting disease Permissible during OLV (40-50 mmHg) to minimize barotrauma. Blood loss; hypovolemia; ↓venous return 2° ↑intrathoracic pressure

POSTOPERATIVE

Complications	Atelectasis Hypoventilation Hypoxia Pneumothorax	Supplemental 0_2 Check breath sounds, chest wall motion, CXR. May require chest tube.
Pain management	Thoracic epidural Ketorolac 0.5 mg/kg iv q 6 h × 5 d; max 15 mg/dose	Lumbar (or caudal if < 8 kg and < 1 yr) epidural catheter may be placed and threaded up to thoracic levels.
Tests	Hct ABG CXR	

DRAINAGE OF EMPYEMA

SURGICAL CONSIDERATIONS

Description: Most empyemas occur in otherwise healthy children when a necrotizing pneumonia causes a parapneumonic effusion that becomes infected. The infected fluid (empyema) has the tendency to become solid over days to weeks. It compresses the diseased lung and responds poorly to antibiotics because it is remote from the circulatory system. Three phases of empyema are recognized, and the key variable determining outcome is fibrin. The early or **exudative phase** occurs when the effusion becomes purulent—liquid pus without fibrin is successfully treated with a chest tube if it is recognized early (uncommon). The second phase, **fibrinopurulent**, occurs over the next days as thick strands of infected fibrin replace exudative fluid. It is the most common phase and is most expeditiously treated by **thoracoscopic ± open**

empyemectomy. The last phase, **organized**, occurs when all exudate has been replaced by thick, infected fibrin, compressing the lung and adhering to both visceral and parietal pleura. Fortunately, this stage is rare in children; tedious **thoracoscopic decortication** may be successful, but often **thoracotomy** is required and the procedure is bloody. Some previously common organisms (e.g., *Haemophilius influenzae*) are decreasing with the advent of pediatric vaccines; *Streptococcus pneumonia*, *Staphylococcus aureus,* and *Streptococcus pyogenes* remain common pathogens, joined more recently by gram-negative rods. Significant bleeding is not uncommon and bronchopleural fistulae, if not already present, may occur when dead lung adheres to debrided overlying fibrin.

Surgical approach: Ipsilateral long-term venous access (peripherally inserted central or subclavian catheter) is placed before or during surgery. In larger children, a BB may protect the healthy lung from pus, which may extrude from the infected side into the trachea during operation. A **2- or 3-port thoracoscopic technique** is most common, aided by hermetic trochars used with 5 mmHg intrathoracic pressure (unless a bronchopleural fistula exists). The first port is placed into a preexisting chest tube site or the largest known pocket of pus/fibrin observed on preop imaging. Gradually, this space is enlarged until the remaining ports can be inserted under direct vision. As fibrin and pus are removed, trapped lung is liberated and the procedure continues somewhat tediously until the entire lung is free and most fibrin is removed. One or two large-bore chest tubes are placed at the end of the procedure.

SUMMARY OF PROCEDURES

	Thoracoscopic	Thoracotomy
Position	Contralateral decubitus	⇐
Incision	3 ports	5th interspace
Special instrumentation	Suction irrigator; chest tube	Rib retractor; suction; chest tube
Unique considerations	5 mmHg capnothorax	–
Antibiotics	Cefuroxime (25 mg/kg) and clindamycin (10 mg/kg)	⇐
Surgical time	1.5 h	2 h
Closing considerations	Local anesthetic	± Epidural catheter
EBL	10-20ml/kg	⇐
Postop care	May be septic for 24 h.	⇐
	Extubation ideal	⇐
Mortality	< 5%	< 10% when used for advanced disease
Morbidity	Air leak	⇐
	Bleeding	⇐
	Sepsis	⇐
	Atelectasis	⇐
	Pneumatocele	⇐
Pain Score	3-4	7-8

PATIENT POPULATION CHARACTERISTICS

Age range	1-17 yr
Male: Female	1:1
Incidence	1/150 pneumonias
Etiology	Bacteria infect pleural effusion.
Associated conditions	Chronic granulomatous disease (uncommon)

ANESTHETIC CONSIDERATIONS

See Anesthestic Considerations for Pediatric Thoracic Surgery, p. 1026.

REPAIR OF PECTUS EXCAVATUM/CARINATUM

SURGICAL CONSIDERATIONS

Description: Pectus excavatum ('funnel chest') is a sternochondral deformity more common in boys and of greater frequency than pectus carinatum ('pigeon chest'). Both may be associated with scoliosis, spontaneous pneumothorax, and Marfan syndrome—for which children of appropriate body habitus should be screened. It is difficult to confirm significant cardiorespiratory compromise in other than very severe excavatum lesions; transient pains are common and psychosocial distress is often the impetus for repair. The timing of repair is variable; some surgeons preferring to operate on younger children (5-6 yr) because of the ease and decreased bleeding, while others prefer doing surgery during adolescence to prevent possible recurrence during puberty.

Surgical approach: The classic **Ravitch** approach involves an omega-shaped chest incision in the supine position. The pectus muscles are detached from the sternum and 3-5 pairs of costochondral cartilages are resected, leaving the perichondrium for subsequent cartilage regeneration (Fig 12.5-4). A transverse osteotomy of the upper sternum corrects its appearance. In some excavatum patients, a metal bar or 'strut' may be placed beneath the sternum but on top of the ribs. If used, the strut is removed 2 yr later in a short operation through a small lateral incision. Hemovac drains are placed beneath the skin to trap bleeding from cut bony surfaces; chest tube(s) are placed if the pleura or pericardium is violated. Significant blood loss from cut surfaces of bones and cartilage occurs in older patients. A newer, quicker approach (**Nuss**), in supine position from the right chest, involves small, bilateral axillary incisions—one on the left and two on the right—for thoracoscopic visualization, as a curvilinear stainless steel bar is placed on top of and then through the ribs (from R → L) and beneath the sternum at the point of maximal sternal depression. The bar travels through both hemithoraces anterior to the heart and lungs; when 'flipped' 180° it exerts powerful forces backwards on the ribs and forward on the sternum. Sometimes fixation devices must be added to the ribs to keep the bar from 'flipping back' into original position. A chest tube is not always necessary; however, very significant pain results, optimally treated with an epidural catheter. There are small risks to the heart and lungs; the rapid change of chest-wall shape also has caused thoracic outlet syndrome.

Usual preop diagnosis: Pectus excavatum; carinatum

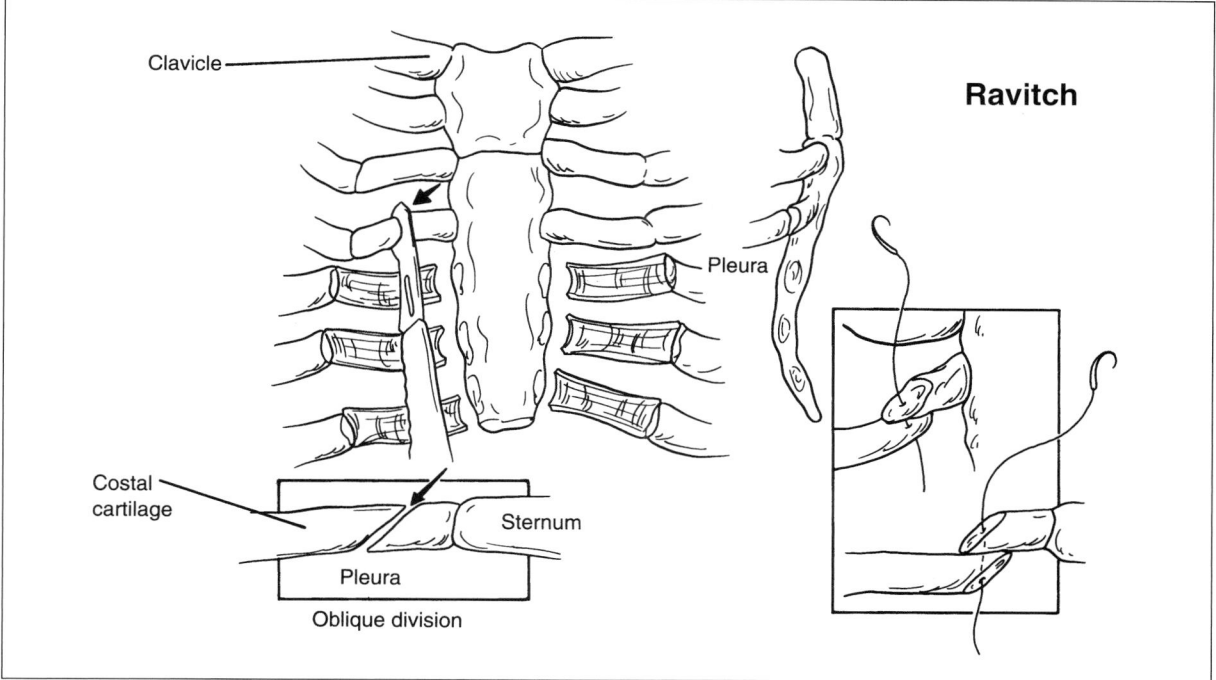

Figure 12.5-4. Ravitoh approach: The costal cartilage immediately above the most cephalad abnormal costal cartilage is divided obliquely from medial to lateral, as shown. This is often at the level of the second costal cartilage, at the manubrial-sternal junction. The divided normal costal cartilages are allowed to overlap, the medial portion being anterior and the lateral being posterior. Suture fixation of the transected cartilage provides immobilization, ensuring sternal support at this level (insert). (Reproduced with permission from Oldham KT, Colombani PM, Foglia RP: *Surgery of Infants and Children.* Lippincott-Raven, 1997.)

SUMMARY OF PROCEDURES

	Ravitch	Nuss
Position	Supine	⇐, R side slightly elevated
Incision	Omega, chest	2 right axilla, 1 left axilla
Special instruments	Periosteal elevators; sternal saw; possible strut	Steel bar; bar bender; stabilizers
Unique considerations	Heart and lungs beneath	Cosmetically superior
Antibiotics	1st generation cephalosporin	⇐
Surgical time	~3 h	≤1 h
Closing considerations	Extubate; epidural, if possible	Epidural very important
EBL	10-20 ml/kg	< 5ml/kg
Postop care	Drains out 1-3 d → home 5 d	→ home 5 d
Mortality	< 2%	⇐
Morbidity	Bleeding	⇐
	Recurrence	Bar 'flips'
	Pneumothorax	Thoracic outlet syndrome
	Cardiac injury	⇐
Pain score	5-6	8-9

PATIENT POPULATION CHARACTERISTICS

Age range	5 yr–adolescent
Male:Female	5-9:1
Incidence	Uncertain
Etiology	Relationship with reactive airway disease
Associated conditions	Marfan syndrome (5%); mitral valve prolapse (5%)

ANESTHETIC CONSIDERATIONS

PREOPERATIVE

Pectus excavatum (a condition in which there is concave depression of the lower sternum) may be associated with CHD and restrictive lung disease. If the deformity is present without cardiac or pulmonary disease, the patient is asymptomatic and the procedure is cosmetic. Surgery usually occurs between 5-10 yr of age. **Pectus carinatum** (a convex lower sternum) usually is repaired for cosmetic reasons only, and usually during the teenage years. Cardiac abnormalities (VSD, PDA, mitral valve anomalies) may be associated with the pectus disorder.

Respiratory	Restrictive lung disease 2° chest-wall deformity may be present. If a longstanding condition, patient may have chronic hypoxemia, with resultant pulmonary HTN and polycythemia. If patient has exercise limitations, there is a need to differentiate between cardiac and pulmonary components. **Tests:** CXR: AP, lateral; PFTs; ABG, if symptomatic
Cardiovascular	In both conditions, CHD should be investigated if present. Pulmonary HTN may be 2° pulmonary overcirculation (e.g., VSD), or chronic hypoxemia. **Tests:** ECG; ECHO
Laboratory	Hct; T&C; electrolytes
Premedication	If patient is an asymptomatic child, midazolam (0.75 mg/kg po up to 20 mg) or diazepam (0.1-0.2 mg/kg po up to 5 mg).

INTRAOPERATIVE

Anesthetic technique: GETA, using a pediatric circle or Bain circuit with warmed, humidified gases. Heating pad on OR table. Maintain body temperature close to 37°C.

Induction	IV or mask induction. With restrictive lung disease, there is ↓FRC, which will shorten the time to alveolar equilibration for the volatile anesthetics. Hypercarbia will aggravate pulmonary HTN; institute early manual hyperventilation. Tracheal intubation, facilitated by neuromuscular blockade (pancuronium 0.1 mg/kg, rocuronium 1 mg/kg, vecuronium 0.1 mg/kg). Use cuffed ETT for patient

Induction, cont.	> 6-8 yr old. With uncuffed ETT, keep air leak to minimum (15-35 cmH$_2$O) to avoid alterations in alveolar ventilation with changes in chest and pulmonary compliance.	
Maintenance	Primarily narcotic-based with air/O$_2$ low-percent volatile agent. Insertion of thoracic lumbar epidural catheter will provide for supplemental anesthesia and treatment of postop pain. Use morphine/hydromorphone-bupivacaine mixture (p. D-3).	
Emergence	Plan for extubation in OR. Ensure adequate reversal of neuromuscular blockade with neostigmine (0.07 mg/kg iv) and glycopyrrolate (0.014 mg/kg iv).	
Blood and fluid requirements	Usually minimal blood and 3rd-space losses IV: 18 or 20 ga × 1 NS/LR @ 3-5 kg/h	With chronic hypoxemia or right-side heart disease, maintain Hct > 30. If otherwise healthy, maintain Hct > 22.
Monitoring	Standard monitors (p. D-1)	Arterial line if pulmonary HTN present.
Positioning	✓ and pad pressure points. ✓ eyes.	Elbow padding to avoid ulnar nerve compression.
Complications	Pneumothorax Atelectasis Subglottic edema	

POSTOPERATIVE

Complications	Respiratory insufficiency 2° splinting, preexisting restrictive pulmonary disease Pneumothorax	
Pain management	Epidural (thoracic or lumbar) or PCA (p. E-3)	Standard epidural infusion (p. E-5). Ketorolac (0.5 mg/kg iv q 6 h × 48 h), in addition to the above measures

References

1. Arn PH, Scherer LR, Haller JA Jr, Pyeritz RE: Outcome of pectus excavatum in patients with Marfan syndrome and in the general population. *J Pediatr* 1989; 115(6):954-8.
2. Chidambaram B, Mehta AV: Currarino-Silverman syndrome (pectus carinatum type 2 deformity) and mitral valve disease. *Chest* 1992; 102(3):780-2.
3. Derveaux L, Ivanoff I, Rochette F, Demedts M: Mechanism of pulmonary function changes after surgical correction for funnel chest. *Eur Respir J* 1988; 1(9):823-5.
4. Gregory GA, ed: *Pediatric Anesthesia*, 4th edition. Churchill Livingstone, New York: 2002.
5. Kandel J, Haller JA: Chest wall and breast. In *Surgery of Infants and Children.* Oldham KT, Colombani PM, Foglia RP, eds. Lippincott-Raven, Philadelphia: 1997, 871-82.
6. Motoyama EK, Davis PJ: *Smith's Anesthesia for Infants and Children*, 6th edition. Mosby-Year Book, St. Louis: 1996, 583-4.

ESOPHAGEAL REPLACEMENT, COLON INTERPOSITION, WATERSTON PROCEDURE, GASTRIC TUBE PLACEMENT

SURGICAL CONSIDERATIONS

Description: Esophageal replacement in children usually is performed for caustic stricture or esophageal atresia (EA) refractory to other therapy. Caustic esophageal strictures—usually in toddlers following lye ingestion—are becoming less common; esophageal replacement is indicated after failed attempts at balloon dilation (BD). Patients with EA may have a primary replacement for known long-gap atresia (Type A), or will have a secondary replacement after failed attempts at anastomosis (all types). There is no good long-term esophageal replacement; a segment of colon, stomach, or (rarely) jejunum is the best surrogate.

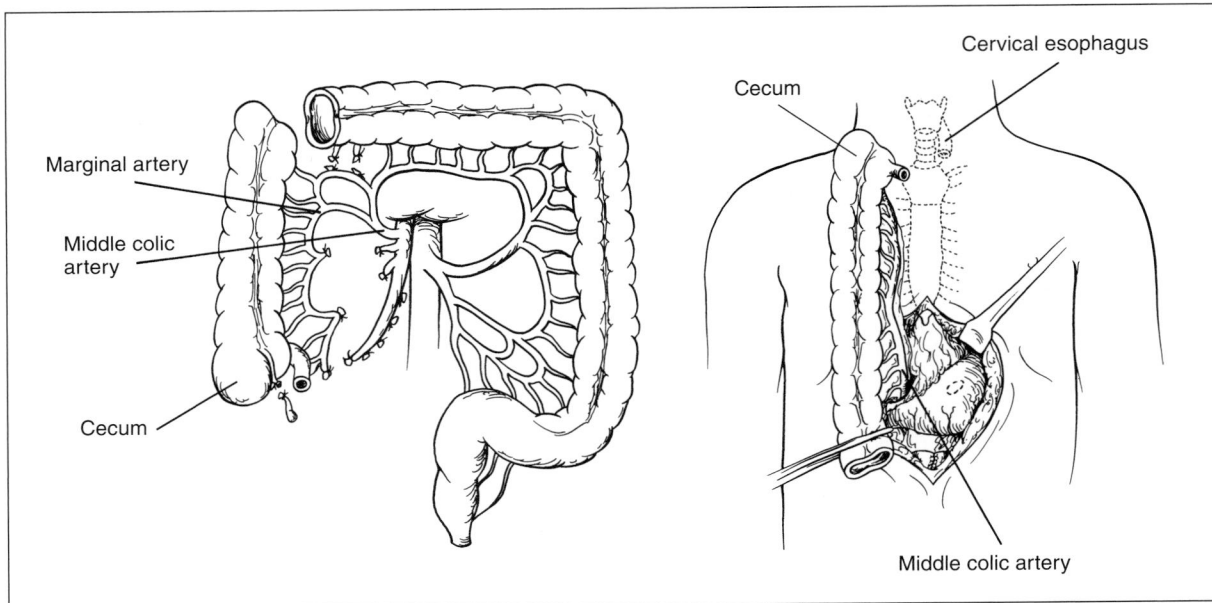

Figure 12.5-5. Esophageal replacement using a right colon interposition in a retrosternal position. (Reproduced with permission from Oldham KT, Colombani PM, Foglia RP: *Surgery of Infants and Children*. Lippincott-Raven, 1997.)

Surgical approach: Depending on anatomy and surgeon preference, the **distal dissection** occurs in the abdomen and/or chest; the **proximal anastomosis** occurs in the chest or neck. Position changes with redraping may be required, depending on the selection of incisions. The esophageal substitute usually is brought through the bed of the esophagus with small risks to the pulmonary vessels, recurrent laryngeal nerves, and brachiocephalic vein. The **retrosternal approach** may be safer but is less optimal in children because of long-term problems with obstruction and emptying.

Variant procedures or approaches: Colon is most frequent substitute, with the transverse colon attached to either the R colon (isoperistaltic) or L colon (reverse peristaltic) being used. When the stomach is used, it may be pulled up entirely from the abdomen through the chest with **gastroesophageal anastomosis** in the neck (**Orringer**); alternatively, a **gastric tube** of greater (common) or lesser curve may be constructed for cervical or thoracic anastomosis. Small bowel is used only when other substitutes are inappropriate—because an additional microvascular anastomosis is needed for graft survival.

Usual preop diagnosis: EA; caustic stricture

SUMMARY OF PROCEDURE

Position	Supine, tilted; or supine, ± lateral
Incision	Abdominal and cervical ± thoracotomy
Special instrumentation	Bougie (upper esophagus)
Antibiotics	Preop: ampicillin 25 mg/kg iv + gentamicin 2.5 mg/kg iv
Surgical time	3-5 h (4-6 h with position change)
EBL	20-40 ml/kg
Postop care	PICU
Mortality	< 5%
Morbidity	Respiratory failure
	Anastomotic leak
	Sepsis
	Stricture
Pain score	7-8

PATIENT POPULATION CHARACTERISTICS

Age range	1-5 yr
Male:Female	2:1
Incidence	~200/yr in U.S.
Etiology	Caustic ingestion; EA
Associated conditions	Caustic stricture; imperforate anus; VACTERL association

ANESTHETIC CONSIDERATIONS

PREOPERATIVE

These patients usually are children presenting with a Hx of caustic substance ingestion and subsequent development of esophageal stricture. They have undergone multiple esophageal dilations under GA. Previous anesthesia records should be obtained. Preop, these patients are admitted for bowel prep and, consequently, may be hypovolemic.

Gastrointestinal	Varying degrees of esophageal reflux may be present. Preop H_2-blocker administration is appropriate (e.g., ranitidine 0.8 mg/kg iv) the night before and morning of surgery. A gastrostomy may be present in some patients. **Tests:** Review prior barium swallow studies and upper GI endoscopy reports; electrolytes.
Hematologic	Anemia due to poor nutrition **Tests:** CBC; T&C
Laboratory	Other tests as indicated from H&P. (✓ parental/directed donor blood availability.)
Premedication	IV may already be in place and midazolam (0.05-0.1 mg/kg iv) can be administered in holding area. Alternatively, midazolam usually can be given po (0.5-0.75 mg/kg) 30 min before surgery.

INTRAOPERATIVE

Anesthetic technique: GETA, using a pediatric circle or Bain circuit with humidified and warmed gases. Heating pad on OR table. Warm room to 78-80°F. An epidural catheter (for postop pain management) may be placed once child is anesthetized and airway is secured.

Induction	IV induction preferred. If reflux concerns present, preoxygenate for 2-3 min and perform rapid-sequence induction and intubation with cricoid pressure (p. B-5). Children > 9 mo of age do not require pretreatment with atropine. In patients < 6-8 yr, intubate trachea with uncuffed ETT that has air leak at 15-35 cmH_2O. Continue neuromuscular blockade with vecuronium or pancuronium (0.1 mg/kg iv) or rocuronium (0.6 mg/kg).
Maintenance	Use air/O_2/isoflurane. Avoid N_2O to minimize increase in size of possible pneumothorax during mediastinal dissection. Appropriate use of NMR with train-of-four monitoring. Epidural catheter is used for opiate/local anesthetic administration (see p. D-5).
Emergence	Plan for extubation in OR.

Blood and fluid requirements	Blood loss mild-to-moderate IV: 22 ga × 2 NS/LR @ ~10 ml/kg/h	Replace 3rd-space losses with NS/LR (~10 ml/kg/h). Replace blood loss ml for ml with albumin 5%. Transfuse to maintain Hct > 22.
Monitoring	Standard monitors (p. D-1) CVP: 4 Fr DLT ± Arterial line (22 ga) Foley catheter Axillary stethoscope	CVP line used for postop TPN (maintain 1 lumen for that purpose); also enables blood draws. Marked arterial waveform variation with ventilation is a sensitive indicator of hypovolemia. ABG/Hct prn.
Positioning	Shoulder roll ✓ and pad pressure points. ✓ eyes.	Beware of tracheal extubation with head extension. Confirm ETT position with laryngoscopy.
Complications	Hypoventilation Hypothermia Pneumothorax Dysrhythmias Aspiration	Suprasternal dissection involves traction on trachea and recurrent laryngeal nerve. Mediastinal pullthrough may damage great vessels and → pneumothorax, manipulation-induced dysrhythmias, impaired chest-wall compliance.

POSTOPERATIVE

Complications	Subglottic edema Hypoventilation Pneumothorax Recurrent laryngeal nerve injury Mediastinitis	Inadequately treated pain → hypoventilation.

Pain management	Epidural analgesia (see p. E-5).	
	Acetaminophen (10-20 mg/kg pr q 4 h prn)	
	Ketorolac (0.5 mg/kg iv up to 30 mg q 6 h × 2 d)	Ketorolac's opiate-sparing effect is of particular benefit.
Tests	CXR	
	Hct	

References

1. Anderson KD: Esophageal substitution. In *Pediatric Surgery*. Holder TM, Ashcraft KW, eds. WB Saunders, Philadelphia: 1980, 284-91.
2. Cywes S, et al. Corrosive strictures of the oesophagus in children. *Pediatr Surg Int* 1993; 8:8-13.
3. Schecter NL, Berde CB, Yaster M, eds: *Pain in Infants, Children, and Adolescents.* Williams and Wilkins, Baltimore: 1993, 357-83.

REPAIR OF CONGENITAL DIAPHRAGMATIC HERNIA

SURGICAL CONSIDERATIONS

Description: Congenital diaphragmatic hernia (CDH) remains a potentially lethal anomaly due to pulmonary HTN, pulmonary hypoplasia, and associated cardiac dysfunction. In utero Dx allows for delivery at (ideally) or transport to a tertiary center with sophisticated ventilatory support techniques. Early NG tube placement is important to minimize distention of the intrathoracic viscera. Surgery transiently worsens pulmonary HTN and may cause 'persistent fetal circulation,' in which fetal circulation reopens to shunt blood around the lungs, causing further hypoxemia, hypercarbia, and acidosis—all stimuli for further pulmonary HTN. Thus, in the sickest newborns, surgery is delayed until after cardiorespiratory stabilization, with an arsenal of supportive measures, including: low-pressure, high-frequency ventilation; passive hypercapnia; oscillating or jet ventilation; NO; and even ECMO, which is becoming less common with the success of the former methods. When ECMO (with anticoagulation) is used, diaphragm repair is performed: **early** during ECMO (less swelling, more bleeding); **late** during ECMO (more swelling, ability to 'come off' if bleeding); or **after** ECMO (less bleeding, less swelling, little recourse if surgery worsens ventilation). (For a description of ECMO, see p. 1203.) When the intestines are reduced from the chest, there is sometimes insufficient room in the abdomen, in which case, an abdominal silo is placed transiently.

Surgical approach: Left-side lesions (Fig 12.5-6) are 7 × more frequent than right; repair usually is performed through a subcostal incision, although some surgeons prefer a thoracic approach to right-side lesions and laparoscopic repair is possible for smaller defects. Small defects cause few ventilation problems and are closed primarily. Larger defects are associated with more challenging ventilation and require thin Gore-Tex augmentation. Recurrent defects may be approached through the abdomen or chest and sometimes require transfer of muscle flaps (serratus anterior). Unless ECMO is used, a chest tube is not necessary.

Variant procedure: In utero therapies for CDH, including tracheal occlusion, have not been shown to improve survival. Although the defect commonly originates in the posterolateral diaphragm (Bochdalek), less common retrosternal defects (Morgagni) present later in life without the same degree of cardiorespiratory compromise.

Usual preop diagnosis: Diaphragmatic hernia; Bochdalek's hernia (posterolateral diaphragm)

SUMMARY OF PROCEDURE

Position	Supine (lateral for thoracic approach)
Incision	Subcostal (posterolateral for thoracic approach)
Special instrumentation	Pre- and postductal arterial monitors
Unique considerations	Reactive pulmonary vasculature
Antibiotics	Preop: ampicillin 25 mg/kg iv + gentamicin 2.5 mg/kg iv
Surgical time	1-2 h
Closing considerations	Assess for changes in ventilation (e.g., PIP, pre- and postductal ABG).

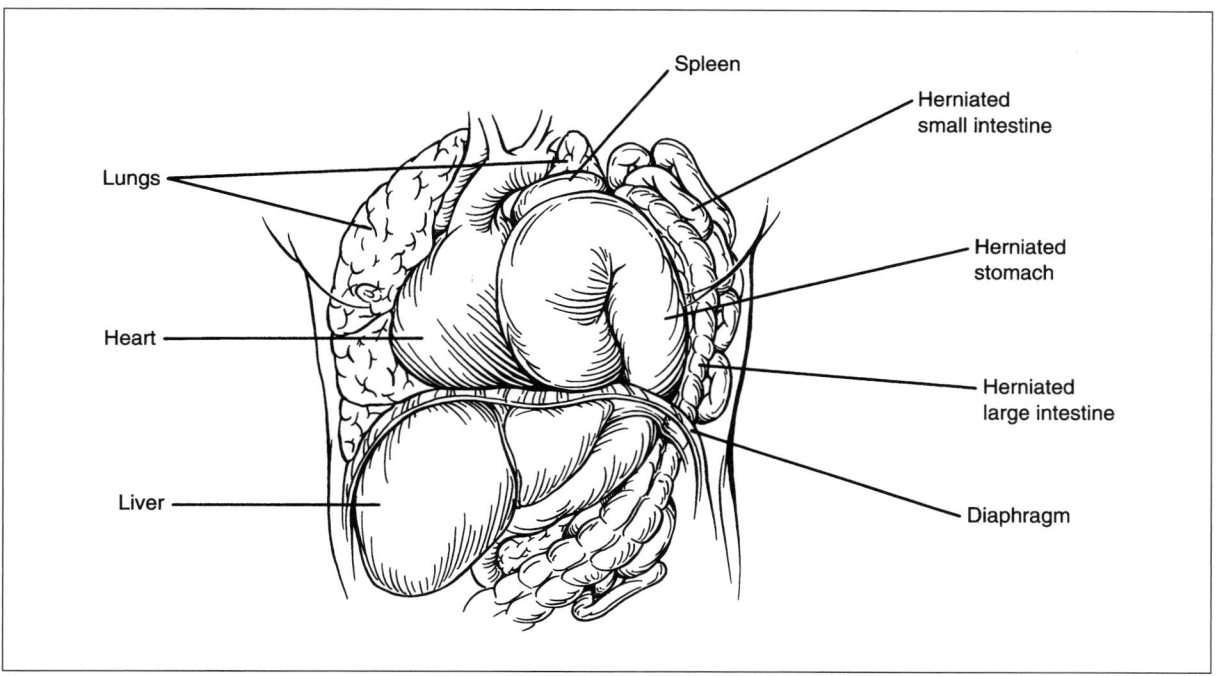

Figure 12.5-6. Left-sided congenital diaphragmatic hernia demonstrating translocation of the abdominal viscera into the left hemothorax and displacement of the mediastinum to the contralateral side. (Reproduced with permission from Oldham KT, Colombani PM, Foglia RP: *Surgery of Infants and Children.* Lippincott-Raven, 1997.)

EBL	5-10 ml/kg
Postop care	Paralysis maintained; hyperventilation; fentanyl infusion @ 2-5 μg/kg/min
Mortality	15-50% without ECMO
	25-30% with ECMO
Morbidity	Pulmonary HTN
	Respiratory failure
	Sepsis
	Intestinal obstruction/dysfunction
Pain score	6-7 (7-8 for thoracic approach)

PATIENT POPULATION CHARACTERISTICS

Age range	Newborn–wk or mo
Male:Female	1-2:1
Incidence	1/4000
Etiology	Unknown
Associated conditions	Malrotation (40-100%); congenital heart disease (e.g., PDA) (15%); renal anomalies (rare); esophageal atresia (rare); CNS abnormalities (e.g., myelomeningocele, hydrocephalus) (rare)

ANESTHETIC CONSIDERATIONS

PREOPERATIVE

These infants present with varying degrees of respiratory distress. Surgery is performed after the child has been stabilized medically. The majority are already mechanically ventilated, sedated, and paralyzed in the NICU prior to anesthesia consultation. The anesthesiologist needs to be aware of the distinction between early and late diaphragmatic hernias. Late events (occurring near or even after delivery) are associated with mature, well developed lungs and minimal problems with ventilation. These babies often can be extubated in the early postop period, facilitated by epidural analgesia. Some infants may be on ECMO (see p. 1203).

Respiratory	The lung on affected side is variably hypoplastic and the lung on the contralateral side is compressed and also may be hypoplastic. Pulmonary hypoplasia is most severe in patients with early herniation, and may be minimal in cases of late (even postnatal) herniation. The prognosis is correlated with magnitude of pulmonary hypoplasia and pulmonary muscular abnormalities present on the contralateral side. There is ↓compliance, → risk for hypoventilation. ↑PIP → ↑risk for pneumothorax. Persistent pulmonary HTN and progressive hypoxemia may be present. **Tests:** CXR; ABG
Cardiovascular	R→L shunting may occur at level of PDA or preductally (e.g., PFO). The degree of R→L shunting may be dramatically increased by ↑pulmonary vasoconstriction (2° ↓PO_2, ↑PCO_2, ↑pH, ↑sympathetic tone) → severe systemic hypoxemia. ↓CO 2° persistent pulmonary HTN and hypoxemia will lead to metabolic acidosis. **Tests:** CXR; ECHO; ABG
Neurological	Myelomeningocele and/or hydrocephalus may be present. Repeated bouts of hypoxemia predispose to intraventricular hemorrhage (IVH) in preterm infant. These areas of hemorrhage have loss of cerebral autoregulation and BP increases are directly transmitted to the microvasculature, with ↑risk of recurrent hemorrhage and edema. **Tests:** Head ultrasound
Hematologic	Hct should be maintained at 35%. HbF has ↑affinity for O_2 and ↓sensitivity to 2,3-DPG. This will aggravate cellular hypoxia in the patient with compromised circulatory status. Confirm that vitamin K was administered at birth. **Tests:** CBC; T&C; PT; PTT
Metabolic	Negligible glycogen stores in neonate; therefore, dextrose hyperalimentation should be initiated early. In patients with CHF, diuretic administration leads to ↓K^+. **Tests:** Electrolytes; glucose; BUN; Cr
Gastrointestinal	Constant NG/OG suction. Gastric distention will worsen ventilation.
Laboratory	Other tests as indicated from H&P.
Premedication	None

INTRAOPERATIVE

Anesthetic technique: GETA, using a pediatric circle or Bain circuit with humidified and warmed gases. Use pressure-limited ventilation (PIP < 30 cmH_2O). Continue NO if administered preop. Maintain body temperature as close to 37°C as possible. Warm room to 75-80°F. Warming blanket on OR table. Consider use of NICU ventilator (e.g., Baby Bird, high-frequency oscillator), particularly if high RR (>30/min) is required.

Induction	Transported from NICU to OR by anesthesia team. If infant is already intubated, confirm paralysis prior to transport. This is to lessen the risk of patient movement and inadvertent extubation. Transport with full monitoring (ECG, pulse oximetry, arterial pressure tracing). Have airway equipment available (Miller 1 laryngoscope blade, ET 3.0-3.5 with stylets, neonatal mask). Resuscitation drugs (e.g., epinephrine 1 and 10 μg/ml) should be drawn up. Syringe with NS/LR flush. Prior to any further anesthetic administration, reestablish all monitoring in OR. Atropine (0.02 mg/kg iv) given prior to opiates to counteract bradycardia. For nonintubated patients, rapid-sequence induction (p. B-5) is appropriate. If necessary to mask ventilate, avoid high inflation pressures, as this may further dilate the bowel. Place an OG tube prior to induction. Avoid N_2O and maintain PIPs as low as possible. For patients with late herniations and healthy lungs, consider caudal/thoracic level epidural instead of iv opioids, and early extubation (OR or NICU); see p. D-5. If surgery is performed on ECMO, give high-dose iv opiods (may be given in ECMO circuit) and muscle relaxant.
Maintenance	Opiate-based anesthetic (fentanyl 10-25 μg/kg iv total) with isoflurane supplementation. Ventilate with air/O_2 to maintain O_2 saturation 95-100%, as measured by preductal ABGs/pulse oximetry. Avoid hypoxia, acidosis, hypothermia, which will ↑ pulmonary vasoconstriction. Keep CO_2 normal or slightly ↑ (permissive hypercapnea). Continue neuromuscular blockade with pancuronium, rocuronium, or vecuronium.
Emergence	Transport back to NICU with full monitoring, airway equipment, and drugs.
Blood and fluid requirements	Blood loss minimal IV: 22-24 ga × 2 NS/LR @ 4 ml/kg/h maintenance	These infants are fluid-restricted in NICU. Continue dextrose-containing solution from NICU. If umbilical venous line not present, dopamine may be infused via peripheral

Blood and fluid requirements, cont.		iv with dextrose solution serving as the carrier fluid. In emergency, NS/LR, albumin 5%, PRBCs (Hct < 50%) may be given via umbilical artery line.
Monitoring	Standard monitors (p. D-1) Right-side precordial stethoscope Arterial line (umbilical artery or radial – 24 ga); if possible, right hand (preductal) ± Umbilical vein line	ABG, Hct, glucose q 30-60 min. Contralateral pneumothorax is detected using a right axillary precordial stethoscope.
	Preductal and postductal pulse oximetry	Changes in pre- and postductal pulse oximetry provide early warning of R→L shunt/pulmonary HTN.
Positioning	✓ and pad pressure points. ✓ eyes.	Arms/iv access sites should be positioned to be visible and easily available.
Complications	Pneumothorax Hypoventilation Hypothermia Metabolic acidosis R→L shunting CHF	With acute deterioration in O_2 sat, pneumothorax on unaffected side is likely. With removal of abdominal contents from thorax, do not attempt to expand lungs vigorously. Hypoplasia, not atelectasis, is the primary problem. Keep PIP < 30 cmH_2O, if possible.

POSTOPERATIVE

Complications	Same as Intraoperative Complications, above.	Those infants whose oxygenation continues to worsen are possible candidates for ECMO, p. 1203. Discuss with NICU team their criteria for initiation of ECMO. High-frequency jet ventilation may be an option prior to ECMO. These children initially may look good postop, only to decompensate in the next 24 h 2° ↑pulmonary HTN ('honeymoon period').
Pain management	Fentanyl (0.5-2.0 μg/kg/h iv) Epidural analgesia	Tachyphylaxis can develop in 24-48 h.
Tests	CXR ABG Hct Glucose Electrolytes	

References

1. Azarow K, Messineo A, Pearl R, et al: Congenital diaphragmatic hernia: A tale of two cities: The Toronto experience. *J Pediatr Surg* 1997; 32:395-400.
2. Bikhazi GB, Davis PJ: Anesthesia for neonates and premature infants. In *Smith's Anesthesia for Infants and Children*, 6th edition. Motoyama EK, Davis PJ, eds. Mosby-Year Book, St. Louis: 1996, 445-74.
3. Cook DR, Marcy JH, eds: *Neonatal Anesthesia*, 1st edition. Appleton Davies, Pasadena: 1988.
4. Falconer AR, Brown RA, Helms P, Gordon I, Baron JA: Pulmonary sequelae in survivors of congenital diaphragmatic hernia. *Thorax* 1990; 45(2):126-9.
5. Goldsmith JP, Karokin EH, eds: *Assisted Ventilation of the Neonate*, 2nd edition. WB Saunders, Philadelphia: 1988.
6. Liu LM, Pang LM: Neonatal surgical emergencies in anesthesiology. *Clin North Am* 2001; 19(2):268-72.
7. Stehling L, ed: *Common Problems in Pediatric Anesthesia*, 2nd edition. Mosby-Year Book, St. Louis: 1992, 7-11.
8. Wilson JM, Lund DP, Lillehei, CW, et al: Congenital diaphragmatic hernia: A tale of two cities: The Boston experience. *J Pediatr Surg* 1997; 32:401-5.
9. Wilson JM, Lund DP, Lillehei CW, Vacanti JP: Congenital diaphragmatic hernia: predictors of severity in the ECMO era. *J Pediatr Surg* 1991; 26(9):1028-33.

PYLOROMYOTOMY FOR PYLORIC STENOSIS

SURGICAL CONSIDERATIONS

Description: Pyloric stenosis due to idiopathic hypertrophy of the muscular layers of the antrum and pylorus occurs in infants 1-3 mo of age, causing projectile vomiting with subsequent dehydration and metabolic alkalosis. Surgical division of the hypertrophied fibers—**pyloromyotomy**—is the treatment of choice. Preop hydration and electrolyte replacement are becoming less frequently needed, as early Dx by ultrasound becomes more common. Aspiration (of food and, especially, barium) is avoided by NG suction.

Surgical approach: The operation is performed through either a RUQ, periumbilical, or three laparoscopic incisions. The serosa and hypertrophic muscle of the pylorus are divided with a scalpel handle or Benson spreader. Careful inspection for a mucosal tear will avoid a subsequent leak, the most common serious complication. Mucosal injury is treated by a simple repair or by closing the entire myotomy and creating a new one at an alternate site. Early discharge is facilitated when iv narcotics are avoided.

Usual preop diagnosis: pyloric stenosis; gastroenteritis; GERD

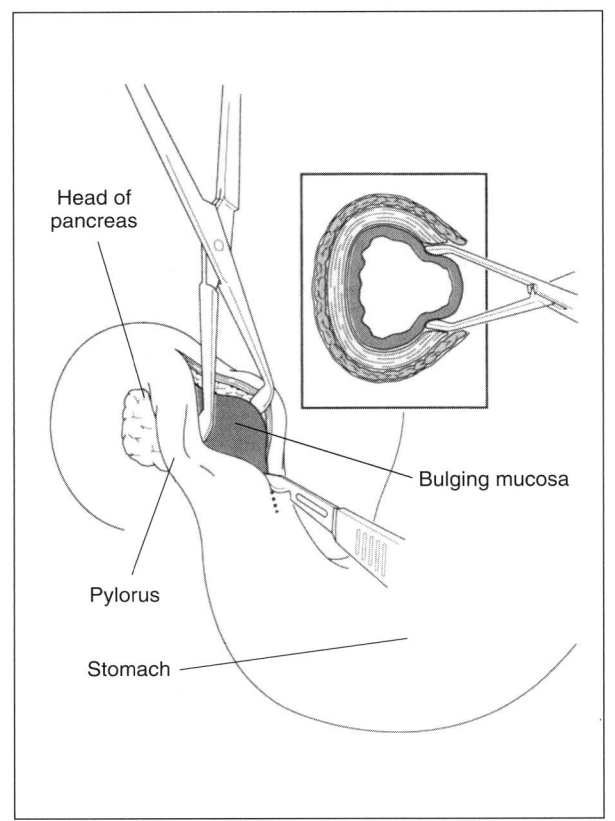

Figure 12.5-7. Ramstedt pyloromyotomy for infantile hypertrophic pyloric stenosis. The cross-sectional view shows herniation of the submucosa into the myotomy site, indicative of an adequate myotomy. (Reproduced with permission from Sato TT, Oldham KT: Pediatric abdomen. In *Surgery: Scientific Principles and Practice*, 3rd edition. Greenfield LJ, et al, eds. Lippincott Williams & Wilkins, 2001.)

SUMMARY OF PROCEDURE

Position	Supine
Incision	Transverse; RUQ; periumbilical, or 3 laparoscopic ports
Special instrumentation	Benson pyloric spreader; arthrotome (laparoscopy)
Intraop antibiotics	Cefazolin 25 mg/kg iv
Surgical time	0.5-1 h
EBL	< 5 ml/kg
Postop care	Cardiac/apnea monitoring
Mortality	0.3%
Morbidity	Duodenal perforation
	Incomplete myotomy with recurrent vomitting
	Dehiscence
	Hernia
Pain score	4-5

PATIENT POPULATION CHARACTERISTICS

Age range	1-12 wk
Male:Female	4:1
Incidence	3/1000 births
Etiology	Unknown
Associated conditions	Has occurred following repair of other congenital anomalies, such as esophageal atresia, omphalocele.

ANESTHETIC CONSIDERATIONS

PREOPERATIVE

Patients with pyloric stenosis are usually term infants that present in the first mo of life with mild-to-moderate dehydration 2° intractable vomiting. Correction of volume deficit and metabolic abnormalities is the first line of treatment. Surgery should proceed only after patients are medically stabilized.

Cardiovascular	Mild-to-moderate dehydration (50-100 ml/kg) is common and this deficit should be replaced with NS over ~12 h. **Tests:** Urinary C1 > 20 mEq/L or plasma C1 >100 mEq/L, when fluid volume restored.
Metabolic	Protracted vomiting → dehydration with hypochloremic hypokalemic metabolic alkalosis. ↓K^+ should be treated once alkalemia is resolved and UO is confirmed. **Tests:** ABGs; electrolytes; Ca^{++}; glucose
Gastrointestinal	Full-stomach precautions (p. B-5)
Laboratory	Hct; other tests as indicated from H&P.
Premedication	None

INTRAOPERATIVE

Anesthetic technique: GETA, using a pediatric circle or Bain circuit with warmed, humidified gases. Warm OR to 75-80° F. Use air/O_2 or N_2O/O_2 mixture to maintain O_2 sat @ 95-100%. Maintain body temperature close to 37°C.

Induction	An iv catheter will be in place prior to induction for preop fluid management. Decompress stomach with NG or OG tube. Atropine (0.02 mg/kg iv, 0.1 mg minimum) commonly given before induction. Preoxygenate 2-3 min. Rapid-sequence induction with cricoid pressure should be performed, using STP (4 mg/kg iv) or propofol (2-3 mg/kg) and succinylcholine (1-2 mg/kg iv) or rocuronium (1 mg/kg). Use awake laryngoscopy if difficulty with intubation is anticipated. Intubate trachea with a 3.5 uncuffed ETT. Should have air leak at 15-35 cmH_2O pressure. Do not wait for return of muscle function before administering vecuronium (0.1 mg/kg iv) or rocuronium (0.6 mg/kg/30 min).	
Maintenance	Volatile agent (isoflurane) and air/O_2 or N_2O/O_2. Avoid opiates to lessen risk of postop apnea. Maintain muscle relaxation. Surgeon can infiltrate wound site with bupivacaine 0.25% (with epinephrine 1:200,000)—not to exceed 2.5 mg/kg (1 ml/kg), for postop pain relief.	
Emergence	Reverse with neostigmine (70 μg/kg iv) and atropine (0.02 mg/kg iv). Prior to extubation, suction stomach contents via NG/OG tube. Extubate when fully awake.	
Blood and fluid requirements	Minimal blood loss IV: 22 ga × 1 NS/LR @ (maintenance): 4 ml/kg/h – 0-10 kg	Minimal 3rd-space loss
Monitoring	Standard monitors (p. D-1)	
Positioning	✓ and pad pressure points. ✓ eyes.	
Complications	Aspiration	ETT in trachea does not prevent aspiration absolutely. Active inspiration and vomiting may permit vomitus to pass around ETT.

POSTOPERATIVE

Complications	Apnea	Pulse oximetry/apnea monitor × 12 h. Differential diagnoses of apnea includes hypoglycemia and hypothermia.
	Hypoglycemia (rare)	Rx for hypoglycemia: dextrose 0.5 g/kg iv
Pain management	Acetaminophen (10-15 mg/kg po/pr q 4 h prn)	For child with severe dehydration and electrolyte abnormalities, ICU admission may be necessary.
Tests	None routinely indicated.	

References

1. Andropoulos DB, Heard MB, Johnson KL, Clarke JT, Rowe RW: Postanesthetic apnea in full-term infants after pyloromyotomy [see comments]. *Anesthesiology* 1994; 80(1):216-9.
2. Goh DW, Hall SK, Gornall P, Buick RG, Green A, Conkery JJ: Plasma chloride and alkalemia in pyloric stenosis. *Br J Surg* 1990; 77(8):922-3.
3. Liu LM, Pang LM: Neonatal surgical emergencies in anesthesiology. *Clin North Am* 2001; 19(2):265-8.
4. Maher M, Hehir DJ, Horgan A, Stuart RS, O'Donnell JA, Kirwan WO, Brady MP: Infantile hypertrophic pyloric stenosis: long-term audit from a general surgical unit. *Ir J Med Sci* 1996; 165(2):115-7.
5. Oldham KT: Introduction to neonatal intestinal obstruction. In *Surgery of Infants and Children*. Oldham KT, Colombani PM, Foglia RP, eds. Lippincott-Raven, Philadelphia: 1997, 1181-2.
6. Scorpio RJ, Tan HL, Hutson JM: Pyloromyotomy: comparison between laparoscopic and open surgical techniques. *J Laparoendosc Surg* 1995; 5(2):81-4.

ABDOMINAL TUMOR: RESECTION OF NEUROBLASTOMA, WILMS' TUMOR, HEPATOBLASTOMA

SURGICAL CONSIDERATIONS

Description: Pediatric abdominal tumors occur most commonly in children 1-4 yr old, may be massive, and usually arise from the sympathetic chain (including adrenal gland), kidney, or liver. Neuroblastoma and Wilms' tumors are the most common; hepatic tumors (including hemangiomas) are less common but challenging. Because they originate in sympathetic tissue, many neuroblastomas produce catecholamines; however, these rarely have hemodynamic consequences.

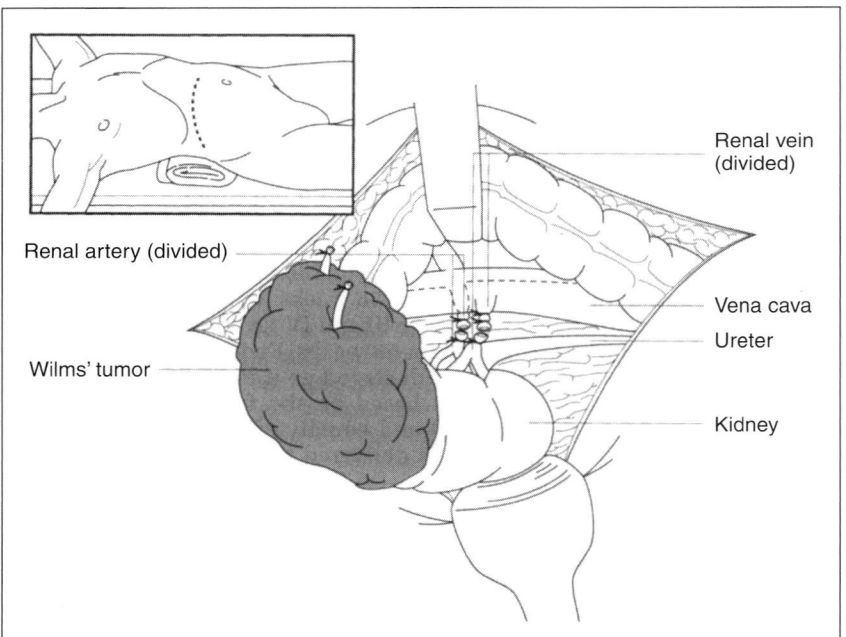

Surgical Approach: At first operation, a central line is placed and very large neuroblastomas and hepatoblastomas are biopsied; definitive resection follows neoadjuvant therapy. Small neuroblastomas, small hepatoblastomas, and even large Wilms' tumors (without vascular extension or bilateral involvement) may be excised primarily. The principles of operation for these tumors are similar, beginning with a generous incision (transverse, midline, or thoracoabdominal), depending on tumor location and surgeon preference. The incision may be extended into the chest if control of the suprahepatic vena cava is necessary. Epidural anesthesia is ideal. Mobilization of the tumor from adjacent structures may precede vascular control when the latter is difficult to obtain early, as is often the case. Tumors encasing

Figure 12.5-8. Operative approach to resection of a right renal Wilms' tumor. Insert shows transverse incision. (Reproduced with permission from Laquaglia MP: Childhood tumors. In *Surgery: Scientific Principles and Practice*, 3rd edition. Greenfield LJ, et al, eds. Lippincott Williams & Wilkins, 2001.)

vessels may be divided to preserve end-organ blood supply. Neuroblastomas tend to invade local structures. Wilms' tumors and hepatoblastomas tend to push aside adjacent structures. Wilms' tumors are bilateral in 10-15% of cases and are prone to vascular extension into the renal vein, IVC, and (rarely) right atrium. Major hepatic resections are sometimes required for hemangiomas that cause CHF or thrombocytopenia (Kassabach-Merritt syndrome).

Usual preop diagnosis: Neuroblastoma; Wilms' tumor; hepatoblastoma

SUMMARY OF PROCEDURES

	Neuroblastoma	Wilms' Tumor	Hepatic Resections
Position	Supine, 15° lift	⇐	⇐
Incision	Transverse, possible thoracic extension (Fig 12.5-8)	⇐	⇐
Special instrumentation	None	Bypass instruments	CUSA; laser; argon beam coagulator
Unique considerations	Rarely, hormonally active; may wrap blood vessels	Atrial tumor; IVC may be obstructed → ⇓⇓CO.	Possible CHF; Plt trapping
Antibiotics	Cefotaxime 25 mg/kg	⇐	⇐
Surgical time	3-6 h	⇐	⇐
Closing considerations	None	⇐	Hypoglycemia
EBL	20-50 ml/kg	⇐	20-100 ml/kg
Postop care	PICU	± PICU	PICU
Mortality	< 5%	⇐	⇐
Morbidity	Intestinal obstruction: 10%	⇐	–
	Postop respiratory atelectasis	⇐	⇐ Hypoglycemia: 10% Bile leak: 5-10%
Pain score	7-8	7-8	7-8

PATIENT POPULATION CHARACTERISTICS

Age range	Few months–school age	⇐	⇐
Male:Female	1:1	⇐	⇐
Incidence	1/10,000	< 1/10,000	⇐
Etiology	Unknown	⇐	⇐
Associated conditions	Beckwith-Wiedemann syndrome; aniridia; hemihypertrophy; HTN (rare)	None	⇐

ANESTHETIC CONSIDERATIONS

PREOPERATIVE

Neuroblastoma, Wilms' tumor (nephroblastoma), and hepatoblastoma commonly present as abdominal masses in infants and children < 4 yr old. Abdominal pain, fever, and ↑BP (2° ↑catecholamines or renal ischemia) are often associated findings. These patients may have received chemotherapy or XRT preop, and the timing of surgery may be based on multiple factors.

Respiratory	There may be respiratory compromise (as a result of a large abdominal mass pushing up on the diaphragm), which may worsen in the supine position. Wilms' tumor commonly metastasizes to the lungs. **Tests:** CXR, if indicated from H&P.
Cardiovascular	↑BP is associated with both Wilms' tumor and neuroblastoma, and volume status should be assessed carefully. Tumor bulk may impede venous return by occluding the IVC. Wilms' tumor may extend through the IVC into the right atrium. These patients may have received doxorubicin, which is associated with cardiomyopathy and CHF (most commonly at doses > 200 mg/m²). Consultation with a pediatric cardiologist may be appropriate.

Renal	Wilms' tumor may present with hematuria and other GU anomalies. Renal function is usually normal. **Tests:** BUN; Cr
Endocrine	Neuroblastomas are associated with ↑catecholamine production. Preop adrenergic blockade (as would be required for a pheochromocytoma) is not necessary. **Tests:** Urine VMA and HVA
Gastrointestinal	Persistent, watery diarrhea (→ hypovolemia, ↓K⁺) is associated with neuroblastoma 2° VIP secretion. Intestinal compression from tumor may ↑ risk of gastric aspiration. A surgical bowel prep may cause additional fluid and electrolyte disturbances. **Tests:** Electrolytes
Hematologic	Severe anemia and thrombocytopenia may be present. Blood should be available because of possible massive intraop blood loss. **Tests:** CBC; T&C. ✓ availability of parental/directed donor blood, if requested. ✓ PT, PTT.
Laboratory	Other tests as indicated from H&P.
Premedication	In patients at risk for gastric aspiration, prophylaxis with metoclopramide (0.1 mg/kg iv) and ranitidine (0.8 mg/kg iv) should be considered. Patients >12 mo may benefit from midazolam (0.5-0.75 mg/kg po) 30 min before surgery.

INTRAOPERATIVE

Anesthetic technique: Combined epidural/GETA, using a pediatric circle or Bain circuit with humidified and warmed gases. Warm OR to 75°-80°F; use warming pad on OR table. Warming all iv fluids may help to maintain body temperature.

Induction	IV catheter insertion before induction may be preferable. An upper extremity or EJ site is preferred due to potential for obstruction of IVC during surgery. A modified rapid-sequence induction is recommended in those patients with a large intraabdominal mass compressing the GI tract. Otherwise, standard pediatric induction (p. D-2) is appropriate. Children < 6-9 mo may benefit from a preinduction dose of atropine (0.2 mg/kg iv) to ablate vagal response to laryngoscopy. In children < 6-8 yr of age, an uncuffed ETT commonly is used; however, there is growing interest in the use of cuffed tubes in infants and children > 2 yr old, as it allows more flexibility in obtaining a close fit and appropriate leak. The appropriate size for the ETT is one that will allow a small leak around the tube when positive pressure is applied (15-35 cmH₂O).
Maintenance	Standard maintenance (see p. D-3). Muscle relaxation is appropriate. HTN associated with tumor manipulation can be treated with SNP (0.5-2.0 μg/kg/min) or labetalol (0.1 mg/kg iv) boluses.
Emergence	In most instances, patient can be extubated at the end of surgery. Suction NG tube and confirm air leak around ETT before extubation. If there is no air leak, consider laryngeal edema and need for continued intubation.

Blood and fluid requirements	Potential for large blood loss/moderate 3rd-space loss
	IV: 18-20 ga × 1-2
	NS/LR @ (maintenance):
	  4 ml/kg/h – 0-10 kg
	  + 2 ml/kg/h – 11-20 kg
	  + 1 ml/kg/h – > 20 kg
	  (e.g., 25 kg = 65 ml/h)
		Tumor resection may be associated with massive blood loss, especially with IVC or renal vein involvement. Avoid placement of iv catheter in lower extremities. 5% albumin may be useful to replace 3rd-space losses (8-10 ml/kg/h). Transfuse to maintain Hct > 23. If > 2 mo of age, dextrose-containing solutions are not required.

Monitoring	Standard monitors (p. D-1) Arterial line: (e.g., 22 ga) CVP line: 4 Fr (subclavian or IJ) Urinary catheter	ABG, Hct, blood glucose should be measured hourly. CVP measurement may be useful to evaluate fluid status. UO monitored and kept at 1 ml/kg/h.
Positioning	✓ and pad pressure points. ✓ eyes.	
Complications	Hypotension HTN PE	↓BP 2° blood loss or IVC obstruction or PE ↑BP 2° tumor or adrenal manipulation 2° tumor embolization usually from IVC →↓BP.

Complications, cont.	Hypothermia Hypoventilation	Abdominal retractors and packing will interfere with ventilation.

POSTOPERATIVE

Complications	Atelectasis Hypoventilation	If supplemental O_2 required, pulse oximetry useful for weaning from O_2.
Pain management	Epidural or iv opiates Ketorolac 0.5 mg/kg iv q 6 × 2 d	See p. E-5 for dosing schedule.
Tests	Hct ABG CXR	If CVP placed.

References

1. Charlton GA, Sedgwick J, Sutton DN: Anaesthetic management of renin-secreting nephroblastoma. *Br J Anaesth* 1992; 69(2):206-9.
2. Creagh-Barry P, et al: Neuroblastoma and anaesthesia. *Paed Anaesth* 1992; 2:147-52.
3. Gregory GA, ed: *Pediatric Anesthesia*, 3rd edition. Churchill Livingstone, New York: 1994, 596-7.
4. Kain ZN, Shamberger RS, Holzman RS. Anesthetic management of children with neuroblastoma. *J Clin Anesth* 1993; 5(6): 486-91.
5. Motoyama EK, Davis PJ, eds: *Smith's Anesthesia for Infants and Children*, 6th edition. CV Mosby-Year Book, St. Louis: 1996. 579-80.
6. Nagabuchi E, Ziegler MM: Neuroblastoma. In *Surgery of Infants and Children*. Oldham KT, Colombani PM, Foglia RP, eds. Lippincott-Raven, Philadelphia: 1997, 593-614.
7. Ritchey ML, Andrassy RJ, Kelalis PP: Pediatric Urologic Oncology. In *Adult and Pediatric Urology*, Vol 3, 3rd edition. Gillenwater JY, Grayhack JT, Howards SS, Duckett JW, eds. Mosby-Year Book, St. Louis: 1996, 2675-93.
8. Shochat SJ: Renal tumors. *Surgery of Infants and Children*. Oldham KT, Colombani PM, Foglia RP, eds. Lippincott-Raven, Philadelphia: 1997, 581-92.
9. Tagge EP, Tagge DU: Hepatoblastoma and hepatocellular carcinoma. *Surgery of Infants and Children*. Oldham KT, Colombani PM, Foglia RP, eds. Lippincott-Raven, Philadelphia: 1997, 633-44.

LAPAROTOMY FOR INTESTINAL PERFORATION, NECROTIZING ENTEROCOLITIS

SURGICAL CONSIDERATIONS

Description: Necrotizing enterocolitis (NEC) is an ischemic/inflammatory condition of the entire GI tract, most commonly affecting the terminal ileum, occurring in stressed, premature infants, often after feeding with formula. It may resolve with conservative management (npo, antibiotics, NG suction) or progress to necrosis and perforation, treated by resection and stoma formation or drainage procedure, according to patient weight and surgeon preference. Isolated ileal perforation—occurring without precedent pneumatosis intestinalis—may be a different disease entity; it is sometimes treated by primary repair. Infants with NEC may be septic, thrombocytopenic, and coagulopathic, with organ dysfunction related to prematurity, and have marginal ventilation. Despite expeditious surgery, several blood volumes may be lost and hypothermia must be prevented. Unstable infants often have surgery performed in the NICU.

Surgical approach: If not already present, central venous access is established at the time of surgery. A transverse laparotomy incision enables inspection of all intestines; dead bowel is resected, a proximal stoma is created in the healthy bowel, and a distal mucous fistula is created to protect potentially viable bowel. Less commonly, a **Hartmann's pouch** is created (distal intestine remains inside without stoma). When proximal bowel is of intermediate viability, a second-look operation is wise.

Variant procedures or approaches: The role of **drainage procedures** is undetermined; some who advocate their use in < 1 kg neonates are less enthusiastic about larger children. It is quick, relatively easy, and attended by little bleeding or hypothermia. Between 60-80% of drained children subsequently will require laparotomy.

Usual preop diagnosis: Perforated NEC

SUMMARY OF PROCEDURES

	Resection	Drainage
Position	Supine	⇐
Incision	Transverse	RLQ
Special instrumentation	None	Penrose drains
Unique considerations	Temperature support	⇐
Antibiotics	Ampicillin 50 mg/kg + gentamicin 2.5 mg/kg + clindamycin 10 mg/kg iv preop	⇐
Surgical time	1-2.5 h	0.5 h
EBL	10-100 ml/kg	1-2 ml/kg
Postop care	NICU	⇐
Mortality	20-25%	16-20%
Morbidity	Respiratory failure Sepsis Stricture Intracranial hemorrhage	⇐
Pain score	6-7	3-4

PATIENT POPULATION CHARACTERISTICS

Age range	Newborn–weeks
Male:Female	> 1:1
Incidence	5-8% NICU admissions
Etiology	Multifactorial, including intestinal ischemia; bacterial colonization; perinatal stress; immaturity; hypoxia; hyperosmolar feeding; splanchnic ischemia
Associated conditions	Prematurity (80-90%); respiratory distress; PDA

ANESTHETIC CONSIDERATIONS

PREOPERATIVE

Most (80-90%) of these patients are premature infants (< 36 wk gestational age) presenting with sepsis and pulmonary insufficiency. In addition to sepsis, significant 3rd-space losses contribute to hypovolemia and metabolic acidosis.

Respiratory Premature infants are at risk for RDS. These infants are usually on mechanical ventilation with ↑FiO_2 prior to surgery. They also are at ↑risk for pneumonia, pneumothorax, and pulmonary edema 2° to sepsis and/or CHF. ✓ ventilator settings and recent ABG in preparation for OR mechanical ventilation.
Tests: CXR; ABG

Cardiovascular Intrinsically labile BP. Inotropes (e.g., dopamine 5-10 μg/kg/min) may be required to maintain adequate CO. Associated cardiac anomalies (e.g., VSD, PDA) can → CHF, further complicating fluid management. Pulmonary overcirculation and intrinsic pulmonary disease contribute to pulmonary HTN.
Tests: CXR; ABG; ECG; ± ECHO

Neurological Intraventricular hemorrhage (IVH) may be 2° to prematurity or birth asphyxia. These hemorrhagic regions have impaired autoregulation, and wide variations in BP (20-30 mmHg) can aggravate ischemia/hemorrhage. In addition, these patients may have a seizure disorder. Should this be the case, ✓ medication list for appropriate anticonvulsant therapy.
Tests: Head ultrasound, if indicated from H&P.

Renal Presence of PDA and previous Rx with NSAID can → impaired renal perfusion and clearance. Aggravating factors are aminoglycoside antibiotics, sepsis, and CHF.
Tests: BUN; Cr

Metabolic Metabolic acidosis 2° to sepsis/CHF will further worsen myocardial function. Neonate has minimal glycogen stores and impaired ability to mobilize calcium.
Tests: ABG; Ca^{++}; glucose; electrolytes

Hematologic	DIC, thrombocytopenia, hemolysis, and T-antigen activation on RBCs are present with overwhelming sepsis, particularly clostridial infections. **Tests:** CBC; PT; PTT; fibrinogen; T-antigen; availability of irradiated, washed RBCs and instrumentation (plasma can contain antibody against T-antigen that causes hemolysis).
Laboratory	Others as indicated from H&P.
Premedication	None

INTRAOPERATIVE

Anesthetic technique: GETA, using a pediatric circle, a Mapleson D circuit, or Bain circuit, each with warmed, humidified gases. Use air/O_2 mixture for ventilation that maintains SpO_2 between 95-100% to minimize risk of retinopathy. Avoid high concentrations of O_2. Consider use of NICU ventilator (e.g., Baby Bird) if patient requires ↑RR or ↑PIPs. Epidural catheter insertion is not recommended in the presence of sepsis.

Induction	These patients usually are intubated. If not, intubate with full-stomach precautions (p. B-5). Give atropine 0.02 mg/kg iv (0.1 mg minimum dose) before laryngoscopy. Preoxygenate for 2 min. Miller 0/1 blade with O_2 side port, if available. Suction NG. Apply cricoid pressure until airway secured. ETT should have leak at 15-35 cmH_2O pressure.	
Maintenance	Narcotic technique (fentanyl 20-30 μg/kg iv total)—avoid myocardial depression from volatile agents. Avoid N_2O (↑bowel size). Muscle relaxation required.	
Emergence	Postop ventilation generally is required. Transport to NICU with full monitoring (ECG, arterial line, pulse oximetry). Have laryngoscope and appropriately sized mask and ETT available. Extra volume (albumin 5% in 20 ml syringes) may be needed during transport.	
Blood and fluid requirements	Anticipate moderate-to-large blood and fluid losses. IV: 22-24 ga × 2 (or 1 + CVP) Continue dextrose-containing solution from NICU. Warm fluids.	Neonates are usually fluid-restricted in NICU to lessen incidence of PDA. 3rd-space losses are usually significant. Rx: ↑ BP with volume before increasing dopamine. Maintain Hct > 35%. Albumin 5% (10 ml/kg iv) boluses as needed. Crystalloid/colloid > 100 ml/kg total not uncommon. Hct, glucose, Ca^{++}, ABG, Plt count, PT/PTT, electrolytes q 30-60 min.
Monitoring	Standard monitors (p. D-1) Arterial line – preferably preductal (RUE) ± CVP line (subclavian, IJ, femoral) 3 Fr	Central line not as important as arterial line for intraop care, but may be useful for administering inotropic drugs.
Positioning	✓ and pad pressure points. ✓ eyes.	
Complications	Hypothermia Metabolic acidosis Hypovolemia Hemolysis 2° blood products (rare) Pneumothorax Hypocalcemia Hypoglycemia	Aggressive volume repletion and maintaining normothermia will prevent or ameliorate metabolic acidosis. Bicarbonate replacement = base deficit × wt (kg) × 0.3 → ↓SVR. Minimized by use of washed PRBCs. ↓O_2 sats, ↑PIPs. ✓ for mucus plugging or mainstem intubation. Frequent blood sampling is necessary. Rx: $CaCl_2$ (10 mg/kg iv) via central line or Ca gluconate (30 mg/kg iv) via peripheral line. Continue 10% dextrose infusion from NICU.

POSTOPERATIVE

Complications	Retrolental fibroplasia Hypovolemia from continued 3rd-spacing Metabolic acidosis/sepsis Pulmonary edema with fluid remobilization	Maintain PaO_2 < 70 mmHg to ↓ incidence of retrolental fibroplasia.

| Pain management | Morphine (0.05-0.10 mg/kg iv) q 1-2 h prn or via continuous infusion for initial 24-48 h | |
| Tests | CBC
Electrolytes
Ca^{++}
Glucose
ABG | CXR, if central line placed. |

References

1. Ade-Ajayi N, Kiely E, Drake D, Wheeler R, Spitz L: Resection and primary anastomosis in necrotizing enterocolitis. *J R Soc Med* 1996; 89(7):385-8.
2. Diaz JH, ed: *Perinatal Anesthesia and Critical Care*. WB Saunders, Philadelphia: 1991.
3. Ein SH, Shandling B, Wesson D, Filler RM: A 13-year experience with peritoneal drainage under local anesthesia for necrotizing enterocolitis perforation. *J Pediatr Surg* 1990; 25(10):1034-7.
4. Grosfeld JL, Molinari F, Chaet M, Engum SA, West KW, Rescorla FJ, Scherer LR III: Gastrointestinal perforation and peritonitis in infants and children: experience with 179 cases over ten years. *Surgery* 1996; 120(4):650-5.
5. Kosloske AN: Necrotizing enterocolitis. In *Surgery of Infants and Children*. Oldham KT, Colombani PM, Foglia RP, eds. Lippincott-Raven, Philadelphia: 1997, 1201-14.
6. Liu LM, Pang LM: Neonatal surgical emergencies in anesthesiology. *Clin North Am* 2001; 19(2):277-9.
7. Luzzatto C, Previtera C, Boscolo R, Katende M, Orzali A, Guglielmi M. Necrotizing enterocolitis: late surgical results after enterostomy without resection. *Eur J Pediatr Surg* 1996; 6(2):92-4.

REPAIR OF BILIARY ATRESIA AND CHOLEDOCHAL CYSTS

SURGICAL CONSIDERATIONS

Description: 'Biliary atresia' is a misnomer, since the pathology seems to be an ascending progressive fibrosis of the biliary tree ultimately manifest by intrahepatic bridging fibrosis and cirrhosis. The obstruction develops postnatally, typically in an otherwise healthy 4- to 6-wk-old girl, though it may be confused with neonatal hepatitis or with the cholestasis seen in sick neonates fed intravenously. Preop studies often are not diagnostic and there is some time pressure because of dismal surgical outcomes when definitive operation is performed after 8-10 wk of age. **Todani** classified choledochal cysts into 5 types. The first type is the most common: a fusiform ballooning of the extrahepatic bile ducts often involving the gallbladder. Cysts are prone to bile stasis, obstruction, and malignant conversion in adulthood. Some are detected when they become symptomatic; an increasing number are detected on antenatal ultrasound.

Surgical approach: Following preop administration of vitamin K, operation for biliary atresia begins through a transverse RUQ incision (or laparoscopically) for liver biopsy and operative cholangiography. Ascent of contrast into the liver and descent into the duodenum excludes biliary atresia and will terminate the operation. Failure to establish patency of the biliary tree is indication to extend the incision to excise the gallbladder and extrahepatic biliary tree. In doing so, the portal vein and hepatic artery are skeletonized up to the base of the liver (called the portal or hepatic 'plate.') (Fig 12.5-9) This region is excised (attended by some bleeding) in the hope that bile will drain from the liver above into a Roux-en-Y loop of jejunum, which is sewn to the undersurface of the liver (**portoenterostomy** or **Kasai procedure**). There is currently little support for early liver transplantation. **Choledochal cyst resection** involves a smaller incision, possible cholangiogram, and dissection similar to the Kasai procedure, but only to a level above the cyst (frequently, the bifurcation of the hepatic ducts). Liver biopsy is not always required and cirrhosis is uncommon. Bleeding may result when an inflamed cyst is adherent to the portal vein or hepatic artery. The distal end of the cyst is ligated, the body of it excised, and the proximal bile duct (usually the common hepatic duct) sewn to a Roux-en-Y limb of jejunum.

Usual preop diagnosis: Biliary atresia; choledochal cyst; obstructive jaundice

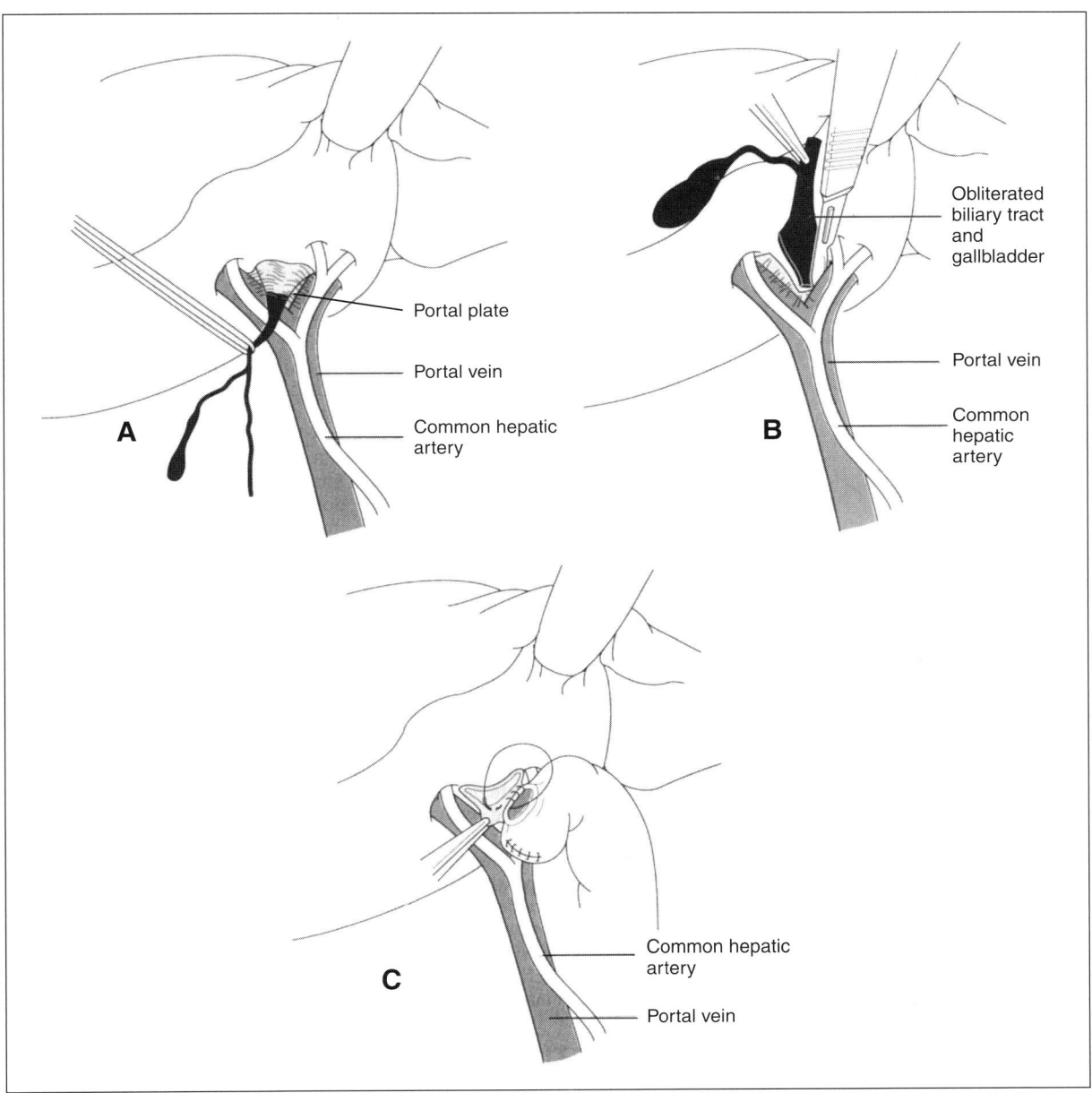

Figure 12.5-9. The essential features of the portoenterostomy for biliary atresia include appropriate mobilization (A) and transection (B) of the fibrous biliary tract remnant. (C) Creation of a Roux-en-Y jejunal conduit with biliary enteric anastomosis completes the procedure. (Reproduced with permission from Sato TT, Oldham KT: Pediatric abdomen. In *Surgery: Scientific Principles and Practice*, 3rd edition. Greenfield LJ, et al, eds. Lippincott Williams & Wilkins, 2001.)

SUMMARY OF PROCEDURE

Position	Supine
Incision	Upper transverse-chevron; right transverse for cholangiogram
Special instrumentation	Cholangiography equipment
Unique considerations	Cholangiogram, if gallbladder patent; ↑glucose requirement (4-8 mg/kg/min)
Antibiotics	Preop: ampicillin 25 mg/kg iv + gentamicin 2.5 mg/kg iv
	Intraop: cephalosporin irrigation (1 g/500 ml NS)
Surgical time	4-6 h (1-2 h if cholangiography/biopsy only)
EBL	10-20 ml/kg (5-10 ml/kg for cholangiogram)
Postop care	PICU
Mortality	< 5%

Morbidity	Bile leak: 10-15%
	Obstruction: 10%
	Sepsis: 5-10%
	Respiratory failure: 5%
Pain score	7-8 (4-5 for cholangiogram)

PATIENT POPULATION CHARACTERISTICS

Age range	6-12 wk
Male:Female	> 1:1
Incidence	1/15,000 births
Etiology	Viral; autoimmune
Associated conditions	**NB:** Asplenia syndrome (5-10%); polysplenia (5-10%)

ANESTHETIC CONSIDERATIONS

PREOPERATIVE

Biliary atresia is a postnatal inflammatory disorder of the hepatobiliary tree involving the intrahepatic biliary radicles → obstructive jaundice. The Kasai procedure is performed when the diagnosis of biliary atresia is made in the first 3-4 mo of life.

Gastrointestinal	Hepatic function preserved initially (i.e., normal albumin synthesis). Cholestatic jaundice usually present. There may be impaired elimination of drugs, particularly NMRs. Glucose homeostasis is usually normal.
Hematologic	Anemia 2° hepatic disease. Impaired vitamin K absorption 2° lack of bile salts. Elevated PT will variably correct with vitamin K administration (phytonadione 1 mg im/iv given during the week before surgery). Have FFP available if PT not corrected after vitamin K. **Tests:** PT; PTT; CBC; T&C
Laboratory	Electrolytes; BUN; Cr; LFTs; albumin; bilirubin, direct and indirect; glucose; others as indicated from H&P. Confirm availability of blood products (PRBCs, FFP). (✓ parental/directed donor blood availability.)
Premedication	None

INTRAOPERATIVE

Anesthetic technique: GETA/epidural, using a pediatric circle with warmed and humidified gases. Warm OR to 75°-80°F; use warming pad on OR table. (Remember: majority of heat loss is radiant).

Induction	Mask induction is appropriate if no iv in place. NMR (e.g., rocuronium 0.6-1 mg/kg) to facilitate tracheal intubation, typically using an uncuffed 3.5-4.0 ETT (with leak at 15-35 cmH$_2$O). Place epidural in lateral position, lumbar or thoracic (preferred) if child is < 12 mo.
Maintenance	Isoflurane/air/O$_2$, supplemented with epidural anesthesia if PT/PTT normal. No N$_2$O, to avoid bowel distention. Continue muscle relaxant to facilitate abdominal closure.
Emergence	Patient usually extubated in OR and transported to PACU or, in the case of prolonged surgery and/or significant blood loss, to PICU with O$_2$ and monitors in place.
Blood and fluid requirements	Moderate blood loss IV: 22 ga × 1-2 NS/LR @ 10 ml/kg/h Albumin 5%	Potential for large 3rd-space losses. Plan 10 ml/kg/h of NS/LR for replacement, and be prepared for sudden blood loss. Use albumin 5%, or NS/LR to replace blood loss; transfuse to maintain Hct > 22%. If dextrose infusion required, give 4-6 mg/kg/min.
Monitoring	Standard monitors (p. D-1) Urinary catheter NG tube Arterial line (22-24 ga) ±CVP line	Hct, blood glucose, ±ABG q 1-2 h and prn. Maintain UO @ 1 ml/kg/h. The presence of ⬆⬆BP variations with respiration is a useful indicator of hypovolemia. CVP may be indicated for blood sampling/intravascular volume monitoring.

Positioning	✓ padding – heels, elbows, occiput.	
	✓ eyes.	
Complications	Hypothermia	In upper abdominal surgery, the retractors and abdominal
	Hypovolemia	packing may limit diaphragmatic excursion, thus requiring
	Hypoventilation	higher PIP to adequately ventilate the patient. ETT leak
	Metabolic acidosis	(PIP) > 20 cmH$_2$O to ensure adequate ventilation.

POSTOPERATIVE

Complications	Hypovolemia	3rd-space losses continue in the immediate postop
	Transfusion-associated disease	period.
	Atelectasis	Postop mechanical ventilation with TV 10-12 ml/kg and
	Cholangitis	PEEP 3-5 cmH$_2$O to minimize atelectasis.
Pain management	Fentanyl (1-2 mg/kg/iv q 1 h prn)	Epidural analgesia if catheter in place (see p. E-5). Marcaine dose should be limited to 0.25-0.3 mg/kg 2° hepatic
	MSO$_4$ (0.05-0.1 mg/kg iv q 2-4 h prn)	clearance and serum protein binding capacity.
Tests	Hct	
	ABG	

References

1. Engelskirchen R, Holschneider AM, Gharib M, Vente C: Biliary atresia—a 25-year survey. *Eur J Pediatr Surg* 1991; 1(3): 154-60.
2. Flake AW: Disorders of the gallbladder and biliary tract. In *Surgery of Infants and Children.* Oldham KT, Colombani PM, Foglia RP, eds. Lippincott-Raven, Philadelphia: 1997, 1405-14.
3. Green DW, Howard ER, Davenport M: Anesthesia, perioperative management and outcome of correction of extrahepatic biliary atresia in the infant: A review of 50 cases in the King's College Hospital Series. *Pediatr Anesth* 2000; 10(6):581-9.
4. Karrer FM, Hall RJ, Stewart BA, Lilly JR: Congenital biliary tract disease. *Surg Clin North Am* 1990; 70(6):1403-18.
5. Karrer FM, Lilly JP: Biliary atresia. In *Surgery of Infants and Children.* Oldham KT, Colombani PM, Foglia RP, eds. Lippincott-Raven, Philadelphia: 1997, 1395-1404.
6. Kasai M, Suzuki H, Ohashi E, Ohi R, Chiba T, Okamoto A: Technique and results of operative management of biliary atresia. *World J Surg* 1978; 2(5):571-9.
7. Katz J, Steward DJ, eds: *Anesthesia and Uncommon Pediatric Diseases*, 2nd edition. WB Saunders, Philadelphia: 1993.
8. Meunier JF, Goujard E, Dubousset AM, et al: Pharmakokinetics of bupivacaine after continuous epidural infusion in infants with and without biliary atresia. *Anesthesiology* 2001; 95(1):87-95.

REPAIR OF ABDOMINAL WALL DEFECTS: OMPHALOCELE/GASTROSCHISIS

SURGICAL CONSIDERATIONS

Description: Omphalocele is a herniation of bowel and sometimes viscera into an enlarged umbilical cord that may be categorized as small (< 2 cm, sometimes called a 'hernia of the cord'); medium (2-5 cm defect); or giant (≥ 6 cm and containing liver). The larger the defect, the more difficult the repair for lack of skin and muscle; primary repair is virtually never possible for giant defects. Omphaloceles are associated with genetic defects (trisomy 21) and may be part of other syndromes (e.g., OEIS, pentalogy of Cantrell, which includes cardiac defects). The surprisingly tough membrane of the umbilical cord protects the intestines from exposure to amniotic fluid. **Gastroschisis** is not associated with chromosomal anomalies or syndromes. It involves a 1-2 cm defect to the right of the umbilicus, through which bowel, and sometimes stomach or gonads, extrude and are exposed to the sclerosing effects of amniotic fluid, causing variable degrees of 'peel' (bowel-wall thickening).

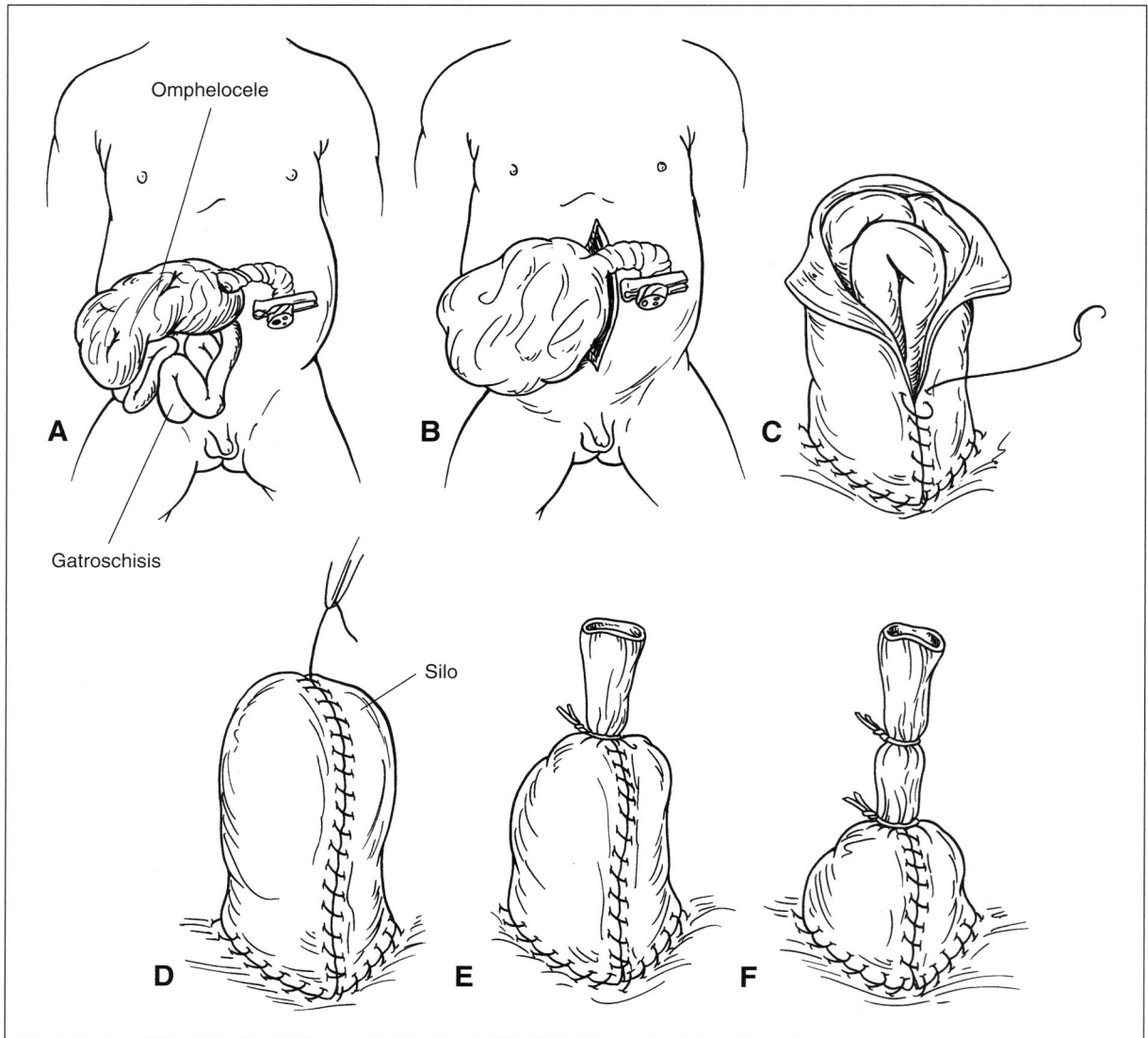

Figure 12.5-10. Management of gastroschisis and omphalocele (both shown together): (A) Gastroschisis defect. (B) Extension of opening with midline incision (optional). (C) Use of silo if primary closure is not possible. (D) Finished silo. (E, F) Staged ligation of silo with reduction of silo contents into abdominal cavity proper. (Reproduced with permission from Oldham KT, Colombani PM, Foglia RP: *Surgery of Infants and Children.* Lippincott-Raven, 1997.)

Surgical approach: Central venous catheter placement precedes or accompanies the initial operation. Enlargement of the defect is sometimes necessary to permit visceral reduction, provided there is sufficient abdominal domain. If not, reduction will cause bowel ischemia and respiratory embarrassment. Some surgeons will use a maximal transduced bladder or stomach pressure (20 mmHg) or maximal PIP (35 mmHg) as an indicator that primary repair is dangerous. In this case, a prosthetic abdominal wall of Silastic is created (or purchased) and applied to the edges of the defect, creating a tubular prominence called a 'silo.' In the NICU this is reduced for 3-10 d, whereupon the abdomen is closed primarily (Fig 12.5-10). Small and medium size omphaloceles are treated similarly. Return of intestinal function will take 3-7 d for omphaloceles and 1-4 wk for gastroschisis.

Variant procedures or approaches: Giant omphaloceles are sometimes treated without initial attempts at definitive surgery. Instead, the amniotic membrane retaining the intestinal contents is treated with daily applications of a sclerosing solution (silver sulfasalazine, tincture of mercurochrome). This causes the membrane to thicken and eventually epithelialize. Many months later, the resulting unsightly bulge may be excised and closure of the abdominal defect attempted without undue respiratory or bowel compromise.

Usual preop diagnosis: Omphalocele; gastroschisis; pentalogy of Cantrell; exstrophy cloaca

SUMMARY OF PROCEDURE

Position	Supine
Incision	Midline
Special instrumentation	None; for staged repair, reinforced Silastic sheeting or pre-made (Bentec) silo
Antibiotics	Preop: ampicillin 25 mg/kg iv + gentamicin 2.5 mg/kg iv
Surgical time	2 h
Closing considerations	Assess respiratory and cardiovascular function after muscle closure by PIP, ABG, MAP. Impaired ventilation and venous return will result from overaggressive attempts at closure.
EBL	5-10 ml/kg
Postop care	Assisted ventilation; volume support (gastroschisis)
Mortality	Omphalocele: 28%
	Gastroschisis: 15-23%
Morbidity	Respiratory failure
	Intestinal ischemia/obstruction
	Infection
Pain score	5-6 (primary); 4-5 (staged repair)

PATIENT POPULATION CHARACTERISTICS

Age range	Newborn
Male:Female	1:1
Incidence	1/3000–1/10,000 live births
Etiology	Unknown
Associated conditions	Gastroschisis: malrotation, intestinal atresia
	Omphalocele: cardiac, renal anomalies
	Trisomy 13, 18, 21
	Beckwith-Wiedemann syndrome (hypoglycemia, macroglossia)
	Pentalogy of Cantrell: omphalocele, sternal, diaphragmatic, pericardial, cardiac anomalies
	Exstrophy cloaca: omphalocele, exstrophy bladder, imperforate anus

ANESTHETIC CONSIDERATIONS

PREOPERATIVE

Newborns with omphalocele/gastroschisis present for urgent surgery. The large exposed surface area of abdominal contents allows substantial evaporative heat and fluid losses. Omphalocele is associated with other congenital anomalies (e.g., VSD, Beckwith-Wiedemann syndrome [infantile gigantism, macroglossia]). The majority of these patients should be medically stabilized in the nursery before coming to the OR.

Respiratory	If premature (< 36 wk gestational age), infant is at ↑risk for RDS. Respiratory insufficiency may be present. **Tests:** CXR; ABG
Cardiovascular	With omphalocele, there is a 20% incidence of cardiac anomalies (VSD, PDA). Presence of murmur. **Tests:** ECHO, if indicated
Gastrointestinal	Intestinal atresia may be present. Hypovolemia from evaporative loss also may be present. Use full-stomach precautions (p. B-5). ✓ administration of antibiotics to prevent peritonitis.
Endocrine	Beckwith-Wiedemann associated with hypoglycemia (term infant glucose—nl = > 36 mg/dL). **Tests:** Glucose; electrolytes
Laboratory	CBC; T&C; PT; PTT; UA

INTRAOPERATIVE

Anesthetic technique: Epidural anesthesia and GETA, using a pediatric circle or Bain circuit with humidified and warmed gases. Maintain body temperature close to 37°C. Use Bair-Hugger and warm room to 78-80°F. (Remember majority of heat loss is radiant.)

Induction	Atropine (0.02 mg/kg iv; minimum dose, 0.1 mg) is given before induction in patients < 9 mo to ablate vagal response to laryngoscopy. Pass an OG tube to decompress stomach. Assure adequate intravascular volume status (capillary refill < 2 sec; warm, pink extremities). Preoxygenate with 100% O_2 for 2-3 min prior to rapid-sequence intubation. STP (4-6 mg/kg iv) or propofol (2-3 mg/kg) and succinylcholine (1-2 mg/kg iv) or rocuronium (1 mg/kg) administered to facilitate tracheal intubation. 3.5 ETT is most appropriate for this age group. Keep air leak around ETT at 15-35 cmH$_2$O. Lower pressure air leak may make ventilation difficult if primary closure of abdomen is accompanied by significant rise in intraabdominal pressure. Epidural catheter inserted via the caudal or lumbar route after intubation. If positioning for the epidural catheter insertion is difficult, do not proceed; insert at the end of the case for postop analgesia.	
Maintenance	Avoid high FiO$_2$. Use air/O$_2$ mixture for ventilation to maintain O$_2$ sat 95-100% and PaO$_2$ < 100. If no epidural is placed, then use a primarily narcotic-based technique with fentanyl (10-25 μg/kg iv total), low-dose isoflurane as needed. Note initial PIP prior to abdominal closure. Maintain neuromuscular blockade to facilitate abdominal closure. If an epidural catheter is available, dose with local anesthetic and opiate (p. D-5) to supplement inhalation iv agent.	
Emergence	Remain intubated postop. Transport to NICU on 100% O$_2$ to increase margin of safety in case of accidental extubation.	
Blood and fluid requirements	Marked 3rd-space fluid loss Minimal-moderate blood loss IV: 22-24 ga × 1-2, upper extremities NS/LR @ 4 ml/kg/h	Continue dextrose-containing solution from NICU. Replace 3rd-space losses (10-15+ ml/kg/h). Replace blood loss with albumin 5% and/or blood ml for ml. Maintain Hct > 30%. Lower extremities usually edematous due to abdominal venous and lymphatic compression.
Monitoring	Standard monitors (p. D-1) Arterial line (24-ga radial) ± CVP – 3 Fr subclavian or 4 Fr IJ ± Intragastric catheter Urinary catheter	ABG pre- and postabdominal closure. Hct, glucose, electrolytes q 60 min. CVP; reserve 1 lumen for postop TPN. Respiratory variation on arterial waveform is sensitive indicator of hypovolemia. May be used to measure pressure during abdominal closure.
Positioning	✓ and pad pressure points. ✓ eyes.	Arms positioned to have ready access to arterial line.
Complications	Hypothermia Hypovolemia Respiratory insufficiency/hypoventilation Atelectasis Volume overload/pulmonary edema	Some institutions monitor intraabdominal pressure during closure. If intragastric pressure is > 20 mmHg and CVP increases by 4 mmHg with initial primary closure, it should be converted to a staged repair. Raised abdominal pressure will cause an acute restrictive ventilatory defect and promote abdominal visceral ischemia.

POSTOPERATIVE

Complications	Respiratory failure Bowel ischemia/necrosis Renal failure Peritonitis Sepsis/metabolic acidosis Pneumothorax RDS Hypothermia	Abdominal 3rd spacing will persist in immediate postop period → ↓intraabdominal pressure → bowel ischemia + ↓renal perfusion. Persistent metabolic and/or respiratory acidosis mandates staged repair.
Pain management	Continuous epidural or iv infusion (p. E-5)	
Tests	ABG Hct Glucose Electrolytes, Ca^{++}	UO maintained at > 0.5 ml/kg/h

References

1. Gregory GA, ed: *Pediatric Anesthesia*, 4th edition. Churchill Livingstone, New York: 2002.

2. Liu LM, Pang LM: Neonatal surgical emergencies in anesthesiology. *Clin North Am* 2001; 19(2):276-7.
3. Motoyama EK, Davis PJ, eds: *Smith's Anesthesia for Infants and Children*, 6th edition. Mosby-Year Book, St. Louis: 1996, 455-7.
4. Novotny DA, Klein RL, Boeckman CR: Gastroschisis: an 18-year review. *J Pediatr Surg* 1993; 28(5):650-2.
5. Sauter ER, Falterman KW, Arensman RM: Is primary repair of gastroschisis and omphalocele always the best operation? *Am Surg* 1991; 57(3):142-4.
6. Schier F, Schier C, Stute MP, Wurtenberger H: 193 cases of gastroschisis and omphalocele—postoperative results. *Zentralbl Chir* 1988; 113(4):225-34.
7. Tracy TF Jr: Abdominal wall defects. In *Surgery of Infants and Children*. Oldham KT, Colombani PM, Foglia RP, eds. Lippincott-Raven, Philadelphia: 1997, 1083-94.
8. Tsakayannis DE, Zurakowski D, Lillehei CW: Respiratory insufficiency at birth: a predictor of mortality for infants with omphalocele. *J Pediatr Surg* 1996; 31(8):1088-90.
9. Yaster M, et al: Hemodynamic effects of primary closure of omphalocele/gastroschisis in human newborns. *Anesthesiology* 1988; 69:84-8.

PULLTHROUGH FOR HIRSCHSPRUNG'S DISEASE

SURGICAL CONSIDERATIONS

Description: Congenital aganglionosis, called **Hirschprung's disease** (HD), begins at the dentate line of the anus and extends proximally for a variable distance. It produces functional obstruction because the involved bowel is tonically contracted. The 'transition zone' to ganglionic bowel occurs in the distal colon in 80% of cases; in 10%, it occurs in the small bowel. Sx range from mild-to-severe constipation, sometimes complicated by toxic enterocolitis. When severe, it may be life-threatening and mandates a rapid **loop colostomy**. Three classical operations (**Swenson, Soave, Duhamel**) and a newer perineal one-stage pullthrough (**POOP**) were developed to remove or bypass the affected bowel (Fig 12.5-11). Today, classic three-stage operations are being reduced to one or two stages, often assisted by laparoscopy.

Surgical Approach: There is enthusiasm for **one-stage neonatal repair**, which avoids a colostomy and may be performed via a perianal incision, sometimes preceded by laparoscopic biopsy to determine the transition zone. Others prefer to biopsy through a LLQ incision initially, bringing out a loop ('levelling') colostomy above the transition zone, identified using frozen sections. Subsequent definitive repair is performed in one stage or two, if a protective proximal stoma needs subsequent closure. Positioning depends on the approach chosen; some surgeons prefer a lower body antibacterial preparation, others position the child in lithotomy position and prepare the abdomen and perineum. Positioning neonates transversely across an operating table rotated 90° affords good surgical access to the perineum and anesthesia access to the head. Significant bleeding is infrequent; operative time often is determined by the delay for frozen sections, which are challenging for most pediatric pathologists. Where skilled pediatric pathologists are unavailable, some surgeons will perform a RUQ transverse colostomy in the hope that the transition zone is distal to it. This is a significantly faster procedure, followed by permanent sections on which ganglia are more easily identified; it is inadequate in 10-20% of 'long-segment' patients.

Usual preop diagnosis: Hirschsprung's disease; congenital aganglionosis; congenital megacolon

SUMMARY OF PROCEDURES

	Preliminary Colostomy	Pullthrough
Position	Supine	Supine → lithotomy
Incision	LLQ transverse	Low transverse
Special instrumentation	None	Staplers
Unique considerations	Frozen section to confirm ganglion cells	No monitors or iv lower extremity; frozen sections
Antibiotics	Preop: ampicillin 25 mg/kg iv + gentamicin 2.5 mg/kg iv	⇐
Surgical time	1-1.5 h	1-2 h (POOP) 3-4 h (Duhamel, Swenson, Soave)
Closing considerations	None	Reprep/drape
EBL	< 5 ml/kg	5-10 ml/kg
Postop care	Cardiac/apnea monitor	PICU
Mortality	With enterocolitis: 10% Without enterocolitis: 0-2%	< 5%

Morbidity	Prolapse	Anastomotic leak: 5%
	Stricture	Wound infection: 4%
	Hernia	Pelvic abscess: 3%
Pain score	4	6-7

PATIENT POPULATION CHARACTERISTICS

Age range	Newborn-18 mo (normally)	1 yr
Male:Female	4:1	⇐
Incidence	1/5000	⇐
Etiology	Unknown	⇐
Associated conditions	Trisomy 21 (5%); GU anomalies (< 5%); neurofibromatoses	⇐

ANESTHETIC CONSIDERATIONS

PREOPERATIVE

Infants (~12 mo of age) with Hirschsprung's disease (congenital aganglionosis) have had prior colostomies and now present for colorectal reanastomosis. They may be mildly malnourished, but otherwise healthy.

GI	Diarrhea may be present with associated malabsorption state. **Tests:** Electrolytes
Laboratory	Hct; T&C
Premedication	Midazolam 0.5-0.75 mg/kg po administered 30 min before induction for child >12 mo.

INTRAOPERATIVE

Anesthetic technique: Combined epidural/GETA, using a pediatric circle with humidified and warmed gases. Warm OR to 75-80°F; use warming pad on OR table.

Induction	Mask induction is preferable, unless iv is already in place. Keep air leak around ETT to 15-35 cmH$_2$O to minimize alterations in ventilation 2° changes in chest and pulmonary compliance. The patient is placed in a lateral decubitus position for lumbar epidural anesthesia (see p. D-5).	
Maintenance	Low-dose volatile agent and air/O$_2$ with muscle relaxation for majority of cases. During last 30 min, N$_2$O can be substituted for air. Epidural anesthesia will provide the majority of analgesia, but not the degree of muscle relaxation that will be necessary. Supplemental muscle relaxants (e.g., pancuronium or vecuronium 0.1 mg/kg), therefore, are required.	
Emergence	The goal is to extubate at end of case. Reverse neuromuscular blockade with neostigmine (0.07 mg/kg iv) and atropine (0.02 mg/kg) or glycopyrrolate (0.01 mg/kg).	

Blood and fluid requirements	Mild blood loss
	IV: 20-22 ga × 1-2 in upper extremities
	NS/LR @ (maintenance):
	  4 ml/kg/h – 0-10 kg
	  + 2 ml/kg/h – 11-20 kg
	  + 1 ml/kg/h – > 20 kg
	  (e.g., 25 kg = 65 ml/h)
		Potential for large 3rd-space losses; plan 10 ml/kg/h of crystalloid for replacement. Use 5% albumin for rapid volume expansion; transfuse to maintain Hct > 23%. As a result of bowel prep, patient may require 10-20 ml/kg iv of NS/LR to offset volume deficit.

Monitoring	Standard monitors (p. D-1) Urinary catheter ± Arterial line (22 ga)	ABG, Hct, blood glucose prn. Maintain UO @ 1 ml/kg/h. Arterial line helpful for monitoring BP, lab draws, and presence of respiratory variations as indicator of volume status.
Positioning	✓ padding, particularly over lateral fibular head (common peroneal nerve). ✓ eyes.	
Complications	Hypothermia Hypovolemia	Majority of heat loss is radiant (skin), but potential for large volume shifts mandates warming fluids.

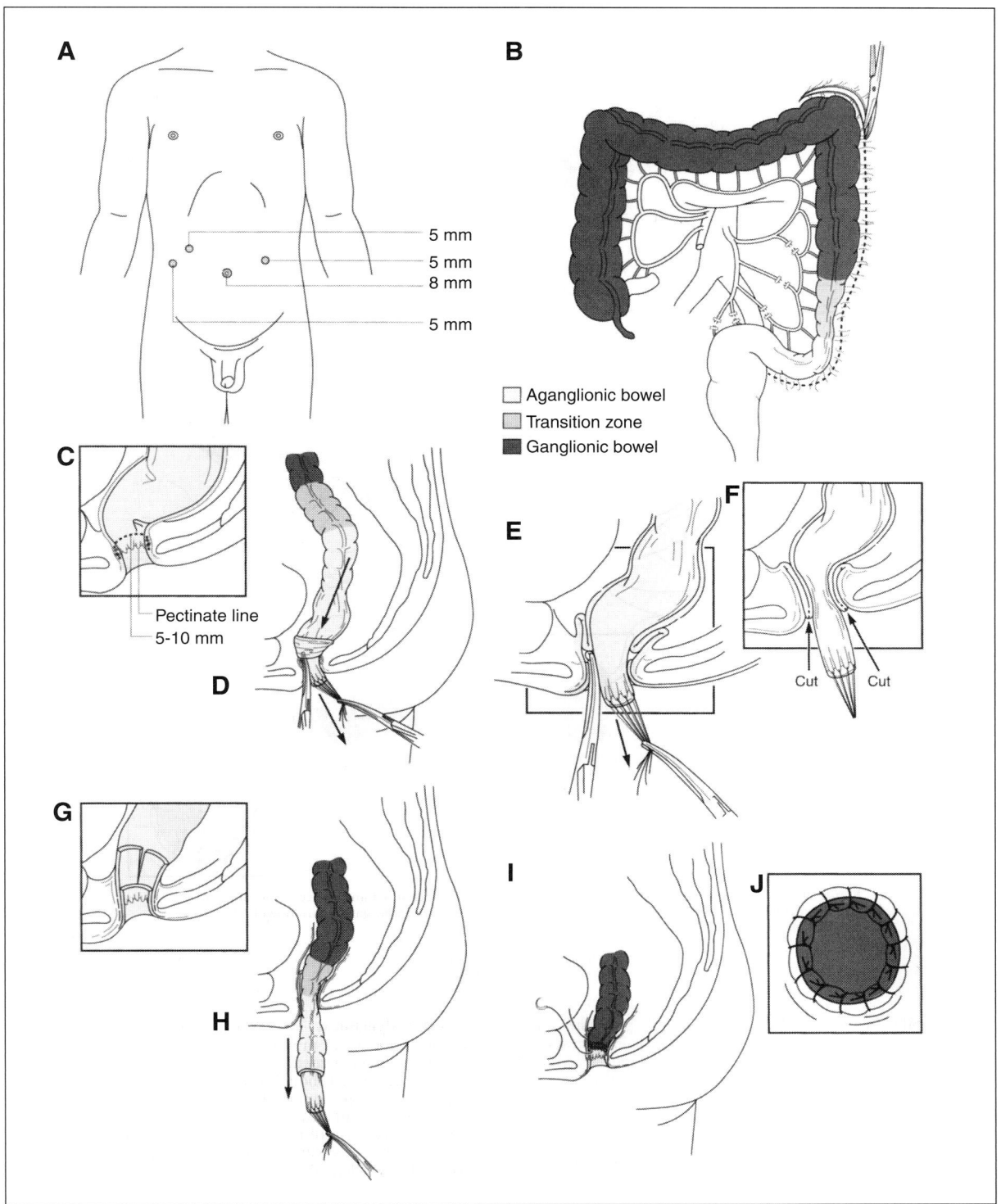

Figure 12.5-11. Laparoscopically assisted pullthrough for Hirschsprung's disease. (A) Sites for operative trocar placement. (B) Division of colon and rectal mesentery with mobilization of proximal colon. (C) Circumferential incision in rectal mucosa 5-10 mm cephalad to the pectinate line. (D) Mucosal traction sutures to facilitate further dissection from rectal muscular cuff. (E) Transanal submucosal dissection is continued cephalad to meet the caudal extent of the transperitoneal rectal dissection. (F) Circumferential incisions of rectal muscular cuff. (G) Rectal muscular cuff is split posteriorly to accommodate the pullthrough segment (segment is not shown here). (H) Rectum and sigmoid colon are pulled through the rectal muscular cuff to the anastomotic sites. (I) Colon is transected at appropriate site with confirmation of ganglion cells by frozen section. (J) Transanal, end-to-end single layer colorectal anastomosis. (Reproduced with permission from Sato TT, Oldham KT: Pediatric abdomen. In *Surgery: Scientific Principles and Practice*, 3rd edition. Greenfield LJ, et al, eds. Lippincott Williams & Wilkins, 2001.)

POSTOPERATIVE

Complications	Hypothermia	
	Hypovolemia	
	Respiratory depression 2° opiates	
Pain management	Continuous epidural	Bupivacaine with epinephrine and morphine will provide analgesia for 8-16 h (see p. E-5).
Tests	Hct	

References

1. Puri P: Hirschsprung disease. In *Surgery of Infants and Children.* Oldham KT, Colombani PM, Foglia RP, eds. Lippincott-Raven, Philadelphia: 1997, 1277-1300.
2. Raffensperger JG, ed: *Swenson's Pediatric Surgery*, 5th edition. Appleton & Lange, Norwalk: 1990, 555-78.
3. Swenson O, Sherman JO, Fisher JH, Cohen E: The treatment and postoperative complications of congenital megacolon: A 25-year followup. *Ann Surg* 1975; 182(3):266-73.

PULLTHROUGH FOR IMPERFORATE ANUS, CLOACA

SURGICAL CONSIDERATIONS

Description: Imperforate anus anomalies are classified as **high** or **low**, depending on whether the distal rectum ends above or below the levator muscle. Usually the rectum terminates as a 'fistula' entering the perineum or pelvic structures anterior to the external anal sphincter. Rarely the rectum ends blindly, often associated with Trisomy 21. If the fistula terminates on the perineum, it is called a 'perineal fistula' or 'anterior anus.' In girls, it often terminates inside the fourchette but outside the hymen, called a 'vestibular' fistula. Fistulas to the vagina or uterus are rare; when they occur, they may be in conjunction with urethral anomalies. This combined structure—including rectum, vagina, and urethra—is called a 'cloaca.' In boys, the fistula often ends in the urethra, occasionally the prostate, and rarely the bladder neck.

Surgical approach: At birth, associated conditions (e.g., VACTERL syndrome, see p. 942) are excluded while one waits 24 h for the appearance of meconium through a sometimes-hard-to-see perineal fistula. The operation is then performed according to the estimated site of the fistula. Low lesions are dilated or repaired; high lesions are treated with a divided RLQ colostomy. Definitive repair of high lesions occurs after months following contrast studies. This operation—called a **perineal sagittal anorectoplasty (PSARP)** or **Pena procedure**—is performed in the prone jackknife position. If the fistula is high, it occasionally will be necessary to turn the patient over for abdominal mobilization of the sigmoid colon. High lesions are also amenable to early **laparoscopic mobilization and pullthrough**. This can be done with low fistulas as well, but dissection of the common wall between the urethra and fistula has not been perfected.

Usual preop diagnosis: Imperforate anus

SUMMARY OF PROCEDURES

	Low Lesions	High Lesions
Position	Supine, lithotomy	Prone, possible turn to spine or lithotomy
Incision	Midline perineal	Midline sacral, transverse abdominal
Special instrumentation	Muscle stimulator	⇐ + Urethral sound; vaginal pack
Unique considerations	None	Pressure points; prone position
Antibiotics	Preop: ampicillin 25 mg/kg iv + gentamicin 2.5 mg/kg iv	⇐
Surgical time	1-1.5 h	3-6 h

	Low Lesions	**High Lesions**
EBL	< 5 ml/kg	5-20 ml/kg
Postop care	Apnea monitor if neonate	PICU
Mortality	≤ 20%, due to associated anomalies	≤ 40%, due to associated anomalies
Morbidity	Anal stenosis: 5-10%	⇐
	Mucosal prolapse: 5%	Intestinal obstruction: 5-10%
		Neurogenic bladder: < 5%
		Urethral stricture: 1-3%
Pain score	3-4	5-6

PATIENT POPULATION CHARACTERISTICS

Age range	Newborn–6 mo	12-18 mo
Male:Female	1.5:1	⇐
Incidence	1/5000	⇐
Etiology	Unknown	⇐
Associated conditions	CHD (common); esophageal atresia (15%); GU anomalies; sacral/spinal cord anomalies; VATER association	⇐

ANESTHETIC CONSIDERATIONS

PREOPERATIVE

Definitive repair is performed via the sacral and/or perineal route at ~12 mo. Children with rectal or anal agenesis without fistula will have had colostomies in newborn period. Other anomalies (e.g., VATER association, VSDs, vertebral anomalies, anal agenesis, tracheoesophageal fistula [TEF]), esophageal atresia (EA), and/or renal or radial bone abnormalities may be present.

Respiratory	If VATER association present, ✓ cervical spine film and neck ROM. Avoid extreme head flexion. If prior TEF repair, concerns as previously noted in Anesthetic Considerations for Repair of Tracheoesophageal Fistula/Esophageal Atresia, p. 1020. **Tests:** CXR; cervical spine film
Cardiovascular	Patients with VATER association have a 20% incidence of CHD (e.g., VSD). Prior cardiology consultation.
Gastrointestinal	Colostomy may be present; thus, anesthesia records may be available for review.
Renal	Renal abnormalities may be present. **Tests:** BUN; Cr; electrolytes
Musculoskeletal	Radial bone deformities may be present. There is no evidence to suggest that VATER patients are at ↑risk for malignant hyperthermia (MH).
Laboratory	Hct; T&C (✓ parental/directed donor blood availability.)
Premedication	Midazolam (0.5-0.75 mg/kg po) 30 min prior to arrival in OR. If < 10 mo old, no premedication is given.

INTRAOPERATIVE

Anesthetic technique: Combined epidural/GETA, using a pediatric circle or Bain circuit with humidified and warmed gases. Warm OR to 75°-80°F; heating pad on OR table.

Induction	Awake intubation if airway management problems anticipated; otherwise, standard pediatric induction (see p. D-2). Secure iv access and administer muscle relaxant (e.g., vecuronium or pancuronium [0.1 mg/kg]) to facilitate ET intubation. Maintain air leak at > 15-35 cmH$_2$O. Lumbar epidural catheter inserted after induction.
Maintenance	Volatile agent/air/O$_2$ with epdiural analgesia (2 ml 0.25% bupivacaine or chirocaine @ start, 1 ml/h maintenance), or morphine (0.1-0.25 mg/kg iv total) or fentanyl (5-10 μg/kg iv total). Maintain neuromuscular blockade as surgically indicated.

Emergence	Usually extubated at end of case. Reverse neuromuscular blockade with neostigmine (0.07 mg/kg iv) and atropine (0.02 mg/kg iv). Ability to flex hips is a sign of adequate reversal.	
Blood and fluid requirements	Moderate blood/3rd-space losses IV: 20-22 ga × 2 NS/LR @ (maintenance): 4 ml/kg/h – 0-10 kg + 2 ml/kg/h – 10-20 kg	Place iv's in upper extremities, since positioning of legs may impede venous flow. Maintain Hct > 22. This age group does not require dextrose infusions. 3rd-space losses ~5 ml/kg/h.
Monitoring	Standard monitors (p. D-1) Urinary catheter ± 24 ga radial arterial line	Maintain UO @ 0.5-1 ml/kg/h. Marked arterial waveform variation with ventilation is a sensitive indicator of hypovolemia. ABG/Hct/glucose prn.
Positioning	✓ and pad pressure points. ✓ eyes.	Patient may be turned during procedure.
Complications	Metabolic acidosis Hypovolemia → ↓BP Hypothermia	Mild metabolic acidosis may occur with significant bleeding, or when 3rd-space losses are replaced with bicarbonate-deficient fluids (NS, albumin 5%, PRBCs).

POSTOPERATIVE

Complications	Subglottic edema Respiratory depression 2° to opiates	
Pain management	Continuous epidural analgesia. Fentanyl (1-2 mg/kg iv q 1 h prn) or morphine (0.05-0.10 mg/kg iv q 1-4 h)	See p. E-5. Aggressive pain management warranted.
Tests	Hct ABG Electrolytes	

References

1. DeVries PA, Pena A: Posterior sagittal anorectoplasty. *J Pediatr Surg* 1982; 17(5):638-45.
2. Paidas C, Pena A: Rectum and anus. In *Surgery of Infants and Children.* Oldham KT, Colombani PM, Foglia RP, eds. Lippincott-Raven, Philadelphia: 1997, 1323-64.
3. Schecter NL, Berde CB, Yaster M, eds: *Pain in Infants, Children, and Adolescents.* Lippincott Williams & Wilkins, Philadelphia: 2002.
4. Smith EI, Tunell WP, Williams GR: A clinical evaluation of the surgical treatment of anorectal malformations (imperforate anus). *Ann Surg* 1978; 187(6):583-92.

REPAIR OF INGUINAL & UMBILICAL HERNIAS, HYDROCELE

SURGICAL CONSIDERATIONS

Description: Inguinal hernia repair (**herniorrhaphy**) and its variant, **hydrocele repair**, are the most frequently performed operations in pediatric surgery. Most pediatric hernias are indirect; they occur when the processus vaginalis (a small pouch of peritoneum dragged down to the scrotum during gonadal descent) fails to obliterate. Infants, particularly the premature, are more likely than toddlers to develop bilateral and incarcerated hernias. Hydroceles are identical to hernias in origin but have a smaller neck and derive their name because this neck is so small that only intraperitoneal fluid, not bowel, can pass through it. Hydroceles tend to close spontaneously (~80%) during the first 2 yr of life; those that fail to resolve are repaired at ~2 yr. Hydroceles are termed 'communicating' when they empty/fill with postural change. Umbilical hernias have a similar tendency to close—but over the first 5 yr of life (~95%)—and are repaired when large (> 2 cm) or persistent. Complications of hernia/hydrocele repair include damage to the vas deferens or testicular vessels, metachronous contralateral hernias (~10%) if just one side is repaired initially, and a very low incidence of infertility when bilateral repairs are undertaken. Bleeding, if any, is minor, recurrence uncommon (≤ 1%) and bowel resection is rarely necessary even when a hernia is incarcerated. Overnight admission for apnea monitoring is suggested in premature children (≤ 48-60 wk corrected age). **Hydrocele repair** complications are similar to those of herniorrhaphy. **Umbilical hernia repairs** have very few complications. Acetaminophen pr at the beginning of the procedure aids postop pain management.

Surgical approach: Inguinal hernias and hydroceles are repaired through a lower lateral abdominal skin crease incision (more recently, laparoscopically), permitting separation of the sac from spermatic cord structures, followed by high ligation ± distal fenestration (in hydroceles). Umbilical hernia repair is performed through a transverse incision in the infraumbilical skin fold, through which the sac is resected from the undersurface of the skin and healthy fascial edges closed.

Usual preop diagnosis: Inguinal hernia; umbilical hernia; hydrocele

SUMMARY OF PROCEDURES

	Inguinal	Umbilical
Position	Supine	⇐
Incision	Inguinal, bilateral	Infraumbilical
Unique considerations	Prematurity	Abdominal compression if hernia large
Antibiotics	None	⇐
Surgical time	40 min	⇐
Closing considerations	Nerve block, caudal	Umbilical block
EBL	5 ml/kg	⇐
Postop care	Apnea monitor; hospitalization for premature infants	None
Mortality	< 1%	⇐
Morbidity	Apnea Recurrence	None
Pain score	3-5	3-5

PATIENT POPULATION CHARACTERISTICS

Age range	Premature–adolescent	> 2 yr
Male:Female	5:1	N/A
Incidence	1-2%	1%
Etiology	Patent processus vaginalis	Persistent umbilical defect
Associated conditions	Gonadal dysgenesis (Rare)	None

ANESTHETIC CONSIDERATIONS

PREOPERATIVE

Hernia repair is most commonly performed in otherwise healthy infants in the first 2 yr of life, often on an outpatient basis. It is also performed on premature infants (< 36 wk gestational age at birth) and other neonates requiring intensive care. Premature infants are particularly prone to inguinal hernias. Postop apnea can occur in infants ≤ 50-60 wk postconceptual age, particularly if the infant was premature, has neurologic disease, or required intensive care in the early neonatal period.

Respiratory	Bronchopulmonary dysplasia (BPD), tracheomalacia, and subglottic stenosis are consequences of prolonged mechanical ventilation and immature lungs at birth. ✓ prior NICU Hx. ↓FRC and ↑PVR make infants with this disease more susceptible to hypoxia. They may require supplemental nasal O_2 on a chronic basis. **Tests:** CXR
Cardiovascular	Prior PDA ligation is possible. These patients may be on diuretic therapy for intrinsic lung disease (e.g., BPD) with resultant decreased intravascular volume. **Tests:** CXR; electrolytes
Neurological	Premature infants may be prone to seizure disorders. Premature infants have immature respiratory centers and may exhibit paradoxical apneic/bradycardic episodes in response to hypoxemia. **Tests:** Anticonvulsant levels

Hematologic	Anemia is common at ~ 3 mo of age and increases risk of postop apnea.
	Tests: Hct; PT; PTT; Plt, as indicated from H&P.
Laboratory	Other tests as indicated from H&P.
Premedication	If > 1 yr of age, midazolam (0.5-0.75 mg/kg po) 30 min prior to arrival in OR.

INTRAOPERATIVE

Anesthetic technique: Typically, GETA, LMA or mask GA (± caudal or ilioinguinal/iliohypogastric block), using a pediatric circle or Bain circuit with warm, humidified gases. An alternative in ex-preterm infants at high risk for postop apnea is spinal anesthesia without GA or iv sedation (p. D-6). Warm OR to 75°-80° F; use warming pad on OR table.

Induction	Mask induction in children with sevoflurane or halothane/N_2O/O_2. Secure iv. If appropriate, position child for placement of caudal anesthetic: bupivacaine 0.25% ± epinephrine 1:200,000 @ 1 ml/kg. If child otherwise healthy and >1 yr old, can proceed with LMA or mask anesthetic; otherwise, tracheal intubation is preferred. Atropine (0.02 mg/kg iv) given prior to laryngoscopy in patients < 9 mo. Intubation may be facilitated with vecuronium (0.1 mg/kg) or rocuronium (1 mg/kg).	
Maintenance	Standard pediatric inhalational anesthetic (p. D-3) is appropriate. With caudal anesthetic or nerve block, decrease amount of volatile anesthetic and avoid or reduce opiates. 2 MAC of inhalational agents at incision is required to avoid laryngospasm in this patient population. Caudal bupivacaine onset time ~15 min.	
Emergence	Reverse neuromuscular blockade with neostigmine (0.07 mg/kg iv) and atropine (0.02 mg/kg iv). Extubate only when fully awake.	

Blood and fluid requirements	Negligible blood loss
	IV: 22-24 ga × 1
	NS/LR @ (maintenance):
	  4 ml/kg/h – 0-10 kg
	  + 2 ml/kg/h – 11-20 kg
		Infants receiving diuretics will require 10-20 ml/kg iv of NS/LR to avoid ↓BP 2° volatile anesthetics. In children < 1 mo old, use dextrose-containing iv solution (e.g., D2.5/LR)

Monitoring	Standard monitors (p. D-1)	Premature infants may become hypoglycemic. ✓ blood glucose during surgery.
Positioning	✓ and pad pressure points. ✓ eyes.	With too-large mask, beware of ocular compression/corneal abrasion.
Complications	Laryngospasm Bronchospasm Hypothermia Pulmonary hypertensive episode Local anesthetic toxicity Hypoglycemia	Rx bronchospasm: albuterol inhaler. Mist O_2 after extubation. Avoid hyperglycemia → diuresis and dehydration.

POSTOPERATIVE

Complications	Apnea/bradycardia Subglottic edema	Can ↓ incidence of apnea/bradycardia by administering caffeine (10 mg/kg iv) intraop or in NICU/PACU.
Pain management	Field block Acetaminophen (10-20 mg/kg po q 4-6 h prn)	If no caudal used, a field block (bupivacaine 0.25% 2-3 ml) at end of surgery reduces pain in the immediate postop period. It is usually performed by the surgeon.
Tests/monitoring	Apnea monitor and pulse oximeter for 12-18 h for premature infants < 60 wk postconception	Caffeine is no substitute for monitoring and attentive parents/nurses.

References

1. Beckerman RC, Brouillette RT, Hunt CE, eds: *Respiratory Control Disorders in Infants and Children.* Williams & Wilkins, Baltimore: 1991, 161-77.
2. Kurth CD, Spitzer AR, Broennle AM, Downes JJ: Postoperative apnea in preterm infants. *Anesthesiology* 1987; 66(4): 483-8.

3. Rescorla FJ: Hernias and umbilicus. In *Surgery of Infants and Children.* Oldham KT, Colombani PM, Foglia RP, eds. Lippincott-Raven, Philadelphia: 1997, 1069-82.

4. Stehling L, ed: *Common Problems in Pediatric Anesthesia*, 2nd edition. Mosby-Year Book, St. Louis: 1992, 69-85.

5. Welborn LG, Hannallah RS, Fink R, Ruttimann VE, Hick JM: High-dose caffeine suppresses postoperative apnea in former preterm infants. *Anesthesiology* 1989; 71(3):347-9.

SURGERY FOR THE UNDESCENDED TESTICLE

SURGICAL CONSIDERATIONS

Description: Also called 'cryptorchidism,' this occurs when a testicle fails to follow the usual pattern of descent. Testicles begin fetal life just inferior to the kidney and, through differential growth, migrate to the base of the ipsilateral hemiscrotum, attached there by the gubernaculum. Problems occur when testicular descent does not occur, occurs partially, or occurs incorrectly. Testicles that are found in the abdomen, inguinal canal, perineum, thigh, suprapubic fat, or contralateral scrotum may be associated with subsequent problems, including infertility and malignant degeneration. Transposition and fixation of the testicles into their normal location (**orchidopexy**), does not eliminate these problems; rather, it places the testicle in a position where it can be more easily evaluated and may mitigate the progressive infertility thought to occur when testicles remain outside the scrotum. Because testicular descent is a dynamic process, cryptorchidism is not addressed until 18-24 mo of life, since a significant portion of initially cryptorchid testes will descend into the scrotum during this time.

Surgical approach: The operation begins in a similar fashion to a hernia repair, as 95% of cryptorchid testes have an associated hernia sac. One exception is if the testicle is thought to be **intraabdominal**. In this circumstance, many surgeons will begin with a laparoscopic abdominal examination, using the vas deferens and testicular vessels to locate the testis. If it is high in the abdomen, it may be brought immediately to the perineum (difficult if the testicular vessels are short), or a two-step **Fowler-Stevens** approach is undertaken. In this approach, the gubernacular vessels supplying the inferior pole of the testis are encouraged to hypertrophy by division of the spermatic vessels, and the testicle is left in the abdomen near the internal ring. At a second operation ~6 mo later, the testicle is brought down, much as in the primary operation following hernia repair. This involves creation of a passage down to the base of the ipsilateral hemiscrotum, through which the testicle is advanced as far as the vas deferens permits. The tough outer layer of the testicle—the tunica albuginea—is then attached to the scrotum in a subcutaneous pocket outside the dartos fascia to discourage migration back up to a high location. There is scant blood loss; however, there is a small risk to testicular viability. Small, high, abnormal testes with short vessels and vas associated with poor gubernacular vessels are deemed better removed than left in a high location where malignant degeneration might go undetected. A caudal block may be preferable to injection of local anesthesia at multiple sites.

Usual preop diagnosis: Undescended testicle; cryptorchidism

SUMMARY OF PROCEDURES

	Orchidopexy	First of Two-stage Repair
Position	Supine	⇐
Incision	Lower groin crease	Laparoscopic or open
Special instrumentation	–	1-3 ports if laparoscopic
Unique considerations	Length of vas and vessels	Length of vas deferens
Antibiotics	None	⇐
Surgical time	1-1.5 h	30 min
EBL	< 5 ml/kg	⇐
Postop care	Home	⇐
Mortality	< 1%	⇐
Morbidity	Bleeding	⇐
	Orchiectomy	
Pain score	4-5	2-3

PATIENT POPULATION CHARACTERISTICS

Age range	18-24 mo
Incidence	1/2,000 births
Etiology	Unknown
Associated conditions	Prematurity; gastroschisis; intersex anomaly; Turner's syndrome (potential for airway, cardiac, and renal problems)

ANESTHETIC CONSIDERATIONS

See Anesthetic Considerations for Pediatric Urology, Inguinoscrotal Procedures, p. 1080.

References:

1. Kogan SJ, Gill B: Cryptorchidism and pediatric hydrocele/hernia. In *Glenn's Urologic Surgery,* 5th edition. Graham SD Jr, Glenn JF, eds. Lippincott Williams & Wilkins, Philadelphia: 1998; 833-42.
2. Rozanski TA, Bloom DA: Male genital tract. In *Surgery of Infants and Children: Scientific Principles and Practice.* Oldham KT, Colombani PM, Foglia RP, eds. Lippincott-Raven, Philadelphia: 1997, 1550-2.

RESECTION OF SACROCOCCYGEAL TERATOMA

SURGICAL CONSIDERATIONS

Description: Occasionally during gestation, a group of cells composing all three germ layers segregates and begins autonomous development as a teratoma. When this occurs just anterior to the coccyx, the tumor may remain small and local, or grow up into the abdomen or down into the peritoneum, attaining sizes as large as the child itself. Although a few centers attempt fetal surgery for very large lesions, in most hospitals the child is delivered by the appropriate route (cesarian delivery for large external lesions) and the mass is addressed in the neonatal period or whenever it is diagnosed thereafter. Most (though not all) sacrococcygeal teratomas (SCTs) are initially benign; however, they may soon transform into malignancy beginning at 2 mo of age.

Surgical approach: Small teratomas are approached prone from the rectum; larger ones, with high blood flow, may first have an intraabdominal procedure to ligate feeding vessels and mobilize the tumor. Once prone, a V-shaped incision is created down to the posterior aspect of the anteriorly displaced anus. Surgical principles of dissection include avoiding entry into the rectum (a colostomy is rarely necessary); meticulous hemostasis, including ligation of the median sacral artery; and removal of the coccyx, from which the tumor arises and may recur. At the end of the procedure, the levator muscles are brought together and the anus is suspended from the presacral fascia. Bleeding can be massive, and adjacent structures (bowel, bladder, and presacral nerve plexus) are distorted and prone to injury.

Usual preop diagnosis: Sacrococcygeal teratoma.

Differential diagnosis: May appear similar to meningomyelocele.

SUMMARY OF PROCEDURE

Position	Prone, sometimes preceded by supine
Incision	Perineal chevron, sometimes preceded by transverse abdominal
Special instrumentation	Hegar dilators
Unique considerations	Intraabdominal blood supply
Antibiotics	Ampicillin 25 mg/kg and gentamicin 2.5 mg/kg

Surgical time	2-5 h
Closing considerations	Extubation depends on duration and blood loss
EBL	20-80 ml/kg
Postop care	NICU, prone
Mortality	Fetal, due to hydrops and high flow state; < 10% neonatal
Morbidity	Bleeding
	Colostomy
	Pelvic nerve damage → bowel and bladder dysfunction
	Recurrence and/or malignant degeneration

PATIENT POPULATION CHARACTERISTICS

Age Range	1-2 mo
Male:Female	1:1
Incidence	1/15,000 births
Etiology	Unknown
Associated conditions	Constipation; heart failure; Currarino's triad; malignant degeneration

ANESTHETIC CONSIDERATIONS

PREOPERATIVE

Sacrococcygeal teratoma is a rare tumor of infancy. Sometimes diagnosed prenatally, it also can present as late as 18-24 mo. Patients may present with urinary obstruction by the tumor mass; lower extremity pain, numbness, or weakness; or bowel obstruction. ~10% may have a sacral anomaly or myelomeningocele.

Respiratory	There may be respiratory compromise as a result of a large abdominal mass pushing up on the abdominal contents and the diaphragm. **Tests:** CXR, if indicated from H&P.
Cardiovascular	Sacrococcygeal teratoma may be associated with high-output cardiac failure due to AV fistulae within the tumor. Consultation with a cardiologist may be appropriate. **Tests:** ECG; ECHO may be necessary.
Renal	Postrenal obstruction may compromise renal function. **Tests:** BUN; Cr
Gastrointestinal	Intestinal compression by the tumor may cause ↑risk of gastric aspiration. **Tests:** Electrolytes
Hematologic	This tumor may be associated with coagulopathy. **Tests:** PT; PTT; INR
Laboratory	Other tests as indicated from H&P.
Premedication	In patients at risk for gastric aspiration, prophylaxis with metoclopramide (0.1 mg/kg iv) and ranitidine (0.8 mg/kg iv) should be considered. Patients > 10 mo may benefit from midazolam (0.5-0.75 mg/kg) po 30 min before surgery. If iv is present, iv midazolam 0.05-0.1 mg/kg may be used (e.g., for 10 kg child, 0.5-1 mg midazolam).

INTRAOPERATIVE

Anesthetic technique: GETA, using a pediatric circle or Bain circuit with humidified and warmed gases. Due to risk of coagulopathy and the possibility of spine malformations, epidural catheter usually is not considered. Warm OR to 75-80°F. Use warming pad on OR table. Warm all iv fluids to help maintain body T.

Induction	Usually an inhalation induction. If an iv is present, then an iv induction is performed. A modified rapid-sequence induction is recommended in those patients with a large intraabdominal mass compressing the GI tract. Otherwise, standard pediatric induction (p. D-2) is appropriate. An uncuffed tube normally is used. The appropriate size for the ETT is one that will allow a small leak around the tube when positive pressure is applied (15-35 cmH$_2$O).
Maintenance	Standard maintenance (see p. D-3). Muscle relaxation is appropriate.

Emergence	Depending on blood loss and fluid requirements, the patient may need to remain intubated at the end of the procedure. If extubation is elected, suction NG and confirm air leak around ETT before extubation. If there is no air leak, consider laryngeal edema and the need for continued intubation.	
Blood and fluid requirements	Potential for large or massive blood loss, as well as large 3rd-space loss	Tumor resection may be associated with massive blood loss, due to large pelvic venous bed, AV fistula, coagulopathy. Close monitoring of Hct is necessary, along with correction of acidosis, CaCl replacement.
Monitoring	Central line Arterial line 22 ga 2 large-bore iv catheters (e.g., 22-18 ga) necessary	

POSTOPERATIVE

Complications	Bleeding Coagulopathy Hypoventilation Laryngeal edema	PICU usually required. Maintain normothermia; correct metabolic acidosis. Postop ventilation requirement due to hypoventilation, laryngeal edema
Pain management	Fentanyl 1 μg/kg/h iv Morphine 0.1 mg/kg/h	Approximate doses; titration required.
Tests	ABG Hct PT/PTT	

References

1. Robinson S, Laussen PC, Brown TCK, et al: Anaesthesia for sacrococcygeal teratoma—a case report and a review of 32 cases. *Anaesth Intens Care* 1992; 20:354-86.
2. Sasaoka N, Kitamura S, Kninouchi K, et al: Perinatal and perianesthetic management of the sacrococcygeal teratoma in a neonate. *Masui* 1998; 47(12):1482-5.

ANESTHESIA FOR MINIMALLY INVASIVE SURGERY IN PEDIATRIC PATIENTS

Gregory B. Hammer

In recent years there has been a significant increase in the practice of minimally invasive surgery in pediatric patients. Specific considerations for these surgeries (as in adult patients) include the effects of pneumoperitoneum on respiratory and cardiac function. ↑abdominal pressure → ↓diaphragmatic excursion, ↑atelectasis, and V/Q mismatch. ↑CO_2 levels can be difficult to control with limited ventilation; thus, manual ventilation may be necessary. There is risk of pneumothorax and pneumomediastinum. Use of Trendelenburg position further decreases FRC and lung compliance, and increases the work of breathing. Cephalad movement of the carina may cause endobronchial intubation. Venous return may be impaired, causing ↓CO. These effects are most pronounced in children < 6 mo old. These children also may be at risk for reversal of L→R shunts through a patent foramen ovale (PFO) or ductus arteriosus.

Minimally invasive procedures that are frequently performed in pediatrics include: hernia repair, cholecystectomy, splenectomy, appendectomy, Nissen fundoplication, thoracoscopy (VATS), laparoscopically assisted bowel resection, and congenital diaphragmatic hernia repair. The general principles for anesthesia for minimally invasive surgery in pediatric patients are as follows.

PREOPERATIVE

1. Pay attention to respiratory and cardiac function. For example, ✓ for any cardiac defects (e.g., L→R shunt, ↓CO). Note baseline lung function (SpO_2, CXR, ABG).

2. ✓ PT/PTT if epidural is considered (usually not placed for laparoscopy or thoracoscopy, but it will be placed at the end of the procedure if the decision is made to do open surgery).

3. Blood should be available for major cases. Although there usually is little blood loss with minimally invasive surgery, the potential for large-vessel disruption exists.

Premedication   In patients at risk for aspiration, prophylaxis with metoclopramide (0.1 mg/kg iv) and ranitidine (0.8 mg/kg iv) should be considered. Patients > 10 mo old may benefit from midazolam (0.5-0.75 mg/kg po) 30 min before surgery.

INTRAOPERATIVE

Anesthetic technique: GETA, using a pediatric circle or Bain circuit with humidified and warmed gases. Warm OR to 70-75°F; use warming pad on OR table. Warming all iv fluids may help to maintain body temperature.

Induction   Inhalation induction using sevoflurane, N_2O, followed by iv placement. If patient is at risk for aspiration, rapid-sequence induction with ET intubation is appropriate. For ET intubation in children < 6-8 yr of age, an uncuffed tube is preferred, with the goal being to attain a seal allowing for a leak of 15-25 cmH_2O. A cuffed tube (usually ½ size smaller than the appropriate uncuffed tube also may be used for children > 2 yr old. If OLV is required, see Anesthetic Considerations for Pediatric Thoracic Surgery, p. 1026, for placement. Note distance of end of ETT from carina. As abdominal girth is increased during CO_2 insufflation, it is common for the tube to advance to an endobronchial position.

Maintenance   Standard maintenance (see p. D-3). Muscle relaxation is appropriate. An OG tube is placed to empty the stomach of any residual premedication and excess air introduced during PPV. Continued communication between anesthesiologist and surgeon is essential. Pay attention to changes in positioning, intraabdominal pressure (nl = 15 cmH_2O), Trendelenburg, airway pressures, BP.

Emergence   In most cases, the patient can be extubated at the end of surgery.

Blood and fluid requirements	IV: 22-20 ga catheter × 1 Maintenance fluids	Potential for 3rd-space and blood loss. See Anesthetic Considerations for Repair of Inguinal and Umbilical Hernias, Hydrocele, p. 1060.
Monitoring	Standard monitors (see p. D-1) ± Arterial line Urinary catheter	Consider arterial line if patient has significant cardiac or respiratory compromise.
Positioning	✓ and pad pressure points. ✓ eyes.	
Complications	↑CO_2 (40-50 mmHg) (common) ↑PIP (common) Endobronchial intubation (common) Difficult ventilating (common) HTN Pneumothorax, pneumomediastinum (rare) Inadvertent cannulation of vessel (rare) CO_2 embolus (rare)	2° Trendelenburg position, ↑abdominal girth. In thoracoscopy, if SLV is used, may need to raise lung and ventilate transiently. → ↓CO. Rx: crystalloid or albumin 10-20 ml/kg.

POSTOPERATIVE

Complications	Respiratory function impairment Bleeding Residual subcutaneous CO_2 Pneumothorax	Respiratory function may still be significantly impaired in the postop period and should be monitored closely.
Pain management	Ketorolac 0.5 mg/kg iv q 6 h MSO_4 0.05-0.1 mg/kg	

References:

1. Bissonnette B, Dalens BJ: *Pediatric Anesthesia.* McGraw-Hill, New York: 2002.
2. Cote CJ, Todres ID, Ryan JF, et al: *A Practice of Anesthesia for Infants and Children.* WB Saunders, New York: 2001.
3. Gregory GA: *Pediatric Anesthesia*, 4th edition. Churchill Livingstone, New York: 2002.
4. Pennant JH: Anesthesia for laparoscopy in the pediatric patient. *Anesth Clin North Am* 2001; 19(1):69-88.

Surgeons

Jeffrey B. Marotte, MD
Linda M. Dairiki Shortliffe, MD

12.6   PEDIATRIC UROLOGY

Anesthesiologists

Cathy R. Lammers, MD, FAAP
Gregory B. Hammer, MD

KIDNEY AND UPPER URINARY TRACT OPERATIONS

SURGICAL CONSIDERATIONS

Description: With the increase in perinatal ultrasonographic detection of renal masses and hydronephrosis, the number of pediatric kidney and upper urinary tract surgeries has increased significantly in the past two decades, and children come to surgery at an earlier age to preserve maximal renal function.

Nephrectomy: While the main indications for nephrectomy in the adult population are renal-cell carcinoma or benign renal tumors (with the exception of Wilms' tumors), most nephrectomies in children are performed for congenital anomalies associated with nonfunctioning or infected kidneys. A nonfunctioning kidney can be the result of obstruction or end-stage reflux nephropathy. Multicystic dysplastic kidneys (MCDK) do not require surgery unless they become symptomatic or increase in size. When a flank/subcostal incision is used, careful positioning of the patient

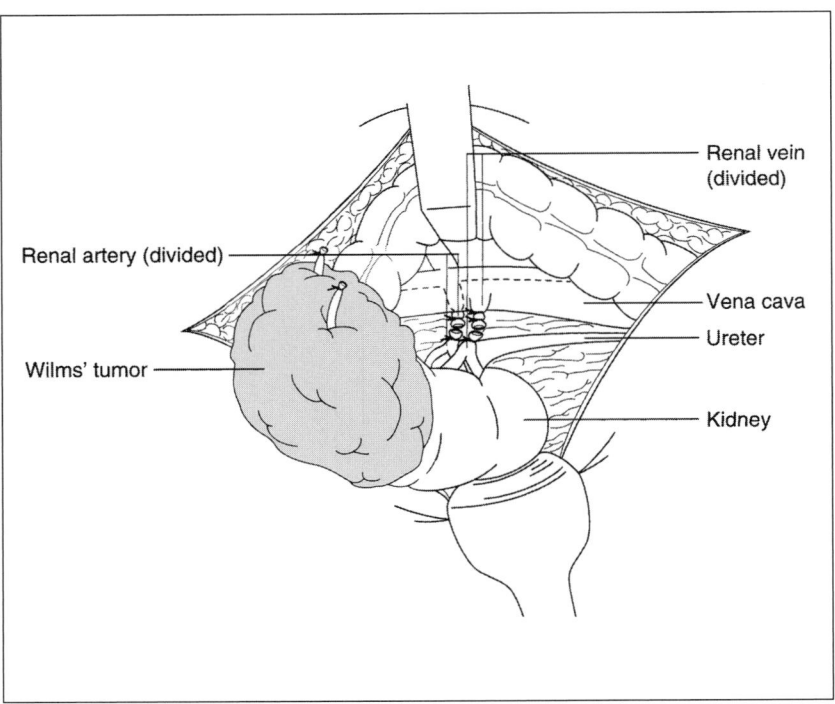

Figure 12.6-1. Anatomy for nephrectomy. (Reproduced with permission from Greenfield LJ, Mulholland MW, Oldham KT, Zelenock GB, Lillemoe KD: *Surgery: Scientific Principles and Practice*, 3rd edition. Lippincott Williams & Wilkins, 2001.)

is crucial. Failure to properly stabilize and secure the patient to the OR table can cause devastating consequences; therefore, efforts must be coordinated to properly position the patient. A rolled sheet or gel pad should be positioned just caudad to the dependent axilla, elevating the thorax to avoid brachial plexus neuropraxia. The dependent lower extremity is flexed at the hip and knee position, while the overlying leg is kept straight. Pillows or padding are placed between the knees. In older children, the kidney bar at the break of the table often is used for maximal exposure of the kidney in the lateral position. The fewest respiratory and circulatory alterations are observed when it is placed directly under the iliac crest. Once the patient is positioned, a transverse incision is made below the 12th rib. The peritoneum is reflected, the upper ureter is dissected to the hilum, and the vessels are ligated. The kidney is excised and the wound is closed.

The lumbodorsal incision (incision parallel to the paraspinous muscle group) is performed with the patient in the prone or lateral position. This has an advantage of being a muscle-splitting, rather than a muscle-cutting incision and, as such, is associated with ↓postop pain and incisional hernias. Some abdominal padding usually is added to raise the lumbodorsal area, and care should be taken to ensure complete pulmonary expansion in this position.

Usual preop diagnosis: MCDK; Wilms' tumor; nonfunctioning kidney; dysplastic kidney; ureteropelvic junction (UPJ) obstruction; ureterocele; and loss of function

Partial nephrectomy: Partial nephrectomies in children usually are performed for a nonfunctioning upper pole of a duplicated system. Ectopic ureters and ureteroceles are frequently the cause of loss of function. Again, these can be approached through either a lumbodorsal or flank incision. If the upper pole is obstructed but functional, a **pyeloureterostomy** from the upper pole ureter to the pelvis of the lower pole may be performed to salvage as much functioning parenchyma as possible. A partial nephrectomy may be performed for bilateral Wilms' tumor or other renal masses through a chevron or midline incision.

Usual preop diagnosis: Nonfunctioning upper pole of a duplex system; ureterocele; ectopic ureter; bilateral Wilms' tumor

Nephroureterectomy: Nephroureterectomy often is performed for the obstructed upper pole of a duplex system 2° a ureterocele or ectopic ureter. After the nephrectomy/partial nephrectomy is performed through a dorsal lumbotomy or flank approach, the ureter is dissected as low as possible (usually to the level of the iliac vessels). The ureteral stump is left open if there is no vesicoureteral reflux, and tied off if there is reflux. If indicated, distal ureterectomy can be performed via a second lower abdominal incision (typically a Pfannensteil's incision). If the initial incision was done in the prone position, the patient will need to be repositioned supine.

Usual preop diagnosis: Nonfunctioning upper pole of a duplex system; ureterocele; ectopic ureter

Pyeloplasty: Fetal hydronephrosis is detected in ~1/300 pregnancies. Pyeloplasty to correct congenital obstruction of the UPJ is a common infant surgical procedure. The hydronephrotic kidney usually is exposed through either a dorsal lumbotomy or a subcostal flank incision; therefore, the patient may be in a prone or modified lateral decubitus position. (See details related to subcostal or lumbodorsal incision, above.) Gerota's fascia is entered and the kidney is mobilized to expose the upper ureter and renal pelvis. The abnormal UPJ usually is excised, followed by an end-to-end anastomosis (**dismembered pyeloplasty** or **Anderson-Hynes pyeloplasty**). At the conclusion of the procedure, a perirenal Penrose drain typically is placed near the new ureteropelvic anastamosis; and, depending on surgeon's preference, a ureteral stent or nephrostomy tube may be used. A urethral catheter may be placed at the beginning of the procedure.

Usual preop diagnosis: Fetal hydronephrosis 2° UPJ obstruction; hydronephrosis

Transureteroureterostomy (TUU): This procedure, in which a ureter is anastomosed to the contralateral ureter, is used when there is problematic drainage of the distal ureter into the bladder. It is sometimes required to salvage a failed reimplantation or to transform a conduit-type diversion to an orthotopic neobladder or augmented native bladder. This technique also can be used to provide drainage in ureteral trauma. A midline, or Pfannenstiel's, incision is used; and the peritoneum is entered. The ureters are dissected and the affected ureter is retroperitonealized and brought to the contralateral side anterior to the great vessels. It is anastomosed to the contralateral ureter end-to-side with absorbable suture. If required, the recipient ureter is then reimplanted into the neobladder or augmented bladder.

Usual preop diagnosis: Failed ureteral reimplant; undiversion; distal ureteral trauma

SUMMARY OF PROCEDURES

	Nephrectomy/pyeloplasty	Nephroureterectomy	TUU
Position	Flank/prone	Supine/flank	Supine
Incision	Dorsal lumbotomy; subcostal; flank; midline	Subcostal flank 2nd incision: Pfannenstiel's	Midline or Pfannenstiel's
Antibiotics	Gentamicin 1.7 mg/kg iv	⇐	⇐
Surgical time	2.5 h	3 h	⇐
EBL	Minimal; if partial nephrectomy, 300 ml	Minimal	⇐
Mortality	< 1%	⇐	⇐
Morbidity	Bleeding: < 5%	⇐	⇐
	Infection: < 5%	⇐	⇐
	Ileus: < 5%	⇐	⇐
			Urinary fistula : < 5%
Pain score	Flank: 10 Lumbotomy: 5	10	10

PATIENT POPULATION CHARACTERISTICS

	Ureteroceles	MCDK	UPJ Obstruction	Wilms' tumor
Age range	Pediatric	Neonates	Neonates, children	Children (average, 4 yr)
Male:Female	1:4	⇐	M > F	M < F in U.S.
Incidence	1:2000	⇐	1:500 birth	1:100,00
Etiology	Congenital	⇐	⇐	Genetic: WT1 gene
Associated conditions	UPJ; VUR; duplicated collecting system	⇐	VUR; renal insufficiency	Hemihypertrophy, aniridia, HTN, Beckwith-Weidemann syndrome

References

1. Kelalis PP, Maizels M, Das S, Kay R, Williams DI: Kidney Reconstruction. In *Atlas of Pediatric Urologic Surgery.* Hinman F Jr, ed. WB Saunders, Philadelphia: 1994, Part II, 112-17, 123-43.
2. Marshall FF, Massad C, Hensle TW, Parrott TS: Kidney Excision. In *Atlas of Pediatric Urologic Surgery.* Hinman F Jr, ed. WB Saunders, Philadelphia: 1994, Part III, 155-88.
3. Richey ML: Pediatric urologic oncology. In *Adult and Pediatric Urology,* Vol 3, 4th edition. Gillenwater JY, Grayhack JT, Howards SS, Mitchell ME, eds. Mosby-Year Book, St. Louis: 2002, 2623-46.
4. Ritchy ML: Pediatric urologic oncology. In *Campbell's Urology,* 8th edition. Walsh PC, Retik AB, Vaughn ED, Wein A, eds. WB Saunders, Philadelphia: 2002, 2649-94.
5. Shaffer BS: Pearls and perils of patient positioning. *AUA Update Series* 1995; 14:178-83.

ANESTHETIC CONSIDERATIONS

PREOPERATIVE

In infants and children, most upper urinary tract surgical procedures are performed to preserve or restore renal function. Patients may present with renal function that varies from minimally abnormal, requiring little or no modification of anesthetic plan, to end-stage renal disease (ESRD) with its associated abnormalities, including hypoproteinemia, chronic anemia, and serum electrolyte disturbances. A careful preop workup is required to determine the presence or absence of abnormal physiologic factors that will affect anesthesia management. For most cases, the workup will have been performed by the patient's physicians before surgery and will provide the rationale for the surgical procedure. Such nonspecific findings as anorexia, headache, nausea, excessive tiredness, alterations in UO, and the presence of edema will alert the clinician to the likelihood of renal failure.

Renal abnormalities often are present as one component of a congenital malformation syndrome (e.g., polycystic kidneys, cerebrohepatorenal syndrome). In formulating the anesthetic plan, drugs eliminated by the kidney (e.g., pancuronium, meperidine, etc.) should be avoided.

Respiratory	An evaluation of pulmonary function, including auscultation of the lungs, may indicate the presence of pulmonary edema (uremic lung) or a pleural effusion. **Tests:** ABG; CXR; pulse oximetry
Cardiovascular	HTN is commonly seen in these patients, who may be taking antihypertensive medications and diuretics. In the severe cases, CHF or pulmonary edema may be present, necessitating the use of cardioactive drugs and diuretics to optimize the patient's clinical condition before surgery. **Tests:** ABG; CXR; digitalis level; electrolytes
Renal	In cases requiring unilateral urinary tract surgery, the opposite kidney is usually normal. In the presence of renal insufficiency, a detailed evaluation of renal function is essential. Chronic metabolic acidosis may be present 2° poor kidney function, electrolyte abnormalities ($\uparrow K^+$, $\downarrow Ca^{++}$, $\uparrow$ or $\downarrow Na^+$), hypovolemia, and/or poor tissue perfusion. Children with ESRD will have been dialyzed before surgery. Preop $K^+ < 6$ mEq/L is usually safe. These patients may have an AV fistula, which must be protected during surgery (padded, no BP cuff). More commonly, a double-lumen central venous catheter will have been placed for hemodialysis (e.g., Penrose catheter or Permacath). **Tests:** UA; UO; serum electrolytes; BUN; Cr; total protein; A/G ratio; ABG
Hematologic	Anemia, bone marrow depression, and coagulopathies are common in patients with poor renal function. An Hct of 15-18 kg/dL is not uncommon. **Tests:** Hb/Hct; PT/PTT; Plt count
Medications	Patients with ESRD will be taking many medications, which may influence the anesthetic plan. For example, chronic steroid therapy → Cushing facies, glycosuria; therefore, ✓ blood sugar and ✓ airway (if difficult, mask ventilation). Patients taking digitalis or diuretics → $\downarrow K^+$ → arrhythmias. Aminoglycosides → prolongation of neuromuscular blockade.
Premedication	Standard preop medication (see p. D-2.)

INTRAOPERATIVE

Anesthetic technique: GETA ± epidural. Warm OR to 70-75° F; use warming pad on OR table.

Induction	Mask induction is preferable, unless iv is already in place. If an indwelling Permacath is to be accessed, heparin should be aspirated from the lumen before use. Succinylcholine should not be used in renal

Induction, cont.	failure patients. In the presence of renal insufficiency, antibiotics (e.g., aminoglycosides) may interfere with the metabolism of muscle relaxants and prolong their effect. Tracheal intubation, facilitated by a NMR (e.g., cisatracurium 0.2-0.3 mg/kg) is appropriate in patients with renal insufficiency. In appropriate patients (normal coags), epidural anesthesia with bupivacaine (see p. D-5) will ★ reduce anesthetic requirements and provide postop analgesia (**NB:** local anesthetic clearance may be impaired). Maintain muscle relaxation with cisatracurium in patients with renal insufficiency; otherwise, intermediate long-acting relaxants are appropriate.	
Maintenance	Standard pediatric maintenance (p. D-3). Moderate hyperventilation may be beneficial ($\rightarrow \downarrow K^+ + \uparrow pH$).	
Emergence	Reverse neuromuscular blockade with neostigmine and atropine or glycopyrrolate.	

Blood and fluid requirements	IV × 1 in upper extremities
	NS @ (maintenance):
	  4 ml/kg/h (1-10 kg)
	  + 2 ml/kg/h (11-20 kg)
	  + 1 ml/kg/h (> 20 kg)
		Usually minimal blood loss; however, renal surgery may be associated with ↑blood loss. Transfuse with whole blood or PRBCs as needed to maintain an adequate Hct (25-30%). Minimal iv flush should be administered in the presence of oliguric renal insufficiency.

Monitoring	Standard monitors (see p. D-1). ± Arterial line	Place arterial line in patients with significant renal failure; ✓ serum electrolytes and ABG frequently.
Positioning	✓ and pad pressure points. ✓ eyes.	✓ eyes frequently if prone or flank positions are used.
Complications	Peripheral nerve injury Eye trauma Hemorrhage	

POSTOPERATIVE

Complications	Hypovolemia Anemia Hypothermia Electrolyte abnormalities Coagulopathy Metabolic/respiratory acidosis	
Pain management	Acetaminophen (see p. E-3). Narcotics by epidural catheter (p. E-5) or PCA (p. E-3)	In renal failure, reduce analgesic doses by 50% to minimize cumulative effects.
Tests	As indicated.	

References

1. Berry F: Anesthesia for genitourinary surgery. In *Pediatric Anesthesia,* 3rd edition. Gregory GA, ed. Churchill Livingstone, New York: 1994.
2. Davis PJ, Hall S. Deshpande JK, Spear RM: Anesthesia for general, urologic and plastic surgery. In *Smith's Anesthesia for Infants and Children,* 6th edition. Motoyama EK, Davis P, eds. Mosby-Year Book, St. Louis: 1996.

TRANSURETHRAL PROCEDURES

SURGICAL CONSIDERATIONS

Description: Transurethral procedures are not as common in pediatric urology as they are in adult urology; however, the instrumentation, general principles, and considerations are similar. The following are the most common pediatric endoscopic procedures: **cystoscopy** and **vaginoscopy,** primarily as diagnostic procedures; or to remove foreign bodies (FBs); **transurethral incision of urethral stricture**, for congenital lesions or complications of urethral surgery; **transurethral incision of posterior urethral valves (PUV); transurethral incision of ureterocele; subureteric injection** for vesicoureteral reflux; and **endoscopic injection** for urinary incontinence.

The positioning and techniques are identical to those in the adult. Careful attention to positioning is required when the pediatric patient is placed in the lithotomy position. The patient can remain supine if a flexible cystoscope is used. Adult leg holders are not appropriate for the majority of children; therefore, special pediatric leg supports are needed to avoid nerve injuries. The most frequent neurological complication is injury to the common peroneal nerve → foot drop and sensory deficit. After the patient is positioned, a lubricated cystoscope or resectoscope (7-18 Fr) is introduced through the urethra. Cystoscopy is used to identify the pathology and to perform ureteral catheterization, with a 3-5 Fr ureteral catheter. In infants, posterior urethral valves may be resected using a small cutting electrode, while a resectoscope is used in older children. With the advent of prenatal ultrasonography, posterior urethral valves (hydronephrosis and azotemia) often are resected in the neonatal period.

Foreign bodies or stones are removed using forceps, after crushing or pulverization with a laser, if necessary; eye protection should be worn by all OR staff if a laser is used. Occasionally, ureteral stents are placed/removed and an intraop retrograde pyeogram is performed to evaluate the upper tract collection system. During cystoscopy, localization of the ureteral orifices may be difficult 2° inflammation, prior bladder surgery, or congenital ectopia. The anesthesiologist may be asked to administer iv indigo carmine (may ↑BP and appear to ↓O_2 sat), which will filter through the kidneys and produce blue urine to assist with locating the ureteral orifices.

While water normally is used as the irrigant during cystoscopy or transurethral procedures in children, fluid absorption toxicity is rare, as opposed to that seen during TURP, because these procedures are short and the prostate and large resections are not involved. Although the risk is low, water absorption toxicity, with subsequent electrolyte imbalance, could occur with transurethral procedures in which unusual venous bleeding is encountered (e.g., incision of urethral strictures).

At times, lidocaine gel injected transurethrally at the completion of the transurethral procedure may be helpful in avoiding immediate urethral irritation.

Usual preop diagnosis: Intravesical FB; bladder calculus; bladder outlet obstruction; urethral stricture; ureterocele; hematuria; urethral/vaginal mass; posterior urethral valves

SUMMARY OF PROCEDURE

Position	Lithotomy
Incision	None
Special instrumentation	Cystoscope, resectoscope, catheters, stents, video camera unit, laser (optional)
Unique considerations	Use of cautery, fluoroscopy, PUV (prematurity or azotemia)
Antibiotics	If infected urine preop, gentamicin 1.7 mg/kg iv
Surgical time	Cystoscopy: 10 min
	Transurethral procedure: 1 h
EBL	Minimal
Postop care	PACU; basic catheter management
Mortality	< 1%
Morbidity	Bleeding
	Urethral stricture
	Infection
	Overdistention in augmented bladder
Pain score	2

PATIENT POPULATION CHARACTERISTICS

Age range	0-18 yr
Male:Female	Posterior urethral valves, strictures: male only
	Ureterocele 1:6
	Vesicoureteral reflux 1:4
Incidence	1/1000–1/5000
Etiology	Posterior urethral valves; vesicoureteral reflux; intravesical FB; bladder calculus; bladder outlet obstruction; urethral stricture; ureterocele
Associated conditions	Spina bifida; paraplegia/quadriplegia; repeat cystoscopies; strictures; bladder stones; latex allergy

ANESTHETIC CONSIDERATIONS

See Anesthetic Considerations for Transurethral Procedures, Open Bladder Procedures, Penile Surgery, Genital Procedures, p. 1077.

References

1. Strand WR, Bloom DA: Pediatric endourology. In *Adult and Pediatric Urology,* Vol 3, 4th edition. Gillenwater JY, Grayhack JT, Howards SS, Mitchell ME, eds. Mosby-Year Book, St. Louis: 2002, 2719-28.
2. Warner MA: Lower extremity neuropathies associated with lithotomy positions. *Anesthesiology* 2000; 93:938-42.

OPEN BLADDER OPERATIONS

SURGICAL CONSIDERATIONS

Description: Open bladder operations commonly performed on children include **ureteral reimplantation** for correction of vesicoureteral reflux, obstructive megaureters, or ureterocele; **vesicostomy (Blocksom);** and **bladder neck operations.**

Ureteral reimplantation: Vesicoureteral reflux (VUR) is one of the most common abnormalities of the urinary tract in children and is present in ~25-50% of those who have UTI. While VUR resolves spontaneously in many children, there are a number of indications for correction of VUR. These include: 1) high-grade VUR, 2) progressive VUR and renal scarring, 3) failure to resolve within several years, 4) other bladder surgery, 5) breakthrough UTIs, and 6) poor medical compliance.

Ureteral reimplantations can be performed using different approaches to the bladder (e.g., extravesical, intravesical, or a combined approach); however, these different approaches require a similar exposure and abdominal incision. Initially, cystoscopy may be performed to plan a potentially complex reimplantation (e.g., duplex systems, ectopia, or periureteral diverticula). A lower abdominal suprapubic (Pfannensteil's) incision (Fig 12.6-2) is usually made, the fascia is opened vertically through the linea alba or the muscle is cut suprapubically, and the bladder is exposed. Sufficient muscle relaxation is required to enable the surgeon to place a self-retaining retractor to expose the bladder. The anesthesiologist also may be asked to limit N_2O to decrease the amount of peritoneal contents bulging toward the bladder surgical field. The bladder is then opened (intravesical approach) and the ureter(s) is (are) reimplanted, or the bladder is mobilized to expose the posterolateral ureter, which is then reimplanted (extravesical approach). When required, ureteral stents are brought to the abdominal skin through the bladder wall.

Obstructive megaureters and ureteroceles are other conditions that may require ureteral reimplantation. The abdominal exposure and indications do not differ significantly from ureteral reimplantation for VUR; however, tailoring of the ureter, by reducing its caliber and excising redundant tissue or plicating it, may be necessary. A procedure on the bladder neck also may be required if a ureterocele extends distally through the bladder outlet. Regional anesthesia techniques—specifically caudal or epidural analgesia—have gained popularity for these procedures. They have been shown to decrease postop pain medication requirements. While the majority of patients void 6-9 h after surgery, there may be ↑risk of urinary retention after a caudal block has been administered. The surgeon's preference on whether an indwelling urethral catheter will be left at the conclusion of the procedure should be discussed before giving the caudal block.

Usual preop diagnosis: VUR; obstructive megaureter; ureterocele

Vesicostomy: Infants and very young children may require bladder drainage until definitive bladder or urethral surgery. A vesicostomy may be performed, allowing the urine to flow continuously from a small, lower abdominal vesicocutaneous fistula. A 2 cm transverse incision is made halfway between the umbilicus and the pubis and the bladder is dissected extraperitoneally to expose the dome. The

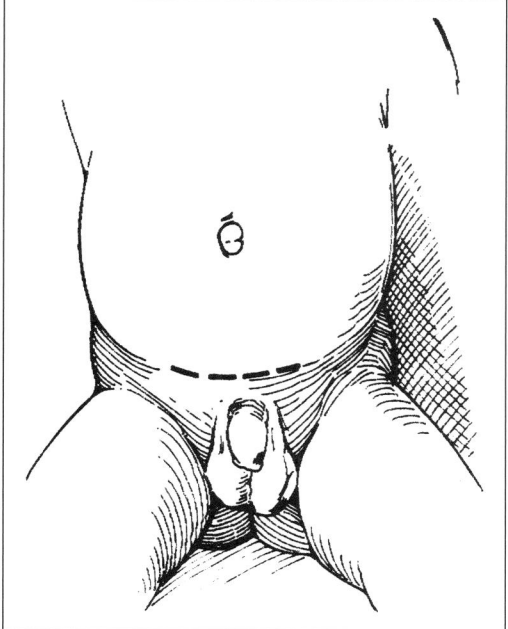

Figure 12.6-2. A Pfannensteil's incision in Langer's lines is a low transverse incision that provides good access to the bladder and other pelvic organs and good cosmesis. (Reproduced with permission from Hinman F: *Atlas of Pediatric Urologic Surgery*, 2nd edition. WB Saunders, 1994.)

bladder is opened at the dome (urachus) and is anastomosed to abdominal skin with absorbable sutures, creating a small (24 Fr) fistula.

Usual preop diagnosis: Posterior or anterior urethral valves; severe VUR; neurovesical dysfunction; prune-belly syndrome

Bladder neck operations: These procedures usually are required in patients with severe anomalies, such as exstrophy, or severe incontinence due to an incompetent bladder neck. These are more complex procedures, with dissection often difficult. The approach to the bladder is similar to that of ureteral reimplantation, using a lower abdominal (Pfannenstiel's) (Fig 12.6-2) incision. The Retzius space is dissected bluntly and the anterior bladder wall and pubic bone exposed. The bladder is opened and the bladder neck dissected and reconstructed. Various techniques to tubularize the anterior bladder wall, elongate the urethra, and increase the outlet resistance have been described. Bilateral ureteral reimplantation and bladder neck suspension can be performed at the same time. One special consideration is latex allergy (see Appendix G).

Usual preop diagnosis: Exstrophy/epispadias complex; spina bifida; neurogenic bladder; incontinence; bladder-neck reconstruction

SUMMARY OF PROCEDURES

	Reimplantation	Vesicostomy	Bladder Neck
Position	Supine	⇐	⇐
Incision	Pfannenstiel's or low midline extraperitoneal	⇐	⇐
Unique considerations	None	⇐	Latex allergy (see Appendix G)
Antibiotics	None unless indicated	⇐	Gentamicin 1.7 mg/kg iv, slowly
Surgical time	1.5 h	45 min	2 h
EBL	Minimal	⇐	200 ml
Postop care	PACU; ± urethral catheter ± stents. Anticholenergics for bladder spasms; belladonna and opioid suppositories, if given, must be monitored with caution because of the potential of oversedation and respiratory depression.	PACU	Urethral catheter 4-7 d; PACU → ward
Mortality	< 1%	⇐	⇐
Morbidity	Infection: < 3%	⇐	⇐
	Bleeding: < 3%	⇐	< 5%
	Urinary retention:	–	Urinary retention
	Unilateral: < 5%		
	Bilateral: 8-10%		
	Ureteral obstruction		⇐
	Persistent reflux		
Pain score	7	4	7

PATIENT POPULATION CHARACTERISTICS

Age range	1 mo–teenage	⇐	⇐
Male:Female	1:4	1:1	⇐
Incidence	1%	⇐	⇐
Etiology	Unknown	Congenital	⇐
Associated conditions	UTI; renal failure	⇐	⇐

ANESTHETIC CONSIDERATIONS

See Anesthetic Considerations for Transurethral Procedures, Open Bladder Procedures, Penile Surgery, Genital Procedures, p. 1077.

References

1. Canning DA, Koo HP, Duckett JW: Anomalies of the bladder and cloaca. In *Adult and Pediatric Urology,* Vol 3, 3rd edition. Gillenwater JY, Grayhack JT, Howards SS, Duckett JW, eds. Mosby-Year Book, St. Louis: 1996, 2445-88.
2. Dixon Walker R: Vesicoureteral reflux and urinary tract infection in children. In *Adult and Pediatric Urology,* Vol 3, 3rd edition. Gillenwater JY, Grayhack JT, Howards SS, Duckett JW, eds. Mosby-Year Book, St. Louis: 1996, 2459-95.
3. King LR: Vesicoureteral reflux, megaureter, and ureteral reimplantation. In *Campbell's Urology,* Vol 2, 6th edition. Walsh PC, Retik AB, Stamey TA, Vaughn ED Jr, eds. WB Saunders, Philadelphia: 1992, 1689-1742.
4. Smith GHH, Duckett JW: Urethral lesions in infants and children. In *Adult and Pediatric Urology,* Vol 3, 3rd edition. Gillenwater JY, Grayhack JT, Howards SS, Duckett JW, eds. Mosby-Year Book, Inc., St. Louis: 1996, 2411-43.
5. Wilton NT. Postoperative pain management for pediatric urologic surgery. In *Urologic Clin North Am* 1995; 22(1):189-201.

PENILE SURGERY

SURGICAL CONSIDERATIONS

Description: Pediatric penile operations usually correct congenital urethral abnormalities or involve circumcision. The most common surgical operation performed in the U.S., **circumcision** consists of the excision of the preputial skin to expose the glans. It can be performed for either religious, ethnic, social, or medical reasons (e.g., phimosis or recurrent balanitis).

Circumcision: Freehand circumcision involves excising preputial skin using two incisions to remove a sleeve of penile skin to fully expose the glans. At times, various clamps (Gomco, Mogen, etc.) can be used to circumcise in the newborn period. Most circumcisions performed in the OR on older children or those with penile skin anomalies will be free-hand excisions of the foreskin. Newer considerations regarding analgesia even in the neonate recommend a penile block for this procedure. In older children being circumcised, both caudal and penile block can offer similar duration of anesthesia (4-8 h). School-age children may, however, be bothered more by leg numbness from the caudal block than their younger counterparts.

Hypospadias is the abnormal opening of the urethral meatus resulting from incomplete development of the urethra. The defect can be located anywhere from the corona of the glans to the perineum. Accordingly, surgical correction can require minimal dissection, as in the **meatal advancement granuloplasty (MAGPI)** procedure. More proximal defects, however, may require extensive dissection and may necessitate a two-staged repair wherein the meatus is brought to the base of the penis at the first stage, then constructed at the apex months later. Postop urethral instrumentation should be avoided because catheterization of the newly formed urethra could cause disruption of the repair. Preputial or meatal skin flaps are used to reconstruct the defect. Removal of excess preputial skin is usually part of the hypospadias repair. **Chordee** is a curvature of the penis due to fibrous tissue. If present, it may require additional surgery on the penis, such as a **Nesbitt plication** or **tunica albuginea plication (TAP).** An artificial erection is obtained by infusion of NS through a 25 ga butterfly needle. The curvature is corrected by incising and plicating the tunica albuginea of the penis with absorbable suture. Stenting of the repair is usually reserved for complicated cases. In very complex redo cases, bladder or buccal mucosa may be needed to create a new urethra. Whether a urethral catheter is placed depends on the extent of the repair. Many distal hypospadias repairs do not require a urethral catheter; in any case, postop urethral instrumentation should be avoided because postop catheterization of the newly formed urethra could cause disruption of the repair. If a penile block is contemplated before operation, consideration must be given to avoiding a penile hematoma or disrupting penile anatomy or blood flow to the dorsal penis. Often at the conclusion of the surgery, a penile block will be performed, and the surgeon may require an additional 3-5 min of anesthesia to properly apply elaborate dressings.

Usual preop diagnosis: Phimosis; circumcision; hypospadias ± chordee; fistula repair; epispadias repair; penile torsion; concealed penis

SUMMARY OF PROCEDURES

	Circumcision	Hypospadias
Position	Supine	⇐
Incision	Circumferential penile	⇐ + ventral penis
Special instrumentation	None	Optical magnification

	Circumcision	Hypospadias
Unique considerations	1% lidocaine with 1:100,000 epinephrine for better hemostasis.	Tourniquet; injectable NS for artificial erection; 1% lidocaine
Antibiotics	None	⇐
Surgical time	30 min	1.5-4 h
EBL	Minimal	< 50 ml
Postop care	Outpatient	Outpatient or ward ± urethral catheter
Mortality	< 1%	⇐
Morbidity	Infection: 2%	⇐
	Hematoma: 2%	⇐
		Urethrocutaneous fistula: 5-20%
Pain score	2	5

PATIENT POPULATION CHARACTERISTICS

Age range	Neonates-children	> 4 mo
Incidence	61%	1:300
Etiology	Acquired	Congenital
Associated conditions	Infection	Cryptorchidism; inguinal hernia; bifid scrotum

ANESTHETIC CONSIDERATIONS

See Anesthetic Considerations for Transurethral Procedures, Open Bladder Procedures, Penile Surgery, Genital Procedures, p. 1077.

References

1. Elder JS: Hypospadias. In *Campbell's Urology,* Vol 3, 8th edition. Walsh PC, Retik AB, Vaughn ED, Wein A, eds. WB Saunders, Philadelphia: 2002, 2334-6.
2. Snodgrass W, Baskin LS: Abnormalities of the genitalia in boys and their surgical management. In *Adult and Pediatric Urology,* Vol III, 4th edition. Gillenwater JY, Grayhack JT, Howards SS, Mitchell ME, eds. Mosby-Year Book, St. Louis: 2002, 2509-32.
3. Wilton NT: Postoperative pain management for pediatric urologic surgery. *Urologic Clin North Am* 1995, 22(1):189-201.

GENITAL PROCEDURES
(CLITOROPLASTY, VAGINOPLASTY, URETHROPLASTY)

SURGICAL CONSIDERATIONS

Description: Masses of the introitus include urethral prolapse, prolapsed ectopic ureterocele, and rhabdomyosarcoma. Genitoplasty usually is performed in female patients with abnormal genitalia, e.g., ambiguous genitalia resulting from abnormal steroidogenesis (congenital adrenal hyperplasia [CAH], danazol exposure) and urogenital sinus or cloacal anomalies.

Urethral prolapse: With the patient in a lithotomy position, a simple circumferential incision is made at the junction between the prolapsed mucosa and the urethral meatus. The prolapsed tissue is excised, and anastomosis is performed with absorbable suture. Introital rhabdomyosarcoma often requires open or transurethral biopsy of the mass, and is usually treated with chemotherapy.

Vaginoplasty/clitoroplasty: These procedures are performed in patients with ambiguous genitalia, and are usually associated with hormonal imbalance (CAH). The initial procedure usually requires reduction of the enlarged clitoris and reconstruction of the labioscrotal folds. With the patient in a lithotomy position, skin incisions are made to allow partial resection of the corporal bodies and glans with nerve sparing. Periclitoral skin flaps are used to reconstruct the clitoris and labial folds. Vaginoplasty is performed through a perineal approach by creating a urethrovaginal septum. The vagina usually can be pulled into its normal position between the urethra and rectum, and anastomosed to perineal skin flaps using absorbable sutures. Vaginoplasty can be performed with clitoroplasty in an infant. If performed later in life (puberty), a vaginoplasty with complex flaps and bowel interposition is necessary. Many of these patients are on long-term corticosteroid replacement therapy and, therefore, preop stress-dosing of steroids may be indicated; if a long, complicated intraabdominal procedure is anticipated, an abdominoperineal approach is required. A loop of sigmoid colon or ileum is isolated, along with its mesentery, and is brought through the perineal incision. It is then anastomosed proximally to the vagina and distally to skin flaps. Also, these procedures may be used for **gender reassignment** if masculinization of the ambiguous genitalia in a genotypic male is not possible.

Usual preop diagnosis: Ambiguous genitalia; CAH; cloacal exstrophy; urogenital sinus persistence; danazol exposure

SUMMARY OF PROCEDURE

Position	Lithotomy
Incision	Perineal
Special instrumentation	Loupes
Unique considerations	Steroid replacement may be necessary (CAH)
Antibiotics	Gentamicin 1.7 mg/kg iv (children)
Surgical time	2-4 h
EBL	10-15 ml
Postop care	± urethral catheter
Mortality	< 1%
Morbidity	Infection: < 5%
	Bleeding: < 5%
	Flap necrosis: < 5%
Pain score	6

PATIENT POPULATION CHARACTERISTICS

Age range	Clitoroplasty: 3-6 mo; vaginoplasty: puberty
Incidence	1:30,000 births (ambiguous genitalia)
Etiology	Congenital
Associated conditions	Hypothalamic-pituitary axis suppression; adrenal hyperplasia; steroid replacement therapy

References

1. Hussman D: Intersex. In *Adult and Pediatric Urology,* Vol 3, 4th edition. Gillenwater JY, Grayhack JT, Howards SS, Mitchell ME, eds. Mosby-Year Book, St. Louis: 2002, 2533-64.
2. Rink R, Kaefer M: Surgical management of intersexuality, cloacal malformations, and other genitalia in girls. In *Campbell's Urology*, Vol 4, 8th edition. Walsh PC, Retik AB, Vaughn ED, Wein A, eds. WB Saunders, Philadelphia: 2002, 2428-68.

ANESTHETIC CONSIDERATIONS FOR TRANSURETHRAL PROCEDURES, OPEN BLADDER PROCEDURES, PENILE SURGERY, GENITAL PROCEDURES

PREOPERATIVE

Typically, infants and children presenting for these procedures are otherwise healthy, with some notable exceptions. **Vesicoureteral reflux** may be associated with renal dysplasia and HTN. The **prune-belly (Eagle-Barrett) syndrome** includes dystrophic abdominal musculature, requiring an evaluation of pulmonary function. **Bladder and cloacal exstrophy** may be accompanied by a spinal cord abnormality (e.g., tethered cord, spina bifida).

Pediatric urology patients with lower urinary tract dysfunction and underlying neurologic disorders (e.g., myelomeningocele), and exstrophy are at risk for developing latex allergy as a result of repeated urethral catheterizations or surgical procedures. (See Special Considerations for Latex Allergy, Appendix G.)

Circumcision and hypospadias repair are most commonly performed in the first 2 yr of life in otherwise healthy children.

Respiratory	Prune-belly syndrome: pulmonary function may be decreased. These patients are at risk for pulmonary aspiration; therefore, precautions to avoid aspiration of gastric contents should be carried out (e.g., Bicitra, ranitidine, cricoid pressure). ✓ Hx for evidence of recurrent pulmonary disease. **Tests:** CXR; others as indicated from H&P.
Renal	Renal anomalies may be present as part of a congenital malformation complex. **Tests:** As indicated from H&P.
Endocrine	Surgery for genital disorders usually are performed to reshape anatomic abnormalities 2° congenital endocrine disorders. Ambiguous genitalia are associated with congenital adrenal abnormalities. They are usually detected in the first month of life and may lead to severe salt-losing crises with ↓Na^+ and ↑K^+. The electrolyte status of these patients must be evaluated in the preop period. Treatment consists of steroid replacement. **Tests:** Electrolytes; blood sugar
Premedication	Preop medication usually is administered if the child is > 12 mo; midazolam po or iv (see p. D-2).

INTRAOPERATIVE

Anesthetic technique: GA (ETT or LMA) using a pediatric circle with humidified and warmed gases. A combined technique with epidural or caudal anesthesia is often used. For small children, warm OR to 70-75°F. Use warming pad on OR table.

Induction	For patients < 10 yr, standard mask induction with sevoflurane or halothane/N_2O/O_2. Older patients may agree to standard iv induction (see p. D-2). For open-bladder and complex genital procedures, an indwelling epidural catheter for intraop and postop pain relief is recommended.	
Maintenance	Standard pediatric maintenance (see p. D-3). With epidural anesthesia, amount of volatile and/or iv anesthetic requirements are diminished.	
Emergence	Typically, no special considerations. Carefully evaluate patient for adequate ventilation prior to extubation in those with prune-belly syndrome.	

Blood and fluid requirements	Minimal blood loss
	IV: 22 or 24 ga × 1
	NS/LR @ (maintenance):
	  4 ml/kg/h (1-10 kg)
	  + 2 ml/kg/h (11-20 kg)
		Complex cases may be associated with significant blood loss. Transfuse with whole blood or PRBC.

Monitoring	Standard monitors (see p. D-1). ± Arterial line	Place arterial line for measurement of arterial gases, Hct and blood glucose if significant blood loss or long case is anticipated.
Positioning	✓ and pad pressure points. ✓ eyes.	With too-large mask, beware ocular compression/corneal abrasion.
Complications	Nerve damage	In lower extremities, if padding is insufficient with lithotomy position

POSTOPERATIVE

Complications	Prune belly: hypoventilation Adrenogenital syndrome: adrenal insufficiency	Assisted ventilation may be required.
Pain management	Acetaminophen Epidural (p. E-5) or PCA (p. E-3) analgesia IV opiates	See p. E-3. Ditropan or ketorolac will ↓ bladder spasm.

References

1. Berry F: Anesthesia for genitourinary surgery. In *Pediatric Anesthesia,* 3rd edition. Churchill Livingstone, New York: 1994.
2. Davis PJ, Hall S, Deshpande JK, Spear RM: Anesthesia for general, urologic and plastic surgery. In *Smith's Anesthesia for Infants and Children,* 6th edition. Motoyama EK, Davis PJ, eds. Mosby-Year Book, St. Louis: 1990.
3. Sheldon CA, Snyder HM III: Principles of urinary tract reconstruction. In *Adult and Pediatric Urology*, Vol 1, 3rd edition. Gillenwater JY, Grayhack JT, Howards SS, Duckett JW, eds. Mosby-Year Book, St. Louis: 1996, 249-50, 2394-5.

INGUINOSCROTAL PROCEDURES

SURGICAL CONSIDERATIONS

Description: Undescended testis (cryptorchidism), hydrocele, and inguinal hernia are common in pediatric urology, and surgery is usually performed on an outpatient basis. Testicular torsion is one of the few true pediatric urologic emergencies because testicular infarction will occur within hours of the torsion. Testicular tumors in children, accounting for 1-2% of all pediatric solid tumors, are more frequently benign than those in adults, and represent the main indication for **radical or simple orchiectomy.**

Orchiopexy: Orchiopexy for a palpable undescended testis is performed through a small inguinal incision. A nonpalpable testis may warrant diagnostic laparoscopy as the initial procedure; otherwise, the external oblique fascia is opened, exposing the inguinal canal. The testis is localized and the cord is dissected to gain adequate length for scrotal fixation, without torsion or tension, to prevent postop ischemia and atrophy. If the testicle is high and adequate inguinal mobilization is not possible, dissection into the retroperitoneum may be required. The scrotal pouch is created by skin incision two-thirds the way down to the scrotum and blunt dissection between the skin and dartos muscle. The testis is fixed with suture material. An initially nonpalpable testis may become palpable with anesthetic relaxation. Both ilioinguinal nerve block and caudal analgesia appear to be equally effective in management of postorchiopexy pain. When inguinal block is contemplated prior to incision, this should be discussed with the surgeon. At times, inguinal infiltration distorts the anatomy and may perforate the hernia sac, thus turning a relatively simple operation into a more complex one. Alternatively, the block may be performed at the end of the procedure or the wound irrigated with 0.25% bupivacaine, which provides excellent postop analgesia and facilitates early discharge from the surgical recovery unit. (Also see Surgery for the Undescended Testicle, p. 1061.)

Testicular torsion is a pediatric urologic emergency. There is no definitive diagnostic imaging study, although Doppler and isotope scans of the testis can be useful. At times, Sx of testicular torsion may be indistinguishable from epididymitis or torsion of the testicular appendages (embryonic remnants). The testis is delivered through a scrotal incision, examined, detorsed, and assessed for viability. If the testis is nonviable, a **simple orchiectomy** is performed. If the testicle is viable, it is fixed in a **scrotal dartos pouch**. The contralateral testis is fixed in a similar fashion. A torsion of a testicular appendage usually is treated medically, with pain control and anti-inflammatory agents. If this condition is discovered at surgical exploration, the diseased tissue is excised, the testis is simply reinserted in the scrotum, and the wound is closed.

Usual preop diagnosis: Cryptorchidism; nonpalpable testis; testicular torsion; torsion of the testicular appendage

Hydrocelectomy–inguinal hernia repair: This procedure is performed through an inguinal incision and dissection of the inguinal canal. The patent processus vaginalis is carefully dissected from the cord structures; the peritoneal sac is ligated at the level of the internal inguinal ring; and the wound is closed after evacuation of the hydrocele liquid. (Also see Repair of Inguinal and Umbilical Hernias, Hydrocele, p. 1058.)

Usual preop diagnosis: Hydrocele; inguinal hernia

Radical orchiectomy: While simple orchiectomy is performed through a scrotal incision, radical orchiectomy (used when testicular cancer is suspected) is performed through an inguinal incision. The external oblique fascia is opened, and the spermatic cord is isolated and clamped at the level of the internal ring. The testis is delivered through the incision and examined. If the testis is felt to contain malignancy, the cord is ligated and divided at the level of the internal inguinal ring. If there is uncertainty in the Dx, a biopsy can be performed.

Usual preop diagnosis: Testicular mass

SUMMARY OF PROCEDURES

	Hydrocelectomy, Hernia Repair	Orchiopexy, Orchiectomy
Position	Supine	⇐
Incision	Inguinal/scrotal	⇐ + Can be extended to reach retroperitoneum ± laparoscopic exploration.
Antibiotics	None	⇐
Surgical time	1 h	⇐
EBL	Minimal	⇐
Postop care	PACU → home	⇐
Mortality	< 1%	⇐
Morbidity	Infection: 1-2%	Testicular atrophy: 7%
	Recurrence: 1%	
Pain score	5	5

PATIENT POPULATION CHARACTERISTICS

Age range	1 yr–puberty	Cryptorchidism: 1-2 yr Torsion: 0-18 yr
Incidence	1-4%	Cryptorchidism: 3% Torsion: 1:4000
Etiology	Congenital	⇐

ANESTHETIC CONSIDERATIONS

PREOPERATIVE

Orchiopexy, orchiectomy, hydrocelectomy, and hernia repair are performed most commonly in otherwise healthy children.

Renal
With phimosis, there may be Hx of UTIs. Possible pyelonephritis. Hematuria requires GU workup.
Tests: UA; renal function (BUN, Cr), as clinically indicated.

Laboratory
Hct; others as indicated from H&P.

Premedication
If > 1 yr of age, consider midazolam (0.5-0.75 mg/kg po) or diazepam (0.1-0.2 mg/kg po up to 10 mg) 1 h before induction. If > 10 yr old: standard premedication (p. D-1).

INTRAOPERATIVE

Anesthetic technique: GETA or LMA/mask anesthetic, using a pediatric circle with humidified and warmed gases. A combined technique with caudal anesthesia often is used for nonendoscopic procedures. For small children, warm OR to 70-75°F. Use warming pad on OR table.

Induction
In younger patients, mask induction is customary before iv placement. If the surgical procedure will be > 30 min, tracheal intubation or LMA is preferred. Intermediate-acting NMR (e.g., vecuronium 0.1 mg/kg iv or rocuronium 1 mg/kg iv) is administered to facilitate tracheal intubation. If appropriate, caudal anesthesia can be obtained using bupivacaine or levobupivacaine 0.25% with epinephrine 1:200,000; 0.75 ml/kg. The addition of clonidine (2 mg/kg) to the caudal block intensifies the analgesia, with minimal sedation. Acetaminophen 30-40 mg/kg pr may be given following intubation.

Maintenance
Standard pediatric maintenance (p. D-3). If no regional block is performed, at least 2 MAC anesthesia is required prior to skin incision to prevent laryngospasm in nonintubated patients. Caudal anesthesia can be used to provide the majority of analgesia in nonendoscopic procedures.

Emergence
If neuromuscular blockade is used, reverse with neostigmine (0.07 mg/kg iv) and atropine (0.02 mg/kg iv) or glycopyrolate (0.01 mg/kg). Extubate when patient is fully awake.

Blood and fluid requirements
Negligible blood loss
IV: 20-22 ga × 1
NS/LR @ maintenance

Pediatric maintenance:
4 ml/kg/h (0-10 kg)
+ 2 ml/kg/h (11-20 kg)
+ 1 ml/kg/h (>20 kg)

Monitoring
Standard monitors (p. D-1)

Positioning
✓ and pad pressure points.
✓ eyes.

Ocular compression/corneal abrasion may occur with oversized mask.

Complications
Laryngospasm

Intravascular local anesthetic administration

Rx: 100% O_2, jaw thrust, positive pressure. If necessary, administer succinylcholine (1-2 mg/kg iv).
Epinephrine in caudal anesthetic (to detect intravascular administration) does not significantly prolong analgesia.

POSTOPERATIVE

Complications
Bleeding

Pain management
Caudal or regional block
Acetaminophen (10-20 mg po/pr q 6 h prn)

Optimal analgesia and presence of parents in PACU will minimize child's agitation/movement/crying.

References

1. Berry FA: Anesthesia for genitourinary surgery. In *Pediatric Anesthesia,* 3rd edition, Gregory GA, ed. Churchill Livingstone, New York: 1994, 571-606.
2. Motoyama EK, Davis PC, eds: *Smith's Anesthesia for Infants and Children*, 6th edition. Mosby-Year-Book, St. Louis: 1996, 512-13.
3. Rozanski TA, Bloom DA: Male genital tract. In *Surgery of Infants and Children.* Oldham KT, Colombani PM, Foglia RP, eds. Lippincott-Raven Publishers, Philadelphia: 1997, 1543-58.
4. Schneck FX, Bellinger MF: *Campbell's Urology,* Vol 4, 8th edition. Walsh PC, Retik AB, Vaughn ED, Wein A, eds. WB Saunders, Philadelphia: 2002.
5. Wilton NT. Postoperative pain management for pediatric urologic surgery. In *Urologic Clin North Am* 1995; 22(1):189-201.

LAPAROSCOPIC PROCEDURES

SURGICAL CONSIDERATIONS

Description: Laparoscopy has become a useful technique for many pediatric urologists. It is used widely to locate the impalpable testis, and has gained popularity for many procedures. Among them are **laparoscopic nephrectomy, partial nephrectomy, nephroureterectomy, adrenalectomy,** and **pyeloplasty**.

A pneumoperitoneum is created by insufflating CO_2 (to a pressure of 14-16 mmHg). A trocar is inserted through a small, 1-cm periumbilical incision and positioned in the peritoneal cavity under direct vision (**Hasson technique**). Other trocars (2, 5, or 10 mm) are then inserted, as necessary, under direct laparoscopic vision, avoiding abdominal wall vessels and internal organs.

Impalpable testis: If diagnostic laparoscopy reveals blind ending vessels, confirming the absence of a testis, the procedure is terminated and no inguinal incision is made. An inguinal testis remnant usually indicates either antenatal testicular ischemia or torsion. If the vessels are seen to enter the inguinal ring, the laparoscopy is ended and inguinal exploration is performed. If the testis is located intraabdominally, it is evaluated for size and location to determine whether to use **orchiectomy** or a one- to two-stage (**Fowler Stevens**) or **laparoscopic orchiopexy**. Laparoscopic ligation of the vessels may be done with placement of the testis into a scrotal pouch (**darto pouch**) in one stage, if adequate cord length permits. In other situations, **laparoscopic or open dissection** in the retroperitoneum may be performed. A second-stage Fowler Stevens is performed to allow adequate collateral vascular development before it is brought into the scrotum. Laparoscopic orchiectomy or **gonadectomy** also may be performed in intersex situations for a dysgenetic (streak), nonviable gonad, or for a gonad in which inadequate cord length exists.

Varicocele ligation: The spermatic veins are isolated from the abdominal wall and are ligated with metallic clips, using the same initial laparoscopic approach as for an undescended testis.

Heminephrectomy, nephroureterectomy, and pyeloplasty: With the patient in the lateral decubitus position, the initial trocar is inserted extraperitoneally on the anterior axillary line just below the 12th rib. Gas dissection is used to open the retroperitoneal space, and kidney dissection is performed. The hilar vessels are ligated with metallic clips. The kidney is then retrieved through the 10-mm port by morcellating it, or the incision can be elongated.

Usual preop diagnosis: Nonpalpable testis; cryptorchidism; varicocele; ambiguous genitalia; UPJ obstruction; infected or nonfunctioning kidney; HTN; multicystic or dysplastic kidney; protein-losing nephropathy in ESRD

SUMMARY OF PROCEDURES

	Undescended Testis/Varicocele	**Renal Surgery**
Position	Supine; 15° Trendelenburg	Lateral decubitus
Incision	5-10 mm umbilical port + 1 or 2 additional ports	4 ports usually necessary
Special instrumentation	Bladder catheterization, NG tube	⇐
Unique considerations	Secure child firmly to avoid movement with table tilting. Intraabdominal pressure of 14-16 mmHg. Lower pressure may be needed if pulmonary mechanics are compromised. Urethral catheter commonly placed.	⇐
Antibiotics	None	⇐
Surgical time	1 h	2.5 h
EBL	Minimal	⇐
Postop care	PACU → home	PACU → ward
Mortality	< 1%	⇐
Morbidity	Overall: 0.6-5%	⇐
	Trocar misplacement: bowel perforation	⇐
	Vascular/organ thermal injury from electro-cautery	⇐
	CO_2 embolus	Bleeding < 5%
	Grounding pad thermal injury	
	Trocar site bleeding	
	Hernia from trocar site	
Pain score	2	4

PATIENT POPULATION CHARACTERISTICS

Age range	10 mo-18 yr
Male:Female	Male (cryptorchidism)
Incidence	3% of newborn boys
Etiology	Congenital
Associated conditions	Renal insufficiency

ANESTHETIC CONSIDERATIONS

Creation of a pneumoperitoneum as part of a laparoscopic procedure impairs ventilation and can restrict venous return. The use of Trendelenburg and lithotomy positions can further worsen the respiratory changes that occur. Anesthetic considerations for pediatric patients undergoing laparoscopic procedures are similar to those in adults (see p. 461).

References

1. Farber GJ, Bloom DA: Pediatric endourology. In *Adult and Pediatric Urology,* Vol 3, 3rd edition. Gillenwater JY, Grayhack JT, Howards, SS, Duckett JW, eds. Mosby-Year Book, St. Louis: 1996, 2739-47.
2. McDougall EM, Gill IS, Clayman RV: Laparoscopic urology. In *Adult and Pediatric Urology,* Vol 1, 3rd edition. Gillenwater JY, Grayhack JT, Howards, SS, Duckett JW, eds. Mosby-Year Book, St. Louis: 1996, 829-912.

Surgeons

Lawrence A. Rinsky, MD
Todd Lincoln, MD
James Chang, MD
Amy L. Ladd, MD

12.7 PEDIATRIC ORTHOPEDIC SURGERY

Anesthesiologists

Komal Kamra, MD
Alice A. Edler, MD

PERCUTANEOUS PINNING OF DISPLACED SUPRACONDYLAR HUMERUS FRACTURE

SURGICAL CONSIDERATIONS

Description: Supracondylar fractures of the humerus are the most common elbow fractures in children; and they probably are the most common pediatric fractures requiring reduction under GA. They have a justifiable reputation for difficulties because they are often associated with complications, including vascular injuries and compartment syndromes, nerve palsies, malreductions, and late deformities. The vast majority of these injuries result from falling on an outstretched hand with an extended elbow—a common childhood event. Although an occasional angulated fracture may be stable after reduction with a splint alone, most displaced supracondylar fractures are treated by **closed reduction and percutaneous pinning**.

Documentation of the neurovascular examination is mandatory immediately before anesthesia and upon awakening. Reduction is obtained by a combination of traction and manipulation; complete muscular relaxation is essential. Usually two small, smooth, crossed pins are inserted under I.I. control. Many surgeons use the intensifier screen as a platform, thus requiring the patient to be at the extreme edge of the OR table. Rarely is the fracture irreducible. In that case, the arm is reprepped and a small, lateral incision is made to openly visualize and reduce the fracture. The same type of smooth pin fixation is then carried out. Prolonged skeletal traction has been used extensively in the past for these fractures; however, it is rarely used now in the U.S.

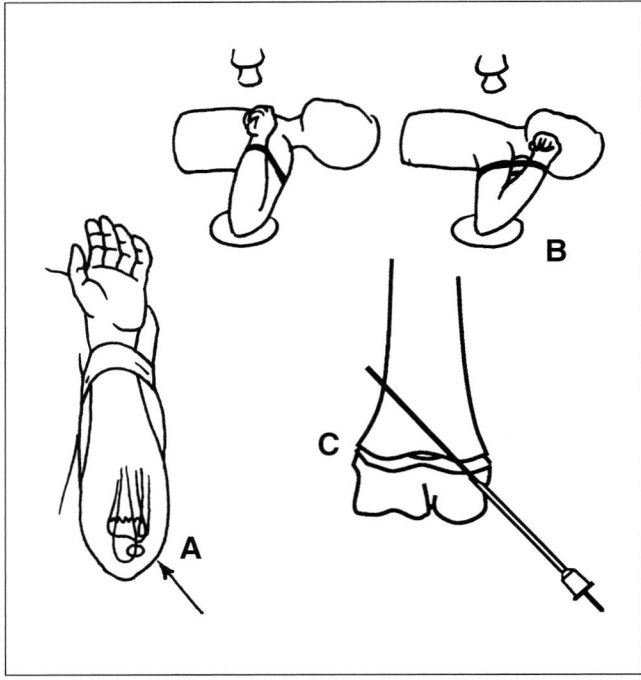

Figure 12.7-1. Percutaneous pinning of supracondylar humerus fracture. (A) The fracture is manually reduced and held with elbow flexed. (B) Fracture reduction is assessed with I.I. (C) The fracture is stabilized with percutaneous K-wires. (Reproduced with permission from Chapman MW: *Chapman's Orthopaedic Surgery*, Vol IV, 3rd edition. Lippincott Williams & Wilkins, 2001.)

Usual preop diagnosis: Acute, displaced, supracondylar fracture of the humerus

SUMMARY OF PROCEDURES

	Percutaneous Pinning	Open Reduction
Position	Usually supine, occasionally prone or lateral	⇐
Incision	None	1″ lateral
Special instrumentation	Power drill, I.I.	⇐
Unique considerations	Full-stomach; compartment syndrome	⇐
Antibiotics	Usually none	Cefazolin 25 mg/kg
Surgical time	30-60 min	30-90 min
Closing considerations	Cast or splint	⇐
EBL	Minimal	⇐
Postop care	PACU → room; close neurovascular monitoring	⇐
Mortality	Rare	⇐
Morbidity	Late angular deformity, especially cubitus varus: 10%	⇐
	Nerve palsy (typically radial nerve) from the fracture itself: 7%	⇐
	Compartment syndrome (Volkmann's contracture): < 0.5% (some degree of vascular spasm or loss of radial pulse much more common)	⇐
	Stiffness, myositis ossificans	⇐
	Ipsilateral fracture	⇐
Pain score	3-5	3-6

PATIENT POPULATION CHARACTERISTICS

Age range	< 10 yr: 84%; most are 5-8 yr
Male:Female	1.6:1
Incidence	Third most common child's fracture (most common is an elbow fracture)
Etiology	Trauma
Associated conditions	Usually normal, healthy child

ANESTHETIC CONSIDERATIONS

See Anesthetic Considerations for Upper Extremity Procedures, p. 1091.

References

1. Bell C, Kain Z: Acute pediatric pain management. In *The Pediatric Anesthesia Handbook*. Mosby, St. Louis: 1997.
2. Dormans JP, Squillante R, Sharf H: Acute neurovascular complications with supracondylar humerus fractures in children. *J Hand Surg* [Am] 1995; 20(1):1-4.
3. Garbuz DS, Leitch K, Wright JG: The treatment of supracondylar fractures in childen with an absent radial pulse. *J Pediatr Orthop* 1996; 16(5):594-6.
4. Gordon JE, Patton CM, Luhmann SJ, Basset GS, Schoenecker PL: Fracture stability after pinning of displaced supracondylar distal humerus fractures in children. *J Pediatr Orthop* 2001; 21(3):313-18.
5. Kasser JR, Beaty JH: Supracondylar fractures of the distal humerus. In *Fractures in Children*. Beaty JH, Kasser JR, eds. Lippincott-Raven, Philadelphia: 2001, 577-624.
6. Otsuka NY, Kasser JR: Supracondylar fractures of the humerous in children. *J Am Acad Orthop Surg* 1997; 5(1):19-26.
7. Pullerits J, Holzman R: Pediatric neuraxial blockade. *J Clin Anesth* 1993; 5(4):342-54.
8. Salem MR, Klowden AS: Anesthesia for orthopaedic surgery. In *Pediatric Anesthesia*, 3rd edition. Gregory G, ed. Churchill Livingstone, New York: 1994, 607-56.
9. Shaw BA, Kasser JR, Emans JB, Rand FF: Management of vascular injuries in displaced supracondylar humerus fractures without arteriography. *J Orthop Trauma* 1990; 4(1):25-9.

CLOSED OR OPEN REDUCTION OF DISPLACED LATERAL CONDYLE HUMERUS FRACTURE

SURGICAL CONSIDERATIONS

Description: The lateral condyle of the distal humerus is a common site of elbow fractures during childhood (second only to supracondylar fractures). Initial radiographs of lateral condyle fractures can look deceptively benign; however, these fractures cross the physis (growth plate) and enter the articular surface, demanding perfect reduction to restore joint surface congruity and to avoid a premature physeal arrest. In addition, the elbow may be rendered unstable and dislocate if the fracture extends into the trochlea of the humerus. Accurate and stable reduction minimizes the risk of nonunion, a well known complication resulting from unsuspected rotation of the fracture fragment and by traction forces of the extensor muscles attaching to this condyle. Unlike supracondylar fractures, neurovascular complications are rare with lateral condyle fractures.

Although minimally displaced fractures are suitable for casting alone, 60% of lateral condyle fractures are displaced significantly and require manipulation and pinning. Casting without manipulation is only indicated for stable fractures displaced < 2 mm. **Closed reduction and percutaneous pinning** under I.I. control is suitable for stable fractures with 2-4 mm displacement. **Open reduction and pinning** is necessary for fractures that are unstable, rotated, or displaced > 4 mm. Complete muscular relaxation is advantageous when performing either a closed or open reduction of the fracture.

Usual preoperative diagnosis: Displaced lateral condyle humerus fracture

SUMMARY OF PROCEDURES

	Closed Reduction/Pinning	Open Reduction/Pinning
Position	Supine	⇐
Incision	None	1-2″ lateral
Instrumentation	Power drill, I.I.	⇐
Unique considerations	None	⇐
Antibiotics	Usually none	Cefazolin 25 mg/kg
Surgical time	30-60 min	45-90 min
Closing considerations	Cast or splint	⇐
EBL	Minimal	⇐
Postoperative care	PACU → room	⇐
Mortality	Rare	⇐
Morbidity	Delayed or nonunion	⇐
	Cubitus valgus (more common) or varus	⇐
	Lateral condylar overgrowth	⇐
	Physeal arrest	⇐
	Osteonecrosis of lateral trochlea	⇐
	Ulnar nerve palsy	⇐
		Avascular necrosis of trochlea
Pain score	3-5	3-6

PATIENT POPULATION CHARACTERISTICS

Age range	5-10 yr; average = 6 yr
Male:Female	Boys > Girls
Incidence	15% of all elbow fractures; more common in summer
Etiology	Trauma
Associated conditions	Usually normal, healthy child

ANESTHETIC CONSIDERATIONS

See Anesthetic Considerations for Upper Extremity Procedures, p. 1091.

References

1. Foster DE, Sullivan JA, Gross RH: Lateral humeral condylar fractures in children. *J Pediatr Orthop* 1985; 5(1):16-22.
2. Mintzer CM, Waters PM, Brown DJ, Kasser JR: Percutaneous pinning in the treatment of displaced lateral condyle fractures. *J Pediatr Orthop* 1994; 14(4):462-5.
3. Thomas DP, Howard AW, Cole WG, Hedden DM: Three weeks of Kirschner wire fixation for displaced lateral condylar fractures of the humerus in children. *J Pediatr Orthop* 2001; 21(5):565-9.

ASPIRATION AND INJECTION OF UNICAMERAL BONE CYST

SURGICAL CONSIDERATIONS

Description: Unicameral bone cysts (UBC) are benign lesions typically located in the metaphyseal regions of long bones, usually in the proximal humerus of a growing child. The cyst is rarely a source of pain until presentation (typically with a minimally displaced fracture). The benign radiographic appearance allows clinicians to follow most lesions without the need for surgical biopsy. Surgical care is indicated when the UBC is of sufficient size and location to cause mechanical weakening of the bone and predispose to a pathologic fracture. The goals of surgical care are to confirm the Dx of UBC and to reestablish the mechanical integrity of the bone. Dx of a UBC is made via percutaneous aspiration of the lesion, using a standard 16-18 ga spinal needle under GA. I.I. guidance helps in needle placement. The presence of clear, straw-colored fluid confirms Dx of UBC. An alternative Dx must be considered if frank blood is aspirated (e.g., from an aneurysmal bone cyst) or if there is no fluid (e.g., from a nonossifying fibroma). Open biopsy is necessary if the Dx of a UBC is not clear. Following aspiration of the UBC, a radiopaque dye is injected into the cyst to verify that the entire cavity is contiguous. If the cystic cavity is loculated by bony trabecula, a **needle** or **percutaneous Kirschner** wire is used to convert the lesion into a unicompartmental space so the subsequent injection will easily access the entire lesion. Scraping the inner cyst walls with a needle also helps to disrupt the cyst lining and is thought to improve the chance of filling in the cavity. The final surgical step is to introduce a second 'venting' needle into the cyst to allow lavage with sterile saline, followed by injection of the cavity with a substance to promote new bone formation. Historically, methylprednisolone has been used, but more recent evidence suggests a higher success rate when autologous bone marrow is injected. **Injectable allograft bone** preparations also can supplement the bone marrow injection. Care must be taken to avoid aspirating from the first needle after the second has been placed, to avoid intraosseous air embolism.

Usual preoperative diagnosis: Unicameral bone cyst

SUMMARY OF PROCEDURES

	Percutaneous	Open
Position	Supine	⇐
Incision	None	Length of cyst
Instrumentation	Spinal needles, Kirschner wires, I.I.	Curettes
Unique considerations	Risk of air embolus	Additional time for intraop pathology evaluation
Antibiotics	Usually none	Cefazolin 25 mg/kg
Surgical time	30-60 min	60-90 min
Closing considerations	None	Cast or splint
EBL	Minimal	⇐
Postop care	PACU → home	PACU → room/home
Mortality	Rare	⇐
Morbidity	Infection	⇐
	Iatrogenic fracture	⇐
	Growth arrest: Rare	⇐
Pain score	0-2	3-6

PATIENT POPULATION CHARACTERISTICS

Age range	5-15 yr; not found in adults
Male:Female	1:3
Incidence	20% of benign bone lesions; most common location is the proximal humerus (67%), followed by the proximal femur (15%)
Etiology	Unknown. Venous obstruction → fluid transudate containing high levels of interleukin-1 and interleukin-6, which stimulate osteoclasts
Associated conditions	Usually normal, healthy child. Initial presentation typically follows a pathologic fracture.

ANESTHETIC CONSIDERATIONS

See Anesthetic Considerations for Upper Extremity Procedures, p. 1091.

References

1. Bensahel H, Jehanno P, Desgrippes Y, Pennecot GF: Solitary bone cyst: controversies and treatment. *J Pediatr Orthop* [Br] 1998; 7(4):257-61.
2. Killian JT, Wilkenson L, White S, Brassard M: Treatment of unicameral bone cyst with demineralized bone matrix. *J Pediatr Orthop* 1998; 18(5):621-4.
3. Rougraff BT, Kling TJ: Treatment of active unicameral bone cysts with percutaneous injection of demineralized bone matrix and autogenous bone marrow. *J Bone Joint Surg* [Am] 2002; 84A(6):921-9.
4. Yandow SM, Lundeen GA, Scott SM, Coffin C: Autogenic bone marrow injections as a treatment for simple bone cyst. *J Pediatr Orthop* 1998; 18(5):616-20.

RELEASE FOR TORTICOLLIS

SURGICAL CONSIDERATIONS

Description: Congenital muscular torticollis is a painless condition associated with a contracture of the sternocleido-mastoid muscle, leading to a head tilt toward the involved side and head rotation toward the opposite side (a 'cocked-robin' posture). It is associated with breech and difficult deliveries, as well as other musculoskeletal disorders, such as meta-tarsus adductus, hip dysplasia, and talipes equinovarus. Multiple theories regarding the etiology of congenital muscular torticollis have been proposed, including fibrosis of the sternocleidomastoid muscle following a peripartum intramuscular bleed, fibrosis resulting from a compartment syndrome of the sternocleidomastoid muscle, intrauterine crowding, and a primary myopathy of the sternocleidomastoid muscle. Eighty percent of cases of torticollis are a result of this congenital contracture of the sternocleidomastoid muscle. Less common etiologies—such as congenital cervical spine malforma-tions (e.g., Klippel-Feil syndrome), neurologic disorders, a cranial or cervical neoplasm, inflammatory conditions (e.g., Grisel's syndrome), or an ocular dysfunction—should also be excluded. Congenital muscular torticollis is seen more frequently on the right side. A persistent torticollis will lead to skull and facial deformities (plagiocephaly). If the child sleeps prone, he will usually lie with the affected side down, resulting in flattening of the face on that side. If the child sleeps supine, flattening of the contralateral skull occurs. This plagiocephaly will become permanent if the torticollis per-sists and is left untreated.

Initial treatment is predominately conservative. For infants < 1 yr, a program of sternocleidomastoid muscle stretching is recommended, with 90% of cases being resolved with this treatment. After age 2 yr, conservative treatment is not likely to be effective. Children with persistent torticollis and an unacceptable amount of facial asymmetry preferably are treated surgically before the age of 3 yr; however, some improvement in facial asymmetry has been shown even in children sur-gically treated up to 8 yr of age.

Surgical options include a **unipolar release**, a **bipolar release, middle-third transection**, or a **complete resection**. Uni-polar release involves division of the distal insertion of the sternocleidomastoid muscle and usually is performed for a mild deformity. Bipolar release entails division of both the sternocleidomastoid origin and insertion, and usually is done for more marked involvement. **Z-plasty** of the clavicular head or transfer of the clavicular head to the sternal head may be done to maintain a more normal cosmetic contour of the neck. Potential surgical complications include injury to the spinal accessory nerve, jugular veins, carotid vessels, and the facial nerve. Postop, patients may perform simple stretch-ing exercises, but they often require bracing to maintain a corrected alignment.

Usual preoperative diagnosis: Congenital muscular torticollis

SUMMARY OF PROCEDURES

	Unipolar	Bipolar
Position	Supine	⇐
Incision	Transverse, 1.5 cm superior to sternum and clavicle over muscle insertion	⇐ + 1 cm distal to mastoid pro-cess behind ear at muscle origin
Unique considerations	Plagiocephaly	⇐
Antibiotics	Cefazolin 25 mg/kg	⇐
Surgical time	30 min	45 min
EBL	Minimal	⇐
Postoperative care	PACU → room/home	⇐
Mortality	Rare	⇐
Morbidity	Hypertrophic scar	⇐
	Loss of normal muscle contour	⇐
		Spinal accessory nerve injury
Pain score	3-5	3-5

PATIENT POPULATION CHARACTERISTICS

Age range	Onset at birth, surgery after age 1 yr
Male:Female	1:1
Incidence	1/100
Etiology	Fibrosis of sternocleidomastoid; possible intrauterine or perinatal muscle compartment syndrome
Associated conditions	Usually normal, healthy child; hip dysplasia in 20%

ANESTHETIC CONSIDERATIONS

See Anesthetic Considerations for Upper Extremity Procedures, p. 1091.

References

1. Ballock RT, Song KM: The prevalence of nonmuscular causes of torticollis in children. *J Pediatr Orthop* 1996; 16(4):500-4.
2. Davids JR, Wenger DR, Mubarak SJ: Congenital muscular torticollis: sequela of intrauterine or perinatal compartment syndrome. *J Pediatr Orthop* 1993; 13(2):141-7.
3. Ferkel RD, Westin GW, Dawson EG, et al: Muscular torticollis: a modified surgical approach. *J Bone Joint Surg* 1983; 65A: 894-900.
4. Wirth CJ, Hagena FW, Wuelker N, Siebert WE: Biterminal tenotomy for the treatment of congenital muscular torticollis. Long-term results. *J Bone Joint Surg Am* 1992; 74(3):427-34.

POLLICIZATION OF A FINGER

SURGICAL CONSIDERATIONS

Description: This procedure is indicated in the infant with congenital absence or hypoplasia of the thumb. A normal finger—usually the index finger—with its tendon, nerve, and vascular supply is shortened and rotated into the position of the thumb (Fig 12.7-2). Tendon transfers are performed to substitute for the absent or hypoplastic thenar muscles. These patients may have many other associated congenital anomalies, which should be ruled out prior to surgery.

Variant procedure or approaches: There are several different surgical techniques, which share the basic transposition and rotation of the finger to the thumb position.

Usual preop diagnosis: Aplastic thumb; hypoplastic thumb; radial club hand; radial longitudinal deficiency

SUMMARY OF PROCEDURE

Position	Supine, with arm extended on hand-surgery table
Incision	Multiple incisions on the hand
Special instrumentation	Pneumatic tourniquet; magnification loupes
Antibiotics	Cefazolin 25 mg/kg (children)
Surgical time	3-4 h
Tourniquet	100 mmHg above systolic; max time = 120 min
Closing considerations	Complex skin flaps are necessary. A plaster splint is placed while the patient is still anesthetized.
EBL	Minimal; performed under tourniquet control.
Postop care	PACU → overnight admission for observation or perfusion to the transposed finger
Mortality	Minimal
Morbidity	Ischemia (loss of digit): Rare
	Skin flap necrosis: Moderately common
Pain score	1-2

PATIENT POPULATION CHARACTERISTICS

Age range	1-2 yr is ideal time for surgery. Procedure should be done before patient begins school.
Male:Female	1:1
Incidence	Overall, about 1/20,000 live births require a variant of this procedure.

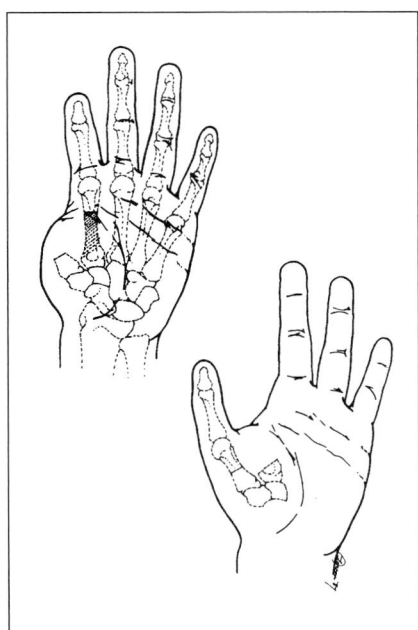

Figure 12.7-2. Pollicization of a finger. (Reproduced with permission from Chapman MW: *Chapman's Orthopaedic Surgery*, 3rd edition. Lippincott Williams & Wilkins, 2001.

Etiology	Unknown; also associated with thalidomide ingestion.
Associated conditions	Associated congenital anomalies of the upper extremity, esophagus, spine, and lower extremities Absence of radius (radial club hand), common Various forms of syndactylies, common Abnormalities of the hematopoietic system (Fanconi's syndrome), cardiovascular system (ASDs in Holt-Oram syndrome), spine, and GI system, along with hypothyroidism, are frequently associated.

ANESTHETIC CONSIDERATIONS

See Anesthetic Considerations for Upper Extremity Procedures, p. 1091.

Reference

1. Light TR: Amputations of the hand. In *Chapman's Orthopaedic Surgery*, 3rd edition. Vol II. Chapman MW, ed. Lippincott Williams & Wilkins, Philadelphia: 2001, 1454-5.

SYNDACTYLY REPAIR

SURGICAL CONSIDERATIONS

Description: Syndactyly refers to congenital failure of separation of two or more fingers. It is complete if it extends to the ends of the fingers; incomplete syndactyly extends short of the finger ends. A **simple syndactyly repair** joins fingers by only skin and fibrous tissues. A **complex syndactyly repair** signifies fusion of adjacent phalanges or interposition of accessory phalanges, with frequent abnormalities of the neurovascular structures. Surgical separation is performed in the first few years of life for functional, as well as aesthetic reasons. The technique involves creation of a dorsal, proximally based skin flap to recreate the web. A zigzag dorsal and palmar incision is then created, separating from the distal end in a proximal direction. The digital nerve and arteries are dissected proximally as far as possible. Primary closure is almost never possible, and supplemental full-thickness skin graft harvested from the groin is used to complete the closure. Usually only one site is done at a time per hand; and, never should both sides of a digit be released, because of risk to the vascular supply. It is not always possible to save all the bony elements. Patients with conditions such as Apert syndrome must undergo careful evaluation of the airway.

Usual preop diagnosis: Syndactyly of fingers; bifid finger, thumb/finger

SUMMARY OF PROCEDURE

Position	Supine
Incision	Zigzag between digits; skin graft donor site from groin
Special instrumentation	Magnification loupes always necessary. Tourniquet is mandatory.
Unique considerations	Groin skin also must be taken for graft closure.
Antibiotics	Usually none
Surgical time	2-4 h
Closing considerations	Above-the-elbow cast or splint to keep incision away from mouth and other hand of the infant or child
EBL	< 20 ml

Postop care	PACU → home, if simple syndactyly
Mortality	None associated with procedure.
Morbidity	Partial slough of flaps or skin graft requiring revision
	Scarring and some stiffness of fingers
	Angulatory deformities late, occasionally depending on degree of involvement of the skeleton and joint
Pain score	1-3

PATIENT POPULATION CHARACTERISTICS

Age range	6 mo-5 yr
Male:Female	2:1
Incidence	1/2000 births (the most common significant congenital hand anomaly)
Etiology	Family Hx (10-40%); failure of differentiation in the 6th-8th wk of intrauterine life
Associated conditions	Polydactyly, accessory phalanges; Apert syndrome; Poland syndrome

ANESTHETIC CONSIDERATIONS

See Anesthetic Considerations for Upper Extremity Procedures, below.

References

1. Bauer TB, Tondra JM, Trusler HM: Technical modification in repair of syndactylism. *Plast Reconstr Surg* 1956; 17:385-92.
2. Chang J, Danton TK, Ladd AL, Hentz VR: Reconstruction of the hand in Apert's syndrome: a simplified approach. *Plast Reconstr Surg* 2002; 109(2):465-70.
3. Ezaki M, Kay SP, et al: In *Green's Operative Hand Surgery*. Green DP, Hotchkiss RN, Pederson WC, eds. Churchill Livingstone, Philadelphia: 1993, 325+.

ANESTHETIC CONSIDERATIONS FOR UPPER EXTREMITY PROCEDURES

(Procedures covered: percutaneous pinning, displaced supracondylar humerus fracture; closed/open reduction, displaced lateral condylar humerus fracture; aspiration/injection, unicamera/bone cyst; torticollis release; pollicization of finger; syndactly release)

PREOPERATIVE

The majority of children presenting for repair of upper extremity fractures are otherwise healthy. Most of these patients present for repair of a traumatic injury; thus, the preop workup is routine. Some arm procedures, such as repair of a compound fracture, require immediate attention and necessitate emergency surgery and full-stomach considerations (see p. B-5).

Laboratory	Tests as indicated from H&P.
Premedication	Standard premedication (see p. D-2).

INTRAOPERATIVE

Anesthetic technique: GETA, since small children rarely tolerate regional anesthesia alone. In the older patient, regional anesthesia may be appropriate, and can reduce the risk of aspiration pneumonitis associated with GA in the patient with a full stomach. A combined technique offers the advantages of reduced anesthetic requirements and postop pain relief; however, regional anesthesia is relatively contraindicated in patients with neurovascular damage.

General anesthesia:

Induction	Standard induction (see p. D-2) except in acute-trauma patients, where rapid-sequence induction is appropriate (see p. B-5).
Maintenance	Standard maintenance (see p. D-3).
Emergence	Management of emergence and extubation should be routine, except in difficult airway cases, which require awake extubation. Skin closure is frequently followed by application of a splint; patient should remain anesthetized during splinting procedure.

Regional anesthesia:

Anesthetics and doses	See Table 12.7-1.

<table>
<tr><td colspan="3">**Table 12.7-1. Maximum Recommended Doses of Local Anesthetics for Regional Anesthesia**</td></tr>
<tr><td>**Drug**</td><td>**Mg/kg (with epinephrine)**</td><td>**Duration (min)**</td></tr>
<tr><td>Lidocaine</td><td>5 (7)</td><td>45-180</td></tr>
<tr><td>Bupivicaine</td><td>2.5 (3)</td><td>180-600</td></tr>
<tr><td>Tetracaine</td><td>1.5</td><td>180-600</td></tr>
<tr><td>2-Chloroprocaine</td><td>8 (10)</td><td>30-60</td></tr>
<tr><td>Procaine</td><td>8 (10)</td><td>60-90</td></tr>
</table>

Interscalene block	Phrenic nerve block → hemidiaphragm paralysis is an inevitable consequence of the interscalene block. Major complications (e.g., total spinal or pneumothorax) resulting from interscalene block, are very rare; therefore, this technique is suitable for outpatients. Interscalene block is contraindicated in patients with contralateral recurrent laryngeal nerve or phrenic nerve palsy.
Axillary block	The medial aspect of the upper arm is innervated by the intercostobrachial nerve (T2) and requires a separate subcutaneous field block in the axilla, especially when a tourniquet is used. The lateral cutaneous nerve of the forearm, a sensory branch of the musculocutaneous nerve supplying sensation to the lateral forearm, is frequently missed by the axillary approach to the brachial plexus. Thus, a block of this nerve at the elbow is sometimes necessary. The dose volume of local anesthetic required varies with the height and weight of the child. As a rule, the child's body surface area can be used as an approximate proportion of the usual adult volume (e.g., a 1.7 M^2 adult will require 40 ml of local anesthetic; a 1 M^2 patient requires 20-25 ml). Care must be taken to avoid local anesthetic overdose (see Table 12.7-1).
Supplemental sedation	Supplemental sedation may be accomplished with use of propofol by continuous infusion (50-150 μg/kg/min).
Blood and fluid requirements	Minimal blood loss IV: 20 ga × 1 NS/LR @ 1.5-3 ml/kg/h	IV catheter should be placed in the contralateral upper extremity.
Monitoring	Standard monitors (see p. D-1).
Positioning	✓ and pad pressure points. ✓ eyes.
Interscalene block complications	Total spinal Epidural anesthesia IV injection (Sz/dysrhythmias) Stellate ganglion block (Horner's syndrome) Laryngeal nerve block Phrenic nerve block Pneumothorax	Resuscitative equipment, including airway management tools, should be immediately available.
Axillary block complications	Inadequate block Intravascular injection Peripheral nerve damage Axillary hematoma Axillary artery thrombosis Pneumothorax	Very minimal doses of local anesthetic can cause CNS toxicity if reverse flow occurs during an intraarterial injection. Axillary thrombosis and pneumothorax are extremely rare.

POSTOPERATIVE

Pain management	PCA (see p. E-3). ± Regional block	Combined regional-GA provides excellent postop pain management.
Tests	None routinely indicated.	

POSTERIOR SPINAL INSTRUMENTATION AND FUSION

SURGICAL CONSIDERATIONS

Description: Posterior spinal instrumentation refers to implanted metal rods affixed to the spine to correct and internally splint the deformed spine. Originally designed for scoliosis, posterior spinal instrumentation is commonly performed simultaneously with **spinal fusion** for a variety of diagnoses, including fracture, tumor, degenerative changes, and developmental spinal deformity. Although posterior spinal instrumentation with the ratcheted **Harrington rod** gained widespread usage in the 1970s, it is no longer used by spinal surgeons. The current standard is a hook-rod system, such as the **Cotrel-Duboussett** (C-D), the **Texas Scottish Rite Hospital** (TSRH), the **Miami Modular Orthopaedic Spinal System** (MOSS) and the **Universal Spine System** (USS). Regardless of the surgeon's choice of instrumentation, the spine is approached by an extensive midline posterior incision, in which a subperiosteal exposure (typically T2-5 down to L1-4) is used to elevate all the paraspinous muscles as far laterally as the tips of the transverse processes. Typically, 4-8 hooks are affixed to the posterior spinal elements (lamina, pedicles, or transverse processes) on both the concave and convex sides of the spine (Figure 12.7-3). These points of spinal fixation are then joined to two contoured rods. By compressing along the convex surfaces and distracting along the concave surfaces, some degree of rotational correction is possible. Some spine surgeons advise the patient to wear a brace for the initial months following surgery; however, body casts are no longer necessary.

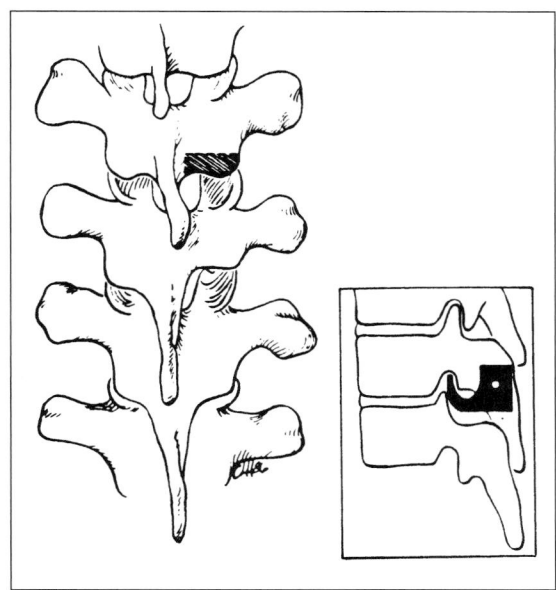

Figure 12.7-3. Placement of a standard pedicle hook, in a hood-rod device. (Reproduced with permission from Chapman MW, ed: *Operative Orthopaedics*, 3rd edition. Lippincott Williams & Wilkins, 2001.)

Sublaminar wire loops (Fig 12.7-4) are commonly used instead of the hook-rod method of spinal instrumentation when treating neuromuscular spinal deformity (e.g., cerebral palsy, muscular dystrophy, myelomeningocele, or spinal muscular atrophy). This alternative construct provides more points of fixation to the spine and eliminates the need for postop bracing. When a large degree of pelvic obliquity is a component of the patient's deformity, the instrumentation often is extended into the iliac wings (Fig 12-7.5).

Somatosensory evoked potentials (SSEP) and **motor evoked potentials** (MEP) are used routinely in centers where spinal deformity correction surgery is common. Close coordination among the surgeon, spinal cord monitoring personnel, and anesthesiologist is necessary to properly recognize adverse intraop spinal events and to minimize the occurrence of false-positive findings. Many spine surgeons also request that an intraop wake-up test be performed to further verify spinal cord function.

Usual preop diagnosis: Scoliosis (usually idiopathic or neuromuscular); kyphosis (increased round back); reconstruction for tumor, trauma, and other

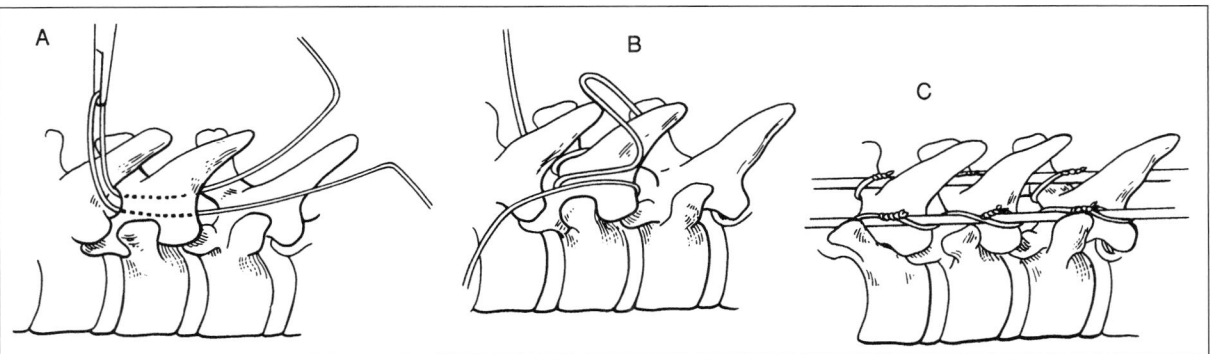

Figure 12.7-4. An example of passing and attaching sublaminar wires. (Reproduced with permission from Chapman MW, ed: *Operative Orthopaedics*, 3rd edition. Lippincott Williams & Wilkins, 2001.)

SUMMARY OF PROCEDURE

Position	Prone (on spinal frame or bolsters); avoid abdominal, elbow, and ocular compression.
Incision	Posterior midline; optional separate iliac crest bone graft
Special instrumentation	Rods, hooks, pedicle screws, wires
Unique considerations	'Wake up' test and/or SSEPs; frequently, induced ↓BP is requested; prolonged prone positioning places brachial plexus and ulnar nerve at risk.
Antibiotics	Cefazolin 1-2 g iv
Surgical time	2-6 h
Closing considerations	Greatest blood loss typically toward the end of procedure. Avoid hypotension after instrumentation is implanted.
EBL	1200-3000 ml
Postop care	ICU: 1-2 d
Mortality	0-0.5%
Morbidity	Acute ileus: Very common
	Genitourinary infection: 5-7%
	Hematoma, massive bleeding: 1-5%
	Pneumothorax, pneumonia, atelectasis, etc: 1-5%
	Hook dislodgement requiring reoperation: 0-2%
	Wound infection: 0-2%
	Superior mesenteric artery syndrome: 0-1%
	Thromboembolism: < 1%
	Spinal cord injury and/or root injury: 0.6%
	Delayed:
	Pseudarthrosis: 0-5%
	Late rod fracture: 0-5%
	Progression of spinal deformity: 0-2%
Pain score	7-9

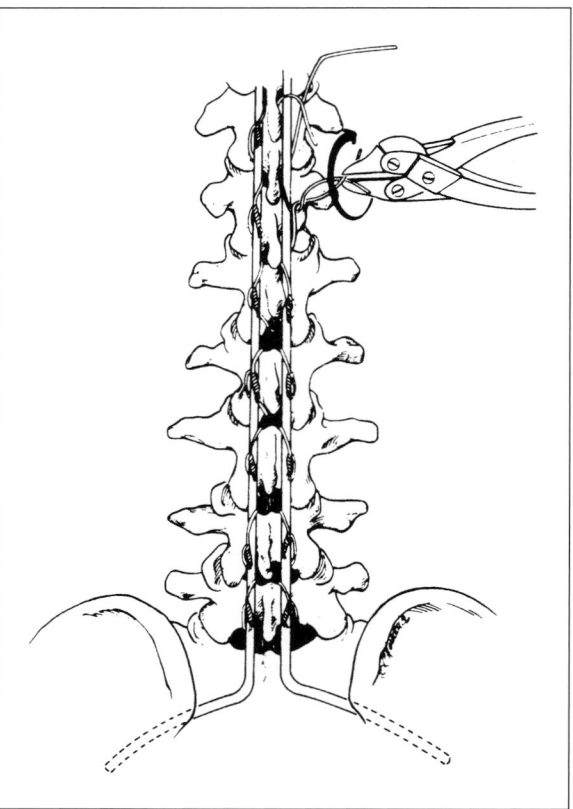

Figure 12.7-5. Positioning rods in pelvis; sublaminar wires being tightened. (Reproduced with permission from Chapman MW, ed: *Operative Orthopaedics*, 3rd edition. Lippincott Williams & Wilkins, 2001.)

PATIENT POPULATION CHARACTERISTICS

Age range	Usually 8-40 yr
Male:Female	1:5
Incidence	1-2/10,000
Etiology	Idiopathic (50-75%); neuromuscular (20-30%); associated with syndromes such as osteochondral dystrophies, osteogenesis imperfecta, etc. (5%); congenital scoliosis (2-5%)

Associated conditions	Neuromuscular:
	  Freidrich's ataxia (myocarditis and other cardiovascular anomalies; sudden death)
	  Myelomeningocele (latex allergy, chronic UTI, hydrocephalus)
	  Muscular dystrophy (muscle weakness, cardiomyopathy, dysrhythmias, succinylcholine → prolonged muscle contraction, ↑sensitivity to respiratory depressant effect of barbiturates, opiates, and benzodiazepines)
	  Cerebral palsy (GERD, ↓airway protective reflexes, ↑postop pulmonary complications, malnourishment, Sz, medication may interfere with Plt function)
	  Higher incidence of MH
	Connective tissue disease:
	  Ehlers-Danlos and Marfan syndromes (avoid ↑BP → aortic dissection; ↑risk of pneumothorax).
	  Osteogenesis imperfecta (position and intubate with great care).
	  Congenital osteochondral dystrophies

ANESTHETIC CONSIDERATIONS

See Anesthetic Considerations for Spinal Reconstruction and Fusion, p. 789.

References

1. Bridwell KHL: Spinal instrumentation in the management of adolescent scoliosis. *Clin Orthop* 1997; (335):64-72.
2. Drummond DS: A perspective on recent trends for scoliosis correction. *Clin Orthop* 1991; (264):90-102.
3. Dubousset J, Cotrel Y: Application technique of Cotrel-Dubousset instrumentation for scoliosis deformities. *Clin Orthop* 1991; (264):103-10.
4. Heller KD, Wirtz DC, Siebert CH, Forst R: Spinal stabilization in Duchenne muscular dystrophy: principles of treatment and record of 31 operative treated cases. *J Pediatr Orthop* [Br] 2001; 10(1):18-24.
5. Thomson JD, Banta JV: Scoliosis in cerebral palsy: an overview and recent results. *J Pediatr Orthop* [Br] 2001; 10(1):6-9.

ANTERIOR SPINAL FUSION FOR SCOLIOSIS ± INSTRUMENTATION

SURGICAL CONSIDERATIONS

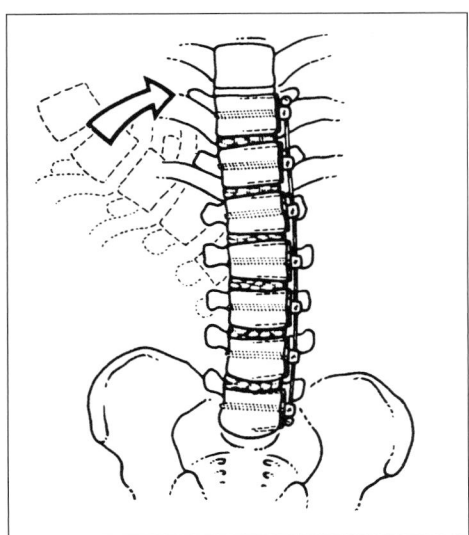

Figure 12.7-6. Dwyer instrumentation used to make spinal correction. (Reproduced with permission from Crenshaw AH, ed: *Campbell's Operative Orthopaedics*, 8th edition. Mosby-Year Book: 1992.)

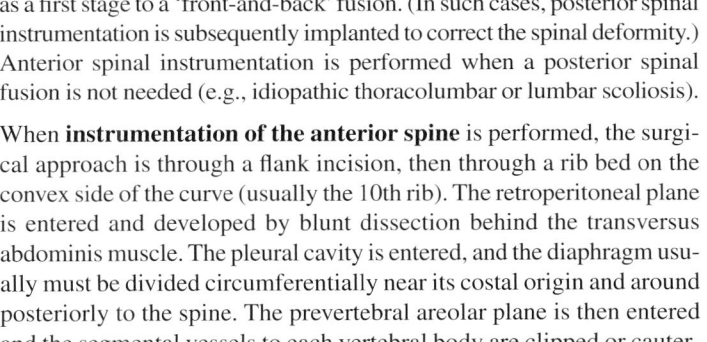

Figure 12.7-7. Instrumentation from T10-L3 (Zielke). (Reproduced with permission from Chapman MW, ed: *Operative Orthopaedics*, 3rd edition. Lippincott Williams & Wilkins, 2001.)

Description: Anterior spinal fusion is performed through a transthoracic and/or retroperitoneal approach to the vertebral bodies, in which the intervertebral discs are removed and a bone graft is placed between the vertebral bodies. The disc removal ('release') loosens the spine and allows greater deformity correction than posterior-only procedures. Often, no instrumentation is used anteriorly when the anterior fusion is performed as a first stage to a 'front-and-back' fusion. (In such cases, posterior spinal instrumentation is subsequently implanted to correct the spinal deformity.) Anterior spinal instrumentation is performed when a posterior spinal fusion is not needed (e.g., idiopathic thoracolumbar or lumbar scoliosis).

When **instrumentation of the anterior spine** is performed, the surgical approach is through a flank incision, then through a rib bed on the convex side of the curve (usually the 10th rib). The retroperitoneal plane is entered and developed by blunt dissection behind the transversus abdominis muscle. The pleural cavity is entered, and the diaphragm usually must be divided circumferentially near its costal origin and around posteriorly to the spine. The prevertebral areolar plane is then entered and the segmental vessels to each vertebral body are clipped or cauterized in the midline. The psoas muscle is elevated off the lateral aspects of the vertebral bodies. Each disc in the fusion area (usually 3-5 discs) is excised back to the posterior longitudinal ligament. Next, vertebral screws (e.g. **Texas Scottish Rite Hospital** [TSRH], **Miami Modular Orthopaedic Spine System** [MOSS], **Universal Spine System** [USS] instrumentation) are inserted transversely across the appropriate bodies and joined at their heads by a rod (Figs 12.7-6 and 12.7-7). Bone graft (typically from the rib harvested during the surgical approach) is placed within each discectomy level. A chest tube is placed before closure of the thoracic cavity.

Usual preop diagnosis: Idiopathic or neuromuscular scoliosis

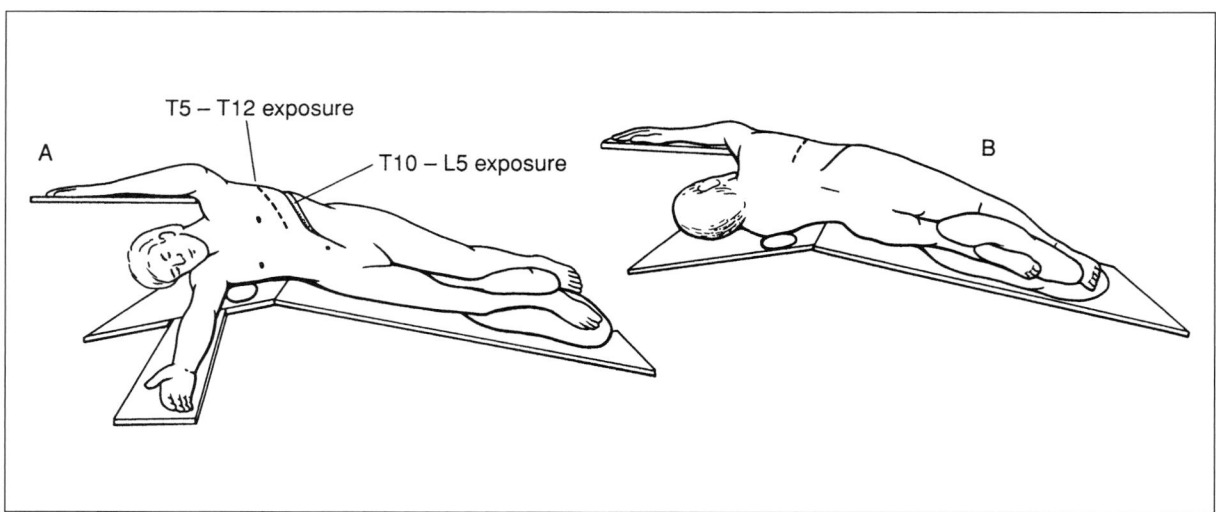

Figure 12.7-8. Lateral decubitus position (diagrammatic) for anterior spinal procedures: (A) anterior view; (B) posterior view. Roll is placed under axilla to minimize axillary artery compression. Skin incision for exposure of T5-T12 is shown with the dotted line. (Reproduced with permission from Chapman MW, ed: *Operative Orthopaedics*, 3rd edition. Lippincott Williams & Wilkins, 2001.)

SUMMARY OF PROCEDURES

	Fusion with Instrumentation	Release (No Instrumentation)
Position	Full lateral decubitus (Fig 12.7-8)	⇐
Incision	Flank: over rib at top vertebra in the curve (usually T9-T11)	⇐
Special instrumentation	Screws, staples, rods	None
Unique considerations	Flex OR table at thoracolumbar junction until disc removal and deformity correction. Procedure often followed by posterior spinal fusion. Proximity of great vessels → potential for major bleeding. Patients with neuromuscular scoliosis often have poor generalized nutrition. SSEP/MEP often used to monitor spinal cord function.	⇐ Uninstrumented release is always followed by posterior spinal fusion with instrumentation.
Antibiotics	Cefazolin 25 mg/kg iv	⇐
Surgical time	3-4 h	2-3 h
Closing considerations	Chest tube always used; hypotension, if used electively, must be reversed before closure.	⇐
EBL	500-2000 ml	250-2000 ml
Postop care	ICU 1-2 d	⇐
Mortality	0-2%, depending on underlying conditions	⇐
Morbidity	Overall: 30%, depending on underlying condition	20%
	Ileus and atelectasis: ~50%	⇐
	UTI: 10-25% (common in spina bifida)	⇐
	Minor transient root weakness, or paraesthesia: 10-20%	1-5%
	Partial sympathectomy: Common	⇐
	Late kyphosis above instrumentation: 5-10%	–
	Nonunion and hardware failure: 5%	–
	Massive blood loss: 2-5%	⇐
	Respiratory failure: 1-2%	⇐
	Pneumonia: 1%	⇐
	Paraplegia (acute anterior spinal artery syndrome): < 1%	⇐
	Thromboembolism: Rare (< 5% in children)	⇐
Pain score	5-8	4-7

PATIENT POPULATION CHARACTERISTICS

Age range	5-35 yr
Male:Female	Idiopathic: 1:10
	Neuromuscular: 1:1
Incidence	< 0.1/1000
Etiology	Idiopathic scoliosis; neuromuscular disease (especially cerebral palsy, spina bifida, polio, myopathies, muscular dystrophies); other genetic bone dysplasias; Marfan syndrome (occasionally)
Associated conditions	See Associated Conditions for Posterior Spinal Instrumentation and Fusion, p. 1094.

ANESTHETIC CONSIDERATIONS

(See Anesthetic Considerations for Spinal Reconstruction and Fusion, p. 789.)

References

1. Betz RR, Harms J, Clement DH III, Lenke LG, Shufflebarger HL, Jesenszky D, Beele B: Comparison of anterior and posterior instrumentation for correction of adolescent thoracic idiopathic scoliosis. *Spine* 1999; 24(3):225-39.
2. Betz RR, Shufflebarger H. Anterior versus posterior instrumentation for the correction of thoracic idiopathic scoliosis. *Spine* 2001; 26(9):1095-1100.
3. Hammmerberg KW, Rodts MF, DeWald RL: Zielke instrumentation. *Orthopedics* 1988; 11(10):1365-71.
4. Kaneda K, Shono Y, Satoh S, Abumi K: New anterior instrumentation for the management of thoracolumbar and lumbar scoliosis. Application of the Kaneda two-rod system. *Spine* 1996; 21(10):1250-61.

PELVIC OSTEOTOMY

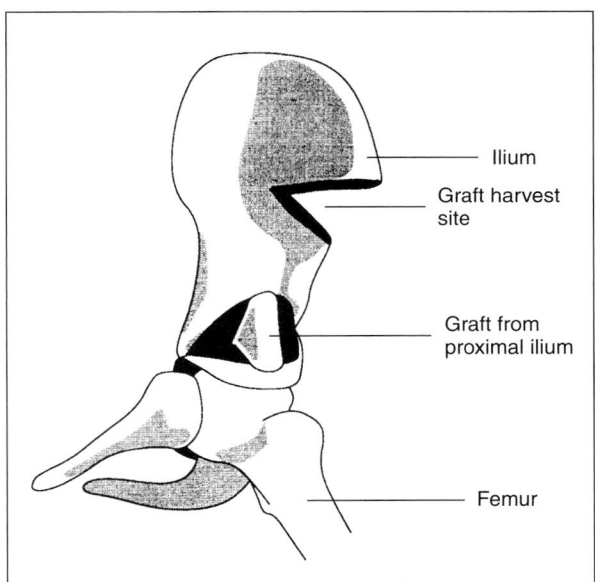

Figure 12.7-9. Pemberton osteotomy: A triangular graft is cut from the proximal ilium, and the graft is carefully wedged into the osteotomy site. (Reproduced with permission from Chapman MW: *Chapman's Orthopaedic Surgery*, Vol IV, 3rd edition. Lippincott Williams & Wilkins, 2001.)

SURGICAL CONSIDERATIONS

Description: Pelvic osteotomy is used to improve hip instability in cases of congenital or developmental hip dysplasia and dislocation by 'deepening' the shallow acetabulum.[7] It is frequently performed in conjunction with open reduction, and occasionally with femoral osteotomy. The surgical approach is made along the iliac crest, always exposing the external (gluteal) surface of the pelvis, and sometimes the internal (iliac) surface. The pelvis is osteotomized closely above the acetabulum, and sometimes through the pubis and ischium as well, depending on the direction of rotation and reorientation desired. Pelvic osteotomies either reorient an intact acetabular hyaline cartilage surface or are designed as salvage procedures to enlarge the acetabulum by fibrocartilage metaplasia (see Acetabular Augmentation, Chiari, p. 1099). **Salter's innominate osteotomy** is the classic reorientation osteotomy, in which a complete cut of the supraacetabular iliac bone allows rotation through the symphysis pubis.[5,11] **Pemberton's operation** is a slightly more difficult incomplete iliac osteotomy, rotating on the triradius cartilage (Fig 12.7-9), which is at the center of the acetabulum in young children.[4] The **Steel**,[8] '**Dial**' or **Eppright osteotomies** are the most difficult reorientation procedures. In each, the acetabulum is freed totally from any bony contact with the remainder of the pelvis and rotated into better position.[7]

Usual preop diagnosis: Acetabular dysplasia due to congenital or developmental hip dislocation

SUMMARY OF PROCEDURES

	Salter	**Pemberton**	**Steel, Dial**
Position	Supine	⇐	⇐
Incision	Oblique or longitudinal anterior hip	⇐	⇐
Special instrumentation	Steinmann pins	Special curved, custom osteotomes	Steinmann pins
Unique considerations	Frequently follows previous unsuccessful open-hip surgery.	⇐	⇐ + Additional ischial incision
Antibiotics	Usually, cefazolin 25 mg/kg iv	⇐	⇐
Surgical time	1.5-2 h	2-3 h	2-4 h
Closing considerations	Hip spica	⇐	⇐
EBL	100-300 ml	⇐	200-600 ml
Postop care	PACU → room; care as needed for spica cast	⇐	⇐
Mortality	Minimal	⇐	⇐
Morbidity	Avascular necrosis of the hip: 5-6%	–	–
	Persistent hip subluxation: ~5%	⇐	⇐
	Infection: < 1%	⇐	⇐
	Sciatic or perineal palsy: < 0.1%	⇐	⇐
	Excess bleeding from superior gluteal artery: Rare	⇐	Occasional
	Ileus: Rare	⇐	Occasional
Pain score	2-5	2-5	3-6

PATIENT POPULATION CHARACTERISTICS

Age range	18 mo-6 yr, if dislocated 18 mo-10 yr, if only subluxated	18 mo-7 yr	> 12 yr
Male:Female	1:2	⇐	⇐
Incidence	0.1/1000	< 0.1/1000	< 0.01/1000
Etiology	Congenital and/or developmental hip dysplasia: 98% Perthes disease: 1%	⇐	⇐
Associated conditions	Torticollis: < 1%	⇐	⇐
	Other joint contractures in cases of neuromuscular dislocation: < 1%	⇐	⇐

ANESTHETIC CONSIDERATIONS

See Anesthetic Considerations for Pediatric Orthopedic Surgery of the Pelvis and Lower Extremities, p. 1121.

References

1. Ganz R, Klaue K, Vinh TS, Mast JW: A new periacetabular osteotomy for the treament of hip dysplasias. *Clin Orthop Rel Res* 1998; 232:26-36.
2. Millis MB, Kaelin AJ, Schluntz K, Curtis B, Hey L, Hall JE: Spherical acetabular osteotomy for the treatment of acetabular dysplasia in adolescents and young adults. *J Pediatr Orthop* [Br] 1994; 3:47-53.
3. Millis MB, Kim YJ: Rationale of osteotomy and related procedures for hip preservation: a review. *Clin Orthop* 2002; (405):108-21.

4. Pemberton PA: Pericapsular osteotomy of the ilium for the treatment of congenitally dislocated hips. *Clin Orthop* 1974; 98:41-54.
5. Salter RB, Duboi JP: The first fifteen years' personal experience with innominate osteotomy in the treatment of congenital dislocation and subluxation of the hip. *Clin Orthop* 1974; 98:72-103.
6. Sanchez-Sotelo J, Trousdale RT, Berry DJ, Cabanela ME: Surgical treatment of developmental dsyplasia of the hip in adults: I. Nonarthroplasty options. *J Am Acad Orthop Surg* 2002; 10(5):321-33.
7. Staheli LT: Surgical management of acetabular dysplasia. *Clin Orthop* 1991; 264:111-21.
8. Steel HH: Triple osteotomy of the innominate bone. *J Bone Joint Surg* [Am] 1973; 55(2):343-50.
9. Tonnis D, Arning A, Block M, Heinecke A, Kalchschmidt K. Triple pelvic osteotomy. *J Pediatr Orthop* [B] 1994; 3:54-67.
10. Vitale MG, Skaggs DL: Developmental dysplasia of the hip from six months to four years of age. *J Am Acad Orthop Surg* 2001; 9(6):401-11.
11. Waters P, Kurica K, Hall J, Micheli LJ: Salter innominate osteotomies in congenital dislocation of the hip. *J Pediatr Orthop* 1988; 8(6):650-5.

ACETABULAR AUGMENTATION (SHELF) & CHIARI OSTEOTOMY

SURGICAL CONSIDERATIONS

Description: Acetabular augmentation is a 'salvage' procedure used to deepen the hip socket when a realignment osteotomy of the pelvis and/or femur would not adequately cover the femoral head.[6,9] This is accomplished by securing strips of cortical cancellous bone graft onto the proximal surface of the hip capsule. The surgical approach is anterior to the hip, elevating the gluteal muscles subperiosteally from the outer surface of the ilium. The reflected head of the rectus femoris tendon is elevated, and a domed-shaped slot is created just above the capsular attachment to the ilium. Abundant cortical cancellous strips of bone graft are then harvested from the upper two-thirds of the outer wall of the ilium. These bone grafts have a natural curve and lie on the convexity of the hip capsule. No internal fixation, other than suture repair, is used to hold the bone graft in place. This creates a large bony augmentation (shelf) over the uncovered femoral capsule.

Variant procedure or approaches: The bone graft may be taken as a large, sculpted, solitary, cortical cancellous strut or wedge, or more commonly, as curved 'shavings' anchored in a dome-shaped slot just above the hip capsule. In the **Chiari procedure**,[1,2,3,5] a complete dome-shaped osteotomy allows lateral displacement of the ilium just above the proximal hip capsule (Fig 12.7-10). The line of the osteotomy corresponds more or less with the slot of the shelf procedure. In either case, the result is abundant bony coverage over the hip capsule, which undergoes metaplasia into fibrocartilage.

Usual preop diagnosis: Acetabular dysplasia (shallow socket) due to congenital hip dislocation or developmental neurologic subluxation

SUMMARY OF PROCEDURES

	Acetabular Augmentation	Chiari Osteotomy
Position	Supine or slightly tilted up (reverse Trendelenburg)	⇐ or lateral decubitus
Incision	Oblique or longitudinal; anterior hip region	⇐
Special instrumentation	Usually no internal fixation; I.I. or intraop x-ray	Two large screws or pins; I.I. or intraop x-ray
Antibiotics	Cefazolin 25 mg/kg iv	⇐
Surgical time	1.5-3 h	⇐
Closing considerations	Unilateral or 1.5 spica cast mandatory	Spica cast (optional)
EBL	100-500 ml	200-800 ml
Postop care	PACU → room. Care as necessary for cast.	⇐
Mortality	Minimal	⇐

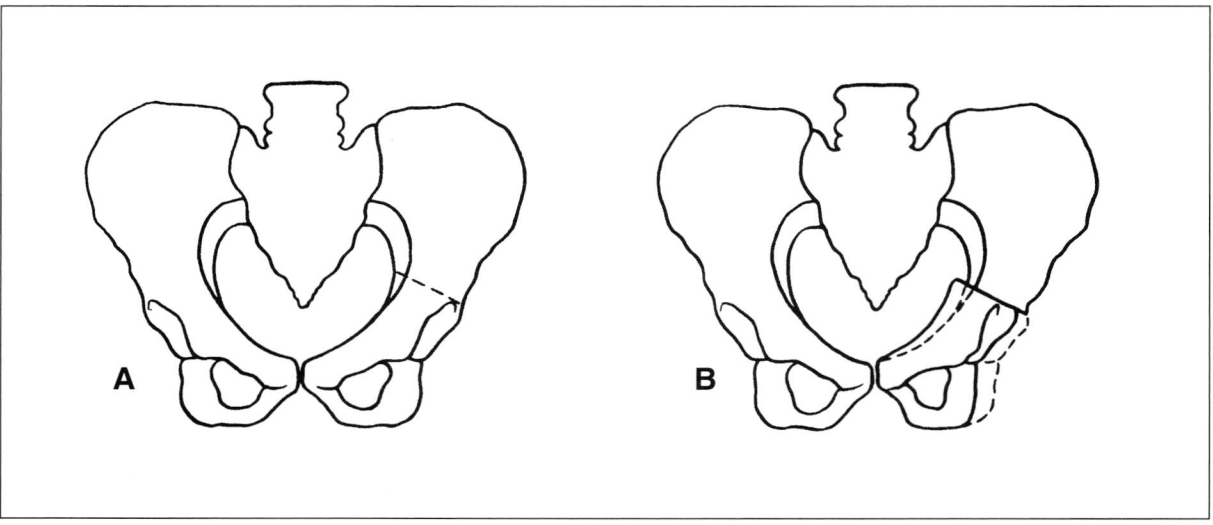

Figure 12.7-10. Chiari osteotomy: (A) Line of osteotomy. (B) Completed osteotomy. (Reproduced with permission from Crenshaw AH, ed: *Campbell's Operative Orthopaedics*, 8th edition. Mosby-Year Book, 1992.)

	Acetabular Augmentation	**Chiari Osteotomy**
Morbidity	Lateral femoral cutaneous nerve dysfunction: 30-50%[6-9]	Sciatic or peroneal palsy: 2%
	Infection: 1%	Possible need[1,2,3,5] for later C-section: Rare
Pain score	4-6	4-6

PATIENT POPULATION CHARACTERISTICS

Age range	6-35 yr
Male:Female	1:1.5
Incidence	< 0.1/1000 in general population; in neuromuscular population (e.g., cerebral palsy, poliomyelitis residuals): ≤ 5-10%
Etiology	Neuromuscular hip subluxation with shallow acetabulum; residual shallow acetabulum (poor coverage from congenitally dislocated hip)
Associated conditions	Cerebral palsy; polio; spina bifida; myopathy; congenital atrophies; Charcot-Marie Tooth disease

ANESTHETIC CONSIDERATIONS

See Anesthetic Considerations for Pediatric Orthopedic Surgery of the Pelvis and Lower Extremities, p. 1121.

References

1. Betz RR, Kumar SJ, Palmer CT, MacEwen GD: Chiari pelvic osteotomy in children and young adults. *J Bone Joint Surg* [Am] 1988; 70(2):182-91.
2. Calvert PT, Augaust AC, Albert JS: The Chiari pelvic osteotomy. A review of the long-term results. *J Bone Joint Surg* [Br] 1987; 69(4):551-5.
3. Chiari K: Medial displacement osteotomy of the pelvis. *Clin Orthop* 1974; 98:55-69.
4. Fong HC, Lu W, Li YH, Leong JC: Chiari osteotomy and shelf augmentation in the treatment of hip dysplasia. *J Pediatr Orthop* 2000; 20(6):740-4.
5. Morrissy RT: *Atlas of Pediatric Orthopaedic Surgery*. JB Lippincott, Philadelphia: 1992, 201-10.
6. Staheli LT, Chew DE: Slotted acetabular augmentation in childhood and adolescence. *J Pediatr Orthop* 1992; 12(5):569-80.
7. Summers BN, Turner A, Wynn-Jones CH: The shelf operation in the management of late presentation of congenital hip dysplasia. *J Bone Joint Surg* [Br] 1988; 70(1):63-8.
8. White RE Jr, Sherman FC: The hip shelf procedure. A long-term evaluation. *J Bone Joint Surg* [Am] 1980; 62(6):928-32.
9. Zuckerman JD, Staheli LT, McLaughlin JF: Acetabular augmentation for progressive hip subluxation in cerebral palsy. *J Pediatr Orthop* 1984; 4(4):436-42.

OBER FASCIOTOMY, YOUNT-OBER RELEASE

SURGICAL CONSIDERATIONS

Description: **Ober's fasciotomy** is performed to release flexion, abduction, and external rotation contracture at the hip.[1-4] This contracture usually occurs as a result of profound flaccid paralysis → prolonged positioning in a so-called 'frog' position of 90° flexion, abduction, and lateral rotation at the hips. This results in tightening of the iliotibial (IT) band (the greatly thickened lateral aspect of the fascia lata) and related structures. The operation is performed through an anterolateral incision just distal to the iliac crest. All of the fascial investments of the tensor, sartorius, and, at times, the rectus femoris and gluteus medias and minimus are divided, while preserving any normal-appearing muscle fibers. The limb is stretched into progressively more adduction and extension, until a neutral position can be obtained. The **Yount procedure** is added when the knee also is contracted in a flexed mode due to tightness of the IT band. The Yount procedure consists of further resection of a segment of the IT band and a lateral intermuscular septum through a separate distal mid-lateral longitudinal incision just above the knee. An oblique segment of the IT band and septum are removed and not repaired.

Usual preop diagnosis: Flaccid paralysis and 'frog'-type contracture due to poliomyelitis, myelomeningocele, or myopathy

SUMMARY OF PROCEDURES

	Ober Fasciotomy	Yount-Ober Release
Position	Supine; both legs must be prepped and draped to well above the iliac crest area for intraop stretching.	⇐
Incision	Oblique iliac crest	Mid-lateral longitudinal above knee joint, ~10 cm
Unique considerations	Patients with sensory and motor loss have a tendency to get pressure sores.	⇐
Antibiotics	Usually none	⇐
Surgical time	1 h/side	30 min/side
Closing considerations	Bilateral above-knee casts	⇐
EBL	< 150 ml	< 50 ml
Postop care	PACU → room; extensive physical therapy program of stretching exercises. Myopathic patients at risk for postop respiratory compromise.	⇐
Mortality	Minimal	⇐
Morbidity	Hematoma: ~1%	⇐
	Fracture of atrophied bone postop: < 1%	⇐
	Infection: < 1%	⇐
	Pressure sores from positioning or casts: < 1%	⇐
Pain score	3-4	3-4

PATIENT POPULATION CHARACTERISTICS

Age range	2-15 yr
Male:Female	1:1
Incidence	Extremely rare in U.S.-born children; however, polio is seen commonly in southeast Asian and Latin-American immigrants.
Etiology	Polio; myelomeningocele; myopathy or dystrophy
Associated conditions	Other contractures; incontinence; pressure sores in myelomeningocele

ANESTHETIC CONSIDERATIONS

See Anesthetic Considerations for Pediatric Orthopedic Surgery of the Pelvis and Lower Extremities, p. 1121.

References

1. Beaty JH: Paralytic disorders. In *Campbell's Operative Orthopaedics*, 8th edition. Crenshaw AH, ed. Mosby-Year Book, St. Louis: 1992, 2412-16.

2. Irwin CE: The iliotibial band, its role in producing deformity in poliomyelitis. *J Bone Joint Surg* [Am] 1949; 31:141-52.

3. Ober FR: The role of the iliotibial band and fascia lata as a factor in the causation of low-back disabilities and sciatica. *J Bone Joint Surg* [Am] 1936; 18:105-19.

4. Yount CC: The role of the tensor fasciae femoris in certain deformities of the lower extremities. *J Bone Joint Surg* [Am] 1926; 8:171-82.

HIP, OPEN REDUCTION ± FEMORAL SHORTENING

SURGICAL CONSIDERATIONS

Description: **Open reduction of the hip** replaces a congenitally or developmentally dislocated femoral head into the anatomic acetabulum, usually after an unsuccessful attempt to reduce the hip by closed means.[1-4,6,7] It often is preceded by traction and always is followed by spica cast. A developmental dislocation presents with a more normal acetabulum and occurs around birth or later. Teratologic congenital dislocation of the hip occurs early in utero; and, as a result, is a high-riding dislocation with a poorly developed acetabulum, presenting much more difficulty in obtaining and maintaining reduction. The most common surgical approach is through an anterior groin incision. The hip capsule is exposed circumferentially, after division and tagging of the origins of the rectus, femoris, and sartorius muscles, and retraction of the tensor and gluteal muscles. The capsule is opened in an oblique fashion, the ligamentum teres is excised, and any obstacle to reduction is removed. The iliopsoas tendon is lengthened; then the capsule is repaired in a 'vest-over-pants' imbrication, with the hip

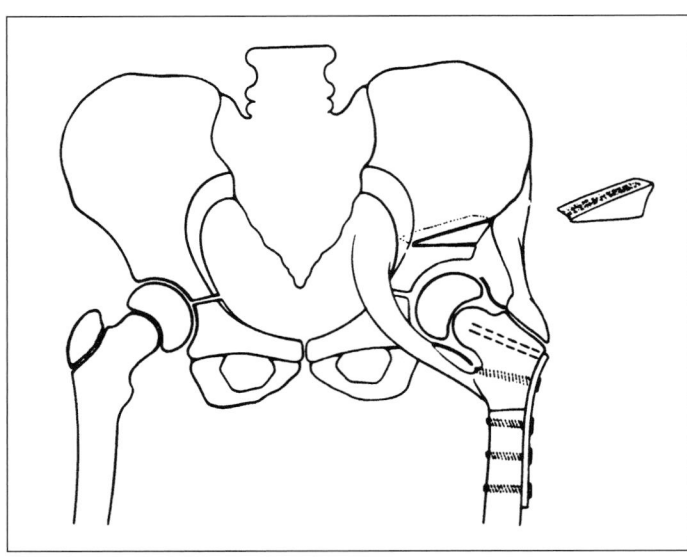

Figure 12.7-11. Open reduction with femoral shortening. (Reproduced with permission from Crenshaw AH, ed: *Campbell's Operative Orthopaedics*, 8th edition. Mosby-Year Book, 1992.)

reduced under direct visualization (Fig 12.7-11). A medial approach through the adductor region can be used in very young children (< 18 mo), but does not allow a capsular repair.[3] If femoral shortening is necessary, the surgical excision is either extended anterolaterally, or a separate lateral incision is made longitudinally over the proximal femur.

Variant procedure or approaches: Most children < 2 yr old can simply have the hip repositioned—closed or open—and subsequently have normal hip development. In older children, especially with a high dislocation, a segment of the femur is removed subtrochanterically to allow reduction without pressure (thus allowing 'descent' of the femoral head). If the acetabulum is very shallow, a pelvic osteotomy may be added.

Usual preop diagnosis: Developmental dislocation of hip; teratologic congenital dislocation of hip

SUMMARY OF PROCEDURES

	Open Reduction	Open Reduction + Femoral Shortening
Position	Supine	⇐
Incision	Oblique groin ('bikini') or medial longitudinal over joint	⇐ + Anterolateral thigh over joint
Special instrumentation	None	Plates and screws
Unique considerations	Preliminary arthrogram and, often, attempted closed reduction. I.I. is used.	⇐
Antibiotics	Usually cefazolin 25 mg/kg iv	⇐

	Open Reduction	**Open Reduction + Femoral Shortening**
Surgical time	1.5-3 h	2-4 h
Closing considerations	Hip spica cast applied on child's spica frame.	⇐
	★ **NB**: Do not wake patient until last radiograph is taken, in case cast has to be reapplied.	
EBL	< 100 ml	100-400 ml
Postop care	PACU → room; care as necessary for spica cast	⇐
Mortality	Minimal	⇐
Morbidity	Avascular necrosis of femoral head	⇐
	Stiffness and late arthritis	⇐
	Limb-length discrepancy	⇐
	Marked scrotal or labial swelling: Temporary	⇐
	Redislocation	⇐
	Infection	⇐
Pain score	2-4	3-5

PATIENT POPULATION CHARACTERISTICS

Age range	Closed reduction: 3 mo-3 yr
	Open reduction: 6 mo-10 yr
	Open reduction femoral shortening: 2-14 yr
Male:Female	1:5 (approximate)
Incidence	1:10,000
Etiology	Genetic background; breech presentation; first-born girl
Associated conditions	Arthrogryposis; Larsen's disease; myelomeningocele; chromosomal anomalies; congenital torticollis; cerebral palsy

ANESTHETIC CONSIDERATIONS

See Anesthetic Considerations for Pediatric Orthopedic Surgery of the Pelvis and Lower Extremities, p. 1121.

References

1. Coleman SS: *Congenital Dysplasia and Dislocation of the Hip.* Mosby-Year Book Inc, St. Louis: 1978.
2. Ferguson AB: Primary open reduction of congenital dislocation of the hip using a median adductor approach. *J Bone Joint Surg* [Am] 1973; 55:671-89.
3. Galpin RD, Roach JW, Wenger DR, Herring JA, Birch JG: One-stage treatment of congenital dislocation of the hip in older children, including femoral shortening. *J Bone Joint Surg* [Am] 1989; 71(5):734-41.
4. Morrissy RT: *Atlas of Pediatric Orthopaedic Surgery.* JB Lippincott, Philadelphia: 1992, 137-54.
5. Moseley CF: Developmental hip dysplasia and dislocation: management of the older child. *Instr Course Lect* 2001; 50:547-53.
6. Rab GT: Surgery for developmental dysplasia of the hip. In *Chapman's Orthopaedic Surgery*, 3rd edition. Chapman MW, ed. Lippincott Williams & Wilkins, Philadelphia: 2001, 4241-58.
7. Schoenecker PL, Strecker WB: Congenital dislocation of the hip in children. Comparison of the effects of femoral shortening and of skeletal traction in treatment. *J Bone Joint Surg* [Am] 1984; 66(1):21-7.
8. Wenger, DR, Lee CS, Kolman B: Derotational femoral shortening for developmental dislocation of the hip: special indications and results in the child younger than 2 years. *J Pediatr Orthop* 1995; 15(6):768-79.

ADDUCTOR RELEASE OR TRANSFER, PSOAS RELEASE

SURGICAL CONSIDERATIONS

Description: The adductor tendon origins and/or the iliopsoas insertion are frequently released in spastic and other neurologic conditions (especially cerebral palsy) that cause crossing of the legs ('scissoring').[1,2,5,7] The goal is to allow greater abduction by decreasing the strength of the adductors and flexors. The releases also are performed for other causes of hip contracture due to developmental hip dislocation, juvenile arthritis, etc. The procedure is always performed on a supine patient through a groin incision, in which the tendons (usually the adductor longus, brevis, and gracilis) are isolated by blunt dissection and divided by electrocautery. In the classic procedure popularized by **Banks** and **Green**, the anterior branch of the obturator nerve is divided on the surface of the adductor brevis to effect more permanent adductor weakness. **Neurectomy** is now less popular because of the fear that the denervated muscle will fibrose into a worse scar. The iliopsoas tendon may be released at its insertion on the lesser trochanter, in the base of the adductor incision; or, just the tendinous portion of the combined iliopsoas may be released at the pelvic rim, which produces a more modest degree of the flexor lengthening. Some surgeons transfer the adductor longus and gracilis muscles proximally and laterally, suturing them to the ischium to convert the adductors to hip extensors by changing their mechanics.[5,7] Theoretically, this is desirable; but it has not proven to be more effective overall than simple adductor release, and is a more complicated procedure.

Usual preop diagnosis: Adduction and flexion contracture of the hip with subluxation due to cerebral palsy, acquired encephalopathy, or progressive neurologic disorder

SUMMARY OF PROCEDURES

	Adductor Release	Adductor Transfer	Psoas Release
Position	Supine	Supine or lithotomy	⇐
Incision	Medial proximal groin, longitudinal or transverse	Transverse medial groin	Anterior groin
Unique considerations	Frequently bilateral; often poor hygiene, especially if severe contracture; proximity to perineum	⇐	⇐
Antibiotics	± Cefazolin 25 mg/kg iv	⇐	⇐
Surgical time	1 h	1.5 h	1 hr
Closing considerations	Bilateral leg casts or double spica cast	⇐	⇐
EBL	< 100 ml	⇐	⇐
Postop care	PACU → room; care as necessary for spica cast	⇐	⇐
Mortality	Minimal	⇐	⇐
Morbidity	Hematoma, drainage Infection: < 1% Recurrence of adduction deformity	⇐	⇐
Pain score	2-4	2-4	2-4

PATIENT POPULATION CHARACTERISTICS

Age range	2-20 yr
Male:Female	1:1
Incidence	0 in general population; ≤ 30% of cerebral palsy patients (0.6-5.9/1,000)
Etiology	Cerebral palsy (90%); slowly progressive degenerative neurologic conditions (8-10%); head injury and drowning (1-2%)
Associated conditions	Multiple other contractures; GERD; poor general nutrition; mental retardation

ANESTHETIC CONSIDERATIONS

See Anesthetic Considerations for Pediatric Orthopedic Surgery of the Pelvis and Lower Extremities, p. 1121.

References

1. Banks HH, Green WT: Adductor myotomy and obturator neurectomy for the correction of adduction contracture of the hip in cerebral palsy. *J Bone Joint Surg* [Am] 1960; 42:111-26.
2. Bleck EE: The hip in cerebral palsy. *Orthop Clin North Am* 1980; 11(1):79-104.
3. Kalen V, Bleck EE: Prevention of spastic paralytic dislocation of the hip. *Dev Med Child Neurol* 1985; 27(1):17-24.
4. Miller F, Cardoso Dias R, Dabney KW, Lipton GE, Triana M: Soft-tissue release for spastic hip subluxation in cerebral palsy. *J Pediatr Orthop* 1997; 17(5):571-84.

5. Reimers J, Poulsen S: Adductor transfer versus tenotomy for stability of the hip in spastic cerebral palsy. *J Pediatr Orthop* 1984; 4(1):52-4.
6. Rinsky LA: Surgery for cerebral palsy. In *Chapman's Orthopaedic Surgery*, 3rd edition. Chapman MW, ed. Lippincott Williams & Wilkins, Philadelphia: 2001, 4485-4504.
7. Root L, Spero CR: Hip adductor transfer compared with adductor tenotomy in cerebral palsy. *J Bone Joint Surg* [Am] 1981; 63(5):767-72.

PINNING OF SLIPPED CAPITAL FEMORAL EPIPHYSIS (SCFE)

SURGICAL CONSIDERATIONS

Description: During the rapid growth period of adolescence, the shearing stress of the body weight on the proximal femoral growth plate may cause the femoral head (capital epiphysis) to gradually move relative to the femoral neck physis (growth plate). The displacement occurs over weeks-to-months, with the head appearing to move posteriorly and inferiorly on the neck. **In situ pinning** (no reduction) is the most common treatment.[2,5,8,9] The goal is to prevent further slipping and subsequent arthritis by causing closure of the growth plate. The procedure must be performed under radiographic control (usually I.I.), using a variety of threaded pins or screws, which are passed through the neck into the femoral head. Currently, the favored technique uses one stout cannulated screw, which is passed percutaneously over a guide wire from the anterolateral aspect of the proximal femur. Traditionally, a small lateral incision was used at the base of the trochanter, with 2-4 pins placed; however, screws now in use are strong enough so that one is adequate for most chronic slips. More importantly, one screw can be placed 'dead center' in the femoral head, avoiding the frequent complication of having a pin penetrate the joint.

Variant procedure or approaches: Although most slips are chronic, occasionally following mild trauma, an acute slip will supervene. Following severe trauma, a previously normal hip with an open physis (growth plate) may suffer an acute displacement, but this is rare. In such acute slips, some degree of reduction may be possible, and two pins are usually necessary. Because pin-related complications are common, some surgeons prefer to close the growth plate by open drilling and curettement, with bone grafting across the cartilaginous plates.[1] This is performed through an anterior incision, opening the hip capsule widely from an oblique groin incision. No pins are used, but an iliac bone graft is placed across the physis. A body spica cast is frequently needed. Once the physis is closed, if there is severe residual deformity, a corrective osteotomy is performed in the trochanteric region (see Proximal Femoral Osteotomy, Southwick procedure, p. 1108).

Usual preop diagnosis: Acute or chronic SCFE

SUMMARY OF PROCEDURES

	Pinning of SCFE	**Variant Open Epiphysiodesis**
Position	Supine	⇐
Incision	Short, proximal thigh or stab incision	Anterolateral groin
Special instrumentation	Guide wires; cannulated screws; I.I.; ± fracture table	I.I. (recommended)
Unique considerations	Frequently bilateral (≤ 20%); often obese	⇐
Antibiotics	Cefazolin 1 g iv	⇐
Surgical time	0.5-2 h	1-3 h
Closing considerations	None	Frequently needs spica cast
EBL	Negligible	200-500 ml
Postop care	PACU → room	⇐ + Body spica cast, occasionally
Mortality	Minimal	⇐
Morbidity	Unsuspected pin penetration: ≤ 37%[5]	⇐
	Avascular necrosis: ≤ 33% (in acute slip cases)	⇐
	Chondrolysis, hip stiffness: 1-28%	⇐
	Fracture after pin removal: < 1%	⇐
	Infection: < 1%	⇐
Pain score	2-3	2-3

PATIENT POPULATION CHARACTERISTICS

Age range	10-16 yr
Male:Female	2-3:1
Incidence	1-3/100,000 (higher in African-Americans)
Etiology	Excessive loading of the growth plate (obesity or increased angle of inclination of the physis)
	Insufficient tensile strength of collagen and proteoglycans around the femoral neck
	Increased thickness of the physis as from excessive growth hormone, hypogonadism, hypothyroidism, hyperparathyroidism, renal osteodystrophy, almost any other significant endocrinopathy
	Radiation therapy
Associated conditions	Obesity; endocrinopathies; renal osteodystrophy

ANESTHETIC CONSIDERATIONS

See Anesthetic Considerations for Pediatric Orthopedic Surgery of the Pelvis and Lower Extremities, p. 1121.

References

1. Aadalen RJ, Weiner DS, Hoyt W, Herndon CH: Acute slipped capital femoral epiphysis. *J Bone Joint Surg* [Am] 1974; 56(7): 1473-87.
2. Asnis SE: The guided screw system in slipped capital femoral epiphysis. *Contemp Orthop* 1985: 11:27-31.
3. Dobbs MB, Weinstein SL: Natural history and long-term outcomes of slipped capital femoral epiphysis. *Instr Course Lect* 2001; 50:571-5.
4. Lee FY, Chapman CB: In situ pinning of hip for stable slipped capital femoral epiphysis on a radiolucent operating table. *J Pediatr Orthop* 2003; 23(1):27-9.
5. Lehman WB, Menche D, Grant A, Norman A, Pugh J: The problem of evaluating *in situ* pinning of slipped capital femoral epiphysis: an experimental model and a review of 63 consecutive cases. *J Pediatr Orthop* 1984; 4(3):297-303.
6. Loder RT: Unstable slipped capital femoral epiphysis. *J Pediatr Orthop* 2001; 21(5):694-9.
7. Loder RT, Aronsson DD, Dobbs MB, Weinstein SL: Slipped capital femoral epiphysis. *Inst Course Lect* 2001; 50:555-70.
8. Morrissy RT: *Atlas of Pediatric Orthopaedic Surgery*. JB Lippincott, Philadelphia: 1992, 212-44.
9. O'Brien ET, Fahey JJ: Remodeling of the femoral neck after *in situ* pinning for slipped capital femoral epiphysis. *J Bone Joint Surg* [Am] 1977; 59(1):62-8.

FLEXIBLE INTRAMEDULLARY NAILING OF LONG-BONE FRACTURES

SURGICAL CONSIDERATIONS

Description: For decades, long-bone fractures in children have been treated by closed methods, such as traction, manipulation, and casting. Recent progress in orthopedic instrumentation and techniques have broadened treatment options, and flexible intramedullary nailing of long-bone fractures in children ≥ 6 yr have become an increasingly popular choice to promote early mobility, avoid cumbersome casts, and achieve successful fracture union.

Flexible titanium nails have been used in France since the 1980s, and have gained popularity in the U.S. since the late 1990s. This method is applicable to both lower- and upper-extremity fractures. Casting is unnecessary in many cases because of the balanced dynamic forces exerted by the elastic memory of the implanted precontoured nails. This is particularly appealing when treating femur fractures that otherwise would require spica casting and prolonged immobility. This technique results in a high rate of fracture union, promoted by the implant load-sharing characteristics with a modulus of elasticity that is close to bone, thereby avoiding stress shielding. The flexible nailing technique for treatment of femur fractures in children also avoids the risk of avascular necrosis of the femoral head because of a more distal entry point on the bone, compared to standard rigid intramedullary nails that enter the medullary canal at the base of the femoral neck, where the primary vascular supply to the femoral head is located.

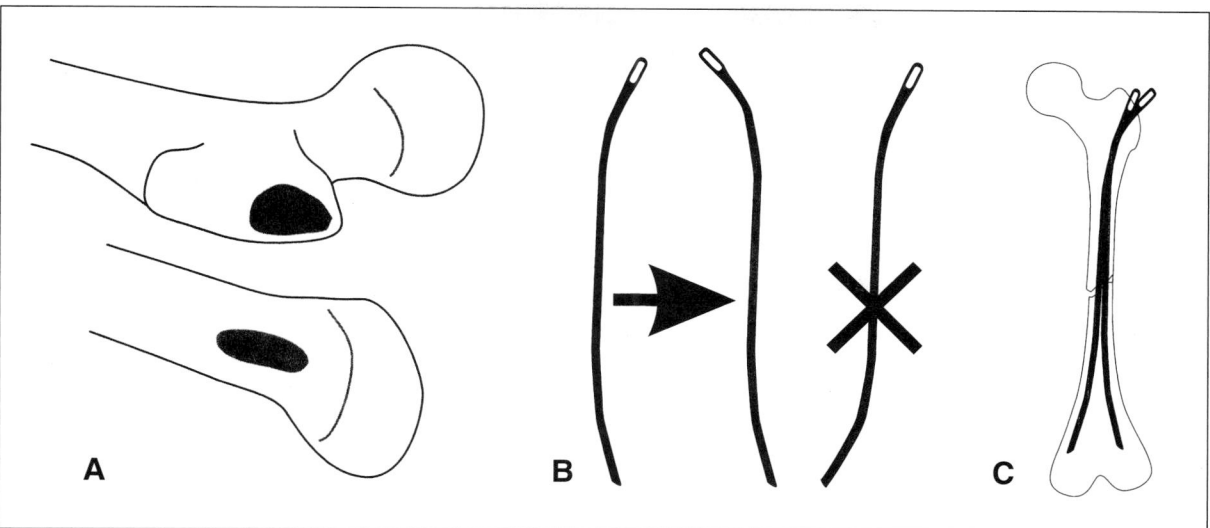

Figure 12.7-12. Intramedullary nailing. (A) Nail entry site through greater trochanter (antegrade) or distal metaphysic (retrograde). (B) Nails are contoured before insertion. (C) Fracture stabilized with two antegrade nails. (Reproduced with permission from Chapman MW: *Chapman's Orthopaedic Surgery*, Vol IV, 3rd edition. Lippincott Williams & Wilkins, 2001.)

The child usually is placed supine on a radiolucent operating table, although some surgeons opt to use a fracture table when treating femur fractures with this method. The surgeon performs a closed reduction of the fracture with I.I. assistance, proceeding to an open incision and reduction only if an acceptable fracture reduction cannot be achieved with closed techniques. Once the fracture is aligned, a small incision for each nail is made on the extremity proximal to the physis at the knee. A drill is used to create an entry point in the cortex of the bone, and each nail is contoured before insertion through this entry point. No intramedullary reaming is performed before nail insertion. The rare need for cast application is judged by intraop imaging for rotational and angular stability.

Usual preop diagnosis: Fracture

SUMMARY OF PROCEDURES

	Closed Reduction	Open Reduction
Position	Supine; may be performed on fracture table if femoral.	⇐
Incision	2-3 cm at entry site for each nail	Incision at fracture site and 2-3 cm at entry site for each nail
Instrumentation	Intramedullary nails, power drill, I.I.	⇐
Unique considerations	Blood loss from fracture; muscle relaxation may be necessary to obtain reduction.	⇐
Antibiotics	Cefazolin 25 mg/kg	⇐
Surgical time	45-60 min	60-90 min
Closing considerations	May supplement with cast.	⇐
EBL	Minimal	50-200 ml
Postoperative care	PACU → room	⇐
Mortality	Rare, except in multitrauma	⇐
Morbidity	Nonunion, malunion	⇐
	Shortening	⇐
	Infection	⇐
	Painful instrumentation	⇐
Pain score	4-7	4-7

PATIENT POPULATION CHARACTERISTICS

Age range	6-14 yr
Male:Female	2.6:1
Incidence	19/100,000 for femoral shaft
Etiology	Trauma
Associated conditions	Usually normal, healthy child

ANESTHETIC CONSIDERATIONS

See Anesthetic Considerations for Pediatric Orthopedic Surgery of the Pelvis and Lower Extremities, p. 1121.

References

1. Hedlund R, Lindgren U: The incidence of femoral shaft fractures in children and adolescents. *J Pediatr Orthop* 1986; 6(1): 47-50.
2. Hinton RY, Lincoln A, Crockett MM, Sponseller P, Smith G: Fractures of the femoral shaft in children. Incidence, mechanisms, and sociodemographic risk factors. *J Bone Joint Surg* [Am] 1999; 81(4):500-9.
3. Mazda K, Khairouni A, Pennecot GF, Bensahel H: closed flexible intramedullary nailing of femoral shaft fractures in children. *J Pediatr Orthop* 1997; 6(3):198-202.
4. Vrsansky P, Bourdelat D, Al Faour: Flexible stable intramedullary pinning technique in the treatment of pediatric fractures. *J Pediatr Orthop* 2000; 20(1):23-7.

PROXIMAL FEMORAL OSTEOTOMY

SURGICAL CONSIDERATIONS

Description: Femoral osteotomy is performed in the inter- or subtrochanteric area to redirect the proximal femur more superiorly (valgus) or inferiorly (varus) and/or for rotational correction of excessive medial/femoral torsion (anteversion). A plate and screws are commonly used, but an **external fixator** and/or spica cast may be placed instead. The usual surgical approach is directly and laterally over the proximal shaft of the femur, beginning at the greater trochanter. The deep fascia is split and the underlying vastus muscle is elevated subperiosteally to expose the femoral shaft. Normally, a power saw is used to make the osteotomy; and, depending on the correction desired, there are a variety of internal fixation devices which can be used.

Variant procedure or approaches: Different named plates (e.g., AO blade, Coventry screw, Richards screw, Wagner, etc.) may be used to affix the proximal to the distal femoral segments.[4,6] A 1-4 cm segment of femur may be removed in cases of superior hip dislocation to allow soft-tissue relaxation and descent of the femoral head into the socket. Most proximal femoral osteotomies are performed in the subtrochanteric area, but some are performed in the intertrochanteric or base of the neck (**Kramer compensating**).[3] The **Southwick osteotomy** is a more complicated example of a subtrochanteric osteotomy, which corrects for three directions (varus, lateral rotation, and extension).[6]

Usual preop diagnosis: Developmental hip subluxation; excessive hip anteversion; residual deformity from Perthes disease; coxa vara; slipped capital femoral epiphysis (SCFE); residual deformity

SUMMARY OF PROCEDURES

	Varus Derotation Osteotomy + Plate and Screws	External Fixator	Southwick or Kramer
Position	Supine	⇐	⇐
Incision	Lateral thigh or, occasionally, long anterior thigh	⇐	⇐
Special instrumentation	Plate and screws; power drill and saw; I.I.	External fixator; multiple pins; I.I.	Plate and screws; power drill and saw; I.I.
Unique considerations	Fracture or radiolucent table	⇐	⇐
Antibiotics	± Cefazolin 25 mg/kg iv	⇐	⇐
Surgical time	1.5-2.5 h	⇐	2-4 h

	Varus Derotation Osteotomy + Plate and Screws	External Fixator	Southwick or Kramer
Closing considerations	Spica cast, frequently	± Spica cast	Spica cast, occasionally
EBL	250-750 ml	⇐	500-1000 ml
Postop care	PACU → room. Spica cast; nonweight-bearing ~6 wk; no full weight-bearing, 3 mo.	⇐	⇐
Mortality	Minimal	⇐	⇐
Morbidity	Persistent hip dysplasia: 5-20% (depending on etiology)	⇐	⇐
	Excess blood loss from a perforating branch of the profunda femoris: < 1%	⇐	⇐
	Infection: < 1%	⇐	⇐
	Loss of fixation, instrument failure: < 1%	⇐	⇐
	Nonunion: < 1%	⇐	⇐
	Persistent hip stiffness: < 1%	⇐	⇐
	Avascular necrosis: Rare	⇐	⇐
Pain score	6-8	6-8	6-8

PATIENT POPULATION CHARACTERISTICS

Age range	2-21 yr
Male:Female	1:1
Incidence	Depending on Dx
Etiology	Coxa varum, coxa valgum due to muscle imbalance; hip dislocation; excessive medial femoral torsion (anteversion); osteochondrodystrophies (dwarfing syndromes); Perthes disease; SCFE
Associated conditions	Cerebral palsy; myelomeningocele, neuromyopathies; congenital hip dislocation; occasionally, hypothyroidism as a cause of SCFE

ANESTHETIC CONSIDERATIONS

See Anesthetic Considerations for Pediatric Orthopedic Surgery of the Pelvis and Lower Extremities, p. 1121.

References

1. Beauchesne R, Miller F, Moseley C: Proximal femoral osteotomy using the AO fixed-angle blade plate. *J Pediatr Orthop* 1992; 12(6):735-40.
2. Hau R, Dickens DR, Nattrass GR, O'Sullivan M, Torode IP, Graham HK: Which implant for proximal femoral osteotomy in children? A comparison of the AO (ASIF) 90 degree fixed-angle blade plate and the Richards intermediate hip screw. *J Pediatr Orthop* 2000; 20(3)336-43.
3. Kramer WG, Craig WA, Noel S: Compensating osteotomy at the base of the femoral neck for slipped capital femoral epiphysis. *J Bone Joint Surg* [Am] 1976; 58(6):796-800.
4. Morrissy RT: *Atlas of Pediatric Orthopaedic Surgery.* JB Lippincott, Philadelphia: 1992, 264-304.
5. Raney EM, Grogan DP, Hurley ME, Ogden MJ: The role of proximal femoral valgus osteotomy in Legg-Calve-Perthes disease. *Orthopedics* 2002; 25(5):513-17.
6. Southwick WO: Osteotomy through the lesser trochanter for slipped capital femoral epiphysis. *J Bone Joint Surg* [Am] 1967; 49(5):807-35.

EPIPHYSIODESIS

SURGICAL CONSIDERATIONS

Description: Epiphysiodesis is performed in skeletally immature adolescents to eliminate or retard growth of the longer limb in cases of leg-length discrepancy (anisomelia). The timing of the procedure[1,7] is critical, based on the child's bone age and discrepancy, which are plotted on a graph or computer program. The procedure is most commonly performed through small incisions (1") about the knee, centered on the growth plate (physis) of the distal femur or proximal tibia. The original **Phemister technique**[8] (Fig 12.7-13) is an approach in which a 3/4"-1 1/4" square or rectangular block of bone is removed using a box chisel centered on the physis, visualized directly. The bone block is rotated 90° or 180° and reinserted, causing a bony bridge across the physis. **Blount**[2] subsequently used stout, reinforced staples to bracket the physis and 'lock it.' This provides a theoretical advantage of reversibility (i.e., if staples are removed, growth may resume if the procedure was performed at too early an age). More recently, a **percutaneous technique** of simply drilling directly across the cartilaginous physeal growth plate, causing a bony bridge, has been used. This is accomplished through small stab incisions, under I.I. control.[6]

Usual preop diagnosis: Limb-length discrepancies of 2-5 cm in adolescents (willing to accept a slight diminution in adult stature)

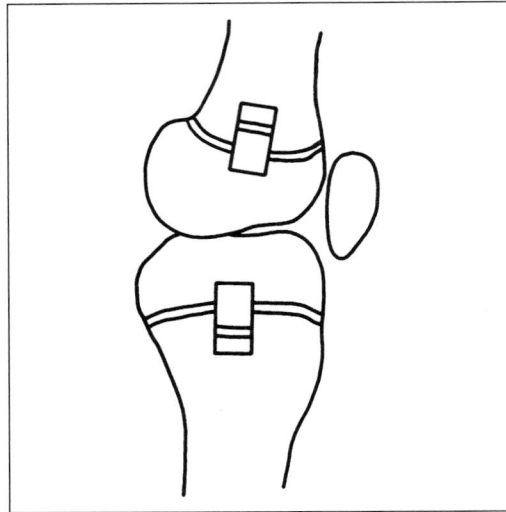

Figure 12.7-13. Phemister method of epiphysiodesis (block of bone reversed, then reinserted to form osseous bar). (Reproduced with permission from Chapman MW: *Chapman's Orthopaedic Surgery*, Vol IV, 3rd edition. Lippincott Williams & Wilkins, 2001.)

SUMMARY OF PROCEDURES

	Open Epiphysiodesis	Percutaneous Epiphysiodesis	Epiphyseal Stapling
Position	Supine, with tourniquet	Supine	Supine, with tourniquet
Incision	3-4 cm longitudinal incision, medial and laterally centered incisions over distal femoral and/or proximal tibial epiphysis	1 cm, same area as open epiphysiodesis	4-5 cm, same area as open epiphysiodesis
Special instrumentation	Box chisel	Drill point and sleeve	Heavy, reinforced staples
Unique considerations	Tourniquet used	I.I control mandatory; tourniquet (optional)	⇐
Antibiotics	± Cefazolin 25 mg/kg iv	⇐	⇐
Surgical time	1 h	⇐	⇐
Closing considerations	Cylinder cast or knee immobilizer	⇐	⇐
EBL	< 50 ml	⇐	⇐
Postop care	PACU → room; crutches for comfort	⇐	⇐
Mortality	Minimal	⇐	⇐
Morbidity	Under- or overcorrection with regard to length: 5-10%	⇐	⇐
	Wound problems: < 5%	⇐	⇐
	Asymmetric growth arrest → valgus or varus deformity: 2-5%	⇐	⇐
	Anterior or lateral compartment syndrome: 1%	–	–
	Fracture: 1%	–	–
	Peroneal palsy: < 1%	–	–
Pain score	3-5	2-3	3-5

PATIENT POPULATION CHARACTERISTICS

Age range	9-14 yr (adolescents, usually healthy with limb-length discrepancy 2-6 cm)
Male:Female	1:1
Incidence	< 1/1000
Etiology	Idiopathic hemihypertrophy; neurologic (e.g., polio, hemiplegia); congenital deformities of the lower extremities (e.g., congenitally short femur, fibular hemimelia); osteomyelitis; development of tumorous conditions (e.g., enchondromatosis); traumatic growth plate injuries occurring near puberty; epiphyseal problems related to hip (slipped epiphysis, sequelae of Perthes disease); Klippel-Trenaunay-Weber syndrome
Associated conditions	Other contractures in neurologic conditions (e.g., polio); neurofibromatosis, AV fistulae; Wilms' tumor (rare)

ANESTHETIC CONSIDERATIONS

See Anesthetic Considerations for Pediatric Orthopedic Surgery of the Pelvis and Lower Extremities, p. 1121.

References

1. Blair VP III, Walker SJ, Sheridan JJ, Schoenecker PL: Epiphysiodesis: a problem of timing. *J Pediatr Orthop* 1982; 2(3): 281-4.
2. Blount WP, Clarke GR: Control of bone growth by epiphyseal stapling. *J Bone Joint Surg* [Am] 1949; 31:464-78.
3. Bowen JR, Torres RR, Forlin E: Partial epiphysiodesis to address genu varum or genu valgum. *J Pediatr Orthop* 1992; 12(3):359-64.
4. Johnston CE II, Beuche MJ, Williamson B, Birch JG: Epiphysiodesis for management of lower limb deformities. *Instr Course Lect* 1992; 41:437-44.
5. Kemnitz S, Moens P, Fabry G: Percutaneous epiphysiodesis for leg length discrepancy. *J Pediatr Orthop* [Br] 2003; 12(1): 69-71.
6. Liotta FJ, Ambrose TA II, Eilert RE: Fluoroscopic technique vs Phemister technique for epiphysiodesis. *J Pediatr Orthop* 1992; 12(2):248-51.
7. Moseley CF: A straight line graft for leg length discrepancies. *Clin Orthop* 1978; 136:33-40.
8. Phemister DB: Operative arrestment of longitudinal growth of bones in the treatment of deformities. *J Bone Joint Surg* 1933; [Am] 15:1-15.
9. Scott AC, Urquhart BA, Cain TE: Percutaneous vs modified Phemister epiphysiodesis of the lower extremity. *Orthopedics* 1996; 19(10):857-61.
10. Stanitski DF: Limb-length inequality: assessment and treatment options. *J Am Acad Orthop Surg* 1999; 7(3):143-53.

SOFIELD PROCEDURE

SURGICAL CONSIDERATIONS

Description: The **Sofield procedure**, or **'fragmentation rodding,'** is most commonly performed for deformity of the long bone, and to prevent recurrent fracture, usually a result of osteogenesis imperfecta.[1-3,6,7] The procedure involves exposure of at least one end and a varying amount of the bony shaft. If the deformity is severe, the entire shaft is exposed via a longitudinal incision, usually laterally. The bone is divided (osteotomized) into the minimum number of segments that will allow a straight intramedullary rod to traverse the segments (usually 2-4 osteotomies). The construct is justly referred to as a 'shish kebab.' It is needed less frequently in the upper extremities.

Variant procedure or approaches: Because a growing bone will elongate beyond the end of a simple intramedullary rod after 1-2 yr, the resulting unsupported portion of the bone will be liable to fracture or new deformity. To obviate this problem, **Bailey** and **Dubow** developed an **elongating rod system**,[1] consisting of an outer tubular rod sleeve (the female portion) and an inner obturator portion (male). Both ends of the telescoping rod are anchored in the ends of the bones. The system elongates much like a car radio antenna and decreases the need for frequent revisions. The surgical technique is, however, identical to any fragmentation rodding, except that both ends of the bone must be exposed.

Usual preop diagnosis: Osteogenesis imperfecta; fibrous dysplasia (occasionally); rickets; congenital pseudarthrosis of the tibia

SUMMARY OF PROCEDURE

Position	Supine
Incision	Lateral for femur; anterolateral for tibia
Special instrumentation	± I.I. table
Unique considerations	Tendency to hyperthermia; other bones may fracture in more severe cases, even as a result of a BP cuff. If dentinogenesis imperfecta is present, extreme care should be taken during intubation to prevent tooth trauma. In these patients, neck motion is often limited.
Antibiotics	Cefazolin 25 mg/kg iv
Surgical time	1-1.5 h/tibia; 1.5-2.5 h/femur (often done sequentially on the same day)
Closing considerations	Double spica cast if femur is rodded.
EBL	Depending on patient age and size, as well as use of a tourniquet for the femur, 50-250 ml; for the tibia, 50-100 ml
Postop care	PACU → room; avoid trauma to teeth, mouth, or other bones in PACU.
Mortality	< 1% (usually related to severe restrictive lung disease, in the most severely involved cases[1-3,6])
Morbidity	Intraop hyperthermia: Common
	Intraop fracture of other bones or teeth
	Late rod migration: Common
	Late refracture: Common
	Nonunion: Rare
	Exuberant callus simulating osteosarcoma: Rare
	Infection: < 1% of rodding
	Radial nerve palsy (in cases of humerus or radius rodding)
Pain score	2-3 (It is surprising how little discomfort these children have, especially the 2nd or 3rd time a bone is rodded.)

PATIENT POPULATION CHARACTERISTICS

Age range	2-25 yr
Male:Female	1:1
Incidence	1/20,000 (osteogenesis imperfecta); other etiologies much less common
Etiology	Congenital (hereditary deficit in collagen synthesis), most commonly as autosomal dominant or spontaneous mutation: All cases
Associated conditions	Dentinogenesis imperfecta; diminished vital capacity due to associated kyphoscoliosis; ↓hearing due to otosclerosis and impingement of the 8th cranial nerve; pelvic distortion causing chronic constipation; basilar impression and other C-spine abnormalities[5] causing brain stem compression or even hydrocephalus (rare)

ANESTHETIC CONSIDERATIONS

See Anesthetic Considerations for Pediatric Orthopedic Surgery of the Pelvis and Lower Extremities, p. 1121.

References

1. Bailey RW, Dubow HI: Evolution of the concept of an extensible nail accommodating to normal longitudinal bone growth: clinical considerations and implications. *Clin Orthop* 1981; 159:157-70.
2. Gamble JG, Strudwick WJ, Rinsky LA, Bleck EE: Complications of intramedullary rods in osteogenesis imperfecta: Bailey-Dubow rods versus non-elongating rods. *J Pediatr Orthop* 1988; 8(6):645-9.
3. Marafioti RL, Westin GW: Elongating intramedullary rods in the treatment of osteogenesis imperfecta. *J Bone Joint Surg* [Am] 1977; 59(4):467-72.
4. Peluso A, Cerullo M: Malignant hyperthermia susceptibility in patients with osteogenesis imperfecta. *Paediatr Anaesth* 1995; 5(6):398-9.
5. Pozo JL, Crockard HA, Ransford AO: Basilar impression in osteogenesis imperfecta. A report of three cases in one family. *J Bone Joint Surg* [Br] 1984; 66(2):233-8.

6. Rodriquez RP, Bailey RW: Internal fixation of the femur in patients with osteogenesis imperfecta. *Clin Orthop* 1988; 159: 126-33.
7. Stockley I, Bell MJ, Sharrad WJ: The role of expanding intramedullary rods in osteogenesis imperfecta. *J Bone Joint Surg* [Br] 1989; 71(3):422-7.
8. Sofield HA, Millar EA: Fragmentation, realignment and intramedullary rod fixation of deformities of the long bones in children. A ten-year appraisal. *J Bone Joint Surg* [Am] 1959; 41:1371-91.
9. Wilkinson JM, Scott BW, Clarke AM, Bell MJ: Surgical stabilization of the lower limb in osteogenesis imperfecta using the Sheffield Telescopic Intramedullary Rod System. *J Bone Joint Surg* [Br] 1998; 80(6):999-1004.

LIMB LENGTHENING

SURGICAL CONSIDERATIONS

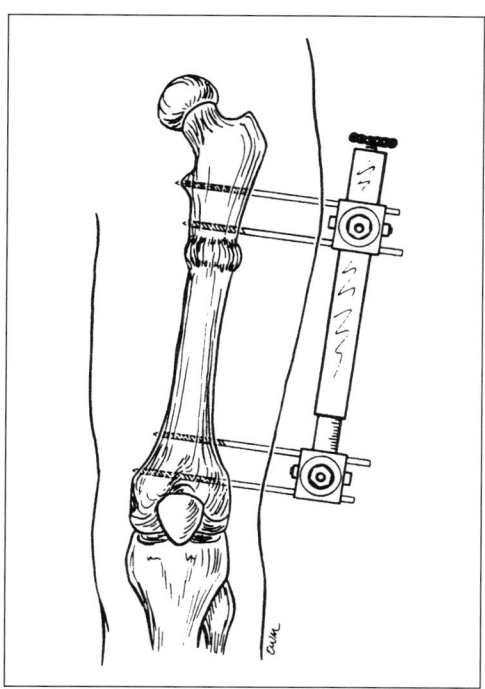

Figure 12.7-14. Wagner apparatus for leg lengthening. (Reproduced with permission from Chapman MW, ed: *Operative Orthopaedics*, 2nd edition. JB Lippincott, 1993.)

Description: Limb lengthening usually is performed in the lower extremity for congenital or acquired leg-length discrepancies of at least 5 cm. Lesser discrepancies are dealt with by bone shortening or epiphysiodesis of the long side. The basic principles include: (1) application of an adjustable, external fixator; (2) 'low-energy,' transverse bone cut (osteotomy without use of a power saw) through a small, longitudinal incision over the involved bone; (3) preservation of the periosteal sleeve; (4) gradual lengthening, usually 1 mm/day in fractional adjustments; and (5) when desired limb length is obtained, either use bone graft and plate acutely, or leave until the bone gap fills in and stabilizes (average 38 d/cm gained).[3]

Limb lengthening dates back to the early 1900s; but it fell into disfavor because of the high rate of major complications.[1] **Wagner** improved the technique by introducing a simplified, unilateral, large-pin fixator, but performed the osteotomy in the midshaft and began lengthening immediately[3,7] (Fig 12.7-14). This technique usually requires a bone graft and later plating as a second operation, to obtain healing. **DeBastiani** uses a similar large-pin fixator (**Orthofix**), but performs the osteotomy more toward the end of the bone (metaphysis), and waits a week before beginning the lengthening.[3] Spontaneous healing is usual. **Ilizarov** introduced a more complex, but more adaptable, small-pin transfixation system with a circular fixator.[2] In a similar fashion, the Ilizarov method stretches the healing callus (callostasis). Typically, 4-10 cm/bone are gained with any of the above techniques.

Usual preop diagnosis: Congenital or acquired anisomelia (limb-length discrepancy) due to overgrowth or growth retardation > 5 cm

SUMMARY OF PROCEDURES

	Wagner	Orthofix	Ilizarov
Position	Supine	⇐	⇐
Incision	Longitudinal midshaft	Longitudinal proximal shaft (metaphyseal)	⇐
Special instrumentation	I.I.; Wagner device (Fig 12.7-13); large bone pins	I.I.; Orthofix device; large bone pins	Ilizarov frame ('Erector set'); multiple 1.5-1.8 mm small-diameter wires
Unique considerations	Acute lengthening may cause ↑BP.	–	Frame should be prepped prior to surgery because of 'fiddle factor.'

	Wagner	Orthofix	Ilizarov
Antibiotics	Cefazolin 25 mg/kg iv	⇐	⇐
Surgical time	1-2 h	⇐	2-4 h
EBL	< 100 ml	⇐	⇐
Postop care	PACU → room; early initiation of physical therapy and/or CPM machine	⇐	⇐
Mortality	Minimal	⇐	⇐
Morbidity	While device remains in place, at least one of the following complications is usual; frequently, several occur before healing is complete:	⇐	⇐
	Joint stiffness or localized pin infection: Very common - 50% (temporary)	⇐	⇐
	Edema, swelling, pressure sores: Common	⇐	⇐
	Joint subluxation: Common	⇐	⇐
	Psychological decompensation due to pain: Common	⇐	⇐
	Premature consolidation: Common	⇐	⇐
	Skin necrosis: Common	⇐	⇐
	Wound infection: Common	⇐	⇐
	Localized osteomyelitis: Common	⇐	⇐
	Axial deviation of the bone: Common	⇐	⇐
	Delayed union, nonunion, late fracture: Common	⇐	⇐
	Pin penetration of a vessel or nerve: Rare	⇐	⇐
	Compartment syndrome: Rare	⇐	⇐
	Sudeck's atrophy: Rare	⇐	⇐
Pain score	7-8	7-8	7-8

PATIENT POPULATION CHARACTERISTICS

Age range	10-30 yr
Male:Female	1:1
Incidence	Dependent on underlying Dx (common in polio)
Etiology	Congenital deficiencies of the lower extremities (e.g., proximal focal femoral deficiency, congenitally short femur, fibular hemimelia, etc.); osteomyelitis, traumatic growth plate injury, fracture; asymmetric neurologic conditions (e.g., polio or cerebral palsy); congenital hemihypertrophy
Associated conditions	Hip and knee contractures; in cases of polio, other deformities, and weaknesses; AVM; congenital or developmental hip dislocation

ANESTHETIC CONSIDERATIONS

See Anesthetic Considerations for Pediatric Orthopedic Surgery of the Pelvis and Lower Extremities, p. 1121.

References

1. Abbott LC: The operative lengthening of the tibia and fibula. *J Bone Joint Surg* [Am] 1927; 9:128-52.
2. Aronson J: Limb-lengthening, skeletal reconstruction, and bone transport with the Ilizarov method. *J Bone Joint Surg* [Am] 1997; 79(8):1243-58.
3. DeBastiani G, Aldegheai R, Renzi-Briviol, Trivella G: Limb lengthening by callus distraction (callotasis). *J Pediatr Orthop* 1987; 7(2):129-34.

4. Murray JH, Fitch RD: Distraction Histiogenesis: Principles and Indications. *J Am Acad Orthop Surg* 1996; 4(6):317-27.
5. Noonan KJ, Leyes M, Forriol F, Canadell J: Distraction osteogenesis of the lower extremity with use of monolateral external fixation. A study of two hundred and sixty-one femora and tibiae. *J Bone Joint Surg* [Am] 1998; 80(6):793-806.
6. Wagner H: Operative lengthening of the femur. *Clin Orthop* 1978; 136:125-42.

PATELLAR REALIGNMENT

SURGICAL CONSIDERATIONS

Description: Patellar realignment encompasses over 100 procedures designed to prevent lateral subluxation and dislocation of the patella. These disorders include a spectrum of malalignments of the patella, ranging from simple excess lateral tilt, recurrent partial subluxation, and recurrent episodic dislocation, to irreducible chronic dislocation.[9] As such, the surgical procedures also encompass a spectrum of complexities, depending on the degree of instability. Nowadays, an arthroscopic inspection often is performed first. The basic principles of the repair include both proximal and distal realignment.[2-9] **Proximal realignment** includes: (1) lateral release, which is the division of the contracted lateral patellar retinacular joint capsule and other tight lateral tissue—the first step in all surgical repair—(2) medial tightening, including reefing and/or advancement of the medial capsule and vastus medialis muscle insertion; and (3) distal realignment, consisting of redirection of the patellar tendon more medially (and sometimes more anteriorly).

Variant procedure or approaches: **Arthroscopic or open lateral release** is the simplest and first-step procedure. It may be sufficient when there is only subluxation and not true dislocation; and it has the advantage of being an outpatient procedure. For frank dislocation, an open 'proximal realignment' also includes the medial tautening. If this is not sufficient to hold the patella centralized, and if the patient has open epiphyses (< 16 yr), the lateral half of the patellar tendon may be released (distal realignment) and reattached medially (**Roux-Goldthwait**); or the patella may be held medially by tenodesing the semitendinosis tendon to it.[1,8] In skeletally mature patients, the bony insertion of the patellar tendon is osteotomized and transferred medially (**Trillat**)[4] or anteriomedially (**Macquet**).[7] The **Hauser procedure** of distal and medial transfer of the tibial tubercle has had a very poor long-term outcome and is seldom performed.

Usual preop diagnosis: Lateral patellar subluxation; recurrent dislocation; congenital or chronic lateral patellar dislocation

SUMMARY OF PROCEDURES

	Proximal Realignment	Trillat	Macquet
Position	Supine, with tourniquet	⇐	⇐
Incision	Anterior transverse or longitudinal or oblique, about the knee, or arthroscopic	Anterior longitudinal	Transverse or oblique
Special instrumentation	None	Single bone screw	⇐
Unique considerations	Tourniquet	⇐	May use iliac or bank bone graft.
Antibiotics	Optional, cefazolin 25 mg/kg iv	Usually, cefazolin 25 mg/kg iv	⇐
Surgical time	1.5 h	1-2 h	⇐
Closing considerations	Cylinder cast	⇐	Skin closure may be difficult, depending on elevation of tibial tubercle.

	Proximal Realignment	Trillat	Macquet
Postop care	PACU → home, if arthroscopic	PACU → room	⇐
EBL	< 100 ml	⇐	⇐
Mortality	Minimal	⇐	⇐
Morbidity	Recurrence: 5-10%	⇐	⇐
	Late stiffness or ↑knee pain: 5%	⇐	⇐
	Superficial wound dehiscence or infection: ≤ 5%	> 5%	≤ 5%
	Anterior compartment syndrome of the leg (Hauser procedure): 1-5%	⇐	⇐
	Deep infection: 1-2%	⇐	⇐
	Peroneal palsy: < 1%	⇐	⇐
Pain score	4-6	4-6	4-6

PATIENT POPULATION CHARACTERISTICS

Age range	2-20 yr (most commonly, 13-20 yr)
Male:Female	1:3[2]
Incidence	Subluxation: Very common
	Recurrent dislocation: Rare
	Congenital dislocation: Very rare[9]
Etiology	Generalized ligamentous laxity; familial tendency; congenital hypoplasia at a lateral femoral condyle; abnormal attachment or contracture of the IT band; medial femoral torsion or genu valgum; trauma
Associated conditions	Diffuse hyperlaxity syndromes (Ehlers-Danlos, Marfan, etc.); nail patella syndrome (hypoplastic nails and dislocated radial heads, as well as hypoplastic patellae)

ANESTHETIC CONSIDERATIONS

See Anesthetic Considerations for Pediatric Orthopedic Surgery of the Pelvis and Lower Extremities, p. 1121.

References

1. Baker RH, Carroll N, Dewar FP, Hall JE: The semitendinosus tenodesis for recurrent dislocation of the patella. *J Bone Joint Surg* [Br] 1972; 54(1):103-9.
2. Bowker JH, Thompson EB: Surgical treatment of recurrent dislocation of the patella. A study of forty-eight cases. *J Bone Joint Surg* [Am] 1964; 46:1451-61.
3. Chrisman OD, Snook GA, Wilson TC: A long-term prospective study of the Hauser and Roux-Goldthwait procedures for recurrent patellar dislocation. *Clin Orthop* 1979; 144:27-30.
4. Cox JS: Evaluation of the Roux-Elmslie-Trillat procedure for knee extensor realignment. *Am J Sports Med* 1982; 10(5): 303-10.
5. Fondren FB, Goldner JL, Bassett FH III: Recurrent dislocation of the patella treated by the modified Roux-Goldthwait procedure. A prospective study of forty-seven knees. *J Bone Joint Surg* [Am] 1985; 67(7):993-1005.
6. Hughston J, Walsh WM: Proximal and distal reconstruction of the extensor mechanism for patellar subluxation. *Clin Orthop* 1979; 144:36-42.
7. Maquet P: Mechanics and osteoarthritis of the patellofemoral joint. *Clin Orthop* 1979; 144:70-3.
8. Morrissy RT: *Atlas of Pediatric Orthopaedic Surgery.* JB Lippincott, Philadelphia: 1992, 425-38.
9. Tachdjian MO: *Pediatric Orthopaedics.* WB Saunders, Philadelphia: 1990, 1551-95.
10. Trillat A, DeJour H, Louette A: Diagnostic et traitement des subluxations récidivantes de la rotule. *Rev Chir Orthop* 1964; 50:813-24.
11. Wall JJ: Compartment syndrome as a complication of the Hauser procedure. *J Bone Joint Surg* [Am] 1979; 61(2):185-91.

TENDON TRANSFER, LENGTHENING (POSTERIOR TIBIAL)

SURGICAL CONSIDERATIONS

Description: Extremity tendons may be lengthened (for contracture) or transferred to change the muscle force vector and compensate for paralysis or paresis of other muscle groups.[2] Originally used for the treatment of poliomyelitis sequelae, these lengthenings and transfers are now used for a variety of deformities 2° more common neuromuscular disorders, such as cerebral palsy, muscular dystrophies, Charcot-Marie-Tooth disease, traumatic nerve palsies, etc. Basic principles are that the muscles to be transferred should be at least grade 4/5 strength, and that the loss of normal function should be well compensated. The posterior tibial muscle (PTM) is a representative example, but many extremity muscles have one or more described lengthenings or transfers. Such procedures frequently are combined with other transfers or fusions.

For moderate spastic ankle varus, the simplest procedure, **PTM lengthening**, is accomplished by an intramuscular myotendinous 'slide.' This refers to simply cutting the tendinous fibers well within the distal muscle belly and leaving a small gap in the tendon, while the surrounding muscle fibers remain intact. An alternative for spastic varus is the **split posterior tibial transfer** of the PTM.[2,6] Four short, 2-3 cm incisions are used to expose and dissect $^1/_2$ of the posterior tibia tendon at its insertion on the navicular. Then, $^1/_2$ of the tendon is passed proximally up its sheath to a second incision just posterior to the distal tibial shaft medially. The freed $^1/_2$ tendon is passed laterally to the peroneal tendon sheath just distal to the lateral malleolus, where, through a final incision, the tendon is anastomosed to the peroneus brevis.

For complete flaccid foot drop (e.g., peroneal nerve palsy), the entire posterior tibial tendon is transferred.[6,7] First, it is detached at its medial insertion, delivered proximally at the distal tibia posteriorly, passed **anteriorly** through a window in the interosseous membrane, and then subcutaneously passed to the mid-dorsal surface of the foot, where it is fixed into the middle cuneiform by a pull-out stitch.

Usual preop diagnosis: Flaccid or spastic developmental deformity, such as varus or valgus foot neuromuscular disease

SUMMARY OF PROCEDURES

	Lengthening	Split Transfer	Anterior Transfer
Position	Supine	⇐	⇐
Incision	Longitudinal posteromedial calf	Medial foot; posteromedial calf; lateral ankle; lateral foot	Medial foot; posteromedial calf; anterior ankle; dorsal foot
Special instrumentation	None	Tendon passer	Pull-out suture; buttons
Unique considerations	Underlying neurologic disease. Usually added to other procedures (e.g., Achilles tendon lengthenings).	⇐	⇐
Antibiotics	Usually none	⇐	⇐
Surgical time	30 min	1 h	⇐
Closing considerations	Below-knee cast	⇐	⇐
EBL	< 20 ml	< 50 ml	⇐
Postop care	PACU or room	⇐	⇐
Mortality	Rare	⇐	⇐
Morbidity	Over- or undercorrection	⇐	⇐
	Hematoma	⇐	⇐
	Drainage: < 1%	⇐	⇐
Pain score	1-3	3-4	3-4

PATIENT POPULATION CHARACTERISTICS

Age range	3-30 yr
Male:Female	1:1
Incidence	Dependent on Dx
Etiology	Poliomyelitis; cerebral palsy, spina bifida; traumatic peroneal nerve injury; neuropathies, myopathies (e.g., Charcot-Marie-Tooth disease)
Associated conditions	Multiple other contractures

ANESTHETIC CONSIDERATIONS

See Anesthetic Considerations for Pediatric Orthopedic Surgery of the Pelvis and Lower Extremities, p. 1121.

References

1. Barnes MJ, Herring JA: Combined split anterior tibial-tendon transfer and intramuscular lengthening of the posterior tibial tendon. Results in patients who have a varus deformity of the foot due to spastic cerebral palsy. *J Bone Joint Surg* [Am] 1991; 73(5):734-8.
2. Green NE, Griffin PP, Shiavi R: Split posterior tibial-tendon transfers in spastic cerebral palsy. *J Bone Joint Surg* [Am] 1983; 65(6):748-54.
3. Greene WB: Cerebral palsy. Evaluation and management of equinus and equinovarus deformities. *Foot Ankle Clin* 2000; 5(2):265-80.
4. Hoffer MD, Barakat G, Koffman M: 10-year follow-up of split anterior tibial tendon transfer in cerebral palsied patients with spastic equinovarus deformity. *J Pediatr Orthop* 1985; 5(4):432-4.
5. Miller G, Hsu JD, Hoffer MM, Rentfro R: Posterior tibial tendon transfer: a review of the literature and analysis of 74 procedures. *J Pediatr Orthop* 1982; 2(4):363-70.
6. Morrissy RT: *Atlas of Pediatric Orthopaedic Surgery.* JB Lippincott, Philadelphia: 1992, 645-68.
7. Richards BM: Interosseous transfer of tibialis posterior for common peroneal nerve palsy. *J Bone Joint Surg* [Br] 1989; 71(5):834-7.
8. Rinsky LA: Surgery for cerebral palsy. In *Chapman's Orthopaedic Surgery*, 3rd edition. Chapman MW, ed. Lippincott Williams & Wilkins, Philadelphia: 2001, 4485-504.
9. Woo R: Spasticity: orthopedic perspective. *J Child Neurol* 2001; 16(1):47-53.

TRIPLE ARTHRODESIS AND GRICE PROCEDURE (EXTRAARTICULAR SUBTALAR ARTHRODESIS)

SURGICAL CONSIDERATIONS

Description: Triple arthrodesis is used to realign the hind foot of skeletally mature patients with significant fixed or flexible deformities of multiple etiologies. The technique involves denuding the cartilaginous surfaces of the talonavicular, talocalcaneal (subtalar), and calcaneocuboid joints and fusing them. The approach is always through an oblique lateral sinus tarsi incision and often an additional short medial incision over the talonavicular joint. For supple (passively correctable) deformities, the fusion is performed easily in situ. Fixed deformities are more difficult; but, basically, any deformity (valgus, varus, planus, cavus, etc.) can be corrected by resecting appropriate wedges of bone. Fixation is usually internal with pins, screws, or staples, in addition to an external cast.

Variant procedure or approaches: Because the triple arthrodesis removes growth cartilage, it is unsuitable in growing children (< 12-14 yr). **Grice** developed an **extraarticular subtalar fusion**[3] which can be performed as early as age 3. It is basically a block of autologous bone graft placed between the talus and the calcaneus to stabilize a valgus heel. Tibial, fibular or, preferably, iliac autologous graft is used through the same lateral sinus tarsi incision as for a triple arthrodesis.

Usual preop diagnosis: Varus or cavovarus foot deformities; severe valgus or equinovalgus

SUMMARY OF PROCEDURES

	Triple Arthrodesis	Grice Procedure
Position	Supine, slightly tilted up on the operative side	⇐
Incision	2″ oblique over the sinus tarsi; optional medial incision	⇐
Special instrumentation	Pins, screws, or rods	Pin or screw
Unique considerations	Intraop x-ray to confirm pin position	Iliac or tibial autologous graft
Antibiotics	Usually, cefazolin 1 g iv	Cefazolin 25 mg/kg iv
Surgical time	1-2 h	1.5 h
Closing considerations	Above-the-knee cast	⇐

	Triple Arthrodesis	Grice Procedure
EBL	< 100 ml	< 50 ml
Postop care	PACU → room	⇐
Mortality	Rare	⇐
Morbidity	Superficial skin slough	⇐
	Superficial infection	⇐
	Nonunion of at least one arthrodesis site (usually talonavicular)	⇐
	Aseptic necrosis of the talus: Rare	⇐
Pain score	6-8	4-5

PATIENT POPULATION CHARACTERISTICS

Age range	> 12 yr (triple arthrodesis); 3-10 yr (Grice)
Male:Female	1:1
Incidence	< 1% (depends on diagnosis and severity of deformity)
Etiology	Neuromuscular imbalance (most cases); congenital malformations (e.g., coalitions, severe pes planus); incompletely treated or overcorrected clubfoot; postfracture of calcaneus or talus
Associated conditions	Poliomyelitis; cerebral palsy (↑GERD, ↓airway protective reflexes, ↑postop pulmonary complications); myelomeningocele; Charcot-Marie-Tooth disease (↑sensitivity to muscle relaxants); congenital tarsal coalition

ANESTHETIC CONSIDERATIONS

See Anesthetic Considerations for Pediatric Orthopedic Surgery of the Pelvis and Lower Extremities, p. 1121.

References

1. Dennyson WG, Fulford GE: Subtalar arthrodesis by cancellous grafts and metallic internal fixation. *J Bone Joint Surg* [Br] 1976; 58(4):507-10.
2. Duncan JW, Lovell WW: Hoke triple arthrodesis. *J Bone Joint Surg* [Am] 1978; 60(6):795-8.
3. Grice DS: An extra-articular arthrodesis of the subastragalar joint for correction of paralytic flat feet in children. *J Bone Joint Surg* [Am] 1952; 34:927-40.
4. Mann RA, Mann JA: Arthrodesis of the foot and ankle. In *Chapman's Orthopaedic Surgery*, 3rd edition. Chapman MW, ed. Lippincott Williams & Wilkins, Philadelphia: 2001, 3057-72.
5. Morrissy RT: *Atlas of Pediatric Orthopaedic Surgery*. JB Lippincott, Philadelphia: 1992, 589-99.

SURGICAL CORRECTION OF CLUBFOOT

SURGICAL CONSIDERATIONS

Description: **Turco** popularized the one-stage surgical correction of resistant (uncorrected by casting) clubfoot (talipes equinovarus) in 1971.[11] The orthopedic literature, however, is replete with reports of varying techniques for surgical correction of clubfoot. The three components of the deformity are: (1) hindfoot equinus (back of the heel is up); (2) varus (rolled inwardly); and (3) forefoot adductus (medial deviation). Beyond this, however, there exists considerable disagreement as to the pathologic anatomy, ideal skin incision, position, and which structures to release. Most surgeons vary the degree of release in proportion to the degree of deformity, often performing release of the same deep structures through totally different skin incisions. The most important structures released include: the entire posterior capsule of the ankle and subtalar joint; capsule of the subtalar, talonavicular, and calcaneal cuboid joints; tendo-Achilles, posterior tibial tendon, and usually the toe flexors; and origin of the abductor, halluces, and the plantar fascia. The navicular is repositioned on the talus and usually held with a small pin.

Variant procedure or approaches: **Turco's procedure**[10,11] is essentially a posteromedial procedure only and is performed through one incision on the medial aspect of the foot. **Crawford**[3] described a much more extensile approach through an incision (**Cincinnati**) that runs from anteromedial, around the back of the tendo-Achilles, and then anterolateral to the calcaneal cuboid joint. This approach is also used by **McKay**,[6] **Simons**[8,9] and others for a more complete release. If there is severe equinus deformity, however, the incision is difficult to close posteriorly when the foot is brought up. **Carroll**[2] accomplishes much the same correction using a separate medial and posterolateral incision.

Usual preop diagnosis: Resistant idiopathic clubfoot; secondary clubfoot due to paralysis

SUMMARY OF PROCEDURES

	Turco	Cincinnati/McKay/Simons	Carroll
Position	Supine	Prone or supine	Supine
Incision	Straight medial foot	Transverse from the navicular bone medially-posteriorly across the heel cord, then laterally to the cuboid	Medial zigzag and posterolateral longitudinal
Special instrumentation	Usually loupe magnification; small K wires to hold reduction	⇐	⇐
Unique considerations	Tourniquet mandatory and often bilateral	⇐	⇐
Antibiotics	Cefazolin 25 mg/kg iv	⇐	⇐
Surgical time	1-2 h/foot	⇐	⇐
Closing considerations	Well padded, loose-fitting, above-the-knee cast × 10-14 d	⇐	⇐
EBL	< 30 ml	⇐	⇐
Postop care	PACU → room	⇐	⇐
Mortality	Rare	⇐	⇐
Morbidity[6-11]	Mild, persistent deformity: Very common Hematoma: 2% Superficial infection: 1-2% Avascular necrosis Overcorrection valgus, planus Pressure changes of the navicula Wound dehiscence or necrosis Transection of posterior tibial nerve or artery branch: Rare (except in previously multiple-operated patient)	⇐	⇐
Pain score	2-5	2-5	2-5

PATIENT POPULATION CHARACTERISTICS

Age range	3 mo-6 yr
Male:Female	2:1 (idiopathic type)
Incidence	1.2/1000 live births (idiopathic type)
Etiology	Genetic, or hereditary effects; neuromuscular defects of the calf muscles; primary defect of formation of the talus and/or other tarsal bones; shortened ligaments and muscles
Associated conditions	Arthrogryposis (difficult intubation; ± VSD, other CHD); Larsen's syndrome (difficult intubation, ± ↑ICP); Freeman-Sheldon syndrome (difficult intubation); osteochondral dystrophies (e.g., diastrophic dwarfism); spinal dysraphism; tethered spinal cord; congenital constricting bands; poliomyelitis

ANESTHETIC CONSIDERATIONS

See Anesthetic Considerations for Pediatric Orthopedic Surgery of the Pelvis and Lower Extremities, p. 1121.

References

1. Beat JH: Congenital anomalies of the lower extremity. In *Campbell's Operative Orthopaedics*, 8th edition. Crenshaw AH, ed. Mosby-Year Book, St. Louis: 1992, 2075-91.
2. Carroll NC: Congenital clubfoot: pathoanatomy and treatment. *AAOS Instr Course Lect* 1987; 36:117-21.
3. Crawford AH, Marxen JL, Osterfeld DL: The Cincinnati incision: a comprehensive approach for surgical procedures of the foot and ankle in childhood. *J Bone Joint Surg* [Am] 1982; 64(9):1355-8.
4. Cummings RJ, Davidson RS, Armstrong PF, Lehman WB: Congenital clubfoot. *J Bone Joint Surg* [Am] 2002; 84A(2)290-308.
5. Lichtblau S: A medial and lateral release operation for clubfoot. *J Bone Joint Surg* [Am] 1973; 55(7):1377-84.
6. McKay DW: New concept of and approach to club foot treatment: Section II – correction of the club foot. *J Pediatr Orthop* 1983; 3(1):10-21.
7. Morrissy RT: *Atlas of Pediatric Orthopaedic Surgery*. JB Lippincott, Philadelphia: 1992, 523-8.
8. Simons GW: Complete subtalar release in clubfeet: Part I – a preliminary report. *J Bone Joint Surg* [Am] 1985 67(7):1044-55.
9. Simons GW: Complete subtalar release in clubfeet: Part II – comparison with less extensive procedures. *J Bone Joint Surg* [Am] 1985; 67(7):1056-65.
10. Turco VJ: Resistant congenital club foot - one-stage posteromedial release with internal fixation. A follow-up report of a fifteen-year experience. *J Bone Joint Surg* [Am] 1979; 61(6A):805-14.
11. Turco VJ: Surgical correction of the resistant club foot. One-stage posteromedial release with internal fixation: a preliminary report. *J Bone Joint Surg* [Am] 1971; 53(3):477-97.

ANESTHETIC CONSIDERATIONS FOR PEDIATRIC ORTHOPEDIC SURGERY OF THE PELVIS AND LOWER EXTREMITIES

(Procedures covered: pelvic osteotomy; acetabular augmentation & Chiari osteotomy; Ober fasciotomy; Yount Ober release; hip, open reduction; adductor release and/or transfer; psoas release; pinning of SCFE; femoral osteotomy; epiphysiodesis; Sofield procedure; limb lengthening; tendon transfer or lengthening; triple arthrodesis, Grice procedure; correction of clubfoot)

PREOPERATIVE

Children undergoing orthopedic procedures of the lower extremities typically fall into two groups: (1) posttrauma but otherwise healthy; and (2) those with a variety of chronic medical problems, including cerebral palsy, congenital hip dislocation, limb deformities, osteogenesis imperfecta, juvenile rheumatoid arthritis, epidermolysis bullosa, and various myopathies and muscular dystrophies. The anesthesiologist should review the anesthetic implications of these various syndromes or diseases (see Table 12.7-2). Many of these patients will have cardiac, respiratory, endocrine, and metabolic derangements, as well as airway abnormalities that may affect anesthetic management. In addition, the surgical procedures may run the gamut from a simple syndactyly repair of the fingers with little blood loss, to pelvic osteotomies (in small children) with blood loss approaching patient blood volume. Patients presenting for SCFE repair are frequently mesomorphically similar. Many SCFE patients are obese and require anesthtic techniques that minimize the risk of aspiration.[10]

Respiratory   Patient's preop activity level is a good indication for baseline respiratory function. Careful assessment is necessary as associated anomalies may affect airway or lungs. Chronic otitis 2° eustachian tube dysfunction is common. Postpone surgery (~2 wk) if Sx of acute URI (e.g., runny nose, fever, sore throat, cough) are present.
Tests: As indicated from H&P (although PFTs are not currently recommended as a routine part of the preanesthetic evaluation of the scoliosis patient).

Cardiovascular   Some pediatric patients with congenital musculoskeletal anomalies presenting for orthopedic procedures have coexisting cardiovascular anomalies. Although this is not common, preop review of patient's H&P is essential. Patients should not be accepted for orthopedic surgery and anesthesia until they are in the best possible physical and emotional condition. For children with CHD or who require cardiac medication, it is advisable to consult with a pediatric cardiologist before surgery.
★ **NB:** The consequences of VAE may be disastrous (e.g., cerebral or myocardial embolization) in patients with R→L shunt lesions. All iv lines, injection ports, and syringes should be air-free.
Tests: ECG; Hct; baseline O_2 sat; chest radiograph, as necessary

Neurological   For patients with cerebral palsy presenting for orthopedic surgery, preop understanding of their intellectual functional capacity is necessary. Information about patient's behavioral or intellectual abilities is usually best obtained from parents or guardian. If patient is on seizure-control medication, it is recommended that the medication be continued until surgery. ✓ levels.

Table 12.7-2. Preop Anesthesia Considerations for Pediatric Orthopedic Diseases

Pediatric orthopedic patients may present with a spectrum of congenital and acquired problems. Congenital malformations and deformations include clubfoot, developmental dislocation of hip, and congenital limb deficiencies. Acquired conditions include trauma, infections, and growth disturbance.

A variety of patients with neuromuscular disorders present for orthopedic procedures and constitute special challenges to the anesthesiologist (e.g., cerebral palsy, spina bifida, muscular dystrophy). Other syndromes and chronic conditions with orthopedic manifestations include osteogenesis imperfecta, juvenile rheumatoid arthritis, and epidermolysis bullosa. The anesthesiologist should review and understand the anesthetic implications of these various syndromes.

Disease	Anesthetic Considerations
Achondroplasia	± Unstable spine: preop neuro and ortho exams are critical. Careful positioning necessary; prevent compression of cervicomedullary junction by placing a bolster under shoulders. Difficult iv access. ± GERD 2° obesity. Anticipate difficult mask fit and intubation. Possible choanal stenosis/narrow nasopharynx; may preclude nasal airway/nasal intubation and placement of NG tube. Smaller ETTs are needed. ± Restrictive lung disease and chronic respiratory infections common.
Apert syndrome	C-spine fusion and small nasopharynx. Hypoplastic maxilla, prominent mandible/cleft palate. Difficult laryngoscopy and ET intubation. ± Tracheal stenosis/abnormal tracheal cartilage. Possible choanal stenosis/atresia; may preclude nasal airway, nasal ETT, and NG tube placement. Difficult vascular access. ± Craniosynostosis → ↑ICP. ± CHD.
Arthrogryposis	Poor cervical mobility; TMJ ankylosis; possibility of difficult intubation. IV access and positioning difficult 2° flexion or contracture deformity. 10% incidence of CHD.
Cerebral palsy	Communication difficulties. Scoliosis → restrictive lung disease. ± GERD. ↑sensitivity to succinylcholine. ↑resistance to NMRs. MAC decreased. Contractures → restricted access for examination and positioning. ± Malnutrition. ± Latex allergy. Difficult iv access.
Juvenile rheumatoid arthritis	Poor cervical mobility; TMJ ankylosis; possibility of difficult intubation. ± Restrictive pulmonary disease. ± Restrictive pericarditis and tamponade.
Klippel-Feil syndrome	Limited C-spine mobility → difficult intubation. Impaired renal drug excretion.
Marfan syndrome	Atlantoaxial instability: evaluate C-spine before laryngoscopy. Care in positioning needed. May require larger than normal doses of spinal epidural anesthesia 2° height. Aortic dilatation → aortic insufficiency ± aortic dissection/aneurysm. Avoid ↑BP. Anticipate difficult intubation 2° narrow palate. Lung cysts → pneumothorax.
Muscular dystrophy	Possible cardiomyopathy: avoid cardiac depressant drugs. ↑sensitivity to muscle relaxants. MH susceptibility. ↓gastric emptying and weak laryngeal reflexes. Avoid succinylcholine. May have MVR and cardiac conduction abnormalities. May require postop ventilation.
Myopathies	Avoid all muscle relaxants and respiratory depressants. Postop ventilation may be necessary.
Osteogenesis imperfecta	Bones fracture easily (e.g., with BP cuff): use extreme care in positioning and intubation. Hypermetabolic fever may occur during anesthesia. Plt dysfunction; difficult airway. Use atropine with caution as it may exacerbate pyrexia. CHD may require antibiotic prophylaxis. ± Difficult airway. ± Restrictive lung disease. Deafness may make communication difficult.
Septic arthritis	Infection/systemic toxicity slows gastric emptying; requires rapid-sequence intubation (p. B-5). Dehydration 2° ↑T and ↓fluid intake → hypovolemia/hemodynamic instability. Rx: adequate fluid resuscitation with balanced salt solution.

References

1. Baum VC, O'Flaherty JE: *Anesthesia for Genetic, Metabolic, and Dysmorphic Syndromes of Childhood.* Lippincott Williams & Wilkins, Philadelphia: 1999.
2. Bernstein R, Rosenberg AD: *Manual of Orthopedic Anesthesia and Related Pain Syndromes.* Churchill Livingstone, New York: 1993.
3. Tetzloff JE, ed: *Clinical Orthopedic Anesthesia.* Butterworth-Heinemann, Boston: 1995.
4. Wedel DJ: *Orthopaedic Anesthesia.* Churchill Livingstone, New York: 1993.
5. Wongprasartsuk P, Stevens J: Cerebral palsy and anesthesia. *Paed Anaesth* 2002; 12:296-303.

Neurological, cont.	All patients who require Ober fasciotomy or Yount release will have profound weakness of lower extremities, if not of the entire body. Must be careful in choice of muscle relaxant (generally avoid depolarizing agents). Many patients with muscular dystrophy present for repeated orthopedic procedures. Patients with congenital muscular dystrophy (especially Duchenne's or Becker's) can have significant associated cardiac dysfunction. A pediatric cardiologist should be involved in the preanesthetic evaluation of their LV function, size, LV ejection fraction, shortening fraction, and ECHO exam.[5] It is important to note that asymptomatic carriers of these X-linked muscular dystrophies can have associated ECHO and ECG abnormalities.[7]
Hematologic	Complications of blood loss remain a major anesthetic consideration in pelvic osteotomies, especially in small children or those who have ↑bleeding 2° osteogenic bone or bleeding disorders. There is no hard-and-fast rule for an acceptable amount of blood loss before transfusion therapy begins; each case must be individualized. Patients who need ↑O_2-carrying capacity (e.g., congenital heart disease, sickle cell anemia (SSA), evidence of V/Q mismatch from preexisting pulmonary disease) will require transfusion at lower levels of blood loss than otherwise healthy children. Blood transfusion therapy must be considered after the loss of 15-20% of the patient's total blood volume. Predonation is limited by age, size, and level of cooperation with blood-collecting techniques. Hemodilution is not used frequently in pediatrics. Cell salvaging can introduce both intracellular and surgical debris back into circulation.[9]
Laboratory	Tests as indicated from H&P.
Premedication	Premedication for separation anxiety (e.g., midazolam) and facilitating induction. Care must be taken if premedication is used in patients with respiratory or cardiac dysfunction. Dosage must be individualized (see p. D-2). Children with valvular disease, prosthetic valves, and/or most forms of CHD, as well as postcardiac-correction patients, should receive antibiotics for bacterial endocarditis prophylaxis preop.[12]

INTRAOPERATIVE

Anesthetic technique: As indicated in the preop considerations, these patient populations cover a vast spectrum, from fit and healthy children to those suffering from a variety of clinical syndromes with airway and cardiorespiratory problems. Thus, anesthesia needs to be tailored to the individual patient. Some older children may benefit from regional anesthesia with sedation. Others may do well with a combined regional/GA technique, while still others with difficult airways may require awake FOL (p. B-6). The following sections address some (not all) of these concerns.

Induction	**Normal:** standard pediatric (< 12 yr) (see p. D-2) or adult induction (see p. B-2).
	Difficult airway: a mask induction and FOL during spontaneous respiration should be considered. Alternatives include use of LMA/intubating LMA, FOL or light wand stylet, retrograde wire intubation, and tracheostomy.
	Muscle abnormalities: these patients may be very sensitive to muscle relaxants, have gastric hypomotility, and may be predisposed to MH. Induction should be accomplished by nontriggering agents (e.g., propofol 1-2 mg/kg and rocuronium 0.5-1 mg/kg) if necessary for intubation. Succinylcholine usually is contraindicated in these patients. Dantrolene must be available, but it need not be administered prophylactically. A study of MH patients showed that 32 out of 89 had preexisting musculoskeletal abnormalities.[2]
	Cardiorespiratory compromise: inhalational induction, when administered cautiously, may be used safely in this group of patients. Intramuscular (e.g., ketamine 4-8 mg/kg im) inductions are usually safe and effective in neonates and infants with severe cardiac disease.
Maintenance	**Normal**: standard pediatric maintenance (see p. D-3).
	Muscle abnormalities: maintenance of anesthesia with a nontriggering agent (e.g., N_2O, opiates) and short-acting NMRs is prudent. A peripheral nerve stimulator should be used to monitor muscle relaxation, as the effects of muscle relaxants may be unexpectedly prolonged.
	Cardiorespiratory compromise: the maintenance of anesthesia in this group most commonly is accomplished by use of inhalational agents, additional narcotics, or other iv agents, depending on patient tolerance and postop plans for ventilatory management.
Emergence	**Normal:** if muscle relaxant used, reverse with neostigmine (0.07 mg/kg) and glycopyrrolate (0.01 mg/kg iv) or edrophonium (0.5 mg/kg) and atropine (0.015 mg/kg iv). Make sure patient is awake and able to protect airway. A vital capacity of > 15 ml/kg is considered an adequate sign of recovery of respiratory reserve.[15]

Emergence, cont.	**Muscle abnormalities:** Anticipate postop respiratory impairment. Suction airway carefully. The response to neostigmine is unpredictable and may precipitate myotonia. Continued postop mechanical ventilation may be required.	
	Cardiorespiratory compromise: Tourniquet release may cause significant ↓CO and ↓BP, requiring temporary inotropic support. Otherwise, emergence as in normal patients.	

Regional anesthesia: Used in patients undergoing lower extremity surgery.

Caudal epidural	In young children, the epidural space can be reached easily by the caudal epidural approach, with less risk of dural puncture than with thoracic or lumbar epidural approaches. There is minimal risk of cord injury at the level of the sacrococcygeal ligament; therefore, GA or heavy sedation is not often required to prevent the child from moving.[1] The dural sac, however, can extend to the level of the third or fourth sacral vertebra in the newborn; therefore, care must be taken to avoid an inadvertent intrathecal injection. Bupivacaine provides reliable, long-lasting anesthesia and postop analgesia when given via the caudal epidural route. Bupivacaine 0.25% with epinephrine 1:200,000 (1 ml/kg) provides 3-6 h of anesthesia for all procedures below the umbilicus. In infants (< 2.5 kg), a more dilute solution is used (0.125% or 0.175%) and the volume can be increased to remain below the toxic dose range. Intraop anesthesia with bupivacaine 0.25% with epinephrine 1:200,000 is given as a bolus with volumes determined by level desired (0.05 ml/kg/segment, not to exceed 1 ml/kg).[13] If no more than 1 ml/kg of 0.25% bupivacaine is given, the plasma levels will be within a safe range.	
Continuous epidural infusion	Use bupivacaine 0.1-0.125% at rate of 0.1 ml/kg/h in patients < 5 yr; thereafter, patients may require 0.05-0.15 ml/kg/h.	

Blood and fluid requirements	IV: 22 ga or greater × 1-2
	NS/LR @:
	  4 ml/kg/h: 0-10 kg
	  + 2 ml/kg/h: 11-20 kg
	  + 1 ml/kg/h: >20 kg (e.g., 25 kg = 65 ml/h)
	Warm fluids.
	Humidify gases.
		There may be rapid fluid shifts in pediatric patients undergoing orthopedic procedures. Close monitoring and adequate fluid replacement will ensure hemodynamic stability. In hip or pelvis surgery, blood loss may be substantial, and adequate iv access is important as blood transfusion may be required.

Control of blood loss	Tourniquet: 120-min limit	Use of pneumatic tourniquets has become common practice in peripheral orthopedic procedures. They reduce intraop blood loss; however, they cause pain and, upon removal, release products of anaerobic metabolism.[4]
Monitoring	Standard monitors (see p. D-1). ± Arterial line ± CVP line Temperature	Most pediatric patients presenting for extremity surgery do not require invasive monitoring. An arterial or CVP line may be helpful, depending on patient's medical condition, length of surgery, and anticipated blood loss.
Positioning	✓ and pad pressure points. ✓ eyes.	Patients with osteogenesis imperfecta or osteoporosis are at risk for fractures and joint dislocations and require special care in positioning.
Complications	MH	Early Sx of MH include: tachycardia, tachypnea, unstable BP, dysrhythmias, cyanotic mottling of skin, rapid rise in T (1°/15 min), discolored urine, metabolic acidosis, respiratory acidosis, hyperkalemia, myoglobinuria. Rx: stop surgery and anesthesia immediately; hyperventilate with 100% O_2; administer dantrolene sodium iv (starting dose = 1-2 mg/kg q 5-10 min; maximum cumulative dose = 10 mg/kg) by rapid infusion. Procainamide (15 mg/kg) over 15 min may be required for dysrhythmias. Initiate cooling, correct acidosis and hyperkalemia. Maintain UO of at least 2 ml/kg/hr. Monitor patient in ICU until danger of subsequent episodes is over (24 h).

POSTOPERATIVE

Complications   MH   For MH considerations, see above.
Respiratory insufficiency

Pain management   PCA (see p. E-3).
Parenteral opiates
Spinal/epidural opiates

References

1. American Heart Association: Prevention of bacterial endocarditis. AHA Committee on *Rheumatic Fever, Endocarditis and Kawasaki Disease of the Council on Cardiovascular Disease in the Young. JAMA* 1990; 264(22):2919-22.
2. Bell C, Kain Z: Acute pediatric pain management. In *The Pediatric Anesthesia Handbook.* Mosby, St. Louis: 1997.
3. Britt BA, Kalow W: Malignant hyperthermia: a statistical review. *Can Anaesth Soc J* 1970; 17(4):293-315.
4. Brownell AK, Paasuke RT, Elash A, Fowlow SB, Seagram CG, Diewold RJ, Friesen C: Malignant hyperthermia in Duchenne muscular dystrophy. *Anesthesiology* 1983; 58(2):180-2.
5. Brustowicz RM, et al: Metabolic responses to tourniquet release in children. *Anesthesiology* 1987; 67(5):792-4.
6. Ceviz N, Alehan F, Alehan D, Ozme S, Akcoren Z, Kale G, Topaloglu H: Assessment of left ventricular systolic and diastolic functions in children with merosin-positive congenital muscular dystrophy. *Int J Cardiol* 2003; 87(2-3):129-33.
7. Glassman SD, Rose SM, Dimar JR, Puno RM, Campbell MJ, Johnson JR: The effect of postoperative nonsteroidal anti-inflammatory drug administration on spinal fusion. *Spine* 1998; 23(7):834-8.
8. Grain L, Cortina-Borja M, et al: Cardiac abnormalities and skeletal muscle weakness in carriers of Duchenne and Becker muscular dystrophies and controls. *Neuromuscul Disord* 2001; 11(2):186-91.
9. Howell TK, Patel D: Plasma paracetamol concentrations after different doses of rectal paracetamol in older children. A comparison of 1 g vs. 40 mg × kg(-1). *Anaesthesia* 2003; 58(1):69-73.
10. Lemos J, Helay W: Blood transfusion on orthopedic operations. *J Bone Joint Surg* 1996; 78:1260-70.
11. Loder RT, Aronson DD, Greenfield ML: The epidemiology of bilateral slipped capital femoral epiphysis. A study of children in Michigan. *J Bone Joint Surg* [Am] 1993; 75(8):1141-7.
12. Melacini P, Fanin M, Danieli GA, Fasoli G, Villanova C, Angelini C, Vitiello L, Miorelli M, Buja GF, Mostacciulo ML, et al: Cardiac involvement in Becker muscular dystrophy. *J Am Coll Cardiol* 1993; 22(7):1927-34.
13. Pullerits J, Holzman R: Pediatric neuraxial blockade. *J Clin Anesth* 1993; 5(4):342-54.
14. Salem MR, Klowden AJ: Anesthesia for Orthopedic Surgery. In *Pediatric Anesthesia*, 4th edition. Gregory GA, ed. Churchill Livingstone, New York: 2001, 617-62.
15. Shimada Y, Yoshiya I, Tanaka K, Yamazaki T, Kumon K: Crying vital capacity and maximal inspiratory pressure as clinical indicators of readiness for weaning of infants less than a year of age. *Anesthesiology* 1979; 51(5):456-9.
16. Tait AR, Knight PR: The effects of general anesthesia on upper respiratory tract infections in children. *Anesthesiology* 1987; 67(6):930-5.
17. Takasaki M, Dohi S, Kawabata Y, Takahashi T: Dosage of lidocaine for caudal anesthesia in infants and children. *Anesthesiology* 1977; 47(6):527-9.

SURGERY FOR EPIDERMOLYSIS BULLOSA

SURGICAL CONSIDERATIONS

Description: Epidermolysis bullosa (EB) is a disabling inherited condition affecting the skin and submucosa. Recessive dystrophic EB is the most common type requiring surgical treatment. Children develop lesions associated with minimal trauma, which most commonly result in contractures of the hands and feet, mouth, and esophagus. Special care is required in handling patients with EB, since minor trauma from iv or ECG lead placement can cause severe blistering. Hand surgery typically involves opening up the contracted fingers by removing the cocoon of epidermis. The defects are grafted with full-thickness skin grafts, typically taken from the abdomen. Following sedation or anesthesia, the affected extremity is gently sponged with dilute chlorhexidine solution. A tourniquet is not applied since it is typically not required. A wrist block is administered by the surgeon. The cocoon of scar tissue is removed, the fingers manipulated to expose the defects, and a full-thickness skin graft is harvested. Generous Bactroban ointment and nonadhesive dressings are placed on the hand and a well padded cast is applied at the end of the procedure. Adhesive tape is avoided throughout the procedure.

Usual preop diagnosis: EB

SUMMARY OF PROCEDURE

Position	Supine
Incision	As necessary to relieve skin contractures on the hands
Antibiotics	Cefazolin 20-40 mg/kg iv
Surgical time	1-2 h. Positioning, iv placement and sedation/anesthesia are time-consuming, often longer than the procedure itself.
EBL	< 100 ml
Postop care	PACU → home. Return in 2 wk for intraop removal of cast, dressing change, and first splint application. Splinting and special gloves are the mainstay of postop treatment.
Mortality	None associated with procedure
Morbidity	Trauma from positioning and monitoring → new blisters
Pain score	7-9 (similar to 2nd-degree burns)

PATIENT POPULATION CHARACTERISTICS

Age range	1-20 yr; older patients with precancerous or cancerous hand lesions
Male:Female	2-3:1
Incidence	Extremely rare
Etiology	Inherited
Associated conditions	Malnutrition; esophageal strictures; generalized skin contractures; malignant transformation of skin lesions

ANESTHETIC CONSIDERATIONS

PREOPERATIVE

EB is a heterogenous group of rare hereditary disorders characterized by blister formation in the skin in response to minor trauma, friction, or pressure. The most minor form of EB is EB simplex, in which the blisters heal without scarring. The junctional form often is diagnosed at birth, with blisters caused by the physical trauma of delivery. These patients develop severe scarring and have a short life expectancy. Patients with the recessive dystrophic form may have strictures of the oropharynx, larynx, and esophagus. Patients may be on long-term corticosteroid treatment. Periop hydrocortisone treatment may be required to compensate for adrenal suppression.

Airway	A careful airway evaluation is essential, since these patients may have a difficult airway 2° mucous membrane and skin involvement in the area of the oropharynx, face, and neck. Patients with EB also may have limited mouth opening and neck movement as the result of scarring and contractures. Poor dentition: ✓ for loose teeth.
Skin	Because of the fragility of skin and mucous membranes in patients with EB, the anesthetic plan should be designed to prevent even the slightest trauma to skin and mucous membranes.
Gastrointestinal	The most common sites of involvement are the oropharynx, esophagus, and anus. Dysphagia, esophageal stricture and constipation are common, and are the major causes of morbidity, nutritional deficiencies, and growth retardation. Esophageal dilatation, insertion of NG feeding tubes, gastrostomy, and colonic interposition have been performed in patients with EB.[3] Esophageal stricture increases the risk of regurgitation and aspiration, and precautions to avoid aspiration should be taken (e.g., Na citrate, ranitidine [1 mg/kg po], metoclopramide [150 μg/kg po]).
Musculoskeletal	Skin lesions can be painful, and some patients will be on chronic opiate medication for pain management.
Hematologic	Chronic blood loss from denuded skin can → anemia and hypoalbuminemia. **Tests:** CBC
Laboratory	Other tests as indicated from H&P.
Premedication	Adequate premedication is essential to minimize movement during induction. An orally administered combination of midazolam (0.5 mg/kg) and ketamine (3 mg/kg) facilitates the atraumatic placement of iv lines in the OR. Glycopyrrolate 10 μg/kg can be given as antisialagogue. EMLA cream can be applied without adhesive dressing.

INTRAOPERATIVE

Patients are placed on sheepskin to cushion pressure points. The following should be available: Albolene liquefying cleanser, Surg-O-Flex (flexible tubular bandage), Vaseline gauze, Zeroform, Kerlix, Webril, cotton umbilical tape, and Coban wrap. No adhesive tape is used. Adhesive portions of ECG leads and electrocautery dispersion plates are removed; the leads and plates are secured to patients, using Webril or Surg-O-Flex. BP cuffs are applied over multiple layers of cotton padding. Carefully trim the adhesive off the pulse oximetry probe, wrap around the palm or finger, and wrap Coban around the probe. Alternatively, use adult clip-on probe. Anesthesia masks, ETTs, temperature probes, and all attached monitoring equipment are lubricated with Albolene. Venipuncture can be difficult, and the iv lines are secured with Vaseline gauze and Coban.

Anesthetic technique: GETA is the preferred method of anesthesia when upper airway manipulation is required or airway protection is compromised. Anticipate difficult airway. Use smaller ETT to avoid formation of laryngeal bullae. ETT and laryngoscope blade should be well lubricated. Smaller than normal LMA has been used, with the shaft and cuff lubricated. Secure tube with umbilical tape. James, et al, reported 309 anesthetics performed on 73 patients with recessive dystrophic EB without the occurrence of laryngeal bullae, postop stridor, or 'airway embarrassment.'[9] The safety of GETA, however, is not well documented in junctional EB patients, where columnar epithelium can be involved. Avoid succinylcholine 2° risk of ↑K^+ 2° muscle atrophy. NMRs prolong duration of action 2° ↓muscle mass and changes in volume of distribution 2° hypoalbuminemia, which results from ill health and poor nutritional status.

IV anesthesia: Ketamine has been utilized for patients with EB undergoing surgical procedures. For iv anesthesia, use a loading dose of midazolam 0.1-0.2 mg/kg with ketamine 0.25-0.5 mg/kg, followed by a continuous infusion of ketamine (1 mg/kg/h) and midazolam (0.1 mg/kg/h). Glycopyrrolate can be used as an antisialagogue in these patients. Alternatively, propofol (50-100 µg/kg/h) with remifentanil (0.05-0.1 µg/kg/h) infusions may be used. Titrate both medications according to patient's response to the surgical stimulation.

Local anesthesia: At our institution, local anesthetic infiltration has not been associated with any serious sequelae; however, Kubota, et al, have recommended against the use of local anesthetic infiltration.[11]

Regional Anesthesia: In some patients with EB, regional anesthesia techniques allow maintenance of airway patency, involve minimal epidermal/dermal damage, and can offer prolonged postop pain relief. Brachial plexus anesthesia,[9,10] epidural anesthesia,[2,14,15] and spinal anesthesia[2,5,14] have been used successfully in patients with EB.

Emergence   Adequate postop analgesia and parental presence in the PACU may help prevent excessive struggling and skin trauma during emergence and recovery. Plastic O_2 delivery masks should be avoided as they have sharp edges. Avoid rectal route for pain management, as it may cause perianal trauma and blistering. Acetaminophen, ketorolac, and opiates can be used for postop analgesia. Pruritus, a common side effect of opiates, should be treated promptly.[6,16]

References

1. Ames WA, Mayou BJ, Williams K: Anaesthetic management for epidermolysis bullosa. *Br J Anaesth* 1999; 82:746-51.
2. Broster T, Placek R, Eggers G: Epidermolysis bullosa: anesthetic management for cesarean section. *Anesth Analg* 1987; 66:341-3.
3. Campiglio GL, Pajardi G, Rafanelli G: A new protocol for the treatment of hand deformities and recessive dystrophic epidermolysis bullosa (13 cases). *Ann Chir Main Memb Super* 1997; 16(2): 91-100, discussion 101.
4. Ergun G, Lin A, Dannenberg A, Carter D: Gastrointestinal manifestations of epidermolysis bullosa: a study of 101 patients. *Medicine* 1992; 71(3):121-7.
5. Farber N, Troshynski T, Turco G: Spinal anesthesia in an infant with epidermolysis bullosa. *Anesthesiology* 1995; 83:1364-7.
6. Griffin R, Mayou B: The anesthetic management of patients with dystrophic epidermolysis bullosa. *Anaesthesia* 1993; 48: 810-15.
7. Herod J, et al: Epidermolysis bullosa in children: pathophysiology, anaesthesia and pain management. *Paediatr Anesth* 2002; 12:388-97.
8. Iohom G, Lyons B: Anaesthesia for children with epidermolysis bullosa: a review of 20 years' experience. *EU J Anesthesiology* 2000; 18:745-54.
9. James I, Wark H: Airway management during anesthesia in patients with epidermolysis bullosa dystrophica. *Anesthesiology* 1982; 56(4):323-6.
10. Kelly R, Koff H, Rothaus K, Karter D, Artosio J: Brachial plexus anesthesia in eight patients with recessive dystrophic epidermolysis bullosa. *Anesth Analg* 1987; 66:1318-20.
11. Kubota Y, Norton M, Goldenberg S, Robertazzi R: Anesthetic management of patients with epidermolysis bullosa undergoing surgery. *Anesth Analg* 1961; 40(2):244-50.
12. Ladd AL, Kibele A, Gibbons S: Surgical treatment and postoperative splinting of recessive dystrophic epidermolysis bullosa. *J Hand Surg* [Am] 1996; 21(5):888-97.

13. Patch MR, Woodey RD: Spinal anaesthesia in a patient with epidermolysis bullosa dystrophica. *Anaesth Inten Care* 2000; 28:446-8.

14. Spielman F, Mann E: Subarachnoid and epidural anaesthesia for patients with epidermolysis bullosa. *Can Anaesth Soc J* 1984; 31(5)549-51.

15. Yee C, Gunter J, Manley C: Caudal epidural anesthesia in an infant with epidermolysis bullosa. *Anesthesiology* 1989; 70: 149-51.

16. Yonker-Sell A, Connolly L: Twelve-hour anaesthesia in a patient with epidermolysis bullosa. *Can J Anaesth* 1995; 42(8): 735-9.

Surgeons

Lonny L. Ross, MD, FRCSC
Stephen A. Schendel, MD, DDS, FACS
Lawrence M. Shuer, MD (*Craniosynostosis*)

12.8 SURGERY FOR CRANIOFACIAL MALFORMATIONS

Anesthesiologists

Louise Furukawa, MD
Gregory B. Hammer, MD

SURGICAL CORRECTION OF CRANIOSYNOSTOSIS

SURGICAL CONSIDERATIONS

Description: Premature fusion of cranial sutures, or **craniosynostosis**, causes various well recognized patterns of cranial vault and facial deformities. Rarely, these are related to conditions such as Crouzon, Apert, Saethre-Chotzen, and Pfeiffer syndromes. Single or multiple sutures can be involved, the most common being the sagittal suture. This condition is called **scaphocephaly**, in which the cranial vault is bitemporally narrow, with AP elongation. **Anterior or posterior plagiocephaly** involves a single coronal suture or lambdoid suture and is characterized by flattening of the forehead on the affected side. **Oxycephaly** ('tower-head deformity') involves bilateral coronal sutures, with a flat, high forehead, whereas **brachycephaly** also involves the cranial base sutures, and results in bitemporal bulging, midfacial hypoplasia, an anterior open bite, and hypertelorism. These patients may have severe sleep apnea and can pose a challenge for airway management. **Trigonocephaly** (triangular head shape) (Fig 12.8-1), with a keel-shaped forehead and hypoteloric tendency, involves the metopic suture.

Surgical correction of these craniofacial anomalies requires a combined plastic surgery and neurosurgery team approach involving the release or resection of the affected suture and simultaneous correction of the asymmetric skull by **bone-flap repositioning or advancement**. Frontal/orbital abnormalities are addressed with **bifrontal craniotomy** and **floating forehead advancement**, along with advancement of the supraorbital bar (**fronto-orbital advancement**) (Fig 12.8-2). For example, in plagiocephaly, because of the unilateral coronal synostosis, the frontal bone is retruded and the superior orbital rim is elevated and retruded on this side. Craniectomy is performed, the forehead is removed, the involved coronal suture is resected, and the supraorbital bar is cut above the orbit and down to the lateral orbital wall across the midline. The bar is bent, advanced on the involved side—sometimes up to 1.5 cm—and fixed in this position. Additional bone strips are taken from the posterior cranium and split for use as graft material; the other bone pieces are replaced and fixed with either wires, suture, or restorable plates.

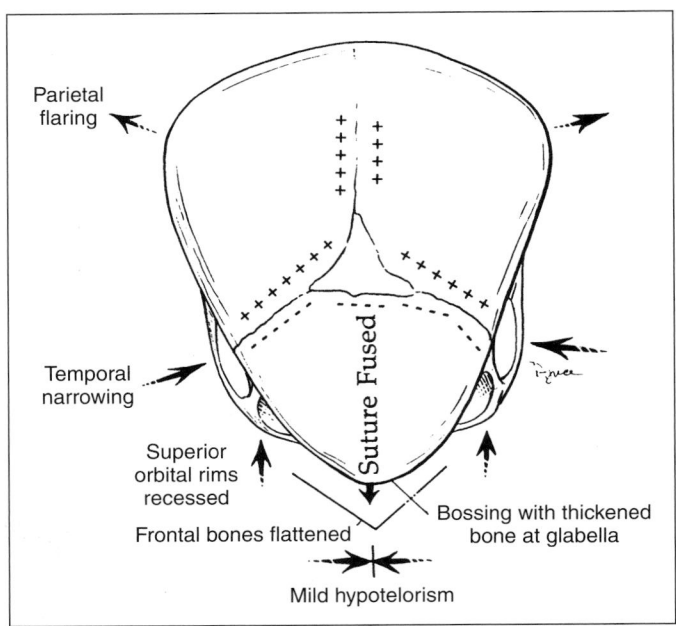

Figure 12.8-1. Skull shape abnormalities in metopic synostosis: Regions of reduced bone deposition (- - -). Regions of compensatory increased bone deposition (+ + +). (From Belfrey ME, Pershing JA, et al: Surgical Treatment of Metopic Synostosis. In *Neurosurgical Clinics of North America*. Pershing JA, Jane JA, eds. WB Saunders, 1991.)

Patient positioning, type of headrest, and incision all vary, depending on location of the suture abnormality. If the deformity is mostly posterior (e.g., a sagittal or plagiocephaly case), a prone approach with biparietal or midsagittal incision can be used. Resection of the involved suture and **barrel staving** of the cranium, with grafting for reshaping, works well. Reconstruction as above usually is accomplished at ~3-6 mo of age. Brain mass doubles in size the first 6 mo and triples by age 3 yr, when ~80% of the brain growth is completed (the driving force for cranial vault growth).

All procedures are extradural. Dural tears, if they occur, are repaired to prevent CSF leak and CNS infection.

In the syndromic cases, the cranial synostosis deformity is treated similarly to the procedure described, usually before the age of 12 mo, with a view to midfacial advancement at maturity of the primary dentition either by **LeFort III or monobloc advancement**. (See LeFort Osteotomies, p. 902, and Major Secondary Craniofacial Surgical Procedures, p. 1134.)

Postsurgical orthopedic distraction devices like the **Delaire mask** also can be used to encourage midfacial growth. The syndromic cases may require repeat craniotomy and reshaping at a young age if signs of ↑ICP appear. Other synostotic cases also should be monitored for ↑ICP and the need for urgent secondary craniotomy. Marchac and Renier detected ↑ICP in 13% of single-suture synostosis and 42% of multisuture synostosis.[5] ↑ICP may increase the risk of dural breach during craniotomy 2° cranial bone resorption and thinning.

Blood loss can be significant at first incision through the vessel-rich scalp. Rainey clips are applied immediately to minimize blood loss. In anticipation of major blood loss, transfusion should be started with the first incision. Severe life-threatening

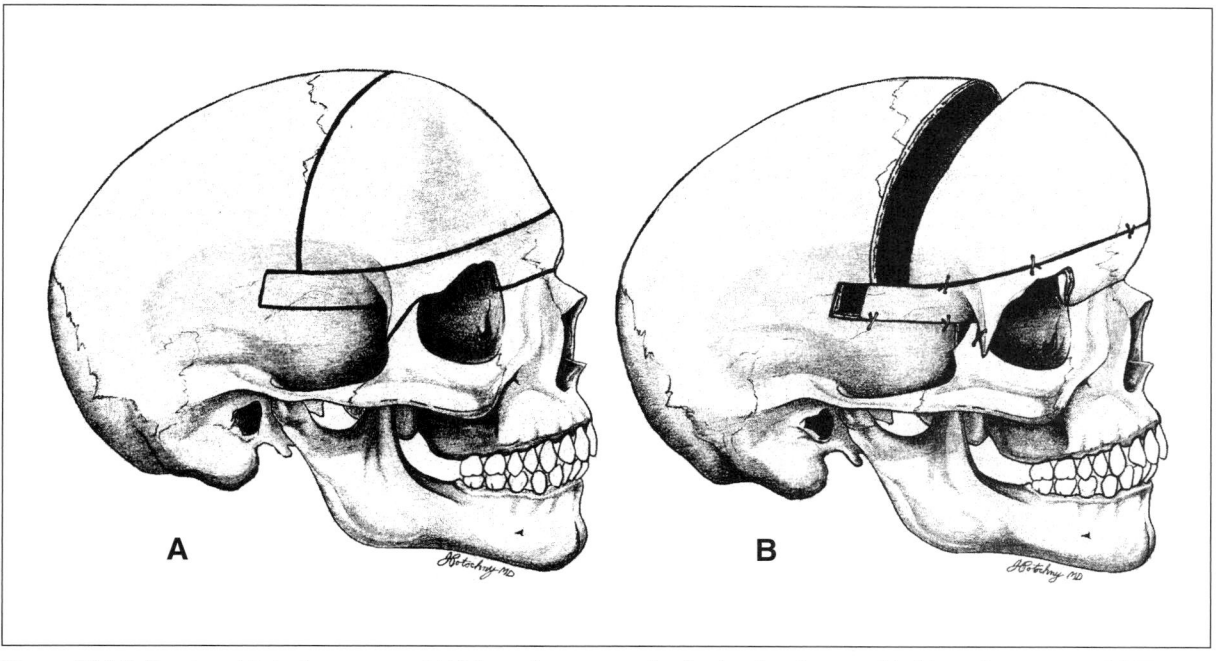

Figure 12.8-2. Fronto-orbital advancement. (A) Lines of osteotomy for forehead and supraorbital bar advancement. (B) Fronto-orbital advancement in a tongue-in-groove manner and fixation with wires. (Reproduced with permission from Aston SJ, Beasley RW, Thorne CH, eds: *Grabb and Smith's Plastic Surgery*, 5th edition. Lippincott-Raven, 1997.)

blood loss can occur if the sagittal sinus is breached, and neurosurgical repair must be accomplished quickly. Elevation of the bone flaps usually causes diffuse bleeding, which is stopped easily with irrigated bipolar cautery and thrombin-soaked sponges. It is useful to have the patient in the reverse Trendelenburg position from the start. Diffuse bleeding at the cut bone edges and over the bone surfaces can be further controlled with bone wax. Focal bleeding from around the orbit and in the temporal fossa region subperiosteally also can be controlled with bone wax. A LeFort/monobloc component to the surgery increases blood loss, especially during the initial mobilization of the facial segment. Local anesthetic with epinephrine injected, and/or on sponge packs for pressure, will control the diffuse mucosal bleeding. BP control is also paramount. Electrocautery and Ligaclips to larger vessels (e.g., descending palatine pedicles) may be necessary.

Variant procedure or approaches: In older children (> 2 yr), split cranial bone grafts may be required to correct defects caused by bone-flap advancement. Excision of skull segments is commonly accompanied by rigid fixation.

Usual preop diagnosis: Craniosynostosis (sagittal, coronal, metopic, lambdoid); syndromes such as Apert and Crouzon syndromes; ↑ICP

SUMMARY OF PROCEDURE

Position	Usually supine; prone for correction of lambdoidal suture synostosis or posterior sagittal synostosis. If entire cranial vault reshaping (multiple sutures), special padded occipital-cheek headrest, since pin fixation is not safe until > 2 yr.
Incision	Usually bicoronal, biparietal, Meisterschnitt, midsagittal
Special instrumentation	Horseshoe headrest, usually pediatric; occasionally, Gardiner tongs; Midas Rex craniotome; resorbable plates and screws
Unique considerations	Control of ICP – spinal drain may be placed. Blood in room, if transfusion anticipated.
Antibiotics	Pediatric: cefazolin 25 mg/kg q 8 h, or vancomycin 10-15 mg/kg q 6 h, and cefotaxime 25-50 mg/kg q 6 h for oropharyngeal contamination and following dural tears
Surgical time	2-6 h
Closing considerations	Blood loss with Rainey clip removal. Full head-wrap dressing causes head/neck movement → bucking.
EBL	200-800 ml; may be formidable.
Postop care	ICU: 1-2 d (further transfusion often necessary in 1st 2 h to replace drain losses)
Mortality	0.6-1.6%

Morbidity	Major complications: 14.3%
	Bone infection: 3-7%
	Meningitis
	CSF leak: 4.5%
	↑ICP
	Air embolus: < 1%
	Blindness: < 1%
	Massive bleeding: < 1%
	Venous thrombosis
	Neurologic injury: Rare
Pain score	4

PATIENT POPULATION CHARACTERISTICS

Age range	2-24 mo (primary correction)
Male:Female	1:1
Incidence	Non syndromic: 1/10,000 births (most sporadic; few familial patterns)
	Crouzon syndrome: 1/25,000
	Apert syndrome: 1/100,000
Etiology	Idiopathic; however, some are associated with specific genetic conditions (e.g., Crouzon and Apert syndromes). Other cases may be 2° ↓ brain growth.
Associated conditions	Hydrocephalus; ↑ICP; mental retardation; airway problems; ocular abnormalities; exotropia (29% Crouzon or Apert syndromes); lagophthalmus; exorbitism

---

ANESTHETIC CONSIDERATIONS

PREOPERATIVE

Patients may have craniofacial anomalies—particularly Apert and Crouzon syndromes—which are associated with mid-face hypoplasia and difficult intubation. Hence, detailed preop airway evaluation is necessary. Children with single-suture craniosynostosis are usually healthy. Surgery is often performed between 3-6 mo of age, preferably when the infant weighs > 5 kg.

Respiratory	Patients with long-standing upper airway obstruction due to choanal atresia, mandibular and maxillary hypoplasia, or other causes, may have chronic hypoventilation and hypoxia and may experience episodes of apnea. If the patient has Sx of acute URI, delay elective surgery at least 2 wk. The presence of fever, cough, and abnormal chest auscultation necessitates radiographic evaluation and pediatric consultation.
	Tests: As indicated from H&P.
Airway	Be aware of other congenital anomalies affecting the patient's airway, such as Apert, Klippel-Feil, Goldenhar, Pierre Robin, Treacher Collins, or Crouzon syndromes. Review any previous anesthetic records for patient to gain insights into appropriate airway management (e.g., FOI may be necessary). Consider elective tracheostomy under local anesthesia in patients with severe airway abnormalities.
Cardiovascular	Consider the coexistence of congenital cardiopulmonary anomalies, particularly in patients with Apert syndrome (autosomal dominant trait, craniosynostosis, syndactyly of hands and feet). Preop evaluation of a patient with a known or suspected heart defect should include thorough H&P, ECG, Hct, baseline O_2 sat, and CXR. For children with Sx of cardiac dysfunction or those requiring cardiac medication, it is advisable to consult with a pediatric cardiologist to optimize the patient's condition prior to surgery.
	Tests: Preop ECG indicated for patients with CHD; others as indicated from H&P.
Neurological	If only the sagittal suture is involved, ICP is usually normal. If more than one suture is involved, brain growth will be impaired, the patient will be developmentally retarded, and intracranial HTN may be present.
Hematologic	Surgery in early infancy (< 9 mo) is common; thus, allowable blood loss is small; blood transfusion usually is required.
	Tests: Hct; PT; PTT; T&C blood.

Laboratory	Other tests as indicated from H&P.
Premedication	Patients < 12 mo old usually do not require premedication. Antibiotic prophylaxis for CHD (e.g., ampicillin 25 mg/kg + gentamicin 2.5 mg/kg iv).

INTRAOPERATIVE

Anesthetic technique: GETA. Anticipate possible difficult airway. Heat OR to 78-80°.

Induction	Surgery for craniectomies is extradural. Either mask induction with N_2O and inhalational agent or iv induction is suitable for the infant with a normal airway. For a difficult airway, intubation may be facilitated by using a FOI while patient is awake or anesthetized and spontaneously ventilating. In rare situations, tracheostomy, under sedation and local anesthesia, may be necessary. Consider suturing ETT to prevent accidental extubation.
Maintenance	Maintenance anesthesia with inhalational agent, or balanced anesthesia and long-acting muscle relaxant, should be adequate. Surgery may be prolonged. Control of ICP may be necessary (see below). A remifentanil infusion 100-500 ng/kg/min provides profound intraop analgesia and rapid awakening.
Emergence	Prompt awakening to allow neurological evaluation is an important goal.

Blood and fluid requirements	Anticipate large blood loss.
	IV: 18 ga × 1-2
	LR @:
	  4 ml/kg/h – 0-10 kg
	  + 2 ml/kg/h – 11-20 kg
	  + 1 ml/kg/h – > 20 kg
	  (e.g., 25 kg = 65 ml/h)
	Warm all fluids.
	Humidify gases.
		Have 1-2 U PRBC or whole blood available. Use LR for replacing deficit, maintenance, and 3rd-space fluid loss. Replace blood loss with colloid and PRBC ml for ml. Significant blood loss begins with scalp incision; allowable blood loss is small, so that it is important to begin transfusion early before hypovolemia occurs.[2] EBV for an infant in this age group is 75 ml/kg. A good rule is to infuse a volume of blood equal to 10% of EBV prior to incision in the healthy infant. Avoid NS (acidosis, ↑bleeding) in children < 5 yr. Beware of ↑K^+ and ↓Ca^{++} associated with massive transfusion.

Control of ICP	Hyperventilation Osmotic diuretic Loop diuretic	In some cases, it may be desirable to ↓ ICP. This can be accomplished by ↑ventilation ($PaCO_2$ = 25-30 mmHg), diuretics (furosemide 1 mg/kg iv).
Monitoring	Standard monitors (see p. D-1). ± Arterial line ± CVP line ± Precordial Doppler[4] ± Urinary catheter	Arterial cannulation for continuous monitoring of ABG, Hct, electrolytes, etc. ↑K^+ and ↓Ca^{++} are most common following transfusion with whole blood or FFP. VAE has been reported during craniectomies in infants; hence, a precordial Doppler and CVP line will be helpful. CVP may be particularly helpful in the infant with marginal cardiovascular status for volume assessment and drug administration.
Positioning	✓ and pad pressure points. ✓ eyes.	Positioning depends on surgical approach; most are performed with patient prone; however, use of the head-up position is not uncommon.
Complications	Oculocardiac reflex (OCR) → ↓↓HR and ↓↓BP VAE	Notify surgeons and Rx with atropine 0.02 mg/kg iv. Be prepared to make prompt Dx of VAE (↓$ETCO_2$, change in Doppler sounds, ↑ETN_2 ↓O_2 sat, ↓BP, ↑HR) and Rx: notify surgeons, flood wound, ± head down, aspirate CVP, ± vasopressors.

POSTOPERATIVE

Complications	Hypovolemia with ↓BP Hypothermia	Inadequate volume replacement may result in ↓BP. ✓ Hct to establish need for further fluid or blood therapy.
Pain management	Parenteral narcotics (see p. E-3).	
Tests	Followup Hct postop	Transfuse to keep Hct ≥ 30%.

References

1. Chiaretti A, Pietrini B: Safety & efficacy of remifentanil infusion in craniosynostosis repair in infants. *Ped Neurosurg* 2002; 36(1):55-6.
2. Davies DW, Munro IR: The anesthetic management and intraoperative care of patients undergoing major facial osteotomies. *Plast Reconstr Surg* 1975; 55(1):50-5.
3. Harris MM, Yemen TA, Davidson A, Strafford MA, Rowe RW, Sanders SP, Rockoff MA: Venous embolism during craniectomy in supine infants. *Anesthesiology* 1987; 67(5):816-19.
4. Krane EJ, Domino KB: Anesthesia for Neurosurgery. In: *Smith's Anesthesia for Infants and Children*, 6th edition. Motoyama EK, Davis PJ, eds. Mosby-Year Book, St. Louis: 1996, 541-70.
5. Marchac D, Renier D, Jones BM: Experience with the "Floating Forehead." *Br J Plast Surg* 1988; 41(1):1-15.
6. Muhling J: Surgical treatment of craniosynostosis. In *Maxillofacial Surgery*. Booth PW, Schendel SA, Hausamen J-E, eds. Churchill Livingstone, Edinburgh: 1999, 877-88.
7. Palmisano BW, Rusy LM: Anesthesia for plastic surgery. In *Pediatric Anesthesia*, 4th edition, Gregory GA, ed. Churchill Livingstone, NY: 2002, 707-45.
8. Posnick JC: Surgical management of Crouzon, Apert and related syndromes. In *Maxillofacial Surgery*. Booth PW, Schendel SA, Hausamen J-E, eds. Churchill Livingstone, Edinburgh: 1999, 863-75.
9. Tessier P: Relationship of craniostenoses to craniofacial dysostoses and to faciostenoses: a study with therapeutic implications. *Plast Reconstruct Surg* 1971; 48(3):224-37.

MAJOR SECONDARY CRANIOFACIAL SURGICAL PROCEDURES

SURGICAL CONSIDERATIONS

Description: These procedures usually are performed on children ≥ 5 yr. There are two basic approaches. The first involves advancement of the upper face and frontal bone, frequently described as a **monobloc** (Fig 12.8-3) or **frontofacial advancement**. The second variation, called **facial bipartition** or **periorbital osteotomy**, is for correction of telorbitism (widely spaced eyes), usually accomplished by a combined extra- and intracranial approach, using both plastic and neurosurgery teams.

Variant procedure or approaches: Many different variations of the above-named procedures can be performed; however, from an anesthetic standpoint, they are not significantly different. The use of **cranial bone grafts** and **rigid fixation** have shortened these somewhat lengthy procedures. Other bone grafts, however, from ribs and iliac crest, are occasionally required. These procedures frequently last ≥ 6 h and blood loss can be very heavy. Reconstruction of the forehead and orbital area following a tumor excision, for example, uses a similar approach, but requires additional bone grafts.

Usual preop diagnosis: Craniofacial malformations; craniofacial deformities; telorbitism or hypertelorism; craniofacial dysostosis

SUMMARY OF PROCEDURES

	Monobloc/Frontofacial Advancement	Facial Bipartition, Periorbital Osteotomies
Position	Supine	⇐
Incision	Bicoronal, oral	Bicoronal, infraorbital
Special instrumentation	Horseshoe headrest, usually pediatric; disimpaction forceps; Midas Rex craniotome; resorbable plates and screws; mini/micro titanium plates and screws; ± distraction device to supplant bone grafting and rigid fixation.	⇐
Unique considerations	Control of ICP: spinal drain may be placed, hyperventilation. Blood in room for anticipated transfusion.	⇐
Antibiotics	Pediatric: cefazolin 25 mg/kg q 8 h or vancomycin 10-15 mg/kg q 6 h, and cefotaxime 25-50 mg/kg q 6 h for oropharyngeal contamination and following dural tears	⇐
Surgical time	4-10 h	⇐

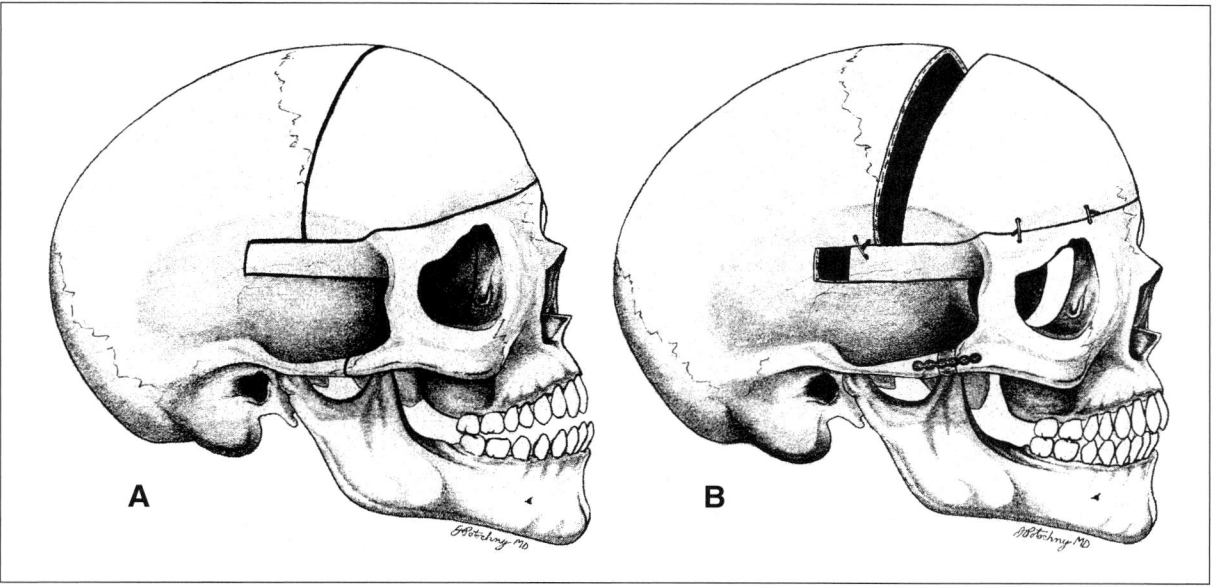

Figure 12.8-3. Monobloc advancement. (A) Lines of osteotomy for monobloc osteotomy. (B) Advancement of midface, orbits, and frontal bone, and stabilization with bone grafts and miniplates. (Reproduced with permission from Aston SJ, Beasley RW, Thorne CH, eds: *Grabb and Smith's Plastic Surgery*, 5th edition. Lippincott-Raven, 1997.)

	Monobloc/Frontofacial Advancement	Facial Bipartition, Periorbital Osteotomies
Closing considerations	Blood loss with Rainey clip removal for suturing. Full head-wrap dressing → head/neck movement → bucking.	⇐
EBL	400-800 ml; may be formidable	⇐
Postop care	ICU: 1-2 d; Monitor Hct.	⇐
Mortality	0.6-1.6%	⇐
Morbidity	Major complications: 14.3%	⇐
	Bone infection: 3-7%	⇐
	Meningitis	⇐
	Infection rates higher if:	⇐
	Adults rather than children (10 ×)	⇐
	Longer OR times and longer hospital stay	⇐
	Tracheostomy	⇐
	Foreign body (plates/screws/other alloplast)	⇐
	Anterior fossa entered	⇐
	Large dead space (e.g., in adult nongrowing brain)	⇐
	CSF leak: 4.5%	⇐
	↑ICP	⇐
	Air embolus: < 1%	⇐
	Blindness: < 1%	⇐
	Massive bleeding: < 1%	⇐
	Venous thrombosis	⇐
	Neurological injury: Rare	⇐
Pain score	6	6

PATIENT POPULATION CHARACTERISTICS

Age range	3-20 yr
Male:Female	1:1
Incidence	Crouzon syndrome: 1/25,000
	Apert syndrome: 1/100,000
Etiology	Congenital (80%); occasionally trauma or tumor (20%)
Associated conditions	Depends greatly on the syndrome or disease entity. See Craniosynostosis, p. 1130.

ANESTHETIC CONSIDERATIONS

PREOPERATIVE

Craniofacial syndromes often are associated with maxillofacial deformities, mandibular abnormalities and challenging airway management.[1]

Respiratory	Patients with long-standing upper airway obstruction due to choanal atresia, mandibular and maxillary hypoplasia, etc., may have chronic hypoventilation and hypoxia, and may have apnea episodes. If Sx of acute URI, delay elective surgery at least 2 wk. The presence of fever, cough, and abnormal chest auscultation necessitates radiographic evaluation and pediatric consultation. **Tests:** As indicated from H&P.
Airway	Be aware of other congenital anomalies affecting the airway, such as Apert, Goldenhar, Klippel-Feil, Pierre Robin, Treacher Collins, or Crouzon syndromes. Review any previous anesthetic records for insights into airway management (e.g., need for FOI). Consider elective tracheostomy under local anesthesia in patients with severe airway abnormalities.
Cardiovascular	Frequency of CHD is increased in patients with craniofacial abnormalities. Preop evaluation of patient with known or suspected heart defect should include H&P, ECG, Hct, baseline O_2 sat, and CXR. For children with Sx of cardiac dysfunction or those requiring cardiac medication, it is advisable to consult with a pediatric cardiologist to optimize patient's condition prior to surgery. **Tests:** Preop ECG indicated for patients with CHD; others as indicated from H&P.
Neurological	Neurologic deficits, if any, should be documented preop.
Laboratory	Hb/Hct; therapeutic drug levels for patients taking anticonvulsants.
Premedication	Premedication is helpful for patients > 1 yr – oral midazolam 0.5-0.75 mg/kg or oral ketamine 6 mg/kg about 30-60 min before induction.

INTRAOPERATIVE

Anesthetic technique: GETA, with special consideration given to associated CHD, pulmonary, and airway problems.

Induction	In an otherwise healthy patient, inhalational induction with subsequent placement of iv lines is appropriate. Muscle relaxants facilitate intubation but should be used only when adequate mask ventilation can be assured. An oral RAE ETT is useful for this procedure and should be secured carefully in place (often by suturing). Intubation in a patient with airway abnormalities may be facilitated by using a FOI with patient awake or lightly anesthetized and spontaneously ventilating. In rare situations, tracheostomy, under sedation and local anesthesia, may be necessary.[3,5]
Maintenance	Standard pediatric maintenance (see p. D-3). Consider use of remifentanil infusion (100-500 ng/kg/min) for supplemental analgesia and to facilitate rapid awakening.
Emergence	Extubate trachea when patient is awake and protective airway reflexes have returned. Patients with reactive airway disease may require deep extubation.

Blood and fluid requirements	Anticipate large blood loss.
	IV: 18 ga × 1-2
	NS/LR @:
	  4 ml/kg/h – 0-10 kg
	  + 2 ml/kg/h – 11-20 kg
	  + 1 ml/kg/h – > 20 kg
	  (e.g., 25 kg = 65 ml/h)
	Warm fluids.
	Humidify gases.
		The goal of intraop fluid therapy is to replace preop deficits, intraop fluid, electrolyte, and blood losses, while providing maintenance fluids. Half of the calculated deficit (hours fasting × hourly maintenance fluid requirement) generally is replaced during the 1st h of anesthesia and the balance over the next 1-2 h. Surgical manipulation of tissue will cause 3rd-space fluid loss proportional to the degree of surgical trauma and tissue exposure. It may range from 0-10 ml/kg/h.

Control of blood loss	Deliberate ↓BP	Deliberate ↓BP can be accomplished by use of SNP, esmolol, or potent inhalational agents titrated to effect (MAP 50-60 mmHg).
Monitoring	Standard monitors (see p. D-1). Arterial line ± CVP line	Arterial line is essential for monitoring BP during deliberate ↓BP and for ABGs and blood chemistries.
Control of ICP	Hyperventilation Mannitol	For some procedures, it is essential to reduce intracranial volume to facilitate surgical access. If prolonged brain retraction is required, postop cerebral edema may ensue.

Control of ICP, cont.	Loop diuretics	
	CSF drainage (> 1 yr)	
Positioning	✓ and pad pressure points.	Positioning head above the heart facilitates venous drainage, but also increases the incidence of VAE. Do not hyperextend or hyperflex the head and neck. Flexion of the neck will move the ETT downward (mainstem intubation); extension will move the ETT upward (cuff leak).
	✓ eyes.	
Complications	Displacement of ETT	Suture ETT to alveolar ridge.
	Oculocardiac reflex (OCR) → ↓↓HR, ↓BP	Notify surgeon. Rx: atropine 0.02 mg/kg.
	VAE	VAE should be suspected if sudden ↑ETN$_2$, ↓ETCO$_2$, ↓O$_2$ sat, ↓BP, ↑HR. Notify surgeon, flood surgical field with NS, support patient hemodynamically and D/C N$_2$O.
	Major blood loss	

POSTOPERATIVE

Complications	↑ADH secretion	SIADH or DI may follow brain manipulation and may require pharmacologic intervention for Rx.
	Diabetes insipidus (DI)	
	Cerebral edema	Cerebral edema may → ↑ICP (headache, N/V, ↓mental status, etc.)
	Pneumothorax	Pneumothorax (Sx = ↑respirations, wheezing, ↓BP, ↓CO, ↓O$_2$ sat) may occur 2° rib resection for bone graft. ✓ CXR.
	Bleeding	
Pain management	PCA (see p. E-3).	
Tests	Hct	

References

1. Christianson L: Anesthesia for major craniofacial operations. *Int Anesthesiol Clin* 1985; 23(4):117-30.
2. David DJ, Cooter RD: Craniofacial infection in 10 years of transcranial surgery. *Plast Reconstruct Surg J* 1987; 80(2):213-23.
3. MacLennan FM, Robertson GS: Ketamine for induction and intubation in Treacher Collins syndrome. *Anesthesia* 1981; 36(2):196-8.
4. Posnick JC: Surgical management of Crouzon, Apert and related syndromes. In *Maxillofacial Surgery*. Booth PW, Schendel SA, Hausamen J-E, eds. Churchill Livingstone, Edinburgh: 1999, 863-75.
5. Rasch DK, Browder F, Barr M, Greer D: Anaesthesia for Treacher Collins and Pierre Robin syndromes: a report of three cases. *Can Anaesth Soc J* 1986; 33(3P+1):364-70.
6. Williams JK, Longaker MT: Surgical complications of craniofacial surgery. In *Maxillofacial Surgery*. Booth PW, Schendel SA, Hausamen J-E, eds. Churchill Livingstone, Edinburgh: 1999, 905-16.

CLEFT LIP REPAIR—UNILATERAL/BILATERAL

SURGICAL CONSIDERATIONS

Description: Cleft lip may be either unilateral or bilateral, associated frequently with clefts of the alveolus and palate. Surgical repair involves the design and execution of geometric flaps on the medial and lateral sides of the cleft and primary repair of the cleft nasal deformity. The most common unilateral technique is the **rotation advancement flap of Millard** (Fig 12.8-4). Multiple bilateral lip repairs have been described, some repairing both sides simultaneously and some one side at a time (Fig 12.8-5). Technique depends on the amount of prolabial and lateral element tissue available. Recently, **primary nasal repair** has been coupled with these bilateral procedures. These nasal repairs involve extensive mobilization of the alar cartilages and transfer of tissue up into the cleft nasal vestibule and floor, with nasal stents often placed. All of these factors can decrease or occlude nasal airway breathing. Although only a minority of neonates have been found to be true nasal obligatory breathers, this should be kept in mind for those postop patients with respiratory distress.

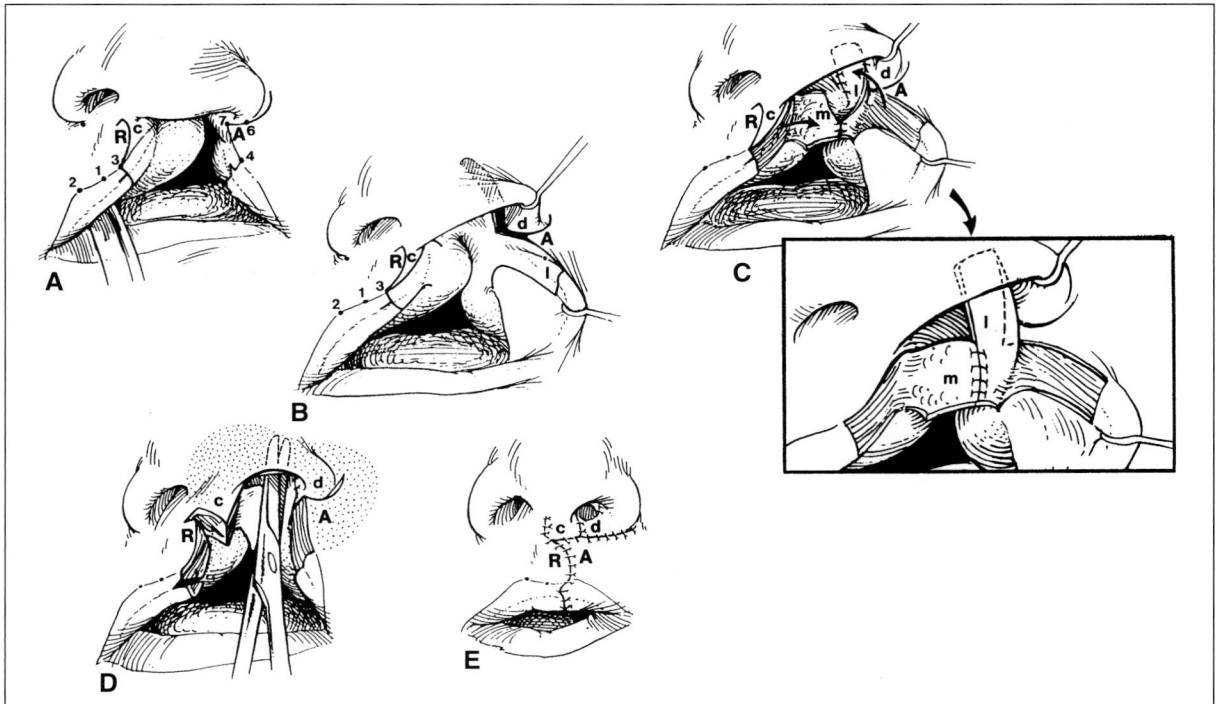

Figure 12.8-4. Step-by-step unilateral complete cleft rotation advancement: m = medial mucosal flap; l = lateral mucosal flap. (Reproduced with permission from Aston SJ, Beasley RW, Thorne CH, eds: *Grabb and Smith's Plastic Surgery*, 5th edition. Lippincott-Raven, 1997.)

Variant procedure or approaches: Other approaches commonly performed are those of the **Davies-** or **Tennison**-type (Z-plasty) lip repairs (Fig 12.8-6). In large clefts, a lip adhesion may be performed as an initial stage several months before the actual definitive correction of the cleft lip. This procedure basically involves creating a wound on either side and suturing the muscles, mucosa, and skin together. The procedure itself is very short (~45 min). **Presurgical orthopedic devices** may be placed and manipulated, instead of a lip adhesion, to bring a wide, bony cleft into better opposition for a tension-free complete repair. These are custom-fitted and may be fixed with pins to the palate. They are removed in the OR at time of repair.

Usual preop diagnosis: Cleft lip/palate

SUMMARY OF PROCEDURE

Position	Supine; table rotated either 90° or 180°, with oral RAE or anode tube toward chin; patient's head at the edge of head of bed; shoulder roll; neck extended; entire face exposed; scleral shields
Incision	Medial and lateral cleft margins into the nose and in the maxillary vestibule on the cleft side
Special instrumentation	★ Throat pack (**NB: ✓** removal before extubation); oral RAE or anode tube.
Unique considerations	Local anesthesia with epinephrine injected **after** lip and nose markings complete. Pediatric patients should wake up in an unagitated state, as undue crying may place excessive tension on repair. Immediate elbow restraints for children × 2 wk.
Antibiotics	Cefazolin 25 mg/kg iv
Surgical time	1.5 h (bilateral usually ¹/₂ h longer) Lip adhesion: 45 min
Closing considerations	Nasal stent; swelling and ointment may occlude nasal airway; smooth emergence important.
EBL	5-10 ml (higher with palatoplasty)
Postop care	Elbow restraints × 2 wk; PACU → room overnight → home POD 1.
Mortality	Minimal
Morbidity	Infection
	Wound breakdown
	Hypertrophic scars
Pain score	4

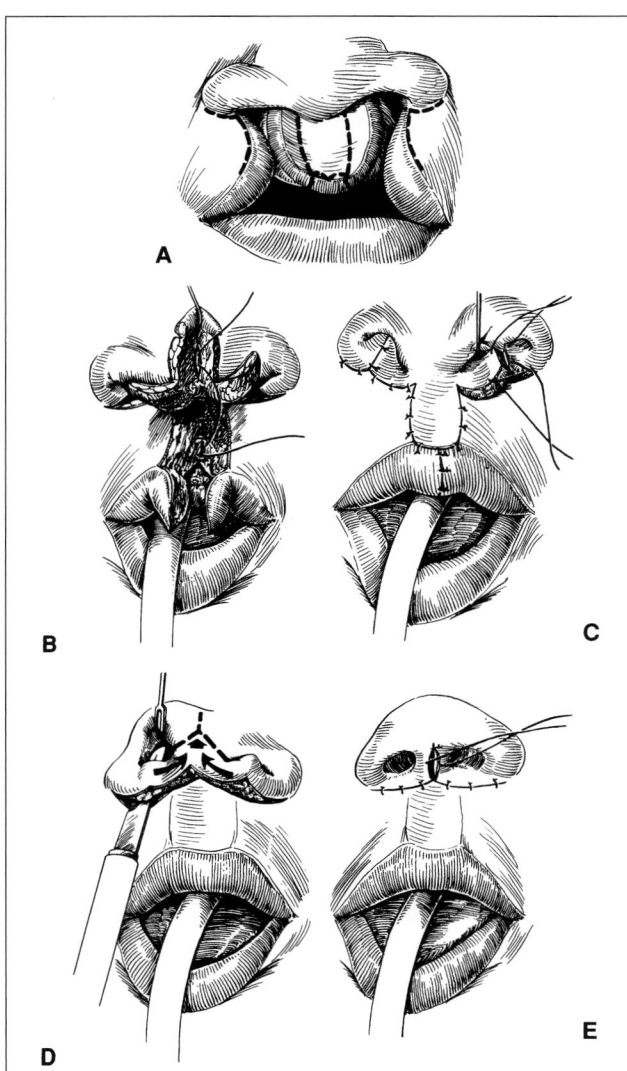

← **Figure 12.8-5.** Banked fork-flap procedure. In the first stage (A-C), bilateral straight line repairs are done after the prolabium is divided vertically into three forks. The central limb is used to construct the center of the lip. The lateral forks are 'banked' at the alar bases for later use in constructing a columella. At the second stage (D-E), bipedicle flaps from the nasal floor, which include the banked forks, are used in combination with a membranous septum incision to elongate the columella and increase tip projection. (Reproduced with permission from Aston SJ, Beasley RW, Thorne CH, eds: *Grabb and Smith's Plastic Surgery*, 5th edition. Lippincott-Raven, 1997. After Millard DR Jr: Closure of bilateral cleft lip and elongation of columella by two operations at infancy. *Plast Reconstr Surg* 1971; 47:324-31.)

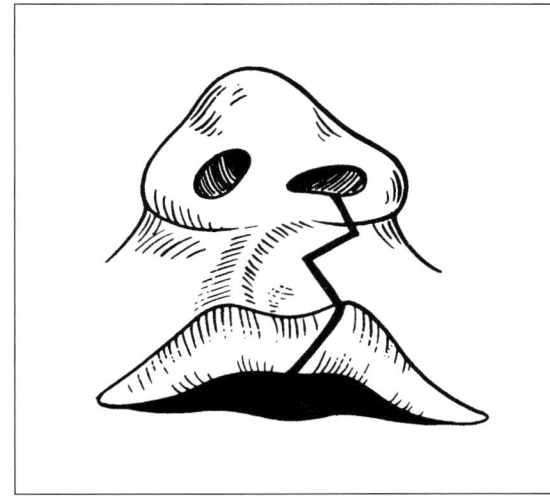

↑ **Figure 12.8-6.** Z-plasty closure of lip. (Reproduced with permission from McCarthy JG, ed: *Plastic Surgery*. WB Saunders: 1990).

PATIENT POPULATION CHARACTERISTICS

Age range	1 wk-6 mo
Male:Female	2:1 – cleft lip and palate. Isolated cleft palate more common in females.
Incidence	1/750 for Caucasians; more common in Asians; less in African Americans. Left cleft more common than right; both more common than bilateral, in the ratio of 6:3:1.
Etiology	Multifactorial, including both genetic and environmental aspects
Associated conditions	Associated anomalies are seen in ~29% of cleft lip cases, and may include major chromosomal deletions and/or duplications, along with possible severe mental retardation and CHD.

ANESTHETIC CONSIDERATIONS

See Anesthetic Considerations for Lip and Nose Surgery, p. 1147.

Reference

1. Grayson BH, Cutting CB: Presurgical nasoalveolar orthopedic molding in primary correction of the nose, lip, and alveolus of infants born with unilateral and bilateral clefts. *Cleft Palate Craniofac J* 2001; 38(3):193-8.
2. Gundlach KKH: Etiology, prevalence, growth and trends in cleft lip, alveolus and palate. In: *Maxillofacial Surgery*. Booth PW, Schendel SA, Hausamen J-E, eds. Churchill Livingstone, Edinburgh: 1999, 991-1003.

3. Mommaerts Y: The traditional 'Millard' approach to lip and palate repair. In *Maxillofacial Surgery*. Booth PW, Schendel SA, Hausamen J-E, eds. Churchill Livingstone, Edinburgh: 1999, 1029-45.

4. Schendel SA: Unilateral cleft lip repair—State of the art. *Cleft Palate-Craniofac J* 2000; 37(4):335-41.

5. Sullivan WG: Respiratory distress following cleft lip repair: the role of obligatory nasal breathing in the infant. *Ann Plast Surg* 1988; 20(6):590-2.

6. Winters JC, Hurwitz DJ: Presurgical orthopedics in the surgical management of unilateral cleft lip and palate. *Plast Reconstruct Surg J* 1995; 95(4):755-64.

PALATOPLASTY

SURGICAL CONSIDERATIONS

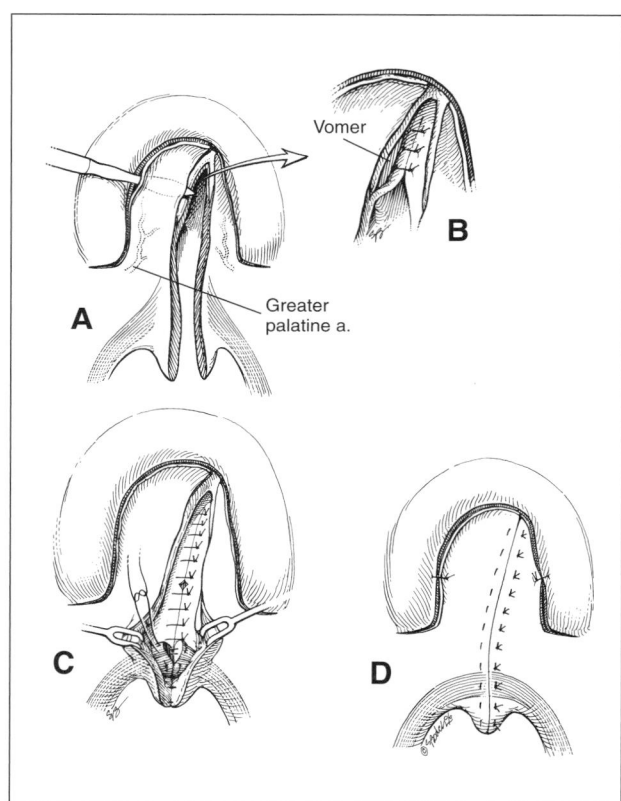

Figure 12.8-7. Palatoplasty technique. (A) Cleft palate closure after healing of gingivoperiosteoplasty at 11-12 mo of age. Bilateral, unipedicled mucoperiosteal flaps, based on the greater palatine arteries, are elevated. (B) Anteriorly, the nasal floor is repaired by suturing the vomerine mucosa to the nasal mucosa on the cleft side. (C) The levator muscles are dissected free from the oral and nasal mucosa and released from the posterior edge of the hard palate. The levator muscles are approximated to each other in the midline. (D) The oral mucosa is reapproximated in the midline with interrupted horizontal mattress sutures. (Reproduced with permission from Aston SJ, Beasley RW, Thorne CH, eds: *Grabb and Smith's Plastic Surgery*, 5th edition. Lippincott-Raven, 1997.)

Description: Cleft palate can be seen as either an isolated condition or in conjunction with clefting of the lip. The mildest form of cleft palate is the submucous, or occult cleft, in which there is no visible cleft but, rather, a nonunion of the soft-palate muscles. This is followed by the incomplete soft-palate cleft and, finally, the complete cleft, which includes soft and hard palates and may extend through the alveolar portion of the maxilla. Repair involves mobilizing the lateral soft tissue and moving it toward the midline to close the cleft and elongate the palate, if necessary. The most important goal of cleft-palate repair is the attainment of normal speech. Children with unrepaired or inadequately repaired clefts develop nasal-sounding speech patterns termed 'rhinolalia.' Cleft-palate repair, therefore, usually is done when the child is 9-18 mo old, before consequential speech development. In addition to closing the cleft itself, an important goal of palate repair is normal anatomic approximation of the levator palati muscles, which are responsible for oronasal valving in speech and swallowing. The cleft palate is closed by elevating the mucoperiosteum from the underlying bones and approximating it in the midline (**von Langenbeck technique**) (Fig 12.8-7) or using a V-Y type of retrodisplacement and closure (**Wardill-Kilner technique**). In either method, the levator muscles are specifically dissected and the levator sling is reconstructed. A layered closure usually is accomplished, including repositioning of the uvular muscles.

There are several different approaches to the muscle reconstruction in the soft palate, generally termed **intravelarveloplasties**. Z-plasty of the soft palate, also called a **Furlow procedure**, (Fig 12.8-8) has been used to lengthen the palate and reorient the palatal muscles across the cleft. The other procedures basically involve direct closure of the muscles and a push-back to lengthen the palate.

Usual preop diagnosis: Cleft palate

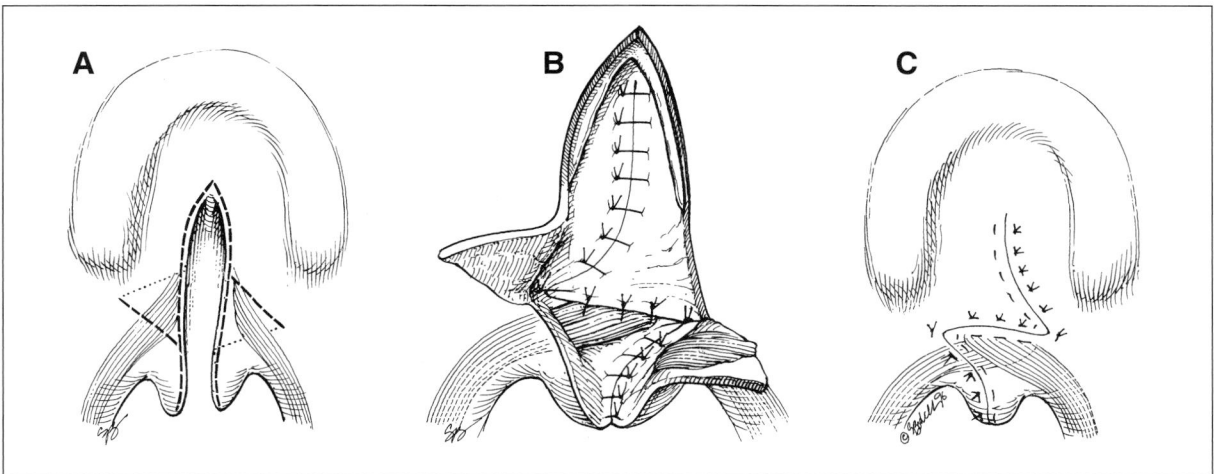

Figure 12.8-8. Double opposing Z-plasty closure of an isolated cleft palate. (A) Design of the incisions. (B) Muscle included in the posteriorly based flap. (C) Final result with recreation of the levator sling. (Reproduced with permission from Aston SJ, Beasley RW, Thorne CH, eds: *Grabb and Smith's Plastic Surgery*, 5th edition. Lippincott-Raven, 1997.)

SUMMARY OF PROCEDURE

Position	Supine; table rotated 90°-180° with oral RAE tube extending down the midline of the lower jaw and taped to the chin.
Incision	Edges of the cleft palate and, possibly, the alveolar and pterygomandibular raphe areas.
Special instrumentation	Dingman mouth gag (when setting the gag, communication between surgeon and anesthetist allows ETT compression to be noted early); usually, a headlight; oropharyngeal pack
Unique considerations	The gag may be released intermittently to allow reperfusion of the tongue; each manipulation may affect the ETT. Minimal-to-moderate amount of blood in the oropharynx at end of procedure—should be carefully suctioned. Also, there may be some respiratory difficulties on emergence. Traction with a tongue suture often proves helpful in restoring patient's airway (maintained 24 h). Usually, oral or nasopharyngeal airways should not be placed in children.
Antibiotics	Cefazolin 25 mg/kg q 5-6 h (up to 1 g) × 5 d
Surgical time	1-1.5 h
Closing considerations	Child should not wake up crying and hypertensive. Tongue suture may be placed prior to ★ extubation. **NB:** Dingman gag will stick to the ETT; therefore, holding the tube with a forceps deep in the oropharynx and careful removal of the gag avoids accidental extubation.
EBL	50 ml
Postop care	Elbow restraints; PACU → room; → home next d. OG tube placed, suctioned, and removed.
Mortality	Rare
Morbidity	Recurrent bleeding (requiring early return to OR): Rare
	Hematoma under palate
	Dehiscence of palate
Pain score	4

PATIENT POPULATION CHARACTERISTICS

Age range	6-18 mo
Male:Female	1:3 (isolated cleft palate)
Incidence	1/1,000
Etiology	Failure of fusion of the palatal shelves from anterior to posterior. (Can be due to a persistent high-tongue position in utero, increased facial width, reduced facial mesenchyme and/or drugs such as steroids, anticonvulsants, and benzodiazepines, or infection.)
Associated conditions	Multiple associated conditions. Most common is the Pierre Robin syndrome, in which cleft palate is found in association with glossoptosis and a micrognathic retruded mandible. These children frequently have airway obstruction and, even at an older age, may have sleep apnea.[1] Other associations include Klippel-Feil syndrome, Treacher Collins syndrome, CHD, chronic URI, chronic otitis media, subglottic stenosis.

ANESTHETIC CONSIDERATIONS

See Anesthetic Considerations for Lip and Nose Surgery, p. 1147.

Reference

1. Gorlin RJ, Cohen MM, Hennekam RCM: *Syndromes of the Head and Neck*, 4th edition. Oxford University Press, NY: 2001.
2. Gundlach KKH: Etiology, prevalence, growth and trends in cleft lip, alveolus and palate. In: *Maxillofacial Surgery*. Booth PW, Schendel SA, Hausamen J-E, eds. Churchill Livingstone, Edinburgh: 1999, 991-1003.
3. Kirschner RE, Wang P, Jawad AF, et al: Cleft-palate repair by modified Furlow double-opposing Z-Plasty: *The Children's Hospital of Philadelphia Experience, Plastic and Reconstructive Surgery* 1999; 104(7):1998-2014.
4. Mommaerts Y: The traditional 'Millard' approach to lip and palate repair. In *Maxillofacial Surgery*. Booth PW, Schendel SA, Hausamen, J-E, eds. Churchill Livingstone, Edinburgh: 1999, 1029-45.

PHARYNGOPLASTY

SURGICAL CONSIDERATIONS

Description: Following the initial repair of palatal clefts, some children or young adults demonstrate continued hypernasal speech patterns, a condition called 'velopharyngeal incompetence.' This can be 2° a short soft palate, a large nasopharynx, or a soft palate that has inadequate movement either 2° scarring or due to neurogenic problems. The typical repair would be a superiorly based **pharyngeal flap** (Fig 12.8-9) to the soft palate.

Variant procedure or approaches: The **Jackson modification of the Orticochea flap** uses the posterior tonsillar pillars, which consist of the palatopharyngeus muscle and overlying mucosa, to create a competent oronasal sphincter (Fig 12.8-10). The flaps are based superiorly and repositioned horizontally to meet above and behind the soft palate. Although they act to augment the posterior pharyngeal wall, they also are intended to maintain their innervation and, therefore, augment sphincter activity. A posterior pharyngeal wall implant also may be placed.

Usual preop diagnosis: Velopharyngeal incompetence

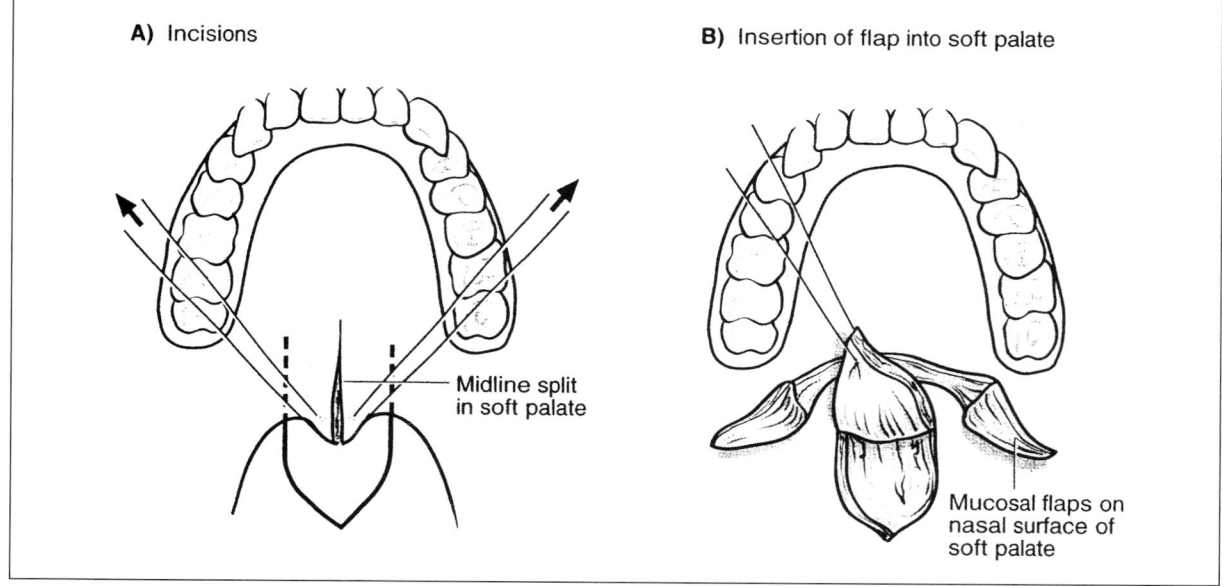

Figure 12.8-9. Pharyngeal flap, superiorly based. (Reproduced with permission from Booth PW, Schendel SA, Hausamen J-E, eds: *Maxillofacial Surgery*. Churchill Livingstone, 1999.)

SUMMARY OF PROCEDURE

Position	Supine, table rotated 90° or 180°; oral RAE tube extending down the midline chin and taped in position.
Incision	Involves incisions in soft and hard palates and in the posterior pharyngeal wall.
Special instrumentation	Dingman mouth gag (caution with removal and manipulation re ETT); headlight
Unique considerations	Avoid oral or nasopharyngeal airways or nasal suctioning.
Antibiotics + other meds	Cefazolin 25 mg/kg q 6-8 h (up to 1 g) × 3 d; periop steroids, depending on preop airway.
Surgical time	1-1.5 h
Closing considerations	Pediatric patients should not become hypertensive (↑bleeding). There will be some nasopharyngeal drainage; thorough oral suctioning is important.
EBL	50-100 ml
Postop care	Avoid postop oral or nasopharyngeal airways or nasal suctioning. Be aware of possible occlusion of nasopharynx with flap and bleeding. Tongue suture can be placed for 24 h.
Mortality	Rare
Morbidity	Recurrent bleeding Hematoma under palate Dehiscence of palate Nasopharyngeal obstruction Secondary sleep apnea
Pain score	4

PATIENT POPULATION CHARACTERISTICS

Age range	3-11 yr most common
Male:Female	1:1
Incidence	~15% of children undergoing cleft palate repair will need some type of secondary palatal lengthening procedure after 3 yr.
Etiology	Short and scarred palate; neurogenic palate; palate-to-pharyngeal ratio that is too small
Associated conditions	Sleep apnea; Pierre Robin sequence, with glossoptosis and micrognathia; Treacher Collins syndrome; microtia with craniofacial malformation; subglottic stenosis; CHD. Of special interest: some patients with cleft palate may have **velocardiofacial syndrome**. These children may have **medially displaced internal carotid arteries**, placing these major arteries in harm's way during dissection along the posterior pharyngeal wall.

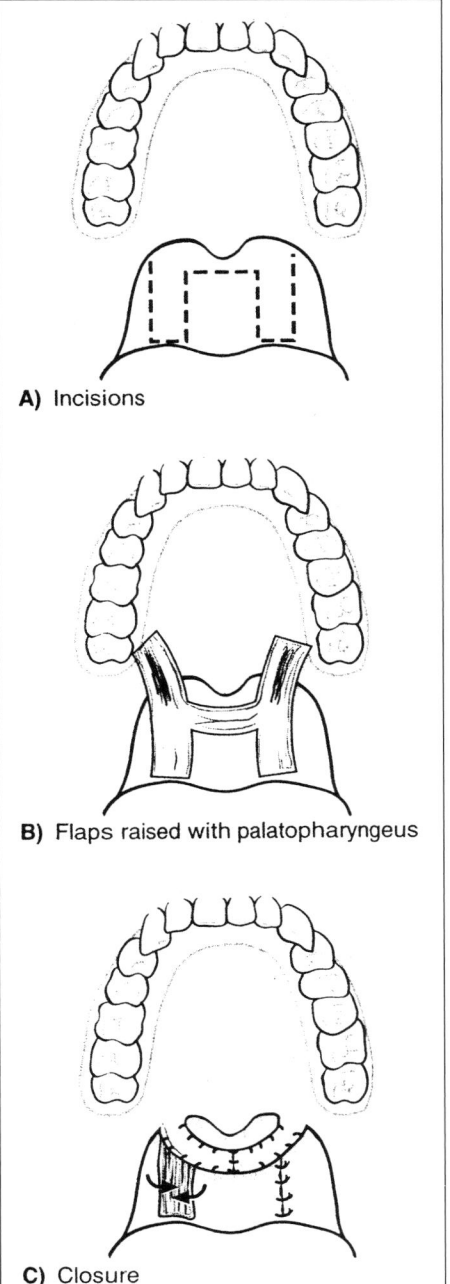

A) Incisions

B) Flaps raised with palatopharyngeus

C) Closure

Figure 12.8-10. Sphincter pharyngoplasty. (Reproduced with permission from Booth PW, Schendel SA, Hausamen J-E, eds: *Maxillofacial Surgery*. Churchill Livingstone, 1999.

ANESTHETIC CONSIDERATIONS

See Anesthetic Considerations for Lip and Nose Surgery, p. 1147.

References

1. Boorman JG, Bharathwaj S: Secondary palatal surgery and pharyngoplasty. In *Maxillofacial Surgery*. Booth PW, Schendel SA, Hausamen J-E, eds. Churchill Livingstone, Edinburgh: 1999, 1083-99.

2. Jackson IT: Sphincter pharyngoplasty. *Clin Plastic Surg* 1985; 12(4):711-17.
3. Markus AF, Precious DS: Secondary surgery for cleft lip and palate. In *Maxillofacial Surgery*. Booth PW, Schendel SA, Hausamen J-E, eds. Churchill Livingstone, Edinburgh: 1999, 1057-72.

Also see References for Cleft Lip, p. 1139.

ALVEOLAR CLEFT REPAIR WITH BONE GRAFT

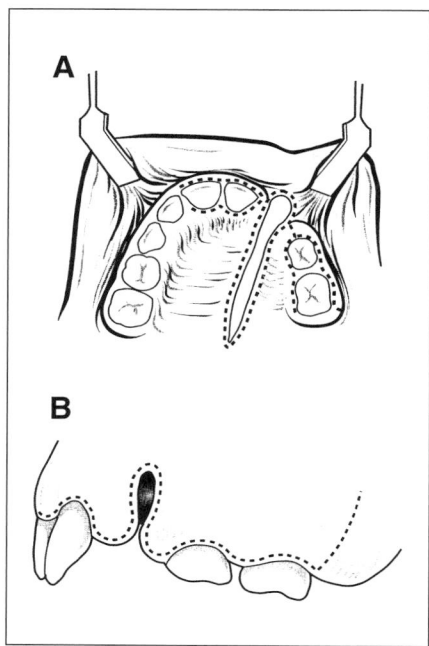

Figure 12.8-11. Gingivoalveoloplasty (GAP). Gingival and mucosal incisions are shown on the palate (A) and vestibular (B) surfaces, extending along the cleft borders. (Reproduced with permission from Booth PW, Schendel SA, Hausamen J-E, eds: *Maxillofacial Surgery*. Churchill Livingstone, 1999.

SURGICAL CONSIDERATIONS

Description: Alveolar cleft occurs as both bony and soft-tissue defects in the alveolar portion of the maxilla in the position of the lateral incisor tooth; thus, an oral/nasal fistula exists with this deformity. The size of the cleft is variable; it may be unilateral or bilateral and is associated with cleft lip and palate. The alveolar segments are often collapsed such that orthodontic expansion is required before bone graft and repair. These devices are maintained to stabilize the graft in situ for a 3-mo healing period. The surgical procedure involves raising mucosal-gingival-periosteal flaps, advancing them, and performing a layered closure, starting with the nasal floor and working toward the oral cavity. A bone graft is placed in between these two layers to consolidate the upper arch. Cancellous bone usually is taken from the iliac crest or corticocancellous bone from the outer table of the skull.

Most commonly, the bone is harvested from the ilium. This can be accomplished via limited access and a trephine or via an open technique. depending on the amount of bone required. This portion of the procedure, especially by open technique can add 50-100 ml of blood loss. Most nasal and lip revision surgery should be put off until the alveolus is reconstructed, since this is the base on which the lip and nose sit.

Variant procedure or approaches: In young children, the alveolar cleft procedure may be performed without the use of bone grafts at the time of lip or hard palate closure (**gingivoalveoloplasty**, Fig 12.8-11), with the hope that preop alignment of the clefted alveolus and periosteal creation of new bone will fill the bony defect and allow subsequent normal tooth eruption. This is not always complete, and some of these children will need later bone grafting at age 7-8 yr, before eruption of the permanent canine teeth.

Usual preop diagnosis: Congenital alveolar cleft

SUMMARY OF PROCEDURE

Position	Supine; table rotated 90°-180° ± roll under hip (bone harvest)
Incision	Oral, with the addition of iliac crest incision or scalp incision, either parasagittal or coronal
Special instrumentation	Throat pack; Dingman mouth gag; headlight. Two instrument setups used, to prevent cross-contamination from oral to iliac surgical sites.
Unique considerations	Important to ensure that the hip iliac crest bone graft site is on the opposite side from the anesthesiologist if the table is rotated only 90°. Midline oral RAE tube to chin. Care when manipulating Dingman, as it sticks to ETT.
Antibiotics	Cefazolin 25 mg/kg (up to 1 g) iv preop
Surgical time	1.5-2.5 h
Closing considerations	★ **NB:** Ensure that throat pack has been removed. Pediatric patients should not wake up in agitated state. Noncleft-side oral mouth gag and gentle oral suctioning permissible; avoid nasal suctioning, especially from the cleft side.
EBL	100-200 ml
Postop care	PACU → ward; walking POD 1 or 2 post-iliac graft.

Mortality	Rare
Morbidity	Bone graft loss: 2-10%
	Infection: 2-10%
	Refistulization: 2-10%
	Prolonged hip discomfort (bone graft donor site)
	Bleeding—oral or at bone donor site
Pain score	6

PATIENT POPULATION CHARACTERISTICS

Age range	8-12 yr
Male:Female	2:1
Incidence	Unknown
Etiology	Multifactorial, including both genetic and environmental aspects
Associated conditions	Associated anomalies are seen in ~29% of cleft lip cases; and may include major chromosomal deletions and/or duplications, with the possibility of severe mental retardation, CHD.

ANESTHETIC CONSIDERATIONS

See Anesthetic Considerations for Lip and Nose Surgery, p. 1147.

References

1. Brusati R, Mannucci N: Primary repair of the lip and palate using the Delaire philosophy. In *Maxillofacial Surgery*. Booth PW, Schendel SA, Hausamen J-E, eds. Churchill Livingstone, Edinburgh: 1999, 1005-28.
2. Stassen LFA: Alveolar bone grafting—how I do it. In *Maxillofacial Surgery*. Booth PW, Schendel SA, Hausamen J-E, eds. Churchill Livingstone, Edinburgh: 1999, 1047-55.
3. Wolfe SA, Kawamoto HK: Taking the iliac bone graft: A new technique. *J Bone Joint Surg* [Am] 1978; 60-A(3):411.

Also see References for Cleft Lip, p. 1139.

SECONDARY CLEFT LIP/NASAL SURGERY

SURGICAL CONSIDERATIONS

Description: Secondary deformities of the nose and lip develop following the initial repair of either bilateral or unilateral cleft lip deformities. These subsequent deformities depend on the extent of the initial congenital anomaly, the quality of the surgical repair, and resulting oral/facial function. Revision can vary from a minimal scar revision (Fig 12.8-12), to a complete opening and reconstruction of the lip and nose, with or without ancillary procedures such as **septorhinoplasty ± cartilage grafting, forked flaps** (Fig 12.8-13), **fascial lip augmentation, or Abbe-Estlander flap** (lip-switch flap) (Fig 12.8-14).

Occasionally, the individual born with a cleft lip and palate is severely deficient in tissue of the upper lip. This occurs most frequently in the bilateral condition. Correction involves switching tissue from the midline of the lower lip to the central portion of the upper lip, maintaining a pedicle of soft

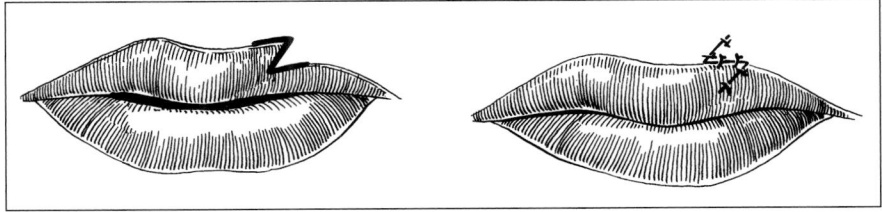

Figure 12.8-12. Z-plasty to correct notching of the vermillion border. (Reproduced with permission from Aston SJ, Beasley RW, Thorne CH, eds: *Grabb and Smith's Plastic Surgery*, 5th edition. Lippincott-Raven, 1997. Originally from Millard DR Jr: *Cleft Craft: The Evolution of Its Surgery*. Little, Brown, 1976.)

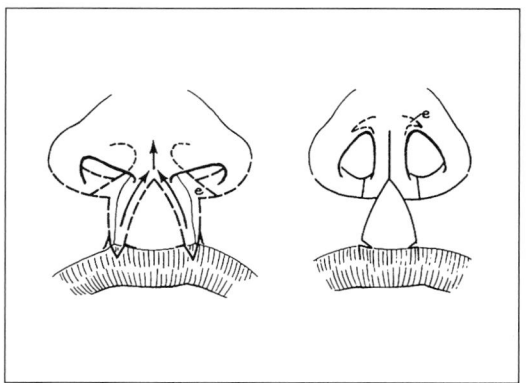

Figure 12.8-13. Short columella associated with the bilateral cleft nose, elongated by forked flaps. (Reproduced with permission from Aston SJ, Beasley RW, Thorne CH, eds: *Grabb and Smith's Plastic Surgery*, 5th edition. Lippincott-Raven, 1997.)

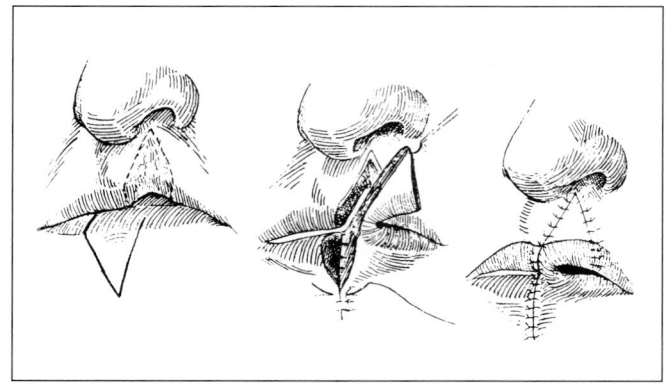

Figure 12.8-14. Abbe-Estlander flap. Note lips sutured together. (Reproduced with permission from Converse JM, ed: *Reconstructive Plastic Surgery*, Vol 3, 2nd edition. WB Saunders Co: 1977.)

tissue between the lips, which usually contains the labial artery on one side. This pedicle normally is cut between 7-11 d. The redundant tissue in the mid portion of the upper lip is transferred to the columellar portion of the nose at the same time, which elongates this section (Fig 12.8-14). To avoid disruption of the flap, the older child should be cautioned to avoid wide mouth opening in the postop period.

Usual preop diagnosis: Secondary cleft deformity

SUMMARY OF PROCEDURE

Position	Supine, table rotated 90°-180°; oral RAE; nasal RAE tube when working on lips only (especially if lips are held closed by a flap pedicle, making extubation more difficult).
Incision	Variable, in lip or nasal areas. (See Figs 12.8-12, 13, 14.)
Special instrumentation	Throat pack; possibly rhinoplasty instruments; oral RAE tube; head light; loupe magnification.
Unique considerations	Procurement of a cartilage graft is usually from the nasal septum or ear; thus, the head may need to be turned to one side and this area also prepped. Elbow restraints for children. A switch flap leaves the lips connected at their mid-portion by a thin, easily damaged, soft-tissue pedicle; therefore, the patient should wake up unagitated.
Antibiotics	Cefazolin 25 mg/kg (up to 1 g) iv preop
Surgical time	Variable, depending on the extent of revision: 0.5-3 h
Closing considerations	★ **NB:** Remove throat pack.
EBL	Minimal-75 ml
Postop care	May be obligatory mouth breathing post-rhinoplasty, or lips may be held mostly closed by the pedicle and swelling of a lip-switch flap; consider oral-pharyngeal airway; avoid wide mouth opening. PACU → room; elbow restraints in young children.
Mortality	Rare
Morbidity	Infection
	Wound breakdown
	Flap necrosis: < 1% (with lip switch)
	Bleeding
Pain score	3-5 (depending on extent of procedure)

PATIENT POPULATION CHARACTERISTICS

Age range	2-50 yr
Male:Female	1:1
Incidence	20-60% of patients with primary clefts
Etiology	Unsatisfactory outcome of previous lip/nose surgery
Associated conditions	Associated anomalies are seen in ~29% of the clefts and may include major chromosomal deletions or duplications, with a possibility of severe mental retardation.

ANESTHETIC CONSIDERATIONS

See Anesthetic Considerations for Lip and Nose Surgery, below.

References

1. Palmisano BW: Anesthesia for plastic surgery. In: *Pediatric Anesthesia*, 3rd edition, Gregory GA, ed. Churchill Livingstone, NY: 1994, 699-741.
2. Sadove AM, Eppley BL: Correction of secondary cleft lip and nasal deformities. *Clin Plastic Surg* 1993; 20(4):793-801.
3. Talmant JC: Cleft rhinoplasty. In *Maxillofacial Surgery*. Booth PW, Schendel SA, Hausamen J-E, eds. Churchill Livingstone, Edinburgh: 1999, 1133-71.

ANESTHETIC CONSIDERATIONS FOR LIP AND NOSE SURGERY

(Procedures covered: cleft lip repair; palatoplasty; pharyngoplasty; alveolar cleft repair with bone graft; secondary cleft lip/nasal surgery)

PREOPERATIVE

The anesthesiologist should be aware of the parent's feelings about their child with a congenital malformation. The whole family needs to be treated with sensitivity and compassion. Cleft lip closure may be carried out as early as the first wk of life in the healthy neonate; however, many surgeons and anesthesiologists find the 'rule of ten' helpful: the child should have an Hb >10 g, be 10 wk old, and weigh 10 lbs. The hard palate usually is closed between the ages of 1-5 yr; however, the soft palate should be closed prior to speech development (12-15 mo). **Palatoplasty** and **pharyngoplasty** usually are carried out from 1-15 yr. Patients with these midline facial defects are most likely to have other associated anomalies, including CHD, subglottic stenosis, and Pierre Robin or Treacher Collins syndromes.

Respiratory	Careful assessment is necessary as associated anomalies may affect airway or lungs. Chronic otitis 2° eustachian tube dysfunction is common. Treat with antibiotics before surgery. Postpone surgery (~2 wk) if Sx of acute URI present (e.g., runny nose, fever, sore throat, cough). Chronic aspiration may be associated with cleft lip/palate. **Tests:** as indicated from H&P.
Airway	Be aware of other congenital anomalies affecting the airway, such as Apert, Goldenhar, Klippel-Feil, Pierre Robin, or Treacher Collins syndromes. Review any previous anesthetic records for insights into airway management. Consider fiber optic intubation (FOI) in patients with suspected difficult airway. Also consider elective tracheostomy under local anesthesia in patients with severe airway abnormalities. Patients with severe subglottic stenosis may require preop tracheostomy.
Cardiovascular	CHD is frequently associated with cleft palate. Preop evaluation of a patient with a known or suspected heart defect should include thorough H&P, ECG, Hct, baseline O_2 sat, and CXR. For children with Sx of cardiac dysfunction or those requiring cardiac medication, it is advisable to consult with a pediatric cardiologist to optimize the patient's condition prior to surgery. **Tests:** Preop ECG indicated for patients with CHD; others as indicated from H&P.
Nutritional	Infants with cleft lip/palate may have problems with oral feeding. Assess nutritional status from physical exam and by comparison to expected growth for age. ★ **NB:** NPO after midnight for solids. Patients should continue to have clear liquids up until 2 h preop.
Neurological	Delayed development of speech is common in the older child with cleft palate. Some of these children may be hearing impaired. Preop preparation and discussion is important to minimize the impact of these communication problems.
Psychological	Many patients with orofacial congenital malformations require multiple procedures; emotional support and psychological assessment of these patients are essential.
Hematologic	High incidence of iron deficiency anemia; T&C for 1 U PRBC (cleft palate). **Tests:** Hct
Laboratory	Other tests as indicated from H&P.
Premedication	< 1 yr old rarely needs premedication; > 1 yr old, either oral midazolam (0.75 mg/kg) or oral ketamine (6 mg/kg) ~30 min preop is adequate.

INTRAOPERATIVE

Anesthetic technique: GETA

Induction	Typically, an inhalational induction (sevoflurane or halothane ± N_2O/O_2) while patient is breathing spontaneously. Airway obstruction is best treated with an oral airway. Anticipate difficult laryngoscopy if large, prepalatal cleft present. Intubate with oral RAE tube and secure in midline of lower lip. In patients with difficult airways, FOI is the technique of choice. Avoid muscle relaxants for difficult intubations until ETT is placed.
Maintenance	Standard pediatric maintenance (see p. D-3) ± muscle relaxant. Airway is shared with the surgeons. The Dingman mouth gag is used for surgical exposure and may inadvertently compress the ETT or cause an endobronchial intubation. Monitor PIP before and after placement of Dingman. Flexion of the neck also may cause endobronchial intubation. Extension of the neck may cause complete or partial extubation. Adequacy of ventilation should be checked after every position change. Bilateral breath sounds should be equal after final positioning. ETT should be sutured to the alveolar ridge. In palatoplasty, the palate is infiltrated with epinephrine (in lidocaine usually) →↓blood loss + ↑dysrhythmias (halothane > sevoflurane). ↑$PaCO_2$ →↑dysrhythmias.
Emergence	★ Pharyngeal (throat) packs are usually placed to prevent aspiration of blood. **NB:** Packs must be removed before extubating the trachea. Consider laryngoscopy to inspect airway and remove blood and clots before extubation. A tongue stitch is useful postop following cleft palate surgery. It may be used to pull the tongue forward to relieve postop respiratory obstruction. Extubation in the lateral (tonsillar) position is useful in promoting drainage of blood and secretions.

Blood and fluid requirements	IV: 18-20 ga × 1
	NS/LR @:
	  4 ml/kg/h – 0-10 kg
	  + 2 ml/kg/h – 11-20 kg
	  + 1 ml/kg/h – > 20 kg
	  (e.g., 25 kg = 65 ml/h)
		Blood loss replaced by 3:1 crystalloid or 1:1 colloid (e.g., 5% albumin or 6% hetastarch). Rarely, a blood transfusion may be indicated for hemorrhage.

Monitoring	Standard monitors (p. D-1)	
Positioning	✓ and pad pressure points. ✓ eyes.	
Complications	Obstructed ETT →↑PIP Mucous plugging Hemorrhage	✓ ETT to see that it is not partially or completely obstructed by mouth gag. ✓ bilateral breath sounds.

POSTOPERATIVE

Complications	Retained throat pack Airway edema → croup Hemorrhage Obstructive sleep apnea	✓ for retained throat pack if there are Sx of airway obstruction in immediate postop period. Rx of postintubation croup consists of cool, humidified, 100% O_2 mask, or nebulization 2.25% racemic epinephrine (0.5 ml in 3 ml NS). Racemic epinephrine is given for its vasoconstrictor, rather than its bronchodilator, effect. If posterior pharyngeal edema is present, consider dexamethasone 0.5 mg/kg iv.

Pain management	Acetaminophen 20 mg/kg
	  (suppository/po)
	Morphine 0.05-0.1 mg/kg iv
	  q 2-3 h prn
		Avoid oversedation in patients with Abbe-Estlander repair 2° airway obstruction.

Tests	Hct, if indicated.	Others as indicated.

OTOPLASTY

SURGICAL CONSIDERATIONS

Description: There are a number of congenital ear malformations. The two most frequently encountered in the OR are **prominent ear** and **microtia**. Both conditions can be unilateral or bilateral.

Prominent ears are usually an isolated finding. The ear is examined in thirds to determine where the prominence lies, and the surgery is tailored to correct the specific excesses. The antihelical fold is usually flattened and requires reshaping. The prominence of the ear, as measured by its projection from the mastoid process, is decreased accordingly. This usually involves an elliptical skin incision in the posterior ear area, dissection over the mastoid, and one, or a combination of three techniques—mattress sutures, cartilage scoring, and/or resection.

Variant procedure or approaches: All procedures are similar, with minor differences in suturing and amount of resected tissue. In addition to the posterior incisions, an anterior incision can be used in some approaches.

Microtia is within the congenital anomaly spectrum of hemifacial microsomia, and the associated facial malformation may include a small asymmetric jaw, creating a difficult intubation. Reconstruction is most often accomplished

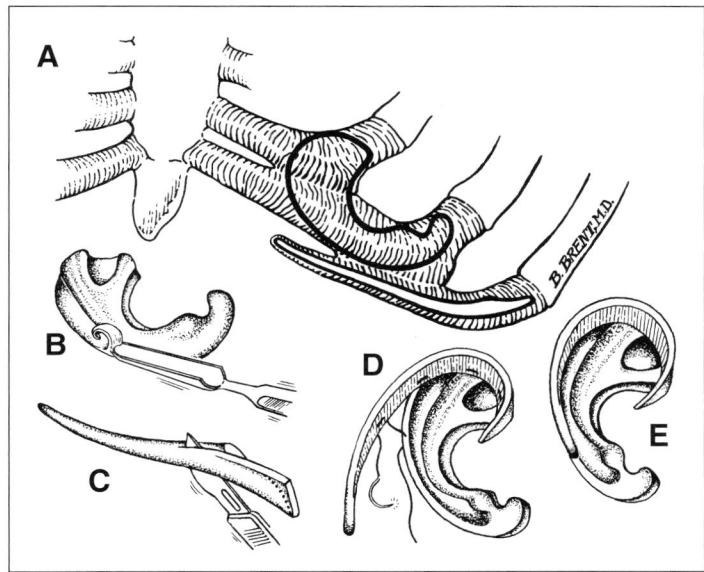

Figure 12.8-15. Fabricating an ear framework from costal cartilage. (A) Donor site: the contralateral thorax. The helical rim is obtained from a 'floating' rib cartilage, the main pattern from the synchondrosis of two cartilages. (B) Sculpting the main block. (C) Thinning the 'floating' rib cartilage to produce a delicate helical rim. (D) Affixing the rim to the main framework block. (E) Completed framework. (Reproduced with permission from Aston SJ, Beasley RW, Thorne CH, eds: *Grabb and Smith's Plastic Surgery*, 5th edition. Lippincott-Raven, 1997.)

with autologous rib graft as a multistaged procedure. This donor site comes with the attendant risks of pneumothorax and hemothorax (Fig 12.8-15). Stage one is the creation of a cartilaginous framework, with placement into a cutaneous pocket symmetric with the normal ear, if present (Fig 12.8-16). Stage one is accomplished once the rib cartilage has grown to sufficient size—usually, ~6-7 yr of age. Stage two requires transposition of the lobule 3 mo after stage one. Stage three is the elevation with skin graft of the framework from the head posteriorly. Stage four is the creation of a tragus and conchal excavation.

Variant procedure or approaches: Recently, **porous polyethylene implants** have been used to avoid donor-site morbidity, and **temporoparietal fascial flaps** provide coverage to avoid alloplastic extrusion.

Usual preop diagnosis: Ear malformation; prominent ears; microtia; anotia

SUMMARY OF PROCEDURE

Position	Supine; table rotated either 90° or 180°; oral intubation
Incision	Posterior ear; occasionally anterior ear; microtia, stage-dependent; and chest wall
Unique considerations	Head turned from side-to-side during operation.
Antibiotics	Cefazolin 25 mg/kg (up to 1 g) iv preop
Surgical time	2-4 h (depends on unilateral vs bilateral); 1st stage microtia much longer
Closing considerations	Ear dressing requires 5-10 min at end of procedure. Delicate vacuum test-tube drainage system in 1st stage microtia repair fixed to head dressing.
EBL	10-100 ml
Postop care	PACU → room
Mortality	Rare
Morbidity	**Protruding ears:**
	Hematoma formation: < 1%
	Infection: < 1%
	Asymmetrical ear reduction: < 1%
	Suture extrusion < 1%

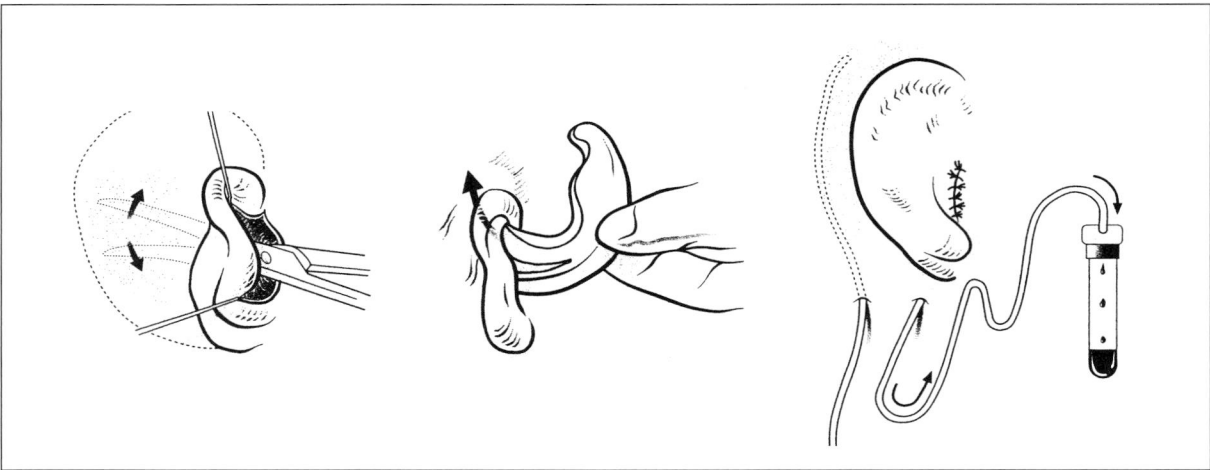

Figure 12.8-16. The cutaneous 'pocket.' The vestigial native cartilage is excised, then a skin pocket is created. To provide tension-free accommodation of the framework, the dissection is carried out well beyond the proposed auricular position. Using two silicone catheters, the skin is coapted to the framework by means of vacuum tube suction. (Reproduced with permission from Booth PW, Schendel SA, Hausamen J-E, eds: *Maxillofacial Surgery*. Churchill Livingstone, 1999.)

Morbidity, cont.	**Microtia:**
	Pneumothorax or hemothorax
	Hematoma, infection, and skin loss: 1.6% (total)
	Overgrowth: $\leq 41\%$
Pain score	4

PATIENT POPULATION CHARACTERISTICS

Age range	6+ yr
Male:Female	2:1
Incidence	Unknown
Etiology	**Microtia:** 9.2% bilateral; 32% left vs 58% right; 4.9% recurrence within immediate family
	Protrusion: Also seen among family members. Most are bilateral.
Associated conditions	**Protruding ears:** none known
	Microtia: Brachial arch deformities: bone/soft tissue deficit, 36.5%; facial nerve weakness, 15.2%; cleft lip ± palate, 4.3%; macrostomia, 2.5%; urogenital defects, 4%; cardiovascular malformations, 2.5%; other, 1.6%

ANESTHETIC CONSIDERATIONS

See Anesthetic Considerations for Ear Surgery, Chapter 3.0 Otolaryngology, p. 162.

References

1. Brent B: Ear reconstruction. In *Maxillofacial Surgery*. Booth PW, Schendel SA, Hausamen J-E, eds. Churchill Livingstone, Edinburgh: 1999, 1419-28.
2. Brent B: Technical advances in ear reconstruction with autogenous rib cartilage grafts: Personal experience with 1200 cases. *Plastic Reconstruct Surg J* 1999; 104(2):319-38.

13.0 OUT-OF-OPERATING ROOM PROCEDURES

Surgeons

Charles DeBattista, MD (*Electroconvulsive therapy*)
Joan K. Frisoli, MD, PhD (*TIPS*)
Stephen T. Kee, MD (*Tracheobronchial stenting, RF ablation*)
L. Bing Liem, DO (*DC cardioversion, ICD*)
Michael P. Marks, MD (*Interventional neuroradiology*)
Erik J. Sirulnick, MD (*DC cardioversion, ICD*)
Daniel Y. Sze, MD, PhD (*Image-guided procedures*)

13.1 OUT-OF-OPERATING ROOM PROCEDURES—ADULT

Anesthesiologists

Jay B. Brodsky, MD
John L. Chow, MD, MS
J. Kent Garman, MD, MS, FACC
Leland H. Hanowell, MD
Richard A. Jaffe, MD, PhD
Stanley I. Samuels, MB, BCh, FFARCS
Richard C. Shinaman, MD

ANESTHESIA FOR OUT-OF-OPERATING ROOM PROCEDURES

GENERAL COMMENTS

Advances in the fields of radiology, cardiology, and neurology have led to an increase in the number of anesthesia procedures performed away from the OR. In line with these changes, the ASA has provided guidelines for the safe delivery of anesthesia at locations remote from the OR environment.

Anesthetic considerations for out-of-OR locations (modified from ASA Guidelines[1]) include:

- Primary and backup O_2 sources (e.g., piped O_2 + 1 full E cylinder)
- Adequate and reliable suction
- Adequate and reliable scavenging system (for inhalational anesthesia)
- Self-inflating hand resuscitator bag with ability to deliver at least 90% O_2
- Adequate anesthetic drug supplies and equipment
- Adequate monitoring equipment to allow adherence to the "Standards of Basic Anesthetic Monitoring"[2]
- Sufficient electrical outlets connected to an emergency power supply
- Wet locations (e.g., cysto, arthroscopy, labor, and delivery) should be equipped with either an isolated electrical source or circuits with ground-fault interrupters.
- Adequate illumination for patient observation and monitoring equipment (flashlight backup)
- Sufficient space for expeditious access to patient, machine, and support equipment
- Emergency cart with defibrillator immediately available
- Immediate access to skilled anesthesia support personnel

References

1. Guidelines for Non-Operating Room Locations. American Society of Anesthesiologists, Park Ridge, IL: 1997.
2. Standards for Basic Anesthesia Monitoring. American Society of Anesthesiologists, Park Ridge, IL: 1998.

ELECTROCONVULSIVE THERAPY (ECT)

PROCEDURAL CONSIDERATIONS

Description: **Electroconvulsive therapy (ECT)** is the transcutaneous application of small electrical stimuli to the brain to produce generalized seizures for the treatment of selected psychiatric disorders, such as severe depression. There are several important aspects of ECT that are of relevance to the anesthesiologist. The first is the uncontrolled motor activity associated with generalized seizures. Prior to introduction of GA, the most common injuries associated with ECT were compression fractures of the vertebral bodies and broken limbs from violent tonic clonic motor activity. Even with complete paralysis, the masseter muscles are directly stimulated to contract during seizure induction. As a result, the most common malpractice claims in ECT involved dental injuries.

A second consequence of ECT induction is that the electrical stimulus can cause contraction of cranial musculature and a brief dilation of meningeal blood vessels, resulting in postictal headaches in up to 40% of patients. Patients < 50 yr and those with a Hx of migraine headaches appear most at risk for post ECT headaches that may occasionally require aggressive pain management. Finally, ECT may be a significant hemodynamic stressor. Initially, central parasympathetic centers are activated, resulting in bradydysrhythmias in ~30% of patients. Brief sinus pauses are not uncommon. The initial parasympathetic effects are followed by sympathetically mediated increases in HR and BP up to 20-30% above baseline. In some patients, MAP may even double. These cardiovascular responses can persist even after the procedure is completed.

The optimal position for ECT is supine. Occasionally, the head is kept slightly raised to help maintain an adequate airway and decrease anxiety. Patients typically come to ECT quite anxious about the procedure. ECT is generally performed in a PACU, or specialized ECT suite. The electrical stimulus is applied through plastic adhesive leads or metal leads prepared with a contact gel. These leads are usually applied to the forehead in a bitemporal or right unilateral placement. Monitoring typically includes a two-lead electroencephalogram (EEG) and frequently an electromyogram (EMG) to measure motor activity. A BP cuff is inflated to act as a tourniquet and prevent neuromuscular blockade in the distal limb. Thus, an arm or leg can be used to measure motor duration of the seizure. A special ECT device is used to generate the appropriate electrical stimulus. Seizures are typically 30-90 sec in duration, and the entire procedure—from the induction of anesthesia to patient awakening—is generally < 15 min. The recovery period averages 45-90 min and allows for monitoring of vital signs, as well as the opportunity for the postictal confusion to clear. Patients can wake up mildly confused-to-frankly delirious and require close nursing supervision. Treatments are typically performed every other day, and the average number of treatments is 6-12 in the management of major depression.

The most common morbidities associated with ECT include headaches and myalgias. Postictal confusion is the rule and some anterograde and retrograde memory loss occurs in all patients. Memory loss is typically confined to the preop and postop settings; however, there may be a cumulative memory loss with subsequent ECT treatments within a given series. In most patients, memory loss recovers in 1-3 wk following treatment. In rare instances, autobiographical memory loss has been reported for months or years after an ECT series has been completed. Long-term memory loss appears to be more common with bilateral lead placement. ECT-related mortality is estimated at approximately 4/10,000. Cardiac events account for 67% of all ECT-related deaths, with malignant arrhythmias and MIs accounting for most fatalities. Pulmonary events (obstruction, pulmonary edema, or emboli) account for most additional mortality. Cerebrovascular infarctions or hemorrhages have rarely been reported with ECT.

Usual preop diagnosis: Depression; mania; catatonia; refractory psychosis

SUMMARY OF PROCEDURE

Position	Supine
Incision	None
Special instrumentation	Seizure generator & electrodes; EEG/EMG monitors
Unique considerations	Requires complete muscle relaxation to prevent injury. Bite block required to prevent dental injury. Tourniquet (BP cuff) applied before administration of muscle relaxant.
Antibiotics	None
Procedure time	Setup: 5-10 min
	Treatment: < 10 min (seizure duration 25-280 sec)
Postop care	PACU → room or home
Mortality	4/10,000
Morbidity	HA/myalgias: Common
	Confusion/memory loss: Common
	Cardiac dysrhythmias: 10-40% (brief asystole common)
	MI: Rare
	Pulmonary edema/pulmonary aspiration: Rare
	CVA: Rare
Pain score	2-3 (HA)

PATIENT POPULATION CHARACTERISTICS

Age range	≥ 18 yr. Some states (e.g., Texas) forbid ECT in minors, and ECT is rarely performed in adolescents; however, patients in their 90s are sometimes candidates for ECT. There is a preponderance of geriatric patients on many ECT services.
Male:Female	1:2
Incidence	The lifetime prevalence of major depression (the primary indication for ECT) is ~17%; 26% of women and 12% of men are affected. < 1% of patients with major depression undergo ECT; and approximately 400,000 ECT procedures are performed in North America annually.
Associated conditions	Substance abuse (30% of all depressed patients meet criteria for alcohol or drug abuse); panic attacks (30% of depressed patients); psychotic symptoms (14% of patients); HTN and sinus tachycardia; dehydration; self-inflicted trauma

ANESTHETIC CONSIDERATIONS

PREOPERATIVE

Patients presenting for ECT often have failed to respond to antidepressants; however, most will continue to take psychotherapeutic agents. Many of the older patients will be taking other medications for coexisting medical conditions. Drug interactions are an important consideration for the anesthesiologist (see Drug Interactions, p. F-1). The most commonly used antidepressants are listed in Table 13.1-1.

Anesthesia for ECT may seem to be a benign procedure; however, these cases—which seldom take > 20 min—can prove very challenging, especially in the geriatric population. ECT can place significant stress on the cardiovascular system; therefore, particular care should be taken to evaluate and optimize the patient's pretreatment cardiovascular status. ECT usually takes place in remote locations, so the anesthesiologist must ensure that the location is properly equipped and complies with ASA Guidelines for Out-of-OR Procedures (see p. 1154).

Respiratory	These patients will require airway management and PPV. Hence, preop assessment of the airway must focus on the ease of mask ventilation and the potential need for ET intubation (e.g., airway compromise or severe GERD).
Cardiovascular	A recent MI (< 3 mo) is a contraindication to ECT. Relative contraindications include aortic aneurysm, angina, CHF, and thrombophlebitis. The presence of dysrhythmias, a pacemaker, or ICD is not a contraindication for ECT. For the patient with a pacemaker, a means (e.g., a magnet) should be available to convert the pacemaker to an asynchronous mode. **Tests:** As indicated from H&P.
Gastrointestinal	Patient should be npo. Patients with Sx of GERD should be pretreated with Na citrate (30 ml po), ranitidine (50 mg iv) and metoclopramide (10 mg iv). ET intubation should be considered for all patients at risk for aspiration.
Neurological	ECT is relatively contraindicated in the presence of ↑ICP, and recent CVA (< 3 mo), intracranial mass lesions or recent intracranial surgery (< 3 mo).
Endocrine	Presence of a pheochromocytoma is a contraindication to ECT. < 1% of hypertensive patients will have a pheochromocytoma, Sx of which may be confused with a psychiatric disorder.
Genetic	✓ for family Hx of pseudocholinesterase deficiency. Mivacurium (0.15 mg/kg) is a suitable alternative to succinylcholine. **Tests:** Dibucaine number (nl ≥ 80) and serum cholinesterase level, if indicated from H&P.
Hepatic	Hepatotoxicity has been associated with use of MAOI. **Tests:** Consider LFTs for patients on chronic MAOI therapy.
Orthopaedic	In patients susceptible to bone fracture (e.g., severe osteoporosis, osteoporosis imperfecta), an increased succinylcholine dosage (1.5 mg/kg) is given to ensure profound muscle relaxation. Patients with severe rheumatoid arthritis may have unstable C-spine, and extreme care should be taken during positioning of head and neck.

Table 13.1-1 Commonly Used Antidepressant Medications

Tricyclic	**MAOI**	**SSRI**	**SNRI and other Antidepressants**
amitriptyline (Elavil, others)	isocarboxazid (Marplan)	fluoxetine (Prozac)	venlafaxine (Effexor)
amoxapine (Asendin)	phenelzine (Nardil)	paroxetine (Paxil)	nefazodone (Serzone)
desipramine (Norpramin)	tranylcypromine (Parnate)	sertraline (Zoloft)	sibutramine (Meridia)
doxepin (Sinequan)	St. John's wort	fluvoxamine (Luvox)	mirtazapine (Remeron)
imipramine (Tofranil)	selegiline	citalopram (Celexa)	bupropion (Wellbutrin)
maprotiline (Ludiomil)		escitavopram (Lexapro)	trazodone (Desyrel)
nortriptyline (Pamelor)	**Lithium**		
protriptyline (Vivactil)	(Often used as an adjunctive agent/mood stabilizer in depression)		
trimipramine (Surmontil)			

MAOI = monoamine oxidase inhibitor
SSRI = selective serotonin reuptake inhibitor
SNRI = selective norepinephrine/serotonin reuptake inhibitor

Ophthalmologic   Retinal detachment is a relative contraindication to ECT. Succinylcholine should be avoided in patients with glaucoma treated with cholinesterase-inhibitors (e.g., echothiophate). Mivacurium (0.15 mg/kg) is a suitable alternative.

Pregnancy   Pregnancy is not a contraindication for ECT (even in the third trimester). After the 4th mo, the need for full-stomach precautions requires rapid-sequence induction and ET intubation (see p. B-5). Left uterine displacement should be maintained during treatment. Monitor fetal heartbeat.

Psychiatric Drugs   Patients receiving tricyclic antidepressants (TCAs) may have an exaggerated pressor response to direct-acting sympathomimetic drugs, with the potential for tachycardia, dysrhythmias, and hyperthermia. The response to indirect-acting sympathomimetic drugs (e.g., ephedrine) may be attenuated in these patients. TCAs also will increase the effects of anticholinergic drugs (e.g., glycopyrrolate, atropine). Patients receiving MAOIs will exhibit exaggerated responses to indirect-acting sympathomimetic drugs (e.g., ephedrine). Additionally, in these patients succinylcholine metabolism is inhibited (↑NMB), and meperidine is contraindicated (↑↑BP, ↑Sz, ↑↑T). It is probably unnecessary to discontinue TCAs or MAOIs prior to ECT, as long as these interactions can be avoided. Lithium should be discontinued for at least 3 d prior to ECT to avoid delayed recovery and subsequent posttreatment agitation and confusion. Lithium also is associated with ↑NMB (succinylcholine and pancuronium). SSRIs have been associated with prolonged ECT-induced seizure duration, and adverse behavioral/neurological effects following haloperidol administration (use droperidol and metoclopramide with caution). No adverse interactions have been reported between anesthetic agents and SSRIs or SNRIs.

Laboratory   Tests as indicated from H&P.

Premedication   Although usually not required, some patients may benefit from an antisialagogue (glycopyrrolate 0.2 mg iv). Patients with Hx of postop N/V will benefit from a prophylactic antiemetic (e.g., ondansetron 4 mg iv). Patients with postseizure muscle pain and headache may benefit from ketorolac (30 mg iv). Some patients will require 500-1000 mg caffeine iv to decrease seizure threshold. The caffeine effect should be manifest in 5 min. Verapamil (not adenosine, which is blocked by caffeine) should be available to control supraventricular tachycardia (0.07-0.25 mg/kg over 2 min). Esmolol and diltiazem are alternative drugs for control of HR.

INTRAOPERATIVE

Anesthetic technique: A review of previous anesthetic records is very helpful in formulating the anesthetic plan and in anticipating physiological changes unique to each patient. Usually brief iv anesthesia (mask oxygenation and ventilation) with profound muscle relaxation is required to prevent patient injury during seizures. Prior to induction, a tourniquet (BP cuff) is applied to the non-iv arm and inflated to a pressure above systolic. This prevents neuromuscular blockade distal to the cuff and permits direct monitoring of seizure activity. Preop BP control (e.g., labetalol 5-20 mg, diltiazem 10-20 mg iv, or esmolol 0.5-1 mg/kg iv in increments) is often necessary.

Induction   Preoxygenation should be attempted in all patients. In some patients who are intolerant of a mask, a less intrusive blow-by technique may be tried. Anesthesia is induced with either STP (1.5-3 mg/kg), sodium methohexital (0.5-1 mg/kg), or etomidate (0.1-0.2 mg/kg). Propofol (1-1.5 mg/kg) may be used, but may shorten seizure duration. Remember that TCAs and MAOIs can increase sleep time. After tourniquet inflation, succinylcholine (1 mg/kg) is injected to induce paralysis. Hyperventilation is carried out to enhance seizure activity. A bite block is placed and then the patient is ready for ECT. In barbiturate-tolerant patients, remifentanil (1-3 µg/kg) has been used as a means of reducing the barbiturate dose, thereby permitting adequate seizure duration. Patients receiving remifentanil need minimal postseizure BP control.

Maintenance   Given the brevity of this procedure, maintenance of anesthesia is rarely a concern; however, occasionally a second or third treatment may be necessary if the seizures are of inadequate duration (< 25 sec) and quality. In this case, a subsequent dose (10-30 mg) of succinylcholine may be needed. Assisted ventilation is necessary until spontaneous ventilation resumes. Of major concern during the seizure period is the hypertensive response. Some patients may need to be treated prior to induction of anesthesia with either labetalol (5-20 mg iv) or esmolol (10 mg q 1 min) to control HR/BP. SNP (5-50 µg/bolus iv) is useful to control BP in refractory cases.

Emergence   Patients should be awake within 5-10 min postseizure and often are disoriented. Small doses of midazolam (e.g., 0.25-0.5 mg iv) may help to control agitation. ASA guidelines for postanesthesia care should be followed (see p. 1154).

Blood and fluid requirements	No blood loss IV: 20 ga × 1 NS/LR @ TKO	
Monitoring	Standard monitors (p. B-1) Tourniquet EEG EMG	Seizure activity is usually monitored by a psychiatrist observing the tourniqueted limb, and by measuring EMG and EEG activity. (These monitors are usually an integral part of the ECT seizure generator.)
Positioning	Supine	
Complications	Dysrhythmias	Brief periods of asystole and profound bradycardia are not uncommon (usually related to parasympathetic overactivity). Treatment is rarely necessary.
	Tachydysrhythmias	Responds well to esmolol (10-15 mg iv) or lidocaine (1 mg/kg iv), although treatment is usually unnecessary.
	↑BP	↑BP readily responds to esmolol (10-30 mg), or labetalol (5-20 mg). In refractory cases, 10-50 μg of SNP may be necessary.
	Dental damage Pulmonary edema Aspiration	Use of bite block is essential. Dental damage is not prevented by muscle relaxation (direct electrical stimulation of facial and jaw muscles).

POSTOPERATIVE

Complications	HA, myalgias	Rx: ketorolac 30 mg iv
	N/V	Rx: ondansetron 4 mg iv
	Disorientation	Rx: midazolam 0.25-0.5 mg iv
	Memory impairment	
	MI/ischemia	
	Dysrhythmias	
	Pulmonary edema/aspiration	
	↑BP	Prolonged ↑BP is unusual and may suggest the need for further workup.

References

1. Ding Z, White PF: Anesthesia for electroconvulsive therapy. *Anesth Analg* 2002; 94:1351-64.
2. Martin DE, Kettl P: Anesthesia for electroconvulsive therapy. In *Alternate-Site Anesthesia: Clinical Practice Outside the Operating Room.* Russell GB, ed. Butterworth-Heinemann, Boston: 1997, 243-68.

INTERVENTIONAL NEURORADIOLOGY

PROCEDURAL CONSIDERATIONS

The indications for endovascular therapy for the brain and spine have grown extensively with the technical strides made during the past decade. Endovascular therapy is now widely used in the treatment of arteriovenous malformations (AVMs), arteriovenous fistulas (AVFs), tumors, and aneurysms. It also is used broadly for revascularization of the cerebral circulation in states of acute stroke or chronic intermittent ischemia. Many of these procedures can be performed with the patient awake; however, GA or deep sedation often is used in uncooperative patients and to minimize patient movement during procedures that require careful catheter and device control for safe operation. These procedures can be divided into three broad categories: 1) embolization, 2) aneurysm therapy, and 3) cerebral revascularization.

Embolization: This therapy may be used for a variety of lesions, including AVMs in the brain; dural AVFs; Vein of Galen malformations; vascular neoplasms, such as meningiomas, hemangiomas, glomus tumors, and juvenile nasal angiofibromas; and for treatment of epistaxis.

Embolization of AVM usually is performed as an adjunct to radiosurgery or neurosurgery, although in selected cases, embolization may be the definitive treatment. Brain AVMs are generally parenchymal lesions with multiple feeding pial arteries and draining veins. The goal of embolization is to reduce the size and shunt burden presented by the AVM before either radio- or neurosurgery. Liquid embolic agents are preferred, with the most widely used being n-butyl cyanoacrylate. Embolization often is preceded by physiologic testing, which may include the superselective injection of amobarbital into the portion of the intracranial circulation being considered for embolization.

Dural arteriovenous fistulas may involve the dural sinuses, most commonly in the area of the cavernous, transverse, and sigmoid sinuses. Because of their location, these malformations usually are supplied from meningeal vessels. A cavernous sinus fistula also may develop as a direct large-hole fistula between the internal carotid artery and the cavernous sinus. The embolization process for these dural-based lesions differs somewhat from the technique used for pial-based brain AVMs. Arterial embolization may be used, but venous occlusion with either balloons or coils is often the preferred treatment. Embolization of meningeal arteries may be preceded by clinical testing for cranial nerve deficits. This usually is accomplished with the superselective injection of lidocaine before embolization. If arterial embolization is utilized, liquid or particulate embolics may be used. Particle embolization employs polyvinyl alcohol particles (PVA) or the more recently introduced trisacryl gelatin microspheres.

Vein of Galen malformations are congenital lesions that may present in infants or children. Presenting symptoms include CHF, hydrocephalus, and neurodevelopmental delay. These lesions often require a staged approach, and present a special challenge in the neonate or infant. In general, arterial embolization is performed as the initial endovascular approach and a liquid embolic agent (n-butyl cyanoacrylate) is used. In some cases, this may be augmented by a venous approach, with embolization using platinum coils.

Tumor embolization usually is performed as an adjunct to the surgical resection of highly vascular tumors (e.g., hemangiomas, hemangioblastomas, glomus tumors, and juvenile nasal angiofibromas). Generally, arterial embolization of meningeal supply vessels is done before surgery, using PVA or trisacryl gelatin microspheres. Physiologic testing with superselective injection of lidocaine often precedes embolization.

Aneurysm therapy: Endovascular therapy is the treatment of choice for many intracranial aneurysms, and consists of either direct intraaneursymal obliteration with detachable platinum coils or occlusion of the parent artery to produce thrombosis of the aneurysm. Narrow-necked aneurysms may be treated using a microcatheter to introduce thrombosing coils directly into the aneurysm; however, wide-necked aneurysms are more difficult to treat using this technique. Balloon remodeling often is used for treatment of wide-necked aneurysms. This technique involves placing a balloon over the ostium of the aneurysm. The balloon is intermittently inflated with each coil insertion to prevent coil prolapse into the parent vessel. Recently, fenestrated stents have become available to treat wide-necked aneurysms. These are introduced into the parent vessel over the ostium of the aneurysm, which is then coiled through the fenestrations. Parent vessel occlusion is still used for some giant fusiform aneurysms. It generally is done in a two-step process, with clinical and neurophysiological monitoring. Test occlusion is initially performed with a balloon-tipped catheter, followed by permanent occlusion, using detachable balloons and/or coils.

Cerebral Revascularization: These procedures may be used in the setting of acute ischemic stroke or for the treatment of fixed atherosclerotic lesions. Acute stroke thrombolysis is performed up to 6 h after the onset of symptoms in the middle and anterior circulations (carotid territory) and up to 36 h after the onset of symptoms in the vertebrobasilar territory. Atherosclerotic stenosis in the cerebrovascular circulation (e.g., cervical carotid, extracranial vertebral artery) usually is treated with primary stenting (without prior angioplasty). Distal protection devices (e.g., balloon or basket devices) have been shown to reduce the thromboembolic complication rate and are likely to be adopted for routine use in the future. More distal lesions and intracranial lesions are treated either with angioplasty alone or are stented.

SUMMARY OF PROCEDURES

	Embolization	Aneurysm Therapy	Cerebral Revascularization
Position	Supine	⇐	⇐
Incision	Femoral artery, catheterization	⇐	⇐
Unique considerations	BP control; AVM; anticoagulation; EP monitoring	BP control; ± EP monitoring; anticoagulation	⇐
Antibiotics	None	⇐	⇐

	Embolization	Aneurysm Therapy	Cerebral Revascularization
Procedure time	2-5 h	2-4 h	⇐
Closing considerations	Femoral artery compression or closure device	⇐	⇐
EBL	Minimal	⇐	⇐
Postop care	Ward or ICU × 24-48 h	ICU	Ward or ICU
Mortality	1-2% (brain AVMs)	⇐	⇐
Morbidity	Overall: ~5%	⇐	⇐
	Thromboembolic stroke	⇐	⇐
	Hemorrhage (AVM, AVF)	SAH	Vessel rupture/dissection
Pain score	1-2	1-2	1-2

PATIENT POPULATION CHARACTERISTICS

Age range	Neonatal-elderly
Male:Female	1:1
Etiology	Congenital; acquired (traumatic, infectious, degenerative, etc.)
Associated conditions	SAH ± vasospasm; ↑ICP; HTN/CAD/PVD; blood dyscrasia

ANESTHETIC CONSIDERATIONS

PREOPERATIVE

Patients presenting for diagnostic neuroradiologic procedures frequently may require only local anesthesia and sedation. The newer nontoxic and low osmolality contrast agents have improved patient comfort and tolerance of these procedures while minimizing adverse reactions. Patients presenting for interventional neuroradiological procedures (e.g., embolization or stenting) are likely to experience more discomfort and, therefore, may require GA in order to tolerate the often lengthy procedures. The advantages of GA, however, must be balanced against the potential need for intraop neurological monitoring (e.g., speech, vision, and mental status) that requires the patient to be awake and cooperative. In this set of circumstances, close consultation between the neuroradiologist and anesthesiologist is required in formulating the anesthesia plan.

Respiratory	Access to the airway may be limited; therefore, examination should focus on the need for elective ET intubation. Patients with chronic cough may require GA to ensure immobility. **Tests:** As indicated from H&P.
Cardiovascular	Patients with recent intracranial hemorrhage may demonstrate ECG abnormalities, which need to be differentiated from new ischemic heart disease (ECHO, cardiac enzymes). **Tests:** ECG; other tests as indicated from H&P.
Neurological	Symptoms vary with the location, size, and type of lesion. Aneurysms seldom produce neurological symptoms unless they leak or rupture, whereas tumors are commonly associated with symptoms of ↑ICP (HA, N/V, altered mental status, papilledema). Patients with recent cerebral hemorrhages are likely to be medicated with calcium channel blockers (e.g., nimodipine, nicardipine) to ↓arterial vasospasm. Patients with ↑ICP or cranial trauma usually will need GA with intubation and mechanical ventilation.
Premedication	Preop sedation may mask the Sx of ↑ICP or intracranial hemorrhage. Patients at high risk for contrast-media reactions (e.g., patients with previous contrast reaction, allergy to iodine or seafood) should receive prophylactic treatment consisting of prednisone, 50 mg po q 6 h × 3, starting 18 h before the study, and diphenhydramine, 50 mg po/im, 1 h before the procedure.

INTRAOPERATIVE

Anesthetic technique: MAC (p. B-4) may be adequate for patients undergoing diagnostic procedures and necessary for patients requiring neurological assessment during more invasive procedures; otherwise, GETA.

Induction	Standard induction (p. B-2). Patients with ↑ICP should be hyperventilated to an $ETCO_2$ of 30 mmHg. In patients with vascular lesions that may leak or rupture, BP responses to laryngoscopy and intubation should be blunted (e.g., remifentanil 3-5 $\mu g/kg$).

Maintenance	Standard maintenance (p. B-3). Muscle relaxation is usually mandatory to control ventilation and minimize the chance of movement. Hyperventilation may be necessary to ↓ ICP and may also enhance the quality of the angiogram.	
Emergence	Prompt awakening is important to permit neurologic evaluation. Metoclopramide (10 mg iv) and ondansetron (4 mg iv) are useful to ↓ postop N/V. Extubate when airway reflexes have returned. Continuous control of BP may be necessary during emergence phase. Patients typically are transported to ICU.	
Blood and fluid requirements	IV: 18 ga × 1-2 NS/LR @ 3-5 ml/kg/h	
Monitoring	Standard monitors (see p. B-1). Arterial line Urinary catheter	BP can be monitored from femoral line placed by radiologist. Place urinary catheter if procedure is lengthy (> 3 h).
	± EPs	Keep inhalation agents < 0.5 MAC to minimize interference with EP monitoring. Supplement with remifentanil infusion, if necessary.
Control of BP	Isoflurane (if no EP monitoring) Esmolol (50-200 μg/kg/min) SNP (0.2-2 μg/kg/min) Maintain normovolemia.	BP control may be necessary during intracranial catheter manipulation, embolization, and postembolization. Close communication with the radiologist is important. SNP/esmolol may be infused through a second peripheral iv.
Positioning	✓ and pad pressure points. ✓ eyes.	X-ray table may not be well padded → nerve damage.

Complications, contrast-related	Common reactions:
	  N/V
	  Itching
	  Urticaria
	  Sensation of warmth
	  Pain
	  Anxiety
	  Rash
		These reactions occur in > 5% of patients, and may require no treatment apart from reassurance or a mild anxiolytic. Mild allergic reactions may be treated with diphenhydramine 25-50 mg iv. Monitor patients for progression of Sx, suggesting the need for more aggressive therapy.

	Neurotoxic Sx:
	  Hemiplegia
	  Blindness
	  Aphasia
	  ↓consciousness
		These reactions may be related to the hyperosmolarity of the agent. If persistent, procedure should be terminated. Rx may require steroids and vasopressors to improve perfusion. In the anesthetized patient, these Sx will be masked.

	Major allergic reactions:
	  Bronchospasm
	  ↓BP
	  Cardiac arrest
	  Pulmonary edema
	  Laryngeal edema
	  Dysrhythmias
		Epinephrine (0.25-0.5 mg iv) should be given immediately. Rx of **anaphylaxis** includes: eliminate antigens (e.g., contrast agent, latex, etc.); secure airway; administer 100% O_2, iv fluids, epinephrine, diphenhydramine. Supplemental Rx may include steroids (e.g., hydrocortisone 5 mg/kg), atropine, $NaHCO_3$, and epinephrine infusion.

Complications, other	Hemorrhage	Aneurysmal rupture or AVM bleeding may require immediate transport to OR for surgical repair.
	Vasospasm	Rx: vasodilators (e.g., NTG) or papaverine delivered by catheter, or balloon angioplasty.
	Occlusion of vessel	2° catheter injury of vessel wall. Rx: angioplasty. (Recanalization and stenting may be used for thrombotic occlusions.)

POSTOPERATIVE

Complications	Neurologic deficits	CT scan for evaluation, as prompt neurosurgical intervention may be required.
	Vasospasm	May require Ca^{++} channel blocker (e.g., nimodipine). Consult with neurosurgeon.

References

1. Bader MK: The complexity of caring for patients with ruptured cerebral aneurysm: case studies. *AACN Clinical Issues* 1997; 8(2):182-95.
2. Brilstra EH, Rinkel GJE, van der Graaf Y, van Rooij WJ, Algra A: Treatment of intracranial aneurysms by embolization with coils. *Stroke* 1999; 30:470-6.
3. Cardella JF, Waybill PN: Interventional radiology: diagnostic and interventional vascular applications. In *Alternate-Site Anesthesia: Clinical Practice Outside the Operating Room.* Russell GB, ed. Butterworth-Heinemann, Boston: 1997, 115-32.
4. Gobin YP, Laurent A, Merienne L, et al: Treatment of brain arteriovenous malformations by embolization and radiosurgery. *J Neurosurg* 1996; 85:19-28.
5. Guimaraens L, Sola MT, Matali A, et al: Carotid angioplasty with cerebral protection and stenting: report of 164 patients (194 carotid percutaneous transluminal angioplasties). *Cerebrovascular Diseases* 2002; 13:114-9.
6. Hashimoto T, Gupta DK, Young WL: Interventional neuroradiology-anesthetic considerations. *Anesth Clinics North Am* 2002; 20:347-59.
7. International subarachnoid aneurysm trial (ISAT) of neurosurgical clipping versus endovascular coiling in 2143 patients with ruptured intracranial aneurysms: a randomised trial. *Lancet* 2002; 360:1267-74.
8. Lai YC, Manninen PH: Anesthesia for cerebral aneurysms: a comparison between interventional neuroradiology and surgery. *Can J Anaesth* 2001; 48:391-5.
9. Liu AY, Paulsen RD, Marcellus ML, Steinberg GK, Marks MP: Long-term outcomes after carotid stent placement for treatment of carotid artery dissection. *Neurosurg* 1999; 45:1368-73.
10. Marks MP, Marcellus M, Norbash AM, Steinberg GK, Tong D, Albers GW: Outcome of angioplasty for atherosclerotic intracranial stenosis. *Stroke* 1999; 30:1065-9.
11. The n-BCA Trial Investigators: N-butyl cyanoacrylate embolization of cerebral arteriovenous malformations. Results of a prospective, randomized, multi-center trial. *AJNR* 2002; 23:748-55.
12. Phatouros CC, Higashida RT, Malek AM, et al: Carotid artery stent placement for atherosclerotic disease: rationale, technique and current status. *Radiology* 2000; 217:26-41.
13. Pollice PA, Yoder MG: Epistaxis: a retrospective review of hospitalized patients. *Otolaryngol Head Neck Surg* 1997; 117(1):49-53.
14. Qureshi AI, Suri MF, Khan J, Kim SH, Fessler RD, Ringer AJ, Guterman LR, Hopkins LN: Endovascular treatment of intracranial aneurysms by using Guglielmi detachable coils in awake patients: Safety and feasibility. *J Neurosurg* 2001; 94(6):880-5.
15. Russell GB: Anesthesia and interventional radiology. In *Alternate-Site Anesthesia: Clinical Practice Outside the Operating Room.* Russell GB, ed. Butterworth-Heinemann, Boston: 1997, 157-70.
16. Young WL, Pile-Spellman J, Bey-Hacein L, et al: Invasive neuroradiologic procedures for cerebrovascular abnormalities: anesthetic considerations. *Anesth Clinics North Am* 1997; 15:631-53.

DIRECT CURRENT (DC) CARDIOVERSION

PROCEDURAL CONSIDERATIONS

Description: Direct current (DC) cardioversion is a treatment for cardiac arrhythmias that uses a brief, dosed discharge of electricity across the heart. This biphasic waveform energy is more efficient, requiring 20-170 J, than monophasic waveform, which requires 50-360 J. Effective depolarization of a critical mass of the heart terminates the arrhythmia, allowing NSR to resume. The electrical shock is delivered across the chest wall, using two external paddles placed in one of the standard positions (i.e., the anterior-posterior (A-P), basilar-apical, or apical-posterior). The pulse is delivered synchronous to the QRS, thus avoiding the vulnerable period for inducing malignant tachyarrhythmias. Shock to treat ventricular fibrillation is applied emergently and asynchronously (thus, the term 'defibrillation'). To avoid discomfort, cardioversion should always be performed with the patient under deep sedation or brief GA. It is unacceptable to deliver this therapy to an awake patient.

Usual preop diagnosis: Atrial fibrillation (AF); atrial flutter; other supraventricular tachyarrhythmias; ventricular tachyarrhythmias

SUMMARY OF PROCEDURE

Position	Supine with defibrillator pads positioned A-P, basilar-apical, or apical-posterior
Unique considerations	Adequate anticoagulation (INR = 2-3) in patients with AF
Antibiotics	None
Procedure time	≤ 30 min
Postop care	Monitoring of cardiac rhythm in treatment room
Mortality	0.1%
Morbidity	Skin burns: < 15% (1st degree); 2% (2nd degree); lesser incidence with biphasic waveform
	Embolic event: 2% (↑risk with mitral valve disease)
	Acute pulmonary edema: 1%
	More serious arrhythmia: 1%
	Myocardial damage: Incidence unknown, but estimated to be very low–proportional to delivered energy.
Pain score	2-3

PATIENT POPULATION CHARACTERISTICS

Age range	All ages
Male:Female	3:1
Incidence	100,000/yr in the U.S.
Etiology	Reentry substrates (e.g., atrial flutter and fibrillation, ventricular tachycardia) from hypertensive heart disease, remote MI, cardiomyopathy; idiopathic
Associated conditions	LV dysfunction; CAD; cardiomyopathy; HTN; valvular disease; COPD; obesity; CVA; acute MI; pulmonary edema

ANESTHETIC CONSIDERATIONS

PREOPERATIVE

In general, patients presenting for cardioversion fall into one of two categories: elective or emergent. The presence or absence of hemodynamic instability will define the category. In the emergency patient, full-stomach precautions may be necessary (see p. B-5). Elective cardioversions usually are carried out on patients who have failed drug therapy.

Respiratory	Preop evaluation of the airway should focus on the need for elective ET intubation (patients with GERD, difficult mask fit, or airway compromise).
Cardiovascular	Relative contraindications to elective cardioversion include digitalis toxicity (toxic = > 3 ng/ml), ↓K⁺, inadequate anticoagulation, presence of β-blockade, AV block. The presence of significant CHF, CAD, or valvular disease may predispose this patient population to ↓↓BP in response to anesthetic agents. Consider use of etomidate (0.1-0.2 mg/kg). Patients at ↑risk for embolization include those with Hx of embolization within 2 yr, mitral stenosis, intraarterial thrombus, CHF, or hyperthyroidism. In these patients, ensure adequate anticoagulation (PT 1.5-2 × baseline, INR 2.0-3.0). It has been suggested that NTG patches near the electrodes be removed prior to cardioversion to avoid risk of explosion. **Tests:** ECG; TEE (✓ for thrombus and size of atrium); digitalis level (toxic = > 3 ng/ml → refractory VF following cardioversion); electrolytes; INR.
Endocrine	Hyperthyroidism → AF
Gastrointestinal	Full-stomach precautions (see p. B-5) may be necessary in the emergency patient.
Neurological	✓ Hx for TIAs or CVAs → ↑risk of embolic event. Pre- and postprocedure neurologic exams should be done.
Hematologic	✓ need for anticoagulation (see above).
Laboratory	Other tests as indicated from H&P.
Premedication	Usually not needed. For the emergency patient, take full-stomach precautions (p. B-5).

INTRAOPERATIVE

Anesthetic technique: Brief GA with mask oxygenation and ventilation

Induction	Preoxygenate patient. For hemodynamically fragile patients, etomidate (0.1-0.2 ml/kg iv) is perhaps ★ the agent of choice (**NB**: etomidate-induced clonus → ECG artifact). For the hemodynamically stable patient, use propofol (1.0-1.5 mg/kg iv slowly) until loss of lid reflex. Additional analgesia may be provided by remifentanil (1-2 μg/kg iv), thereby reducing anesthetic requirements.	
Maintenance	Occasionally necessary to repeat cardioversion. Additional small doses of propofol, etomidate, or remifentanil may be required.	
Emergence	Patients should awaken rapidly with full recovery of airway reflexes. Outpatients are usually discharged to home within 1-2 h.	
Blood and fluid requirements	No blood loss IV: 20 ga × 1 NS/LR @ TKO	
Monitoring	Standard monitors (see p. B-1).	Avoid placement of ECG electrodes in precordial area.
Positioning	Hospital bed, supine	Procedure takes place at patient's bedside.
Complications	Loss of airway	Use airway manipulation ± artificial airways; be prepared to intubate.
	VF	Use ACLS protocols.
	↑↑BP/myocardial ischemia	Cardioversion → catecholamine surge → acute MI in susceptible patient population.
	Severe bradycardia	Rx: Atropine (e.g., 0.4 mg iv)
	Thermal injury	Ensure good electrode/skin contact.
	↓CO	2° anesthetic drugs or myocardial stunning from cardioversion. Rx: inotropic support (e.g., ephedrine)

POSTOPERATIVE

Complications	Recall	Especially in hemodynamically fragile patients. Discuss possibility with patient in advance.
	Systemic embolization	Neurological exam should be repeated postcardioversion.
	↓BP/↓CO/CHF	Atrial contraction may not be effective following cardioversion → ↓CO/↓BP.
	New dysrhythmia	
Pain management	Minimal	Myalgias not uncommon; consider ketorolac.
Tests	ECG	Verify NSR.

References

1. Braunwald E, Zipes DP, Libby P, Zipes DD: *Heart Disease: A Textbook of Cardiovascular Medicine*, 6th edition. WB Saunders, Philadelphia, 2001.
2. Dell'Orfano JT, Naccarelli GV: Update on external cardioversion and defibrillation. *Curr Opin Cardiol* 2001; 16(1):54-7.
3. Ewy GA: The optimal technique for electrical cardioversion of atrial fibrillation. *Clin Cardiol* 1994; 17(2):79-84.
4. Gale DW, Grissom TE, Mirenda JV: Titration of intravenous anesthetics for cardioversion: a comparison of propofol, methohexital, and midazolam. *Crit Care Med* 1993; 21(10):1509-13.
5. Hullander RM, Leivers D, Wingler K: A comparison of propofol and etomidate for cardioversion. *Anesth Analg* 1993; 77(4): 690-4.
6. Kerber RE: Transthoracic cardioversion of atrial fibrillation and flutter: standard techniques and new advances. *Am J Cardiol* 1996; 78(8A):22-6.
7. Stoneham, MD: Anesthesia for cardioversion. *Anaesthesia* 1996; 57:565-70.
8. Trohman RG, Parrillo JE: Direct current cardioversion: indications, techniques, and recent advances. *Crit Care Med* 2000; 28(10Suppl):N170-3.

IMPLANTATION OF CARDIOVERTER-DEFIBRILLATOR (ICD)

PROCEDURAL CONSIDERATIONS

Description: The implantable cardioverter-defibrillator (ICD) is an effective device for the prevention of premature death from ventricular tachycardia (VT) or ventricular fibrillation (VF). The results of randomized trials involving survivors of cardiac arrest and those considered at risk for sudden death showed the superiority of ICD therapy over conventional medical therapy in lowering the incidence of sudden death and overall mortality. The most recent trial—MADIT II—showed the device therapy to be advantageous over standard medical therapy in patients with low LVEF (< 30%). Over the past decade, significant advances have occurred in ICD technology. The devices have decreased dramatically in size (now at 30-40 ml), along with substantial increases in functionality. Newer devices can incorporate the full capabilities of a permanent pacemaker for bradycardia support and resynchronization therapy, as well as hemodynamic monitoring. Therapies for atrial tachyarrhythmias (atrial tachycardia and fibrillation) are also available in select devices (e.g., Medtronic GEM AT). The more efficient biphasic waveform, which results in a much lower defibrillation threshold (DFT) and, hence, lowers required energy delivery and storage, is now standard for all ICDs, allowing for further miniaturization. Implantation of these small ICDs results in mortality and morbidity rates very similar to those associated with standard pacemaker implantation.

The device system consists of a small pulse generator and transvenous leads that are designed to record ventricular depolarizations and deliver a shock via coils or patches. ICD terminates VT/VF by sensing these rhythms and responding with an appropriate countershock. The most common ICD implantation uses endocardial leads inserted percutaneously (transvenous approach) via pectoral (or, rarely, abdominal) subcutaneous/submuscular pulse generator placement. In the unusual circumstances of difficult endocardial access or high DFT (> 25 J), additional leads can be placed either in the coronary sinus or subcutaneously. Very rarely would the leads (in the form of patches) be applied epicardially via a thoracotomy approach.

In the **transvenous approach**, the insertion of leads and pulse generator requires minimal anesthesia; however, during testing of defibrillation efficacy, VF is induced once or twice, and sometimes more frequently. Thus, in addition to continuous monitoring of VS and cardiac rhythm, the anesthesiologist should pay special attention to the patient's hemodynamic

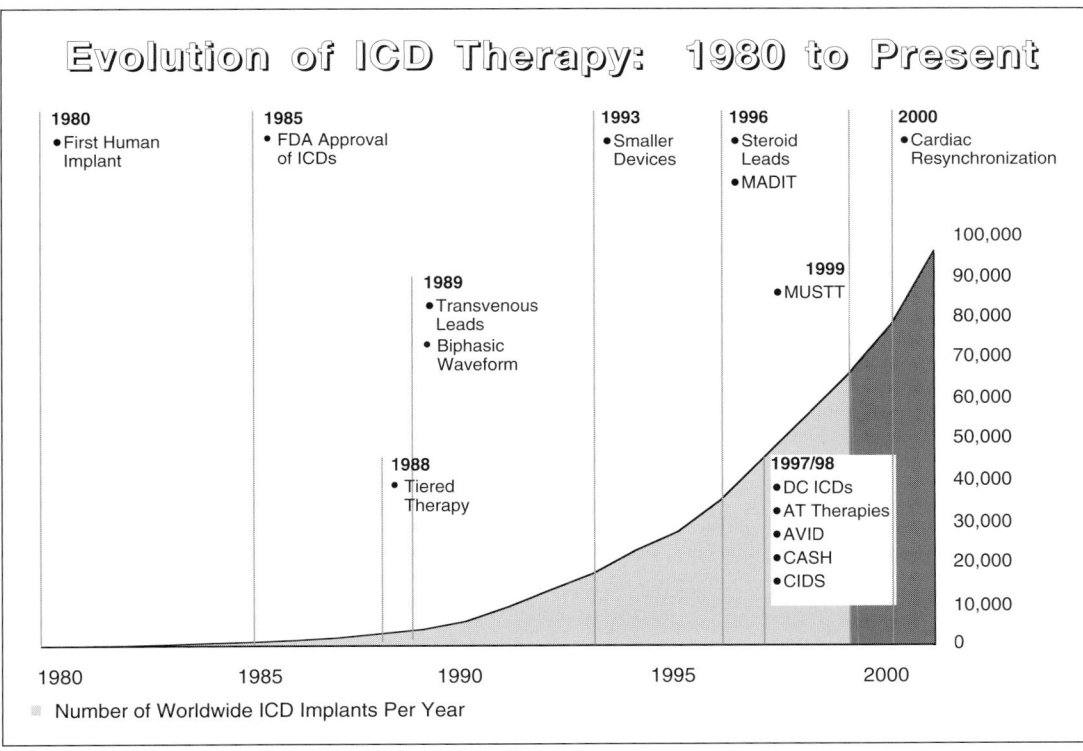

Figure 13.1-1. The annual implantation rate of ICDs is rising as the units become easier to implant and the indications for their use broadens. (Reproduced with permission from Medtronic, Inc. Minneapolis MN.)

stability prior to VF induction and after the defibrillation. In the event of failed defibrillation by the programmed first shock, a somewhat prolonged VF may occur. In the case of repeated DFT testing, it is customary to give at least 5-min intervals between VF inductions to allow for sufficient hemodynamic recovery. In patients with significant LV dysfunction, ↓BP is not uncommon, but caution should be taken with fluid administration. If recovery from ↓BP is slow, complications such as pneumo/hemothorax or pericardial effusion/tamponade should be considered. In the absence of a PA catheter (which would interfere with ICD lead positioning), accurate assessment of hemodynamic status is limited. Thus, meticulous attention should be directed at arterial pressure, HR, and oxygenation status. Finally, it is not uncommon to encounter acute atrial fibrillation (AF) from induction and conversion of VF.

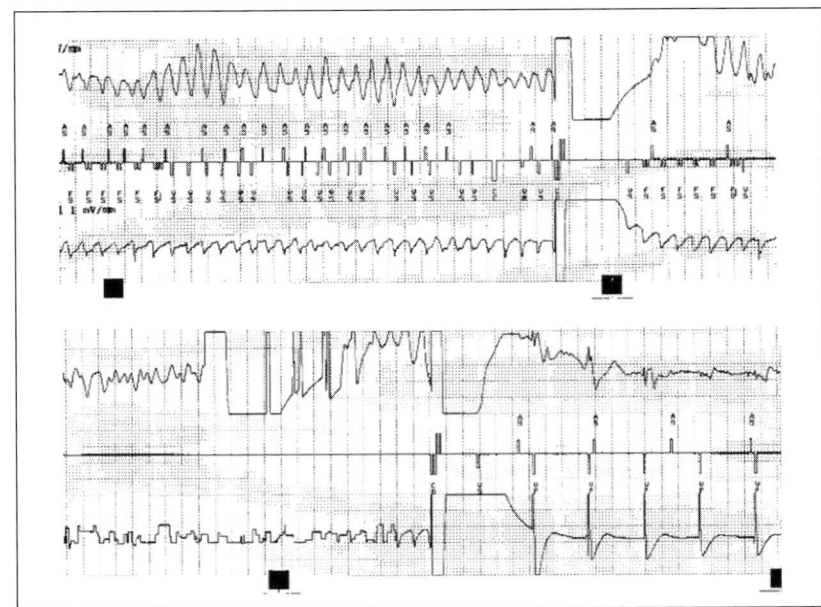

Figure 13.1-2. Induced VF (with underlying AF) is shown on top panel, whereby the first (24-J) shock failed to terminate VF but terminated AF (as indicated by the ICD annotation). The second shock (34-J) terminated VF, resulting in V-paced rhythm with underlying sinus and AV block. Total down-time during VF was 16 sec. Down-time is dependent on the detection time and charge time, which, in turn, depend on the energy programmed.

Fortunately, a cardioversion can be applied easily, using the ICD itself or relying on the external rescue system (external cardioversion).

Usual preop diagnosis: Documented, induced, or high-risk ventricular fibrillation

SUMMARY OF PROCEDURE

Position	Supine with defibrillator pads positioned A-P or basilar-apical
Incision	Left pectoral or abdominal
Special instrumentation	ICD pulse generator, lead(s), and testing system (manufacturer-specific)
Unique considerations	Multiple inductions of VT/VF with associated ↓CO, ↓BP
Antibiotics	Standard iv antimicrobial for staphylococcus/streptococcus organism
Surgical time	1-2 h (more for ICD with cardiac resynchronization [CRT])
Closing considerations	Routine subcutaneous/submuscular pocket closure
EBL	5-20 ml
Postop care	Monitoring of arrhythmia, pocket bleeding/hematoma, pneumothorax
Mortality	0.1% (transvenous); ≤ 5% (thoracotomy)
Morbidity	New-onset arrhythmias: ≤ 5%
	Pneumothorax: ≤ 5% (transvenous)
	Pericardial effusion/tamponade: ≤ 1% (transvenous)
Pain score	3 (6-9, thoracotomy)

PATIENT POPULATION CHARACTERISTICS

Age range	5-90 yr
Male:Female	4:1
Incidence	50,000/yr in the U.S.
Etiology	Reentry substrates from remote MI and cardiomyopathy; congenital anomalies (e.g., Long-QT and Brugada syndromes)
Associated conditions	LV dysfunction; CAD; cardiomyopathy; HTN; valvular disease; COPD; obesity; AF; CVA; anoxic encephalopathy

ANESTHETIC CONSIDERATIONS FOR ICD AND PACEMAKER PLACEMENT

PREOPERATIVE

Patients presenting for **ICD placement** may be divided into three populations, based on symptomatology, associated pathology, and probable outcome: (1) **Supraventricular dysrhythmias** (e.g., Wolff-Parkinson-White [WPW] syndrome): usually young and otherwise healthy patients. May be associated with Ebstein's anomaly (tricuspid valve defect → RV failure), mitral valve disease, or CAD. Low periop mortality (1%). (2) **Ventricular dysrhythmias:** usually older patients with significant ventricular dysfunction (EF = 10-35%) and other pathologies, such as CAD or cardiac failure. These patients have either survived an episode of VT/VF or are otherwise at risk for sudden death. (3) **Congestive heart failure (CHF)** without significant dysrhythmias, usually 2° dilated cardiomyopathy. These patients have very low EFs (10-25%), left bundle branch block, and Hx of failed conventional means of CHF treatment. The ICD device is implanted in these patients to provide paced 'resynchronization' of the contractions of the LV and RV. This requires a third-pacer lead placed into the coronary sinus to pace the LV independently of the RV. In this case, the device is not placed primarily for its defibrillator function, but for its ability to pace both ventricles synchronously (biventricular pacing). Patients presenting for **permanent pacemaker insertion** may have a variety of dysrhythmias, including sick sinus syndrome (SSS), heart blocks (2nd and 3rd degree), and tachycardias refractory to medication.

Respiratory	May have associated pulmonary disease 2° smoking.
	Tests: CXR; consider PFT, as indicated from H&P.
Cardiovascular	**ICD:** ICD patients are left on full medication, since it usually is impossible to wean them from antidysrhythmic medications before surgery. In most studies, patients have a mean LV EF of 35% and a New York Heart Association functional class of II or III.
	Supraventricular dysrhythmias: Look for precipitating factors in the dysrhythmia, and any methods that have been used to terminate the dysrhythmia. Usually, drug therapy is terminated before surgery to make a dysrhythmia inducible. Note type of drugs used to terminate a dysrhythmia.
	Ventricular dysrhythmias: Ask about any methods that have been used to terminate dysrhythmia. Look for associated conditions, including CAD, CHF, cardiomyopathy, LV aneurysm, HTN, mitral insufficiency, diabetes. Generally, these patients have poor LV function with ↑sensitivity to myocardial depressants. It is important to note that they may be on combinations of antidysrhythmics. Many of these drugs have significant negative inotropic effects. Of special note is amiodarone, which has been associated with intractable bradydysrhythmias, refractory vasodilation, and difficulty in weaning from CPB.
	Pacemaker: The anesthesiologist should be aware that there is an NASPE code (North American Society of Pacing and Electrophysiology) that describes pacemaker function with a 3- to 5-letter code. The first letter refers to the heart chamber that is paced and the second to the chamber that is sensed. These first two letters can be A (atrial), V (ventricular), or D (dual). The third letter indicates whether there is a triggering (T) or inhibiting (I) function, or both (D). For example, a VVI notation indicates that the ventricle is paced and sensed and there is inhibition by native beats. A fourth and fifth letter may be used to describe programmability and dysrhythmia control, respectively.
	Tests: ECG: ✓ dysrhythmia, ischemia, electrophysiologic report. ECHO: ✓ ventricular function, wall motion abnormalities, valvular problems. Cardiac angiography: ✓ ventricular function, CAD, valvular disease, LV aneurysm.
Renal	Patients with poor ventricular function may have associated renal compromise. Electrolyte abnormalities (K^+, Mg^{++}) may be associated with ↑cardiac irritability and should be corrected preop.
	Tests: BUN; Cr; electrolytes
Hematologic	Hb/Hct; coag tests (PT, PTT, Plt)
Laboratory	Other tests as indicated from H&P.
Premedication	For adults: midazolam 0.5-2.0 mg iv, with careful observation and supplemental O_2

INTRAOPERATIVE

Anesthetic technique: Local anesthesia with sedation, GA with LMA, or GETA, as indicated. Placement of most ICDs and pacemakers is done in the cardiac catheterization suite. ICDs are very small and are implanted in the same position as a pacemaker. If patients are orthopneic due to their CHF, or if the procedure is projected to be long, GA is often preferable. Also, elderly patients may become disoriented with sedation and, thus, may require GA.

Induction	Exact type of induction depends on the patient's medical condition. Sedation can be provided with small doses of midazolam (1-2 mg) ± fentanyl (25-50 μg) titrated to effect. An alternative technique is to use a propofol infusion (e.g., 25-75 μg/kg/min). Since local anesthesia is provided by the surgeon, the procedure usually is not painful and does not require postop pain control. It is important to avoid oversedating these patients, since they will tend to become disoriented and uncooperative. Even if local anesthesia with sedation is provided for the placement of leads and the device, a brief period of GA is always required for device testing. This can be provided easily with mask ventilation and induction with propofol (e.g., 1 mg/kg iv) or etomidate (e.g., 0.1 mg/kg iv), similar to anesthesia for cardioversion procedures. For those patients requiring GA for the entire procedure, induction with STP (2-4 mg/kg), propofol (1-2 mg/kg), or etomidate (0.1-0.3 mg/kg) is often used. Muscle relaxants are not required unless intubation is planned. Narcotics usually are not required since local anesthesia is used.	
Maintenance	As previously discussed, verification of correct lead placement involves the induction of ventricular fibrillation or tachycardia and the testing of the device's capability to restore NSR. External defibrillation should be available at all times, as should antidysrhythmics (e.g., lidocaine and amiodarone). While the device is tested, the patient should be breathing 100% O_2. Multiple testing cycles can result in depressed LV function, and inotropes may be needed.	
Emergence	These patients are extubated (if GETA or LMA used). Recovery is in the PACU. If, however, multiple test shocks are needed or the heart displays evidence of injury (need for inotropes, ST segment abnormalities), then extubation may need to be deferred to ICU.	
Blood and fluid requirements	IV: 16-18 ga × 1 NS/LR @ 6-8 ml/kg/min	Care should be taken to minimize iv fluids in CHF patients.
Monitoring	Standard monitors (see B-1). ± Arterial line ± CVP/PA External defibrillation Temperature	 A CVP or PA catheter may be placed according to LV function. ICD patients generally require only an arterial line. Because antidysrhythmics may affect the testing procedure, they should be avoided when possible. Defibrillation or cardioversion are treatments of choice. Normothermia should be maintained.
Positioning	Supine ✓ and pad pressure points. ✓ eyes.	
Complications	Pneumohemothorax Pericardial effusion/tamponade HTN/CHF Coronary sinus rupture	 Rarely, cardiac rupture may occur during lead extraction. Coronary sinus rupture has been reported during biventricular lead placement.

POSTOPERATIVE

Complications	Recurrent dysrhythmias Hemorrhage Ischemia	
Pain management	Usually managed with oral analgesics.	
Tests	CXR ECG Electrophysiologic testing Electrolytes	✓ line/lead placement, r/o pneumohemothorax. ✓ for ischemia, dysrhythmias.

References

1. Abraham WT, Fisher WG, Smith AL, Delurgio DB, Leon AR, Loh E, Kocovic DZ, Packer M, Clavell AL, Hayes DL, Ellestad M, Trupp RJ, Underwood J, Pickering F, Truex C, McAtee P, Messenger J: MIRACLE Study Group. Cardiac resynchronization in chronic heart failure. *N Engl J Med* 2002; 346(24):1845-53.

2. Cox JL: Anatomic electrophysiologic basis for the surgical treatment of refractory ischemic ventricular tachycardia. *Ann Surg* 1983; 198(2):119-29.
3. Craney JM, Gorman LN: Conscious sedation and implantable devices. Safe and effective sedation during pacemaker and implantable cardioverter defibrillator placement. *Crit Care Nurs Clin North Am* 1997; 9(3):325-34.
4. Kupersmith J: The past, present, and future of the implantable cardioverter defibrillator. *Am J Med* 2002; 113(1):82-4.
5. Kusumoto FM, Goldschlager N: Device therapy for cardiac arrhythmias. *JAMA* 2002; 287(14):1848-52.
6. Lappas DG, Hogue CW Jr, Cain ME, Cox JL: Anesthesia for electrophysiologic procedures. In *Cardiac Anesthesia*, 3rd edition. Kaplan JA, ed. WB Saunders, Philadelphia: 1993, 780-818.
7. Matthews EL, Atlee JL, Luck JC, Martin DE: Anesthesia for patients with electrophysiologic disorders. In *A Practical Approach to Cardiac Anesthesia*, 2nd edition. Hensley FA Jr, Martin DE, eds. Little, Brown, Boston: 1995, 392-415.
8. Swygman C, Wang PJ, et al: Advances in implantable cardioverter defibrillators. *Curr Opin Cardiol* 2002; 17(1):24-8.
9. Vijayakumar E: Anesthetic considerations in patients with cardiac arrhythmias, pacemakers, and AICDs. *Int Anesthesiol Clin* 2001; 39(4):21-42.

TRANSJUGULAR INTRAHEPATIC PORTOSYSTEMIC SHUNT (TIPS)

PROCEDURAL CONSIDERATIONS

Description: Hepatic cirrhosis is a progressive disease which eventually results in portal HTN and the development of varices at a variety of sites. Bleeding from esophageal varices is a serious complication of portal HTN, occurring in 25% of patients within 1 yr of diagnosis (~50% mortality). Prior to 1989, surgically placed shunts were used to direct high-pressure portal blood into the systemic venous circulation in patients with recurrent bleeding after endoscopic sclerotherapy or banding. The **transjugular intrahepatic portosystemic shunt (TIPS)** procedure has almost completely replaced surgical shunts.

TIPS is, as the name suggests, a percutaneous shunt between the portal and systemic circulations. The shunt is created between the hepatic vein and portal vein within the liver parenchyma, maintained by placement of metallic stents. This creates a low-resistance conduit to decompress the portal circulation, thereby decreasing variceal blood flow and ascites formation. Although it can be performed with conscious sedation, balloon dilation of the tract is extremely painful, typically requiring GA.

TIPS was developed initially by Rosch in dog studies in 1969. The first percutaneous portosystemic shunts were performed in humans using an angioplasty balloon in 1982, but the tract closed due to elastic recoil of the cirrhotic liver tissue. Palmaz and Richter performed the first successful TIPS in humans in 1989, using metallic stents to maintain the patency of the tract. Since then, TIPS has become the procedure of choice for patients who fail sclerotherapy and banding. In addition, it addresses another common problem associated with cirrhosis: refractory ascites.

Through the right IJ, a 10 Fr sheath is placed in the upper IVC. A catheter/guidewire combination is used to select the right hepatic vein. A wedged hepatic venogram using CO_2 is performed. Injection of iodinated contrast can result in rupture of the liver capsule and exsanguination. The wedged venogram refluxes contrast through the sinusoids and into the portal vein, thereby providing a map. The catheter is exchanged over a stiff wire for a metallic introducer/needle, either a Colapinto or Rosch-Uchida transjugular needle (Cook Inc., Bloomington IN). This device is curved at the tip and can be steered to puncture the right portal vein (Fig 13.1-3A). It is then rotated anteriorly and medially, so that the tip is pointed toward the portal vein bifurcation, and the needle is advanced 3-4 cm into the hepatic parenchyma toward the hepatic hilum. Suction is applied to the needle as it is slowly withdrawn until blood is aspirated. Contrast is then injected to identify the vascular structure that has been entered. If it is the portal vein, a guidewire is advanced into the splenic vein (Fig 13.1-3B), and the needle is exchanged for a 65 cm 5 Fr diagnostic catheter, typically a pigtail.

Portal venous pressures are measured and the pressure gradient between the portal vein and right atrium determined. Following a portal venogram, the catheter is exchanged for an angioplasty balloon, and the tract dilated (Fig 13.1-1C). A self-expanding stent (Wallstent, Schneider, Minneapolis, MN), is then positioned across the tract and deployed (Fig 13.1-1D). As most TIPS patients are future transplant candidates, care is taken to position the stent within the portal vein-to-hepatic vein tract, without encroaching on either the superior mesenteric vein or the IVC. The stent is then dilated to a diameter of 8-12 mm, using an angioplasty balloon. If necessary, a second stent is deployed to cover any remaining unstented tract. Following stent placement, the portal venogram and pressure gradients are remeasured. Ideally, the pressure gradient following shunting should be between 6-12 mmHg. If the gradient is too high, there is a risk of rebleeding; if too low, there is overshunting of blood, thus bypassing the entire portal venous system and increasing the risk of encephalopathy and liver failure. After successful completion of the shunt, all devices, including the right jugular sheath, are removed, and hemostasis is achieved. Patients are closely monitored in an ICU or step-down unit for 24-48 h.

Usual preop diagnosis: Bleeding esophageal varices (as a result of portal HTN); ascites; Budd-Chiari and hepatorenal syndromes

SUMMARY OF PROCEDURE

Position	Supine
Incision	Right IJ access
Special instrumentation	Rosch-Uchida or Colapinto needle set; angioplasty balloons; endovascular stents
Unique considerations	May need FFP.
Antibiotics	Cefazolin 1 g iv
Procedure time	2-6 h
EBL	0-3000 ml
Postop care	ICU or step-down unit; careful fluid management
Mortality	Emergency: 50-100%
	Child's A: 4% ⎫
	Child's B: 11% ⎬ See Table 13.1-2
	Child's C: 25% ⎭
Morbidity	Encephalopathy: 18-30%
	Late liver failure: 10-25%
	Shunt occlusion: 10%/yr
	Liver capsule puncture → intraperitoneal hemorrhage (continue procedure to decompress portal venous system → ↓bleeding).
	Hepatic artery puncture: may require embolization.
	Allergic reactions (see Contrast-related complications, p. 1161).
	MI (related to ↑CVP)
	Renal failure (usually transient)
Pain score	7-8 (first few h only)

Table 13.1-2. Child's Classification

	Class A	Class B	Class C
Ascites	None	Controlled	Uncontrolled
Bilirubin	< 2.0	2.0-2.5	> 3.0
Encephalopathy	None	Minimal	Advanced
Nutritional status	Excellent	Good	Poor
Albumin	> 3.5	3.0-3.5	< 3.0
Operative mortality	2%	10%	50%

(Adapted with permission from Baker RJ, Fischer JE: *Mastery of Surgery*, 4th edition. Lippincott Williams & Wilkins, 2001.)

ANESTHETIC CONSIDERATIONS
PREOPERATIVE

Patients presenting for TIPS procedures have portal HTN usually 2° end-stage liver disease (ESLD), which will affect the function of a variety of organ systems, as described below.

Respiratory   Abdominal distension → atelectasis → ↑pulmonary shunting → hypoxemia (hepatopulmonary syndrome in ESLD).

Encephalopathy → hyperventilation → ↓PaCO$_2$ (respiratory alkalosis with chronic acidosis as compensation). Pulmonary effusion may be present in 5-10% of patients.

Tests: ✓ CXR (for Sx of atelectasis); ABG and PFT, if indicated.

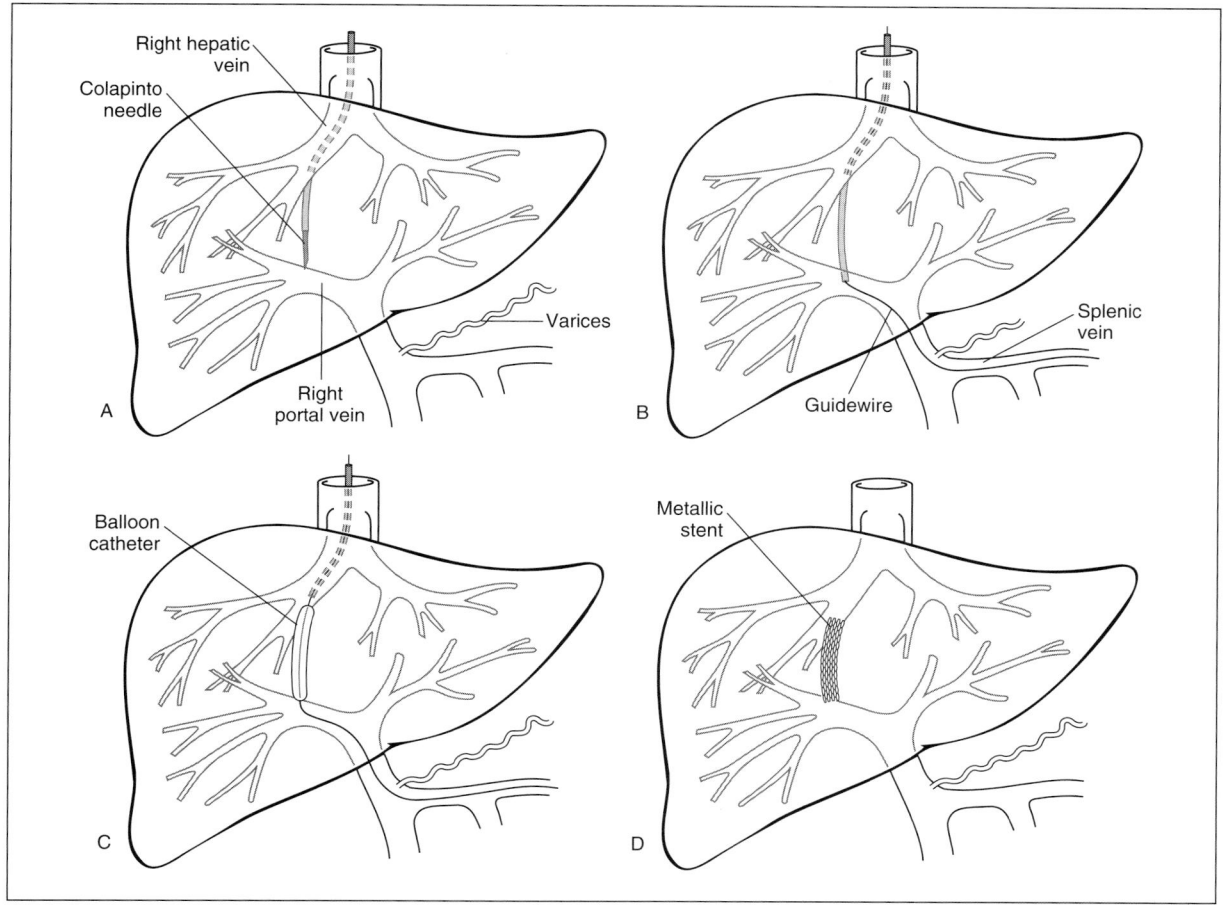

Figure 13.1-3. TIPS placement: (A) Sheathed Colapinto needle is advanced out of hepatic vein into portal vein branch. Varices are present. (B) Guide wire is advanced through the needle sheath into splenic vein. (C) Parenchymal liver tract is dilated using a balloon angioplasty catheter. (D) The metallic stent is deployed within the shunt tract. (Redrawn with permission from Haskal ZJ, Ring F: *Current Techniques in Interventional Radiology.* Cope C, ed. Current Science, Philadelphia, 1994.)

Cardiovascular	Cardiomyopathy (ETOH) and CAD (tobacco) occur at higher incidence in this patient population. Diuretic therapy → hypovolemia + ↓K$^+$ (furosemide) or ↑K$^+$ (spironolactone). Hyperdynamic circulation 2° to ↓peripheral resistance + ↓cardiac reserve are common findings, and correlate with poor postop outcome. **Tests:** ECG; electrolytes; cardiac ECHO, if indicated from H&P.
Neurological	Symptoms of hepatic encephalopathy range from mild confusion to coma. These patients may be very sensitive to narcotics and sedatives. A characteristic finding in liver failure is asterixis (liver flap). Hypernatremia and hypoglycemia may mimic hepatic encephalopathy. **Tests:** As indicated from H&P.
Hepatic	Drug metabolism may be markedly reduced; anticipate prolonged effect with sedative and narcotic drugs. Drugs with particularly prolonged action include midazolam, meperidine, ranitidine and lidocaine. Apparent resistance to pancuronium and all muscle relaxants is most likely due to an increased volume of distribution. Succinylcholine effects may be prolonged in patients with severe ESLD (2° ↓plasma cholinesterase). **Tests:** Bilirubin; PT; albumin; LFTs
Gastrointestinal	Ascites →↑intraabdominal pressure →↑risk of aspiration. Full-stomach precautions and rapid-sequence induction are recommended (see p. B-5). Portal HTN → variceal bleeding. If possible, avoid esophageal instrumentation (e.g., TEE, esophageal stethoscope, etc.). Gastritis and peptic ulceration may be present.

Renal	Oliguric renal failure may complicate ESLD (hepatorenal syndrome). This may be reversible if liver failure improves. Differential Dx includes prerenal azotemia and acute tubular necrosis. ★ **NB**: bilirubin metabolites interfere with creatinine measurement and may mask ↑creatinine levels. **Tests:** BUN; Cr; electrolytes
Endocrine	Hypoglycemia may be present in cases of severe cirrhosis. ESLD patients may have ↓ response to catecholamines. **Tests:** Glucose
Hematologic	Patients may be anemic 2° GI bleeding. The majority of patients will exhibit coagulopathy 2° ↓hepatic synthetic function (all factors except VIII and fibrinogen) and ↓Plt. Patients may require vitamin K (if coagulopathy is present and time permits), FFP (if PT > 2 sec above baseline), or Plt transfusion (if Plt < 100 K) before procedure; these products should be readily available. **Tests:** CBC; Plt; PT; others as indicated from H&P.
Premedication	Patients with significant ascites will require full-stomach precautions (see p. B-5). ★ **NB**: benzodiazepines should be used with caution in liver failure patients.

INTRAOPERATIVE

Anesthetic technique: In some patients (and at some centers), sedation with local anesthesia may be satisfactory; however, balloon dilation of the intrahepatic tract can be exceedingly painful. Remember, these patients may be very sensitive to narcotics → respiratory arrest. GETA is often necessary to provide adequate analgesia and airway protection.

General anesthesia

Induction	Rapid-sequence induction (see p. B-5) is necessary in patients with encephalopathy, abdominal distention and recent variceal bleeds (blood in the stomach).	
Maintenance	Standard maintenance (see p. B-3). If muscle relaxation is to be maintained, low-dose vecuronium (0.15 mg/kg) or cisatracurium (3 μg/kg/min infusion) may be used to maintain muscle relaxation.	
Emergence	Extubate when the patient is awake and protective laryngeal reflexes are present. Patient should be transferred to PACU accompanied by anesthesiologist.	
Blood and fluid requirements	Potential for large blood loss IV: 14-16 ga × 1-2 FFP available Plt available 2-4 U PRBC available NS/LR (as appropriate)	Glucose-containing solutions may be required for patients with hepatic failure ± CHF. ✓ blood glucose levels frequently. Vasopressor response may be impaired.
Monitoring	Standard monitors (see p. B-1).	Ventricular arrhythmias can be provoked by hepatic vein catheterization.
Positioning	✓ and pad pressure points. ✓ eyes.	Radiology tables usually are not well padded → nerve damage.
Complications	Portal vein rupture Liver capsule perforation Complete heart block CHF	Intraabdominal hemorrhage may be massive and require emergency surgery. Patients with preexisting LBBB may require a pacemaker pre-TIPS (2° risk of RBBB during procedure). Shunt → ↑↑venous return → CHF

POSTOPERATIVE

Complications	Portal vein thrombus ↑encephalopathy Sepsis Bleeding Fluid/electrolyte disturbance	May mimic symptoms of PE or MI. 2° ↓hepatic portal blood flow May require hemodynamic support (e.g., dopamine) Stent insertion → ↑venous return → ↑diuresis → electrolyte/ fluid imbalance.
Pain management	IV opiates	

References

1. Cardella JF, Waybill PN: Interventional radiology: diagnostic and interventional vascular applications. In *Alternate-Site Anesthesia: Clinical Practice Outside the Operating Room.* Russell GB, ed. Butterworth-Heinemann, Boston: 1997, 115-32.
2. Cejna M, Peck-Radosavljevic M, Thurnher S, Hittmair K, Schoder M, Lammer J: Creation of transjugular intrahepatic portosystemic shunts with stent-grafts: initial experiences with a polytetrafluoroethylene-covered nitinol endoprosthesis. *Radiology* 2001; 221:437-46.
3. Cello JP, Ring EJ, Olcott EW, et al: Endoscopic sclerotherapy compared with percutaneous transjugular intrahepatic portosystemic shunt after initial sclerotherapy in patients with acute variceal hemorrhage. A randomized, controlled trial [see comments]. *Ann Intern Med* 1997; 126(11):858-65.
4. Colapinto RF, Stronell RD, Gildiner M, et al: Formation of intrahepatic portosystemic shunts using a balloon dilatation catheter: preliminary clinical experience. *AJR Am J Roentgenol* 1983; 140(4):709-14.
5. Freedman AM, Sanyal AJ, Tisnado J, et al: Complications of transjugular intrahepatic portosystemic shunt: a comprehensive review. *Radiographics* 1993; 13(6):1185-210.
6. Huonker M, Schumacher YO, Ochs A, Sorichter S, Keul J, Rossle M: Cardiac function and haemodynamics in alcoholic cirrhosis and effects of the transjugular intrahepatic portosystemic stent shunt. *Gut* 1999; 44(5):743-8.
7. Kerlan RK Jr, LaBerge JM, Gordon RL, et al: Inadvertent catheterization of the hepatic artery during placement of transjugular intrahepatic portosystemic shunts. *Radiology* 1994; 193(1):273-6.
8. LaBerge JM, Ring EJ, Gordon RL, et al: Creation of transjugular intrahepatic portosystemic shunts with the Wallstent endoprosthesis: Results in 100 patients. *Radiology* 1993; 157(2):413-20.
9. LaBerge JM, Somberg KA, Lake JR, et al: Two-year outcome following transjugular intrahepatic portosystemic shunt for variceal bleeding: results in 90 patients. *Gastroenterology* 1995; 108(4):1143-51.
10. Nicoll A, Fitt G, Angus P, et al: Budd-Chiari syndrome: intractable ascites managed by a trans-hepatic portacaval shunt. *Australas Radiol* 1997; 41(2):169-72.
11. Richter GM, Palmaz JC, Noldge G, et al: The transjugular intrahepatic portosystemic stent-shunt. A new nonsurgical percutaneous method. *Radiologe* 1989; 29(8):406-11.
12. Rosch J, Hanafee W, Snow H: Transjugular portal venography and radiologic portacaval shunt: an experimental study. *Radiology* 1969; 92:1112-14.
13. Rosch J, Keller F: Transjugular intrahepatic portosystemic shunt: present status, comparison with endoscopic therapy and shunt surgery, and future prospectives. *World J Surg* 2001; 25:337-46.
14. Russell GB: Anesthesia and interventional radiology. In *Alternate-Site Anesthesia: Clinical Practice Outside the Operating Room.* Russell GB, ed. Butterworth-Heinemann, Boston: 1997, 157-71.
15. Semba CP, Saperstein L, Nyman U, et al: Hepatic laceration from wedged venography performed before transjugular intrahepatic portosystemic shunt placement [see comments]. *J Vasc Interv Radiol* 1996; 7(1):143-6.

IMAGING AND IMAGE-GUIDED PROCEDURES

PROCEDURAL CONSIDERATIONS

Description: Projectional imaging includes x-ray fluoroscopy, and cross-sectional imaging includes computed tomography (CT), ultrasound (US), and magnetic resonance imaging (MRI). These techniques have become indispensable in modern diagnosis. In addition, a growing number of invasive procedures are being performed using cross-sectional imaging for guidance, not only for diagnostic purposes but also for therapeutic purposes. Indications include Dx of primary or metastatic tumors; tumor staging; Dx of benign processes, such as infections; drainage of fluid collections; local regional treatment of tumors, endovascular treatment of hemorrhage, aneurysms, and dissections; percutaneous treatment of urinary and biliary obstructions; and placement of venous access devices. Selection of imaging modality depends on ease of identification of the target lesion and resolution of surrounding and intervening structures. Patient compliance is crucial to success, because image resolution and spatial accuracy require the patient to be immobile during image acquisition and the procedure itself. In compliant adults, most of these procedures may be done using conscious sedation. For procedures in the pediatric population, as well as for more invasive procedures in adults, GA is frequently necessary.

Diagnostic imaging: Pediatric: CT scans are performed in a large, ring-shaped gantry, through which the patient is passed on an automated table. US is performed with a hand-held transducer attached to a console. Diagnostic MRI scans are performed primarily in a large, circumferential magnet with a cylindrical center bore, also incorporating an automated table. In general, conscious sedation is sufficient to ensure pediatric patient compliance for diagnostic CT, US, or MRI, but occasionally GA is necessary. **Adults:** Almost all CT, US, and MRI studies are performed without anesthesia. Approximately 5% of adult patients are too claustrophobic to complete an MRI study. Some of these may benefit from sedation, but use of GA is rare.

Image-guided procedures: Pediatric: Procedures performed on the pediatric patient routinely require GA. X-ray fluoroscopy-guided procedures—including angiography, angioplasty, stent placement, arterial embolization, thrombolysis, venography, renal and adrenal vein sampling, transvenous biopsy, gastrostomy and gastrojejunal tube placement, ureteral stent placement, biliary drainage, bronchial dilation, and placement of venous access devices (Broviacs, ports, and PICCs)—are performed in a cath-angio lab, which frequently is OR-certified. Procedures usually entail real-time x-ray imaging, requiring all personnel in the room to wear protective lead garments. For CT- and US-guided biopsies and fluid drainage, initial lesion localization images are obtained after initiation of anesthesia and immobilization of the patient. A skin entry site is then selected and marked, based on coordinates determined from the initial images. Biopsies may require multiple needle passes, either coaxially through a large-bore guiding needle, or separately without such a guide. With CT, confirmation of needle position requires interruption of the procedure to acquire images, while with US, real-time images are obtained. Ideally, adequacy of biopsy sample is determined by an on-site cytopathologist. Fluid drainage may be simple aspiration or, more frequently, will result in placement of an indwelling drainage catheter. **Adults:** x-ray fluoroscopy, CT- and US-guided procedures, such as biopsies, fluid drainage, and tissue ablation, are routinely performed under conscious sedation. More invasive and painful procedures, such as stent-graft repair of aneurysms and dissections and radiofrequency (RF) ablation of unresectable tumors (see p. 1182), frequently require GA, spinal, or epidural anesthesia. The required site of access and the positioning of the operators should be considered before the procedure. Position of the ETT and central lines can be immediately confirmed using fluoroscopy. Occasionally, iv injection of iodinated contrast medium is necessary, and adverse reactions—such as urticaria, airway edema, hormone release (e.g., from pheochromocytoma, etc.), or anaphylaxis—may occur.

The developing field of MRI-guided procedures—sometimes referred to as interventional MRI (iMRI) or magnetic resonance-guided therapy (MRT)—reflects the emergence of new magnet geometries, allowing physician access to the patient during imaging. These geometries may be C-arm configurations, parallel discs above and below the patient, or dual rings where the patient is placed either through the apertures of the rings or perpendicularly between the rings. Faster image-acquisition pulse sequences are allowing near-real-time feedback. In addition to guiding biopsies and drainage, this technology enables more aggressive procedures, such as craniotomies or percutaneous tumor ablations, to be performed with immediate feedback showing the progress of excision or ablation. Clearly, many of these procedures require GA and, accordingly, require MRI-compatible monitoring and anesthetic equipment. For safety, the anesthesiologist also is subject to the same restrictions that apply to patients, so having a pacemaker, ICD, ferromagnetic aneurysm clips, or a metallic foreign body in the orbit precludes that person's suitability to perform these cases. Hybrid systems also are being marketed, combining MRI and x-ray fluoroscopy, CT and x-ray fluoroscopy, or CT and positron emission tomography (PET). These may involve overlapping precautions and risks.

Usual preop diagnosis: Tumor, primary or metastatic; lymphadenopathy; abscess, effusion, empyema, pseudocyst, or other fluid collection; arterial occlusive disease; aneurysm or pseudoaneurysm; trauma; DVT; cirrhosis

SUMMARY OF PROCEDURES

	CT/X-ray Fluoroscopy	US	MRI/MRT
Position	Supine, prone or lateral decubitus	⇐	⇐ + sitting
Unique considerations	Metallic objects should be kept out of the CT imaging field. Exit the procedure room during scanning to avoid radiation exposure, or use protective lead garment. Contrast reaction possible.	No ionizing radiation. Room lights are frequently dimmed for better viewing of the screen.	All equipment, including monitors, valves, anesthesia machine, O_2 tanks, laryngoscopes, etc., must be nonferromagnetic. Other metals should be removed from the imaging field to avoid artifact.
Antibiotics	Indicated for open procedures or when draining infected fluid collections, including abscesses, empyemas, obstructed biliary or urinary systems.	⇐	⇐
Procedure time	≥ 1 h	⇐	⇐
EBL	Procedure-dependent; may be internal hemorrhage.	⇐	⇐

	CT/X-ray Fluoroscopy	US	MRI/MRT
Postop care	PACU → room	⇐	⇐
Mortality	Rare	⇐	⇐
Morbidity	Hemorrhage Infection Organ injury/perforation Pneumothorax	⇐	⇐
Pain score	1	1	Procedure-dependent

PATIENT POPULATION CHARACTERISTICS

Age range	All
Male:Female	1:1
Incidence	Common

Associated conditions	**Fluid collections:** Patients may present with fever, sepsis, pain, or ileus. Mass effect, such as with empyema or pericardial effusion, may also affect respiratory or cardiovascular function. Instrumentation or relief of mass effect may induce a vasovagal response. Some infections (echinococcus, entamoeba, methicillin-resistant staphylococcus aureus [MRSA], vancomycin-resistant enterococci [VRE]) may require special precautions, such as respiratory isolation, gown/glove standards, and pre- and post-procedure equipment sterilization.
	Solid tumors: Mass effect may result in obstruction of airways, blood vessels, GI/biliary tract, or urinary tract, or neural impingement. HTN may be seen with significant renal compression and, occasionally, with neuroendocrine tumors. Hematopoietic, hepatic, or renal compromise may result in coagulopathy or Plt dysfunction.
	Vascular pathologies: Aggressive anticoagulation and/or antiplatelet therapy may be used intraop. Restoration of arterial flow to kidneys may → rapid ↓ of renin production and BP. Thrombolysis of venous occlusions can → PE. Placement of central vascular access catheters can cause air embolism or cardiac arrhythmias from right atrial irritation.

ANESTHETIC CONSIDERATIONS

PREOPERATIVE

The adult patient population requiring anesthesia services for cross-sectioned imaging is medically quite diverse; however, many have in common the inability or unwillingness to lie still during the scanning procedure. Some of these patients are very ill, requiring the services of an anesthesiologist to maintain cardiorespiratory stability. Adult patients should be npo for 6 h preprocedure (elective). In general, US and CT scans present fewer problems for the anesthesiologist than MRI. Regardless of the method of anesthesia chosen, these patients must lie perfectly still, the airway must be protected, and IPPV may be required. Thus, children, the mentally retarded, and claustrophobic, uncooperative, or critically ill patients may all require GA.

Respiratory	As a result of limited access to the patient's airway, the preop examination should focus on the need for elective ET intubation to protect the airway. ET intubation and mechanical ventilation also may be required in trauma patients, the critically ill, or patients with GERD or sleep apnea.
Cardiovascular	Presence of a cardiac pacemaker or ICD is a contraindication to MRI, as are PA catheter thermistors or pacing wires.
Neurological	Patients with ↑ICP or cranial trauma usually need GA with mechanical ventilation and intubation. The presence of aneurysm clips and/or coils may be a contraindication to MRI (✓ with surgeon or radiologist). Some of the newer aneurysm clips are nonferromagnetic and are, therefore, MRI-compatible.
Musculoskeletal	The presence of spinal instrumentation, metal plates, pins, screws, joint replacements, or other prostheses is usually not a contraindication to MRI.
Premedication	Midazolam 1-5 mg iv (titrated to effect) may be appropriate in the very anxious adult patient; alternatively, lorazepam 1-2 mg po/sl 1 h before procedure.

UNIQUE CONSIDERATIONS FOR MRI/MRT

The MRI/MRT suite poses many challenges to the anesthesiologist. Because of the high magnetic fields involved in MRI, any equipment containing ferromagnetic components—such as ECG monitors, anesthesia machines, etc.—cannot go near the magnet. Thus, MRI-compatible equipment is mandatory in the area of the MRI scanner. The magnetic field will destroy information on credit card/access card magnetic strips, and may damage pagers as well as mechanical devices, including wrist watches and infusion pump motors. (A microdrip infusion set is a suitable replacement for an infusion pump.)

Noise	May be very distressing for some patients and may average 95 dB in a 1.5-T scanner. Exposure to noise levels of this magnitude should not exceed 2 h/d. Ear plugs or earphones with music can be helpful.
Thermal injury	Thermal injury is caused by induced currents in metal implants or in looped conductors in contact with the skin.
Projectile effect	The magnet has a strong attraction for ferromagnetic objects that can become lethal missiles; therefore, all objects, such as pens, scissors, iv poles, O_2 cylinders, keys, stethoscopes, etc., must be removed prior to entering the scanning room.
Implanted/foreign material	There are several reports describing problems that may occur with cardiac pacemakers (failure to pace), aneurysm clips (hemorrhage) and intravascular wires (induced currents). Metal workers may be at special risk for ocular damage 2° imbedded particles.
Contrast agent	Currently, gadolinum chelates are the only agents in use and have a higher safety margin than iodinated contrast agents. Adverse reactions, however, occur in ~2% of patients, and include HA, nausea, dizziness, hemodynamic instability, and dysrhythmias.

INTRAOPERATIVE

Anesthetic technique: Typically, iv/po sedation, often without the services of an anesthesiologist. Patients unwilling or unable to cooperate will require GA.

IV sedation	In patients with a normal airway and no Hx of GERD, sedation can be carried out most easily using a propofol infusion (25-100 μg/kg/min), ± midazolam (0.025-0.10 mg/kg) titrated to effect. ★ **NB:** Infusion pumps may be damaged by the magnet. (A microdrip infusion is a useful alternative.)

General anesthesia:

Induction	Standard induction (p. B-2) on an MRI gantry (typically in the magnet anteroom). The anesthetized patient is then transported into the magnet.
Maintenance	Standard maintenance (p. B-3). Most commonly, a propofol infusion provides satisfactory sedation for the procedure (see pump considerations, above). Since continuous muscle relaxation is usually not required, spontaneous ventilation may be safest.
Emergence	Emergence and extubation are often accomplished after the patient has been moved to the adjacent anteroom, where additional airway and other support equipment are readily available. The patient should be recovered in the PACU, which may be some distance from the MRI suite. Appropriate monitoring and personnel should accompany the patient.
Blood and fluid requirements	No blood loss IV: 20 ga × 1 NS/LR @ TKO
Monitoring	Standard monitors (see p. B-1).	Monitoring in the MRI/MRT suite presents special problems, discussed below.
Monitoring, MRI	ECG	ECG may be distorted by magnetic fields. Use MRI-compatible electrodes. Twist leads together to avoid creating loops (↓artifacts, ↓burns). V5 and V6 are least likely to develop artifacts.
	Pulse oximetry	MRI-compatible oximeters are available. Locate probe outside bore of the magnet (e.g., toe). Avoid burn injury 2° induced current in looped leads.
	BP (NIBP)	Replace all ferrous connections on cuff and tubing with nylon connectors. Use tubing extensions to keep apparatus away from the field.

Monitoring, MRI, cont.	± Arterial Line	If an arterial line is medically indicated, keep the transducer close to the patient to avoid recording artifacts. Use MRI-compatible transducers and connectors. Recording equipment should have radiofrequency filters.
	Precordial/esophageal stethoscope	Often unsatisfactory because of magnet noise. An MRI-compatible, infrared, wireless stethoscope is available.
	Temperature	MRI-compatible T monitors are available, although usually not necessary for adults (short procedure).
	Capnography	MRI-compatible capnographs are available. Long sample lines will distort waveforms, and $ETCO_2$ concentration may not be accurate; however, this is still useful for measuring RR and relative changes in $ETCO_2$.
	PA catheter	PA catheters with thermistors or pacing wires are an absolute contraindication to MRI.
	Urinary catheter	Catheters with T probes must be removed to avoid electrical or burn hazards.
	Verbal/visual	The patient and the monitors may be viewed directly (in procedure room) or through a screened window. Contact should be maintained throughout the procedure.
Positioning	✓ and pad pressure points. ✓ eyes.	CT and MRI gantries may be poorly padded → potential nerve injury.
Complications	Contrast-related	Gadolinum → local and systemic reactions (see Contrast-related complications, p. 1161).
	Loss of airway	Patient must be promptly extracted from the magnet bore and moved beyond the range of the magnet to permit use of emergency intubation and resuscitation equipment.
	Psychological	Panic attacks and claustrophobia occur in 5-10% of patients. Use of a blindfold may be helpful in selected patients. Heavy sedation or even GA may be necessary.
	Hearing loss	Temporary hearing loss and tinnitus may be expected in 43% of patients. Prevent by using ear plugs. GA ↑ risk of hearing damage 2° stapedius muscle relaxation.
	Thermal injury	Results from induced current, heating of oximeter probe, and looping cables.

POSTOPERATIVE

Complications	Hearing loss	See discussion above.
	Thermal injury	See discussion above.

References

1. Barth KH, Matsumoto AH: Patient care in interventional radiology: A perspective. *Radiology* 1991; 178:11-17.
2. Brown TR, Goldstein B, Little J: Severe burns resulting from magnetic resonance imaging with cardiopulmonary monitoring. Risks and relevant safety precautions. *Am J Phys Med Rehab* 1993; 72:166-7.
3. Douglas BR, Charboneau JW, Reading CC: Ultrasound-guided intervention: expanding horizons. *Radiol Clin North Am* 2001; 39:415-28.
4. Hagspiel KD, Kandarpa K, Jolesz FA: Interventional MR imaging. *J Vasc Interv Radiol* 1997; 8:745-58.
5. Holshouser BA, Hinshaw DB, Shellock FG: Sedation, anesthesia, and physiological monitoring during magnetic resonance imaging: evaluation of procedures and equipment. *J Magn Reson Imaging* 1993; 3:553-8.
6. Johnson JC, Blackburn TW, Russell GB: Anesthesia for computed tomography. In *Alternate-Site Anesthesia: Clinical Practice Outside the Operating Room.* Russell GB, ed. Butterworth-Heinemann, Boston: 1997, 83-100.
7. Jolesz FA, Kahn T: Interventional MRI: State of the art. *Appl Radiol* 1997; 26:8-13.
8. Jorgensen NH, Messick JM, Gray J, Nugent M, Berquist TH: ASA monitoring standards and magnetic resonance imaging. *Anesth Analg* 1994; 79:1141-7.
9. Kettenbach J, Kacher DF, Koskinen SK, Silverman SG, Nabavi A, Gering D, Tempany CM, Schwartz RB, Kikinis R, Black PM, Jolesz FA: Interventional and intraoperative magnetic resonance imaging. *Ann Rev Biomed Eng* 2000; 2:661-90.
10. Malviya S, Voepel-Lewis T, Eldevik OP, Rockwell DT, Wong JH, Tait AR: Sedation and general anaesthesia in children undergoing MRI & CT: adverse events and outcomes. *Br J Anaesthesia* 2000; 84(6):743-8.

11. McBrien ME, Winder J, Smyth L: Anaesthesia for magnetic resonance imaging: a survey of current practice in the UK and Ireland. *Anaesthesia* 2000; 55(8):737-43.
12. Meilstrup JW, Van Slyke MA, Russell GB: Ultrasound-guided interventional diagnosis and therapy. In *Alternate-Site Anesthesia: Clinical Practice Outside the Operating Room.* Russell GB, ed. Butterworth-Heinemann, Boston: 1997, 225-42.
13. Morcos SK, Thomsen HS: Adverse reactions to iodinated contrast media. *Eur Radiol* 2001; 11:1267-75.
14. Mueller PR, vanSonnenberg E: Interventional radiology in the chest and abdomen. *N Engl J Med* 1990; 322:1364-74.
15. Murphy KJ, Brunberg JA: Adult claustrophobia, anxiety, and sedation in magnetic resonance imaging. *Magn Reson Imaging* 1997; 15:51-4.
16. Russell GB, Taekmann JM, Cronin AJC: Anesthesia and magnetic resonance imaging. In *Alternate-Site Anesthesia: Clinical Practice Outside the Operating Room.* Russell GB, ed. Butterworth-Heinemann, Boston: 1997, 69-82.
17. Sandner-Kiesling A, Schwarz G, Vicenzi M, Fall A, James RL, Ebner F, List WF: Side-effects after inhalational anaesthesia for paediatric cerebral magnetic resonance imaging. *Paediatr Anaesth* 2002; 12(5):429-37.
18. Van Slyke MA, Wise SW, Spain JW: Computerized patient imaging. In *Alternate-Site Anesthesia: Clinical Practice Outside the Operating Room.* Russell GB, ed. Butterworth-Heinemann, Boston: 1997, 35-68.
19. Zorab JS: A general anaesthesia service for magnetic resonance imaging. *Eur J Anaesth* 1995; 12:387-95.

TRACHEOBRONCHIAL STENTING

SURGICAL CONSIDERATIONS

Description: Tracheobronchial stenting may be performed for both benign and malignant strictures of upper and lower airways that are unsuitable for surgical reconstruction. The general condition of the patient (e.g., comorbidity, recent thoracic surgery, or limited life span) or certain characteristics of the stricture (e.g., active disease, airway inflammation, extensive length, or multifocality) may prohibit reconstructive surgery. Strictures of the trachea are most commonly due to prolonged intubation or neoplasm. Less common causes include radiation stenosis, polychondritis, tracheomalacia, and, in children, extrinsic strictures 2° vascular malformations.

Before the introduction of lung transplantation, bronchial stenoses were almost invariably due to underlying cancer, and were usually amenable to surgical resection or dilatation. Stenting was reserved for cases of advanced malignancy in patients who were not surgical candidates. Bronchial stenosis is a relatively common complication of lung transplantation, occurring in single-lung, double-lung, and heart/lung transplant recipients. It is believed that this complication is 2° the lack of bronchial artery supply, with resulting airway ischemia. These ischemic stenoses occur at the bronchial suture line and in the more distal airway, and have been reported to occur in ~10% of patients undergoing transplantation.

Stent types: There are two primary types of airway stents: silicone-based and metallic, with both bare and covered metallic prostheses available.

Silicone stents: Silicone-based stents are available both as straight, short tubes and as bifurcated Y-shaped devices. Straight stents are flanged on both ends to prevent dislodgement, and can remain in place in patients for extended periods. The selection of the correct size and length is critical. The stent must be long enough to enable its flanges to anchor the stent within the stricture; short enough to avoid compromise of a lobar bronchus distally or the trachea proximally; and of satisfactory diameter to maintain the caliber of the airway. The main advantage of silicone stents is that they are easily removed, either when the patient's ventilatory status has recovered sufficiently, or when reconstructive surgery is possible. Silicone stents that can accommodate a bifurcation, such as the carina, are available, and may be used to maintain patency of the distal trachea and both mainstem bronchi.

Silicone-based (Silastic) stents do have disadvantages. Stenotic airways need to be predilated before stent insertion, whereas metallic stents can be placed within a narrow airway lumen and subsequently dilated. Silicone stents frequently become occluded with mucus plugs and granulation tissue or tumor overgrowth; therefore, regular bronchoscopic examination and treatment are necessary to keep the airway clear. In general, silicone stents must be placed under GA because of the need for rigid bronchoscopic instrumentation.

Metallic stents: The main advantages of metallic stents (e.g., Gianturco Z, Wallstent, Palmaz) are the ease of insertion, an extremely thin wall that rapidly becomes embedded in the airway, and the large gaps in the wall that allow normal ciliary function and reduced mucus impaction. The procedure can be performed using flexible bronchoscopy in the interventional room, under deep sedation. The main disadvantage of metallic stents is the inability to remove or reposition these devices once deployed. Stents become firmly embedded in the wall of the airway and incorporated into the epithelium in < 6 wk. Removal can be accomplished by using pincers to grip the wall of the stent and applying a twisting motion to pull the stent away from the wall. Potential complications from this maneuver are catastrophic and, in our experience, once these devices are placed, they are permanent. Another problem associated with metallic stents is the development of granulation tissue either at the ends of the stents or through the interstices. This requires careful follow-up by repeat bronchoscopy and may require subsequent procedures, such as bronchoplasty, restenting, and laser tissue ablation.

Because of the flexibility and low profile of the deployment systems used for metal stents, it is feasible to place them under conscious sedation; however, our practice is to utilize GA for tracheal stent placement to reduce patient movement due to the coughing that occurs with tracheal irritation. Most bronchial interventions can be performed without full GA.

Insertion Techniques: Silicone stents have low inherent radial force, and strictures should be dilated before stenting. Rigid bronchoscopy is necessary to allow dilation and subsequent stent placement. Dilation can be performed with the Holinger bronchoscope, which is insinuated into the stricture and advanced with a corkscrew motion. Gum-tipped Jackson dilators and various angioplasty balloons also can be used. In patients with tracheal stomas, a T-tube stent can be inserted either via the stoma or the mouth. This extends up to the vocal cords and down as far as the carina. In patients without tracheal stomas, either Y-tubes or straight stents are inserted in a similar fashion. The stent is mounted on the rigid scope, which is advanced across the stricture and then withdrawn, leaving the stent in place. A biopsy forceps is used to advance a limb of the Y-tube into the other bronchus. Placement of stents above the carina in this fashion is relatively straightforward, and the stents can be removed and repositioned until a satisfactory result is achieved. With more distal bronchial stents, the operator's vision is somewhat obscured and deployment is more difficult.

For insertion of **metallic stents**, imaging is used to determine the optimal length and diameter of the stent. For tracheal stenosis, care must be taken during intubation, as the stricture often is close to the vocal cord. Flexible bronchoscopy is used for stent placement, with a soft-tipped guidewire being advanced through either the scope or the ETT into the distal airway. In the rare case where the stricture is too narrow and tight to allow passage of a small, flexible bronchoscope, the guidewire is passed, and the lesion is stented based on reconstructed CT images. Using fluoroscopy, the stent is positioned across the stricture.

Usual preop diagnosis: Bronchial compression 2° carcinoma; post-transplantation; relapsing polychondritis; sarcoidosis

SUMMARY OF PROCEDURE

Position	Supine
Incision	None
Special instrumentation	Bronchoscope (usually flexible); self-expanding metallic stent (covered and uncovered); balloon-expandable, short metallic stent
Unique considerations	May have to pull the end of the tracheal tube back to the level of the vocal cords to adequately treat the entire trachea.
Antibiotics	Not usually administered.
Procedure time	1-2 h
EBL	0
Postop care	ICU or step-down unit
Mortality	1-5%
Morbidity	Tracheobronchial irritation (usually temporary)
	Stent malposition → bronchial occlusion or vocal-cord paralysis
Pain score	2-4 (first few h only)

ANESTHETIC CONSIDERATIONS

PREOPERATIVE

Respiratory compromise due to airway obstruction may pose a significant management challenge. A thorough preop workup is necessary before anesthesia. Although many of these patients have end-stage pulmonary malignancy and present for palliative therapy, some may present emergently with impending airway obstruction that precludes a complete preop workup. The choice of anesthesia is primarily a function of the types of stent used, the comfort of the physician placing the stent with respect to the type of anesthesia used, and the comorbid condition of the patient. In general, silicone stent placement which requires prior airway dilation with rigid bronchoscopy will necessitate GA. Metallic stents can be placed without the need for preceding airway dilatation; therefore, either topical anesthesia, with or without conscious sedation, or GA can be used. Improvements in FEV$_1$, FVC, and PEF are expected after pulmonary stenting.

Respiratory Patients with upper or lower airway stricture may present with cough, stridor, dyspnea, and fatigue. Airway obstruction can be classified as dynamic or fixed, depending on whether the obstruction varies with the respiratory cycle. Stridor that worsens during inspiration suggests an extrathoracic dynamic obstruction, while expiratory stridor is associated with intrathoracic dynamic obstruction. Other physical findings may include bronchospasm (in COPD patients), clubbing, or cyanosis. Preop fiber optic bronchoscopic examination and/or high-resolution, thin-section CT scans will help to define the location, size, and extent of the obstruction. In patients suspected of having tracheomalacia, scans are performed at maximal inspiration and maximal expiration to unmask subtle areas of narrowing exacerbated by ↑ intrathoracic pressure on inspiration. Using this information, the appropriate size for an ETT can be estimated and potential problems with tracheal intubation can be anticipated.
Tests: CXR; PFTs with flow/volume loops (see Fig 5-14, Anesthetic Considerations for Mediastinoscopy, p. 233); CT scans preferably with 3-dimensional reconstructions

Cardiovascular Directed at any underlying disease process. Restoration of intravascular volume before induction of GA is important in patients with hypovolemia 2° chronic malnutrition from malignancy.
Tests: As indicated from H&P.

Musculoskeletal Patients with lung cancer may have myasthenic syndrome (Eaton-Lambert) with ↑ resistance to depolarizing muscle relaxants and ↑ sensitivity to NMRs. Post-lung transplant patients on certain immunosuppressive therapies (e.g., cyclosporine) may have prolonged muscle blockade from NMRs.

Hematologic Blood cross-match not necessary unless high risk of hemorrhage from injury (e.g., rigid bronchoscopy used in patients with friable tumors). Maintaining adequate O$_2$-carrying capacity is important in patients with poor pulmonary reserve.
Tests: CBC; others as indicated from H&P.

Laboratory Other tests as indicated from H&P.

Premedication Standard premedication (p. B-2). Patients in respiratory distress are extremely anxious. Careful titration of anxiolytic medications is necessary to avoid oversedation that might impair ventilation. An antisialagogue (e.g., glycopyrrolate 0.2 mg iv) will help minimize secretions and improve visualization through the bronchoscope. Post-lung transplant patients may be steroid-dependent and stress-dose steroid supplement may be required.

INTRAOPERATIVE

Anesthetic technique: Be prepared for an airway emergency. Preparations should be made for emergency rigid bronchoscopy and/or tracheostomy below the lesion. A variety of laryngoscope blades and ETTs of all sizes, including small, uncuffed (5-6 mm) tubes, should be readily available. Endoscopic evaluation of the airway must be performed in a spontaneously breathing patient. Muscle relaxation must be avoided until a detailed examination is completed and the operator is certain an airway can be maintained subsequently. Vocal-cord paralysis, which can mimic tracheal stenosis, can be obscured by muscle relaxation.

Topical anesthesia Anesthetize palate, pharynx, larynx, vocal cords, and trachea with 5-7 ml lidocaine (4%), using nebulizer, or have patient gargle equal volume of viscous lidocaine (4%). Caution must be exercised to avoid overdosing the patient with local anesthesia.

Conscious sedation Can be achieved by titrating low-dose midazolam (0.5-2 mg) or propofol (10-100 µg/kg/min), with or without a short acting-opioid (e.g., fentanyl 25-50 µg; remifentanil 0.05-0.1 µg/kg/min) to avoid respiratory depression or untoward hemodynamic changes.

Induction Preoxygenate for 3-5 min before induction. Patients may be unable to lie flat 2° respiratory distress. The goal of induction is to maintain spontaneous ventilation until the airway is secured. Mask induction with sevoflurane or an awake FOL with topical anesthesia are appropriate. Optimally, the ETT is positioned ~1 cm above the lesion. Flexible bronchoscopy of the distal airways is then performed through the stricture, and the distal extent of the stricture relative to the carina is identified. In patients with a stricture near the vocal cords, the use of an LMA is a viable option. Avoid muscle relaxation; if necessary, however, consider small dose of succinylcholine. Standard iv induction (p. B-2) may be possible in some patients with a small obstruction and no significant clinical symptoms. Low-density helium-oxygen mixtures (Heliox) have the clinical advantage of reducing airway

Induction, cont.	resistance to flow past the obstruction. Heliox, however, is not readily available in most institutions and, therefore, is not used routinely.
Maintenance	100% FiO_2 with sevoflurane or TIVA using propofol (25-100 μg/kg/min) and remifentanil (0.05-0.5 μg/kg/min) infusions. Once the airway is secured, muscle relaxation can be given to avoid movement or coughing during the procedure. Succinylcholine drip (0.25-1 g/250 ml NS, titrated to effect; avoid phase II block by keeping dose < 5-6 mg/kg), or short-acting (mivacurium 0.1 mg/kg iv) or intermediate-acting (cisatracurium 0.1 mg iv or vecuronium 0.1 mg/kg iv) muscle relaxant may be used. Manual IPPV through side-arm of rigid bronchoscope or via the swivel connector if fiber optic bronchoscope is used. High-flow (up to 20 L/min) O_2 or O_2 flush (barotrauma risk) may be required to compensate for leak if rigid bronchoscope is used, → ↓ anesthetic concentration. Hyperventilate patient in preparation for periods of apnea. Low-frequency jet ventilation (50 psi at 10/min with I:E 1:2-4) via a Sander's injector is an alternative. Barotrauma and dynamic lung hyperinflation are potential problems with this approach.
Emergence	Patient must be fully awake before extubation with no residual neuromuscular blockade. Emergence can be 'stormy.' Patient may cough violently to clear secretions and blood. A smooth emergence may be facilitated by early suctioning of the airway, use of an antisialagogue and lidocaine (1 mg/kg iv) to decrease airway reactivity. Continue O_2 supplementation.

Blood and fluid requirements	IV: 18 ga × 1 NS/LR @ 1-2 ml/kg/h	Transfusion unnecessary except to optimize O_2-carrying capacity or to treat hemorrhage.
Monitoring	Standard monitors (p. B-1) ± Arterial line	$ETCO_2$ not accurate during rigid bronchoscopy because of dilution effect at sample port. Depending on patient's comorbidities.
Positioning	Supine ✓ and pad pressure points. ✓ eyes.	
Complications	Hypoxemia Hypercarbia Dysrhythmias Hypertension Bronchospasm Stent dislodgement Bleeding Tracheobronchial injury Aspiration of debris	Suction secretions/blood; airway instrumentation may have to be interrupted and bronchoscope removed to improve oxygenation and ventilation. Commonly 2° inadequate ventilation. ↑ TV and RR. Most likely 2° hypercarbia or stimulation. Ensure adequate ventilation and sedative/anesthesia. Rx: bronchodilator (e.g., albuterol puff) From coughing or movement. Ensure adequate anesthesia and muscle relaxation. Common with rigid bronchoscope. Requires frequent suctioning. Major hemorrhage may require thoracotomy using DLT or BB to isolate and/or tamponade bleeding site. Transfusion. Patient may need to be kept intubated after the procedure.

POSTOPERATIVE

Complications	Airway edema Airway obstruction Stent fracture/migration Pneumothorax Secretion retention	Rx with corticosteroids (dexamethasone 6-8 mg IV) and/or racemic epinephrine nebulizer. Impending airway obstruction will require reintubation. From secretion retention or stent dislodgement. Rigorous suction. Reintubation or restenting. May require emergent reintubation or restenting. Obtain CXR. May require chest tube placement if > 20%.
Pain management	None	

References:

1. Baraka AS, Siddik SS, Taha SK, et al: Low frequency jet ventilation for stent insertion in a patient with tracheal stenosis. *Can J Anaesth* 2001; 48(7):701-4.

2. Bolliger CT, Probst R, Tschopp K, Soler M, Perruchoud AP: Silicone stents in the management of inoperable tracheobronchial stenoses. Indications and limitations. *Chest* 1993; 104(6):1653-9.

3. Brodsky JB: Anesthesia for pulmonary stent insertion. *Curr Opin Anaesthesiol* 2003; 16:65-7.

4. Hautmann H, Bauer M, Pfeifer JK, and Huber RM: Flexible bronchoscopy: A safe method for metal stent implantation in bronchial disease. *Ann Thorac Surg* 2000; 69(2):398-401.

5. Monnier P, Mudry A, Franz S, et al: The use of the covered Wallstent for the palliative treatment of inoperable tracheobronchial cancers: A prospective, multicenter study. *Chest* 1996; 110(5):1161-8.

6. O'Sullivan GJ, Kee ST, Semba CP, Dake, MD: Techniques in stenting the tracheobronchial tree. *Tech in Int Rad* 1999; 2:19-32.

7. Rousseau H, Dahan M, Lauque D, Carre P, Didier A, Bilbao I, Herrero J, Blancjouvant F, Joffre F: Self-expandable prostheses in the tracheobronchial tree. *Radiology* 1993; 188(1):199-203.

8. Slonim SM, Razavi M, Kee S, Semba CP, Dake MD: Transbronchial Palmaz stent placement for tracheo-bronchial stenosis. *J Vasc Interv Radiol* 1998; 9(1 Pt 1):153-60.

9. Van De Putte P, Martens P: Anaesthetic management for placement of a stent for high tracheal stenosis. *Anaesth Intens Care* 1994; 22(5):619-21.

RADIOFREQUENCY ABLATION

SURGICAL CONSIDERATIONS

Description: Radiofrequency ablation (RFA) was pioneered in 1920 by Harvey Cushing for the creation of small lesions within the CNS. Since then, the technique has been refined so that precise control of lesion size can be achieved by measuring the temperature and electrical resistance within the tissues being treated. Ablating neural tissue with RF is successful in treating pain from trigeminal neuralgia, facet osteoarthritis, and failed-back syndrome. RFA is the treatment of choice for many symptomatic cardiac arrhythmias and small, painful osteoid osteomas. The clinical efficacy of RFA in these areas has been clearly established. In contrast, experience with newer techniques is limited due to the lack of large clinical trials and recent technological advances.

Mechanism of tissue destruction: In RFA, an alternating current operating in the frequency of radio waves (460-480 kHz) is emitted from the tip of an electrode or needle placed directly into tissues. This alternating current causes the local ions to vibrate, producing heat and inducing cell death by coagulative necrosis. The cytotoxic T threshold is 50°C; however, with RFA, temperatures can exceed this, and actually reach the boiling point of water (100°C). Until recently, a major limitation of RFA was the small lesion size it created. Within the past several years, technical advances in RF systems have improved such that heat lesions > 5 cm in diameter can be created with a single treatment. This ability makes RFA well suited for the treatment of primary and secondary malignancies in the liver, as well as other sites in patients who are not suitable for open surgery.

Techniques of radiofrequency ablation: Grounding pads are placed on the patient's thighs; if a single RF treatment probe is used, at least two and, preferably, four pads (96-cm^2 surface area each) or the equivalent (minimum total surface area = ~200 cm^2) must be used. If a three-probe cluster is used, at least four RF grounding pads or their equivalent (~400 cm^2 surface area) must be used. The grounding pads and the treatment probes are connected to the RF generator. When the generator is activated, current flows between the conductive electrode tip and the grounding pads (or 'dispersive electrode'). The increase in the tissue T is proportional to the current density. Since the density is highest near the conductive electrode tip, coagulation is induced in the tissue surrounding the treatment probe. The linear extent (depth) of the resulting coagulation is determined by the length of the uninsulated probe tip, while the diameter of coagulation necrosis produced around the probe tip depends on the duration of treatment. Based on our experience using perfusion probes and pulsed current technique, areas of the tissue up to 4.5 cm diameter may be induced with a single probe and up to 7.3 cm diameter with clustered probes.

The lesion to be treated is identified and characterized by ultrasound or CT, which is used to guide the RF probe to the distal margin of the lesion. The generator is activated and output is gradually increased to a predetermined maximum, based on tip exposure and probe configuration (single vs clustered probes). Maximum power (90-120 Watts) is applied to the treatment probe cluster until tissue impedance rises. At this point, the power is turned off for 60 sec, then increased to maximum until once again impedance is seen to rise. Ultrasound monitoring of the RF site may be carried out throughout the ablation; however, it usually is limited due to the production of tissue water vapor that interferes with the transmission of the sound waves. CT can be used occasionally to check the stable position of the needle. Final tissue temperatures usually range from 60°-90°C.

Lesion size varies according to the size of the electrode, the current, duration of the treatment, and local blood flow. Tumor cells adjacent to large blood vessels may not be treated thoroughly due to the heat-sink effect of flowing blood, which carries away the RF energy as fast as it is deposited. Alternatively, cirrhotic livers with extensive fibrosis and ↓blood flow may need fewer treatments because of larger achievable coagulation diameters.

Lung RF: Recently, RF energy has been used to attempt ablation of certain primary and secondary lung tumors. The work that has been done to date has been performed in patients whose disease extent offers few therapeutic options. The results, therefore, have been understandably mixed; however, there has been a satisfying lack of major complications reported. Pneumothorax is seen in ~30% of cases (similar to rates reported during lung biopsy); and, while transcranial Doppler has demonstrated microbubbles in the brain during ablation, there have been no reported sequelae. The same basic technique is used, although lower energies are applied, since there is less solid tissue in the lung, and high levels of impedance are reached sooner.

Bone RF: RF has been applied to both benign and malignant bone tumors. The first use was for the thermocoagulation of small, painful, benign bone tumors called osteoid osteomas, which occur predominantly in pediatric patients and arise within the cortex of long bones. The cause of these tumors is unknown. Nocturnal pain that is relieved with anti-inflammatory drugs is the classic presentation. Pain is related to prostaglandin production within the cells of the small, central, vascularized tumor nidus. Most of these tumors require removal either by surgical or percutaneous methods, although occasionally, they spontaneously regress. Surgical removal is the most extensive treatment and requires cortical osteotomy, with the accompanying risks of anesthesia, surgical wound complication, and incomplete removal. RF ablation can be performed under iv sedation or GA, using CT guidance. Patients typically leave the hospital several h after the procedure. The lesion is initially localized with CT, and a safe percutaneous route is planned to avoid vital neurovascular structures. A core of bone is removed with a bone-cutting biopsy needle. Once the overlying dense cortex has been traversed to the center of the osteoid osteoma, a conventional (non-internally cooled) RF electrode is placed within the center. The internally cooled RF electrodes are not needed in this application because the area of treatment is almost always < 10 mm in diameter. A single grounding pad is placed on the skin of the opposing surface from the electrode placement. CT confirms satisfactory positioning, and the RF generator connected to the electrode is activated. A 6-min RF energy application with T maintained at 90°C is almost always sufficient to destroy the small central nidus of prostaglandin-producing cells. The electrode is removed and a small bandage is applied to the skin. Patients typically have 1-2 d of postprocedure pain that differs from the pain of osteoid osteoma. Relief of the osteoid osteoma pain almost always occurs within the first 24-48 h. Cure with one session can be as high as 90%, and retreatment can be performed if the first treatment is not immediately successful or if the patient's pain returns in the future. Follow-up imaging is usually unnecessary since the small, ablated area does not cause significant bone weakening. The ablated region of bone typically undergoes demineralization after ~6 wk. Healing of the thermocoagulation defect is slow and radiographic changes may take as long as 1 yr. No significant complications have been reported in the literature.

Preliminary studies in **malignant bone tumor treatment** with RF show promise. Previously irradiated foci of tumor, whether primary or metastatic, that are still biologically active can be treated locally with internally cooled RF electrodes. Pain reduction, control of hemorrhage, and local tumor eradication can be performed in both the axial and appendicular skeletons. In areas where tumor abuts vital structures, such as the spinal cord, RF may not be effective, since local thermal injury may not be desirable. Spinal RF can be performed in the vertebral body when the cortex between the electrode and the spinal canal is intact.

The treatment of bone tumors with direct cytotoxic therapy using a minimally invasive, CT-guided procedure may provide a cost-effective means for local tumor control. In certain patients, RF alone may provide a means for tumor eradication. In larger tumors, a combination of RF and external-beam radiotherapy may improve local recurrence rates. In theory, thermocoagulation of the central, less vascular tumor (often not effective with radiation) with RF may help improve the effectiveness of radiation treatment of the peripheral, well oxygenated tumor. This is being evaluated currently at several centers. Regarding RF and its ability to treat large areas of tumor within bone, the technology is present, but the clinical applications are still being defined. Larger, multicenter trials are being devised to evaluate the efficacy of pain control in sites of metastatic disease. In primary bone malignancies, minimally invasive strategies are far from clinical implementation, since the majority of patients undergo standard surgical removal and reconstruction. In nonsurgical candidates, RF may provide a minimally invasive alternative for local tumor eradication.

Usual preop diagnosis: Primary or metastatic hepatic malignancy; primary or metastatic pulmonary malignancy; osteoid osteoma.

SUMMARY OF PROCEDURE

Position	Supine or prone
Incision	Over the site to be accessed
Special instrumentation	RFA probes and generator
Unique considerations	Mild ↑T during procedure; ↑pain as ablation continues.
Antibiotics	None usually; occasionally, ciprofloxacin 500 mg iv
Procedure time	2-4 h
EBL	None
Postop care	Step-down unit
Mortality	< 5%
Morbidity	Postprocedure pain at site
	Hepatic hemorrhage: Rare, due to cauterizing nature of procedure
	Pneumothorax (during hepatic dome lesion ablation, pulmonary ablation)
	Hepatic abscess (↑incidence in patients with previous biliary manipulation)
Pain Score	5-8 (first few h only)

PATIENT POPULATION CHARACTERISTICS

Age range	Adults
Male:Female	M > F
Incidence	Uncommon
Etiology	Pain (trigeminal neuralgia, facet osteoarthritis; metastatic cancer); primary malignancies
Associated conditions	Lung cancer; cancers of the neck; polychondritis; prolonged ICU stay; lung transplantation

---

ANESTHETIC CONSIDERATIONS

Patients presenting for RF ablation range from those with end-stage lung cancer to otherwise healthy chronic-pain patients. In addition, analgesic/anesthetic requirements are highly variable, depending on the size and location of the target lesions. Close communication between the various care providers is essential to achieving a positive outcome.

Respiratory	Access to the airway may be limited in the typical interventional radiology suite; thus, a patient with a potentially difficult airway may require elective intubation. Appropriate airway adjuncts (LMAs, light wand, fiber optic cart, etc.) should be readily available. Intraop risks include the possibility of pneumothorax, so needle decompression supplies also should be available. Lung cancer patients presenting for tumor ablation may have compromised pulmonary function and require objective assessment of pathophysiology with PFTs and/or ABG analysis. **Tests:** PFTs, ABG, as indicated from H&P.
Cardiovascular	HTN and CHF are seen frequently in elderly patients presenting for RF procedures. These patients often have a severe disease process, which may be complicated by other significant comorbidities. The potential for cardiac ischemia should be evaluated carefully. Preop beta blockade and antihypertensive therapy may be required. **Tests:** ECG, ECHO, noninvasive stress testing as indicated from H&P.
Neurological	A thorough neurological exam is important to document neurological deficits that are present before the procedure.
Hepatic	Patients may have coagulation defects and mental status changes 2° systemic liver disease. The potential for severe hemorrhage from vascular injury, the risk of aspiration, and the lack of cooperation (encephalopathy) should all be taken into account when planning the anesthesia. Patients with severe liver disease also may exhibit hepatopulmonary or hepatorenal syndrome manifested as hypoxemia or renal failure. Consider the need for preop correction of coagulation and fluid status. **Tests:** LFTs; ammonia; INR
Endocrine	The possibility of endocrine and metabolic derangements should be assessed. Lung cancer patients may have electrolyte problems 2° SIADH, while patients with liver disease are prone to developing hypoglycemia. **Tests:** As indicated from H&P.

Hematologic	Consider the possibility of chronic anemia or hypercoagulability 2° neoplastic disease. Chemotherapy or systemic disease may have depressed bone marrow function and altered the activity of WBCs and Plts. **Tests:** Hct, Plt count, or CBC, as indicated by H&P.
Premedication	Sedation must be adjusted according to patient requirements. Small doses of midazolam, titrated to minimal sedation, is most reasonable (0.5-1 mg increments). Patients with end-stage disease often require very little premedication.

INTRAOPERATIVE

Anesthetic technique: Sedation or GA, depending on the size and location of lesions. Most ablations are well tolerated with MAC; however, large lesions may require GA. The out-of-OR site often involves working in cramped quarters with poor access to anesthesia equipment. Nevertheless, the ASA standards of monitoring should be followed.

MAC: MAC cases are performed with fentanyl (25-150 μg) and midazolam (0.5-2 mg) boluses, combined with a propofol infusion (25-100 μg/kg/min). The substitution of remifentanil (0.02-0.1 μg/kg/min) for fentanyl allows rapid titration of analgesia for the brief periods of intense stimulation.

Induction	Standard induction (p. B-2), preceding placement of an ETT or LMA.	
Maintenance	Standard maintenance (p. B-3). Since procedures are of an unpredictable duration, short-acting muscle relaxants (e.g., mivacurium 0.2 mg/kg, rocuronium 0.6 mg/kg) are advised. Propofol (25-100 μg/kg/min) and remifentanil (0.02-0.1 μg/kg/min) are an appropriate combination that easily can be titrated to effect. Persistent intraop HTN may be treated with labetolol (5-25 mg) or hydralazine (5-20 mg).	
Emergence	Standard emergence (p. B-4). Short-acting analgesics (e.g., fentanyl 25-150 μg) should be used in outpatients. Prophylactic treatment with antiemetics (metoclopramide 10 mg and granisetron 100 μg iv) may be beneficial, since there is a high incidence of PONV.	
Blood and fluid requirements	IV: 20-14 ga × 1-2 NS/LR: 3-5 ml/kg/h	Larger access needed for hepatic lesions.
Monitoring	Standard monitors (p. B-1) ± Arterial line ± Urinary catheter	Foley for longer procedures (> 2 h)
Positioning	✓ & pad pressure points ✓ eyes.	Radiology tables often poorly padded.
Complications	Hemorrhage	Blood or colloid should be readily available, if the need is anticipated. Large retroperitoneal hemorrhage can develop, yet not be appreciated until blood loss is extensive
	Pneumothorax Hemothorax	Needle decompression and/or thoracostomy tube placement may be necessary during thoracic or high hepatic procedures.
	Electrical shock	Electrocautery devices can produce serious injury if not properly grounded.
	Thermal injury Hyperthermia	Patients may develop rapid T increases 2° direct heating of large lesions.

POSTOPERATIVE

Complications	PONV	Common.
	Hemorrhage	Occult blood loss may continue for several h after the procedure is terminated.
Pain management	Standard pain management (p. C-2)	Postprocedure pain is usually well tolerated.
Tests	Postprocedure HCT, as indicated.	

References

1. Amin Z, Donald JJ, Masters A, Kant R, Steger AC, Bown SG, Lees WR: Hepatic metastases: interstitial laser photocoagulation with real-time US monitoring and dynamic CT evaluation of treatment. *Radiology* 1993; 187(2):339-47.

2. De Giovanni JV: Treatment of arrhythmias by radiofrequency ablation. *Arch Dis Childhood* 1995; 73(5):385-7.

3. Eagle KA, Berger PB, Calkins H, Chaitman BR, Ewy GA, Fleischmann KE, Fleisher LA, Froehlich JB, Gusberg RJ, Leppo JA, Ryan T, Schlant RC, Winters WL Jr: *ACC/AHA Guideline Update for Perioperative Cardiovascular evaluation for Noncardiac Surgery*: A Report of the American College of Cardiology/American Heart Association Task Force on Practice Guidelines (Committee to Update the 1996 Guidelines on Perioperative Cardiovascular Evaluation for Noncardiac Surgery), 2002.

4. Erb TO, Hall JM, Ing RJ, Kanter RJ, Kern FH, Schulman SR, Gan TJ: Postoperative nausea and vomiting in children and adolescents undergoing radiofrequency catheter ablation: a randomized comparison of propofol- and isoflurane-based anesthetics. *Anesth Analg* 2002; 95(6):1577-81.

5. Goldberg SN, Solbiati L, Hahn PF, Cosman E, Conrad J, Fogle R, Gazelle GS: Large-volume tissue ablation with radiofrequency by using a clustered, internally cooled electrode technique: laboratory and clinical experience in liver metastases. *Radiology* 1998; 209:371-9.

6. Le Groupe de Rythmologie de la Societe Francaise de Cardiologie: Complications of radiofrequency ablation: A French experience. *Arch Mal Coeur Vaiss* 1996; 89(12):1599-605.

7. Murakami R, Yoshimatsu S, Yamashita Y, Matsukawa T, Takahasi M, Sagara K: Treatment of hepatocellular carcinoma: Value of percutaneous microwave coagulation. *AJR* 1995; 164:1159-64.

8. Rhim H, Yoon KH, Lee JM, Cho Y, Cho JS, Kim SH, Lee WJ, Lim HK, Nam GJ, Han SS, Kim YH, Park CM, Kim PN, Byun JY: Korean Study Group of Radiofrequency Ablation. Major complications after radio-frequency thermal ablation of hepatic tumors: spectrum of imaging findings. *Radiographics* 2003;23(1):123-34.

9. Rosenthal DI, Hornicek FJ, Wolfe MW, Jennings LC, Gephart MC, Mankin HJ: Changes in the management of osteoid osteoma. *J Bone Joint Surg* 1998; 80:815-21.

10. Rossi S, Buscarini E, Garbagnati F, DiStasi M, Quaretti P, Rago M, Zangrandi A, Andreola S, Silverman DE, Buscarini L: Percutaneous treatment of small hepatic tumors by an expandable RF needle electrode. *AJR* 1998; 170:1015-22.

11. Sabo B, Dodd G, Halff G, Naples J: Anesthetic considerations in patients undergoing percutaneous radiofrequency interstitial tissue ablation. *AANA Journal* 1999; 67(5):467-8.

12. Seki T, Wakabayashi M, Nakagawa T, Itho T, Shiro T, Kunieda K, Sato M, Uchiwama S, Inoue K: Ultrasonically guided percutaneous microwave coagulation therapy for small hepatocellular carcinoma. *Cancer* 1994; 74:817-25.

13. Solbiati L, Ierace T, Goldberg SN, Livraghi T, Rizatto G, Mueller PR, and Gazelle GS: Percutaneous US-guided RF tissue ablation liver metastases: Long-term follow up. *Radiology* 1997; 202:195-203.

14. Vogl TJ, Muller PK, Hammerstingl R, Weinhold N, Mack MG, Philipp C, Deimling M, Beuthan J, Pegios W, Reiss H, et al: Malignant liver tumors treated with MR imaging-guided laser-induced thermotherapy: technique and prospective results. *Radiology* 1995; 196:257-65.

Authors

Sarah S. Donaldson, MD, FACR (*Radiation therapy*)
Anne M. Dubin, MD (*Pediatric cardiac catheterization*)
Jeffrey A. Feinstein, MD, MPH (*Pediatric cardiac catheterization*)
Gary E. Hartman, MD (*ECMO*)
Stanton B. Perry, MD (*Pediatric cardiac catheterization*)
Michael V. Sattah, MD (*Radiation therapy*)
Kalyani R. Trivedi, MD (*Pediatric cardiac catheterization*)

13.2 OUT-OF-OPERATING ROOM PROCEDURES—PEDIATRIC

Anesthesiologists

M. Gail Boltz, MD (*Pediatric cardiac catheterization*)
Gregory B. Hammer, MD (*Oncology, endoscopy, imaging*)
Cathy R. Lammers, MD, FAAP (*Oncology, endoscopy, imaging*)
Chandra Ramamoorthy, MD (*Pediatric cardiac catheterization*)
Glyn D. Williams, MBChB, FFA (*Radiation therapy*)

PEDIATRIC RADIATION THERAPY

PROCEDURAL CONSIDERATIONS

Michael V. Sattah and Sarah S. Donaldson

Description: Modern pediatric radiation therapy (XRT) requires that the patient be in a stable and reproducible position for daily treatment. Sharply defined beams with secondary collimation are used to irradiate the tumor volume and to spare normal tissue. Patient movement may undermine techniques for sparing normal tissue and, while movement cannot be completely prevented, it must be minimized. In very young children, it is often impossible to prevent movement and achieve adequate cooperation for radiation treatment. In such cases, daily anesthesia is required. Close cooperation of the radiation oncology and anesthesia teams allows for safe and reproducible daily treatment.[10] In general, children older than 3 or 4 yr can be persuaded to lie still for radiation therapy. Children from 2.5-4 yr may cooperate during the treatment (which is usually < 15 min), but not for the treatment planning and simulation, in which an immobilization-stabilization device is made (often requiring 1-1.5 h). In most infants and young children (< 2.5 yr), anesthesia is essential.[6]

The optimal position for XRT also must be optimal for the anesthesiologist. Ideally, the area to be treated is determined using 3-dimensional conformal techniques to optimize treatment and to minimize normal tissue exposure. This requires an imaging study (e.g., CT scan), with the patient in the same position as will be used during the radiation treatment. A series of radiographs are taken at the treatment-planning appointment, which typically lasts 1-1.5 h and requires GA. It is essential that there be no patient movement between exposures; if the patient moves, the entire procedure must be repeated. After examining the radiographs, the area to be scanned is determined, and then the patient is transported (anesthetized) to the CT suite for a 3-dimensional treatment-planning CT scan. Thereafter, the specific area can be determined and individual beam-shaping devices made.

One or two days following the initial planning session, the patient has a verification procedure, which usually is of shorter duration—often requiring only 30 min of anesthesia time. The verification procedure consists of a series of radiographs using the beam-shaping devices, which simulate the treatment to be given. When this procedure is successfully completed, the anesthetized patient is moved to the treatment room. The child is put in the identical position achieved during the planning/verification procedures, and treatment is administered.

The first day or two, and weekly thereafter, a verification x-ray (called a 'port film') is taken to confirm the accuracy of the treatment field. The treatment itself is of only a few min duration for each field; ideally, the entire procedure is completed within 15-30 min. A course of treatment may be only a few d, or may last for 5-6 wk, generally with treatment given 5 × per wk. Occasionally, multiple (2-3) treatments per d are given at 4-8 h (usually 6 h) intervals. At the initial appointment, the patient's optimal position is determined, an immobilization device is constructed, and measurements are taken. The immobilization device is usually a body cradle or cast, and often a head/face mask is made for head and neck or brain treatment. Initially, temporary marks or Band-Aids are used; however, when the final positioning has been determined, a more permanent mark, such as a tattoo, is applied. Often, a head holder with tape or Velcro and/or a belt or mask is applied to ensure the position for XRT.[9]

In managing certain brain tumors (e.g., medulloblastoma, high-grade intratentorial ependymoma, germ cell tumors, and CNS leukemia), **cranial spinal irradiation** (CSI) is used. This procedure requires that the patient be placed in the prone position with the head flexed as much as possible to minimize a cervical lordosis. This positioning, however, creates special difficulties for the anesthesiologist. If the child is intubated for the setup, the radiation stabilization device must allow space for the ETT. If the child is not intubated, there must be adequate access to the airway.

Fractionation: Pediatric protocols have been testing the efficacy of giving multiple fractions (treatments) of radiation 2-3 times per d, usually at 6-h intervals, to allow higher total radiation doses to be administered with possible less normal-tissue morbidity. These schemes have been or are being evaluated for children with: brain stem gliomas; supratentorial glial tumors; medulloblastoma and other posterior fossa tumors; soft-tissue sarcomas, including rhabdomyosarcoma; some bone tumors, including Ewing's sarcoma; and total body irradiation (TBI) in preparation for bone marrow transplantation. Until proven to be of increased efficacy, such schemes should remain part of large protocol studies. The timing of radiotherapy may be at 4-, 6-, or 8-h intervals 2-3 × per d, depending on the protocol. These studies provide several challenges for anesthesiologists, radiotherapists, and parents. Radiotherapy under anesthesia, however, has been successfully administered to infants undergoing multiple fractions per d.[9] Attention must be given to potential malnutrition and/or dehydration from prolonged periods of npo status.

Total body irradiation (TBI): Although most TBI techniques are administered with the patient standing, infants and small children must lie prone and supine for the treatment. This positioning requires sedation and/or anesthesia. Retching and vomiting, sometimes provoked by the radiation, present an additional challenge for proper radiotherapy technique, as well as for anesthetic management. Anesthesia for high-dose TBI has been accomplished with inhalation anesthetics and mechanical ventilation and with ketamine anesthesia.[8]

Radiosurgery: The technique of using stereotactically localized radiosurgery with a highly collimated radiotherapy photon beam, as generated from a linear accelerator, is currently being employed for select patients with small CNS tumors or base-of-skull tumors. There is increasing enthusiasm for this technique for infants and children with recurrent posterior fossa and cerebral tumors, craniopharyngiomas, optic nerve and chiasmal gliomas, and small AVMs. Radiosurgery requires 6-10 h of continuous anesthesia while a patient undergoes application of a metal frame, CT localization, and multiport radiotherapy treatment. Newer techniques, using image guidance, now allow frameless radiosurgery and fractionated radiotherapy. These approaches require close coordination between the anesthesiologist, neurosurgeon, and radiotherapist.[1]

Usual preop diagnosis: Leukemia; retinoblastoma; most of the solid tumors of childhood

SUMMARY OF PROCEDURE

	Standard XRT	TBI	Radiosurgery
Position	Supine or prone	Supine and prone	Supine or prone
Unique considerations	If prone: head flexed for maximal straightening of the C-spine.	May be repeated 2-3 × d at 4-6 h intervals.	Halo frame placement at CT
Anesthesia time	Planning: 30-120 min Treatment: < 15 min	< 20 min	6-10 h
Postop care	PACU → home	PACU → room	PACU → room or home

PATIENT POPULATION CHARACTERISTICS

Age range	Usually ≤ 4 yr
Male:Female	1:1
Incidence	NA
Associated conditions	**Brain tumors:** ↑ICP is of concern in these patients. Postradiation edema following the first few treatments may further ↑ ICP, with potential for brain stem herniation. Some children with brain stem tumors are particularly difficult to anesthetize, perhaps because of disruption of nerve pathways in those areas of the brain stem that are affected by anesthetics.[10]
	Diabetes insipidus (DI): It is often impossible to withhold fluids for 4-6 h prior to radiotherapy in an infant with symptomatic polydipsia from DI.
	Neuroblastoma: Neuroblastomas are capable of secreting catecholamines and related substances; hence, there is a potential for paroxysmal HTN during anesthesia induction. In these children, the principles of anesthetic management are similar to those for pheochromocytoma.[4]
	Retinoblastoma:[4,7,8] It is imperative that the patient be properly immobilized with no movement, as even a mm of change, as occurs with a sigh, may cause unnecessary radiation to the radiosensitive lens and anterior chamber. Optimal anesthesia prevents nystagmus and motion of the head. Even minimal lateral or rotary nystagmus may increase the risk of cataract induction. A course of radiotherapy for retinoblastoma may involve 20-25 GA procedures in 4-5.5 wk.

ANESTHETIC CONSIDERATIONS

Glyn D. Williams

PREPROCEDURE

Reassurance, play therapy, and friendly orientation to the XRT suite can reduce the number of children requiring anesthesia for XRT; however, the majority of children < 3 yr old will require anesthesia.[6] A detailed preanesthesia visit is essential as this is the prime opportunity to gain the confidence of both child and parents. The importance of npo status needs to be stressed repeatedly to the parents, discussing the potential danger of vomiting during treatment. Written instructions regarding preop protocols are extremely helpful in this context. For children with cancer, prolonged preop fasting for XRT once or twice daily could severely compromise an already marginal nutritional intake. Infants, children, and adolescents can safely drink clear liquids until 2 h before induction. Milk and solid foods should be withheld for an age-appropriate time interval

(4-8 h). Reassessment before each anesthetic is recommended because the patient's medical status may change during the course of radiation therapy. Some children will have Sx of ↑ICP, which must be taken into account when designing an anesthetic plan. Many patients will have recent exposure to cytotoxic/immunosuppressive chemotherapy.[6]

Respiratory	Patients with Sx of URI (runny nose, cough, fever) are commonly seen during XRT treatment and may pose problems for the anesthesia team. If the infection is acute, XRT probably should be delayed for a few d or until symptoms abate. Fortunately, most of the children can be managed without the use of an ETT, which might otherwise cause excessive secretions and postop laryngospasm. As always, the benefit of Rx must be balanced against the risks of anesthesia (induction laryngospasm, retained secretions, atelectasis/bronchospasm, and postop laryngospasm). **Tests:** As indicated from H&P.
Neurological	Patients with intracranial tumors may have ↑ICP. Sx include irritability, HA, N/V, and papilledema. Suspicion of ↑ICP probably mandates ET intubation and controlled ventilation to induce hypocarbia.
Laboratory	Tests as indicated from H&P.
Premedication	Usually unnecessary in this patient group. Reliance on sedation or restraints is ill-advised and will lead to frustration on the part of the child, parents, technologists, and physicians. Inappropriate sedation may cause respiratory and cardiovascular depression, and → prolonged period of recovery.

INTRAPROCEDURE

In one report describing 512 children receiving XRT, the diagnoses were: primary CNS tumor (28%), retinoblastoma (26%), neuroblastoma (18%), acute leukemia (9%), rhabdomyosarcoma (7%), Wilms' tumor (5%), Langerhans' cell histiocytosis (4%), and other (3%). The total number of treatments ranged from 1-65 (mean ± SD, 24 ± 16); 22% of patients received more than one treatment/d, and the prone position was required during 19% of therapy courses. Children ranged in age from 20 d-11 yr, (mean ± SD, 2.6 ± 1.8 yr).[6]

Anesthetic technique: Provision of anesthesia to children at sites remote from the OR is often challenging.[11] During XRT, control of patient movement must be precise and absolute so the radiation oncologist can irradiate the lesion while minimizing radiation dose to uninvolved normal tissue. There are no prospective randomized trials demonstrating the superiority of one anesthetic technique over another for XRT. Anesthetic goals include: (a) patient immobility; (b) good patient acceptance; (c) rapid onset; (d) brief duration of action; (e) prompt recovery; (f) minimal interference with eating, drinking, and playing; (g) avoidance of tolerance to the anesthetic agent(s) (tachyphylaxis); and (h) maintenance of a patent airway in a variety of body positions.[6] A number of techniques have been described, including inhalation, iv, and im techniques.[12] Ketamine is a potent sialogogue and can cause nystagmus, which prevents precision radiation of retinoblastomas. It may → prolonged or unpleasant emergence and is best avoided in patients with ↑ICP. Thiopental, methohexital, and propofol are popular choices for intravenous induction.[6,11] Inhalational agents require an anesthetic machine, and scavenging of anesthetic gases is problematic if an insufflation technique is used. Choice of anesthetic technique may be limited by equipment or logistical issues if the requirements of pediatric anesthesia were not considered when the XRT suite was constructed.

Induction	**IV:** Propofol (1.5-3.5 mg/kg) slowly, titrated to effect, followed by heparinized saline flush. Intubation is usually unnecessary, except for patients with ↑ICP or those with potential for airway obstruction. **Inhalation:** Mask induction with sevoflurane is appropriate in children without iv access, and may be preferred by some children. Again, intubation is usually unnecessary. The airway may be maintained by extension of the neck and use of a head holder.[2] Alternatively, an LMA may be inserted to maintain airway patency. It is essential that this same degree of head flexion/extension be maintained for each daily treatment. An immobilization device may be molded, with the requirements for anesthesia kept in mind. If extreme neck flexion is required, ET intubation may be necessary.
Maintenance	**IV:** Propofol (50-200 μg/kg/min) by continuous infusion. The airway usually can be well maintained by careful positioning and the use of a head strap. Supplemental O_2 should be administered via nasal prongs, mask, or LMA. **Inhalation:** Maintain anesthesia with sevoflurane in O_2, usually delivered by mask, LMA, or insufflation.
Emergence	**IV:** Flush iv with heparinized saline to prevent clotting. Patients will awaken rapidly following cessation of propofol infusion or inhaled agents. Extubation should be accomplished when the patient is fully awake, unless there is the possibility of ↑ICP, in which case a deep extubation is appropriate. This is important as there is frequently a long journey between the XRT department and PACU. Antiemetics should be considered.

Blood and fluid requirements	IV: usually permanent access NS/LR: infusion not usually required	Many children receiving radiotherapy have a central venous access line, placed for long-term administration of chemotherapy.
		A planned course of anesthesia for radiotherapy, in itself, is an acceptable indication for placement of a central venous access line, even in the absence of plans for chemotherapy. Alternatively, an indwelling iv catheter with a heparin-lock for repeated iv injections has been effective in outpatient anesthesia for pediatric radiotherapy.
Monitoring	Standard monitors (see p. D-1).	A critical problem is the lack of access to the patient and monitors during XRT. A video camera with a zoom lens can focus on the visual displays of the monitors; and a second camera is trained on the patient. A small marker may be placed on the chest so that the rise and fall of chest motion is easily seen.[10] Respiration also may be observed by direct visualization through a leaded-glass viewing port.
Positioning	✓ and pad pressure points. ✓ eyes.	
Complications	Airway obstruction	Respiratory obstruction occasionally occurs; it responds to either nasopharyngeal or oropharyngeal airways. In rare instances, ET intubation may be required for persistent airway obstruction.
	Patient movement	Deepen anesthesia.

POSTPROCEDURE

Complications	Cerebral edema	In patients with ↑ICP, XRT can provoke an acute ↑ICP, with consequent ↑HA, ↑N/V, ↓consciousness → cardiac arrest. These patients should be monitored × 24 h post Rx.
	Central line sepsis	Patients may be immunocompromized following chemotherapy. Attention to sterility during access of the central venous line is important because repeated use by multiple anesthesiologists ↑ risk of catheter contamination. Aseptic preparation of anesthetic iv medications, especially propofol, is important.
	PONV	Many patients have chemotherapy-induced nausea, which may be aggravated by anesthesia, XRT, and stress.
Pain management	Standard approaches	Radiation treatments are not associated with pain, but they may be useful in relieving pain associated with neoplastic disease.

References

1. Bauman GS, Brett CM, Ciricillo SF, Larson DA, Sneed P, Stalpers LJA, Edwards M, Wara WM: Anesthesia for pediatric stereotactic radiosurgery. *Anesthesiology* 1998; 89(1):255-7.
2. Browne CH, Boulton TB, Crichton TC: Anaesthesia for radiotherapy. A frame for maintaining the airway. *Anaesthesia* 1969; 24(3):428-30.
3. Casey WF, Price V, Smith HS: Anaesthesia and monitoring for paediatric radiotherapy. *J R Soc Med* 1986; 79(8):454-6.
4. Donaldson SS, Egbert PR: Retinoblastoma. In *Principles and Practice of Pediatric Oncology*. Pizzo PA, Poplack DG, eds, JB Lippincott, Philadelphia: 1989, 555-68.
5. Donaldson SS, Shostak CA, Samuels SI: Technical and practical considerations in the radiotherapy of children. *Front Radiat Ther Oncol* 1987; 21(1):256-69.
6. Fortney JT, Halperin EC, Hertz CM, Schulman SR: Anesthesia for pediatric external beam radiation therapy. *Int J Rad Oncol Biol Phys* 1999; 44(3):587-91.
7. Harnett AN, Hungerford JL, Lambert GD, Hirst A, Darlison R, Hart BL, Trodd TC, Plowman PN: Improved external beam radiotherapy for the treatment of retinoblastoma. *Br J Radiol* 1987; 60(716):753-60.
8. Lo JN, Buckley JJ, Kim TH, Lopez R: Anesthesia for high-dose total body irradiation in children. *Anesthesiology* 1984; 61(1):101-3.

9. Menache L, Eifel PJ, Kennamer DL, Belli JA: Twice-daily anesthesia in infants receiving hyper-fractionated irradiation. *Int J Radiat Oncol Biol Phys* 1990; 18(3):625-9.

10. Murray WJ: Anesthesia for external beam radiotherapy. In *Pediatric Radiation Oncology,* Halperin EC, Kun LE, Constine LS, Tarbell NJ, eds. Raven Press, New York: 1989, 399-407.

11. Roy WL: Anaesthetizing children in remote locations: necessary expeditions or anaesthetic misadventures? *Can J Anaesth* 1996; 43(8):764-8.

12. Singapuri K, Russell GB: Anesthesia and radiation therapy. In *Alternate-Site Anesthesia: Clinical Practice Outside the Operating Room.* Russell GB, ed. Butterworth-Heinemann, Boston: 1997, 365-80.

PEDIATRIC CARDIAC CATHETERIZATION AND ELECTROPHYSIOLOGY

PROCEDURAL CONSIDERATIONS

Kalyani R. Trivedi, Anne M. Dubin, Stanton B. Perry, and Jeffrey A. Feinstein

Cardiac catheterization and electrophysiology testing have evolved over the recent decades from purely diagnostic tools to combined diagnostic and therapeutic procedures. Although the use of anesthesiologists and GA varies from institution to institution, higher levels of sedation are required at a minimum for critically ill patients, those requiring complex interventional strategies, small children who must remain totally still, and when TEE is used for image-guided therapy. A thorough review of diagnostic and interventional cardiac catheterization and electrophysiology is not possible in this chapter, and the interested reader is referred to the multiple textbooks available on the subject.[2,6,13,19]

The placement of anesthesia equipment for these procedures must allow for: (1) proper positioning of the patient, (2) easy access to the head and neck and/or groin for the physician performing the procedure, and (3) rotation and angulation of the imaging equipment. The goal of sedation in all of these procedures is to provide a nontraumatic, safe environment for the patient. Many patients can be cared for adequately and safely using conscious sedation; however, there is a subset of pediatric patients who may require GA. This group may include patients with complex congenital heart disease, ventricular dysfunction, or airway abnormalities.[7] It is important to understand that certain anesthetic agents may alter cardiac conduction, making arrhythmia inducibility more difficult. Catecholamine-dependent arrhythmias, such as an automatic atrial tachycardia, may be impossible to induce with the patient under GA.[11] Furthermore, the arrhythmia itself may complicate anesthetic care, by causing sudden decreases in BP due to excessively rapid rates. In patients undergoing radiofrequency ablation (RFA) (see p. 1182) in areas close to other critical structures of the heart, GA may be necessary to keep the patient motionless during application of energy.

VASCULAR ACCESS

The modified **Seldinger technique** of cannulating blood vessels percutaneously is used to establish vascular access for cardiac catheterization. (The femoral, IJ, and subclavian veins are most commonly used for venous access.) Transhepatic access to the IVC has been used safely and successfully in patients without femoral venous access. The femoral artery is most commonly used, although the carotid and axillary arteries may be used for specific procedures or when there is bilateral femoral artery occlusion. In newborns, the umbilical artery and vein may be used. Access may be especially difficult in patients who have undergone multiple previous procedures. In the most severe cases, **reconstructive transcatheter techniques**, including **balloon angioplasty** and **stent implantation** to rehabilitate the vessels, have been used to allow future catheter-based diagnostic and therapeutic interventions.

Infiltration of the skin and the subcutaneous tissues with a local anesthetic agent to reduce pain is used when the procedure is being performed under conscious sedation. With GA, infiltration of a local anesthetic agent may be deferred to the end of the procedure to alleviate pain and discomfort at vascular access sites during recovery.

HEMODYNAMIC DATA

O_2 sat measurements are made routinely in the various cardiac chambers, vena cavae, and great vessels. These measurements are used to calculate the systemic flow (CO, Q_s), pulmonary flow (Q_p), the ratio of the pulmonary-to-systemic flow (Q_p:Q_s), and PVR and SVR.

It is ideal to obtain the data with the patient awake and breathing spontaneously in room air. This is rarely possible in pediatric patients. The use of light anesthesia and sedation during the diagnostic part of the study facilitates acquisition of data in as near normal state as is possible. It is important to recognize and limit effects on intracardiac and intrapulmonary pressures and systemic and pulmonary resistances when the procedure is done under GA with IPPV. At a minimum, and when tolerated, baseline hemodynamic measurements should be performed with an FiO_2 as close to 0.21 as possible. In some cases, additional diagnostic information may be collected to study the effects of O_2, NO, vasodilators or inotropes, exercise and balloon occlusion of intracardiac or extracardiac shunts on the CO, pulmonary flow, and PVR and SVR.

From O_2 sat, dissolved O_2 (PO_2), and Hb measurements, the O_2 content (ml/dl) of the mixed venous blood and systemic arterial blood is used to calculate systemic AV O_2 content difference. Pulmonary AV O_2 content difference is similarly estimated by calculating the O_2 content of pulmonary venous and arterial blood. Systemic (Q_s) and pulmonary flow (Q_p) can then be derived using the **Fick principle:**

$$\text{Flow (Q)(L/min)} = \frac{O_2 \text{ consumption (ml/min)}}{\text{AV } O_2 \text{ difference (ml of } O_2/\text{L of blood)}}$$

When the partial pressure of dissolved O_2 is < 100, the PO_2 portion of the equation can be negated and the flow can be calculated using the O_2 consumption and sat measurements alone.

$$\text{Pulmonary Flow } (Q_p) = \frac{O_2 \text{ Consumption}}{\text{Pulmonary vein sat} - \text{Pulmonary artery sat}}$$

$$\text{Systemic Flow } (Q_s) = \frac{O_2 \text{ Consumption}}{\text{Systemic artery sat} - \text{Mixed venous sat}}$$

Based on Ohm's law, which states V = IR, where V = voltage (or pressure drop) across a circuit, I = the current (or flow) through the circuit, and R = the resistance in the circuit, SVR and PVR can be calculated as follows:

$$PVR = (PA_p - LA_p)/Q_p$$

$$SVR = (Ao_p - RA_p)/Q_s$$

Where PA_p = pulmonary artery pressure; LA_p = left atrial pressure; Ao_p = aortic pressure; and RA_p = right atrial pressure; pulmonary vascular resistance = PVR; systemic vascular resistance = SVR.

ANGIOGRAPHY

Biplane cineangiography is performed to delineate intracardiac or vascular anatomy and to evaluate ventricular function. Images are obtained by injection of radiographic contrast agents through angiographic catheters positioned in appropriate locations. The angiograms may be performed in postero-anterior and lateral projections or by angling the cameras to obtain cranial, caudal, left anterior, or right anterior oblique projections. Based on the site of injection and the information required, the injection may be performed with a power injector, delivering large amounts of contrast quickly, or by hand.

INTERVENTIONAL PROCEDURES

Valvuloplasty

Aortic valvuloplasty: A retrograde approach from the femoral artery generally is used, although an antegrade and transseptal approach from the femoral vein is preferred by some. In either approach, following hemodynamic evaluation and angiographic estimate of the aortic valve annulus, a wire is positioned across the valve and a balloon catheter is advanced over the wire and positioned across the aortic valve. The balloon is then inflated and deflated quickly. The inflation of the balloon leads to a transient loss of CO, ↓SBP, and occasionally may be accompanied by ↓HR. These hemodynamic changes recover quickly on balloon deflation. While complications of aortic valvuloplasty are rare, the anesthesiologist must be 'prepared for the worst,' which includes annular rupture and the creation of significant aortic regurgitation.[16,21]

Pulmonic valvuloplasty: After femoral venous or IJ access is obtained, the technique for balloon dilation of the pulmonary valve is nearly identical to that outlined above for the aortic valve. Loss of CO and ↓HR are seen during the time of balloon inflation with this intervention as well. While annular rupture also is a potential complication of this procedure, the creation of pulmonary insufficiency is of less concern and better tolerated than aortic insufficiency.[15,18]

Angioplasty

A number of transcatheter treatment options are available for management of **pulmonary artery stenoses**, including **balloon angioplasty** and **endovascular stent implantation**. Angioplasty has been shown to be highly effective in anatomically appropriate cases with a low complication rate. Hemodynamic and angiographic assessment of the lesion is obtained, followed by selection of an optimal balloon catheter, based on both the size of the stenosis and surrounding 'normal' tissue. Using the same 'over-the-wire technique,' a balloon is advanced and centered over the stenosis. Hemo-dynamic and angiographic data are assessed following each intervention. A high index of suspicion for complications—including dissection or pulmonary artery tear, obstructive intimal flaps, thrombi, and reperfusion pulmonary edema—is justified, as management may require ventilatory manipulations and/or emergent cardiovascular resuscitation.[3]

Balloon angioplasty of coarctation of the aorta may be performed for treatment of native or recurrent coarctation. Angi-ography of the aorta is performed to delineate the coarctation and estimate the dimension of the coarctated segment and the adjacent aorta. As with other angioplasty techniques, the balloon size is based on the dimensions of the stenotic area and surrounding vessel. Transient loss of lower body perfusion and ↓HR are to be expected, as with balloon valvuloplasty, on inflation of the balloon. Pressure and angiographic data are obtained to determine adequacy of results and absence of complications. There is a 4-5% incidence of intimal tear and dissection that, in most cases, are nonprogressive. Rarely, aortic disruption may require emergent surgical repair.[15]

Endovascular stent placement

Stent implantation in the pulmonary arteries or for aortic coarctation is used to maintain vessel diameter and decreased gradients in patients unresponsive to balloon dilation. Stents are mounted on balloon catheters and the balloon/stent com-bination is advanced over a previously placed wire. A long sheath (originating in the groin or neck) is placed across the area of narrowing to prevent the stent from slipping off the balloon catheter as it makes its way through the heart or vessels. After the stent has been properly positioned, the long sheath is withdrawn to expose the balloon/stent combination. The balloon is inflated to expand the stent and appose it to the vessel wall. Placement of long sheaths, particularly through the right ventricular outflow tract (RVOT), can be difficult and may result in transient bradyarrhythmias and loss of CO.[22]

Closure of congenital defects

Atrial septal defects (ASDs): As many as 80-85% of secundum ASDs may be amenable to device closure in the cath lab. Most devices currently used include a left atrial disc with an occlusive membrane, a central spool or connecting pin, and a right atrial disc with an occlusive membrane. The membrane occludes flow through the defect and, within months, the device becomes incorporated into the septum due to endothelialization. A sizing balloon inflated across the defect per-mits estimation of the stretched diameter. A long sheath is then placed across the defect over a wire. The device attached to the delivery cable is loaded in the long sheath and advanced to the left atrium. The left atrial disc is opened, the device is withdrawn until the left atrial disk is in contact with the atrial septum; then, the right atrial disc is opened, effectively 'sandwiching' the atrial septum between the two disks. TEE is used to guide placement of the device. Intracardiac ECHO has been introduced recently and offers ECHO guidance without the requirement of GA.[9,24]

Ventricular Septal Defect (VSD): Closure with a device can be performed in the cath lab for isolated or multiple mus-cular VSDs, as well as perimembranous defects. The technique requires establishment of a continuous AV guide wire loop across the defect. Most often, the wire course is from the femoral vein, through the right atrium, into the RV, across the VSD, out the aortic valve, around the aorta, and out the femoral artery. The device is then deployed via a long sheath placed across the VSD through the RV aspect. Hemodynamic compromise may be seen with tension on the wire if aortic or tricuspid insufficiency is induced. Transient arrhythmias are routine while crossing the VSD and deploying the device. Great care must be taken to avoid entrapment in the mitral, aortic, and tricuspid valves during device deployment. In addi-tion to fluoroscopy, TEE is used to guide placement of the device. Improvements in the devices developed more recently have significantly reduced the cath lab morbidity of this procedure.[5]

Coil occlusion: Aortopulmonary collaterals, AVMs, Blalock-Taussig (B-T) shunts, venous collaterals, coronary artery fistulae, and patent ductus arteriosi (PDA) have all been successfully occluded using the technique of coil embolization. The embolization coils consist of a metal wire, either stainless steel or platinum, ± Dacron strands, and are available in multiple sizes, lengths, and shapes. While PDA or coronary artery fistula embolization may obviate the need for surgery, most embolizations serve to either reduce the cardiac workload by decreasing the amount of shunting or simplify a planned surgical procedure.[20]

The technique for coil closure of collaterals or other communications is straightforward. A catheter is placed in the vessel to be occluded and a selective angiogram is done to delineate the anatomy and diameter of the vessel to be closed. Coils that are slightly larger than the diameter of the vessel are used, since the vessel will distend when the coil is deployed. Using a long 'pusher' wire, the coil is advanced through the catheter and deployed in the vessel. Repeat angiography is performed to confirm complete closure. If residual flow remains, additional coils are placed. Coil dislodgement and embo-lization to a distal blood vessel is the most common complication. In general, the errant coil can be retrieved in the cath lab without much difficulty and a new coil of a larger size placed to occlude the vessel.

OTHER PROCEDURES

Endomyocardial biopsy is commonly performed for rejection surveillance in patients following cardiac transplantation. It also may be performed in patients presenting with acute onset of cardiomyopathy for histopathological Dx of myocarditis. The preferred site for obtaining cardiac biopsy is the RV aspect of the intraventricular septum. The specimen is obtained with a biopsy forceps advanced to the RV through a long sheath. It is usual to obtain 4-5 specimens to improve the diagnostic gain, as the histopathological changes can be patchy. Complications of endomyocardial biopsy include cardiac perforation and tricuspid valve damage. GA is required in patients with compromised airway and/or cardiopulmonary status from lymphoproliferative disease or obesity 2° to steroid therapy.

A variety of other transcatheter therapeutic procedures may be performed in the cardiac cath suite. **Rashkind balloon atrial septostomy, static balloon septoplasty, Brockenbrough transseptal needle puncture**, and **radiofrequency-assisted perforation** of the pulmonary valve or the atrial septum are all less commonly used than the procedures described above, but routinely are undertaken in high-volume cath labs.[4]

ELECTROPHYSIOLOGY STUDY (EPS)

Patients with atrial or ventricular arrhythmias may require either diagnostic or therapeutic interventions in the cath lab. EP studies are catheterization procedures in which intracardiac electrical signals are recorded via specialized catheters that can both record electrical activity and stimulate the heart. These studies often are used to make a Dx of the mechanism of arrhythmia, assess the hemodynamic impact of the arrhythmia, assess efficacy of pharmacologic therapy, and map the location of abnormal conduction pathways or automatic foci.[23] While routine studies usually take 2-3 h, some may be quite lengthy.

Radiofrequency ablation (RFA) is a procedure in which abnormal electrical conducting pathways or automatic electrical foci (identified by EPS) are destroyed, using the application of RF energy delivered through a deflectable electrode catheter (see p. 1182). This procedure was first described in pediatric surgery in 1991, but has rapidly become a preferred therapeutic option for supraventricular tachycardia in this population.[10] On some occasions, RF lesions must be placed close to other critical structures in the heart (e.g., AV node).

With advances in technology and an increased understanding of high-risk pediatric patient populations, **transvenous pacemaker** (see p. 284) and **implantable cardioverter defibrillator (ICD)** (see p. 1165) placements are becoming more common in the pediatric population. Pacemaker placement has become more common as data have accumulated regarding the risk of sudden death in patients with congenital complete heart block, as well as increased survival with postop heart block.[14] New indications for ICD placement in patients with long QT syndrome, congenital heart disease, and hypertrophic cardiomyopathy have increased the number of ICD implantations in the last 5 yr.[1] These procedures are commonly performed in the cath lab under GA.

ANESTHETIC CONSIDERATIONS

M. Gail Boltz and Chandra Ramamoorthy

PREOPERATIVE

Pediatric patients presenting for interventional cardiology range from those requiring simple diagnostic procedures to those requiring complex interventional procedures (balloon angioplasty or stenting). These patients can present a challenge, given their abnormal cardiac anatomy and physiology. Many of them must undergo repeated catheterizations and will have had multiple anesthetic experiences. All patients must receive a thorough preanesthetic H&P, emphasizing cardiorespiratory function and coexisting congenital anomalies that may predict difficult airway management. Children should follow the same npo protocol as they would for surgery (see NPO Guidelines, p. D-1).

Respiratory	URIs must be evaluated carefully. If Sx are limited to nasal congestion, the procedure can be carried out. Sx of lower respiratory tract involvement—including fever, productive cough, or wheezing—warrant postponement for 2-3 wk unless the procedure is urgent. Room air saturation less helpful in cyanotic children for URI assessment.
Cardiovascular	Review prior catheterizations, echocardiograms, ECGs, and cardiology evaluations. Cardiac transplant recipients can demonstrate HTN 2° cyclosporine use and can develop progressive coronary artery stenosis in their grafts. Antibiotics are given to patients as required for SBE prophylaxis or for those undergoing interventional procedures.
Immunology	Cardiac transplant recipients can develop lymphoproliferative disease, which results in redundant lymphoid tissue in the pharynx and epiglottis → possible airway obstruction. Careful evaluation of the airway is required.

Gastrointestinal	Chronic steroid use → significant obesity → difficult airway management; reflux.
Renal	Cardiac transplant recipients can have renal dysfunction 2° antirejection medications or HTN. Additionally, cyclosporine →↑K⁺.
Laboratory	Tests as indicated from H&P. Most patients will require electrolytes and Hct; however, sometimes these labs can be deferred until after induction and vascular access is acquired. Some interventional procedures require a T&C, with blood available in the room.
Premedication	Usually not needed because parents can accompany child into the catheterization suite and be present during induction. Some children (> 6 mo), however, who have had many prior studies may be anxious and require oral premedication with midazolam 0.5-0.75 mg/kg.

INTRAOPERATIVE

Anesthetic technique: MAC with sedation is preferred for measuring hemodynamic parameters in children because GA will distort these values; however, some patients require GA. Some interventional procedures (e.g., stenting or coiling) require a motionless field or may be too long for mild sedation. Patients who require venous access via the IJ vein may not tolerate lying still for long periods of time. Critically ill neonates require intubation and controlled ventilation. Patients with moderate-to-severe pulmonary HTN can be managed with sedation. Some older children with studies of shorter duration using groin access may tolerate incremental iv sedation with local anesthesia.

MAC: Sedation can be managed with propofol/ketamine or propofol/remifentanil infusion, as long as the patient remains normocarbic and normoxic. Hypercapnia affects hemodynamic catheterization values.

Induction	Standard inhalation or iv induction (see p. D-2). The choice of anesthetic drugs must include careful consideration of their effects on myocardial function, pulmonary resistance, and respiration.
Maintenance	GETA with volatile agents (e.g., sevoflurane) or iv infusion (e.g., propofol, remifentanil, ketamine). Most catheterizations require the patient to be maintained on room air for accurate O_2 sat and pressure measurements. EPS studies are best managed with iv propofol 50-150 μg/kg/min, since this agent has the least ability to induce dysrhythmias. Recent studies, however, demonstrate that sevoflurane or isoflurane (1 MAC or lower) also may be acceptable. Most cardiologists request heparin 50-100 U/kg for patients with arterial sheaths in place and any interventional procedures. Heparin 50 U/kg is repeated every 90 min. NTG, Ca⁺⁺ channel blockers, or NO may be requested by the cardiologist to evaluate the reversibility of pulmonary HTN.
Emergence	Do not allow child to emerge before hemostasis has been achieved at the access site. Use of remifentanil infusion may provide analgesia during the procedure, yet allow for a rapid emergence. Consider remifentanil for patients with pulmonary HTN, where a smooth emergence is essential to prevent a hypertensive crisis. Interventional procedures and EPS/ablations require overnight ICU admission for observation. Most other patients can recover in PACU.

Blood and fluid requirements	IV: 20-22 ga × 1 NS/LR PRBCs Fluid warmer	A second volume iv may be desirable for interventional cases. The cardiologist also will have a venous access line that can be used if necessary. Avoid volume overload. Interventional procedures may → tearing of vessels and/or myocardium and can cause abrupt hemorrhage; therefore, blood must be available in the room. Neonates can lose significant blood during access and sampling and also may require transfusion. Follow serial Hct.
Monitoring	Standard monitors, including Bair-Hugger ± Arterial line ± Foley catheter	If arterial access is required, discuss with the cardiologist. Frequently, the femoral artery is cannulated for the catheterization and may be available for use; however, access may be limited at crucial times (e.g., stenting or coiling), so a peripheral arterial line may be desirable. For cases of long duration, consider Foley catheter placement. Monitor temperature.
Positioning	✓ and pad pressure points. ✓ eyes.	Supine, arms flexed above head to allow fluoroscopy of chest. All ECG leads and monitoring wires must be cleared from axilla and chest to allow fluoroscopy.
Complications	Airway obstruction	Rx: Airway support, oral/nasal airway, LMA. Intubate if needed.

Complications, cont.	Arrhythmias	Usually self-limiting; determine etiology (e.g., catheter or wire).
	Hemorrhage	Rx: Fluid resuscitation with crystalloid, 5% albumin and/or blood; vasopressors as needed.
	Hypoxemia	Rx: Airway support; increase FiO_2. Intubate and ventilate as needed.
	Pulmonary hypertensive crisis	Rx: 100% O_2, administer iv opioid, systemic vasopressors. Consider NO and/or nebulized prostacyclin.
	Hypothermia	Rx: Forced-air warming device, heat lamp. Increase environmental temperature.
	Contrast reaction/anaphylaxis	Rx: Support airway, 100% FiO_2, intubate if needed: epinephrine, volume resuscitation, steroid, antihistamine.
	Air embolism	Rx: 100% FiO_2; identify and occlude source; Trendelenburg; fluid resuscitation; vasopressor support. Aspirate air from central access if possible.

POSTOPERATIVE

Complications	Hematoma at access site Ischemic limb Emergence delirium	
Pain management	Infiltrate access sites with local anesthetic.	Postop analgesia usually not required.
Tests	CXR, if indicated.	

References

1. Alexander ME, Walsh EP, Saul JP, et al: Value of programmed stimulation in patients with congenital heart disease. *J Cardiovasc Electrophysiol* 1999; 10(8):1033-44.
2. Baim DS, Grossman W: *Grossman's Cardiac Catheterization, Angiography, and Intervention*, 6th edition. Lippincott Williams & Wilkins, Philadelphia: 2001.
3. Baker CM, McGowan FX Jr, Keane JF, Lock JE: Pulmonary artery trauma due to balloon dilation: recognition, avoidance and management. *J Am Coll Cardiol* 2000; 36(5):1684-90.
4. Benson LN, Nykanen D, Collison A: Radiofrequency perforation in the treatment of congenital heart disease. *Catheter Cardiovasc Interv* 2002; 56(1):72-82.
5. Chessa M, Carminati M, Cao QL, Butera G, Giusti S, Bini RM, Hijazi ZM: Transcatheter closure of congenital and acquired muscular ventricular septal defects using the Amplatzer device. *J Invasive Cardiol* 2002; 14(6):322-7.
6. Freedom RM, Mawson JB, Yoo SJ, Benson LN: *Congenital Heart Disease Textbook of Angiography*. Futura Publishing, Armonk, NY: 1997.
7. Friedman RA, Walsh EP, Silka MJ, Calkins J, Stevenson WG, Rhodes LA, Deal BJ, Wolff GS, DeMaso DR, Hanisch D, Van Hare GF: NASPE Expert Consensus Conference: Radiofrequency Catheter Ablation in Children with and without Congenital Heart Disease. Report of the Writing Committee. *PACE* 2002; 25:1000-17.
8. Hamid RKA: Anesthesia for nonsurgical procedures in children: cardiac catheterization and electrophysiology studies. In *Pediatric Cardiac Anesthesia*, 3rd edition. Appleton-Lange, Norwalk, CT: 1997, 165-80.
9. Hijazi Z, Wang Z, Cao Q, Koenig P, Waight D, Lang R: Transcatheter closure of atrial septal defects and patent foramen ovale under intracardiac echocardiographic guidance: feasibility and comparison with transesophageal echocardiography. *Catheter Cardiovasc Interv* 2001; 52(2):194-9.
10. Kugler JD, Danford DA, Houston K, et al.: Radiofrequency catheter ablation for paroxysmal supraventricular tachycardia in children and adolescent without structural heart disease. The Pediatric EP Society Radiofrequency Catheter Ablation Registry. *Am J Cardiol* 1997; 80(11):1438-43.
11. Lai LP, Lin JL Wu MH, Wang WJ, Huang CH, Yeh, HM, Tseng YZ, Lien WP, Huang SKS: Usefulness of intravenous propofol anesthesia for radiofrequency catheter ablation in patients with tachyarrhythmias: Infeasibility for pediatric patients with ectopic atrial tachycardia *PACE* 1999; 22(9):1358-64.
12. Lavoie J, Walsh EP, Burrows FA, et al: Effects of propofol or isoflurane anesthesia on cardiac conduction in children undergoing radiofrequency catheter ablation for tachydysrhythmias. *Anesthesiology* 1995; 82:884-7.
13. Lock JE, Keane JF, Perry SB: *Diagnostic and Interventional Catheterization in Congenital Heart Disease*, 2nd edition. Kluwer Academic Publishers, Nowell, MA: 2000.
14. Maron BJ, Shen WK, Link MS, et al.: Efficacy of implantable cardioverter-defibrillators for the prevention of sudden death in patients with hypertrophic cardiomyopathy. *N Eng J Med* 2000; 342(6):365-73.
15. McCrindle BW: Independent predictors of long-term results after balloon pulmonary valvuloplasty. Valvuloplasty and Angioplasty of Congenital Anomalies (VACA) Registry Investigators. *Circulation* 1994; 89(4):1751-9.

16. McCrindle BW, Blackstone EH, Williams WG, Sittiwangkul R, Spray TL, Azakie A, Jonas RA: Are outcomes of surgical versus transcatheter balloon valvotomy equivalent in neonatal critical aortic stenosis? *Circulation* 2001; 104(12 Suppl 1): 1152-8.

17. McCrindle BW, Jones TK, Morrow WR, Hagler DJ, Lloyd TR, Nouri S, Latson LA: Acute results of balloon angioplasty of native coarctation versus recurrent aortic obstruction are equivalent. Valvuloplasty and Angioplasty of Congenital Anomalies (VACA) Registry Investigators. *J Am Coll Cardiol* 1996; 28(7):1810-7.

18. McCrindle BW, Kan JS: Long-term results after balloon pulmonary valvuloplasty. *Circulation* 1991; 83(6):1915-22.

19. Perry SB, Keane JF, Lock JE: Interventional catheterization in pediatric congenital and acquired heart disease. *Am J Cardiol* 1988; 61(14):109G-17G.

20. Perry SB, Rome J, Keane JF, Baim DS, Lock JE: Transcatheter closure of coronary artery fistulas. *J Am Coll Cardiol* 1992; 20(1):205-9.

21. Satou GM, Perry SB, Lock JE, Piercey GE, Keane JF: Repeat balloon dilation of congenital valvar aortic stenosis: immediate results and midterm outcome. *Catheter Cardiovasc Interv* 1999; 47(1):47-51.

22. Shaffer KM, Mullins CE, Grifka RG, O'Laughlin MP, McMahon W, Ing FF, Nihill MR: Intravascular stents in congenital heart disease: short- and long-term results from a large single-center experience. *J Am Coll Cardiol* 1998; 31(3):661-7.

23. Van Hare GF, Lesh MD, Scheinman M et al.: Percutaneous radiofrequency catheter ablation for supraventricular arrhythmias in children. *J Am Coll Cardiol* 1991; 17(7):1613-20.

24. Vogel M, Berger F, Dahnert I, Ewert P, Lange PE: Treatment of atrial septal defects in symptomatic children aged less than 2 years of age using the Amplatzer septal occluder. *Cardiol Young* 2000; 10(5):534-7.

25. Yaster MY, Krane EJ, Kaplan RF: Diagnostic evaluation of congenital heart disease. In *Pediatric Pain Management and Sedation Handbook*. Mosby Yearbook, St. Louis: 1997.

26. Zimmerman AA, Ibrahim AE, et al: The effects of halothane and sevoflurane on cardiac electrophysiology in children undergoing radiofrequency catheter ablation. *Anesthesiology* 1997; 87:A1066.

PEDIATRIC ONCOLOGIC PROCEDURES

Cathy R. Lammers and Gregory B. Hammer

Pediatric oncology patients must endure multiple painful procedures, including bone marrow aspirations, biopsies, lumbar punctures, and removal of central venous access ports. All of these procedures can be performed in a procedure room with sedation or GA.

PREPROCEDURE

A thorough preanesthetic H&P should be performed in all cases and the usual npo protocol applied (see p. D-1). Prior treatment with chemotherapeutic agents should be identified for evaluation of toxic side effects (see below).

Respiratory	Surgeries for patients with Sx of URI (e.g., cough, fever) are usually postponed. Some chemotherapeutic agents have been associated with pulmonary toxicity: bleomycin (2-5%), BNCU (20-50%), busulfan (2.5-11.5%), cyclophosphamide (rare), methotrexate (rare). **Tests:** As indicated from H&P.
Cardiovascular	Some chemotherapeutic agents have been associated with cardiac toxicity: cyclophosphamide, doxorubicin, Adriamycin, radiation (cardiomyopathy); doxorubicin, m-AMSA (dysrhythmias). **Tests:** Consider a functional cardiac study if patient received a chemotherapeutic agent associated with cardiac toxicity (most will already have had a study done at this stage of their treatment).
Hematologic	Bone marrow suppression with all cytotoxic drugs. **Tests:** As indicated.
Laboratory	Many patients will have had a recent CBC. In general, no additional labs are required.
Premedication	Usually not required because a parent can accompany child into procedure room; however, most children will have venous access and can be given small doses of midazolam if necessary. Consider midazolam syrup 0.5-0.75 mg/kg po for the particularly anxious child without iv access in place. For children without venous access, a peripheral iv may be placed (± premedication). Prior to this, application of EMLA or ELA Max cream (1 h, or 20 min, respectively) provides topical anesthesia of the skin at the lumbar puncture or bone-marrow aspiration site, as well as the peripheral iv site.

INTRAPROCEDURE

Anesthetic technique: GA (LMA or mask) or MAC in the appropriate patient

Induction	Most children have a central venous access line in place for their oncology treatment protocol; thus, induction can proceed with iv propofol 2-3 mg/kg. Infrequently, mask induction is performed.	
Maintenance	The oncologist infiltrates the area with lidocaine. For Broviac catheter removals, heparin must be removed from the catheter and discarded before use for induction. A sufficient bolus of propofol (e.g., 0.5-1 mg/kg) must be given just prior to pulling the catheter. Additional iv usually is not warranted, since the procedure is normally < 10 min. Occasionally, the catheter may break during attempted removal, and the surgeon will have to make a skin incision to allow for removal of the internal fragment. In such cases, a peripheral iv may be inserted quickly to facilitate administration of additional propofol, or mask anesthesia may be given. If the SpO_2 decreases, blow-by O_2 with gentle head and neck positioning are generally sufficient.	
Emergence	Allow child to awaken in procedure room. Consider ondansetron 0.1 mg/kg for patients receiving intrathecal chemotherapy during their lumbar puncture. Most patients should be recovered in the PACU.	
Blood and fluid requirements	No blood loss	IV central line may be in situ.
Monitoring	Standard monitors (see p. D-1).	
Positioning	Lateral, fetal position (lumbar punctures) Supine or prone (bone marrow aspiration/biopsy) Supine for Broviac removal	
Complications	Airway obstruction Retained central venous catheter	Head and neck reposition, jaw thrust. Rx may require open surgical procedure.
Pain management	Acetaminophen	Lumbar punctures are not generally painful afterwards, whereas bone marrow aspirations and biopsies, especially, can be. Acetaminophen po is usually sufficient for analgesia. Rectal route should be avoided, unless adequate Plt and WBC counts are confirmed.

References

1. Cote CJ: Anesthesia outside the operating room. In *A Practice of Anesthesia for Infants and Children.* Cote CJ, Ryan JF, Todres ID, et al, eds. WB Saunders, Philadelphia: 1993.
2. Martin TM, Nicolson SC, Bargas MS: Propofol anesthesia reduces emesis and airway obstruction in pediatric outpatients. *Anesth Analg* 1993; 76(1):144-8.
3. McDowall RH, Scher CS, Barst SM. Total intravenous anesthesia for children undergoing brief diagnostic or therapeutic procedures. *J Clin Anesth* 1995; 7(4):273-80.

UPPER/LOWER GI ENDOSCOPY

Cathy R. Lammers and Gregory B. Hammer

Children presenting for upper and/or lower GI endoscopy may have a wide variety of congenital and acquired abnormalities of the GI tract. Examples include repaired tracheoesophageal fistula (TEF) with residual esophageal dysmotility, presence of a foreign body, and various congenital lesions. Patients presenting for gastrostomy tube placement may have encephalopathy 2° cerebral palsy, with associated seizure disorder and muscle contractures. Severe GERD may be present, with the associated risk of pulmonary aspiration following induction of anesthesia. Many GI endoscopy procedures are done without anesthesia. Requests for anesthesia are dependent on the gastroenterologist's preference, as well as the severity of the patient's underlying illnesses. All patients must receive a thorough preanesthesia H&P. Children should follow the same npo protocol used for surgery (see p. D-1).

ANESTHETIC CONSIDERATIONS

Gastroenterology   Carefully question the parents for Sx of GERD or esophageal dysfunction resulting in retained food within the esophagus. The stomach and bowel will be insufflated with CO_2 during the procedure, increasing the likelihood of reflux.

Neurologic   Patients with seizure disorders that are well controlled do not need to have recent anticonvulsant levels documented. If spasticity 2° cerebral palsy is present, special attention to careful evaluation of the airway is warranted; vascular access may be difficult.

Laboratory   As indicated from H&P. Usually none.

Premedication   If inhalation induction is planned, premedication may not be required because a parent can accompany the child into the procedure room. Consider midazolam 0.5-0.75 mg/kg po for particularly anxious children and for those in whom iv induction is planned. EMLA cream or ELA Max (4% lidocaine) should be applied at least 1 h or 20 min, respectively, in advance for topical anesthesia before iv placement.

INTRAPROCEDURE

Anesthetic technique: Upper endoscopy and gastrostomy tube placement generally require GETA 2° ↑risk of pulmonary aspiration (2° GERD and insufflation of CO_2). In children > 3-4 yr, the indication for tracheal intubation in the absence of Hx of GERD is less clear. Placement of the endoscope in the mouth precludes the ability to use a mask or LMA. Alternatively, an iv sedation technique with propofol (50-100 μg/kg/min), spontaneous respiration, and supplemental O_2 via nasal cannula or blow-by can be used if the risk of aspiration is considered low. For lower GI endoscopy procedures (e.g., colonoscopy), iv sedation may be preferable.

Induction   For upper GI endoscopies, if Hx of severe GERD is present, an iv catheter is placed prior to induction of anesthesia. A modified, rapid-sequence intubation is performed with preoxygenation, cricoid pressure, STP (4-6 mg/kg) or propofol (2-3 mg/kg), and rocuronium 1 mg/kg. If the risk of aspiration is relatively low, a standard pediatric iv or mask induction is appropriate (see p. D-2). Alternatively, iv sedation may be performed with propofol (75-150 μg/kg/min), ± remifentanil (0.05-0.10 μg/kg/min), by continuous infusion. ETT should be well secured to the side of the mouth.

Maintenance   GETA with inhalational agents or iv infusion of propofol ± remifentanil. Alternatively, iv sedation as above. Young children may have tracheal compression caused by passage of the relatively large endoscope into the esophagus. Careful observation and/or holding the ETT prevents inadvertent extubation during removal of the endoscope.

Emergence   Emergence in procedure room. Transport to PACU for recovery.

Blood and fluid requirements   No blood loss
IV: 22 or 24 ga × 1
NS/LR @ maintenance

Monitoring   Standard monitors (see p. D-1).

Positioning   ✓ and pad pressure points.   Lateral decubitus for upper and lower endoscopy.
✓ eyes.   Supine for G-tube placement.

Complications   Airway obstruction
Hypoxemia 2° gastric insufflation
Pulmonary aspiration
GI perforation
Inadvertent extubation   2° endoscopist working in the mouth and pharynx

POSTPROCEDURE

Pain management   G-tube placements require postop analgesia.   Gastroenterologist infiltrates local anesthetic at the site.

Rectal acetaminophen (35-40 mg/kg)   Following induction for upper GI endoscopies
Morphine 0.1-0.2 mg/kg or fentanyl   Usually provides adequate analgesic in the immediate post-
2-3 μg/kg intraop   op period.

References

1. Balsells F, Wyllie R, Kay M, Steffen R: Use of conscious sedation for lower and upper gastrointestinal endoscopic examinations in children and adults: a twelve-year review. *Gastrointest Endosc* 1997; 45(5):375-80.
2. Cote CJ: Anesthesia outside the operating room. In *A Practice of Anesthesia for Infants and Children.* Cote CJ, Ryan JF, Todres ID, et al, eds. WB Saunders, Philadelphia: 1993.
3. Haight M, Thomas DW: Pediatric gastrointestinal endoscopy. *Gastroenterologist* 1995; 3(3):181-6.
4. Squires RH, Morriss F, Schluterman S, et al: Efficacy, safety, and cost of intravenous sedation versus general anesthesia in children undergoing endoscopic procedures. *Gastrointest Endosc* 1995; 41(2):99-104.

CROSS-SECTIONAL IMAGING (CT, MRI)

Cathy R. Lammers and Gregory B. Hammer

PREPROCEDURE

All patients must receive a thorough preanesthesia H&P. Children should follow the same npo protocol as they would for surgery (see p. D-1). For MRI, thorough questioning regarding metal implants is essential. Any questions regarding appropriateness of specific metal implants should be directed to the radiologist.

Respiratory	URIs must be evaluated carefully. If Sx are limited to nasal congestion, the study may proceed. Sx of lower tract involvement—including fever, productive cough or wheezing—warrant postponement for 2-3 wk unless the study is urgent.
Cardiovascular	Pacemakers are a contraindication for MRI. Prosthetic heart valves may be a contraindication (identify the type of valve present and consult with radiologist). Fresh surgical clips (e.g., recent PDA ligation) also may represent a contraindication for MRI.
Neurologic	Head CT or MRI may be performed in patients with primary seizure disorders or brain tumors. Review seizure medications and ✓ serum levels if appropriate. Recent drug levels may not be necessary in children with well controlled or stable seizure disorders. If ↑ICP or ↓intracranial compliance are present (e.g., 2° tumors or hydrocephalus), the anesthesia plan should include tracheal intubation with controlled ventilation. Metal clips or coils are usually contraindications for MRI. For children with head trauma, concurrent injuries involving the C-spine may be present.
Laboratory	As indicated from H&P. Usually none required.
Premedication	If inhalation induction is planned, premedication may not be required because a parent can accompany child into induction area (either inside CT scan or in outer induction area of MRI). Consider midazolam 0.5-0.75 mg/kg po for particularly anxious children and for those in whom iv induction is planned.

INTRAPROCEDURE

Unique considerations for MRI: See Adult Out-of-OR Procedures, p. 1176.

Anesthetic technique:

CT scans—many children undergo noninvasive CT scans with po sedation without involvement of anesthesia service. For more complex cases requiring the presence of an anesthesiologist, the procedure may be performed with iv sedation or GA. Most commonly, noninvasive CT scans are performed under iv sedation with a continuous infusion of propofol (100-200 μg/kg/min). Alternatively, incremental doses of midazolam (0.025-0.10 mg/kg) may be given. For patients undergoing invasive CT-guided procedures (needle biopsy, placement of drainage tubes, such as thoracostomy tube, etc.), GETA is usually performed. Techniques include spontaneous breathing with inhalational anesthesia and/or propofol infusion or iv anesthesia (propofol ± remifentanil infusion) and controlled ventilation.

MRI—iv sedation or GA may be performed. A deeper level of anesthesia is needed compared with noninvasive CT because MRI requires the child to be motionless for up to 1-2 h. IV propofol infusion may be administered by gravity via a microdrip device, or inhalational anesthesia may be given with MRI-compatible anesthetic machines. Hypothermia frequently occurs in small children anesthetized for 1-2 h in the MRI scanner. The cooling fan for the magnet can sometimes be turned off to decrease heat loss (discuss with MRI technician). One blanket over patient is usually permissible. The iv, airway circuit and monitors require extensions.

Induction	Standard pediatric iv or mask induction can be accomplished in the CT scanner room or for MRI in a special induction area outside the MRI scanner. LMA placement for MRI with inhalational anesthesia facilitates a patent airway and capnograph monitoring. After induction and stabilization of the airway, the patient and all personnel entering the MRI scanner should undergo a second check for removal of metal objects and equipment. A metal object, such as a manometer, laryngoscope blade, or O_2 tank can be propelled toward the magnet with sufficient speed and force to result in serious or fatal injury to the patient and/or health care provider. The patient then will be transported into the scanner.
Maintenance	For iv technique, use propofol infusion pump in CT scanner and microdrip infusion set in MRI (e.g., add 10 ml propofol solution to 90 ml iv fluid to yield propofol concentration of 1 mg/ml [60 drops]; therefore, 1 drop per sec delivers 1 mg/min, or 100 μg/kg/min for a 10-kg child). Most infusion pumps need to remain a specific distance from the MRI scanner. The appropriate distance can be determined and is dependent on the degree of shielding on each particular magnet. Typically, these patients do not require muscle relaxants, and spontaneous breathing is appropriate unless controlled ventilation is required to treat ↑ICP.
Emergence	Transport MRI patient back to induction room for emergence (where airway equipment is available). Although these patients usually are recovered in PACU, children having short procedures with propofol anesthesia who are wide awake in the CT or MRI holding area following the study may be recovered there.

Blood and fluid requirements	No blood loss IV, if required: 22 or 24 ga × 1 NS/LR @ maintenance	
Monitoring	Standard MRI-compatible monitors (see p. D-1 for discussion of monitoring considerations).	For infants, use a child-size NIBP cuff on the leg. The length of tubing required significantly alters the values on infant-size cuffs.
Positioning	✓ and pad pressure points. ✓ eyes.	Ear protection for MRI
Complications	Hypothermia	See adult MRI Unique Considerations and Complications, p. 1176.
	Burn injury IV contrast reaction Airway obstruction Hearing loss (MRI)	From inappropriate placement of pulse oximeter probe or ECG wires in MRI. Avoid coiling of wires and use only monitors approved for MRI. Ear plugs should be placed routinely during MRI.

POSTPROCEDURE

Pain management	Noninvasive procedures are painless. IV fentanyl or morphine appropriate for invasive procedures

References

1. Cote CJ: Anesthesia outside the operating room. In *A Practice of Anesthesia for Infants and Children.* Cote CJ, Ryan JF, Todres ID, et al, eds. WB Saunders, Philadelphia: 1993.
2. Jorgensen NH, Messick JM, Gray J, Nugent M, Berquist TH: ASA monitoring standards and magnetic resonance imaging. *Anesth Analg* 1994; 79:1141-7.
3. Levati A, Colombo N, Arosio EM, Savoia G, et al: Propofol anesthesia in spontaneously breathing pediatric patients during magnetic resonance imaging. *Acta Anaesth Scand* 1996; 40:561-5.
4. Young AE, Brown PN, Zorab JS: Anesthesia for children and infants undergoing magnetic resonance imaging: a prospective study. *Eur J Anaesthesiol* 1996; 13:400-3.

EXTRACORPOREAL MEMBRANE OXYGENATION (ECMO)

Gary E. Hartman

PROCEDURAL CONSIDERATIONS

Description: **Extracorporeal membrane oxygenation (ECMO)** for prolonged periods (3-21 d) allows cardiopulmonary support for newborns and children with reversible respiratory failure. The most common indications are meconium aspiration and pulmonary HTN associated with congenital diaphragmatic hernia. The procedure is performed in the NICU with OR techniques. Patients are given anticoagulants prior to cannulation. Subsequently, repair of the diaphragmatic hernia also may be performed in the NICU on ECMO support before decannulation. (Fig 13.2-1 shows ECMO schematic.)

The potential detrimental effects of the diaphragmatic repair on respiratory function can be managed with increased circuit flow. ECMO also has been helpful in some newborns with cardiopulmonary failure following correction of congenital cardiac defects. Vascular access is accomplished with one (venovenous) or two (venoarterial) cannulas. The IJ vein is cannulated in both methods with the tip of the cannula in the right atrium. In venoarterial ECMO, the common carotid artery is used with the tip of the cannula at the aortic arch. The wound is closed around the cannulas, which are secured to the infant's scalp.

Usual preop diagnosis: Meconium aspiration; diaphragmatic hernia; Bochdalek's hernia

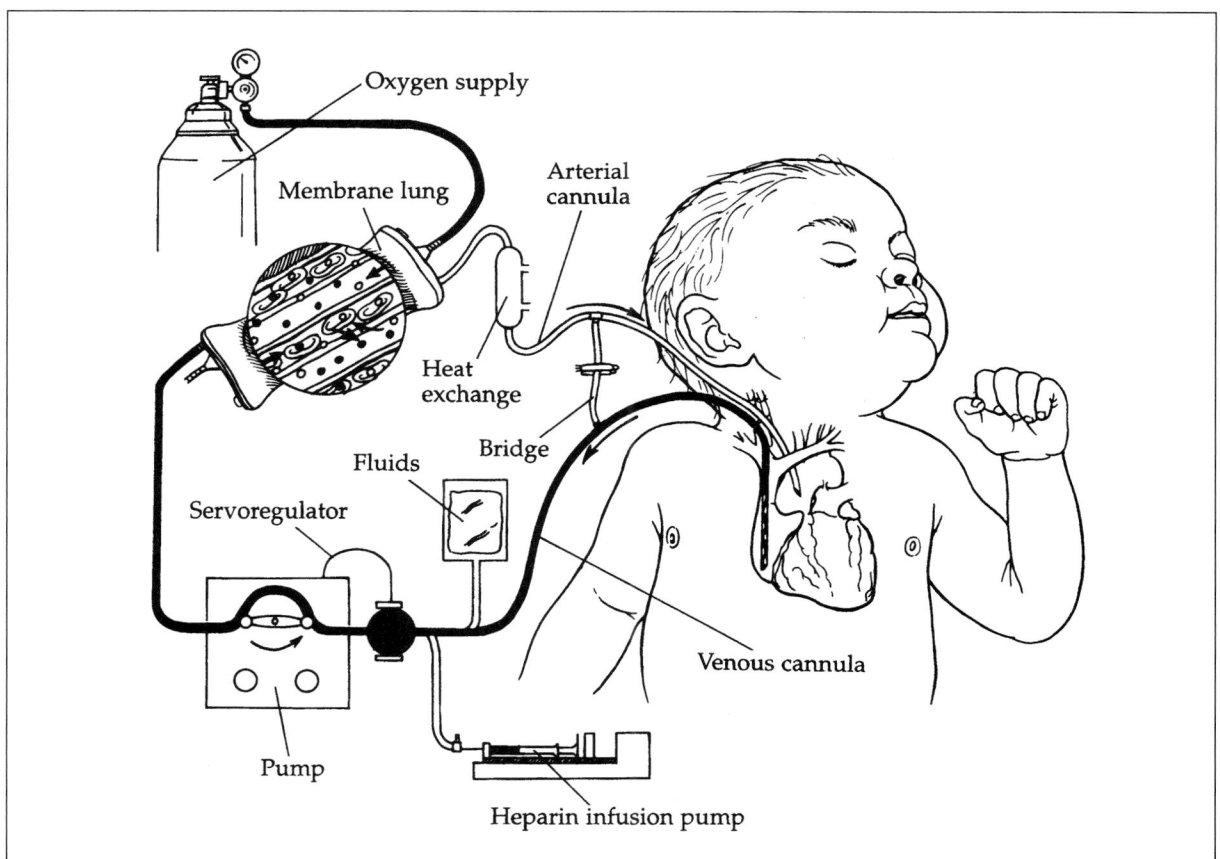

Figure 13.2-1. ECMO circuit. Venous blood is withdrawn by gravity through a servoregulator to prevent pump from actively siphoning venous return. A pump delivers blood back to the arterial cannula after it passes through the membrane oxygenator and heat exchanger. Venous return is from the right atrium, arterial infusion is into the aortic arch in double cannula (venoarterial) or right atrium (venovenous) techniques. (Reproduced with permission from Baker RJ, Fischer JE: *Mastery of Surgery,* Vol I, 4th edition. Lippincott Williams & Wilkins, 2001.)

SUMMARY OF PROCEDURE

Position	Supine
Incision	Subcostal, right neck incision
Special instrumentation	ECMO circuit (Fig 13.2-1)
Unique considerations	Anticoagulation
Antibiotics	Preop: ampicillin 25 mg/kg iv + gentamicin 2.5 mg/kg iv
	Intraop: cefazolin irrigation (1 g/500 ml NS)
Surgical time	1-2 h
Closing considerations	Assess for changes in ventilation (e.g., PIP, pre- and postductal ABG).
EBL	> 5-10 ml/kg
Postop care	Paralysis maintained; fentanyl infusion @ 2-4 μg/kg/h
Mortality	25-30%
Morbidity	Respiratory failure
	Sepsis
Pain score	6-7

PATIENT POPULATION CHARACTERISTICS

Age range	Newborn–weeks or months
Male:Female	1-2:1
Incidence	1/4000 live births
Etiology	Unknown
Associated conditions	For diaphragmatic hernia: malrotation (40-100%); congenital heart disease (15%); renal anomalies; esophageal atresia; CNS abnormalities

References

1. Falconer AR, Brown RA, Helms P, Gordon I, Baron JA: Pulmonary sequelae in survivors of congenital diaphragmatic hernia. *Thorax* 1990; 45(2):126-9.
2. Stolar CJH: Congenital diaphragmatic hernia. In *Surgery of Infants and Children.* Oldham KT, Colombani PM, Foglia RP, eds. Lippincott-Raven Publishers, Philadelphia: 1997, 883-96.
3. Wilson JM, Lund DP, Lillehei CW, Vacanti JP: Congenital diaphragmatic hernia: predictors of severity in the ECMO era. *J Pediatr Surg* 1991; 26(9):1028-33.

Surgeons

David A. Berman, MD (*Laser skin resurfacing*)
Vernon J. Adams, Jr, DMD (*Dental rehabilitation*)
Azeem K. Lakha, DMD (*Dental implants*)

14.0   OFFICE-BASED ANESTHESIA

Anesthesiologist

Terri D. Homer, MD

INTRODUCTION—ANESTHESIOLOGIST'S PERSPECTIVE

Terri D. Homer

DEFINITION OF OFFICE-BASED ANESTHESIA

The assumption in this chapter is that office-based anesthesia (OBA) is distinct from outpatient anesthesia in a freestanding surgery facility. OBA is used in many medical specialties, including most dental subspecialties, dermatology, plastic surgery, ophthalmology, otolaryngology, and gynecology. The procedures described in this chapter are but a small sampling of the ways in which anesthesia is used in medical/dental offices. Anesthesiologists who carry out anesthetic procedures in the office setting may be sole practitioners or part of a group of anesthesiologists who have a 'division' or rotation devoted to OBA. Although anesthesia practiced in an office carries the same risks, burdens of responsibility, and skill requirements as in a fully-equipped surgical center, in the office setting, oftentimes there will be no anesthesia machine, and the anesthesiologist may be expected to arrange for O_2, suction, monitoring, and emergency equipment. This unique challenge for the anesthesia provider includes: qualifying personnel and the facility, equipping the office, selecting appropriate patients, providing safe and effective anesthesia/analgesia, and properly preparing and recovering the patients.

STATE REGULATIONS REGARDING OFFICE-BASED ANESTHESIA

Many states have laws listing strict requirements for medical facilities where anesthesia is provided for surgical procedures. Some states have regulations based on the type of surgical procedure performed. Others regulate and credential the facility based on the type of anesthesia used (i.e., GA, iv, local). Still others base regulations on the type of facility itself. In California, for example, dental offices are regulated differently than medical offices. For many years, the California Dental Board has regulated anesthesia in the dental or oral surgery office by credentialing the anesthesia provider and/or the office facility itself. An oral surgeon, dentist, or physician issued a GA permit by the Dental Board goes through a credentialing process by two examiners that includes direct observation of an anesthesia case, demonstration of emergency drills, and examination of required monitoring and resuscitation equipment on site. The permit allows the holder to provide GA in any dental office. The Dental Board also issues 'Conscious Sedation' permits to those dental practitioners who qualify and want to use this technique.

EQUIPMENT NEEDED FOR OFFICE-BASED ANESTHESIA

As mentioned above, 'office-based anesthesia' assumes the absence of an anesthesia machine and other sophisticated equipment that is readily available in a surgical center. In some respects, however, this setting is analogous to other out-of-OR locations. The ASA Guidelines for Nonoperating Room Anesthetizing Locations[1] covers all types of out-of-OR facilities, and these recommendations should be followed. Appropriate monitoring—including pulse oximetry, ECG, and BP—is required. Many portable monitors have $ETCO_2$ monitoring capability, which may be useful for the spontaneously ventilating, sedated patient. A precordial stethoscope is quite useful for monitoring respirations, especially in the dental patient, in whom airway obstruction is a frequent occurrence during the procedure. Also in accordance with the ASA guidelines, full resuscitation equipment, an adequate source of O_2 (and backup O_2), a functioning suction, adequate lighting and electrical outlets (with backup battery source), and a telephone with immediate access to a hospital ER also must be available. In the credentialed medical facility, these items will already be present. In the dental facility, they may or may not be present. It is the responsibility of the anesthesia provider to make sure these items are available in the facility before administering an anesthetic.

ANESTHETIC GOALS IN THE OFFICE SETTING

Typically, the primary anesthetic goal in the office setting is to provide moderate-to-deep sedation; however, the definition of 'sedation' in this setting varies considerably. For example, in the pediatric patient having dental restoration work, 'conscious sedation' often is not adequate. In the patient having dental implants, minimal or moderate sedation may be all that is required as the oral surgeon may need the patient's cooperation at times during the procedure. A patient undergoing full-face laser resurfacing most likely will require deep sedation, since this procedure can be quite painful. Because sedation is a continuum and individual patient responses vary, the anesthesia provider must be prepared to resuscitate any patient receiving sedation in the office.[3]

PATIENT SELECTION

As in all medical facilities, the patient's safety is of paramount importance. In the office setting, the ability to achieve a successful outcome is dependent first of all on appropriate patient selection. The patients presenting for OBA will fall into several categories, depending on the procedure and the patient's age and medical condition. An 'appropriate patient' can be an ASA 1 or 2 patient. They may even be an ASA 3, if: (1) their medical problems are stable and well controlled with medication, and (2) the office procedure itself will not pose an undue risk to them.

PREOPERATIVE PREPARATION

An important role of the anesthesiologist is to educate the patient (or patient's parents, as appropriate) about the office anesthesia experience. A preop phone call discussing the patient's medical Hx, past anesthesia experience (in a hospital, surgicenter, or dental office), npo requirements, the anesthesia technique(s) to be used, postanesthesia expectations, and fees is essential. A written packet describing some of this information can be given to the patient in advance.

Safe and accepted npo requirements on the day of the procedure are as follows:

- A light breakfast, up to 6 h before the appointment.
- Clear liquids (including Gatorade, Jell-O, fruit popsicles) up to 3 h before the appointment.
- The patient's usual medications should be continued on the day of the procedure.

RECOVERY AND DISCHARGE

In a medical or dental office, often there is no separate recovery area designated as such. It is common practice for the patient to be recovered by the anesthesiologist in the treatment room until they can open their eyes and maintain a normal airway without assistance. At that point, any iv or monitors that may have been used can be removed. If it is a pediatric patient, the parents may be brought into the room, although recovery remains under the supervision of the anesthesiologist. Office anesthesia patients can be discharged when they are well oriented, their pain and nausea are controlled, and they have a responsible adult to accompany them. They may still feel drowsy, but this should not prevent them from being able to walk with assistance.

Discharge instructions regarding appropriate postop activities should be given to the responsible adult with the patient. Generally, patients are asked to adhere to the following instructions upon discharge:

- NPO except clear liquids in the first 2 h after arriving at home. (Unless the ride is > 1 h, we ask the patient not to drink anything in the car on the way home from the procedure facility.)
- A light meal after the first 2 h, if the patient wishes.
- Adults should take it easy the rest of the day and have a responsible adult companion for at least 4 h postprocedure.
- No driving for 24 h.
- Children should stay home for the rest of the day postprocedure, under the direct supervision of a responsible adult.

The anesthesiologist also should give the responsible party (parent, friend, other relative) his/her pager or cell phone number in the event they need to contact the anesthesiologist after patient discharge.

References

1. *ASA Guidelines for Nonoperating Room Anesthetizing Locations.* American Society of Anesthesiologists, 1994.
2. *ASA Guidelines for Office-Based Anesthesia.* American Society of Anesthesiologists, 1999.
3. *Continuum of Depth of Sedation, Definition of General Anesthesia and Levels of Sedation and Analgesia.* American Society of Anesthesiologists, 1994.

LASER SKIN RESURFACING

SURGICAL CONSIDERATIONS

David A. Berman

Description: Laser skin resurfacing treats a variety of skin conditions, including acne scars, traumatic scars, wrinkles, and pre-cancers (actinic keratoses). Usually, CO_2 or erbium:yag lasers are used. Because these lasers deliver a tremendous amount of heat to the skin surface, previous attempts at using nerve blocks and local infiltration with lidocaine were generally inadequate for complete analgesia; thus, either iv sedation or GA is used. Facial nerve blocks usually are performed to supplement iv sedation (added analgesia). After a Betadine prep, anesthetic eye drops are used, followed by the insertion of protective metal corneal shields. The laser resurfacing then begins, with 2-3 laser passes performed at various energy levels. Commonly, two resurfacing lasers may be used during one procedure. Afterwards, the newly exposed dermal layer is covered in a protective and soothing facial dressing, although many practitioners dress the treated area with an emollient cream or Vaseline only. (For discussion of specific safety issues on use of lasers, see Facial Laser Resurfacing, p. 881.)

Usual preop diagnosis: Acne scars; traumatic scars; wrinkles; solar keratoses (precancers).

SUMMARY OF PROCEDURE

Position	Supine, with shoulder roll. Surgeon at head of table.
Antibiotics	None during procedure. Antivirals and antibiotics started 1 d before procedure, and continued for 1-2 wk following.
Surgical time	45 min for full-face laser resurfacing; less for regional areas
Postop care	Supine position, maintenance of facial dressing, occasional ice packs, antiviral medications, antibiotics
Mortality	None reported.
Morbidity	Bacterial infection
	Herpes simplex virus reactivation
	Delayed re-epithelialization
	Hypertrophic or keloid scar formation
	Corneal abrasion
	Delayed healing with redness
	Hyperpigmentation and hypopigmentation
Pain Score	3-5

PATIENT POPULATION CHARACTERISTICS

Age Range	18-85 yr
Male:Female	1:4
Incidence	Number of cases performed by members of the American Academy of Cosmetic Surgery/yr in U.S.: men, 2,936; women, 12,457. (Stats for 2002, with only 5% of members responding.)
Etiology	Acne; sun damage; traumatic incident resulting in scars

ANESTHETIC CONSIDERATIONS

PREOPERATIVE

A full-face laser resurfacing procedure is quite painful and can be very stressful to the patient; thus, local anesthesia is often inadequate. For these procedures, it is important to make sure that the patient with chronic HTN and/or other cardiovascular or respiratory disease is being adequately treated for these problems before undergoing laser resurfacing. A preop ECG (taken within the last yr) is recommended for those patients > 60 yr old or those being treated for HTN.

Premedication	In the adult patient, an oral premed can be given, if necessary, before the patient arrives in the office for the procedure. Diazepam 10-20 mg, or lorazepam 0.5-1.0 mg po 1 h before the appointment will help relax the severely anxious patient.

INTRAOPERATIVE

Anesthetic technique: MAC and/or GA

MAC/GA	During full-face laser resurfacing, the patient will need to be under deep iv sedation, unless the surgeon is willing to use a large amount of local anesthetic. Usually, a combination of intermittent doses of midazolam (1-2 mg iv), meperidine (25 mg iv), ketamine (25-30 mg iv q 1 h prn), and propofol (25-50 μg/kg/min iv) will provide an adequate anesthetic state. If a nasal airway is inserted, nasal O_2 can be used—if the cannula is placed deep in the airway—at low flows. Otherwise, O_2 should be used only between facial passes of the laser. Again, the patient is not electively intubated, but an LMA may be needed if it is difficult to maintain a patent airway. Usually, patients having this procedure will require at least 75-150 mg meperidine (or its equivalent drug) to relieve the painful burning caused by $\geq$ 3 passes of the CO_2 or erbium laser. These patients will shiver and sustain HTN and tachycardia unless an adequate level of analgesia is achieved. Because of the narcotic requirement, they should have prophylactic antiemetics during the procedure. Dexamethasone (8 mg iv) and metoclopramide (15 mg iv) are a good combination. In addition, im promethazine (25 mg) is very effective.
Blood and fluid requirements	IV: 20 ga × 1 NS/LR @ 4-6 ml/kg/h
Monitoring	Standard monitors (see p. B-1).

Positioning	✓ and pad pressure points.
	✓ eyes (eye shields in place).
Complications	Laser fire

Use intermittent, low-flow O_2. Consider wrapping foil around cannula.

POSTOPERATIVE

Complications	PONV
Pain management	Oral analgesics (see p. C-2).
Recovery and discharge	The patient recovering from a full-face laser procedure usually has received a lot of potent anesthetic medication in a short period of time. They require at least 45-60 min to recover in the office. Vital signs should be stable (↓BP and tachycardia must be treated). Pain and nausea also should be under control. These patients must be accompanied by a responsible adult who can stay with them at home for a few h after the procedure. A follow-up phone call to the patient by the anesthesiologist that evening is very helpful and appreciated.

OFFICE DENTAL REHABILITATION UNDER DEEP IV SEDATION

SURGICAL CONSIDERATIONS

Vernon Adams

Description: Dental rehabilitation includes the restoration of good dental health by removal of caries and decayed teeth, replacement of crowns or bridges, root canals, and periodontal treatment. Prior to treatment, the patient is placed in a supine position with a shoulder roll and the head immobilized. A throat pack is placed and a mouth prop inserted. The throat pack should be placed more anteriorly than normal since, in general, the patient will not be intubated. Dental rehabilitation is usually done in phases, starting with the operative phase. A rubber dam is placed to surgically isolate the teeth that will be treated. All dental caries are removed, the restorations are placed, and all debris is irrigated and suctioned away from the rubber dam, which is then removed. This sequence is repeated in quadrants as needed. Once the operative phase of treatment is completed, the next phases—e.g., taking impressions for various appliances or dental prosthetics, dental extractions, or a dental prophylaxis—are undertaken, as necessary. Great care must be taken in maintaining the airway when taking impressions, as the bulk of impression material can compromise airway management.

Usual preop diagnosis: In-office dental rehabilitation usually focuses on treatment of the patient who is disabled from being treated in a conventional setting for primarily behavioral/emotional reasons. These include dentophobia; pediatric patients who are excessively apprehensive and/or combative or who have a significant amount of dental caries; 'special needs' pediatric patients—autistic, mentally retarded, developmentally delayed—and patients with mild-to-moderate forms of cerebral palsy.

SUMMARY OF PROCEDURE

Position	Supine, with shoulder roll, head extended; surgeon at head of table (turned 90°)
Incision	Gingival or intraoral mucosa
Special instrumentation	Dental setup
Unique considerations	Nasal airway recommended; throat pack placed; forward displacement of tongue is important for airway management.
Antibiotics	None used routinely.
Surgical time	60-120 min
EBL	Minimal
Postop care	Recover in lateral position.
Mortality	Rare
Morbidity	Biting of lips or tongue 2° local anesthesia: 1%
	Bleeding: 1%
	Infection: < 1%
	Delayed Bleeding: Rare
Pain Score	1-2; higher for certain procedures (e.g., extraction of impacted tooth)

PATIENT POPULATION CHARACTERISTICS

Age range	13 mo +
Male: Female	1:1
Incidence	20,000/yr in U.S.
Etiology	Poor oral hygiene and/or dietary habits; lack of continuing periodic dental care

ANESTHETIC CONSIDERATIONS

PREOPERATIVE

In the pediatric dental office, the patients presenting for iv sedation are those who cannot cooperate due to age (too young) or to a preexisting mental or physical disease. Examples include a 20-mo-old child with multiple 'bottle caries,' an 8-yr-old autistic child, or a 14-yr-old with cerebral palsy. Obviously, the anesthetic treatment plan must be tailored to the patient's individual needs. These patients must be screened in advance for clinical conditions that would put them at undue risk for problems 2° the anesthetic. Specifically, a patient with any cardiac, respiratory, endocrine, or neurologic problem must be evaluated. If the clinical problem is mild, stable, and under good control, the patient may be considered for anesthesia in the office. Examples of such conditions include mild nonsteroid-dependent asthma, corrected congenital heart disease, or a stable Sz disorder. The child with Down syndrome may pose a very difficult problem in this setting, since airway obstruction can occur easily under deep iv sedation. Also, these patients frequently have concurrent congenital heart disease. Any child with a Hx of obesity, snoring, and/or sleep apnea can present a problem under iv sedation, due to airway obstruction. The child with a current or recent URI always poses a dilemma. Although there is controversy on this issue, these children generally should have their procedures postponed, since their chances of sustaining periop respiratory problems are higher than normal.

Premedication   Because there is no possibility of an inhalation induction in the office setting, as described here, the pediatric patient should receive adequate sedation as an 'induction' that will allow placement of an iv with little or no emotional trauma. There are several options available for preprocedure sedation. In the older child (> 8 yr) who is psychologically mature, an iv can be placed without premedication. In a dental office that is equipped with N_2O, the patient can breathe a high-flow N_2O/O_2 mix through a nasal mask for 10 min before iv placement. If the patient accepts the mask, this technique can help lessen the patient's fear of the iv. The use of a 30 ga needle for infiltration of buffered local anesthetic and, sometimes, the use of EMLA cream (placed 30 min in advance) also can be very helpful.

Oral premedication is used commonly in children 4-8 yr old. Midazolam (0.5-0.7 mg/kg; maximum = 20 mg) mixed in liquid acetaminophen, given in the office 20 min before the procedure, can provide adequate sedation. In some, the addition of oral ketamine 2-3 mg/kg to the midazolam solution may result in a better sedating effect, especially in older pediatric patients.

For those children who cannot cooperate with an oral premed (too young or emotionally or physically unable to do so), an im premedication is very effective. This can be administered 5 min before the procedure, in the treatment room, with the parents present. Ketamine 3 mg/kg, midazolam 0.2 mg/kg, atropine 0.02 mg/kg (or glycopyrrolate 0.01 mg/kg) can be mixed in the same syringe and given in the anterior thigh with a 23 ga needle. This has the benefits of rapid uptake and reliable achievement of an adequate level of amnesia and sedation. Because of the rapid onset, the anesthesiologist must be prepared to begin monitoring the patient immediately after injection. Additionally, the parents usually require some reassurance as they watch their child become sedated so rapidly.

INTRAOPERATIVE

Anesthetic technique: MAC. These patients are not intubated electively. A flexible LMA can be used for airway management, if needed. Following sedation, the patient is placed in the dental chair, with the head positioned to maintain an open airway. A shoulder roll may be needed to help with head extension. Monitoring—including pulse oximeter, ECG, BP cuff, and precordial stethoscope—is attached. O_2 is supplied, and $ETCO_2$ can be measured through a nasal cannula. An iv is started if not previously placed. A nasal airway is positioned with care (to avoid epistaxis) after the dental x-rays are taken. To prevent aspiration, a throat pack with a piece of dental floss attached—which remains outside the mouth—is placed, and minimal irrigation with constant suctioning is used. A rubber dam acts as a barrier between the teeth and the back of the throat. The anesthesiologist must be constantly vigilant in maintaining an open airway in these patients in the face of an oral procedure. Placing a flexible LMA may make airway management easier without interfering with the dental procedure. A propofol infusion can be started at a rate of 100-150 μg/kg/min. Administration of a small amount of meperidine (e.g., 5-15 mg iv) may be useful in alleviating emergence delirium, especially if there is not adequate local anesthesia. Routine use of prophylactic antiemetics is recommended. In children, the use of metoclopramide (0.2 mg/kg) with dexamethasone (0.1 mg/kg) is very effective as a prophylactic antiemetic combination.

Emergence	No special considerations, except that throat packs must be removed.
Blood and fluid requirements	IV: 20-22 ga × 1 NS/LR @ 4-6 ml/kg/h
Monitoring	Standard monitors (see p. B-1)
Positioning	✓ and pad pressure points. ✓ eyes.

POSTOPERATIVE

Complications	PONV	These patients may swallow blood, with consequent PONV.
Pain management	Oral analgesics (see p. C-2).	
Recovery and discharge	In the dental office, there may not be a separate, designated recovery area. Usually, the pediatric patient is recovered by the anesthesiologist in the treatment room for at least 30 min, or until the patient is opening his/her eyes and maintaining a normal airway without assistance. At this point, the iv and monitors can be removed and the patient can continue recovering in the parents' arms, under the supervision of the anesthesiologist. The patient may need to stay another 30 min, or until he/she opens his eyes without prompting, recognizes his parents, and has no nausea. Postop instructions given to the parents include: no outside or unsupervised activities for the rest of the day, no drinking or eating in the car on the way home, clear liquids for the first 1-2 h, followed by light food. The anesthesiologist should give the parents his/her pager or cell phone number so they can call with any questions that arise after they are at home. Regardless, a follow-up phone call from the anesthesiologist is always a good policy.	

DENTAL IMPLANTS AND BONE GRAFTING

SURGICAL CONSIDERATIONS

Description: A dental implant consists of a tooth-root-shaped titanium post that is used to support a crown, bridge, or denture. Dental implants are inserted surgically into the mandibular or maxillary alveolar bone where teeth are missing. Single implants may be done with local anesthesia, but multiple or complex procedures are best accomplished with iv sedation. After the local anesthetic is administered, a mucoperiosteal flap is raised over the edentulous alveolus and the bone is exposed. Precise drill holes are made in the bone and the implants are screwed or tapped into place. Bone grafting may be necessary around the implants to fill in defects and is carried out using autologous, allogenic, xenogenic, or synthetic materials. In most cases, the gum tissue is closed over or around the implant. The bone is allowed to heal around the implant and 2-6 mo later the implant can be used to attach crowns, bridges, or dentures. In cases where there is insufficient bone, a bone graft is necessary **before** implants can be placed. Typically, bone grafts are allowed to heal for 6 mo before implant insertion. Most minor grafting procedures are accomplished in the dental office under iv sedation and local anesthesia. Major grafts requiring extraoral donor sites may have to be done under GA via nasal ETT intubation.

Usual preop diagnosis: Acquired or congenital absence of dentition

SUMMARY OF PROCEDURE

Position	Supine, with head tilted back, using an articulating headrest in the dental chair
Incision	Intraoral mucoperiosteal flaps
Special instrumentation	Precordial stethoscope

Unique considerations	Throat packs are used to prevent aspiration of teeth, crowns, blood, and irrigation fluids. Ensure that they are removed at the end of the case.
Antibiotics	Prophylactic antibiotics, given orally before surgery
Surgical time	1-3 h
EBL	25-100 ml
Mortality	Rare
Morbidity	Infection: 1%
	Bleeding: Rare
	Delayed Bleeding: Rare
	Aspiration: Rare
Pain Score	1-4, depending on procedure

PATIENT POPULATION CHARACTERISTICS

Age range	17+ yr
Male: Female	1:1
Incidence	Becoming more common as technology improves
Etiology	Tooth loss

ANESTHETIC CONSIDERATIONS

PREOPERATIVE

Many patients having dental implant procedures are elderly and/or have multiple medical problems. The anesthesiologist should be consulted in advance about these patients so that questions about their medical conditions can be answered and a current list of medications can be obtained. Sometimes the patient's primary care physician needs to be contacted to discuss details of medical Hx. If chronic medical conditions are stable, patients often can receive 'conscious sedation' and monitoring by the anesthesiologist for this procedure in the office.

Premedication   Usually not necessary

INTRAOPERATIVE

Anesthetic technique: MAC. These patients are not intubated electively. In the adult patient having dental implants, the maintenance of a lightly sedated state is achieved using a combination of iv midazolam, fentanyl (or meperidine), and small amounts of ketamine (20-30 mg/dose). A pulse oximeter, ECG, BP cuff, precordial stethoscope or $ETCO_2$ monitor, and nasal O_2 should be in place. Glycopyrrolate (0.1-0.2 mg) should be given to decrease secretions. Dexamethasone 8 mg and metoclopramide 15 mg are useful as an antiemetic combination. Usually, the oral surgeon needs the patient's cooperation at some point during the procedure; therefore, propofol is not an ideal drug to use. It can be given, however, in small doses to the patient who requires more than the other drugs for sedation. Occasionally, the adult patient in this setting will require a nasal airway.

Emergence	No special considerations, except that throat packs must be removed at end of procedure.
Blood and fluid requirements	IV: 20-22 ga × 1
	NS/LR @ 4-6 ml/kg/h
Monitoring	Standard monitors (see p. B-1)
Positioning	✓ and pad pressure points.
	✓ eyes.

POSTOPERATIVE

Complications	PONV	These patients may swallow blood, with consequent PONV.
Pain management	Oral analgesics (see p. C-2).	
Recovery and discharge	See Recovery and Discharge for Office Dental Rehabilitation	

Anesthesiologists

Frederick G. Mihm, MD
Myer H. Rosenthal, MD, FACCP

15.0 EMERGENCY PROCEDURES FOR THE ANESTHESIOLOGIST

INTRODUCTION

Even when working with a surgeon, the anesthesiologist is sometimes faced with the need to perform certain minor, but very important invasive procedures. In these cases, the procedures may be for life-threatening events. Some of the most important of these procedures are presented in this chapter.

EMERGENCY CRICOTHYROTOMY

Clinical situation: Typically, this is a hypoxic patient with obstructed airway (not involving direct tracheal trauma), who cannot be mask ventilated or intubated.

Emergency 'Stab' Cricothyrotomy[5]

Equipment
- Scalpel with #11 blade
- Tracheal hook
- Tracheostomy tubes: #6, #7
- ETTs: #6, #7
- Umbilical or twill tape for securing tube
- 10 ml syringe for inflating cuff
- Prep solution
- 2% lidocaine
- Suction device (Yankauer or Tonsil Tip)
- Lubricant (lidocaine jelly or KY jelly)

Procedure
1. Prep skin.
2. Palpate cricothyroid membrane.
3. Make transverse incision through skin and cricothyroid membrane with single stab[5] (Fig 15-1).
4. Reverse scalpel, place handle into wound, and turn 90° to expand incision.
5. Pass tracheostomy tube (or standard ETT) into trachea.
6. Inflate cuff on tracheostomy/ETT.
7. Ventilate patient.
8. Secure tube.

Emergency 'Guidewire' Cricothyrotomy

Equipment
- Melker Emergency Cricothyrotomy Set (Cook Critical Care), or equivalent
- Scalpel with #15 blade
- 6 ml syringe half-filled with NS
- 18 ga introducer needle
- 18 ga iv catheter/needle
- Amplatz extra-stiff guidewire 0.038″
- Curved dilator
- Airway catheter
- Umbilical or twill tape

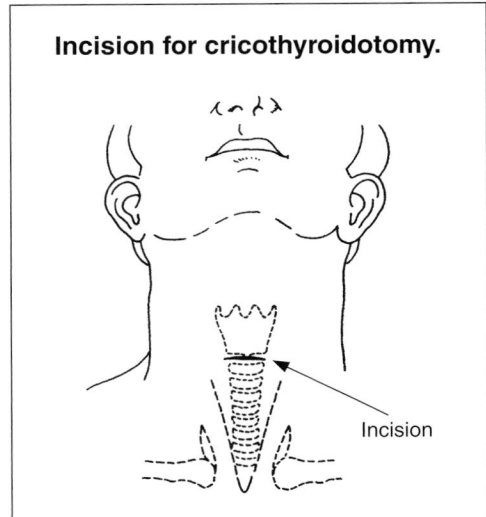

Incision for cricothyroidotomy.

Incision

Figure 15-1.

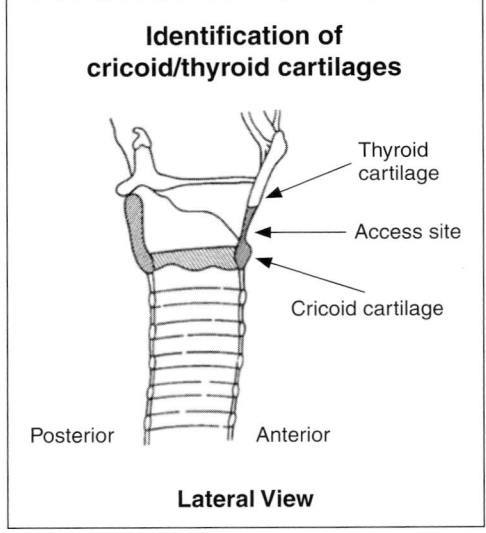

Identification of cricoid/thyroid cartilages

Thyroid cartilage

Access site

Cricoid cartilage

Posterior   Anterior

Lateral View

Figure 15-2.

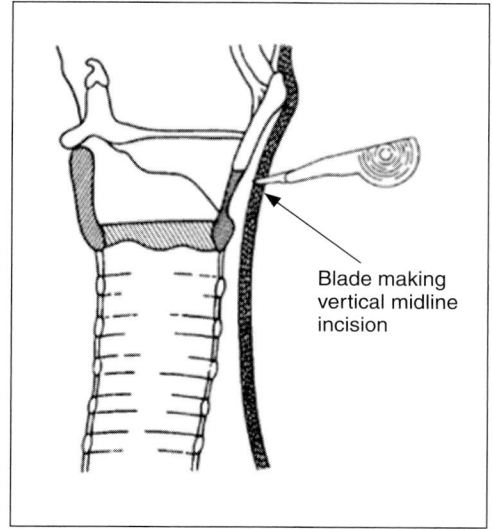

Figure 15-3.

Blade making vertical midline incision

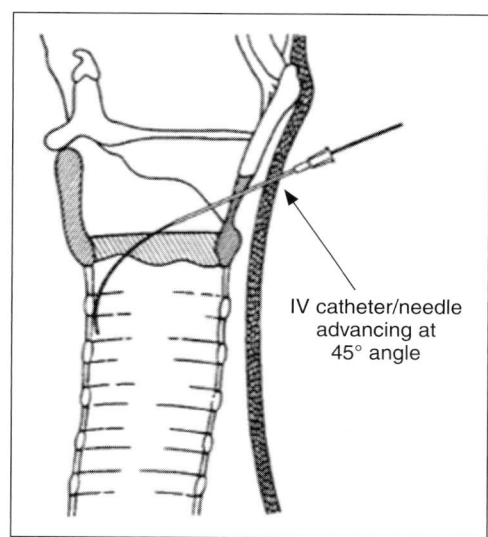

Figure 15-4.

IV catheter/needle advancing at 45° angle

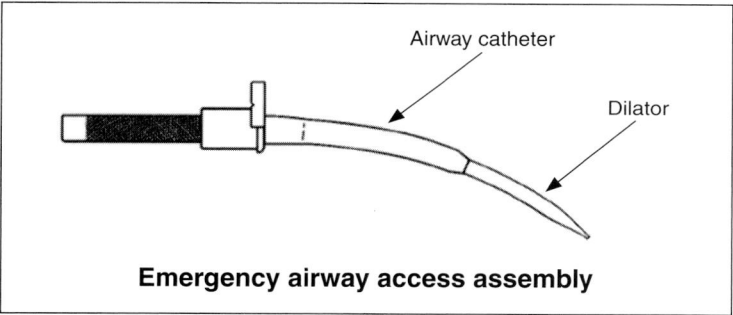

Airway catheter

Dilator

Emergency airway access assembly

Figure 15-5.

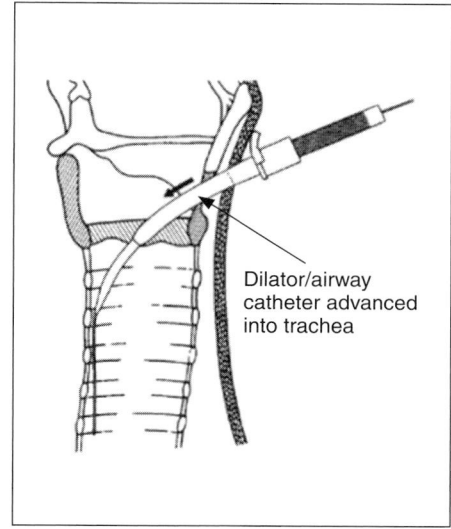

Dilator/airway catheter advanced into trachea

Figure 15-6.

Emergency 'Guidewire' Cricothyrotomy, cont.

Procedure

1. Identify cricothyroid membrane between cricoid and thyroid cartilages (Fig 15-2).
2. Stabilize cricothyroid membrane and make a vertical midline incision with #15 blade (Fig 15-3).
3. Attach syringe to iv catheter and needle, and advance at a 45° caudad angle through incision until air bubbles can be aspirated (tracheal lumen). (See Fig 15-4).
4. Remove syringe and needle, leaving catheter in place.
5. Advance soft end of guidewire into catheter several cm past end of catheter.
6. Remove catheter.
7. Assemble emergency airway device (Fig 15-5) by inserting the dilator through the airway catheter until the handle stops against the connector of the airway catheter.
8. Advance the dilator/airway catheter assembly over the guidewire into the trachea, keeping proximal end of guidewire visible at all times (Fig 15-6).
9. Remove guidewire and dilator, leaving airway catheter in place.
10. Ventilate patient.
11. Secure airway with umbilical or twill tape around the neck.

PERICARDIOCENTESIS

Clinical situation: The patient typically has severe ↓BP unexplained by any other causes (e.g., anesthetic drugs, autoPEEP, tension pneumothorax) and consistent with acute cardiac tamponade (↓BP, ↑HR, ↓pulse pressure, ↑CVP) ± equalization of pressures (RAP ~RVEDP ~PAD ~PAOP) ± confirmation by TEE.

Equipment
- 10 ml syringe
- 18 ga spinal needle

Procedure[2]
1. Identify xiphoid process and point 1″ below and 1″ left of midline (Fig 15-7).
2. Prep skin below xiphoid.
3. Attach needle to syringe and direct needle under rib toward left shoulder (Fig 15-8).
4. If pericardial fluid is withdrawn, BP will ↑ immediately.

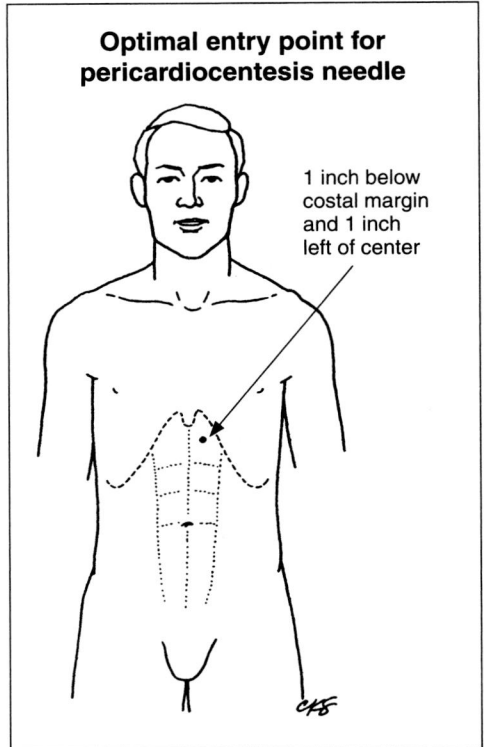

Optimal entry point for pericardiocentesis needle

1 inch below costal margin and 1 inch left of center

Figure 15-7.

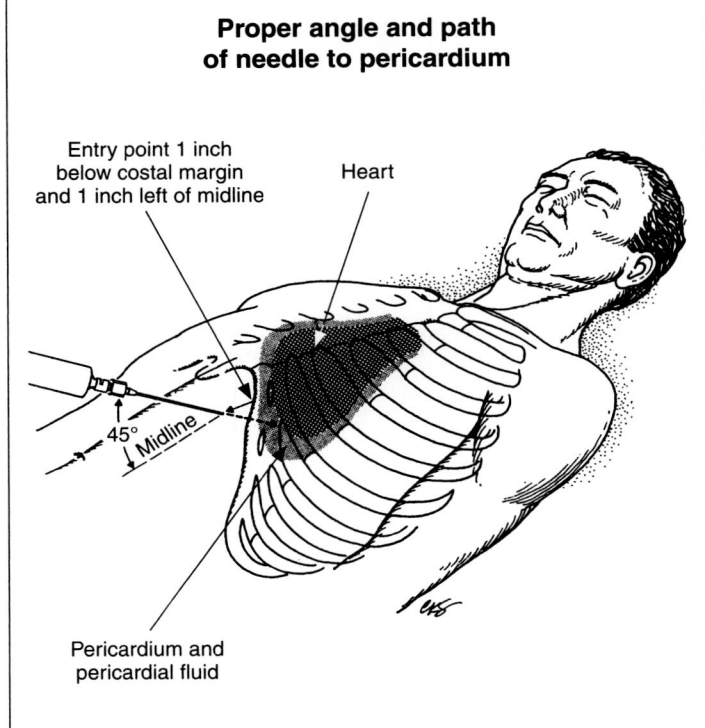

Proper angle and path of needle to pericardium

Entry point 1 inch below costal margin and 1 inch left of midline

Heart

45° Midline

Pericardium and pericardial fluid

Figure 15-8.

ARTERIAL CUTDOWN

Clinical situation: A patient requires arterial catheterization for BP/blood gas monitoring, following failed percutaneous attempts, or with coagulopathy.

Equipment
- Prep solution
- Wrist board
- 2% lidocaine
- Curved hemostat
- Curved pickups
- Scalpel with #10 and #11 blades
- Gauze
- 2-0 suture
- Needle driver

Radial artery cutdown procedure[3,4]
1. Position wrist in extension on arm board.
2. Prep and drape wrist.
3. Infiltrate skin and deep tissues down to the bone on either side of the vessel with lidocaine (1-2%, 2-3 ml).
4. Make 1 cm transverse incision ~2 cm proximal to wrist crease and just lateral to flexor carpi radialis tendon (Fig 15-9).
5. Using blunt dissection with the hemostat (in the direction of the vessel), identify the artery.
6. Blunt dissect just under artery and pass sutures around the vessel (do not ligate vessel) both distally and proximally (Fig 15-10).
7. Use traction on the distal suture to stabilize artery for cannulation.[1]
8. After cannulation, remove sutures and close incision. (For cleaner wound closure, pass catheter through skin rather than directly into wound.)
9. Suture catheter to skin.

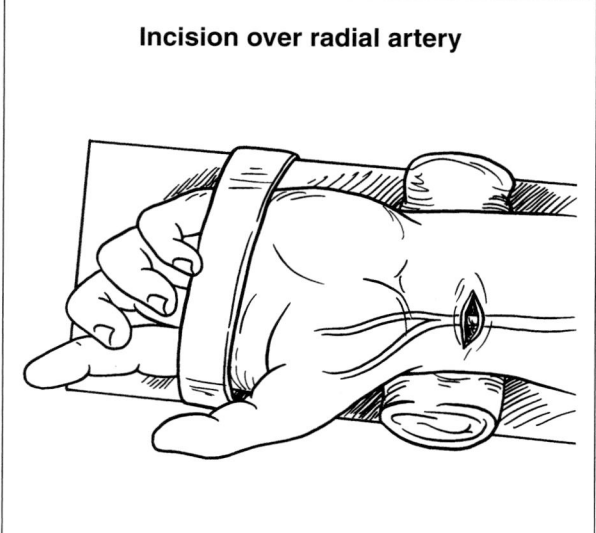

Incision over radial artery

Figure 15-9.

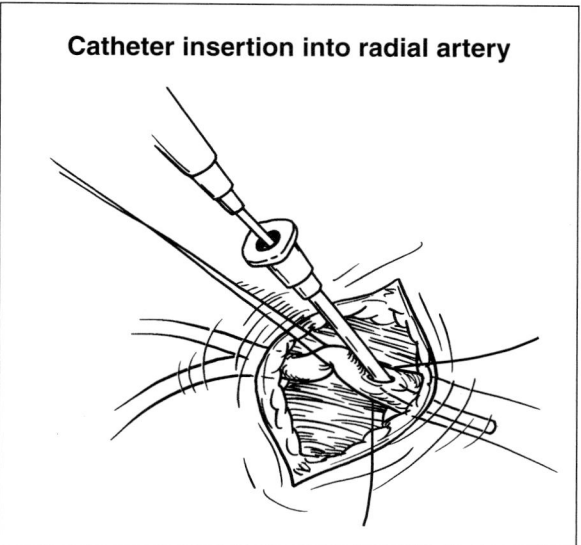

Catheter insertion into radial artery

Figure 15-10.

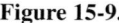

EMERGENT NEEDLE/CATHETER THORACOSTOMY

Clinical situation: A patient is experiencing severe hypotension and hypoxemia unexplained by any other cause (e.g., autoPEEP, cardiac tamponade) and consistent with acute tension pneumothorax ($\uparrow P_{aw}$, $\downarrow$movement of involved chest, $\downarrow$breath sounds/$\uparrow$resonance to percussion, compared to uninvolved side), and cardiovascular Sx related to $\uparrow$thoracic pressures → $\downarrow$preload ($\downarrow$BP, $\uparrow$HR, $\downarrow$pulse pressure, $\uparrow$CVP artifactually).

★ **NB**: Release of the pressure that has built up in the chest is a life-saving maneuver. A large-bore chest tube does not need to be placed emergently. The much simpler needle/catheter thoracostomy is effective and less demanding for the nonsurgeon.

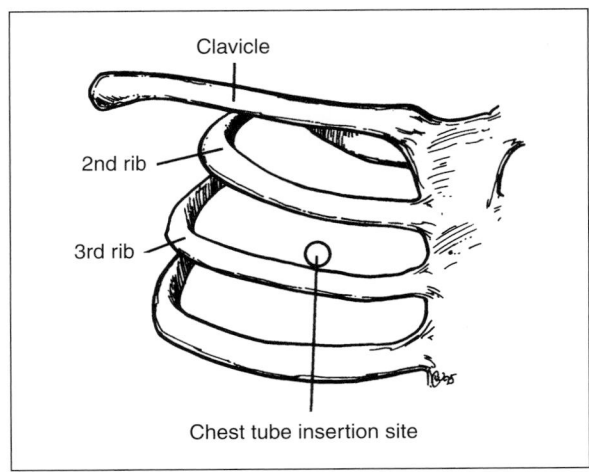

Figure 15-11.

Equipment	One of the following:
	• 16 ga needle
	• 16 ga iv catheter/needle
	• 16 ga single-lumen CVP kit

Procedure

1. Identify the 2nd intercostal space by first identifying the Angle of Louis (union of manubrium and sternum); then move laterally to find the insertion of the 2nd rib. The interspace directly below this rib is the 2nd intercostal space. (See Fig 15-11.)
2. Wipe skin with alcohol.
3. Use needle to enter the interspace anteriorly in line with a line drawn down from the clavicle at the junction of the middle and medial 1/3 sections. (This should be ~3cm from the sternal margin.)
4. With entry into the pleural space, there should be an audible rush of air and immediate hemodynamic improvement in the patient.

(Note: A more permanent chest tube will still need to be placed (i.e., the patient no longer has a tension pneumothorax, but still has a pneumothorax.) This can be done in a more controlled situation by someone skilled in that procedure.)

References:

1. Barftlett R, Munster A: An improved technique for prolonged arterial cannulation. *N Engl J Med* 1968; 279:92-3.
2. Danforth J: Pericardiocentesis. In *Clinical Procedures in Anesthesia and Intensive Care*. Benumof JL, ed. JB Lippincott, Philadelphia: 1992, 561-75.
3. Grassmick B: Venous and arterial access. In *Manual of Critical Care Procedures*. Victor L, ed. Aspen Publishers, Rockville MD: 1989, 47.
4. Mackersie R: Venous and arterial cutdown. In *Clinical Procedures in Anesthesia and Intensive Care*. Benumof JL, ed. JB Lippincott, Philadelphia: 1992, 391-403.
5. Shackford S: Tracheostomy and cricothyrotomy. In *Clinical Procedures in Anesthesia and Intensive Care*. Benumof JL, ed. JB Lippincott, Philadelphia: 1992, 215-26.

Figure Sources:

Figure 15-1 reproduced with permission from Shackford S: Tracheostomy and cricothyrotomy. In *Clinical Procedures in Anesthesia and Intensive Care*. Benumof JL, ed. JB Lippincott, 1992.

15-2, 15-3, 15-4, 15-5, 15-6 from the author.

Figures 15-7, 15-8 reproduced with permission from Danforth J: Pericardiocentesis. In *Clinical Procedures in Anesthesia and Intensive Care*. Benumof JL, ed. JB Lippincott, 1992.

Figures 15-9, 15-10 reproduced with permission from Hirschl RB, Heiss K: Cardiopulmonary critical care and shock. In *Surgery of Infants and Children*. Oldham KT, Colombani PM, Foglia RP, eds. Lippincott-Raven, 1997.

Figure 15-11 adapted with permission from Baker RJ, Fischer JE: Mastery of Surgery, 4th edition. Lippincott Williams & Wilkins, 2001.

Authors

Sandra Leigh Bardas, RPh, BS (*Drug interactions*)
Stephen P. Fischer, MD (*Lab and diagnostic studies*)
Raymond R. Gaeta, MD (*Standard perioperative pain management*)
Brenda Golianu, MD (*Pediatric pain management*)
Julie Good, MD (*Pediatric pain management*)
Alvin Hackel, MD (*Latex allergy considerations*)

APPENDICES

Gregory B. Hammer, MD (*Pediatric anesthetic protocols, pain management*)
Richard A. Jaffe, MD, PhD (*Adult anesthetic protocols*)
Cathy R. Lammers, MD, FAAP (*Latex allergy considerations*)
C. Philip Larson, Jr., MD, CM (*Adult anesthetic protocols*)
Sean Mackey, MD, PhD (*Adult perioperative pain management*)
Stanley I. Samuels, MB, BCh, FFARCS (*Adult anesthetic protocols*)
Clifford A. Schmiesing, MD (*Prophylactic perioperative beta blockade*)

APPENDIX A: PREOPERATIVE CONSIDERATIONS

PREOPERATIVE LABORATORY TESTING AND DIAGNOSTIC STUDIES

Stephen P. Fischer

The value and utility of preop diagnostic studies have become central issues in evaluating cost-effective health care in the surgical patient. It is estimated that up to $3 billion is spent in the U.S. annually on preop laboratory and diagnostic studies. Unnecessary testing is inefficient and expensive, and it requires additional technical resources. Inappropriate studies may lead to evaluation of 'borderline' or false-positive laboratory abnormalities. This may result in unnecessary OR delays, cancellations, and potential patient risk through additional testing and follow-up.

Surgical patients require preop lab and diagnostic studies that are consistent with their medical histories, the proposed operative procedures, and the potential for blood loss. Preop lab and diagnostic testing should be ordered for specific clinical indications rather than simply because the patient is about to undergo a certain surgical procedure.

The following preop diagnostic guidelines provide basic recommendations. They are **not** intended as absolute or standard requirements. Practice guidelines should be modified based on clinical needs and individual practice, to ensure the highest quality of anesthesia and surgical patient care.

SUMMARY OF PREOP STUDIES

Chest x-ray (CXR) — **Overview:** A preop CXR should be used to assess the presence of acute, progressive, or chronic changes in cardiac/pulmonary disease. The decision to obtain a preop CXR should be individualized and based on clinical indications (see Table A-1). CXRs should not be part of a routine preop screening protocol.

Clinical indications: Pneumonia; pulmonary edema; atelectasis; aortic aneurysm; mediastinal or pulmonary masses; tracheal deviation; pulmonary HTN; cardiomegaly; advanced COPD and blebs; dextrocardia; pulmonary embolism

Electrocardiogram (ECG) — **Overview:** ECGs evaluate cardiac rhythm/conduction disturbances, ischemia, myocardial infarction, hypertrophy, and metabolic and electrolyte disorders.

Clinical indications: Patients with suspected or known Hx of CAD; patient age > 50; HTN; chest pain; CHF; diabetes; cerebral vascular disease and PVD; syncope or presyncope; dizziness; SOB; DOE; PND; palpitations; leg/ankle edema; abnormal valvular murmurs

Liver function test (LFT) — **Overview:** LFTs establish the absence or presence of hepatic injury and the degree of hepatic reserve in disease states. LFTs consist of: AST(SGOT), ALT(SGPT), GGTP, alkaline phosphatase, serum albumin, bilirubin.

Clinical indications: Patients with suspected or known Hx of hepatitis (viral, alcohol, drugs); infiltration (tumor, immunologic); cirrhosis; portal HTN; gallbladder or biliary tract disease; jaundice; intravascular hemolysis

Renal function testing — **Overview:** Renal function testing measures glomerular filtration and the magnitude of renal tubular dysfunction. These tests include: serum creatinine and BUN.

Clinical indications: Renal function testing is indicated for patients with HTN; increased fluid overload (CHF/peripheral edema/ascites) associated with cardiac, hepatic, or renal impairment; dehydration; diabetes; nausea, emesis, or anorexia; polyuria; nocturia; oliguria; anuria; high-risk surgery in patients with low CO syndrome; hematuria; costovertebral angle pain; renal transplant Hx; renal disease; dialysis.

Hemoglobin (Hb), Hematocrit (Hct), CBC — **Overview:** The decision to obtain a preop Hb, Hct, or CBC should be individualized and based on clinical indications, medical Hx, and the proposed surgical procedure. Hb/Hct or CBC should not be part of a routine preop screening protocol.

Clinical indications: Hematological disorder; bleeding/coagulopathy Hx; malignancy; chemotherapy; radiation therapy (CBC); renal disease; anticoagulant and steroid therapy; surgical procedures with high blood loss (> 1500 ml); highly invasive or trauma surgery; malabsorption/poor nutrition status; CNS disease.

Pregnancy testing	**Overview:** The decision to obtain a preop pregnancy test should be based on clinical Hx and examination. Several assays are available (serum hCG, urine hCG); β-hCG detectable in maternal urine and blood 8-9 d post conception.
	Clinical indications: Sexually active; time of last menstrual period; presence or absence of birth control method; patient intuition
Coagulation testing	**Overview:** Coagulation testing, or clotting function studies, should be obtained in patients with known or suspected coagulopathies as indicated from H&P and drug therapies. Tests include: prothrombin time (PT), partial prothrombin time (PTT), INR, platelet (Plt) count.
	Clinical indications: Bleeding disorder Hx; anticoagulants or other drugs affecting coagulation; critical-risk surgeries with significant blood loss expected; hepatic disease; malabsorption/poor nutrition
Urine analysis	**Overview:** Assessment of renal function, infection, intravascular volume status, metabolic disorders
	Clinical indications: There are no routine anesthesia preop requirements for a urine analysis.

References

1. Fischer SP: Medical assessment of the surgical patient. In *Fundamentals of Surgery*. Appleton and Lange, Stamford, CT: 1997, 19-30.
2. Fischer SP: Preoperative evaluation of the neurosurgical patient. In *International Anesthesia Clinics*. Little, Brown, Boston: 1996.
3. Friedman LS, Maddrey WC: Surgery in the patient with liver disease. *Med Clin North Am* 1987; 71(3):453-76.
4. MacPherson D: Preoperative laboratory testing: should any tests be "routine" before surgery? *Med Clin North Am* 1993; 77(2):289-308.
5. Mangano DT, Goldman L: Preoperative assessment of patients with known or suspected coronary artery disease. *N Engl J Med* 1995; 333(26):1750-6.
6. Pasternak LR: Preanesthesia evaluation of the surgical patient. *ASA Refresher Courses in Anesthesiology* 1996; 24:205-19.
7. Roizen MF, Cohn S: Preoperative evaluation for elective surgery—what laboratory tests are needed? In *Advances in Anesthesia*, Vol 10. Stoelting RK, ed. Mosby-Year Book, St. Louis: 1993, 25-47.
8. Schiff RL, Emanuele MA: The surgical patient with diabetes mellitus: guidelines for management. *J Gen Intern Med* 1995; 10(3):154-61.

Table A-1. Diagnosis-Based Preop Testing											
Preop Diagnosis	**ECG**	**CXR**	**Hct/Hb**	**CBC**	**Lytes**	**Renal**	**Glucose**	**Coag**	**LFTs**	**Drug levels**	**Ca⁺**
Cardiac disease:											
Chronic atrial fib	X									X^2	
CHF	X	±				±					
HTN	X	±			X^1	X					
MI history	X				±						
PVD	X										
Stable angina	X				±						
Valvular heart disease	X	±									
CNS disorders:											
Seizures	X			X	X		X			X	
Stroke	X			X	X		X			X	
Tumor	X			X							
Vascular/aneurysms	X	X									
Coagulopathies				X				X			
Endocrine disease:											
Addison's disease				X	X		X				
Cushing's disease				X	X		X				
Diabetes	X				±	X	X				
Hyperparathyroidism	X		X		X						X
Hyperthyroidism	X		X		X						X
Hypoparathyroidism	X				X						X
Hypothyroidism	X		X		X						
Hematological disorders				X							
Hepatic disease:											
Alcohol/drug-induced								X	X		
Infectious hepatitis								X	X		
Tumor infiltration								X	X		
Malabsorption/poor nutrition	X			X	X	X	X	±			
Malignancy				X							
Morbid obesity	X	±					X				
Pulmonary disease:											
Asthma	(PFT only if symptomatic; otherwise no tests required)										
Chronic bronchitis	X	±		X							
Emphysema	X	±								X^3	
Renal disease			X		X	X					
Select drug therapies:											
Anticoagulants			X					X			
Aspirin/NSAID	(No tests)										
Chemotherapy				X							
Digoxin (digitalis)	X				±					X	
Dilantin										X	
Diuretics					X	X					
Phenobarbital										X	
Steroids				X			X				
Theophylline										X	

X = OBTAIN   ± = CONSIDER
[1] Patients on diuretics   [2] Patients on digoxin   [3] Patients on theophylline

PROPHYLACTIC PERIOPERATIVE BETA BLOCKADE

Clifford A. Schmiesing

Several recently published studies suggest an improvement in outcomes following prophylactic periop beta-blocker (PPBB) therapy in patients at risk for CAD while undergoing major noncardiac surgery.[6,8,10,11,12] In a randomized, multicenter study, Poldermans, et al, found that periop administration of the β-1 selective β-blocker bisoprolol reduced the incidence of both death from cardiac causes and nonfatal MI in high-risk patients undergoing major vascular surgery. The combined incidence of these cardiac events was 34% in the standard-care group, vs only 3.4% in the bisoprolol group.[8] Wallace, et al, demonstrated that prophylactic periop administration of atenolol in patients at high risk for CAD undergoing major elective noncardiac surgery significantly reduced the incidence of postop myocardial ischemia.[12] Follow-up analysis of both Polderman's and Wallace's study groups suggested a reduced risk of death in patients treated periop with β-blocker therapy for as long as 2 yr after surgery).[6,7] The American Heart Association (AHA), American College of Cardiology (ACC), and the American College of Physicians (ACP) have endorsed the use of PPBB therapy in select patient groups.[2,3] In a recent report, the Agency for Healthcare Research and Quality (AHRQ) included PPBB in its list of 11 patient safety practices (out of > 79 reviewed), wherein research evidence supported reduced patient risk from hospitalization, critical care, and surgery, and merit wider implementation.[4]

Despite reports of significantly improved outcomes in patients treated with PPBBs, several important points are worth noting. These recommendations are all based on relatively small numbers of studies and of patients. The benefit of PPBB therapy appeared greatest in those at greatest risk—patients with positive dobutamine stress tests undergoing major vascular surgery, who represent only a small fraction of patients undergoing surgical procedures. Subsequent reanalysis of the Polderman's high-risk cohort of 1,351 patients scheduled for major vascular surgery showed that, in those few patients with markedly positive dobutamine stress tests, PPBB therapy did not result in improved outcomes and was associated with a very high rate of periop morbidity that was similar to patients in the standard care group.[2] This appears to underscore the continued importance of careful preop assessment, cardiac risk stratification, selective preop cardiac stress testing, and, in some (rare) instances, revascularization before major elective noncardiac surgery. At the other end of the spectrum, the benefit of PPBB in patients at low risk for CAD and/or those undergoing low-risk surgery has not been extensively studied, but appears to be small.[2,3] The major studies of PPBB have initiated therapy at least 1 wk before surgery and continued it for at least 1 wk following surgery. It is unclear if β-blocker therapy given for shorter durations will have the same effect. The comparative effectiveness of the β-1 selective blocking agents vs the nonselective agents in reducing periop death and cardiac ischemia has not been studied specifically.

PPBB is generally well tolerated even in the elderly and in patients with compensated underlying COPD and CHF, although certain contraindications must be considered before initiating therapy.[5,8,12] Several institutions have developed preprinted order forms to help clinicians implement PPBB in appropriate patients.[9] The PPBB order forms in use at Stanford Hospital (see pp. A-5, 6) provide general inclusion and exclusion criteria to help identify patients most likely to benefit from PPBB, based on the criteria of Wallace and Mangano.[12] Preprinted order forms can increase the use of PPBB by clinicians.[9]

PPBB, while very promising, should not replace the careful, thorough preop assessment and selective use of functional cardiac testing for identification of very high-risk cardiac patients. In this population, PPBB may not provide adequate protection from complications of periop myocardial ischemia.

References

1. American College of Physicians: Guidelines for Assessing and Managing Periopertive Risk from Coronary Artery Disease Associated with Noncardiac Surgery. *Ann Int Med* 1997; 127(4):309-12.
2. Boersma E, Poldermans D, Bax J, et al: Predictors of cardiac events after major vascular surgery: role of clinical characteristics, dobutamine echocardiography, and β-blocker therapy. *JAMA* 2001; 285(14):1865-73.
3. Eagle KA, Berger PB, Calkins H, et al: ACC/AHA guideline update for perioperative cardiovascular evaluation for noncardiac surgery: a report of the American College of Cardiology/American Heart Association Task Force on Practice Guidelines [American College of Cardiology web site: http://www.acc.org/clinical/guidelines/perio/update/pdf/perioupdate.pdf. (Accessibility verified January 28, 2003.)
4. Evidence Report/Technology Assessment No. 43: Making health care safer; a critical analysis of patient safety practices. Agency for Health Care Research and Quality. U.S. Dept of Health and Human Services. 2101 East Jefferson St. Rockville MD 20852. Web site: www.ahrq.gov.
5. Gottlieb SS, McCarter RJ, Vogel RA: Effect of beta-blockade on mortality among high-risk and low-risk patients after myocardial infarction. *N Engl J Med* 1998; 339(8):489-97
6. Mangano DT, Layug E, Wallace A, et al: Effect of atenolol on mortality and cardiovascular morbidity after noncardiac surgery. *N Engl J Med* 1996; 335(23):1713-20.
7. Poldermans D, Boersma E, Bax J, et al: Bisoprolol reduces cardiac death and myocardial infarction in high-risk patients as long as 2 years after successful major vascular surgery. *Eur Heart J* 2001; 22(15):1353-8.

8. Poldermans D, Boersma E, Bax J, et al: The effect of bisoprolol on perioperative mortality and myocardial infarction in high-risk patients undergoing vascular surgery. *N Engl J Med* 1999; 341(24):1789-94.
9. Pollard JB, Chow RC, Hansen JR: Effectiveness of preprinted order forms in promoting perioperative β-blocker use. *Am J Health Sys Pharm* 2002; 59(4):359-60.
10. Raby KE, Brull SJ, Timimi F, et al: The effect of heart rate control on myocardial ischemia among high-risk patients after vascular surgery. *Anesth Analg* 1999; 88(3):477-82.
11. Urban MK, Markowitz SM, Gordon MA, et al: Postoperative prophylactic administration of β-adrenergic blockers in patients at risk for myocardial ischemia. *Anesth Analg* 2000; 90(6):1257-61.
12. Wallace A, Layug B, Tateo I, et al: Prophylactic atenolol reduces postoperative myocardial ischemia. *Anesthesiology* 1998; 88(1):7-17.

SAMPLE ORDER FORM

Orders • Prophylactic Perioperative Beta Blockade (PPBB) Protocol

PHYSICIAN: Please initial or complete all applicable orders. Please date, time, and sign the Order Form at the bottom.

_____ 1. **Baseline ECG** before initiating therapy, unless recent (< 1 mo) ECG already in chart.

_____ 2. **In Post Anesthesia Care Unit (PACU):**

   a. Metoprolol _____ [2.5-5 mg] iv q _____ [10] min prn HR > _____ [70-80] bpm, up to total dose of _____ mg.

   b. Call physician on pager #: _____ if HR remains > _____ after total dose.

_____ 3. **On Postop Unit:**

   a. If npo, metoprolol _____ [2.5-10 mg] iv in 50 ml D5W q 6 h. Infuse over 10-15 min.

   • Check BP and HR 15 min after iv infusion completed.

   • Automatically convert from iv dose to po dose when patient is taking fluids.

   b. If taking fluids, metoprolol _____ [25-50 mg] po q 12 h.

   c. Check BP and HR before each dose of metoprolol.

   Hold metoprolol for HR < _____ [< 55] bpm or SPB < _____ [< 100] mmHg.

   d. Call physician if HR remains > _____ [> 70] bpm.

   e. D/C metoprolol after 7 d (combined iv and po doses).

NOTE: Authorization for dispensing in accordance with the hospital formulary system is given unless checked in this box.

❏ _____ M.D.

_____   _____
      Date   Time

[ ] Figures in brackets are suggested values.

_____   _____
      Pager   Print Name

SAMPLE SUPPLEMENT INFORMATION FORM

Prophylactic Perioperative Beta Blockade (PPBB) Considerations

■ **All patients scheduled for major elective noncardiac surgery requiring general anesthesia and a hospital stay qualify.** Patients for emergency surgery, hemodynamically unstable patients, and renal transplant patients need to be assessed individually.[1] These guidelines are intended to provide supplemental information for use with the Prophylactic Perioperative Beta Blockade (PPBB) Protocol Order Form.

■ **Consider PPBB for patients within at least one of the following categories:**
  - ❏ Known coronary artery disease
  - ❏ Atherosclerotic vascular disease
  - ❏ Diabetes
  - ❏ Any two of the following:
    - Age > 65 yr
    - Hypertension
    - Current smoker
    - Hyperlipidemia

■ **Patients within any of the following categories *should not* receive PPBB:**
  - ❏ Known sensitivity to beta-blockers
  - ❏ Acute congestive heart failure
  - ❏ Acute bronchospasm
  - ❏ Acutely hemodynamically unstable patients
  - ❏ Hypotension
  - ❏ Significant bradycardia or high-grade heart block

■ **Care must be taken with administration to patients with Hx of asthma or COPD.**

■ **Drug Choice:** Atenolol, bisoprolol, and metoprolol may be used. They are all long-acting, Beta-1 selective, and have similar efficacy in the prevention of death after myocardial infarction.

■ **How should PPBB be initiated?**
  - ❏ **Preop:** If HR > 60 bpm and SBP > 100 mmHG, then oral dosing with twice daily metoprolol (25-50 mg), bisoprolol (5-10 mg), or atenolol (50-100 mg) once daily can be started several d before surgery. Target HR is > 50 and < 70 bpm.
  - ❏ **In holding area *before* surgery:** If HR > 60 bpm and SBP > 100 mmHg, metoprolol 2.5-5.0 mg iv can be given while monitoring HR and BP. For maximal beta blockage, consider additional dose(s) every 10 min if HR remains > 70 bpm and SBP > 100 mmHg. Target HR is > 50 and < 70 bpm.
  - ❏ **During surgery:** If HR > 60 bpm and SBP > 100 mmHg, metoprolol 2.5-5.0 mg iv q 10 min may be given 30 min before emergence. Target HR for maximal beta blockade is < 70 bpm. Alternatively, esmolol infusion may be titrated to maintain HR < 70 during emergence.
  - ❏ **PACU or ICU *after* surgery:** If HR > 60 bpm and SBP > 100 mmHg, metoprolol 2.5-5.0 mg iv may be given while monitoring HR and BP. For maximal beta blockade, consider additional dose(s) q 10 min if HR remains > 70 bpm and SBP > 100 mmHg. Target HR is > 50 and < 70 bpm. Consider use of PPBB Protocol Order Form.
  - ❏ **Postop care:** If the patient is to be kept npo, metoprolol 2.5-10 mg iv q 6 h dosing should be continued with target > 50 and < 70 bpm, while maintaining SBP > 100 mmHg. When patient is able to take oral medications, the patient may be switched to twice daily oral metoprolol (25-50 mg), once daily atenolol (50-100 mg) or bisoprolol (5-10 mg) with dosage adjusted to keep HR > 50 and < 70 bpm and SBP > 100 mmHg. Consider use of PPBB Protocol Order Form.

■ **PPBB should be continued for at least 7 d postop.** Patients with Hx of CAD may benefit from indefinite beta blockade therapy.

---

[1] These guidelines provide basic recommendations. They are not intended as absolute or standard requirements. Practice guidelines should be modified based on clinical needs and individual practice to ensure the highest quality of patient care.

APPENDIX B: STANDARD ADULT ANESTHETIC PROTOCOLS

Stanley I. Samuels, Richard A. Jaffe, C. Philip Larson, Jr.

STANDARD MONITORS (NONINVASIVE)

Blood pressure (BP)	Usually noninvasive (oscillometric) technique. Match cuff width to arm size to avoid inaccurate BP.
Capnometry/capnography	Measurement of $ETCO_2$/display of wave form
Gas analyzer (e.g., Raman, IR, mass spectometry)	Measurement of respired gases and anesthetics
Electrocardiogram (ECG)	5-lead preferred
Esophageal or precordial stethoscope	Breath and heart sounds monitored; dysrhythmias and $\downarrow$BP may be detected.
Nerve stimulator	Monitor status of neuromuscular blockade
Oxygen analyzer	Measurement of FiO_2
Pulse oximetry	Measurement of O_2 saturation of hemoglobin
Temperature	Nasal, esophageal, bladder, rectal, tympanic, or skin
Visual observation of patient	Skin color, pupils, temperature, edema, sweating, movement
Ventilator function monitors	PIP, TV, disconnect alarm, etc.

STANDARD ANESTHETIC MANAGEMENT (ADULT ASA 1 & 2)

★ **NB:** The following sections are guidelines only (for an otherwise healthy 70 kg adult). Specific drugs and drug dosages should be individualized, based on the physiological and pharmacological status of the patient, including factors such as age, weight, concurrent medication, and comorbidities.

PREMEDICATION

Light	Diazepam 5-10 mg	po 1 h preop
	Lorazepam 1-2 mg	po 1 h preop
	Hydroxyzine 25-100 mg	po 1 h preop
Moderate	Midazolam 1-2 mg iv	Prior to induction (in patient holding area or OR)
	± Fentanyl 25-100 μg iv	Monitor for respiratory depression.
Heavy	Diazepam 10 mg	po 1-2 h preop
	+ Morphine 0.1 mg/kg	} im 30-60 min preop
	+ Scopolamine 0.2-0.4 mg	

INDUCTION TECHNIQUES

Preinduction
1. ✓ anesthesia machine, suction, airway equipment, drugs.
2. Attach monitors and verify function.
3. Administer 100% O_2 by mask × 1-3 min.
4. Administer supplemental sedation/analgesia (as appropriate).
   e.g.: fentanyl   1-3 μg/kg iv
   ± midazolam   0.03-0.1 mg/kg iv

Induction agents
Thiopental   3-5 mg/kg iv
Propofol   1.5-2.5 mg/kg iv (in increments) **NB:** Pain on injection ★
Etomidate   0.2-0.4 mg/kg iv **NB:** Pain on injection; myoclonus   ★

	Drugs	**Doses**	**Onset**	**Duration**
Muscle relaxants for intubation	Succinylcholine:	1.0 mg/kg	30-60 sec	4-6 min
	If given after defasciculating dose of NMR	1.5 mg/kg	30-60 sec	4-6 min
	Infusion	1 g/250-500 NS (titrated to effect)	+ 60 sec	While infusing (phase II block possible)
	Vecuronium	0.1 mg/kg	2-3 min	24-30 min
		0.2 mg/kg (rapid onset)	< 2 min	45-90 min
	Pancuronium	0.1 mg/kg	3-4 min	40-65 min
	Mivacurium	0.1-0.2 mg/kg	1-2 min	6-10 min
	Cisatracurium	0.2 mg/kg	2 min	40-80 min
	d-tubocurarine (dTC)	0.5 mg/kg	3-5 min	30 min
	Pipecuronium	0.07-0.09 mg/kg	2-3 min	45-120 min
	Rocuronium	0.6-1.2 mg/kg	45-90 sec	30-120 min

MAINTENANCE TECHNIQUES

Inhalational anesthesia	30-100% O_2 + 0-70% N_2O + Isoflurane (MAC in 100% O_2 = 1.15%) titrated to effect Alternatively, for short procedures or for the last hour of long procedures, use sevoflurane (MAC = 1.7%) or desflurane (MAC = 6%)
Balanced anesthesia	30-100% O_2 + 0-70% N_2O + Meperidine 0.5-1.5 mg/kg/3-4 h (intermittent bolus) or morphine 0.05-0.15 mg/kg/3-4 h (intermittent bolus) or fentanyl 1-10 μg/kg prn response to surgical stimulation or remifentanil 0.05-2 μg/kg/min prn response to surgical stimulation + Isoflurane ~0.5% or propofol 50-200 μg/kg/min Alternatively, for short procedures or for the last hour of long procedures, use sevoflurane (MAC = 1.7%) or desflurane (MAC = 6%).

Total intravenous anesthesia (TIVA)[1]

30% O_2 in N_2O (continue 70% N_2O until end of procedure)

+ Remifentanil infusion* (infusion off 2-5 min before end of surgery)	Induction infusion Maintenance	@ 0.5-1 μg/kg/min × 1-2 min @ 0.05-0.2 μg/kg/min
+ Propofol bolus + infusion (infusion off 2-5 min before end of surgery)	Induction bolus Maintenance	1-1.5 mg/kg @ 40-80 μg/kg/min

30% O_2 in air

+ Remifentanil infusion* (infusion off 5 min before end of surgery)	Induction infusion Maintenance 10 min before end surgery	@ 0.5-1 μg/kg/min × 1-2 min @ 0.1-0.35 μg/kg/min @ 0.05-0.1 μg/kg/min
+ Propofol bolus + infusion (infusion off 2-3 min before end of surgery)	Induction bolus Maintenance 10 min before end surgery	1-1.5 mg/kg @ 60-90 μg/kg/min @20-40 μg/kg/min

* No residual analgesia: postop pain management depends on type of surgery, and analgesic requirements may be substantial.
[1] Steven Shafer, MD (TIVA).

If continued muscle relaxation is required during the above maintenance techniques, several options are available. Always use a nerve stimulator to assess block before redosing.

Short-acting	Mivacurium	0.1 mg/kg/10-20 min or 1-15 μg/kg/min
Intermediate	Vecuronium Rocuronium Cisatracurium	0.025 mg/kg/30 min 0.6 mg/kg/30 min 0.2 mg/kg/40 min
Long-acting	Pancuronium Pipecuronium	0.02 mg/kg/60-90 min 0.015 mg/kg/60-90 min

EMERGENCE

1.	**Reversal of muscle relaxant**	As surgical conditions permit, reverse residual muscle relaxant (when at least 1 twitch is present in train-of-four) with one of the following: Neostigmine 0.05-0.07 (maximum dose) mg/kg iv + glycopyrrolate 0.01 mg/kg iv, or Edrophonium 0.5-1.0 (maximum dose) mg/kg iv + atropine 0.015 mg/kg iv.
2.	**Analgesia**	If remifentanil was used during surgery, supplemental analgesics will be necessary and should be given before emergence.
3.	**Nausea prophylaxis**	Metoclopramide (10 mg iv), and/or ondansetron (4 mg iv), dolasetron (12.5 mg iv), or granisetron (100 μg iv). The use of droperidol (0.625 mg iv) is controversial. Consider OG tube placement and suction to empty stomach.
4.	**O_2**	D/C N_2O/volatile agents and administer 100% O_2.
5.	**Suction**	Suction oropharynx thoroughly.
6.	**Extubation**	Extubate after protective airway reflexes have returned, the patient is breathing spontaneously, and is able to follow commands.

MONITORED ANESTHESIA CARE (MAC)

1. Standard monitoring with regular verbal contact.

2. Nasal O_2 (qualitative measurement of $ETCO_2$ can be accomplished by attaching a sampling catheter to the nasal cannula).

3. If the initial local anesthetic injection will be painful (e.g., retrobulbar block), then a brief period of analgesia, sedation, and amnesia can be induced with:

		Advantages:	Disadvantages:
A.	Midazolam (0.5-2 mg) 3-5 min before injection + Ketamine (10-20 mg) 3 min before injection ± alfentanil 3-7 μg/kg 2 min before injection or remifentanil 0.5 μg/kg 1-2 min before injection or	Profound amnesia and analgesia. Usually no apnea and airway reflexes maintained. Patient able to cooperate.	Patient not 'asleep.' Timing is important. Possible ↑BP and HR.
B.	STP (1-3 mg/kg) ± fentanyl (25-50 μg/)	Patient 'asleep'	Possible apnea with loss of airway. ↓BP Patient unresponsive.

4. Light-to-moderate levels of sedation (± analgesia) can be maintained using a **propofol infusion** (25-100 μg/kg/ min), or with intermittent bolus injections of midazolam (0.25-1mg) ± fentanyl (10-25 μg) or with a remifentanil infusion (0.025-0.07 μg/kg/min), titrated to effect. Monitor closely for respiratory depression.

RAPID-SEQUENCE INDUCTION OF ANESTHESIA
(FULL-STOMACH PRECAUTIONS)

1. ↓ gastric volume/acidity	Ranitidine 50 mg iv at least 30-60 min before induction
	Metoclopramide 10 mg iv 30-60 min before induction
	0.3 M sodium citrate 30 ml po immediately before induction
2. **Induction**	Preoxygenation ≥ 3 min
	± Defasciculate: e.g., vecuronium 1 mg iv 3-5 min before succinylcholine
	Cricoid pressure (Sellick maneuver) by assistant
	Etomidate 0.1-0.4 mg/kg
	or
	STP 3-5 mg/kg
	or
	Ketamine 1 mg/kg
	or
	Propofol 1.5-2.5 mg/kg
	+ Succinylcholine 1.5 mg/kg for intubation (stylet ETT). If succinylcholine contraindicated, consider rocuronium (1.2 mg/kg).
3. **Intubation**	Intubate when patient is fully relaxed.
	Watch chest movement and auscultate for equal BBS.
	✓ expired CO_2 on monitor.
	Listen over stomach.
	Secure ETT and release cricoid pressure.
	Pass NG tube and suction stomach contents.
4. **Failed intubation protocol**	See Anesthetic Considerations for Cesarean Section, Obstetric Surgery, p. 664.
5. **Maintenance**	As indicated by patient's condition and type of surgery.
6. **Extubation**	Extubate when patient is awake and with active laryngeal protective reflexes. Remember, some may require postop ICU care until safe extubation can be assured.

SPECIAL PEDIATRIC CONSIDERATIONS

1. The same principles apply in children requiring surgery, and in those who may have full stomachs. Consider emptying the stomach with an OG tube prior to induction in patients with pyloric stenosis or with high-grade intestinal obstruction following po barium. If iv is placed, continue as indicated above. If iv access is difficult, O_2/sevoflurane induction with cricoid pressure, succinylcholine (2-4 mg/kg im) will permit intubation and minimize risks of gastric aspiration.

2. Awake intubation in neonates and sick infants may be the safest method.

AWAKE FIBER OPTIC INTUBATION PROTOCOL

C. Philip Larson, Jr.

Premedication

If not contraindicated, patients should receive mild-to- moderate sedation with meperidine 0.5 mg/kg or fentanyl 0.3-0.5 μg/kg and midazolam 1-2 mg iv.

Topical anesthesia

When premedication has been established, the oropharynx is sprayed vigorously ~6 times over a span of 10 min, using lidocaine 4% solution. Initially, the spray is directed at the front of the tongue; gradually, it is directed further back in the throat, until the entire oropharynx is numb. In reality, the lateral recesses of the oropharynx need not be anesthetized topically because both fiber optic laryngoscope (FOL) and ETT are confined to the midline of the mouth.

Tracheal anesthesia

Next, a transtracheal injection of cocaine or lidocaine 4% (4 ml) is made through the cricothyroid membrane, using a 5-ml syringe and a 23-ga, $^3/_4$-inch needle. So that this injection can be made as rapidly as possible, it is important to use a small syringe, making certain that the connection between syringe and needle is tight. The patient is instructed not to cough until the injection is complete. Since this may be impossible for some patients, it is important that the operator's hand be fixed firmly against the patient's upper chest to assure that needle movement is minimized and that the full injection is made into the trachea. When the injection is complete, the patient is urged to cough vigorously.

Laryngoscopy

Once the mouth and trachea are anesthetized with local anesthetic, an oral airway with a central orifice (e.g., Tudor-Williams airway) is placed in the midline of the mouth. A 7 mm orotracheal tube, without connector attached, is placed over a FOL. With the operator at the patient's side near the waist, the FOL is introduced through the hole in the airway and advanced to end of airway. At this point, the epiglottis should be visible. The tip of the fiber optic scope is flexed toward the operator about 15-20°, which should bring arytenoid cartilages and laryngeal opening into view. The scope is advanced into the larynx so that tracheal rings can be visualized. Often, the carina also can be visualized. The laryngoscopist also can place the scope in the airway by darkening the room and using the scope as a light wand, directing the light externally to the sternal notch and advancing it down the trachea. If a wire-reinforced tube is desired, use a Patel or Ovassapian airway instead of the Tudor-Williams airway for guidance, as these airways can be removed with the tube connector in place.

Intubation

The scope is placed on the patient's chest and, holding it so that it is not advanced further, the orotracheal tube is advanced gently into the trachea. To facilitate passage of the orotracheal tube past the arytenoid cartilages and into the larynx, it is often necessary to rotate the tube counterclockwise 90°—or even as much as 180°—several times as it is being advanced. Using this rotational movement, the operator should never need to push hard on the tube to position it in the larynx. Once the tube is in place, the FOL and oral airway are removed, and the 15-mm connector is reattached to the tube. To verify that the tube is properly positioned, a device can be attached to the connector that will make a distinct whistle as the patient exhales. Alternatively, $ETCO_2$ confirms proper placement. The orotracheal tube is then firmly taped in place at one side of the mouth.

APPENDIX C: STANDARD PERIOPERATIVE PAIN MANAGEMENT

Sean Mackey and Raymond R. Gaeta

INTRODUCTION

Pain during the periop period has recently become an area of significant focus. Of the > 25 million surgical procedures performed in this country each year, > 75% of patients experience pain, and > 80% of those experience moderate-to-extreme pain.[5] These observations have led, in part, to the adoption of the new Joint Commission Pain Standards recognizing the rights of patients to appropriate assessment and management of their own medical needs.

The primary goals of periop pain control traditionally have been the humanitarian notion of reducing pain and suffering and improvement in function. Poor pain control leads to problems, such as a decreased ability to ambulate, which increases the risk of thromboembolic phenomenon and fatal PE. Inadequate pain control after abdominal and thoracic surgeries leads to splinting, atelectasis, and risk of pneumonia. Furthermore, activation of the neuroendocrine stress response to surgical pain stimulates the anterior pituitary gland, releasing a cavalcade of stress hormones and catecholamines, which have been shown to have deleterious effects on postop outcomes. These effects include weight loss, fatigue, immunosuppression, thromboembolism and hypercoagulability, dysrhythmias, urinary retention, and impaired pulmonary function.[2] As an additional consequence, the continuous afferent barrage of nociceptive signals induces changes in the spinal cord and brain, leading to a phenomenon of central hypersensitization or 'wind-up,' which is thought to play a role in the perpetuation of pain after surgery and even the transformation of acute pain states into chronic ones.[6] As we understand more of the effects of pain on organ function and the CNS during the periop period, we realize that, through optimal pain control, not only can we impact pain and suffering, but also improve the overall morbidity and mortality of our surgical patients.

MULTIMODALITY ANALGESIA

Acute pain specialists have not been particularly successful in eliminating a patient's postop pain using a single analgesic agent or technique. Instead, we have found that we can enhance patient satisfaction by using small amounts of multiple agents, each working to reduce nociception at different points along the pain processing pathways—a concept called '**multimodality analgesia**.' By utilizing small amounts of opiates, COX-2 inhibitors, and neural blockade together, side effects have been reduced and pain control and patient satisfaction improved. This concept is most effective when integrated with a periop rehab approach to surgery, which involves teams of surgeons, anesthesiologists, rehabilitation specialists, nurses, pharmacists, and other health care providers, all working together. It requires that the patient be given appropriate preop education, excellent periop nociceptive blockade and attenuation of the neuroendocrine stress response, postop exercise, and early enteral nutrition.[1]

PREEMPTIVE ANALGESIA

An important component of multimodality analgesia is the notion of preemptive analgesia. This concept has been well known to the basic science researchers, but has caused much confusion, and often disappointment, in clinical practice. Part of the problem lies in how the term has been used in the past—often applied only to the provision of an analgesic agent preop or preincision. In fact, while the term does imply an intervention before surgery, it has much more stringent requirements. Specifically, it implies providing antinociceptive measures preop and postop to prevent the establishment of central sensitization caused by incisional and inflammatory injuries. Preincisional, long-acting neural blockade and administration of NSAIDs or COX-2Is have been shown to significantly reduce postop pain and opiate requirements, as compared with initiating therapy after surgery. Clinical researchers also have demonstrated improvements in postop rehab of patients by using preemptive analgesia, particularly in lower-extremity orthopedic surgery. Preemptive analgesia also may reduce the development of chronic pain syndromes following surgery, due to reduction in central hypersensitization.[4]

THE NEW ANALGESIC PARADIGM

This concept utilizes preemptive and multimodal administration of COX-2Is, neural blockade, and sustained-release opiates to replace the current overreliance on potent, short-duration opiates for postop pain management. The combination of COX-2Is, which reduce nociceptive sensitization both peripherally and centrally with a high degree of safety, and neural conduction blockade can significantly reduce pain scores, parenteral opiate dose requirements, and dose-dependent adverse events. When used in conjunction with a structured postop rehab program, these techniques can lead to decreased patient morbidity and mortality, increased patient satisfaction, decreased recovery time, and shorter hospitalization.[1,3]

References

1. Kehlet H: Acute pain control and accelerated postoperative surgical recovery. *Surg Clin North Am* 1999; 79(2).
2. Kehlet H: Manipulation of the metabolic response in clinical practice. *World J Surg* 2000; 24:690-5.
3. Kirsh E, Worwag E, Sinner M, Chodak G: Using outcome data and patient satisfaction surveys to develop policies regarding minimum length of hospitalization after radical prostatectomy. *Urology* 2000; 56(1):101-7.
4. Kissin I: Preemptive analgesia. *Anesthesiology* 2000; 93(4):1138-43.
5. Warfield CA, Kahn CH: Acute pain management. Programs in U.S. hospitals and experiences and attitudes among U.S. adults. *Anesthesiology* 1995; 83(5):1090-4.
6. Woolf CJ, Salter MW: Neuronal plasticity: increasing the gain in pain. *Science* 2000; 288(5472):1765-9.

STANDARD ADULT POSTOP ANALGESICS AND ANTIEMETICS

Analgesics	Morphine	2 mg/10 min, up to 10 mg iv
	Meperidine	10 mg/10 min, up to 150 mg iv; not to exceed (NTE) 600 mg/d
	Hydromorphone	0.5-1 mg/10-20 min, up to 6 mg
	Fentanyl	12.5-35 μg/5 min, up to 200 μg iv
	Ketorolac	30 mg iv slowly; then 15 mg q 6 h × 3 d max
Antiemetics	Metoclopramide	5-10 mg iv
	Ondansetron	4 mg iv – repeat if necessary after 30 min.
	Dolasetron	12.5 mg iv
	Granisetron	100 μg iv

EPIDURAL ANALGESIA

	Lumbar Epidural		Thoracic Epidural	
Loading dose	**Morphine**	**Hydromorphone**	**Morphine**	**Hydromorphone**
Lower extremities	2-3 mg	0.4-0.6 mg	–	–
Pelvis	3-4 mg	0.5-0.8 mg	1-3 mg	0.15-0.4 mg
Abdomen	5-7 mg	0.5-1 mg	2-3.5 mg	0.2-0.6 mg
Thorax	7-8 mg	0.5-1 mg	2-3.5 mg	0.4-0.8 mg
Infusion	**Morphine**	**Hydromorphone**	**Morphine**	**Hydromorphone**
Lower extremities	0.3-0.5 mg/h	0.1-0.2 mg/h	–	–
Pelvis	0.3-0.5 mg/h	0.1-0.2 mg/h	0.1-0.3 mg/h	0.1-0.15 mg/h
Abdomen	0.4-0.7 mg/h	0.2-0.3 mg/h	0.2-0.5 mg/h	0.1-0.2 mg/h
Thorax	0.5-1.0 mg/h	0.2-0.3 mg/h	0.2-0.6 mg/h	0.15-0.2 mg/h

Special considerations:

1. Concentrations of opioids used for epidural infusions (in preservative-free solution):
   - Morphine, 0.15 mg/ml
   - Hydromorphone, 0.05 mg/ml
2. Ketorolac may impair hemostasis. Use for breakthrough pain, following consultation with the surgical team.

EPIDURAL ANESTHESIA/POSTOP ANALGESIA

Surgical Site	**Epidural Catheter Location**	**Initial Bolus of 0.5% Bupivacaine**	**Infusion Rate of 0.125% Bupivacaine**
Thoracic or upper abdomen	T6-T8	4-6 ml	5-10 ml/h
Lower abdomen	T10	10 ml	15 ml/h
Hip or knee	L2-3	8 ml	10 ml/h

Special considerations:

1. Give initial bolus dose before incision. Then, if patient hemodynamically stable, give 1/2 bolus dose 30 min before end of surgery.

2. In recovery room, ✓ sensory level. If no sensory block, ✓ whether catheter is functioning with 8 ml 2% lidocaine bolus. (✓ vital signs.) If thoracic epidural starts with 2 ml, redose with 2 ml q 5-10 min, up to 8 ml.

3. Start infusions: If catheter is functional, as evidenced by loss of sensation, start: local anesthetic + opioid infusions (see table, above).

4. Best results: Local anesthetics and opioids are mixed in line using two separate infusion pumps. Thus, if either causes side effects, one can be stopped without the other.

PATIENT-CONTROLLED ANALGESIA (PCA) FOR INTRAVENOUS ADMINISTRATION

Loading dose	Morphine	Titrate to comfort
	Hydromorphone	Titrate to comfort
	Fentanyl	Titrate to comfort
Basal rate	Morphine	0.5-1 mg/h
	Hydromorphone	0.1-0.2 mg/h
	Fentanyl	5-10 μg/h
PCA lock-out dose and time	Morphine	1-2 mg q 10-15 min
	Hydromorphone	0.1-0.2 mg q 10-15 min
	Fentanyl	5-10 μg q 10-15 min

Typical orders:

1. Call anesthesiologist with any questions about PCA.
2. Check respiratory rate q 1 h while PCA in use.
3. Call anesthesiologist if respiratory rate < 10/min. If rate < 6/min, treat with naloxone 0.1-0.2 mg iv (may repeat, to 0.6 mg), push and assist ventilation while waiting for anesthesiologist.
4. Encourage patient to ambulate 4-6 h after surgery (unless contraindicated).
5. After PCA D/C'd, start po pain medications (per surgeon).
6. If patient required a large loading dose, the PCA lockout dose may need to be increased. Expect patient to need about $^1/_3$ loading dose q h. Change PCA dose or lockout time to permit this dosing.

PATIENT-CONTROLLED EPIDURAL ANALGESIA (PCEA)

Loading dose	Morphine	2-3 mg
	Hydromorphone	0.5-1.0 mg
	Fentanyl	50-75 μg
Basal rate	Morphine	0.2-0.5 mg/h
	Hydromorphone	0.08-0.12 mg/h
	Fentanyl	5-10 μg/h
PCA lock-out dose and time	Morphine	0.1-0.2 mg q 10-15 min
	Hydromorphone	0.02-0.06 mg q 10-15 min
	Fentanyl	5-10 μg q 10-15 min

Special considerations:

1. For thoracic epidural, decrease all doses by one-third ($^1/_3$); if high thoracic, decrease by $^1/_2$.
2. Concentrations of opioids for epidural infusion (in preservative-free solution).

   • Morphine   0.15 mg/ml
   • Hydromorphone   0.05 mg/ml
   • Fentanyl   10 μg/ml

3. Bupivacaine (0.125% @ 5-8 ml/h) may be added to the above regimen for supplemental analgesia. Typically, the bupivacaine infusion is stopped on POD 1 to facilitate early ambulation. Thoracic epidural local anesthetic may be continued if it does not interfere with ambulation.

TYPICAL ORDERS FOR POSTOP EPIDURAL/SPINAL ANALGESIA

I. EPIDURAL MEDICATIONS

_____ **1. Epidural Infusion – Opiate**
- ☐ Hydromorphone (Dilaudid) 0.05 mg/ml concentration @ _____ mg/h = _____ ml/h
- ☐ Morphine sulfate 0.15 mg/ml concentration @ _____ mg/h = _____ ml/h
- ☐ Fentanyl (Sublimaze) 10 μg/ml concentration @ _____ μg/h = _____ ml/h
- ☐ Range: May vary infusion between _____ /h to _____ /h prn pain.

_____ **2. Epidural Infusion – Anesthetic**
- ☐ Bupivacaine 0.125% concentration @ _____ ml/h
- ☐ Bupivacaine 0.25% concentration @ _____ ml/h
- ☐ Turn off bupivacaine on POD #1 @ 5 am.

_____ **3 Epidural Bolus – Opiate**
- ☐ Hydromorphone (Dilaudid) _____ mg q _____ h in 10 ml preservative-free NS (PFNS)
- ☐ Morphine sulfate _____ mg q _____ h in 10 ml PFNS

_____ **4. Breakthrough Pain**
- ☐ Fentanyl [_50-100_] μg via epidural q _[1]_ h prn pain in 10 ml PFNS
- ☐ Call MD if ≥ 2 doses in [_2_] h.
- ☐ Ketorolac (Toradol) [_15_] mg iv q 6 h × [_3_] d (for a maximum of 12 doses)

II. NURSING CARE

_____ **1. Vital Signs**
- ☐ For opiates: T, P, BP q 4 h; RR q 2 h; then q 8 h, if stable.
    Continuous O$_2$ sats × 24 h; then D/C if O$_2$ sats > 90% on room air.
- ☐ For anesthetics: BP & P q 2 h; then q 4 h, if stable.
    Orthostatic BP before ambulation × 24 h.

_____ **2.** Label tubing, pump, infusion as "epidural." Place sign over bed; cover "Y" ports on tubing.

_____ **3.** Place naloxone (Narcan) and syringe at bedside.

_____ **4.** Administration of any additional opiates, sedatives, or antiemetics must be approved by anesthesiologist.

_____ **5.** Assess patient's pain (0-10 scale: 0 = no pain; 10 = worst pain imaginable) and level of sedation (awake, drowsy, asleep, unresponsive), along with VS.

_____ **6.** D/C Epidural Protocol when epidural D/C'd.

III. SIDE EFFECTS MANAGEMENT

_____ **1. Respiratory depression:** For RR < 6 or O$_2$ sat < 86% (on 2 separate occasions < 5 min apart): Administer naloxone (Narcan) 0.1 mg-0.2 mg iv STAT; may repeat, to total of 0.6 mg. Administer O$_2$ 10 L/min via nonrebreathing mask. TURN OFF INFUSION. CALL ON-CALL MD STAT.

_____ **2. Excessive somnolence/sedation:**
    Administer naloxone (Narcan) 0.1 mg-0.2 mg iv STAT; may repeat, to total of 0.6 mg. Administer O$_2$ 10 L/min via nonrebreathing mask. TURN OFF INFUSION. CALL ON-CALL MD STAT.

_____ **3. Nausea/Vomiting:**
- ☐ Metoclopramide (Reglan) [_10 mg_] iv q 4-6 h prn
- ☐ Ondansetron [_4 mg_] q 6 h prn
- ☐ Nalbuphine (Nubain) [_2.5-5.0 mg_] iv q 4 h prn

_____ **4. Pruritus:**
- ☐ Nalbuphine (Nubain) [_2.5-5.0 mg_] iv q 2-4 h prn
- ☐ Diphenhydramine (Benadryl) [_10-25 mg_] iv q 4 h prn

[ ] indicates suggested dosage

APPENDIX D: STANDARD PEDIATRIC ANESTHETIC PROTOCOLS

Gregory B. Hammer

STANDARD PEDIATRIC MONITORS (NONINVASIVE)

Blood pressure (BP)	
Capnometry/capnography	Measurement of $ETCO_2$/display of wave form
Gas analyzer (e.g., Raman, IR, or mass spectroscopy)	Measurement of respired gases and anesthetics
Electrocardiogram (ECG)	5-lead preferred
Esophageal or precordial stethoscope	Breath and heart sounds monitored; dysrhythmias and ↓BP detected
Nerve stimulator	Monitor status of neuromuscular blockade
Oxygen analyzer	Measurement of FiO_2
Pulse oximetry	Measurement of O_2 saturation; 2 pulse oximeters in neonates—1 preductal; 1 postductal
Temperature	Nasal, esophageal, rectal, or skin
Visual observation of patient	Skin color, pupils, temperature, edema, sweating, movement
Ventilator function monitors	PIP, TV, disconnect alarm, etc.

STANDARD PREOP FASTING (NPO) GUIDELINES

- All solid foods and nonclear liquids (e.g., milk, infant formula, orange juice) should be withheld after midnight before scheduled surgery.

- All clear liquids (and breast milk) should be given up to 3 h before scheduled surgery. Because breast milk has a relatively short transit time through the stomach, and to simplify—therefore, to increase compliance with—these guidelines, breast milk is considered a clear liquid.

- In practice, nonemergency cases may proceed 6 h after solids and nonclear liquids and 2 h after clear liquids and breast milk have been ingested.

STANDARD PEDIATRIC ANESTHETIC MANAGEMENT

★ **NB:** The following sections are guidelines only. Specific drugs and drug dosages should be individualized, based on the physiological and pharmacological status of the patient, including factors such as age, weight, medication, and concurrent diseases.

PREMEDICATION

- In general, patients < 9 mo of age do not need premedication—only atropine 0.01-0.02 mg/kg iv or 0.02 mg/kg im before intubation if no contraindication. Minimum iv atropine dose = 100 μg

- Older children (9 mo-10 yr) can be premedicated successfully by using oral midazolam (0.5-0.75 mg) in syrup, grape Kool-Aid, or cherry-flavored Tylenol elixir (10-15 mg/kg) 20-30 min before surgery.

- For patients > 35-40 kg, oral lorazepam (0.03-0.05 mg/kg) or diazepam (0.1-0.15 mg/kg) may be given 60 min before surgery with a sip of water.

INDUCTION TECHNIQUES

Preinduction
1. ✓ anesthesia machine, suction, airway equipment, drugs.
2. Attach monitors and verify function.
3. Premedication: < 6-9 mo—consider atropine 0.01-0.02 mg/kg iv before laryngoscopy to prevent vagally mediated bradycardia.

Induction

Routes of administration:
1. Intramuscular: ketamine hydrochloride 3-5 mg/kg (with atropine 0.02 mg/kg)
2. IV: STP   4-7 mg/kg
    Propofol   2-3 mg/kg
3. Inhalational: halothane (MAC = 0.87% [neonates], and 1-2% [infants], or sevoflurane (MAC = 3.3% [neonates and younger infants], and 2.5% [older infants and children], in N_2O (up to 70%)/O_2. Increase inspired concentration of halothane incrementally every 3 breaths (up to 4%); sevoflurane (up to 7%). Monitor BP and HR closely.

Muscle relaxation
1. Succinylcholine (controversial*): 1-2 mg/kg iv or 2-4 mg/kg im
2. Vecuronium or pancuronium: 0.1 mg/kg iv
3. Rocuronium 0.6-1 mg/kg iv
4. Cisatracurium 0.1 mg/kg iv
5. Deep halothane or sevoflurane + anesthesia

Laryngoscope

Blade	Age
Miller 0	Neonate
Miller 1	6-9 mo
Wis-Hipple 1.5	9 mo-3 yr
Macintosh 2	1-4 yr
Macintosh 3 or Miller 2	> 4 yr

* Succinylcholine may trigger MH in susceptible patients or cause cardiac arrest in myopathic patients; therefore, many pediatric anesthesiologists avoid the use of succinylcholine.

TYPICAL ETT SIZE AT DIFFERENT AGES

Age	Wt	ETT Size
Newborn	3-4 kg	3.0
≤ 6-8 mo	6-8 kg	3.5
≤ 8-16 mo	10-12 kg	4.0
2-3 yr	13-15 kg	Thereafter use formula:
6 yr	20 kg	4 + (age/4) = ETT size (to allow for a slight
9 yr	30 kg	leak when positive pressure is applied).
12 yr	40 kg	

★ **NB:** This is a guide only; prepare an ETT one size larger and one size smaller than the ETT size selected. ✓✓ ET placement of tube by auscultation of breath sounds bilaterally. ✓ depth of carina by auscultation over left axilla as ETT is slowly advanced. Withdraw and secure ETT 2 cm from position where diminution of breath sounds was first noted. Positive pressure leak between 30-40 cmH$_2$O is desirable. Leaks < 30 cm result in volume loss and difficulty in providing appropriate ventilation during critical phases intraop or postop. Conversely, leaks > 40 cmH$_2$O carry a higher risk of subglottic edema and/or stenosis. Cuffed ETTs may be used, provided that leak is maintained < 40 cmH$_2$O.

MAINTENANCE TECHNIQUES

Inhalational anesthesia

30-100% O$_2$ + 0-70% N$_2$O. In preemies and for cases where N$_2$O is contraindicated, air may be used to lower FiO$_2$. + Isoflurane, halothane, or sevoflurane, titrated to effect

★ **NB**: Warm and humidify all gases. Warm room to 75-80° F for infants; 70-75° F for children.

Balanced anesthesia

30-100% O$_2$
+ 0-70% N$_2$O
+ ~0.5% isoflurane
or propofol (50-200 μg/kg/min)

+ morphine (0.05 mg/kg/h) or
fentanyl (1-3 μg/kg/h)

If continued muscle relaxation is required during the above maintenance techniques, several options are available. Always use a nerve stimulator to assess block before redosing.

Short-acting	Mivacurium	0.1 mg/kg → 6-10 min
Intermediate	Vecuronium	0.01 mg/kg → 25-30 min
	Rocuronium	0.6 mg/kg/30 min
	Cisatracurium	0.1 mg/kg/30 min
Long-acting	Pancuronium	0.1 mg/kg → 40-65 min

EMERGENCE

1. **Reversal of muscle relaxant**

As surgical conditions permit, reverse residual muscle relaxant (when at least 1 twitch is present in train-of-four) with one of the following:
• Neostigmine 0.05-0.07 (maximum dose) mg/kg iv + glycopyrrolate 0.01 mg/kg iv, or
• Edrophonium 0.5-1.0 (maximum dose) mg/kg iv + atropine 0.01 mg/kg iv.

2. **Nausea prophylaxis**

Metoclopramide 0.1 mg/kg iv (~1 h before emergence) or
Ondansetron 0.1 mg/kg

3. **O$_2$**

D/C N$_2$O/volatile agents and administer 100% O$_2$.

4. **Suction**

Suction oropharynx thoroughly.

5. **Extubation**

Laryngeal spasm is common in children; therefore, it is usual to extubate them when they are awake, moving all limbs, and breathing adequately. Infants and children with full stomachs or difficult airways must be extubated when they are fully awake. The pharynx should be suctioned thoroughly prior to extubation. If laryngeal spasm occurs, Rx with 100% O$_2$ and CPAP or PPV. If spasm fails to resolve and hypoxemia occurs, give succinylcholine 0.1-0.5 mg/kg and administer PPV. Consider reintubation if hypoxemia fails to resolve quickly. Consider atropine 0.01-0.02 mg/kg iv before succinylcholine, to preempt bradycardia.

PEDIATRIC EPIDURAL ANESTHESIA

Epidural anesthesia may be combined with GA for infants and children undergoing surgery involving the lower extremities, abdomen, chest, or spine. Single-dose ('single-shot') techniques may be used, or epidural catheters may be placed for longer procedures and to facilitate postop epidural analgesia (see below). Bupivacaine 0.25% ± epinephrine 1:200K is most commonly used intraop. For patients admitted following surgery, opioids (e.g., hydromorphone [Dilaudid]) are generally added, together with bupivacaine 0.1% (see p. E-5). Use saline-filled syringe for loss-of-resistance to minimize chances of VAE.

TECHNIQUES AND DOSAGES

1. **Caudal**
   - Single-shot: 22 ga iv catheter (< 5 yr), 20 ga iv catheter (> 5 yr), or 21-23 ga iv catheter may be inserted via sacrococcygeal membrane.
     - A test dose with 0.1-0.2 ml/kg lidocaine or bupivacaine + epinephrine 1:100K or 1:200K is given.
     - Initial dose: 0.5 ml/kg for lower extremity/perineal/genital procedures
                                1.0 ml/kg for abdominal procedures
   - Catheter technique: in patients < 10 kg, first dilate the epidural space with 5-10 U NS; then, a 20 ga epidural catheter may be inserted through 18 ga Critikon iv catheter and advanced so that tip is located near level of incision (e.g., ~17 cm from skin to T4 in infant). If resistance is met, it may be necessary to pull the catheter back slightly, together with the needle (to avoid shearing catheter), or repeat procedure.
     - Initial dose: 0.5 ml/kg

2. **Lumbar**
   - 17 or 18 ga epidural needle inserted via L3-4 or L4-5 interspace for single-shot injection or placement of 20 ga epidural catheter.
   - Use loss-of-resistance technique with fluid-filled syringe (air may cause VAE).
   - Good estimate of depth to epidural space is 1 mm/kg, up to ~30 kg.
   - Catheter should be threaded ~4 cm (maximum) beyond tip of needle.
   - A test dose with 0.1-0.2 ml/kg lidocaine or bupivacaine + epinephrine 1:100K or 1:200K is given.
   - Initial dose: 0.5 ml/kg for lower abdominal procedures
                            1.0 ml/kg for upper abdominal and thoracic procedures

3. **Thoracic**
   - The technique described for lumbar epidural catheter placement may be used between T6 and T12 in children.
   - A test dose with 0.1-0.2 ml/kg lidocaine or bupivacaine + epinephrine 1:100K or 1:200K is given.
   - Initial dose: 0.5 ml/kg
   - Local anesthetic-dosing guidelines same as above (note that volume will be ~$^1/_3$ less than with caudal approach.

For indwelling catheter techniques, hourly maintenance doses of $^1/_3$-$^1/_2$ the initial dose may be given.
For continuous infusion, maximum rate for bupivacaine is 0.5 mg/kg/h.

PEDIATRIC SPINAL ANESTHESIA AND ANALGESIA

Spinal anesthesia is used primarily for procedures such as inguinal herniorrhaphy in former preterm infants at risk for postop apnea following GA. By avoiding GA, the incidence of postop apnea is reduced, but not eliminated. In most patients arriving in the OR without iv access, an iv may be inserted in a lower extremity immediately following placement of the spinal anesthetic, as little change in BP or HR occurs in infants < 6 mo of age.

After standard monitors are applied, the infant is placed in a supine or lateral decubitus position. Care is taken to avoid neck flexion, which may cause airway obstruction. The skin is infiltrated with 1% lidocaine using a 27 or 30 ga needle. Lumbar puncture is performed with a 22 ga 1.5" spinal needle to an average depth of 1.5 cm from skin. The most commonly used local anesthetic for spinal anesthesia in infants is tetracaine 1.0%, mixed with an equal volume of 10% dextrose in a dose of 0.8-1.0 mg/kg. Epinephrine 1:1000 0.01 ml/kg is added. This dose usually provides adequate anesthesia for 90-120 min for inguinal herniorrhaphy.

Complications include high spinal anesthesia requiring tracheal intubation. PDPH is very uncommon in children < 12 yr of age, and probably rare in infants.

References:

1. Alifimoff JK, Cote CJ: Regional anesthesia. In *A Practice of Anesthesia for Infants and Children.* Cote CJ, Ryan JF, Todres ID, Goudsouzian NG, eds. WB Saunders, Philadelphia: 1993, 429-49.
2. Sethna NF, Berde CB: Pediatric regional anesthesia. In *Pediatric Anesthesia,* 4th edition. Gregory GA, ed. Churchill Livingstone, NY: 2002, 267-316.
3. Yaster M, Krane E, Kaplan R, Cote C, Lappe D: *The Pediatric Pain and Sedation Handbook.* Mosby-Year Book, St. Louis: 1997.

APPENDIX E: STANDARD PEDIATRIC POSTOPERATIVE PAIN MANAGEMENT

Julie Good and Brenda Golianu

Traditionally, children have been undermedicated for their pain because of difficulty with assessment, concerns for safety, and lack of understanding of the physiologic consequences of untreated pain. Evidence to suggest that it is not only safe, but also 'good medicine' to treat children's procedural pain is increasing. It is now known, for example, that infants have adverse behavioral cardiorespiratory and neuroendocrine responses to pain.[1]

Pain assessment

Unlike most adults, infants and children < 7 yr have difficulty understanding and using a Visual Analog Scale (VAS). A frequently used tool for assessing pain in children 3-7 yr old is the Wong-Baker Faces Scale (Fig E-1). For infants and non-verbal children, observational scales that rely on behavioral and/or physiologic parameters are often used (e.g., the FLACC Pain Scale, Fig E-2, PIPP, NIPS, CHEOPS, CRIES), although the 'gold-standard' of pain measurement is to solicit a direct subjective report from the child whenever possible.

Oral medications

For simple outpatient procedures, such as tonsillectomy, hernia repair, circumcision, or closed reduction of a fracture, a weak oral opiate, in combination with acetaminophen, is appropriate (see chart for dosing examples, p. E-3).

Intravenous medications

PCA: IV PCA can be considered in patients > 5 yr who are expected to remain hospitalized overnight, especially in those who are unlikely to tolerate oral intake in the initial hours after surgery (see initial dosing chart, p. E-3). When the patient begins oral medications, D/C the basal rate but continue to provide the lockout dose for several more h to be sure that the child is tolerating the oral medication.

Adjuvant medications

In addition to opiates, several adjuvant medications are useful in the periop period. **Lorazepam** (Ativan) 0.025 mg/kg iv q 6 h is useful in preventing spasms and lessening fear in an unfamiliar environment. It is important to remember that lorazepam has a half-life of up to 16 h and doses can be additive.

Another useful adjuvant is **ketorolac** (Toradol) 0.5 mg/kg, up to a maximum of 15 mg iv q 6 h, up to 72 h. Ketorolac is not recommended in patients with poor renal function or following surgeries where there is a large bleeding surface or complex bone repair. Ketorolac has been shown to cause delay in bony fusion in animal models, but conflicting information has been presented in humans. It also has been reported to cause acute renal failure with prolonged use. Given these concerns, it is helpful to observe hydration status, Plt count, and Cr, and discuss the use of this medication with the surgical team.

Other adjuvants to consider include **acetaminophen** po (10 mg/kg/dose) or pr (20 mg/kg/dose). An initial loading dose of 30-40 mg/kg pr administration for postop pain may be helpful. **Ibuprofen** 10 mg/kg po dose also may be used. Medications to manage side effects, such as pruritis, N/V, constipation, and respiratory depression are presented in detail on the PCA order form, p. E-4.

Epidural pain management

In children, it is generally considered safer to place epidurals after induction of GA to avoid movement during placement. For children 0-12 mo, a **caudal technique** can be used. The patient is placed in the lateral decubitus position, the caudal anatomy is identified, and an 18 ga iv catheter is used

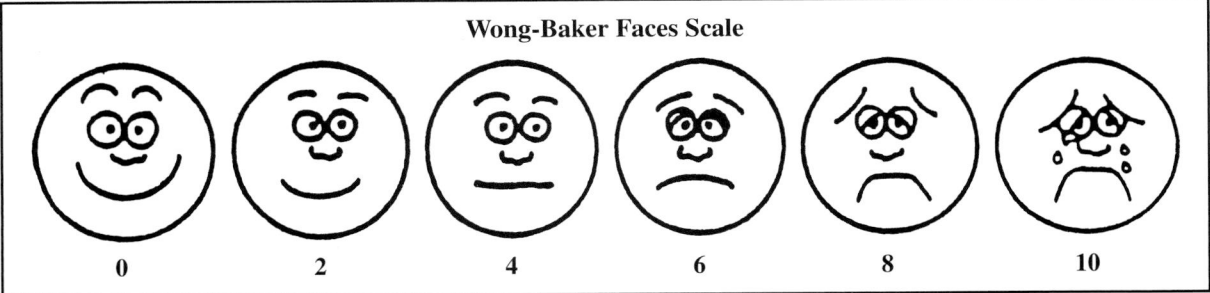

Wong-Baker Faces Scale

| 0 | 2 | 4 | 6 | 8 | 10 |

Fig. E-1. Wong-Baker Faces Scale used in pain assessment in children (and other patients developmentally from 3-7 yr old). The higher the score, the greater the child's pain. (After Wong DL, Baker CM: Pain in children: comparison of assessment scales. *Pediatr Nurs* 1988; 14:9.)

FLACC Pain Scale (For Non-Verbal Patients)			
Categories	**Scoring**		
	0	**1**	**2**
Face	No particular expression or smile	Occasional grimace or frown, withdrawn, disinterested	Frequent-to-constant quivering chin, clenched jaw
Legs	Normal position or relaxed	Uneasy, restless, tense	Kicking, or legs drawn up
Activity	Lying quietly, normal position, moves easily	Squirming, shifting back and forth, tense	Arched, rigid or jerking
Cry	No cry (awake or asleep)	Moans and whimpers; occasional complaint	Crying steadily, screams or sobs, frequent complaints
Consolability	Content, relaxed	Reassured by occasional touching, hugging, or being talked to; distractible	Difficult to console or comfort
Each of the five categories (F) Face, (L) Legs, (A) Activity, (C) Cry, and Consolability is scored from 0-2, which results in a total score between 0 and 10.			

Figure E-2. FLACC Pain Scale for pain assessment in non-verbal patients. By Merkel S, Voepel-Lewis T, Shayevitz JR, Malviya S.

Epidural pain management, cont.

to enter the caudal space. The catheter is advanced and aspirated. The space is then dilated with 5-8 ml of preservative-free NS. A 20 ga epidural catheter is then advanced to the desired location, or until obstruction is felt (~10-15 cm). The catheter is taped securely with a moisture-resistant dressing. A test dose is given (lidocaine 1.5% with 1:200,000 epinephrine; 0.1 ml/kg + 0.8 ml for the dead space of the catheter). **Lumbar** and **thoracic epidurals** can be placed in children > 10-12 mo. **Contraindications** for epidural catheters include infection at the local site, coagulopathy, low Plt, sepsis, progressive neurologic deficit, and refusal of family.

Epidural placement should be checked by syringe aspiration before starting the infusion. Return of any bloody fluid or > 0.5 ml clear aspirant necessitates further evaluation before use of the catheter for pain control. Patients with indwelling epidural catheters may receive postop analgesia with either continuous infusion alone or continuous infusion with intermittent bolus dosing (patient-controlled epidural analgesia [PCEA]). Similar to PCA, PCEA can be used in ages ≥ 5-7 yr. Typical starting infusions are discussed in the table below. Medication doses will depend on patient's age, location of surgical pain, catheter insertion level, and catheter tip location.

A bolus dose equivalent to the hourly volume of infusion may be given when a patient is uncomfortable. Increase the infusion by 10% to maintain the new level of analgesia. Infusion should not exceed 0.3 ml/kg/h in children ≤ 6 mo, or 0.5 ml/kg/h in older patients. If inadequate analgesia persists after 2 dosing increases, it may be appropriate to abandon this form of treatment in favor of systemic analgesia.

References

1. Anand KJ, Carr DB: The neuroanatomy, neurophysiology, and neurochemistry of pain, stress, and analgesia in newborns and children. *Ped Clin North Am* 1989; 36(4):795-822.
2. Williams DG, Patel A, Howard RF: Pharmacogenetics of codeine metabolism in an urban population of children and its implications for analgesic reliability. *Br J Anaesth* 2002; 89(6):839-45.

STANDARD PEDIATRIC POSTOP ANALGESICS AND ANTIEMETICS

Analgesics	Lortab Elixir	7.5 mg Hydro + 500 mg APAP/15 ml	0.15 mgHydro/kg q 6 h (e.g., 1.5 mg ≅ 3 ml for 10 kg child)
	Vicodin	5 mg Hydro + 500 mg APAP/TAB	⎫ Dose based on maximum acetaminophen
	Lorcet	10 mg Hydro + 650 mg APAP/TAB	⎬ allowed for weight (up to 15 mg/kg/dose)
	Norco	10 mg Hydro + 325 mg APAP/TAB	⎭ q 4-6 h, but not to exceed 75 mg/kg/d
	Tylenol #2	15 mg Cod + 300 mg APAP/TAB	
	Tylenol #3	30 mg Cod + 300 mg APAP/TAB	
	Tylenol #4	60 mg Cod + 300 mg APAP/TAB	
	Tylenol with codeine elixir	12 mg Cod + 120 mg APAP/5 ml	0.5-1 mg/kg Cod q 6 h (e.g., 5-10 ≅ mg 2-4 ml for 10 kg child)

Hydro = Hydrocodone; APAP = Acetaminophen; Cod = Codeine

Antiemetics	Metoclopramide*	0.1 mg/kg, may repeat × 1 iv
	Ondansetron	0.1 mg/kg iv

*NB: Increased incidence of extrapyramidal reactions.

Notes:

Codeine preparations are not recommended as a first-line analgesic because a substantial portion of the population cannot convert codeine to morphine, an action that is necessary to derive analgesic effect from the drug.

To prevent irreversible liver damage, it is important to D/C or supervise all other use of acetaminophen when prescribing the above medications, so as not to exceed the maximum dose of 75 mg/kg/d acetaminophen.

PATIENT-CONTROLLED IV ANALGESIA (PCA)

In a setting with trained nursing supervision, PCA can be used safely by children ≥ 5 yr old (about the age they are able to play video games). The lockout time usually is set at 10 min, but can be as short as 5 min for fentanyl. Common PCA medications and recommended starting doses in opiate-naive patients are listed below.

Common PCA Medications

Medication	Loading dose	Basal Rate	Patient-controlled bolus
Morphine (1 or 5 mg/ml)	0.03 mg/kg	0.01 mg/kg/h	0.02-0.03 mg/kg
Hydromorphone (100 μg/ml)	5 μg/kg	1 μg/kg/h	2 μg/kg
Fentanyl (50 μg/ml)	0.3 μg/kg	0.1 μg/kg/h	0.2-0.3 μg/kg

Continuous iv infusion: When PCA is not practical (e.g., in children unable to understand PCA), continuous iv infusion of opiates may be used. Morphine infusion of 10-30 μg/kg/h results in serum concentrations of 10-22 ng/ml and provides adequate analgesia. A common technique is to initiate iv morphine infusion with 1 mg/kg of morphine in 100 ml of D5W at 1 ml/h (the effective infusion rate is 10 μg/kg/h); the infusion rate is slowly increased to provide adequate pain relief.

Typical Orders for IV PCA are on p. E-4.

TYPICAL ORDERS FOR PATIENT-CONTROLLED IV ANALGESIA (PCA)

Patient's Name: _____ Medical Record No.: _____

Weight (kg): _____ Allergies: _____

Drug	Recommended Concentration	Loading Dose	Mode (select one)			PCA Dose	Lockout Interval	Basal Rate
			PCA Only	Continuous	PCA + Continuous			
Morphine	1 mg/ml	0.03 mg/kg*				0.02–0.03 mg/kg*	6–10 min	0.01 mg/kg/h*
Hydromorphine	100 μg/ml	5 μg/kg*				2 μg/kg*	6–10 min	1 μg/kg/h*
Fentanyl	50 μg/ml	0.3 μg/kg*				0.2–0.3 μg/kg*	6–10 min	0.1 μg/kg/h*

Physician: Check all orders that apply: *Recommended starting dose for opiate-naive patients.*

Nursing Care:

❑ 1. For renewed or changed PCA orders only, continue PCA Nursing Care as previously ordered.

❑ 2. Do not administer any other opioids, benzodiazepines, sedatives, or antiemetics unless approved by:
Service _____ Pager No.: _____

☒ 3. Continuous O_2 sat monitor. For SaO_2 < 94%, administer O_2 per nasal cannula to maintain $SaO_2 \geq 94\%$.

☒ 4. Assess and record at least q 2 h: RR, O_2 sat, and level of pain, using appropriate tool.
(0-10 Scale, Wong-Baker Faces Scale, FLACC Scale, or PIPP Scale)

☒ 5. Assess and record at least q 4 h: HR, BP, and T.

☒ 6. Bag and mask at bedside.

❑ 7. Assess for bladder retention. If no void for _____ h (since surgery or last void), may straight cath prn × 2.

Medications:

❑ 1. For renewed or changed PCA orders only, continue prn medications for PCA as previously ordered.

❑ 2. Metoclopramide (Reglan) _____ mg iv q 6 h prn N/V (0.1 mg/kg/dose; max 15 mg).

❑ 3. Ondansetron (Zofran) _____ mg iv q 8 h prn N/V (0.1 mg/kg/dose; max 4 mg).

❑ 4. Diphenhydramine (Benadryl) _____ mg iv q 6 h prn pruritus (0.5 mg/kg/dose; max 50 mg).

❑ 5. Nalbuphine (Nubain) _____ mg iv q 4 h prn pruritus (0.05 mg/kg/dose; max 20 mg).

❑ 6. If no stool by _____ (POD 3), administer:

    ❑ 1 pediatric glycerin suppository pr 1 or 2 × daily prn (ages 2-6 yr).

    ❑ Bisacodyl 5 mg (1/2 suppository) pr daily prn (ages 6-11 yr).

    ❑ Bisacodyl 10 mg (1 suppository) pr daily prn (ages > 11 yr).

    ❑ If no stool within 24 h of beginning treatment, notify physician listed above.

❑ 7. If unable to arouse or SaO_2 < 85%, turn off PCA pump, administer O_2 and/or ambu-bag, stimulate patient, administer naloxone _____ mg (0.001 mg/kg) q 1-2 min (obtain naloxone from floor stock) as needed to restore LOC, and STAT page physician.

❑ 8. Other medications: _____

Date:	Time:	Physician's Signature:	Pager:	Noted by:		Date/Time:
Orders signed				RN:		Date/Time:

POSTOPERATIVE EPIDURAL ANALGESIA

Patients with indwelling epidural catheters may receive postop analgesia with either continuous infusion alone or continuous infusion with intermittent bolus-dosing (patient-controlled epidural analgesia [PCEA]). The infusate may be either local anesthetic with an opioid, local anesthetic alone, or opioid alone. At Stanford, the most commonly used epidural infusate for continuous infusion is bupivacaine 0.1% with hydromorphone 3 μg/ml. In patients receiving PCEA, bupivacaine 0.1% with hydromorphone 25 μg/ml is often used (see Typical Orders for Continuous Epidural Analgesia and Epidural PCA, pp. E-7, E-6).

At Stanford, patients receiving epidural analgesia are managed by the Pediatric Pain Service.

Hydromorphone (Dilaudid): The usual bolus dose is 10 μg/kg, although a reduced dose may be given when the epidural catheter tip is near the level of the incision. The duration of action is 6-12 h.

When opioid epidural analgesia is indicated, hydromorphone is most commonly used because:

(a) It causes less itching and nausea, compared with morphine.

(b) It is more water soluble than fentanyl (therefore, ↑ spread, ↓ systemic absorption).

(c) It is less water soluble than morphine (thereby minimizing late respiratory depression).

STARTING DOSES FOR EPIDURAL INFUSION

Age	Starting dose
0-6 mo	hydromorphone 3 μg/ml + 0.1% bupivacaine @ 0.1-0.15 ml/kg/h
6 mo-3 yr	hydromorphone 3 μg/ml + 0.1% bupivacaine @ 0.1-0.15 ml/kg/h
3-7 yr	hydromorphone 3-5 μg/ml + 0.1% bupivacaine @ 0.1-0.15 ml/kg/h
≥ 7 yr	hydromorphone 5-10 μg/ml + 0.1% bupivacaine @ 0.1-0.15 ml/kg/h + 0.05 ml/kg/h PCEA dose q 30 min lockout

Notes:

In general, use a lower concentration of opiate infusion for neonates and, when spread is desired (for surgeries with incisions that cross multiple dermatomes or when catheter placement is below the level of anticipated pain), a higher concentration in larger adolescents or in epidurals located in the thoracic/upper lumbar region.

References

1. Alifimoff JK, Cote CJ: Pediatric regional anesthesia. In *A Practice of Anesthesia for Infants and Children*. Cote CJ, Ryan JF, Todres ID, Goudsouzian NG, eds. WB Saunders, Philadelphia: 1993, 429-49.
2. Yaster M, Krane E, Kaplan R, Cote CJ, Lappe D: *The Pediatric Pain and Sedation Handbook*. Mosby-Year Book, St. Louis: 1997.

TYPICAL ORDERS FOR CONTINUOUS EPIDURAL ANALGESIA

Patient's Name: _____ Medical Record No.: _____

Weight (kg): _____ Allergies: _____

Drug and Concentration (*Check one*)	Basal Rate (0.15 ml/kg/h) (maximum 0.3 ml/kg/h for 0-6 mo)
❏ Hydromorphone 3 µg/ml with bupivacaine 0.1% →	Epidural infusion rate _____ ml/hr
❏ Hydromorphone 3 µg/ml with bupivacaine 0.1% → **and** Clonidine 0.5 µg/ml	Epidural infusion rate _____ ml/hr
❏ Hydromorphone 3 µg/ml with chirocane 0.1% →	Epidural infusion rate _____ ml/hr

Physician: Check all orders that apply:

Nursing Care:

❏ 1. Do not administer any other opioids, benzodiazepines, sedatives, or antiemetics unless first approved by Pain Management Service.

☒ 2. Maintain iv access until epidural catheter D/C'd.

☒ 3. Check epidural site q d and notify Pain Management Service if site is soiled, red, or tender.

☒ 4. Check lower extremities q 8 h while awake, and notify Pain Management if numbness or weakness exist.

☒ 5   Continuous O_2 sat monitor. For $SaO_2 < 94\%$, administer O_2 per nasal cannula to maintain $SaO_2 \geq 94\%$.

☒ 6. Assess and record at least q 2 h: RR, O_2 sat, and level of pain, using appropriate tool.
(0-10/Numeric Scale, Wong-Baker Faces Scale, FLACC Scale, or PIPP Scale)

☒ 7. Assess and record at least q 4 h: HR, BP. Check orthostatic BP before ambulating.

☒ 8. Assess for bladder retention. If no void for _____ h (since surgery or last void) may straight cath prn × 2.

☒ 9. Bag and mask at bedside.

Medications:

❏ 1. Metoclopramide (Reglan) _____ mg iv q 6 h prn N/V (0.1 mg/kg/dose; max 15 mg).

❏ 2. Ondansetron (Zofran) _____ mg iv q 6 h prn N/V (0.1 mg/kg/dose; max 4 mg).

❏ 3. Diphenhydramine (Benadryl) _____ mg iv q 6 h prn pruritus (0.5 mg/kg/dose; max 50 mg).

❏ 4. Nalbuphine (Nubain) _____ mg iv q 4 h prn pruritus (0.05 mg/kg/dose; max 20 mg).

❏ 5. If no stool by _____ (POD 3), administer:
   ❏ 1 pediatric glycerin suppository pr 1-2 × daily prn (2-6 yr).
   ❏ Bisacodyl 5 mg (½ suppository) pr daily prn (6-11 yr).
   ❏ Bisacodyl 10 mg (1 suppository) pr daily prn (> 11 yr).
   ❏ If no stool within 24 h of beginning treatment, notify physician listed above.

❏ 6. If unable to arouse or SaO_2 is < 85%, turn off PCA pump, administer O_2 and/or ambu-bag, stimulate patient, administer naloxone (Narcan) _____ mg (0.001 mg/kg) q 1-2 min (obtain naloxone from floor stock) as needed to restore LOC, and STAT page Pain Management Service.

❏ 7. Other medications: _____

Date: Time: Orders signed	Physician Signature: Pager:	RN Signature: Date/Time:

TYPICAL ORDERS FOR PATIENT-CONTROLLED EPIDURAL ANALGESIA (PCEA)

Patient's Name: _____ Medical Record No.: _____

Weight (kg): _____ Allergies: _____

Drug & Concentration	Mode	Basal Rate*	Epidural PCA Dose*
		(0.1-0.15 ml/kg/h)	(0.05 ml/kg/h)
Hydromorphone 5 μg/ml with bupivacaine 0.1%	PCA + Continuous		
Hydromorphone 10 μg/ml with bupivacaine 0.1%	PCA + Continuous		
Hydromorphone 5 μg/ml with bupivacaine 0.1% **and** Clonidine 0.5 μg/ml	PCA + Continuous		
	PCA + Continuous		

*When using Bupivacaine 0.1%, Basal Rate and Epidural PCA Dose combined may **not** exceed 0.5 ml/kg/h (0.3 ml/kg/h in ≤ 6 mo).

Physician: Check all orders that apply:

Nursing Care:

❑ 1. **For renewed or changed Epidural PCA orders only, continue Epidural PCA Nursing Care as previously ordered.**

☒ 2. Do not administer any other opioids, benzodiazepines, sedatives, or antiemetics unless first approved by Pain Management Service.

☒ 3. Maintain iv access until epidural catheter is D/C'd.

☒ 4. Check epidural site q 8 h while awake, and notify Pain Management Service if site is soiled, red, or tender.

☒ 5. Check lower extremities q 8 h while awake, and notify Pain Management if numbness or weakness exist.

☒ 6. Assess and record at least q 4 h: HR and BP. Check orthostatic BP before ambulating.

☒ 7. Assess and record at least q 2 h: RR, SaO_2, and level of pain, using appropriate tool.
(0-10 Scale, Wong-Baker Faces Scale, FLACC Scale, or PIPP Scale)

☒ 8. Bag and mask at bedside.

☒ 9. Continuous O_2 sat monitor. For SaO_2 < 94%, administer O_2 per nasal cannula to maintain SaO_2 ≥ 94%.

❑ 10. Assess for bladder distention. If no void for _____ h (since surgery or last void), may straight cath prn × 2.

☒ 11. For any pain management issues, notify Pain Management Service.

Medications:

❑ 1. **For renewed or changed Epidural PCA orders only, continue prn medications for Epidural PCA as previously ordered.**

❑ 2. If unable to arouse or SaO_2 < 85%, D/C infusion, administer O_2 and/or ambu-bag, stimulate patient, administer naloxone _____ mg iv (0.001 mg/kg) q 1-2 min (obtain naloxone from floor stock), as needed, to restore LOC, and **STAT page** Pain Management.

❑ 3. Metoclopramide (Reglan) _____ mg iv q 6 h prn N/V (0.1 mg/kg/dose; max 15 mg).

❑ 4. Ondansetron (Zofran) _____ mg iv q 8 h prn N/V (0.1 mg/kg/dose; max 4 mg).

❑ 5. Diphenhydramine (Benadryl) _____ mg iv q 6 h prn pruritus (0.5 mg/kg/dose; max 50 mg).

❑ 6. Nalbuphine (Nubain) _____ mg iv q 4 h prn pruritus (0.05 mg/kg/dose).
(Use communication slip to order a dose from pharmacy when needed.)

❑ 7. If no stool by _____ (POD 3), administer:
    ❑ 1 pediatric glycerin suppository pr once or twice daily prn (ages 2-6 yr)
    ❑ Bisacodyl 5 mg (½ suppository) pr daily prn (ages 6-11 yr)
    ❑ Bisacodyl 10 mg (1 suppository) pr daily prn (ages > 11 yr)
    ❑ If no stool within 24 h of beginning treatment, notify Pain Management Service.

❑ 8. When Epidural PCA is D/C'd, D/C all prn medications for Epidural PCA.

❑ 9. Other Medications: _____

Date:	Time:	Physician Signature:	Pager:	Noted by:	Date/Time:
Orders signed				RN Signature:	Date/Time:

APPENDIX F: TABLE OF DRUG INTERACTIONS

Sandra Leigh Bardas

This table is intended only as an advisory overview of potential interactions between various drug classes that patients may be taking preop and the drugs used in anesthetic practice. It is not intended to be a comprehensive list. In view of the constant flow of new drug information, the reader is strongly urged to check the primary literature of each drug and tailor drug usage to the specific clinical situation. An excellent source for the predictive values of drug interactions due to altered metabolism include references for inhibitors, inducers, and substrates of the Cytochrome P450 Enzymes.

Preop Drug or Drug Class	Anesthetic Drug or Drug Class	Interaction	Clinical Management
Albuterol	inhalation anesthetics	↑risk of dysrhythmia	Monitor rhythm.
Alteplase	nitroglycerin	Impaired thrombolytic effect	Avoid combination.
Aminoglycosides	succinylcholine	↑depolarizing blockade	Delay administration of aminoglycoside for as long as possible after recovery. Support respiration.
	fluorinated inhalation agents	↑potential for nephrotoxicity 2° to fluoride	Monitor renal function postop.
	NMR (nondepolarizing muscle relaxants)	↑blockade, possible prolonged respiratory depression	Support respiration.
Amiodarone	fentanyl	↓HR, ↓BP, sinus arrest	Monitor hemodynamic function. Administer inotropic, chronotropic, and pressor agents as indicated. Large doses of vasopressors may be required. Bradycardia usually not responsive to atropine.
	inhalation anesthetics	Enhanced myocardial depression and conduction defects	Monitor HR and rhythm.
Amphetamines	opiate agonists	↑analgesia	Titrate dose of opiate.
Amphotericin B	NMR	↑toxicity 2° to hypokalemia	Monitor K^+.
Antacids	oral medications	Delayed drug absorption 2° to delayed gastric emptying	Avoid administration within 2 h of each other.
Antibiotics, polypeptide (bacitracin, capreomycin, colistmethate, polymixin B)	NMR	↑blockade, possible prolonged respiratory depression	Support respiration.

Preop Drug or Drug Class	Anesthetic Drug or Drug Class	Interaction	Clinical Management
Anticholinergics, including drugs with an anticholinergic adverse effect profile	opiate agonists	Potential for central or peripheral anticholinergic syndrome	Monitor for effects.
Anticholinesterases	succinylcholine	Blockade may be prolonged or antagonized	Monitor for therapeutic effect.
Anticholinesterases (including ophthalmics)	NMR	↓blockade	Titrate dose of NMR to therapeutic effect.
Anticholinesterase inhibitors, cholinergic agents (tacrine, donepezil)	succinylcholine	↑blockade	Titrate to therapeutic effect. Monitor and support respiration.
Aprotinin	NMR	Prolonged or recurring apnea	Monitor respiratory status.
Azathioprine	NMR	May ↓ or reverse blockade	Titrate NMR to therapeutic effect.
Azithromycin	alfentanil	↑effect of alfentanil	Titrate dose of alfentanil. Monitor and support respiration.
Azole antifungal agents	alfentanil	Inhibition of alfentanil metabolism	Monitor for respiratory depression. Consider lower dosage.
	midazolam	Prolonged CNS depression	Titrate midazolam to effect. Consider lower dosage
Barbiturate anesthetics	opiate agonists	Synergy	Monitor for CNS depression.
Barbiturates	inhalation anesthetics	↑respiratory depression	Monitor and support respiration.
	ketamine	↑respiratory depression	Monitor and support respiration.
	opiate agonists	↑respiratory depression	Monitor and support respiration.
Benzodiazepines	opiate agonists	↓BP	Monitor and support BP.
	NMR	May prolong or antagonize blockade	Monitor and support respiration.
	barbiturates	Synergy	Titrate doses.

Preop Drug or Drug Class	Anesthetic Drug or Drug Class	Interaction	Clinical Management
Benzodiazepines, cont.	bupivacaine	Sz threshold raised, masking signs of toxicity	Monitor for symptoms of bupivacaine toxicity.
β-adrenergic agonist	anticholinesterase inhibitors (central)	↓BP + ↓HR	Monitor HR and BP.
	inhalation anesthetics	Potentiation of cardiovascular effects	Monitor BP, HR, rhythm.
β-blockers	NMR	May prolong or antagonize blockade	Monitor and support respiration.
	lidocaine	↓lidocaine clearance	Infuse slowly to prevent high peak levels.
	epinephrine	↑BP + ↓HR	Avoid combination. Consider discontinuation of nonselective β-blocker 3 d preop.
Botulinum toxins	NMR	↑blockade	Titrate NMR to therapeutic effect.
Bupivacaine	chloroprocaine	Enhanced bupivacaine toxicity	**Avoid combination!**
Calcium channel blockers	fentanyl	↓BP	Monitor and support BP.
	NMR	↑blockade	Titrate NMR to therapeutic effect.
	inhalation anesthetics	↑potential for cardiovascular depression → ↓BP, ↓HR, asystole	Monitor and support cardiovascular function.
	dantrolene	Can precipitate hyperkalemia and cardiovascular collapse	Avoid combination.
Calcium channel blockers (diltiazem)	alfentanil	↑anesthetic effect.	Monitor and support respiration.
Carbamazepine	NMR	↓blockade	Titrate NMR to therapeutic effect.
	diltiazem, verapamil	Potential for CNS toxicity	Monitor for symptoms of CNS toxicity.
	midazolam	↓effect of midazolam due to enzyme induction	Titrate midazolam to effect.
Cimetidine	lidocaine	↑potential for lidocaine toxicity	Monitor for Sx.

Preop Drug or Drug Class	Anesthetic Drug or Drug Class	Interaction	Clinical Management
Cimetidine, cont.	opiate agonists	↑CNS depression	Monitor and support respiration.
	succinylcholine	↑blockade	Titrate to therapeutic effect. Monitor and support respiration.
Clarithromycin	alfentanil, fentanyl	↑effect of opiate	Titrate dose of opiate. Monitor and support respiration.
	midazolam	↑CNS depression	Titrate dose of midazolam.
Clindamycin	NMR	↑blockade	Avoid combination if possible. Monitor and support respiration. Anticholinesterases or Ca⁺⁺ may be beneficial.
Clonidine	esmolol	Attenuation or reversal of anti-hypertensive effect	Monitor BP.
Clonidine, epidural	local anesthetics	Prolonged sensory and motor blockade	Titrate dose of local anesthetics.
Corticosteroids	NMR	Altered effectiveness of blockade	Titrate NMR to therapeutic effect.
	anticholinesterases	Possible antagonism of reversal agents	Monitor and support respiration.
Cyclophosphamide	succinylcholine, mivacurium	↑blockade	Titrate to therapeutic effect. Monitor and support respiration.
Cyclosporine	NMR	↑blockade	Titrate to therapeutic effect. Monitor and support respiration.
Digoxin	esmolol	↑digoxin toxicity	Monitor for symptoms of toxicity.
	NMR	Precipitate new dysrhythmias or potentiate existing dysrhythmias	Monitor rhythm.
	succinylcholine	Precipitate new dysrhythmias or potentiate existing dysrhythmias	Monitor rhythm.
Dobutamine	inhalation anesthetics	Ventricular arrhythmias	Monitor HR and rhythm.
Erythromycin	alfentanil, fentanyl	↑effect of opiate	Titrate dose of opiate. Monitor and support respiration.
	midazolam	↑CNS depression	Titrate dose of midazolam.

Preop Drug or Drug Class	Anesthetic Drug or Drug Class	Interaction	Clinical Management
Esmolol	NMR	↑blockade	Titrate NMR to therapeutic effect.
Estrogens	succinylcholine	↑blockade	Titrate NMR to therapeutic effect.
Ethanol	alfentanil	Chronic alcohol consumption → pharmacodynamic tolerance	Titrate dose of alfentanil.
	barbiturates	Acute ingestion → CNS depression; chronic ingestion → tolerance	Avoid combination as tolerance is unpredictable.
	benzodiazepines	Acute ingestion → CNS depression; chronic ingestion → tolerance	Titrate dose of benzodiazepines.
Fluvoxamine	ropivacaine	Inhibition of CYP1A2 metabolism	Monitor for ropivacaine toxicity.
Furazolidone	sympathomimetics	↑pressor sensitivity due to MAOI activity of furazolidone	**Avoid combination!** In hypertensive crisis, consider phentolamine.
	meperidine	Risk of MAOI/meperidine interaction	**Avoid combination!**
Guanethidine	sympathomimetics	↑direct-acting agents (epinephrine, phenylephrine); ↓indirect-acting agents (ephedrine, dopamine)	Use combination with caution. Titrate dosages. Monitor BP.
Imipenem	NMR	↑blockade	Titrate NMR to therapeutic effect.
Inhalation anesthetics, halogenated	NMR	↑blockade	Titrate dose of both agents.
Isoniazid (INH)	enflurane	Fast acetylators of INH facilitate defluorination of enflurane → high output renal failure	Monitor renal function postop.
	halothane	↑hepatotoxicity	Avoid giving rifampin-INH after halothane anesthesia.
	meperidine	↓BP, ↑CNS depression	Use combination with caution.

Preop Drug or Drug Class	Anesthetic Drug or Drug Class	Interaction	Clinical Management
Ketamine	halothane	↓BP, ↓CO	Use combination with caution.
	NMR	↑blockade	Titrate NMR to therapeutic effect.
Labetolol	inhalation anesthetics	↓BP, possible myocardial depression	Monitor BP.
Lidocaine & other local anesthetics	NMR	Possible ↑blockade	Monitor and support respiration.
Linezolid	meperidine	Risk of MAOI/meperidine interaction	**Avoid combination!**
Lithium	NMR	↑blockade	Titrate NMR to therapeutic effect. Monitor and support respiration.
	succinylcholine	↑blockade	Titrate succinylcholine to therapeutic effect. Monitor and support respiration.
Loop diuretics (including furosemide)	NMR	Blockade may be prolonged or antagonized; possibly dose-dependent, ↓K⁺ → ↑blockade	Titrate NMR to therapeutic effect. Monitor and support respiration.
Macrolide antibiotics, including erythromycin, clarithromycin, azithromycin	NMR	Case reports of potentiation of blockade	Titrate NMR to therapeutic effect. Monitor and support respiration.
Magnesium, parenteral	NMR	↑blockade	Titrate NMR to therapeutic effect. Monitor and support respiration.
Mercaptopurine	NMR	May ↓ or reverse blockade	Titrate NMR to therapeutic effect.
Methyldopa	naloxone	Naloxone may precipitate a mild ↑BP	Monitor BP.
	ephedrine	↓ephedrine effect	Consider alternative pressor agent.
Metoclopramide	succinylcholine	↑blockade	Titrate succinylcholine to therapeutic effect. Monitor and support respiration.
Monoamine oxidase inhibitor (MAOI); selective MAO Type B may have a lower risk	meperidine	Agitation, Sz, diaphoresis, hyperpyrexia, coma, apnea	**Avoid combination!** Although other opiate agonists may not have these associated problems, monitoring is prudent.

Preop Drug or Drug Class	Anesthetic Drug or Drug Class	Interaction	Clinical Management
MAOI, cont.	sympathomimetics (including local anesthetic/epinephrine combinations, and cocaine)	Indirect- or mixed-acting sympatho-mimetic may cause severe HA, hyperpy-rexia, or hypertensive crisis. (Direct-acting sympathomimetics appear to interact minimally.)	**Avoid combination!** Treat ↑BP with phentolamine.
	succinylcholine, mivacurium	↑blockade	Titrate succinylcholine to therapeutic effect. Monitor and support respiration.
Muscle relaxants, skeletal (including methocarbamol)	anticholinesterases	Possible severe muscle weakness	Monitor neuromuscular blockade. Titrate dose of anticholinesterase.
Nifedipine	fentanyl	↓BP with high dose fentanyl	Monitor BP. Titrate dose of fentanyl.
Nitrates, including NTG	pancuronium	↑blockade	Titrate NMR to therapeutic effect. Monitor and support respiration.
Omeprazole	midazolam	Possible enhanced ataxia or sedation due to ↓clearance of midazolam	Monitor for prolonged effect of midazolam.
Opiate agonists	NMBs	↑potential for opiate toxicity	Titrate dose of opiate.
	propofol	↓BP	Titrate dose of each agent.
Oxytocic drugs (including oxytocin, ergotamine, methylergonovine)	sympathomimetics	↑BP 2° to synergistic vasoconstrictive effects	Titrate dosage. Monitor BP.
Phenothiazines	phenylephrine	↓α-adrenergic effects	Use alternative pressor agent.
	opiate agonists	↓analgesic effect	Titrate opiate to effect.
Phenoxybenzamine	local anesthetics	↑absorption of local anesthetic	Titrate dose; possibly add epinephrine to local anesthetic.
Phenytoin (including fosphenytoin)	midazolam	Enzyme induction	Titrate midazolam to effect. May need to ↑ dosage.
	NMR	Reduced duration of blockade	Consider cisatracurium. Titrate NMR to therapeutic effect.
Piperacillin (including piperacillin/ tazobactam sodium)	NMR	↑blockade	Titrate NMR to therapeutic effect. Monitor and support respiration.
Probenecid	thiopental	↑CNS depression	Titrate dose of thiopental.

Preop Drug or Drug Class	Anesthetic Drug or Drug Class	Interaction	Clinical Management
Procaine, procainamide	NMR	↑blockade	Titrate NMR to therapeutic effect. Monitor and support respiration.
	succinylcholine	↑blockade 2° to competition for pseudocholinesterases	Titrate NMR to therapeutic effect. Monitor and support respiration.
Propofol	alfentanil	Alfentanil may enhance the adverse effects of propofol	Monitor for opisthotonos and/or Sz.
	atracurium	Bronchospasm	Anaphylactoid-type reaction
	succinylcholine	↓HR	Monitor HR. Consider atropine premed when propofol precedes succinylcholine.
	vecuronium	↑blockade	Titrate NMR to therapeutic effect. Monitor and support respiration.
Protease inhibitors	fentanyl	↑fentanyl levels due to CYP3A4 enzyme inhibition	Monitor respiration.
	midazolam	↑midazolam levels	Titrate midazolam to effect. Contraindicated with amprenavir and ritonavir.
Quinine, quinidine	NMR	↑blockade	Titrate NMR to therapeutic effect. Monitor and support respiration.
	succinylcholine	↑blockade	Use this combination with caution.
Ranitidine	NMR	Possible resistance to NMR	Titrate dosage. Consider another NMR.
Reserpine	sympathomimetics	↑direct-acting agents; ↓indirect-acting agents	Monitor BP.
Rifampin	halothane	↑risk of hepatotoxicity	Avoid administration of rifampin-INH after halothane anesthesia.
	midazolam	Enzyme induction	Titrate midazolam to effect. May need to ↑ dosage.
	alfentanil	↑clearance of alfentanil	Titrate alfentanil to effect. Increased dosage may be needed.
Selective serotonin reuptake inhibitors (SSRIs)	opiate agonists	Unknown mechanism	Monitor for serotonin syndrome.
	sympathomimetic amines	Potential for serotonin syndrome	Monitor for serotonin syndrome.

Preop Drug or Drug Class	Anesthetic Drug or Drug Class	Interaction	Clinical Management
Selegiline MAO Type B inhibitor	meperidine	Risk of MAOI/meperidine interaction	**Avoid combination!**
Sildenafil	nitrates	Severe ↓↓BP	Half-life of 4 h may be prolonged by drug interactions, renal or hepatic impairment. Avoid combination, especially in elderly.
Succinylcholine	anticholinesterases	↑blockade	Use combination with caution. Titrate NMR to therapeutic effect. Monitor and support respiration.
Tetracycline	NMR	↑blockade	Titrate NMR to therapeutic effect. Monitor and support respiration.
Theophylline	halothane	↑catecholamine-induced dysrhythmias	Use alternative inhalation agent.
	ketamine	Sz	Use combination with caution.
	NMR	Resistance to blockade	Titrate NMR to effect.
	midazolam	↓midazolam effectiveness	Titrate midazolam to effect.
	propofol	Possibly antagonized sedation	Titrate propofol to effect.
Thiazide diuretics	NMR	↑blockade may be 2° to hypokalemia	Correct hypokalemia. Titrate NMR to effect.
Thiopental	succinylcholine	Possible disseminated intravascular coagulation	Use large veins. Flush tubing with saline. Wait 2-3 min between administration.
Thiotepa	NMR	↑blockade	Titrate NMR to therapeutic effect. Monitor and support respiration.
Tricyclic antidepressants	sympathomimetics	↑direct-acting agents; ↓indirect-acting agents	Monitor BP and rhythm. Effect unlikely in dose administered as infiltration with local anesthetics.
	fentanyl	Potentiation of fentanyl	Titrate opiate agonist to effect.
Trimethaphan	NMR	↑blockade	Titrate NMR to therapeutic effect. Monitor and support respiration.
	succinylcholine	↑blockade	**Avoid combination!** Use nitroprusside instead.
Vancomycin	NMR	↑blockade	Titrate NMR to therapeutic effect. Monitor and support respiration.

Preop Drug or Drug Class	Anesthetic Drug or Drug Class	Interaction	Clinical Management
Vancomycin, cont.	succinylcholine	↑blockade	Avoid administering vancomycin in the postanesthesia period.
Verapamil	etomidate	↑respiratory depression, apnea	Monitor and support respiration.
	midazolam	Deep and prolonged sedation	Monitor CNS and respiratory status.
	NMR	↑blockade	Titrate NMR to therapeutic effect. Monitor and support respiration.

HERBAL AGENTS

It may be difficult to accurately predict the potential for drug interactions, because the majority of people neglect to inform health care providers of their consumption of herbal agents, natural remedies, alternative or complimentary medicines, nutritional supplements, and illicit substances. The significance of the potential interaction is also difficult to assess due to variations of botanical species, the different parts of plants that are used, assay of active ingredient(s), and product formulation. Herbs that alter hemostasis should be D/C'd 14 d before surgical, dental, or invasive procedures.

Plant	Precautions for Anesthesia and Surgery
Bilberry (*Vaccinium myrtillus)*	May alter hemostasis.
Black cohosh (*Cimicifuga racemosa*)	Potential for enhanced ↓BP.
Cat's Claw (*Uncaria tomentosa*)	May alter hemostasis.
Cayenne (*Capsicum annum*)	Has biological effect of ↑catecholamine secretion.
Chamomile, German (*Matricaria chamomilla*)	May enhance CNS depression.
Coleus (*Coleus forskohlii*)	May alter hemostasis. Has potential for enhanced ↓BP.
Devil's claw (*Harpagophytum procubens*)	May have chronotropic and inotropic effects. May alter hemostasis.
Dong quai (*Angelica sinensis*)	May alter hemostasis. May cause vasodilation.
Ephedra ma huang (*Ephedra sineca*)	Potent sympathomimetic may cause cardiac arrhythmias.
Evening primrose (*Oenothera biennis*)	May alter hemostasis.
Fenugreek (Trigonella foenum-graecum)	May alter hemostasis.

Plant	Precautions for Anesthesia and Surgery
Feverfew (*Tanacetum parthenium*)	May alter hemostasis.
Fish oils	May alter hemostasis.
Garlic (*Allium sativum*)	May inhibit Plt aggregation; potential for enhanced ↓BP.
Ginger (*Zingiber officinale*)	May → prolonged bleeding time; possible ↑catecholamine secretion; cardioactive in large and prolonged doses.
Ginkgo (*Ginkgo biloba*)	Selective antagonist of Plt aggregation; may cause vasodilation.
Ginseng, American (*Panax quinquefolius*)	May alter hemostasis.
Ginseng, Panax (*Panax ginseng*) root	Dose-dependent effects on BP. May cause tachycardia. May alter hemostasis.
Ginseng, Siberian (*Eleutherococcus senticosus*)	May alter hemostasis. Use barbiturates with caution. May affect BP.
Golden Seal (*Hydrastis Canadensis*)	May alter hemostasis. Potential for enhanced ↓BP and bradycardia.
Grapefruit	Cytochrome P450 (CYP3A4) inhibition. Onset of midazolam may be delayed and action increased.
Grape seed (*Vitis vinifera*)	May alter hemostasis.
Hawthorn (*Crataegus oxyacantha*)	High doses may cause ↓BP & CNS depression.
Kava kava (*Piper methysticum*)	Synergy with midazolam.
Licorice (*Glycyrrhiza glabra*)	May alter hemostasis.
Melatonin	May enhance CNS depressants.
Passion flower (*Passiflora spp*)	Synergy with CNS depressants.
Red clover (*Trifolium pratense*)	May alter hemostasis.
Reishi (*Ganoderma lucidum*)	May alter hemostasis.
Schisandra (*Schizandra chinensis*)	Inducer of Cytochrome P450 enzyme system.
St. John's wort (*Hypericum perforatum*)	May have some MAOI activity. May reduce midazolam levels due to enzyme induction. Delayed emergence from anesthesia with propofol.
Tumeric (*Curcuma longa*)	May alter hemostasis.
Valerian (*Valeriana officinalis*)	Potentially synergistic with opiates & CNS depressants, including thiopental.
Yohimbe (*Corynanthe yohimbe*) (*Pausinystalia yohimbe*)	May cause CNS stimulation. May have cardiovascular effects.

APPENDIX G: SPECIAL CONSIDERATIONS FOR LATEX ALLERGY

Cathy R. Lammers and Alvin Hackel

Sensitization to latex can occur in patients with a Hx of multiple surgical procedures. Repeated exposure to latex → increased risk for Type I IgE-mediated latex allergic reactions and life-threatening anaphylaxis. Patients at risk for latex allergy include those with myelomeningocele and those who have had multiple neurologic, orthopedic, and urologic procedures. Patients with food allergies to kiwi, banana, avocado, and chestnuts have been shown to have cross-reactivity with latex. In these high-risk patients, latex-avoidance protocols are recommended, as this may decrease the incidence of subsequent intraop allergic reactions. Skin-prick tests are available to identify patients with a high titer of IgE to latex, but this is not predictive for the development of an allergic reaction.

Health care workers comprise ~5-10% of latex allergy cases. Occupational exposure can be minimized by avoiding powdered latex gloves and limiting the use of latex-containing gloves. Applying lotion to hands before using latex gloves facilitates the transfer of latex proteins to hands and should be avoided.

Hospitals and ORs have decreased the use of products that contain latex to the extent that some are essentially latex-free. Anesthesia carts can be assembled with latex-free products, reducing the risk of latex sensitization for all patients and negating the need for a special 'latex-free cart.' At the very least, a latex-safe environment is recommended for patients with Hx of myelomeningocele and/or latex allergic reaction. The latex content of commonly used materials can be identified from external labeling, package inserts, or directly from the manufacturers. Even minimal latex exposure (e.g., an injection through a latex port of iv tubing or opening a package of powdered latex gloves) has resulted in anaphylaxis.

Prophylaxis for latex-sensitive patients:

- Prophylaxis consists of diphenhydramine (0.5 mg/kg), ranitidine (0.5 mg/kg iv), and hydrocortisone (1-2 mg/kg iv) q 8 h × 24 h before surgery and 24 h after surgery.
- Consider continuing prophylaxis through the patient's entire hospital admission.
- Prophylaxis is controversial. Some authors recommend it, while others have demonstrated no difference in the incidence of anaphylaxis following prophylactic treatment. Others express concern that prophylaxis may mask the early signs of allergic reaction.

To prepare a latex-safe environment:

- Consider isolation room for preop and postop care.
- Notify OR nurses, anesthesia technicians, and surgical staff of the need for a latex-free room.
- Place a sign on the door stating: 'LATEX-FREE ROOM.'
- Schedule the latex-allergic patient as the first case of the day to minimize the presence of airborne latex particles.
- Set up the room with latex-free materials (e.g., bag, bellows, ECG electrodes, pulse oximeter clip, iv tubing without latex ports, vinyl gloves, vinyl BP cuffs, clear micropore tape).
- Avoid bouffant surgical hair caps and shoe covers that contain latex bands.
- Wrap latex tubing on stethoscope, BP cuff, or tourniquet with Webril or cotton gauze.
- Removal of rubber stoppers from drug vials (instead of withdrawing through the stopper) remains controversial, but probably does not represent a significant allergen exposure.[2]

Diagnosis of anaphylaxis or latex allergy:

- Skin: urticaria at site of contact with latex product or generalized urticaria.
- Respiratory: bronchospasm, wheezing, ↑PIP, ↓O_2 sat, ↓$ETCO_2$.
- Cardiac: ↓BP, ↑HR, cardiac arrest.

Treatment of anaphylaxis:

- 100% O_2 and manually ventilate if needed.
- Epinephrine 0.1-1 μg/kg iv initially, with rapid escalation as needed to support BP.
- Administer iv fluid to ↑ preload and support BP; may require an epinephrine infusion (0.05-0.1 μg/kg/min).
- Consider isoproterenol infusion if resistant to epinephrine.
- Stop administration of any suspected medications and remove latex products. (Instruct surgical staff to change to nonlatex gloves and remove any latex products from surgical field).

- Administer steroids (hydrocortisone 100 mg iv for adults or 2 mg/kg for pediatric patient) and antihistamine (diphenhydramine 50 mg or 0.5 mg/kg iv).
- Continue steroids and diphenhydramine for 24-48 h or until symptoms resolve.
- Consider drawing blood within 2 h of reaction to send for tryptase level (mediator released from mast cells during degranulation).
- Refer patient to allergist to follow up on Dx. Skin prick test or RAST can be performed (after the acute reaction resolves) to specifically test for latex allergy. Neither test is 100% sensitive. Patients with a Hx of latex anaphylaxis should be advised to wear a Medic Alert bracelet.

References

1. ASA Committee for Occupational Health of Operating Room Personnel: Latex allergy considerations for anesthesiologists. 2001. Available at http://www.asahg.org/ProfInfo/latexallergy.html.
2. Blum RH, Rockoff MA, Holzman RS, et al: Overreaction to latex allergy? *Anesth Analg* 1997; 84:467-8.
3. Hamann CP, Kick SA: What the practicing urologist should know about latex allergies. *AUA Update Series* 1994; 13:110-15.
4. Hirshman CA: Latex anaphylaxis. *Anesthesiology* 1992; 77:223-4.
5. Holtzman RS: Clinical management of latex-allergic children. *Anesth Analg* 1997; 85(3):529-33.
6. Holtzman RS: Latex allergy: an emerging operating room problem. *Anesth Analg* 1993; 76:635-41.
7. Michael T, Niggemann B, Moers A, Seidel U, Wahn U, Scheffner D: Risk factors for latex allergy in patients with spina bifida. *Clin Exp Allergy* 1996; 26(8):934-9.
8. Pollard RJ, et al: Latex allergy in the operating room: case report and a brief review of the literature. *J Clin Anesth* 1996; 8(2): 161-7.
9. Porri F, Pradal M, Lemiere C, Birnbaum J, Mege JL, Lanteaume A, Charpin D, Vervloet D, Camboulives J: Association between latex sensitization and repeated latex exposure in children. *Anesthesiology* 1997; 86(3):599-602.
10. Rao AM et al: Syringes and latex allergy. *Anaesthesia* 1997; 52(5):506.
11. Spears FD, et al: Anaesthesia for the patient with allergy to latex. *Anaesth Intensive Care* 1995; 23(5):623-5.
12. Vassallo SA, et al: Allergic reaction to latex from stopper of a medication vial. *Anesth Analg* 1995; 80(5):1057-8.
13. Yunginger JW, Jones RT, Fransway AF, et al: Latex allergen contents of medical and consumer rubber products. *J Allergy Clin Immunol* 1993; 91:241.

APPENDIX H: ACRONYMS AND ABBREVIATIONS

~: approximately
↓BP: hypotension
2°: secondary to

A-a: alveolar-arterial
AAA: abdominal aortic aneurysm
ABC: argon beam coagulator
ABG: arterial blood gas
ACAS: Asymptomatic Carotid
  Atherosclerosis Study
ACE: angiotensin converting enzyme
ACL: anterior cruciate ligament
ACLS: advanced cardiopulmonary
  life support
ACT: activated clotting time
ACTH: adrenocorticotropic hormone
ADH: antidiuretic hormone
  (vasopressin)
AEC: airway exchange catheter
AF: atrial fibrillation
A/G: albumin/globulin
AH: autonomic hyperreflexia
AI: aortic insufficiency
ALCAPA: anomalous left coronary
  artery from pulmonary artery
ALT: alanine amino transferase
  (SGPT)
AOVM: angiographically occult
  vascular malformations
A-P: anterior-posterior
AR: aortic regurgitation
ARDS: adult respiratory distress
  syndrome
AS: aortic stenosis
ASA: American Society of
  Anesthesiologists
ASD: atrial septal defect
AST: aspartate amino transferase
  (SGOT)
ATG: antithymocyte globulin
ATLS: Advanced Trauma Life-
  Support System
AV: arteriovenous
A-V: atrioventricular
AVF: arteriovenous fistula
AVM: arteriovenous malformation
AVN: avascular necrosis
AVR: aortic valve replacement

BAEP: brainstem auditory evoked
  potential
BAER: brain stem auditory evoked
  response
BB: bronchial blocker
BBS: bilateral breath sounds

BD: balloon dilation
BE: base excess
β-HCG: β-human chorionic
  gonadotrophin
BMI: body mass index
BMR: basal metabolic rate
BNCU: chemotherapy agent
BOR: branchio-oto-renal (syndrome)
BP: blood pressure
BPD: bronchopulmonary dysplasia
BPF: bronchopleural fistula
bpm: beats per minute
BRCA: breast cancer gene
BSA: body surface area
BSO: bilateral salpingo-
  oophorectomy
B-T: Blalock-Taussig (operation)
BUN: blood urea nitrogen
BVH: biventricular hyperplasia
Bx: biopsy

C-section: cesarean section
C-spine: cervical spine
Ca^{++}: calcium
CABG: coronary artery bypass
  graft(ing)
CAD: coronary artery disease
CAH: congenital adrenal hyperplasia
CAJ: cricoarytenoid joint
CBC: complete blood count
CBF: cerebral blood flow
CBV: cerebral blood volume
CCAM: congenital cystic adenoid
  malformation
CCU: coronary care unit
CD: Chrohn's disease
CDDP: combination of
  chemotherapy agents
CDH: congenital diaphragmatic
  hernia
CEA: carotid endarterectomy
CHD: congestive heart disease
CHF: congestive heart failure
CI: cardiac index
CK: creatinine kinase
CLO: congenital lobar
  overdistension
cm: centimeter
CMC: carpometacarpal (joint)
cmH_2O: centimeters of water
$CMRO_2$: cerebral O_2 consumption
CN: cranial nerve
CNS: central nervous system
CO: cardiac output
CO_2: carbon dioxide

COPD: chronic obstructive
  pulmonary disease
CP: cerebral palsy
CPAP: continuous positive airway
  pressure
CPB: cardiopulmonary bypass
CPD: citrate-phosphate-dextrose
CPK: creatinine phosphokinase
CPM: continuous passive motion
CPP: cerebral perfusion pressure
CPR: cardiopulmonary resuscitation
Cr: creatinine
CRI: chronic renal insufficiency
CRT: cardiac resynchronization
  therapy
CSE: combined spinal-epidural
CSF: cerebrospinal fluid
CSI: cranial spinal irradiation
CT: computed tomography
CTR: carpal tunnel release
CTS: carpal tunnel syndrome
CUSA: Cavitron ultrasonic aspirator
CV: cardiovascular
CVA: cerebrovascular accident
CVP: central venous pressure
CXR: chest x-ray

d: day(s)
D5W: dextrose 5% in water
D&C: dilation and curettage
D&E: dilation and evacuation
DBP: diastolic blood pressure
DC: direct current
D/C: discontinue
DCR: dacryocystorhinostomy
DDAVP: desmopressin acetate
DFT: defibrillation threshold
DHCA: deep hypothermic cardiac
  arrest
DI: diabetes insipidus
DIC: disseminated intravascular
  coagulation
DIP: distal interphalangeal (joint)
DJD: degenerative joint disease
DKA: diabetic ketoacidosis
dL: deciliter(s)
DL: direct laryngoscopy
DL_{CO}: carbon monoxide diffusion
  capacity
DLT: double lumen tube
DM: diabetes mellitus
DO_2: oxygen delivery
DOE: dyspnea on exertion
DORV: double outlet right ventricle
DP: dorsalis pedis

DPG: diphosphoglycerate angiography
dTC: d-tubocurarine
DTR: deep tendon reflex
DVT: deep venous thrombosis
Dx: diagnosis

EA: esophageal atresia
EAC: endoaortic clamp catheter
EACA: epsilon aminocaproic acid
EARC: endoaortic return cannula
EB: epidermolysis bullosa
EBL: estimated blood loss
EBV: estimated blood volume
EC-IC: extracranial-intracranial
ECG: electrocardiogram
ECHO: echocardiogram
ECMO: extracorporeal membrane oxygenation
ECT: electroconvulsive therapy
ED: emergency department
EDAS: encephaloduro-arteriosynangiosis
EEA: end-to-end anastomosis
EEG: electroencephalogram
EF: ejection fraction
EJ: external jugular
EMG: electromyogram
EMLA: eutectic mixture of local anesthetic
ENT: ear-nose-throat
EP: evoked potentials
EPS: electrophysiologic studies
EPV: endopulmonary vent
ER: emergency room
ERCP: endoscopic retrograde cholangiopancreatography
ERV: expiratory reserve volume
ESC: endocoronary sinus catheter
ESLD: end-stage liver disease
ESRD: end-stage renal disease
ESS: endoscopic sinus surgery
ET: endotracheal
ETCO$_2$: end tidal CO$_2$
ETN$_2$: end tidal N$_2$
ETOH: alcohol
ETT: endotracheal tube
EVD: endovascular drain (extraventricular catheter)

FAP: familial adenomatous polyposis
FAST scan: focussed assessment by sonography for trauma
FB: foreign bodies
FDP: flexor digitorum profundus (tendon)
FDS: flexor digitorum superficialis (tendon)

FDT: forced duction test
FESS: functional endoscopic sinus surgery
FEV$_1$: forced expiratory volume (in 1 sec)
FFP: fresh-frozen plasma
FHR: fetal heart rate
FIGO: International Federation of Gynecologists & Obstetricians
FiO$_2$: fraction of inspired oxygen
FNA: fine needle aspiration
FOB: fiber optic bronchoscopy
FOI: fiber optic intubation
FOL: fiber optic laryngoscopy
Fr: French (size)
FRC: functional residual capacity
FSP: fibrin-split products
FTSG: full-thickness skin graft
FTT: failure to thrive
FVC: forced vital capacity

g: gram(s)
ga: gauge
GA: general anesthesia
GCS: Glasgow coma scale
GE: gastroesophageal
GERD: gastroesophageal reflux disease
GETA: general endotracheal anesthesia
GFR: glomerular filtration rate
GGTP: liver enzyme
GH: growth hormone
GI: gastrointestinal
GIA: gastrointestinal anastomosis
GIFT: gamete intrafallopian transfer
GM-CSF: granulocyte macrophage colony-stimulating factor
Gn-RH: gonadotropin-releasing hormone
GSW: gunshot wound
GTD: gestational trophoblastic disease
GU: genitourinary

h: hour(s)
HA: headache
H&P: history and physical examination
Hb: hemoglobin
Hb/Hct: hemoglobin/hematocrit
HbA: adult hemoglobin
HbF: fetal hemoglobin
HCC: hepatocellular carcinoma
HCG: human chorionic gonadotropin
HCO$_3$: bicarbonate
Hct: hematocrit
HD: Hirschprung's disease

HELLP: hemolysis, elevated liver enzymes, and low-platelet count
HFV: high-frequency ventilation
Hg: mercury
HIV: human immune deficiency virus
HLHS: hypoplastic left heart syndrome
HM: hyoid myotomy
Ho:YAG: holmium-yag laser
HPV: hypoxic pulmonary vasoconstrictive (reflex)
HR: heart rate
HSV: highly selective vagotomy
HTN: hypertension
HVA: homovanillic acid
Hx: history

IABP: intraaortic balloon pump
IBD: inflammatory bowel disease
IC: inspiratory capacity
ICD: implantable cardioverter-defibrillator
ICP: intracranial pressure
ICU: intensive care unit
ID: inside diameter
I:E: inspiratory: expiratory
IgE: immunoglobin E
IHSS: idiopathic hypertrophic subaortic stenosis
I.I.: image intensifier
IIC: intermediate intensive care
IJ: internal jugular (vein)
im: intramuscular
IMA: internal mammary artery
IMF: intermaxillary fixation
iMRI: interventional magnetic resonance imaging
INH: isonicotinic acid (isoniazid)
INR: International Normalized Ratio
IOFB: intraocular foreign body
IOL: intraocular lens
IOP: intraocular pressure
IORT: intraoperative radiation therapy
IPAA: ileal pouch anal anastomosis
IPG: implantable generator
IPPV: intermittent positive pressure ventilation
IRDS: infant respiratory distress syndrome
ISS: injury severity score
IT: iliotibial
ITP: idiopathic thrombocytopenic purpura
IUP: intrauterine pressure
iv or IV: intravenous
IVC: inferior vena cava

IVF: in vitro fertilization
IVH: intraventricular hemorrhage
IVP: intravenous pyelogram
IVS: intact ventricular septum

J: Joule
JET: junctional ectopic tachycardia
JI: jejunoileal
JVD: jugular venous distention

K⁺: potassium
KCl: potassium chloride
kg: kilogram(s)

L: liter
LA: left atrium
LAD: left anterior descending
LAE: left atrial enlargement
LAP: left atrial pressure
LAVH: laparoscopy-assisted vaginal hysterectomy
LBBB: left bundle branch block
LDH: lactate dehydrogenase
LE: lower extremity
LEEP: loop electrosurgical excision procedure
LFT: liver function test
LGL: Lowen-Ganong-Levine (syndrome)
LH-RH: luteinizing hormone-releasing hormone
LHSV: laparoscopic highly selective vagotomy
LIMA: left internal mammary artery
LINAC: linear accelerator
LLETZ: large loop excision of transitional zone
LLQ: left lower quadrant
LMA: laryngeal mask airway
LMG: laser midline glossectomy
LMP: last menstrual period
LP: lumbar puncture
LR: lactated Ringer's (solution)
LRD: living related donor
LSC: laparoscope approach
LTA: lidocaine tracheal anesthesia
LUQ: lower left quadrant
LV: left ventricle/ventricular
LVAD: left ventricular assist device
LVEDP: left ventricular end-diastolic pressure
LVEF: left ventricular ejection fraction
LVH: left ventricular hypertrophy
LVOT: left ventricular outflow tract
LVOTO: left ventricular outflow tract obstruction
LVRS: lung volume reduction surgery

m: meter(s)
M: molar
MAC: monitored anesthesia care
MAGPI: meatal advancement granuloplasty
MAO-B: monoamine oxidase-B
MAOI: monoamine oxidase inhibitor (antidepressant)
MAP: mean arterial pressure
MAPCAS: major aortopulmonary collaterals
MCA: middle cerebral artery
MCKD: multicystic kidney dysplasia
MDI: multidirectional instability
MEA: multiple endocrine adenopathy
MED: microendoscopic lumbar discectomy
MEN: multiple endocrine neoplasia
MEP: motor-evoked potential
mEq: milliequivalent
mEqK⁺: milliequivalency of potassium
metHb: methemoglobin
mg: milligram(s)
Mg⁺⁺: magnesium
MgSO₄: magnesium sulfate
MH: malignant hyperthermia
MI: myocardial infarction
MICAB: minimally invasive coronary artery bypass
MICABG: minimally invasive coronary artery bypass graft(ing)
µg: microgram(s)
MIDCAB: minimally invasive direct coronary bypass
MIDCABG: minimally invasive direct coronary bypass graft(ing)
MIF: maximum inspiratory force
min: minute(s)
ml: milliliter(s)
MLT: microlaryngeal tube
mm: millimeter(s)
MMEF₂₅₋₇₅: maximum mid-expiratory force
mmHg: millimeters of mercury
mo: month(s)
MOGA: mandibular osteotomy and genioglossal advancement
MR: mitral regurgitation
MRA: magnetic resonance angiography
MRI: magnetic resonance imaging
MRT: magnetic resonance-guided therapy
MS: mitral stenosis
MSRA: methicillin-resistant staphylococcus aureus

MUF: modified ultrafiltration
MUGA: multi-unit gated acquisition (scan)
MUPIT: Martinez Universal Perineal Interstitial Template
MV: minute ventilation
MVA: motor vehicle accident
MVD: microvascular decompression
MVO₂: mixed venous oxygen content
MVP: mitral valve prolapse

Na⁺: sodium
NaHCO₃: sodium bicarbonate
NB: nota bene (note well)
Nd:YAG: neodymium-yag laser
NEC: necrotizing enterocolitis
ng: nanogram(s)
NG: nasogastric (tube)
NIBP: noninvasive blood pressure
NICU: neonatal intensive care unit
NIF: negative inspiratory force
nl: normal
NLD: nasolacrimal duct
NMB: neuromuscular blocker
NMR: nondepolarizing muscle relaxant
NO: nitric oxide
NOE: naso-orbital ethmoid
NPH: neutral protamine Hagedorn (insulin)
npo: nothing by mouth
NS: normal saline (solution)
NSAID: nonsteroid anti-inflammatory drug
NS/LR: normal saline/lactated Ringer's (solution)
NSR: normal sinus rhythm
NTE: not to exceed
NTG: nitroglycerin
NTP: nitroprusside
N₂O: nitrous oxide
N/V: nausea & vomiting

OA: osteoarthritis
OATS: osteochondral autograft transfer system
OCR: oculocardiac reflex
OD: outside diameter
OEIS: omphalocele extrophy imperforate anus spinal defect
OG: orogastric (tube)
OLV: one-lung ventilation
OPCAB: off-pump coronary artery bypass
OPCABG: off-pump coronary artery bypass graft(ing)
OPLL: ossification of the posterior longitudinal ligament

OR: operating room
ORIF: open reduction and internal fixation
ORR: oculorespiratory reflex
OSA: obstructive sleep apnea
O_2: oxygen
O_2 sat: oxygen saturation

P: pulse
PA: pulmonary artery
$PaCO_2$: partial pressure of CO_2 (arterial)
PACU: post anesthesia care unit
PAD: pulmonary artery diastolic
PADP: pulmonary artery diastolic pressure
PAK: pancreas after kidney (transplant)
PAOP: pulmonary artery occlusion pressure
PaO_2: partial pressure of oxygen (arterial)
PAP: pulmonary artery pressure
PAR: postanesthesia room
PAWP: pulmonary artery wedge pressure
PCA: patient-controlled analgesia
PCEA: patient-controlled epidural analgesia
PCL: posterior cruciate ligament
PCO_2: partial pressure of carbon dioxide
PCV: parietal cell vagotomy
PCWP: pulmonary capillary wedge pressure
PDA: patent ductus arteriosus
PDPH: postdural puncture headache
PE: pulmonary embolus
PEEP: positive end-expiratory pressure breathing
PEF: peak expiratory flow
PET: positron emission tomography
$PetCO_2$: end-tidal CO_2 partial pressure
PFNS: preservative-free normal saline
PFO: patent foramen ovale
PFT: pulmonary function test
PGE: prostaglandin E
PICC: peripherally inserted central catheter
PICU: pediatric intensive care unit
PID: pelvic inflammatory disease
PIH: pregnancy-induced hypertension
PIP: peak inspiratory pressure
PKP: penetrating keratoplasty

PLIF: posterior lumbar interbody fusion
Plt: platelet
PND: paroxysmal nocturnal dyspnea
po: by mouth
POC: product of conception
POD: postoperative day
PONV: postoperative nausea & vomiting
POOP: perineal one-stage pullthrough
POPE: postobstructive pulmonary edema
PO_2: partial pressure of oxygen
PPH: postpartum hemorrhage
PPI: proton pump inhaler
ppm: parts per million
PPTL: postpartum tubal ligation
PPV: positive pressure ventilation
pr: per rectum
PRBC: packed red blood cell
prn: as needed
PS: pulmonic stenosis
PSARP: perineal sagittal anorectoplasty
PT: prothrombin time
PTCA: percutaneous transluminal coronary angioplasty
PTM: posterior tibial muscle
PTS: post-tourniquet syndrome
PTT: partial thromboplastin time
PUD: peptic ulcer disease
PUV: posterior urethral ablation
PVA: polyvinyl alcohol
PVB: paravertebral block
PVC: premature ventricular contraction
PVD: peripheral vascular disease
PVOD: pulmonary vascular occlusive disease
PVR: pulmonary vascular resistance

q: every
qd: every day
Q_P/Q_S: pulmonary-to-systemic flow ratio
QRS: QRS complex of ECG
qs: quantum satis (sufficient quantity)

RA: radial artery
RAD: right axis deviation
RAE: right atrial enlargement
RAP: right atrial pressure
RAST: radioallergosorbent test
RBBB: right bundle branch block
RBC: red blood cell
RC: rotator cuff

RCA: right coronary artery
RDS: respiratory distress syndrome
RF: radiofrequency
RFA: radiofrequency ablation
RFT: renal function test
RIND: reversible ischemic neurological deficit
RLQ: right lower quadrant
r/o: rule out
ROM: range of motion
ROP: retinopathy of prematurity
RR: respiratory rate
RSD: reflex sympathetic dystrophy
RSI: rapid-sequence induction
RSV: respiratory syntial virus
RUE: right upper extremity
RUQ: right upper quadrant
RV: right ventricle
RVE: right ventricular enlargement
RVEDP: right ventricular end-diastolic pressure
RVESV: right ventricular end-systolic volume
RVH: right ventricular hypertrophy
RVOT: right ventricular outflow tract
RVOTO: right ventricular outflow tract obstruction
Rx: treatment

SA: sinoatrial (node)
SAB: subarachnoid block
SAD: subacromial decompression
SAH: subarachnoid hemorrhage
SAM: systolic anterior motion
SBE: subacute bacterial endocarditis
SBO: small-bowel obstruction
SBP: systolic blood pressure
sc: subcutaneous
SCD: sequential compression device
SCFE: slipped capital femoral epiphysis
SCT: sacrococcygeal teratoma
sec: second(s)
SGOT: serum glutamic-oxaloacetic transaminase
SGPT: serum glutamate pyruvate transaminase
SI: sacroiliac
SIADH: syndrome of inappropriate antidiuretic hormone
SICU: surgical intensive care unit
sl: sublingual
SLAP: superior labral anterior or posterior
SLE: systemic lupus erythematosus
SLH: subtotal laparoscopic hysterectomy

SMA: superior mesenteric artery
SMV: superior mesenteric vein
SNP: sodium nitroprusside
SOB: short(ness) of breath
S/P: status post
SPK: simultaneous kidney/pancreas (transplant)
SpO$_2$: oxygen saturation measured by pulse oximetry
SSA: sickle cell anemia
SSEP: somatosensory evoked potential
SSRI: selective serotonin reuptake inhibitor
SSS: sick sinus syndrome
S-T: wave of ECG
ST-T: ST-T wave of ECG
STA: superficial temporal artery
STP: sodium thiopental
STSG: split-thickness skin graft
SV: stroke volume
SVC: superior vena cava
S$_v$O$_2$: venous O$_2$ saturation
SVR: systemic vascular resistance
SVT: supraventricular tachycardia
Sx: signs and symptoms
Sz: seizure

T: temperature
T&C: type and cross-match
T&S: type and screen
T/A: tonsillectomy/adenoidectomy
TAAA: thoracoabdominal aortic aneurysm
TAB: therapeutic abortion
TAH: total abdominal hysterectomy
TAPVC: total anomalous pulmonary venous connection
TB: tuberculosis
TBI: total body irradiation
TBSA: total body surface area
TCA: tricyclic antidepressant
TCD: transcranial Doppler
TE: tangential excision
TEA: thromboendarterectomy
TEE: transesophageal echocardiogram(graphy)
TEF: tracheoesophageal fistula
TEG: thromboelastogram
TET: tubal embryo transfer

TGA: transposition of great arteries
TGV: transposition of the great veins
TIA: transient ischemic attack
TID: 3 times per day
TIPS: transjugular intrahepatic portosystemic shunt
TIVA: total intravenous anesthesia
TKO: to keep open
TL: thoracolumbar
TLC: total lung capacity
TLH: total laparoscopic hysterectomy
TLIF: transforaminal interbody fusion
TMJ: temporomandibular joint
TMJD: temporomandibular joint dysfunction
TOF: tetralogy of Fallot, train of force
TPN: total parenteral nutrition
TR: tricuspid regurgitation
TRAM: transverse rectus abdominus muscle (flap)
TSA: total shoulder arthroplasty
TSH: thyroid-stimulating hormone
TT: thrombin time
TTP: thrombotic thrombocytopenic purpura
TUMT: transurethral microwave thermotherapy
TUNA: transurethral needle ablation
TUR: transurethral resection
TURBP: transurethral resection of bladder tumor
TURP: transurethral resection of the prostate
TUVP: transurethral vaporization of the prostate
TV: tidal volume
TVOR: transvaginal oocyte retrieval
TVT: tension-free vaginal tape procedure
TW airway: Tudor-Williams airway
TWR: total wrist replacement
Tx: transplant

U: unit(s)
UA: urinalysis
UAC: umbilical artery catheter
UBC: unicameral bone cyst

UC: ulcerative colitis
UE: upper extremity
UO: urine output
UPJ: ureteropelvic junction
UPPP: uvulopalatopharyngoplasty
URI: upper respiratory infection
US: ultrasound
UTI: urinary tract infection
UVC: umbilical vein catheter
UW: University of Wisconsin (solution)

V&A: vagotomy and antrectomy
V&P: vagotomy and pyloroplasty
VA: ventriculoatrial
VAE: venous air embolism
VALH: vaginally assisted laparoscopic hysterectomy
VAT: video-assisted thoracoscopy
VATS: video-assisted thoracoscopic surgery
VBG: vertical banded gastroplasty
VC: vital capacity
Vd: volume of distribution
VF: ventricular fibrillation
VIP: vasoactive intestinal peptide
VIP-oma: vasoactive intestinal peptide-secreting tumor
VLAP: visual laser ablation of the prostate
VMA: vanillylmandelic acid
VO$_2$: oxygen consumption
VP: ventriculoperitoneal
VPI: velopharyngeal insufficiency
V/Q: ventilation-perfusion ratio
VRE: vancomycin-resistant enterococci
VS: vital signs
VSD: ventricular septal defect
VT: ventricular tachycardia
VUR: vesicoureteral reflux

WBC: white blood cell
WPW: Wolff-Parkinson-White (syndrome)
W/U: work-up

XRT: x-ray therapy

yr: year(s)

SUBJECT INDEX

Note: Page numbers followed by *f* indicate figures.

A

Abbe-Estlander flap for lip/nose
    deformities, 1145-8, 1146*f*
Abdomen, acute, 472-5
Abdominal aorta surgery, 327-31, 328*f*
Abdominal aortic aneurysm, 313-16;
    anesthesia, 327-31
Abdominal compartment syndrome, 582
Abdominal dehiscence repair, 506-9
Abdominal suspension, 654-7
Abdominal trauma, 582-9
    damage control, 582-3
    exploratory/staging laparotomy, 496-9
    hepatic, splenic injuries, 583-4
    vascular injuries, 585-9
Abdominal tumor resection, 1040-3
Abdominal wall defects repair, 1049-53
Abdominal wall laxity, 889-92
Abdominal-transsacral resection, 431-2;
    anesthesia, 436-8
Abdominoplasty, 889-92; anesthesia,
    890-1; flap, incisions, excision, 889*f*
Abortion
    spontaneous, surgery for, 643-7
    therapeutic/D&E, 633-4, 635-6
Abscess
    biopsy, drainage, low extremities, 864
    imaging for, 1174-8
Accucise cutting electro-wires, 697-9
Acetabular augmentation (shelf), 1099-
    1100; anesthesia, 1121-5
Acetabular dysplasia, 802-3, 803*f*, 1007-
    1100
Acetabular growth plate trauma, 812
Acetabular insufficiency, 802-3, 806-8
Acetabulum
    biopsy, abscess drainage, 861-4
    osteomyelitis, septic arthritis, 861
Acetabulum fracture
    repair, 799-801, 800*f*, 801*f*, 901*f*
    ORIF for, 796-797, 799-801, 806-8
Acetaminophen, in pediatric pain
    management, E-1, E-3
Acetazolamide, in ophthalmology, 126
Achalasia, 382-3, 387-90; 458-9, 461-3
Achilles tendon, 835-7; 852
Achondroplasia, 1122
Achondroplastic dwarfism, 144
Acoustic neuroma, 27; 187-92
Acromegaly, 44, 45, 492
Acromial fracture, surgery for, 773-8
Acromial impingement, 762-4, 766-9
Acromioclavicular arthritis, arthroscopic
    surgery, 760-2, 766-9
Acromioclavicular joint
    arthritis, 762-4, 766-9
    separation, 773-4, 776-8
Acromion, hooked, 762-4, 766-9
ACTH, ectopic, in adrenal surgery, 532
ACTH-secreting tumor, 44
Actinomycin D, toxic effects, 598
Addison's disease, 524
    preop testing indications, A-3

Adductor tendon release/transfer, 1103-4;
    anesthesia, 1121-5
Adenocarcinoma, 431-2; 530-5
Adenoid pathology, 226-29; 956-9
Adenoidectomy, 143-6; anesthesia, 144-6
    pediatric, 956-9; anesthesia, 957-8
Adenoma, laparotomy, 640-41, 644-6
    tubular, rectal surgery, 431-2
Adenomyosis, hysterectomy for, 690-3
Adhesions, 415-18; 647-51
Adjuvant medications, in pediatric postop
    pain management, E-1
Adrenal adenoma, adrenalectomy, 530-5
Adrenal gland, 467*f*
    tumor, adrenalectomy for, 530-5
Adrenal hyperplasia, congenital, 1076-8
Adrenal tumor, adrenalectomy for, 530-5
Adrenal vein sampling, 1174
Adrenalectomy, 530-5, anatomy, 530*f*,
    incisions, 531*f*; anesthesia, 533-5
    laparoscopic, 466-9, 467*f*, 531-5, 532*f*;
    anesthesia, 467-8
    pediatric, 1081-2
Adrenocongenital syndrome risk, 1078
Adriamycin, anesthetic concerns, 1198
Adson's approach, 337-8
Aesthetic surgery, 867-94
Aganglionosis, congenital, 1053-6
Ahmed implant (glaucoma), 117
Air embolism, in hysteroscopy, 639
Airway compromise
    in awake pediatric patient, 1023
    management of in trauma, 568-9
    in surgery for sleep disorders, 198
    in thyroidectomy, 525
    in upper respiratory abscess/cyst, 964
Airway control, ABCs, for trauma, 568
Airway, difficult
    in epidermolysis bullosa surgery, 1126
    in pediatric lip/nose surgery, 1147
    in pediatric orthopedics, 1123
Airway edema
    in pediatric lip/nose surgery, 1147
    tracheal resection for, 229
    in tracheobronchial stenting, 1181
Airway emergency preparation, 228
Airway establishment, tracheostomy for,
    182-5; anesthesia, 183-5
Airway exchange catheter (AEC), 85
Airway fire, 150
    in bronchoscopy, esophagoscopy,
    laryngoscopy, 152, 235
    in thoracic laser resection, 239
    in tracheostomy, 185
Airway loss, in imaging procedures, 1177
Airway/lung access conflicts
    in head and neck surgery, 140
    in pediatric otolaryngology, 954
    in thoracic surgery, 206
Airway management
    head and neck surgery, 141, 149
    trauma surgery, 568-9; 589 (pediatric)
Airway obstruction
    in adenoidectomy/tonsillectomy, 958

    bronchoscopy/laryngoscopy for, 959-
    63
    emergency tube thoracostomy, 569-71
    in laryngectomy, 176
    in mandibular surgery, 908
    in maxillofacial surgery, 902
    in out-of-OR XRT, 1191
    in pediatric trauma, 589-90
    in spinal neurosurgery, 86
    in thoracic laser resection, 239
    in tracheobronchial stenting, 1181
    tracheostomy for, 182-5
Airway trauma during intubation, 214
Airway, upper, approaches to, 193-8
Alarplasty, alar reduction, 878-81
Albumin, use in laparotomy for ovarian
    cancer, 600
Albuterol, drug interactions, F-1
Alcohol/drug-induced hepatic disease,
    preop testing indications, A-3
Alcoholic cirrhosis, 547-58
Alcoholic hepatitis, 345-8
Alfentanil, drug interactions with, F-2,
    F-3, F-4, F-5, F-8
All-arterial revascularization, 266
Alteplase, drug interactions, F-1
Alveolar cleft repair, 1144-5, 1147-8
Alveolar microlithiasis, proteinosis, 252-5
Alveolus, neoplastic disease, 177-8
Ambiguous genitalia, 1076-8, 1081-2
Amicar, used in CPB, 265
Aminoglycosides, drug interactions, F-1
Amiodarone, drug interactions, F-1
Amphetamines, drug interactions, F-1
Amphotericin B, drug interactions, F-1
Amputation. *See* specific sites.
Amygdalohippocampectomy, 66-7
Anal fistulotomy/fistulectomy, 433-4;
    anesthesia, 436-8
Anal gland infection, surgery, 433-4
Anal incontinence, in procidentia, 429
Analgesia
    adult emergence, B-4; postop, C-2
    centrally acting, 783
    intrathecal, indwelling system, 61
    multimodality, periop, C-1
    pediatric, E-1-E-7
    preincisional, preemptive, C-1
Anaphylaxis
    in interventional neuroradiology, 1161
    with latex allergy, Dx and Rx, G-1, G-2
Anastomotic leaks, enteric fistulae, 416
Anatomic pulmonary resection, bronchial
    injury, 579-80; anesthesia, 580-2
Anderson and D'Alonzo classification of
    odontoid fractures, 73
Anderson-Heinz pyeloplasty, 709-10;
    anesthesia, 710-12; pediatric, 1069
Anemia
    complications in liver transplant, 553
    hemolytic, 463-6, 497
Anesthesia dolorosa, 109
Anesthetic protocols, standard adult
    pain management, C-1-C-5

perioperative maintenance, B-1-B-6
preoperative, A-1-A-6
Anesthetic protocols, standard pediatric
pain management, perioperative, D-4-
D-5; postoperative, E-1-E-7
perioperative maintenance, D-2-D-5
preoperative, D-1
Aneurysm. Also *see* specific sites.
anterior, posterior circulation, 4-13
cerebral, craniotomy for, 4-13
dissecting, repair, 317-22
endovascular stent-grafting, 313-16
imaging, image-guided, 1174-8
LV, 271, 267-70; in CABG, 268
neuroradiology therapy for, 1156-62
skull base surgery for, 187-92
Angina, preop testing indications, A-3
Angiographically occult vascular
malformation (AOVM), 15-21
Angiography, 1174; pediatric, 1193
Angiomyolipoma, 530-5, 706-11
Angioplasty, pediatric, 1174, 1193-4
Angle classification of mandibular
occlusion, 903f
Aniridia, 1041, 1069
Anisomelia, 1110-11, 1113-15
Ankle
amputation (Syme's), 849-50, 863-4
arthritis, arthrodesis for, 847-8
arthroscopy—portals, anatomy, 845f
arthrotomy, 846-7, 863-4
capsulotomy (posterior), 852
disarticulation with closure, 849-50
fracture, ORIF for, 843, 863-4
fusion, 847-8, 863-4
ligaments, instability, 848-9, 863-4
tendon lengthening/transfer, 851-2
trauma, infection, 849-50, 863-4
arthroscopy for, 845-6, 863-4
Anoplasty, posterior (Parks), for fecal
incontinence, 435-8
Anorectal anatomy, 421f
Anorectal atresia, 408
Anorectoplasty, perineal sagittal, for
imperforate anus, 1056-8
Anotia, otoplasty for, 162-3, 1149-50
Anovulation, laparotomy for, 640-41
Antacids, drug interactions with, F-1
Anterior capsule-labral repair, 760-2
Antibiotic therapy, chronic, permanent
vascular access for, 351-4
Anticholinergic syndrome, 126
Anticholinergics, drug interactions, F-2
Anticholinesterase inhibitors, drug
interactions with, F-2, F-3
Anticholinesterases, drug interactions
with, F-2, F-4, F-7, F-9
Anticoagulants, preop testing, A-3
Anticoagulation reversal, in CPB, 265
Antidepressants commonly used, 1156
Antiemetics; adult, C-2; pediatric, E-3
Antineoplastics, toxic effects, 598, 599
Antinociceptive measures, as preemptive
analgesia, C-1
Antireflux procedure, 458-9, 461-3
Antrectomy and vagotomy, 396-9

Anus, imperforate, 1056-8
Aorta. (Also *see* specific sites.)
ascending
dissections, 317-22, 318-21
rupture, repair, 577-8, 580-2
thoracic, aneurysms, 310-13
descending, lesions, 320
Aortic aneurysms (Also *see* Aneurysm
and specific sites.)
endovascular stent-grafting for, 313-16
Aortic arch injury, repair, 577-8, 580-2
lesions, 320
Aortic atresia, surgery for, 1008-11
Aortic cannulation, in CPB, 262
Aortic coarctation repair, 984-7
Aortic cross-clamping, 987
Aortic dissections
classification systems, 317f
repair, 317-22; anesthesia, 318-21
Aortic insufficiency, 272-5
Aortic node dissection, 594f
Aortic regurgitation, 273, 274, 301
Aortic root pressure, 301
Aortic rupture, repair, 577-8, 580-2
Aortic stenosis (AS), 272-5
Aortic valvuloplasty, pediatric, 1193
Aortoiliac occlusive disease, 327-31
Aortoiliac stenosis, severe, 327-31
Aortopulmonary collaterals, 1194
Apert syndrome, 1091, 1136
complications in anesthesia, 1147
craniosynostosis for, 1130-4
LeFort osteotomies for, 902-4
pediatric surgery, 936-8, 1122
Apnea. *See* Obstructive sleep apnea.
Appendectomy
in staging laparotomy for gynecologic
cancer, 595-7
laparoscopic, 472-5, 472f
minimally invasive, pediatric, 1065
open, 407-8, 407f; anesthesia, 408-10
Appendicitis, 407-10, 472-5, 1065
Apron flap incision, 173, 174f
Aprotinin
drug interactions with, F-2
used in CPB, 265
Aqueductal stenosis, 49
Arachnoid cyst, ventriculostomy, 945-8
ARDS, in chest trauma surgery, 581
Arm
adduction, impingement of
subacromial bursa, 207f, 762f
fractures and nonunion, 778-80
surgery, 778-80; anesthesia, 779-80
tendon transfers, 778-80
tumor excision, biopsy, 778-80
Arnold-Chiari malformation, 51, 940
Arom and Emery partial sternotomy in
mitral/aortic valve surgery, 300
Arterial anastomosis, in replantation
microsurgery, 913-16
Arterial bypass, 331-5
Arterial conduits, in CABG, 266
Arterial cutdown, 1217, 1217f
Arterial embolectomy, 335-6
Arterial embolization, 1156-62, 1174

Arterial insufficiency, acute, 335-6
Arterial occlusive disease, 1174-8
Arterial switch operation, 996, 1006-8
Arteriotomy, 102
Arteriovenous access for hemodialysis,
349-51; anesthesia, 352-4
Arteriovenous canal defect, 976, 977
Arteriovenous (AV) fistula, 349-54
craniotomy (pediatric) for, 943-5
dural, neuroradiology for, 1159
endovascular therapy, 1158-62
prosthetic graft for, 349-51, 350f
Arteriovenous hemodialysis access with
prosthetic graft, 350f
Arteriovenous malformation (AVM), 67,
1194
craniotomy for, 15-21
embolization, neuroradiology, 1156-62
endovascular therapy for, 1158-62
high-flow/low-flow, 15-21
microsurgical resection for, 15-21
Arteritis, sympathectomy for, 339-41
Arthritis. *See* specific sites.
Arthritis, posttraumatic, 737-8, 769-73,
810
Arthritis, rheumatoid
arthrodesis for, 737-8
with atlantoaxial instability, 73
glenohumeral shoulder arthroplasty for,
769-73, anesthesia, 770-2
hip, arthroplasty for, 810; anesthesia,
813-15
with impingement of cord, 42-3
joint arthroplasty for, 736-7, 740-3
pannus formation, 43f
with tenosynovitis, 735-6
ulnar, 734-5, 740-3
wrist, TWR for, 738-9, 740-3
Arthritis, rheumatoid, juvenile
hip, 810, 812-15
knee procedures, 836
preop anesthesia, 1122
Arthrodesis
ankle, 847-8; anesthesia, 863-4
hip, 811-12; anesthesia, 813-15
triple, 1118-19; 1121-5
wrist, 737-8; anesthesia, 740-3
Arthrogryposis, 1103, 1120, 1122
Arthroplasty
interphalangeal joint, 736-7, 740-3
knee, 826-7; anesthesia, 835-7
metacarpophalangeal joint, 736-7
Arthroscopic screw fixation, distal radius,
carpus, metacarpals, 753-5
Arthroscopy
ankle, 845-6, 845f; anesthesia, 863-4
knee, 833; anesthesia, 835-7
shoulder, 760-2; anesthesia, 766-9
TMJ, 200-1; anesthesia, 203-4
wrist, 749-50; anesthesia, 751-2
Arthrotomy
ankle, 846-7; anesthesia, 863-4
hip joint, 812-13
knee, 834; anesthesia, 835-7
TMJ, 200-1; anesthesia, 203-4
Arytenoid resection, 175f

ASA Guidelines for Non-Operating
    Room Locations, 1154, 1206
Ascites, 343-5, 346-8; 1169-73, 1170-2
ASD. *See* Atrial septal defect.
Asian eyelid, plastic surgery for, 874-8
Aspiration
    in bronchopulmonary lavage, 253
    intractable, laryngectomy for, 173-6
    in repair of TEF, EA, 1018
Aspirin, preop testing indications, A-3
Asplinia syndrome, 1048
Asthma
    PPBB precautions, A-6
    preop testing indications, A-3
    refractory, lavage for, 252-5
Asymmetric septal hypertrophy, 282-4
Atelectasis, 253, 588
Atenolol, use in prophylactic periop beta
    blockade, A-4, A-6
Atherosclerosis, 13-15, 21, 295-9, 302,
    322-7
Atkin's approach, upper extremity
    sympathectomy, 339-41
Atlantoaxial fusion, C1, C2, 75-7, 83-7
Atlantoaxial instability, 73
Atracurium, drug interactions with, F-8
Atrial fibrillation (AF), 13-15, 1166
    DC cardioversion for, 1162-4
    preop testing indications, A-3
Atrial flutter, 1162-4
Atrial septal defect (ASD), 972-5, 972f
    closure, 972, 976, 1194
    ostium primum/secundum, 973-8
    repair, anterolateral thoracotomy, 972
    robotic approach, 972
Atrial septectomy for TGA, 996
Atrial switch operations for TGA, 996
Atrioventricular (A-V) canal defect
    palliative repair, 976
    pediatric surgery, 975-8
    pulmonary artery banding, 976, 976f
Atropine
    cautions in pediatric orthopedics, 1122
    in ophthalmic procedures, 126
    in pediatric anesthesia, D-2
    in pediatric neurosurgery, 940
Atypical mycobacterial adenitis, 1014-16
Augmentation cystoplasty, 715-17
Augmentation mammoplasty, 884-5
Autistic patient, anesthesia in, 1210-11
Autonomic hyperreflexia (AH), 699, 924,
    925, 926
Avascular necrosis, 810, 848
AVM: *See* Arteriovenous malformation.
Awake craniotomy, 26-27
Awake intubation, 247
    fiber optic (FOI), B-6
Axillary block
    in flexor tendon repair, 746, 747
    in lower extremity fractures, 754, 755
    in upper extremity orthopedics, 1092
    in wrist procedures, 741, 742
Axillary lymph node dissection, 516-8
Azathioprine
    drug interactions with, F-2

in heart/lung transplant, 364, 369, 372
Azithromycin, drug interactions, F-2, F-6
Azole antifungal agents, drug interactions
    with, F-2
Azzolina bidirectional cavopulmonary
    anastomosis, 1003-6

B
Bacitracin, drug interactions with, F-1
Back pain, microdiscectomy for, 782-4
Baclofen infusion, spasticity surgery, 69
Baerveldt implant (glaucoma), 117
Bailey and Dubow rod system, 1111-13
Bailey cardiac transplantation, 1009
Balanced anesthesia, adult, B-3; pediatric,
    D-3
    in lung wedge resection, 216
Balloon angioplasty, pediatric, 1192-4
Balloon atrial septostomy, 996, 998
Balloon catheters, transurethral, 697-9
Balloon dilatation
    for esophageal replacement, 1031-4
    with esophagoscopy, 959
    radial, 1016-17
    with stent placement, 985
Balloon-tipped catheter, in OLV, 1026
Bankart repair, 760-2; anesthesia, 766-9
Banked fork flap procedure, 1139f
Banks and Green adductor release, 1104
Barbiturates, drug interactions, F-2, F-5
Bard shunt, 102
Bariatric surgery, laparoscopic, 477-9,
    478f; anesthesia, 401-3
Barnett ileostomy, 412
Barrel staying, facial anomalies, 1130-4
Barrett's esophagus, 385-90, 392-4, 456-7
Barton's fracture of distal radius, 753-5
Basal joint arthritis operations, 739-43
Basilar artery stenosis/occlusion, 23
Basilar impression, 42-3, 42f, 45-7, 73
Bassini repair for inguinal hernia, 504
Becker's disease, in anesthesia, 1123
Beckwith-Weidemann syndrome, 1041,
    1051, 1069
Beck's triad, in chest trauma, 576
Belsey Mark IV repair, 384-5, 387-90
Benzodiazepines, drug interactions with,
    F-2, F-3, F-5
Bernese periacetabular osteotomy, 803f
Beta adrenergic agonist, drug interactions
    with, F-2
Beta blockade, prophylactic, A-4-A-6
Beta blockers, drug interactions, F-2
Betadine/amphotericin B, in organ
    procurement, 560
Betaxolol, in ophthalmic procedures, 126
Bextra, in lumbar discectomy, 783
Biceps function trauma, 778-80
Bicipital tendinitis, surgery for, 762-4
Bicoronal approach, face fractures, 900f
Bicoronal skin incision, 40f
Bidirectional cavopulmonary
    anastomosis, for tricuspid atresia,
    1003-6; anesthesia, 1005-6

Bidirectional Glenn procedure, 1003-6,
    1009-11
Bier block
    in flexor tendon repair, 746, 747, 748
    in wrist procedures, 741, 742, 751-2
Bifrontal craniotomy
    for craniofacial anomalies, 1130-4
    for CSF leak, 40-1; anesthesia, 45-7
Bilateral sagittal-split mandibular
    osteotomy, for sleep-disorders, 194
Bilateral salpingo-oophorectomy (BSO)
    for gynecologic cancers, 594-7, 618-
        21
    with hysterectomy, 648
    laparoscopic, 684-6, 692-3
Bilateral subcostal incision, 531f
Bilberry (*Vaccinium myrtillus*),
    precautions with anesthesia, F-10
Bile duct
    distal, strictures, surgery, 448-54
    obstruction, surgery, 448-50
    reconstruction, liver transplant, 549
    strictures, endoscopic stenting, 450
    tumor excision, 450-1, 452-4
Biliary atresia, anatomy, 1047f
    liver transplant for, 547-52
    pediatric portoenterostomy, 1046-9
Biliary cirrhosis, liver transplant, 547-52
Biliary drainage, 448-50, 452-4
    endoscopic, transhepatic, 448-50
    image-guided, 1174
Biliary tract surgery, 445-54
    cancer surgery, 448-50
    choledochal cyst excision/anastomosis,
        451-2
    open cholecystectomy, 446-7
Billroth I, II, anatomy, 393f
    in gastrectomy, 392
    in reconstruction, for PUD, 396
Biopsy. (Also *see* specific sites.)
    needle, 496, 861
    incisional, excisional, 861
    transvenous, image-guided, 1174
    using VATS for, 240-3
    with ventriculostomy, 945-8
    wedge, 496
Biplane cineangiography, 1193
Bipolar TURP, 700
Bisoprolol, in prophylactic beta blockade,
    A-4, A-6
Black cohosh (*Cimicifuga racemosa*),
    precautions with anesthesia, F-10
Bladder
    calculus, 1071-3
    cancer, 696-9, 712-15
    contracted, 715-17
    diverticulum, cystectomy for, 712-15
    endometriosis, surgery, 684-6
    exstrophy, 1077
    perforation, 699
Bladder neck operations
    exstrophy/epispadias complex, spina
        bifida, 1074-5
    neurogenic, incontinence,
        reconstruction, 1073, 1074

pediatric, 1074-5; anesthesia, 1077-8
substitution, 712, anatomy, 713*f*
vesicle neck, 655-7
Bladder operations (except neck)
cystectomy, 712-15; 716-17
open, 715-17; anesthesia, 716-17
open, pediatric, 1073-5, 1077-8
Bladder outlet obstruction, 699-703
pediatric procedures, 1071-3
Blalock and Hanlon septectomy, 996
Blalock and Park repair, 984
Blalock-Taussig (B-T) shunts, 988, 1003-6, 1194
Bleb rupture, excision, stapling, clamp/suture, thoracotomy, 246-9
Bleeding esophageal varices, 343-8
TIPS for, 1169-73
Bleomycin
in esophageal procedures, 388
in staging laparotomy, 497
toxic effects, 598, 599
Blepharoplasty, 120, 874-6, 874*f*; anesthesia, 876-8
laser techniques, 875
Blind intubation
light-wand, in otolaryngology, 144
in neck trauma surgery, 575
Blind nasal intubation
in esophageal procedures, 388
in maxillofacial surgery, 900
nasotracheal, in trauma surgery, 568
Bloc-Potts bowel clamps, 414*f*
Block. *See* specific types, sites.
Blocksom vesicostomy, 1073-5
Blood loss, control
in bronchoscopy, 238
in burn wounds, 928, 932
in craniofacial neurosurgery, 938
in heart/lung transplantation, 368
laparoscopic hysterectomy for, 690-3
in liver transplantation, 547
in pancreatic surgery, 492
in pelvic exenteration, 616-17
post-CPB, 264*f*
in retained placenta, 677, 678
in suction curettage, 612
in thoracolumbar neurosurgery, 98
Blood pressure (BP) management
in carotid endarterectomy, 106
in CPB, 265
in craniotomy, 8, 11, 20, 29-30
Blood pressure, standard monitoring—
adult, B-1; pediatric, D-1
Blood product utilization chart, 992
Blood volume control, 36, 588
Blount epiphysiodesis, 1110-11
Blow-by O$_2$, in DL, 962
Bochdalek's hernia, 1034-7, 1203-4
Bone. (Also *see* specific sites.)
cancer, patient considerations, 863-4
fixation, in replantation, 913-16
flap, craniofacial anomalies, 1130-4
graft, 802-3, 806-8, 844-5
marrow
aspiration, pediatric, 1198-9

suppression, 599; RFA in, 1183
tumor, XRT for, 1188-92
Botulinum toxin, drug interactions, F-2
injection, for achalasia, 458-9
Bowel injury
damage control, 582-3, 586-9
in laparotomy, hysterectomy, 619
Bowel obstruction, 427
Bowel resection, 595
laparoscopic, 469-72, trocar, 469*f*
in pediatrics, 1065
Bowel, small. *See* Small bowel.
Bowers hemiresection, 734-5
Boyle-Davis mouth gag, 144
Brachial plexus surgery, 775-8, 775*f*
Brachytherapy, 624, 1130-4
Brachytherapy for prostate cancer, 726-7, 726*f*; anesthesia, 727
Bradycardia, in heart transplant, 362
Bradydysrhythmia, 284-7
Brain
biopsy, stereotactic surgery for, 53-6
endovascular therapy for, 1158-62
metastasis in, 27
relaxation, in bifrontal craniotomy, 41
shrinkage, 39
Brain stem
gliomas, radiation therapy, 1188-92
stereotactic surgery, 53-6
tumor, craniotomy for, 26-30
vascular malformation, 15-21
Brain volume control, 8, 11, 19, 29-30
Brain-dead organ donors
anesthetic considerations in, 563-5
reflex hypertensive responses in, 564
Branchial cleft
cyst/fistula resection, 1014-16
cyst and tract removal, 963-5
Branchio-oto-renal (BOR) syndrome, 963
Breast augmentation, 884-5; anesthesia, 887-8; implant positions, 884*f*
Breast biopsy
diagnostic, excisional, open, 512-15
hook-wire localization, 512-15
sentinel lymph node, 513-5
Breast cancer surgery, 516-8
microsurgical reconstruction, 911
post-XRT, 916-22
Breast reconstruction, 916-22
after mastectomy, 516-8
autologous grafts, 917-22
autologous myocutaneous flaps, 516
expander/implant, 917, 917*f*, 919-20
subglandular and subpectoral, 884*f*
latissimus myocutaneous flap, 917-22
TRAM flaps, 917-22
Breast reduction, 885-6; anesthesia, 887-8
inferior pedicle technique, 885, 886*f*
Breast surgery, 511-18
axillary lymph node dissection, 516-8
breast-conserving, 516-18
ductoscopy, 512
lift, 887; anesthesia, 887-8
mastectomy, 511-18
mastopexy for ptosis (droop), 887-8

Brescia-Cimino fistula, 349-51, 350*f*
Brokenbrough transseptal needle
puncture, 1195
Bronchial alveolar lavage, 960
Bronchial compression, 1178-82
Bronchial dilation, image-guided, 1174
Bronchial fibrosis, anesthetic
considerations, microsurgery, 912
Bronchial foreign body removal, 959-63
Bronchial injury repair, 579-82
Bronchial lesion, bronchoscopy, 959-63
Bronchial stricture, bronchoscopy, 235-8
Bronchiectasis, 365-73
Bronchitis, chronic, preop testing, A-3
Broncho-pleural-cutaneous fistula, 247
Bronchogenic carcinoma, 231-5
Bronchogenic cyst, 1025*f*
Bronchopleural fistula, 222-6
Bronchopulmonary dysplasia, 1059
Bronchopulmonary lavage, 252-5
Bronchoscopy, 146-53
diagnostic, in cricoid split, 966
in DLT positioning, 211*f*
with esophagoscopy, 150
fiber optic (FOB), 209, 213, 235-8
flexible, 235-8, 959-63
laser, 235-8
pediatric, 959-60; anesthesia, 961-3
rigid, 147*f*, 150, 151*f*, 235-8
in laser resection, 239
pediatric, 235*f*; 959-60; 961-3
Bronchospasm, 1181
Brook's wiring technique, C-spine, 75*f*
Brooke ileostomy, 410-12, 410*f*
Broviac catheter
in pediatric oncology, 1199
for permanent vascular access, 351-4
placement, image-guided, 1174
Brow resuspension, 872-6
Browlift, for ptosis, droop, 872-8, 873*f*
endoscopic, 872-6
Brugada syndrome, 1166
Budd-Chiari syndrome, 343-5, 1169-73
Bullae, excision, stapling, clamp,
thoracotomy for, 246-9
Bupivacaine
adult epidural anesthesia/analgesia,
C-2; PCEA, C-3
drug interactions with, F-2
pediatric epidural anesthesia, D-4, E-5
Burch abdominal approach, for urinary
incontinence, 655-7
Burn injuries—chemical, electrical,
thermal, 928-32
patient transport considerations, 931
physiologic impairments, 930-2
Probit Survival Curve, 929*f*, 930*f*
wound classification, 930
Burn surgery, 927-32; anesthesia, 930-2
debridement, 928-32
excision (tangential, fascial), 928-32
free skin graft, 928-32
patient positioning, 928
Burr hole
in deep brain stimulation, 59

microvascular decompression, 38*f*
placement, in craniotomy, 32*f*

C

C-section. *See* Cesarean section.
CABG. *See* Coronary artery bypass graft surgery.
Calcium channel blockers, drug interactions with, F-2
Caldwell-Luc approach, 156
Callostasis, 1113
Camitz opponensplasty, 750-2
Cannulation, in CPB, 259, 262
Cantholysis (ectropion), 118, 122-3
Canthotomy, 118, 122-3
Capillary telangiectasias, 15
Capnometry/capnography, monitoring, adult, B-1; pediatric, D-1
Capreomycin, drug interactions, F-1
Capsular plication, for multidirectional instability (MDI), 760-1
Capsular release, frozen shoulder, 760-1
Capsular shift for shoulder dislocation, instability, 765-6; anesthesia, 766-9
Capsular shrinkage, arthroscopic, 760-1
Capsulorrhaphy, thermal, for shoulder procedures, 760-1, 765-9
Capsulotomy
    for ankle, posterior, 852
    for hip, 812-13
    of joints, with tendolysis, 748-9; anesthesia, 751-2
    reverse, in prostatectomy, 703*f*
Carbamazepine, drug interactions, F-2
Carboplatin, in gynecology, 597, 598
Cardiac arrest
    deep hypothermic, in TAAA, 325
    emergency tube thoracostomy, 569-71
Cardiac arrhythmia
    DC cardioversion for, 1162-4
    treated with RFA, 1182-6
Cardiac catheterization, pediatric, out-of-OR, 1192-8; anesthesia, 1195-7
Cardiac disease, preop testing, A-3
Cardiac laceration repair, in chest trauma, 576-7; anesthesia, 580-2
Cardiac surgery, 259-90 (Also *see* specific procedures.)
    minimally invasive, 291-306
Cardiac tamponade, 288, 289, 568
    emergency tube thoracostomy, 569-71
Cardiac toxicity, in chemotherapy, 1198
Cardiomyopathy, 360-5
Cardiopulmonary bypass (CPB), 259-65
    alpha-stat vs pH-stat management, 263
    anticoagulation, 262, 263
    bleeding, treatment of, 264*f*
    in CABG, 266
    circuit, 260*f*, 261*f*
    coagulation, 265
    in heart, lung transplant, 362-3
    patient preparation for, 262
    physiologic response to, 262
    termination, weaning, 262, 263, 265
    transition onto, 262-3

Cardiovascular surgery, 257-373 (*See* specific procedures.)
    pediatric, 971-1011
Cardioversion, DC, 1162-4
Cardioverter-defibrillator (ICD) implantation, 1165-9
Carotid artery disease, 102*f*
    in cerebral embolectomy, 13-15
Carotid artery injury repair, 577-8
Carotid artery stenosis, 23, 102-8
Carotid bifurcation, exposure, 308*f*
Carotid endarterectomy, 308*f*, 309*f*
    neurosurgical, 102-8; anesthesia, 103-7
    vascular, 308-10, anesthesia, 103-7
Carpal instability, arthrodesis, 737-8
Carpal tunnel release (open, endoscopic), 750-51, 750*f*
Carpal tunnel syndrome, 750-52, 753
Carpometacarpal (CMC), degenerative arthritis of, 739-43
Carpometacarpal synovitis, joint dislocation, trauma, 739-43
Carpus fractures, dislocations, 753-5
Carroll's procedure for clubfoot, 1119-20
Carvon, anesthetic considerations in lumbar discectomy, 783
CASS study, 267
Cat-scratch disease, 1014
Cataract extraction, intraocular lens insertion, 114-15, 124-6
    in-the-bag lens insertion, 114*f*
Catatonia, ECT for, 1154-8
Catheter
    emergent thoracostomy, 1218*f*
    epidural techniques, pediatric, D-4
    indwelling, pediatric, D-4
    for permanent vascular access, 351-4
    positioning for pediatric shunt, 945-8
    retained, ventriculostomy for, 945-8
    ventricular, insertion, 49*f*
Cat's Claw (*Uncaria tomentosa*), precautions with anesthesia, F-10
Cauda equina syndrome, 357, 437, 508
Caudal agenesis, surgery for, 941-3
Caudal epidural anesthesia
    in pediatric orthopedic surgery, 1123
    in pediatric pain management, E-1-E-2
    pediatric, single-shot, D-4
Causalgia, sympathectomy for, 336-8
Caustic ingestion, 1031-4
Cavernous malformation, 15
Cavopulmonary procedure for tricuspid atresia, 1003-6
Cavovarus foot, 1118-19, 1121-5
Cayenne (*Capsicum annum*), precautions with anesthesia, F-10
CBC preop testing, indications, A-1
Celebrex, anesthetic considerations, 783
Central line sepsis, in XRT, 1191
Central venous access port removal, pediatric, 1198-9
Cerebellar pontine angle, 26, 188-92
Cerebral artery stenosis/occlusion, 23
Cerebral edema, 639, 1191
Cerebral embolectomy, 13-15, 14*f*
Cerebral infarct, craniotomy for, 4-13

Cerebral oximetry, 105
Cerebral palsy, 812, 852, 951, 1094, 1100, 1103-4, 1109, 1114, 1117, 1119, 1122, 1210
Cerebral perfusion monitoring, 105-6
Cerebral revascularization, in neuroradiology, 1156-62
Cerebrohepatorenal syndrome, 1070
Cervical artery—stenosis, occlusion, 21
Cervical bleeding, D&C for, 632-3
Cervical cancer, 621-4
Cervical cerclage (elective, emergent), 674-6; anesthesia, 675-6
Cervical disc disease, 81
Cervical discectomy, anterior, 77
Cervical dysplasia, 605-8
Cervical incompetence, 674-6
Cervical instability, 78
Cervical laceration repair, 672-4
Cervical laminectomy/foraminotomy, 80-2
Cervical mass resection, 1014-16
Cervical myelopathy, 78, 81
Cervical plating, posterior, 80
Cervical radiculopathy, 80-2
Cervical spine (C-spine)
    abnormalities, 1112
    injuries, in trauma surgery, 580, 587
    transarticular screw fixation, 75-7, 83-7
    wiring techniques, 75-7, 80-2, 83-7
Cervical spine, mid/lower, 76*f*, 79*f*
    anterior fusion/fixation, 77-9, 83-7
    corpectomy/fusion, 77-9, 83-7
    fractures, anterior fusion/fixation, 77-9; anesthesia, 83-7
    posterior fusion/fixation, 80-2, 83-7
    screw-plate fixation, 77-9, 83-7
Cervical spine, upper (C1-C2), 76*f*
    anterior fusion/fixation, 72-4, 83-7
    plating, 75
    posterior fusion/fixation, 75-7, 83-7
    rod and wiring, 75-7, 83-7
Cervical stenosis, 632-3
Cervical structures, zones, anatomy, 573*f*
Cervicomedullary junction, transoral approach, 42-3, anatomy, 42*f*, 45-7
Cervicothoracic junction (CTJ), anterior approach, 82-7; pathology, 81
Cervix
    conization, 605-8; excision, 606*f*
    laser, 606-8
    laceration repair, 672-4
    laser therapy, 608-9
Cesarean section
    anatomy, incisions, 660*f*
    classic/lower-segment, 660-5; anesthesia, 661-5
Chamberlain procedure, 231-5, 1022
Chamomile (*Matricaria chamomilla*), precautions with anesthesia, F-10
Charcot-Marie Tooth disease, 1100, 1117, 1119
CHARGE association, 968, 969
Chemical instillation for transurethral therapy, 697-9

Chemotherapeutic agents
  effects in anesthetic planning, 517-8
  in staging laparotomy, 497, 498
  toxicities, 598
Chemotherapy
  in chest-wall reconstruction, 921-2
  permanent vascular access for, 351-4
  platinum-based, in ovarian cancer, 597
  preop testing indications, A-3
Cherney rectus muscle detachment, 648
Chest drainage, lobectomy, 210
Chest trauma, 576-82
  anesthesia for prcedures, 580-2
  blunt, repair, 579-80
  cardiac laceration repair, 576-7
  great vessels, repair, 577-8
  penetrating, 569-71, 579-80
  pericardial window, 576-7
  pneumonectomy/lobectomy, 579-80
  tamponade release, 576-7
  tracheobronchial repair, 579-80
Chest wall
  reconstruction, 920-1
  resection, 218-19; anesthesia, 220-1
Chest x-ray (CXR), preop, clinical
    indications for, A-1
Chevron incision, midline extension, 552f
Chiari I, II malformations, 51, 938-9
Chiari osteotomy for acetabular dysplasia,
    1099-1100, 1100f, 1121-5
Child's classification, 1170
Child's procedure, 488-9, 491-4
Chin augmentation, osteotomy,
    genioplasty, 905-8, implants, 905f
Chitwood micro-mitral approach, 300
Cholelithiasis, cholecystectomy, 459-63
Chloroprocaine, drug interactions, F-3
Choanal atresia, 1136; repair, 968-9
Cholangiocarcinoma, 450-4
Cholangiography, 446-8, 452-4
  + cholecystectomy, 459-61
Cholangitis, primary sclerosing, 547-52
Cholecystectomy
  laparoscopic, 459-63; anatomy, 460f;
    anesthesia 461-2
  ± common duct exploration, 459-
    63
  minimally invasive, pediatric, 1065
  open, 446-8, 447f; anesthesia, 452-4
Cholecystitis, surgery, 446-8, 459-63
Cholecystojejunostomy, 448-50;
    anesthesia, 452-4
Choledochal cyst
  excision, anastomosis, 451-4
  pediatric, portoenterostomy for, 1046-9
  resection, 1056
Choledochoduodenostomy, 448-50, 452-4
Choledochojejunostomy, 448-50, 452-4
  in liver transplantation, 549
Choledocholithiasis, 446-8, 459-63
Choledochoscopy, 446-8, 452-4
Cholelithiasis, 446-8, 452-4
Cholesteatoma surgery, 160-3, 187-92
Cholesterol granuloma surgery, 187-92
Cholinergic agents, drug interactions, F-2
Chordee, with hypospadias, 1075-8

Chordoma, 42f, transoral approach, 42-3
Chromopertubation, for infertility, 643
Chronic obstructive pulmonary disease
    (COPD)
  in abdominal aorta surgery, 328, 329
  PPBB precautions, A-6
  infrainguinal arterial bypass for, 331-5
  lung transplant for, 255-6
  lung-volume reduction, 249-52
Chvostek's sign, 529
Cicatricial ectropion, entropion, 118-19
Cimetidine, drug interactions, F-2-F-3
  use in peptic ulcer disease, 396
Cincinnati procedure for clubfoot, 1119-
    20; anesthesia, 1121-5
Circle of Willis, location, 5f
Circulatory arrest (also see CPB), with
    deep hypothermia, for intracranial
    aneurysms, 4-13
Circumcision, 1075-6; anesthesia, 1077-8
Cirrhosis
  alcoholic, 547-58
  hepatic, TIPS for, 1169-73
  imaging for, 1174-8
  portal HTN surgery for, 345-8
Cisatracurium
  adult intubation, B-2; muscle
    relaxation, B-3
  pediatric muscle relaxation, D-2, D-3
Cisplatin
  in staging laparotomy, 497, 498
  toxic effects, 598, 599
Clagett procedure, empyema, 223-6
Clamp and suture technique
  in excision of blebs, bullae, 246-9
  lung wedge resection, 215
Clamshell incision, 206, 207f, 255
Clarithromycin, drug interactions with,
    F-4, F-6
Clatworthy shunt for portal HTN, 343-5;
    anesthesia, 346-8
Clavicle
  distal, resection, 760-2, 766-9
  fractures, surgery for, 773-4, 776-8
Cleft deformity, secondary, 1145-8
Cleft lip, 1150
  LeFort osteotomies for, 902-4
  repair, unilateral/bilateral, 1137-40
Cleft palate, 906
  intravelar veloplasties for, 1140-2
  LeFort osteotomies for, 902-4
  repair, 1137-40, 1140f, 1147-8
Cleft rotation advancement repair, 1137-
    40, 1138f; anesthesia, 1147-8
Clindamycin, drug interactions, F-4
Clitoroplasty, 1076-7; anesthesia, 1077-8
Clivus, inferior exposure, 42f
Cloaca, pullthrough, 1056-8
Cloacal exstrophy, 1076-8
Clonidine, drug interactions, F-4
Clonidine patch, control of HTN, 110
Clostridia, 805
Cloward cervical spine fusion, wrist
    arthrodesis, 738
Clubfoot, surgical correction, 1119-20;
    anesthesia, 1121-5

CNS disorders, preop testing, A-3
CNS tumor, XRT for, 1188-92
Coagulation management in liver
    transplantation, 556
Coagulation, preop testing, A-2
Coagulation therapy
  in heart/lung transplantation, 368
  with TEG, in liver transplantation, 558
Coagulopathies, preop testing, A-3
Coarctation of aorta, 6, 996
  balloon angioplasty, endovascular
    stenting, pediatric, 1194
  end-to-end repair, 984-7, 984f
  left posterolateral thoracotomy, 984-7
  prosthetic interposition tube graft, 984
  subclavian artery flap repair, 984-7
  surgery for, 984-7; anesthesia, 985-7
Codeine, in pediatric analgesia, E-3
Cohen-Edwards truncus, 1000, 1001f
Coil occlusion
  for aortopulmonary, venous collaterals,
    AVMs, B-T shunt, 1194
  for coronary artery fistulae, PDA, 1194
Colapinto needle, in TIPS, 1169, 1171f
Colectomy, 423-5; anesthesia, 427-9
  abdominal + ileorectal anastomosis,
    424
  hemi, right/left, 424
  segmental, 423-5
  sigmoid, 424
  trocar placement for, 469f
Coleus (Coleus forskohlii), precautions
    with anesthesia, F-10
Colistmethate, drug interactions, F-1
Colitis, segmental colectomy, 423-5
Collateral blood flow monitoring, 102
Collateral ligament reconstruction, 830-1;
    anesthesia, 835-7
Collecting system, double
  nephrectomy for, 706-9, 710-11
  with ureterocele, MCDK, 1069
Colles' fracture, 734-5, 753-5
Colon, 424f
  cancer, segmental colectomy, 423-5
  diverticulum, colectomy for, 423-5
    stomal repair, 426-9
  infections, perforation, 423-5
  injuries, damage control, 582-3
  pullthrough, 1055f
Colon interposition
  in esophageal replacement, 1031-4,
    1032f
  with proctocolectomy, 421-3
  with total esophagectomy, 385-90
  volvulus, 423-5, 427-9
Colon obstruction, repair/segmental
    colectomy, 423-5; anesthesia, 427-9
Colon resection, 423-5; anesthesia, 427-9
Colorectal surgery, 419-38 (See specific
    procedures.)
  laparoscopic, 420
  proctocolectomy, 420-3, 427-9
Colostomy, 426-7; anesthesia, 427-9
  for Hirschsprung's disease, 1053-6
Colpopexy, abdominal, for vaginal vault
    prolapse, 640-1; anesthesia, 644-6

Colporrhaphy, 640, 652-4, 656-7
Combined epidural/GA
    in intestinal, peritoneal procedures, 417
    in operations for morbid obesity, 402
    in operations for PUD, 398
    in pancreatic surgery, 492-3
    in staging laparotomy, 498
    in stomal closure, 428
Combined spinal/epidural (CSE)
    anesthesia
    in C-section, 664
    in cervical/vaginal laceration, 673
    in D&C, D&E, 635
    in hysterectomy, 650
    in hysteroscopy, 638
    for urinary incontinence, 656
'Commando resection,' neck, 169
Common bile duct
    exploration, 446-8, 452-4
        laparoscopic, 459-63, 460*f*
    obstruction, 448-50, 452-4
Common duct stone, 397-9, 406
Compartment syndrome
    leg, fasciotomy for, 858-61
    intrauterine, perinatal muscle, 1088
    patellar realignment, 831
    supracondylar humerus fracture, 1084
    thigh, fasciotomy, 857-61
    tibia fracture/nonunion/malunion,
        841-2
Complete transposition of the great
    arteries (TGA) surgery, 996-1000
Completion axillary dissection, for node-
    positive axillas, 513
Computed tomography (CT), 1173-8;
    anesthesia, 1175-7; 1201-2
Concorde position, 17*f*
Conduit insertion for truncus arteriosus—
    allograft, artificial, 1000, 1001*f*
Congenital defects, closure of, 1194
Congenital diaphragmatic hernia (CDH),
    repair, 1034-7, anatomy, 1035*f*
    ECMO for, 1203-4
    in utero therapy, 1034
    lung resection for, 1024-7
    respiratory concerns, 1035, 1036
Congenital lobar overdistention (CLO)
    (emphysema), resection for, 1024-7
Congenital webs/cysts, 147
Congestive heart disease (CHD)
    cyanotic, pediatric surgery for, 988-92
    heart transplantation for, 360-5
Congestive heart failure (CHF)
    with DORV, surgery for, 1006-8
    ICD placement for, 1167
    mitral valve replacement/repair, 275-9
    pediatric, 943
    preop testing indications, A-3
    valve replacement, 272-5
Conization of the cervix, 605-8;
    anesthesia, 607-8
Conjunctival transposition, 123
Connective-tissue disorder, hand/wrist,
    736-7
Conn's syndrome, 53-5

Conscious sedation, for infertility
    procedures, 642, 646
Constipation, 423-5, 430
Constrictive pericarditis, 287-90
Continuous iv infusion, in pediatric
    postop analgesia, E-3
Contrast-media complications
    in imaging procedures, 1177
    in neuroradiology, 1160, 1161
COPD. *See* Chronic obstructive
    pulmonary disease.
Cornea
    dystrophy, surgery for, 115-16
    edema, surgery for, 115-16
    scar, 115-16
    transplant, 115-16; anesthesia, 124-6
Coronal flap in nasal surgery, 156*f*
Coronal incision, in browlift, 873*f*
Coronal synostosis, craniosynostosis,
    1130-4
    pediatric, 936-8
Coronary artery bypass (CAB), 292*f*
    endo and port-access procedures, 303
    monitoring, complications, 304
Coronary artery bypass graft (CABG)
    surgery, 266-70; anesthesia, 267-70
    graft materials, 266
    minimally invasive, 295-9
    off-pump, 295-9; anesthesia, 297-8
Coronary artery circulation, anterior, 266*f*
Coronary artery disease, 329
    CABG for, 266-70; anesthesia, 267-70
    heart transplantation for, 360-5
    infrainguinal arterial bypass, 331-5
    port-access coronary revascularization
        for, 293-5; anesthesia, 301-6
Coronary artery fistulae, 1194
Coronary revascularization
    left IMA dissection, anastomosis, 294*f*
    port-access, 293-5; anesthesia, 301-6
Coronary sinus, 972-5, 972*f*, 1168
Coronary vein ligation, portal HTN, 345
Corpus callosotomy, 66
Cortical stimulation, 61-4
Corticosteroids
    drug interactions with, F-4
    in heart, lung transplant, 364, 369, 372
Cosmetic facial surgery, 867-82
Costotransversectomy, 89-91
COX-2 inhibitors
    anesthetic considerations in lumbar
        discectomy, 783
    in multimodality analgesia, C-1
    in preemptive analgesia, C-1
Coxa valgum, varum, 1109
CPB. *See* Cardiopulmonary bypass.
Crafoord end-to-end repair of aortic
    coarctation, 984
Cranial dysostosis, surgery for, 936-8
Cranial fossa, anterior, fracture, 41
Cranial nerve
    compression (vascular), 109
    microvascular decompression, 37-50
Cranial spinal irradiation (CSI) for CNS
    leukemia, 1188

Craniectomy
    for brain tumor, 26
    for intracranial aneurysms, 4
    linear, pediatric, 937
    in microvascular decompression, 38
    subtemporal, for epilepsy, 66
Craniocervical decompression, for Chiari
    malformation, 51; anesthesia, 83-7
Craniocervical occipitocervical fusion,
    75-7; anesthesia, 83-7
Craniofacial deformities, malformations
    (congenital), surgery for, 1129-50
    dysmorphism, 936-8
    dysostosis, 1134-7
    facial bipartition, 1134-7
    major secondary surgery for, 1134-7
    monobloc, frontofacial advancement,
        1134-7
    pediatric neurosurgery for, 936-8
    periorbital osteotomies, 1134-7
Craniofacial neurosurgery, pediatric, 936-
    8; anesthesia, 937-8
Craniofacial reconstructive surgery, 895-
    908; OR setup, 900*f*
Craniopharyngioma, 27, 44
Cranioplasty, 31
Craniosynostosis
    fronto-orbital advancement, 1131*f*
    pediatric, correction of, 1130-4
    sagittal, coronal, metopic,
        lambdoidal—surgery for, 936-8
    skull shape abnormalities, 1130*f*
Craniotomy
    awake, 26-7
    bifrontal, 40-1; anesthesia, 45-7
    for cerebral embolectomy, 6-15
    for cribriform plate tumor, 40-1
    for EC-IC bypass, 21-26, 21*f*, 22*f*
    frontal, for epilepsy, 66
    frontotemporal (pterional), 4
    for intracranial aneurysms, 4-13
    intracranial vascular malformations,
        15-21; anesthesia, 17-21
    middle/posterior fossa, 187-92, 188*f*,
        191*f*
    occipital, temporal, for epilepsy, 66
    for skull tumor, 31; anesthesia, 28-30
    for subdural hematoma, 33*f*
    translabyrinthine, 187-92, 191*f*
    for trauma, 26-30, 32-7
    for vein of Galen malformation, 943-5
Crawford inclusion technique, 121*f*, 322-
    7, 323*f*
Crawford's classification of aortic
    aneurysms, thoracoabdominal, 322*f*
Crawford's procedure for clubfoot, 1119-
    20, 1121-5
Cricoarytenoid joint involvement, in
    shoulder surgery, 766
Cricoid cartilage exposure, 174*f*
Cricoid split, for subglottic stenosis,
    pediatric, 966-8; anesthesia, 966-7
Cricothyroidostomy, needle, 589
Cricothyroidotomy, in trauma surgery,
    568, incision, tube insertion, 568*f*
Cricothyrotomy, 182-5; anesthesia, 183-5

dilator/catheter advancement, 1215*f*
emergency, 1214-15
  airway access assembly, 1215*f*
  'guidewire,' 1214-15, 1214*f*
  in pediatric trauma, 589
  'stab' emergency, 1214
  in trauma surgery, 569
Crohn's disease, 416, 433
  proctocolectomy for, 420-3, 427-9
  segmental colectomy for, 423-5
  small-bowel resection for, 413-14
  stomal repair, 426-7
Cross-clamping
  in abdominal aortic aneurysm, 330
  ascending aortic lesions, 320-1
  in TAAA repair, 326
Cross-sectional imaging, 1173-8
  pediatric, 1201-2
Crouzon syndrome
  craniofacial surgery for, 936-8
  craniosynostosis for, 1130-4
  LeFort osteotomies for, 902-4
Crowe-Davis mouth gag, 956
Cruciate ligament
  arthroscopy for, 833, 835-7
  reconstruction, 830-1, 835-7
Cryotherapy
  hemorrhoids, 434
  retinal tears, 135
Cryptic AVM, 15
Cryptoglandular fistula surgery, 433-4
Cryptorchidism surgery, 1061-2, 1080-1
  laparoscopic procedures, 1079, 1081-2
CSF flow pathways, obstruction, 48*f*
CSF leak, craniotomy for, 40-1, 45-7
CT. *See* Computed tomography.
CT-guided phenol sympathetic block, 339
Cul-de-sac incision, strabismus, 950
Culdotomy, for myomas, 689-93
Currarino's triad, 1063
Cushing triad, 28
Cushing's disease, 44; preop testing
  indications, A-3
Cushing's response, 947
Cushing's syndrome
  in adrenal surgery, 532, 533-5
  in pancreatic surgery, 492
Cyanotic spells, (CHD), pediatric, 988-92
Cyclopentolate, in ophthalmology, 126
Cyclophosphamide
  anesthetic concerns, 1198
  drug interactions, F-4
  toxic effects, 598, 599
Cyclosporine
  drug interactions, F-4
  in heart, lung transplant, 360, 364, 365,
    369, 372
Cyst
  aspiration, ventriculostomy, 945-8
  drainage, stereotactic surgery, 53-6
  subarachnoid, 49
Cyst-enteric bypass, choledochal, 451-2;
  anesthesia, 452-4
Cystadenoma resection, 490-4
Cystectomy (simple, partial, radical),
  712-15; anesthesia, 714-15

anatomy, male and female, 713*f*
  ovarian, 640-1; anesthesia, 644-6
Cystic adenomatoid malformation
  (CCAM), resection, 1024-7, 1025*f*
Cystic fibrosis
  heart/lung transplantation, 365-73
  lavage for, 252-5
  lung transplant for, 255-6
  in rectal prolapse, 430
Cystic hygroma, 1014-16, 1023
Cystic neoplasms, 488-9
Cystitis
  chronic, operations for, 715-17
  hemorrhagic, interstitial
    endoscopic diagnostics for, 696-7;
      anesthesia, 698-9
    radiation-induced, 712-15
    therapeutic transurethral procedures,
      697-9
Cystocele
  in rectal prolapse, 430
  repair, 728-30; anesthesia, 729-30
  surgery for, 652-4, 652*f*, 656-7
Cystoplasty, augmentation, 715-17
Cystoscopy, 696-7; anesthesia, 698-9
  in bladder (male, female), 696*f*
  pediatric, 1071-3; anesthesia, 1077-8
Cytopenia, in staging laparotomy, 498
Cytoreductive surgery, 595

D
d-tubocurarine, in adult intubation, B-2
D&C. *See* Dilatation and curettage.
D&E. *See* Dilatation and evacuation.
Dacryocystorhinostomy (DCR), 129-130;
  anesthesia, 124-126
Danazol exposure, 1076-8
Dandy-Walker malformation, 49
Dantrolene, drug interactions with, F-3
Darling definition of TAPVC drainage
  patterns, 993
Darrach procedure, 734-5; anesthesia,
  740-3; anatomy, incision, 734*f*
  modified, for rheumatoid wrist, 735-6
Dartos pouch
  in pediatric laparoscopy, 1081-2
  scrotal, testicular torsion, 1079-81
Darvocet, in lumbar discectomy, 783
Daunorubicin, toxic effects, 598, 599
Davies Z-plasty, 1137-40, 1147-8
DeBastiani, large-pin fixator/osteotomy,
  1113-5; anesthesia, 1121-5
Debridement
  ankle—trauma, infection, arthritis,
    845-6; anesthesia, 863-4
  knee arthroscopy, 833; arthrotomy,
    834; anesthesia, 835-7
Decompressive laminectomy, 80, 93
Decubitus ulcer, 912, 922, 925
Deep brain stimulation, 59-60, 62-4
Deep hypothermic cardiac arrest
  in aortic dissection repair, 320
  in TAAA repair, 325
Deep venous thrombosis (DVT)
  acute, venous surgery for, 341-3
  imaging for, 1174-8

in knee procedures, 826, 828
  in proctocolectomy, 421
  in thoracic surgery, 207
Defibrillation threshold (DFT), 1165
DeGeorge syndrome, 989, 1001, 1002
Dehydration, Sx, 692; 1039
Delaire mask, in craniosynostosis, 1130
Deliberate occlusion, cervical artery, 21
Delivery complications, 690-3
Delorme procedure for rectal prolapse,
  429-30; anesthesia, 436-8
Deltopectoral incision, 769*f*, 778
Dens, removal by drill, 42*f*
Dental damage, in ECT, 1157
Dental surgery
  bone grafting 201-4; 1211-12
  extractions, 201-4
  implants, 201-4, 1211-12
  Office-based, 1209-12
  OR-based, 199-204
  restorative, 201-4
Dental rehabilitation
  'special needs' patients, 1209-11
  under deep iv sedation, 1209-11
Dentinogenesis imperfecta, 1112
Dentophobia, 1209
Dentoskeletal dysplasia, 902-4, 906-8
Depression, ECT for, 1154-8
Dermal sinus tract, pediatric, 941-3
Developmental neurologic subluxation, 1099
Developmental venous anomalies, 15
Deviated septum, surgery for, 153-5
Devil's claw (*Harpagophytum
  procubens*), precautions with
  anesthesia, F-10
Dong quai (*Angelica sinensis*),
  precautions with anesthesia, F-10
Dextran reaction, 912, 921-2
Diabetes, 125, 351
  preop testing indications, A-3
Diabetes insipidus (DI)
  complications in organ donors, 563
  infrainguinal arterial bypass for, 331-5
Diabetes melitis (DM)
  with ESRD, 539-42
  infrainguinal arterial bypass for, 331-5
Diabetic gangrene, 852-3
Diabetic retinopathy, 135, 136
Diagnosis-based preop testing, A-3
Diagnostic neuroradiology, 1160-1
Diagnostic studies, preop, A-1-A-2
Dial osteotomy, for pelvic reconstruction,
  1097-9; anesthesia, 1121-5
Dialysis, anesthetic concerns, 541, 542
Diaphragmatic paralysis, 172
Diarrhea, in rectal prolapse, 430
Diastematomyelia correction, 941-3
Diastrophic dwarfism, 1120
Diazepam, premedication—adult, B-2;
  pediatric, D-2
Difficult airway. *See* Airway, difficult.
Difficult iv access, pediatric, 589-90
Digit
  amputation, tendolysis for 748-9, 751-2
  amputation level, 853*f*
  traumatic, 755-8

fracture, burn, injury, contracture, dislocation—tendolysis for 748-9
nerve laceration, repair, 745-6
replantation, 755-8
Digital fasciectomy, 744, 746-8
Digoxin (digitalis)
  drug interactions with, F-4
  preop testing indications, A-3
Dilantin, preop testing indications, A-3
Dilatation and curettage (D&C), 632-3, 632f, 640; anesthesia, 635-6
  for cervical stenosis with dysmenorrhea, obstruction, menstrual flow, 632-3
  for pregnancy termination, 632-3
  for uncontrolled uterine/cervical bleeding, 632-3
Dilatation and evacuation (D&E) 2nd trimester, 633-4; anesthesia, 635-6
  uterine aspiration, 633f
Dilaudid, in pediatric postop epidural analgesia, E-5
Diltiazem, drug interactions, F-2, F-3
Dingman mouth gag, 956, 968, 969, 1143, 1144, 1147
Direct current (DC) cardioversion, 1162-4; anesthesia, 1163-4
  contraindications, 1163
Direct laryngoscopy (DL), 146-53, for stridor, 961-2
Direct-trocar insertion, laparoscopy, 684-5
Disc
  degeneration, 81, 787-94
  herniation, 81, 782-4
Dismembered pyeloplasty, 709-10, 709f pediatric, 1069
Dissecting aneurysms, 317-22
Dissociative anesthetic, 876-7
Distal clavicle resection (Mumford procedure), 760-2; anesthesia, 766-9
Distal interphalangeal (DIP) arthrodesis, in flexor tendon repair, 745
Distal interphalangeal (DIP) arthroplasty, 736-7; anesthesia, 740-3
Distal revascularization, lumbar sympathectomy for, 336-8; anesthesia, 332-4
Distraction, in-wrist visualization, 749
Distraction osteogenesis, internal, external, 903-4; anesthesia, 906-8
  incision, instrumentation, 907f
Diuretics, preop testing indications, A-3
Diverticulectomy, esophageal, 379-81
  anesthesia, 387-90
  laparoscopic, 379
Diverticulitis, 416, 466-9
Diverticulum (Also see specific sites.)
  Meckel's, excision, 408, 408-10
  pharyngoesophageal (Zenker's), 379-81, stapling of, 378f
DL. See Direct laryngoscopy.
DLT. See Double-lumen tube.
Dobutamine, drug interactions, F-4
Docetaxel, toxic effects, 598

Dohlman procedure, for Zenker's diverticulum, 379-81
Dolasetron, for adult antiemetics, C-2
Dolstad modified hysterectomy, 622
Donazepril, drug interactions, F-2
Dopamine-responsive dystonia, 59
Doppler, transcranial, 106
Dor fundoplication, laparoscopic, 456-7; anesthesia, 461-3
DORV. See Double-outlet right ventricle.
Double-lumen tube (DLT)
  assessment of positioning, 211f
  in bronchopulmonary lavage, 253
  in excision of blebs/bullae, 248
  in OLV, pediatric surgery, 1026
  in VATS, 240
Double-opposing z-plasty closure of cleft palate, 1141f
Double-outlet right ventricle (DORV), surgery for, 1006-8, types, 1007f
  arterial switch operation for, 1006-8
  intraventricular baffle-to-pulmonary valve repair, 1006-8
  intraventricular tunnel repair, 1006-8
  ± pulmonary stenosis, 1006-8
  + subaortic/subpulmonic VSD, 1006
Down syndrome, 954, 957, 977
  airway complications in, 144
  in dental patients, 1210-11
Doxorubicin
  anesthetic concerns, 1198
  in breast surgery, 517
  toxic effects in oncology, 598, 599
Drainage implants (glaucoma), 117
Drug abuse, considerations in anesthesia for orthopedic procedures, 863
Drug interaction table, F-1-F-10. (See specific medications.)
  with herbal agents, F-10-F-11
Drug therapies, preop testing, A-3
Duchenne's disease, 1123
Duct stone, duodenotomy for, 406
Ductal sling, with aortic coarctation, 985
Ductoscopy, for breast, 512
Ductus arteriosus, concerns in minimally invasive pediatric surgery, 1064
Duhamel pullthrough for Hirschsprung's disease, 1053-6
'Dumbbell' tumor, mediastinal, 1022
Duodenal mobilization for abdominal vascular injuries, 585-6
Duodenal perforation, oversew, 394-5; anesthesia, 397-9
Duodenal rupture, laparotomy, 496-9
Duodenal ulcer, 396-9, 406
Duodenostomy, 392-4, anatomy, 393f
Duodenotomy, 406; anesthesia, 397-9
Duplex system, nonfunctioning upper pole, 1069-71
Dupuytren's contracture, 744, 746-8
DVT. See Deep venous thrombosis.
Dwarfing syndromes, 1109
Dwyer instrumentation for spinal correction, 1095f
Dwyer's approach, in anterior spinal reconstruction/fusion, 792

Dysmenorrhea, D&C for, 632-3
Dysmorphism, craniofacial, 936-8
Dyspareunia, 652-4, 656-7
Dysplasia
  cervical, conization for, 605-8
  fibrous, in skull tumor, 31
Dysraphism, spinal, correction, 941-3
Dysrhythmias, 1157 (ECT), 1181
Dystonia musculorum deformans, 60
Dysvascular limb amputation, 854-7

E
Eagle-Barrett syndrome, 1077
Ear
  canals, small size, 954-6
  deformed, 160-3
  infections, chronic, 954-6
  malformations, congenital, 1149-50
  prominent, protruding, 1149-50
Ear reconstruction, grafts, flaps, implants, 1149-50; anesthesia, 162-3
  cutaneous 'pocket,' 1150f
  fabrication of framework, 1149f
Ear surgery, 160-3; anesthesia, 162-3
  drum repair, 160-3, anatomy, 161f
  myringotomy/tympanostomy tube placement, 954-6; anesthesia, 955-6
  otoplasty, 1149-50; anesthesia,162-3
Ear-to-ear scalp incision, for facial fracture surgery, 898
Eating inability, 411
Eaton-Lambert syndrome, 211, 224
Ebstein's anomaly, 279, 1167
EC-IC bypass, 21-6; anesthesia, 24-6
ECG. See Electrocardiogram.
Echothiophate, in ophthalmology, 126
Eclampsia, in C-section, 662
ECMO, 1203-4; circuit, 1203f
Ectopic pregnancy
  laparoscopic surgery, 687-8, 692-3
  laparotomy, 639-41, 644-6
Ectropion repair, 118-19; anesthesia, 124-6
Edrophonium, in pediatric muscle relaxant reversal, D-3
EEG. See electroencephalogram.
Effusion, image-guided, 1174-8
Ehlers-Danlos syndrome, 6, 1094, 1116
Eisenmenger's syndrome, 255-6, 365-73, 979
Elastosis, facelift for, 869-71
Elbow fractures, pediatric, closed/open reduction for, 1085-6, 1091-2
Electrical burns, surgery for, 928-32
Electrical shock, in RFA, 1185
Electrocardiogram (ECG)
  monitoring, adult B-1; pediatric, D-1
  preop, clinical indications, A-1
Electroconvulsive therapy (ECT), 1154-8; anesthesia, 1156-8
Electrodes
  in spinal cord stimulation, 61-4
  surface, depth, for epilepsy, 66
Electroencephalograph (EEG)
  in aortic dissection repair, 320
  in carotid endarterectomy, 105

Electrolyte abnormalities, in pancreatic surgery, 492
Electrophysiology
    monitoring, in craniotomy, 26
    pediatric, 1192-8; anesthesia, 1195-7
Eleventh-rib extrapleural-retroperitoneal approach, spine surgery, 87
Elliptocytosis, 497
Eloesser flap, 223-6
Embolectomy
    arterial, 335-6; anesthesia, 332-4
    cerebral, craniotomy for, 6-15
    with Fogarty catheter, 341f
Embolization
    of intracranial artery, catheter, 13-15
    in neuroradiology, 1156-62
    risks, in DC cardioversion, 1163
Emergence—adult, B-4; pediatric, D-2
Emergency airway access assembly, for cricothyrotomy, 1215f
Emergency procedures for anesthesiologists, 1213-18
    arterial cutdown, 1217
    cricothyrotomy, 1214-15
    needle/catheter thoracostomy, 1218
    periocardiocentesis, 1216
Emergency revascularization, 268
Emergency tube thoracostomy, 569-71
Emphysema, 210-11, 247
    heart/lung transplant for, 365-73
    lung transplant for, 255-6
    lung-volume reduction, 249-52
    preop testing indications, A-3
    resection for, 1024-7, anatomy, 1025f
Empyema
    drainage/thoracoplasty, 222-6, 1027-8
        long-term venous access, 1028
    imaging for, 1174-8
    thoracoscopic ± open empyemectomy for, 1027-8
    thoracotomy for, 1027-8, 1026-7
    VATS for, 240-3
En bloc resection, pelvic, 613-18
En bloc vulvectomy, 601-5, 601f
Encephalitis, 67
Encephalo-duro-arterio-synangiosis, 22
Encephalocele, intracranial, 40-1
Enchondromatosis, 1111
End stoma closure, 426-9
End-stage heart disease, transplant for, 365-73
End-stage liver disease, 1170
    transplant for, 547-58, 559-60
End-stage lung disease
    transplant for, 255-6, 365-73
End-stage reflux nephropathy, 1068
End-stage renal disease (ESRD)
    pediatric, 1070, 1081-2
    transplant for, 538-9, 539-42
End-stage renal failure
    hemodialysis for, 349-51
    permanent vascular access, 351-4
End-stage valvular heart disease, 360-5
End-to-end repair of aortic coarctation, 984-7, 984f
End-to-side portacaval shunt, 343-8, 344f

Endarterectomy, carotid, 102-8, 308-10
Endoaortic clamp (EAC), 293
    + port-access procedures, 303, 304
Endocardial cushion defects, 975-8
Endocoronary sinus catheter (ESC)
    + port-access procedures, 302-3
Endocrine diseases, preop testing, A-3
Endocrine surgery
    laparoscopic (adrenalectomy), 466-8
    open, 520-35
Endometrial cancer
    hysterectomy/BSO for, 618-21
    Stage II cancer, hysterectomy, 621-4
Endometrial cavity exam with hysteroscopy, 636-9
Endometrial lining curettage, 632f
Endometrioma, rectal surgery for, 431-2
Endometriosis,
    bladder, GI/GU, 684-6
    ovarian, 684-6
    peritoneal, 684-6
    surgery for, 640-1, 647-51, 690-3
Endomyocardial biopsy, for posttransplant rejection surveillance, 1195
Endopulmonary vent (EPV), 303
Endorectal advancement flap, 433-4
Endoscopic common bile duct stone removal (ERCP), 446
Endoscopic diagnostic transurethral procedures, 696-7; anesthesia, 698-9
Endoscopic procedures, pediatric, 1071-3; anesthesia, 1077-8
Endoscopic retrograde cholangiopan-creatography, 460
Endoscopic sinus surgery (ESS), 157-60
Endotracheal tube. See ETT.
Endovascular drain (EVD), and port-access procedures, 303
Endovascular stent implantation, out-of-OR, pediatric, 1193-4
Endovascular stent-grafting, 312-16
Endovascular therapy
    for brain and spine, 1158-62
    embolization, aneurysm therapy, cerebral revascularization, 1156-62
Enflurane, drug interactions with, F-5
Enteral feeding, 410-12
Enteric fistula closure, 416-18
Enteric incontinence, 435-8
Enteritis, radiation, 413-14, 416-18
Enterocele, anatomy, 652f
    laparotomy for, 639-41, 644-6
    repair, 640-1, 652-4, 656-7
Enterocystoplasty, 715-17
Enterolysis, 415; anesthesia, 416-18
Enterostomy, 410-11; anesthesia, 411-12
Enterovesical fistula repair, 715-17
Entropion repair, 119-20, 124-6
Enucleation, 131-2, 124-6
Eosinophilic granuloma, 31
Ephedra, precautions with anesthesia, F-10
Ephedrine, drug interactions, F-3, F-6
Epidermolysis bullosa (EB), recessive dystrophic, simplex, 1126
    surgery, 1125-8; anesthesia, 1126-7

Epididymal cyst, 723-5
Epidural anesthesia/analgesia
    in C-section, 663, 665
    adult (lumbar, thoracic), C-2, C-4
    pediatric (caudal, lumbar, thoracic), D-4
        contraindications, E-2
        postop, E1-E-2, E-5, E-6
Epidural catheter
    indwelling, pediatric, E-5
    locations, adult, C-2
Epidural hematoma, in craniotomy, 32
Epidural infusion, pediatric, postop, E-5
    continuous, in orthopedics, 1123
Epidural motor cortex stimulation, 61
Epiglottic cancer, 151
Epiglottitis, intubation for, 186-7
Epilepsy
    extratemporal, temporal, 64-5
    in intracranial venous malformation, 16
    temporal lobectomy for, 66-9
    vagal nerve stimulation for, 64-5
Epinephrine
    drug interactions with, F-3, F-6, F-8
    in pediatric epidural anesthesia, D-4
Epinephrine-containing wetting solution injection for liposuction, 892
Epiphrenic diverticulum, 379-81, 379f
Epiphyseal stapling for limb-length discrepancies, 1110-11, 1121-5
Epiphysiodesis (open, percutaneous, Phemister), 1105-6, 1110-11, 1121-5
Epispadias repair, 1075-6, 1077-8
Eppright osteotomy, for pelvic reconstruction, 1097-9, 1121-5
Equinovalgus, severe, 1118-19, 1121-5
ERCP, 484
    failure, 448-50; anesthesia, 452-4
Ergonovine maleate
    use in suction curettage, 612
    use in therapeutic abortion, 633
Ergotamine, drug interactions with, F-7
Erythromycin, drug interactions, F-4, F-6
Erythropoietin, recombinant, in pediatric craniofacial surgery, 936
Eschar excision, 928-32
ESLD. See End-stage liver disease.
Esmolol, drug interactions with, F-4, F-5
Esophageal atresia (EA) 408, 1019f
    failed anastomosis, dilation, 1031-4
    gastrostomy for, 1018-21, 1019f
Esophageal dilation, 959-63
    balloon, 959
    in laparoscopic fundoplication, 456
Esophageal diverticulectomy, 379-81; anesthesia, 387-90
Esophageal foreign body, stricture, esophagoscopy for, 959-63
Esophageal fundoplication, laparoscopic, 456-7; anesthesia, 461-3
Esophageal motility disorder, 379
    GI endoscopy, pediatric, 1199-1200
Esophageal perforation (spontaneous, instrumental), 381-2
    cervical, thoracic drainage, 381-2
    esophagostomy for, 377, 387-90

Esophageal replacement, 1031-2; anatomy, 1032*f*; anesthesia, 1033-4 colon interposition, Waterston, gastric tube anastomosis, 1031-4, 1032*f* dissection, anastomosis, 1032 gastroesophageal anastomosis (Orringer), 1032
Esophageal spasm, 381-3, 387-90
Esophageal stethoscope monitoring, adult, B-1; pediatric, D-1
Esophageal stricture, caustic, 1031-4 dilation for, 1016-17
Esophageal surgery, 377-90
Esophageal varices, bleeding, 1016-17 decompression, shunts, 343-5, 346-8 TIPS for, 1169-73, 1170-2
Esophagectomy, 385-90; anesthesia, 387-90 with colonic interposition, 385-90 transhiatal, 386-90, 392 VATS for, 240
Esophagitis, fundoplication for, 456-7
Esophagogastrectomy, 385-90, 386*f*
Esophagogastric fundoplasty, 384-5, 387-90 anastomosis and gastric drainage, 387*f* intrathoracic anastomosis, 386*f*
Esophagogastric reflux, 384-5
Esophagogastroduodenoscopy, 1016-17
Esophagomyotomy, 382-3, 383*f*, 387-90
Esophagoscopy, 146-53 pediatric, 959-63, 1016-17 rigid, head and neck surgery, 150
Esophagostomy, 377, 378*f*, 387-90
Esophagus, surgery for, 377-90 Barrett's, 385-90 cancer, esophagectomy for, 385-90 nutcracker, 382-3, 387-90 strictures, esophagectomy for, 385-90
Estrogen, drug interactions with, F-5 in uterine cancer, 619
Ethanol, drug interactions with, F-5
Ethmoidectomy. 155*f*, 156, 178-9
ETOH abuse, in anesthetic planning for head/neck surgery, 149
Etomidate, 1164 in adult induction, B-2 drug interactions with, F-10 in heart/lung transplantation, 367
ETT blockage, in epiglottitis, 187 damage, in maxillofacial surgery, 902 difficult insertion/reinsertion, 185 dislodgement/kinking in adenoidectomy/tonsillectomy, 958 in neck mass resection, 1015 in upper respiratory abscess, 965 placement, by auscultation of breath sounds bilaterally, pediatric, D-3 securing, 190, 965 verification of positioning, 209, 211*f*
ETT, laser, 150
ETT, nasal, damage, 902-3
ETT, tube sizes in head/neck surgery, 140 pediatric, by age, 1017, D-3

in thoracic surgery, 206
Evan's syndrome, 465
Evening primrose (*Oenothera biennis*), precautions with anesthesia, F-10
Ewing's sarcoma, 218; XRT, 1188-92
Exomphalos, 408
Exorbitism, 1132
Exostoses (leg, foot), biopsy for, 861
Exotropia, 1132
Exploratory laparotomy peritoneal, 496-9; anesthesia, 497-9 for uterine cancer, 618-21
Exstrophy, cloaca, repair, 1049-53
Exstrophy/epispadias complex, 1074
Exstrophy imperforate anus spinal defect (OEIS), 1049
Extensor tendon repair, 735-6, 748-9 microsurgery, 913-16 tendolysis, 748-9; anesthesia, 751-2 tenosynovitis, operations for, 735-6
External fixator for hip subluxation, anteversion, SCFE, 1108-9, 1121-5
Extraanatomic graft, 328
Extraarticular subtalar arthrodesis, 1118-19; anesthesia, 1121-5
Extracorporeal membrane oxygenation (ECMO), 1203-4
Extracranial neurosurgery, 101-11
Extracranial-intracranial revascularization (EC-IC bypass), craniotomy, 21-6
Extralobar sequestration, 1025
Extrathoracic muscle flap, 222*f*
Extubation—adult, B-4; pediatric, D-3 accidental, 187, 952 in RSI, B-5
Eye, anatomy, 134*f* injury, in laser therapy, 609 painful blind, tumor, 131
Eye positioning, under GA, 950
Eye surgery, 113-37. (Also *see* Ophthalmic surgery and specific procedures.) pediatric, 949-52
Eyelid procedures Asian, plastic surgery for, 874-6, 876-8 closure of full-thickness defect, 122*f* ectropion of, 118-19 entropion of, 119-20, 124-6 lidlift, 874-6; anesthesia, 876-8 lower, flap elevation, 874*f* ptosis (drooping), 120-1, 874-8
Eyelid reconstruction, 122-6 canthotomy and cantholysis, 122-3 frozen sections, 122 grafting techniques, 122-3 Moh's technique 122-3

F
Face aging concerns, 868 anatomic layers, 868*f* bone anomalies, surgery for, 1134-7 cosmetic surgery, 867-82 fractures, 897-902
Face masks, high-filtration, 882
Facelift, 869-71; anesthesia, 876-8

+ laser resurfacing, precautions, 870 nerve and sensory injuries, 871, 869 poor cosmetic results, 871 SMAS, platysma flap, 869*f* 'wet' techniques, 870
Facial bipartition for craniofacial malformations, 1134-7
Facial deformities, disproportions LeFort osteotomies, distraction osteogenesis for, 902-4, 906-8 mandibular osteotomies/genioplasty for, 905-8
Facial fracture surgery, 896-902 bicoronal approach, 900*f* flap closure for CSF leak, 897 OR set-up, 900*f* primary bone grafting, 897
Facial nerve, inferior approach, 165*f* paralysis, 187-92
Facial skeleton reconstruction, 896*f*
Facial/skin laser resurfacing, 881-2; anesthesia, 876-8, 1208-9 airborne contaminants in, 882 hazards—fire, ocular, reflectivity, 882 safety issues, 882
Facial trauma, surgery for, 897-902
Failed intubation in C-section, 664 protocol, in RSI, B-5
Failed-back syndrome, RFA, 1182-6
Failure to thrive (FTT), 988-92
Fallopian tube cancer, staging laparotomy, 594-7 occlusion, fimbrioplasty for, 643
False tracheal passage/disruption, 185
Familial adenomatus polyposis, 420-3 ileostomy, 412-13
Familial cancer syndromes, 595
Familial cavernous malformation syndrome, 17
Fanconi's syndrome, 1090
Fascial excision, burn wound, 928-32
Fascial lip augmentation, 1145-8
Fasciectomy (palmar, digital), 744; anesthesia, 746-8
Fasciocutaneous flaps, in pressure-sore reconstruction, 923
Fasciotomy—leg/thigh, 857-9; anesthesia, 859-61
FAST scan, in chest trauma, 580
Fast-track anesthesia, 587, 973-4
Fasting, preop pediatric guidelines, D-1
Fat filum terminale, correction, 941-3
Fecal incontinence, 430, 435-8
Feeding G-tube for EA repair, 1018
Feldene, in lumbar discectomy, 783
Felty's syndrome, 497
Femoral canal bulging, 505-6, 508-9
Femoral hernia repair, 505-6, 508-9 anatomy, incision, 505*f*
Femoral neck fracture, 808-10, 815-17 ORIF for, 815-17, 863-4
Femoral shaft repair intramedullary nailing, 820-1, 863-4 ORIF with plate for, 819-20, 863-4

Femoral shortening, for hip dislocation, 1102-3; anesthesia, 1121-5

Femoral thrombosis, 341-4

Femoral torsion, medial, 1108-9

Femoro-femoral (fem-fem) CPB, 293*f*

Femur
malignant tumor, surgery, 805-6
mass, infection, osteomyelitis, biopsy for, 861, 863-4
traumatic amputation, 805-8, 852-7

Femur, distal
nonunion/malunion, 818-19, 863-4

Femur fractures, nonunion/malunion arthroplasty, 808-10, 813-15
closed reduction/external fixation, 823-4; anesthesia, 863-4
closed reduction/percutaneous pinning, 815-16; anesthesia, 863-4
intramedullary nailing, 820-1, 863-4
ORIF for, 815-17; anesthesia, 863-4
with plate for, 819-20
prosthetic replacement, 815-17

Femur, proximal
fractures, ORIF for, 815-17, 815*f*; anesthesia, 863-4
nonunion/malunion, 822-23, 863-4
osteotomy for osteoarthritis, 822-23; anesthesia, 863-4

Fenestration procedures, 945-8

Fenfluramine, effects of in anesthesia for abdominoplasty, 890

Fentanyl
in adult anesthesia, B-2, B-3
postop analgesia, C-2; PCA, PCEA, C-3
drug interactions with, F-1, F-3, F-4, F-7, F-8, F-9
in MAC, B-4
in pediatric balanced anesthesia, D-3 PCA, E-3
in septal myectomy/myotomy, 283

Fenugreek (*Trigonella foenum-graecum*), precautions with anesthesia, F-10

Fetal death, 1025; anesthesia-related, 480-2

Fetal distress, C-section for, 660-5

Fetal surgery for large CCAMs, 1025

Feverfew (*Tanacetum parthenium*), precautions with anesthesia, F-11

Fiber optic bronchoscopy (FOB), 235-8; anesthesia, 237-8
assessment of DLT positioning, 211*f*
in lobectomy/pneumonectomy, 213

Fibromuscular dysplasia, 6

Fibrosis, in microsurgery, 912

Fibrosis syndromes, in strabismus, 951

Fibrous dysplasia, 31
rodding for, 1111-13, 1121-5

Fibula flap, in microsurgery, 911

Fibula transection, in amputation, 855*f*

Fibular hemimelia, 1111, 1114

Fick principle, 1193

Field block, for hernia, hydrocele, 1060

Filum lipoma, pediatric, 941-3

Fimbrioplasty repair of fallopian tube occlusion, 643

Fine-needle aspiration cytology, for breast biopsy, 512-13; anesthesia, 514-15

Finger/thumb
bifid, repair, 1090-2
pollicization, 1089-92, 1089*f*
replantation microsurgery, 913-16
trauma, in D&C, D&E, 636

Fire, airway, in tracheostomy, 185

Fire hazards, in laser surgery, 882, 962

Fish oils, precautions with anesthesia, F-11

Fistula-in-ano, surgery for, 433-4

Fistulectomy, anal, 433-4, 436-8

Fistulotomy, anal, 433-4, 436-8

FLACC Pain Scale, E-2

Flail chest, 569-71

Flank incision, 531*f*, 708*f*, 788*f*

Flaps (*See* specific types and donor sites.)
for lip/nose deformities, 1145-8
for microsurgical reconstruction, 911
in pressure-sore reconstruction, 923*f*

Fletcher-suit applicators for perineal implants, 624*f*

Flexible bronchoscopy, 235-8

Flexible LMA, 144. (Also *see* LMA.)

Flexor digitorum profundus tendon avulsion, 745-6

Flexor digitorum superficialis, 745-6

Flexor tendon
injury zone classification, 745*f*
laceration repair, 745-6
nerve injuries, 745
replantation microsurgery, 913-16
tendolysis repair, 748-9, 751-2

Flieringa ring, corneal transplant, 115

Floating thrombi (hip level), 341-3

Flow volume loop, 233*f*, 1023

Flowthow approach, lumbar sympathectomy, 336

Fluid collection, 1174-58

Fluid overload, 639, 693

Fluorinated inhalation agents, drug interactions with, F-1

Fluoroscopy, 1174-8

Fluorouracil, toxic effects, 598

Fluvoxamine, drug interactions, F-5

FOB. *See* Fiber optic bronchoscopy.

Focal cartilage lesions, 760-1

Fogarty catheter, 341*f*, 342

Fontan lateral tunnel operation, 1003-6, 1004*f*; anesthesia, 1005-6

Fontan procedure for HLHS, 1010-11

Foot
flaccid, drop, 1117-18, 1121-5
fracture, ORIF, irrigation and debridement, 843, 863-4
muscle contracture, 851-2
tendon lengthening/transfer, 851-2; anesthesia, 863-4
tumor, infection, biopsy, 861, 863-4
varus/cavovarus, arthrodesis/Grice procedure, 1118-19, 1121-5

Foraminotomy, 80

Forbes-Albright syndrome, 44

Forced duction testing (FDT) in strabismus surgery, 950

Forearm AV fistula, loop graft, for hemodialysis, 349-54

Foregut, cyst duplication, 1021-4

Forehead
advancement, 1130-4
lift, 872-6, 873*f*; anesthesia, 876-8

Foreign body
in bronchus, 147
esophageal, removal, 959-63
pediatric, 1016-17, 1071, 1072
GI endoscopy for, 1199-1200
in lung, removal, 235-8
perforation, with enteric fistulae, 416

Forked flaps, for lip/nose deformities, 1145-8; incisions, anatomy, 1146*f*

Fornix incision for strabismus, 950

Fosphenytoin, drug interactions with, F-7

Four-compartment fascial decompression, leg, 859

Four-corner (capitate-hamate-triquetral-lunate) intercarpal arthrodesis, 737-8

Four-gland hyperplasia, 526

Four-part proximal humerus fracture, arthroplasty for, 769-73

Fowler-Stevens approach for undescended testicle, 1061

Fowler-Stevens orchiopexy, 1081-2

Fractionation, in XRT, 1188-92

Fragmentation rodding, for long-bone, 1111-13; anesthesia, 1121-5

Frame-based stereotaxy, 52-6, 59-60, 62-4

Frameless craniotomy, 53-6

Frameless stereotaxy, 44, 52-6; anesthesia, 55-6, OR layout, 53*f*

Free bone flap, in craniotomy, 26

Free flap reconstruction, microsurgery, 910-13
commonly used flaps, 911, 910*f*
survival, 910

Free graft technique, pterygium, 123

Free mammary graft, in CABG, 266

Free reflux, surgery for, 384-5

Free skin graft for burn wound, 928-32

Freeman-Sheldon syndrome, 1120

Freidrich's ataxia, 1094

Frey's syndrome, 164

Frontalis sling, ptosis repair, 121, 121*f*

Fronto-orbital advancement—osteotomy, tongue-in-groove, wiring, 1131*f*

Frontofacial advancement for upper face and frontal bone anomalies, 1134-7

Frostbite, 336-8

Frozen shoulder, 760-1

Fulguration of bleeding vessels, 698

Full-stomach precautions, 127, B-5

Functional end-to-end anastomosis for small bowel, 413-14

Functional endoscopic sinus surgery (FESS), 157-8; anesthesia, 158-60

Functional neck dissection, 168-73

Functional neurosurgery, 54-6, 57-70

Functional restoration procedures, 909-26

Functional side-to-side shunt, for portal HTN, 343-5; anesthesia, 346-8

Fundoplication
laparoscopic, Nissen, Toupet (partial), 456-7; anesthesia, 461-3

open, Nissen, 384-5; 387-90
'Funnel chest.' *See* Pectus excavatum.
Furazolidone, drug interactions, F-5
Furlow procedure for cleft palate, 1140-2, 1141*f*; anesthesia, 1147-8
Furosemide, drug interactions with, F-7
in craniotomy for trauma, 36

G

Galactorrhea-amenorrhea syndrome, 44
Gallbladder, 446-7, 447*f*, 452-4
Gallie wiring technique, C-spine, 75*f*
Gallstone ileus, 415
Gallstones, duodenotomy for, 406
in pancreatitis, 484, 486
Gamete intrafallopian transfer (GIFT), 644
Gamma stretch reflex, 70
Ganglion, wrist, cyst excision, 743
Ganglionectomy, 336
Ganglioneuroma, 229-30, 232-5
Gangrene (diabetic, gas), 852-3
Garlic (*Allium sativum*), precautions with anesthesia, F-11
Gas analyzer monitoring—adult, B-1; pediatric, D-1
Gas-fluid exchange, retinal, 134-7
Gastrectomy (total, hemi), 392-4, 397-9
Gastric fundus, 457*f*
Gastric hypersecretion, malignancy, 392-4
Gastric outlet obstruction, 396-9
Gastric perforation, oversew, 394-5; anesthesia, 397-9
Gastric reflux, complications in esophageal procedures, 388
Gastric tube anastomosis for esophageal replacement, 1031-4
Gastric ulcers, 392-4
Gastric volume/acidity, in RSI, B-5
Gastrinoma, in pancreatic surgery, 492
Gastritis, diffuse, hemorrhagic, 392-4
Gastrocystoplasty, 715-17
Gastroenteritis, pediatric, 1038-40
Gastroesophageal junction cancer, 385-90, 392-4
Gastroesophageal reflux disease. *See* GERD.
Gastrointestinal. *See* GI.
Gastrojejunal tube placement, 1174
Gastrojejunostomy, 393*f*, 491*f*
Gastroplasty, vertical banded, 399-403, 399*f*; anesthesia, 401-3
in laparoscopic bariatric surgery, 477-9; anesthesia, 401-3
Gastroschisis repair, 1049-53, 1050*f*
Gastrostomy
Janeway, 403-4; anesthesia, 411-12
percutaneous endoscopic, 403-4, 411-12
Stamm, 403-4; anesthesia, 411-12
for TEF, EA repair, 1018-21
tube placement, 1174, 1199
Gaucher's disease, 345-8
Gender reassignment surgery, 1076
Gengraf, in heart transplantation, 360
Genioglossal muscle, exposure, 195*f*

Genioplasty for chin deformity, 905-8, with internal fixation, 905*f*
Genital procedures, pediatric, 1076-8
clitoroplasty, vaginoplasty, urethroplasty, 1076-8
Genitalia, abnormal, 1076-8
Genitalia, ambiguous, 1076-8, 1081-2
Genitourinary endometriosis, 684-6
Genu valgum, 1116
GERD, 961
bronchoscopy/esophagoscopy, 959-63
in GI endoscopy, 1199-1201
laparoscopic fundoplication, 456-7
in pancreatic surgery, 492
pediatric pyloromyotomy, 1038-40
Germ-cell tumor, 229, 1188-92
Gestational trophoblastic disease, 610-13
GI distention compromise of respiration in repair of TEF, EA, 1018
GI endometriosis, 684-6
GI hemorrhage, 423-5
GI stromal tumor, 501-2
GI, upper/lower, endoscopy, pediatric, 1199-1201
Giant intracranial aneurysms, 10-13
Gianturco Z stent, 1178
GIFT, for infertility, 644
Gigantism, infantile, 1051
Ginger (*Zingiber officinale*), precautions with anesthesia, F-11
Gingivoalveoloplasty, for alveolar cleft, 1144-5, 1144*f*; anesthesia, 1147-8
Ginkgo (*Ginkgo biloba*), precautions with anesthesia, F-11
Ginseng, precautions with anesthesia, F-11
Girdlestone procedure (hip resection), 808-10; anesthesia, 813-15
Glasgow Coma Scale (GCS), 34, 35
Glaucoma
goniotomy for, 117
implants for, 117-18
trabeculectomy for, 116-18
Glenn bidirectional shunt
for HLHS, 1009-11
for tricuspid atresia, 1003-6
Glenohumeral instability, 760-2, 766-9
Glenohumeral shoulder arthroplasty, 769-73, incision, 769*f*; anesthesia, 770-2
Glial scar, 67
Glioblastoma, glioma, 27
Globe, ruptured/lacerated, 126-9
Glomerulonephritis, 351
Glomus tumor, 161, 187-92
Glossectomy (partial, total), 177-8
laser midline (LMG), 193-8
Glossopharyngeal neuralgia, 37-40
Glossoptosis, 1141, 1143
Glucose, in brain ischemia, 105
Gluteal flap, in microsurgery, 911
Glycerol injection, for trigeminal neuralgia, 108-11
Glycopyrrolate, in EB surgery, 1127
Goiter
substernal, excision of, 229-30
thyroidectomy for, 521-6

Golden Seal (*Hydrastis Canadensis*), precautions with anesthesia, F-11
Goldenhar syndrome, 1136, 1147
Gonadal dysgenesis, 1059
Gonadectomy, laparoscopic, 1081-2
Goniotomy (glaucoma), 117
Gorlin's syndrome, in gynecology, 595
Gracilis flap, in microsurgery, 911
Gracilis myocutaneous flaps, for vaginal/perineal reconstruction, 613
Grade IIIC injuries with neurovascular severance, 852-3
Graft (tube, Y, extraanatomic), in abdominal aneurysm surgery, 328
Granisetron, for adult antiemetics, C-2
Granulocyte macrophage colony-stimulating factor (GM-CSF), for alveolar proteinosis, 253
Granuloma, cholesterol, 187-92
Grape seed (*Vitis vinifera*), precautions with anesthesia, F-11
Grapefruit, precautions with anesthesia, F-11
Graves disease
with strabismus, 951
thyroidectomy for, 521-6
Great vessel injury, repair, 577-8, 580-2
Grice extraarticular subtalar fusion, for foot deformities, 1118-19, 1121-5
Grisel's syndrome, in torticollis, 1088
Groin
hernias—anatomy, sites, 718*f*
node dissection, unilateral, 602
pain/lump in, 504-5, 508-9
Groshong catheter, for permanent vascular access, 351-4
Growth hormone-secreting tumor, 44
Guanethidine, drug interactions, F-5
Guidewire cricothyrotomy, 1214-15
Guillotine amputation
above knee, 852-4; anesthesia, 855-7
below knee, 854-5; anesthesia, 855-7
Guillotine tonsillectomy technique, 143
Gynecologic oncology, 593-629
laparoscopic surgery, 627-9, 692-3
Gynecologic surgery, 591-657, 683-93
laparoscopy for, 683-93
Gynecology/infertility surgery, 631-57

H

Haemophilus influenza, 186-7
Hairy-cell leukemia, 465
Halothane
deep, pediatric muscle relaxation, D-2
drug interactions, F-5, F-6, F-8, F-9
in pediatric inhalational anesthesia, D-2, D-3
in pediatric neurosurgery, 940
Hand
joint replacement, 736-7, 740-3
replantation, 755-8
microsurgery, 913-16
traumatic amputation, 755-8
zones of injury, 745, 745*f*
Hand surgery, 733-58

Hand-assisted donor nephrectomy, laparoscopic, 544; anesthesia, 546
Hanlon atrial septectomy for TGA, 996
Harrington rod technique, 90, 1093-5
Hartmann's pouch in laparotomy for intestinal perforation, NEC, 1043
Hartmann's procedure, 426
Hassab procedure, portal HTN, 345-8
Hasson technique, laparoscopic
    cholecystectomy, 459
    fundoplication, 456-7
    pediatric, 1081-2
Haultain procedure for uterine reinversion, 680; anesthesia, 680-1
Hauser procedure, for patellar realignment, 1115
Hawthorn *(Crataegus oxyacantha)*, precautions with anesthesia, F-11
Hayes-Martin maneuver, submandibular gland excision, 166
Head and neck surgery, 139-98
Head
    injury, craniotomy for, 32-7
    microsurgical reconstruction, flaps, 911
    shape abnormalities, 1130-4
Headache—migraine, vascular, 16
Hearing loss
    conductive, surgery for, 160-3
    in imaging procedures, 1177
Heart
    block, pacemaker for, 284-7
    cannulation, in CPB, 259
    failure, 1009, 1063
    nonbeating, in trauma surgery, 571-2
Heart disease, end-stage
    transplant for, 360-5; 365-73
    radiation exposure, in microsurgical reconstruction, 912
Heart surgery, 257-373. (Also *see* Cardiac surgery.)
Heart transplantation, adult, neonatal, 360-5; anesthesia, 361-4
    heart procurement, 560-5
    + lung transplantation, 365-73
Helicobacter pylori, in PUD, 396
Heliox, tracheobronchial stenting, 1180-1
Heller's myotomy, 382-3, 387-90
    laparoscopic, 458-9, 461-3
    VATS for, 240-3
Hemangioblastoma, 27
Hemangioma, 31, 442, 1023, 1041
Hematocrit (Hct) preop testing, A-1
Hematologic diseases/disorders, 345-8
    preop testing indications, A-3
Hematoma
    with airway compromise, 525
    epidural, in craniotomy, 32
    in facial cosmetic surgery, 877
    intracerebral, in craniotomy, 32
    risk, complications in facelift, 869-70
    subdural, 32; 32f; precautions, 33f
Hematuria
    endoscopic diagnostics for, 696-7
    pediatric procedures, 1071-3
Hemiarthroplasty, shoulder, 769-73
Hemicolectomy (right, left), 424

Hemifacial spasm, 37-40
Hemigastrectomy, 392-4, 397-9
    limb-length discrepancies, 1111, 1114
    pediatric abdominal tumors, 1041
Hemihypertrophy, 1069
Hemilaminectomy, with TLIF, 95
Hemilaryngectomy, 173-6
Hemimegalencephaly, 67
Heminephrectomy, laparoscopic, 1081-2
Hemivulvectomy, 602-5
Hemodialysis, arteriovenous access for, 349-51; anesthesia, 352-4
Hemodynamic instability, in replantation microsurgery, 915
Hemoglobin (Hb) preop testing, A-1
Hemolytic anemia
    splenectomy for, 499-501
        laparoscopic, 463-6
    in staging laparotomy, 497
Hemophilia, in knee procedures, 835-7
Hemoptysis, bronchoscopy for, 235-8
Hemorrhage, abdominal, control, 582-3
Hemorrhagic cystitis, 712-15
Hemorrhagic shock, 796
Hemorrhoid, 434-5; anesthesia, 436-8
    laser, nonexcisional treatment, 434
    prolapse, surgery for, 434-5
    symptomatic, bleeding, 434-8
Hemorrhoidectomy (Whitehead, circumferential, Lord procedures), 434-5; anesthesia, 436-8
Hemothorax
    in chest trauma surgery, 580
    emergency tube thoracostomy, 569-71
    in esophageal procedures, 388
    in RFA, 1185
Hemovac drains, 1029
Heparinization, systemic, in anesthesia for giant intracranial aneurysms, 12
Hepatectomy, in liver transplant, 547-8
Hepatic bifurcation, 450-4
Hepatic cirrhosis, 1169-73
Hepatic diseases, preop testing, A-3
Hepatic failure, transplant for, 547-58
Hepatic fibrosis, congenital, 345-8
Hepatic malignancy, RFA for, 1182-6
Hepatic portoenterostomy (Kasai), 1046-9
Hepatic resection, 440-1, 442-4
    partial right lobectomy, left lateral segmentectomy, 440-4
    right/left lobectomy, trisegmentectomy, 440-4
Hepatic surgery, 439-44
Hepatic trauma injuries, repair, 441-2
    splenic, 583-4; anesthesia, 586-9
Hepatic tumor resections, 1040-3
Hepatic vein occlusion, 345-8
Hepaticoduodenal ligament occlusion, 440
Hepaticojejunostomy, 491f
Hepatitis
    alcoholic, 345-8
    B, C, transplant for, 547-52
    infectious, preop testing, A-3
Hepatoblastoma, resection, 1040-3
Hepatocellular carcinoma, 547-52

Hepatorenal syndrome, 1169-73
Hepatorrhaphy, 441-2; anesthesia, 442-4
Herbal agents, precautions for anesthesia and surgery, F10-F-11
Hernia, *See* specific site (e.g., femoral, groin, inguinal) or type.
    predisposing factors, 508
'Hernia of the cord' (omphalocele), 1049
Hernia repair (Also *see* Herniorrhaphy.)
    minimally invasive, pediatric, 1065
    strangulated, small-bowel resection for, 413-14, 416-18
    totally extraperitoneal, transabdominal preperitoneal, 475-7
Herniated disc, 93-4, 97-9
Herniated lumbar disc, 782-4
Herniorrhaphy
    femoral, 505-6; anesthesia, 508-9
    inguinal, 504-5; anesthesia, 508-9; 718-21; anesthesia, 720-1
    pediatric 1058-61; anesthesia, 1059-60
Hess and Hunt Grading System for Aneurysmal SAH, 4, 6
Hiatus (hiatal) hernia, 384-5
Hickman catheter, for permanent vascular access, 351-4
High ligation and stripping, varicose veins, 355-8; anesthesia, 356-8
High-flow AVM, 15-21
High-frequency ventilation, 225, 228
High-spinal anesthetic technique, in secundum ASD surgery, 973
Highly selective vagotomy, 394
Hill procedure, 384-5, 385f, 387-90
Hill-Sachs lesions, OATS for, 760-1
Hindfoot equinus, with clubfoot, 1119
Hindquarter amputation, 805-8
Hip
    adduction/flexion contracture, 1103-4
    anteversion, 1108-9, 1121-5
    arthritis, arthrosis, 808-15, 822-3
    contracture, release, 1103-4
    deformity, 1108-9; anesthesia, 1121-5
    disarticulation, 805-8, 853f
    flaccid paralysis, 'frog'-type contracture, 1101-2
    loose bodies, 812-15
    malignant tumor, 805-8
    shallow socket, 1099
    subluxation, 1108-9, 1121-5
        recurrent, 811-12, 813-15
    synovitis, chronic, 812-15
    traumatic amputation, 805-8
    uncontrollable infection, 805-8
Hip dislocation, 808-15
    chronic, 808-10, 813-15
    congenital, 810
    pediatric, 1099-1100, 1102-3, 1097-9, 1121-5
Hip dysplasia, 812
    developmental, 802-3, 803f, 806-8
    pediatric, 1088, 1098
Hip surgery, 795-824
    acetabular augmentation, Chiari osteotomy, 1099-1100, 1121-5
    amputation, 805-6; anesthesia, 806-8

arthrodesis, 811-15; cobra plate, 811*f*
arthroplasty (total, Girdlestone), 808-
    10; anesthesia, 813-15
    revision procedures, 808-10
    unipolar, bipolar approaches, 808-10
capsulotomy, 812-13
external fixator, 1108-9, 1121-5
joint arthrotomy, 809*f*, 812-13,
Ober fasciotomy, Yount-Ober release
    for contracture, 1101-2
open reduction ± femoral shortening,
    1102-3, 1102*f*, 1121-5
osteotomy, 822-3, anesthesia, 863-4
    Bernese periacetabular osteotomy,
        803*f*
    with bone graft for dysplasia, 802-3,
        806-8
    for dislocation, 1097-9, 1121-5
prosthesis, malpositioned, loose,
    arthroplasty for, 808-10, 813-15
resection, arthroplasty, 808-10;
    anesthesia, 813-15
screw, dynamic, placement, 816*f*
synovectomy, 812-13, 813-15
trochanteric osteotomy, 811-15
Hirschsprung's disease, 1055*f*
colostomy, loop/primary, 1053-6
one-stage neonatal repair, 1053
pullthrough for, 1053-6, 1055*f*
transanal, anastomosis, 1055*f*
Histiocytoma, excision of, 501-2
Histiocytosis, in craniotomy, 31
HLHS. *See* Hypoplastic left heart
    syndrome.
Hodgkin's disease, 465, 496-9
Holinger bronchoscope, 1179
Holt-Oram syndrome, 973, 1090
Hook-rod construction
    in posterior spinal instrumentation/
        fusion, 1093-5; anesthesia, 789-93
    in thoracic spine surgery, 90
Hook-wire localization, breast biopsy,
    512-13; anesthesia, 514-15
Hooked acromion, 762-4, 766-9
Horner's syndrome, 339, 518, 780, 1022
House-Urban retractor, 189*f*
Human chorionic gonadotropin, 641
Humerus fractures
    lateral condyle, closed/open reduction
        for, 1085-6; anesthesia, 1091-2
    proximal, 773-4; anesthesia, 776-8
    4-part fracture, 769-73
    supracondylar, displaced, closed
        reduction, 1084-5, 1091-2
    percutaneous pinning, 1084-5, 1084*f*;
        anesthesia, 1091-2
Hunting procedure for uterine reinversion,
    680; anesthesia, 680-1
Hurst esophageal dilators, 959
Hydrocele
    pediatric, 1079-81
    repair, 1058-61; anesthesia, 1059-60
    scrotal, 723-5, incisions, 724*f*
Hydrocelectomy
    for hydrocele, 723-5; anesthesia, 724-5

for inguinal hernia, 1079-81
Hydrocephalus, 49, 938-9, 1010, 1132
    loculated multicompartmental, 945-8
    obstructive, 945-8
    pediatric procedures, 943-8
    ventricular shunt for, 47-50
Hydrocodone, in pediatric analgesia, E-3
Hydromorphone
    adult analgesia, C-2; PCA/PCEA, C-3
    lumbar/thoracic epidural analgesia, C-2
    pediatric PCA, E-3; epidural, E-5
Hydronephrosis
    endoscopic diagnostics for, 696-9
    nephrectomy for, 706-9, 1068-71
    pyeloplasty for, 1069-71
Hydrops fetalis, with CCAM, 1025
Hydrotherapy, for burn wounds, 928
Hydroxyzine, in adult premedication, B-2
Hygroma, subdural, 49
Hyoid bone cyst, 520*f*
Hyoid myotomy and suspension, 194-8,
    196*f*; anesthesia, 196-8
Hypaque dye, in interstitial perineal
    implant, 625
Hyperadrenocorticism, 532, 533-5
Hyperaldosteronism, 530-5
Hypercalcemia, in parathyroidectomy, 528
Hypercapnia, in bronchoscopy, 238
Hypercarbia, in tracheobronchial stenting,
    1181
Hypercortisolism, 530-5
Hypercyanotic episodes, with TOF, 989
Hyperemesis gravidarum, 611
Hypergastrinemia, 392-4
Hyperhidrosis
    sympathectomy for, 339-41
    VATS for, 240-3
Hypermenorrhea, 639-41, 644-6
Hyperosmolar feeding, 1044
Hyperparathyroidism, 526-30
    minimally invasive surgery, endoscopic
        techniques for, 526
    parathyroidectomy for, 526-30
    preop testing indications, A-3
Hypersplenism
    laparoscopic splenectomy for, 463-6
    shunt procedures for, 343-5, 346-8
    staging laparotomy for, 497
Hypertelorism, 1134-7
Hypertension (HTN)
    in facelift, necklift, 869
    infrainquinal arterial bypass for, 331-5
    laparoscopy (pediatric), 1081-2
    preop testing indications, A-3
Hypertension, portal, 343-8
    esophageal transection for, 345-8
    TIPS for, 1169-73, 1170-2
Hypertension, pulmonary, 255-6
    risk, surgery for sleep disorders, 197
Hypertensive response, control of, in
    aortic dissection repair, 319
Hyperthermia, in RFA, 1185
Hyperthyroidism
    preop testing indications, A-3
    thyroidectomy for, 521-6

Hypertrophy, asymmetric septal, 282-4
Hyperventilation, in craniotomy, 36
Hypocalcemia, 492, 525, 529
Hypocarbia, in craniotomy for trauma, 36
Hypoglycemia, 493
Hypokalemia, 492; Sx, 692
Hypomastia, 884-5, 887-8
Hypopharyngeal diverticulum, 379-81
Hypopharyngeal tumor, 147
Hypopharynx, visualization of, 146
Hypoplasia, 996, 1116
    mandibular, maxillary, 1136
    thumb, 1089-90, 1091-2
Hypoplastic left heart syndrome, 995,
    1008-11
    Fontan procedure for, 1010-11
    Glenn procedure for, 1010-11
    heart transplant for, 360-5
    Norwood operation for, 1010-11
Hypospadias, surgery for, 1075-6, 1077-8
Hypotension, controlled/deliberate
    in neurosurgery, 98
    in organ donors, 562
    in otolaryngology, 142
    in pelvis/hip procedures, 807
Hypotensive anesthesia, 140
Hypothermia
    in craniotomy, 8, 19
    deep (with CPB), in anesthesia for
        giant intracranial aneurysms, 11
    deliberate, in craniotomy, 26
    in gynecologic procedures, 596, 693
    in MRI, 1201
    in pressure-sore reconstruction, 925
    in secundum ASD surgery, 974-5
    in trauma surgery, 581, 585, 587, 588
Hypothyroidism, 524-5
    preop testing indications, A-3
Hypoventilation, in bronchoscopy, 238
Hypovolemia, 6, 492
Hypovolemic shock, 589-90
Hypoxemia, 214, 238, 253
    during OLV, 389
    in pediatric extubation, D-3
    in tracheobronchial stenting, 1181
Hypoxia, with NEC, 1044
Hyskon, use in hysteroscopy, 637
Hysterectomy
    abdominal, 647-51; anesthesia, 649-51
    + BSO, for uterine cancer, 618-21
    emergent obstetrical, for postpartum
        hemorrhage, 666-7
    for endometriosis, 684-6, 692-3
    laparoscopic, 690-2; anesthesia, 692-3
    modifications—Stallworthy, Dolstad,
        Novak, Rutledge, Wertheim, 622
    radical, 621-4, 621*f*; anesthesia, 622-3
    ± salpingo-oophorectomy, 690-3
    supracervical, anesthesia for, 661-5
    total, uterine rupture, 668-9
    total, subtotal, 666-7
    total abdominal, 647-51
    vaginal, 647-51, 648*f*
Hysteroscopy, 636-7, 637*f*; anesthesia,
    638-9

I

Iatrogenic bowel injury, 416
Iatrogenic endovascular catheter, 13-15
Iatrogenic injury, 448-50, 452-4
Iatrogenic lumbar instability, 96-9
Ibuprofen, in pediatric pain management, E-1
ICD. *See* Implantable cardioverter-defibrillator.
ICHD, five-position code, 285
Idiopathic hypertrophic subaortic stenosis (IHSS), 283
Idiopathic hypertrophy of muscle of antrum/pylorus in infants, 1038
Idiopathic pancreatitis, 484
Idiopathic thrombocytopenic purpura (ITP), 463-6, 497
Ileal conduit in cystectomy, 712, 713*f*
Ileal pouch and anastomosis (IPAA), with proctocolectomy, 421-3
Ileostomy
    Brooke, 410-11, 410*f*, 411-12
    continent, with proctocolectomy, 421-3
    end, with proctocolectomy, 421-3
    malfunctioning, 412-13
    pouch (Kock), 412-13, 412*f*
    proximal loop, 426-7, 427-9
Iliac crest bone, biopsy, 496*f*
Iliac crest flap, in microsurgery, 911
Iliac grafting for tibia nonunion/malunion, 844-5; anesthesia, 863-4
Iliac thrombosis, 341-3
Iliac vessel injury, 585
Iliac wing fractures, 796
Iliofemoral thrombophlebitis, 354-5
Ilizarov pin fixator
    for limb lengthening, 1113-5, 1121-5
    for tibia fracture, 842
Image intensifier (I.I.), 799
Image-guided navigation, craniotomy, 26
Imaging and image-guided procedures, 1173-8; anesthesia, 1175-7
    cross-sectional (CT, MRI), 1201-2
    intraop complications, 1177
Imipenem, drug interactions with, F-5
Immune thrombocytopenic purpura, 497-501
Imperforate anus
    with esophageal replacement, 1032
    laparoscopic mobilization/pullthrough, 1056
    pullthrough for lesions, 1056-8
Implantable cardioverter-defibrillator (ICD), 1165-9, 1165*f*
    pediatric, 1195; anesthesia, 1195-7
    in functional neurosurgery, 60, 62
Impotence, penile prosthesis for, 721-3
In utero therapies for CHD, 1034
In vitro fertilization, 643-4, 646-7, 687
Incisions (Also *see* specific procedures.)
    bicoronal, 40*f*
    chevron with midline extension, 552*f*
    clamshell, 206, 207*f*, 255
    ear-to-ear scalp, facial surgery, 898
    flank, 708*f*, 788*f*

low midline abdominal, 703*f*
low transverse, 660*f*
lower quadrant curvilinear, 538*f*
maxillary, 179*f*
median sternotomy, 206*f*, 573
midline, 561*f*
muscle-sparing, 207, 208-9
perineal, midline, transverse curvilinear, 704*f*
Pfannenstiel's, 703*f*
prone, 27; modified, 17*f*
radial artery cutdown, 1217*f*
Stallard-Wright, 132
thoracoabdominal, left, 323*f*, 386*f*
thoracotomy, left, 379*f*
three-incision vulvectomy, 602*f*
transverse, 521*f*
vertical, 183*f*
Y-shaped, 52*f*
Incisional biopsy (leg, foot), 861, 863-4
Incisional hernia repair, 506-7, 508-9
Inclusion technique for TAAA repair, 322-7, anatomy, 323*f*
Incontinence
    anal, in procidentia, 429
    fecal, enteric, 435-8
    fecal, in rectal prolapse, 430
    pediatric, operations for, 1074
Indigo carmine
    in laparoscopic hysterectomy, 690
    in pediatric transurethral procedures, 1072
    reaction, in prostatectomy, 706
Indomethacin, for PDA, 981, 982
Induction
    adult standard, B-2
    blind nasal, in esophageal procedures, 388
    in heart/lung transplant, 367
    pediatric, im, iv, inhalational, D-2-D-3
    in RSI, B-5
Indwelling epidural catheter, E-5
Infant respiratory distress syndrome (IRDS), in subglottic stenosis, 967
Infantile gigantism, 1051
Infantile hypertrophic pyloric stenosis, 1038-40
Infectious granulomata, 231-5
Inferior sagittal mandibular osteotomy/ genioglossal advancement (MOGA), 193-8
Inferior vena cava injury, 585-9
Infertility surgery, 631-57; anesthesia, 644-6
    fimbrioplasty, pelvic laparotomy/ laparoscopy, salpingolyis, 643
    GIFT, 644
    hysteroscopy, 636-7; anesthesia, 638-9
    laparotomy, myomectomy, 639-41; anesthesia, 644-6
    ovariolysis, chromopertubation, 643
    TET, 644
    transvaginal oocyte retrieval, 641-3
    tubal reanastomosis/cannulation, metroplasty, Strassman, 644

Inflammatory bowel disease, 411, 415
    ileostomy (Kock) pouch for, 412-13
    proctocolectomy for, 420-3, 427-9
    segmental colectomy, 423-5, 427-9
Infracardiac drainage for TAPVC, 993
Infraclavicular block
    in arm surgery, 779, 780
    in flexor tendon repair, 746, 747
    in fractures of distal radius, carpus, metacarpals, 754, 755
    in wrist procedures, 741, 742
Infracolic omentectomy for gynecologic cancer, 594-7; anesthesia, 595-7
Infrainguinal arterial bypass, 331-5; anesthesia, 332-4
Infrared coagulation, for hemorrhoid, 434
Infrarenal vena cava ligation, 586
Infratentorial brain tumor, 26-30
Inguinal hernia, 504*f*, 718*f*
Inguinal hernia surgery/repair
    Bassini, McVay's, Shouldice, mesh, patch repair, 504
    herniorrhaphy, 504-5, 718-21, 719*f*
    open, 504-5; anesthesia, 508-9
    laparoscopic, 475-7, 1079-81
    pediatric, 1058-61, 1079-81
Inguinal ligation of spermatic vein, 718-21, 719*f*; anesthesia, 720-1
Inguinal lymphadenectomy, 601*f*, 602*f*
Inguinal orchiectomy, groin dissections, 718-21
Inguinal orchiopexy, 718-21
Inguinal region, anatomy, 475*f*
Inguinofemoral lymphadenectomy, 718-21; anesthesia, 720-1
Inguinoscrotal procedures, pediatric, 1079-81; anesthesia, 1080
Inhalational anesthesia
    adult, B-3
    drug interactions with, F-1, F-2, F-3, F-4, F-6
    halogenated, drug interactions, F-5
    in out-of-OR XRT, 1190-1
    pediatric, D-2, D-3
Innominate artery injury repair, 577-8
Insulinoma, in pancreatic surgery, 492
Intact ventricular septum (IVS), 996
Intercarpal arthrodesis (partial wrist fusion), 737-8; anesthesia, 740-3
    scaphocapitate, lunotriquetrel, four-corner, 737-8
Intercarpal instability, 749-50
Intercarpal ligament tears, 749-50
Intermaxillary fixation (IMF), of facial fractures, 897-9
Intermittent apnea, in airway management, 150
Interphalangeal joint arthroplasty, proximal, distal, 736-7, 740-3
Interscalene block
    in arm surgery, 779, 780
    in glenohumeral arthroplasty, 771, 772
    in shoulder surgery, 767
    in upper extremity pediatric orthopedic surgery, 1092

Intersex anomaly, 1062, 1081-2
Interspinous wiring, C-spine, 80-2, 80f
Interstitial perineal implants, 624-7
    laparoscopy/laparotomy-guided, 624-7
Interstitial pulmonary fibrosis, 365-73
Intertrochanteric fracture, 815-17
Interventional cardiology, pediatric, 1192-
    8; anesthesia, 1195-7
Interventional MRI (iMRI), 1174
Interventional neuroradiology, 1158-62
Intestinal adhesions, 410-11
Intestinal atresia, 1051
Intestinal bleeding, bowel resection for,
    466-9
Intestinal fistulae, small-bowel resection
    for, 413-14, 416-18
Intestinal neoplasms, 466-9, 467-8
Intestinal obstruction
    from adhesions, 410-12
    enterolysis for, 415, 416-18
    laparoscopic bowel resection, 466-9
Intestinal perforation drainage, 1043-6
Intestinal surgery, 405-18
Intimal flap, stroke, 106
Intimal tear repair, 317-22, 317f
Intraabdominal adhesions, 415, 416-18
Intraabdominal hemorrhage, 584
Intraabdominal trauma, 582-3, 586-9
Intraabdominal tumor excision, 497-9,
    416-18, 501-2
Intraarticular infection, wrist, 749-50
Intraaxial tumors, 27
Intracapsular cataract extraction, 114-15;
    anesthesia, 124-6
Intracerebral hematoma, craniotomy, 32
Intracerebral hemorrhage, 4-13
Intracranial aneurysms, 4-13, 5f, 6-13
    giant, 10-13
Intracranial arterial occlusion, 13-15
Intracranial artery catheter embolization,
    13-15
Intracranial hemorrhage (pediatric), 943-5
Intracranial neurosurgery, 4-56
Intracranial pressure (ICP)
    in craniofacial surgery, 1132, 1133
    increase, Sx of, 947
    pediatric, 936
Intracranial tumor, primary, 187-92
Intracranial vascular malformation, 15-21
Intramedullary fixation (IMF) in
    mandibular osteotomy, 905, 906
Intramedullary lipoma, 941-3
Intramedullary nailing
    femoral shaft, 820-1; anesthesia, 863-4
    simple and locked fixation, 820f
    long-bone fractures (pediatric), closed/
        open reduction, 1106-8, 1121-5
    tibia, 841; anesthesia, 863-4
Intramuscular induction, pediatric, D-2
Intraocular lens, insertion, 114-115, 114f;
    anesthesia, 124-126
    dislocation, 135
Intraocular pressure, control, 117f
Intraocular tumor, 131
Intraosseous access, infusion in pediatric
    trauma, 589-90, 590f

Intraosseous compression wires, in thumb
    joint procedures, 740
Intraparietal hernia, 718f
Intrapleural anesthesia in VATS, 242
Intrarenal collecting system, 697
Intraspinal tumor, 90
Intrathecal analgesia, in C-section, 665
Intrathecal pump, neurosurgery, 61-4
Intrathoracic vena cava repair, 577-8
Intrauterine myelomeningocele repair,
    pediatric, 939
Intravascular injection, arm surgery, 780
Intraventricular tumor/mass, pediatric,
    945-8
Intravesical foreign body removal, 1071-
    3; anesthesia, 1077-8
Introitus masses, 1076-8
Intubation
    awake, in excision of blebs/bullae, 247
    awake FOI, B-6
    complications, in chest trauma, 580, 581
    IV, pediatric, D-2
    muscle relaxants for, adult, B-2
    orotracheal, in trauma surgery, 568
    in RSI, B-5
    in stereotactic frame, 28
    tracheal, with C-spine fractures, 4
Intubation, blind techniques
    nasal, light wand, in neck trauma, 575
    nasal, in maxillofacial surgery, 900
    nasotracheal, in trauma surgery, 568
Intubation, difficult
    in craniofacial surgery, 1132
    in craniotomy for tumor, 28
    in head and neck surgery, 140
Intubation, emergency oral, 900
Intubation, ET, with laryngoscopy,
    bronchoscopy, 150
Intubation, failed, 664
    protocol, in RSI, B-5
Intussusception, 413-14, 416-18
Ipsilateral long-term venous access for
    empyema drainage, 1028
Iridectomy, 117
Irving technique for PPTL, 669-71
Ischemia
    in CABG, 268, 269
    functional, of claudication, 331
    intestinal, splanchnic, 1044
    in surgery for TGA, 998
    sympathectomy for, 339-41
Ischemic colitis, 423-5, 427-9
Ischemic heart disease, 360-5
Ischial pressure sores, 923-6
Islet cell tumors, 488-9
Isoflurane
    in adult anesthetic maintenance, B-3
    in craniotomy for trauma, 35
    in pediatric balanced and inhalational
        anesthesia, D-3
    use in suction curettage, 611
Isolated-inflow disease, 327-31
Isoniazid (INH), drug interactions, F-5
Isoperistaltic valve construction, 412
Isosulfan blue vital dye, in sentinel node
    biopsy, 513-5

Isovolemic hemodilution, 11
IV access, difficult, (pediatric), 590
IV anesthesia
    in EB surgery, 1127
    fast-track, in ASD surgery, 973
    in out-of-OR XRT, 1190-1
IV medications, in pediatric postop pain
    management, E-1
Ivor Lewis approach, 385-90, 392

J

Jackson dilators, in tracheobronchial
    stenting, 1178-82
Jackson modification flap, velopharnygeal
    incompetence, 1142-4, 1147-8
Jackson-Pratt drains, vulvectomy, 602
Janeway gastrostomy, 403-4, 411-12
Janzekovic's excision for burns, 928-32
Jatene arterial switch for TGA, 996
Javid shunt, 102
Jaw deformities, congenital, 906
Jaw thrust maneuver, 589
Jaw wiring/banding, 901, 908
Jejunal reservoir, in gastrectomy, 392
Jejunoileal bypass for morbid obesity,
    400-3, 400f, 477-9
'Jersey finger', repair, 745-6
Jet ventilation, 150, 151f, 237, 962
Johnson uterine reinversion, 680-1
Joint Commission Pain Standards, C-1
Joint replacement, hand, 736-7, 740-3
Jones tube, 129, 130f
Jowling, facelift for, 869-71
Juvenile rheumatoid arthritis. *See*
    Arthritis, rheumatoid.
'J' stripper, for osteotomy, 905f

K

K-wire stabilization, 72f, 1084f
Kaneda rod system, 91
Kasai procedure, 1046-9
Kassabach-Merritt syndrome, 1041
Kava kava (*Piper methysticum*),
    precautions with anesthesia, F-11
Kelly urethral plication, for urinary
    incontinence, 654-7
Keratoconus, 115-16
Keratoses, 1207-9
Ketamine
    drug interactions with, F-2, F-6, F-9
    in EB surgery, 1127
    low-dose, 493, 498
    in pediatric im induction, D-2
    in septal myectomy/myotomy, 283
Ketorolac
    for adult postop analgesia, C-2
    in pediatric esophageal replacement,
        1034
    in pediatric pain management, E-1
Kidney donor nephrectomy, 707-11
Kidney
    anatomy, 707f
    dysplastic, 1068-71, 1081-2
    hypoplastic, 706-11
    infected, pediatric, 1081-2
    multicystic, pediatric, 1081-2

nonfunctioning, 708, 1068-71, 1081-2
polycystic, 1070
tumor, benign, 706-11
vessel injury, 585
Kidney operations
excision, 706-11
pediatric, 1068-71; anesthesia, 1070-1
salvage surgery, 585
Kidney procurement, 560-5
donor nephrectomy, 545-7
Kidney transplantation, 538-46, 538*f*;
anesthesia, 541-2
cadaveric, live-donor, 538-9, 541-2
graft rejection, 545-7
LQ curvilinear incision, 538*f*
+ pancreas transplant, 539-42
Kienbock's disease, 737-8
Killian's triangle, 379*f*
Kirklin DORV repairs, 1006
Kirklin VSD closure, 979
Kirschner wires
in repair of fractures of distal radius,
carpus, metacarpals, 753-5
in thumb joint procedures, 740
Klatskin tumor, 450-4
Klein subcutaneous infiltration mixture
for facelift, 869
Klippel-Feil syndrome, 1122, 1132, 1136,
1141, 1147
Klippel-Trenaunay-Weber syndrome, 1111
Knee
fusion failure, nonunion/malunion, 828
infection, fracture, sprain, 834
joint, anatomy, 830*f*, 832*f*
Knee amputation
above, 852-4; anesthesia, 855-7
below, 854-5, 855*f*; anesthesia, 855-7
disarticulation amputation levels, 853*f*
Knee arthritis
arthroscopy for, 833
+ arthrosis, loose/malpositioned
prosthesis, infection, 826-7
degenerative, ± deformity, 840-1
septic, failed/infected, 827-8
Knee surgery, 825-37; anesthesia, 835-7
arthrodesis, 827-8
arthroplasty, 826-7
arthroscopy, with meniscectomy and/or
debridement, 833; anesthesia, 835-7
arthrotomy, with debridement/
synovectomy, 834
fasciotomy, anterior compartment, 831
ligament repair/reconstruction, 830-1
ORIF, 840-1; anesthesia, 863-4
replacement, total, 826-7
resection/excision arthroplasty, 826-7
revision, 826-7
tendon rupture, repair, 835
in trauma patients, 835-7
trauma repair/reconstruction, 830-1
Kocher clamp, 414*f*
Kocher incision, 521
Kocher maneuver, 343-4, 486
Kocher-Langenbeck approach, 801*f*
Kock pouch, 412-13, 412*f*
with proctocolectomy, 421-3

Kostuik-Harrington rod system, 91
Kramer osteotomy, 1108-9, 1121-5
Kraske approach, rectal surgery, 431-2
Krupin implant (glaucoma), 117
Kussmaul's sign, 288
Kyphosis, 1093-5
Kyphotic deformity correction, 81

L
L-asparaginase, in staging laparotomy,
497, 498
L-Dopa-induced dyskinesia, 60
Labetalol, drug interactions, F-6
prophylaxis for control of BP, 110
Laboratory testing/diagnostics, preop,
A-1-A-2
Labral tear, arthroscopy, debridement,
760-2, 766-9
Lagophthalmus, 1132
Laks procedure for tricuspid atresia, 1004
Lambdoid synostosis, 1130-4
Lambdoidal craniosynostosis, 936-8
Laminectomy, 89*f*, 91*f*; lumbar, 93-4
Laminotomy, 80; lumbar, 93-4
Langenbeck technique for cleft palate,
1140-2, 1140*f*; anesthesia, 1147-8
Laparoscopic procedures
adrenalectomy, 466-9, 467*f*, 531-5,
532*f*
appendectomy, 472-5, 472*f*
bariatric surgery, 401-3, 477-9, 478*f*
bowel resection, 469-72, 469*f*
cholecystectomy ± common duct
exploration, 459-63
colorectal surgery, 420
contraindications to laparoscopy, 461
esophageal fundoplication, 456-7
general surgery, 455-82
Heller's myotomy ± antireflux
procedure, 458-9; anesthesia, 461-3
inguinal hernia repair, 475-7
nephrectomy, 707-9, 708*f*, 710-11
live-donor, 543-4, 543*f*, 546
nonobstetric surgery in pregnancy,
480-2
in pregnancy, advantages,
disadvantages, 480
splenectomy, 463-6; anesthesia, 465-6
transperitoneal, lumbar spine, 91
Laparoscopic procedures, gynecologic
assessment of adnexal masses,
diagnosis of ovarian cancer, 627-8
in gynecologic oncology, 627-9, 692-3
for gynecologic surgery, 683-93
hysterectomy, 647, 690-2, 692-3
with BSO, 684-6
interstitial brachytherapy implants, 627
lymphadenectomy with vaginal
hysterectomy, 627-8
myomectomy, 688-90, 692-3
pelvic, for infertility, 643
second-look evaluation for ovarian
cancer, 627-8
surgery for ectopic pregnancy, 687-8;
anesthesia, 692-3
staging of endometrial cancer, 627-8

Laparoscopic procedures, pediatric
anesthesia, 461-2, 1081
dissection in retroperitoneum, 1081-2
heminephrectomy, varicocele ligation,
renal surgery, 1081-2
mobilization/pullthrough for
imperforate anus, 1056
nephrectomy, nephroureterectomy,
adrenalectomy, 1081-2
pyeloplasty, orchiopexy, orchiectomy,
gonadectomy, 1081-2
Laparoscopically assisted procedures
bowel resection (pediatric), 1065
vaginal hysterectomy (LAVH), 690-3
vaginal hysterectomy/BSO, 618-21
Laparoscopy-guided interstitial perineal
implants, 624-7; anesthesia, 626
Laparotomy
for enterocele, presacral neurectomy,
pelvic pain, 639-41
for myomata, ovarian cysts, ectopic
pregnancy, vaginal vault prolapse
639-41
pelvic, 639-41; anesthesia, 644-6
rapid, in abdominal injuries, 582
second-look, ovarian cancer, 597-601
Laparotomy, exploratory
peritoneal surgery, 496-9
for uterine cancer, 618-21
Laparotomy, staging
for fallopian tube cancer, 594-7
for ovarian cancer, 594-7
for peritoneal surgery, 496-9
for primary peritoneal cancer, 594-7
Laparotomy-guided interstitial perineal
implants, 624-7
Larsen's disease, 1103
Larsen's syndrome, 1120
Laryngeal lesion excision, 960-3
Laryngeal mask airway (LMA), in
otolaryngology, 142. (Also *see*
LMA.)
Laryngeal nodules, 960-1
Laryngeal obstruction, 186-7
Laryngeal papilloma, 960-1
Laryngeal tumor, 147
Laryngeal web, polyps, 960-1
Laryngectomy (total, near-total,
supraglottic, hemi, vertical partial),
173-6, 175*f*
with glossectomy, 177
Laryngomalacia, 960-3
Laryngoscope blades, pediatric, D-2
Laryngoscopy, 146-53; anesthesia, 148-52
in awake FOI, B-6
flexible, diagnostic direct, micro,
pediatric, 960-1; anesthesia, 961-3
scope placement, 147*f*
Laryngospasm
in myringotomy/tympanostomy tube
placement, 956
in pediatric extubation, D-3
in tonsillectomy, 145
Laryngotracheal anesthesia device, 84-5
Laryngotracheoplasty, for subglottic
stenosis, 966-8

Larynx, exposure, anatomy, 174*f*
  cancer, 173-6
  visualization, flexible bronchoscopy
    for, 959-60; anesthesia, 961-3
Laser resurfacing, 1207-9
  facial, 881-82; anesthesia, 876-8, 1208-9
  hazards—ocular, fire, reflectivity, 882
  office-based, 1207-9
Laser surgery/resection
  ablation, peritoneal endometriosis, 685
  airway management, 150
  blepharoplasty, 875
  in bronchoscopy, 235-8
  conization of cervix, 606-8
  facelift, precautions, 870
  fire hazards, in otolaryngology, 962
  precautions in thoracic resection, 239
  midline glossectomy, 193-8, 194*f*
  otolaryngology, anesthesia, 140
  papillomas, precautions, 150
  pediatric otolaryngology, precautions, 954
  safety issues, 882
  thoracic surgery, 238-40
Laser therapy
  for hemorrhoids, 434
  to vulva, vagina, cervix, 608-9
Lateral canthotomy/cantholysis, 118
Lateral condyle humerus fracture, closed/
    open reduction with pinning, 1085-6; anesthesia, 1091-2
Lateral epicondylitis, 778-80
Lateral extracavitary approach
  lumbar/lumbosacral surgery, 91*f*
  posterior thoracic spine surgery, 89-90, 89*f*, 97-99
Lateral pelvic/perirenal hematoma,
    hemorrhage, 585
Lateral position
  in craniotomy for tumor, 27
  decubitus, 1096*f*
  in thoracic surgery, 206, 207*f*
  in ureter, renal pelvis surgery, 711
Lateral tarsal strip procedure (entropion),
    119-20; anesthesia, 124-6
Lateral thoracotomy
  for excision of mediastinal tumor, 229
  for mediastinal masses, 1021-4
Latex allergy
  anaphylaxis, Dx and Rx, G-1, G-2
  cross-reactive food allergies, G-1
  in health care workers, G-1
  in pediatric transurethral surgery, 1077
  prophylaxis, G-1
  special considerations for, G-1-G-2
  in spinal abnormalities, 1094
  Type I IgE-mediated, G-1
  in urethral pathology, 1072
Latex-safe environment, G-1
Latissimus dorsi flap, microsurgery, 911
Latissimus myocutaneous flap, in breast
    reconstruction, 917-20, 918*f*
Lavage, bronchopulmonary, unilateral,
    252-5; anesthesia, 253-5
Lecompte maneuver, for TGA, 996

Ledderhose's disease, 744
LeFort fractures, 897, 897*f*, 898-902
LeFort movement technique with
    mandibular osteotomy, 905
LeFort osteotomies, 902-4, 903*f*, 906-8
  LeFort I, 194, 196*f*, 897*f*, 902-4
  LeFort II, 897*f*, 902-4
  LeFort III, 1130-4
Left IMA dissection, 294*f*
Left IMA-to-left anterior descending
    artery anastomosis, 294*f*
Left ventricular (LV) aneurysm,
    aneurysmectomy, 267-70, 268, 271
Left ventricular deconditioning, 999
Left ventricular outflow tract obstruction
    (LVOTO), A-V canal defect, 976
Leg
  compartments, cross-section, 859*f*
  muscle, impaired pumping action,
    venous surgery for, 354-5
  scissoring, 1103-4
  tendon rupture, 835-7
  tumor, infection, 805-8, 861, 863-4
Leg procedures
  biopsy (needle, incisional, excisional),
    861; anesthesia, 863-4
  fasciotomy for compartment syndrome,
    vascular trauma, 858-9, 859-61
  four-compartment fascial
    decompression, 859
  tendon repair, 835; anesthesia, 835-7
  uncontrollable infection, surgery for,
    805-6; anesthesia, 806-8
  upper-leg surgery, 795-824
Leg-length discrepancy, intramedullary
    nailing, 820-1; anesthesia, 863-4
Leiomyomata, 690-2, 692-3
Lesions (cervical, lateral, midline),
    resection, 1014-16
Lesions, therapeutic, locations, 59*f*
Leukemia
  chronic, in staging laparotomy, 497
  pediatric, XRT for, 1188-92
Lewis and Varco TAPVC repair, 993
Licorice (*Glycyrrhiza glabra*),
    precautions with anesthesia, F-11
Lid-splitting procedure (eye), 119-120
Lidlift, 874-6; anesthesia, 876-8
Lidocaine
  drug interactions with, F-3, F-6
  in pediatric caudal, lumbar, thoracic
    epidural anesthesia, D-4
  precautions, inguinal operations, 720
Life-threatening injuries, 570
Ligation
  of PDA, 981
  of perforators (venous), 354-5, 356-8
  of spermatic vein, incision for, 719*f*
Light wand intubation, neck trauma, 575
Lillehei, Varco VSD repair, 979
Limb-length discrepancy surgery
  anesthesia, 1121-5
  epiphyseal stapling for, 1110-11
  instrumentation fixation, 1113-15
  lengthening, pediatric, 1113-15
Limbal incision for strabismus, 950

Limited thoracotomy
  in lung wedge resection, 215
  in mitral valve surgery, 300-6
Linezolid, drug interactions, F-6
Lingual cysts, locations, 520*f*
Lingualplasty, 193-8, anatomy, 194*f*
Linton approach, venous surgery, 354
Lip surgery
  LeFort osteotomies for cleft lip, 902-4
  pediatric, 145-8
  secondary deformities, 1145-8
Lip-switch flaps, for secondary lip/nose
    deformities, 1145-8
Lipectomy, in necklift, 870
Lipodystrophy, 889-92
Lipoid pneumonitis, lavage for, 252-5
Lipoma, filum, intramedullary, 941-3
Lipoma (leg, foot), biopsy for, 861
Lipomyelomeningocele, 941-3
Liposuction, 892-4; anesthesia, 893-4
  with abdominoplasty, 889
  high-volume, contraindications, 893
  preaspiration injection of epinephrine-
    containing wetting solution, 892
  with reduction mammoplasty, 885
  submental, in necklift, 870
  ultrasonic, 892
Lithium, drug interactions, F-6
  with ECT, 1157
  in stabilizing depression, 1156
Lithotomy position, 635, 638
Lithotripsy, 446
Live-donor nephrectomy, laparoscopic
    and open, 543-4; anesthesia, 546
Liver disease
  alcoholic, 345-8
  end-stage, 547-52, 553-8
Liver function test (LFT), preop, clinical
    indications, A-1
Liver injuries, anatomy, 583*f*
  damage control, 582-3, 586-9
  portal triad occlusion, Pringle
    maneuver, 583, 583*f*
  repair, 583-4; anesthesia, 586-9
Liver resection, 440-1, 440*f*
  anesthesia, 442-4
  partial right lobectomy, left lateral
    segmentectomy, 440-2
  right/left lobectomy, trisegmentectomy,
    440-1
Liver surgery, 439-44; anesthesia, 442-4
Liver transplantation, 547-52; anesthesia,
    553-8
  anastomoses, incision, Roux-en-Y
    loop, 552*f*
  anhepatic phase, 548-9
  coagulation management, 556, 558
  hyperdynamic state of patients, 553
  liver procurement, 560-5, 562-5
  living-donor, 442, 559-60
  neohepatic phase, 554-5
  orthotopic, 549
  pediatric, 552*f*
  postrevascularization stage, 549
  preanhepatic phase, 554
  reperfusion syndrome, 555-8

without venovenous bypass, 550*f*
Liver tumor, 440-4
LMA, flexible
    in head and neck surgery, 142, 144
    in-office dental rehabilitation, 1210-11
    vs ETT, in hernia procedure, 508
Lobar emphysema, 1025*f*
Lobar overdistention, congenital, 1024-7
Lobectomy, 208-215; anesthesia, 210-15
    in chest trauma, 579-80, 580-2
    fiber optic bronchoscopy, 213
    hepatic resections, 440-4
    lung isolation, 213
    OLV in, 213-14
    pulmonary complication risks, 212
    temporal, for epilepsy, 64, 66-9
    thoracoscopic, neonatal, 1025
    VATS for, 240
Local anesthesia
    in facelift, subcutaneous infiltration
        mixtures, 869
    in pediatric orthopedic surgery, 1092
    toxicity, 780, 891
    transtracheal, 237
Local anesthetics, drug interactions with,
        F-6, F-7
Localization
    neuroanatomic, 54
    stereotactic, for craniotomy, 17
Loculated multicompartmental
        hydrocephalus, 945-8
Long-bone deformities, surgery for
    anesthesia, 1121-5
    fragmentation rodding, 1111-13
    Sofield procedure for, 1111-13
Long-bone fractures, intramedullary
        nailing, 1106-8; anesthesia, 1121-5
Long-gap atresia, 1031-4
Long-QT syndrome, 1166
Loop cholecystojejunostomy, 448-50;
        anesthesia, 452-4
Loop diuretics, drug interactions, F-6
Loop electrosurgical excision procedure
        (LEEP), cervix conization, 605-8
Loop stoma closure, 426-7
Lorazepam
    in adult premedication, B-2
    in pediatric pain management, E-1
    in pediatric premedication, D-2
Lorcet, in pediatric analgesia, E-3
Lord procedure, hemorrhoidectomy, 434
Lortab elixir, in pediatric analgesia, E-3
Loss-of-resistance technique, D-4
Lower extremities
    amputation levels, 853*f*
    cancer, infection, trauma, microsurgical
        reconstruction, flaps, 911
    orthopedic procedures, 840-64
    PVD, gangrene, trauma, tumor,
        amputation for, 852-4, 855-7
    salvage, severely ischemic, 331
    tumor excision, 861, 863-4
Lower GI hemorrhage, 423-5, 427-9
Lower-limb ischemia, 336-8
Lower-limb venous thrombosis, 341-4
Ludwig's angina, 183

Lumbar anesthesia
    epidural analgesia, adult, C-2
    pediatric, D-4, E-2
Lumbar canal stenosis, 93-4, 97-9
Lumbar disc herniation/degeneration,
        93-4, 97-9
Lumbar discectomy, posterior, minimally
        invasive, 782-4; anesthesia, 783-4
Lumbar fusion/instrumentation, posterior,
        94-6; anesthesia, 97-9
Lumbar interbody fusion
    anterior, 91
    posterior, 95-9
    transforaminal, 95-9
Lumbar laminectomy, laminotomy, 93-4
Lumbar/lumbosacral spine surgery,
        anterior, 91-3; anesthesia, 97-9
Lumbar microdiscectomy, 782-4
Lumbar percutaneous discectomy, 782-4
Lumbar puncture, pediatric, 1198-9
Lumbar radiculopathy
    microdiscectomy for, 782-4, 783-4
    posterior surgery for, 93-4, 97-9
Lumbar root decompression, 782-4
Lumbar segmental instability, 96-9
Lumbar spine neurosurgery, 91*f*
    anterior, 91-3; anesthesia, 97-9
    anterior/posterior instrumentation, 96-9
    posterior, 93-4; anesthesia, 97-9
Lumbar spine orthopedic surgery, 789-9,
        788*f*, 789-94
Lumbar spondylosis, 93-4, 97-9
Lumbar sympathectomy, 336-8, 337*f*;
        anesthesia, 332-4
    Adson's approach, 337-8
    Flowthow approach, 336
    posterior/Royle approach, 337-8
Lumbar/thoracic junction fractures,
        reconstruction/fusion, 784-7, 789-94
Lumbar transpedicular fixation and short-
        segment fusion, 782-4; anesthesia,
        783-4
Lumbosacral spine, anterior
        reconstruction and fusion, 787-9;
        anesthesia, 789-94
Lumpectomy
    breast-conserving, 516-8
    with breast biopsy, 512-13, 514-15
Lung
    anatomy, segmental, 209*f*
    bilateral procedures, 207*f*
    compromised function, 211*f*
    foreign body, bronchoscopy for, 235-8
    infection, trauma, developmental
        abnormalities, surgery for, 208-15
    isolation, in lobectomy/
        pneumonectomy, 213
    lesion, wedge resection, 215-18, 215*f*
    masses, localized, VATS for, 240-3
    resection, neonatal, 1024-5, 1026-7
    RFA, 1183
    thoracic, exposure to radiation, 912
Lung cancer surgery, 208-15
    bronchoscopy for, 235-8
    chest-wall resection, 218-21
    mediastinoscopy, 231-5

wedge resection, 215-18
Lung disease, end stage, 255-6, 365-73
Lung transplantation
    + heart, 365-73
    single/bilateral sequential, 365-9;
        anesthesia, 370-3
    single/double, 255-6
Lung-volume reduction surgery (LVRS),
        249-52; anesthesia, 250-2
    endoscopic, 249-52
    in lung/heart transplant, 359-73, 365-9
    with VATS, 240-3
Lunotriquetral dissociation, 749-50
Lunotriquetrel intercarpal arthrodesis,
        737-8
Luque loop fixation, C-spine, 81*f*
Luque rectangle/contoured rod and
        wiring, upper C-spine, 75-7, 83-7
Luque rods, mid/lower C-spine, 80
LVOTO. *See* left ventricular outflow tract
        obstruction.
Lymph node
    axillary, dissection, 516-8
    biopsy, incision, 513*f*
    dissection, with gastrectomy, 392, 719
    with radical hysterectomy, 621
    mediastinal, sites, 233*f*
    sentinel, biopsy; anesthesia, 514-15
Lymphadenectomy
    bilateral inguinal, 601-5, 601*f*
    cervical, in neck dissection, 168-73
    limited pelvic, with prostatectomy, 703
    with nephrectomy, 707
    pelvic, 601-5; anesthesia, 603-5; 712
    unilateral, 602-5, 602*f*, 603-5
Lymphadenopathy
    image-guided procedures, 1174-8
    mediastinoscopy for, 231-5
Lymphangioleiomyomatosis, 365-73
Lymphatic malformations, neck, 1014-16
Lymphatic mapping, vulvectomy, 602
Lymphazurin, in sentinel node biopsy,
        513-5
Lymphoma
    adrenalectomy for, 530-5
    excision, 1014
    laparoscopic splenectomy for, 463-6
    mediastinal, biopsy/resection, 1021-4
    mediastinal, excision, 229-30, 232-35
Lymphomatous disorder, laparotomy for,
        496-9
Lymphoscintigraphy, 513-4

M
m-AMSA, anesthetic concerns, 1198
ma huang (*Ephedra sineca*), precautions
        with anesthesia, F-10
MAC, B-4
    in colorectal surgery, 437
    dental procedures, in-office, 1210-12
    laser skin resurfacing, 1208-9
Macquet procedure for patellar
        realignment, 1115-16, 1121-5
Macroglossia, 1051
Macrolide antibiotics, drug interactions
        with, F-6

Macromastia, 885-8
Macular degeneration, 135, 136
Macular epiretinal membranes, 135
MADIT trial on ICD use, 1165
Magnesium, drug interactions, F-6
Magnetic resonance imaging (MRI),
    1173-8; anesthesia, 1175-7
  pediatric anesthesia, 1201-2
  unique anesthetic considerations, 1176
Magnetic resonance-guided therapy
    (MRT), 1174-5; anesthesia, 1175-6
Magnuson-Stack operations for shoulder
    instability, 765-6
Main-stem bronchial repair, 579-82
Maintenance, anesthetic techniques
  adult, B-3
  pediatric, D-3
  RSI, B-5
Major aortopulmonary collaterals
    (MAPCAS), in unifocalization, 990
Malabsorption/poor nutrition, preop
    testing indications, A-3
Malabsorptive procedures for morbid
    obesity, 399-403; anesthesia, 401-3
Malignancy, preop testing, A-3
Malignant hyperthermia, 951, 952, 1124
Mallinkrodt Laser-Flex tube, 150
Maloney esophageal dilators, 959
Mammary hypertrophy, 885-8
Mammoplasty
  augmentation, 884-5; anesthesia, 887-8
  reduction, 885-6; anesthesia, 887-8
  + inferior pedicle technique, 886f
Mandible, anatomy, 89f
  deficiency, retrocclusion, 903f
  deformities (retruded, prognathic,
    malocclusion), osteotomy for, 905-8
  distraction technique, 906, 907f
  fractures, 897-902; frequency, 898f
  hypoplasia, 1136
Mandibular genioplasty, 905-8
Mandibular osteotomy, 905-8, 905f
  bilateral sagittal-split, for OSA, 194
  rigid fixation, 905
  Risdon, sagittal ramus split,
    Obwegesser, 905-8
Mandibular osteotomy and genioglossal
    advancement (MOGA), inferior
    sagittal, 193-8, anatomy, 195f
Mandibulectomy, with glossectomy, 177
Mania, ECT for, 1154-8
Mannitol, in craniotomy for trauma, 36
Manual compression, hepatic, 583, 584
MAP control, in trauma craniotomy, 36
Mapping, in craniotomy, 61
Marfan syndrome, 6, 1029, 1094, 1116
  in aortic dissection, 318
  in pediatric orthopedics, 1122
  in port-access procedures, 301
  in TAAA repair, 322, 324
Marshall-Marchetti-Krantz (MMK)
    operation, 729-30
  abdominal approach for urinary
    incontinence, 654-7, 656-7
Martinez Universal Perineal Interstitial
    Template (MUPIT), 624, 625

Mason approach, rectal surgery, 431-2;
    anesthesia, 436-8
Mastectomy (total, simple, radical,
    modified radical, partial), 516-18
  breast reconstruction, 916-20, 921-2
  ± reconstruction, 516-18
  skin-sparing, 516
Mastoidectomy (simple, radical, modified
    radical), 161-3
  pediatric, contraindications, 954
Mastopexy, 887; anesthesia, 887-8
Maxilla, 155f, 903f
  advancement, with bone grafts, 903
  deformities, osteotomy for, 902-4
  fractures, repair, 897-902
  hypoplasia, 1136
  maxillectomy, 178-82
  mobilization with Rowe forceps, 903
  occlusion, Angle classification, 902, 903f
  osteotomy, 902-3
  sinus, neoplastic disease, 178-82
Maxillectomy, (partial, total), 178-82,
    179f; anesthesia, 180-1
  plate and screw fixation, 196f
Maxillofacial surgery, 897-902, OR setup,
    900f; anesthesia, 899-902
Maxillomandibular osteotomy and
    advancement (MMO), 194-8,
    anatomy, 196f; anesthesia, 196-8
Mayfield headrest, 40f
Mayfield-Kees skeletal fixation, 29, 35
Mayfield pin fixation system, 26
Maylard muscle-splitting technique, 648
McBurney incision, appendectomy, 407
McCall's culdoplasty, for vaginal apex
    support, 653
McCash technique, palmar disease, 744
McDonald cerclage, 674-6
McGovern nipple, choanal atresia, 968
McIvor mouth gag, in adenoidectomy/
    tonsillectomy, 956
McKay procedure for clubfoot, 1119-20;
    anesthesia, 1121-5
McVay's repair, inguinal hernia, 504
Meatal advancement granuloplasty
    (MAGPI), for hypospadias, 1075-8
Mechanical back pain syndrome, 95
  instrumentation for, 96-9
Mechlorethamine, toxic effects in
    gynecologic oncology, 598
Meckel's diverticulum, excision, 408-10
Meconium aspiration, 1203-4
Median nerve
  compression (wrist), release, 750-51
  laceration repair, 745-6
Median sternotomy
  chest trauma, 576-7, 580-2
  complications in, 920-21
  excision of mediastinal tumor, 229
  in lobectomy, 209
  in lung wedge resection, 215
  in LVRS, 249-52
  mediastinal masses, 1021-4
  in pericardiectomy, 287-90
  right-neck injuries, 573
  in thoracic surgery, 206f

Mediastinal cysts/tumors, 1022f
Mediastinal lesions, 149
Mediastinal lymph nodes, 231-5, 233f
Mediastinal mass lesions, 1021-4
Mediastinal tumor, excision, 229-30
  + lymphomas, thyroid tumors,
    teratomas, thymomas, 1023-4
Mediastinitis, 921
Mediastinoscopy (anterior, transthoracic),
    231-5, 231f, 233f; anesthesia, 232-4
Mediastinotomy, anterior, 3rd rib, 1022
Mediport device, for permanent vascular
    access, 351-4
Medpore implants, for nose
    augmentation, 878
Medulloblastoma, 27
  pediatric XRT for, 1188-92
Megacolon, congenital, 1053-6
Meisterschnitt incision, 1131
Melatonin, precautions with anesthesia,
    F-11
Meloplasty, 869-71; anesthesia, 876-8
Memory loss in ECT, 1155
Meniere's disease, surgery for, 187-92
Meningioma, 44; surgery for, 187-92
  in craniotomy, 27, 31
Meningocele, 936-8
Meningocele manqué, 941-3
Meningomyelocele. 812, 951
Meniscectomy, with knee arthroscopy,
    833; anesthesia, 835-7
Meniscus tear, arthroscopy, arthrotomy
    for, 833-4; anesthesia, 835-7
Menstrual flow obstruction, 632-3
MEP. See Motor evoked potentials.
Meperidene
  in adult anesthesia, B-3; postop, C-2
  drug interactions with, F-5, F-6, F-9
  for sphincter of Oddi spasm, 453
Mercaptopurine
  drug interactions with, F-6
  toxic effects in oncology, 598
Mesenteric fibroma, excision of, 501-2
Mesenteric vascular occlusion, 413-14
Mesial temporal sclerosis, 67
Mesocaval shunt, for portal HTN, 343-5,
    344f; anesthesia, 346-8
Metacarpal fractures/dislocations, 753-5
Metacarpophalangeal joint arthroplasty,
    736-7; anesthesia, 740-3
Metaplasia, myeloid, 497
Metastatic breast cancer, anesthetic
    implications, 517-8
Metatarsal amputation, 850-1, 863-4
Metatarsus adductus, 1088
Methocarbamol, drug interactions, F-8
Methotrexate, 498
  toxic effects in oncology, 598
Methyldopa, drug interactions, F-6
Methylene blue dye, 526, 527
Methylene blue-tinged NS, 150
Methylergonovine, drug interactions, F-7
Methylmethacrylate cement, 372, 815
Methylmethacrylate dental splint, 194
Metoclopramide
  for adult antiemetics, C-2

drug interactions with, F-6
in patients with bowel obstruction, 428
for pediatric nausea prophylaxis, D-3
for pediatric postop antiemetics, E-3
in RSI, full-stomach precautions, B5
Metopic craniosynostosis, 936-8
Metopic synostosis, craniosynostosis,
1130-4; anesthesia, 1132-4
skull shape abnormalities, 1130f
Metoplasty, for infertility, 644
Metoprolol, use in prophylactic periop
beta blockade, A-6
Miami Modular Orthopaedic Spinal
System (MOSS)
in pediatric surgery, 789-93, 1093-5
in scoliosis correction, 789-93, 1095-7
MICAB. See Minimally invasive
coronary artery bypass.
MICABG. See Minimally invasive
coronary artery bypass grafting.
Microendoscopic lumbar discectomy,
93-4
Microgenia, 905-8
Micrognathia, 1002, 1141, 1143
Microlaryngoscopy, 960-3
Microsomia, hemifacial, 906, 1149-50
Microsurgery
airway management for, 150
replantation, 913-16
Microsurgery free-flap reconstruction,
910-13; anesthesia, 911-13
congenital anomalies, burns, 910-13
flaps—locations, 910f; types, 911
Microtia, 1143, 1149-50
Microvascular decompression
burr holes, opening, incision, 38f
cranial nerve, 37-40; anesthesia, 39-40
for trigeminal neuralgia, 61-4
Midazolam
in adult premedication, B-2; MAC, B-4
drug interactions with, F-2, F-3, F-4,
F-7, F-8, F-9, F-10
in pediatric premedication, D-2
in septal myectomy/myotomy, 283
Middle cerebral artery, 14f, 22f
Middle fossa approach, 188f
with House-Urban retractor, 189f
Middle fossa craniotomy, 187-92, 191f
Midesophageal diverticulum, 379-81
Midface hypoplasia, 1132
Midface lift, 869-71; anesthesia, 876-8
Midline cervical lesions, 1014-16
Midline incisions, 531f, 704f
Midline inframesocolic/supramesocolic,
hemorrhage, hematoma, 585-6
Midtarsal amputation, 851
'Mill wheel' murmur, 172
Millard rotation advancement flap, cleft
lip repair, 1137-40, 1147-8
Minilaparotomy, 688-90, 691, 692-3
Minimally invasive surgery
cardiac, 291-306; acronyms, 292
coronary artery bypass grafting
(MICABG), 295-9, 296f, 297f
hernia repair, pediatric, 1064-5
posterior lumbar discectomy, 782-4

Miosis (abnormal response to darkness),
855
Mithramycin, in staging laparotomy, 497,
498
Mitomycin, toxic effects in gynecologic
oncology, 598
Mitral atresia, 973; + HLHS, 1008-11
Mitral commissurotomy, 276
Mitral insufficiency, 275-9
Mitral regurgitation, 275-9
Mitral stenosis, 973
in mitral valve repair, 277, 278
rheumatic calcific, 275-9
Mitral valve disease, 300-6
Mitral valve prolapse, 275-9, 1030
Mitral valve stenosis/insufficiency, 275-9
Mitral valve surgery
anesthesia, 301-5
limited thoracotomy for, 300-6
port access approach, 300-6
upper sternotomy approach, 300
Mivacurium F-7
in adult intubation, B-2; muscle
relaxation, B-3
drug interactions with, F-4,
in pediatric muscle relaxation, D-3
Miya hook, in vaginal sacrospinous
suspension, 653, 654
Modified Thiersch procedure, for fecal
incontinence, 435-6, 436-8
Modified ultrafiltration (MUF), in
secundum ASD surgery, 975
Moh's technique, eyelid reconstruction,
122-3, 124-6
Molar pregnancy, 610f
Mole (small and large), removal, 610-13
Molteno implant (glaucoma), 117-18,
117f, 124-6
Monitored anesthesia care. See MAC.
Monitors, noninvasive—adult, B-1;
pediatric, D-1
Monoamine oxidase inhibitor (MAOI),
1156; in ECT, 1157
drug interactions with, F-6-7
Monobloc advancement
craniofacial anomalies, 1130-4, 1135f
upper face and frontal bone anomalies,
1134-7
Monogenic syndromes, 937
Morbid obesity
laparoscopic procedures, 401-3, 477-9
patient positioning, 478f
trocar location, 478f
malabsorptive procedures, 399-403
open operations, 399-403
patient positioning, 401f
partitioning procedures, 399-403
preop testing indications, A-3
special anesthetic considerations, 891
Morcellation
of myoma, 689-90; anesthesia, 692-3
uterine, 691
Morphine
in adult anesthetic maintenance, B-3
in adult PCA/PCEA, C-3
for adult postop analgesia, C-2

in adult premedication, B-2
infusions, for lumbar and thoracic
epidural analgesia, C-2
in pediatric balanced anesthesia, D-3
in pediatric PCA, E-3
Moschowitz procedure, 640-1, 644-6
MOSS. See Miami Modular Orthopaedic
Spinal System.
Motor cortex stimulation, epidural, 61
Motor evoked potentials (MEP)
in aortic dissection repair, 320
in pediatric spinal surgery, 1093
Motor imbalance, 851-2
Mouth diseases, 168-73, 177-8
Mouth gag
in otolaryngology, 145
McIvor, Crowe-Davis, Dingman, in
tonsillectomy/adenoidectomy, 956,
958
Moyamoya disease, 21, 23
MRI. See Magnetic resonance imaging.
Multicystic dysplastic kidneys (MCDK),
1068-71; patient population, 1069
Multidirectional instability (MDI), 760-1
Multimodality analgesia, periop, C-1
Multiorgan procurement, 560-5
Multiple endocrine neoplasia (MEN) 1 or
2A, in parathyroidectomy, 526, 527
Multiple endocrine syndrome, 492
Multiple sclerosis
neurosurgery for, 69-70
plaque, 109
surgical analgesia for, 61-4
Multiple-trauma patient, 570
Mumford procedure for distal clavicle,
760-2; anesthesia, 766-9
Muscle relaxants (skeletal), drug
interactions with, F-7
Muscle relaxation
in adult intubation, B-2
continued—adult, B-3; pediatric, D-3
in head and neck surgery, 140
pediatric, standard, D-2
in pediatric otolaryngology, 954
reversal—adult, B-4; pediatric, D-3
Muscle-sparing incision, 207, 208-9
Muscular dystrophy, 1094, 1117, 1122,
1123
Musculocutaneous flaps, in pressure-sore
reconstruction, 923
Mustard atrial switch operation for TGA,
996
Myasthenia gravis
sensitivity to muscle relaxants, 245
thymectomy for, 243-6
in thyroidectomy, 523
Myasthenic syndrome, 211, 224
Mycobacterial adenitis, 1014-16
Myectomy, septal, 282-4
Myelocystocele, pediatric, 941-3
Myelofibrosis, 465
Myelomeningocele, 1094, 1103, 1109,
1119
closure, pediatric, 938-41
intrauterine, repair, pediatric, 939
in rectal prolapse, 430

Myeloproliferative disorders, 497, 499-501
Myelotomy, 69
Myocardial infarction, preop testing, A-3
Myocardial O₂ balance, in CABG, 269
Myodesis, in above-knee amputation, 852
Myoglobinemia, 85, 860
Myoma
    laparotomy, myomectomy, 639-41
    removal—culdotomy, morcellation, minilaparotomy, 689-90
    uterine, hysterectomy for, 647-51
Myomectomy, 640-1; anesthesia, 644-6
    laparoscopic, 688-90; anesthesia, 692-3
Myoplasty, above-knee amputation, 852
Myositis ossificans, 1084
Myotomy
    laparoscopic, 379
    septal, 282-4; anesthesia, 283-4
Myringotomy, tympanostomy tube placement, 954-6; anesthesia, 955-6
Myxedema coma, in thyroidectomy, 524-5
Myxomatous degeneration, 276

N

N₂O
    in pediatric balanced, inhalational anesthesia, D-3
    in strabismus surgery, 951
    in TIVA, B-3
Nager's syndrome, 906
Nail patella syndrome, 1116
Nail/plate device, femoral ORIF, 815
Nail/rod device, femoral ORIF, 815
Naloxone, drug interactions with, F-6
Naprosyn, narcotics, considerations in lumbar discectomy, 783
Nasal airway obstruction, 143
Nasal cavity, 155f
Nasal deformities
    developmental, posttraumatic, 154-5, 158-60, 878-81
    deviation, surgery for, 153-5
    secondary, 1145-6
Nasal fractures, repair, 897-902
Nasal intubation, in neck trauma, 575
Nasal neoplasia, 178-82
Nasal repair + cleft lip repair, 1137
Nasal surgery, 153-5; anesthesia, 154-5
    Alarplasty, 878-81
    augmentation, 878-82
        materials, donor sites, 878
    cosmetic, 153-5, 158-60, 878-81
        +functional restoration of airway, 153-5
    for deformities, 878-81
    pediatric, 1147-8
    for polyps, endoscopic, open, 155-60
    rhinoplasty, 153-5, 878-81
    septoplasty, 153-5, 878-81
    septorhinoplasty, 153-5
    tip depressor muscle release, 879
NASCET Collaborators, 308
Naso-orbital-ethmoid (NOE) fractures, 897-902

Nasolacrimal duct obstruction, 129-30
Nasopharyngeal cancer, 377, 387-90
National Pediatric Trauma Registry, 589
Nausea prophylaxis, adult, B-4; pediatric, D-3
Navigation, surgical
    in endoscopic sinus surgery, 157
    image-guided
        in craniotomy, 16, 26
        sinus, 157
    neuronavigation, computer-assisted, 44
Near-total laryngectomy, 173-6
Near-total pancreatectomy, 488-9, 489f
NEC. *See* Necrotizing enterocolitis.
Neck
    abscess incision/drainage, 964-5
        pediatric (retropharyngeal, parapharyngeal, peritonsillar), 964-5
    aging concerns, 868
    cancer, infection, 911
    stabilization, in trauma surgery, 569
    'turkey gobbler,' necklift for, 869-71
    zones, 572, 573f, anatomy, 573f
Neck surgery
    dissection for lesion/mass, 1014-16
        functional (modified radical, radical), 168-73; anesthesia, 170-2
    with glossectomy, 177
    microsurgical reconstruction, flaps, 911
    submandibular gland excision, 166, 168
Neck resection
    'commando,' composite, 169
    of mass, 1014-16; anesthesia, 1014-15
Neck trauma, 911
    exploratory surgery for, 572-4, 574-5
Necklift, 869-71; anesthesia, 876-8
    with liposuction, lipectomy, platysma muscle modification, 870
Necrotizing enterocolitis (NEC)
    drainage, 1043-6; anesthesia, 1044-6
    perforated, laparotomy for, 1043-6; anesthesia, 1044-6
Necrotizing fasciitis, thigh/leg, 857-8
Needle biopsy
    breast aspiration, core, 512-13, 514-15
    leg, foot, 861; anesthesia, 863-4
    in staging laparotomy, 496
Needle/catheter thoracostomy, emergent, 1218, chest tube insertion, 1218f
Needle cricothyroidostomy, in pediatric trauma, 589
Needle localization, breast, 512-15
Neonatal lung resection, 1024-5, 1026-7
Neoplasia, 147; surgery for, 155-7
    anal fistulotomy, 433-4
    ear, surgery for, 160-3
    in submandibular gland excision, 167
Neostigmine, in pediatric muscle relaxant reversal, D-3
Nephrectomy (simple, partial, radical), 706-9; anesthesia, 710-11
    anatomy, 543f
    for kidney vessel injury, 585
    incisions, 1068
    kidney transplant (early, late), 545-7

    laparoscopic, 707-9, 708f, 710-11
    live-donor, laparoscopic and open, 543-4 anesthesia, 546
    partial, 1068-71; laparoscopic, 1081-2
    patient positioning, 1068
    pediatric, 1068-71, 1068f
    posttransplantation, 546
Nephroblastoma, pediatric, 1040-3
Nephropathy, end-stage reflux, 1068
Nephroscopy, 696-7; anesthesia, 698-9
Nephroureterectomy, 708-9; 1069-71
    laparoscopic, 1081-2
    with partial nephrectomy, 1069-71
Nerve injury, in neck dissection, 172
Nerve palsy, 1084
Nerve stimulator, monitoring, adult, B-1; pediatric, D-1
Nerve-root compression, 93-4, 97-9
    mid/lower C-spine, 80-2
    thoracic spine, 90
Nerve-root irritation, 784
Nesbitt plication for hypospadias, 1075-8
Neural blockade
    in multimodality analgesia, C-1
    as preemptive analgesia, C-1
Neural tissue ablation with RFA, 1182
Neuralgia (glossopharyngeal, trigeminal), 37-40
Neurectomy, for hip contracture, 1104
Neuritis, vestibular, 187-92
Neuroanatomic localization, 54
Neuroblastoma, surgery for, 1021-4
    olfactory, craniotomy for, 40-1
    patient population, 1189
    pediatric, resection, 1040-3
Neuroenteric cyst, 941-3
Neurofibromatoses, 1054
Neurogenic bladder, 1074
Neurogenic claudication, 93-4, 97-9
Neurological deficits, progressive, 4-13
Neuroma, acoustic, 187-92
Neuromuscular hip subluxation, 1100
Neuroradiology, interventional, 1158-62
Neurosurgery, 1-111 (Also *see* specific procedures.)
    extracranial, 101-11
    functional, 54-6, 57-70
    intracranial, 4-56
    pediatric, 933-48
    spinal, 71-99
Nifedipine, drug interactions, F-7
Nissen fundoplication, 384-5, 385f; anesthesia, 387-90
    laparoscopic, 456-7, 456f
    minimally invasive, in pediatrics, 1065
Nitrates, drug interactions with, F-7, F-9
Nitroglycerin, drug interactions, F-1, F-7
NMR, drug interactions, F-1, F-2, F-3, F-4, F-5, F-6, F-7, F-8, F-9,
Nociceptive sensitization reduction, C-1
Nodules, laryngoscopy for, 960-1
Non-shunt procedures for portal HTN, 345-6; anesthesia, 346-8
Noncommitted VSD, 1006, 1007f
Norco, in pediatric analgesia, E-3
Normasol, in liver transplantation, 555

Norwood operation for HLHS, 1009-11
Nose (Also *see* Nasal surgery.)
 crooked, 'saddle,' 154-5, 158-60, 878-81
 neoplastic disease, 178-82
 secondary deformities, 1145-4
 tip deformities, 878-81
Novak modified hysterectomy, 622
NPO pediatric guidelines, D-1
NSAIDs
 anesthetic considerations in lumbar discectomy, 783
 as preemptive analgesia, C-1
 preop testing indications, A-3
Nuss approach to pectus excavatum/carinatum, 1029-31
'Nutcracker' esophagus, 382-3, 387-90
Nutrition, poor, preop testing, A-3

O

Ober fasciotomy, 1101-2; anesthesia, 1121-5
Ober-Yount release, 1101-2, 1121-5
Obesity, liposuction for, 892-4
Obstetric surgery, 659-81 (*See* specific procedures.)
Obstetrical palsy, 775-8
Obstructive jaundice, 1046-9
Obstructive pulmonary artery disease, 331-5
Obstructive sleep apnea (OSA), 193-8
 adenoidectomy/tonsillectomy, 143-6, 956-9
 in morbidly obese patient, 401, 402
 in mandibular deformity, 906, 907
Obwegesser osteotomy for mandibular deformities, 905-8, 905*f*
Occipitocervical plate/rod fixation, upper C-spine, 76-7, 83-7
Occlusive vascular disease, types, 332
Occult airway compromise, 149
Occult postop bleeding, 181
Occult spinal dysraphism, 941-3
Octopus 2 coronary artery stabilizer, 296*f*
Ocular abnormalities, 1132
Ocular anatomy, 117*f*
Ocular hazards in laser resurfacing, 882
Oculocardiac reflex (OCR), 902, 951-2
Odontoid
 excision, transoral, high cervical, 73
 fracture, 42-3, 45-7, 73
 transoral approach, 42-3, anatomy, 42*f*
Off-pump coronary artery bypass grafting (OPCABG), 295-9; anesthesia, 297-8
 incisions, 296*f*
 OR configuration, 297*f*
Office-based anesthesia, 1205-12
 anesthetic goals of, 1206
 equipment required, 1206
 facility regulations, 1206
 patient recovery, discharge, 1207
 patient selection, 1206
 preop preparation, 1207
Olecranon osteotomy, arm surgery, 778
Olfactory neuroblastoma, 40-1
Oligodendroglioma, 27

Oliguria, in heart transplant, 364
OLV. *See* One-lung ventilation.
Omental pelvic carpet/sling, in pelvic exenteration, 613-18
Omental transposition, 222
Omentectomy
 with gastrectomy, 392
 infracolic, 594-7
Omentum-to-brain transposition, 23-6
Omeprazole, drug interactions, F-7
Omphalocele repair, 1049-53
Oncologic procedures, pediatric, out-of-OR, anesthesia, 1198-9
Oncology, gynecologic, 593-629
Ondansetron, antiemetic—adult, C-2; pediatric, D-3, E-3
One-lung ventilation (OLV)
 in bronchopulmonary lavage, 253
 in lobectomy/pneumonectomy, 213-14
 in lung transplantation, 371
 in LVRS, 249-52
 in pediatric thoracic surgery, 1026
 in TAAA repair, 324
 in thoracoplasty, empyema, 225
ONLAY hernia repair, 475
Oocyte retrieval, transvaginal, 641-3
Oophorectomy, 640-1; anesthesia, 644-6
 bilateral, 684-6; anesthesia, 692-3
 salpingo, 595-7; laparoscopic, 690-3
Oophoropexy, 621
OPCABG. *See* Off-pump coronary artery bypass grafting.
Open reduction and internal fixation (ORIF) for fracture, dislocation
 acetabulum, 796-7, 799-801, 806-8
 ankle, foot, 843; anesthesia, 863-4
 carpus, metacarpals, 753-5
 femoral neck, 816
 femoral shaft with plate, 819-20, 863-4
 femur, distal, 818-19, 863-4
 femur, proximal, 815-17, 863-4
 patella, 829; anesthesia, 835-7
 pelvis, 796-7; anesthesia, 806-8
 radius, distal, 753-5
 tibia, distal, 843; anesthesia, 863-4
 tibial plateau, 840-1; anesthesia, 863-4
Ophthalmia, 131
Ophthalmic drugs, systemic effects, 126
Ophthalmic surgery, 113-37 (Also *see* specific procedures.)
 under MAC, 124-6
 pediatric, 949-52, 951-2
Opiate agonists, drug interactions with, F-1, F-2, F-4, F-7, F-8
Opiates
 dose reduction with preemptive and multimodality analgesia, C-1
 sustained-release, in multimodality analgesia, C-1
Opioid epidural analgesia, pediatric, E-5
Opioid-based anesthetic techniques, in head and neck surgery, 141-2
OPLL, 78
Opponensplasty, Camitz, for carpal tunnel tendon transfer, 750-2
Oral airway, 237

Oral anesthetic medications, drug interactions with, F-1
 in pediatric pain management, E-1
Oral bone grafting/extractions, 201-2; anesthesia, 203-4
Oral pathology, 201-2, 203-4
Oral secretions, adenoidectomy/tonsillectomy, 957-8
Oral surgery, 201-2; anesthesia, 203-4
Orbital anatomy, 155*f*
Orbital mass, 132-3
Orbital/zygomatic fractures, 897-902
Orbitotomy (anterior, lateral, medial), 132-3; anesthesia, 133
Orchiectomy (simple, radical), 1079-81
 laparoscopic, 1081-2
 metastatic prostate cancer, 723-5
Orchiopexy (orchidopexy), 718-21, 1079-81
 laparoscopic, 1081-2
 for undescended testicle, 1061-2; anesthesia, 1080-1
Organ donor
 brain-dead, anesthetic considerations, 563-5
 cardiovascular complications, 562-3
 living, liver transplant, 442, 559-60
 nephrectomy in, 543-4, 546
 non-heart-beating, 561
Organ procurement, intraop complications
 in brain-dead donors, 564-5
 cardiovascular, 562-4
 diabetes insipidus, 563, 564
 hyperglycemia, hypothermia, hypotension, hypovolemia, 562, 564
 neurogenic shock, 564
 pulmonary dysfunction after brain death, 562
Organ procurement, preservation, 560-5
 anesthesiologist's administrative aspects, 562
 flushing, 560; rapid-flush, 561
 incision and exposure, 561*f*
Organogenesis, drug exposure during, 675
Oriental cholangiohepatitis, 448-50
ORIF. *See* Open reduction and internal fixation.
Oropharyngeal tumor, 147
Oropharynx cancer, 168-73
Orotracheal intubation, in trauma, 568-9
Orringer gastroesophageal anastomosis for esophageal replacement, 1032
Orthofix, for limb lengthening, 1113-15
Orthotopic liver transplant, 549
Ortiochea flap for velopharyngeal incompetence, 1142-4, 1147-8
Ortner's syndrome, 276
OSA. *See* Obstructive sleep apnea.
Osseointegrated implants, 201-2
Osseous genioplasty, 905-8, 905*f*
Osserman scheme, 243
Osteoarthritis
 arthrodesis for, 737-8
 facet, treated with RFA, 1182-6
 femoral, osteotomy for, 82223
 hip, arthroplasty for, 810

knee, 835
shoulder, arthroplasty for, 769-73
Osteochondral autograft transfer system (OATS) for focal cartilage, Hill-Sachs lesions, 760-1
Osteochondral dystrophies, 1094, 1109, 1120
Osteogenesis imperfecta, 1094, 1122
   Sofield procedure, fragmentation rodding for, 1111-13, 1121-5
Osteoid osteoma, RFA for, 1182-6
Osteoma, in craniotomy, 31
Osteomyelitis
   limb-length discrepancies, 1111, 1114
   pelvis, acetabulum, 861, 863-4
   pyogenic/TB of spine, reconstruction/fusion, 784-7, 789-94
      anterior thoracic surgery, 87-89
Osteoplastic flap, 26; bilateral, 156f
Osteosarcoma, in craniotomy, 31
Osteotomy
   + bone graft augmentation of pelvis, 802-3; anesthesia, 806-8
   Chiari, 1099-1100, 1121-5
   Dial, 1097-9, 1121-5
   Eppright, 1097-9, 1121-5
   femoral (proximal), 1108-9, 1121-5
      Kramer, 1108-9, 1121-5
   LeFort, 902-4; anesthesia, 906-8
   pelvic, pediatric, 1097-9, 1121-5
   Pemberton, 1097f
   periorbital, 1134-7
   Salter's innominate, 1097-9, 1121-5
   Southwick, 1108-9, 1121-5
   Steel, 1097-9; anesthesia, 1121-5
   transverse sternal, 219
   wedge, 219-21, 219f
Ostium primum ASD + A-V canal defect, surgery for, 975-8
Ostium secundum defect, surgery for, 972-5, 972f
Otitis media
   chronic, 1141
   complications in anesthesia for pediatric lip/nose surgery, 1147
   serous and acute, 954-6
   surgery for, 160-3
Otolaryngology, 139-98 (See specific procedures.)
Otolaryngology, pediatric, 953-70
   anesthesiologist/surgeon cooperation, airway competition, 954
   laser precautions, 954
   spontaneous ventilation, muscle relaxation, 954
   tube positioning, 954
Otoplasty, 1149-50; anesthesia, 162-3
   cutaneous 'pocket,' 1150f
   fabrication of ear framework, 1149f
Out-of-OR procedures, 1151-1204
   adult, 1153-86
   pediatric, 1187-1204
Ovarian cancer
   hysterectomy, laparoscopic, 690-3
   laparoscopic surgery, 627-9, 692-3

second-look/reassessment, 597-601
   staging laparotomy, 594-7
Ovarian cysts, 639-41, 644-6
Ovarian endometriosis, 684-6, 692-3
Ovariolysis, for infertility, 643
Ovassapian airway, 237
Overlapping sphincteroplasty, for fecal incontinence, 435-6, 436-8
Oversew operations, gastric or duodenal perforation, 394-5; anesthesia, 397-9
Oxycephaly, 1130-4
OxyContin, anesthetic considerations in lumbar discectomy, 783
Oxygen analyzer monitoring, adult, B-1; pediatric, D-1
Oxytocic drugs, drug interactions, F-7
Oxytocin
   in D&E, D&C, 633, 635
   drug interactions with, F-7
   hazards in uterine reinversion, 681
   infusion, in suction curettage, 612

P

Pacemaker
   five-position code (ICHD), 285
   insertion, 284-7, 1167-8
   transvenous placement, 1195-7
Paclitaxel, toxic effects, 598, 599
Pain management
   adult, C-1-C-4
   central origin, surgical analgesia for, 61-4
   pediatric, E-1-E-7
   reduction with preemptive and multimodality analgesia, C-1
   Rx with functional neurosurgery, 57-70
   stereotactic surgery for, 53-6
Painful shoulder syndrome, 170
Palate
   cleft, 1140-2, 1140f, 1147-8
   collapse, obstruction, 193-8
   LeFort osteotomies for, 902-4
   soft, reconstructive surgery for, 193-8
Palatopharyngoplasty + tonsillectomy, 143
Palatoplasty, for cleft palate, 1140-2, 1140f; anesthesia, 1147-8
Pallidotomy, 54, 59-60, 59f, 62-4
Palmar fasciectomy, 744, 746-8
Palmar hyperhidrosis, 339-41
Palmaz stent, tracheobronchial, 1178
Pancreas, anatomy, 489f
   abscess drainage, 484-5
   cancer, pancreatectomy, 488-9
      resection, 490-4
   distal, resection, 489f
   drainage, with simultaneous kidney/pancreas transplant, 540f
   ductal system anatomy, 397f
   transected, 496-9
Pancreas transplantation
   after kidney transplant (PAK), 539-42
   anesthesia, 541-2
   pancreas/kidney, 539-42
   pancreas procurement, 560-5

Pancreatectomy (distal, subtotal, near-total), 488-9, 489f; anesthesia, 491-4
   regional, total, 490-1; anesthesia, 491-4
Pancreatic divisum, 397-9, 406
Pancreatic duct
   dilation, 486-7, 491-4
   obstruction, 397-9, 406
Pancreatic pseudocyst, 485-6, 491-4
Pancreatic surgery, 483-94
   anesthesia, 491-4
   resection, 490-4
Pancreaticoduodenectomy, for bile duct tumor, 450
Pancreaticojejunostomy, 486-7, 491f; anesthesia, 491-4
Pancreatitis
   acute, 486
   alcoholic, 406
   biliary tract drainage, 448-50, 452-4
   chronic, 488-9
   operative drainage, 484-5, 484f, 491-4
   pancreaticojejunostomy, 486-7, 491-4
   with pseudocyst, 485-6
   resection for, 490-1; anesthesia, 491-4
Pancreatoduodenectomy, 486-7, anatomy, 491f; anesthesia, 491-4
   in Whipple resection, 490-4
Pancuronium
   in adult intubation, B-2
   in adult muscle relaxation, B-3
   drug interactions with, F-7
   in pediatric muscle relaxation, D-3
   in septal myectomy/myotomy, 283
Panendoscopy, 147
   in head and neck surgery, 149, 150
   in laryngoscopy/bronchoscopy/esophagoscopy, 152
Panfacial fracture treatment protocol, 896f
Panic attacks, 1155
Pannus formation, removal, 43f
Panvertebral disorders, C-spine, 81
Papilloma
   choroid plexus, in craniotomy, 27
   inverting, 157-60, 178-82
   laryngoscopy for, 960-1
   laser resection precautions, 150
Papillomatosis, respiratory, 235-8
Paraaortic lymph node dissection for gynecologic cancer, 594-7, 595-7
Paracolostomy hernia repair, 426-9
Paralytic ileus, in uterine cancer, 619
Paralytics, in facelift, 869
Parametrial anatomy, 621f
Parametrial disease, 690-3
Parapharyngeal abscess, 964-5
Paraplegia, 1072, 923-4
Parasitic diarrheal illness, acute, 430
Parastomal hernia repair, 426-9
Parasymphyseal fracture, 897
Parathormone assay, 526
Parathyroid gland, 527f
   adenoma, 526-30
   carcinoma, 526-30
   exploration, incision for, 526f
   four-gland visualization, 526

Parathyroidectomy, 526-30, 527f
  anesthesia, 528-9
  endoscopic, 526-7
Paravaginal repair, 652-4
Paravertebral block (PVB), in breast
    surgery, 517, 518
Parenchyma, in/out of brain, 27
Parenchymal laceration repair, 579-82
Parietal cell vagotomy (PCV), for PUD,
    396-9, 396f; anesthesia, 397-9
Parkinson's disease
  deep brain stimulation, 59-60, 62-4
  stereotactic surgery, 53-6
Parkland technique for PPTL, 669-71
Parks anoplasty for fecal incontinence,
    435-6; anesthesia, 436-8
Parotid gland, surgery, 163-6, 164f, 165f
Parotidectomy (superficial, supraneural,
    total, radical), 163-6; anesthesia,
    167-8
  pediatric, muscle relaxation,
    contraindications, 954
Partial anomalous pulmonary venous
    return, with ASD, 973
Particle embolization, neuroradiology,
    1156-62
Passion flower (*Passiflora spp*),
    precautions with anesthesia, F-11
Patella
  arthroscopic, open, lateral release,
    1115-16; anesthesia, 1121-5
  dislocation, recurrent, 831-2, 835-7;
    1115-16, 1121-5
  fractures, ORIF for, 829, 835-7
  hypoplastic, 1116
  realignment, 831-2; anesthesia, 835-7
    proximal, distal, 1115-16, 1121-5
  retinaculum anatomy, 832f
  subluxation, chronic, 831-2, 835-7
    lateral, 1115-16, 1121-5
Patellofemoral joint, severe degenerative
    arthritis, ORIF for, 829, 835-7
Patent ductus arteriosus (PDA), 982f
  coil occlusion for, 981, 1194
  pediatric surgery for, 981-4
  repair, in A-V canal defect, 976
  robotic approach, 981
  with TGA, 996-1000
  thoracoscopic clip ligation for, 981
Patent foramen ovale (PFO), 972
  anesthetic concerns in minimally
    invasive pediatric surgery, 1064
Patent processus vaginalis, 1059
Patient-controlled analgesia (PCA)
  adult, C-3
  pediatric, E-1, E-3, E-4
Patient-controlled epidural analgesia
    (PCEA)
  adult, C-3; pediatric, E-2, E-7
Patil-Syracuse face mask, 237
PCA. *See* Patient-controlled analgesia.
PDA. *See* Patent ductus arteriosus.
Pectoralis major muscle flap, in chest-
    wall reconstruction, 921-2
Pectus excavatum/carinatum repair, 219-
    21, 219f; anesthesia, 219-21

  pediatric, 1029-31; anesthesia, 1030-1
  Ravitch approach, 1029-31, 1029f
Pediatric anesthetic considerations
  anesthetic protocols, D-1-D-5
  emergence, D-3
  epidural analgesia, postop, E-5
  epidural, techniques and dosage, D-4
  extubation, D-3
  induction, D-2-D-3
  lumbar, D-4
  maintenance techniques, D-3
  management, standard, D-2-D-5
  muscle relaxation, D-2; reversal, D-3
  nausea prophylaxis, D-3
  noninvasive monitors, D-1
  pain management, standard, E-1-E-7
  postop analgesics, antiemetics, E-3
  premedication, D-2
  spinal anesthesia, analgesia, D-5
  thoracic epidural anesthesia, D-4
Pediatric surgery, 933-1150 (Also *see*
    specific procedures.)
  cardiac catheterization and
    electrophysiology, 1192-8, 1195-7
  cardiovascular, 971-1011
  craniomalformations, 1129-1150
  general ssurgery, 1013-66
  neurosurgery, 935-48
  oncologic procedures, 1198-9
  ophthalmology, 949-52
  orthopedic, 1083-1128
  otolaryngology, 953-70
  out-of-OR procedures, 1187-1204
  radiation therapy (XRT), 1188-92
  thoracic, 1026-7
  urology, 1067-82; anesthesia, 1077-8
Pediatric trauma, 589-90
  airway patency restoration, 589
  airway/vascular access, 589-90
  blunt injuries, 589
  intraosseous access, 589, 590f,
    saphenous cutdown, 590
  needle cricothyroidostomy, 589,
    cricothyrotomy, 589
Pedicle hook, in posterior spinal
    instrumentation and fusion, 1093-5,
    placement, 1093f
Pedicle screw plate fixation, mid/lower
    C-spine, 81
Pedicle screw stabilization, posterior
    lumbar, 95-9
Pelvic blood vessels, 704f
Pelvic exenteration (total, en bloc), 613-18
  anterior, posterior, 613-18
  sagittal section of pelvis, 613f
  urinary and fecal diversions, 615f
Pelvic inflammatory disease (PID)
  in ectopic pregnancy, 687
  in endometriosis surgery, 684
  in infertility, 643
  lid, in pelvic exenteration, 614
  mass, staging laparotomy for, 594-7
Pelvic lymph node dissection, 594-7
  surgical anatomy, 704f
Pelvic relaxation syndrome, 647-54,
    656-7

Pelvic surgery, orthopedic, 795-824
  amputations, 805-8
  arthrodesis, 804-8
  biopsy, abscess drainage, 861, 863-4
  fractures, nonunion/malunion, ORIF
    for, 796-797; anesthesia, 806-8
  nonunion, pelvis/acetabulum, 796-7
  osteotomy, bone graft augmentation,
    802-3; anesthesia, 806-8
    pediatric, 1097-9; anesthesia, 1121-5
  traumatic amputation, 805-8
Pelvis
  anatomy (male, female), with
    cystectomy excision areas, 713f
  anteroposterior compression or external
    rotation injury, 796f
  female, laparoscopic view, 685f
  fractures, displaced/unstable, 798-9,
    806-8
  floor muscle atrophy, 435-8
  infection, 619; 690-3
  instability, 804-8
  lateral compression/ internal rotation,
    796f
  malignant tumor surgery, 805-8
  muscle weakness, rectal prolapse, 430
  osteomyelitis, 861, 863-4
  pain, adhesions, 639-41, 690-3
  posterior, anterior schematic, 796f
  principal injury patterns, 796f
  prolapse repair, 728-30
  relaxation, 640-41, 644-6
  renal operations, 709-12
  uncontrollable infection, 805-8
  unstable vertical shear disruption, 796f
  wall, right lateral, anatomy, 704f
Pemberton osteotomy, pediatric,1097-9,
    anatomy, 1097f; anesthesia, 1121-5
Pena procedure for imperforate anus,
    1056-8
Penectomy, 721-3; anesthesia, 722-3
Penetrating keratoplasty (PKP), 115-16;
    anesthesia, 124-6
Penile surgery, 721-3, 721f
  anesthesia, 722-3
  cancer, inguinal operations for, 719
  penectomy, penile prosthesis, 721-3
Penile surgery, pediatric, 1075-6
  anesthesia, 1077-8
  fistula repair, 1075-6
  repair of concealed penis, 1075-6
  torsion repair, 1075-6
Penis
  anatomy, 721f
  concealed, 1075-6
  prosthesis insertion, 721-3
  skin squamous-cell carcinoma, 721-3
  torsion in, 1075-6
Penrose catheter, 1070
Penrose drains, 800f
Pentalogy of Cantrell, 1049, 1050, 1051
Pentalogy of Fallot, 988
Peptic ulcer disease (PUD)
  gastrectomy for, 392-4
  operations for, 396-9
  parietal cell vagotomy (PCV), 396-9

vagotomy and antrectomy, 396-9
vagotomy and pyloroplasty, 396-9
Peptic ulcer, perforated
    nonoperative management of, 395
    oversew procedures for 394-5, 397-9
Percocet, anesthetic considerations in
    lumbar discectomy, 783
Percutaneous balloon compression, for
    trigeminal neuralgia, 108
Percutaneous coil embolization, PDA, 981
Percutaneous discectomy, lumbar, 782-4
Percutaneous endoscopic gastrostomy
    (PEG), 403-4; anesthesia, 411-12
Percutaneous epiphysiodesis, pediatric,
    1110-11; anesthesia, 1121-5
Percutaneous nephrostomy, 697-9
Percutaneous pinning
    closed/open reduction, lateral condyle
        humerus fracture, 1085-6, 1091-2
    distal radius, carpus, metacarpals
        fractures, 753-5
    femoral neck fracture, 816
    supracondylar humerus fractures,
        1084-5, 1084f; anesthesia, 1091-2
Percutaneous procedures for trigeminal
    neuralgia, 108-11
Percutaneous radiofrequency rhizotomy,
    for spasticity, 69-70, 942-3
Pereyra suspension, for urinary
    incontinence, 655-7
Perforative diverticulitis, 416
Perforator (venous) ligation, 354-8
Perianal fistula, 433-4, 436-8
Peribulbar block, in ophthalmic surgery,
    125, 950
Pericardial decompression, in chest
    trauma, 576-7; anesthesia, 580-2
Pericardial effusion, 288
Pericardial window, 287
    in chest trauma, 576-7, 580-2
    subxiphoid, 576-7, 580-2
Pericardiectomy, 287-90
Pericardiocentesis, 1216, 1216f
    in chest trauma, 576-7, 580-2
Pericarditis, constrictive, 287-90
Perihepatic packing, 584
Perineal operations, 726-7, 704f
    anesthesia, 727
    artificial urinary sphincter, 726-27
    brachytherapy, 726-7
    one-stage pullthrough (POOP), 1053-6
    rectosigmoidectomy, 429-30, 436-8
    sagittal anorectoplasty, 1056-8
    transperineal prostate seed
        implantation, 726-7
    transurethral incision/dilation, 726-7
    trauma surgery, 435-8
    urethroplasty, urethrectomy, 726-27
Periodontal treatment, in-office, under
    deep iv sedation, 1209-11
Perioperative pain management, C-1-C-4
Perioperative beta blockade, prophylactic,
    A-4-6
Periorbital fat, 874-6, 876-8
Periorbital osteotomies, for craniofacial
    malformations, 1134-7

Peripheral artery embolism, 335-6
Peripheral subcutaneous AV fistula,
    349-54
Peripheral vascular disease (PVD)
    in ankle amputation, 850
    infrainquinal arterial bypass, 331-5
    in port-access procedures, 302
    preop testing indications, A-3
Peripherally inserted central catheter
    (PICC), image-guided, 1174
Periportal fibrosis, 343-8
Peritonsillar abscess, 143, 964-5
Periventricular cyst, 945-8
Permacath DL catheter, for permanent
    vascular access, 351-4
    in kidney, upper urinary tract surgery,
        pediatric, 1070
Permanent vascular access, 351-4
Permissive hypercapnia, 1036
Peroneal nerve injury, 634, 636, 1117
Persistent fetal circulation, 1034
Perthes disease, 1098, 1109, 1111
Pes planus, 1119
Peutz-Jeghers syndrome, 595
Peyronie's disease, 744
Pfannenstiel's incision
    access to bladder/pelvic organs, 1073f
    in prostatectomy, 703f
Pfeiffer syndrome, 1130
Phantom limb pain, 853
Pharyngeal flap for velopharnygeal
    incompetence, 1142-4, 1147-8
Pharyngeal incisions, 1143f
Pharyngeal obstruction, 195-8
Pharyngectomy, 173
Pharyngoesophageal (Zenker's)
    diverticulum, 379-81, 387-90
Pharyngoplasty
    anesthesia, 1147-8
    sphincter, 1142-4, 1143f
    for velopharyngeal incompetence,
        1142-4
Pharynx, visualization of, 146
Phemister epiphysiodesis, 1110-11, 1110f
Phenobarbital, preop testing, A-3
Phenothiazines, drug interactions, F-7
Phenoxybenzamine, drug interactions, F-7
Phentermine, effects of in anesthesia for
    abdominoplasty, 890
Phenylephrine, drug interactions, F-7
    in ophthalmic procedures, 126
Phenytoin, drug interactions, F-7
Pheochromocytoma, 229, 528
    adrenalectomy for, 530-5
    contraindication to ECT, 1156
Phimosis, 1075-8, 1080
Photodynamic therapy, bronchoscopy,
    235
PICC placement, image-guided, 1174
Pickwickian syndrome, 890
Pierre Robin sequence, 1141, 1143
Pierre Robin syndrome, 906, 1132, 1136
    in pediatric lip/nose surgery, 1147
'Pigeon chest.' See Pectus carinatum.
Piggyback liver transplant, 548, 549, 551f
Pigmented villonodular synovitis, 812-15

Pinch graft, for fecal incontinence, 435-8
Pinning of slipped capital femoral
    epiphysis (SCFE), 1105-6;
    anesthesia, 1121-5
'Pinocchio nose,' 878-81
Pipecuronium, in adult intubation, B-2;
    muscle relaxation, B-3
Piperacillin, drug interactions with, F-7
Pitocin, in D&E, D&C, 633, 635
Pituitary tumor, 44-7, 44f
Placenta abruptio, previa, 662
Placenta, retained, 677-9
Plagiocephaly, 1130-4
Plasmalyte A, liver transplant, 555, 558
Plasmapheresis, in thymectomy, 244
Plastic surgery, 865-932
Plating systems, anterior lumbar/
    lumbosacral, 91
Platinum-based chemotherapy, 597
Platybasia, 42-43, 45-7
Platysma flap, in facelift, 869f
Platysma muscle modification, necklift, 870
Platysmal bands, 869-71
Pleural abrasion, 246
Pleural disease, effusion, 240-3
Pleural scarring, 301
Pleurectomy, with excision of blebs/
    bullae, 246
Pleurodosis, talc, 240-3
Pneumatic dilation for achalasia, 458-9
Pneumatic retinopexy, 135
Pneumonectomy, 208-215; anesthesia,
    210-15
    in chest trauma, 579-82
    with drainage of empyema, 223
    fiber optic bronchoscopy in, 213
    lung isolation, 213
    OLV in, 213-14
    pulmonary complication risks, 212
    VATS for, 240
Pneumonitis
    with bronchoalveolar lavage, 959-63
    with intractable aspiration, 173
    lipoid, lavage for, 252-5
Pneumoperitoneum
    in laparoscopic procedures, 462, 1082
    effects on respiratory/cardiac function,
        pediatric, 1064-5
    in infertility operations, 645
Pneumoplasty, reduction, 250
Pneumothorax
    in adrenal surgery, 534
    in arm surgery, 780
    in bronchopulmonary lavage, 253
    in chest trauma surgery, 580
    in esophageal procedures, 389
    in in vitro fertilization, 647
    in neck dissection, 172
    in parathyroidectomy, 529
    in RFA, 1185
    recurrent, VATS for, 240-3
    spontaneous, 1029, 240-3, 246-9
    Sx, in ureter/renal pelvis surgery, 711
    tube thoracostomy for, 569-71
Pneumothorax, tension
    in excision of blebs/bullae, 248

in trauma, 568
tube thoracostomy for, 569-71
in VATS, 242
Poland syndrome, 885, 916-22, 1091
Poliomyelitis, 1100, 1111, 1114, 1117, 1120
Pollicization of finger, 1089-90, 1089*f*; anesthesia, 1091-2
Polychondritis, 1178-82
Polycystic kidney disease, 6, 1070
Polycythemia vera, 465
Polydactyly, with syndactyly, 1091
Polyethylene articulations for wrist prostheses, 738-9
Polymyxin B, drug interactions, F-1
Polyposis, familial adenomatus, 412-13, 420-3, 427-9
Pomeroy technique for PPTL, 669-71
Port placement, image-guided, 1174
Port-access procedures
anesthesia, 301-6
mitral valve surgery, 300-6
contraindications, 301-2
coronary revascularization, 293-5
CPB system, 293*f*
special anesthetic concerns, 302-3
Portacath, for permanent vascular access, 351-4
Portacaval shunt, for portal HTN, 343-8
Portal hypertension, 343-8
shunt/non-shunt procedures, 345-8
Sugiura operation, Hassab procedure, esophageal transection, 345-8
TIPS for, 1169-73; anesthesia, 1170-2
Portal triad, 343-8, 583*f*, 584
Portazygous disconnection, for portal HTN, 345
Portoenterostomy, Kasai procedure, pediatric, 1046-9; anesthesia, 1048-9
Portosystemic shunt, 343-8
Positions, patient (Also *see* specific procedures.)
Concorde, 17*f*
lateral, 27, 207*f*
lateral decubitus, 1096*f*
prone, 27; modified, 17*f*
rose, 143*f*
semisitting, 17*f*
sitting, 27
supine, 18*f*, 27
Positron emission tomography (PET), 1174-5; anesthesia, 1175-6
Postbypass hemorrhage, 363
Postdural puncture headache (PDPH), 609, 645
Posterior cervical lateral plating, 80
Posterior fossa
craniotomy (suboccipital), translabyrinthine, 187-92, OR set-up, 191*f*
tumors, XRT for, 1188-92
Posterior fusion/fixation
mid/lower C-spine, 80-2, 83-7
upper C-spine, 75-7, 83-7
Posterior lumbar fusion/instrumentation, 94-6; anesthesia, 97-9

Posterior lumbar interbody fusion (PLIF), 95-9
Posterior mediastinal lesions, 1022
Posterior spinal instrumentation/fusion
pediatric, 1093-5; anesthesia, 789-93
sublaminar wire attachment, 1093*f*
rod, sublaminar wires, 1094*f*
Posterior spine surgery, 93-4; anesthesia, 97-9
Posterior urethral valves (PUV), 1071-3
Postoperative anesthesia
adult, C-2, C-4
pediatric, E-1-E-7
Postpartum hemorrhage (PPH), management, 661-5, 666-7
Postpartum tubal ligation (PPTL), 669-71
Pomeroy, Parkland, Irving, Uchida techniques, 669-71
Posttransplant lymphoproliferative disease, 961
Posttraumatic pain syndromes, 339-41
Potts shunt, for tricuspid atresia, 1003-6
PPTL. *See* Postpartum tubal ligation.
Precordial stethoscope monitoring—adult, B-1; pediatric, C-1
Preemptive analgesia, C-1
Pregnancy
in cervical conization, 607, 608
+ delivery, complications, 690-3
fetal loss, recurrent, 636-9
ectopic, 639-41, 644-6, 687-8, 692-3
nonobstetric surgery during, 480-2
patient special considerations, 480-2
prematurity, 1043, 1044-5, 1062
preop testing, clinical indications, A-2
ruptured tubal, 687
termination, D&C for, 632-3
Pregnancy-induced hypertension (PIH), 662
Preincisional analgesia, C-1
Premedication for surgery—adult, B-2; pediatric, D-2
in awake FOI, B-6
Preoperative anesthesia, general, A-1-A-6
fasting (NPO) guidelines, D-1
laboratory testing, diagnostics, A-1-A-2
Prepontine space aneurysm, 188-92
Prepyloric ulcer disease, 396-9
Presacral neurectomy for pelvic pain, 639-41; anesthesia, 644-6
Pressure-equalizing (PE) tube placement, 954-6; anesthesia, 955-6
Pressure-sore reconstruction, 923-6; flap designs, 923*f*; anesthesia, 924-6
Preterm labor, 644
Pringle maneuver, 440, 442, 583*f*, 584
Probenecid, drug interactions with, F-7
Probit Survival Curve for burn victims, 929*f*, 930*f*
Procainamide, drug interactions, F-8
Procaine, drug interactions, F-8
Procidentia, 429-30, 436-8
Proctectomy (simple, radical), 703-6
Proctocolectomy
anesthesia, 427-9

+ continent ileostomy (Kock pouch), 421-3
+ end ileostomy, 421-3
restorative, with ileal pouch anal anastomosis (IPPA), 420-3
total, 420-3
Proctoscopy, rigid, 431-2, 436-8
Prognathic mandible, 905-8
Prognathic occlusion, 903*f*
Progressive neurologic deficits, 16, 943-5
Prolactin-secreting tumor, 44-7
Proliferative vitreoretinopathy (PVR), 134
Prominent ears, 162-3, 1149-50
Prone position, 27; modified, 17*f*
Prophylactic periop beta-blocker (PPBB), A-4-A6
Propofol
in adult induction, B-2; maintenance, B-3
bolus/infusion, in TIVA, B-3
drip, in strabismus surgery, 951
drug interactions with, F-7, F-8, F-9
in pediatric induction, D-2; balanced anesthesia, D-3
Propofol infusion
in adult MAC, B-4
pump for CT, pediatric, 1202
in TIVA, B-3
Prostate cancer
endoscopic diagnostics, 696-9
metastatic, 723-5
open operations, 703-6
radioactive seed implantation, 726-7
TURP, 699-703
Prostate gland enlargement, 699-703
Prostate hypertrophy, 696-9, 703-6
Prostate operations, open, 703-6
Prostate resection
visual laser ablation, transurethral vaporization, thermotherapy, 700
with thermocoagulation, 700-1
transurethral, 699-703
Prostatectomy
open, in TURP, 699-703
radical-retropubic, radical-perineal, 703-6
retropubic, 703-6, 703*f*
suprapubic, 703
Prosthetic interposition tube graft repair of aortic coarctation, 984
Protease inhibitors, drug interactions, F-8
Protein-losing nephropathy, 1081-2
Proteinosis, alveolar, 252-5
Proton pump inhibitor (PPI), 396
Pruitt-Inahara shunt, 102
Prune-belly syndrome, 1073-4, 1077, 1078
Pseudoaneurysm, 1174-8
Pseudoarthrosis of tibia, 1111-13
Pseudocyst, 1174-8
Pseudoxanthoma elastica, 6
Psoas hitch procedure, 716
Psoas release, 1103-4, 1121-5
Psychiatric drugs, 1156; in ECT, 1157
Psychiatric syndromes, 53-6

Psychological complications
    in breast surgery, 518
    in imaging procedures, 1177
Psychosis, refractory, 1154-8
Psychotherapeutic agents, anesthetic
        considerations in ECT, 1156
Pterygium
    conjunctival transposition, 123
    excision, 123-4; anesthesia, 124-6
    free-graft, 123
Ptosis repair, 120-1, 124-6
    frontalis sling, 121
Pubic rami fracture, 796
PUD. *See* Peptic ulcer disease.
Pudendal neuropathy, 430, 435-8
Puestow pancreaticojejunostomy, 486-7,
        anatomy, 487*f*; anesthesia, 491-4
'Puff' sign, 86
Pullthrough
    Hirschsprung's disease, 1053-6
    imperforate anus, cloaca, 1056-8
Pulmonary alveolar proteinosis, 252-5
Pulmonary artery banding
    for A-V canal defect, 976, 976*f*
    for tricuspid atresia, 1004
    in VSD repair, 979
Pulmonary artery clamping, in lung
        transplant, 371, 372
Pulmonary artery stenosis, 1193-4
Pulmonary artery/vein injury, 577-8
Pulmonary aspiration
    in pediatric transurethral surgery, 1078
    Sx, in pelvis/hip trauma patients, 806
Pulmonary atresia, 996
Pulmonary cysts, congenital, 1024-7
Pulmonary diseases, preop testing, A-3
Pulmonary edema, 186, 369, 639
Pulmonary embolism (PE), in laparotomy,
        hysterectomy/BSO, 619
Pulmonary fat embolus, 806, 863
Pulmonary fibrosis
    in chest-wall reconstruction, 921
    lung transplant for, 255-6
Pulmonary hypertension
    in heart transplant, 364
    heart/lung transplant for, 365-73
    lung transplant for, 255-6
    refractory, in surgery for TAPVC, 995
Pulmonary hypertensive crisis, 1003
Pulmonary infiltrates, 240-3
Pulmonary insufficiency, 1044
Pulmonary lesion, 215-18
Pulmonary malignancy, 1182-6
Pulmonary obstruction, 235-8
Pulmonary resection, 208-215; anesthesia,
        210-15, spirometric criteria for, 208
    for bronchial injury, 579-80, 580-2
Pulmonary sequestration, 1025*f*
Pulmonary stenosis, 973, 996, 1006-8
Pulmonary TB, 222-3, 224-6
Pulmonary toxicity with chemotherapy,
        1198
Pulmonary vascular occlusive disease
        (PVOD), with ASD, 972
Pulmonary vascular resistance (PVR), in
        tricuspid valve repair, 281

Pulmonary wedge resection, 230
Pulmonary-to-systemic flow ratio, 973
Pulmonic valvuloplasty, pediatric, 1193
Pulse generator, implantable, 60
Pulse oximetry monitoring—adult, B-1;
        pediatric, D-1
    in CHD surgery, 1037
Pulsed-current technique in RFA, 1182
Pump system, in functional neurosurgery,
        62
Putti-Platt operation for shoulder
        instability, 765-6
PVD. *See* Peripheral vascular disease.
Pyelography, retrograde, 696-7, 698-9
Pyelolithotomy, for ureter and renal pelvis
        calculi, 709-10; anesthesia, 710-12
Pyelonephritis, 351
Pyeloplasty
    Anderson-Heinz, 709-12, 1069
    dismembered, 709-12, 709*f*; 1069
    for fetal hydronephrosis, 1069-71
    laparoscopic, 1081-2
    for ureteropelvic junction stenosis,
        709-10; anesthesia, 710-12
Pyeloureterostomy, for ectopic ureters,
        ureteroceles, 1068-71
Pyloric stenosis in infants, 1038-40
Pyloromyotomy
    + esophagectomy, 385
    for pyloric stenosis, infants, 1038-40
    Ramstedt, for infantile pyloric stenosis,
        anatomy, 1038*f*
Pyloroplasty
    + esophagectomy, 385
    + oversew, duodenal perforation, 394
    + vagotomy, for PUD, 396-9
Pyogenic osteomyelitis, 87-89, 97-99

Q

Quadriplegia, 923-4, 1072
Quinidine, drug interactions with, F-8
Quinine, drug interactions with, F-8

R

Racine adaptor, bronchoscopy, 147*f*, 150
Radial artery cutdown, 1217, 1217*f*
Radial balloon dilation, for esophageal
        foreign body/stricture, 1016-17
Radial bone abnormalities, 1057
Radial club hand, 1089-90, 1091-2
Radial forearm flap, in microsurgery, 911
Radial longitudinal deficiency, 1089-92
Radiation
    anesthetic concerns, 1198
    for cystitis, 712-15
    for enteritis, 413-14, 416-18
    exposure, in uterine cancer, 619
    injuries, chest-wall, 920-2
        in craniotomy for EC-IC bypass, 21
    for necrosis, 218-19, 220-1
    for stenosis, 1178-82
Radiation implants for cervical, vaginal,
        vulvar cancer, 624-7; anesthesia, 626
Radiation therapy
    complications, 433-4

in radical vulvectomy, 601
    pediatric, 1188-92; anesthesia, 1189-91
Radioactive dust inhalation, 252-5
Radioactive seed implantation for prostate
        cancer, 726-7
Radioactive tracers, 526
Radiocarpal arthritis, 737-8, 740-3
Radiofrequency ablation (RFA), 1182-6
    pediatric, out-of-OR, 1195
Radiofrequency probes, for sleep-
        disordered breathing surgery, 195-8
Radiofrequency rhizotomy
    for spasticity, 69-70; anesthesia, 942-3
    for trigeminal neuralgia, 108-11
Radiofrequency-assisted perforation of
        pulmonary valve, atrial septum,
        1195
Radiolunate arthrodesis, 737-8, 740-3
Radiopancarpal arthrodesis, 737-8, 740-3
Radioscapholunate arthrodesis, 737-8;
        anesthesia, 740-3
Radiosurgery, 54-6; anesthesia, 55-6
    ablation, stereotactic, 61
    pediatric, 54-6
    in pediatric XRT, 1189-92
Radiotherapy, for cervical, vaginal, vulvar
        cancer, 624-7; anesthesia, 626
Radioulnar distal joint
    osteoarthritic degeneration, 734-5
    synovitis, subluxation, 735-6
Radius, distal—fractures, dislocation
    arthroscopy for, 749-50
    ORIF for, 753-5
    resection, 734-5
Rainey clips, in craniosynostosis
        correction, 1130
Ramstedt pyloromyotomy, 1038*f*
Ranitidine
    drug interactions with, F-8
    in full-stomach precautions, B-5
    in PUD, 396
Rapid-sequence induction (RSI) of
        anesthesia, B-5
Rashkind balloon atrial septostomy, 1195
    for TGA, 996, 998
Rastelli conduit procedure
    for TGA/VSD, 997
    for TOF surgery, 988
    for truncus arteriosus, 1002
Ravitch approach to pectus excavatum/
        carinatum, 1029-31, 1029*f*
Ray amputation, 851, level, 853*f*
Raynaud's phenomenon, 332-4, 336-8
Raz bladder neck suspension for urinary
        incontinence, 728-30
RC. *See* Rotator cuff.
Reconstructive surgery, facial, nonfacial,
        865-932
Reconstructive transcatheter techniques
        for vascular rehabilitation, 1192
Rectal cancer, 613-18
Rectal prolapse, 429-30, 436-8
    Delorme procedure, 429-30
    full-thickness, 429-30
    perineal rectosigmoidectomy, 429-30
    rectopexy, 429-30

Ripstein, 429-30
sigmoid resection, 429-30
sling, 429-30
Rectal surgery, 431-2; anesthesia, 436-8
abdominal-transsacral resection,
Kraske approach, 431-2, 436-8
removal, with proctocolectomy, 421-3
rigid proctoscopy, 431-2, 436-8
transanal excision, rigid proctoscopy,
431-2; anesthesia, 436-8
transsacral/transsphincteric excision,
Mason approach, 431-2, 436-8
Rectal ulcer, 431-2
Rectocele, 430
repair, 652-4, 652f; 728-30
Rectopexy, 429-30; anesthesia, 436-8
Rectosigmoidectomy, perineal, 429-30;
anesthesia, 436-8
Rectovaginal anatomy, 621f
Rectum pullthrough in Hirschsprung's
disease, 1055f
Rectus abdominis muscle flap
in chest-wall reconstruction, 921-2
in pelvic exenteration, 613-14
Rectus diastasis, 889-92
Red clover (Trifolium pratense),
precautions with anesthesia, F-11
Reduction mammoplasty, 885-8
Reduction pneumoplasty, 250
Reflex sympathetic dystrophy (RSD)
in palmar fasciectomy, 744
sympathectomy for, 339-41
VATS for, 240-3
Reflux, esophagogastric, 384-5
Refractory psychosis, 1154-8
Regional CBF (rCBF), 105
Regurgitation, risk factors, 692
Reishi (Ganoderma lucidum), precautions
with anesthesia, F-11
Relafen, anesthetic considerations in
lumbar discectomy, 783
Remifentanil infusion
in MAC, B-4
in TIVA, B-3
Renal collecting system carcinoma, 707-9
Renal disease, end-stage
kidney/pancreas transplant, 539-42
kidney transplant for, 538-9, 541-2
Renal disease, preop testing, A-3
Renal failure
in chest trauma surgery, 581
end-stage
hemodialysis for, 349-54
permanent vascular access for, 351-4
in gynecologic staging laparotomy, 596
Renal fascias, anatomy, 707f
Renal function preop testing, A-1
Renal function preservation, 1070
Renal pelvis
cancer, endoscopic diagnostics, 696-9
operations, 709-12
stone, 709-10
Renal transplantation, 442, 559-60
Renal ultrafiltration, in pelvic
exenteration, 616
Renal vein sampling, image-guided, 1174

Renal-cell carcinoma, 706-11, 1068-71
Rendu-Osler-Weber syndrome, 6, 17
Renovascular HTN, 706-9, 710-11
Reperfusion syndrome, in liver transplant,
555
Replantation
digit, hand, 755-8
microsurgery for finger, hand,
extremities, 913-16
scalp, 914; anesthesia, 915-16
Replogle tube (indwelling), 1018
Resection arthroplasty, hand, 736-7;
anesthesia, 740-3
Resectoscope, in TURP, 699-703
inserted in bladder, 700f
Reserpine, drug interactions with, F-8
Respiratory failure
pediatric, ECMO for, 1203-4
tracheostomy for, 182-5
Respiratory insufficiency, in carotid
endarterectomy, 106
Respiratory special concerns
in surgery for CHD, 1035, 1036
in tracheobronchial stenting, 1179-80
Retinal detachment, 134-7
Retinal surgery, 134-7
gas-fluid exchange, 134-7
retinopexy, 135
scleral buckling, 134-7
tear, surgery for, 134-7
vitrectomy, 134-7
Retinoblastoma, 1188-92
Retinopathy, 135, 136
Retrobulbar block, in ophthalmology,
125, 950
Retrolingual collapse, enlargement,
obstruction, 193-8
Retropalatal collapse, 193-8
Retroperitoneal tumor, 416-18, 497-9,
501-2
Retroperitoneum, anatomy, 530f
Retropharyngeal abscess, 964-5
Retrorectal tumor, 431-2
Revascularization
all-arterial, 266
emergency, in CABG, 268
RFA. See Radiofrequency ablation.
Rhabdomyolysis
in above/below-knee amputation, 855
in fasciotomy, thigh/leg, 860
Rhabdomyosarcoma, 218, 1076-8, 1188-
92
Rheumatoid arthritis. See Arthritis,
rheumatoid.
Rheumatoid synovitis, wrist, 749-50
Rhinoplasty, 153-5; anesthesia, 158-60
open/closed techniques, 878-81, 880f
dorsal, 878-81
reduction, augmentation, 878-81
tip, 878-81
Rhinorrhea, bifrontal craniotomy, 41
Rhizotomy, radiofrequency. See
Radiofrequency rhizotomy.
Rhytidectomy, 869-71; anesthesia, 876-8
Rib resection, drainage of empyema, 223
Rickets, 1111-13

Rifampin, drug interactions with, F-8
Right ventricle (RV)
dysfunction, heart/lung transplant, 369
failure, tricuspid valve repair, 281
Rigid bronchoscopy, 151f, 235-8
Ripstein procedure, for rectal prolapse,
429-30; anesthesia, 436-8
Risdon osteotomy, for mandibular
deformities, 905-8
Rocuronium
in adult intubation, B-2; muscle
relaxation, B-3
in pediatric muscle relaxation, D-2,
D-3
Rod and wiring
posterior spinal instrumentation, 1094f
upper C-spine, 75-7, 83-7
Rod systems, anterior lumbar/
lumbosacral, 91
Root canal, under deep iv sedation,
1209-11
Ropivacaine, drug interactions, F-5
Rosch-Uchida transjugular needle, in
TIPS, 1169
Rose position, 143f
Rossetti modified esophageal
fundoplication, 456-7, 461-3
Rotation advancement flap (Millard) in
cleft lip repair, 1137-40, 1147-8
Rotator cuff arthropathy, 769-73
Rotator cuff (RC) tear, surgery for, 762-4
anesthesia, 766-9
arthroscopic surgery, 760-2, 766-9
repair, direct lateral open, mini-open,
deltoid-splitting approaches, 763
Roux-en-Y bile duct reconstruction, in
liver transplant, 549
Roux-en-Y cholecystojejunostomy, 448-
50; anesthesia, 452-4
Roux-en-Y gastric bypass
for morbid obesity, 400-3, 400f; 477-9
Roux-en-Y jejunal conduit, in
portoenterostomy, 1047f
Roux-en-Y loop of jejunum
in bile duct tumor excision, 450
in drainage of pancreatic pseudocyst,
485-6, 485f
in gastrectomy, 392
Roux-en-Y loop of small intestine, in
liver transplantation, 552f
Roux-en-Y pancreaticojejunostomy, 486-
7, anatomy, 487f; anesthesia, 491-4
Roux-Goldthwait procedure for patellar
realignment, 1115-16, 1121-5
Rowe disimpaction forceps, 903
Royle approach, lumbar sympathectomy,
337-8
Rubber-band ligation, hemorrhoids, 434
Rubens/iliac crest flap, microsurgery, 911
Rutledge modified hysterectomy, 622

S
Sacrococcygeal teratoma, 1062-4
Sacroiliac (SI), posterior ligaments, 796f
Sacroiliac joint arthritis/arthrosis, 804-8
dislocation, anterior, 796

Sacrum fractures, 796
Saethre-Chotzen syndrome, 1130
Sagittal craniosynostosis, 936-8
Sagittal ramus split osteotomy, for
    mandibular deformities, 905-8, 905f
Sagittal synostosis, 1130-4
SAH. *See* Subarachnoid Hemorrhage
Salpingectomy, 640; total, for ectopic
    pregnancy, 687-8; anesthesia, 692-3
Salpingo-oophorectomy
    bilateral, unilateral, 595-7
    laparoscopic, 690-3
Salpingolyis, for infertility, 643
Salpingostomy, 640
Salter's innominate osteotomy, pelvic
    reconstruction, 1097-9, 1121-5
Samter's disease, 158
Sanders Injection System, 237
Sanders jet ventilation, 151f; 962
Sano modified homograft conduit, 1011
Saphenous cutdown, pediatric, 590
Sarcoidosis
    heart/lung transplantation, 365-73
    laparoscopic splenectomy, 465
    portal HTN surgery, 345-8
    tracheobronchial stenting, 1178-82
Sarcoma
    intraabdominal, retroperitoneal, 501-2
    soft-tissue, XRT for, 1188-92
Satinsky clamp, for abdominal vascular
    injuries, 585
Savary/Gilliard esophageal dilators, 959
Scalp
    avulsion, replantation, 913-16
    resuspension ± resection, 872-6
Scalp flap, in craniotomy, 15
Scaphocapitate intercarpal arthrodesis,
    737-8
Scaphoid, rotatory subluxation, 749-50
Scapholunate dissociation, 749-50
Scapular flap, in microsurgery, 911
Scapular fractures, 773-4, 776-8
Scapulothoracic dissociations, 773-4
SCFE. *See* Slipped capital femoral
    epiphysis.
Scheuermann's kyphosis, 97-9; 784-7
Schisandra (*Schizandra chinensis*),
    precautions with anesthesia, F-11
Schistosomiasis, 345-8
Schwannoma, 187-92, 229-30, 232-5
Sciatic nerve injury, in hip surgery, 815
Sclera excision, 123f
Scleral buckle or mass, strabismus, 951
Scleral buckling, 134
Scleral fixation ring, 115
Scleroderma, 336-8
Sclerosing cholangitis
    bile duct excision for, 450-1, 452-4
    primary, liver transplant for, 547-52
Sclerotherapy, for hemorrhoid, 434
Scoliosis, 942, 1029
    anterior spinal fusion ±
        instrumentation, 1095-7
    anterior spinal reconstruction, 787-94
    anterior thoracic surgery, 87-9

idiopathic, 784-7, 789-94
    release, repair, 1095-7, 1095f
    posterior spinal instrumentation/fusion,
        789-93, 1093-5
Scopolamine, in adult premedication, B-2
Screw fixation
    distal radius, carpus, metacarpals, 753-5
    upper C-spine, 72f
Screw-plate fixation, mid/lower C-spine,
    77-9, 83-7
Scrotal dartos pouch, 1079-81
Scrotal incisions, 724f
Scrotal operations, 723-5
    anesthesia, 724-5
    hydrocelectomy, 723-5
    orchiectomy, 723-5
    reduction of testicular torsion, 723-5
    spermatocelectomy, 723-5
    testicular prosthesis insertion, 723-5
    vasvasostomy, 723-5
Sitting position, 85-6
Second-look/reassessment laparotomy for
    ovarian cancer, 597-8, 598-601
Segmental colectomy, 423-5, 427-9
Segmental lumbar instability, 94
Segmental tubal resection, for ectopic
    pregnancy, 687-8; anesthesia, 692-3
Segmentectomy
    in hepatic resection, 440-1, 442-4
    for neonatal lung resection, 1025
Seizures
    in intracranial venous malformation, 16
    precautions in ECT, 1157
    preop testing, indications for, A-3
Seldinger technique
    bypass for liver transplant, 549
    cannulating blood vessels, 1192
Selective norepinephrine/serotonin
    reuptake inhibitors (SNRI), 1156
Selective serotonin reuptake inhibitor
    (SSRI), 1156, 1157
    drug interactions with, F-8
Selective vagotomy, 396f
Selegiline, drug reactions with, F-9
Sella turcica, 44-7
Sellick's maneuver, abdominal trauma, 587
Semisitting position, craniotomy, 17f
Senning atrial switch for TGA, 996
Sentinel lymph node, biopsy, 513-15,
    513f
Sepsis syndrome, 860
Septal defects
    ASD, 972-5, 976
    VSD, 979-81
Septal deviation, 153-5, 158-60, 878-81
Septal hypertrophy, asymmetric, 282-4
Septal myectomy/myotomy, 282-4
Septic arthritis
    acetabulum, 861, 863-4
    knee, 827-8, 835-7
    pediatric orthopedic preop anesthetic
        considerations, 1122
Septoplasty, 153-5; anesthesia, 157; 878
Septorhinoplasty 153-5
    ± cartilage grafting, for secondary
        lip/nose deformities, 1145-8

Sequestration, intralobar/extralobar, 1024-
    7, 1025f
Serratus anterior flap, in microsurgery,
    911
Seton use with fistulotomy, 433-4;
    anesthesia, 436-8
Sevoflurane
    adult anesthetic maintenance, B-3
    pediatric, muscle relaxation,
        inhalational anesthesia, D-2
    in pediatric neurosurgery, 940
    in strabismus surgery, 951
Shallow cone of cervix, 606-8
Sheehan's syndrome, 667
Shelf augmentation for acetabular
    dysplasia, 1099-1100, 1121-5
Shirodkar cerclage, 674-6
'Shisk kebab' construct in Sofield
    procedure, 1111
Shock, in abdominal trauma, 582
Short-segment fusion, lumbar, 782-4
Short-stature syndrome, 144
Shoulder girdle procedures, 773-4, 776-8
    sling, sling-and-swathe immobilization,
        773-4
Shoulder
    arthritis, 769-73
    avascular necrosis, osteoarthritis, 769-
        73
    dislocation, instability, 765-9
    frozen, capsular release for, 760-1
    joint, anterior, surgical anatomy, 761f
        cross-section anatomy, 763f
    separation, 762-4
    traumatic instability, 765
Shoulder surgery, 759-80
    arthroplasty, 769-73
    arthroscopy, 760-2; anesthesia, 766-9
    glenohumeral arthroplasty, 769-73
    hemiarthroplasty, 769-73
    instability (multidirectional, traumatic),
        stabilization (reconstructive, open,
        arthroscopic), 765-9
        Magnuson-Stack, Putti-Platt
        operations, 765-6
    open surgery for dislocation, 765-9
    replacement, 769-73
    separation, surgery for, 762-4, 766-9
    special anesthetic considerations in
        arthritic patients, 766-7
Shouldice repair for inguinal hernia, 504
Shunts
    for carotid endarterectomy, 309f
    malfunction, pediatric, 945-8
    for portal HTN (total, selective), 343-8
    for tricuspid atresia, 1003-6
    ventricular, 47-50; anesthesia, 50
Shunts for portal hypertension
    anesthesia, 346-8
    Clatworthy, 343-5
    end-to-side, 343-5, 344f
    mesocaval, 343-5, 344f
    portacaval, 343-8, 344f
    portarenal, 343-8
    portosystemic, 343-8
    side-to-side, 343-8, 344f

splenorenal, 343-8, 344f
Warren, 344-5
Sialoadenitis, chronic,166-8
Sick sinus syndrome (SSS), 284-7
Sickle cell disease, 497
Side-to-end anastomosis, hemodialysis, 349-51, 350f; anesthesia, 352-4
Side-to-side anastomosis for small bowel, 413-14
Sigmoid colectomy, 424
Sigmoid resection, 429-30, 436-8
Silastic stents, tracheobronchial, 1178-82
Silastic wrist prostheses, 738-9, 740-3
Sildenafil, drug reactions with, F-9
Silicone rubber prostheses, in thumb joint procedures, 740
Silicone stents, tracheobronchial, 1178-82
Simons procedure for clubfoot, 1119-20
Simultaneous kidney/pancreas transplant (SPK), 539-41, 540f
Single-lung transplant, 365
Single-lung ventilation. *See* One-lung ventilation.
Single-shot caudal epidural, D-4
Single-shot spinal anesthesia, 334, 357, 508
Sinus, 155f
frontal fractures, 897, 898-902
infections, tumor, 157-60
Sinus surgery
endoscopic, 157-8; anesthesia, 158-60
external, 155-157; anesthesia, 158-60
Sinus venosus ASD, 972-5, 972f
Sinusitis, chronic, 157-60
Sinusoidal occlusion, 345-8
Sistrunk procedure, for thyroglossal duct cyst, 963; anesthesia, 964-5
Sitting position, in craniotomy, 27
Skeletal fixation, tibia, 844-5
Skin graft for burn wound, 928-32
Skin resurfacing, laser, office-based, 1207-9; anesthesia, 1208-9
Skin-only flaps, in pressure-sore reconstruction, 923
Skull base surgery, 187-92
right middle fossa approach, 188f
Skull base tumor, 26
Skull fracture, 32
Skull shape abnormalities, 1130f
Skull tumor, 28-30, 31
SLAP lesions, 760-2, 766-9
Sleep apnea, with cleft palate, 1141 (Also *see* Obstructive sleep apnea.)
Sleep-disordered breathing, 193-8
Sling-and-swathe immobilization for shoulder girdle trauma, 773-4
Sling procedures
for nonfunctioning urethra, 728-30
for rectal prolapse, 429-30, 436-8
for urinary incontinence, 655-7, 728f
Slipped capital femoral epiphysis (SCFE), external fixator for, 1108-9; anesthesia, 1121-5
Small bowel
injuries, damage control, 582-3, 586-9

resection, with anastomosis, 413-14; anesthesia, 416-18
stapled, functional anastomosis, 413-14
Small-pin fixators for tibia fracture, 842
Smith's fracture of distal radius, 753-5
'Sniff' position, for morbid obesity operations, 401f
Snoring, 143
Soave pullthrough for Hirschsprung's disease, 1053-6
Soave-Kapandji radioulnar procedure, 734-5
Sodium citrate, in full-stomach precautions, B-5
Sofield procedure, for long bone, 1111-13; anesthesia, 1121-5
Somatosensory evoked potential (SSEP), 6, 320, 1093
Southwick osteotomy, for proximal femur, 1108-9, 1121-5
Spastic developmental deformity, 1117-18, 1121-5
Spasticity, surgery, 69-70, 942-3
treatment, 59
Spermatic cord exposure, 719f
Spermatocelectomy, for spermatocele, epididymal cyst, 723-5
Sphenoidectomy, transseptal, 156
Spherocytosis 463-6, 498
splenectomy for, 499-501
Sphincter deficiency, intrinsic, 654-7
Sphincter of Oddi spasm, 453
Sphincter pharyngoplasty, 1142-4; anesthesia, 1147-8
Sphincter stretch (Lord procedure), 434
Sphincterectomy
for common bile duct stones, 446
endoscopic, open, transduodenal, for biliary drainage, 448-50, 452-4
for choledochal cyst, 452
for fecal incontinence, 435-8
Sphincterotomy, endoscopic
for biliary drainage, 448-50, 452-4
for choledochal cyst, 452
Spina bifida, 430, 946, 1072, 1100, 1117
bladder neck operations for, 1074
neurosurgery for, 936-8
Spinal anesthesia/analgesia, 663
adult, C-4; pediatric, D-5
single-shot, hernia procedure, 508
Spinal cord
abnormality, pediatric, 1077
compression, 78, 81, 90; 89-91, 97-99
injury, 69-70
stimulation, 61-4
tethered, 941-3
Spinal dysraphism, correction, 941-3
associated with clubfoot, 1120
occult, 941-43
Spinal neurosurgery, 71-99
cervical, mid/lower/upper anesthesia, 83-7
anterior fusion/fixation, 72-74
posterior fusion/fixation, 75-76
cervicothoracic, anterior, 82-86, 97-9

lumbar/sacrolumbar
anesthesia, 97-9
anterior, endoscopic, 91-3
combined anterior/posterior instrumentation, 96-7
posterior procedures, 93-6
thoracic
anesthesia, 97-99
anterior surgery, 87-9, 89f
combined anterior/posterior instrumentation, 96-7
posterior surgery, 89-91, 91f
thoracoscopic, 87
Spinal RFA, 1183
Spinal single-shot anesthesia, 508
in vascular surgery, 334
in venous surgery, 357
Spinal surgery (orthopedic), 781-94
anterior reconstruction
bone grafts, metal implants, bone cement, 785-6
+ fusion for osteomyelitis, 784-7; anesthesia, 789-94
for neoplastic disease, 787-9, 789-94
for segmental instability, 789-94
lumbar/sacrolumbar, anterior reconstruction/fusion, 787-9, 788f; anesthesia, 789-94
retroperitoneal approach (anterior), patient positioning, 785f
thoracic/thoracolumbar, anterior reconstruction /fusion, 784-7
cervicothoracic approach, 784-7
transdiaphragmatic approach (anterior), 785-7, patient positioning, 785f
transthoracic approach (anterior), 785, surgical anatomy, 785f
Spinal surgery, pediatric
abnormalities, correction of, 941-3
anterior spinal fusion ± instrumentation for scoliosis, 1095-7, 1121-5
posterior instrumentation/fusion (Pemberton, Salter, Steel, Dial), 1093-9, 1096f; anesthesia, 789-93
pedicle hook, 1093f
rod position, 1094f
sublaminar wiring, 1993f
Spine (Also *see* Cervical spine, Lumbar spine.)
abnormalities, pediatric, 941-3
endovascular therapy for, 1158-62
fractures, 87-9, 97-99
neoplastic, metastatic diseases, 789-94
osteomyelitis, 784-7, 789-94
scoliosis. *See* Scoliosis.
segmental instability, 787-94
three-column model (Denis), 95f
tumor, 87-9, 93-4
Spirometric criteria for pulmonary resection, 208
Spleen, anatomy, 463f
injuries, repair, 582-4, 586-9
trauma, 499-501, 583-4, 586-9
vein occlusion, 345-8
Splenectomy, 499-501; anatomy, 500f; anesthesia, 497-9

with gastrectomy, 392
hand-assist device, 464
laparoscopic, 463-6, 464f
for portal HTN, 345
for splenic injuries, 584, 586-9
in staging laparotomy, 496
Splenic salvage, 400-1, anesthesia, 584
Splenomegaly, complications, 497
Splenorenal shunt, for portal HTN, 343-8
distal, 344-5, 344f; anesthesia, 346-8
Splenorrhapy, 500-1, 500f
Split posterior tibial transfer, for spastic
varus, 1117-18; anesthesia, 1121-5
Spondylolisthesis, 93-9
Spondylolysis, 93-9
Spontaneous pneumothorax, 1029
excision, 246-9
VATS for, 240-3
Spontaneous ventilation, in pediatric
otolaryngology, 954
Sprotte needle, for spinal anesthesia, 650
Squamous-cell carcinoma
head and neck, 147
resection for, 226-9
SSEP. *See* Somatosensory evoked potentials.
St. John's wort (*Hypericum perforatum*),
precautions with anesthesia, F-11
Stab avulsion technique, varicose veins,
355-8; anesthesia, 356-8
Stab cricothyrotomy, emergency, 1214
Staging laparotomy, for gynecologic
cancer, 594-7; anesthesia, 595-7
Stallard-Wright incision, orbitotomy, 132
Stallworthy modified hysterectomy, 622
Stamey procedure for urinary
incontinence, 654-7; 728-30, 728f
Stamm gastrostomy, 403-4, 411-12
Standards of Basic Anesthetic Monitoring,
1154
Stapedectomy, stapedotomy, 160-3
Stapling procedures, 215-18, 215f
in excision of blebs, bullae, 246-9
Static balloon septoplasty, 1195
Steel osteotomy for pelvic reconstruction,
1097-9; anesthesia, 1121-5
Stein-Leventhal syndrome, 619
Stent
tracheobronchial
dislodgement, 1181
fracture/migration, 1181
insertion techniques, 1179
placement, image-guided, 1174
types—silicone-based, metallic 1178
self-expanding (in TIPS), 1169-70
for vascular rehabilitation, 1192
Stent-graft
deployment, anesthetic management
during, 315, 316
migration, endovascular, 316
Stenting, transhepatic, endoscopic, for
bile duct stricture, 450
Stereotactic neurosurgery, 52-6, 59-50,
62-4
craniotomy, for AVMs, 15
localization, 17
OR set-up, 53f

Stereotactic radiosurgery
ablation, 61-4
in craniotomy for intracranial vascular
malformations, 15
Stereotaxy, image-guided, frameless, 53-6
Also *see* Frameless stereotaxy.
Sterilization (female), 669-71
Sternal dehiscence, infection, 920-2
Sternal notch, 573f
Sternocleidomastoid muscle transection,
in neck dissection, 168
Sternotomy
complete, in thymectomy, 243-6
in tracheal resection, 226-9
Sternotomy, median
in chest trauma, 576-7, 580-2
in lobectomy, 209
in lung wedge resection, 215
in LVRS, 249-52
for mediastinal masses, 1021-4
for mediastinal tumor excision, 229
in mitral valve surgery, 300
in pericardiectomy, 287-90
in thoracic surgery, 206f
Steroidogenesis, abnormal, 1076-8
Steroids
complications in laparotomy for
ovarian cancer, 599
preop testing, indications for, A-3
Stoma
closure (colostomy, loop, end), 426-9
continent + proctocolectomy, 422
stenosis, 426-0
Stomach
injuries, 411-12, 582-3, 586-9
surgery, 391-404 (Also *see* specific
procedures.)
Stomach-to-duodenal loop, 396
Stomach-to-jejunal loop, 393f, 396
Stone disease, 448-50, 452-4
Stone extraction, transurethral, 697-9
STP
in adult MAC, B-4
in pediatric iv induction, D-2
Strabismus surgery, 950-2
adjustable suture technique, 950
complications in anesthesia, 951, 952
Straddling atrioventricular valves, 996
Straight graft, for hemodialysis, 349-54
Strangulated hernia, 413-14, 416-18
Strassman procedure, bicornuate uteri,
644
Stress urinary incontinence, 652, 654-7,
728-30
Strictures, airways, 1178-82
Stridor
at rest, in airway management, 149
diagnostic laryngoscopy for, 960-2
in laryngectomy, 176
in neck mass resection, 1015
Stroke
carotid endarterectomy for, 102-8
in cerebral embolectomy, 13-15
in craniotomy for EC-IC bypass, 21
preop testing, indications for, A-3
Stump pressure, in endarterectomy, 105

Sturge-Weber syndrome, 67
Sub-tenon's anesthesia, for ophthalmic
surgery, 124, 950
Subacromial bursa, anatomy, 762f
Subacromial decompression, 760-4, 766-9
Subacromial impingement, 760-4, 766-9
Subaortic VSD, 1006, 1007f
Subarachnoid cyst, 49
Subarachnoid hemorrhage, 4-13, 16
Subclavian artery flap repair of aortic
coarctation, 984
Subclavian artery/vein injury, 577-8
Subcondylar fractures, 897-902
Subcostal transabdominal incision, for
nephrectomy, 708f
Subcutaneous dissection, in facelift,
869-71
Subcutaneous emphysema, 462
Subdural hematoma, 32f; precautions, 33f
Subdural hygroma, 49
Subfascial ligation of perforators, 354
Subgaleal dissection of forehead, 873f
Subglottic edema, 964, 1015
Subglottic hemangioma, cysts, 960-1
Subglottic lesions, 149
Subglottic stenosis, 966-8, 1059
Sublaminar wiring
in posterior spinal repair, 193f
in spinal hook-rod repair 1093-5
Submandibular gland excision, 166-8;
exposure, anatomy, 166f
Submucosal collagen injection for
nonfunctioning urethra, 728-30
Subphrenic abscess drainage, 416-18,
502-3, anatomy, 503f
Subpulmonary VSD, 1006, 1007f
Subscapularis release, 765-6
Subtemporal craniectomy, for epilepsy, 66
Subtotal laparoscopic hysterectomy
(SLH), 690-3
Subtrochanteric fracture, 815-17, 863-4
Subureteric injection for vesicoureteral
reflux, 1071-3
Subxiphoid pericardial window, in chest
trauma, 576-7; anesthesia, 580-2
Succinylcholine
in adult intubation—bolus, infusion,
B-2
drug interactions with, F-1, F-2, F-4,
F-5, F-7, F-8, F-9, F-10
in EB surgery, avoidance, 1127
in pediatric muscle relaxation, D-2
in strabismus surgery, 951
Suction curettage
1st trimester, for therapeutic abortion,
633-4; anesthesia, 635-6
for gestational trophoblastic disease,
610-13; anesthesia, 611-12
of molar pregnancy, 610f
Suction on emergence—adult, B-4;
pediatric, D-3
Sufentanil, in septal myectomy/myotomy,
283
Sugiura operation for portal HTN, 345-8
Superficial musculoaponeurotic system
(SMAS) of the face, 869-71, 869f

Superficial temporal artery (STA)-to-middle cerebral artery (MCA) branch anastomosis, 22-6, 22*f*
Superior labral anterior-posterior. *See* SLAP.
Superior vena cava compression, 1021
Superior vena cava syndrome, 234, 1023
Supine position
    in craniotomy, 27, 18*f*
    in morbid obesity operations, 401*f*; risks, 403
Suppurative thrombophlebitis, 341-3
Supracardiac drainage for TAPVC, 993
Supraclavicular block, in arm surgery, 779, 780
Supracondylar amputation level, 853*f*
Supracondylar humerus fracture, displaced, 1084-5, 1084*f*, 1091-2
Supracristal (subarterial) defects, 979
Supraglottic laryngectomy, 173-6, 175*f*
Supraglottic tumor, soft-tissue, 151
Supraglottoplasty, pediatric, 960-2
Suprahyoid transection, 174*f*
Supraomohyoid neck dissection, 168
Supraperiosteal dissection of the forehead, 873*f*
Suprasternal fossa cyst, 520*f*
Supratarsal fold absence, 874-8
Supratentorial brain tumor, 26-30
Supratentorial glial tumors, 1188-92
Supraventricular dysrhythmias, 1167
Supraventricular tachyarrhythmias, 1162-4
Surgical analgesics, neurosurgical, 61-4; anesthesia, 62-4
Suture closure for ASD, 972-5
SVC. *See* Superior vena cava.
Swanson joint replacement, hand, 736
Swenson pullthrough for Hirschsprung's disease, 1053-6
'Swiss cheese' ventricular septum, 979
Syed Neblett applicator, for interstitial perineal implants, 624, 625
Syme's amputation, 849-50, 853*f*; anesthesia, 863-4
    level of bone transection, 849*f*
Sympathectomy
    lumbar, 336-8; anesthesia, 332-4
    upper dorsal, VATS for, 240-3
    upper extremities, 339-41
Sympathomimetics, drug interactions with, F-5, F-7, F-8, F-9
Symphysis pubis, fracture/dislocation, 796, fibrocartilage, 796*f*
Syncope, 272, 282
Syndactyly
    with aplastic thumb, 1090
    finger repair, 1090-2
Synostosis (metopic, sagittal, coronal, lambdoid), 1130-4
Synovectomy
    of hip, 812-13; anesthesia, 813-15
    with knee arthrotomy, 834, 835-7
    + thumb joint reconstruction, 739-43
Synovitis of CMC joint, 739-43
Syringomyelia, 51, 90

T
TAAA. *See* Thoracoabdominal aorta aneurysms.
Tachyrhythmia, 1162-4
Tacrine, drug reactions with, F-2
Talipes equinovarus, 1119-25
Talus, avascular necrosis, 848
Tamponade release, chest trauma, 576-7
TAPVC. *See* Total anomalous pulmonary venous connection.
Tarsal strip procedure (ectropion), 118-19, 118*f*
Taussig-Bing DORV, 1006-8
Taxol, toxic effects in gynecologic oncology, 598, 599
Tazobactam sodium, drug interactions with, F-7
Technetium-labeled sulfur colloid (TSC), in sentinel node biopsy, 513-15
TEE
    in aortic dissection/aneurysm, 317, 320
    in cardiac surgery, 262
    in mitral valve repair, 278
TEF. *See* Tracheoesophageal fistula.
Telorbitism, 1134-7
Temperature monitoring—adult, B-1; pediatric, D-1
Temporal lobectomy, 64; anesthesia, 66-9
Temporomandibular joint (TMJ), 906
    ankylosis, derangement, subluxation, arthroscopy/arthrotomy for, 200-1; anesthesia, 203-4
Tendolysis of flexor or extensor tendon, 748-9; anesthesia, 751-2
'Tennis elbow,' 778-80
Tennison Z-plasty for cleft lip/palate repair, 1137-40; anesthesia, 1147-8
Tenosynovectomy (dorsal, radical), 735-6. 735*f*; anesthesia, 740-3
Tension pneumothorax. *See* Pneumothorax, tension.
Tension-band intraosseous wire, cortical graft, for thumb joint, 740
Tension-free vaginal tape (TVT), for urinary incontinence, 655-7
Tensor facia lata flap, microsurgery, 911
Teratodermoid, 229-30, 232-5
Teratoma, pediatric, 1021-4, 1062-4
Tessier procedure for face surgery, 936
Testicular cancer, 718-21, 1079-81
Testicular prosthesis insertion, 723-5
Testicular torsion
    pediatric surgery for, 1079-81
    reduction, 723-5
Testis
    absent, prosthesis insertion, 723-5
    nonpalpable, laparoscopy for, 1081-2
    orchiectomy for, 1079-81
    undescended, 1061-2
    orchiopexy for, 718-21, 1079-81
'TET' spells, associated with TOF, treatment modalities, 989
Tetracycline, drug interactions, F-9
Tetralogy of Fallot (TOF), 988*f*
    in A-V canal defect correction, 976
    challenges in unifocalization, 990

surgery for neonates, infants, adults, 988-92
    with CPB, 988-92
Texas Scottish Rite Hospital (TSRH) hook-rod system, 789-93, 1093-5
    in scoliosis correction, 1095-7
TGA. *See* Transposition of the great arteries.
Thalamic deep brain stimulation, 61
Thalamic vascular malformation, 15-21
Thalamotomy, 54, 59-60, 59*f*, 62-4
Thalamus, ventrolateral, anatomy, 58*f*
Thalassemia, 497
The Critical Pathway for the Organ Donor, 562
Theophylline, drug interactions, F-9
    preop testing, indications for, A-3
Therapeutic abortion (TAB), 633-6
Therapeutic lesions, locations, 59*f*
Therapeutic transurethral procedures (except TURP), 697-8; anesthesia, 698-9
Thermal capsulorrhaphy for shoulder repair, 760-6; anesthesia, 766-9
Thermal injury
    in imaging procedures, 1177
    in RFA, 1185
Thiazide diuretics, drug interactions, F-9,
Thiersch operation (pinch graft), for fecal incontinence, 436; anesthesia, 436-8
Thigh
    amputation levels, 853*f*
    anterolateral flap, in microsurgery, 911
    compartment syndrome, crush injury, necrotizing fasciitis, 857-61
    cross-section, compartments, 857*f*
    fasciotomy, 857-8; anesthesia, 859-61
Thioguanine
    in staging laparotomy, 498
    toxic effects, gynecologic oncology, 598
Thiopental
    in adult induction, B-2
    drug interactions with, F-7, F-9
Thiotepa, drug interactions with, F-9
Third-ventricle fenestration, 945-8
Third-rib anterior mediastinotomy, 1022
Thoracic anesthesia, pediatric, D-4
Thoracic aorta
    dissections, 317-22, 577-8, 580-2
    rupture, 577-8, 580-2
Thoracic aortic aneurysm
    ascending, transverse arch, descending, 310-13
    port-access procedures, 301
    stent-grafting for, 313-16
Thoracic epidural anesthesia—adult, C-2; pediatric, E-2
Thoracic injuries, emergency tube thoracostomy for, 569-71
Thoracic outlet syndrome, 1029
Thoracic radiculopathy, 90
Thoracic spine (neurosurgery)
    instrumentation, 89-91, 89*f*, 96-9
    laminectomy, 89-91, 97-9
Thoracic surgery
    drainage of empyema, 223-6

general surgery, 205-56 (Also *see* specific procedures.)

laser resection, 238-40

myelopathy (neurosurgical), 90

pediatric, 1026-7

pulmonary complication risks, 212

Thoracic vena cava injury, 577-8, 580-2

Thoracoabdominal aorta aneurysms (TAAA), 322-7, anatomy, 323*f*

inclusion repair technique, 322-7

classification, 324

no-clamp technique, 323

Thoracoabdominal incision, 531*f*

Thoracolumbar neurosurgical procedures, anesthesia, 97-9

Thoracolumbar transdiaphragmatic approach, spine surgery, 87

Thoracoplasty, 222-3, 224-6

pedicled muscle flap, 222

Thoracoscopy

clip ligation for PDA, 981

lobectomy, neonatal, 1025

for mediastinal masses, 1022

port placement, 241*f*

segmentectomy, neonatal lung, 1025

spine surgery, 87

for TEF, EA repair, 1018-21

video-assisted, 229, 1065

Thoracostomy

chest tube insertion, emergent, 1218*f*

emergency tube, 569-71

needle/catheter, emergent, 1218

tube, drainage of empyema, 223-6

tube incision, anatomy, 570*f*

Thoracotomy

anterior, thoracic surgery, 206*f*

anterolateral, pericardiectomy, 287-90

in ED, 571-2

lateral, 229, 1021-4

left anterior/anterolateral, in chest trauma, 576-7, 577*f*, 580-2

left anterolateral, 571-2

in lung wedge resection, 215

open, drainage of empyema, 223

posterolateral approach, 206*f*, 208

repair of TEF, EA, 1018-21

right, for mitral valve surgery, 300*f*;

in tracheal resection, 226-9

Three-incision vulvectomy, 602-5, 602*f*

Throat pack retention, 145, 958, 1147

Thrombectomy, venous, 341-4

Thrombi, floating, 341-4

Thromboelastograph (TEG)

coagulation therapy, 558

in liver transplantation, 556, 557*f*

variables and values, 557

Thrombolysis

image-guided, 1174

intravenous/endovascular, 13

Thrombophlebitis

in laparotomy, hysterectomy/BSO, 619

portal vein, 343-5, 346-8

suppurative, femoral, iliac, lower-limb venous surgery for, 341-4

thigh, 858

Thrombosis. *See* specific sites.

Thrombotic thrombocytopenic purpura (TTP), 463-6, 497

Thumb

aplastic, hypoplasia, pollicization for, 1089-90; anesthesia, 1091-2

arthroplasty/stabilization, 739-43

carpometacarpal joint fusion, 739-43

Thumb/finger, bifid, repair, 1090-2

Thumb joint arthrodesis, arthroplasty, 739-40; anesthesia, 740-3

Thymectomy, 243-6; anesthesia, 244-6, transcervical, 243-6

Thymic tumor, 229-30

Thymoma

excision, 229-30, 232-5

mediastinoscopy for, 231-5

thymectomy for, 243-6

Thyroglossal cyst removal, 963-5

Thyroglossal duct cyst excision, 520-1, 520*f*; anesthesia, 523-6

remnants, resection of, 1014-16

Thyroid

cancer, 521-6

disease, with strabismus, 951

lamina resection, in laryngectomy, 175*f*

nodule, 521-6

perichondrium, anatomy, 175*f*

tumor, pediatric, 1021-4

Thyroid gland, anatomy, exposure, vascular relationships, 174*f*, 522*f*

Thyroid storm, 524, 525

Thyroidectomy, 521-6; anesthesia, 523-5

minimally invasive approaches, 521

patient positioning, 522*f*

transverse incision, 521*f*

TIA. *See* Transient ischemic attack

Tibia

distal, fractures, ORIF, 843, 863-4

external fixation, 842, 863-4

posterior tendon repair, 835-7

proximal, fracture, osteotomy, 840-4

shortening, external fixation, 842, 863-4

tendon lengthening, 852, 1117-18; anesthesia, 1121-5

tendon transfer, 1117-18

transection, in amputation, 855*f*

Tibial nonunion/malunion

anesthsia, 863-4

intramedullary nailing, 841

repair, with iliac graft, skeletal fixation, 844-5

with shortening, external fixation, 842

Tibial plateau fracture, nonunion/ malunion, 840-1, 863-4

Tibial tubercle transfer, 831-2, 835-7

Tic douloureux, 37-40, 109-11

Timolol, in ophthalmic procedures, 126

Tinnitus, 37-40

TIPS, 1169-73; stages, 1171*f*

Tissue destruction in RFA, 1182

Titanium nails, for long-bone intramedullary nailing, 1106

TIVA

in adult anesthetic maintenance, B-3

in bronchoscopy, 151, 237

in esophagoscopy, 151

in laryngoscopy, 151

in thoracic laser resection, 239

TMJ. *See* Temporomandibular joint.

Todani classification of choledochal cysts, 1046

Toe gangrene, infection, necrosis, amputation for, 850-1, 863-4

TOF. *See* Tetralogy of Fallot.

Tongue, 906

neoplastic disease of, 177-8

Tongue-splitting transmandibular approach, upper C-spine, 73-4

Tonsil

asymmetric enlargement, 956-9

bleeding, 145

cancer, neck dissection for, 168-73

hypertrophy, 956-9

Tonsillectomy, 143-146, 143*f*

pediatric, 956-9; anesthesia, 957-8

Tooth crowns, bridges, replacement, 1209-11

Topical anesthesia

in awake FOI, B-6

in ophthalmic surgery, 125

Toradol, pediatric pain management, E-1

Torticollis, 60, 1103

muscular release (unipolar, bipolar), 1088-9; anesthesia, 1091-2

middle-third transection, complete resection, 1088-9, 1091-2

Total abdominal hysterectomy (TAH), 594, 647-51; anesthesia, 649-51

Total anomalous pulmonary venous connection (TAPVC), 973, 993*f*

to coronary sinus, 993*f*

to left innominate vein, 993*f*

to right atrium, 993*f*

Total anomalous pulmonary venous drainage, return, 993-6

Total body irradiation (TBI), 1188-92

Total intravenous anesthesia. *See* TIVA.

Total knee replacement (TKR), 826-7; anesthesia, 835-7

Total laparoscopic hysterectomy, 690-3

Total parental nutrition (TPN), permanent vascular access for, 351-4

Total shoulder arthroplasty, 769-73

Total wrist replacement (TWR), 738-9; anesthesia, 740-3

Toupet procedure (partial fundoplication), 384-5; anesthesia, 387-90

laparoscopic, 456-7, 456*f*, 461-3

Tourniquet considerations in anesthesia, 742, 885, 864, 915

'Tower-head' deformity, 1130-4

TPN. *See* Total parental nutrition.

Trabeculectomy, 116-18; anesthesia, 124-6

Trachea

disruption, 185

lesion, 959-63

reconstruction, 227*f*

stricture, 235-8

tumor, 226-9

visualization (bronchoscopy), 959-63

Tracheal anesthesia, in awake FOI, B-6
Tracheal fibrosis, in microsurgical
 reconstruction, 912
Tracheal intubation
 with acute fractures of C-spine, 4
 spinal neurosurgery, 86
Tracheal resection, 226-29
 airway emergency preparation, 228
 sternotomy, right thoracotomy, 226-29
Tracheobronchial injury, 579-82, 1181
Tracheobronchial stenting, out-of-OR,
 1178-82
 anesthesia, 1179-81
 intraop complications, 1181
 respiratory concerns, 1179-80
 stent types, 1178
Tracheobronchial tree, classic
 abnormalities, 1025f
Tracheobronchoscopy, in chest trauma,
 579-80; anesthesia, 580-2
Tracheoesophageal fistula (TEF),
 pediatric, 1018-21, 1019f
 aspiration and GI distention, 1018
 GI endoscopy, out-of-OR, 1199-1200
Tracheomalacia, 525, 1059, 1178-82
Tracheostomy, 182-5, 183f; anesthesia,
 183-5
 with glossectomy, 177
 in laryngectomy, 173, 176
 in neck dissection, 169
 pediatric, 970; anesthesia, 183-5
 for pharyngeal obstruction, 195-8
 in trauma surgery, 569
 tube insertion, 568f
 vertical incision for, 183f
Train-of-four, in esophageal foreign body/
 stricture removal, 1017
TRAM flap
 in breast reconstruction, 917-20, 918f
 in chest-wall reconstruction, 921-2
 in microsurgical reconstruction, 911
Transabdominal preperitoneal (TAPP)
 hernia repair, 475-7
Transanal excision, 431-2, 436-8
Transantral ethmoidectomy, 156
Transcranial Doppler (TCD), in carotid
 endarterectomy, 106
Transduodenal sphincteroplasty, for
 biliary drainage, 448-50, 452-4
Transesophageal echocardiography. See
 TEE.
Transesophageal varix ligation, 345
Transforaminal lumbar interbody fusion
 (TLIF), 95-9
Transgastric varix ligation, 345
Transhepatic stenting, for stricture, 450
Transient ischemic attack (TIA), 13-15, 21
 carotid endarterectomy for, 102-8
 craniotomy for, 4-13
Transitional malformation, 15
Transjugular intrahepatic portosystemic
 shunt, 1169-73 (Also see TIPS.)
Translabyrinthine craniotomy, 187-92,
 OR setup, 191f; anesthesia, 190-2
Transluminal endovascular stent-grafting,
 313

Transmetatarsal amputation, 850-1, level,
 853f; anesthesia, 863-4
Transodontoid screw fixation, 73-4, 83-7
Transoral odontoid excision, 72-4
Transpalatal exposure, 72-4
Transpedicular decompression, 89f
Transpedicular fixation, lumbar, 782-4
Transperitoneal instrumentation, lumbar/
 lumbosacral spine, 91-3, 97-9
Transplantation. See specific sites.
Transport, for special-needs patients
 burn patients, 931
 critically ill neonates, 995, 998
 pediatrics in CHD surgery, 1036
Transposition of the great arteries (TGA),
 995; surgery for, 996-1000
Transsphenoidal resection of pituitary
 tumor, 44-7; anesthesia, 45-7
Transtracheal local anesthesia, in
 bronchoscopy, 237
Transureteroureterostomy (TUU), 709-12
 710f; 1069-71
Transurethral microwave thermotherapy
 (TUMT), 700-3
Transurethral procedures (Also see
 specific procedures.)
 diagnostic (endoscopic) procedures,
  696-7; anesthesia, 698-9
 incision and dilation, 726-7
 incision of urethral stricture, PUV,
  ureterocele, 1071-3
 pediatric, 1071-3; anesthesia, 1077-8
 strictures, incision and dilation, 697-9
 therapeutic (except TURP), 697-9
 TURP, 699-703
Transurethral resection (TUR), 697-9
Transurethral resection of the prostate
 (TURP), 699-703; anesthesia, 701-2
 with resectoscope, 700f
Transurethral vaporization of the prostate
 (TUVP) with resectoscope, roller
 ball electrode, 700
Transvaginal oocyte retrieval (TVOR),
 641-2; anesthesia, 642-3
Transverse arch thoracic aortic
 aneurysms, 310-13
Transverse curvilinear perineal incision,
 704f
Trauma
 assessment/airway management, 568-9
 craniotomy for, 32-7
 emergency tube thoracostomy, 569-71
 general surgery, 567-90
 growth plate injury, 1111, 1114
 imaging and image-guided procedures
  for, 1174-8
 intubation (orotracheal, blind
  nasotracheal, cricothyroidotomy),
  568
 lower extremity injuries, 863-4
 neck stabilization, 569
 pediatric airway/vascular access, 589-
  90
 replantation microsurgery, 913-16
Traumatic injuries, blunt, emergency tube
 thoracostomy for, 569-71

Traumatic injuries, penetrating
 abdominal vascular injuries, 585-9
 chest, 569-71
 damage control, 582-3
 of great vessels, 578
 hepatic, splenic, 583-4, 586-9
 neck 572, 573
Treacher Collins syndrome, 906, 907,
 1132, 1136, 1141, 1143
 complications in anesthesia for
  pediatric lip/nose surgery, 1147
Trendelenburg position
 concerns in minimally invasive
  pediatric surgery, 1064, 1065
 in laparotomy, hysterectomy/BSO, 618
 in postpartum tubal ligation, 669
 reverse, in head and neck surgery, 140
 steep, in infertility operations, 645, 646
 in vaginal hysterectomy, 650
Triangular fibrocartilage tears, 749-50
Triceps-splitting approach, 778
Tricuspid atresia, 973, anatomy, 1004f
 bidirectional Glenn shunt for, 1003-6
 Fontan procedure for, 1003-6
 pediatric surgery for, 1003-6
 RA → RV connection, 1004
 ventriculoarterial concordance
  relationship, 1003
Tricuspid regurgitation, 279-82
Tricuspid valve, failure/atresia, 1003-6
 repair, 279-82
Tricyclic antidepressants, 1156
 drug interactions with, F-9
 in ECT, 1157
Trigeminal nerve pathology, 61-4
Trigeminal neuralgia
 microvascular decompression, 37-40
 percutaneous procedures, 108-11
 treated with RFA, 1182-6
Trigonocephaly, 1130-4
Trillat procedure for patellar realignment,
 1115-16; anesthesia, 1121-5
Trimethaphan, drug interactions, F-9
Triple arthrodesis, for varus/cavovarus
 foot, 1118-19, 1121-5
Triple wire technique, C-spine, 80, 81f
Trisegmentectomy, in hepatic resection,
 440-1; anesthesia, 442-4
Trismus, 144, 898
Trisomy, 1019, 1051, 1054, 1056
Trochanteric osteotomy for hip, 811-15
Trophoblastic disease, 687
Trousseau's sign, 529
Truncal vagotomy, 396f
Truncus arteriosus, 1000-3, 1001f
 anatomic classification, Collett and
  Edwards, 1000
 in critically ill neonate, 995
 nonvalved artificial conduits, aortic
  allograft and valve conduits, 1000
 special considerations for, 1000.
Tubal cannulation for infertility, 644
Tubal disease, ectopic pregnancy, 640-1
Tubal embryo transfer, 644
Tubal ligation, postpartum, 669-71
Tubal pregnancy, ruptured, 687

Tubal reanastomosis, 644
Tubal resection
  partial, 640
  segmental, 687-8; anesthesia, 692-3
Tube, endotracheal. *See* ETT.
Tube positioning, in pediatric
  otolaryngology, 954
Tube section in OLV for pediatric thoracic
  surgery, 1026
Tube thoracostomy, 570*f*
  drainage of empyema, 223-6
Tuberculosis (TB), pulmonary, 222-6
Tuberculous osteomyelitis, 87-9, 97-9
Tuberous sclerosis, 67
Tubular (rectal) adenoma, 431-2
Tumeric (*Curcuma longa*), precautions
  with anesthesia, F-11
Tumor. *See* specific sites.
  biopsy, pediatric, out-of-OR, 1198-9
  CNS, preop testing indications, A-3
  debridement, bronchoscopy for, 235-8
  debulking, peritoneal, 501-2
  embolization, neuroradiology, 1156-62
  imaging and image-guided procedures
    for, 1174-8
  pediatric, XRT for, 1188-92
TUMT. *See* Transurethral microwave
  thermotherapy.
Tunica albuginea plication (TAP) for
  hypospadias, 1075-8
Turbinate, 155*f*, reduction, 157
Turco's procedure for clubfoot, 1119-25
'Turkey gobbler' neck, 869-71
Turner's syndrome, 1062
TURP syndrome, 702
TURP. *See* Transurethral resection of the
  prostate.
TVOR. *See* Transvaginal oocyte retrieval.
Tylenol
  ± codeine, in pediatric analgesia, E-3
  in pediatric premedication, D-2
Tympanic membrane perforation, 160-3
Tympanomeatal flap, 160-3
Tympanoplasty, 160-3
Tympanostomy tube placement, 954-6;
  anesthesia, 955-6
Tympanotomy, exploratory, 160-3

U

Uchida technique, PPTL, 669-71
Ulcer. *See* specific sites.
Ulcerative colitis, 420-3, 427-9
Ulna
  resection/Darrach procedure for, 734-5,
    734*f*; anesthesia, 740-3
  translation of carpus, fusion for, 737-8
Ulnar impingement syndrome
  arthroscopy for, 749-50
  resection procedures for, 734-5
Ultram, anesthetic considerations in
  lumbar discectomy, 783
Ultrasound, 1173-8; anesthesia, 1175-7
Umbilical hernia repair, 1058-61
Unicameral bone cyst aspiration,
  injection, 1086-7; anesthesia, 1091-2

United Network for Organ Sharing
  (UNOS), 562
Universal Spine System (USS), in
  pediatric surgery, 789-93, 1093-7
Upper airway resistance syndrome, 193-8
Upper extremity orthopedic procedures,
  pediatric; anesthesia, 1091-2
Upper extremity sympathectomy. *See*
  Sympathectomy.
Upper/lower GI endoscopy, pediatric,
  1199-1201; anesthesia, 1200-1
Upper respiratory infection (URI), 957,
  964, 1141
  airway complications, 144
  anesthesia for, 955
  considerations in pediatric XRT, 1190
  in patients for PE tube placement, 955
Upper-arm straight graft, hemodialysis,
  349-51, 352-4
Ureter
  cancer, 696-7, 698-9, 707-9
  ectopic, 1070-1
  resection, 708, 709-10
  stone, 709-12
  trauma (lower) operations, 715-17
  trauma (upper), transureteroureter-
    ostomy, 1069-71
  tumor, 709-12
  upper, operations, 709-12
Ureteral reimplantation, 715-17
  failed, transureteroureterostomy for,
    1069-71
  vesicoureteral reflux, obstructive
    megaureters, ureterocele, 1073-5,
    1077-8
Ureteral stent placement, image-guided,
  1174
Ureteral undiversion, 1069-71
Ureterocele
  ectopic, prolapsed, 1076-8
  nephrectomy, nephroureterectomy,
    partial nephrectomy for, 1068-71
  pediatric procedures for, 1071-3
  ureteral reimplantation for, 1073-5
Ureterolithotomy, 709-12
Ureteropelvic junction obstruction
  endoscopic diagnostics for, 696-7
  pediatric procedures for, 1069, 1081-2
Ureteropelvic junction stenosis, 709-10
Ureteroscopy, 696-7; anesthesia, 698-9
Urethra
  diverticulum excision, 728-30
  fistulae, 1056
  nonfunctioning, 728-30
  prolapse, pediatric, 1076
  sling procedure 654-7
Urethral cancer, tumor, mass
  endoscopic diagnostics, 696-9
  pediatric procedures, 1071-3
  urethrectomy for, 726-7
Urethral plication, Kelly, for urinary
  incontinence, 654-7
Urethral stricture
  endoscopic diagnostics for, 696-9
  operations for, 726-7

pediatric transurethral procedures for,
  1071-3
Urethrectomy (partial, total), 726-27
Urethropexy, for urinary incontinence,
  655-7
Urethroplasty, 1076-7, 1077-8
  for urethral strictures, 726-7
Urethroscopy, 696-7; anesthesia, 698-9
Urinary diversion, after cystectomy, 712
Urinary/fecal diversions after total pelvic
  exenteration, 615*f*
Urinary incontinence
  artificial urinary sphincter for, 726-7
  MMK operation for, 729-30
  pediatric, endoscopic injection, 1071-3
  in rectal prolapse, 430
  stress, 654-7
Urinary sphincter, artificial, 726-7
Urinary tract, anatomy, 707*f*
  injury, in laparotomy, hysterectomy/
    BSO, 619
  stones, tumors, 696-9
  upper, pediatric, 1068-71
Urine analysis, preop, indications, A-2
Urology, 695-730 (Also *see* specific
  procedures.)
Uterine artery embolization, management
  of, 666-7; anesthesia, 661-5
Uterine aspiration, 633*f*
Uterine bleeding, abnormal
  D&C for, 632-3, 635-6
  hysteroscopy for, 636-7, 638-9
Uterine cancer
  exploratory laparotomy for, 618-21
  hysterectomy/BSO for, 618-21
Uterine devascularization, in postpartum
  hemorrhage, 661-5, 666-7
Uterine morcellation, laparoscopic, 691
Uterine segment incision, 660*f*
Uteropelvic junction (UPJ) obstruction,
  1068-71
Uterosacral ligament suspension, for
  vaginal apex support, 653-4
Uterus
  gravid, rupture, 666-7
    repair, 668-9; anesthesia, 661-5
  inversion (complete, incomplete), 679-
    81; anesthesia, 680-1
    manual reinversion, Hunting and
      Haultain procedures, 679-81
  myomata, fibroids, 688-90, 692-3
    hysterectomy for, 647-51
  prolapse, 652-4, 656-7, 690-3
    in C-section, 662
UTI, in laparotomy, hysterectomy/BSO
  for uterine cancer, 619
Uvula, reconstructive surgery for, 193-8
Uvulopalatal flap (UPF), 193-8, 194*f*
Uvulopalatopharyngoglossoplasty
  (UPPGP), 193-8; anesthesia, 196-8
Uvulopalatopharyngoplasty (UPPP), 193-
  8, 193*f*; anesthesia, 196-8

V

V/Q mismatch, in abdominal trauma
  surgery, 587

VA shunt, 48-50
VACTERL association, 942, 1019, 1032, 1056
Vagal nerve stimulation (VNS), 64-5
Vagal reflex, in neck dissection, 172
Vagal stimulation
  in D&C, D&E, 636
  in vaginal hysterectomy, 651
Vaginal cancer/mass
  pediatric procedures for, 1071-3
  pelvic exenteration, 613-18
  Stage I hysterectomy, 621-4
Vaginal hysterectomy, 647-51, 648*f*, 652
  with BSO, laparoscopic, 618-21
Vaginal surgery
  clitoroplasty, 1076-8
  colporrhaphy, 652-4; anesthesia, 656-7
  general operations, 728-30; anesthesia, 729-30
  lacerations, repair, 672-4; anesthesia, 673-4
  laser therapy, 608-9
  sacrospinous suspension, 652-4; anesthesia, 656-7
  sling operations, 728-30
  urethroplasty, 1076-8
  for urinary incontinence, 654-7, 728-30
  vaginoplasty, 1076-8
  vesicovaginal fistula repair, 728-39
Vaginal vault prolapse, 639-41, 644-6
Vagotomy, with oversew for duodenal perforation, 394, types, 396*f*
Vagotomy and antrectomy (V&A), for PUD, 396-9; anesthesia, 397-9
Vagotomy and pyloroplasty (V&P), for PUD, 396-9; anesthesia, 397-9
Valerian (*Valeriana officinalis*), precautions with anesthesia, F-11
Valgus
  deformity, ORIF, 840-1, 863-4
  foot neuromuscular disease, tendon transfer/lengthening, 1117-18, 1121-5
  severe, triple arthrodesis and Grice procedure for, 1118-19, 1121-5
Valvular disease, 272-5
Valvular heart disease, preop testing, indications for, A-3
Valvuloplasty (aortic, pulmonic, pediatric), 1193
  in venous surgery, 354
Vancomycin, drug reactions with, F-9-10
Vaporization (electrocautery or laser) for prostate resection, 700
Varco VSD repair, 979
Varicocele, operation for, 718-21
  ligation, laparoscopic, 1081-2
Varicose vein
  chronic primary, surgery for, 354-5
  high ligation, stab avulsion, 355-8
  stripping, 355-8; anesthesia, 356-8
Varix ligation, transesophageal, transgastric, for portal HTN, 345
Varus deformity, 840-1, 863-4

Varus foot neuromuscular disease, 1117-19, 1121-5
Varus (proximal femur) derotation osteotomy + plates/screws, 1108-9; anesthesia, 1121-5
Vascular access
  pediatric cardiac catheterization, 1192
  pediatric trauma, 589-90
  permanent, 351-4; anesthesia, 352-4
Vascular aneurysms, CNS, preop testing, indications for, A-3
Vascular injuries
  abdominal, 585-9; regions, 585
  lateral pelvic/perirenal hematoma or hemorrhage, 585-6
  midline inframesocolic hemorrhage or hematoma, 585-6
Vascular malformations, 53-6
  neck, 1014-16
Vascular rehabilitation, transcatheter techniques, balloon angioplasty, stent implantation, 1192
Vascular surgery, 307-58 (Also *see* specific procedures.)
Vasectomy, 725
Vasoconstriction, in replantation microsurgery, prevention, 913
Vasospastic disorders, 336-8, 339-41
Vasovasostomy for infertility, 723-5
VATER association, 942, 1019, 1057
VATS. *See* Video-assisted thoracoscopic surgery.
Vecuronium
  in adult intubation, B-2; muscle relaxation, B-3
  drug interactions with, F-8
  in pediatric muscle relaxation, D-2, D-3
Vein excision, 341-3; anesthesia, 332-4
Vein of Galen
  aneurysm, craniotomy for, 943-5
  malformation (congenital), craniotomy for, 943-5; anesthesia, 944-5
  interventional neuroradiology for, 1156-62
Vein stripping/transposition, 354-8
Velocardiofacial syndrome, 1143
Velopharyngeal incompetence, 1142-4
Venography, 1174
Veno-occlusive disease, 345-8
Venorrhaphy, lateral, for iliac vessel injury, 585
Venotomy, 357
Venous access devices, 1174
Venous air embolism (VAE)
  in craniofacial surgery, 1132, 1133
  in neck dissection, 172
Venous angiomas, 15
Venous cannulation, in CPB, 262
Venous collaterals, 1194
Venous insufficiency, 354-8
Venous occlusion with balloons or coils, in neuroradiology, 1158
Venous return obstruction, 354-5
Venous surgery
  thrombectomy, vein excision, 341-4

vein stripping/perforator ligation, 354-8
  thrombectomy, 332-4
  valve transplant, 354-5
Venovenous bypass, in liver transplantation, 547-58, circuit, 548*f*
Ventilation
  high-frequency, in thoracoplasty, drainage of empyema, 225, 228
  jet, 150, 151*f*, 237, 962
  spontaneous, in pediatric otolaryngology, 954
Ventilator function monitoring—adult, B-1; pediatric, D-1
Ventricular catheter insertion, 49*f*
Ventricular chamber hypoplasia, 996
Ventricular dysrhythmias, in ICD placement, 1167
Ventricular fibrillation
  ICD placement for, 1165-9
  induced, recordings, 1166*f*
Ventricular septal defect (VSD), 973, 996
  anatomy, locations, 979*f*
  classifications, 1007*f*
  closure, in A-V canal defect, 976
  with DORV, 1006, 1007*f*9
  patch closure, 1001*f*
  pediatric surgery for, 979-81, closure, 1194
  postinfarction, in CABG, 268
  pulmonary artery banding, 97
Ventricular shunt procedures, 47-50
Ventricular tachycardia (VT), 1165-9
Ventricular tachyrhythmia, 1162-4
Ventriculoarterial concordance, 1003
Ventriculoatrial (VA) shunt, 48-50
Ventriculoperitoneal (VP) shunt, 47-50
Ventriculoscopy
  pediatric, 945-8; anesthesia, 947-8
  third, endoscopic, 945-8
Ventrolateral thalamus, anatomy, 58*f*
Verapamil, drug interactions, F-3, F-10
Veress needle placement, 456-7, 459
Vertebral artery stenosis/occlusion, in craniotomy for EC-IC bypass, 23
Vertebral fractures, 787-94
Vertebral osteomyelitis, TB, 787-94
Vertical banded gastroplasty, 399-403, 399*f*; anesthesia 401-3
  laparoscopic, 477-9; anesthesia, 401-3
Vesical neck suspension for urinary incontinence, 728-30
Vesicostomy, 1073-5; anesthesia, 1077-8
  for neurovesical dysfunction, prune-belly syndrome, 1073-5
  for urine drainage, posterior/anterior urethral valves, VUR, 1073-5
Vesicoureteral reflux, 715-17, 1069
  complications, 1077
  subureteric injection for, 1071-3
  ureteral reimplantation for, 1073-5
Vesicovaginal fistula repair, 715-17
  vaginal approach, 728-3
Vestibular neuritis, 187-92
Vestibular schwannoma, 187-92
Viaspan, in organ procurement, 560

Vicodin
    anesthetic considerations in lumbar
       discectomy, 783
    in pediatric postop analgesia, E-3
Video thoracoscopy, 229, 246
Video-assisted thoracoscopic urgery
       (VATS), 240-3; port placement, 241f
Villous adenoma, 431-2
Vinblastine
    in staging laparotomy, 497
    toxic effects, 598, 599
Vioxx, anesthetic considerations in
       lumbar discectomy, 783
VIP-oma, 492
Visual monitoring of patient—adult, B-1;
       pediatric, D-1
Vitrectomy, 134-7
Vitreous hemorrhage, opacification, 135
Vocal cord
    anatomy, exposure, 174f, 175f
    polyps, 151
    resection, in laryngectomy, 175f
    in skull base surgery, 190, 191
    surgery for, 150
Volkmann's contracture in supracondylar
       humerus fracture, 1084
Voltaren, anesthetic considerations in
       lumbar discectomy, 783
Volvulus, 415
    colon, segmental colectomy, 423-5
    obstruction of small bowel, 413-14
Von Hippel-Lindau disease, 17
VP shunt, 47-50
VSD. *See* Ventricular septal defect.
Vulva
    cancer, 601-5, 613-18
    laser therapy, 608-9
    reconstruction, 602
Vulvectomy, en bloc, radical, 601-5, 601f;
       anesthesia, 603-5

W

Wagner large-pin fixator for limb
       lengthening, 1113-15, 113f; 1121-5
Wake-up testing
    in anterior spinal reconstruction and
       fusion, 792
    in functional neurosurgery, 68

Waldhause subclavian artery flap for
       repair of aortic coarctation, 984
Wallstent
    in TIPS, 1169
    in tracheobronchial stenting, 1178
Wardill-Kilner technique for cleft palate,
       1140-2; anesthesia, 1147-8
Warren shunt, 344-5; anesthesia, 346-8
Washout acidosis, in abdominal vessel
       injury, 586
Water absorption toxicity, in pediatric
       transurethral procedures, 1072
Waterston procedure for esophageal
       replacement, 1031-4
Waterston shunt for tricuspid atresia,
       1003-6
Weber-Ferguson incision, 178, 179
Wedge biopsy, in staging laparotomy, 496
Wedge resection, lung lesion, 215-18,
       215f; anesthesia, 216-17; 230
Weight control drugs
    in abdominoplasty, 890
    in liposuction, 893
Wertheim modified hysterectomy, 622
Wetting solutions, liposuction, 892, 893
'Wet' techniques, facelift, 870
Whipple resection, 490-4
    for pancreatitis, 486-7; 491-4
Whitacre needle, in spinal anesthesia, 650
Whitehead hemorrhoidectomy, 434
Whitesides and Kelly anterolateral
       retropharyngeal approach, 72f
Wilms' tumor
    bilateral, 1068-71
    nephrectomy for, 707-9, 1068-71
    in patients having XRT, 1190
    pediatric, resection, 1040-3, 1040f,
       1069
Wilson's disease, 547-58
Wire localization breast biopsy, 512-15
Wiring techniques, C1/C2, 75-7, 83-7
Wolff-Parkinson-White syndrome, 1167
Wong-Baker Faces Scale, E-1f
Wound dehiscence
    in laparotomy, hysterectomy, 619
    repair, 506-7; anesthesia, 508-9
Wrist
    arthritis, 738-9, 740-3
    dislocations (perilunate, lunate), 753-5

fusion (total, partial), 737-8, 740-3
    ganglion excision, 743, 746-8
    prostheses (Silastic, metal,
       polyethylene), 738-9, 740-3
Wrist arthrodesis (total, radiopancarpal,
       radiolunate, radioscapholunate,
       intercarpal), 737-8, 740-3
    bilateral, 738-9; anesthesia, 740-3
    patient positioning, 741, 742
Wrist arthroscopy, 749-50, 751-2
Wrist replacement, total, 738-9, 740-3
Wrist, rheumatoid
    dorsal stabilization, 735-6, 740-3
    extensor synovectomy of, 735-6, 740-3
    with synovitis, intraarticular infection,
       fractures, dissociation, 749-50

X

X-ray fluoroscopy, 1174; anesthesia,
       1175-7
XRT. *See* Radiation therapy.

Y

Y graft, in abdominal aorta surgery, 328
Y-tubes, in tracheobronchial stenting,
       1178-82
Yacoub arterial switch for TGA, 996
Yohimbe (*Corynanthe yohimbe*,
       Pausinystalia yohimbe), precautions
       with anesthesia, F-11
Yount-Ober release, 1101-2, 1121-5

Z

Z plating, anterior lumbar/lumbosacral, 91
Z-plasty
    clavicular head in torticollis release,
       1088
    cleft lip/palate, 1137-40, 1139f, 1141f;
       anesthesia, 1147-8
    notching of vermillion border, 1145f
    palmar/digital fasciectomy, 744
    secondary lip/nose deformities, 1145-8
Zenker's diverticulum, formation, 379f
    surgery for, 378f, 379-81, 387-90
Zielke instrumentation from T10-L3, for
       spinal correction, 1095f
Zollinger-Ellison syndrome, 492
    gastrectomy for, 392-4
Zygomatic fractures, 897-902